Pathology
of the
HUMAN
PLACENTA

FIFTH EDITION

Kurt Benirschke, MD

Peter Kaufmann, MD

Rebecca Baergen, MD

Pathology
of the
HUMAN
PLACENTA

FIFTH EDITION

With 745 Illustrations, 170 in Full Color

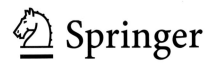 Springer

Kurt Benirschke, MD
8457 Prestwick Drive
La Jolla, CA 92037
USA

Peter Kaufmann, MD
Department of Anatomy
RWTH Aachen
D-52057 Aachen
Germany

Rebecca Baergen, MD
New York-Presbyterian Hospital–Weill
  Medical College of Cornell University
New York, NY 10021
USA

Library of Congress Control Number: 2005928850

ISBN 10: 0-387-26738-7   e-ISBN 0-387-26742-5
ISBN 13: 978-0-387-26738-8 e-ISBN 978-0-387-26742-5

Printed on acid-free paper.

Printed in China.   (BS/EVB)

9 8 7 6 5 4 3 2 1

springer.com

Preface

Most obstetricians and pediatricians would agree that the examination of the placenta often helps to explain an abnormal neonatal outcome. As early as in 1892, Ballantyne wrote,

> *A diseased foetus without its placenta is an imperfect specimen, and a description of a foetal malady, unless accompanied by a notice of the placental condition, is incomplete. Deductions drawn from such a case cannot be considered as conclusive, for in the missing placenta or cord may have existed the cause of the disease and death. During intrauterine life the foetus, the membranes, the cord and the placenta form an organic whole, and disease of any part must react upon and affect the others.*

Similar thoughts were succinctly detailed in Price's (1950) discussion of his concept of the prenatal biases as they affected twins. His contribution also admonishes us that placental study is a *sine qua non* for a more perfect understanding of fetal development. Despite all this understanding of the past and appreciation for placental disease, great resistance still exists to perform the task of placental examination routinely. For many pathologists, therefore, the placenta has remained a mysterious organ.

This book had its beginning in 1967 when Shirley G. Driscoll and Kurt Benirschke wrote the volume on placental pathology for the *German Handbook of Pathology*, the "Henke-Lubarsch." Because there seemed to be a need for wider dissemination of the text, this book was reprinted by Springer-Verlag New York but soon became unavailable. Since then, a number of books on placental pathology have been written, in French, English, and German (Philippe, Baldwin, Fox, Lewis and Perrin, Lavery, Gall, Kraus et al., Naeye, Becker and Röckelein, Vogel, Kaplan, and Joshi), and much more interest has been accorded this so readily available but poorly studied organ. The journal *Placenta* has become a significant outlet for results from sophisticated placental studies. Regular trophoblast conferences are being held in Rochester, New York, and European and international meetings were organized. Much other new information has been obtained, and the continuing enigma of placental nonrejection has been tackled by numerous investigators. In addition, the availability of the placenta for biochemical study has stimulated many cell biologists and molecular biologists to use this organ as a convenient source of human tissue. Genetic information now adds to our understanding of the complexity of placental function and other issues. Also, because much interest is developing in comparative placentation, a new Web site may be found at http://medicine.ucsd.edu/cpa.

This fifth edition is being written because so many new findings have come from systematic study in the last few years that updating seemed necessary. Moreover, there is a great need to have documentation for legal purposes as the placenta has become an important aspect of medicolegal adjudication of circumstances around the time of birth. The organization of the previous edition also left some topics uncovered that are now being corrected. Many changes have been made throughout the book. Not only was the text updated, but also a more complete index was created, the order of chapters is presented more logically, and tables are presented more usefully. The text was written with MSWord. A complete set of diskettes with the references can be made available from the authors, if the reader desires.

I (K.B.) am indebted to many people, foremost to my wife for her understanding and patience with me and with this task; the publishers and many of its staff members have been gracious and patient; my colleagues at the university, and other persons who have all helped gather data, are gratefully acknowledged. Many students and colleagues have graciously read most chapters and they have made many helpful suggestions and corrections, for which I am appreciative. There are some colleagues, however, whose inspiration have helped more than others: Marjorie Grafe; the dysmorphologists Kenneth L. Jones, his wife Marilyn, and their numerous fellows as well as neonatologist Frank Mannino; and ultrasonographer Dolores Pretorius, who continues to challenge me and requires that I provide explanations for perinatal deaths and abnormalities. Having examined all placentas of all deliveries in the institutions with which I was affiliated over the past five decades, I have gathered a large amount of material to digest. Most of all, however, I am grateful to Dr. Geoffrey Altshuler, Oklahoma City, for many stimulating discussions and endless patience with me and his friendship.

P.K. gratefully acknowledges the scientific cooperation of many former and present coworkers: Mario Castellucci, Ayse Demir, Hans-Georg Frank, Hitoshi Funayama, Gabriele Gaus, Berthold Huppertz, Mahmed Kadirov, Sonja Kertschanska, Gaby Kohnen, Georg Kosanke, Azizbek Nanaev, Frank Reister, and the late Gertfried Schweikhart. Many of my data are based on their material, their findings, and their ideas. Also, many colleagues and friends from other laboratories have contributed by discussion and by offering technical help. In this respect I am particularly grateful to Ramazan Demir, Gernot Desoye, Jean-Michel Foidart, John Kingdom, Hubert Korr, Rudolf Leiser, Peter Ruck, Hobe Schröder, Tullia Todros, and the late Elizabeth Ramsey. In many cases it is virtually impossible to differentiate between their and my ideas.

These chapters do not only require scientific inspiration but also much artistic, technical, and secretarial work. The artistic help of Wolfgang Graulich and the photographic assistance of Gaby Bock as well as of Helga Kriegel are gratefully acknowledged. The histologic and electron-microscopic pictures are based on material processed by Marianne von Bentheim, Barbara Ihnow, Michaela Nicolau, Lian Shen, and Uta Zahn. Perfect secretarial assistance was provided by Jutta Ruppert.

The collaboration of all these coworkers and friends was the basis for my contribution. Last but not least, I am very much indebted to my wife for her support and understanding.

Kurt Benirschke, MD
La Jolla, California

Peter Kaufmann, MD
Aachen, Germany

Rebecca Baergen, MD
New York, NY

References

Baldwin, V.J.: Pathology of Multiple Pregnancy. Springer-Verlag, New York, 1994.

Ballantyne, J.W.: The Diseases and Deformities of the Foetus. Vol. I. Oliver and Boyd, Edinburgh. 1892.

Becker, V. and Röckelein, G.: Pathologie der weiblichen Genitalorgane I. Pathologie der Plazenta und des Abortes. Springer-Verlag, Heidelberg, 1989.

Benirschke, K. and Driscoll, S.G.: The Pathology of the Human Placenta. Springer-Verlag, New York. 1967.

Fox, H.: Pathology of the Placenta. 2nd Edition. W.B. Saunders Co. Philadelphia. 1997.

Gall, S.A.: Multiple Pregnancy and Delivery. Mosby, St. Louis, 1996.

Joshi, V.V.: Handbook of Placental Pathology. Igaku-Shoin, New York, 1994.

Kaplan, C.G.: Color Atlas of Gross Placental Pathology. Igaku-Shoin, New York, 1994.

Kraus, F.T., Redline, R.W., Gersell, D.J., Nelson, D.M. and Dicke, J.M.: Placental Pathology. Atlas of Nontumor Pathology. AFIP, Washington, DC, 2004.

Lavery, J.P., ed.: The Human Placenta. Clinical Perspectives. Aspen Publishers, Rockville, Maryland. 1987.

Lewis, S.H. and Perrin, V.D.K., eds.: Pathology of the Placenta. Churchill Livingstone, New York. 1999.

Naeye, R.L.: Disorders of the Placenta, Fetus, and Neonate. Mosby Year Book, St. Louis, Missouri, 1992.

Philippe, E.: Pathologie Foeto-Placentaire. Masson, Paris. 1986.

Price, B.: Primary biases in twin studies: review of prenatal and natal differences-producing factors in monozygotic pairs. Amer. J. Hum. Genet. **2**:293–352, 1950.

Vogel, M.: Atlas der morphologischen Plazentadiagnostik. Springer-Verlag, Heidelberg, 2nd Edition, 1995.

Contents

1
Examination of the Placenta

Macroscopic Examination

Most placentas are normal, as are most babies. Therefore, an examination of all placentas may not be warranted, although this has been advocated repeatedly. Practical guidelines, including indications for the examination have been published by the College of American Pathologists (Langston et al., 1997). This reference describes in tabular form the major abnormalities and their association with clinical features. Booth et al. (1997) inquired what reasons constituted the submission of a placenta for examination and found, regrettably, that it was cesarean section delivery. This is hardly a good reason, as will be seen. A large number of surgical deliveries are repeat sections and have little impact on perinatal problems for which placental examination might be useful. Altshuler and Hyde (1996), on the other hand, found that 92% of placentas for which an examination was requested by obstetrician or neonatologist had relevant pathology. Salafia and Vintzileos (1990) made a strong plea for the study of all placentas by pathologists. We concur with this view, as the sporadic examination does not provide sufficient training for young pathologists and it does not allow the "routine" pathologist to obtain sufficient background knowledge as to what constitutes a truly normal placenta. Another reason for the examination of all placentas is today's litigious climate; it makes study of placentas highly desirable (see Chapter 26). Furthermore, it has been shown repeatedly that a placental examination is needed to understand the causes of perinatal deaths. This was demonstrated, especially for stillbirths, by the study of Las Heras et al. (1994). The most important lesions were found in the umbilical cord (18%), with inflammatory lesions being second. Altshuler (1999) wrote a searching essay on the placenta-related epidemiology from his vast experience in these matters. Because placentas differ widely in shape, size, and in appearance, the novice must become familiar with this spectrum of placental shapes. To do so, a large number of placentas must be examined routinely. In hospitals with large numbers of deliveries, however, it may be prudent to select placentas for examination by the pathologist.

Storage

To facilitate the practice of saving placentas for a week, storage is required so that placentas are available when needed. The American College of Obstetricians and Gynecologists (ACOG), on the other hand, has suggested, surprisingly, that the routine study of the placenta is not warranted (ACOG, 1991), a decision with which we strongly disagree. Placentas should **not** be frozen prior to examination, as this obliterates the most useful histologic characteristics and makes even the macroscopic examination more difficult. We believe that formalin fixation has a similar unwanted effect. It is best to store the delivered placentas in containers, such as plastic jars. We have found ice cream cartons, made from Styrofoam, the most convenient and least expensive. Cardboard containers absorb the fluids, and the placentas tend to stick to them. These containers can also be readily labeled and stored in a refrigerator at 4°C. In this state, the placenta is preserved for a meaningful examination for many days. Autolysis is minimal. We cannot agree with the opinion of Naeye (1987) that this storage causes significant artifacts that render a subsequent examination difficult. Indeed, the immediate fixation of the organ in formalin, recommended by others (Bartholomew et al., 1961) as a good means to evaluate the extent of infarction, makes the placenta more difficult to evaluate critically, aside from the storage problems, expense, and odor. Prior fixation also makes tissue culture, bacteriologic examination, and other procedures more difficult or impossible. For maximal convenience, it is a good idea to have a refrigerator with seven shelves, labeled Monday through Sunday, and to discard the normal placentas from one shelf when the next similar weekday arrives. In this way, all placentas from problem births will be available for study.

The placenta loses some weight during storage. In part, the loss is due to evaporation, but most weight is lost by leakage of blood and serum occasioned by the weight of placental tissue resting on other portions. The quantity of weight loss depends on the length of storage and the degree of edema, but the edema is not great in the normal placenta. It is most significant in the edematous placentas of hydrops. We have observed a 180-g fluid extravasation from a 740-g placenta within 1 day from a hydropic placenta. The freshly examined placenta is thus softer, bloodier, and thicker than one that has been stored. On the other hand, it must be noted that the placenta gains weight when it is stored in formalin, particularly during the first day of fixation. Not all organs increase in weight uniformly after such fixation, as the detailed report by Schremmer (1967) specified. The placenta, according to this author, gains between 0.7% and 23.0%, with an average of +9.9%. It is among the organs with the largest deviations in weight gain after fixation. Our own findings are summarized in the graph shown in Figure 1.1.

Selection

Placentas from all prematurely delivered infants and all twins should be examined routinely, at least macroscopically, and many of them require histologic study as well. In addition, many circumstances arise during the first few days of life of an infant where the neonatologist is interested in placental findings. These often help to clarify whether a particular disease had a prenatal onset. Furthermore, there are some maternal conditions that warrant placental examination, for example preeclampsia, the condition known as lupus anticoagulant, diabetes, fever, and many more. In our routine study of placentas, the obstetricians and neonatologists alert us as to which placentas they believe warrant more scrutiny, and thus

perhaps 5% to 10% of all placentas undergo histologic examination in our hands.

Photography

A photographic record is often desirable and is useful for many purposes. Most pathology laboratories are equipped with cameras that can take Kodachrome color pictures, which are then valuable for teaching purposes. It has been our experience, however, that colors tend to disappear, and certainly these photographs cannot generally be retrieved years later when they may be of interest in litigation or review of material. Nowadays, digital photography has become such a routine procedure and storage of the digital images has become so easy that much more photography of specimens is desirable and practiced. The photographic task is generally quickly accomplished. Colleagues have often been amused by this recommendation, but they agree that a good picture is worth a lot of words, especially when it comes to litigation.

Examination

Detailed protocols for the examination of the placenta have been presented in the past (Snoeck, 1958; Benirschke, 1961a,b; Gruenwald, 1964; Fox, 1997). Some protocols were designed to allow an unbiased examination of the placenta and record keeping by the many different medical centers of the Collaborative Study so that, ultimately, correlations could be made regarding fetal outcome. Our routine procedure now is to select for histologic study those that appear abnormal or whose perinatal circumstances demand such an examination. The selection process just outlined has been helpful, and we have rarely missed a placenta that was of importance. Other recommendations for a "triage" of placental study and other

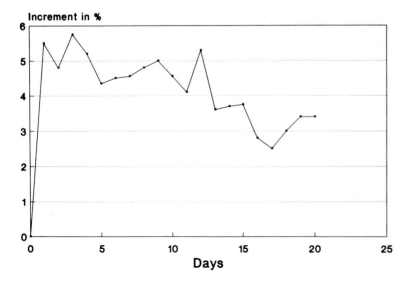

FIGURE 1.1. Weight gain of placenta (trimmed, without cord or membranes) after formalin fixation.

FIGURE 1.2. Instruments found to be most practical for the placental examination: scissors, forceps, "dipstick" to measure the thickness of placental tissue, and a long, stiff knife.

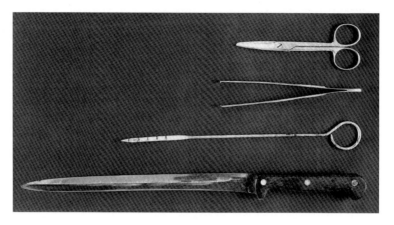

ramifications come from a joint conference held in 1990 (Travers & Schmidt, 1991). That volume provides useful information on many aspects of placental pathology.

The tools for the examination are simple (Fig. 1.2). They consist of a ruler, a long and sharp knife, a toothed forceps, a pair of scissors, and a scale. Our ruler is permanently mounted over the cutting board, thus enabling rapid measurement of the length of the umbilical cord and the placenta's diameter. A butcher's scale with removable bucket that weighs items up to 2 kg is also available. The long knife, best obtained from a butcher supply house, is sharpened just before examination.

The placenta is removed from its container. At this time one often perceives rather characteristic odors. For instance, when a mother has recently eaten garlic, the intense smell of its diallyl sulfides is readily apparent. Also, in infected placentas the fetid smell of *Escherichia coli* and the rather sweeter smell of *Listeria monocytogenes* can be distinguished by an experienced pathologist. Storage in the refrigerator enhances the growth and hence the recognition of these organisms.

The shape of the placenta is then ascertained by stretching it flat on the cutting board. Is it normally round or oval? Are there accessory (succenturiate) lobes? Is a question now answered? One finds that, during the delivery, the membranes have generally inverted over the maternal surface (Schultze procedure) and rarely are they found in the position they held in utero (Duncan) (Pritchard et al., 1985). They are then inverted by the examiner so that they assume the in utero configuration, and one next ascertains the completeness of the membranes. It is also noted at this time if the tear that allowed the infant to escape from its membranous enclosure extends to the edge of the placenta or if free membranes extend beyond the edge. If there is **any** margin of intact membranes, this placenta could not have been a placenta previa, provided it was from a vaginal delivery. If the edge of the membranous tear is far from the placental border (often the case with circumvallate placentas), a fundal

position can be deduced. Torpin and Hart (1941) made the point that when the minimally disturbed sac is immersed in a bucket of water the sac assumes the configuration of the uterus, and that its position before birth can be reasonably accurately determined by this study. At this time it is prudent to inspect the color and appearance of the fetal surface of the placenta. Normally it is shiny, and the subjacent blood is seen as a clear blue hue, particularly in the immature organ. When chorioamnionitis is present, the membranes become opaque by the interposition of leukocytes, and the surface usually loses its sheen. Greenish discoloration betrays either meconium (slimy) or hemosiderin deposition.

Next the membranes are cut off the edge of the placenta with the knife. If one anticipates making sections of the placenta for histologic study, it is wise to follow a routine protocol for doing it, as it enhances subsequent interpretation. Therefore, it is recommended that one get used to doing it one way, once and for all. It is preferable to cut the membranes off in such a manner that one knows the point of rupture; then, when sections are made, the membrane roll is prepared in such a fashion that the point of rupture is in the center of the roll with the amnion inward (Fig. 1.3). This method of preparing a roll of membranes (the "jelly roll"), in order to obtain a maximum amount of membranes with decidua capsularis, was first described by Zeek and Assali (1950). In immature placentas, there may be a large amount of decidua, and it is often ragged. In more mature organs the decidua atrophies and often it degenerates. Occasionally, one finds an intrauterine device in this decidua capsularis, usually at the edge of the placenta and associated with old clot and debris (Figs. 1.4 and 1.5). Frequently, there are areas of brown to green discoloration in the membranes that are from former hemorrhages, or they may have been induced by amniocentesis.

In many placentas that come from patients after labor, in contrast to those after cesarean section, the amnion is disrupted or sheared off the underlying chorion. In fact,

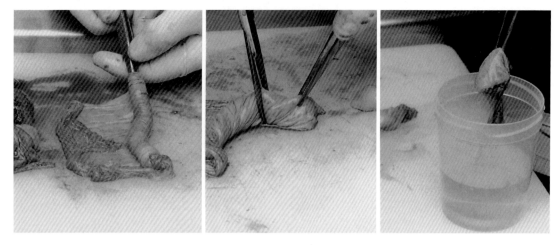

FIGURE 1.3. Rolling of membranes for fixation and later sectioning. It is best to prepare them in a standardized fashion, for example, amnion inside, starting at the site of rupture and proceeding toward the edge of the placenta, as shown at left. A segment is then taken from a well-rolled portion (center) and is fixed for a day (right) before trimming.

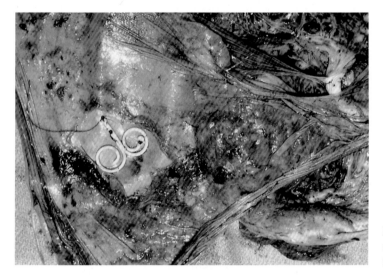

FIGURE 1.4. Edge of the placenta (right) with an intrauterine device embedded in degenerating decidua (partly removed) and old blood clot.

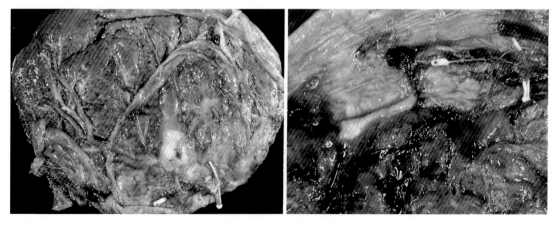

FIGURE 1.5. Intrauterine devices at the placental margin at term (left) and in a slightly immature (right) pregnancy. Note the attending hemorrhagic degeneration of the adjacent tissues.

the amnion may be totally detached. Often, though, there is milky, white vernix caseosa that has dissected underneath the amnion; it is readily moved about by pressure. It has no significance. Moreover, the membranes near the edge of the placenta frequently contain the remnant of the yolk sac, a small white to yellow oval disk that is located underneath the amnion. The yolk sac of early stages of development can now be visualized ultrasonographically. Measurements have shown that the size of the yolk sac is variable, and that it is not a useful prognosticator of fetal well-being (Reece et al., 1988). Occasionally, one sees remnants of tiny vessels traversing from it to the insertion of the cord, or even within the cord.

The color of the membranes is noted, as are the surface characteristics. A slimy feeling is often the result of meconium discharge, as is a green color. The length of time of meconium discharge can be estimated by the presence of green discoloration in different layers. When it is only in the amnion, this suggests a short time interval; when meconium is found also in the chorion after the amnion is stripped off, a longer interval has passed since discharge (Miller et al., 1985). We found that after 1 hour the meconium macrophages are visible within the amnion; after 3 hours they may be seen in the chorionic membrane. At even later times it reaches the decidua capsularis. Greenish or brownish discolorations in immature placentas are more often due to blood breakdown products (hematoidin, hemosiderin) following hemolysis, rather than due to meconium. Hemosiderin can be stained with the Prussian blue method for iron, and the bilirubin of meconium stains (poorly) with bile stains. The very immature fetus cannot discharge meconium, lacking the hormonal maturation for intestinal propulsion (Lucas et al., 1979). The surface of the membranes, the amnion, is normally shiny. Around the insertion of the cord, one may find squamous metaplasia in the form of concentric nodules that are hydrophobic (Fig. 1.6). They are normal

features. Amnion nodosum, usually represented by a finely granular, dull appearance of the amnionic surface, correlates with oligohydramnios. One must be cognizant of whether the amnion is present at all and, if not, whether amnionic bands exist. Also, often some blood has dissected underneath the amnion during delivery or especially when fetal blood has been aspirated for diagnostic tests from the fetal surface blood vessels.

The placenta is next measured, and then the cord is examined. Is it central, eccentric, marginal, or membranous (velamentous) in its insertion? What is its length, and is it spiraled? We now believe that the length of the umbilical cord is determined primarily by fetal movements and that excessive spiraling implies unusual fetal motions (Moessinger et al., 1982). There may be a genetic component to the spiraling and the length, as the umbilical cords of some animals have different and consistent lengths; but this characteristic is so far unknown for human umbilical cords. Are there knots, thrombi, or discolorations? Can any other unusual features be detected? The cord is then severed from the bulk of the placenta, and its cut surface is studied at several locations. The most important observation to be made here is whether there are three vessels and if other unusual features are present. A single umbilical artery (SUA) is the commonest abnormality. One must also appreciate that there is almost always an anastomosis (Hyrtl's anastomosis) between the two umbilical arteries, which is usually found near the point of insertion on the placental surface (Priman, 1959). Thus, counting the number of vessels is best done farther away from the insertion. When a velamentous insertion of the cord is found, the examiner must pursue the ramifications of the fetal vessels after they leave the site of cord insertion, at times finding thrombi, and particularly in membranous vessels. These vessels may be disrupted, as in vasa previa, and acute exsanguination of the fetus is common in such circumstances.

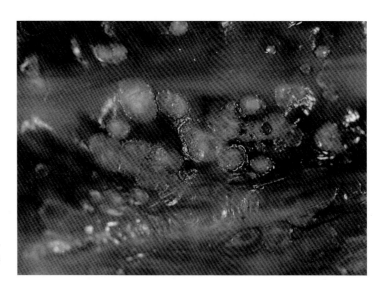

FIGURE 1.6. Squamous metaplasia of amnion in concentric patches, usually found near the insertion of the umbilical cord. The plaques are water-repellent.

The weight of the remaining disk is ascertained. It is generally useless to know the weight of the entire organ, including cord and membranes. Correlations with fetal weight and development can be made only by knowing the "net" weight of placental tissue (Walker, 1954; Gruenwald & Minh, 1961). Excessive amounts of maternal, retroplacental clots must also have been removed before weighing. Note again that the weight of formalin-fixed placentas is greater than that of fresh organs (Fig. 1.1) (Schremmer, 1967). Variations in normal placental weight are common. They reflect mostly the length of storage and the amount of fetal blood content.

When studying the fetal surface of the placenta, one notes its color and the possible presence of granular excrescences. Most importantly, however, one must carefully inspect the fetal vessels, which are carried in the chorion; the amnion has no blood vessels. In nearly all placentas, one can recognize the fetal arteries as those vessels that cross over the veins (Hyrtl, 1870; Bacsich & Smout, 1938; Boe, 1953; Crawford, 1962). It will be observed that the terminal branches of arteries dip singly into a cotyledon; and next to it, a vein emerges to return the blood to the cord (Fig. 1.7). One often finds thrombi in these vessels in placentas of abnormal newborns. They appear as white-yellow streaks on the vessel's surface and are usually not completely occlusive. When they are, an area of hemolysis is often seen adjacent to the thrombosis. Thrombi may also calcify. They must be sampled for histologic study.

The fetal surface of the mature placenta is often described as being "bosselated" or "tessellated," meaning that tiny white elevations are present underneath the chorion, giving the surface a mosaic, irregular pattern. These protrusions represent accumulations of fibrin in the intervillous space and they increase in number with advancing maturity. Larger patches of fibrin also exist; at

times they have a liquefied center, but they are assumed to be of little significance (Geller, 1959). In our experience, however, larger subchorionic thrombi are abnormal and occasionally associated with fetal growth restriction. Cysts from the subchorionic extravillous trophoblast cells ("X-cells") may bulge on the surface and contain a clear, slightly viscid mucoid substance. At times it is discolored with blood. Finally, the insertion of the membranes is observed. Was it at the edge, or was there a ring of "circumvallation"?

When the placenta is turned over then, thus exposing the maternal surface, the first need is to identify possible areas of abruptio placentae. When an abruption is fresh, one may not be able to differentiate it from the normally present postpartum maternal blood clot that adheres. Within a few hours, though, the blood dries, becomes firmer and stringy, and then changes color to brown and eventually it may become greenish. In such cases, the placenta underneath the clot is usually infarcted or it is at least compressed. Abruptios are common, and most are clinically silent. Most are located at the margin of the placenta; and on occasion one finds old clot behind the membranes. Calcification on the maternal surface is then sought: small yellow-white granules in the decidua basalis and septa. Calcifications vary a good deal in quantity; they are usually found only in mature organs. The quantity has no clinically important correlations (Fujikura, 1963a,b; Jeacock et al., 1963), but clinicians have paid much attention to the recognition of calcification. It may be detected by sonography and has served as a method to "grade" (age) the placenta (Fisher et al., 1976). This is rarely done now as it has not been found to be helpful. At this point one also observes the cotyledons, the major subdivisions of the placental tissue. They increase in size and differentiation with advancing gestation, being absent early. One needs to ascertain now whether all of the

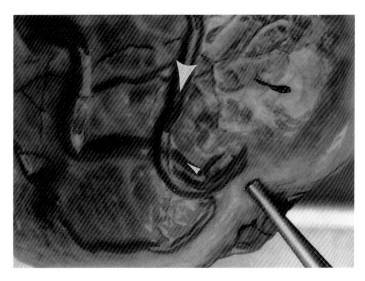

FIGURE 1.7. Entrance of fetal vessels on the chorionic plate into the cotyledon. One artery (large arrowhead) brings the fetal blood; the vein (small arrowhead) next to it returns it to the fetus.

placental "floor" is present or whether there are missing cotyledons. If no cotyledonary subdivisions exist in the mature placenta, then the floor is often too thick and it may be infiltrated with an excess amount of fibrin. This condition is known as maternal floor infarction (MFI) and is best noted at this time (Naeye, 1985).

Long, parallel cuts are now made with the long knife and, most importantly, the color of the villous tissue is observed. The red color of the villous tissue is almost wholly determined by its content of fetal blood. Thus, a congested placenta (as in maternal diabetes, for instance) is dark, and that of an anemic, hydropic, exsanguinated, or erythroblastotic fetus is pale, and it is usually also much more friable. Such a placenta is also commonly thicker, 3 to 5 cm, in contrast to the normal placenta, which averages 2.0 to 2.5 cm at term.

It is normal to find "holes" in the center of many placental cotyledons (Fritschek, 1927). Such holes were filled, in vivo, with maternal blood and represent the areas of first blood distribution into the intervillous space from the maternal injection jet. Intervillous thrombi, often located in these spaces, may be dark when fresh; alternatively, they are composed of layered white fibrin when older. The intervillous thrombi differ from infarcts in that they displace villous tissue. Furthermore, infarcts are granular in contrast, because they are composed of dead villous tissue. Fresh infarcts are red, and older ones are yellow to white. When sectioning the placenta, one also finds that the intercotyledonary septa contain some calcium, and often they contain some cystic spaces filled with trophoblastic secretion, the same clear mucoid material as contained in surface cysts. They too arise from extravillous trophoblast cells. Occasionally, one encounters round tumors of a solid nature, chorioangiomas. "Gitterinfarcts" or "Netzinfarcts," because they appear to form a network of fibrin, accompany maternal floor infarction. They may be prominent, appear as dense fibrin patches throughout the organ, and have great clinical significance. It is a good practice to estimate the total amount of infarction and to record it; in fact, it is ultimately of some importance and may have medicolegal implications in infants with growth retardation. Single marginal infarcts are common and do not correlate with either fetal or maternal conditions. Other lesions are occasionally seen. Thus, some lesions that appear grossly as "infarcts" may turn out to be choriocarcinoma on histologic study (Driscoll, 1963).

Placentas of Multiple Births

Placentas of multiple births are important records for infants and pediatricians alike, and they are routinely examined. A recording of the membrane relation between twins, triplets, and so on is mandatory. For meaningful analysis it is necessary that the umbilical cords be labeled with sutures or clamps by the obstetrician, in the order of births. The most important decisions to be made in examining placentas of multiple births are (1) the number of membranes that divide the sacs (two or four) and (2) the types of vascular anastomoses that are generally present only in monochorionic twin placentas (Schatz, 1886). Fraternal (dizygotic) twins essentially *always* have diamnionic/dichorionic (DiDi) placentas. Fused placentas, however, are not always monochorionic. They may be DiDi and they may be diamnionic/monochorionic (DiMo). Finally, there may be no "dividing membranes" between the fetuses, as in the monoamnionic/monochorionic twin placenta (MoMo). All monochorionic twin placentas belong to monozygotic (MZ; identical) twins. The time at which MZ twins separated one from another during the early embryonic stages presumably determines the type of placentation that ultimately develops, and this can thus be estimated from an examination of the membrane relation. It is easiest, but not necessarily best, to separate the dividing membranes from each other. If there are four distinctive leaves, it is a DiDi placenta, whereas if only two membranes are apposed it is a DiMo placenta. Equally readily, the diagnosis of a DiDi twin placenta is made by ascertaining that the dividing membranes are opaque and contain remnants of old vessels or other debris (old decidua, degenerated villi). Also, in DiDi placentas one usually finds a ridge at the site where the membranes meet over the placenta. It is caused by the buckling of tissues from the collision of the two expanding placental tissue masses. The dividing membranes of DiMo placentas, in contrast, are transparent. The diagnosis of membrane relationship is easiest and most permanently established by a histologic section of a membrane roll of this tissue, or by a T-shaped section that includes this area (Fig. 1.8).

The location of the cord insertion is especially important in twin placentas, as it is much more frequently marginal or membranous than in singletons; this may reflect some problems in early placental development. Moreover, the absence of one umbilical artery (single umbilical artery, SUA) is more common in multiple births (Heifetz, 1984).

After the membrane relation is established, the "vascular equator," that is, the area where the two chorionic vascular districts meet, is examined. In DiDi placentas, there is **never** a confluence of fetal blood vessels; if one were found, it would be exceptional and would be the basis for the exceedingly rare blood chimerism in fraternal twins. It must be cautioned here that ascertainment of a DiDi relation does *not* make the diagnosis of fraternal twins. Approximately one third of identical twins have this placentation (discussed in greater detail in Chapter 25). In monochorionic placentas (DiMo, MoMo), there are almost always some anastomoses, particularly in the prematurely delivered placentas. These anastomoses have

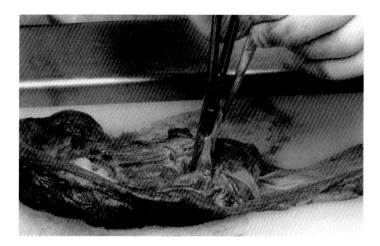

FIGURE 1.8. Preparation of a "T section" of the meeting point of the dividing membranes in twin placentas.

a great influence on the well-being of the developing fetus (Benirschke, 1961b; Bejar et al., 1988). They take three forms: artery to artery (AA), vein to vein (VV), and artery to vein (AV). The latter is doubtless the most important and is the basis for the twin-to-twin transfusion syndrome (TTTS). It must here be remembered that arteries lie on top of veins and that they are thus readily identified macroscopically. An arteriovenous (AV) anastomosis carries the blood of one twin, through a cotyledon in a one-way direction, from one twin to the other. Often the various types of anastomoses coexist, and the consequences for fetal development may be different depending on the arrangements that are present. When in doubt, one injects the vessels in question with colored water or milk, all being readily available in obstetrical suites. Only the most sophisticated studies require injection with plastics (Panigel, 1962). Injection of vessels has presented some problems for novices. First it must be remembered that most placentas have suffered some disruption during delivery, especially the immature twin placentas. Thus, only small, selected districts should be injected, and this should be done only after the umbilical cords have been cut off in order to reduce resistance. Before injecting one should seek to identify by careful inspection those areas that seem most profitable for the injection study. Large interarterial anastomoses (common) may be identified by one's ability to push blood back and forth from one side to the other. When one attempts to demonstrate the areas that reflect shared cotyledons, as in the transfusion syndrome, one best uses a 20-mL syringe and a large (15-gauge) blunt needle. This is inserted into an arterial branch a short distance away from the prospective site and gradually one then fills the area with water or milk. The cotyledon will first rise and, when completely filled, it will empty into the vein that drains the cotyledon. It is also advisable to make a drawing or photograph of the anastomotic arrangements among

multiple placental vascular districts, just to have them available for the record.

Examination of the maternal surface and of other parameters of the placentas of twins follows that of the regular protocol. It must be borne in mind that when the blood content of twins differs considerably it may be reflected in the macroscopic placental examination as well. One portion of such a twin placenta may be severely congested and larger, with the other being pale and smaller. This condition is present when only one AV anastomosis exists. Here, in the classical mechanism of the transfusion syndrome, one twin constantly loses blood through this one-way AV shunt, whereas the other becomes plethoric. Usually, it leads to hydramnios, premature birth, and disparate birth weights of these "identical twins." It must be recognized, however, that differences in neonatal hemoglobin content of monochorionic twins may also occur acutely, when large AA and VV anastomoses exist. Thus, after the delivery of one twin, the other twin may "bleed" through anastomoses if the cord of the delivered twin is not promptly clamped. Likewise, when one such twin dies in utero, significant shifts of blood may occur from the live twin through such large anastomoses into the relaxed vascular bed of the deceased twin. Finally, it is our practice to dissect the two halves of the twin placenta at the site of the vascular equator in order to determine the placental weight of each twin. Higher multiple births are handled the same way.

Fixation

The pathologist is used to fixing tissues for histologic study in 10% formalin solution (a 1:10 dilution of the commercial 40% formaldehyde) and there is no need to make an exception with the placenta. For **routine histopathology** we prefer Bouin's solution, however, because it makes embryonic and placental tissue considerably harder and allows one to trim the tissue more readily before embedding. After a membrane roll is made with the help of the forceps, it is also much easier to trim this jelly roll when Bouin's solution, rather than formalin, has been used. Bouin's solution is made by preparing a saturated solution (1.2%) of picric acid in water and adding 40% formaldehyde solution and glacial acetic acid in proportions of 15:5:1. After overnight fixation, the tissue is ready to be trimmed. The solution has the additional benefit of decalcifying fetal tissues. Prolonged storage of tissues in Bouin's solution makes them very hard.

Carnoy solution is a useful alternative if immediate fixation is required directly after delivery and if obstetricians refuse the use of formaldehyde in the vicinity of the delivery room. This fixative is composed of 60 mL absolute ethanol, 30 mL chloroform, and 10 mL glacial acetic acid. It guarantees good structural preservation, provided that the thickness of the tissue blocks does not exceed 3 to 4 mm.

Many other fixatives have been used. Jiricka and Preslickova (1974) made a detailed study of seven solutions and evaluated the effect for the staining characteristics with different dyes. They found that none is ideal for all purposes, so the fixative must be chosen that gives the best results for a specific reason. The authors presented this information in tabular form, and the article must be consulted if optimal results are to be obtained.

Ideally, the sectioned slices, when Bouin-fixed, are immersed in a saturated lithium carbonate solution before embedding. This step is not absolutely required, but it helps to remove extraneous pigments. Moreover, some intervillous blood is lysed, and pigments derived from blood ("formalin pigment," acid hematin) are more frequently present when lithium carbonate is omitted. Note, however, that occasionally the use of Bouin's fixation is disadvantageous. For instance, Altshuler and Hyde (1985) reported that infection with fusobacteria was less readily appreciated after Bouin's fixation than when formalin was used. Furthermore, Bouin's solution is not useful for fixation when the purpose is to conduct immunohistochemical or in situ hybridization studies (Gleich, personal communication, 1989). Today many **immunohistochemical studies** can be carried out on paraffin sections, such as the demonstration of most cytoskeletal proteins, extracellular matrix molecules, and several proliferation markers (Frank et al., 1994). For all these purposes we suggest the fixation in 4% neutral buffered formaldehyde solution for a maximum of 24 hours followed by paraffin embedding not exceeding 60°C. Possible flow cytometry is also more readily done with such material.

Another important issue is the manner of tissue handling prior to fixation. The time and the mode of cord clamping (Bouw et al., 1976), the ischemic period before onset of fixation (Voigt et al., 1978; Kaufmann, 1985), as well as the composition of the fixative (Kaufmann, 1980)

may well influence the distention of the fetal vascular bed and the width of the intervillous space (see tables in Chapters 15, 17, 18, and 19). We recommend particularly for all studies concerning the pathology of the fetoplacental vessels (e.g., in cases with Doppler high resistance index) that a strictly standardized sampling and fixation protocol be used. If this is not done, false impressions of such conditions as chorangiosis may be obtained.

Other techniques may also require special handling, as for instance in the studies by Becker and Bleyl (1961) on toxemia. They employed fluorescence microscopy of villi to understand their different composition in this disease.

It is the recommended practice to save at least one section of umbilical cord, a membrane roll, and three pieces of placental tissue for histologic examination. Of course, having more sections of umbilical cord available for histological study is ideal, as an inflammatory response, thrombi, and other features are not always uniformly distributed throughout the length of the umbilical cord. Preparing more than one piece of placental tissue for histologic study is also desirable because so many areas of the placenta show histologic variations. Thus, one can much better determine the existence of inflammatory lesions and is less apt to overlook changes that are not ascertained macroscopically. Moreover, one must obtain sections from the more normal portions of the placenta as well. Although the pathologist is used to sampling abnormal areas for histologic study, it is not desirable to take only abnormal areas of the placenta. Indeed, almost all infarcts are histologically alike, and since they also have a typical macroscopic appearance, they are rarely worth the trouble of histologic study, except that the sections provide verifiable evidence of the existence of infarcts. It is much more important to save normal-appearing placental tissue for microscopy. One must sample both the fetal and maternal surfaces in order to include some fetal surface blood vessels. Because it is generally impossible to anticipate from macroscopic inspection whether chronic villitis and many other lesions exist, it is better to preserve too much than too little in the fixative. It goes without saying that unusual-appearing areas must also be sampled.

For histologic examination, we prefer the hematoxylin and eosin (H&E) stain. On many occasions, however, it is useful to employ special stains, such as elastica preparations, bacterial and spirochete stains, periodic acid-Schiff (PAS) preparations, and specific immunohistochemical stains that disclose the presence of viruses (e.g., cytomegalovirus and herpes antigens) as well as specific proteins [e.g., human chorionic gonadotropin (hCG), human placental lactogen (hPL), major basic protein (MBP), cytokeratin, vimentin, fibrin, proliferation markers] (see Chapter 3). These tests have given much insight into the distribution of various placental tissue components, the

REPORT OF PLACENTAL EXAMINATION

NAME of PATIENT:..........................   Path. #.............
                                                              Unit #.............

HISTORY:..
....
....
INFANT:..
....
<u>Macroscopic:</u>

WEIGHT (disk only)..........g Formalin-fixed.......Fresh.......
SIZE.....×...... ×.....cm
CORD: INSERTION: Central..... Eccentric:........cm from margin

                  Marginal....Velamentous.....Vasa previa...........
      Vessels: 3...2... Thrombosis: Yes...No...Knots:..........Twists: Right...Left....
MEMBRANES: Marginal..... Circumvallate..... Color: Green.....Opaque.....Normal.....
      Point of rupture from margin:......cm
      Amnion nodosum.........
SURFACE VESSELS:...
TWINS: Yes....No......   HIGHER MULTIPLES:...
      DiDi.....DiMo.....MoMo....
Describe..Anastomoses...
MATERNAL SURFACE: Intact: Yes....No.... Calcification: Marked....normal....no...
      Color:.......... (Normal?).......(Pale?)........
      Abruptio: Yes.... No...... Size........cm Old.....Recent.......
CUT SURFACE: Infarct..... % of total placenta.... Old..... Recent....
TUMORS..
OTHER...

<u>Microscopic</u>:...
....
....

<u>DIAGNOSIS:</u>

                                          ....
                                       Pathologist

Pictures taken? Yes.......(Color......B&W.......Digital.....) No........

FIGURE 1.9. Example of a report form to use during placental examination.

sites of hormone production, and the involvement by organisms as well as other pathologic processes. The report form that we use during placental examination is reproduced in Figure 1.9.

Special Procedures

The placenta can serve as a good source of tissue for **chromosome analysis**. This is especially true when the fetus is macerated. One proceeds best by disinfecting the amnion with some alcohol and then stripping the amnion off a portion of placental surface. For the purpose of taking the biopsy from chorion, sterile instruments are recommended. A small piece of chorion, ideally with a bit of fetal surface vessel, is best for the purpose of establishing a tissue culture. The biopsies are placed into tissue culture medium with antibiotics and transferred to the laboratory. Touch preparations of amnionic surface or from the undersurface of the amnion may be useful for the **identification of bacteria or leukocytes**. It is of parenthetic interest that Jauniaux and Campbell (1990) showed that many structural abnormalities of the placenta can already be anticipated from sonography.

References

ACOG: Placental Pathology. Committee Opinion. **102**:1–2, 1991.

Altshuler, G.: Placental pathology clues for interdisciplinary clarification of fetal disease. Trophobl. Res. **13**:511–525, 1999.

Altshuler, G. and Hyde, S.: Fusobacteria: an important cause of chorioamnionitis. Arch. Pathol. Lab. Med. **109**:739–743, 1985.

Altshuler, G. and Hyde, S.: Clinicopathologic implications of placental pathology. Clin. Obstet. Gynecol. **39**:549–570, 1996.

Bacsich, P. and Smout, C.F.V.: Some observations on the foetal vessels of the human placenta with an account of the corrosion technique. J. Anat. **72**:358–364, 1938.

Bartholomew, R.A., Colvin, E.D., Grimes, W.H., Fish, J.S., Lester, W.M. and Galloway, W.H.: Criteria by which toxemia of pregnancy may be diagnosed from unlabeled formalin-fixed placentas. Amer. J. Obstet. Gynecol. **82**:277–290, 1961.

Becker, V. and Bleyl, U.: Placentarzotte bei Schwangerschaftstoxicose und fetaler Erythroblastose im fluorescenzmikroskopischen Bilde. Virchows Arch. (Pathol. Anat.) **334**:516–527, 1961.

Bejar, R., Wozniak, P., Allard, M., Benirschke, K., Vaucher, Y., Coen, R., Berry, C., Schragg, P., Villegas, I. and Resnik, R.: Antenatal origin of neurologic damage in newborn infants. I. Preterm Infants. Amer. J. Obstet. Gynecol. **159**:357–363, 1988.

Benirschke, K.: Examination of the placenta. Obstet. Gynecol. **18**:309–333, 1961a.

Benirschke, K.: Twin placenta and perinatal mortality. New York State J. Med. **61**:1499–1508, 1961b.

Boe, F.: Studies on vascularization of the human placenta. Acta Obstet. Gynecol. Scand. (Suppl. 5) **32**: 1–92, 1953.

Booth, V.J., Nelson, K.B., Dambrosia, J.M. and Grether, J.K.: What factors influence whether placentas are submitted for pathologic examination? Amer. J. Obstet. Gynecol. **176**: 567–571, 1997.

Bouw, G.M., Stolte, L.A.M., Baak, J.P.A. and Oort, J.: Quantitative morphology of the placenta. 1. Standardization of sampling. Eur. J. Obstetr. Gynecol. Reprod. Biol. **6**:325–331, 1976.

Crawford, J.M.: Vascular anatomy of the human placenta. Amer. J. Obstet. Gynecol. **84**:1543–1567, 1962.

Driscoll, S.G.: Choriocarcinoma: An "incidental finding" within a term placenta. Obstet. Gynecol. **21**:96–101, 1963.

Fisher, C.C., Garrett, W. and Kossoff, G.: Placental aging monitored by gray scale echography. Amer. J. Obstet. Gynecol. **124**:483–488, 1976.

Fox, H.: Pathology of the Placenta. 2nd edition. Saunders, London, 1997.

Frank, H.G., Malekzadeh, F., Kertschanska, S., Crescimanno, C., Castellucci, M., Lang, I., Desoye, G. and Kaufmann, P.: Immunohistochemistry of two different types of placental fibrinoid. Acta Anat. **150**:55–68, 1994.

Fritschek, F.: Über "leere" Placentarhohlräume. Anat. Anz. **64**: 65–73, 1927.

Fujikura, T.: Placental calcification and maternal age. Amer. J. Obstet. Gynecol. **87**:41–45, 1963a.

Fujikura, T.: Placental calcification and seasonal difference. Amer. J. Obstet. Gynecol. **87**:46–47, 1963b.

Geller, H.F.: Über die Bedeutung des subchorialen Fibrinstreifens in der menschlichen Placenta. Arch. Gynäkol. **192**:1–6, 1959.

Gruenwald, P.: Examination of the placenta by the pathologist. Arch. Pathol. **77**:41–46, 1964.

Gruenwald, P. and Minh, H.N.: Evaluation of body and organ weights in perinatal pathology. II. Weight of body and placenta of surviving and of autopsied infants. Amer. J. Obstet. Gynecol. **82**:312–319, 1961.

Heifetz, S.A.: Single umbilical artery. A statistical analysis of 237 autopsy cases and review of the literature. Perspect. Pediatr. Pathol. **8**:345–378, 1984.

Hyrtl, J.: Die Blutgefässe der Menschlichen Nachgeburt unter Normalen und Abnormen Verhältnissen. Braumüller, Vienna, 1870.

Jauniaux, E. and Campbell, S.: Ultrasonographic assessment of placental abnormalities. Amer. J. Obstet. Gynecol. **163**: 1650–1658, 1990.

Jeacock, M.K., Scott, J. and Plester, J.A.: Calcium content of the human placenta. Amer. J. Obstet. Gynecol. **87**:34–40, 1963.

Jiricka, Z. and Preslickova, M.: The effect of fixation on staining of placental tissue. Z. Versuchstierk. **16**:127–130, 1974.

Kaufmann, P.: Der osmotische Effekt der Fixation auf die Placentastruktur. Verh. Anat. Ges. **74**:351–352, 1980.

Kaufmann, P.: Influence of ischemia and artificial perfusion on placental ultrastructure and morphometry. Contrib. Gynecol. Obstet. **13**:18–26, 1985.

Langston, C., Kaplan, C., MacPherson, T., Manci, E., Peevy, K., Clark, B., Murtagh, C., Cox, S. and Glenn, G.: Practice guidelines for examination of the placenta. Developed by the placental pathology practice guideline development task force of the College of American Pathologists. Arch. Pathol. Lab. Med. **121**:449–476, 1997.

Las Heras, J., Micheli, V. and Kakarieka, E.: Placental pathology in perinatal deaths. Modern Pathol. **7** (1):abstract 26 (p. 5P), 1994.

Lucas, A., Christofides, N.D., Adran, T.E., Bloom, S.R. and Aynsley-Green, A.: Fetal distress, meconium, and motilin. Lancet **i**:718, 1979.

Miller, P.W., Coen, R.W. and Benirschke, K.: Dating the time interval from meconium passage to birth. Obstet. Gynecol. **66**:459–462, 1985.

Moessinger, A.C., Blanc, W.A., Marone, P.A. and Polsen, D.C.: Umbilical cord length as an index of fetal activity: Experimental study and clinical implications. Pediatr. Res. **16**: 109–112, 1982.

Naeye, R.L.: Maternal floor infarction. Hum. Pathol. **16**:823–828, 1985.

Naeye, R.L.: Functionally important disorders of the placenta, umbilical cord, and fetal membranes. Hum. Pathol. **18**: 680–691, 1987.

Panigel, M.: Placental perfusion experiments. Amer. J. Obstet. Gynecol. **84**:1664–1683, 1962.

Priman, J.: A note on the anastomosis of the umbilical arteries. Anat. Rec. **134**:1–5, 1959.

Pritchard, J.A., MacDonald, P.C. and Gant, N.F.: Williams Obstetrics, 17th ed. Appleton Century Crofts, Norwalk, CT, 1985.

Reece, E.A., Scioscia, A.L., Pinter, E., Hobbins, J.C., Green, J., Mahoney, M.J. and Naftolin, F.: Prognostic significance of the human yolk sac assessed by ultrasonography. Amer. J. Obstet. Gynecol. **159**:1191–1194, 1988.

Salafia, C.M. and Vintzileos, A.M.: Why all placentas should be examined by a pathologist in 1990. Amer. J. Obstet. Gynecol. **163**:1282–1293, 1990. (See discussion Amer. J. Obstet. Gynecol. **165**:783–784, 1991.)

Schatz, F.: Die Gefässverbindungen der Placentakreisläufe eineiiger Zwillinge, ihre Entwicklung und ihre Folgen. Arch. Gynäkol. **27**:1–72, 1886.

Schremmer, B.-N.: Gewichtsveränderungen verschiedener Gewebe nach Formalinfixierung. Frankfurt. Z. Pathol. **77**: 299–304, 1967.

Snoeck, J.: Le Placenta Humain. Masson & Cie, Paris. 1958.

Torpin, R. and Hart, B.F.: Placenta bilobata. Amer. J. Obstet. Gynecol. **42**:38–49, 1941.

Travers, H. and Schmidt, W.A.: College of American Pathologists Conference XIX on the Examination of the Placenta. Arch. Pathol. Lab. Med. **115**:660–731, 1991. (This is a composite of many articles by numerous authors).

Voigt, S., Kaufmann, P. and Schweikhart, G.: Zur Abgrenzung normaler, artefizieller und pathologischer Strukturen in reifen menschlichen Plazentazotten. II. Morphometrische Untersuchungen zum Einfluss des Fixationsmodus. Arch. Gynäkol. **226**:347–362, 1978.

Walker, J.: Weight of the human fetus and of its placenta. Cold Spring Harbor Symp. Quant. Biol. **19**:39–40, 1954.

Zeek, P.M. and Assali, N.S.: Vascular changes in the decidua associated with eclamptogenic toxemia of pregnancy. Amer. J. Clin. Pathol. **20**:1099–1109, 1950.

2
Macroscopic Features of the Delivered Placenta

The full-term, delivered placenta is, in more than 90% of the cases, a disk-like, flat, round to oval organ. In nearly 10% it has abnormal shapes, such as placenta bilobata, placenta duplex, placenta succenturiata, placenta zonaria, and placenta membranacea (Torpin, 1969). The average diameter is 22 cm, the average thickness in the center of the delivered organ 2.5 cm, and the average weight 470 g (see Chapter 28, Table 28.1). The respective measurements show considerable interindividual variation and strongly depend on such factors as the mode of birth, timing of cord clamping (see Chapter 28, Table 28.8), and time elapsed between delivery and examination.

Fetal Surface

The **fetal (chorionic or amnionic) surface**, facing the amnionic cavity, has a glossy appearance because of the intact epithelial surface of the amnion. This membrane covers the **chorionic plate**, including the **chorionic vessels**. The latter branch is a star-like pattern positioned centrifugally from the cord insertion over the fetal surface (Fig. 2.1, left). Where arteries and veins cross, the arterial branches are usually closer to the amnion; they cross the veins on their amnionic aspect. Wentworth (1965) reported that only about 3% show the opposite condition. According to Boyd and Hamilton (1970), the superficial position of one or few venous branches at points of arteriovenous crossing is not unusual.

In the vicinity of the larger chorionic vessels, the chorionic plate normally has an opaque appearance because an increased number of collagen fibers accompany the vessels. Those areas of the chorionic plate located between the chorionic vessels are mostly transparent and are dark lilac to black because maternal blood in the intervillous space shines through. Opaque spots (bosselations) or large opaque areas independent of chorionic vessels usually point to large subchorionic deposits of Langhans' fibrinoid.

Near the **placental margin**, where the most peripheral branches of the chorionic vessels bend vertically toward the marginal villous trees, the transparency of the chorionic plate decreases, resulting in a largely incomplete, opaque **subchorial closing ring** that is a result of increased amounts of cytotrophoblast and collagen fibers (see Chapter 9). It connects the placenta with the membranes. In the case of a particularly broad and prominent subchorial closing ring, the specimen is called a placenta marginata. A placenta circumvallata is formed when the closing ring is peripherally undergrown by villous trees. In such cases, it does not represent the outermost margin of the placenta; rather, the membranes insert superficially from the fetal surface of the placenta.

Placental shape and cord insertion are sometimes regarded as structurally impressive but functionally unimportant parameters. Becker (1989) stressed that both are influenced by the intrauterine position of the placenta. According to Schultze (1887), the location of the cord insertion represents the epicenter of implantation. Eccentric or marginal cord insertion thus points to an eccentric implantation on the anterior or posterior uterine wall, which causes asymmetrical development of the organ for mechanical and nutritional reasons.

Maternal Surface

The **uterine (maternal) surface** of the placenta is opaque, as it is an artificial surface originating from laminar degenerative processes within the **junctional zone** that led to the separation of the organ. This separation process subdivides the junctional zone between placenta and uterine wall into

- the **basal plate,** which is attached to the placenta and represents the maternal, uterine surface of the organ; and
- the **placental bed,** which remains in utero.

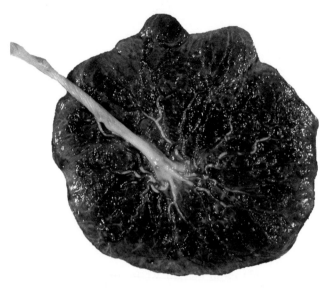 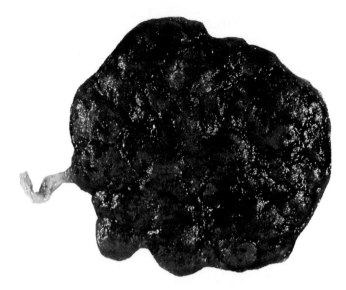

FIGURE 2.1. Apical (left) and basal (right) views of a freshly delivered, mature human placenta. Note the slightly eccentric insertion of the umbilical cord, which is the most usual location. The chorionic arteries (white because of postpartum injection of milk) cross over the corresponding veins (dark). The basal surface (right) is subdivided into placental lobules of varying size by an interrupted net of dark grooves. × 0.4.

The basal plate and the maternal surface of the placenta could not be identified before placental separation in the in situ specimens that were fixed before the onset of labor (see Chapter 4, Fig. 4.7). It is composed of a heterogeneous mixture of trophoblastic and decidual cells embedded into prevailing amounts of extracellular debris, fibrinoid, and blood clot.

An incomplete system of grooves subdivides the basal surface of the placenta into 10 to 40 slightly elevated areas called **maternal cotyledons** (lobes or lobules) (Fig. 2.1, right; Fig. 2.2). Internally, these grooves correspond to the **placental septa**, folds of the basal plate, which project into the intervillous space (see Fig. 4.7). In histologic sections, the septa can often be seen to be indented at their basal surfaces. It is likely that these grooves and the respective basal indentations of the septa are the postpartal results of tearing at sites of minor mechanical resistance, as the basal central parts of the septa are often characterized by

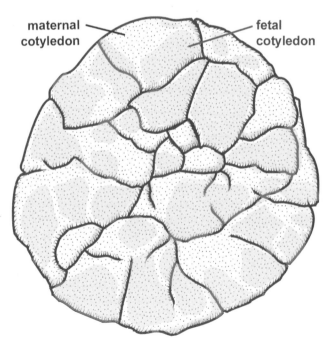

maternal cotyledon

fetal cotyledon

FIGURE 2.2. Basal view of the placenta, drawn in combination with a radiograph of the same placenta after injection of a radio-paque medium into the fetal vessels. The borderlines of the placental lobules (maternal cotyledons, red stippled) are marked by red lines corresponding to the grooves. The radiographic projections of 29 villous trees are represented by blue stippled areas. This combination demonstrates a fairly good harmony of villous trees and maternal lobes. One to three villous trees (fetal cotyledons) are projected on one lobe (maternal cotyledon). (*Source:* Kaufmann & Scheffen, 1992, with permission; based on photographs by Boyd & Hamilton, 1970.)

necrotic zones, clefts, and local pseudocysts. Despite their possibly artifactual genesis, the grooves delineate the lobes and mark the position of the septa. As is described in Chapter 9, the scpta must not be misunderstood as separating structures that subdivide the intervillous space into chambers; rather, they are irregular pillars or short sails that only trace the lobular borders.

The lobes show fairly good harmony with the position of the **fetal cotyledons.** From the chorionic plate at term, 60 to 70 villous stems arise, each branching into one villous tree (or fetal cotyledon) (see Fig. 4.7 and Chapter 7, Fig. 7.18). Thus, according to Boyd and Hamilton (1970) and Kaufmann (1985), each lobe is occupied by one or several villous trees. When a radioangiograph of the villous trees is projected onto a basal view of the same placenta (Fig. 2.2), the borderlines of the lobes usually coincide with the borderlines of single villous trees or small groups of trees. Small marginal lobes are likely to be occupied by only a single villous tree and thus correspond to what Schuhmann and his group (1981) described as representing a **placentone**.

The Terms **Fetal Placenta** and **Maternal Placenta**

In describing human placentation, terms such as **fetal placenta** and **maternal placenta** must be avoided because they are misleading and often cause misinterpretation. This point may become important as soon as morphologically inexperienced biochemists, endocrinologists, and others isolate respective parts of the organ, then place trust in their putative and designated origin, and draw functional conclusions.

A typical example is the questionable interpretation that maternal tissues (decidua) may produce human placental lactogen (hPL). The basal plate, often erroneously referred to as **"maternal placenta,"** is not exclusively composed of maternal cells but rather represents a colorful mixture of trophoblastic (fetal) and endometrium-derived (maternal) cells. And only the fetal, trophoblastic cells secrete hPL.

A corresponding warning is necessary regarding the placental bed. It is often thought to represent only the maternal remains of the placental site after separation of the placenta. Trophoblastic streamers deeply invade the endometrium, however, and even penetrate the myometrium. They remain in utero long after delivery and can be found as fetal admixtures in the placental bed.

The term "fetal placenta" is also inappropriate. With the possible exception of central parts of the chorionic plate, there are no placental structures for which the pure fetal composition can be ensured. The marginal zone of the chorionic plate contains decidua, and the same is true for parts of the cell islands and septa. Because the latter may be attached to the villous trees, one is never certain that preparations of it are devoid of maternal tissues, even if we disregard maternal blood and fibrinoid deposits that are partly maternal blood clot products.

References

Becker, V.: Plazenta. In, Pathologie der Plazenta und des Abortes. V. Becker and G. Röckelein, eds., pp. 1–155. Springer-Verlag, Berlin, 1989.

Boyd, J.D. and Hamilton, W.J.: The Human Placenta. Heffer, Cambridge, 1970.

Kaufmann, P.: Basic morphology of the fetal and maternal circuits in the human placenta. Contrib. Gynecol. Obstet. **13**: 5–17, 1985.

Kaufmann, P. and Scheffen, I.: Placental development. In, Neonatal and Fetal Medicine-Physiology and Pathophysiology, Vol. 1. R. Polin and W. Fox, eds., pp. 47–55. Saunders, Orlando, 1992.

Schuhmann, R.: Plazenton: Begriff, Entstehung, funktionelle Anatomie. In, Die Plazenta des Menschen. V. Becker, T.H. Schiebler and F. Kubli, eds., pp. 199–207. Thieme Verlag, Stuttgart, 1981.

Schultze, B.S.: Über velamentöse und placentale Insertion der Nabelschnur. Arch. Gynäkol. **30**:47–56, 1887.

Torpin, R.: The Human Placenta. Thomas, Springfield, IL, 1969.

Wentworth, P.: Some anomalies of the foetal vessels of the human placenta. J. Anat. **99**:273–282, 1965.

3
Microscopic Survey

For the beginner in placental histology and histopathology, paraffin sections of the organ look confusing because they contain not only a broad variety of differently structured villi but many nonvillous structures as well. This chapter introduces those basic histologic features that leap to the eye when inspecting a paraffin section and thus provides a quick orientation for the inexperienced reader. For this purpose we have selected a collection of conventional photographs from routine histologic sections, of routine quality. Labeling of the figures is explained in the text. For further reading concerning the various structures, we refer the reader to later chapters. For quantitative data, see Chapter 28, Table 28.1.

Ideally, the routine histologic examination of the human placenta requires vertically oriented sections that cover all placental structures from the chorionic plate, via the intervillous space down to the basal plate (Figs. 3.1 and 3.2). Such sections are easily obtained from most second and third trimester placentas, as well as from the rare in situ specimens obtained by hysterectomy in the first trimester (Fig. 3.1). Tissue biopsies from legal interruptions are in most cases less ideal for good survey pictures; usually the basal plate together with neighboring tissues such as septa, anchoring villi, and cell columns are either absent or at least difficult to identify because they are destroyed and mixed up among the villi.

Typical Histologic Features of the First Trimester Placenta

Complete and well-preserved survey sections of the first trimester placenta, such as this vertical section of an in situ specimen from the 6th week postmenstruation (p.m.) (Fig. 3.1A), cover the following structures: chorionic plate (Fig. 3.1B), intervillous space surrounding the placental villi (Fig. 3.1C–F), cell islands (Fig. 3.1G), and the basal plate (Fig. 3.1J–M) from which a septum (Fig. 3.1H) protrudes into the intervillous space; some anchoring villi are connected via cell columns to the septum (Fig. 3.1H) or to the basal plate (Fig. 3.1I).

In Figure 3.1A, the **intervillous space** (see Intervillous Space as Related to the Villous Trees in Chapter 7) is the diffuse space that is surrounded by the chorionic plate on the one side and the basal plate on the other. From the 13th week on, it contains ample maternal blood, the volume of which increases to about 100 to 200 mL at term. Up to the 12th week p.m. only little maternal blood has been found in the intervillous space; limited maternal circulation of the intervillous space is probably caused by intraluminal plugs of trophoblast cells within the uteroplacental vessels (see Basal Plate in Chapter 9). The maternal blood flows around the villous trees, cell islands, septa, and fibrinoid deposits. In early pregnancy, the mean width of the intervillous space (between neighboring villi) usually amounts to several hundred micrometers.

In Figure 3.1B, the histologic specimens of the first trimester **chorionic plate** (see Chorionic Plate in Chapter 9) is devoid of amnion as this membrane is only superficially attached to the chorionic plate and is usually removed during preparation. Occasionally, pieces of amnion can be found curled up or upside down somewhere at the section's margin. As it is a regular constituent of most third trimester survey sections, the chorionic plate is discussed in the next part of this chapter (see Typical Histologic Features of the Third Trimester Placenta; Fig. 3.2A,B).

If the amnion is missing, as it is in this case, the surface of the chorionic plate (toward the fetus) is covered by an inconspicuous, incomplete layer of mesothelium. It follows a thick layer of chorionic mesoderm in which the chorionic branches of the umbilical vessels are embedded. Toward the intervillous space, the surface is covered in the early stages by a layer of syncytiotrophoblast, which with progressing pregnancy is replaced by fibrinoid (Fig. 3.2C).

Figure 3.1C: The tree-like arranged placental villi arise from the chorionic plate and protrude into the intervillous space, the villous trophoblastic surface being bathed directly by maternal plasma or blood. The trophoblastic surface of the villi is composed of an outer continuous layer of **villous syncytiotrophoblast** beneath which is a discontinuous layer of **villous cytotrophoblast** (Langhans' cells) (see Villous Cytotrophoblast in Chapter 6). The villous cytotrophoblast represents the proliferating stem cells for the syncytiotrophoblast that forms the decisive maternofetal transport barrier. The relative number of Langhans' cells decreases toward term.

The stroma of the villi is composed of the **fetal vessels**, which are embedded in a mixture of fixed connective tissue cells, macrophages, and connective tissue fibers. Throughout the first 2 months of pregnancy, **nucleated red blood cells** are a regular finding inside the fetal villous vessels (see Nucleated Red Blood Cells in Chapter 12).

In Figure 3.1D, very early in gestation, the **central stems** of the villous trees show signs of fibrosis around larger central vessels that gradually achieve the structural characteristics of arteries and veins. The superficial stromal layer has an unfibrosed, reticular appearance (see Development of Stem Villi in Chapter 7; also see Figs. 7.4 and 8.3 to 8.6). Arrows indicate the syncytial sprouts (Fig. 3.1F). Before the 8th week p.m., even the largest villi show a homogeneous mesenchymal stroma that is mostly not fibrosed and is devoid of the reticular structure; arteries and veins are absent also (see Figs. 8.1 and 8.2).

Figure 3.1E: Most of the large, bulbous villi of the first and second trimesters are the **immature intermediate villi** with reticular stroma and without stromal fibrosis. The fixed connective tissue cells surround channel-like spaces within the reticular stroma (Fig. 3.1J; see Immature Intermediate Villi in Chapter 7). These channels contain stromal macrophages (Hofbauer cells) that are easily identifiable by their rounded shape and their vacuolated or granular cytoplasm (see Hofbauer Cells in Chapter 6).

In Figure 3.1F, the peripheral branches of the immature intermediate villi are the **mesenchymal villi** (see Mesenchymal Villi in Chapter 7). They usually have diameters of 60 to 200 mm, are characterized by a dense cellular stroma, and do not possess many fetal vessels or collagen fibers. Peripherally, the mesenchymal villi extend into **syncytial sprouts** (see Development of the Mesenchymal Villi in Chapter 7), representing syncytiotrophoblastic, multinucleated structures. Very often the sprouts appear as dark cross sections (Fig. 3.1D) that seemingly do not contact villous surfaces.

Syncytial or trophoblastic sprouts are the first steps in the formation of new villi. They are invaded by mesenchymal stroma and by fetal capillary sprouts and thus transform into mesenchymal villi. Later, the mesenchymal villi grow in size and achieve the typical structure of immature intermediate villi (see Development and Fate of Immature Intermediate Villi in Chapter 7). For a description of the structural aspects of syncytial knotting and sprouting, see Syncytial Knotting in Chapter 15; for histopathologic significance see Control of Villous Development in Chapter 7, and Chapter 14.

In Figure 3.1G, a **cell island** as globular accumulation of extravillous trophoblast cells adheres to several villi (see Cell Islands in Chapter 9). They are directly continuous with villous cytotrophoblast in places where the villous syncytiotrophoblast is interrupted. Parts of the surfaces of these islands may be covered with plaques of syncytiotrophoblast. The extravillous trophoblast cells are usually embedded in matrix-type fibrinoid (see the following discussion, and Fibrinoid in Chapter 9). Cell islands are the still proliferating remainders of the free-floating primary villi from early pregnancy stages that never have been excavated by villous stroma.

In Figure 3.1H, a placental septum protrudes as veil-like extension of the basal plate into the intervillous space. They are rudimentary walls that are unable to completely subdivide the intervillous space into separate chambers. Structurally they show the same composition as the basal plate, as they contain mostly extravillous trophoblast cells and sometimes also some decidual cells. Very often, anchoring villi can be seen attached to the septa. In this stage of pregnancy they belong to the mesenchymal or immature intermediate type of villi. Cross sections of tips of septa look like cell islands and can be confused with the latter. For further information see Septa and Cell Islands in Chapter 9.

Figure 3.1I: **Anchoring villi** are peripheral villi that are connected to the basal plate or placental septa (see Fig. 3.1H) via cell columns. They stabilize the position of the villous trees in the maternal intervillous bloodstream. For development see Early Villous Stages in Chapter 5. **Cell columns** are the trophoblastic feet of the anchoring villi. In early stages of pregnancy they consist of several layers of proliferating extravillous cytotrophoblast serving as a proliferative source of villous as well as of basal plate cytotrophoblast (see Extravillous Trophoblast in Chapter 9).

Figure 3.1J: The **basal plate** is the bottom of the intervillous space and represents that part of the maternofetal junctional zone that adheres to the delivered placenta (see Basal Plate in Chapter 9). The basal portion of the maternofetal junctional zone, which adheres to the myometrium and remains in utero after delivery, is called the placental bed. The basal plate is composed of an admixture of extravillous trophoblast cells, various endometrial stromal cells, decidual cells, uteroplacental vessels, and endometrial glands, all embedded in ample fibrinoid that makes up the glossy to fibrillar ground substance.

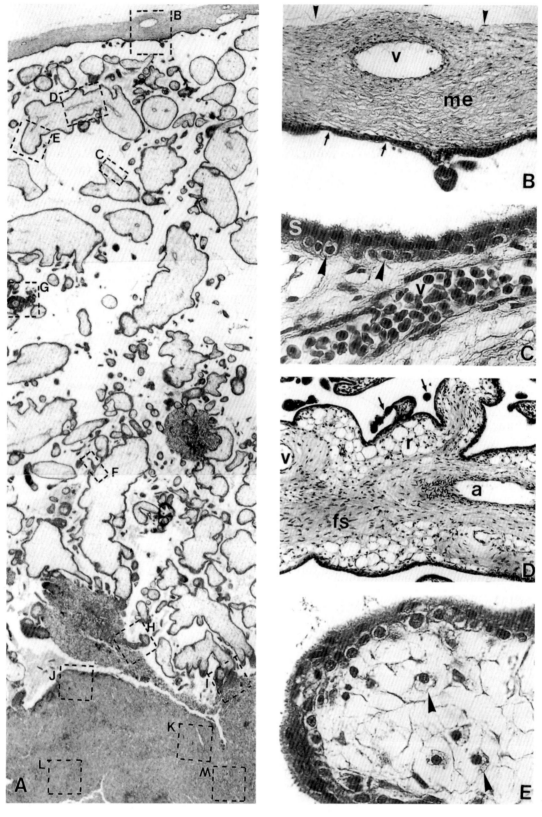

FIGURE 3.1. Typical features of the first trimester placenta as seen in paraffin sections following hematoxylin and eosin (H&E) staining. All specimens are from the 6th week postmenstruation (p.m.), except when otherwise stated. For details, see the text. A: Vertical survey section of an in situ specimen, 6th week p.m. The marked frames refer to the following detailed pictures. ×20. B: Chorionic plate. v, vein; arrowheads, mesothelium; me, chorionic mesoderm; arrows, incomplete layer of syncytiotrophoblast. ×100. C: Surface of an immature intermediate villus with trophoblast and a fetal vessel (V) containing nucleated red blood cells. s, syncytiotrophoblast; arrowheads, cytotrophoblast. ×400. D: Transitional form of an immature intermediate villus to become a stem villus (18th week p.m.). a, artery; v, vein; r, reticular stroma; fs, fibrous stroma; arrows, sprouts. ×100. E: Immature intermediate villus showing characteristic reticular stroma with macrophages (arrowheads). ×400.

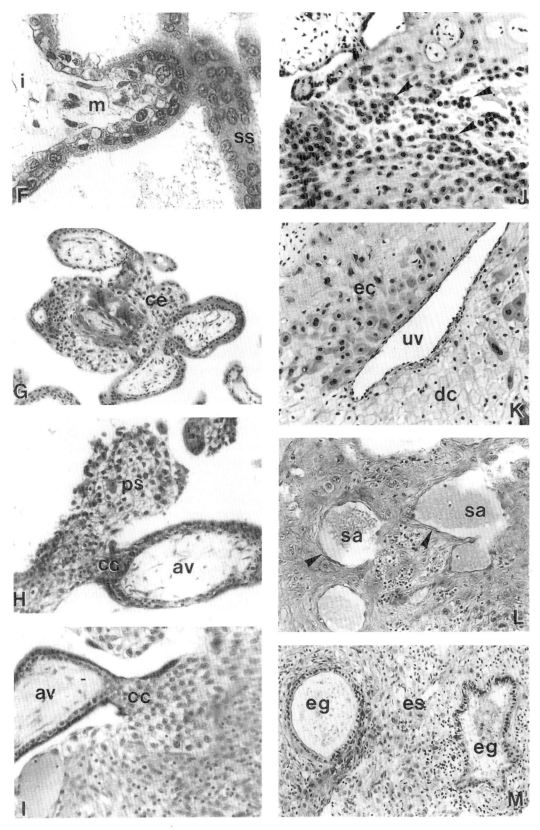

FIGURE 3.1. F: Mesenchymal villus (m) arising from an immature intermediate villus (i) and extending into syncytial sprouts (ss). ×400. G: Cell island (ce) attached to some villi. ×100. H: Placental septum (ps) connected to a villus (av) by a cell column (cc). ×200. I: Anchoring villus (av) connected to the basal plate by a cell column (cc). ×200. J: Surface of the basal plate showing extravillous trophoblast cells (arrowheads) embedded in fibrinoid (10th week p.m.). ×100. K: Deep part of the basal plate showing a uteroplacental vein (uv) surrounded by extravillous cytotrophoblast (ec) and decidua (dc) (37th week p.m., similar to the first trimester situation). ×140. L: Multiple cross sections across a spiral artery (sa), the wall of which is replaced by fibrinoid (arrowheads). ×100. M: Endometrial glands (eg) of the junctional zone embedded in endometrial stroma (es). ×200. For further details see the text.

Extravillous trophoblast cells (see also Fig. 3.1K) is the summarizing term for all trophoblast cells located outside the villi—in the chorionic plate, cell islands, septa, basal plate, cell columns, and membranes. Apparent inhomogeneities within the population are mostly the result of different stages of proliferation and differentiation. Those cells resting on the basal lamina facing the chorionic mesoderm (chorionic plate, membranes) or the villous stroma (cell columns, cell islands) are the proliferating stem cells (Langhans' cells), whereas the nonproliferating extravillous trophoblast cells, which have lost contact to the basal lamina represent more highly differentiated, invasive daughter cells of the former (see Extravillous Trophoblast in Chapter 9). Histologically, extravillous trophoblast cells appear as rounded to polygonal or spindle-shaped cells that may be isolated or grouped in strings; they differ from decidual cells in that, in paraffin sections, most of the cell bodies show nuclear cross sections (see Figs. 3.1K and 3.2L).

In Figure 3.1K, **decidual cells** are enlarged endometrial stromal cells that have elongated, partly branched bodies. Neighboring decidual cells are usually arranged in parallel, resulting in a peculiar histologic appearance. All the cellular sections in one area have the same shape, which is round, ellipsoid, or longitudinal (see Fig. 3.2L), depending on the sectional angle. Because the cell body is elongated, cross sections of the ovoid nuclei are rarely found (see Decidua in Chapter 9). **Uteroplacental** veins are endothelial tubes, surrounded by few regressive medial and adventitial cells, embedded in decidua and extravillous trophoblast cells; the latter rarely invade the venous walls and never the venous lumina (see Uteroplacental Vessels in Chapter 9).

In Figure 3.1L, **uteroplacental arteries (spiral arteries)** traverse the basal plate in spiral turns and connect the maternal uterine arteries to the intervillous space. Because of their shape, usually several cross sections are found close together (see Uteroplacental Vessels in Chapter 9). In contrast to the uteroplacental veins, the endothelial lining of the uteroplacental arteries is largely replaced by intravascular trophoblast, a special form of extravillous trophoblast. These cells may form large plugs that narrow or even occlude the arterial lumen (not shown). Arterial media and also the adventitia are replaced by trophoblast cells and fibrinoid, the latter substance also forming the immediate surrounding of most arteries.

In Figure 3.1M, in the depth of the basal plate, remainders of **endometrial glands** can be found. These are regular findings throughout the first 2 months of pregnancy, forming round to star-shaped lumina lined by cubical epithelium. They are surrounded by endometrial stroma or decidualized endometrial stromal cells. In subsequent stages of pregnancy, the glands disintegrate and only degenerative epithelial remainders may be found (see Decidua in Chapter 9).

Typical Histologic Features of the Third Trimester Placenta

Third trimester sections of the placenta, such as this vertical survey section of a mature placenta (Fig. 3.2A), are more difficult to examine as the villi are smaller and often stick so closely together that it is difficult to find the intervillous space in between. This section covers the chorionic plate (Fig. 3.2C), including the amnion (Fig. 3.2B), different types of villi (Fig. 3.2D–G), fibrinoid deposits in various locations (Fig. 3.2C,F,H–L), anchoring villi with rudimentary cell columns (Fig. 3.2I), cell islands (Fig. 3.2J), septa (Fig. 3.2K), and the basal plate (Fig. 3.2L).

In Figure 3.2A, in contrast to the first trimester situation, the width of the **intervillous space** is highly variable with large "subchorionic lakes" below the chorionic plate and narrow intervillous clefts between the terminal villi. In the normal term placenta, the mean width of the clefts including the subchorionic lakes is between 16 and 32 mm (see Intervillous Space as Related to the Villous Trees in Chapter 7). A generally much wider intervillous space indicates deficiency of terminal villi as in persisting villous immaturity (e.g., rhesus incompatibility) and in cases of excessive nonbranching angiogenesis (e.g., early-onset intrauterine growth restriction, early-onset IUGR) (see Chapter 15). A generally much tighter intervillous space is usually correlated with increased numbers of highly branched terminal villi as, for example, in cases of excessive branching angiogenesis (e.g., late-onset IUGR, often combined with preeclampsia) (see Chapter 15).

Figure 3.2B: The **amnion** covers the chorionic plate toward the amnionic cavity. It consists of a single layer of cubical to columnar cells that participate in the turnover of the amnionic fluid (see Amnion in Chapter 11). Seemingly multilayered segments of the amnionic epithelium represent oblique or tangential sections across the surface in most cases. In addition, nearly 50% of mature placentas also possess foci of real squamous metaplasia of the amnionic epithelium that may become up to 15 cellular layers in thickness (see Amnion in Chapter 11). Underneath the amnionic epithelium is a thin layer of amnionic mesoderm (about 15 to 30 mm in thickness). It is only loosely connected with the next layer, the chorionic mesoderm, via the spongy or intermediate layer, a reticular zone showing larger clefts (Fig. 3.2C). Because of unstable connection, the amnion may start gliding or may even become lost during preparation.

In Figure 3.2C, the third trimester **chorionic plate** is a multilayered structure. It consists of the spongy layer with numerous clefts, followed by the compact layer of chorionic mesoderm that is separated from the Langhans' fibrinoid stria by a rudimentary basement membrane. On the lower side of this basement membrane, highly variable amounts of extravillous cytotrophoblast can be found. During early pregnancy they form a complete and usually multilayered stratum; in later pregnancy, this layer becomes rarefied. Some of the cells deeply invade the fibrinoid (see Chorionic Plate in Chapter 9). Attached to or embedded into the fibrinoid one finds numerous stem villi, representing the first branches of villous trunci branching off from the chorionic plate nearby (see upper third of Fig. 3.2A). The chorionic plate represents the cover of the intervillous space, which follows directly below.

Figure 3.2D: The villous trees measure 1 to 4 cm in diameter. Their central branches are made up of **stem villi** (see Chapter 7, Fig. 7.26). These are the large-caliber villi that range from 80 to several thousand micrometers in diameter (see Stem Villi in Chapter 7). The highest concentration of stem villi and the largest calibers are found near the chorionic plate. Histologically, they are characterized by one or several arteries and veins or arterioles and venules with clearly visible muscular walls and are surrounded by a fibrous stroma that contains few paravascular capillaries (see Paravascular Capillary Net of Stem Villi in Chapter 7). Near term, the trophoblastic cover is focally or largely replaced by fibrinoid (see Perivillous Fibrinoid in Chapter 6). This process is more pronounced in larger stem villi.

In Figure 3.2E, immature forerunners of the stem villi, the **immature intermediate villi** can be seen. They are easily identifiable by their large caliber and their pale staining. Larger arteries and veins are usually absent, as are larger amounts of collagen fibers. The prevailing structure within the stroma is a reticularly arranged loose connective tissue with few fetal vessels. It is composed of net-like arranged fixed connective tissue cells that surround round spaces, the so-called stromal channels (see Immature Intermediate Villi in Chapter 7), which contain the Hofbauer cells (macrophages) (see Hofbauer Cells in Chapter 6). The latter are characterized by their rounded cell body and their numerous vacuoles or lysosomes.

Immature intermediate villi are the dominating villous type in early pregnancy (Fig. 3.1D,E). At term pregnancy, they usually persist in small groups (<10% of the total villous volume) in the centers of the villous trees. They are absent in hypermature placentas and their number is increased with persisting immaturity of the placenta (see Persisting Villous Immaturity and Rhesus Incompatibility in Chapter 15).

In Figure 3.2F, **mature intermediate villi** are slender, multiply curved branches of stem villi that exhibit diameters ranging from 60 to about 100 mm. They differ from stem villi by the absence of both stromal fibrosis and fetal stem vessels (arterioles and venules) with a media identifiable by light microscopy. Their stroma is composed of slender fetal capillaries embedded into a loose connective tissue that is rich in cells but poor in fibers (see Mature Intermediate Villi in Chapter 7). Longitudinal sections of mature intermediate villi are easily identifiable, whereas cross sections can easily be confused with terminal villi (see the following discussion).

Figure 3.2G: **Terminal villi** are the grape-like terminal side branches of the mature intermediate villi (see and Terminal Villi in Chapter 7 and Fig. 7.10). Their diameters range from 40 to about 80 mm. The dominating structures within the loose stroma are sinusoidally dilated and highly coiled fetal capillaries (see Sinusoids of Terminal Villi in Chapter 7). Typically, they bulge against the trophoblastic surface and transform this into extremely thin vasculosyncytial membranes that are devoid of nuclei.

The terminal villi, together with mature intermediate villi, represent the main exchange area of the third trimester placenta. Mature intermediate villi with slender capillaries and terminal villi with dilated sinusoids are easily discernible in placentas following early cord clamping and immediate fixation. Placentas that were fixed late after delivery and have lost larger amounts of fetal blood show the collapse of sinusoids, so that the terminal villi can no longer be discriminated from mature intermediate villi, which have slender capillaries.

A typical cross-sectional feature of terminal villi, and to a certain degree also of other villous types, is the **syncytial knotting** (Tenney-Parker changes). This designation is the usual term applied to an increased appearance of seemingly polypoid trophoblastic outgrowths at the villous surfaces and to the trophoblastic bridges connecting neighboring villi. Only a small percentage of respective structures represents real trophoblast protrusions and real bridges in the third trimester (see Syncytial Knotting in Chapter 15). Rather, the vast majority are flat sections across trophoblastic surfaces of irregularly shaped and branched villi. Toward term, as well as under hypoxic conditions, the outer shape of terminal villi becomes more irregular, thus increasing the chance of trophoblastic flat sectioning (syncytial knotting).

In Figure 3.2H, **fibrinoid** is an acellular, intensely staining, eosinophilic material that is mostly related to the intervillous space (Fig. 3.2C,D,F,H). When it replaces the trophoblastic cover of villi, as shown in this figure, it is called perivillous fibrinoid. In other villi, it may replace the stroma beneath a largely intact trophoblastic surface (intravillous fibrinoid, villous fibrinoid necrosis; Fig. 3.2F). Other sites of fibrinoid deposition are a prominent fibrinoid layer below the chorionic plate (Langhans' fibrinoid, Fig. 3.2C), a corresponding layer at the surface of the basal plate (Rohr fibrinoid, Fig. 3.2I,L), the Nitabuch fibrinoid in the depth of the maternofetal junctional zone (Fig. 3.2L), and the extracellular matrix of cell islands (Fig. 3.2J) and septa (Fig. 3.2K).

Despite the fact that fibrinoid appears to be homogeneous histologically, it is composed of two completely different materials: (1) **fibrin-type fibrinoid** (see

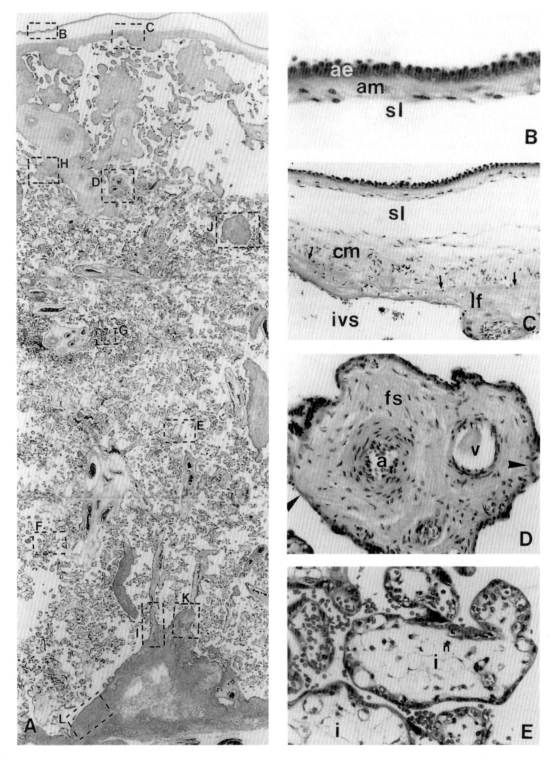

Figure 3.2. Typical features of the third trimester placenta as seen in paraffin sections following H&E staining. All specimens are from the 40th week p.m. For details see the text. A: Vertical survey section. The marked frames refer to the following detailed pictures. ×10. B: Amnion. ae, amnionic epithelium; am, amnionic mesoderm; sl, spongy layer. ×120. C: Chorionic plate, covered by the amnion. lf, Langhans' fibrinoid stria; arrows, basement membrane; cm, chorionic mesoderm; ivs, intervillous space. ×60. D: Peripheral stem villus. fs, fibrous stroma; a, artery; v, vein; arrowheads, syncytiotrophoblast. ×180. E: Two immature intermediate villi (i) surrounded by some mature intermediate and terminal. villi. ×180.

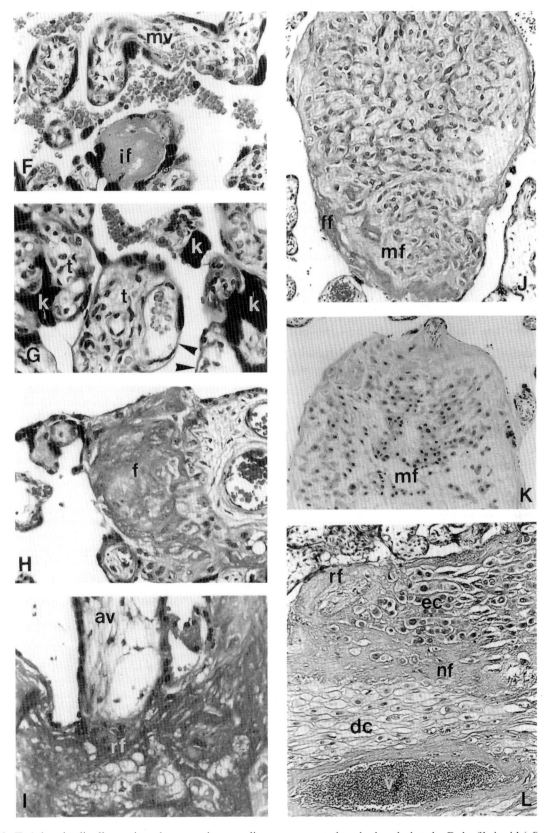

FIGURE 3.2. F: A longitudinally sectioned mature intermediate villus (mv) together with some terminal villi and a villous fibrinoid necrosis (if). ×180. G: A group of terminal villi (t) showing considerable syncytial knotting (k). ×360. H: A small stem villus, the trophoblastic cover of which is partly replaced by a thick plug of perivillous fibrinoid (f). ×180. I: An anchoring villus (av), connected to the basal plate by Rohr fibrinoid (rf) as the originally connecting cell column has vanished. ×180. J: Cell island. mf, matrix-type fibrinoid. ×90. K: Tip of a placental septum. ×90. L: Basal plate with obvious layering. rf, Rohr fibrinoid; nf, Nitabuch fibrinoid; dc, decidual cells; ec, extravillous cytotrophoblast; v, vein. ×90. For further details see the text.

Fig. 3.5C), a blood clotting product that is free of extravillous trophoblast cells and usually in contact with the intervillous space; and (2) **matrix-type fibrinoid** (see Fig. 3.5D), which embeds varying numbers of extravillous trophoblast cells and is itself a secretory product of these cells. Both substances may be deposited close together or separately (see Fibrinoid in Chapter 9).

Figure 3.2I: With the increasing development of free-floating villi that takes place in the course of the last trimester, **anchoring villi** become less prominent. They are still connected to the basal plate or to septa by **cell columns** (see Fig. 3.1H,I). As the proliferative activity of the columnar cytotrophoblast slows down, the cells are rarefied to one layer that is sometimes even incomplete. In some cases, extravillous trophoblast may be completely replaced by matrix-type fibrinoid so that the stroma of the anchoring villus directly borders Rohr's fibrinoid of the basal plate. Some cell columns maintain their proliferative activity and thus act as growth zones for the anchoring villi as well as for the basal plate, even near term (see Extravillous Trophoblast in Chapter 9).

Figure 3.2J: **Cell islands** increase in size throughout pregnancy by means of the continuous proliferation of their extravillous trophoblast cells. Also, the amount of fibrinoid embedding these cells increases steadily by apposition of fibrin-type fibrinoid from the intervillous space and by secretion of matrix-type fibrinoid from the trophoblast cells. Large cell islands may contain central cavities, or "cysts." They must be considered the result of degeneration of trophoblast cells and subsequent liquefaction. Occasionally, cell islands may contain some decidual cells in addition to extravillous trophoblast cells. Such islands can be interpreted either as cross sections of placental septa or as disrupted parts of such. For an understanding of their development see Early Villous Stages in Chapter 5; for the structure, see Cell Islands in Chapter 9.

Figure 3.2K: **Placental septa** are the result of folding of the basal plate, probably supported by tension of anchoring villi (see Septa in Chapter 9). They are rudimentary pillar-shaped structures, insufficient to subdivide the intervillous space into separate chambers. They are attached to the basal plate at their base (Fig. 3.2A) and are usually composed of extravillous trophoblast and decidual cells, both embedded in much fibrinoid. Sometimes large cysts, similar to those of the cell islands, can be found (see Cysts and Breus' Mole in Chapter 9). These sites of minor mechanical resistance during delivery usually give rise to deep basal tears of the placenta, the grooves delineating the placental lobes (see Chapter 2, Figs. 2.1 and 2.2). The septal tips (Fig. 3.2K) are composed mostly of extravillous trophoblast and matrix-type fibrinoid and are surrounded by fibrin-type fibrinoid. Their cross sections are hardly distinguishable from cell islands.

Only in a few exceptional places is the **basal plate** of the term placenta as clearly layered as depicted in Figure 3.2L, showing a superficial stria of Rohr fibrinoid, followed by extravillous cytotrophoblast, a layer of Nitabuch fibrinoid, and a compact decidual layer. In the latter, an uteroplacental vein is embedded. In most cases, however, there is no clearly defined fetomaternal border but rather extravillous cytotrophoblast, decidual cells, uteroplacental vessels, and glandular residues intermingled with ample fibrinoid and having no identifiable order (see Basal Plate in Chapter 9). In such cases, immunohistochemical markers may facilitate orientation (see the following discussion). For a consideration of the uteroplacental vessels and intraarterial trophoblast, see the description of the first trimester placenta, above.

IMMUNOHISTOCHEMICAL MARKERS

Structural orientation in histologic sections can be considerably facilitated by immunohistochemical markers. Some of those may even be applied to paraffin sections, provided that the tissue has been fixed with formalin only. We prefer fixation in a 4% neutrally buffered formaldehyde solution (10% formalin solution) for a maximum of 24 hours and at temperatures below 60°C during the paraffin embedding. Correspondingly prepared paraffin blocks may be used even years later for many immunohistochemical reactions (intermediate filaments, extracellular matrix proteins, proliferation markers, etc.).

The following immunohistochemical reactions may be useful for routine histologic examination of placental paraffin sections. All of them work with human material; some even cross-react with the respective molecules in several animal placentas.

Anticytokeratin stains epithelial structures such as amnionic epithelium, villous syncytio- and cytotrophoblast, and extravillous cytotrophoblast. In particular, for the discrimination between extravillous cytotrophoblast (Fig. 3.3A; also see Figs. 3.5A and 3.7A) and decidual cells (Fig. 3.3B; also see Fig. 3.5B) or intraarterial trophoblast (Fig. 3.3A) and maternal endothelium (Fig. 3.3C), it is a useful marker. We prefer a "pan-cytokeratin" antibody directed against cytokeratins 10, 17, and 18, which stains all cellular epithelial elements and additionally myofibroblasts and some vascular smooth muscle cells. Syncytiotrophoblast is only partly stained. Anticytokeratin 7 is a more specific trophoblast marker that does not cross-react with contractile mesenchymal dells. This antibody reproducibly stains villous and extravillous cytotrophoblast, but rarely villous syncytiotrophoblast or multinucleated trophoblastic giant cells.

Antivimentin stains all mesenchyme-derived cells, such as connective tissue cells, macrophages, decidual cells, smooth muscle cells, and endothelial cells. We use it as control on paraffin sections that are parallel to those stained for cytokeratin. Placental cells should be positive either for cytokeratin (epithelial origin, such as trophoblast, amnion, gland cells) or vimentin (mesenchymal origin, such as connective tissue, decidua, smooth muscle cells endothelium). It is a useful tool to identify decidual cells (Fig. 3.3B; also see Fig. 3.5B) as opposed to extravillous trophoblast cells (Fig. 3.3A; also see Fig. 3.5A) or to discriminate maternal endothelium from intraarterial trophoblast (Fig. 3.3C).

Anti-factor VIII–related antigen (the former anti–von Willebrand factor) is a marker that is largely specific for most endothelial cells. Application of this antibody provided proof that the intervillous space in the adjacency of venous openings is lined by maternal endothelium (Fig. 3.3C). It does not always work on paraffin sections. The much more reliable marker for endothelial cells in paraffin sections is **anti–CD 34** (the monoclonal antibody QBend10) which detects a

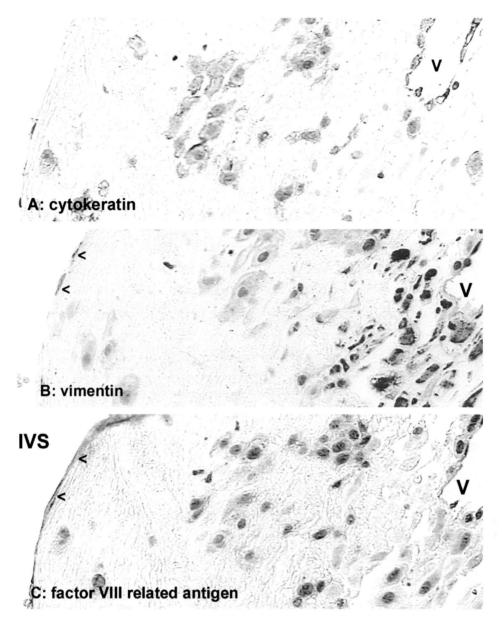

FIGURE 3.3. Serial sections of a superficial part of the mature basal plate bordering the intervillous space (IVS) and showing a colorful mixture of extravillous trophoblast cells with decidual cells as well as a uteroplacental vessel (V). Immunohistochemistry using three different marker antibodies allows easy discrimination of cell types. A: Anticytokeratin, an epithelial marker, binds to evenly spread extravillous trophoblast cells as well as to the trophoblast cell lining of the uteroplacental vessel (brown). The surface of the basal plate remains unstained. B: Antivimentin, a mesenchymal marker, stains the decidual cells (brown) as well as the endothelial lining of the basal plate (arrowheads). The luminal lining of the uteroplacental vessel (V) remains unstained since it consists of trophoblast rather than of endothelium. C: Staining with antibodies to factor VIII–related antigen, an endothelial marker, reveals that the surface of this part of the basal plate is covered by (maternal) endothelium (brown, arrowheads). All other cellular constituents of the basal plate including the luminal lining of the uteroplacental vessel remain unstained. ×230. (Courtesy Dr. Sonja Kertschanska, Aachen.)

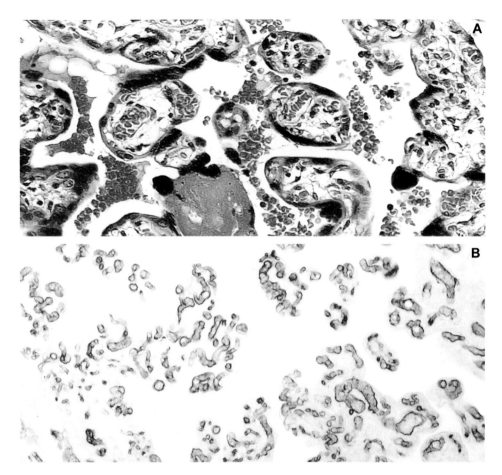

FIGURE 3.4. Endothelial markers facilitate identification of fetal capillaries within placental villi. A: Hematoxylin and eosin staining of term placental villi allows easy identification of villous shapes and of the trophoblastic surface. Discrimination of stromal components such as fibroblasts, macrophages, and endothelium is largely impossible. B: The antibody QBend10 (anti-CD34) specifically stains endothelial cells (brown) of the villous vessels and enables easy discrimination of the fetoplacental vessel bed. Term placenta. ×145.

cell surface marker specific for endothelium and its progenitor cells (Fig. 3.4).

Antifibrin can be used as a specific marker for fibrin-type fibrinoid as a blood clotting product (Fig. 3.5C). Specific detection of fibrin can only be achieved when an antibody is available (e.g., Immunotech, clone E8) that does not cross-react with the nearly universally present fibrinogen.

Anti-oncofetal fibronectin BC-1 (directed against the III-7 domain of oncofetal fibronectins containing the ED-B sequence) and **FDC-6** (directed against the O-glycosylated III-CS region of oncofetal fibronectins) are specific markers for matrix-type fibrinoid as shown for BC-1 in Figure 3.5D. Different from other fibronectin antibodies, they cross-react with neither fibrin-type fibrinoid nor connective tissue.

Anti–γ-smooth muscle actin in placental tissues is largely specific for vascular smooth muscle cells and myofibroblasts. It is a useful tool to identify the vessel walls of fetal villous arteries and arterioles as well as of veins and venules. It may be used as marker for different types of stem villi (Fig. 3.6A) and their immature forerunners, the immature intermediate villi, as both villous types are the only villi having these stem vessels.

The more easily available **anti–α-smooth muscle actin** (Fig. 3.6B) has a staining pattern that is largely comparable to anti–γ-smooth muscle actin. The antibody detects, however, also earlier stages of myofibroblast differentiation and vascular pericytes. As the latter are also present in mature intermediate and terminal villi, this antibody is less useful for the discrimination of different villous types.

Anti-CD68 and **anti-CD14** (antibody leuM3) (see Chapter 6, Fig. 6.27) are the most consistent immunohistochemical markers of macrophages, the Hofbauer cells. They detect monocyte differentiation antigens. Application of these antibodies to placental villi demonstrates that a much larger share of villous stromal cells are in fact macrophages (see Fig. 6.27) than had been expected from ultrastructural and enzyme histochemical studies. Like most antibodies directed against cell-surface receptors, these antibodies preferably should be applied to unfixed cryostat sections. However, with some care they may also work on paraffin sections.

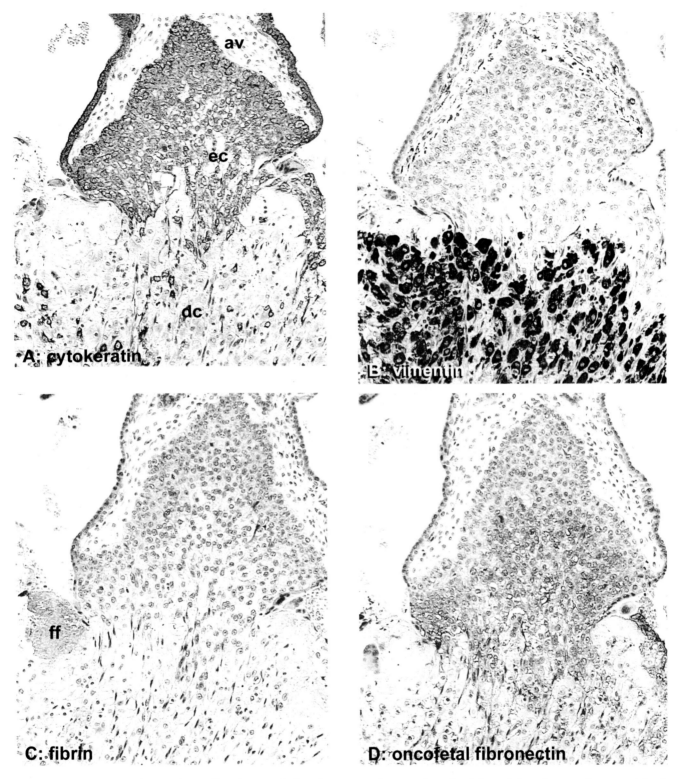

FIGURE 3.5. Serial sections of a cell column of the first trimester placenta. A: Anticytokeratin stains the villous trophoblastic surface as well as extravillous trophoblast (brown, ec) that forms a compact layer at the border to the anchoring villus (av) and invades the basal plate (below). dc, decidual cells. B: Antivimentin staining of a parallel section reveals that most of the basal plate cells are of mesenchymal origin (decidual cells, brown). The trophoblast cells (slender blue nuclei) invade the decidual layer. Also villous stromal cells (above) are of mesenchymal origin and therefore are immunostained. C: Antifibrin binds to a deposit of fibrinoid (fibrin-type fibrinoid, reddish, ff) that is closely related to the intervillous space and devoid of extravillous trophoblast cells. D: In contrast, anti-oncofetal fibronectin (antibody BC-1) binds to the reticular fibrinoid deposits (matrix-type fibrinoid, brownish) around the invading extravillous trophoblast cells and decidua cells. ×105. (Courtesy of Dr. Hans-Georg Frank, Aachen.)

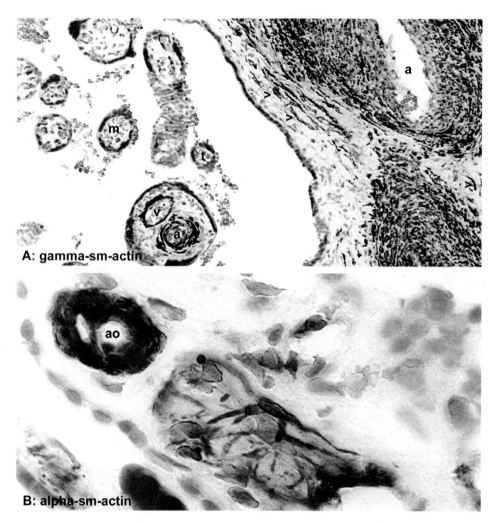

FIGURE 3.6. A: Anti–γ-smooth muscle actin specifically stains smooth muscle cells (brown) of arteries/arterioles (a) and veins/venules (v) of stem villi as well as highly differentiated myofibroblasts (arrowheads), which are characteristic for the extravascular stroma of only the largest stem villi (>300 mm caliber). The stroma of mature intermediate (m) and terminal villi (t) remains unstained. The trophoblastic cover of the villi appears blue from nuclear counterstaining with hematoxylin. ×165. B: The closely related α-smooth muscle actin can be detected immunohistochemically in media smooth muscle cells of an arteriole (brown, ao), in stromal myofibroblasts (brown), and additionally in vascular pericytes (p) identifiable by their characteristic spider-like shapes. ×1080. (Courtesy of Dr. Gaby Kohnen, Aachen.)

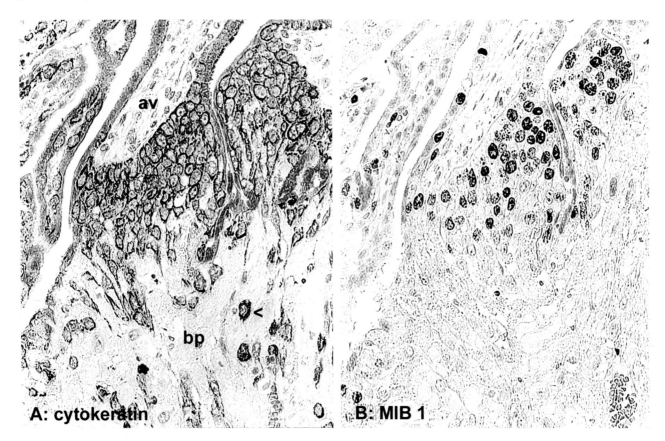

FIGURE 3.7. Serial paraffin sections of a cell column (brown) connecting an anchoring villus (above, av) to the basal plate (bottom, bp). The comparison of anticytokeratin staining of the extravillous cytotrophoblast (brown in part A) with MIB-1 staining of proliferating trophoblast cells (brown in part B) reveals that only extravillous trophoblast cells located close to the basal lamina separating cell column and anchoring villus undergo mitosis. In contrast, those invasive daughter cells (arrowhead in A) that have left the cell column and deeply invaded the basal plate are no longer proliferative (unstained in B). In conclusion, those cells resting on the basal lamina are the proliferating stem cells of all extravillous trophoblast cells. ×150. (Courtesy of Dr. Gaby Kohnen, Aachen.)

The antibodies **Ki-67**, **MIB-1**, and **anti-PCNA** (clones PC10, 19A2, 19F4) bind to nuclear proteins that are expressed in proliferating cells. Ki-67 is only applicable on cryostat sections. MIB-1 is its analogue for carefully fixed paraffin sections; it can be applied also on cryostat sections. Anti-PCNA can be used only for paraffin material. Ki-67/MIB-1 binds only to cells in the mitotic cycle. Because of its longer biologic half-life PCNA (proliferating-cell nuclear antigen) can also be detected in cells that have already left the cell cycle up to 24 hours earlier. These antibodies are useful markers to distinguish proliferating stem cell populations from differentiated ones and identifying growth zones (Fig. 3.7)

4
Placental Types

Throughout pregnancy, the viviparous vertebrates develop a system of membranes that surround the fetus. The apposition or fusion of these fetal membranes with the uterine mucosa, for purposes of maternofetal physiologic exchange, initiates the formation of the placenta. To put it differently, the fetus is surrounded by the fetal membranes, to which it is connected by the umbilical cord (Fig. 4.1). The sac of membranes lies in the uterine cavity and has contact with the endometrium over almost its entire surface. The maternofetal contact zone, thus provided by membranes and endometrium, represents the placenta.

This nonspecific definition points to the great **structural and functional variability of the organ**. There is probably no other organ that exhibits such a large degree of species differences as the placenta. When comparing species, the outer shape and inner structure can vary to such a degree that nonplacentologists who are familiar with the structure of only the human placenta probably cannot identify any other type as a placenta at all. There is only one structural component that all placental types have in common, namely, the existence of two separate circulatory systems—the maternal system and the fetal system. Under normal conditions, the vessels of both systems remain separated by several tissue layers throughout pregnancy. Even the origin of these separating tissue layers, making up the so-called placental barrier or interhemal membrane, varies. These may be derived from fetal tissues such as (1) the blastocyst wall (trophoblast), which following fusion with the fetal mesenchyme is called the chorion; (2) the allantois, which is the extracorporeal embryonic urinary bladder; or (3) the yolk sac, an extracorporeal vesicular extension of the gut (Fig. 4.2). Each of these membranes is complemented by the amnion, which forms a second, fetally derived, membranous sac surrounding the embryo. In some cases, these fetal constituents are complemented by maternal tissues, that is, remainders of the endometrium.

The placenta is unique among all other organs in that it conducts the **functional activities** of most fetal organs

(except the locomotor apparatus and the central nervous system) from its early beginning on throughout its development. The following fetal functions are partially or completely accomplished by the placenta during pregnancy as a substitute for still immature embryonic and fetal organs:

1. Gas transfer (later the function of the lung)
2. Excretory functions, water balance, pH regulation (later the function of the kidney)
3. Catabolic and resorptive functions (later the function of the gut)
4. Synthetic and secretory functions of most endocrine glands
5. Numerous metabolic and secretory functions of the liver
6. Hematopoiesis of the bone marrow (during early stages of pregnancy)
7. Heat transfer of the skin
8. Immunologic functions (to a largely unknown degree)

It is very unlikely that these numerous functional requirements can be fulfilled by a phylogenetic development of an identical structural solution for all species, as species exhibit tremendous variation in size, length of pregnancy, litter size, and living conditions. The logical result of this situation has been the development of numerous placental types, differing from each other with respect to outer shape, kind of maternofetal interdigitation, structure of the maternofetal barrier, and maternofetal blood flow interrelations. As a basis for a better understanding of the human placenta, we present only a brief overview of the so-called **allantochorial placentas**. This group comprises all those placentas that develop from the blastocyst wall and become fetally vascularized from the allantois, the embryonic bladder (see Fig. 4.2). This placental type is the most common among mammals and is also represented in the human. For more detailed information we refer to the fundamental monographs on comparative

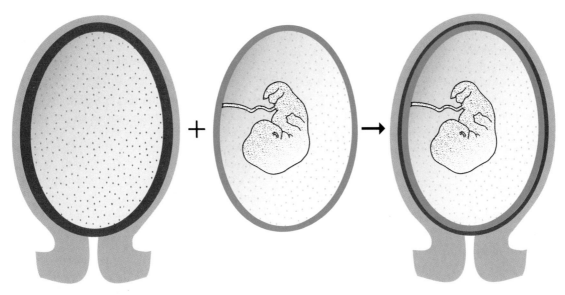

FIGURE 4.1. A placenta is formed when the fetal membranes (blue, central figure) come into close contact by apposition or fusion with the endometrial lining (red, left figure) of the uterus. This theoretically most simple type of a placenta, namely a placenta diffusa with a smooth contact area as shown on the right figure, is not known to exist. (*Source*: Modified from Kaufmann, 1981, with permission.)

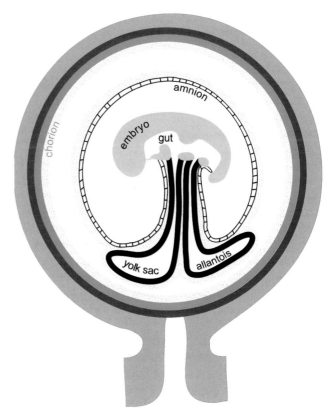

FIGURE 4.2. Synoptic representation of the fetal membranes (black, blue) that may contribute to the formation of a placenta. Maternal tissues are colored red and brown. The trophoblast (blue), as derivative of the blastocyst wall, together with the fetal mesenchyme (gray, dotted), forms the chorion, which is the main exchange membrane of most mammals. The chorion does not develop its own vessels but rather becomes vascularized either by the allantois (black) (→ chorioallantoic placenta) or by the yolk sac (black) (→ choriovitelline placenta). In some species, the chorion is replaced locally by the yolk sac (black) (→ yolk sac placenta). The amnion (black) is unvascularized and never replaces the chorion; rather, it serves as an additional, inner membrane that separates the chorion or yolk sac from the amnionic fluid.

placentology by Björkman (1970), Steven (1975), Ramsey (1982), and Mossman (1987), and to the reviews by Wimsatt (1962), Enders (1965), and Kaufmann (1981).

Among the numerous possibilities for classifying the allantochorial placentas (Amoroso, 1952; Wimsatt, 1962; Steven, 1975; Kaufmann, 1981; Ludwig 1981; King, 1982; Ramsey, 1982; Mossman, 1987; Dantzer et al., 1988), the following characteristics proved to be the most successful for characterizing the organ structurally and, to a limited degree, functionally:

1. Outer shape and surface extension around the chorionic sac
2. Kind and intensity of interdigitation of maternal and fetal tissues
3. Number, kind, and structure of tissue layers separating maternal and fetal blood
4. Spatial arrangement of maternal and fetal vessels or of blood flow directions, respectively

It is impossible to cite here the vast comparative placentologic literature covering the various placental types. Rather, for each placental type or for each group of animals, we refer to one or two detailed publications that may serve as characteristic illustrations.

Placental Shapes

The extent of maternofetal and fetomaternal transfer depends largely on the size of the maternofetal contact area available for exchange (Kaufmann, 1981; Ludwig, 1981; Schröder, 1982). The smooth contact area of the chorion (derivative of the blastocyst wall, and outer layer of the fetal membranes) with the endometrium seems to be insufficient to meet the fetal demands, even if the contact is established over the entire surface of the chorionic sac (as depicted in Fig. 4.1). This placental type does not exist in mammals. Rather, all mammals increase the placental exchange area by interdigitation of the opposing maternal and fetal tissue surfaces. In most cases, the surface enlargement by interdigitation is so intense that enough exchange surface can be provided even if interdigitation takes place only on a limited surface area of the chorionic sac. This interdigitating part is called the **placenta**, whereas those parts of the chorionic sac that maintain a more or less planar apposition to the uterine surface are called smooth chorion, chorion laeve, paraplacenta, or simply outer **fetal membranes**. Each animal order or suborder has a typical shape and surface extension of its placenta.

In the light of phylogeny, it is interesting to note that most of these typical placental shapes have been observed as more or less rare malformations in the human as well. It is still a matter for discussion, however, whether placental shapes of certain animal orders and the respective human malformations are really comparable results of placental development rather than mere products of external similarity in shapes.

In comparative placentology the following placental shapes have been defined:

- Maternofetal interdigitation extending over the entire surface of the chorionic sac is called **placenta diffusa** (placenta membranacea) (Fig. 4.3). This type is seen in Perissodactyla (Amoroso, 1952), Cetacea (Wislocki & Enders, 1941), Suidae (MacDonald & Bosma, 1985), Tylopoda (Ramsey, 1982), and some lower primates (Ramsey, 1982). According to Torpin (1969), it may occur rarely in the human as well (see Chapter 13). In all other cases, maternofetal interdigitations are locally restricted and highly concentrated.
- Many such spot-like regions of intense maternofetal interdigitations, such as those in ruminants (Björkman, 1969), are called **placenta cotyledonaria** or placenta multiplex (Fig. 4.3). To our knowledge, a corresponding malformation has not been described for the human.
- In carnivores (Björkman, 1970), Sirenia (Wislocki, 1935), Hyracoidea (Mossman, 1937), and Proboscidea (Mossman, 1937), the placenta forms a ring-like zone in the chorionic sac surrounding the fetus like a girdle, the **placenta zonaria**, placenta annularis, or girdle-like placenta (Fig. 4.3). The incidence of a corresponding kind of maldevelopment in the human is much less than 0.1%. It has been interpreted as a result of implantation in the uterine cervix, where the fetal membranes establish intense contact with the uterine wall in a ring-like fashion (Torpin, 1969).
- Several lower and higher primates (Luckett, 1970; Ramsey, 1982), as well as the *Tupaia* (Kaufmann et al., 1985; Luckhardt et al., 1985) as a possible phylogenetic link between insectivores and lower primates, develop two disk-like areas of intimate contact, the **placenta bidiscoidalis** (Fig. 4.3). In the human it is represented by the placenta duplex (0.1%). Incomplete subdivision of the placental disk in the human is described as placenta bilobata or placenta bipartita (2–8%). The placenta succenturiata in the human (0.5–1%) shows an asymmetrical complete or incomplete subdivision into a large and a small disk. All three types of placental malformation in the human have been described as being a result of lateral implantation in the corner between the anterior and posterior walls of the uterus (Torpin, 1969).
- The highest degree of concentration of maternofetal interdigitation is realized in the **discoidal placenta** (Fig. 4.3), which provides only a single disk-like zone of intimate maternofetal contact. This most common type of placenta exists in rodents (Enders, 1965; Kaufmann & Davidoff, 1977; Ramsey, 1982), the great apes (Ludwig & Baur, 1971), and the human (Boyd & Hamilton, 1970).

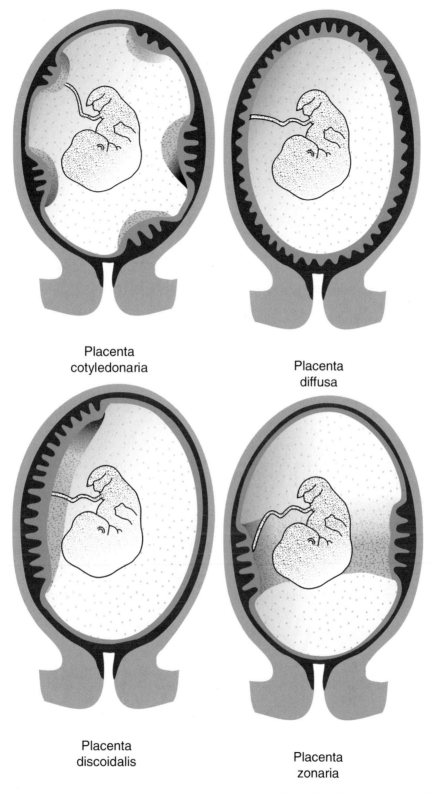

Placenta
cotyledonaria

Placenta
diffusa

Placenta
discoidalis

Placenta
zonaria

FIGURE 4.3. Instead of the smooth contact area shown in Figure 4.1, all known placental types show interdigitations between maternal (red) and fetal (blue) components. Depending on the extent of these interdigitations, several placental shapes are described. For details see text. (*Source*: Modified from Kaufmann, 1981, with permission.)

Types of Maternofetal Interdigitation

If that part of the surface area of the chorionic sac in which maternofetal interdigitation takes place is reduced, it must be compensated for by an increased intensity of the interdigitations. This results in five different types of maternofetal interdigitation:

- The simplest form of interdigitation, consequently, is combined with the large-surfaced diffuse placenta: It is called the **folded type of placenta** (Fig. 4.4A) and is characterized by poorly branching, ridge-like folds of the chorion that fit into corresponding grooves of the uterine mucosa. Examples are seen in the pig (MacDonald & Bosma, 1985) and some lower primates (Ramsey, 1982) that have a diffuse placenta.
- A generally similar but more complex construction is typical for the **lamellar type of placenta** (Fig. 4.4B). This type is found in the carnivores (Leiser & Kohler, 1984). In this case, the ridges multiply branch into complicated systems of slender chorionic lamellae, oriented in parallel to each other and separated by correspondingly branching endometrial folds.
- Even more exchange surface per placental volume is provided by a tree-like branching pattern of the chorion, resulting in the placental villous tree. The villi fit into corresponding endometrial crypts or are directly surrounded by maternal blood. This **villous type of placenta** (Fig. 4.4D) exists in ruminants (Steven, 1975; Kaufmann, 1981) and in higher primates (Boyd & Hamilton, 1970; King & Mais, 1982).
- An intermediate stage between the lamellar and the villous condition is represented by the **trabecular type of placenta** (Fig. 4.4C). It has been described for some platyrrhine monkeys, such as *Callithrix* (Luckett, 1974; Merker et al., 1987). This placental type is characterized by branching folds from which leaf-like and finally finger-like villi branch off.
- The most common and most effective kind of interdigitation can be found in the **labyrinthine type of placenta** (Fig. 4.4E). It has been described so far only in placentas that have a discoidal or bidiscoidal shape. It is the

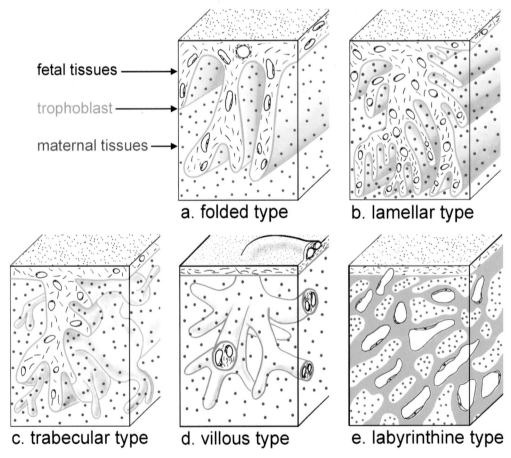

FIGURE 4.4. Types of interdigitation between maternal and fetal tissues. Maternal tissue or maternal blood (red); fetal trophoblast (blue); fetal capillaries and fetal connective tissue (black). For details, see text. (*Source*: Modified and extended from Kaufmann, 1981, with permission.)

typical interdigitation for the placentas of rodents (Kaufmann & Davidoff, 1977), lagomorphs (Mossman, 1937), insectivores (Malassine & Leiser, 1984), bats (Wimsatt & Enders, 1980), and some lower monkeys (Ramsey, 1982; Kaufmann et al., 1985; Mossman, 1987). As the characteristic feature, a tissue block of trophoblast is penetrated by web-like channels that are filled with maternal blood or fetal capillaries.

Maternofetal Barrier

The two preceding systems of classification are merely structurally descriptive ones. Grosser (1909, 1927) initiated a more functional system of classification, describing structure and composition of the so-called placental barrier. This system was later extended by Enders (1965). Although often criticized because it fails to consider structural variation within the same placenta, this system still has its merits, "if for no other reason than that it serves as a ready reminder of the different components that need to be analyzed before drawing functional conclusions" (King, 1982). The terms **maternofetal barrier** and **placental barrier** are traditional descriptions of the tissue layers separating maternal and fetal circulations in the placenta. These terms are still in use despite the fact that they are somewhat misleading (King, 1982). Increasing knowledge of placental physiology has taught us that synthetic, secretory, and transport functions of the placenta are as important aspects of this organ as the barrier role, separating the maternal and the fetal circulations.

As an alternative, the term **interhemal membrane** is in use because it avoids any functional connotation for the separating layers. However, the use of the term **membrane** for a complex layer composed of several cells, rather than for the unit membrane of a cell, is also misleading.

The following types of maternofetal barrier have been classified:

- In the most complete case of a placental barrier—in the Artiodactyla (Wooding et al., 1980), the Perissodactyla (Amoroso, 1952; Ramsey, 1982), and some prosimians (Mossman, 1987)—the fetal chorion directly faces the intact endometrial epithelium. The blastocyst did not invade the endometrium, but only remained attached to it. This condition is called the **epitheliochorial placenta**. Maternal and fetal blood is separated by six tissue layers (Fig. 4.5): maternal capillary endothelium, maternal endometrial connective tissue, and maternal endometrial epithelium, and three layers of fetal origin-trophoblast, chorionic connective tissue, and fetal endothelium. From the six layers, the trophoblast or the maternal epithelium may fuse syncytially.

Sometimes even hybrid syncytia are formed by fusion of trophoblastic (fetal) and uterine epithelial (maternal) cells, as in ruminants (Wooding, 1992).

- By stepwise removal of maternal tissue layers the maximum barrier, consisting of six layers, can be reduced during invasion of the blastocyst. If invasion stops after destruction of the uterine epithelium, the **syndesmochorial placenta** (Fig. 4.5) is obtained. Originally, sheep and goats were said to possess this type. More recently, the existence of this five-layer barrier has been refuted (Kaufmann, 1981; Ramsey, 1982). Sheep and goats seem to display an epitheliochorial or synepitheliochorial condition (Wooding, 1992; Wooding et al., 1980), like all other Artiodactyla.

- Deeper invasion with subsequent removal of endometrial connective tissue, establishing a direct apposition of trophoblast and maternal endothelium, results in the development of the **endotheliochorial placenta** (Fig. 4.5). This placental barrier is characteristic for all carnivores (Björkman, 1970), and it is represented in some insectivores (Malassine & Leiser, 1984), lower primates (Kaufmann et al., 1985), and bats (Ramsey, 1982).

- As the next and final step of invasion, the maternal vessels are eroded and finally completely destroyed by the invasive trophoblast. The trophoblastic surfaces now directly face the maternal blood. The respective placental type is called the **hemochorial placenta** (Fig. 4.5). It has been described, for instance, for all rodents and lagomorphs, for some insectivores, bats, and Sirenia, and for the higher primates including the human (Enders, 1965; Ramsey, 1982). Depending on the number of trophoblastic epithelial layers, Enders (1965) has proposed a more detailed subdivision into **hemotrichorial** (rat: Enders, 1965; mouse: Björkman, 1970; hamster; Carpenter, 1972), **hemodichorial** (beaver: Fischer, 1971; rabbit: Enders, 1965; human in the first trimester: Boyd & Hamilton, 1970), and **hemomonochorial** (caviomorph rodents, e.g., the guinea pig: Kaufmann & Davidoff, 1977; human placenta at term: Boyd & Hamilton, 1970).

- Some authors (see Wimsatt, 1962) have described less common types of placentas in insectivores and bats in which even fetal tissue components are subjected to destruction, resulting in **endothelioendothelial** and even **hemoendothelial** conditions. In most cases, these descriptions have not been based on ultrastructural studies and thus need to be corroborated.

Generally speaking, maternofetal and fetomaternal diffusional transfer depend on the thickness of the separating layers, whereas the number and kind of the layers of the barrier influence facilitated transport, active transport, and vesicular transfer. This statement, however, does not imply that all layers to the same extent contribute to the **barrier function**. When stating that three to six tissue layers make up the placental barrier, this does not necessarily mean that a corresponding number of cells must

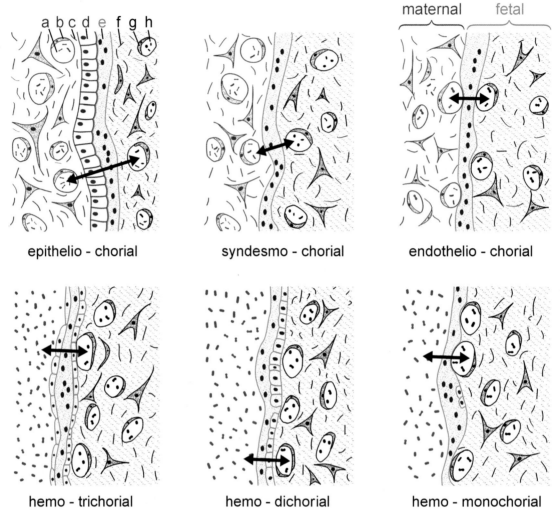

FIGURE 4.5. Tissue layers of the maternofetal barrier according to the Grosser classification. a, maternal blood (red dots); b, maternal endothelium (red); c, endometrial connective tissue (red); d, endometrial epithelium (red); e, trophoblast (blue); f, fetal connective tissue (black); g, fetal endothelium (black); h, fetal blood (black dots). The fetal components of the placental barrier (e–g) are collected under the term **chorion**. The maternal components are reduced step by step until the chorion comes into direct contact with the maternal blood (a, red dots). The trophoblast (blue), normally consisting of a syncytium (e), may be covered on one side (hemodichorial) or on both sides (hemotrichorial) by cytotrophoblast. In most species, the trophoblast fuses syncytially. In some species, mostly those with epitheliochorial placentation, either the maternal epithelium fuses syncytially instead of the trophoblast, or both epithelia remain cellular. For further details, see text. (*Source*: Modified and extended from Kaufmann, 1981, with permission.)

be passed transcellularly by each transported molecule. This situation is only mandatory for the trophoblast, which in most species with invasive implantation is a syncytium that can be passed only transcellularly by transport mechanisms such as diffusion, facilitated transfer, active transport, and vesicular transfer. In both connective tissue layers, however, transport may easily take place paracellularly by diffusion. For smaller molecules, the same is valid for the uterine epithelium (so far as it is cellular in nature) and for both endothelia. These epithelial and endothelial linings offer limited paracellular transfer to small molecules along the lateral intercellular clefts. As a consequence, the syncytiotrophoblast in most placentas, including that of the human, is the decisive barrier that limits or supports transplacental transfer processes.

According to Fick's law of diffusion, **exchange efficiency**, that is the net amount of substance crossing the membrane, depends (*inter alia*) on the concentration difference of the substance across the mem-

brane, as well as on the area and thickness of the membrane. Thus, reduction of the distance between maternal and fetal blood is of decisive importance for the maternofetal diffusional exchange. It makes the Grosser classification valuable for determining diffusional efficiency of the organ. It is, however, important to note that this is valid only for passive diffusion (oxygen, carbon dioxide, water) (Schröder, 1982; Faber & Thornburg, 1983). For most transport mechanisms, the product of exchange surface available and the activity of the uptake mechanisms (carrier molecules, enzymes, and receptors for active and vesicular transport) are the limiting factors, not the barrier thickness. The latter situation is comparable to an escalator, the capacity of which is limited by width and speed rather than by length. It is valid for transplacental transport processes, such as facilitated diffusion (e.g., glucose), active transport (e.g., ions and many amino acids), and vesicular transport (peptides, proteins, lipids). As a consequence, we must conclude that the applicability of the Grosser classification is limited to the interpretation of the capacity of the placenta for passive diffusion. The findings by Dantzer et al. (1988) make it likely that primarily the fetal demands determine placental size during transplacental oxygen diffusion.

Maternofetal Blood Flow Interrelations

Similar advantages but also similar limitations as discussed for the Grosser classification are valid for the placental classification according to the geometric arrangement of maternal and fetal capillaries or blood flows in the exchange area (Bartels & Moll, 1964; Faber, 1969; Moll, 1972, 1981; Martin, 1981; Schröder, 1982; Faber & Thornburg, 1983; Dantzer et al., 1988). The relative efficiencies of various types of the following theoretical exchanges for the diffusion of, for example, oxygen, have been calculated. Physiologists have defined several theoretical models of diffusional exchangers and calculated their efficiency for diffusional transfer. The results have been compared with real structural and functional findings in various mammals:

- The **concurrent flow exchanger** (Fig. 4.6) is the most inefficient system. Its fetal and maternal capillaries are thought to be arranged in parallel, having identical blood flow directions. Obviously it is not represented in placentas of mammals (Martin, 1981).
- Also, with the **countercurrent flow exchanger**, maternal and fetal capillaries are arranged in parallel but with blood flow in opposite directions (Fig. 4.6). This is the most effective vascular arrangement for passive diffusion. It is nearly perfectly realized in the placentas of all rodents (Kaufmann & Davidoff, 1977; Dantzer et al., 1988) and lagomorphs (Mossman, 1926). Accordingly, these animals exhibit small placentas compared to their fetal weight (fetoplacental weight relations up to 20:1).
- The remaining theoretical and real exchange systems have an intermediate position between concurrent and countercurrent exchangers regarding their efficiency. Among them, for placentology the most important ones are the **simple crosscurrent flow** (Fig. 4.6) (carnivores: Leiser & Kohler, 1984; Dantzer et al., 1988), **double crosscurrent flow** (Fig. 4.6) (lower primates: Luckhardt et al., 1985; pig: Dantzer et al., 1988).
- Last but not least also the **multivillous flow exchanger** (Fig. 4.6) (ruminants: Dantzer et al., 1988; higher primates and human: Moll, 1981) have an intermediate position regarding efficiency.

The importance of this classification system for the fetal oxygen supply is stressed by the fact that the animals showing a less efficient vessel arrangement have a poorer fetoplacental weight relation at term (pig: 9:1; cat: 8:1; human: 6:1) compared to the highly effective, small rodent placentas (up to 20:1) (Dantzer et al., 1988).

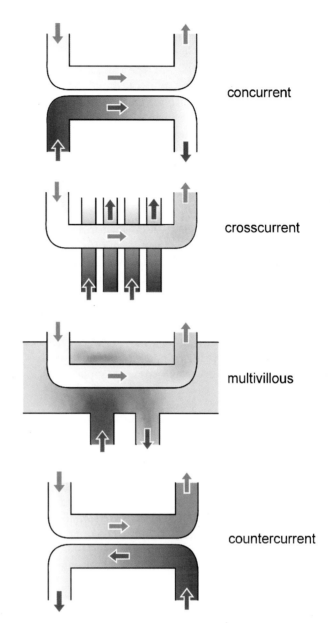

FIGURE 4.6. Idealized arrangement of the fetal (lilac arrows) and maternal (red arrows) bloodstreams of different placental exchange types, according to, Faber (1969), Moll (1972), and Martin (1981). The intensity of blue color in the venous limbs of the fetal vessel loops (upper right vessel of each single drawing) illustrates the efficiency of the various exchangers in diffusional exchange (for example, oxygen). For further details, see text. (*Source*: Dantzer et al., 1988, with permission.)

Placental Types and Phylogeny

The foregoing systems of placental classification have been accused of being merely structurally descriptive but functionally more or less irrelevant, since both

"primitive" and **"highly developed" placentas** produce healthy offspring. This reproach is supported by several facts:

- The pig seems to have one of the most primitive placentas possible: a diffuse, epitheliochorial, folded, crosscurrent placenta (Dantzer et al., 1988).
- By contrast, the guinea pig placenta is thought to be one of the most highly developed ones, belonging to the discoidal, labyrinthine, hemomonochorial, counter-current type (Kaufmann & Davidoff, 1977).

The seemingly primitive pig placenta, however, guarantees embryonic development as satisfactorily as does the highly sophisticated guinea pig placenta for its embryos; and probably nobody would state that the reproductive qualities of the guinea pig are superior to that of the pig. One therefore must be careful when describing a placenta as "primitive" or "highly developed." Independent of the simplicity or complexity of their structure, all placentas fulfill their biologic tasks, when necessary compensating for missing complexity simply by increased mass, as this is the case when comparing pig and guinea pig.

Schröder (1993) has stressed another interesting view to explain the phylogenetic variabilities of placental sizes and efficiencies:

- Animals with a rather short gestational period as compared to neonatal weight have relatively **large daily fetal growth rates**. If such species want to produce their large fetuses within a short time with a small placenta (e.g., myomorph rodents), their choice of placental type is restricted to the high-efficiency type, such as labyrinthine and hemochorial with countercurrent flow.
- With **low daily fetal growth rates**, however, it does not really matter which placental type and efficiency are available to the species; all grades of efficiencies are possible ranging from the villous, synepitheliochorial, multivillous sheep placenta, via the villous, hemomonochorial, multivillous human placenta, to the labyrinthine, hemomonochorial, countercurrent capybara placenta.

Unquestioned is the importance of the classification systems when looking for **in vivo models for the human**. The delivered human term placenta has been easily available for many kinds of research. For nearly all in situ studies, however, we need animal experiments. The only placentas that are directly comparable to those of the human are the placentas of the great apes. For several reasons (expense and protection of rare species) they provide no real alternatives for placental research. Thus, one has to work with laboratory animals with placentas that are largely different from those of the human. The classification systems described here provide a certain orientation regarding differences and similarities between the various animal models and the human placenta. Moreover, as stated by King (1982), they remind us that we must take into consideration the differences before drawing functional conclusions.

When inspecting Table 4.1, one realizes that there is no evident relationship between placental classification and taxonomy. Some orders such as the carnivores, lagomorphs, and rodents seem to be homogeneous regarding placental structure. Others, such as insectivores and primates, may even give us the impression that several animals have acquired their respective placental types by chance. Perhaps this is the result of the special situation of the placenta, which has been developed for single use over a limited life span. Most placentas show considerable excess capacity, which makes a considerable difference when evaluating efficiency. It is an important consideration in pathology: The human placenta, which compared to the fetus, is rather large, can compensate for 50% tissue degeneration, and perhaps even more, without severe disturbance of pregnancy. In animals with relatively small placentas compared to their fetus, such as the guinea pig or the tupaia, fetal death is the normal result as soon as only a small amount of placental parenchyma is destroyed (Van der Heijden, 1981).

Human Placenta

According to these classification systems, the human placenta is discoidal, villous, and hemochorial in structure. The arrangement of its maternal and fetal blood flows is in accord with the multivillous type of exchange system.

These basic structural characteristics are realized by the following design: The human placenta at term is a local, disk-like thickening of the membranous sac (Fig. 4.7) that is achieved by splitting the membranes into two separate sheets, the chorionic plate and the basal plate (Fig. 4.7). Both sheets enclose the intervillous space, as cover and bottom. The intervillous space is perfused with maternal blood, which circulates, without its own vessel wall, directly around the trophoblastic surfaces of the placental villi. The villi are complex tree-like projections of the chorionic plate into the intervillous space. Inside the villi are fetal vessels that are connected to the fetal circulatory system via the chorionic plate and the umbilical cord. At the placental margin, the intervillous space is obliterated so that the chorionic plate and the basal plate fuse with each other and thus form the chorion laeve.

Table 4.1. Placental classification at term in various animal orders

Order/species	Placental shape	Fetomaternal interdigitation	Placental barrier	Fetomaternal blood flow interrelations	Neonatal/placental weight ratio
Marsupialia					
Opossum	Discoidal	Folded	Epitheliochorial	—	—
Insectivora					
Sorex	Discoidal	Labyrinthine	Endotheliochorial	—	—
European mole	Discoidal	Labyrinthine	Endotheliochorial	—	—
Pacific mole	Diffuse	Labyrinthine	Hemochorial	—	—
Primates					
Tupaia	Bidiscoidal	Labyrinthine	Endotheliochorial	Double cross-current	18:1
Galago	Diffuse	Folded	Epitheliochorial	—	—
Marmoset	Bidiscoidal	Trabecular	Hemomonochorial	Multivillous	—
Rhesus monkey	Bidiscoidal	Villous	Hemomonochorial	Multivillous	—
Great apes	Discoidal	Villous	Hemomonochorial	Multivillous	—
Human	Discoidal	Villous	Hemomonochorial	Multivillous	—
Chiroptera					
Microchiroptera	Discoidal	Labyrinthine	Endotheliochorial	—	—
Molossidae	Discoidal	Labyrinthine	Hemodichorial	—	—
Lagomorpha					
Rabbit	Discoidal	Labyrinthine	Hemodichorial	Countercurrent	6:1
Hare	Discoidal	Labyrinthine	Hemodichorial	—	—
Rodentia					
Guinea pig	Discoidal	Labyrinthine	Hemomonochorial	Countercurrent	20:1
Chinchilla	Discoidal	Labyrinthine	Hemomonochorial	Countercurrent	30:1
Hamster	Discoidal	Labyrinthine	Hemotrichorial	Countercurrent	—
Beaver	Discoidal	Labyrinthine	Hemodichorial	—	—
Mouse	Discoidal	Labyrinthine	Hemotrichorial	Countercurrent	—
Rat	Discoidal	Labyrinthine	Hemotrichorial	Countercurrent	10:1
Cetacea					
Dolphin	Diffuse	Villous	Epitheliochorial	—	—
Carnivora					
Dog	Zonary	Lamellar	Endotheliochorial	—	—
Cat	Zonary	Lamellar	Endotheliochorial	Simple cross-current	8:1
Bear	Zonary	Lamellar	Endotheliochorial	—	—
Hyena	Zonary	Villous/labyrinthine	Hemomonochorial	—	—
Sirenia					
Manatee	Zonary	Labyrinthine	Hemochorial	—	—
Pholidota					
Pangolin	Diffuse	Villous	Epitheliochorial	—	—
Proboscidea					
Elephant	Zonary	Villous	Endotheliochorial	—	—
Hyracoidea					
Hyrax	Zonary	Labyrinthine	Hemochorial	—	—
Edentata					
Sloth	Discoidal	Labyrinthine	Endotheliochorial	—	—
Armadillo	Discoidal	Villous	Hemochorial	—	—
Perissodactyla					
Horse	Diffuse	Villous	Epitheliochorial	—	—
Rhinoceros	Diffuse	Villous	Epitheliochorial	—	—
Artiodactyla					
Pig	Diffuse	Folded	Epitheliochorial	Double cross-current	9:1
Alpaca	Diffuse	Folded/villous	Epitheliochorial	—	—
Sheep	Cotyledonary	Villous	Epitheliochorial	Multivillous	10:1
Goat	Cotyledonary	Villous	Epitheliochorial	Multivillous	10:1
Cow	Cotyledonary	Villous	Epitheliochorial	Multivillous	—

The data were assembled from the following publications: Wimsatt (1962), Enders (1965), Björkman (1970), Starck (1975), Ramsey (1982), Mossman (1987), Dantzer et al. (1988).

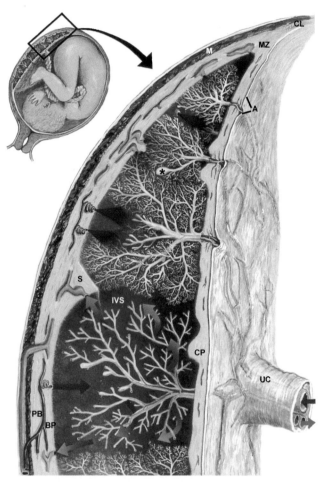

FIGURE 4.7. The mature human placenta in situ is composed of the chorionic plate (CP) and the basal plate (BP) surrounding the intervillous space (IVS) as cover and as bottom, respectively. The fetally vascularized villous trees project from the chorionic plate into the intervillous space and are directly surrounded by the maternal blood that circulates through the intervillous space. The loose centers of villous trees, arranged around the maternal arterial inflow area, are frequent features. M, myometrium; CL, chorion laeve; A, amnion; MZ, marginal zone between placenta and fetal membranes, with obliterated intervillous space and ghost villi; *, cell island, connected to a villous tree; S, placental septum; UC, umbilical cord. (*Source*: Kaufmann & Scheffen, 1992, with permission.)

References

Amoroso, E.C.: Placentation. In, Marshall's Physiology of Reproduction. 3rd Ed. A.S. Parkes, ed., pp. 127–316. Longmans Green, London, 1952.

Bartels, H. and Moll, W.: Passage of inert substances and oxygen in the human placenta. Pflügers Arch. Gesamte Physiol. **280**:165, 1964.

Björkman, N.: Light and electron microscopic studies on cellular alterations in the normal bovine placentome. Anat. Rec. **163**:17–30, 1969.

Björkman, N.: An Atlas of Placental Fine Structure. Bailliere, Tindall & Cassell, London; Williams & Wilkins, Baltimore, 1970.

Boyd, J.D. and Hamilton, W.J.: The Human Placenta. Heffer, Cambridge, 1970.

Carpenter, S.J.: Light and electron microscopic observations on the morphogenesis of the chorioallantoic placenta of the golden hamster (Cricetus auratus): days seven through nine of gestation. Am. J. Anat. **135**:445–476, 1972.

Dantzer, V., Leiser, R., Kaufmann, P. and Luckhardt, M.: Comparative morphological aspects of placental vascularization. Trophoblast Res. **3**:235–260, 1988.

Enders, A.C.: A comparative study of the fine structure in several hemochorial placentas. Am. J. Anat. **116**:29–68, 1965.

Faber, J.J.: Application of the theory of heat exchangers to the transfer of inert materials in placentas. Circ. Res. **24**:221–234, 1969.

Faber, J.J. and Thornburg, K.L.: Placental Physiology. Structure and Function of Fetomaternal Exchange. Raven Press, New York, 1983.

Fischer, T.V.: Placentation in the American beaver (Castor canadensis). Am. J. Anat. **131**:159–184, 1971.

Grosser, O.: Vergleichende Anatomie und Entwicklungsgeschichte der Eihäute und der Placenta mit besonderer Berücksichtigung des Menschen. Braumüller, Vienna, 1909.

Grosser, O.: Frühentwicklung, Eihautbildung und Placentation des Menschen und der Säugetiere. Deutsche Frauenheilkunde, Geburtshilfe, Gynäkologie und Nachbargebiete in Einzeldarstellungen, Vol. 5. R.T. Jaschke, ed. Bergmann, Munich, 1927.

Kaufmann, P.: Functional anatomy of the non-primate placenta. Placenta Suppl. **1**:13–28, 1981.

Kaufmann, P. and Davidoff, M.: The guinea pig placenta. Adv. Anat. Embryol. Cell Biol. **53**:1–90, 1977.

Kaufmann, P. and Scheffen, I.: Placental development. In, Neonatal and Fetal Medicine-Physiology and Pathophysiology, Vol. 1. R. Polin and W. Fox, eds., pp. 47–55. Saunders, Orlando, 1992.

Kaufmann, P., Luckhardt, M. and Elger, W.: The structure of the tupaia placenta. II. Ultrastructure. Anat. Embryol. (Berl.) **171**:211–221, 1985.

King, B.F.: Comparative anatomy of the placental barrier. Bibl. Anat. **22**:13–28, 1982.

King, B.F. and Mais, J.J.: Developmental changes in rhesus monkey placental villi and cell columns. Anat. Embryol. (Berl.) **165**:361–376, 1982.

Leiser, R. and Kohler, T.: The blood vessels of the cat girdle placenta. Observations on corrosion casts, scanning electron microscopical and histological studies. II. Fetal vasculature. Anat. Embryol. (Berl.) **170**:209–216, 1984.

Luckett, W.P.: The fine structure of the placental villi of the rhesus monkey (Macaca mulatta). Anat. Rec. **167**:141–164, 1970.

Luckett, W.P.: Comparative development and evolution of the placenta in primates. Contrib. Primatol. **3**:142–234, 1974.

Luckhardt, M., Kaufmann, P. and Elger, W.: The structure of the tupaia placenta. I. Histology and vascularisation. Anat. Embryol. (Berl.) **171**:201–210, 1985.

Ludwig, K.S.: Vergleichende Anatomie der Plazenta. In, Die Plazenta des Menschen. V. Becker, T.H. Schiebler, and F. Kubli, eds. pp. 1–12. Thieme, Stuttgart, 1981.

Ludwig, K.S. and Baur, R.: The chimpanzee placenta. In, The Chimpanzee, Vol. 4. G.H. Bourne, ed., pp. 349–372. University Park Press, Baltimore, 1971.

MacDonald, A.A. and Bosma, A.A.: Notes on placentation in Suina. Placenta **6**:83–92, 1985.

Malassine, A. and Leiser, R.: Morphogenesis and fine structure of the near-term placenta of Talpa europaea: I. Endothelio-chorial labyrinth. Placenta **5**:145–158, 1984.

Martin, C.B.: Models of placental blood flow. Placenta Suppl. **1**:65–80, 1981.

Merker, H.-J., Bremer, D., Barrach, H.-J. and Gossrau, R.: The basement membrane of the persisting maternal blood vessels in the placenta of Callithrix jacchus. Anat. Embryol (Berl.) **176**:87–97, 1987.

Moll, W.: Gas exchange in concurrent, countercurrent and cross-current flow systems. The concept of the fetoplacental unit. In, Respiratory Gas Exchange and Blood Flow in the Placenta. L.D. Longo and H. Bartels, eds., pp. 281–294. DHEW Publ. No. (NIH) 73–361, Department of Health, Education and Welfare, Washington, D.C., 1972.

Moll, W.: Theorie des plazentaren Transfers durch Diffusion. In, Die Plazenta des Menschen. V. Becker, T.H. Schiebler and F. Kubli, eds., pp. 129–139. Thieme, Stuttgart, 1981.

Mossman, H.W.: The rabbit placenta and the problem of placental transmission. Am. J. Anat. **37**:433–497, 1926.

Mossman, H.W.: Comparative morphogenesis of the fetal membranes and accessory uterine structures. Carnegie Contrib. Embryol. **26**:129–246, 1937.

Mossman, H.W.: Vertebrate Fetal Membranes: Comparative Ontogeny and Morphology; Evolution; Phylogenetic Significance; Basic Functions; Research Opportunities. Macmillan, London, 1987.

Ramsey, E.M.: The Placenta. Human and Animal. Praeger, New York, 1982.

Schröder, H.: Structural and functional organization of the placenta from the physiological point of view. Bibl. Anat. **22**:4–12, 1982.

Schröder, H.: Placental diversity: transport physiology diversity. Keynote Lecture, 5th Meeting of the European Placenta Group, Manchester, UK, 1993.

Starck, D.: Embryologie. Thieme, Stuttgart, 1975.

Steven, D.H., ed.: Comparative Placentation. Academic Press, New York, 1975.

Torpin, R.: The Human Placenta. Thomas, Springfield, 1969.

Van der Heijden, F.L.: Compensation mechanisms for experimental reduction of the functional capacity in the guinea pig placenta. I. Changes in the maternal and fetal placenta vascularization. Acta Anat. (Basel) **111**:352–358, 1981.

Wimsatt, W.A.: Some aspects of the comparative anatomy of the mammalian placenta. Am. J. Obstet. Gynecol. **84**:1568–1594, 1962.

Wimsatt, W.A. and Enders, A.C.: Structure and morphogenesis of the uterus placenta, and paraplacental organs of the neotropical disc-winged bat Thyroptera tricolor spix (Microchiroptera: Thyropteridae). Am. J. Anat. **159**:209–243, 1980.

Wislocki, G.B.: The placentation of the manatee (Trichechus latirostris). Mem. Mus. Comp. Zool. Harvard **54**:159–178, 1935.

Wislocki, G.B. and Enders, R.K.: The placentation of the bottlenosed porpoise (Tursiops truncatus). Am. J. Anat. **68**:97–125, 1941.

Wooding, F.B.P.: The synepitheliochorial placenta of ruminants: binucleate cell fusion and hormone production. Placenta **13**:101–113, 1992.

Wooding, F.B.P., Chamber, S.G., Perry, J.S., George, M. and Heap, R.B.: Migration of binucleate cells in the sheep placenta during normal pregnancy. Anat. Embryol. (Berl.) **158**:361–370, 1980.

5
Early Development of the Human Placenta

For many years, understanding placental pathology was thought to demand only a limited knowledge of implantation and early placental development, because disturbances of these early steps of placentation seemed to cause abortion rather than affecting placental structure and function. Increasing experience with assisted fertilization, however, has taught us that an increased percentage of these cases show impaired fetal and neonatal outcome such as an increased incidence of intrauterine growth retardation and retroplacental hematoma, as well as increased perinatal mortality (Beck & Heywinkel, 1990). The causal connections are still unknown, although the authors give some arguments that placental causes must be considered. It must be speculated that improper conditions during implantation handicap early development and finally result in the inappropriate functioning of the fetoplacental unit.

Basic information concerning early development may be of increasing importance and thus is presented in this chapter. The pathologically interesting interactions between the site of implantation and the shape of the placenta are considered in Chapter 13.

Prelacunar Stage

According to the general definition of the placenta given earlier, the development of the placenta begins as soon as the fetal membranes establish close and stable contacts with the uterine mucosa, that is, as soon as the blastocyst implants. To deal with the molecular mechanisms of implantation in detail would be beyond the scope of this chapter. For this purpose we refer the reader to the literature (Loke et al., 1995; Yoshimura et al., 1995, 1998; Aplin, 1996, 2000; Rao & Sanfilippo, 1997; Simon et al., 1998; Bentin-Ley & Lopata, 2000; Loke & King, 2000; Sunder & Lenton, 2000; Merviel et al., 2001a,b; Lindhard et al., 2002).

The first step of implantation is called apposition. In the human it takes place around day 6 to 7 postcoitus (p.c.) (day 1 p.c. = the first 24 hours after conception). During this stage, the implanting blastocyst is composed of 107 to 256 cells (Hertig, 1960; Boyd & Hamilton, 1970). It is a flattened vesicle, measuring about $0.1 \times 0.3 \times 0.3\,mm$ in diameter. Most of the cells make up the outer wall (**trophoblast**) surrounding the blastocystic cavity (Fig. 5.1A). Generally speaking, the trophoblast is the forerunner of the fetal membranes, including the placenta. The inner cell mass, a small group of larger cells that form the **embryoblast**, is apposed to the inner surface of the trophoblastic vesicle. The embryo, umbilical cord, and amnion are derived from these cells. Moreover, both embryoblast-derived mesenchyme and embryoblast-derived blood vessels contribute to the formation of the placenta.

In most cases, the blastocyst is oriented in such a way that the embryonic pole (that part of the blastocyst bearing the embryoblast at its inner surface) is attached to the endometrium first (Boyd & Hamilton, 1970). Accordingly, this part of the circumference is also called the implantation pole. Rotation of the blastocyst in such a way that the embryonic pole and the implantation pole are not identical results in abnormal cord insertion. Thus, in moderate cases we find an eccentric or marginal insertion of the cord; in severe cases a velamentous cord insertion may be the consequence (see Chapter 12). The usual implantation site is the upper part of the posterior wall of the uterine body, near the midsagittal plane. According to Mossman (1937, 1987), this region is homologous with the antimesometrial wall of a bicornuate uterus, where primary attachment takes place in most mammals.

In all species, implantation is introduced by attachment of the apical plasma membranes of the blastocystic trophoblast to the apical plasma membranes of the uterine epithelium. This phenomenon has been described by Denker (1990) as a cell biologic paradox because

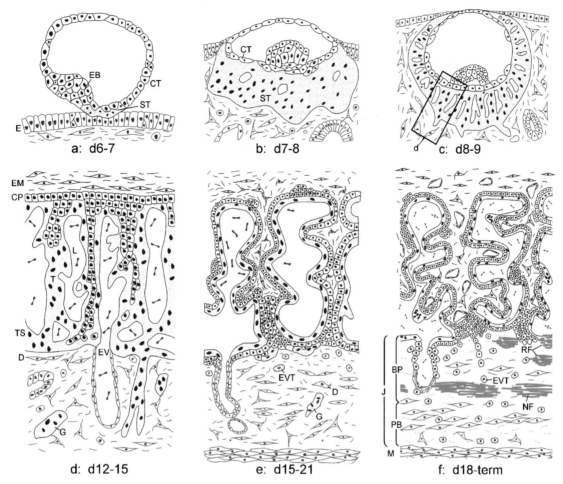

FIGURE 5.1. Simplified drawings of typical stages of early placental development. a,b: Prelacunar stages. c: Lacunar stage. d: Transition from lacunar to primary villous stage. e: Secondary villous stage. f: Tertiary villous stage. Note that the basal segments of the anchoring villi (e,f) remain merely trophoblastic, finally forming cell columns. All maternal tissues are in red, and all fetal tissues are in blue. Fibrinoid of mixed, maternal, and fetal origin are in lilac. E, endometrial epithelium; EB, embryo-blast; CT, cytotrophoblast; ST, syncytiotrophoblast; EM, extra-embryonic mesoderm; CP, primary chorionic plate; T, trabeculae and primary villi, L, maternal blood lacunae; TS, trophoblastic shell; EV, endometrial vessel; D, decidua; RF, Rohr's fibrinoid; NF, Nitabuch's or uteroplacental fibrinoid; G, trophoblastic giant cell; EVT, extravillous cytotrophoblast; BP, basal plate; PB, placental bed; J, junctional zone; M, myometrium. (*Source:* Modified from Kaufmann & Scheffen, 1992, with permission.)

apical plasma membranes of epithelia are normally known to be nonadhesive. Adhesiveness is a normal quality of basolateral epithelial plasma membranes, which are thus attached both to each other and to their basal laminae.

The blastocyst and the endometrium show this usual epithelial behavior throughout the entire preimplantation phase so long as the blastocyst moves in the fallopian tube and uterine cavity. Apical adhesiveness of both epithelia, the trophoblast and endometrium, is apparently achieved for only a short, specific phase, which has been called the implantation window (Psychoyos, 1988). This phase is used for attachment of the blastocyst. To find or to generate this window is the most important prerequisite for successful implantation following in vitro fertilization.

With the noninvasive types of implantation, the epitheliochorial placentation (e.g., pig, horse, some ruminants), implantation is arrested at the stage of attachment. Invasion with destruction of either epithelial surface does not follow. In contrast, in most mammals more intimate types of maternal–fetal contacts are established by invasion. In the human, implantation is also an invasive process. Knowledge of structural details, however, is largely lacking, as appropriate human material is rare and is usually poorly preserved when it is available. Numerous studies in animals have revealed the existence of three types of invasive implantation (Schlafke & Enders, 1975; Denker, 1990):

1. **Displacement type.** This type is observed in rodents. The blastocyst is attached to the apical plasma membrane of the uterine

epithelium. These cells degenerate thereafter and detach from the basal lamina. The subsequent penetration of the basal lamina is initiated by the underlying decidual cells, rather than by penetrative activities of the trophoblast itself.

2. **Fusion type.** The apical plasma membrane of the attached trophoblast fuses with the apical membranes of the uterine epithelial cells and forms a mixed syncytium, derived from maternal and trophoblastic cells. This syncytium then actively penetrates the basal lamina and endometrial connective tissue, and finally it erodes the maternal blood vessels. This mode of invasion has been described for the rabbit. According to Larsen (1970), it may also be present in the human.

3. **Intrusive type.** This type is the usual one in carnivores. Small extensions of syncytiotrophoblast intrude into the intercellular clefts between the uterine epithelial cells, opening the intercellular junctions between the epithelial cells. At the same time, new junctions between trophoblast and uterine epithelium are formed. In some species, even a local formation of mixed syncytia composed of maternal and trophoblastic origin has been observed. Based on the results of investigations by Larsen (1970), this mechanism of implantation may also pertain for the human.

Lacking respective human findings, further structural details and mechanisms of the implantation process are not discussed here. For this purpose, we refer the reader to the comparative anatomy literature (for reviews, see Finn, 1977; Denker, 1977, 1990; Pijnenborg et al., 1981; Denker & Aplin, 1990).

During attachment and after invasion of the endometrial epithelium, the trophoblastic cells of the implanting embryonic pole of the blastocyst show increased proliferation that results in a double-layered trophoblast (Heuser & Streeter, 1941). The outer of the two layers, directly facing the maternal tissue, is transformed to a **syncytiotrophoblast** by fusion of neighboring trophoblast cells. The remaining cellular components of the blastocyst wall, which have not yet achieved contact to maternal tissues, remain temporally unfused and are called **cytotrophoblast** (Fig. 5.1A). Throughout the following days and with progressive invasion, additional parts of the blastocyst surface come into close contact with maternal tissues, followed by trophoblastic proliferation with subsequent fusion. The mass of syncytiotrophoblast increases and achieves considerable thickness at the implantation pole, as the cytotrophoblast lying underneath continues to proliferate and fuses syncytially. The mass increases further by expanding over the surface of the implanting blastocyst as implantation progresses. At the implantation pole, this is not a smooth-surfaced mass; rather, it is covered with branching, finger-like extensions that deeply invade the endometrium. This first stage, lasting from day 7 to day 8 p.c., during which time the syncytiotrophoblast (except for its basal extensions) is a rather solid mass, was defined as representing the prelacunar period by Wislocki and Streeter (1938).

The syncytiotrophoblast has lost its generative potency during fusion. The cytotrophoblast acts as a stem cell that guarantees growth of the trophoblast by continuous proliferation, with subsequent fusion (see Chapter 6). The syncytiotrophoblast is formed by cellular fusion (i.e., syncytium), rather than by nuclear division without subse-

quent cytoplasmic division (i.e., plasmodium). Therefore, Bargmann and Knoop (1959) suggested that the term **plasmodiotrophoblast** (often used in the literature) be abandoned and replaced by **syncytiotrophoblast.**

The syncytiotrophoblast is a continuous system, not interrupted by intercellular spaces, and composed of neither individual cells nor individual syncytial units. Terms such as **syncytial cells** and **syncytiotrophoblasts,** which are widely used in the literature, are inappropriate. The few available reports that point to the existence of vertical cell membranes that subdivide the syncytium into syncytial units (e.g., Tedde et al., 1988 a,b) have an accidental rather than a real basis (see Chapter 6).

Lacunar Stage

On day 8 p.c., small intrasyncytial vacuoles appear in the increasing syncytiotrophoblastic mass at the implantation pole. The vacuoles quickly grow and become confluent, forming a system of **lacunae** (Fig. 5.1B,C). The separating lamellae and pillars of syncytiotrophoblast are called the **trabeculae.** Their appearance marks the beginning of the lacunar or trabecular stage of placentation, which lasts from day 8 to day 13 p.c. Lacuna formation starts at the implantation pole. With advancing implantation, the syncytiotrophoblastic mass expands over the entire blastocystic surface. In all those places where it exceeds a certain critical thickness, new lacunae become evident, so that the lacunar system extends all over the blastocyst within a few days.

This process lasts until day 12 p.c., when the blastocyst is so deeply implanted that the uterine epithelium closes over the implantation site (Boyd & Hamilton, 1970). At this time, the outer surface of the blastocyst is completely transformed to syncytiotrophoblast. At its inner surface, it is covered by a locally incomplete layer of cytotrophoblast. Because trophoblastic proliferation and syncytial fusion have started at the implantation pole, the trophoblastic wall is considerably thicker at this point compared to the antiimplantation pole. This difference in thickness is never made up by the thinner parts during the subsequent developmental steps. The thicker trophoblast of the implantation pole is later transformed to the placenta, whereas the opposing thinner trophoblastic circumference only initially attempts to establish the same structure; later it shows regressive transformation to the smooth chorion, the membranes. All data of placental development given in this volume refer to the situation at the implantation pole.

Lacunar formation subdivides the trophoblastic covering of the blastocyst into three layers (Fig. 5.1C,D): (1) primary chorionic plate, facing the blastocystic cavity; (2) lacunar system together with the trabeculae; and (3) trophoblastic shell, facing the endometrium.

The **primary chorionic plate** is composed of a more or less continuous stratum of cytotrophoblast, which in some places is double- or even triple-layered. Toward the lacunae, the cytotrophoblast is covered by syncytiotrophoblast (Fig. 5.1D). On day 14 p.c., mesenchymal cells spread around the inner surface of the cytotrophoblast layer. There they transform to a loose network of branching cells, the **extraembryonic mesenchyme**. In the older literature, this mesenchyme had been thought to be of trophoblastic origin (Hertig, 1935; Wislocki & Streeter, 1938; Hertig & Rock, 1941, 1945, 1949). When reevaluating the Carnegie collection of early human ova, Luckett (1978) found proof that these primitive connective tissue cells were derived from the embryonic disk. Later, Luckett's findings were supported by Enders and King (1988), who studied the mesenchymal development in early macaque development.

Below the primary chorionic plate is the **lacunar system**. The lacunae are separated from each other by septa or pillars of syncytiotrophoblast, the trabeculae (Fig. 5.1C). Originally, these trabeculae were merely syncytiotrophoblastic in nature. Around day 12 p.c., however, they are invaded by cytotrophoblastic cells (Fig. 5.1D), which are derived from the primary chorionic plate. Within a few days the cytotrophoblast spreads over the entire length of the trabeculae. Where the peripheral ends of the trabeculae join together, they form the outermost layer of the trophoblast, the trophoblastic shell (Hertig & Rock, 1941; Boyd & Hamilton, 1970). In the beginning, this is a merely syncytiotrophoblastic structure, but as soon as the cytotrophoblast reaches the shell via the trabeculae (about day 15 p.c.), the former achieves a more heterogeneous structure (Fig. 5.1E). The syncytiotrophoblast establishes the bottom of the lacunae. It is followed by a more or less complete and sometimes multilayered zone of cytotrophoblast. Below the latter and facing the endometrial connective tissue, one again can find discontinuous syncytiotrophoblastic elements.

During the early stages of implantation, erosion of the maternal tissues occurred under the lytic influence of the syncytial trophoblast. Now the appearance of proliferating and migrating cytotrophoblast at the bottom of the shell starts **trophoblast invasion**, a key event during implantation and placentation that is responsible not only for further invasion of the blastocyst but also for adaptation of the maternal vessels to pregnancy conditions and for anchorage of the developing placenta (Boyd & Hamilton, 1970; Pijnenborg et al., 1981; Enders, 1997). In the course of this process, numerous syncytial elements can be observed far removed from the trophoblastic shell, in the depth of the uterine wall. Boyd and Hamilton (1970) suggested that they were remnants of the originally merely syncytiotrophoblastic shell. More recent publications have provided evidence that these so-called syncytiotrophoblastic or multinuclear giant cells are derived from invading cytotrophoblast that later fused (Park, 1971; Robertson & Warner, 1974; Pijnenborg et al., 1981).

The endometrial stroma undergoes remarkable changes throughout this process. The presence of eroding trophoblast, by being a mechanical irritant and by hormonal activity, causes the endometrial stromal cells to proliferate and to enlarge, thus giving rise to the **decidual cells** (Kaiser, 1960; Dallenbach-Hellweg & Sievers, 1975; Welsh & Enders, 1985). Further structural and functional details are presented in Chapter 9.

The invasive activities of the basal syncytiotrophoblast from day 12 p.c. on cause disintegration of the maternal endometrial vessel walls. Blood cells, leaving the leaky capillaries at that time, are found inside the lacunae (Boyd & Hamilton, 1970). The detailed mechanisms of this phenomenon are still a mystery of early implantation. Studies on rabbit implantation showed subepithelial capillary coiling and dilatation as the initial process, resulting in increased capillary permeability and stromal edema (Hafez & Tsutsumi, 1966; Finn, 1977; Hoos & Hoffman, 1980). This is followed by disintegration of the walls of capillary loops, a process that is likely to be induced by the trophoblast nearby (Larsen, 1961; Denker, 1980; Steven, 1983). At the same time, the disintegrating capillaries are surrounded by the basally expanding syncytiotrophoblast, which replaces the capillary walls in stepwise fashion (Leiser & Beier, 1988). It thus forms new lacunae.

In the next developmental step, the newly formed lacunae fuse with the already preexisting lacunae and thus establish the maternal perfusion of the entire lacunar system. Further invasion of the trophoblast, with progressive incorporation of the capillary limbs down to their arteriolar beginnings and their venular endings, provides the anatomic basis for the final formation of separate arterial inlets into the lacunar system as well as venous outlets.

Throughout the first steps of development, the maternal blood in the lacunae, which is propelled only by capillary pressure, moves sluggishly. With deeper invasion of the endometrium, the spiral arteries are also eroded, resulting in a higher intralacunar blood pressure and in the first real maternal circulation of the placenta.

Note that these views are based largely on studies performed in animals with labyrinthine placentas. Morphologic (Hustin et al., 1988) and clinical studies in the human (Doppler ultrasound, endoscopy) (Schaaps & Hustin, 1988) have suggested that efficient maternal blood flow in the normal human placenta is established only after the 12th week of pregnancy (see Chapter 9). This finding is surprising, in particular because the structural processes of lacuna formation look similar to those in labyrinthine placentas. Further studies are required to solve this problem.

Early Villous Stages

Shortly after the first appearance of maternal erythrocytes in the lacunae, on about day 13 p.c., increased cytotrophoblastic proliferation with subsequent syncytial fusion in the trabeculae takes place. As a result, not only can longitudinal trabecular growth be observed but also blindly ending syncytial side branches form and protrude into the lacunae (Fig. 5.1D,E). With increasing length and diameter, these **primary villi** are invaded by cytotrophoblast. Both processes mark the beginning of the villous stages of placentation. Further proliferative activities, with branching of the primary villi, initiate the development of primitive **villous trees**, the stems of which are derived from the former trabeculae (Fig. 5.1E). When the latter keep their contact to the trophoblastic shell, they are called **anchoring villi**. At the same time, the lacunar system, by definition, is transformed into the **intervillous space**.

Only 2 days later mesenchymal cells derived from the extraembryonic mesenchyme layer of the primary chorionic plate begin to invade the villi, transforming them into **secondary villi** (Fig. 5.1E). Within a few days, the mesenchyme expands peripherally to the villous tips and near the basis of the anchoring villi (Wislocki & Streeter, 1938; Hertig & Rock, 1945; Boyd & Hamilton, 1970).

The expanding villous mesenchyme does not reach the trophoblastic shell, which during these early stages of placentation remains free of fetal connective tissue. Rather, the basal segments of the trabeculae persist until the late stages of pregnancy on the primary villous stage, consisting of clusters of cytotrophoblast that are surrounded by a thin and partly incomplete sheet of syncytiotrophoblast. These cytotrophoblastic feet of the trabeculae or anchoring villi (Fig. 5.1E,F) are called **cell columns**. They are places of longitudinal growth of anchoring villi as well as sources of extravillous trophoblast (see Chapter 9). A similar phenomenon can be found in some free-floating villi. If the villous tips are not invaded by villous mesenchyme, they also persist on the primary villous stage as merely trophoblastic structures. Thus, briefly, cytotrophoblast shows nearly explosive proliferation transforming the villous tips into **trophoblastic cell islands** (see Chapter 9). The function of these cell islands is still uncertain.

The earlier theories of an additional in situ delamination of mesenchyme from villous cytotrophoblast (Hertig, 1935; Wislocki & Streeter, 1938; Hertig & Rock, 1945) have been refuted by Dempsey (1972), King (1987), and Demir et al. (1989). Their electron microscopic studies, performed on human and rhesus monkey placentas, showed that cytotrophoblast and villous mesenchyme are always clearly separated from each other by a complete basal lamina, which is never transgressed by a delaminating cytotrophoblast that might transform to mesenchyme, as was once thought to be the case.

With a few days' delay and beginning between days 18 and 20 p.c., the first **fetal capillaries** can be observed in the mesenchyme. They are derived from hemangioblastic progenitor cells (see Chapter 6, Fig. 7.21), which locally differentiate from the mesenchyme (King, 1987; Demir et al., 1989). The same progenitor cells give rise to groups of **hematopoietic stem cells**, which are always surrounded by the early endothelium and are thus positioned within the primitive capillaries (Fig. 7.22e). The appearance of cross sections of capillaries in the villous stroma marks the development of the first **tertiary villi**. Until term, all fetally vascularized villi (comprising most of the villi) can be subsumed under this name. Henceforth, only cell columns and cell islands, as well as transitory developmental stages of new villous formation (trophoblastic and villous sprouts), correspond to primary or secondary villi. At about the same time the fetal vascularization of the villi begins, the fetally vascularized allantois (Fig. 5.2) reaches the chorionic plate and fuses with the latter. Allantoic vessels develop into the chorionic plate and, according to Benirschke (1965), even into the larger villi. There they come into contact with the locally formed intravillous capillary segments. A complete fetoplacental circulation is established around the beginning of the 5th week p.c., as soon as enough capillary segments are fused with each other to form a regular capillary bed. Intravascular hematopoiesis can be observed during the following weeks, restricted to newly sprouting villi with de novo produced capillaries in most cases.

The expansion of the early villous trees takes place in the following way (Castellucci et al., 1990): at the surfaces of the larger villi, local cytotrophoblast proliferation with subsequent syncytial fusion causes the production of syncytial (trophoblastic) sprouts (see Chapter 7, Fig. 7.12). These sprouts are structurally comparable to the early primary villi and are composed of only trophoblast. Most of the syncytial sprouts degenerate again, probably the result of inappropriate local conditions; only some are invaded by villous mesenchyme and are thus transformed into the so-called villous sprouts (see Fig. 7.13). They correspond structurally to the secondary villi of the first steps of placentation. Formation of fetal vessels within the stroma (see Figs. 7.22 and 7.14), with subsequent growth in length and width, is characteristic of the transformation into new mesenchymal villi. Along their surfaces, new sprouts are again produced. (For further details, see Chapter 7.)

Assuming that there is already an intervillous circulation in the human placenta, fetal and maternal blood come into close contact with each other as soon as an intravillous (i.e., fetal) circulation is established. The two bloodstreams are always separated by the **placental barrier** (see Fig. 6.1D), which is composed of the follow-

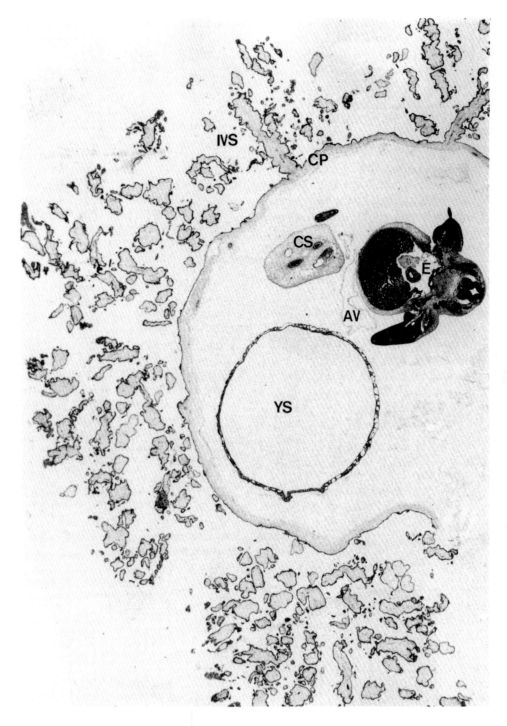

FIGURE 5.2. Semithin section across embryo and placenta of the 4th week after conception. Underneath the embryo (E) one can identify the connective stalk (CS) as precursor of the cord, the yolk sac (YS), and a small amnionic vesicle (AV). The chorionic cavity is surrounded by the chorionic plate (CP); from the latter, numerous placental villi protrude into the surrounding intervillous space (IVS). The basal plate is missing in this specimen, as it remained in utero, attached to the endometrium. ×9.5. (*Source: Kaufmann, 1990, with permission.*)

ing layers: (1) a continuous layer of syncytiotrophoblast covering the villous surface and thus lining the intervillous space; (2) an initially (first trimester) complete, but later (second and third trimesters) discontinuous layer of cytotrophoblast (Langhans' cells); (3) a trophoblastic basal lamina; (4) connective tissue; and (5) fetal endothelium, which is surrounded only by an endothelial basal lamina in the last trimester.

Throughout the subsequent periods of development, the tertiary villi undergo a complex process of differentiation that results in various villous types that differ from each other in terms of structure and function (see Chapter 7). This differentiation process is paralleled by qualitative and quantitative changes of the placental barrier: The syncytiotrophoblast is reduced in thickness from more than 20 mm to a mean of 3.5 mm. The cytotrophoblast is rarefied and, at term, it can be found in only 20% of the villous surface. The mean villous diameter decreases because the newly formed villous types are generally smaller than those preceding. Because of this latter process, the intravillous position of the fetal capillaries comes closer to the villous surface with advanced maturation. In many places, the capillary basal lamina may even fuse with that of the trophoblast (see Fig. 6.7A), thus considerably reducing the barrier in thickness and number of layers.

In summary, all these factors result in a reduction of the mean maternofetal diffusion distance from 50 to 100 mm in the second month to between 4 and 5 mm at term. The evident functional and pathogenetic importance of these phenomena makes it advisable to discuss the villous differentiation in more detail in Chapter 7.

References

Aplin, J.D.: The cell biology of human implantation. Placenta. **17**:269–275, 1996.

Aplin, J.D.: The cell biological basis of human implantation. Baillieres Best Pract. Res. Clin. Obstet. Gynaecol. **14**:757–764, 2000.

Bargmann, W. and Knoop, A.: Elektronenmikroskopische Untersuchungen an Plazentazotten des Menschen. Bemerkungen zum Synzytiumproblem. Z. Zellforsch. **50**:472–493, 1959.

Beck, L. and Heywinkel, E.: Berechtigte und unberechtigte Befürchtungen in der Reproduktionsmedizin. Gynäkologe **23**:249–251, 1990.

Benirschke, K.: In, Fetal Homeostasis, Vol. I. R.M. Wynn, ed., p. 328. New York Academy of Sciences, New York, 1965.

Bentin-Ley, U. and Lopata, A.: In vitro models of human blastocyst implantation. Baillieres Best Pract. Res. Clin. Obstet. Gynaecol. **14**:765–774, 2000.

Boyd, J.D. and Hamilton, W.J.: The Human Placenta. Heffer, Cambridge, 1970.

Castellucci, M., Scheper, M., Scheffen, I., Celona, A. and Kaufmann, P.: The development of the human placental villous tree. Anat. Embryol. (Berl.) **181**:117–128, 1990.

Dallenbach-Hellweg, G. and Sievers, S.: Die histologische Reaktion des Endometrium auf lokal applizierte Gestagene. Virchows Arch. Pathol. Anat. **368**:289–298, 1975.

Demir, R., Kaufmann, P., Castellucci, M., Erbengi, T. and Kotowski, A.: Fetal vasculogenesis and angiogenesis in human placental villi. Acta Anat. (Basel) **136**:190–203, 1989.

Dempsey, E.W.: The development of capillaries in the villi of early human placentas. Am. J. Anat. **134**:221–238, 1972.

Denker, H.-W.: Implantation: the role of proteinases, and blockage of implantation by proteinase inhibitors. Adv. Anat. Embryol. Cell. Biol. **53**:3–123, 1977.

Denker, H.-W.: Embryo implantation and trophoblast invasion. In, Cell Movement and Neoplasia. M. de Brabander, ed., pp. 151–162. Pergamon Press, Oxford, 1980.

Denker, H.-W.: Trophoblast-endometrial interactions at embryo implantation: a cell biological paradox. Trophoblast Res. **4**: 1–27, 1990.

Denker, H.-W. and Aplin, J.D., eds.: Trophoblast invasion and endometrial receptivity: novel aspects of the cell biology of embryo implantation. Trophoblast Res. **4**:1–462, 1990.

Enders, A.C.: Cytotrophoblast invasion of the endometrium in the human and macaque early villous stage of implantation. Trophoblast Res. **10**:83–95, 1997.

Enders, A.C. and King, B.F.: Formation and differentiation of extraembryonic mesoderm in the rhesus monkey. Am. J. Anat. **181**:327–340, 1988.

Finn, C.A.: The implantation reaction. In, Biology of the Uterus. R.M. Wynn, ed., pp. 245–308. Plenum Press, New York, 1977.

Hafez, E.S.E. and Tsutsumi, Y.: Changes in endometrial vascularity during implantation and pregnancy in the rabbit. Am. J. Anat. **118**:249–282, 1966.

Hertig, A.T.: Angiogenesis in the early human chorion and in the primary placenta of the macaque monkey. Contrib. Embryol. Carnegie Inst. **25**:37–81, 1935.

Hertig, A.T.: La nidation des oeufs humains fecondes normaux et anormaux. In, Les Fonctions de Nidation Uterine et Leurs Troubles. J. Ferin and M. Gaudefroy, eds., pp. 169–213, Masson, Paris, 1960.

Hertig, A.T. and Rock, J.: Two human ova of the previllous stage having an ovulation age of about eleven and twelve days respectively. Contrib. Embryol. Carnegie Inst. **29**:127–156, 1941.

Hertig, A.T. and Rock, J.: Two human ova of the pre-villous stage, having a developmental age of about seven and nine days respectively. Contrib. Embryol. Carnegie Inst. **31**:65–84, 1945.

Hertig, A.T. and Rock, J.: Two human ova of the pre-villous stage, having a developmental age of about eight and nine days respectively. Contrib. Embryol. Carnegie Inst. **33**:169–186, 1949.

Heuser, C.H. and Streeter, G.L.: Development of the macaque embryo. Contrib. Embryol. Carnegie Inst. **29**:15–55, 1941.

Hoos, P.G. and Hoffman, L.H.: Temporal aspects of rabbit uterine vascular and decidual responses to blastocyst stimulation. Biol. Reprod. **23**:453–459, 1980.

Hustin, J., Schaaps, J.P. and Lambotte, R.: Anatomical studies of the uteroplacental vascularization in the first trimester of pregnancy. Trophoblast Res. **3**:49–60, 1988.

Kaiser, R.: Über die Rückbildungsvorgänge in der Decidua während der Schwangerschaft. Arch. Gynäkol. **192**:209–220, 1960.

Kaufmann, P.: Placentation und Placenta. In, Humanembryologie. K.V. Hinrichsen, ed., pp. 159–204. Springer-Verlag, Heidelberg, 1990.

Kaufmann, P. and Scheffen, I.: Placental development. In, Neonatal and Fetal Medicine-Physiology and Pathophysiology. R. Polin and W. Fox, eds., pp. 47–56. Saunders, Orlando, 1992.

King, B.F.: Ultrastructural differentiation of stromal and vascular components in early macaque placental villi. Am. J. Anat. **178**:30–44, 1987.

Larsen, J.F.: Electron microscopy of the implantation site in the rabbit. Am. J. Anat. **109**:319–334, 1961.

Larsen, J.F.: Electron microscopy of nidation in the rabbit and observations on the human trophoblastic invasion. In, Ovoimplantation. Human Gonadotrophins and Prolactin. P.O. Hubinont, F. Leroy, C. Robyn and P. Leleux, eds., pp. 38–51. S. Karger, Basel, 1970.

Leiser, R. and Beier, H.M.: Morphological studies of lacunar formation in the early rabbit placenta. Trophoblast Res. **3**:97–110, 1988.

Lindhard, A., Bentin-Ley, U., Ravn, V., Islin, H., Hviid, T., Rex, S., Bangsboll, S. and Sorensen, S.: Biochemical evaluation of endometrial function at the time of implantation. Fertil. Steril. **78**:221–233, 2002.

Loke, Y.W. and King, A.: Immunology of implantation. Baillieres Best Pract. Res. Clin. Obstet. Gynaecol. **14**:827–837, 2000

Loke, Y.W., King, A. and Burrows, T.D.: Decidua in human implantation. Hum. Reprod. **10**:14–21, 1995.

Luckett, W.P.: Origin and differentiation of the yolk sac and extraembryonic mesoderm in presomite human and rhesus monkey embryos. Am. J. Anat. **152**:59–97, 1978.

Merviel, P., Challier, J.C., Carbillon, L., Foidart, J.M. and Uzan, S.: The role of integrins in human embryo implantation. Fetal Diagn. Ther. **16**:364–371, 2001a.

Merviel, P., Evain-Brion, D., Challier, J.C., Salat-Baroux, J. and Uzan, S.: The molecular basis of embryo implantation in humans. Zentralbl. Gynäkol. **123**:328–339, 2001b.

Mossman, H.W.: Comparative morphogenesis of the fetal membranes and accessory uterine structures. Carnegie Contrib. Embryol. **26**:129–246, 1937.

Mossman, H.W.: Vertebrate Fetal Membranes: Comparative Ontogeny and Morphology; Evolution; Phylogenetic Significance; Basic Functions; Research Opportunities. Macmillan, London, 1987.

Park, W.W.: Choriocarcinoma: A Study of Its Pathology, pp. 13–27. Heinemann, London, 1971.

Pijnenborg, R., Robertson, W.B., Brosens, I. and Dixon, G.: Trophoblast invasion and the establishment of haemochorial placentation in man and laboratory animals. Placenta **2**:71–92, 1981.

Psychoyos, A.: The "implantation window": can it be enlarged or displaced? Excerpta Med. Int. Congr. Ser. **768**:231–232, 1988.

Rao, C.V. and Sanfilippo, J.S.: New understanding in the biochemistry of implantation: Potential direct roles of luteinizing hormone and human chorionic gonadotropin. Endocrinologist. **7**:107–111, 1997.

Robertson, W.B. and Warner, B.: The ultrastructure of the human placental bed. J. Pathol. **112**:203–211, 1974.

Schaaps, J.P. and Hustin, J.: In vivo aspect of the maternal-trophoblastic border during the first trimester of gestation. Trophoblast Res. **3**:3–48, 1988.

Schlafke, S. and Enders, A.C.: Cellular basis of interaction between trophoblast and uterus in implantation. Biol. Reprod. **12**:41–65, 1975.

Simon, C., Moreno, C., Remohi, J. and Pellicer, A.: Cytokines and embryo implantation. J. Reprod. Immunol. **39**:117–131, 1998.

Steven, D.H.: Interspecies differences in the structure and function of trophoblast. In, Biology of Trophoblast. Y.W. Loke and A. Whyte, eds., pp. 111–136. Elsevier, Amsterdam, 1983.

Sunder, S. and Lenton, E.A.: Endocrinology of the peri-implantation period. Baillieres Best Pract. Res. Clin. Obstet. Gynaecol. **14**:789–800, 2000.

Tedde, G., Tedde-Piras, A. and Berta, R.: A new structural pattern of the human trophoblast: the syncytial units. In, Abstracts of the 11th Rochester Trophoblast conference, abstract 117, 1988a.

Tedde, G., Tedde-Piras, A. and Fenu, G.: Demonstration of an intercellular pathway of transport in the human trophoblast. In, Abstracts of the 11th Rochester Trophoblast Conference, abstract. 77, 1988b.

Welsh, A.O. and Enders, A.E.: Light and electron microscopic examination of the mature decidual cells of the rat with emphasis on the antimesometrial decidua and its degeneration. Am. J. Anat. **172**:1–29, 1985.

Wislocki, G.B. and Streeter, G.L.: On the placentation of the macaque (Macaca mulatta) from the time of implantation until the formation of the definitive placenta. Contrib. Embryol. Carnegie Inst. **27**:1–66, 1938.

Yoshimura, Y., Shiokawa, S., Nagamatsu, S., Hanashi, H., Sawa, H., Koyama, N., Katsumata, Y. and Nakamura, Y.: Effects of beta-1 integrins in the process of implantation. Horm. Res. **44**:36–41, 1995.

Yoshimura, Y., Miyakoshi, K., Hamatani, T., Iwahashi, K., Takahashi, J., Kobayashi, N., Sueoka, K., Miyazaki, T., Kuji, N. and Tanaka, M.: Role of beta(1) integrins in human endometrium and decidua during implantation. Horm. Res. **50**:46–55, 1998.

6
Basic Structure of the Villous Trees

M. Castellucci and P. Kaufmann

Nearly the entire maternofetal and fetomaternal exchange takes place in the placental villi. There is only a limited contribution to this exchange by the extraplacental membranes. In addition, most metabolic and endocrine activities of the placenta have been localized in the villi (for review, see Gröschel-Stewart, 1981; Miller & Thiede, 1984; Knobil & Neill, 1993; Polin et al., 2004).

Throughout placental development, different types of villi emerge that have differing structural and functional specializations. Despite this diversification, all villi exhibit the same basic structure (Fig. 6.1):

- They are covered by **syncytiotrophoblast**, an epithelial surface layer that separates the villous interior from the maternal blood, which flows around the villi. Unlike other epithelia, the syncytiotrophoblast is not composed of individual cells but represents a continuous, uninterrupted, multinucleated surface layer without separating cell borders (Fig. 6.1C; see Fig.6.21, and Chapter 7, Fig. 7.11).
- Beneath the syncytiotrophoblast is an interrupted layer of **cytotrophoblast**, which consists of single or aggregated cells, the Langhans' cells, which are the stem cells of the syncytiotrophoblast; they support the growth and regeneration of the latter.
- The **trophoblastic basement membrane** separates syncytiotrophoblast and cytotrophoblast from the stromal core of the villi.
- The **stroma** is composed of varying numbers and types of connective tissue cells, connective tissue fibers, and ground substance.
- Additionally, the stroma contains **fetal vessels** of various kinds and calibers. In the larger stem villi, the vessels are mainly arteries and veins; in the peripheral branches, most fetal vessels are capillaries or sinusoids.

Syncytiotrophoblast

Syncytium or Multinucleated Giant Cells?

The syncytiotrophoblast is a continuous, normally uninterrupted layer that extends over the surfaces of all villous trees as well as over parts of the inner surfaces of chorionic and basal plates. It thus lines the intervillous space. Systematic electron microscopic studies of the syncytial layer (e.g., Bargmann & Knoop, 1959; Schiebler & Kaufmann, 1969; Boyd & Hamilton, 1970; Kaufmann & Stegner, 1972; Schweikhart & Kaufmann, 1977; Wang & Schneider, 1987) have revealed no evidence that the syncytiotrophoblast is composed of separate units. Rather, it is a single continuous structure for every placenta. Only in later stages of pregnancy, as a consequence of focal degeneration of syncytiotrophoblast, fibrinoid plaques may isolate small islands of syncytiotrophoblast from the surrounding syncytial continuum; this happens mainly at the surfaces of chorionic and basal plates. Therefore, terms such as *syncytial cells* and *syncytiotrophoblasts*, widely used in experimental disciplines, are inappropriate and should be avoided. Their use points to a basic misunderstanding of the real nature of the syncytiotrophoblast.

Where the syncytiotrophoblast due to degenerative processes is interrupted, the gap is filled by fibrin-type fibrinoid (see Chapter 9). A few reports (Tedde et al., 1988a,b) have pointed to the existence of **vertical cell membranes** that seemingly subdivide the syncytium into syncytial units. These extremely rare findings have an accidental rather than a real basis. They represent the likely results of a syncytiotrophoblastic repair mechanism (Figs. 6.1, 6.2B, and 6.3). That is, after syncytial rupture, apical and basal plasmalemmas fuse at either side of the

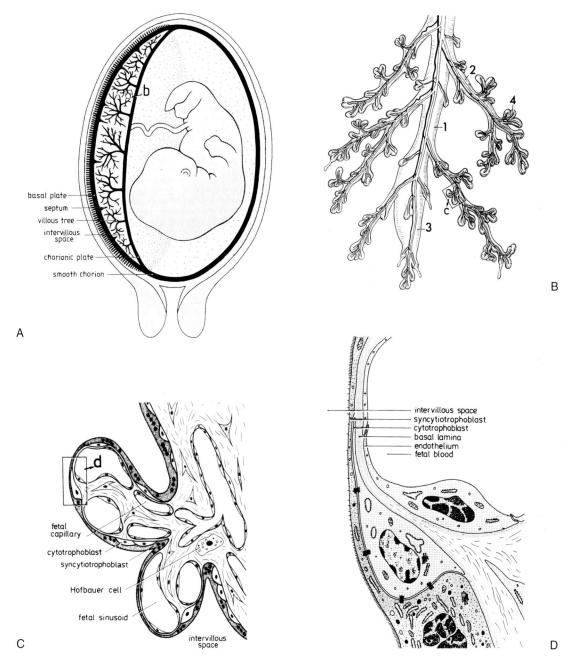

basal plate
septum
villous tree
intervillous space
chorionic plate
smooth chorion

A

B

fetal capillary
cytotrophoblast
syncytiotrophoblast
Hofbauer cell
fetal sinusoid
intervillous space

C

intervillous space
syncytiotrophoblast
cytotrophoblast
basal lamina
endothelium
fetal blood

D

FIGURE 6.1. Basic morphology of human placental villi. A: Simplified longitudinal section across the uterus, placenta, and membranes in the human. The chorionic sac, consisting of placenta (left half) and membranes (right half), is black. B: Peripheral ramifications of the mature villous tree, consisting of a stem villus (1), which continues in a bulbous immature intermediate villus (3); the slender side branches (2) are the mature intermediate villi, the surface of which is densely covered with grapelike terminal villi (4). C: Highly simplified light microscopic section of two terminal villi, branching off a mature intermediate villus (right). D: Schematic electron microscopic section of the placental barrier, demonstrating its typical layers. (*Source:* Modified from Kaufmann, 1983, with permission.)

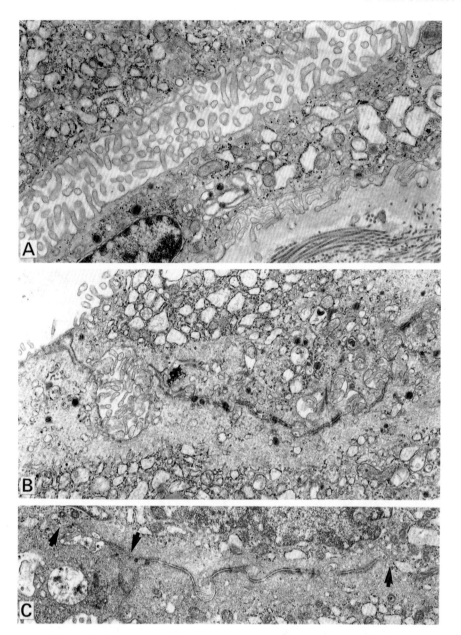

FIGURE 6.2. Remains of cell membranes in the syncytiotropho-blast result from two mechanisms: fusion of neighboring villous surfaces forming bridges and repair of disrupted syncytial surfaces. A: As a first step of formation of syncytial bridges between adjacent villi, the opposing microvillous membranes interdigitate. The identical initial step occurs as a first step of wound repair when the disrupted ends of syncytiotrophoblast become covered by microvillous membranes, which subsequently come into contact and interdigitate. ×14,500. B: Follow-up stage of that depicted in part A. The interdigitating syncytial surfaces have largely lost their microvilli and now establish a smooth intercellular cleft bridged by numerous desmosomes that vertically traverse the syncytiotrophoblast. (See the survey picture in Figure 6.3.) ×11,000. C: As the next step of repair, the newly developed separating cell membranes show disintegration (arrows) so that the newly formed intrasyncytial cleft becomes focally bridged by syncytioplasm. After complete disintegration of membranes and desmosomes, the syncytial villous cover is again continuous. ×13,800. (*Source:* Cantle et al., 1987, with permission.)

wound, thus avoiding further loss of syncytioplasm. Afterward, either a fibrinoid plug closes the wound, or the disconnected parts of the syncytium again come into close contact to form a lateral intercellular cleft bridged by desmosomes. Later, fusion occurs by disintegration of the separating membranes (Fig. 6.2). Transitory stages of this process may be misinterpreted as borders of syncytial units.

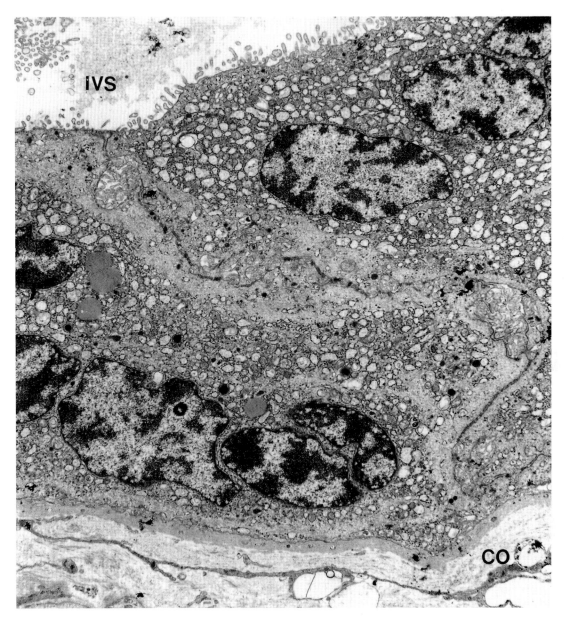

FIGURE 6.3. Survey electron micrograph of the section shown in Figure 6.2B demonstrates that in intermediate stages of syncytial repair the villous syncytial trophoblast can be traversed by vertical "intercellular" clefts connecting the intervillous space (IVS) with the connective tissue core (CO) of the villi. Such intrasyncytial membranes must not be misinterpreted as stable intercellular clefts subdividing the syncytium in smaller syncytial units. ×7000.

Many authors have described **remainders of intercellular junctions** within the syncytiotrophoblast (Carter, 1963, 1964; Boyd & Hamilton, 1966; Burgos & Rodriguez, 1966; Metz et al., 1979; Reale et al., 1980; Wang & Schneider, 1987). Some investigators have interpreted these junctions as vestiges of a former cellular state of the syncytium or as proof of recent cytotrophoblastic contribution to the syncytiotrophoblast (Carter, 1963, 1964; Boyd & Hamilton, 1966). In a systematic study of these junctions, Metz et al. (1979) as well as Reale et al. (1980) have described zonulae and maculae occludentes that were mostly located in apical membrane infoldings, as well as numerous isolated desmosomes, without contact to any surface membranes. The structural evidence has been supported by recent immunohistochemical data that show zonula occludens type 1 (ZO-1) as well

as occludin in the apical part of syncytiotrophoblast (Marzioni et al., 2001). The authors of the publications considered above hypothesized that these junctions represent stages of several dynamic processes: for example,

- remainders of cytotrophoblastic fusion with the overlying syncytium,
- establishment of intervillous contacts by partial or complete syncytiotrophoblastic surface fusion,
- repair of syncytial disruption, or
- decomposition of temporary surface invagination of the syncytiotrophoblast.

The syncytiotrophoblast must be seen as a highly dynamic layer that is qualified for ameboid movements. Disconnection with subsequent refusion and the formation of invaginations and bridges seem to be regular phenomena.

We not only find the ultrastructural remains of this process but also can easily observe it in vitro; when we (1) carefully trypsinize villi from full-term placentas, (2) remove mesenchymal cells by means of CD9-antibodies, (3) remove cytotrophoblast by means of a hepatocyte growth factor-activator-inhibitor (HAI-1) antibody (Pötgens et al., 2003), and (d) let the remaining isolated tissues adhere on culture dishes, we obtain a nearly pure population of mononucleated fragments of syncytiotrophoblast. These small CD105-positive mononucleated trophoblast elements, which result in large numbers during any attempt of trophoblast isolation, should not be misinterpreted as cytotrophoblast (Pötgens et al., 2003), even though they are cytokeratin-positive and each adherent syncytial fragment is surrounded by a plasmalemma (Huppertz et al. 1999). Within 1 or 2 further days of culture, the fragments start refusion, then again forming islands of syncytiotrophoblast.

Syncytial Plasmalemmas and Microvilli

With deference to the intentions of this chapter, we consider here only briefly some aspects of the plasma membranes of the syncytiotrophoblast. Sideri et al. (1983) have pointed to differences between the syncytiotrophoblastic brush-border membrane (BBM; facing the maternal blood) and the basal plasma membrane (BPM; facing adjacent cytotrophoblast or the basal lamina) of the syncytiotrophoblast. Both plasmalemmas exhibit different densities of intramembranous proteins. Vanderpuye and Smith (1987) presented a useful review of the relevant data. Later studies have confirmed these differences between BBM and BPM. They showed that receptors for calcitonin (Lafond et al., 1994) and calcitonin gene-related peptide (Lafond et al., 1997), as well as muscarinic (Pavia et al., 1997) and transferrin receptors (Verrijt et al., 1997) are different in number, affinity, and distribution of their subtypes in BBM and BPM. In addition, some G-protein subunits (Mabrouk et al., 1996) and protein kinase C isoforms (Ruzycky et al., 1996) showed different distributions in the two membranes.

Microvilli nearly completely cover the syncytiotrophoblastic surface and represent an enormous maternofetal contact zone (see Fig. 6.14). At term, the presence of microvilli multiplies the total villous surface area of about 12 m^2 (see Chapter 28, Table 28.5) by a factor of about 7.67 (Teasdale & Jean-Jacques, 1986; see also Mayhew, 1985). Because of their localization at the maternal–fetal border, the microvilli have engendered much immunologic and cell biologic interest. Two summarizing articles provide details (Smith et al., 1977; Truman & Ford, 1984).

Morphologic studies of microvillus structure and its functional significance have been published by Boyd et al. (1968b), Herbst and Multier (1970), Wainwright and Wainwright (1974), Truman et al. (1981), King (1983), Al-Zuhair et al. (1983, 1987), Mazzanti et al. (1994), and Jaggi et al. (1995). Most of the histochemical studies concerning the composition of the microvillous membrane focused on the glycocalix. They describe its polysaccharide composition and discuss the immunologic relevance of the polysaccharides (Bradbury

et al., 1969, 1970; Rovasio & Monis, 1973; Liebhart, 1974; Martin et al., 1974; Okudaira & Hayakawa, 1975; Nelson et al., 1976; Wada et al., 1977, 1979; Kelley et al., 1979; King, 1981; Wasserman et al., 1983a,b; Fisher et al., 1984; Parmley et al., 1984; Maubert et al., 1997). Various lectin-binding sites have been described by Whyte (1980), Gabius et al. (1987), Hoyer and Kirkeby (1996), and Lang et al. (1994a,b).

Cytochemical demonstration of **membrane-bound enzymes** studied in the transmission electron microscope (TEM) comprise alkaline phosphatase (Hempel & Geyer, 1969; Borst et al., 1973; Hulstaert et al., 1973; Kameya et al., 1973; Jemmerson et al., 1985; Matsubara et al., 1987c), galactosyltransferase (Nelson et al., 1977), α-amylase (Fisher & Laine, 1983), protein kinases (Albe et al., 1983), Ca-ATPase (Matsubara et al., 1987b), cyclic 3,5-nucleotide phosphodiesterase (Matsubara et al., 1987d), 5-nucleotidase (Matsubara et al., 1987a), and nicotinamide adenine dinucleotide phosphate diaphorase (Matsubara et al., 1997).

The analysis of **surface receptors involved in transplacental transfer** has achieved even more importance for our understanding of transplacental transport (King, 1976; Ockleford & Menon, 1977; Wood et al., 1978a,b; Galbraith et al., 1980; Johnson & Brown, 1980; Brown & Johnson, 1981; Green & Ford, 1984; Malassine et al., 1984, 1987; Alsat et al., 1985; Parmley et al., 1985; Bierings, 1989; Yeh et al., 1989; for a review see Alsat et al., 1995).

The vast literature on **receptors for hormones and growth factors** has been discussed repeatedly (Adamson 1987; Blay & Hollenberg, 1989; Ohlsson, 1989; Mitchell et al., 1993; Alsat et al., 1995) and cannot be reviewed here. For further reading on some particular subjects we refer the reader to the following publications: insulin receptor (Nelson et al., 1978; Jones et al., 1993; Desoye et al., 1994, 1997); insulin-like growth factor II (IGF-II) (Daughaday et al., 1981; Nissley et al., 1993); interleukin-6 receptor (Nishino et al., 1990); parathyroid hormone receptor (Lafond et al., 1988); vascular endothelial growth factor (Cheung, 1997); calcitonin receptor (Lafond et al., 1994); calcitonin gene-related peptide (Lafond et al., 1997); and colony-stimulating factor and its receptor (CSF-1R: Adamson, 1987; Aboagye-Mathiesen et al., 1997).

Special attention has been paid to the epidermal growth factor receptor (EGFR) a gene-product of the proto-oncogene c-erbB-1 (Rao et al., 1984, 1985; Chegini & Rao, 1985; Maruo & Mochizuki, 1987; Maruo et al., 1987, 1996; Morrish et al., 1987, 1997; Chen et al., 1988; Yeh et al., 1989; Mühlhauser et al., 1993; Evain-Brion and Alsat, 1994), and the closely related proto-oncogene product c-erbB-2 (Mühlhauser et al., 1993; Lewis et al., 1996; Aboagye-Mathiesen et al., 1997):

- Epidermal growth factor receptor is present in the syncytiotrophoblast as well as in the villous and extravillous cytotrophoblast (Bulmer et al., 1989; Ladines-Llave et al., 1991; Mühlhauser et al., 1993). Its ligand, epidermal growth factor (EGF) is detectable in amnionic fluid, umbilical vessels, and placental tissue (Scott et al., 1989). Maruo et al. (1996) found evidence that it is expressed by syncytiotrophoblast. The question of placental production sites is still open. Morrish et al. (1987) have pointed out that this growth factor induces morphologic differentiation of trophoblast together with increased production of human chorionic gonadotropin (hCG) and human placental lactogen (hPL) in vitro. It obviously has no effect on trophoblast proliferation (Maruo et al., 1996).

- Structurally related to the EGF receptor is the gene product of the proto-oncogene c-erbB-2. It represents the only member of the HER receptor family that neither has a direct and specific ligand nor has it kinase activity (for review, see Casalini et al., 2004). Rather, it seems to play a major coordinating role since the other receptors of the HER family act by heterodimerization with c-erbB-2 upon activation by their specific ligand. It seems to be important in human cancer. In some types of malignant tumors, c-erbB-2 protein product and EGFR are both overexpressed, and this correlates with a reduction in patient relapse-free interval and with overall survival (Slamon et al., 1987; Wright et al., 1989). These data suggest that the two receptors may contribute to the development and maintenance of the malignant phenotype. Interestingly, in the human placenta, which shares some aspects with invasive tumors, this coexpression is present in villous syncytiotrophoblast, which, however, and contrary to invasive tumor cells, is nonproliferative; on the other hand, in the proliferating cells of the extravillous trophoblast, only EGFR is expressed, whereas c-erbB-2 characterizes the differentiating and no longer proliferating cells (Mühlhauser et al., 1993).

Syncytiotrophoblastic Cytoskeleton

Ockleford et al. (1981b) have speculated that in addition to the skeletal structures of the villous stroma there must be other mechanical factors responsible for the maintenance of the complex shape of the villi. They described a superficially arranged complex system of intrasyncytial filaments that largely occupies the superficial layer of the syncytiotrophoblast. They suggested the term **syncytio-skeletal layer** for this zone. Numerous other authors have contributed to our knowledge of the syncytial cytoskeleton as well (Vacek, 1969; Scheuner et al., 1980; Ockleford et al., 1981a,c; King, 1983; Khong et al., 1986; Beham et al., 1988; Mühlhauser et al., 1995; Berryman et al., 1995).

The **syncytial cytoskeleton** is composed of actin, tubulin, and intermediate filament proteins as cytokeratins and desmoplakin (Ockleford et al., 1981b; King, 1983; Beham et al., 1988; Mühlhauser et al., 1995; Berryman et al., 1995). The microtubules are arranged in a coarse, open lattice-like network that is oriented parallel to the syncytial surface. They are intermingled with microfilaments that form an apparently disordered meshwork. Actin filaments interact with ezrin, and microfilaments of this meshwork pass into the microvilli, where they display a distinct polarity, with their S1 arrowheads pointing away from the microvillous tips.

Different from intestinal microvilli, the rootlets of the microvillous filaments are short and interact with other filaments of the terminal web almost immediately after emergence from the microvilli. The overall impression of this system, reported by King (1983), is that of a poorly developed terminal web. Beham et al. (1988) and Mühlhauser et al. (1995) found immunohistochemical evidence for the presence of cytokeratin and desmoplakin in the apical zone. The presence of the latter intermediate filament protein is in agreement with the occasional appearance of desmosomes in this zone. Both intermediate filaments were also found in the basal zone of the syncytioplasm (Beham et al., 1988), where King (1983) also detected actin.

Specialized Regions of the Villous Surface

Dempsey and Zergollern (1969) and Dempsey and Luse (1971) have subdivided the syncytiotrophoblast into three zones: an outer absorptive zone in which organelles related to vesicular uptake are accumulated as well as large parts of the cytoskeleton (syncytioskeletal layer; Ockleford et al., 1981b), a middle secretory zone containing most organelles, and a basal zone with few organelles. Structural changes and variations in the thickness of the middle zone are responsible for regional specializations that become evident in the second half of pregnancy.

During earlier stages of pregnancy, the syncytiotrophoblast is a mostly homogeneous layer with evenly distributed nuclei (Boyd & Hamilton, 1970; Kaufmann & Stegner, 1972). The distribution of cellular organelles is homogeneous and does not suggest a marked structural and functional differentiation inside this layer. From the 15th week on, this situation gradually changes (Kaufmann & Stegner, 1972). At term, structural diversification results in a highly variable pattern of mosaic areas of different structure and histochemical attributes (Amstutz, 1960; Fox, 1965; Burgos & Rodriguez, 1966; Hamilton & Boyd, 1966; Schiebler & Kaufmann, 1969; Alvarez et al., 1970; Dempsey & Luse, 1971; Kaufmann & Stark, 1973; Martin & Spicer, 1973b; Kaufmann et al., 1974b; Jones & Fox, 1977) (Figs. 6.4 to 6.6). This mosaic pattern, however, lacks sharp demarcations because all specialized areas are part of one single continuous syncytium.

Several types of syncytiotrophoblast can be classified regarding the thickness of the syncytiotrophoblast, the distribution of its nuclei, the kind and number of its organelles, and its enzymatic activities. As will be dealt with later in this chapter, these specialized regions of syncytiotrophoblast obviously correspond to different stages of the trophoblastic apoptosis cascade, which starts with syncytial fusion resulting in thick nucleated syncytiotrophoblast with ample rough endoplasmic reticulum and ends with extrusion of syncytial knots containing apoptotic nuclei.

Syncytiotrophoblast with Prevailing Rough Endoplasmic Reticulum

Syncytiotrophoblast with prevailing rough endoplasmic reticulum in early stages of pregnancy is the only type of syncytiotrophoblast. At term, it is still the most common type. Its thickness varies between about 2 and 10 μm, depending on whether it contains nuclei or is devoid of them. The surface is covered by more or less densely packed microvilli. In addition to vesicles and all types of lysosomes, numerous mitochondria, Golgi fields, and ample rough endoplasmic reticulum characterize the cytoplasm. After conventional postpartum fixation, the latter is vesicular (Figs. 6.2 and 6.3) (Boyd et al., 1968a). With optimal fixation, as from aspiration biopsy during cesarean section from a placenta in situ that is still being maternally perfused (Schweikhart & Kaufmann, 1977),

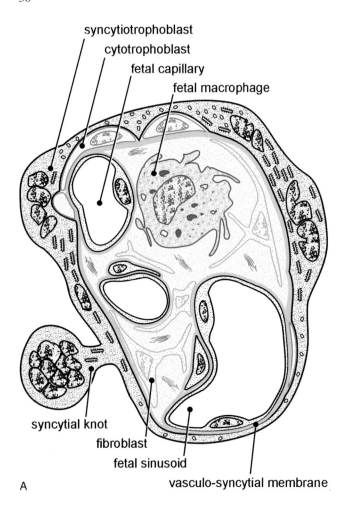

syncytiotrophoblast
cytotrophoblast
fetal capillary
fetal macrophage

syncytial knot
fibroblast
fetal sinusoid
vasculo-syncytial membrane

A

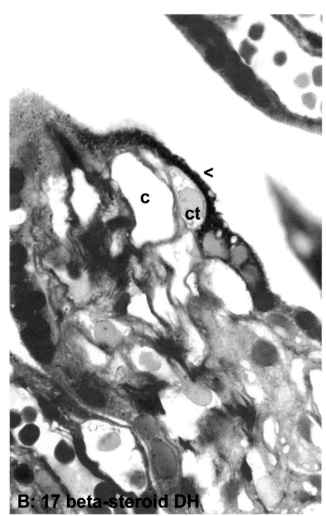

B: 17 beta-steroid DH

FIGURE 6.4. A: Simplified drawing of a cross section of a terminal villus demonstrating the structural variability of its syncytiotrophoblastic cover. B: Semithin section demonstrating the histochemical activity of 17β-hydroxysteroid dehydrogenase (black). As a prominent indicator of syncytiotrophoblastic specialization, this enzyme has maximum activity in and around a syncytial lamella (arrowhead) covering villous cytotrophoblast (ct). Note the close relationship between cytotrophoblast, 17β-steroid dehydrogenase-positive trophoblast and fetal capillary (c). ×800. (*Source:* Kaufmann et al., 1974b, with permission.)

the rough endoplasmic reticulum is composed of slender cisternae oriented in parallel (Fig. 6.7A). The degree of dilatation depends on the delay of fixation (Kaufmann, 1985).

Several publications have presented structural aspects of this type of syncytiotrophoblast (Boyd et al., 1968a; Dempsey & Zergollern, 1969; Schiebler & Kaufmann, 1969; Dempsey & Luse, 1971; Martin & Spicer, 1973a; Ockleford, 1976). The functional interpretation is based on enzyme histochemical data. Most enzymes found, are related to energy metabolism (Fig. 6.5). In addition, relevant activities of glutamate dehydrogenase, α-glycerol-phosphate dehydrogenase, nonspecific esterase, acid phosphatase, alkaline phosphatase, nicotinamide adenine dinucleotide phosphate diaphorase, and proteases were found (Wielenga & Willinghagen, 1962; Wachstein et al., 1963; Velardo & Rosa,

1963; Lister, 1967; Hoffman & Di Pietro, 1972; Hulstaert et al., 1973; Kaufmann et al., 1974b; Gossrau et al., 1987; Matsubara et al., 1997). The immunohistochemical proof of 11b-hydroxysteroid dehydrogenase was interpreted as an enzymatic barrier, preventing maternal glucocorticoids from passing into the fetal circulation where they might have adverse effects (Yang, 1997). In addition, superoxide dismutase and xanthine oxidase were detected in the syncytiotrophoblast and were thought to be involved in degrading superoxide, thus playing a role in the maintenance of uterine quiescence (Myatt et al., 1997; Telfer et al., 1997; Watson et al., 1997). These studies make it likely that this type of syncytium is involved in more complex active maternofetal transfer mechanisms, including catabolism and resynthesis of proteins and lipids.

Immunocytochemical studies have provided evidence that **synthesis of proteo- and peptide hormones** takes place here. These include:

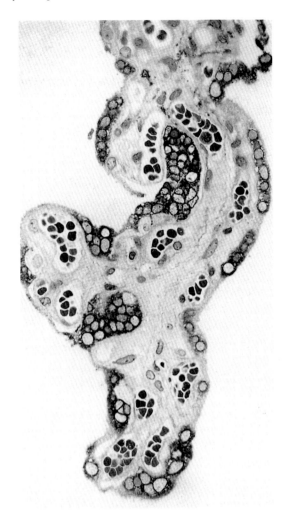

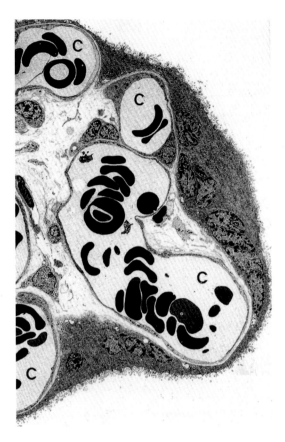

FIGURE 6.6. Transmission electron microscopic section of a terminal villus. Note that the structural specialization of the syncytiotrophoblast depends on its spatial relation to the fetal capillaries (C). In nearly all places where the capillaries bulge against the villous surface, the syncytiotrophoblast is attenuated to thin lamellae (vasculosyncytial membranes) devoid of nuclei. The nuclei accumulate between the lamellae and form syncytial knots. ×1350. (*Source:* Castellucci & Kaufmann, 1982a, with permission.)

FIGURE 6.5. Semithin section with histochemical demonstration of lactate dehydrogenase. The enzyme activity is bound to the vicinity of syncytial nuclei, whereas syncytium devoid of nuclei does not exhibit enzyme activity. ×420. (*Source:* Schiebler & Kaufmann, 1981, with permission.)

- human chorionic gonadotropin (hCG) (Dreskin et al., 1970; Hamanaka et al., 1971; Genbacev et al., 1972; Kurman et al., 1984; Beck et al., 1986; Frauli & Ludwig, 1987c; Morrish et al., 1987; Sakakibara et al., 1987; Hay, 1988);
- human chorionic somatotropin (hCS) or hPL (Kim et al., 1971; De Ikonicoff & Cedard, 1973; Dujardin et al., 1977; Kurman et al., 1984; Beck et al., 1986; Fujimoto et al., 1986; Morrish et al., 1988; Jacquemin et al., 1996);
- other human growth hormones (hGHs) such as hGH-V and hGH-N (Liebhaber et al., 1989; Alsat et al., 1997), human prolactin (hPRL) (Bryant-Greenwood et al., 1987; Sakbun et al., 1987; Unnikumar et al., 1988);
- oxytocin (Unnikumar et al., 1988);
- leptin (Masuzaki et al., 1997; Senaris et al., 1997; Castellucci et al., 2000a);
- erythropoietin (Conrad et al., 1996);
- corticotropin-releasing hormone (CRH) (Warren and Silverman, 1995);
- parathyroid hormone-related protein (PTHrP) (Dunne et al., 1994; Emly et al., 1994);
- b-endorphin and b-lipotropin (Laatikainen et al., 1987);
- pregnancy-specific glycoprotein (Zhou et al., 1997); and
- various placental proteins such as SP1 (Gosseye & Fox, 1984; Beck et al., 1986).

Syncytiotrophoblast with Prevailing Smooth Endoplasmic Reticulum

Syncytiotrophoblast with prevailing smooth endoplasmic reticulum are small spot-like areas, dispersed in the syncytiotrophoblast equipped with rough endoplasmic reticulum (Figs. 6.4A, 6.7, and 6.8), and showing gradual transitions to the latter. They are usually equipped with mitochondria of the tubular type. The structural similarity to endocrine cells active in steroid metabolism (Gillim et al., 1969; Crisp et al., 1970) is striking. Focally increased activities of 3b-hydroxysteroid dehydrogenase and

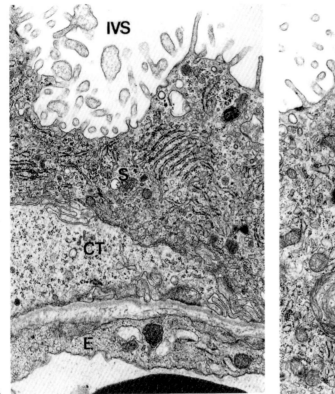

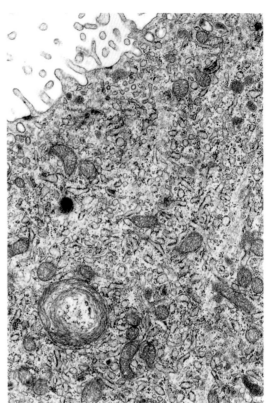

A

B

FIGURE 6.7. A: Transmission electron micrograph of syncytiotrophoblast with well-developed rough endoplasmic reticulum, probably active in protein metabolism. IVS, intervillous space; S, syncytiotrophoblast; CT, cytotrophoblast; E, fetal endothe-lium. ×14,000. (*Source:* Schiebler & Kaufmann, 1981, with permission.) B: Electron micrograph of syncytiotrophoblast with well-developed smooth endoplasmic reticulum. Such areas are probably involved in steroid metabolism. ×14,800.

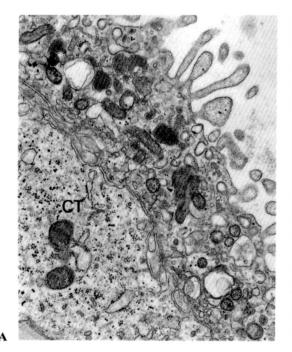

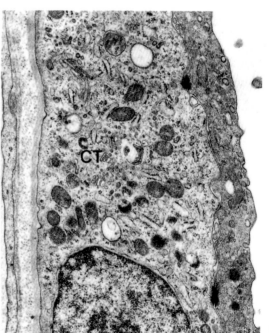

A

B

FIGURE 6.8. A: Transmission electron micrograph of a thin syncytiotrophoblastic lamella covering villous cytotrophoblast (CT). The syncytiotrophoblast of this type is well equipped with dense bodies and vesicles. As can be deduced from its enzymatic activity, such areas are probably involved in endocrine activity. ×22,000. B: Transmission electron micrograph of a thin syncy-tiotrophoblastic lamella covering cytotrophoblast (CT). This lamella is devoid of microvilli and dense bodies. Its cytoplasm is characterized only by vesicles. Following enzyme histochemi-cal reactions (see Fig. 6.4B), it exhibits high activities of 17β-hydroxysteroid dehydrogenase and thus participates in steroid metabolism. ×14,500.

17β-hydroxysteroid dehydrogenase in just these areas (Fig. 6.4B) underline the assumption that these are steroidally active areas (Kaufmann & Stark, 1973; Kaufmann et al., 1974b).

Vasculosyncytial Membranes

Vasculosyncytial membranes or epithelial plates (Figs. 6.4A, 6.6, and 6.9) were first identified by Bremer (1916) and later defined in more detail by Amstutz (1960). They are thin syncytiotrophoblastic lamellae, measuring 0.5 to about 1 μm in thickness; free of nuclei and poor in organelles, they are directly apposed to sinusoidally enlarged parts of the fetal capillaries (Schiebler & Kaufmann, 1969; Fox & Blanco, 1974). One can conclude from the structural features that the expanding fetal sinusoids bulge against the villous surface and completely displace the syncytial nuclei as well as most of the syncytial organelles. Capillary basement membrane and trophoblastic basement membrane may come into such close contact that they fuse (Figs. 6.1 and 6.9A). In agreement with the view, that pressure by the sinusoids displaces the syncytial nuclei, accumulations of nuclei and organelles may be observed directly lateral to the vasculosyncytial membranes; they are called syncytial knots (Figs. 6.4A, 6.6, and 6.10A).

Function: Some further findings are helpful for the functional interpretation. The density of microvilli at the surface of the vasculosyncytial membranes is sometimes considerably reduced (Fig. 6.9) (Leibl et al., 1975; however, compare King & Menton, 1975). There is some evidence that some growth factors particularly involved in angiogenic processes, such as placental growth factor (PlGF) (Khaliq et al., 1996) and hepatocyte growth factor (HGF) (Kilby et al., 1996), are particularly expressed in and around vasculosyncytial membranes. High activities of hexokinase and glucose-6-phosphatase were found histochemically, whereas enzymes of the energy metabolism are largely inactive (Fig. 6.5). With respect to structure and enzymatic equipment, we conclude that these areas are especially involved in diffusional transfer of gases and water as well as in the facilitated transfer of glucose.

Slightly thicker vasculosyncytial membranes are equipped with more organelles. In addition, they show hydrolytic enzymes such as alkaline phosphatase (Kameya et al., 1973), 5-nucleotidase, and adenosine triphosphatase (ATPase) (Schiebler & Kaufmann, 1981). These sites are presumably concerned with active transfer (e.g., amino acids, electrolytes) rather than serving merely passive transfer processes.

When one is studying optimally fixed terminal villi of the term placenta, the vasculosyncytial membranes amount to 25% to 40% of the villous surface (Sen et al., 1979), depending on the maturational status of the villi. After delayed fixation this value may be considerably smaller because of fetal vascular collapse and trophoblastic shrinkage (see Chapter 28, Tables 28.6 and 28.9) (Voigt et al., 1978).

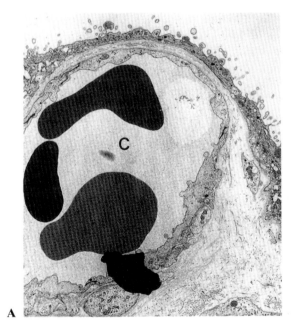

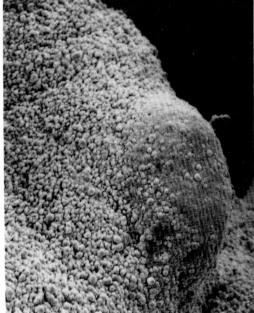

FIGURE 6.9. A: Transmission electron micrograph of a vasculosyncytial membrane. Note the extremely thin syncytial lamella that extends over the fetal capillary (C), the former being characterized by only a few organelles and a reduced number of microvilli. ×4800. B: Scanning electron micrograph of a vasculosyncytial membrane comparable to that depicted in part A. It is viewed here from the intervillous space (black) at the villous surface. The protrusion of the villous surface caused by the underlying capillary is clearly visible. It is largely devoid of microvilli. ×3300. (*Source:* Schiebler & Kaufmann, 1981, with permission.)

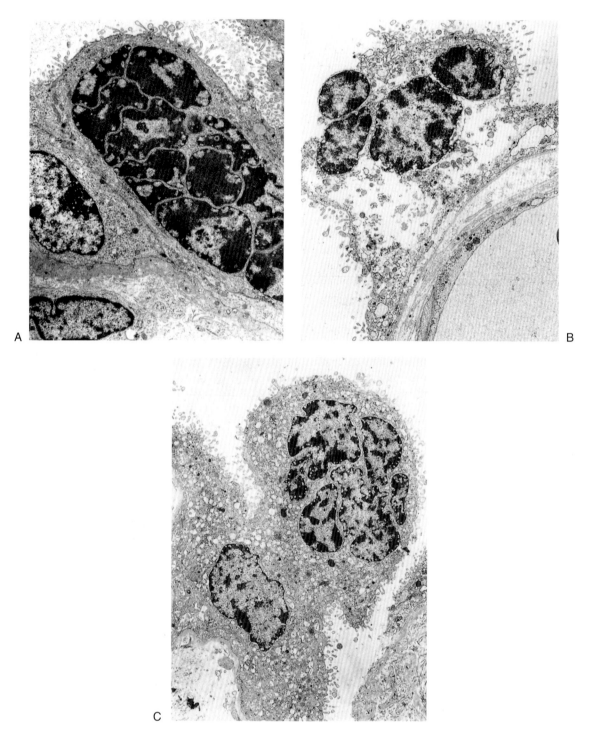

FIGURE 6.10. A: Transmission electron micrograph of a syncytial knot characterized by clustered nuclei that are rich in condensed chromatin, suggesting an apoptotic character. ×5000. (*Source:* Cantle et al., 1987, with permission.) B: Electron micrograph of a sprout-like structure that shows obvious signs of degeneration. The nuclei exhibiting condensed chromatin point to an earlier stage of apoptosis, whereas dissolution of plasmalemma and cytoplasm suggest necrotic events. This combination of two contrasting kinds of cellular death (secondary necrosis) can often be found in syncytiotrophoblast. ×5100. C: Transmission electron micrograph of a syncytial sprout from a mature placenta that, because of its appearance, is likely to represent a tangential section of the villous surface (see Chapter 15, Figs. 15.1 to 15.5). Most knots and sprouts observed in the mature placenta belong to this type of sectional artifact and should be called syncytial knotting or Tenney-Parker-changes. ×4600. (*Source:* Schiebler & Kaufmann, 1981, with permission.)

Syncytial Lamellae Covering Langhans' Cells

The syncytial lamellae covering Langhans' cells are comparable to the vasculosyncytial membranes in structure and thickness. In most cases, they are direct continuations of the vasculosyncytial membranes, as the thin syncytial lamellae of the latter extend from the bulging capillaries to the neighboring bulging Langhans' cells (Figs. 6.4 and 6.8). They are normally characterized by increased numbers of dense bodies (lysosomes? secretory granules?) found in both the syncytiotrophoblast and the underlying cytotrophoblast. Histochemically, they often show an intense reaction for 17β-hydroxysteroid dehydrogenase (Fig. 6.4B) (Kaufmann & Stark, 1973; Kaufmann et al., 1974b).

Function: These zones start developing at about the 15th week postmenstruation (p.m.), in parallel to the development of vasculosyncytial membranes and fetal sinusoids. It may be helpful for the functional interpretation that from the same date onward also the maternal plasma concentrations of 17β-hydroxysteroid dehydrogenase and the maternal urinary estriol excretion increase (see Kaufmann & Stark, 1973).

Syncytial Knots, Sprouts, and Bridges

Syncytial knots, sprouts, and bridges are a very heterogeneous group of syncytiotrophoblastic specializations, all of which have remarkable accumulations of nuclei in common (Hamilton & Boyd, 1966; Boyd & Hamilton, 1970) (see Chapter 15). Since their number increases in many pathologic placentas, they have raised much interest and caused much speculation. The interpretation comprises local hyperplasia of the syncytium (Baker et al., 1944); the results of trophoblastic degeneration (Tenney & Parker, 1940; Merrill, 1963); structural expression of placental insufficiency (Becker & Bleyl, 1961; Kubli & Budliger, 1963; Werner & Bender, 1977); structural expression of ischemia, hypoxia, or hypertension (Wilkin, 1965; Tominaga & Page, 1966; Alvarez, 1970; Alvarez et al., 1972; Gerl et al., 1973); and the results of fetal malperfusion of placental villi (Fox, 1965; Myers & Fujikura, 1968).

Studies by Küstermann (1981), Burton (1986a,b), Cantle et al. (1987), and Kaufmann et al. (1987a) have provided evidence that

- the vast majority of these structures are in fact results of tangential sectioning of the villous surfaces (→ **syncytial knots**, **syncytial buds**, and most **syncytial bridges**).
- There is, however, a limited amount of true syncytiotrophoblastic outgrowth, representing the first steps of villous sprouting (→ **syncytial sprouts**).
- Other true aggregations of syncytial nuclei represent sites of extrusion of aged, dying nuclei (→ **apoptotic knots**).

Syncytial knots are characterized by a multilayered group of aggregated nuclei that bulge only slightly on the trophoblastic surface. If they exhibit the same structural and histochemical features as the surrounding syncytiotrophoblast, they are likely to be only representations of tangential sections (syncytial knotting, Tenney-Parker changes; see Chapter 15). The vast majority of nuclear aggregates within the placenta are such syncytial knots.

Boyd and Hamilton (1970) have described islands of multinuclear syncytiotrophoblast located in the villous stroma and referred to them as **syncytial buds** or "stromal trophoblastic buds." It is very likely that these also are tangential sections of indenting villous surfaces or places of villous branching (Küstermann, 1981). Therefore, the old question whether these trophoblastic elements may "invade" fetal vessels (Salvaggio et al., 1960; Boyd & Hamilton, 1970) is no longer relevant.

There has been intense discussion concerning **syncytial bridges**, which began with their first description by Langhans (1870) and continued with reports by Stieve (1936, 1941), Ortmann (1941), Peter (1943, 1951), Hörmann (1953), Schiebler and Kaufmann (1969), Boyd and Hamilton (1970), Kaufmann and Stegner (1972), and Jones and Fox (1977). Most are sectional artifacts that must be interpreted as the results of tangential sectioning of villous branchings (see Chapter 15, Figs. 15.1 to 15.6) (Küstermann, 1981; Burton, 1986a; Cantle et al., 1987). Placentas with tortuously malformed villi, such as those in maternal anemia or severe preeclampsia, may exhibit so many bridges in histologic sections that a net-like appearance is achieved (see Figs. 15.15 and 15.16). In light of these findings, one may argue that reports on villi, arranged as a three-dimensional network (Stieve, 1941; Schiebler & Kaufmann, 1981) have been three-dimensional misinterpretations of tangential sections of tortuous villi. The famous diagram of the human placenta with villi in a net-like arrangement by Stieve (1941) was refuted by Peter (1951), based on reconstructions of wax plates.

Only the studies of Burton (1986a,b, 1987) and Cantle et al. (1987) made clear that there are real bridges in addition to those of artifactual genesis (Fig. 6.11). Hörmann (1953), Kaufmann and Stegner (1972), Jones and Fox (1977), and Cantle et al. (1987) presented evidence that real bridges are the result of fusion of adjacent villous surfaces that occur as soon as these come into prolonged intimate contact. Intermediate stages can be found as soon as slender intercellular gaps are formed between neighboring villous surfaces and become bridged by desmosomes. Later, the separating membranes disintegrate, causing the formation of a real syncytial bridge. Using radioangiographic and morphologic methods, vascularization of such bridges has been observed resulting in fetal intervillous vascular connections (Peter, 1951; Lemtis, 1955; Boyd & Hamilton, 1970). Unlike Stieve

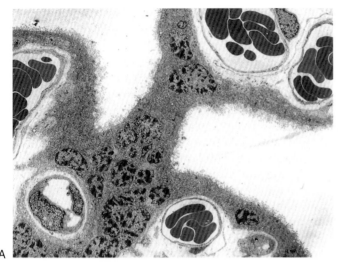
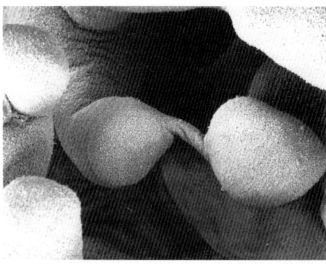

A   B

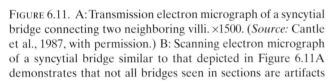

FIGURE 6.11. A: Transmission electron micrograph of a syncytial bridge connecting two neighboring villi. ×1500. (*Source:* Cantle et al., 1987, with permission.) B: Scanning electron micrograph of a syncytial bridge similar to that depicted in Figure 6.11A demonstrates that not all bridges seen in sections are artifacts and caused by tangential sectioning. Such real bridges are probably caused by local contacts of neighboring villous surfaces with subsequent syncytial fusion. ×890. (*Source:* Cantle et al., 1987, with permission.)

(1941), who postulated a net-like fetal vascular system that connects all villi, the authors cited provided evidence that such connections are rare exceptions. Whether the syncytial bridges have any mechanically supporting effects on the villous tree or are accidental structures without significance is a matter of speculation.

Apoptotic knots are structurally similar, but are characterized by more densely packed nuclei, separated from each other by slender strands of cytoplasm that is devoid of most organelles. The small nuclei show a more or less condensed chromatin (Fig. 6.10A) (Martin & Spicer, 1973b; Jones & Fox, 1977; Schiebler & Kaufmann, 1981) and sometimes even evidence of apoptotic or aponecrotic nuclear changes (Huppertz et al., 1998, 2002) (see following discussion on Trophoblast Differentiation and Apoptosis Cascade). The surrounding cytoplasm usually exhibits degenerative changes.

Martin and Spicer (1973b) as well as Dorgan and Schultz (1971) demonstrated that the life span of syncytiotrophoblast is limited (see Quantitation of Trophoblast Turnover, below, for calculations of syncytial life span). Thus, the presence of local degenerative changes caused by normal aging must be expected. Based on such views, Martin and Spicer (1973b), Jones and Fox (1977), Schiebler and Kaufmann (1981), and Cantle et al. (1987) described syncytial nuclear accumulations as sites where

aged syncytial nuclei are accumulated and later pinched off together with some surrounding cytoplasm (Fig. 6.10; se also Fig. 6.18). Huppertz et al. (1998) provided evidence that the nuclei of such sprouts represent various stages of apoptosis, thus suggesting that trophoblastic "sprouting" in fact is the syncytiotrophoblastic correlate of the formation of apoptotic bodies. We suggest the term **apoptotic knotting** (see Trophoblast Differentiation and Apoptosis Cascade).

Iklé (1961, 1964), Wagner et al. (1964), and Wagner (1968) found such segregated parts of the syncytiotrophoblast in the maternal uterine venous blood. According to Iklé's calculations in pregnancy weeks 6 and 20, about 150,000 such sprouts per day were shed into the maternal circulation. Syncytiotrophoblast fragments are nearly exclusively found in uterine venous blood, rather than in other peripheral veins (Wagner et al., 1964). This finding suggests that most of these deported sprouts are eliminated by phagocytosis in the lung; however, to our best knowledge this process has not yet been analyzed in detail. Excess shedding leading to pulmonary embolism has been reported by Schmorl (1893), Marcuse (1954), and Atwood and Park (1961).

Larger, mushroom-like aggregates of syncytial nuclei are historically called **syncytial sprouts** (Figs. 6.10B and 6.12) (Langhans, 1870; Boyd & Hamilton, 1970). In the past, this term has been applied for all mushroom-like or drumstick-shaped multinucleated syncytial protrusions. Meanwhile the term should no longer cover those structures, which are merely sectional artifacts caused by flat-sectioning of villous surfaces (Küstermann, 1981; Burton, 1986a; Cantle et al., 1987) (see the discussion of syncytial knots earlier in this section). Rather it should be restricted to those protrusions that represent true expressions of villous sprouting. They can be identified by large, ovoid, loosely arranged nuclei that possess little heterochromatin and never show signs of apoptosis. The nuclei are surrounded by ample free ribosomes and well-developed rough endoplasmic reticulum. During early pregnancy (Fig. 6.1; see Chapter 7, Fig. 7.12), true syncytial sprouts are regular findings. In term placentas, they are found only in small groups on the surfaces of immature intermediate and mesenchymal villi in the centers of the villous trees.

From studies of villous development (Castellucci et al., 1990c, 2000b) it has become evident that sprouts of this type are really an expression of villous sprouting. Their concentration in the centers of the villous trees is in agreement with Schuhmann's (1981) view that the centers are growth zones for the villous trees.

In conclusion, when observing accumulations of syncytial nuclei in sections of placental villi, three different types of genesis should be considered:

1. In all stages of pregnancy, and in particular in the third trimester placenta, nearly all syncytial bridges and buds as well as many knot-like and sprout-like structures are results of **flat sectioning across syncytiotrophoblastic surfaces**. We suggest the term **syncytial knotting** or **Tenney-Parker changes** (see Three-Dimensional Interpretation of Two-Dimensional Sections in Chapter 15).

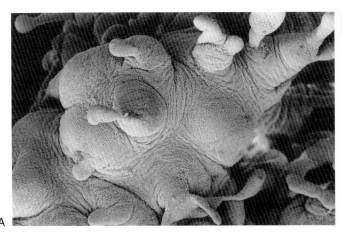
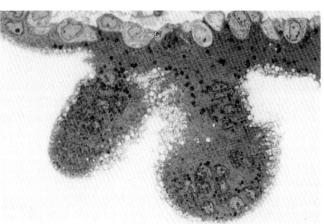

A   B

FIGURE 6.12. A: Scanning electron micrograph from the 8th week postmenstruation (p.m.) of gestation, showing local accumulations of mushroom-like true syncytial sprouts arising from broad villous protrusions. The latter probably represent the initial steps of the formation of new villi; they are common features in the early placenta but are rare at term. ×180. (*Source:* Cantle et al., 1987, with permission.) B: Semithin section from the 9th week of gestation, showing two true syncytial sprouts, comparable to those depicted in part A. Note the unevenly dispersed nuclei and compare with the aggregated and pyknotic nuclei of the apoptotic knots and Tenney-Parker changes depicted in Fig. 6.10. ×870. (*Source:* Cantle et al., 1987, with permission.)

2. In all stages of pregnancy, a minority of knot-like and sprout-like structures characterized by nuclei with highly condensed chromatin, partly showing typical apoptotic annular chromatin condensation, are sites of **shedding of apoptotic nuclei** into the maternal circulation. The term **apoptotic knotting** is recommended (see Trophoblastic Apoptosis, below, and Chapter 15).

3. Throughout the first half of pregnancy, a limited number of syncytial sprouts are early stages of real **trophoblastic sprouting**; these are characterized by loosely arranged, large ovoid syncytial nuclei. In later pregnancy they are extremely rare. Only for these structures do we suggest the term syncytial sprouting (cf. Development of Mesenchymal Villi in Chapter 7; see also Chapter 15).

Transtrophoblastic Channels

The syncytiotrophoblast is thought to be an uninterrupted maternofetal barrier composed of two plasmalemmas with an intermediate layer of syncytial cytoplasm. Therefore, every substance passing the syncytiotrophoblast from the maternal to the fetal circulation was thought to do so under the control of this syncytiotrophoblast layer. The existence of pericellular pathways is still unacceptable to many placentologists. Exchange of respective data during a 1986 workshop on transtrophoblastic channels, held at the second meeting of the European Placenta Group in Rolduc/Aachen, caused considerable controversy lasting until today.

Transport experiments by Stulc et al. (1969) provided the first evidence for the existence of water-filled routes, so-called pores or channels, across the rabbit placenta. Their radius was calculated to be approximately 10 nm. This finding has been confirmed for the guinea pig placenta by Thornburg and Faber (1977) and by Hedley and Bradbury (1980).

However, it took several years to find the structural correlates. Application of lanthanum hydroxide as an extracellular tracer via the maternal or fetal circulation resulted in the demonstration of membrane-lined channels in the isolated guinea pig placenta (Kaufmann et al., 1987b, 1989), in the postpartally perfused human placenta (Kertschanska & Kaufmann, 1992; Kertschanska et al., 1994, 1997), and in the rat placenta (Kertschanska et al., 2000). These channels have a luminal diameter from 15 to 25 nm and extend as winding, branching structures from the apical or basal surface into the syncytiotrophoblast. Because of their winding structure, they have never been traced in full length across the trophoblast. The release of the tracer into the maternal circulation, when applied via the fetal circulation and vice versa, makes it likely that at least some of these channels pass the syncytiotrophoblast in full length.

Function: The functional meaning of the transtrophoblastic channels has been elucidated by further experiments. In the fully isolated, artificially perfused guinea pig placenta, hydrostatic and colloid osmotic forces cause fetomaternal fluid shifts (Schröder et al., 1982). Fetal venous pressure elevation of 5 to 17 mm Hg was enough to shift 30% to 50% of the arterial perfusion volumes into the maternal circulation. We detected, ultrastructurally, initially slender and later bag-like dilated channels that passed the syncytiotrophoblast in full length, as routes for the fluid shift (Kaufmann et al., 1982). As soon as the fetal venous pressure was reduced to normal values, the fluid shift ceased and the bag-like channels disappeared. These experiments have been successfully repeated in the isolated human placental lobule (Kertschanska & Kaufmann 1992; Kertschanska et al., 1997). The reversibility of the events refuted the possibility that the channels were of traumatic origin. The only possible explanation is the existence of channels that can be dilated under condition of pressure increase. It is likely that the channels traced with lanthanum hydroxide are identical to those dilated experimentally under the conditions of fluid shift and those postulated in transfer experiments by the physiologists mentioned (for review, see Stulc, 1989). Similar basal invaginations or intrasyncytial vacuoles such as those found under the experimental conditions of fluid shift are sometimes observed in freshly delivered human placentas. It is still open to question if this phenomenon is an expression of active fetomaternal fluid shift during labor.

Functionally, the transtrophoblastic channels are possible sites of transfer for water-soluble, lipid-insoluble molecules with an effective molecular diameter of about 1.5 nm (Thornburg & Faber, 1977; Stulc, 1989). Under the conditions of fetomaternal fluid shift caused by fetal venous pressure increase or fetal decrease of osmotic pressure, they may dilate to such an extent that all molecules, independent of size and solubility, may pass (Kaufmann et al., 1982; Schröder et al., 1982; Kertschanska & Kaufmann, 1992; Kertschanska et al., 1994, 1997).

Another functional aspect may be important. The embryo and fetus have problems of eliminating surplus water. Simple renal filtration with subsequent urination does not necessarily solve this problem, as the urine is delivered into the amnionic fluid and is still inside the fetoplacental unit. On the other hand, excessive fetal hydration causes an increase of fetal venous pressure and a decrease of fetal osmotic pressure. Both factors have been experimentally proved to dilate channels, allowing fetomaternal fluid shift and equilibration of the surplus water. Thus, pressure-dependent dilatation and closure of the channels may act as an important factor in fetal osmoregulation and water balance.

TROPHOBLASTIC BLEBBING

When studying the syncytiotrophoblastic surface of human placental villi by electron microscopy, many authors have reported the existence of fungiform, membrane-lined protrusions of the apical syncytioplasm. These are largely or completely devoid of organelles. Their diameter normally ranges from 2 μm to about 15 μm (Ikawa, 1959; Hashimoto et al., 1960a,b; Arnold et al., 1961; Geller, 1962; Rhodin & Terzakis, 1962; Lister, 1964; Nagy et al., 1965; Strauss et al., 1965; Herbst et al., 1968, 1969; Knoth, 1968; Kaufmann, 1969). Numerous studies have shown that these protrusions are not a specific feature of syncytiotrophoblast but, rather, common features of most epithelia and sometimes of other cellular types (for review, see Kaufmann, 1975a). They are produced under degenerative conditions (Kaufmann, 1969; Stark & Kaufmann, 1971, 1972) and are likely to correspond to "blebs" observed during apoptotic processes (for review, see Kerr et al., 1995). Blockage of glycolysis by several enzyme inhibitors results in increased development of blebs; experimental substitution of glycolysis below the point of blockage results in suppression of their formation (Kaufmann et al., 1974a; Thorn et al., 1974). Hypoxia or experimental blockage of oxidative phosphorylation does not induce their production (Thorn et al., 1976).

After the protrusions have reached a certain size, they are pinched off into the maternal circulation. The only pathologic importance attributed to the blebs is related to placental infarction. Pronounced production of plasma protrusions in the guinea pig placenta was induced by experimental blockage of glycolysis, which led to obstruction of the maternal placental blood spaces by massive blebbing (Kaufmann, 1975b). The disintegration of the blebs induced blood clotting. The result was experimental infarction. Similar events have been described for the human placenta (Stark & Kaufmann, 1974). Assuming that this experimentally induced trophoblastic blebbing also is related to apoptotic events. The underlying molecular mechanism of blood clotting may be a phosphatidylserine flip in the respective plasmalemma from the inner to the outer leaflet. Externalization of phosphatidylserine was shown to be an early apoptotic event that initiates the coagulation cascade (see Molecular Mechanisms of Syncytial Fusion, below).

Villous Cytotrophoblast (Langhans' Cells)

The villous cytotrophoblast forms a second trophoblastic layer beneath the syncytiotrophoblast. During early pregnancy, this layer is nearly complete (Fig. 6.13) and later becomes discontinuous (see Figs. 6.10A and 6.23A and Chapter 28, Table 28.3). In contrast to earlier reports that described the villous cytotrophoblast to be absent from the mature placenta (Hörmann, 1948; Clavero-Nunez & Botella-Llusia, 1961), it is now well established that the Langhans' cells persist until term. In the mature placenta, they can be found beneath 20% of the villous syncytiotrophoblast (see Chapter 7, Fig. 7.11); the exact figure depends on the villous type, the kind of tissue preservation, and the pathologic state of the organ (see Table 28.6).

One should not deduce from these figures that the number of Langhans' cells is decreasing toward term. When one multiplies the relative numbers (percentages) of Langhans' cells per volume of villous tissue (Table 28.6) with the villous weights (g) per placenta (Table 28.2) during the 12th week p.m. and compares them to the term placenta, one arrives at surprising results. The total amount of Langhans' cells in the 12th week p.m. is about 2 g, as opposed to 12 g at term. In addition, stereologic studies have shown that the absolute number of cells increases steadily until term (Simpson et al., 1992). The real situation is that as the villous surface rapidly expands, the cytotrophoblast cells become widely

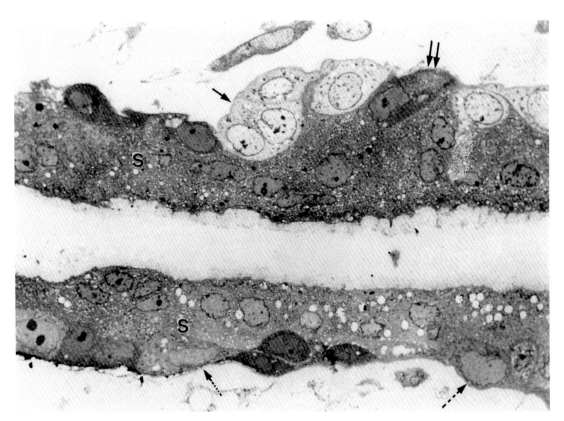

FIGURE 6.13. Semithin section showing two opposing villous surfaces, from the 9th gestational week p.m. Underneath the thick syncytiotrophoblast (S) are nearly complete layers of cytotrophoblast. Its varying staining intensities indicate different stages of differentiation from undifferentiated, proliferating cytotrophoblast (arrow) to highly differentiated cytotrophoblast with signs of syncytial fusion (interrupted arrows). Some of the cytotrophoblastic cells are obviously degenerating (double arrow). ×1270. (*Source:* Kaufmann, 1972, with permission.)

separated and thus less numerous in sectioned material. This change has important consequences for maternofetal immunoglobulin transfer, because unlike the syncytiotrophoblast and endothelial cells, cytotrophoblast cells do not express Fc-γ receptors (Bright & Ockleford, 1993). Transport of immunoglobulins, therefore, may become possible only in later pregnancy when the cytotrophoblastic layer becomes incomplete.

Earlier authors (Spanner, 1941; Stieve, 1941) considered a syncytiotrophoblastic origin of the Langhans' cells. Ortmann refuted this as early as 1942. He pointed out that formation of a syncytium must be regarded as differentiation from cellular precursors, and as an irreversible process. Richart (1961) presented the first proof for this assumption using ³H-thymidine incorporation to demonstrate the absence of DNA synthesis from syncytiotrophoblastic nuclei while it was, however, present in cytotrophoblastic nuclei. Galton (1962), who simultaneously carried out microspectrophotometric DNA measurements of trophoblastic nuclei, supported these data. The cytotrophoblastic contribution to the formation of syncytiotrophoblast has been generally accepted since the detailed ultrastructural evaluation of human placental villi from early pregnancy until full term also structurally demonstrated this process (Boyd & Hamilton, 1966). Hörmann et al. (1969) reviewed the vast literature of subsequent studies in much detail; the early autoradiographic findings were supported and extended by many authors (Pierce & Midgley, 1963; Fox, 1970; Weinberg et al., 1970; Kim & Benirschke, 1971; Geier et al., 1975; Kaufmann et al., 1983). The authors found that ³H-thymidine is incorporated only into the cytotrophoblastic nuclei, never into those of syncytiotrophoblast (see Fig. 6.20A). This fact excludes nuclear replication within the syncytiotrophoblast. Moe (1971), who described mitoses of syncytiotrophoblastic nuclei following in vitro

application of colchicine, has published the only conflicting results. Because no one ever has reproduced these results, they must be regarded as misinterpretation.

Cytotrophoblast Cell Types

During all stages of pregnancy, most of the Langhans' cells possess light microscopic and ultrastructural features that clearly distinguish them from overlying syncytiotrophoblast, the characteristic features of **undifferentiated, proliferating stem cells** (Fig. 6.14). Studies on cyclin D3-expression (DeLoia et al., 1997) suggest that about 50% of these cells are in the cell cycle. Occasional mitoses, ³H-thymidine incorporation, and Ki-67/MIB-1 positivity demonstrate that these are proliferating stem cells (Tedde & Tedde-Piras, 1978; Arnholdt et al., 1991; Kohnen et al., 1993; Kosanke et al., 1998). Another about 40% of cells displays the same undifferentiated phenotype but is immunonegative for cyclin D3. This subset very likely represents G_0-cells.

The cells display an ultrastructurally undifferentiated phenotype with a large euchromatic nucleus and few cell organelles (Kaufmann, 1972; Martin and Spicer, 1973b) (Fig. 6.13). The cytoplasm contains a well-developed Golgi field, few mitochondria, few dilated rough endoplasmic cisternae, and numerous polyribosomes (Figs. 6.14 and 6.15A) (Schiebler & Kaufmann, 1969; Kaufmann, 1972; Martin & Spicer, 1973b). Histochemically, enzymes

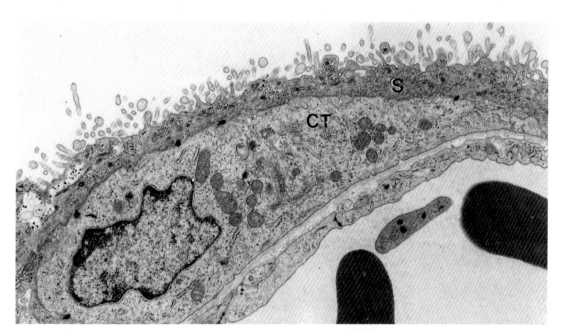

FIGURE 6.14. Transmission electron micrograph of mature placenta shows an undifferentiated cytotrophoblastic cell (CT) lying underneath a thin syncytiotrophoblastic lamella (S). During all stages of pregnancy, most of the villous cytotrophoblast belongs to this type of proliferating or resting stem cell. ×9800. (*Source:* Schiebler & Kaufmann, 1981, with permission.)

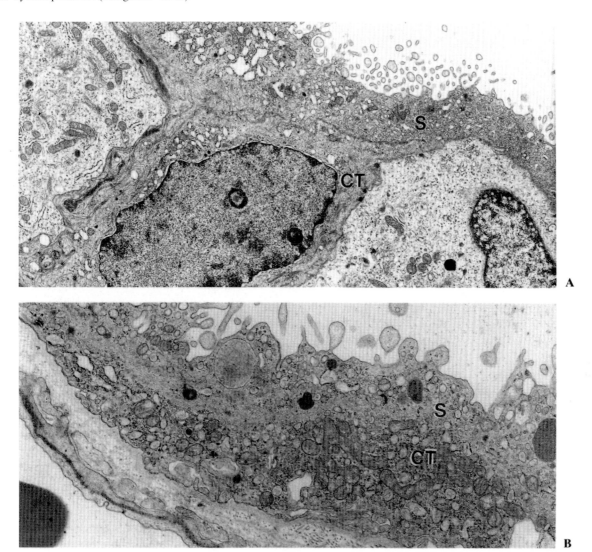

FIGURE 6.15. A: Transmission electron micrograph of mature placenta shows highly differentiated Langhans' cell (CT), shortly before its syncytial fusion with the neighboring syncytiotrophoblast (S). Note the ultrastructural similarity of the two. ×7400. B: Even after syncytial fusion with complete disappearance of the separating cell membranes, the area of the original cytotrophoblast (CT) can be clearly distinguished from the overlying syncytium (S) because of the marked difference in density of cell organelles. Note the accumulation of mitochondria and endoplasmic reticulum transferred into the syncytium by this kind of organellar transplantation into the syncytium. ×14,700.

of the aerobic and anaerobic glycolysis revealed only low activities (see Fig. 6.22) (Kaufmann & Stark, 1972; Kaufmann et al., 1974b).

A few Langhans' cells show **higher degrees of differentiation**, expressed by large amounts of free ribosomes, rough endoplasmic reticulum, and mitochondria (Fig. 6.15A). This finding has usually been interpreted as signs of differentiation toward a later syncytial state (Boyd & Hamilton, 1966; Hörmann et al., 1969; Schiebler & Kaufmann, 1969; Kaufmann, 1972). By light microscopy, these cells may show staining patterns similar to those of syncytiotrophoblast (Fig. 6.13). The enzymes of the

aerobic and anaerobic glycolysis (see Fig. 6.22A) express increasing activities.

As soon as the cytotrophoblast reaches an electron density that is comparable to that of the neighboring syncytium, the first signs of **syncytial fusion** may be observed (Boyd & Hamilton, 1966; Hörmann et al., 1969; Kemnitz, 1970; Kaufmann, 1972; Kaufmann et al., 1977a). Only in severely damaged areas of the villous trees are Langhans' cells observed with an organellar density exceeding that of the overlying syncytiotrophoblast (Figs. 6.16 and 6.17) (Kaufmann et al., 1977a). Syncytial fusion begins with the disintegration of separating cell membranes (Fig. 6.18).

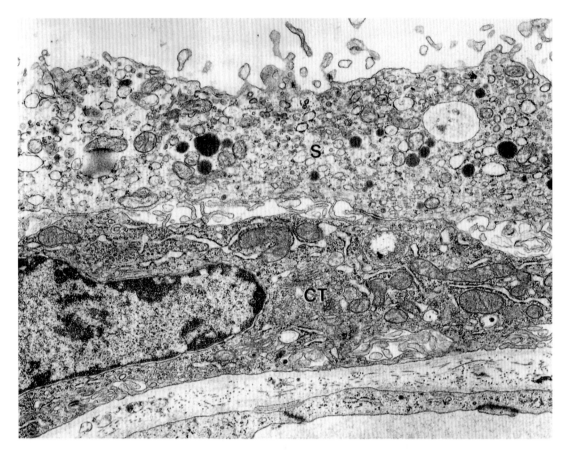

FIGURE 6.16. Transmission electron micrograph of mature placenta shows that the highly differentiated cytotrophoblast (CT) sometimes fails to fuse with the neighboring syncytiotrophoblast (S). Because it lacks regeneration, the latter shows obvious signs of degeneration, such as vesicular hydrops of most organelles, absence of ribosomes, and disintegration of the plasmalemma. Because of continuous differentiation, the nonfusing cytotrophoblast has an unusually large accumulation of organelles. Similar pictures can be seen in extravillous cytotrophoblast, which also lacks syncytial fusion. ×16,800.

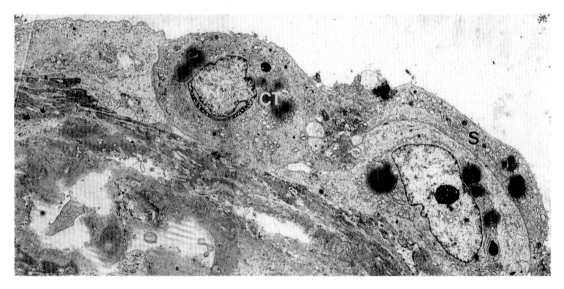

FIGURE 6.17. Survey transmission electron micrograph showing a villus in preeclampsia. If the cytotrophoblast (CT) fails definitely to fuse syncytially, the syncytiotrophoblast (S) degenerates, as demonstrated in Figure 6.16. As a final stage, the syncytiotrophoblast may locally disappear so that hypertrophic cellular trophoblast makes up the villous surface and directly borders the intervillous space (above). In this case, the villous stroma (below) also exhibits severe degenerative changes. ×2800.

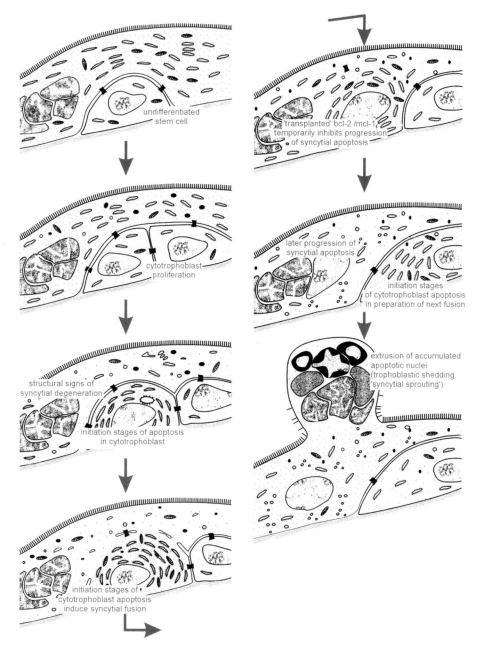

FIGURE 6.18. Cytotrophoblastic contribution to the regeneration of the villous syncytiotrophoblast. As soon as the syncytiotrophoblast shows its first signs of degeneration (loss of ribosomes—blue; degranulation of rough endoplasmic reticulum—blue), the cytotrophoblast begins to proliferate. Some of the daughter cells start differentiation and develop large numbers of organelles. At the same time the initiation stages of apoptosis are started in the cytotrophoblast and the phosphatidylserine flip takes place, which induces syncytial fusion. After disintegration of the separating membranes, the newly formed cytotrophoblast organelles together with high amounts RNA and proteins are transferred into the syncytium and thus regenerate the latter. Apoptosis inhibitors (Bcl-2, Mcl-1) expressed in the cytotrophoblast and transferred into the syncytiotrophoblast by syncytial fusion, temporarily block progression of the apoptosis cascade. The freshly incorporated nucleus can easily be identified for a certain period because of its size and low quantity of heterochromatin. As soon as the syncytial organelles degenerate again, this process starts anew. In this way, large numbers of trophoblastic nuclei accumulate in the syncytiotrophoblast. They are clustered as syncytial knots, protrude as sprout-like structures, and finally are pinched off into the intervillous space. (*Source:* Modified from Kaufmann, 1983, with permission.)

Contractor et al. (1977) have studied this process in detail in the human and Firth et al. (1980) in the guinea pig. The fusion seems to be initiated by establishment of gap junctions that bridge the intercellular space. Connexin 43 is under discussion as the responsible gap junction molecule in the human (Malassine et al., 2003). In vitro data suggest that hCG plays a major role in the stimulation of gap junction communication during human trophoblast fusion and differentiation (Cronier et al., 1997). It is proposed that the major role of the gap junctions is to bring the adjacent plasma membranes into close contact to become the starting points for cell fusion. Experimental studies in pseudopregnant rabbits have shown that the formation of a uterine epithelial syncytium, characteristic for implantation in this species, is also introduced by formation of gap junctions; they establish intercellular coupling and finally induce dissolution of the membranes (Winterhager, 1985). As a second step, plasma bridges between syncytium and cytotrophoblast are formed. From the gap junctions, this process spreads over the contact surface between Langhans' cell and syncytiotrophoblast. According to Contractor (1969) and Contractor et al. (1977), increased numbers of secondary lysosomes are actively involved in disintegration of the plasma membranes.

Freshly fused syncytiotrophoblast can easily be identified by electron microscopy, enzyme histochemistry, and immunohistochemistry (Figs. 6.15B and 6.18; also see Fig. 6.22B). They are characterized by a compact area of accumulated mitochondria, rough endoplasmic reticulum, and free ribosomes. These structures surround a large, ovoid nucleus rich in euchromatin. Such nuclei still may show immunoreactivity for proliferating-cell nuclear antigen (PCNA), a protein related to DNA polymerase δ and usually expressed in proliferating cells (Kohnen et al., 1993); the molecule has a half-life of about 24 hours and may thus persist from the last mitosis, via syncytial fusion, to the syncytial state. Its presence in syncytiotrophoblast must not be misinterpreted as a sign of proliferative activity of the latter.

In accordance with the ultrastructural appearance of freshly fused syncytiotrophoblast, maximal activities of all enzymes of aerobic and anaerobic glycolysis have been shown (Kaufmann & Stark, 1972). The density of organelles and the activities of enzymes considerably exceed that of the overlying syncytiotrophoblast. The density of organelles and enzyme activities decrease soon with spreading over the neighboring parts of the syncytium. Even then, the "new" syncytial area can easily be detected by the unusual size of its nucleus.

According to the results of Martin and Spicer (1973b), the nuclei are the most reliable indicators for the syncytial "age," which is the time elapsed since the syncytial fusion. Prevalence of small, densely stained, obviously pyknotic syncytial nuclei together with reduced numbers of Langhans' cells indicate degenerative changes of the syncytiotrophoblast because of reduced syncytial fusion.

In early stages of pregnancy, also degenerating villous trophoblast cells are regular findings. Between pregnancy weeks 6 and 15, Burton and coworkers (2003) found 0.49% Langhans' cells showing **secondary necrosis** (aponecrosis; abortive forms of apoptosis) and 5.97% Langhans' cells characterized by **primary necrosis**.

NEMATOSOMES

Nematosomes are spherical to ovoid, membrane-free organelles with a diameter of about 1 μm (Fig. 6.19). They consist of helically arranged central strands of filaments to which small electron-dense conglomerates are attached. The latter are thought to consist of storage forms of RNA (Grillo, 1970; Ockleford et al., 1987). Many authors have described nematosomes as regular features of undifferentiated Langhans' cells. They have also been found within other embryonic tissues and in neurons, but never in syncytiotrophoblast. The most detailed review of the relevant literature is that by Ockleford et al. (1987).

Regarding their potential role as RNA storage, studies of apoptosis in villous trophoblast may be of interest. It has been shown that apoptosis is already initiated in cytotrophoblast prior to fusion. Syncytiotrophoblast is already in an advanced stage of apoptosis (Huppertz et al., 1998). In apoptotic tissues transcription is gradually downregulated, and there is evidence that large amounts of RNA already transcribed in the cytotrophoblast are "transplanted" into the syncytium by syncytial fusion. Nematosomes may represent one of such storage forms. No evidence has thus far been found of any relationship between nematosomes and overt gestational pathology and between nematosomes and virus infections in the placenta (Ockleford et al., 1987).

Endocrine Activities of the Villous Cytotrophoblast

In addition to their role as trophoblastic stem cells, endocrine activities have been attributed to the cytotrophoblast. Repeatedly, it has been suggested that Langhans' cells are the source of hCG.

Two arguments have been stressed: the number of Langhans' cells and their proliferative activity seem to parallel the urinary and serum levels of hCG (Gey et al., 1938; Wislocki & Bennett, 1943; Tedde & Tedde-Piras, 1978); trophoblast cultures continue to produce hCG when only cytotrophoblast survives (Stewart et al., 1948). The first deduction is inconclusive, as only the relative rather than the absolute amount of villous cytotrophoblast is so impressive in early pregnancy. As discussed earlier, the absolute number of Langhans' cells increases steadily until term. Also, the second deduction is not convincing. Cytotrophoblast behaves differently under culture conditions; here it acquires stages of differentiation that are not reached in vivo (Nelson et al., 1986; Kao et al., 1988).

Midgley and Pierce (1962), Dreskin et al. (1970), Hamanaka et al. (1971), and Kim et al. (1971) described hCG immunoreactivities mainly within the villous syncytiotrophoblast. Outside the villi, in extravillous tissues where syncytial fusion is rare, extravillous trophoblast locally synthesizes this hormone (see Chapter 9). Gaspard et al. (1980) were the first to point out that α-hCG and β-hCG

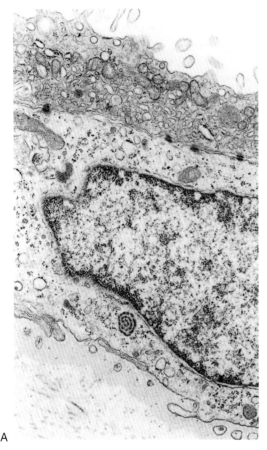

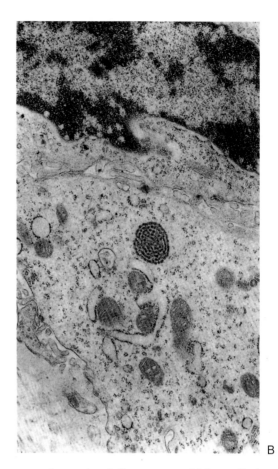

A   B

FIGURE 6.19. A,B: Transmission electron micrographs of undifferentiated villous cytotrophoblast in a human placenta at term. The cells show typical nematosomes consisting of helically arranged strands of filaments to which small electron-dense bodies are attached. The structures resemble coiled strings of beads. A: ×8400; B: ×20,500.

under certain conditions can be found also in the villous cytotrophoblast. The β-hCG subunit, however, was detected in cytotrophoblast only underlying heavily damaged syncytium.

Molecular studies by Hoshina et al. (1982, 1983, 1984) and Kliman et al. (1986, 1987) produced evidence that the ability to secrete hCG and hPL is related to the level of trophoblastic differentiation. Boime et al. (1988) proposed a model for hCG and hPL expression that associates subsequent activation of α-hCG, β-hCG, and hPL genes at different stages of differentiation. Under normal in-vivo conditions, α-hCG is expressed and secreted directly before fusion, β-hCG immediately following fusion, and hPL slightly later. Following discussion with the authors, we suggest, however, that this cascade of gene activation is not tied to the syncytial fusion itself but rather to the process of trophoblastic differentiation. Under normal in vivo conditions, syncytial fusion takes place at the time of α-hCG expression. In pathologic conditions (β-hCG expression by cytotrophoblast; reported by Gaspard et al., 1980), in tissue culture, and under normal conditions in extravillous cytotrophoblast, syncytial fusion but not the sequence of gene expressions may be delayed or completely inhibited.

Only a few reports have considered additional secretory activity of the villous cytotrophoblast. Nishihira and Yagihashi (1978, 1979) reported the production of **somatostatin** in Langhans' cells. Somatostatin is an inhibitor of adenohypophyseal hormones, such as growth hormone and thyroid-stimulating hormone (TSH). These authors discussed a suppressive role of somatostatin on hCG and hPL production by the syncytiotrophoblast.

Other peptides with alleged origin in the villous cytotrophoblast are **corticotropin-releasing factor (CRF)** (Petraglia et al.,1987;Saijonmaa et al.,1988), **gonadotropin-releasing hormone** [GnRH, placental luteinizing hormone releasing factor (LRF)] (Khodr & Siler-Khodr, 1978), neuropeptide Y (NPY) (Petraglia et al., 1989), and inhibin (Petraglia et al., 1987). Reevaluation of the latter two papers (Petraglia et al., 1987, 1989) and repetition of the experiments in cooperation with the author revealed, however, that inhibin and NPY immunoreactivities were clearly localized in the villous capillary walls, and only certain inhibin subunits were found in the trophoblast, too. Korhonen and coworkers (1991) arrived at similar conclusions. In later publications, Petraglia et al. (1991, 1992) have specified their findings for the various inhibin subunits. Regulatory effects of inhibin on the hCG secretion are discussed by Petraglia et al. (1987, 1990) and by Petraglia (1991).

Trophoblast Turnover and Syncytial Fusion

As already discussed above, syncytiotrophoblast lacks ^{3}H-thymidine incorporation and consequently nuclear replication (Richart, 1961; Galton, 1962; Pierce & Midgley, 1963; Fox, 1970; Weinberg et al., 1970; Kim & Benirschke, 1971; Geier et al., 1975; Kaufmann et al., 1983; Huppertz et al., 1999). Therefore, syncytiotrophoblast cannot grow by itself. Rather, syncytial growth and surface expansion throughout pregnancy depend on continuous incorporation of cytotrophoblast by syncytial fusion. As we will show below, syncytial fusion does not only fulfill the syncytiotrophoblastic needs for growth, but rather has additional functional importance.

Quantitation of Trophoblast Turnover

This becomes evident when one compares for an average near-term placenta (1) the number of proliferating trophoblast cells (Kosanke et al., 1998) with (2) the weight gain of syncytiotrophoblast in the respective period (see Tables 28.2 and 28.3). It must be pointed out that the following calculations are partly based on very rough assumptions. The resulting data should be used as very preliminary clues only:

- In the last month of pregnancy, placental villi are covered with a mean of 90g of trophoblast, 77.5g of which are syncytiotrophoblast and 12.5g cytotrophoblast.
- Assuming a mean volume for a villous trophoblast cell to be $1400\,\mu m^3$, 12.5g of cytotrophoblast correspond to 9×10^9 villous trophoblast cells.
- The trophoblastic surface per placenta at term amounts to about $12\,m^2$ (see Table 28.5), and per $10,000\,\mu m^2$ of surface, 70 trophoblast mitoses take place within 4 weeks (Kosanke et al., 1998). From this, we calculate 3×10^9 villous trophoblast mitoses per day and per placenta.
- A low percentage of postmitotic trophoblast cells may degenerate (assumption, 15–20%). We furthermore suppose that the absolute number of villous trophoblast cells is kept largely constant throughout the last trimester (Table 28.3). It follows that about 2.5×10^9 of the trophoblast cells produced daily by mitosis, subsequently will fuse syncytially; this corresponds to a daily generation rate of 3.5g of new syncytiotrophoblast.
- The weight gain of villous syncytiotrophoblast in the last month of pregnancy is 10 to 11g. That equals a daily rate of syncytiotrophoblast growth of about 0.4g.
- Accordingly, only 0.4g of the daily generated 3.5g of syncytiotrophoblast are required to cover the daily expansion of the syncytial surface.
- The remaining about 3.1g, which are generated in excess of the daily growth rate, are shed again as syncytial knots into the maternal circulation. This figure nicely fits to data presented by Iklé (1964); he found a daily shedding rate of about 150,000 "sprouts" (apoptotic knots). Assuming nearly round structures with a mean diameter of 15 to 20μm, this equals 1.5 to 3.5g.
- We know from the structural features described above, that not freshly included nuclei but rather the oldest nuclei are shed as syncytial knots. Based on a total of 77.5g of syncytiotrophoblast at term, a shedding rate of 3.1g/day suggests an average of 25 days between inclusion of a cytotrophoblast nucleus by syncytial fusion and its extrusion via a syncytial knot.
- Accordingly, syncytiotrophoblast generated once, does not live until the end of pregnancy. Rather, the cytotrophoblast is incorporated for a transient period of 25 days only, after which the aged remains of the cells (nuclei and some surrounding cytoplasm) are again extruded by syncytial knots into the maternal.

Why Does Syncytiotrophoblast Survival Depend on Syncytial Fusion?

The importance of syncytial fusion for survival of syncytiotrophoblast is stressed by several observations. The life span of syncytiotrophoblast in culture without syncytial incorporation of cytotrophoblast is limited. Assuming that isolated syncytiotrophoblast has already a mean age of 12.5 days, its complete structural disintegration should be in the same range of nearly 2 weeks. Its functional death happens much earlier: in vitro, syncytiotrophoblast without cytotrophoblastic fusion shows steeply decreasing hormonal production rates within some days and finally dies (Castellucci et al., 1990a; Crocker et al., 2004). Similarly, maximal villous cytotrophoblast proliferation without syncytial fusion, as observed in severe hypoxia in vitro, was accompanied by syncytial degeneration (Fox, 1970). From experimental studies in the rhesus monkey placenta (Panigel & Myers, 1972), it has become evident that loss of villous cytotrophoblast and degenerative changes of the syncytiotrophoblast are usually associated.

Downregulation of transcription following syncytial fusion very likely is the major reason for the limited life span of syncytiotrophoblast. To test this hypothesis, ^{3}H-uridine incorporation into villous trophoblast was studied. The resulting data resembled the results of ^{3}H-thymidine incorporation studies. This RNA precursor was mostly incorporated into the nuclei of cytotrophoblast and stromal cells (Fig. 6.20B) (Kaufmann, 1983; Kaufmann et al., 1983; Huppertz et al., 1999). Syncytiotrophoblast did not show ^{3}H-uridine incorporation levels detectable by autoradiography. Meanwhile, the lack of transcription in syncytiotrophoblast has also been proven specifically for some genes. These include the apoptosis inhibitor *bcl-2* (Huppertz et al., 2003), the protease caspase 8 (Black et al., 2004), and the anion transporter *OAT4* (Black et al., 2004). Downregulation of transcription is a widespread phenomenon after induction of apoptosis (Owens et al., 1991; Leist et al., 1994; Kockx et al., 1998). This does not necessarily imply lacking transcription of all proteins; rather transcription is focused on few genes that are essential for safe execution of apoptosis.

If this were true for the majority of genes in the syncytiotrophoblast, the latter regarding survival and functional activity would depend on continuous supply with cytotrophoblastic RNA through syncytial fusion of cytotrophoblast. In this case, not the rather low requirements of growth expansion of syncytiotrophoblast, but rather the much higher demands of RNA would define the rate of syncytial fusion. One may object that messenger RNA (mRNA) due to universally available ribonuclease (RNAse) has an extremely short half-life, which would not be in agreement with mRNA supply only by cellular fusion. On the other hand, the human placenta is the richest known source for the RNAse inhibitor (RNAsin) (Blackburn & Gavilanes, 1980), which blocks RNA cleavage and thus helps stabilizing mRNA. Moreover, the nematosomes characteristic for the human trophoblast and which are thought to consist of storage forms of RNA (Grillo, 1970; Ockleford et al., 1987) may present means for the preservation of RNA between syncytial fusion and utilization for translation within the syncytiotrophoblast.

In conclusion, it is not only the mass of trophoblast that is required for growth; rather, we suspect that fusion takes place to transfer "consumables" not synthesized in the syncytium itself (e.g., RNA), from the cytotrophoblast into the syncytiotrophoblast to maintain its functional capacity. Only with this continuous regeneration by fusion syncytiotrophoblast is kept functionally active.

Trophoblastic Differentiation and Apoptosis Cascade

Programmed cell death (apoptosis) as opposed to accidental cell death (necrosis) is characterized by typical ultrastructural signs such as annular chromatin condensa-

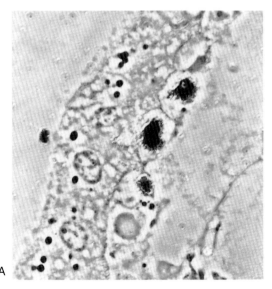

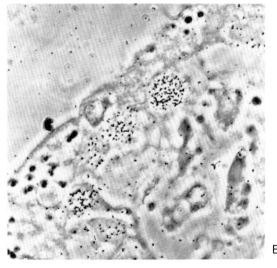

FIGURE 6.20. A: ^{3}H-thymidine incorporation into the villous trophoblast. The black silver grains indicate active DNA synthesis. They have accumulated only over the cytotrophoblastic nuclei (big black spots in the center). The syncytiotrophoblast shows no signs of DNA synthesis. ×1400. (Courtesy of Dr. W. Nagl.) B: ^{3}H-uridine incorporation into the villous trophoblast. Similar to ^{3}H-thymidine incorporation, ^{3}H-uridine, as a precursor of RNA, is mostly incorporated into the cytotrophoblast (fine black grains), indicating that RNA metabolism in the syncytiotrophoblast is downregulated by apoptotic events but fully active in the cellular trophoblast. ×1400. (Courtesy of Dr. W. Nagl.)

tion, loss of microvilli, cytoplasmic dehydration, and membrane blebbing, but preservation of organelle integrity (for review, see Kerr et al., 1995). These features have been observed since the early periods of electron microscopy also in villous syncytiotrophoblast; however, their interpretation and designation as apoptosis took place considerably later. This delay was partly because the term **programmed cell death (apoptosis)** seemed to be not applicable to a tissue, which represents an **acellular**, syncytial continuum.

With a delay of about 25 years, a series of studies of various aspects of apoptosis suggested that villous syncytiotrophoblast undergoes a closely related process of programmed death that involves most but not all the classic features of apoptosis. Aspects studied in the placenta comprise Fas and FasL expression (Runic et al., 1996; Bamberger et al., 1997; Uckan et al., 1997); expression of the tumor necrosis factor-α (TNF-α) receptors p55 and p75 (Yui et al., 1996); Bcl-2 expression (Castellucci et al., 1993c; LeBrun et al., 1993; Sakuragi et al., 1994; Kim et al., 1995; Lea et al., 1997; Marzioni et al., 1998); DNA degradation (TUNEL test) (Yasuda et al., 1995; S.C. Smith et al., 1997a; Kokawa et al., 1998); and annular chromatin condensation (Nelson, 1996).

In a series of studies, different stages of the apoptotic cascade were correlated with differentiation, syncytial fusion, and degeneration of villous trophoblast (Huppertz et al., 1998, 1999, 2001, 2002, 2003; Huppertz & Kaufmann, 1999; Black et al., 2004). In summary, the data suggested that apoptosis starts as early as in the cellular stage of trophoblast differentiation and subsequently is involved in a series of events (Fig. 6.18):

- The p55 receptor for TNF-α, a major inducer of apoptosis, is expressed by villous cytotrophoblast (Yui et al., 1994, 1996). Caspase-8, a so-called initiator caspase that starts the apoptosis cascade becomes activated already in the cellular stage of trophoblast (Huppertz et al., 1999). Moreover, inhibitor proteins (Bcl-2 and Mcl-1) as well as inactive proforms of some of the molecular machinery of later steps of the cascade (pro-caspase-3, inactive transglutaminase) are available in these cells (Huppertz et al., 1998).
- The start of these early stages of the apoptosis cascade seems to be responsible for trophoblast cells leaving the cell cycle and entering the differentiation pathway (for review, see Huppertz et al., 2001). In vitro data by McKenzie et al. (1998) revealed that interactions between (1) increased expression levels of the cyclin-dependent kinase (Cdk) inhibitor Kip1, (2) inactivation of Cdk2, (3) downregulation of cyclin E, and (4) accumulation of active (hypophosphorylated) retinoblastoma gene product (pRb) are responsible for blockage of the S phase of cytotrophoblast and the cells' entrance into the differentiation pathway. This happens only to a small percentage of cells. In a variety of other cells, it was shown that Bcl-2 induces the cells to enter a quiescent G_0/G_1 state and thereby reduces proliferation (Vairo et al., 1996; O'Reilly et al., 1997). Furthermore, Mazel et al. (1996) have shown that elevated levels of Bcl-2 lead to an increase of hypophosphorylated retinoblastoma gene product (pRb), which according to McKenzie et al. (1998) was responsible for blockage of the cell cycle.

- Moreover, the endogenous retroviral envelop protein ERV-3 Env is under discussion because it may commit trophoblast cells to cell cycle arrest (for details, see below) (Rote et al., 2004).
- In some of the cells, which had left the cell cycle and had reached higher levels of differentiation, the flip of phosphatidylserine (PS flip) from the inner to the outer plasmalemmal leaflet occurs (Huppertz et al., 1998). Different molecular steps lead to the PS flip: (1) the activation of initiator caspase-8; (2) the caspase-8-mediated activation of slow floppases or fast scramblases, both of which actively translocate negatively charged phosphatidylserine from the inner to the outer plasmalemmal leaflet; (3) the caspase-8-mediated inactivation of flippases (translocases), which normally would counteract outward flipping of PS from the inner to the outer plasmalemmal leaflet. The net effect of all three processes together is the accumulation of phosphatidylserine in the outer plasmalemmal leaflet (for review, see Huppertz et al., 2001). This PS flip seems to be a prerequisite for syncytial fusion of trophoblast cells (in vitro data by Lyden et al., 1993; Adler et al., 1995; Katsuragawa et al., 1997).
- Consequently, our data suggest that early, but still reversible, stages of apoptosis in highly differentiated trophoblast cells initiate syncytial fusion; parallel expression of the inhibitory proto-oncogene products Bcl-2 and Mcl-1 for 3 to 4 weeks prevents irreversible progression of the apoptotic cascade.
- Inhibition of the apoptosis starter caspase-8 in vitro blocked syncytial fusion and thus demonstrated the importance of these initiation stages of apoptosis for the fusion process.
- Following syncytial fusion, irreversible progression of apoptosis is blocked, so long as sufficient amounts of members of the Bcl-2 family of proteins (Bcl-2: Marzioni et al., 1998; Huppertz et al., 2003; Mcl-1: Huppertz et al., 1998) are present in the syncytiotrophoblast. The data moreover suggest that either the inhibitory protein itself or its mRNA is transferred from the cytotrophoblast into the syncytium by syncytial fusion (Huppertz et al., 2003).
- In apoptotic cells, transcription of mRNA is typically reduced; this was also shown for syncytiotrophoblast (Kaufmann et al., 1983). The RNA of the latter is likely to be transplanted from the cytotrophoblast by syncytial fusion, rather than being synthesized in the syncytium itself (Fig. 6.20B). The data imply that this is also valid for Bcl-2 and Mcl-1 mRNA (Huppertz et al. 2003).
- Consequently, prevention of irreversible apoptotic damage depends on syncytiotrophoblastic availability of inhibitory members of the Bcl-2 protein family; this in turn depends on syncytial fusion of trophoblast cells in regular, but still unknown, intervals.
- As long as fresh cytotrophoblast is incorporated into villous syncytiotrophoblast, syncytial apoptosis does not progress generally but rather only focally. These apoptotic foci in the syncytiotrophoblast are characterized by several features (Huppertz et al., 1998, 1999, 2002): focal loss of immunoreactivities for Bcl-2 and Mcl-1; PS flip; leakiness of the syncytial plasmalemma for propidium iodide; activation of caspase-3; degradation of nuclear proteins such as PARP (poly ADP-ribose polymerase) (involved in DNA repair), lamin B (an intrinsic nuclear pore protein), and topoisomerase IIa (involved in condensation of chromosomes); translocation of TIAR (T-cell restricted intracellular antigen-related protein) (involved in biogenesis and translation of mRNA) from the nucleus to the cytoplasm; activation of transglutaminase II beneath the apical plasmalemma where it prevents loss of proteins through the increasingly leaky membrane.
- The final steps of syncytiotrophoblastic apoptosis comprise DNA degradation with TUNEL positivity and annular chromatin condensation of the nuclei. In most cases, these features are restricted to nuclei in syncytial knots and sprouts, indicating that the apoptotically damaged nuclei are focally accumulated (Fig. 6.21) before shedding into the intervillous space (Yasuda et al., 1995; Nelson, 1996; Huppertz et al., 1998, 2002).

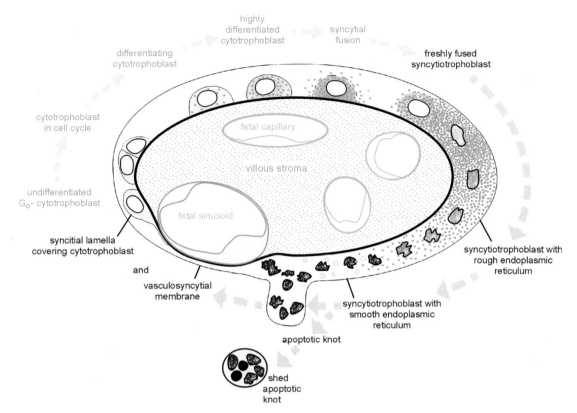

FIGURE 6.21. Schematic representation of trophoblast turnover and trophoblastic apoptosis at the villous surface. Cytotrophoblast nuclei surrounded by high concentrations of ribosomes (blue) are transferred into the syncytiotrophoblast by syncytial fusion. In the course of about 3 weeks the syncytially incorporated nuclei undergo apoptotic changes, accompanied by loss of RNA and degranulation of the surrounding cytoplasm (the density of blue point shading represents density of ribosomes). Finally, the nuclei are accumulated and extruded by apoptotic knotting and shedding. The remaining syncytiotrophoblast is void of nuclei and corresponds to the thin syncytial lamellae of vasculosyncytial membranes and to syncytial lamellae covering villous cytotrophoblast. New syncytial fusion of differentiating cytotrophoblast supplies the syncytiotrophoblast with fresh nuclei, new ribosomes and other organelles. These cyclic events at the villous surfaces are the basis of regional specializations of villous syncytiotrophoblast.

- Interestingly, most of the final steps of apoptosis with accumulation of apoptotic nuclei were observed at or close to villous tips, suggesting that flux of nuclei during the process of apoptosis is a unidirectional process from the villous base to its tip, comparable to that in intestinal villi.
- Since caspase-3 upon activation in the syncytiotrophoblast among others cleaves also cytoskeletal components such as cytokeratins (Huppertz et al., 1998, 2002; Kadyrov et al., 2001), the loss of cytoskeletal anchorage of nuclei may facilitate their movement along the villi and their accumulation at the villous tips. As force causing this unidirectional nuclear movement, one may discuss maternal blood flow in the surrounding intervillous space.
- We never found breakdown of nuclei with formation of typical apoptotic bodies in the syncytiotrophoblast. Rather, accumulated apoptotic and preapoptotic nuclei, surrounded by some cytoplasm and a plasmalemma, are shed as so-called syncytial knots or sprouts. We prefer the term **apoptotic knots**. It is assumed that these are further degraded in the lung (Iklé, 1964; Wagner et al., 1964), presumably by alveolar macrophages (Huppertz et al., 1998), a process that has not yet been studied. The role of this trophoblast deportation for the pathogenesis of preeclampsia is under discussion (Johansen et al., 1999; Huppertz et al., 2002).

Taken together, the above data suggest, that a prolonged form of apoptosis drives the stages of trophoblast differentiation and trophoblast turnover:

1. Initiation stages of apoptosis are responsible for the trophoblast cell's exit from the cell cycle and for its entrance into the differentiation pathway.

2. Activation of the apoptosis initiating caspase-8 induces the phosphatidylserine flip, which is a key signal for syncytial fusion.

3. Upon syncytial fusion, excess expression of apoptosis inhibitors blocks further progression of the apoptosis cascade for 3 to 4 weeks (mean 25 days, see above). Throughout this period, the syncytiotrophoblast fulfills its functions as maternofetal transport barrier and as metabolic center of the placenta.

4. Throughout these 4 weeks of retarded apoptosis so-called differentiation stages of syncytiotrophoblast are driven by apoptotic mechanisms that finally result in the

mosaic pattern of different types of syncytiotrophoblast (see above): Caspase-3 mediated degradation of the cytoskeleton enables nuclear accumulation producing (1) nuclear knots and (2) syncytial lamellae (e.g., vasculosyncytial membranes) void of nuclei. Apoptosis-related continuous loss of RNA leads to degranulation of rough endoplasmic reticulum to the benefit of smooth endoplasmic reticulum.

5. Finally, massive restart of the cascade with activation of endonucleases by caspase-3 induces DNA breakdown and nuclear condensation. This results in extrusion of about 3 g of apoptotic knots per day, consisting of apoptotic nuclei with some surrounding aged syncytioplasm well sealed in plasma membranes.

Molecular Mechanisms of Syncytial Fusion

There are two different types of syncytial fusion of human trophoblast (for review, see Pötgens et al., 2002):

- **Cell–cell fusion** is limited to the periimplantation period and involves trophoblast cells of the blastocyst. As soon as implantation is completed, trophoblast cells do not fuse any longer with each other.
- Rather, extension of the already existing syncytiotrophoblast from now onward takes place by **cell–syncytium fusion**.

One of the critical aspects of all studies on trophoblast fusion is that nearly all in situ studies describing the localization of the various molecules involved are performed on placental villi, and thus on cell-syncytial fusion. By contrast, in vivo models based on trophoblast cells or analogs study cell–cell fusion. Since cell–cell fusion is restricted to implantation and seems to be blocked in subsequent placentation, it is very unlikely that the molecular mechanisms of both events are identical (Pötgens et al., 2002). If this holds true, we also cannot be sure that data obtained on cell–cell fusion in vitro can easily be transferred to such obtained on cell–syncytium fusion in vivo. Several contradictions among the results of both approaches must possibly be explained in this way.

Phosphatidylserine Flip as Fusion Signal

Phosphatidylserine is well accepted as a key player in the syncytial fusion process (for review, see Huppertz et al., 2001). It normally prevails in the inner plasmalemmal leaflet. This asymmetry is maintained by flippases (translocases), which translocate spontaneously outward flipping PS molecules back to the inner leaflet. Accumulation of larger amounts of PS in the outer plasmalemma (PS flip) is the consequence either of degradation of these **flippases** by **caspase-8** or of caspase-8-mediated activation of slow **floppases** and fast **scramblases**, both of which actively translocate phosphatidylserine from the inner to the outer plasmalemma leaflets. Antibodies directed against externalized phosphatidylserine blocked trophoblast fusion in vitro (Adler et al., 1995; Katsuragawa et al., 1997; Rote et al., 1998). The same holds true for the prevention of the PS flip by inhibition of its enzymatic starter, caspase-8 (Black et al., 2004). Also immunohistochemically, the PS flip was shown in fusion-stages of trophoblast cells (Huppertz et al., 1998, 1999).

On the other hand, the PS flip is a ubiquitous phenomenon among apoptotic cells throughout the body (Martin et al., 1995; Bevers et al., 1996); however, most of these cells do not fuse syncytially. Rather, syncytium formation is a strictly regulated event, which in the human occurs only between cells of the same lineage (trophoblast cells, myoblasts, and osteoclasts). This suggests that not only the PS flip, but also additional tissue-specific cell surface signals are required for fusion. Their presence avoids heterofusion with cells of other lineages. Several such fusogenic membrane proteins are currently under discussion (see below). Most of them, however, are continuously expressed in those cells, which are destined to undergo fusion, also in phases of their lives in which they do not fuse. Consequently, a second acute fusion signal is required, which is activated as soon as the cell has reached a degree of differentiation sufficient for syncytial fusion. We suggest that the phosphatidylserine flip may serve as this acute fusion signal.

Junctional and Adhesion Molecules as Fusion Mediators

The formation of gap junctions was shown to precede syncytial fusion (Firth et al., 1980). Therefore, junctional molecules such as connexins are candidates as fusogenic molecules. Antisense inhibition of **connexin 43** expression in primary trophoblast cultures blocked syncytial fusion (Malassiné et al., 2003). The effect of this gap junction molecule is possibly to allow the exchange of cellular messenger molecules that regulate the molecular machinery leading to fusion since blockage of fusion was accompanied by reduced transcription of the syncytin gene, another fusogenic protein (see below).

In addition, the adhesion molecules **cadherin-11** and **E-cadherin** appear to play (opposing) roles in mediating trophoblast fusion (Getsios and MacCalman, 2003).

The ADAM Family of Fusogenic Proteins

A family of proteins called ADAM (**a d**isintegrin and **a m**etalloproteinase domain) is involved in many cell–cell fusion processes (for review, see Wolfsberg & White,

1996). ADAM 1 and 2 (fertilins α and β) were shown to be crucial for sperm–egg fusion in the mouse (Cho et al., 1997, 1998; Evans et al., 1998). The human fertilin gene, however, is dysfunctional so that fertilins are no candidate molecules for any type of cell–cell fusion in the human (Jury et al., 1997, 1998). ADAM 12 (meltrin α) triggers fusion of myoblasts into skeletal muscle fibers (Yagami-Hiromasa et al., 1995; Gilpin et al., 1998; Galliano et al., 2000) and also the formation of osteoclasts (Abe et al., 1999). Meltrin-α mRNA was also detected in the human placenta (Gilpin et al., 1998), but as yet it is not clear whether trophoblast or another cell type (e.g., blood mononuclear cells) was responsible for this expression.

Endogenous Retroviral Envelope Proteins of the HERV Family (Syncytins) and Their Receptors

Retroviruses use fusogenic envelope proteins to attach to and to fuse with host cells. In the course of phylogenesis, certain retroviral proteins have been incorporated into the human genome. Special attention has been attributed to envelope elements of three human endogenous retroviruses (HERV), namely ERV-3 Env, HERV-W Env, and HERV-FRD Env (for review, see Rote et al., 2004).

- Among those, the functional role of the **ERV-3 Env (HERV-R Env) protein** in the placenta is still a mystery. In isolated trophoblast its expression is upregulated during differentiation and in parallel to the expression of the ß-subunit of hCG (for review see Rote et al., 2004). The same authors speculate that expression this retroviral protein commits the trophoblast cells to cell cycle arrest.
- More is known about the fusogenic retroviral envelope protein **HERV-W, named syncytin-1** (Blond et al., 1999; Mi et al., 2000; Lee et al., 2001). Syncytin seems to play a key role in syncytial trophoblast fusion. It was shown to be expressed in human trophoblast and, upon transfection into other cells, induced the formation of syncytia (Blond et al., 2000; Mi et al., 2000). Frendo et al. (2003) showed that syncytin expression was upregulated after stimulating syncytial fusion of primary cytotrophoblast by a cyclic adenosine monophosphate (cAMP) analogue. Furthermore, they showed that antisense inhibition of syncytin in these primary cell cultures actually inhibited fusion.
- A second fusogenic protein of the closely related **HERV-FRD** family was identified in placental tissues recently and named **syncytin-2** (Blaise et al., 2003). It appears to have another receptor. Functional differences as compared to syncytin 1 are not yet known.

Blond et al. (2000) identified the type D mammalian retrovirus receptor (RDR), also known as neutral amino acid transporter system ATB0 (ASCT2 or SLC1A5) (Kekuda et al., 1996; Rasko et al., 1999; Tailor et al., 1999) as a **syncytin receptor**. A second amino acid transporter, ASCT1, was described as an alternative syncytin receptor (Lavillette et al., 1998; Marin et al., 2000, 2003).

Interestingly, also other amino acid transporters are under discussion as candidate fusogenic proteins: CD98 is a subunit of a family of amino acid transporter molecules. Apart from its transporter function, it has been proposed to play a role in cellular differentiation, activation, adhesion, as well as fusion. It has been shown to play a modulating role in cell fusion of monocytes/macrophages into osteoclasts, as well as in virus-mediated cell fusion (reviewed in Devés & Boyd, 2000). Kudo et al. (2003b) have recently shown that reduction of CD98 expression through an antisense oligonucleotide inhibited fusion of BeWo cells. The mechanisms by which CD98 influences cell–cell fusion as well as the question of whether, comparable with ASCT 2, it acts as a receptor for another fusogenic protein, is not yet clear (Devés & Boyd, 2000).

The distribution of syncytin-1 in the human placenta was studied by various means. Syncytin-1 mRNA was detected by Northern blot in the placenta (Mi et al., 2000). By in situ hybridization, mRNA encoding syncytin-1 so far was described only in syncytiotrophoblast of term and preterm placentas (Mi et al., 2000). Immunohistochemical data concerning syncytin-1 localization were quite confusing. Mi et al. (2000) found staining at the basal syncytiotrophoblast membrane, but in some cases also at the apical syncytiotrophoblast membrane. In placentas from pregnancies complicated by preeclampsia syncytin was nearly almost detected in the apical syncytiotrophoblast membrane (Lee et al., 2001). Using the same antibody on first trimester placenta specimens, syncytin-1 immunoreactivities were not only found in villous but also in extravillous trophoblast (Muir et al., 2003). Blond et al. (2000) raised a new recombinant antibody and showed most staining in the syncytiotrophoblast, but there were also areas of positive staining in villous cytotrophoblast. Smallwood et al. (2003) supported these data and additionally found in Western blots that syncytin expression was higher in first trimester compared to term placenta. By contrast, using the same antibody, Frendo et al. (2003) demonstrated anti–syncytin-1 reactivity at the apical syncytiotrophoblast membrane in both first trimester and term placental sections. Using a polyclonal antibody raised by Yu et al. (2002), we found uniform staining in the syncytiotrophoblast of first trimester placental paraffin sections. In the villous cytotrophoblast layer, only a few cells were stained (Pötgens et al., 2004).

Little is known about local distribution of the syncytin receptors ASCT1 and ASCT2. To date, no antibodies against these amino acid transporters/receptors are available, and in situ hybridization on placental sections has not been performed, yet. Functional studies with isolated membrane vesicles suggest that little ASCT1 but high concentrations of ASCT2 are present in the basal syncytiotrophoblast plasmalemma (for review see Jansson, 2001; Cariappa et al., 2003). Unfortunately, preparations of trophoblastic membrane vesicles do not allow any conclusion regarding villous cytotrophoblast.

Molecular Control of Syncytial Fusion

Interaction between syncytins and their receptors is not yet understood. The few, partly contradictory data on localization of syncytin and ASCT cannot exclude the possibility that both syncytins and receptors are constitutively expressed in both the syncytiotrophoblast and the cytotrophoblast. Assuming that both are the only actors realizing syncytial fusion, this would allow uncontrolled fusion of cytotrophoblast with neighboring syncytiotrophoblast, resulting in complete loss of villous cytotrophoblast within a short period of time. Accordingly, in a recent report we showed that both BeWo and JAR cells expressed the mRNA for ASCT2 and syncytin at nearly equal levels; however, unlike BeWo cells, the JAR cells

did not fuse (Borges et al., 2003). Consequently, the simple presence of syncytin and its receptor, or at least the presence of the mRNA of both, is not enough to guarantee fusion.

Rather, whether syncytins and their receptors are part of a complex cascade of events leading to fusion should be investigated (Pötgens et al., 2004). The need for such a complex cascade is underlined by morphologic data reported already above:

- Undifferentiated Langhans' cells are regularly associated with syncytiotrophoblast that is equipped with ample rough endoplasmic reticulum, polyribosomes, and numerous mitochondria (Kaufmann & Stegner, 1972; Jones & Fox, 1991; Martinez et al., 1997) (Figs. 6.7A and 6.14)—thus syncytiotrophoblast without any signs of degeneration or progressing apoptosis.
- With increasing degree of differentiation of the Langhans' cells, in the overlying syncytiotrophoblast the numbers of free and membrane-bound ribosomes as well as mitochondria decrease, to the benefit of smooth endoplasmic reticulum or degenerative/apoptotic features (Figs. 6.15B and 6.18).
- Similar relations are seen in enzyme histochemical preparations (Fig. 6.22). Decreasing syncytial activities of enzymes related to the

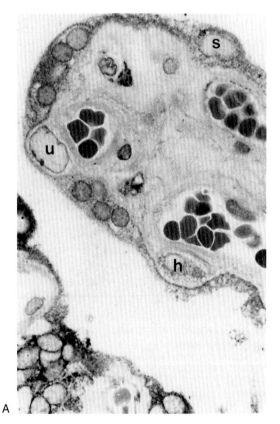
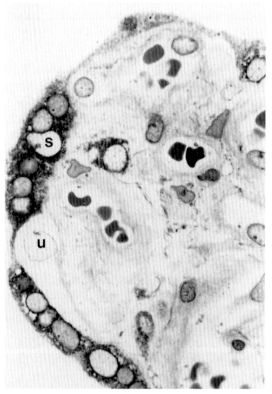

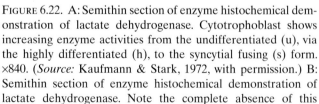

Figure 6.22. A: Semithin section of enzyme histochemical demonstration of lactate dehydrogenase. Cytotrophoblast shows increasing enzyme activities from the undifferentiated (u), via the highly differentiated (h), to the syncytial fusing (s) form. ×840. (*Source:* Kaufmann & Stark, 1972, with permission.) B: Semithin section of enzyme histochemical demonstration of lactate dehydrogenase. Note the complete absence of this

enzyme in an undifferentiated cytotrophoblastic cell (u) compared to the high activity in a cell that is in syncytial fusion (s). The large, bright nucleus of the latter can easily be distinguished from the smaller nuclei of the surrounding older syncytiotrophoblast. ×840. (*Source:* Kaufmann & Stark, 1972, with permission.)

energy metabolism are associated with increasing activities in the cytotrophoblast (Fig. 6.22) (Kaufmann & Stark, 1972).

• Stages of syncytial fusion always involve cytotrophoblast showing the highest degrees of differentiation, and syncytiotrophoblast showing advanced stages of apoptosis, (e.g., complete loss of ribosomes) (Figs. 6.15 to 6.18) (Kaufmann 1972; Kaufmann & Stegner, 1972).

We have concluded that degenerative (progressing apoptotic) changes within the syncytiotrophoblast induce (1) differentiation of the underlying cytotrophoblast (Kaufmann, 1972; Kaufmann & Stark, 1972) and (2) in parallel the initiation stages of cytotrophoblast apoptosis including PS flip, which are thought to be prerequisites of syncytial fusion (Huppertz et al., 1998; Black et al., 2004).

Taken together, according to Pötgens and coworkers (2004) any model of molecular control of syncytial fusion should take into account molecular players which

1. not only represent the ligand-receptor mechanisms that enable firm attachment and finally fusion of the adjacent membranes,
2. but also sense the readiness for fusion of cytotrophoblast, and
3. sense the syncytiotrophoblastic need to incorporate new cytotrophoblast with new organelles and new mRNA.

Re (1): In the ligand-receptor interactions very likely syncytins and receptors, ASCT1 and ASCT2 are involved. Whether also ADAMs and or adhesion molecules are involved, remains open.

Re (2): The readiness to fuse of cytotrophoblast possibly is sensed by the PS flip. Syncytiotrophoblast as a latent apoptotic tissue as visualized by annexin-binding always shows a certain degree of PS flip. In villous cytotrophoblast PS accumulates in the outer plasmalemmal leaflet only after the cell has left the cell cycle, has started the initiation stages of apoptosis and thus has reached a certain degree of differentiation. Additionally, the expression of sufficient levels of ASCT 1 and 2 (or syncytin) may well depend on a sufficient degree of differentiation.

Re (3): The most logical way to report the syncytial need for fusion to the cell surface, would be by lack of respective mRNA and thus by decreasing expression of a protein that is functionally important and at the same time involved in the fusion process (Pötgens et al., 2004). A nice example is the syncytin receptor ASCT2, which acts as amino acid transporter for maternofetal amino acid transfer. This hypothesis depends on the following provisions: First, ASCT2 is expressed by differentiated cytotrophoblast (not yet proven!). Second, syncytin is expressed mainly or exclusively by syncytiotrophoblast. Third, high levels of ASCT2 expression in "young" syncytiotrophoblast would block the coexpressed syncytin for interaction

with ASCT2 in the opposing cell[1]; but decreasing ASCT2 expression in aging/apoptotic syncytiotrophoblast would liberate syncytin for interacting with ASCT2 in the opposing cytotrophoblast and would induce fusion.

The Role of Oxygen and Cytokines in Trophoblast Proliferation and Fusion

Trophoblast proliferation resulting in increased numbers of villous cytotrophoblast cells and in increased syncytiotrophoblast thickness is a striking feature in several pathologic conditions related to hypoxia. Among those are maternal anemia (Piotrowicz et al., 1969; Kosanke et al., 1998), maternal hypertensive disorders (Wigglesworth, 1962), preeclampsia (Jeffcoate & Scott, 1959; Wigglesworth, 1962; Fox, 1964, 1997), and pregnancies at high altitude (Jackson et al., 1985; Mayhew et al., 1990; Mayhew, 1991; Ali, 1997); for review, see Kingdom and Kaufmann (1997). Tissue culture experiments (Fox, 1964; Amaladoss & Burton, 1985; Burton et al., 1989; Castellucci et al., 1990a; Ong & Burton, 1991) have proven the importance of hypoxia for trophoblast proliferation.

A common finding in villous histology illustrates the regulatory influence of local oxygen partial pressure on the turnover of cytotrophoblast. With reduction of the cytotrophoblast layer in the course of pregnancy, the remaining trophoblast cells accumulate in the neighborhood of fetal capillaries, situated near the trophoblastic surface (Fig. 6.23A) (Kaufmann, 1972). Finally, in the term placenta most trophoblast cells are located at the vasculosyncytial membranes, separating the thin syncytial lamella from the fetal capillary (Figs. 6.1D, 6.4, 6.7A, and 6.14; also see Chapter 7, Fig. 7.8). On the first glance, this association appears illogical, as this localization increases the maternofetal diffusion distances at the main sites of diffusional exchange. Reconstructing the oxygen isobars in a respective villous cross section suggests that this finding is a consequence of local oxygen partial pressures (Kaufmann, 1972). As can be seen in Figure 6.23B, the PO_2 gradient is much steeper in places where the fetal capillaries directly face the trophoblast. In this location, the cytotrophoblast is exposed to much lower PO_2 levels than those that are far from the capillaries, indicating that decreased PO_2 stimulates proliferation. Consequently, far from the capillaries, in zones of higher PO_2, the poorly proliferating cytotrophoblast fuses and finally disappears. In contrast, increased proliferation in zones of low PO_2 near the capillaries helps some of the trophoblast cells to persist. This kind of regulation makes sense if we assume that hypoxic conditions damage the syncytiotrophoblast functionally and structurally.

---

[1] Syncytin, as a retroviral envelope protein has the ability to block its own receptors if coexpressed with its receptors in the same cell (Ponferrada et al., 2003; for review see Colman & Lawrence, 2003). Consequently, the mere presence of syncytin in a certain cell or syncytial membrane does not necessarily mean that syncytin is available to interact with a receptor molecule in an opposing cell membrane. If coexpressed on the same side, syncytins and receptors may neutralize each other and may not be available for the respective ligands or receptors in the neighboring membrane. Hence, not the mere presence of both but rather the balance between local syncytin and receptor expression levels may determine whether fusion is initiated or not.

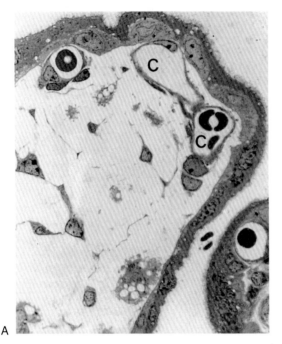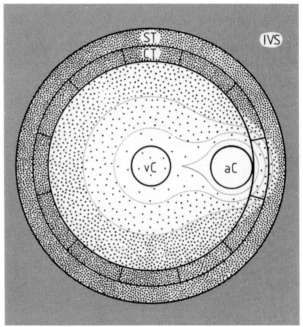

A   B

FIGURE 6.23. A: Semithin section of the 22nd gestational week p.m. In contrast to earlier stages of pregnancy, from this stage onward the fetal capillaries (C) come into a more peripheral position and establish close contacts to the trophoblastic surface of the villus because of the reduced villous diameter. Cytotrophoblast is concentrated in the neighborhood of the capillaries. ×820. (*Source:* Kaufmann, 1972, with permission.) B: Why is cytotrophoblast concentrated near the fetal capillaries? This idealized cross section of a placental villus demonstrates the distribution of the villous cytotrophoblast related to the oxygen tension. The PO_2 is symbolized by the density of dots. The basic assumption is that the PO_2 of the intervillous space (IVS, densely dotted) is highest, whereas the PO_2 in the arterial capillary limb (aC, not dotted) is lowest; despite unlimited oxygen diffusion, this gradient is kept constant so long as the maternal and fetal circulations are intact. If this assumption is true, one expects a steeper PO_2 gradient near the arterial capillary limb (aC) than far from it, as symbolized by the dotting patterns. As becomes evident in this diagram, cytotrophoblast near a capillary is located in zones of lower PO_2, because of its steep gradient, as compared to cytotrophoblast being far away from fetal capillaries and lying in zones of a moderate PO_2-gradient. The stimulating influence of low oxygen tension on cytotrophoblastic mitoses explains the persistence of cytotrophoblast near the capillaries. On the other hand, in zones of elevated PO_2 far from capillaries, retarded mitotic activity and continuous loss of cytotrophoblast by syncytial fusion lead to the disappearance of the cytotrophoblast, as depicted in part A. ST, syncytiotrophoblast; CT, cytotrophoblast; vC, venous capillary limb. (*Source:* Modified from Kaufmann, 1972, with permission.)

Villous oxygenation better than normal, so-called hyperoxia (Kingdom & Kaufmann, 1997), negatively influences trophoblast proliferation. In most placentas, one observes villi with obstructed fetal vessels. This leads to increasing intravillous oxygen partial pressure since the missing fetal circulation no longer extracts oxygen. Loss of villous cytotrophoblast normally accompanies this finding, provided that the maternal circulation is not impaired in these areas. Panigel and Myers (1972) have generated this condition experimentally. These authors ligated the umbilical vessels of one placental disk of the bidiscoidal rhesus monkey placenta. The fetus survived. After disintegration of the fetal villous capillaries in the ligated disk, the authors observed an involution of the villous cytotrophoblast and, finally, degenerative/apoptotic changes of the syncytiotrophoblast. Because the maternal circulation was still intact, the syncytiotrophoblast changes could not be explained as being a consequence of deficient nutrition or hypoxia. Rather, it must be the result of deficient proliferation of cytotrophoblast and deficient syncytial fusion caused by abnormally high intravillous PO_2.

Growth factors and their receptors involved in the regulation of trophoblast proliferation among others comprise the insulin-like growth factors IGF-I and IGF-II and their receptors (Boehm et al., 1989a; Ohlsson, 1989; Ohlsson et al., 1989). In particular, IGF-II is expressed primarily in highly proliferative cytotrophoblast, as for example in cell islands and cell columns, while other cellular components such as villous cytotrophoblast or mesenchymal stromal cells harbor less active IGF-II genes (Ohlsson et al., 1989). Because numerous IGF receptors are expressed in villous cytotrophoblast, it has been suggested that IGF mediates autocrine or short-range paracrine growth control of placental development (Ohlsson et al., 1989). There are only a few data on the interactions between oxygen and IGF action. Owens and coworkers (1994) reported that in sheep the secretion of both IGF-I and IGF-II under hypoxia is decreased, whereas hypoxia increases the secretion of the IGF-inhibiting, IGF-binding proteins (Morrish et al., 1998; Popovici et al., 2001;

Verhaeghe et al., 2001). Epidermal growth factor (EGF) seems to have no effect on trophoblast proliferation (Maruo et al., 1996). The data on transforming growth factor-β (TGF-β) are again confusing: TGF-β, the expression of which is increased by hypoxia (Patel et al., 1994), was found to inhibit (Lysiak et al., 1993; Tse et al., 2002), whereas TGF-α (Lysiak et al., 1993; Filla & Kaul, 1997) stimulates trophoblast proliferation.

Hypoxia-induced trophoblast proliferation would make particular sense as a compensatory mechanism, if hypoxia would also stimulate **trophoblast apoptosis**. This in fact has been reported by Morrish et al. (1998) and by Levy et al. (2000). In addition, in vitro data by Benyo et al. (1997) have shown that villous TNF-α secretion is significantly increased under hypoxic conditions; TNF-α is one of the cytokines capable of inducing trophoblastic apoptosis (see earlier). Its p55 receptor, responsible for the start of the initiation stages of apoptosis, is expressed by villous cytotrophoblast (Yui et al., 1994, 1996). Moreover, the data available show increased trophoblastic apoptosis in pregnancies complicated by preeclampsia and intrauterine growth restriction (IUGR) (Hayakawa et al., 1995; S.C. Smith et al., 1997b), pregnancy complications in the pathogenesis of which abnormal oxygen supply is involved (Kingdom & Kaufmann, 1997).

Data regarding the effects of oxygen on **syncytial fusion** are rare and difficult to interpret. Using cell line BeWo, Kudo et al. (2003a) and Knerr et al. (2003) have demonstrated that under hypoxia syncytin mRNA levels decreased, and were less inducible by forskolin, compared to "normoxia" (20% oxygen). Hypoxia also decreased fusion of BeWo cells (Kudo et al., 2003a). Downregulation of syncytin expression by hypoxia may explain the findings of Lee et al. (2001) that syncytin expression was very low in placentas of preeclamptic pregnancies. It is also our experience from cell culture as well as from evaluation of villous histology that severe degrees of hypoxia completely block syncytial fusion. By contrast, in moderate hypoxia the negative effect of hypoxia may be overridden by the increased availability of cytotrophoblast that is ready to fuse. Cytokines, which were reported to control syncytial fusion, include EGF, which stimulates fusion, and TGF-β, which inhibits fusion (for review, see Morrish et al., 1998). On the other hand, in various tissues, hypoxia increases the expression of TGF-β (Patel et al., 1994), an effect that should again result in inhibitory effects of low oxygen on syncytial fusion.

Recently, Bukovsky and coworkers (2003a,b) have presented new data, which may add to our understanding of the regulation of trophoblast turnover. When studying the expression of estrogen receptors in the human placenta, these authors found that villous cytotrophoblast expresses estrogen receptor α. Upon syncytial fusion in vivo and in vitro, the expression switched to estrogen

receptor ß (Bukovsky et al., 2003a). These data suggest that also estrogens may be involved in proliferation and differentiation of villous trophoblast.

The Impact of Trophoblast Turnover on Syncytiotrophoblast Specialization

The structurally and functionally specialized areas of syncytiotrophoblast described above very unlikely are stable structures. Rather, the comparison of these subtypes of syncytiotrophoblast with the events that take place during trophoblast apoptosis and turnover leads us to suspect that they are an expression of a highly dynamic process of differentiation and degeneration.

Taken together, the data lead us to suggest the following cycle of structural and functional changes within in the villous trophoblastic cover (Fig. 6.21):

- Upon syncytial fusion, syncytiotrophoblast with well-developed rough endoplasmic reticulum, focused on protein metabolism, is generated.
- Within days to a very few weeks, due to missing transcription activity of the syncytial nuclei, the ribosomes are lost and the respective area is transformed into syncytiotrophoblast with smooth endoplasmic reticulum and tubular mitochondria, focused on steroid metabolism.
- As a consequence of progressive apoptotic degradation of the syncytiotrophoblastic cytoskeleton, the aging nuclei are focally aggregated, forming apoptotic knots, which shortly are pinched off from the syncytial surface and are deported into the maternal circulation. The sorting process, which on the one side accumulates the syncytial nuclei and on the other side generates enucleated, thin layers of syncytiotrophoblast, is probably driven by pressure of the underlying fetal capillaries and sinusoids.
- After aggregation and extrusion of the nuclei result enucleated areas of syncytiotrophoblast, which mostly span over (1) fetal sinusoids (vasculosyncytial membranes, specialized in diffusional exchange) or (2) undifferentiated cytotrophoblast in G_0-stage (syncytial lamellae covering cytotrophoblast, possibly specialized in steroid metabolism).
- Formation of the latter structures should be investigated as a signal for the cytotrophoblast to enter the cell cycle, later to differentiate and to fuse.
- By syncytial fusion, the vasculosyncytial membranes and the lamellae covering cytotrophoblast are again equipped with new syncytial nuclei, cell organelles, and RNA so that the turnover cycle can start anew.

As discussed before, the length of such a cycle is estimated to last 3 to 4 weeks.

Also throughout the first 4 months of pregnancy, when the respective syncytiotrophoblast specialization is not demonstrable, similar turnover processes take place within the villous trophoblast (for review, see Huppertz et al., 2002). They are possibly less impressive due to (1) much higher relative numbers of villous cytotrophoblast, (2) higher turnover rates, and (3) reduced villous capillarization as the speculated driving force for nuclear sorting of the differentiation processes within the syncytiotrophoblast, and thus escape electron microscopical and histochemical detection.

Trophoblastic Basement Membrane

The trophoblastic basement membrane separates the trophoblastic epithelium from the villous stroma. It forms a supportive matrix for the cytotrophoblast and, where the latter is lacking, for the syncytiotrophoblast (see Figs. 6.1 and 6.4A). Under normal conditions, the average thickness of the trophoblast basement membrane ranges from 20 to 50 nm. Polarization optical methods as well as fluorescence microscopy by Scheuner (1972, 1975), Scheuner and Hutschenreiter (1972, 1977), and Pfister et al. (1989) have provided basic information about the structural organization and fiber orientation.

The main components of basement membranes of other origin, namely collagen IV, laminin, and heparan sulfate, are also expressed in the basement membrane of the trophoblast (Ohno et al., 1986; Autio-Harmainen et al., 1991; Castellucci et al., 1993a,b). In addition, fibronectin was shown to be present (Virtanen et al., 1988). This molecule has binding sites for various collagens and proteoglycans (Bray, 1978; Duance & Bailey, 1983) and is thought to attach the basal lamina to the connective tissue fibers beneath. Recent analyses of laminin and fibronectin isoforms suggest that the molecular composition changes during maturation of villous trophoblastic and endothelial basement membranes; these changes are particularly obvious in areas of trophoblast proliferation and villous sprouting (Korhonen & Virtanen, 2001). Using lectin histochemistry, Sgambati and coworkers (2002) have added data on oligosaccharide distribution of glycoconjugates with the basal lamina.

Functionally, the basement membrane acts as a support for the trophoblastic epithelium and allows a certain amount of movement. Matrix proteins, such as tenascin, which counteracts the action of fibronectin (Aufderheide & Ekblom, 1988), can possibly unlock the attachment of cytotrophoblast cells. This effect could enable postmitotic Langhans' cells to migrate along the basal lamina to those places where they are needed for syncytial fusion. Accordingly, tenascin is regularly expressed in sites of Langhans' cell mitosis and degenerative syncytiotrophoblastic foci (Castellucci et al., 1991).

Another important function of the basal lamina is to act as a filtration barrier between maternal and fetal circulations. Calcification of the villous trophoblastic basal lamina, a regular finding in intrauterine fetal death, but a rare one with living fetuses (Roberts et al., 2000; Kasznica & Petcu, 2003), may be a hint in this direction. Whether the trophoblastic basal lamina plays a role as a molecular sieve limiting transepithelial (transplacental) transport, as reported for the glomerular basal lamina, remains to be studied.

Connective Tissue

The basic architecture of the villous stroma is constructed of fixed connective tissue cells that form a network; they enmesh connective tissue fibers, and free connective tissue cells (Hofbauer cells) and fetal vessels. Depending on the age of the placenta, on the type of villus, and on the position within the villus, at least five different types of fixed stromal cells have been described (see Fig. 6.26) (Boyd & Hamilton, 1967; Kaufmann et al., 1977b; Castellucci et al., 1980; Castellucci & Kaufmann, 1982a; Martinoli et al., 1984; King, 1987). According to more recent immunohistochemical analyses they represent different stages of a differentiation gradient, ranging from indifferent, proliferating mesenchymal cells (pluripotent stem cells) up to highly differentiated myofibroblasts and possibly even myocytes (Kohnen et al., 1995, 1996; Demir et al., 1997).

Mesenchymal Cells (V Cells)

Mesenchymal cells, or undifferentiated stromal cells, are the prevailing cell type until the end of the second month (Kaufmann et al., 1977b; Martinoli et al., 1984). At all later stages of pregnancy, they are found only in newly formed villi, the mesenchymal villi, and beneath the trophoblastic surface of immature intermediate and stem villi (Kohnen et al., 1996; Demir et al., 1997).

Structure: They are usually small (10–20 μm long and 3–4 μm wide), spindle-shaped cells with little cytoplasm, which are connected to each other by a few thin, long processes. Polyribosomes are the prevailing organelles. Mitotic mesenchymal cells may have much more cytoplasm and form nearly epithelioid cells (see Chapter 7, Fig. 7.14). As cytoskeletal filaments, they usually express only vimentin, but not desmin, sm-actins, or sm-myosin, and are therefore also called **V cells** (Kohnen et al., 1996).

Distribution: In the early stages of pregnancy, these cells make up most of the mesenchymal stroma, which is the primitive forerunner of all other stromal types. Throughout all the later stages of pregnancy, these cells persist in two different locations: first, within mesenchymal villi, the first stages of newly sprouting villi; second, as a small proliferating subset of connective tissue cells beneath the trophoblastic surface of large caliber villi (see Fig. 6.26) (Kohnen et al., 1996; Demir et al., 1997).

Fibroblasts (VD Cells and VDA Cells)

The differentiation of this cell type is closely linked to the development of a new villous type, the immature intermediate villi (see Chapter 7) at the beginning of the third month p.m. At this time, dramatic changes in stromal architecture and cellular composition of villi take place (Kaufmann et al., 1977b; Martinoli et al., 1984). King (1987) reported similar changes for the rhesus monkey placenta.

Structure: Within a few days, starting in the centers of the villi and then slowly spreading toward the villous surface, most of the mesenchymal cells (V cells) acquire desmin as the second cytoskeletal filament and henceforth are characterized as **VD cells** (Kohnen et al., 1995, 1996). Structurally, these cells are very heterogeneous and occasionally have been called reticulum cells (Kaufmann et al., 1977b) or fibroblasts (King, 1987) (Figs. 6.24 and 6.25). The newly formed fibroblasts (VD cells) have elongated, bizarre-shaped cell bodies that measure about 20 to 30 μm in length. From the cell bodies, several long, thin, branching cytoplasmic processes take off.

Serial sections studied by transmission electron microscopy and scanning electron microscopy of immature intermediate villi revealed that the processes are flat sails of cytoplasm (Kaufmann et al., 1977b; Castellucci & Kaufmann, 1982a; Martinoli et al., 1984). They branch in a cone-like pattern, the apex of the cone pointing to the cell body. In sections, these extensions form nets by establishing contacts to the extensions of neighboring cells (see Fig. 7.4C).

In later stages of pregnancy and close to the centrally located fetal stem vessels, these cells additionally may acquire α-sm actin as a third cytoskeletal filament (**VDA cells**), without change in their body shape (Fig. 6.26). This is interpreted as a first step toward differentiation of myofibroblasts (Kohnen et al., 1996) (see following discussion).

Distribution: In three-dimensional preparations of immature intermediate villi, the sail-like processes of several VD cells in series make up longitudinally oriented stromal channels. In cross sections, the latter appear as rounded compartments or chambers 20 to 50 μm in diameter (see Figs. 7.2 and 7.7). Fetal vessels and the connective tissue fibers are fitted into the spaces between the channels, as well as between channels and trophoblastic basement membrane. This reticular structure has been

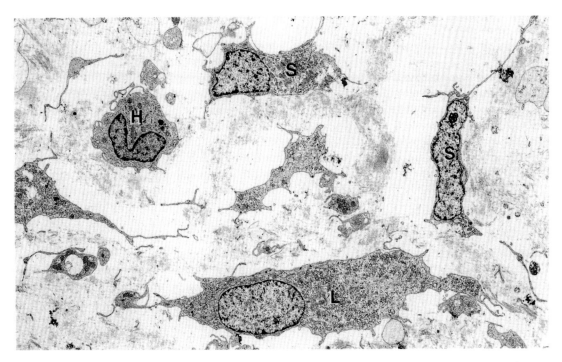

FIGURE 6.24. Transmission electron micrograph shows the typical variety of connective tissue cells in a mature intermediate villus at the 36th week p.m. Small reticulum cells (S) with long, slender, richly branched cytoplasmic extensions, a large reticulum cell (below), and a macrophage (Hofbauer cell, H) are seemingly scattered irregularly among loosely arranged connective tissue fibers. ×2500. (*Source:* Kaufmann et al., 1977a, with permission.)

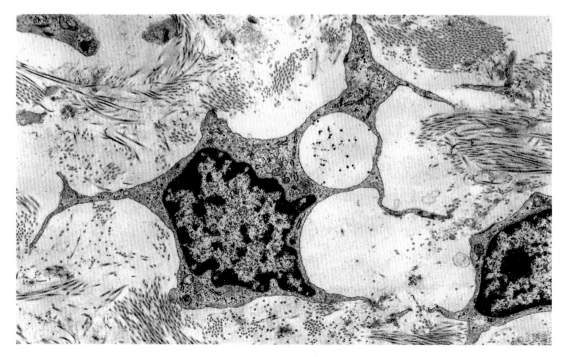

FIGURE 6.25. Electron micrograph of fibroblast with sparse cytoplasm and short but richly branched cytoplasmic extensions, surrounded by bundles of collagen fibers. ×9300.

described in detail by Castellucci and Kaufmann (1982a,b), Castellucci et al. (1984), and Martinoli et al. (1984). It is highly characteristic only for the immature intermediate villi.

In mature intermediate and terminal villi (see Chapter 7) a structurally different subgroup of fibroblasts (VD cells) is found. Fewer and filiform processes but abundant perinuclear cytoplasm characterizes these cells (Fig. 6.24). They do not delimit stromal channels; rather, they are enmeshed in a loose mixture of connective tissue fibers.

Myofibroblasts (VDAG Cells and VDAGM Cells)

A third group of connective tissue cells that are structurally and immunohistochemically different from mesenchymal cells and fibroblasts characterizes the central parts of immature intermediate villi as well as stem villi (Fig. 6.26). They gradually differentiate out of VDA cells so that clear-cut borders among both populations are not always visible.

Structure: The cells have much cytoplasm and are 30 to 100 μm long but only 5 to 8 μm wide. In contrast to the fibroblasts, they have only a few short, filiform, or thick processes. The cytoplasm is rich in rough endoplasmic reticulum, stress fibers, cytoplasmic dense plaques, and caveolae. Locally, the cell body is surrounded by a basal lamina (Demir et al., 1992; Kohnen et al., 1996). These cells obviously correspond to the extravascular contractile cells described in large stem villi by Spanner (1935) as well as Krantz and Parker (1963) and in anchoring villi by Farley et al. (2004). Feller et al. (1985) provided histochemical evidence that these were positive for dipeptidyl-peptidase IV; the isoenzyme pattern of this enzyme is identical with that of myofibroblasts of other origin.

Immunohistochemical analysis of the cytoskeleton of the villous stromal cells (Kohnen et al., 1995, 1996; Demir et al., 1997) revealed a differentiation gradient even within these cells. Those neighboring the VDA cells expressed γ-sm actin in addition to vimentin, desmin, and α-sm actin (**VDAG cells**) (Fig. 6.26). Those directly facing the media of the central stem vessels additionally partly showed expression of sm-myosin (**VDAGM cells**).

Distribution: These same authors demonstrated advancing differentiation of mesenchymal cells via fibroblasts to myofibroblasts (1) from early to later stages of pregnancy, (2) from mesenchymal to stem villi, and (3) from the subtrophoblastic stromal layer to the perivascular stroma (Fig. 6.26). In immature intermediate and stem villi, all stages of differentiation arranged from the

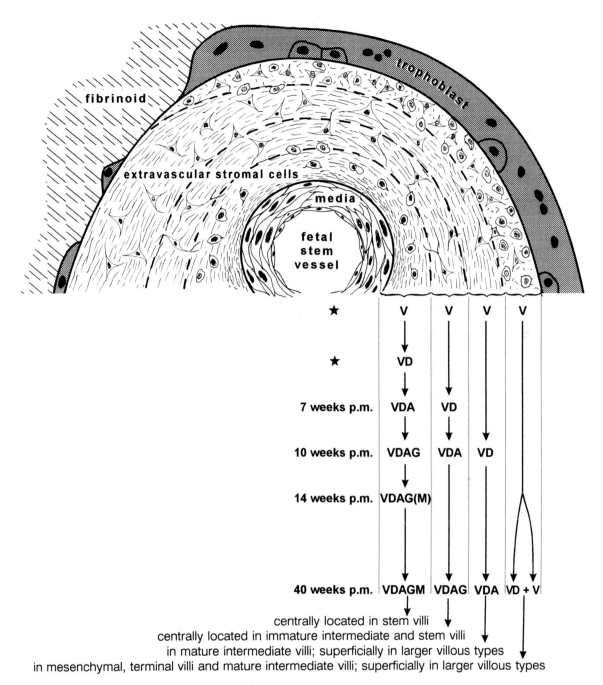

FIGURE 6.26. Representation of stromal differentiation in a stem villus, illustrating the usual differentiation route of villous stromal cells from proliferating mesenchymal precursors to myofibroblasts. A thin subtrophoblastic layer of proliferating mesenchymal cells (V cells) represent the stem cells for the entire extravascular stroma. By proliferation, these cells generate new peripheral layers of stroma and thus contribute to the growing thickness of the villus. More centrally, older and higher differentiated layers of connective tissue cells can be found. V, vimentin; D, desmin; A, α-smooth muscle actin; G, γ-smooth muscle actin; M, smooth muscle myosin. At the bottom, the occurrence of the same stromal cells in other villous types is summarized. (*Source:* Modified from Kohnen et al., 1996, with permission.)

periphery to the center can be observed. The most peripheral, proliferating cells express only vimentin. Slightly more centrally, a layer of cells with the typical shape of fibroblasts, expressing vimentin, α-smooth muscle actin, and desmin, follows. Near the larger vessels, typical myofibroblasts can be seen that express the full range of cytoskeletal antigens and closely resemble smooth muscle cells. The existence of this centripetal differentiation gradient was supported by Kacemi et al. (1999) using a similar panel of immunohistochemical markers.

Function: In contrast to the vascular smooth muscle cells of the central villous stem vessels, the surrounding myofibroblasts are arranged parallel to the longitudinal axis of the villi (Demir et al., 1997). In large stem villi they form a clearly defined perivascular contractile sheath that has been discussed in detail by Graf et al. (1994, 1995). It has been suggested that the contraction of extravascular contractile cells is important for the turgor of the villi (Krantz & Parker, 1963; Graf et al., 1995). Moreover, contraction of longitudinally arranged myofibroblasts within anchoring villi may influence the length of anchoring villi and the width of the intervillous space, thus regulating maternal intravillous blood pressure (Kohnen et al., 1996; Demir et al., 1997). Recently, Farley et al. (2004) have supported this hypothesis. They showed that treatment of isolated anchoring villi with KCl and l-NAME resulted in longitudinal contraction up to 62% and 74%, respectively, over resting tone. Some of the myofibroblasts are positive for nitric oxide synthase (NOS)(Schönfelder et al., 1993), an enzyme that is involved in production of nitric oxide, a potent vasodilator; NOS inhibition in guinea pigs and rats has been shown to result in preeclamptic symptoms, including intrauterine growth retardation (Yallampalli & Garfield, 1993; Chwalisz et al., 1994; Garfield et al., 1994).

Several authors have described immunoreactivities for cytokeratins 6, 8, 17, 18, and 19 in contractile cells (myocytes and myofibroblasts) of placental and embryonic origin (Kasper et al., 1988; Bozhok et al., 1990; Nanaev et al., 1997; Haigh et al., 1999). According to our experience, such cells are particularly frequent in and around vessel walls of large-caliber villi. It is still an open question whether or not all contractile stromal cells coexpress these cytokeratin isoforms, or whether an additional subpopulation of cytokeratin-expressing stromal cells hides among the contractile cells in and around the stem vessels (Haigh et al., 1999). In any case, special care is advisable when using cytokeratin antibodies as a marker for the trophoblastic origin of cells isolated from placental villi.

Matrix Components of the Villous Stroma

Database mining revealed 102 extracellular matrix genes among about 10,000 mRNA species expressed in the human placenta (Chen & Aplin, 2003). Out of these, 23 coded for collagens, 59 for noncollagenous glycoproteins, and 23 for proteoglycans.

Extracellular matrix proteins represent the prevailing matrix molecules. Different types of collagens have been identified in the core of the placental villi by immunohistochemistry, for example, collagen I, III, IV, and VI (Amenta et al., 1986; Autio-Harmainen et al., 1991; Nanaev et al., 1991; Rukosuev, 1992; Castellucci et al., 1993a,b; Frank et al., 1994). In addition, some fibronectin isoforms, tenascin C, fibrillin I, and thrombospondin I, have been detected in the villous stroma (Pfister et al., 1988; Virtanen et al., 1988; Earl et al., 1990; Autio-Harmainen et al., 1991; Castellucci et al., 1991, 1993a,b; Rukosuev, 1992; Frank et al., 1994; Mühlhauser et al., 1996; Chen & Aplin, 2003).

In human placental villi, different from most other organs, molecules such as laminin, collagen IV, and heparan sulfate are not restricted to the basement membranes but are also present throughout the villous stroma or at least in specialized areas of the latter (Yamada et al., 1987; Nanaev et al., 1991; Rukosuev, 1992; Mühlhauser et al., 1996; Chen & Aplin, 2003). The universal presence of these molecules in the extracellular matrix may facilitate remodeling of basement membranes and thus increase morphogenetic and functional flexibility of the various villous cell populations.

Ultrastructural data concerning reticular (precollagen) and collagen fibers have been reported (Enders & King, 1970; Vacek, 1970; Kaufmann et al., 1977b). Precollagen or reticular fibers have a diameter of 5 nm or less. They form seemingly unoriented meshworks without predominant fiber direction. In mesenchymal connective tissue, they are the prevailing fiber type.

The thicker collagen fibers have diameters of 20 to 60 nm. They show the typical 64.9-nm cross-striation. Usually, grouped in twisted bundles of about 100 parallel fibers, they are arranged as a coarse meshwork, running in spiral courses around the fetal vessels (Kaufmann et al., 1977b). The amount of collagenous fibers increases from mesenchymal stroma, via reticular sinusoidal to fibrous stroma (see Figs. 7.3C and 7.7D). Histologically, collagen fibers stain with the usual connective tissue stains and reticular fibers do not.

Proteoglycans are less well studied. Decorin, a small leucine-rich proteoglycan that seems to have a primary function in the organization of the extracellular matrix (Hardingham & Fosang, 1992), has also been detected in the villous stroma (Bianco et al., 1990). Interestingly, the core protein of decorin (whose synthesis is induced by TGF-β) binds and neutralizes TGF-β (Yamaguchi et al., 1990).

Hyaluronan is a high molecular mass polysaccharide that plays a particular role in developmental processes involving cell motility (for review, see Marzioni et al., 2001). In accordance with this view, hyaluronan expression is particularly impressive in newly developing villi (so-called mesenchymal villi, cf. Chapter 7). By contrast, fully developed villi in early stages of pregnancy and all villi in later pregnancy are characterized by moderate hyaluronan content (Marzioni et al., 2001). Interestingly, CD44, the hyaluronan receptor of cells exposed to the extracellular matrix of the villous stroma, shows increasing activity throughout pregnancy (Marzioni et al., 2001).

Matrix-degrading proteolytic enzymes (matrix metalloproteinases) are likely to be involved in remodeling of the villous stroma during placental development. It has been shown that the trophoblast expresses interstitial and type IV collagenolytic activities (Emonard et al., 1990; Moll & Lane, 1990; Librach et al., 1991), and the former has been detected in villous fibroblasts (Moll & Lane, 1990). Autio-Harmainen et al. (1992) detected 70-kd type IV collagenase in endothelial cells and fibroblasts of the villi. Moreover, the exclusive expression of tissue inhibitors of matrix metalloproteinases in the stroma of mesenchymal villi, just those villous types that are most active in villous sprouting and branching, points to the importance of matrix turnover for villous development.

Stromal fibrosis and thickening of basal laminas are considered typical features in many pregnancy pathologies and are often referred to as consequence of hypoxic or ischemic conditions. For review, see Fox (1997). Based on his own experience, Fox, however, has refuted this hypothesis and arrived at the conclusion that oxygen supply that is better than normal increases villous fibrosis (e.g., following intrauterine fetal death). Recent in vitro culture data by Chen and Aplin (2003) suggest a more differentiated reaction pattern that well may explain the above-mentioned discrepancies in the literature. Expression of fibronectins and collagen IV is more strongly upregulated by hypoxia than is expression of collagen I, fibrillin I, and thrombospondin I, whereas expression of laminins and elastin under hypoxia was extremely low.

There is increasing use of extracellular matrix molecules for in vitro studies of the trophoblast. Such molecules influence trophoblast differentiation (Kao et al., 1988; Nelson et al., 1990); they can play a pivotal role in repair mechanisms (Nelson et al., 1990), may participate in modulating hormone and protein production (Castellucci et al., 1990a), and can influence the morphology and proteolytic activity of the trophoblast (Kliman & Feinberg, 1990; Bischof et al., 1991).

Hofbauer Cells (Villous Macrophages)

It is generally agreed that Hofbauer cells are fetal tissue macrophages of the human placenta. Statements concerning their macrophage character are based on morphologic, cytochemical, histochemical, immunologic, and immunohistochemical studies (for reviews, see Bourne, 1962; Boyd & Hamilton, 1970; Castellucci & Zaccheo, 1989; Castellucci et al., 1990b; Vince & Johnson, 1996). Here, we review the main aspects of these cells.

First Descriptions

From the middle of the 19th century, several authors have reported the presence of large cells in the stroma of chorionic villi of the human placenta (Müller, 1847; Schroeder van der Kolk, 1851; Virchow, 1863, 1871; Langhans, 1877; Merttens, 1894; Ulesko-Stroganova, 1896; Marchand, 1898). Kastschenko (1885) first described their precise location in the villous stroma. Virchow (1871), and later Chaletzky (1891) and Neumann (1897), first commented on the particular association of hydatidiform mole with large isolated cells, having clear cytoplasm. This observation led to the term **Chaletzky-Neumann cells,** used in the past by several pathologists. Hofbauer, whose name has come to be associated with these cells, gave a comprehensive description of the cells in normal villi at the beginning of the 20th century (1903, 1905). It is because of these detailed morphologic studies and because of the long-lasting uncertainties about the macrophage nature of these cells that the term **Hofbauer cell** has been widely accepted in the literature.

Morphology

Hofbauer cells were described as frequent, pleomorphic cells of the villous stroma (Fig. 6.28) with round, fusiform, or stellate appearance (Langhans, 1877; Hofbauer, 1903, 1905; Schmidt, 1956; for a review, see Bourne, 1962). Their size depends on the length of their processes. The cells vary from 10 to 30 μm in diameter. Early investigations had already pointed out that the most striking aspects of the Hofbauer cells are their highly vacuolated appearance and their granulated cytoplasm (Virchow, 1863, 1871; Langhans, 1877; Minot, 1889; Merttens, 1894; Hofbauer, 1903, 1905; Graf Spee, 1915; Meyer, 1919; Lewis, 1924). Later studies have pointed out that these cells are characterized by numerous membrane-bound, electron-lucent vacuoles of different sizes, possessing amorphous material of varying density, dense granules (presumably lysosomes), and short profiles of endoplasmic reticulum (Fig. 6.28A,B; see Fig. 7.7B,D) (Hörmann, 1947; Boyd & Hughes, 1955; Rodway & Marsh, 1956; Geller, 1957; Bargmann & Knoop, 1959; Rhodin & Terzakis, 1962; Panigel & Anh, 1964; Boyd & Hamilton, 1967; Fox, 1967a, 1997; Wynn, 1967a,b, 1973, 1975; Enders & King, 1970; Tedde, 1970; Vacek, 1970; Demir & Erbengi, 1984; King, 1987; Katabuchi et al., 1989; for reviews, see Snoeck, 1958; Bourne, 1962; Boyd & Hamilton, 1970; Castellucci & Zaccheo, 1989).

Different phenotypes of Hofbauer cells have been described (Fig. 6.27):

• Enders and King (1970) pointed out that **vacuolated Hofbauer cells** showing large intracytoplasmic vacuoles, containing varying amounts of flocculent precipitate, are numerous, and large during the first half of pregnancy (Fig. 6.28A,B; see Fig. 7.7B).
• As pregnancy progresses, the vacuoles decrease in number and size, and the Hofbauer cells show an increase of intracytoplasmic granules (Figs. 7.7D and 7.11) that are presumably lysosomes (Enders & King, 1970; Castellucci et al., 1980). This **granulated type of Hofbauer cell** can easily be differentiated from the rare mast cells (Fig. 6.28C) because of the metachromasia of the latter.
• **Hofbauer cells largely lacking vacuoles and granules** are present during early pregnancy and have been considered immature Hofbauer cells (Castellucci et al., 1987; Katabuchi et al., 1989). Immunohistochemical studies using macrophage markers, however, have revealed many such undifferentiated Hofbauer cells also in all mature placental villi. This finding is in agree-

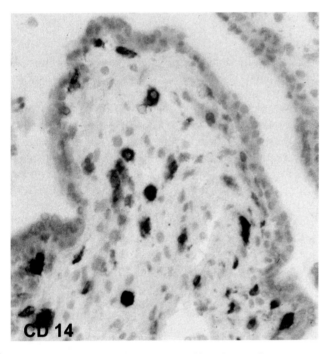

FIGURE 6.27. Cross section of a transitional stage from mesenchymal to immature intermediate villus at the end of the first trimester immunostained with the antibody leu-M3 (anti-CD14), a marker of macrophages. Both the distribution pattern of immunoreactivities and the gradually increasing staining intensities from fibroblast-like phenotypes to macrophage-like phenotypes suggest that fibroblast-like stromal cells may achieve macrophage character. ×170.

ment with immunologic investigations, which consider the vacuolated Hofbauer cells to be the morphologically obvious and fully differentiated member of a much larger mononuclear phagocyte population (Wood, 1980; Frauli & Ludwig, 1987a).

The first three-dimensional visualization of Hofbauer cells, their intracytoplasmic vacuoles, surface aspects, and relationship with other components of the villous core (see Fig. 7.7C) was made possible by combining the cryofracture method with scanning electron microscopy (SEM) (Castellucci et al., 1980; Martinoli et al., 1984). The surface morphology of Hofbauer cells was found to be characterized by spherical or elongated blebs or microplicae (see Fig. 7.7C). These features were irregularly distributed. Other Hofbauer cells showed a ruffled surface, characterized by lamellipodia, which were large, smooth surfaced, and well developed. They sometimes overlapped one another, creating cups or funnel-like structures. Sometimes, Hofbauer cells bearing both lamellipodia and blebs were observed (Castellucci et al., 1980, 1984; Martinoli et al., 1984).

In addition, SEM of chorionic villous stroma during the first half of pregnancy revealed that most of the Hofbauer cells were inside collagen-free intercommunicating stromal channels (see Fig. 7.7C) composed of large sail-like processes of fixed stromal cells (Castellucci et al., 1980, 1984; Castellucci & Kaufmann, 1982a). These channels were particularly well developed in the central region of the core of the chorionic villi and were oriented mostly parallel to the major axis of the villus. Some Hofbauer cells inside the channels had an elongated shape and extended their cellular bodies between intercommunicating channels or between channels and intercellular substance outside the channels (Castellucci et al., 1980, 1984). These morphologic features strongly suggest motility of Hofbauer cells in the villous core.

The channels characterized most of the chorionic villi of the first half of pregnancy (Fig. 6.28A,B; see Fig. 7.7B,C). Toward term, their number was decreased. In the mature placenta, they were found only in villi at the center of the placentones (Fig. 7.7D) (Schuhmann, 1981; Castellucci & Kaufmann, 1982a,b; Castellucci et al., 1990c). During the last trimester of gestation, Hofbauer cells present in villi outside the placentone centers, that is, villi characterized by a core with large amounts of collagen fibers and narrow or absent channels, showed mostly blebs or microplicae at their surface, but rarely lamellipodia (Fig. 6.24; see Fig. 7.11) (Castellucci & Kaufmann, 1982a; Martinoli et al., 1984).

The morphologic features provided the basis for the first functional interpretations:

• The intracytoplasmic vacuoles and large lamellipodia of the Hofbauer cells have been considered **phagocytic**

FIGURE 6.28. A: Transmission electron micrograph: sail-like cytoplasmic processes (arrows) of the small reticulum cells line channel-like stromal cavities within immature intermediate villi. They are filled with some fluid, but are devoid of connective tissue fibers. The latter can only be found in the vicinity of the channels. Suspended in the fluid of the channels, one finds the macrophages (Hofbauer cells, H). ×5300. B: Light microscopic, semithin section of reticular stroma of an immature intermediate villus from the 12th week p.m., showing two Hofbauer cells. Both are located in longitudinally sectioned stromal channels, delimited by long, thin cytoplasmic extensions of fixed stromal cells. The left Hofbauer cell belongs to the highly vacuolated type that prevails in early pregnancy. The right cell shows fewer vacuoles and is characterized by its rounded appearance and by numerous bleb-like protrusions on its surface. This cell is in mitosis. ×1000. C: Transmission electron micrograph. As a second type of free connective tissue cells, mast cells are observed in villous tissues. Their prevailing location is in the vicinity of larger fetal vessels of stem villi. This cell type is easily identified by its typical secretory granules. ×16,000.

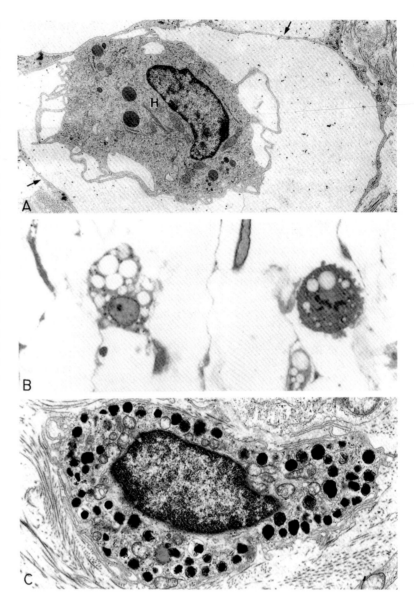

cells involved in the reduction of fetal serum proteins contained in the villous stroma and in the water balance of the early placenta. This function is also likely because the placenta lacks a lymphatic system to return proteins from the interstitial space to the blood vascular system (Enders & King, 1970). Closely related to these concepts is the presence of stromal channels that could allow relatively easy movement of Hofbauer cells along the villous cores of chorionic villi and thus function as a substitute for the lymphatic system (Enders & King, 1970; Castellucci & Kaufmann, 1982a). It must be considered, however, that the motility of Hofbauer cells is hindered, at least in part, in the villi during the last trimester. Here, the stromal channels are mostly narrow or absent (see Figs. 6.24 and 7.11). It is therefore conceivable that the Hofbauer cells assume additional tasks in these villi (Martinoli et al., 1984).

- Moreover, the motility of Hofbauer cells inside the stromal channels might allow these macrophages to exert their role in maintaining **host defense** (Castellucci et al., 1980; Wood, 1980).
- Last but not least, Hofbauer cells are thought to control villous development by (1) remodeling of the villous core by stimulating or inhibiting the proliferation of other mesenchymal cells (Castellucci et al., 1980; Martinoli et al., 1984; King, 1987), (2) controlling villous angiogenesis by secreting angiogenetic cytokines (see Chapter 7), and (3) controlling trophoblast turnover by inducing trophoblast apoptosis and syncytial fusion (see earlier in this chapter).
- Several authors have speculated on questionable endocrine activities of Hofbauer cells (Acconci, 1925; Pescetto, 1952; Rodway & Marsh, 1956). Prosdocimi (1953) suggested hCG synthesis by these cells, and

we detected hCG immunohistochemically within Hofbauer cells (Kaufmann & Stark, 1973); however, it was unlikely that this glycoprotein was synthesized in the cells but, rather, that it was phagocytosed from the surrounding environment. Still, the regular presence of hCG proves to be a useful marker for villous macrophages (Frauli & Ludwig, 1987b); on the other hand, phagocytic activity must be considered when interpreting immunohistochemical findings concerning the presence of proteins in these macrophages, such as hormones and placental proteins.

Occurrence and Distribution

Some initial reports of Hofbauer cells described them to be present in villi that had undergone hydatid degeneration (Virchow, 1871; Chaletzky, 1891; Neumann, 1897); however, for 100 years it has been established that these cells are present in both normal and pathologic conditions (Hofbauer, 1903, 1905, 1925; Graf Spee, 1915; Lewis, 1924; for reviews, see Bourne, 1962; Boyd & Hamilton, 1970; Becker & Röckelein, 1989; Fox, 1997).

Hofbauer cells are first seen in placental villi on day 18 p.c. (Boyd & Hamilton, 1970). In normal pregnancies, they are always present in the villi of immature placentas (Fig. 7.7B,C). It has been claimed that, in placentas from uncomplicated pregnancies, Hofbauer cells either disappear or become scanty after the 4th to 5th month of gestation (see Fox, 1967a, 1997). Geller (1957), Bleyl (1962), Fox (1967a), and several electron microscopy studies have demonstrated, however, that Hofbauer cells are present until term, and not only in immature villi of the center of the placentone (compare Figs. 7.7D and 7.11). The apparent reduction in number as pregnancy progresses occurs because they are compressed and masked by the condensation of the villous stroma (see Fig. 7.11) during placental maturation (Fox, 1967a). This view is supported by Bleyl (1962), who found many Hofbauer cells in villi in which edema is produced by postpartum saline perfusion through the umbilical artery. In normal term placentas, Hofbauer cells can easily be recognized by structural means only in immature intermediate villi. Immunohistochemistry using macrophage markers, however, reveals that a high percentage if not the majority of stromal cells in term placental villi has macrophage character (Fig. 6.28) and thus belongs to the Hofbauer cells.

They are more easily identifiable in many cases of pregnancy pathologies, for example, in placentas from delayed villous maturation, in prematurely delivered placentas, and in cases of maternal diabetes (Horky, 1964; Fox, 1967a, 1997), as well as in rhesus incompatibility (Hörmann, 1947; Thomsen & Berle, 1960; De Cecco et al., 1963; for review, see Fox, 1997). Fox (1967a, 1997) emphasized that villous edema, occurring in the two latter

pathologic conditions by the distention of the villous stroma, can unmask numerous Hofbauer cells.

Hofbauer cells have also been described in placental membranes, in both amnion and chorion laeve (Meyer, 1919; Bautzmann & Schröder, 1955; Schmidt, 1956; Bourne, 1962; for review, see Boyd & Hamilton, 1970).

Origin

The origin of Hofbauer cells has received much attention, starting with the first descriptions (for historical details and reviews, see Geller, 1957; Snoeck, 1958; Bourne, 1962; Wynn, 1967a; Boyd & Hamilton, 1970; Vacek, 1970; Schiebler & Kaufmann, 1981). Numerous theories have been abandoned. These include those proposed by Chaletzky (1891), who derived them from cells of maternal decidua; those by Neumann (1897), who considered them to be derivatives of the syncytium and an expression of malignancy; and those by ten Berge (1922), who supposed them to be derivatives of endothelial cells.

An important finding concerning the origin of Hofbauer cells was Wynn's (1967b) observation, based on sex chromatin staining, that these are fetal cells. This allows different interpretations:

- Most authors now consider Hofbauer cells to be of chorionic mesenchymal origin. That means that these cells gradually differentiate from the fixed stromal cells of the villous core (Fox, 1967a; Wynn, 1967a; Vacek, 1970; Kaufmann et al., 1977b). Morphologic investigations originally have questioned this concept (Martinoli et al., 1984; King, 1987) because no transitional forms between the two cell types have been clearly recognized. There are, however, some observations in the placenta (Demir et al., 1989) and on macrophages in other organs (Sorokin and Hoyt, 1987, 1992; Naito et al., 1989; Mebius et al., 1991; Sorokin et al., 1992a,b), that require one to consider this concept honestly. Hofbauer cells very likely originate from mesenchymal cells during the early stages of pregnancy, before the fetal circulation is established (see Chapter 7, Fig. 7.22).
- Later, once fetal circulation is established, the Hofbauer cells may additionally originate from fetal bone marrow–derived monocytes, as macrophages in other organs do (van Furth, 1982; Castellucci et al., 1987). Indeed, Moskalewski et al. (1975) observed transitional forms between Hofbauer cells and monocytes. Concerning this hypothesis, it must be emphasized that human cord blood contains almost three times as many monocytes at the end of pregnancy as does adult blood (Khansari & Fudenberg, 1984; Santiago-Schwarz & Fleit, 1988). These monocytes show subpopulations with considerable functional heterogeneity (Khansari & Fudenberg, 1984).

- Finally, it has been proposed that Hofbauer cells may have different origins throughout gestation and that they may represent a heterogeneous group of cells (Castellucci et al., 1987). These data related to in vivo (Fig. 6.28B) and in vitro observations, stating that Hofbauer cells can undergo mitotic division (Hofbauer, 1903; Hörmann, 1947; Geller, 1957; Boyd & Hamilton, 1970; Castellucci et al., 1985, 1987; Frauli & Ludwig, 1987b). Mitosis of Hofbauer cells (Fig. 6.28B) may be important for the permanent presence of cell subpopulations with different origins and functions. In addition, the mitotic activity suggests that they may be, in part, an independent self-replicating population, allowing rapid increase in number when required by the local microenvironment (Castellucci et al., 1987).

Immunologic Aspects

Immunologic data indicate that Hofbauer cells are numerous in the chorionic plate and in the villous stroma throughout pregnancy (Wood, 1980; Goldstein et al., 1988; Vince & Johnson, 1996). Studies on isolated Hofbauer cells, as well as immunohistochemical investigations, have provided data that have furthered our knowledge concerning the immunologic role of this cell population. Isolation of Hofbauer cells has usually employed proteolytic enzymes (Moskalewski et al., 1975; Wood et al., 1978a,b; Flynn et al., 1982; Loke et al., 1982; Frauli & Ludwig, 1987a), a combination of enzymatic digestion and density gradient centrifugation (Wilson et al., 1983; Uren & Boyle, 1985; Sutton et al., 1989). Additionally, cell separation methods, based on mechanical action with (Zaccheo et al., 1989) or without (Oliveira et al., 1986) density gradient centrifugation have been used. It has been demonstrated that Hofbauer cells possess Fc receptors for immunoglobulin G (Moskalewski et al., 1975; Wood et al., 1978a,b; Wood, 1980; Johnson & Brown, 1981; Loke et al., 1982; Zaccheo et al., 1982; Uren & Boyle, 1985; Oliveira et al., 1986; Goldstein et al., 1988).

Three different subtypes of leukocyte Fc receptors (FcR) have been identified on the basis of molecular and chemical analysis as well as cloning of cDNA; FcRI (CD64), FcRII (CD32), and FcRIII (CD16) (Stengelin et al., 1988). The three subtypes are expressed on the Hofbauer cells (Goldstein et al., 1988; Kristoffersen et al., 1990; Kameda et al., 1991; Sedmak et al., 1991; Wainwright & Holmes, 1993; Bright et al., 1994), and these receptors have been postulated to serve a protective function by binding maternal antifetal antigen-antibody complexes (Wood, 1980; Johnson & Brown, 1981; Goldstein et al., 1988).

C3b receptor (CR1[CD35]) activity has been shown on isolated Hofbauer cells by only some authors (Wood, 1980; Loke et al., 1982; Oliveira et al., 1986). Others have failed to detect C3b receptors in human placental sections using either tissue hemabsorption techniques with C3b-coated erythrocytes (Faulk et al., 1980), or monoclonal antibodies against C3b receptor (Bulmer & Johnson, 1984; Goldstein et al., 1988). By application of monoclonal antibodies on tissue sections, Goldstein et al. (1988) demonstrated that receptors for the C3bi complement component (CR3 [CD11b/CD18] and CR4 [CD11c/CD18]) are expressed by Hofbauer cells. Moreover, Hofbauer cells are capable of immune and nonimmune phagocytosis (Moskalewski et al., 1975; Wood, 1980; Loke et al., 1982; Wilson et al., 1983; Uren & Boyle, 1985; Oliveira et al., 1986; Zaccheo et al., 1989) and elimination of exogenous antigen-antibody complexes (Wood & King, 1982).

Hofbauer cells also show strong immunostaining for the protease inhibitors α_1-antitrypsin and α_1-antichymotrypsin (Braunhut et al., 1984; Castellucci et al., 1994) suggesting that placental macrophages are involved in villous remodeling and differentiation (Castellucci et al., 1994). Braunhut et al. (1984) failed to demonstrate lysozyme in the cells derived from term placentas when using immunohistochemical methods. Zaccheo et al. (1989) showed that Hofbauer cells from first trimester placentas are capable of secreting lysozyme in vitro. It is at present not clear whether these discrepant results are due to the different techniques used or whether they reflect a functional heterogeneity in lysozyme production between Hofbauer cells from the first trimester and those at term.

Hofbauer cells have been shown to bear Toll-like receptors (TLRs) as TLR4 (Kumazaki et al., 2004). The TLRs are essential for innate immune responses. Indeed, the immune system can be broadly categorized into innate immunity and adaptive immunity. The innate immunity system provides a rapid nonspecific response that acts as the first line of defense against pathogens. Recent reports suggest that innate immune responses are activated by TLRs that recognize certain molecular patterns derived from pathogens and stimulate proinflammatory cytokine gene transcription (Aderem & Ulevitch, 2000; Akira et al., 2001). A protein family that is homologous to Toll has been identified in humans and termed TLR (Rock et al., 1998; Aderem & Ulevitch, 2000). TLR4 has been genetically identified as a mediator of lipopolysaccharide (LPS)-induced signal transduction (Poltorak et al., 1998). Effective TLR4 activation by LPS requires the interaction of LPS with CD14 (see below) and the accessory protein MD-2, which associates with surface TLR4 molecules (Akira et al., 2001). TLR can also be activated by other kinds of molecules such as heat shock proteins (Ohashi et al., 2000) and cellular fibronectin fragments (Okamura et al., 2001). Interestingly, Kumazaki et al. (2004) showed an increased expression of TLR4 in the villous Hofbauer cells of preterm chorioamnionitis, suggesting an important role of the villous Hofbauer cells in the activation of innate immune responses.

It has been established that Hofbauer cells can express class I and II major histocompatibility complex (MHC) determinants (Bulmer & Johnson, 1984; Uren & Boyle, 1985; Sutton et al., 1986; Bulmer et al., 1988; Blaschitz et al., 2001). Concerning the class II MHC determinants, it is well known that they include at least three well-defined subregions: DR, DP, and DQ. First trimester Hofbauer cells are rarely DR- and DP-positive, and DQ antigens are not expressed (Bulmer & Johnson, 1984; Sutton et al., 1986; Bulmer et al., 1988; Goldstein et al., 1988; Lessin et al., 1988; Zaccheo et al., 1989). It may be important that DQ antigens, missing on first trimester cells, are restriction elements for T-cell clones (Thorsby, 1984) and have been implicated in the generation of cytotoxic cells (Corte et al., 1982). Class II MHC antigens are acquired by increasing numbers of placental macrophages from the second trimester on (Edwards et al., 1985; Sutton et al., 1986; Bulmer et al., 1988; Goldstein et al., 1988; Lessin et al., 1988; for a review, see Vince and Johnson, 1996). In term placental tissues, DR-positive villous stromal macrophages are often observed within groups of closely associated chorionic villi (Bulmer & Johnson, 1984; Bulmer et al., 1988). On the other hand, DP and DQ antigens are detected on a small number of Hofbauer cells, mostly located in villi immediately adjacent to the basal plate (Bulmer et al., 1988). In addition, such DP or DQ antigens are not detected in the absence of DR antigens on any placental macrophage (Bulmer et al., 1988). The patchy expression of class II MHC antigens in chorionic villi and the accumulation of DR-, DP-, and DQ-positive cells at the villous decidual junction may indicate areas of enhanced immune stimulation. Although clear evidence is still lacking, these data, and particularly the increasing expression of DR antigens as gestation proceeds, may represent acquisition of antigen-presenting capacity by the Hofbauer cells to fetal lymphocytes. This point may be relevant for fetal responses to transplacental infection.

Goldstein et al. (1988), Nakamura & Ohta (1990), and Lairmore et al. (1993) have shown that Hofbauer cells react strongly with antibodies to the CD4 antigen throughout gestation. This cell-surface glycoprotein is thought to interact with nonpolymorphic determinants of class II MHC molecules (Lamarre et al., 1989). The antigen is present on the T-helper subset of lymphocytes and has been shown to be expressed weakly by blood monocytes, some tissue macrophages, and dendritic cells (Wood et al., 1983, 1985; Buckley et al., 1987). It also functions as the membrane "receptor" for infection of cells by the human immunodeficiency virus (HIV). Lewis et al. (1990) have identified HIV-1 antigen and nucleic acid by immunohistochemical and in situ hybridization techniques in Hofbauer cells of placentas from seropositive patients.

This result has been confirmed in studies of HIV infection of cultured human placental cells where double labeling has demonstrated that the HIV-positive cells are macrophages and not trophoblast (McGann et al., 1994). Thus, the Hofbauer cells could serve as the portal of entry or reservoir for HIV in fetuses of HIV-positive women (Lairmore et al., 1993). The CD4 antigen seems not to be expressed on the surfaces of syncytiotrophoblast (Cuthbert et al., 1992).

One of the most consistent immunohistologic markers of Hofbauer cells throughout gestation is the monoclonal antibody leu-M3 (Fig. 6.27) (Bulmer & Johnson, 1984; Zaccheo et al., 1989). This antibody detects the CD14 monocyte differentiation antigen (Goyert et al., 1986), which is a 55-kd glycoprotein, expressed primarily by monocytes and macrophages (Goyert et al., 1988); it is anchored to the cell membrane by a phosphatidylinositol linkage (Haziot et al., 1988). Its restricted expression on mature cells suggests an important effector function (Goyert et al., 1988). In addition, it has been shown that the gene encoding CD14 is located in a region of chromosome 5 (Goyert et al., 1988) known to encode several growth factors or receptors, including interleukin-3 (IL-3), granulocyte-macrophage colony-stimulating factor (GM-CSF), CSF-1, CSF-1 receptor, and the platelet-derived growth factor receptor. Thus, it has been suggested that the CD14 antigen may also serve as some type of growth factor receptor (Goyert et al., 1988; Ziegler-Heitbrock, 1989), which could be involved in the regulation of the activity of the Hofbauer cells related to the process of villous morphogenesis (Castellucci et al., 1980; Martinoli et al., 1984; King, 1987). CD14 has been found to bind complexes of LPS and LPS-binding protein (Wright et al., 1990). These data suggest that CD14 could play an important role in infections. Some but not all studies have shown that Hofbauer cells express the leukocyte marker CD1 (as recognized by the monoclonal antibody NA1/34), the expression of which is reduced as gestation progresses (Bulmer & Johnson, 1984; Sutton et al., 1986; Goldstein et al., 1988; for a review, see Vince & Johnson, 1996).

Type I interferons (IFN-α, IFN-β) are molecules with multiple biologic activities (reviewed by Russel & Pace, 1987); IFN-α has been found (by immunohistochemical methods) in Hofbauer cells (Howatson et al., 1988; Bulmer et al., 1990); IFN-β has been demonstrated to be produced by isolated Hofbauer cells, particularly in large amounts after priming (Toth et al., 1991). Thus, in vivo the interferon produced by the trophoblast (Toth et al., 1990) could prime placental macrophages and induce these cells to secrete large amounts of interferon. Type I interferons may play important roles in the protection of the fetus against intrauterine infection, in several differentiation processes, and can interact with interferon-γ and other cytokines (Wang et al., 1981;

Taylor-Papadimitriou & Rozengurt, 1985; Hunt, 1989; Toth et al., 1991).

Flynn et al. (1982, 1985), and Glover et al. (1987) showed that placental villous macrophages produce IL-1. Because the antigen presentation correlates with class II antigen expression and IL-1 secretion, the authors suggested that fetal placental macrophages function nearly as efficiently as adult cells for antigen presentation (Glover et al., 1987), which could present a hazard for maintenance of the fetal allograft. They hypothesized that competence for tissue-specific factors or other mediators (Glover et al., 1987) may regulate antigen presentation. In support of this idea is the study by Yagel et al. (1987), which showed that physiologic concentrations of progesterone induced a significant increase in fetal placental macrophage prostaglandin E_2, a potent immunosuppressant. This finding suggested a functional role for fetal placental macrophages in immunosuppression at the fetomaternal surface. Isolated Hofbauer cells consistently demonstrated inhibition or suppression of both mixed lymphocyte reaction (MLR) and cell-mediated lympholysis (CML) (Uren & Boyle, 1990). Therefore, Hofbauer cells may in fact exert a sentinel function that would prevent strong, destructive maternal T-cell responses against the fetus. These data are also in agreement with the observation of Mues et al. (1989), who detected a large number of Hofbauer cells positive for the monoclonal antibody RM3/1. This antibody recognizes an antigen that is strongly induced by dexamethasone, but downregulated by interferon-γ, LPS, and triphorbolacetate on in vitro cultured monocytes. In vivo, RM3/1 macrophage populations are the predominant cells in liver and heart allografts from patients receiving a high-dose corticosteroid medication (Mues et al., 1989). The dominance of a corticosteroid-induced antiinflammatory macrophage phenotype within the placental villous core suggests localized immunosuppression, and it is probably related to the fact that cortisone is a prominent steroid in the human placenta (Murphy, 1979). In this context the observation of Moussa et al. (2001) showing that Hofbauer cells produce a classical chemokine, the macrophage inflammatory protein 1 (MIP1) beta is intriguing.

Interleukin-1 is a well-known stimulus for T-lymphocyte IL-2 production, and therefore placental macrophage-derived IL-1 may stimulate the expression of IL-2 by placental components. Indeed, Boehm et al. (1989b) pointed out that the IL-2 gene is expressed in the syncytiotrophoblast of the human placenta. Interleukin-2 is an important regulator of immune function. If it is produced by the syncytiotrophoblast it would most certainly play a major role in any scheme of immune interaction(s) postulated to exist between the mother and the fetoplacental graft.

Other macrophage cytokines of special interest for villous cell biology are TNF-α and TGF-β; TGF-β and TGF-β mRNA have been isolated from the human placenta (Frolik et al., 1983). This growth factor is a multifunctional peptide involved in immunosuppressive activities and, depending on the cell type, in stimulation or inhibition of cell growth (Miller et al., 1990; Sporn & Roberts, 1990). Concerning the human placenta, Morrish et al. (1991) have shown that it acts as a major inhibitor of trophoblast differentiation and concomitant peptide secretion. Tumor necrosis factor-α binding to its p55 receptor, which is expressed by villous cytotrophoblast, induces trophoblast apoptosis in vitro (Yui et al., 1996). This finding is in agreement with other data that showed that villous trophoblastic apoptosis is started already on the cellular level (Huppertz et al., 1998; for review see Huppertz 2001, 2003).

Other Free Connective Tissue Cells

Most free connective tissue cells of the human placental villi have been identified to be macrophages. There are a few cells, however, without macrophage character, among which are mast cells and plasma cells. Pescetto (1950), Latta and Beber (1953), Mahnke and Jacob (1972), and Durst-Zivkovic (1973) have reported the structural peculiarities of mast cells (Fig. 6.28C). According to these reports, the cells are found mainly in the walls of the large fetal blood vessels of stem villi. Structurally, they correspond to mast cells of other origin. The same is true for plasma cells, the occasional appearance of which in the stroma of stem villi of immature placentas has been reported by Benirschke and Bourne (1958); it is often seen in various types of chronic villitis.

Basic Structure of the Vessel Walls

The fetal placental vessels vary little from the vessels of other organs. Only some peculiarities, which may be considered placenta-specific, shall be listed below (for details, see Kaufmann & Miller, 1988).

Fetal Capillaries

The endothelial cells of capillaries and sinusoids are arranged as a monolayer (Fig. 6.29). During the last trimester, they rest on a basal lamina. The cells are connected to each other by intercellular junctions. Although the rat and mouse placentas display a fenestrated endothelium (Metz et al., 1976; Heinrich et al., 1977), a continuous endothelium is found in the human, guinea pig, and rabbit placenta (Becker & Seifert, 1965; Heinrich et al., 1976, 1977; Kaufmann et al., 1982; Orgnero de Gaisan et al., 1985). Whether it is valid for all segments—from the arterial beginning to the venous end of the long capillary loops—of both the perivascular capillaries and the terminal capillary bed is unresolved. In the human, two types of endothelial cells have been described that differ ultrastructurally (Nikolov & Schiebler, 1973, 1981; Heinrich et al., 1976). Normally, these cell types can be found in the same capillary cross section (Fig. 6.29C). Also, the lectin-binding patterns point to a considerable heterogeneity of the fetal villous endothelium (Lang et al., 1993a, 1994a,b).

The lateral intercellular spaces that separate the single endothelial cells are bridged by intercellular junctions (Fig. 6.29C), which serve as mechanical links between apposed cells and as gates that limit permeability for the paracellular transfer route. In the human placental capillaries and sinusoids, most of these junctions according to their structural features are tight junctions (zonulae occludentes) (Heinrich et al., 1988; Firth & Leach, 1996, 1997; Leach & Firth, 1997). They are known to limit paracellular transfer along the intercellular clefts to molecules of a molecular weight of about 40,000 daltons (molecular diameter about 6 nm) or less. Because of this, the transendothelial transport of immunoglobulin G takes place via plasmalemmal vesicles (Leach et al., 1989). As a second parameter, the molecular charge influences the permeability: This molecular size is valid for cationic probes, whereas anionic molecules of even smaller size may not pass (Firth et al., 1988).

Interestingly, the tight junction molecule occludin was not found in capillaries of peripheral villous exchange vessels but rather within the endothelium of villous stem vessels (Leach et al., 2000). By contrast, the same authors found the tight junction molecule ZO-1 throughout the endothelium of all types of villous vessels. Occludin is not necessarily involved in the permeability features of tight junctions but may be important for their mechanical features. Therefore, this differential expression pattern may simply point to increased plasticity of capillaries and sinusoids in the periphery of villous trees where full functional activity and continuous expansion of the exchange surfaces are required simultaneously.

There exist some hints that the transplacental traffic of smaller molecules is influenced by the capillary endothelium. Mühlhauser et al. (1994) found immunoreactivity of carbonic anhydrase isoenzymes I and II in fetal villous endothelium, which suggests that the capillaries are actively involved in fetomaternal bicarbonate transfer and thus in carbon dioxide removal and fetal pH regulation. During the second and third trimesters, the human villous endothelium acquires insulin receptors that were present in the first trimester only at the intervillous surface of the syncytiotrophoblast (Jones et al., 1993; Desoye et al., 1994, 1997). It is still an open question whether the endothelial receptors bind fetal insulin to regulate maternofetal glucose transfer. Another explanation would be that fetal insulin acts as a growth factor regulating endothelial proliferation and villous angiogenesis according to the fetal demands.

To provide experimental access to fetal villous endothelium and to assess potential organ-specific differences as compared to other systemic endothelium, attempts were made to isolate villous endothelial cells. Lang et al. (1993b, 2001) and Leach et al. (1993, 1994) have developed respective isolation protocols that partly allow differential isolation of villous macro- and microvascular endothelium.

Large Fetal Vessels

The composition of arterial and venous walls of the stem villi largely corresponds to that of the vessels of the chorionic plate and of the umbilical cord (see Chapter 12). In both vessel types, elastic membranes are largely absent. The muscular coats are thinner, and the muscle cells are more dispersed than in corresponding arteries and veins of other organs (Fig. 7.3A).

Nikolov and Schiebler (1973) described numerous myoendothelial contacts. Extensions of smooth muscle cells, as well as of endothelial cells, pass through gaps in the basal lamina into the neighboring layer, where they establish intense intercellular contacts. The attached parts of either cell type are characterized by increased amounts of plasmalemmal vesicles. Nikolov and Schiebler have interpreted this as a "musculoendothelial system" that may have importance for an autonomous, local vasoregulation. Such local regulatory mechanisms of fetal intravillous blood flow must exist, as nerves are absent in the fetoplacental vessel system.

In conventional histologic sections, the arteries and arterioles are often characterized by inappropriately preserved endothelium. It mostly appears to be columnar and the hydropic endothelial cell bodies partly obstruct the lumens. Moreover, deep herniation of muscle cells through gaps in the basal lamina, between or into the endothelial cells, is a usual finding. Such features have been interpreted as results of pathologic processes such as in placentas of HIV-infected mothers (Jimenez et al., 1988). Röckelein and Hey (1985; Hey & Röckelein, 1989) opposed this interpretation. They found endothelial hydrops and myoendothelial herniation to be the results of delayed immersion fixation. It could have been avoided by perfusion fixation of the fetal vascular system. We have shown wide vascular lumina, surrounded by flat endothelium, in large vessels following fetal or maternal perfusion fixation (Fig. 7.3A,B; compare these with the occluded arteriole in the lower right of Fig. 7.7B, obtained from an immersion-fixed specimen).

These considerations do not rule out the possibility that in vivo constrictions or occlusions of the major fetal arteries and arterioles may occur and influence fetal hemodynamics of the placenta. Ample evidence exists that they occur frequently. These findings have achieved major importance in the interpretation of Doppler measurements of umbilical artery flow velocity waveforms (Trudinger et al., 1985; Jimenez et al., 1988; Nessmann et al., 1988). The influence of fixation artifacts must be carefully considered when evaluating factors such as arterial lumen width, endothelial hydrops, and myoendothelial herniation.

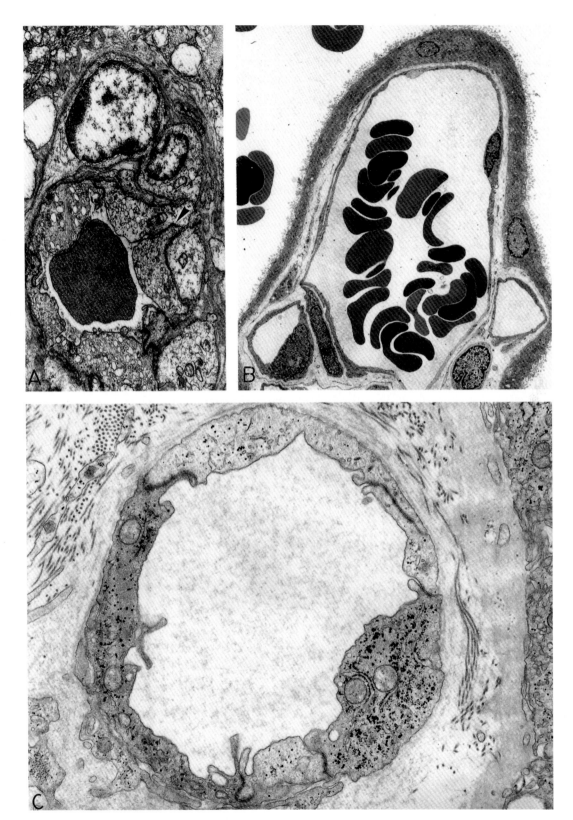

FIGURE 6.29. Comparison of fetal capillaries in delayed versus immediately fixed terminal villi. A: Fetal capillaries with endothelial cells protrude into the lumen and compress the erythrocytes. This phenomenon is best explained by postpartal capillary collapse caused by delayed fixation. In such cases, the tight junctions (arrows) are restricted to the basal parts of the endothelial cell bodies. ×10,300. (*Source:* Demir et al., 1989, with permission.) B: Distended terminal villi are characterized by a mixture of dilated fetal sinusoids with an extremely thin endothelium and neighboring smaller capillary cross sections with the same thin endothelial lining. Such pictures can usually be obtained only from immediately fixed specimens obtained at cesarean section. Even in this well-preserved specimen, angular shapes of the smaller capillaries point to early capillary collapse. ×2000. (*Source:* Demir et al., 1989, with permission.) C: Transmission electron micrograph of fetal vessel cross section at higher magnification demonstrates that the endothelial lining may be composed of differently structured endothelial cells. The functional meaning of this is uncertain. The darker cells, containing numerous filaments, may be contractile and may be involved in peripheral blood flow regulation. It is uncertain whether this vessel is a capillary or a small collecting venule. ×18,000.

Note that the distribution of major fetal vessels throughout the villous trees is not homogeneous. Its density (number of vessel cross sections per surface unit of histologic section) is highest in the centers of the villous trees near the chorionic plate, where the large trunci chorii and rami chorii and their branches prevail; it is lowest in the periphery of the villous trees (placentones), where we find predominantly mature, intermediate, and terminal villi. Thus, without a careful sampling regimen, meaningful results cannot be obtained (Mayhew & Burton, 1988). The principles of sampling and tissue preservation, and of the structural heterogeneity of the organ with artifacts that bias central findings, are further explored in Chapter 28, Tables 28.6, 28.8, 28.9, and 28.10.

Vasomotor Control

Fetal vasoactivity has been described by several authors. Mayer et al. (1959), Sakata (1960), Freese (1966), and Panigel (1968) reported fetal vessel constriction by cinematographic methods. Lemtis (1970) found experimental proof for an uneven blood supply of the various villous trees and interpreted it to result from autonomous regulation and an attempt of adaptation to changing functional demands.

Several substances have been shown to participate in the vasomotor control of the fetoplacental vessels. The most potent vasodilator is the former endothelial-derived relaxing factor (EDRF) (Pinto et al., 1991), which is identical with **nitric oxide (NO)** (Myatt et al., 1991; for review, see Macara et al., 1993). Nitric oxide is formed from the conversion of l-arginine to citrulline by NO synthase (NOS). The activity of the latter enzyme has been found in human placental homogenates (King et al., 1995). The enzyme was found histochemically [reduced nicotinamide dinucleotide phosphate (NADPH) diaphorase], and endothelial NOS (eNOS) and macrophage NOS (mNOS), respectively, have been localized immunohistochemically in the fetal endothelium (Myatt et al., 1993, 1997), villous myofibroblasts (Schönfelder et al., 1993), Hofbauer cells (Myatt et al., 1997), and the syncytiotrophoblast (Myatt et al., 1993, 1997). In cultured trophoblast cells, NOS expression changed with changes in oxygen supply (Seligman et al., 1997).

Data on **carbon monoxide-mediated vasorelaxation** in the placenta are still scarce. From the two hemoxygenases (HOs) involved in CO metabolism, Yoshiki and coworkers (2000) found HO-1 to be constitutively expressed by villous trophoblast cells, whereas HO-2 expression by fetal villous endothelium and smooth muscle cells considerably increased throughout pregnancy (Yoshiki et al., 2000). Other authors described a less differential expression pattern across syncytio- and cytotrophoblast, endothelium, and smooth muscle (McLean et al., 2000; Lash et al., 2003). In preeclampsia expression of HO-2 is locally compromised, suggesting that either vasoregulation or hemoxygenase-related defense mechanisms against oxidate stress may be compromised, too (Lash et al., 2003).

Another vasodilator is **atrial natriuretic peptide**, the receptors of which have been detected in the smooth muscle cells of placental stem vessels (Salas et al., 1991).

Finally, also **calcitonin gene-related peptide** (CGRP) seems to be involved in fetoplacental vascular relaxation. The CGRP receptor was shown to be present in villous endothelium and in the underlying smooth musculature (Dong et al., 2004). In vitro, upon CGRP administration, the same authors were able to show dose-dependent relaxation of placental stem vessels.

Concerning vasoconstrictors, **endothelin-1** has been demonstrated biochemically in the human placenta (Hemsen et al., 1991) and localized to the trophoblast and endothelial cells of villous vessels (Malassine et al., 1993; Marinoni et al., 1995). Endothelin-1 receptor sites have been demonstrated on placental vascular smooth muscle cells, particularly within stem villi (Wilkes et al., 1990; Bourgeois et al., 1997).

Fibrinoid of the Villous Trees

Fibrinoid is a summarizing term for any acellular, eosinophilic, largely homogeneous substance in the placenta (see Fibrinoid in Chapter 9). Disseminated fibrinoid deposition in the intervillous space and the villous trees is a regular finding in every normal placenta. Excess amounts of fibrinoid deposits within and around villi may be pathologic events and are often incompatible with normal fetal outcome.

It is not surprising, then, that pathologists have classified and attempted to define the fibrinoid deposits in this area (Wilkin, 1965; Benirschke & Driscoll, 1967; Fox, 1967b, 1968, 1975; Oswald & Gerl, 1972; Becker, 1981). From an anatomical point of view, the nomenclature used by Fox (1967b, 1968, 1975) seems to be the most appropriate. He differentiated between

- **perivillous fibrin(oid)**, which surrounds more or less altered but still identifiable villi, and
- **intravillous fibrinoid** (subsyncytial fibrinoid, villous fibrinoid necrosis), which primarily affects the villous interior.

Although the two processes may later mix, they appear to have a different pathogenesis, at least in the beginning. Moreover, the composition of both types of fibrinoid is different.

Perivillous Fibrinoid

The perivillous fibrinoid or perivillous fibrin as defined by Fox (1967b, 1975) is probably identical with the microfibrinoid of Oswald and Gerl (1972) and with the gitter-infarct designated by Becker (1981). It probably partly overlaps with the fibrinoid found in the maternal floor infarction, discussed in Chapter 9.

Structure: Perivillous fibrinoid can be found in every term placenta, but Fox (1967b) identified macroscopically such deposits in only 22.3% of normal placentas after 37 weeks of pregnancy. In our own experience, this figure is much too low. A mature placenta, free from macroscopically identifiable perivillous fibrinoid, is a rare exception. Problems may exist only insofar as it might be impossible to differentiate macroscopically among perivillous fibrinoid, intravillous fibrinoid, and old intervillous hematomas. The diameter of perivillous deposits lies in most cases between a few hundred micrometers and some millimeters. Larger deposits that reach a few centimeters usually represent intervillous hematomas and displace villi rather than encasing them. The "placental floor infarction" is easily differentiated because of its large size and normally basal position, being directly connected to the basal plate.

Histologically, perivillous fibrinoid is lamellar in structure (Toth et al., 1973). Immunohistochemically, its superficial layer always represents **fibrin-type fibrinoid** (Frank et al., 1994) (see Chapter 9), which is a blood clot product. This layer may directly contact the trophoblastic lamina of the villi, or it may be followed by the more homogeneous **matrix-type fibrinoid** (see Chapter 9), a secretory product of large trophoblast cells that embeds the latter (Frank et al., 1994).

Perivillous fibrinoid either fills gaps in the syncytiotrophoblastic cover of villi or encases entire villi or even groups of villi. The syncytiotrophoblast of these villi degenerates during the early stages of fibrinoid formation, and in later stages it disappears completely. A thickened trophoblastic basal lamina surrounds the fibrotic villous stroma. Their fetal vessels sometimes remain intact, but in most cases, they obliterate.

The villous cytotrophoblast beneath perivillous fibrinoid may disappear or may show increased proliferation. Like the extravillous trophoblast cells of the basal plate, the cell islands, and the septa, the cells grow to considerable size. Immunohistochemically, they cannot be distinguished from extravillous trophoblast cells of other localizations. They partly lose their connection to the basal lamina and develop in strings or as single cells deep in the fibrinoid (Villee, 1960; Wilkin, 1965; Fox, 1967b), adding by secretion and degeneration additional matrix-type fibrinoid.

This finding suggests that villous cytotrophoblast (Langhans' cells) and extravillous cytotrophoblast do not represent two completely different lines of trophoblast differentiation that separate during the early stages of placentation. Rather it implies that villous trophoblast cells even in late pregnancy can be transformed into extravillous ones, losing their

polarization and secreting matrix-type fibrinoid instead of a basal lamina, as soon as these cells are covered by fibrin-type fibrinoid rather than by villous syncytiotrophoblast.

Origin: Moe and Joergensen (1968) studied aggregates of platelets at the villous syncytial surfaces by electron microscopy and described these aggregates as representing the initial stages of fibrinoid deposition. Also according to Fox (1967b), syncytiotrophoblastic degeneration is only a secondary phenomenon that is introduced by platelet aggregation on the intact syncytial surfaces. The latter process is thought to be caused by a disturbed intervillous circulation.

On the other hand, it is known that collagens (Kunicki et al., 1988), fibronectins (Piotrowicz et al., 1988), and laminin (Sonnenberg et al., 1988) can initiate blood clotting. These molecules are constituents of the trophoblastic basal lamina. Thus, it is reasonable to assume that **focal degeneration of syncytiotrophoblast** with free exposure of the basal lamina to the intervillous blood results in local blood clotting and closure of the trophoblastic defect by a fibrinoid plug. As has been demonstrated by Edwards et al. (1991), it must be discussed how far such fibrinoid plugs are sufficient barriers controlling maternofetal macromolecule transfer.

Also our experimental studies in the pregnant guinea pig (Kaufmann et al., 1974b; Kaufmann, 1975b) led us to assume that, in addition to mere intervillous, circulatory factors, there are intrasyncytial causes for perivillous fibrinoid deposition. Inhibition of intrasyncytial energy metabolism, using monoiodine acetate or sodium fluoride, within minutes after application induced focal ultrastructural degenerative changes in the syncytiotrophoblast, followed by fibrin/fibrinoid deposition in the neighboring maternal blood. This finding is in agreement with older findings by Hörmann (1965), who considered that factors such as hypoxia and acidosis might lead to syncytial degeneration and eventually result in replacement of the syncytium by fibrinoid.

Statistical results published by Fox (1967b, 1975) suggested that perivillous fibrinoid is a more frequent phenomenon in placentas from normal pregnancies than in those involved in pathologic processes. This finding may be an indicator that just the maximal maternal perfusion of the intervillous space predisposes to perivillous fibrin deposition. In agreement with this conclusion, the same author failed to find any local or statistical correlation between perivillous fibrinoid and placental infarction. In general, there seemed to be no influence on fetal well-being.

Even though these findings and theories by Fox are supported by earlier publications (Siddall & Hartman, 1926; Huber et al., 1961), there are many reports that point in another direction. Eden (1897), who was probably also the first author to state that infarcts are the result of maternal vascular occlusion, considered derivation from blood coagulation and degeneration; Sala et al. (1982) found with stereologic techniques that significantly more fibrin was deposited in "venous" ("hypoxic") areas of the placenta, where there is stasis of blood. Huguenin (1909), Wilkin (1965), Boyd and Hamilton (1970), and Toth et al. (1973) considered perivillous fibrinoid to be the result of tropho-blastic degeneration. Boyd and Hamilton (1970) and Wilkin (1965) described fibrinoid deposition below the syncytiotrophoblast, preceding intervillous clotting. Thomsen (1954) reported cases of villous rupture with fetal bleeding into the intervillous space as being responsible for this process.

Intravillous Fibrinoid

Structure: Fox (1968) first described and defined a sepa-rate kind of fibrinoid that appears in the subtrophoblastic space and finally occupies the entire villous stroma. According to his views, as many as 3% of the villous cross sections may be replaced partially or completely by intra-villous fibrinoid during normal pregnancy. The intravil-lous deposition is increased in pregnancies complicated by such conditions as maternal diabetes, Rh-incompati-bility, and preeclampsia.

Composition and nature of the intravillous fibrinoid are still controversially discussed. Based on Liebhart's description (1971) of a primarily intracytotrophoblastic deposition, Fox (1975) concluded that this material cannot be fibrin. In contradistinction to what he has defined to be perivillous "fibrin," he proposed the term **intravillous**

fibrinoid. It seems obvious that an intact syncytiotropho-blastic barrier as well as an intact fetal capillary wall prevent a maternal or fetal fibrin imbibition of the villous interior. On the other hand, Moe (1969a–c) immunohis-tochemically demonstrated fibrinogen and fibrin in the cytotrophoblast. Moreover, several immunohistochemi-cal studies found proof for an intra-villous existence of fibrin and fibrinogen in both the trophoblastic basal lamina (McCormick et al., 1971) and the intravillous fibri-noid (Gille et al., 1974; Faulk et al., 1975), thus supporting earlier respective data (Kline, 1951; McKay et al., 1958; Wigglesworth, 1964). Finally, our own studies concerning the immunohistochemistry of fibrinoids (Frank et al., 1994) gave clear evidence that intravillous fibrinoid may contain both fibrin (fibrin-type fibrinoid) and extracellu-lar matrix molecules such as oncofetal fibronectin, laminin, and collagen IV (matrix-type fibrinoid) (see Origin of Fibrinoids in Chapter 9). Only the question as to a maternal or fetal derivation of the fibrin remained open.

Genesis: The process of intravillous fibrinoid deposi-tion is thought to be initiated by small, subsyncytially positioned nodules that are periodic acid-Schiff (PAS) positive. They later increase in size (Fig. 6.30) and finally

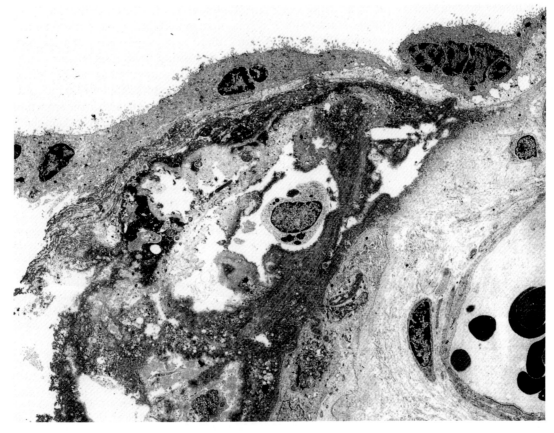

FIGURE 6.30. Intravillous fibrinoid. A large, heterogeneous plaque of fibrinoid intermingled with degenerative cellular remains and white blood cells is deposited between the syncytial covering of the villus and its stromal core. ×2400.

replace the stroma. This view has been supported by Wilkin (1965) and Boyd and Hamilton (1970). As stated by these authors, the originally intact syncytium degenerates only secondarily, if at all.

Liebhart (1971) has described degeneration of the villous cytotrophoblast as the initial process. Some immunologic studies have supported the idea of an extracellular fibrinoid deposition in the villous stroma, independent from cellular degeneration (Gille et al., 1974; Faulk et al., 1975). There has been ample discussion about whether this process is completely independent from the genesis of perivillous fibrinoid (Fox, 1967b) or whether it may be complicated by the latter (Wilkin, 1965; Boyd & Hamilton, 1970; Burstein et al., 1973).

Concerning the etiology of the formation of the intravillous fibrinoid, Fox (1968) discussed an immunologic attack against the villous cytotrophoblast. Wislocki and Bennett (1943) proposed villous degeneration as a result of placental aging to be the primary agent. The histologic and histochemical studies by Burstein and coworkers (1973) have provided some evidence that intravillous fibrinoid and amyloid might be identical, whereas perivillous fibrinoid showed staining patterns that were different from those of amyloid. In agreement with the extraplacental genesis of amyloid, these authors suggested that intravillous fibrinoid is a result of placental degeneration induced by aging and by immunologic processes.

Intravillous fibrinoid, involved in immunologic processes, has been discussed on many occasions. McCormick et al. (1971) described this type of fibrinoid as a result of antigen-antibody reactions in the villous stroma and as resulting in an immunologic barrier between maternal and fetal circulations. Burstein et al. (1963) have even named the villous stroma as an immunologic battlefield, as they found a specific stromal binding of insulin in cases of maternal diabetes mellitus and of anti-D antibodies in cases of Rh incompatibility. Differing slightly from the foregoing and based on experimental studies in healthy pregnant women, Gille et al. (1974) came to the conclusion that immunologic diseases may affect the syncytiotrophoblastic barrier. Consequently, the latter was thought to become permeable for antigen-antibody complexes, which then may become enriched and finally deposited as fibrinoid in the villous stroma.

References

Abe, E., Mocharla, H., Yamate, T., Taguchi Y. and Manolagas, S.C.: Meltrin-alpha, a fusion protein involved in multinucleated giant cell and osteoclast formation. Calcif. Tissue Int. **64**:508–515, 1999.

Aboagye-Mathiesen, G., Zdravkovic, M., Toth, F.D. and Ebbesen, P.: Effects of human trophoblast-induced interferons on the expression of proto-oncogenes c-fms/CSF-1R, EGF-R and c-erbB2 in invasive and non invasive trophoblast. Placenta **18**:155–161, 1997.

Acconci, G.: Mola vesicolare destruente e corioepitelioma. Folia Ginecol. (Genoa) **21**:253–268, 1925.

Adamson, E.D.: Review article: Expression of proto-oncogenes in the placenta. Placenta **8**:449–466, 1987.

Aderem, A. and Ulevitch, R.J.: Toll-like receptors in the induction of the innate immune response. Nature **406**:782–787, 2000.

Adler, R.R., Ng, A.K. and Rote, N.S.: Monoclonal antiphosphatidylserine antibody inhibits intercellular fusion of the choriocarcinoma line, JAR. Biol. Reprod. **53**:905–910, 1995.

Akira, S., Takeda, K. and Kaisho, T.: Toll-like receptors: critical proteins linking innate and acquired immunity. Nat. Immunol. 2:675–680, 2001.

Albe, K.R., Witkin, H.J., Kelley, L.K. and Smith, C.H.: Protein kinases of the human placental microvillous membrane. Exp. Cell Res. **147**:167–176, 1983.

Ali, K.Z.M.: Stereological study of the effect of altitude on the trophoblast cell populations of human term placental villi. Placenta **18**:447–450, 1997.

Alsat, E., Mondon, F., Rebourcet, R., Berthelier, M., Ehrlich, D., Cedard, L. and Goldstein, S.: Identification of specific binding sites for acetylated low density lipoprotein in microvillous membranes from human placenta. Mol. Cell. Endocrinol. **41**:229–235, 1985.

Alsat, E., Marcotty, C., Gabriel, R., Igout, A., Frankenne, F., Hennen, G. and Evain-Brion, D.: Molecular approach to intrauterine growth retardation: an overview of recent data. Reprod. Fertil. Dev. **7**:1457–1464, 1995.

Alsat, E., Guibourdenche, J., Luton, D., Frankenne, F. and Evain-Brion, D.: Human placental growth hormone. Amer. J. Obstet. Gynecol. **177**:1526–1534, 1997.

Alvarez, H.: Proliferation du trophoblaste et sa relation avec l'hypertension arterielle de la toxemie gravidique. Gynecol. Obstet. (Paris) **69**:581–588, 1970.

Alvarez, H., Benedetti, W.L., Morel, R.L. and Scavarelli, M.: Trophoblast development gradient and its relationship to placental hemodynamics. Amer. J. Obstet. Gynecol. **106**:416–420, 1970.

Alvarez, H., Medrano, C.V., Sala, M.A. and Benedetti, W.L.: Trophoblast development gradient and its relationship to placental hemodynamics. II. Study of fetal cotyledons from the toxemic placenta. Amer. J. Obstet. Gynecol. **114**:873–878, 1972.

Al-Zuhair, A.G.H., Ibrahim, M.E.H., Mughal, S. and Mohammed, M.E.: Scanning electron microscopy of maternal blood cells and their surface relationship with the placenta. Acta Obstet. Gynecol. Scand. **62**:493–498, 1983.

Al-Zuhair, A.G.H., Ibrahim, M.E.A., Mughal, S. and Abdulla, M.A.: Loss and regeneration of the microvilli of human placental syncytiotrophoblast. Arch. Gynecol. **240**:147–151, 1987.

Amaladoss, A.S. and Burton, G.J.: Organ culture of human placental villi in hypoxic and hyperoxic conditions: a morphometric study. J. Dev. Physiol. **7**:113–118, 1985.

Amenta, P.S., Gay, S., Vaheri, A. and Martinez-Hernandez, A.: The extracellular matrix is an integrated unit: ultrastructural localization of collagen types I, III, IV, V, VI, fibronectin, and laminin in human term placenta. Collagen Relat. Res. **6**:125–152, 1986.

Amstutz, E.: Beobachtungen Über die Reifung der Chorionzotten in der menschlichen Placenta mit besonderer Berücksichtigung der Epithelplatten. Acta Anat. (Basel) **42**:122–130, 1960.

Arnholdt, H., Meisel, F., Fandrey, K. and Löhrs, U.: Proliferation of villous trophoblast of the human placenta in normal and abnormal pregnancies. Virchows Arch. B Cell Pathol. **60**:365–372, 1991.

Arnold, M., Geller, H. and Sasse, D.: Beitrag zur elektronenmikroskopischen Morphologie der menschlichen Plazenta. Arch. Gynäkol. **196**:238–253, 1961.

Atwood, H.D. and Park, W.W.: Embolism to the lung by trophoblast. J. Obstet. Gynaecol. Br. Emp. **63**:611–617, 1961.

Aufderheide, E. and Ekblom, P.: Tenascin during gut development: appearance in the mesenchyme, shift in molecular forms, and dependence on epithelial-mesenchymal interaction. J. Cell Biol. **107**:2341–2349, 1988.

Autio-Harmainen, H., Sandberg, M., Pihlajaniemi, T. and Vuorio, E.: Synthesis of laminin and type IV collagen by trophoblastic cells and fibroblastic stromal cells in the early human placenta. Lab. Invest. **64**:483–491, 1991.

Autio-Harmainen, H., Hurskainen, T., Niskasaari, K., Höyhtyä, M. and Tryggvason, K.: Simultaneous expression of 70 kilodalton type IV collagenase and type IV collagen a1 (IV) chain genes by cells of early human placenta and gestational endometrium. Lab. Invest. **67**:191–200, 1992.

Baker, B.L., Hook, S.J. and Severinghaus, A.E.: The cytological structure of the human chorionic villus and decidua parietalis. Amer. J. Anat. **74**:291–325, 1944.

Bamberger, A., Schulte, H.M., Thuneke, I., Erdmann, I., Bamberger, C.M. and Asa, S.L.: Expression of the apoptosis-inducing Fas ligand (FasL) in human first and third trimester placenta and choriocarcinoma cells. J. Clin. Endocrinol. Metab. **82**:3173–3175, 1997.

Bargmann, W. and Knoop, A.: Elektronenmikroskopische Untersuchungen an Plazentarzotten des Menschen. Bemerkungen zum Synzytiumproblem. Z. Zellforsch. **50**:472–493, 1959.

Bautzmann, H. and Schröder, R.: Über Vorkommen und Bedeutung von "Hofbauerzellen" ausserhalb der Placenta. Arch. Gynäkol. **187**:65–76, 1955.

Beck, T., Schweikhart, G. and Stolz, E.: Immunohistochemical location of hPL, SP1 and β-hCG in normal placentas of varying gestational age. Arch. Gynecol. **239**:63–74, 1986.

Becker, V.: Gefäße der Chorionplatte und Stammzotten. In, Die Plazenta des Menschen. V. Becker, T.H. Schiebler and F. Kubli, eds. Thieme Verlag, Stuttgart, 1981.

Becker, V. and Bleyl, U.: Placentarzotte bei Schwangerschaftstoxicose und fetaler Erythroblastose im fluorescenzmikroskopischen Bilde. Virchows Arch. Pathol. Anat. **334**:516–527, 1961.

Becker, V. and Röckelein, G., eds.: Pathologie der weiblichen Genitalorgane. Springer-Verlag, Heidelberg, 1989.

Becker, V. and Seifert, K.: Die Ultrastruktur der Kapillarwand in der menschlichen Placenta zur Zeit der Schwangerschaftsmitte. Z. Zellforsch. **65**:380–396, 1965.

Beham, A., Denk, H. and Desoye, G.: The distribution of intermediate filament proteins, actin and desmoplakins in human placental tissue as revealed by polyclonal and monoclonal antibodies. Placenta **9**:479–492, 1988.

Benirschke, K. and Bourne, G.L.: Plasma cells in immature human placenta. Obstet. Gynecol. **12**:495–503, 1958.

Benirschke, K. and Driscoll, S.G.: The Pathology of the Human Placenta. Springer-Verlag, New York, 1967.

Benyo, D.F., Miles, T.M. and Conrad, K.P.: Hypoxia stimulates cytokine production by villous explants from the human placenta. J. Clin. Endocrinol. Metab. **82**:1582–1588, 1997.

Berryman, M., Gary, R. and Bretscher, A.: Ezrin oligomers are major cytoskeletal components of placental microvilli: a proposal for their involvement in cortical morphogenesis. J. Cell Biol. **131**:1231–1242, 1995.

Bevers, E.M., Comfurius, P. and Zwaal, R.F.: Regulatory mechanisms in maintenance and modulation of transmembrane lipid asymmetry: pathophysiological implications. Lupus **5**:480–487, 1996.

Bianco, P., Fisher, L.W., Young, M.F., Termine, J.D. and Robey, P.G.: Expression and localization of the two small proteoglycans biglycan and decorin in developing human skeletal and non-skeletal tissues. J. Histochem. Cytochem. **38**:1549–1563, 1990.

Bierings, M.B.: Placental iron uptake and its regulation. Med. Thesis, University of Rotterdam, 1989.

Bischof, P., Friedli, E., Martelli, M. and Campana, A.: Expression of extracellular matrix degrading metalloproteinases by cultured human cytotrophoblast cells. Effects of cell adhesion and immunopurification. Amer. J. Obstet. Gynecol. **165**:1791–1801, 1991.

Black, S., Kadyrov, M., Kaufmann, P., Ugele, B., Emans, N. and Huppertz, B.: Syncytial fusion of human trophoblast depends on caspase 8. Cell Death Differentiation **11**:90–98, 2004.

Blackburn, P. and Gavilanes, J.G.: The Role of lysine-41 of ribonuclease A in the interaction with RNAse inhibitor from human placenta. J. Biol. Chem. **255**:10959–10965, 1980.

Blaise, S., de Parseval, N., Benit, L. and Heidmann, T.: Genome-wide screening for fusogenic human endogenous retrovirus envelopes identifies syncytin 2, a gene conserved on primate evolution. Proc. Natl. Acad. Sci. USA **100**:13013–13018, 2003.

Blaschitz, A., Hutter, H. and Dohr, G.: HLA Class I protein expression in the human placenta. Early Pregnancy **5**:67–69, 2001.

Blay, J. and Hollenberg, M.D.: The nature and function of polypeptide growth factor receptors in the human placenta. J. Dev. Physiol. (Oxf.) **12**:237–248, 1989.

Bleyl, U.: Histologische, histochemische und fluoreszenzmikroskopische Untersuchungen an Hofbauer-Zellen. Arch. Gynäkol. **197**:364–386, 1962.

Blond, J.-L., Beseme, F., Duret, L., Bouton, O., Bedin, F., Perron, H., Mandrand, B. and Mallet F.: Molecular characterization and placental expression of HERV-W, a new human endogenous retrovirus family. J. Virol. **73**:1175–1185, 1999.

Blond, J.-L., Lavillette, D., Cheynet, V., Bouton, O., Oriol, G., Chapel-Fernandes, S., Mandrand, B., Mallet, F. and Cosset, F.-L.: An envelope glycoprotein of the human endogenous retrovirus HERV-W is expressed in the human placenta and fuses cells expressing the type D mammalian retrovirus receptor. J. Virol. **74**: 3321–3329, 2000.

Boehm, K.D., Kelley, M.F. and Ilan, J.: Expression of insulin-like growth factors by the human placenta. In, Molecular and Cellular Biology of Insulin-Like Growth Factors and Their

Receptors. D. Leroith and M.K. Raizada, eds., pp. 179–193. Plenum, New York, 1989a.

Boehm, K.D., Kelley, M.F., Ilan, J. and Ilan, J.: The interleukin 2 gene is expressed in the syncytiotrophoblast of the human placenta. Proc. Natl. Acad. Sci. U.S.A. **86**:656–660, 1989b.

Boime, I., Otani, T., Otani, F., Daniels-McQueen, S. and Bo, M.: Factors regulating peptide hormone biosynthesis in human placenta. In, Abstracts of the 11th Rochester Trophoblast Conference, Rochester N.Y., p. 1, 1988.

Borges, M., Bose, P., Frank, H.-G., Kaufmann, P. and Pötgens A.J.G.: A two-colour fluorescence assay fort he measurement of syncytial fusion between trophoblast-derived cell lines. Placenta, **24**:959–964, 2003.

Borst, R., Kussäther, E. and Schuhmann, R.: Ultrastrukturelle Untersuchungen zur Verteilung der alkalischen Phosphatase im Placenton (maternofetale Strömungseinheit) der menschlichen Placenta. Arch. Gynäkol. **215**:409–415, 1973.

Bourgeois, C., Robert, B., Rebourcet, R., Mondon, F., Mignot, T.M., Duc-Goiran, P. and Ferre, F.: Endothelin-1 and ETA receptor expression in vascular smooth muscle cells from human placenta: a new ETA receptor messenger ribonucleic acid is generated by alternative splicing of exon 3. J. Clin. Endocrinol. Metab. **82**:3116–3123, 1997.

Bourne, G.: The Human Amnion and Chorion. Lloyd-Luke, London, 1962.

Boyd, J.D. and Hamilton, W.J.: Electron microscopic observations on the cytotrophoblast contribution to the syncytium in the human placenta. J. Anat. **100**:535–548, 1966.

Boyd, J.D. and Hamilton, W.J.: Development and structure of the human placenta from the end of the 3rd month of gestation. J. Obstet. Gynaecol. Br. Commonw. **74**:161–226, 1967.

Boyd, J.D. and Hamilton, W.J.: The Human Placenta. Heffer, Cambridge, 1970.

Boyd, J.D. and Hughes, A.F.W.: Etude des villosites placentaires au moyen du microscope electronique. In, 6th Congress, International Federation of Anatomists, Abstract 32. Masson, Paris, 1955.

Boyd, J.D., Boyd, C.A.R. and Hamilton, W.J.: Observations on the vacuolar structure of the human syncytiotrophoblast. Z. Zellforsch. **88**:57–79, 1968a.

Boyd, J.D., Hamilton, W.J. and Boyd, C.A.R.: The surface of the syncytium of the human chorionic villus. J. Anat. **102**:553–563, 1968b.

Bozhok, J.M., Bannikov, G.A., Tavokina, L.V., Svitkina, T.M. and Troyanovsky, S.M.: Local expression of keratins 8, 17, and 19 in mesenchyme and smooth muscle at early stages of organogenesis in man. Ontogenesis **20**:250–257, 1990.

Bradbury, S., Billington, W.D., Kirby, D.R.S. and Williams, E.A.: Surface mucin of human trophoblast. Amer. J. Obstet. Gynecol. **104**:416–418, 1969.

Bradbury, S., Billington, W.D., Kirby, D.R.S. and Williams, E.A.: Histochemical characterization of the surface mucoprotein of normal and abnormal human trophoblast. Histochem. J. **2**:263–274, 1970.

Braunhut, S.J., Blanc, W.A., Ramanarayanan, M., Marboe, C. and Mesa-Tejada, R.: Immunocytochemical localization of lysozyme and alpha-1-antichymotrypsin in the term human placenta: an attempt to characterize the Hofbauer cell. J. Histochem. Cytochem. **32**:1204–1210, 1984.

Bray, B.A.: Presence of fibronectin in basement membranes and acidic structural glycoproteins from human placenta and lung. Ann. N.Y. Acad. Sci. **312**:142–150, 1978.

Bremer, J.L.: The interrelations of the mesonephros, kidney and placenta in different classes of mammals. Am. J. Anat. **19**:179–209, 1916.

Bright, N.A. and Ockleford, C.D.: Fc-γ receptor bearing cells in human term amniochorion. J. Anat. **183**:187–188, 1993.

Bright, N.A., Ockleford, C.D. and Anwar, M.: Ontogeny and distribution of Fc-γ receptors in the human placenta. Transport or immune surveillance? J. Anat. **184**:297–308, 1994.

Brown, P.J. and Johnson, P.M.: Isolation of a transferrin receptor structure from sodium deoxycholate-solubilized human placental syncytiotrophoblast plasma. Placenta **2**:1–10, 1981.

Bryant-Greenwood, G.D., Rees, M.C.P. and Turnbull, A.C.: Immunohistochemical localization of relaxin, prolactin and prostaglandin synthetase in human amnion, chorion and decidua. J. Endocrinol. **114**:491–496, 1987.

Buckley, P.J., Smith, M.R., Broverman, M.F. and Dickson, S.A.: Human spleen contains phenotypic subsets of macrophages and dendritic cells that occupy discrete microanatomic locations. Amer. J. Pathol. **128**:505–520, 1987.

Bukovsky, A., Cekanova, M., Caudle, M.R., Wimalasena, J., Foster, J.S., Henley, D.C. and Elder, R.F.: Expression and localization of estrogen receptor-alpha protein in normal and abnormal term placentae and stimulation of trophoblast differentiation by estradiol. Reprod. Biol. Endocrinol. **1**:13, 2003a.

Bukovsky, A., Caudle, M.R., Cekanova, M., Fernando, R.I., Wimalasena, J., Foster, J.S., Henley, D.C. and Elder, R.F.: Placental expression of estrogen receptor-beta and its hormone binding variant—comparison with estrogen receptor alpha and a role for estrogen receptor in asymmetric division and differentiation of estrogen-dependent cells. Reprod. Biol. Endocrinol. **1**:36, 2003b.

Bulmer, J.N. and Johnson, P.M.: Macrophage populations in the human placenta and amniochorion. Clin. Exp. Immunol. **57**:393–403, 1984.

Bulmer, J.N., Morrison, L. and Smith, J.C.: Expression of class II MHC gene products by macrophages in human uteroplacental tissue. Immunology **63**:707–714, 1988.

Bulmer, J.N., Thrower, S. and Wells, M.: Expression of epidermal growth factor receptor and transferrin receptor by human trophoblast populations. Am. J. Reprod. Immunol. **21**:87–93, 1989.

Bulmer, J., Morrison, L., Johnson, P.M. and Meager, A.: Immunohistochemical localization of interferons in human placental tissues in normal, ectopic, and molar pregnancy. Amer. J. Reprod. Immunol. **22**:109–116, 1990.

Burgos, M.H. and Rodriguez, E.M.: Specialized zones in the trophoblast of the human term placenta. Amer. J. Obstet. Gynecol. **96**:342–356, 1966.

Burstein, R., Berns, A.W., Hirtata, Y. and Blumenthal, H.T.: A comparative histo- and immunopathological study of the placenta in diabetes mellitus and in erythroblastosis fetalis. Amer. J. Obstet. Gynecol. **86**:66–76, 1963.

Burstein, R., Frankel, S., Soule, S.D. and Blumenthal, H.T.: Ageing in the placenta: autoimmune theory of senescence. Amer. J. Obstet. Gynecol. **116**:271–274, 1973.

Burton, G.J.: Intervillous connections in the mature human placenta: Instances of syncytial fusion or section artifacts? J. Anat. **145**:13–23, 1986a.

Burton, G.J.: Scanning electron microscopy of intervillous connections in the mature human placenta. J. Anat. **147**:245–254, 1986b.

Burton, G.J.: The fine structure of the human placental villus as revealed by scanning electron microscopy. Scanning Electron Microsc. **1**:1811–1828, 1987.

Burton, G.J., Mayhew, T.M. and Robertson, L.A.: Stereological re-examination of the effects of varying oxygen tensions on human placental villi maintained in organ culture for up to 12 h. Placenta **10**:263–273, 1989.

Burton, G.J., Skepper, J.N., Hempstock, J., Cindrova, T., Jones, C.J. and Jauniaux, E.: A reappraisal of the contrasting morphological appearances of villous cytotrophoblast cells during early human pregnancy; evidence for both apoptosis and primary necrosis. Placenta **24**:297–305, 2003.

Cantle, S.J., Kaufmann, P., Luckhardt, M. and Schweikhart, G.: Interpretation of syncytial sprouts and bridges in the human placenta. Placenta **8**:221–234, 1987.

Cariappa, R., Heath-Monnig, E. and Smith, C.H.: Isoforms of amino acid transporters in placental STB: plasma membrane localization and potential role in maternal/fetal transport. Placenta **24**:713–726, 2003.

Carter, J.E.: The ultrastructure of the human trophoblast. Transcripts, 2nd Rochester Trophoblast Conference, C.J. Lund and H.A. Thiede, eds., Plenum, New York, 1963.

Carter, J.E.: Morphologic evidence of syncytial formation from the cytotrophoblastic cells. Obstet. Gynecol. **23**:647–656, 1964.

Casalini, P., Iorio, M. V., Galmozzi, E. and Ménard, S.: Role of HER receptors family in development and differentiation. J. Cellular Physiol. **200**:343–350, 2004.

Castellucci, M. and Kaufmann, P.: A three-dimensional study of the normal human placental villous core: II. Stromal architecture. Placenta **3**:269–285, 1982a.

Castellucci, M. and Kaufmann, P.: Evolution of the stroma in human chorionic villi throughout pregnancy. Bibl. Anat. **22**:40–45, 1982b.

Castellucci, M. and Zaccheo, D.: The Hofbauer cells of the human placenta: morphological and immunological aspects. Prog. Clin. Biol. Res. **269**:443–451, 1989.

Castellucci, M., Zaccheo, D. and Pescetto, G.: A three-dimensional study of the normal human placental villous core. I. The Hofbauer cells. Cell Tissue Res. **210**:235–247, 1980.

Castellucci, M., Schweikhart, G., Kaufmann, P. and Zaccheo, D.: The stromal architecture of immature intermediate villus of the human placenta: functional and clinical implications. Gynecol. Obstet. Invest. **18**:95–99, 1984.

Castellucci, M., Richter, A., Steininger, B., Celona, A. and Schneider, J.: Light and electron microscopy identification of mitotic Hofbauer cells in the human placenta. Arch. Gynecol. **237**(suppl.):235, 1985.

Castellucci, M., Celona, A., Bartels, H., Steininger, B., Benedetto, V. and Kaufmann, P.: Mitosis of the Hofbauer cell: possible implications for a fetal macrophage. Placenta **8**:65–76, 1987.

Castellucci, M., Kaufmann, P. and Bischof, P.: Extracellular matrix influences hormone and protein production by human chorionic villi. Cell Tissue Res. **262**:135–142, 1990a.

Castellucci, M., Mühlhauser, J. and Zaccheo, D.: The Hofbauer cell: the macrophage of the human placenta. In, Immunobiology of Normal and Diabetic Pregnancy. D. Andreani, G. Bompiani, U. Di Mario, W.P. Faulk and A. Galluzzo, eds, pp. 135–144. Wiley, Chichester, 1990b.

Castellucci, M., Scheper, M., Scheffen, I., Celona, A. and Kaufmann, P.: The development of the human placental villous tree. Anat. Embryol. (Berl.) **181**:117–128, 1990c.

Castellucci, M., Classen-Linke, I., Mühlhauser, J., Kaufmann, P., Zardi, L. and Chiquet-Ehrismann, R.: The human placenta: a model for tenascin expression. Histochemistry **95**:449–458, 1991.

Castellucci, M., Crescimanno, C., Schroeter, C.A., Kaufmann, P. and Mühlhauser, J.: Extravillous trophoblast: Immunohistochemical localization of extracellular matrix molecules. In, Frontiers in Gynecologic and Obstetric Investigation. A.R. Genazzani, F. Petraglia and A.D. Genazzani, eds. Parthenon, New York, pp. 19–25, 1993a.

Castellucci, M., Crescimanno, C., Mühlhauser, J., Frank, H.G., Kaufmann, P. and Zardi, L.: Expression of extracellular matrix molecules related to placental development. Placenta **14**:A9, 1993b.

Castellucci, M., Mühlhauser, J., Pierleoni, C., Krusche, C., Crescimanno, C., Beier, H.M. and Kaufmann, P.: BCL-2 expression in the human trophoblast. Ann. Anat. **175**:38–39, 1993c.

Castellucci, M., Theelen, T., Pompili, E., Fumagalli, L., De Renzis G. and Mühlhauser, J.: Immunohistochemical localization of serine-protease inhibitors in the human placenta. Cell Tissue Res. **278**:283–289, 1994.

Castellucci, M., de Matteis, R., Meisser, A., Cancello, R., Monsurro, V., Islami, D., Sarzani, R., Marzioni, D., Cinti, S. and Bischof, P.: Leptin modulates extracellular matrix molecules and metalloproteinases: implications for trophoblast invasion. Mol. Hum. Reprod. **6**:951–958, 2000a.

Castellucci, M., Kosanke, G., Verdenelli, F., Huppertz, B. and Kaufmann, P.: Villous sprouting: fundamental mechanisms of human placental development. Hum. Reprod. Update **6**:485–494, 2000b.

Chaletzky, E.: Hydatidenmole. Thesis, University of Bern, 1891.

Chegini, N. and Rao, C.H.V.: Epidermal growth factor binding to human amnion, chorion, decidua, and placenta from mid- and term pregnancy: quantitative light microscopic autoradiographic studies. J. Clin. Endocrinol. Metabl. **61**:529–535, 1985.

Chen, C.-F., Kurachi, H., Fujita, Y., Terakawa, N., Miyake, A. and Tanizawa, O.: Changes in epidermal growth factor receptor and its messenger ribonucleic acid levels in human placenta and isolated trophoblast cells during pregnancy. J. Clin. Endocrinol. Metab. **67**:1171–1177, 1988.

Chen, C.P. and Aplin, J.D.: Placental extracellular matrix: gene expression, deposition by placental fibroblasts and the effect of oxygen. Placenta **24**:316–325, 2003.

Cheung, C.Y.: Vascular endothelial growth factor: possible role in fetal development and placental function. J. Soc. Gynecol. Invest. **4**:169–177, 1997.

Cho, C., Bunch, D.O., Faure, J.E., Goulding, E.H., Eddy, E.M., Primakoff, P. and Myles, D.G.: Fertilization defects in sperm from mice lacking fertilin beta. Science, **281**:1857–1859, 1998.

Cho, C., Turner, L., Primakoff, P. and Myles, D.G.: Genomic organization of the mouse fertilin beta gene that encodes an ADAM family protein active in sperm-egg fusion. Dev. Genet., 20:320–328, 1997.

Chwalisz, K., Ciesla, I. and Garfield, R.E.: Inhibition of nitric oxide (NO) synthesis induces preterm parturition and preeclampsia-like conditions in guinea pigs. Society for Gynecologic Investigation Meeting, Chicago, IL, 1994.

Clavero-Nunez, J.A. and Botella-Llusia, J.: Measurement of the villus surface in normal and pathologic placentas. Amer. J. Obstet. Gynecol. 86:234–240, 1961.

Colman, P.M. and Lawrence, M.C.: The structural biology of type I viral membrane fusion. Nature Reviews, 4:309–319, 2003.

Conrad, K.P., Benyo, D.F., Westerhausen-Larsen, A. and Miles, T.M.: Expression of erythropoietin by human placenta. FASEB J. 10:760–768, 1996.

Contractor, S.F.: Lysosomes in human placenta. Nature (Lond.) 223:1274–1275, 1969.

Contractor, S.F., Banks, R.W., Jones, C.J.P. and Fox, H.: A possible role for placental lysosomes in the formation of villous syncytiotrophoblast. Cell Tissue Res. 178:411–419, 1977.

Corte, G., Moretta, A., Cosulich, M.E., Ramarli, D. and Bargellesi, A.: A monoclonal anti-DC1 antibody selectively inhibits the generation of effector T cells mediating specific cytolytic activity. J. Exp. Med. 156:1539–1544, 1982.

Crisp, T.M., Dessouky, D.A. and Denys, F.R.: The fine structure of the human corpus luteum of early pregnancy and during the progestational phase of the menstrual cycle. Amer. J. Anat. 127:37–70, 1970.

Crocker, I.P., Tansinda, D.M., Jones, C.J. and Baker, P.N.: The influence of oxygen and tumor necrosis factor-alpha on the cellular kinetics of term placental villous explants in culture. J. Histochem. Cytochem. 52:749–757, 2004.

Cronier, L., Herve, J.C. and Malassine, A.: Regulation of gap junctional communication during human trophoblast differentiation. Microsc. Res. Tech. 38:21–28, 1997.

Cuthbert, P., Sedmak, D., Morgan, C., Lairmore, M. and Anderson, C.: Placental syncytiotrophoblasts do not express CD4 antigen or MRNA [abstract]. Mod. Pathol. 5:91A, 1992.

Daughaday, W.H., Mariz, I.K. and Trivedi, B.: A preferential binding site for insulin-like growth factor II in human and rat placental membranes. J. Clin. Endocrinol. Metabl. 53:282–288, 1981.

De Cecco, L., Pavone, G. and Rolfini, G.: La placenta umana nella isoimmunizzazione anti Rh. Quad. Clin. Ostet. Ginecol. 18:675–682, 1963.

De Ikonicoff, L.K. and Cedard, L.: Localization of human chorionic gonadotropic and somatomammotropic hormones by the peroxidase immunohisto-enzymologic method in villi and amniotic epithelium of human placenta (from six weeks to term). Amer. J. Obstet. Gynecol. 116:1124–1132, 1973.

DeLoia, J.A., Burlingame, J.M., and Karasnow, J.S.: Differential expression of G1 cyclins during human placentogenesis. Placenta 18:9–16, 1997.

Demir, R. and Erbengi, T.: Some new findings about Hofbauer cells in the chorionic villi of the human placenta. Acta Anat. (Basel) 119:18–26, 1984.

Demir, R., Kaufmann, P., Castellucci, M., Erbengi, T. and Kotowski, A.: Fetal vasculogenesis and angiogenesis in human placental villi. Acta Anat. (Basel) 136:190–203, 1989.

Demir, R., Demir, N., Kohnen, G., Kosanke, G., Mironov, V., Üstünel, I. and Kocamaz, E.: Ultrastructure and distribution of myofibroblast-like cells in human placental stem villi. Electron Microsc. 3:509–510, 1992.

Demir, R., Kosanke, G., Kohnen, G., Kertschanska, S. and Kaufmann, P.: Classification of human placental stem villi: review of structural and functional aspects. Microsc. Res. Tech. 38:29–41, 1997.

Dempsey, E.W. and Zergollern, L.: Zonal regions of the human placenta barrier. Anat. Rec. 163:177, 1969.

Dempsey, E.W. and Luse, S.A.: Regional specializations in the syncytial trophoblast of early human placentas. J. Anat. 108:545–561, 1971.

Desoye, G., Hartmann, M., Blaschitz, A., Dohr, G., Hahn, T., Kohnen, G. and Kaufmann, P.: Insulin receptors in syncytiotrophoblast and fetal endothelium of human placenta. Immunohistochemical evidence for developmental changes in distribution pattern. Histochemistry 101:277–285, 1994.

Desoye, G., Hartmann, M., Jones, C.C.P., Wolf, H.J., Kohnen, G., Kosanke, G. and Kaufmann, P.: Location of insulin receptors in the placenta and its progenitor tissues. Microsc. Res. Tech. 38:63–75, 1997.

Devés, R. and Boyd, C.A.R.: Surface antigen CD98(4F2): not a single membrane protein, but a family of proteins with multiple functions. J. Membr. Biol. 173:165–177, 2000.

Dong, Y.L., Vegiraju, S., Chauhan, M., Gangula, P.R., Hankins, G.D., Goodrum, L. and Yallampalli, C.: Involvement of calcitonin gene-related peptide in control of human fetoplacental vascular tone. Am. J. Heart Circ. Physiol. 28:H230-H239, 2004.

Dorgan, W.J. and Schultz, R.L.: An in vitro study of programmed death in rat placental giant cells. J. Exp. Zool. 178:497–512, 1971.

Dreskin, R.B., Spicer, S.S. and Greene, W.B.: Ultrastructural localization of chorionic gonadotropin in human term placenta. J. Histochem. Cytochem. 18:862–874, 1970.

Duance, V.C. and Bailey, A.J.: Structure of the trophoblast basement membrane. In, Biology of Trophoblast. Y.W. Loke and A. Whyte, eds., pp. 597–625. Elsevier, Amsterdam, 1983.

Dujardin, M., Robyn, C. and Wilkin, P.: Mise en evidence immuno-histoenzymologique de l'hormone chorionique somatomammotrope (HCS) au niveau des divers constituants cellulaires du placenta humain normal. Biol. Cell 30:151–154, 1977.

Dunne, F.P., Ratcliffe, W.A., Mansour, P. and Heath, D.A.: Parathyroid hormone related protein (PTHrP) gene expression in fetal and extra-embryonic tissues of early pregnancy. Hum. Reprod. (Oxf.) 9:149–156, 1994.

Durst-Zivkovic, B.: Das Vorkommen der Mastzellen in der Nachgeburt. Anat. Anz. 134:225–229, 1973.

Earl, U., Estlin, C. and Bulmer, J.N.: Fibronectin and laminin in the early human placenta. Placenta 11:223–231, 1990.

Eden, T.W.: A study of the human placenta, physiological and pathological. J. Pathol. Bacteriol. 4:265–283, 1897.

Edwards, D., Jones, C.J.P., Sibley, C.P., Farmer, D.R. and Nelson, D.M.: Areas of syncytial denudation may provide routes for paracellular diffusion across the human placenta. Placenta 12:383, 1991.

Edwards, J.A., Jones, D.B., Evans, P.R. and Smith, J.L.: Differential expression of HLA class II antigens on human fetal and adult lymphocytes and macrophages. Immunology 55:489–500, 1985.

Emly, J.F., Gregory, J., Bowden, S.J., Ahmed, A., Whittle, M.J., Rushton, D.I. and Ratcliffe, W.A.: Immunohistochemical localization of parathyroid hormone-related protein (PTHrP) in human placenta and membranes. Placenta 15:653–660, 1994.

Emonard, H., Christiane, Y., Smet, M., Grimaud, J.A. and Foidart, J.M.: Type IV and interstitial collagenolytic activities in normal and malignant trophoblast cells are specifically regulated by the extracellular matrix. Invasion Metastasis 10:170–177, 1990.

Enders, A.C. and King, B.F.: The cytology of Hofbauer cells. Anat. Rec. 167:231–252, 1970.

Evain-Brion, D. and Alsat, E.: Epidermal growth factor receptor and human fetoplacental development. J. Pediatr. Endocrinol. 7:295–302, 1994.

Evans, J.P., Schultz, R.M. and Kopf, G.S.: Roles of the disintegrin domains of mouse fertilins alpha and beta in fertilization. Biol. Reprod. 59:145–152, 1998.

Farley, A.E., Graham, C.H. and Smith, G.N.: Contractile properties of human placental anchoring villi. Am. J. Physiol. Regul. Integr. Comp. Physiol. 287:R680–R685, 2004.

Faulk, P., Trenchev, P., Dorling, J. and Holborow, J.: Antigens on post-implantation placentae. In, Immunobiology of Trophoblast. R.G. Edwards, C.W.S. Howe and M.H. Johnson, eds. pp. 113–125, Cambridge University Press, Cambridge, 1975.

Faulk, W.P., Jarret, R., Keane, M., Johnson, P.M. and Boackle, R.J.: Immunological studies of human placentae: complement components in immature and mature chorionic villi. Clin. Exp. Immunol. 40:299–305, 1980.

Feller, A.C., Schneider, H., Schmidt, D. and Parwaresch, M.R.: Myofibroblast as a major cellular constituent of villous stroma in human placenta. Placenta 6:405–415, 1985.

Filla, M.S. and Kaul, K.L.: Relative expression of epidermal growth factor receptor in placental cytotrophoblasts and choriocarcinoma cell lines. Placenta 18:17–27, 1997

Firth, J.A. and Leach, L.: Not trophoblast alone: A review of the contribution of the fetal microvasculature to transplacental exchange. Placenta 17:89–96, 1996.

Firth, J.A. and Leach, L.: Structure and permeability in human placental capillaries. A review. Trophoblast Res. 10:205–213, 1997.

Firth, J.A., Farr, A. and Bauman, K.: The role of gap junctions in trophoblastic cell fusion in the guinea-pig placenta. Cell Tissue Res. 205:311–318, 1980.

Firth, J.A., Bauman, K. and Sibley, C.P.: Permeability pathways in fetal placental capillaries. Trophoblast Res. 3:163–177, 1988.

Fisher, S.J. and Laine, R.A.: High alpha-amylase activity in the syncytiotrophoblastic cells of first-trimester human placentas. J. Cell Biochem. 22:47–54, 1983.

Fisher, S.J., Leitch, M.S. and Laine, A.: External labelling of glycoproteins from first-trimester human placental microvilli. Biochem. J. 221:821–828, 1984.

Flynn, A., Finke, J.H. and Hilfiker, M.L.: Placental mononuclear phagocytes as a source of interleukin-1. Science 218:475–477, 1982.

Flynn, A., Finke, J.H. and Loftus, M.A.: Comparison of interleukin-1 production by adherent cells and tissue pieces from human placenta. Immunopharmacology 9:19–26, 1985.

Fox, H.: The villous cytotrophoblast as an index of placental ischaemia. J. Obstet. Gynaecol. Br. Commonw. 71:885–893, 1964.

Fox, H.: The significance of villous syncytial knots in the human placenta. J. Obstet. Gynaecol. Br. Commonw. 72:347–355, 1965.

Fox, H.: The incidence and significance of Hofbauer cells in the mature human placenta. J. Pathol. Bacteriol. 93:710–717, 1967a.

Fox, H.: Perivillous fibrin deposition in the human placenta. Amer. J. Obstet. Gynecol. 98:245–251, 1967b.

Fox, H.: Fibrinoid necrosis of placental villi. J. Obstet. Gynaecol. Br. Commonw. 75:448–452, 1968.

Fox, H.: Effect of hypoxia on trophoblast in organ culture. Amer. J. Obstet. Gynecol. 107:1058–1064, 1970.

Fox, H.: Morphological pathology of the placenta. In, The Placenta and Its Maternal Supply Line: Effects of Insufficiency on the Fetus. P. Gruenwald, ed. Medical Technical Publications, Lancaster, 1975.

Fox, H.: Pathology of the Placenta. 2nd Ed. Saunders, Philadelphia, 1997.

Fox, H. and Blanco, A.A.: Scanning electron microscopy of the human placenta in normal and abnormal pregnancies. Eur. J. Obstet. Gynecol. 4:45–50, 1974.

Frank, H.G., Malekzadeh, F., Kertschanska, S., Crescimanno, C., Castellucci, M., Lang, I., Desoye, G. and Kaufmann, P.: Immunohistochemistry of two different types of placental fibrinoid. Acta Anat. (Basel) 150:55–68, 1994.

Frauli, M. and Ludwig, H.: Demonstration of the ability of Hofbauer cells to phagocytose exogenous antibodies. Eur. J. Obstet. Gynecol. Reprod. Biol. 26:135–144, 1987a.

Frauli, M. and Ludwig, H.: Immunocytochemical identification of mitotic Hofbauer cells in cultures of first trimester human placental villi. Arch. Gynecol. Obstet. 241:47–51, 1987b.

Frauli, M. and Ludwig, H.: Identification of human chorionic gonadotropin (HCG) secreting cells and other cell types using antibody to HCG and a new monoclonal antibody (mABlu-5) in cultures of human placental villi. Arch. Gynecol. Obstet. 241:97–110, 1987c.

Freese, U.E.: The fetal-maternal circulation of the placenta. I. Histomorphologic, plastoid injection, and X-ray cinematographic studies on human placentas. Amer. J. Obstet. Gynecol. 94:354–360, 1966.

Frendo, J.-L., Olivier, D., Cheynet, V., Blond, J.-L., Bouton, O., Vidaud, M., Rabreau, M., Evain-Brion, D. and Mallet, F.: Direct involvement of HERV-W Env glycoprotein in human trophoblast cell fusion and differentiation. Mol. Cell. Biol. 23:3566–3574, 2003.

Frolik, C.A., Dart, L.L., Meyers, C.A., Smith, D.M. and Sporn, M.B.: Purification and initial characterization of a type β transforming growth factor from human placenta. Proc. Natl. Acad. Sci. U.S.A. 80:3676–3680, 1983.

Fujimoto, S., Hamasaki, K., Ueda, H. and Kagawa, H.: Immuno-electron microscope observations on secretion of human placental lactogen (hPL) in the human chorionic villi. Anat. Rec. 216:68–72, 1986.

Gabius, H.-J., Debbage, P.L., Engelhardt, R., Osmers, R. and Lange, W.: Identification of endogenous sugar-binding proteins (lectins) in human placenta by histochemical localization and biochemical characterization. Eur. J. Cell Biol. **44**:265–272, 1987.

Galbraith, G.M.P., Galbraith, R.M., Temple, A. and Faulk, W.P.: Demonstration of transferrin receptors on human placental trophoblast. Blood **55**:240–242, 1980.

Galliano, M.F., Huet, C., Frygelius, J., Polgren, A., Wewer, U.M. and Engvall, E.: Binding of ADAM12, a marker of skeletal muscle regeneration, to the muscle-specific actin-binding protein, alpha -actinin-2, is required for myoblast fusion. J. Biol. Chem. **275**:13933–13939, 2000.

Galton, M.: DNA content of placental nuclei. J. Cell Biol. **13**:183–191, 1962.

Garfield, R.E., Yallampalli, C., Buhimschi, I. and Chwalisz, K.: Reversal of preeclampsia symptoms induced in rats by nitric oxide inhibition with l-arginine, steroid hormones and an endothelin antagonist. Society for Gynecologic Investigation Meeting, Chicago, IL, 1994.

Gaspard, U.J., Hustin, J., Reuter, A.M., Lambotte, R. and Franchimont, P.: Immunofluorescent localization of placental lactogen, chorionic gonadotrophin and its alpha and beta subunits in organ cultures of human placenta. Placenta **1**:135–144, 1980.

Geier, G., Schuhmann, R. and Kraus, H.: Regional unterschiedliche Zellproliferation innerhalb der Plazentone reifer menschlicher Plazenten. Autoradiographische Untersuchungen. Arch. Gynäkol. **218**:31–37, 1975.

Geller, H.F.: Über die sogenannten Hofbauerzellen in der reifen menschlichen Placenta. Arch. Gynäkol. **188**:481–496, 1957.

Geller, H.F.: Elektronenmikroskopische Befunde am Synzytium der menschlichen Plazenta. Geburtsh. Frauenheilkd. **22**:1234–1237, 1962.

Genbacev, O., Robyn, C. and Pantic, V.: Localization of chorionic gonadotropin in human term placenta on ultrathin sections with peroxidase-labeled antibody. J. Microsc. **15**:399–402, 1972.

Gerl, D., Eichhorn, H., Eichhorn, K.-H. and Franke, H.: Quantitative Messungen synzytialer Zellkernkonzentrationen der menschlichen Plazenta bei normalen und pathologischen Schwangerschaften. Zentralbl. Gynäkol. **95**:263–266, 1973.

Getsios, S. and MacCalman, C.D.: Cadherin-11 modulates the terminal differentiation and fusion of human trophoblastic cells in vitro. Dev. Biol. **257**:41–54, 2003.

Gey, G.O., Seegar, G.E. and Hellman, L.M.: The production of a gonadotrophic substance (prolan) by placental cells in tissue culture. Science **88**:306–307, 1938.

Gille, J., Börner, P., Reinecke, J., Krause, P.-H. and Deicher, H.: Über die Fibrinoidablagerungen in den Endzotten der menschlichen Placenta. Arch. Gynäkol. **217**:263–271, 1974.

Gillim, S.W., Christensen, A.K. and McLennan, C.E.: Fine structure of the human menstrual corpus luteum at its stage of maximum secretory activity. Amer. J. Anat. **126**:409–428, 1969.

Gilpin, B.J., Loechel, F., Mattei, M.G., Engvall, E., Albrechtsen, R. and Wewer, U.M.: A novel, secreted form of human ADAM 12 (meltrin alpha) provokes myogenesis in vivo. J. Biol. Chem. **273**: 157–166, 1998.

Glover, D.M., Brownstein, D., Burchette, S., Larsen, A. and Wilson, C.B.: Expression of HLA class II antigens and secretion of interleukin-1 by monocytes and macrophages from adults and neonates. Immunology **61**:195–201, 1987.

Goldstein, J., Braverman, M., Salafia, C. and Buckley, P.: The phenotype of human placental macrophages and its variation with gestational age. Amer. J. Pathol. **133**:648–659, 1988.

Gosseye, S. and Fox, H.: An immunohistological comparison of the secretory capacity of villous and extravillous trophoblast in the human placenta. Placenta **5**:329–348, 1984.

Gossrau, R., Graf, R., Ruhnke, M. and Hanski, C.: Proteases in the human full-term placenta. Histochemistry **86**:405–413, 1987.

Goyert, S.M., Ferrero, E.M., Seremetis, S.V., Winchester, R.J., Silver, J. and Mattison, A.C.: Biochemistry and expression of myelomonocytic antigens. J. Immunol. **137**:3909–3914, 1986.

Goyert, S.M., Ferrero, E.M., Rettig, W.J., Yenamandra, A.K., Obata, F. and Le Beau, M.M.: The CD14 monocyte differentiation antigen maps to a region encoding growth factors and receptors. Science **239**:497–500, 1988.

Graf, R., Langer, J.U., Schoenfelder, G., Oeney, T., Hartel-Schenk, S., Reutter, W. and Schmidt, H.H.H.W.: The extravascular contractile system in the human placenta. Morphological and immunohistochemical investigations. Anat. Embryol. **190**: 541–548, 1994.

Graf, R., Schoenfelder, G., Muehlberger, M. and Gutsmann, M.: The perivascular contractile sheath of human placental stem villi: its isolation and characterization. Placenta **16**:57–66, 1995.

Graf Spee, F.: Anatomie und Physiologie der Schwangerschaft. In, Handbuch der Geburtshilfe, Vol. 1. A. Doederlein, ed., pp. 3–152. Bergmann, Wiesbaden, 1915.

Green, T. and Ford, H.C.: Human placental microvilli contain high-affinity binding sites for folate. Biochem. J. **218**:75–80, 1984.

Grillo, M.A.: Cytoplasmic inclusions resembling nucleoli in sympathetic neurones of adult rats. J. Cell Biol. **45**:100–117, 1970.

Gröschel-Stewart, U.: Plazenta als endokrines Organ. In, Die Plazenta des Menschen. V. Becker, T.H. Schiebler and F. Kubli, eds., pp. 217–233. Thieme Verlag, Stuttgart, 1981.

Haigh, T., Chen, C., Jones, C.J. and Aplin, J.D.: Studies of mesenchymal cells from 1st trimester human placentae: expression of cytokeratin outside the trophoblast lineage. Placenta **20**:615–625, 1999.

Hamanaka, N., Tanizawa, O., Hashimoto, T., Yoshinari, S. and Okudaira, Y.: Electron microscopic study on the localization of human chorionic gonadotropin (HCG) in the chorionic tissue by enzyme labeled antibody technique. J. Electron Microsc. **20**:46–48, 1971.

Hamilton, W.J. and Boyd, J.D.: Specializations of the syncytium of the human chorion. Br. Med. J. **1**:1501–1506, 1966.

Hardingham, T.E. and Fosang, A.J.: Proteoglycans: many forms and many functions. FASEB J. **6**:861–870, 1992.

Hashimoto, M., Kosaka, M., Mori, Y., Komori, A. and Akashi, K.: Electron microscopic studies on the epithelium of the chorionic villi of the human placenta. I. J. Jpn. Obstet. Gynaecol. Soc. **7**:44, 1960a.

Hashimoto, M., Shimoyama, T., Hirasawa, T., Komori, A., Kawasaki, T. and Akashi, K.: Electron microscopic studies on the epithelium of the chorionic villi of the human placenta. II. J. Jpn. Obstet. Gynaecol. Soc. 7:122, 1960b.

Hay, D.L.: Placental histology and the production of human choriogonadotrophin and its subunits in pregnancy. Br. J. Obstet. Gynaecol. 95:1268–1275, 1988.

Hayakawa, S., Watanabe, K. and Satoh, K.: Increased apoptosis and repair hyperplasia of the villous trophoblast in placentae with preeclampsia and IUGR. Placenta 16:A2, 1995.

Haziot, A., Chen, S., Ferrero, E., Low, M.G., Silber, R. and Goyert, S.M.: The monocyte differentiation antigen, CD14, is anchored to the cell membrane by a phosphatidylinositol linkage. J. Immunol. 141:547–552, 1988.

Hedley, R. and Bradbury, M.B.W.: Transport of polar non-electrolytes across the intact and perfused guinea-pig placenta. Placenta 1:277–285, 1980.

Heinrich, D., Metz, J., Raviola, E. and Forssmann, W.G. Ultra-structure of perfusion fixed fetal capillaries in the human placenta. Cell Tissue Res. 172:157–169, 1976.

Heinrich, D., Weihe, E., Gruner, C. and Metz, J.: Vergleichende Morphologie der Placentakapillaren. Anat. Anz. 71:489–491, 1977.

Heinrich, D., Aoki, A. and Metz, J.: Fetal capillary organization in different types of placenta. Trophoblast Res. 3:149–162, 1988.

Hempel, E. and Geyer, G.: Submikroskopische Verteilung der alkalischen Phosphatase in der menschlichen Placenta. Acta Histochem. 34:138–147, 1969.

Hemsen, A., Gillis, C., Larson, O., Haegerstrand, A. and Lundberg, J.M.: Characterization, localization and actions of endothelin in umbilical vessels and placenta of man. Acta Physiol. Scand. 43:395–404, 1991.

Herbst, R. and Multier, A.M.: Les microvillosites a la surface des villosites chorioniques du placenta humain. Gynecol. Obstet. 69:609–616, 1970.

Herbst, R., Multier, A.M. and Hörmann, G.: Die menschlichen Plazentazotten des 2. Schwangerschaftstrimenon im elektronenoptischen Bild. Z. Geburtshilfe Gynäkol. 169:1–16, 1968.

Herbst, R., Multier, A.M. and Hšrmann, G.: Elektronenoptische Untersuchungen an menschlichen Plazentazotten. Zentralbl. Gynäkol. 91:465–475, 1969.

Hey, A. and Röckelein, G.: Die sog. Endothelvakuolen der Plazentagefäße. Physiologie oder Krankheit? Pathologe 10:66–67, 1989.

Hofbauer, J.: Über das konstante Vorkommen bisher unbekannter zelliger Formelemente in der Chorionzotte der menschlichen Plazenta und über Embryotrophe. Wien. Klin. Wochenschr. 16:871–873, 1903.

Hofbauer, J.: Grundzüge einer Biologie der menschlichen Plazenta mit besonderer Berücksichtigung der Fragen der fötalen Ernährung. Braumüller, Vienna, 1905.

Hofbauer, J.: The function of the Hofbauer cells of the chorionic villus particularly in relation to acute infection and syphilis. Amer. J. Obstet. Gynecol. 10:1–14, 1925.

Hoffman, L.H. and Di Pietro, D.L.: Subcellular localization of human placental acid phosphatases. Amer. J. Obstet. Gynecol. 114:1087–1096, 1972.

Horky, Z.: Beitrag zur Funktionsbedeutung der Hofbauer-Zellen (Beobachtungen in der Placenta bei Diabetes mellitus). Zentralbl. Gynäkol. 86:1621–1626, 1964.

Hörmann, G.: Haben die sogenannten Hofbauerzellen der Chorionzotten funktionelle Bedeutung? Zentralbl. Gynäkol. 69:1199–1205, 1947.

Hörmann, G.: Die Reifung der menschlichen Chorionzotte im Lichte ökonomischer Zweckmäßigkeit. Zentralbl. Gynäkol. 70:625–631, 1948.

Hörmann, G.: Ein Beitrag zur funktionellen Morphologie der menschlichen Placenta. Arch. Gynäkol. 184:109–123, 1953.

Hörmann, G.: Die Fibrinoidisierung des Chorionepithels als Konstruktionsprinzip der menschlichen Plazenta. Z. Geburtshilfe Gynäkol. 164:263–269, 1965.

Hörmann, G., Herbst, R. and Ullmann, G.: Die Transformation des Zytotrophoblasten in den Synzytiotrophoblasten. Z. Geburtshilfe Gynäkol. 171:171–182, 1969.

Hoshina, M., Boothby, M. and Boime, I.: Cytological localization of chorionic gonadotropin and placental lactogen mRNAs during development of the human placenta. J. Cell Biol. 93:190–198, 1982.

Hoshina, M., Hussa, R., Patillo, R. and Boime, I.: Cytological distribution of chorionic gonadotropin subunit and placental lactogen messenger RNA in neoplasms derived from human placenta. J. Cell Biol. 97:1200–1206, 1983.

Hoshina, M., Boime, I. and Mochizuki, M.: Cytological localization of hPL and hCG mRNA in chorionic tissue using in situ hybridization. Acta Obstet. Gynaecol. Jpn. 36:397–404, 1984.

Howatson, A.G., Farquharson, M., Meager, A., McNicol, A.M. and Foulis, A.K.: Localization of alpha-interferon in the human feto-placental unit. J. Endocrinol. 119:531–534, 1988.

Hoyer, P.E. and Kirkeby, S.: The impact of fixative on the binding of lectins to N-acetyl-glucosamine residues of human syncytiotrophoblast: a quantitative histochemical study. J. Histochem. Cytochem. 44:855–863, 1996.

Huber, C.P., Carter, J.E. and Vellios, F.: Lesions of the circulatory system of the placenta: a study of 243 placentas with special reference to the developments of infarcts. Amer. J. Obstet. Gynecol. 81:560–572, 1961.

Huguenin, B.: Über die Genese der Fibringerinnungen und Infarktbildungen der menschlichen Placenta. Beitr. Geburtshilfe Gynäkol. 13:339–357, 1909.

Hulstaert, C.E., Torringa, J.L., Koudstaal, J., Hardonk, M.J. and Molenaar, I.: The characteristic distribution of alkaline phosphatase in the full-term human placenta. Gynecol. Invest. 4:24–30, 1973.

Hunt, J.S.: Cytokine networks in the uteroplacental unit: macrophages as pivotal regulatory cells. J. Reprod. Immunol. 16:1–17, 1989.

Huppertz, B. and Kaufmann, P.: The apoptosis cascade in human villous trophoblast. A review. Trophoblast Res. 13:215–242, 1999.

Huppertz, B., Frank, H.G., Kingdom, J.C.P., Reister, F. and Kaufmann, P.: Villous cytotrophoblast regulation of the syncytial apoptotic cascade in the human placenta. Histochem. Cell Biol. 110:495–508, 1998.

Huppertz, B., Frank, H.G., Reister, F., Kingdom, J., Korr, H. and Kaufmann, P.: Apoptosis cascade progresses during turnover of human trophoblast: Analysis of villous cytotrophoblast and syncytial fragments in vitro. Lab. Invest. **79**:1687–1702, 1999.

Huppertz, B., Tews, D.S., and Kaufmann, P.: Apoptosis and syncytial fusion in human placental trophoblast and skeletal muscle. Int. Rev. Cytol. **205**:215–253, 2001.

Huppertz, B., Kaufmann, P. and Kingdom, J.: Trophoblast turnover in health and disease. Mat. Fet. Med. Rev., **13**:103–118, 2002.

Huppertz, B., Kingdom, J., Caniggia, I., Desoye, G., Korr, H., and Kaufmann, P.: Hypoxia favors necrotic versus apoptotic shedding of placental syncytiotrophoblast into the maternal circulation. Implications for the pathogenesis of preeclampsia. Placenta **24**:181–190, 2003.

Ikawa, A.: Observations on the epithelium of human chorionic villi with the electron microscope. J. Jpn. Obstetr. Gynaecol. Soc. **6**:219, 1959.

Iklé, F.A.: Trophoblastzellen im strömenden Blut. Schweiz. Med. Wochenschr. **91**:934–945, 1961.

Iklé, F.A.: Dissemination von Syncytiotrophoblastzellen im mütterlichen Blut während der Gravidität. Bull. Schweiz. Akad. Med. Wissenschaft. **20**:62–72, 1964.

Jackson, M.R., Joy, C.F., Mayhem, T.M. and Haas, J.D.: Stereological studies on the true thickness of the villous membrane in human term placentae: a study of placentae from high-altitude pregnancies. Placenta **6**:249–258, 1985.

Jacquemin, P., Alsat, E., Oury, C., Belayew, A., Muller, M., Evain-Brion, D. and Martial, J.A.: The enhancers of the human placental lactogen B, A, and L genes: progressive activation during in vitro trophoblast differentiation and importance of the DF-3 element in determining their respective activities. DNA Cell Biol. **15**:845–854, 1996.

Jaggi, M., Mehrotra, P.K., Maitra, S.C., Agarwal, S.L., Das, K. and Kamboj, V.P.: Ultrastructure of cellular components of human trophoblasts during early pregnancy. Reprod. Fertil. Dev. **7**:1539–1546, 1995.

Jansson, T.: Amino acid transporters in the human placenta. Pediatric Research **49**:141–147, 2001.

Jeffcoate, T.N.A. and Scott, J.S.: Some observations on the placental factor in pregnancy toxemia. Am. J. Obstet. Gynecol. **77**:475–489, 1959.

Jemmerson, R., Klier, F.G. and Fishman, W.H.: Clustered distribution of human placental alkaline phosphatase on the surface of both placental and cancer cells. J. Histochem. Cytochem. **33**:1227–1234, 1985.

Jimenez, E., Vogel, M., Arabin, B., Wagner, G. and Mirsalim, P.: Correlation of ultrasonographic measurement of the utero-placental and fetal blood flow with the morphological diagnosis of placental function. Trophoblast Res. **3**:325–334, 1988.

Johansen, M., Redman, C.W., Wilkins, T. and Sargent, I.L.: Trophoblast deportation in human pregnancy—its relevance for pre-eclampsia. Placenta **20**:531–539, 1999.

Johnson, P.M. and Brown, P.J.: The IgG and transferrin receptors of the human syncytiotrophoblast microvillous plasma membrane. Amer. J. Reprod. Immunol. **1**:4–9, 1980.

Johnson, P.M. and Brown, P.J.: Fc gamma receptors in the human placenta. Placenta **2**:355–369, 1981.

Jones, C.J.P. and Fox, H.: Syncytial knots and intervillous bridges in the human placenta. An ultrastructural study. J. Anat. **124**:275–286, 1977.

Jones, C.J.P. and Fox, H.: Ultrastructure of the normal human placenta. Electron Microsc. Rev. **4**:129–178, 1991.

Jones, C.J.P., Hartmann, M., Blaschitz, A. and Desoye, G.: Ultrastructural localization of insulin receptors in human placenta. Amer. J. Reprod. Immunol. **30**:136–145, 1993.

Jury, J.A., Frayne, J. and Hall, L.: The human fertilin alpha gene is non-functional: implications for its proposed role in fertilization. Biochem. J. **321**:577–581, 1997.

Jury, J.A., Frayne, J. and Hall, L.: Sequence analysis of a variety of primate fertilin alpha genes: evidence for non-functional genes in the gorilla and man. Mol. Reprod. Dev. **51**:92–97, 1998.

Kacemi, A., Vervelle, C., Uzan, S. and Challier, J.C.: Immunostaining of vascular, perivascular cells and stromal components in human placental villi. Cell. Mol. Biol. (Noisy-le-grand) **45**:101–113, 1999.

Kadyrov, M., Kaufmann, P. and Huppertz, B.: Expression of a Cytokeratin 18 Neo-epitope is a Specific Marker for Trophoblast Apoptosis in Human Placenta. Placenta **22**: 44–48, 2001.

Kameda, T., Koyama, M., Matsuzaki, N., Taniguchi, T., Fumitaka, S. and Tanizawa, O.: Localization of three subtypes of Fc gamma receptors in human placenta by immunohistochemical analysis. Placenta **12**:15–26, 1991.

Kameya, T., Watanabe, K., Kobayashi, T. and Mukojima, T.: Enzyme- and immuno-histochemical localization of human placental alkaline phosphatase. Acta Histochem. Cytochem. **6**:124–136, 1973.

Kao, L.-C., Caltabiano, S., Wu, S., Strauss J.F. III and Kliman, H.J.: The human villous cytotrophoblast: interactions with extracellular matrix proteins, endocrine function, and cytoplasmic differentiation in the absence of syncytium formation. Dev. Biol. (Oxf.) **130**:693–702, 1988.

Kasper, M., Moll, R. and Stosiek, P.: Distribution of intermediate filaments in human umbilical cord: Unusual triple expression of cytokeratins, vimentin, and desmin. Zool. Jahrb. Anat. **117**:227–233, 1988.

Kastschenko, N.: Das menschliche Chorionepithel und dessen Rolle bei der Histogenese der Placenta. Arch. Anat. Physiol. (Leipzig), 451–480, 1885.

Kasznica, J. M. and Petcu, E. B.: Placental calcium pump: clinical-based evidence. Pediatric Pathol. Mol. Med. **22**:223–227, 2003.

Katabuchi, H., Naito, M., Miyamura, S., Takahashi, K. and Okamura, H.: Macrophages in human chorionic villi. Prog. Clin. Biol. Res. **296**:453–458, 1989.

Katsuragawa, H., Kanzaki, H., Inoue, T., Hirano, T., Mori, T. and Rote, N.S.: Monoclonal antibody against phosphatidylserine inhibits in vitro human trophoblastic hormone production and invasion. Biol. Reprod. **56**:50–58, 1997.

Kaufmann, P.: Über polypenartige Vorwölbungen an Zell- und Syncytiumoberflächen in reifen menschlichen Plazenten. Z. Zellforsch. **102**:266–272, 1969.

Kaufmann, P.: Untersuchungen Über die Langhanszellen in der menschlichen Placenta. Z. Zellforsch. **128**:283–302, 1972.

Kaufmann, P.: Über die Bedeutung von Plasmaprotrusionen an reifenden und alternden Zellen. Anat. Anz. Verh. Anat. Ges. **69**:307–312, 1975a.

Kaufmann, P.: Experiments on infarct genesis caused by blockage of carbohydrate metabolism in guinea pig placenta. Virchows Arch. Pathol. Anat. Histol. **368**:11–21, 1975b.

Kaufmann, P.: Vergleichend-anatomische und funktionelle Aspekte des Placenta-Baues. Funkt. Biol. Med. **2**:71–79, 1983.

Kaufmann, P.: Influence of ischemia and artificial perfusion on placental ultrastructure and morphometry. Contrib. Gynecol. Obstet. **13**:18–26, 1985.

Kaufmann, P. and Miller, R.K., eds.: Placental vascularization and blood flow. Basic research and clinical applications. Trophoblast Res. **3**:1–370, 1988.

Kaufmann, P. and Stark, J.: Enzymhistochemische Untersuchungen an reifen menschlichen Placentazotten. I. Reifungs- und Alterungsvorgänge am Trophoblasten. Histochemistry **29**:65–82, 1972.

Kaufmann, P. and Stark, J.: Semidünnschnitt-cytochemische und immunautoradiographische Befunde zum Hormonstoffwechsel der reifen menschlichen Placenta. Anat. Anz. Verh. Anat. Ges. **67**:245–249, 1973.

Kaufmann, P. and Stegner, H.E.: Über die funktionelle Differenzierung des Zottensyncytiums in der menschlichen Placenta. Z. Zellforsch. **135**:361–382, 1972.

Kaufmann, P., Thorn, W. and Jenke, B.: Die Morphologie der Meerschweinchenplacenta nach Monojodacetat- und Fluorid-Vergiftung. Arch. Gynäkol. **216**:185–203, 1974a.

Kaufmann, P., Schiebler, T.H., Ciobotaru, C. and Stark, J.: Enzymhistochemische Untersuchungen an reifen menschlichen Placentazotten. II. Zur Gliederung des Syncytiotrophoblasten. Histochemistry **40**:191–207, 1974b.

Kaufmann, P., Gentzen, D.M. and Davidoff, M.: Die Ultrastruktur von Langhanszellen in pathologischen menschlichen Placenten. Arch. Gynäkol. **22**:319–332, 1977a.

Kaufmann, P., Stark, J. and Stegner, H.E.: The villous stroma of the human placenta. I. The ultrastructure of fixed connective tissue cells. Cell Tissue Res. **177**:105–121, 1977b.

Kaufmann, P., Schröder, H. and Leichtweiss, H.-P.: Fluid shift across the placenta: II. Fetomaternal transfer of horseradish peroxidase in the guinea pig. Placenta **3**:339–348, 1982.

Kaufmann, P., Nagl, W. and Fuhrmann, B.: Die funktionelle Bedeutung der Langhanszellen der menschlichen Placenta. Anat. Anz. Verh. Anat. Ges. **77**:435–436, 1983.

Kaufmann, P., Luckhardt, M., Schweikhart, G. and Cantle, S.J.: Cross-sectional features and three-dimensional structure of human placental villi. Placenta **8**:235–247, 1987a.

Kaufmann. P., Schröder, H., Leichtweiss, H.-P. and Winterhager, E.: Are there membrane-lined channels through the trophoblast? A study with lanthanum hydroxide. Trophoblast Res. **2**:557–571, 1987b.

Kaufmann, P., Firth, J.A., Sibley, C.P. and Schröder, H.: Fetomaternal protein permeability of the placenta-tracer studies using various haeme proteins and lanthanum hydroxide. Gegenbaurs Morphol. Jahrb. **135**:305, 1989.

Kekuda, R., Prasad, P.D., Fei, Y.-J., Torres-Zamorano, V., Sinha, S., Yang-Feng, T.L., Leibach, F.H. and Ganapathy, V.: Cloning of the sodium-dependent, broad-scope, neutral amino acid transporter B0 from a human placental choriocarcinoma cell line. J. Biol. Chem. **271**:18657–18661, 1996.

Kelley, L.K., King, B.F., Johnson, L.W. and Smith, C.H.: Protein composition and structure of human placental microvillous membrane. Exp. Cell Res. **123**:167–176, 1979.

Kemnitz, P.: Die Morphogenese des Zottentrophoblasten der menschlichen Plazenta. Ein Beitrag zum Synzytiumproblem. Zentralbl. Allg. Pathol. **113**:71–76, 1970.

Kerr, J.F.R., Gobé, G.C., Winterford, C.M. and Harmon, B.V.: Anatomical methods in cell death. Methods Cell Biol. **46**:1–27, 1995.

Kertschanska, S. and Kaufmann, P.: Morphological evidence for the existence of transtrophoblastic channels in human placental villi. Placenta **13**:A33, 1992.

Kertschanska, S., Kosanke, G. and Kaufmann, P.: Is there morphological evidence for the existence of transtrophoblastic channels in human placental villi? Trophoblast Res. **8**:581–596, 1994.

Kertschanska, S., Kosanke, G. and Kaufmann, P.: Pressure dependence of so-called transtrophoblastic channels during fetal perfusion of human placental villi. Microsc. Res. Tech. **38**:52–62, 1997.

Kertschanska, S., Stulcova, B., Kaufmann, P. and Stulc, J.: Distensible transtrophoblastic channels in the rat placenta. Placenta **21**:670–677, 2000.

Khaliq, A., Li, X.F., Shams, M., Sisi, P., Acevedo, C.A., Whittle, M.J., Weich, H. and Ahmed, A.: Localisation of placenta growth factor (PlGF) in human term placenta. Growth Factors **13**:243–250, 1996.

Khansari, N. and Fudenberg, H.H.: Functional heterogeneity of human cord blood monocytes. Scand. J. Immunol. **19**:337–342, 1984.

Khodr, G.S. and Siler-Khodr, T.M.: Localization of luteinizing hormone releasing factor (LRF) in the human placenta. Fertil. Steril. **29**:523–526, 1978.

Khong, T.Y., Lane, E.B. and Robertson, W.B.: An immunocytochemical study of fetal cells at the maternal-placental interface using monoclonal antibodies to keratins, vimentin and desmin. Cell Tissue Res. **246**:189–195, 1986.

Kilby, M.D., Afford, S., Li, X.F., Strain, A.J., Ahmed, A. and Whittle, M.J.: Localisation of hepatocyte growth factor and its receptor (c-met) protein and mRNA in human term placenta. Growth Factors **13**:133–139, 1996.

Kim, C.J., Choe, Y.J., Yoon, B.H., Kim, C.W. and Chi, J.G.: Patterns of bcl-2 expression in placenta. Pathol. Res. Pract. **191**:1239–1244, 1995.

Kim, C.K. and Benirschke, K.: Autoradiographic study of the "X cells" in the human placenta. Amer. J. Obstet. Gynecol. **109**:96–102, 1971.

Kim, C.K., Naftolin, F. and Benirschke, K.: Immunohistochemical studies of the "X cell" in the human placenta with anti-human chorionic gonadotropin and anti-human placental lactogen. Amer. J. Obstet. Gynecol. **111**:672–676, 1971.

King, B.F.: Localization of transferrin on the surface of the human placenta by electron microscopic immunocytochemistry. Anat. Rec. **186**:151–159, 1976.

King, B.F.: The distribution and mobility of anionic sites on the surface of human placental syncytial trophoblast. Anat. Rec. **199**:15–22, 1981.

King, B.F.: The organization of actin filaments in human placental villi. J. Ultrastruct. Res. **85**:320–328, 1983.

King, B.F.: Ultrastructural differentiation of stromal and vascular components in early macaque placental villi. Amer. J. Anat. **178**:30–44, 1987.

King, B.F. and Menton, D.N.: Scanning electron microscopy of human placental villi from early and late in gestation. Amer. J. Obstet. Gynecol. **122**:824–828, 1975.

King, R.G., Gude, N.M., Di Iulio, J.L. and Brennecke, S.P.: Regulation of human placental vessel tone: role of nitric oxide. Reprod. Fertil. Dev. **7**:1407–1411, 1995.

Kingdom, J.C.P. and Kaufmann, P.: Oxygen and placental villous development: origins of fetal hypoxia. Placenta **18**:613–621, 1997.

Kliman, H.J. and Feinberg, R.F.: Human trophoblast-extracellular matrix (ECM) interactions in vitro: ECM thickness modulates morphology and proteolytic activity. Proc. Natl. Acad. Sci. U.S.A. **87**:3057–3061, 1990.

Kliman, H.J., Nestler, J.E., Sermasi, E., Sanger, J.M. and Strauss, J.F. III: Purification, characterization and in vitro differentiation of cytotrophoblasts from human term placenta. Endocrinology **118**:1567–1582, 1986.

Kliman, H.J., Feinman, M.A. and Strauss, J.F. III: Differentiation of human cytotrophoblasts into syncytiotrophoblasts in culture. In, Trophoblast Research, vol. 2. R. Miller and H. Thiede, eds., pp. 407–421. Plenum, New York, 1987.

Kline, B.S.: Microscopic observations of development of human placenta. Amer. J. Obstet. Gynecol. **61**:1065–1074, 1951.

Knerr, I., Weigel, C., Linnemann, K., Dötsch, J., Meissner, U., Fusch, C. and Rascher, W.: Transcriptional effects of hypoxia on fusogenic syncytin and its receptor in human cytotrophoblast cells and in ex vivo perfused placental cotyledons. Placenta **24**:A21, 2003.

Knobil, E. and Neill, J.D., eds.: The Physiology of Reproduction, Vol. 2. Raven Press, New York, 1993.

Knoth, M.: Ultrastructure of chorionic villi from a four-somite human embryo. J. Ultrastruct. Res. **25**:423–440, 1968.

Kockx, M. M., Muhring, J., Knaapen, M. W., and de Meyer, G. R.: RNA synthesis and splicing interferes with DNA in situ end labeling techniques used to detect apoptosis. Amer. J. Pathol. **152**:885–888, 1998.

Kohnen, G., Kosanke, G., Korr, H. and Kaufmann, P.: Comparison of various proliferation markers applied to human placental tissue. Placenta **14**:A38, 1993.

Kohnen, G., Castellucci, M., Hsi, B.L., Yeh, C.J.G. and Kaufmann, P.: The monoclonal antibody GB42-a useful marker for the differentiation of myofibroblasts. Cell Tissue Res. **281**:231–242, 1995.

Kohnen, G., Kertschanska, S., Demir, R. and Kaufmann, P.: Placental villous stroma as model system for myofibroblast differentiation. Histochem. Cell Biol. **105**:415–429, 1996.

Kokawa, K., Shikone, T. and Nakano, R.: Apoptosis in human chorionic villi and decidua during normal embryonic development and spontaneous abortion in the first trimester. Placenta **19**:21–26, 1998.

Korhonen, M., Ylanne, J., Laitinen, L., Cooper, H.M., Quaranta, V. and Virtanen, I.: Distribution of the alpha 1-alpha 6 integrin subunits in human developing and term placenta. Lab. Invest. **65**:347–356, 1991.

Korhonen, M. and Virtanen, I.: Immunohistochemical localization of laminin and fibronectin isoforms in human placental villi. J. Histochem. Cytochem. **49**:313–322, 2001.

Kosanke, G., Kadyrov, M., Korr, H. and Kaufmann, P.: Maternal anemia results in increased proliferation in human placental villi. Trophoblast Res. **11**:339–357, 1998.

Krantz, K.E. and Parker, J.C.: Contractile properties of the smooth muscle in the human placenta. Clin. Obstet. Gynecol. **93**:253–258, 1963.

Kristoffersen, E.K., Ulvestad, E., Vedeler, C.A. and Matre, R.: Fc-gamma receptor heterogeneity in the human placenta. Scand. J. Immunol. **31**:561–564, 1990.

Kubli, F. and Budliger, H.: Beitrag zur Morphologie der insuffizienten Plazenta. Geburtsh. Frauenheilkd. **23**:37–43, 1963.

Kudo, Y., Boyd, C.A.R., Sargent, I.L. and Redman, C.W.G.: Hypoxia alters expression and function of syncytin and its receptor during trophoblast cell fusion of human placental BeWo cells: implications for impaired trophoblast syncytialisation in pre-eclampsia. Biochim. Biophys. Acta **1638**:63–71, 2003a.

Kudo, Y., Boyd, C.A.R., Kimura, H., Cook, P.R., Sargent, I.L., Redman, C.W.G. and Ohama, K.: Quantifying the syncytialisation of a human placental trophoblast cell line (BeWo) grown in vitro and effects thereon of manipulation of CD98 expression. Placenta **24**:A58, 2003b.

Kumazaki, K., Nakayama, M., Yanagihara, I., Suehara, N. and Wada, Y.: Immunohistochemical distribution of Toll-like receptor 4 in term and preterm human placentas from normal and complicated pregnancy including chorioamnionitis. Hum. Pathol. **35**:47–54, 2004.

Kunicki, T.J., Nugent, D.J., Staats, S.J., Orchekowski, R.P., Wayner, E.A. and Carter, W.G.: The human fibroblast class II extracellular matrix receptor mediates platelet adhesion to collagen and is identical to the platelet Ia-IIa complex. J. Biol. Chem. **263**:4516–4519, 1988.

Kurman, R.J., Young, R.H., Norris, H.J., Main, C.S., Lawrence, W.D. and Scully, R.E.: Immunocytochemical localization of placental lactogen and chorionic gonadotropin in the normal placenta and trophoblastic tumors, with emphasis on intermediate trophoblast and the placental site trophoblastic tumor. Int. J. Gynecol. Pathol. **3**:101–121, 1984.

Küstermann, W.: Über „Proliferationsknoten" und „Syncytialknoten" der menschlichen Placenta. Anat. Anz. **150**:144–157, 1981.

Laatikainen, T., Saijonmaa, O., Salminen, K. and Wahlström, T.: Localization and concentrations of beta-endorphin and beta-lipotrophin in human placenta. Placenta **8**:381–387, 1987.

Ladines-Llave, C.A., Maruo, T., Manalo, A.S. and Mochizuki, M.: Cytologic localization of epidermal growth factor and its receptor in developing human placenta varies over the course of pregnancy. Amer. J. Obstet. Gynecol. **165**:1377–1382, 1991.

Lafond, J., Auger, D., Fortier, J. and Brunette, M.G.: Parathyroid hormone receptor in human placental syncytiotrophoblast brush border and basal plasma membranes. Endocrinology **123**:2834–2840, 1988.

Lafond, J., Simoneau, L., Savard, R. and Lajeunesse, D.: Calcitonin receptor in human placental syncytiotrophoblast brush border and basal plasma membranes. Mol. Cell Endocrinol. **99**:285–292, 1994.

Lafond, J., St.-Pierre, S., Masse, A., Savard, R. and Simoneau, L.: Calcitonin gene-related peptide receptor in human placental syncytiotrophoblast brush-border and basal plasma membranes. Placenta **18**:181–188, 1997.

Lairmore, M.D., Cuthbert, P.S., Utley, L.L., Morgan, C.J., Dezzutti, C.S., Anderson, C.L., and Sedmak, D.D. Cellular localization of CD4 in the human placenta. Implications for maternal-to-fetal transmission of HIV. J. Immunol. **151**:1673–1681, 1993.

Lamarre, D., Ashkenazi, A., Fleury, S., Smith, D.H., Sekaly, R.-P. and Capon, D.J.: The MHC-binding and gp 120-binding functions of CD4 are separable. Science **245**:743–746, 1989.

Lang, I., Hartmann, M., Blaschitz, A., Dohr, G., Skofitsch, G. and Desoye, G.: Immunohistochemical evidence for the heterogeneity of maternal and fetal vascular endothelial cells in human full-term placenta. Cell Tissue Res. **274**:211–218, 1993a.

Lang, I., Dohr, G. and Desoye, G.: Isolation and culture of fetal vascular endothelial cells derived from human full term placenta. Placenta **14**:A40, 1993b.

Lang, I., Hahn, T., Dohr, G., Skofitsch, G. and Desoye, G.: Heterogeneous histochemical reaction pattern of the lectin Bandeiraea (Griffonia) simplicifolia with blood vessels of human full-term placenta. Cell Tissue Res. **278**:433–438, 1994a.

Lang, I., Hartmann, M., Blaschitz, A., Dohr, G., Kaufmann, P., Frank, H.G., Hahn, T., Skofitsch, G. and Desoye, G.: Differential lectin binding to the fibrinoid of human full term placenta: correlation with a fibrin antibody and the PAF-Halmi method. Acta Anat. **150**:170–177, 1994b.

Lang, I., Hoffmann, C., Olip, H., Pabst, M.A., Hahn, T., Dohr, G. and Desoye, G.: Differential mitogenic responses of human macrovascular and microvascular endothelial cells to cytokines underline their phenotypic heterogeneity. Cell Prolif. **34**:143–155, 2001.

Langhans, T.: Zur Kenntnis der menschlichen Placenta. Arch. Gynäkol. **1**:317–334, 1870.

Langhans, T.: Untersuchungen Über die menschliche Placenta. Arch. Anat. Physiol. Anat. Abt. 188–267, 1877.

Lash, G.E., McLaughlin, B.E., MacDonald-Goodfellow, S.K., Smith, G.N., Brien, J.F., Marks, G.S., Nakatsu, K. and Graham, C.H.: Relationship between tissue damage and heme oxygenase expression in chorionic villi of term human placenta. Amer. J. Heart Circ. Physiol. **284**:H160-H167, 2003.

Latta, J.S. and Beber, C.R.: Cells with metachromatic granules in the stroma of human chorionic villi. Science **117**:498–499, 1953.

Lavillette, D., Maurice, M., Roche, C., Russell, S.J., Sitbon, M. and Cosset, F.-L.: A proline-rich motif downstream of the receptor binding domain modulates conformation and fusogenicity of murine retroviral envelopes. J. Virol. **72**:9955–9965, 1998.

Lea, R.G., al-Sharekh, N., Tulppala, M. and Critchley, H.O.: The immunolocalization of bcl-2 at the maternal-fetal interface in healthy and failing pregnancies. Hum. Reprod. (Oxf.) **12**:153–158, 1997.

Leach, L. and Firth, J.A.: Structure and permeability of human placental microvasculature. Microsc. Res. Tech. **38**:137–144, 1997.

Leach, L., Eaton, B.M., Firth, J.A. and Contractor, S.F.: Immunogold localisation of endogenous immunoglobulin-G in ultrathin frozen sections of the human placenta. Cell Tissue. Res. **257**:603–607, 1989.

Leach, L., Bhasin, Y., Clark, P. and Firth, J.A.: Isolation and characterisation of human microsvascular endothelial cells from chorionic villi of term placenta. Placenta **14**:A41, 1993.

Leach, L., Bhasin, Y., Clark, P. and Firth, J.A.: Isolation endothelial cells from human term placental villi using immunomagnetic beads. Placenta **15**:355–364, 1994.

Leach, L., Lammiman, M.J., Babawale, M.O., Hobson, S.A., Bromilou, B., Lovat, S. and Simmonds, M.J.: Molecular organization of tight and adherens junctions in the human placental vascular tree. Placenta **21**:547–557, 2000.

LeBrun, D.P., Warnke, R.A. and Cleary, M.L.: Expression of bcl-2 in fetal tissues suggests a role in morphogenesis. Amer. J. Pathol. **142**:743–753, 1993.

Lee, X., Keith, J.C., Stumm, N., Moutsatsos, I., McCoy, J.M., Crum, C.P., Genest, D., Chin, D., Ehrenfels, C., Pijnenborg, R., van Assche, F.A. and Mi, S.: Downregulation of placental syncytin expression and abnormal protein localization in preeclampsia. Placenta **22**:808–812, 2001.

Leibl, W., Kerjaschki, D. and Hörandner, H.: Mikrovillusfreie Areale an Chorionzotten menschlicher Placenten. Gegenbaurs Morphol. Jahrb. **121**:26–28, 1975.

Leist, M., Gantner, F., Bohlinger, I., Germann, P. G., Tiegs, G., and Wendel, A.: Murine hepatocyte apoptosis induced in vitro and in vivo by TNF-alpha requires transcriptional arrest. J. Immunol. **153**:1778–1788, 1994.

Lemtis, H.: Über die Architektonik des Zottengefäßapparates der menschlichen Plazenta. Anat. Anz. **102**:106–133, 1955.

Lemtis, H.: Physiologie der Placenta. Bibl. Gynaecol. (Basel) **54**:1–52, 1970.

Lessin, D.L., Hunt, J.S., King, C.R. and Wood, G.W.: Antigen expression by cells near the maternal-fetal interface. Amer. J. Reprod. Immunol. Microbiol. **16**:1–7, 1988.

Levy, R., Smith, S.D., Chandler, K., Sadovsky, Y., and Nelson, D.M.: Apoptosis in human cultured trophoblasts is enhanced by hypoxia and diminished by epidermal growth factor. Amer. J. Physiol. Cell Physiol. **278**:C982–C988, 2000.

Lewis, G.D., Lofgren, J.A., McMurtrey, A.E., Nuijens, A., Fendly, B.M., Bauer, K.D. and Sliwkowski, M.X.: Growth regulation of human breast and ovarian tumor cells by heregulin: evidence for the requirement of ErbB2 as a critical component in mediating heregulin responsiveness. Cancer Res. **56**:1457–1465, 1996.

Lewis, M.P., Clements, M., Takeda, S., Kirby, P.L., Seki, H., Lonsdale, L.B., Sullivan, M.H.F., Elder, M.G. and White, J.O.: Partial characterization of an immortalized human trophoblast cell line, TCL-1, which possesses a CSF-1 autocrine loop. Placenta **17**:137–146, 1996.

Lewis, S.H., Reynolds-Kohler, C., Fox, H.E. and Nelson, J.A.: HIV-1 in trophoblastic and villous Hofbauer cells, and haematological precursors in eight-week fetuses. Lancet **335**:565–568, 1990.

Lewis, W.H.: Hofbauer cells (clasmatocytes) of the human chorionic villus. Bull. Johns Hopkins Hosp. **35**:183–185, 1924.

Librach, C.L., Werb, Z., Fitzgerald, M.L., Chiu, K., Corwin, N.M., Esteves, R.A., Grobelny, D., Galardy, R., Damsky, C.H. and Fisher, S.J.: 92-kD Type IV collagenase mediates invasion of human cytotrophoblasts. J. Cell Biol. **113**:437–449, 1991.

Liebhaber, S.A., Urbanek, M., Ray, J., Ruan, R.S. and Cooke, N.E.: Characterization and histologic localization of human growth hormone-variant gene expression in the placenta. J. Clin. Invest. **83**:1985–1991, 1989.

Liebhart, M.: Some observations on so-called fibrinoid necrosis of placental villi: an electron-microscopic study. Pathol. Eur. **6**:217–220, 1971.

Liebhart, M.: Polysaccharide surface coat (glycocalix) of human placental villi. Pathol. Eur. **9**:3–10, 1974.

Lister, U.M.: Ultrastructure of the early human placenta. J. Obstetr. Gynaecol. Br. Commonw. **71**:21–32, 1964.

Lister, U.M.: The localization of placental enzymes with the electron microscope. J. Obstet. Gynaecol. Br. Commonw. **74**:34–49, 1967.

Loke, Y.W., Eremin, O., Ashby, J. and Day, S.: Characterization of the phagocytic cells isolated from the human placenta. J. Reticuloendothel. Soc. **31**:317–324, 1982.

Lyden, T.W., Ng, A.K. and Rote, N.S.: Modulation of phosphatidylserine epitope expression by BeWo cells during forskolin treatment. Placenta **14**:177–186, 1993.

Lysiak, J.J., Han, V.K.M., and Lala, P.K.: Localization of transforming growth factor alpha in the human placenta and decidua: role in trophoblast growth. Biol. Reprod. **49**:885–894, 1993.

Mabrouk, M. el, Simoneau, L., Bouvier, C. and Lafond, J.: Asymmetrical distribution of G proteins in syncytiotrophoblast brush-border and basal-plasma membranes of human term placenta. Placenta **17**:471–478, 1996.

Macara, L.M., Kingdom, J.C.P. and Kaufmann, P.: Control of fetoplacental circulation. Fetal Maternal Med. Rev. **5**:167–179, 1993.

Mahnke, P.F. and Jacob, C.: Histologische, histochemische und papierchromatographische Untersuchungen an Mastzellen (MZ) der menschlichen Plazenta. Z. Mikrosk. Anat. Forsch. **85**:105–122, 1972.

Malassine, A., Goldstein, S., Alsat, E., Merger, C. and Cedard, L.: Ultrastructural localization of low density lipoprotein bindings site on the surface of the syncytial microvillous membranes of the human placenta. IRCS Med. Sci. **12**:166–167, 1984.

Malassine, A., Besse, C., Roche, A., Alsat, E., Rebourcet, R., Mondon, F. and Cedard, L.: Ultrastructural visualization of the internalization of low density lipoprotein by human placental cells. Histochemistry **87**:457–464, 1987.

Malassine, A., Cronier, L., Mondon, F., Mignot, T.M. and Ferre, F.: Localization and production of immunoreactive endothelin-1 in the trophoblast of human placenta. Cell Tissue Res. **271**:491–497, 1993.

Malassiné, A., Frendo, J.L., Olivier, D., Pidoux, G., Guibourdenche, J. and Mallet, F.: Direct role for HERV-W Env glycoprotein and for connexion 43 in trophoblastic cell fusion demonstrated by antisense strategy. Placenta **24**:A58, 2003.

Marchand, F.: Über das maligne Chorionepitheliom. Berl. Klin. Wochenschr. **35**:249–250, 1898.

Marcuse, P.M.: Pulmonary syncytial giant cell embolism. Obstet. Gynecol **3**:210–213, 1954.

Marin, M., Lavillette, D., Kelly, S.M. and Kabat, D.: N-linked glycosylation and sequence changes in a critical negative control region of the ASCT1 and ASCT2 neutral amino acid transporters determine their retroviral receptor functions. J. Virol. **77**:2936–2945; 2003.

Marin, M., Tailor, C.S., Nouri, A. and Kabat, D.: Sodium-dependent neutral amino acid transporter type 1 is an auxiliary receptor for baboon endogenous retrovirus. J. Virol. **74**:8085–8093, 2000.

Marinoni, E., Picca, A., Scucchi, L., Cosmi, E.V. and Di Iorio, R.: Immunohistochemical localization of endothelin-1 in placenta and fetal membranes in term and preterm human pregnancy. Amer. J. Reprod. Immunol. **34**:213–218, 1995.

Martin, B.J. and Spicer, S.S.: Multivesicular bodies and related structures of the syncytiotrophoblast of human term placenta. Anat. Rec. **175**:15–36, 1973a.

Martin, B.J. and Spicer, S.S.: Ultrastructural features of cellular maturation and aging in human trophoblast. J. Ultrastruct. Res. **43**:133–149, 1973b.

Martin, B.J., Spicer, S.S. and Smythe, N.M.: Cytochemical studies of the maternal surface of the syncytiotrophoblast of human early and term placenta. Anat. Rec. **178**:769–786, 1974.

Martin, S.J., Reutelingsberger, C.P., McGahon, A.J., Rader, J.A., Van Schie, R.C., Laface, D.M. and Green, D.R.: Early redistribution of plasma membrane phosphatidylserine is a general feature of apoptosis regardless of the initiating stimulus: inhibition by overexpression of Bcl-2 and Abl. J. Exp. Med. **182**:1545–1556, 1995.

Martinez, F., Kiriakidou, M. and Strauss, J.F. III: Structural and functional changes in mitochondria associated with trophoblast differentiation: methods to isolate enriched preparations of syncytiotrophoblast mitochondria. Endocrinology **138**:2172–2183, 1997.

Martinoli, C., Castellucci, M., Zaccheo, D. and Kaufmann, P.: Scanning electron microscopy of stromal cells of human placental villi throughout pregnancy. Cell Tissue Res. **235**:647–655, 1984.

Maruo, T. and Mochizuki, M.: Immunohistochemical localization of epidermal growth factor receptor and myc oncogene product in human placenta: implication for trophoblast proliferation and differentiation. Amer. J. Obstet. Gynecol. **156**:721–727, 1987.

Maruo, T., Matsuo, H., Oishi, T., Hayashi, M., Nishino, R. and Mochizuki, M.: Induction of differentiated trophoblast function by epidermal growth factor: relation of immunohistochemically detected cellular epidermal growth factor receptor levels. J. Clin. Endocrinol. Metabol. **64**:744–750, 1987.

Maruo, T., Matsuo, H., Otani, T. and Mochizuki, M.: Role of epidermal growth factor (EGF) and its receptor in the development of the human placenta. Reprod. Fertil. Dev. **7**:1465–1470, 1996.

Marzioni, D., Mühlhauser, J., Crescimanno, C., Banita, M., Pierleoni, C. and Castellucci, M.: BCL-2 expression in the human placenta and its correlation with fibrin deposits. Hum. Reprod. (Oxf.) **13**:1717–1722, 1998.

Marzioni, D., Banita, M., Felici, A., Paradinas, F. J., Newlands, E., De Nictolis, M., Mühlhauser, J. and Castellucci M.: Expression of ZO-1 and occludin in normal human placenta and in hydatiform moles. Molecular Human Reprod. **7**:279–285, 2001.

Marzioni, D., Crescimanno, C., Zaccheo, D., Coppari, R., Underhill, C.B. and Castellucci, M.: Hyaluronate and CD44 expression patterns in the human placenta throughout pregnancy. Eur. J. Histochem. **45**:131–140, 2001.

Masuzaki, H., Ogawa, Y., Sagawa, N., Hosoda, K., Matsumoto, T., Mise, H., Nishimura, H., Yoshimasa, Y., Tanaka, I., Mori, T.

and Nakao, K.: Nonadipose tissue production of leptin: leptin as a novel placenta-derived hormone in humans. Nature Med. **9**:1029–1033, 1997.

Matsubara, S., Tamada, T., Kurahashi, K. and Saito, T.: Ultracytochemical localizations of adenosine nucleotidase activities in the human term placenta, with special reference to 5'-nucleotidase activity. Acta Histochem. Cytochem. **20**:409–419, 1987a.

Matsubara, S., Tamada, T. and Saito, T.: Cytochemical study of the electron microscopical localization of Ca ATPase activity in the human trophoblast. Acta Obstet. Gynaecol. Jpn. **39**:1080–1086, 1987b.

Matsubara, S., Tamada, T. and Saito, T.: Ultracytochemical localizations of alkaline phosphatase and acid phosphatase activities in the human term placenta. Acta Histochem. Cytochem. **20**:283–294, 1987c.

Matsubara, S., Tamada, T. and Saito, T.: Ultracytochemical localizations of adenylate cyclase, guanylate cyclase and cyclic 3',5'-nucleotide phosphodiesterase activity on the trophoblast in the human placenta. Histochemistry **87**:505–509, 1987d.

Matsubara, S., Minakami, H., Takayama, T. and Sato, I.: Cellular and subcellular localization of nicotinamide adenine dinucleotide phosphate diaphorase activity. J. Obstet. Gynaecol. **23**:133–138, 1997.

Maubert, B., Guilbert, L.J. and Deloron, P.: Cytoadherence of plasmodium falciparum to intercellular adhesion molecule 1 and chondroitin-4-sulfate expressed by the syncytiotrophoblast in the human placenta. Infect. Immun. **65**:1251–1257, 1997.

Mayer, M., Panigel, M. and Tozum, R.: Observations sur l'aspect radiologique de la vascularisation fetale du placenta humain isole mainten en survie par perfusion de liquides physiologiques. Gynecol. Obstet. (Paris) **58**:391–397, 1959.

Mayhew, T.M.: The problem of ambiguous profiles of microvilli between apposed cell surfaces: a stereological solution. J. Microsc. **139**:327–330, 1985.

Mayhew, T.M.: Scaling placental oxygen diffusion to birthweight: studies on placentae from low- and high-altitude pregnancies. J. Anat. **175**:187–194, 1991.

Mayhew, T.M. and Burton, G.J.: Methodological problems in placental morphometry: apologia for the use of stereology based on sound sampling practice. Placenta **9**:565–581, 1988.

Mayhew, T.M., Jackson, M.R. and Haas, J.D.: Oxygen diffusive conductances of human placentae from term pregnancies at low and high altitudes. Placenta **11**:493–503, 1990.

Mazel, S., Burtrum, D., and Petrie, H. T.: Regulation of cell division cycle progression by bcl-2 expression: A potential mechanism for inhibition of programmed cell death. J. Exp. Med. **183**:2219–2226, 1996.

Mazzanti, L., Staffolani, R., Cester, N., Romanini, C., Pugnaloni, A., Belmonte, M.M., Salvolini, E., Brunelli, M.A. and Biagini, G.: A biochemical-morphological study on microvillus plasma membrane development. Biochem. Biophys. Acta **1192**:101–106, 1994.

McCormick, J.N., Faulk, W.P., Fox, H. and Fudenberg, H.H.: Immunohistological and elution studies of the human placenta. J. Exp. Med. **91**:1–13, 1971.

McGann, K.A., Collman, R., Kolson, D.L., Gonzalez-Scarano, F., Coukos, G., Coutifaris, C., Strauss, J.F. and Nathanson, N.: Human immunodeficiency virus type 1 causes productive infection of macrophages in primary placental cell cultures. J. Infect. Dis. **169**:746–753, 1994.

McKay, D.G., Hertig, A.T., Adams, E.C. and Richardson, M.V.: Histochemical observations on the human placenta. Obstet. Gynecol. **12**:1–36, 1958.

McKenzie, P. P., Foster, J. S., House, S., Bukovsky, A., Caudle, M. R. and Wimalasena, J.: Expression of G1 cyclins and cyclin-dependent kinase-2 activity during terminal differentiation of cultured human trophoblast. Biol. Reprod. **58**:1283–1289, 1998.

McLean, M., Bowman, M., Clifton, V., Smith, R. and Grossman, A.B.: Expression of the heme oxygenase-carbon monoxide signaling system in human placenta. J. Clin. Endocrinol. Metab. **85**:2345–2349, 2000.

Mebius, R.E., Martens, G., Brevé, J., Delemarra, F.G.A. and Kraal, G.: Is early repopulation of macrophage-depleted lymph node independent of blood monocyte immigration? Eur. J. Immunol. **21**:3041–3044, 1991.

Merrill, J.A.: Common pathological changes of the placenta. Clin. Obstet. Gynecol. **6**:96–109, 1963.

Merttens, I.: Beiträge zur normalen und pathologischen Anatomie der menschlichen Placenta. Z. Geburtshilfe Gynäkol. **30**:1–22, 1894.

Metz, J., Heinrich, D. and Forssmann, W.G.: Ultrastructure of the labyrinth in the rat full term placenta. Anat. Embryol. **149**:123–148, 1976.

Metz, J., Weihe, E. and Heinrich, D.: Intercellular junctions in the full term human placenta. I. Syncytiotrophoblastic layer. Anat. Embryol. **158**:41–50, 1979.

Meyer, A.W.: On the nature, occurrence and identity of the plasma cells of Hofbauer. J. Morphol. **32**:327–349, 1919.

Mi, S., Lee, X., Li, X.-P., Veldman, G.M., Finnerty, H., Racie, L., LaVallie, E., Tang, X.-Y., Edouard, P., Howes, S., Keith, J.C. and McCoy J.M.: Syncytin is a captive retroviral envelope protein involved in human placental morphogenesis. Nature **403**:785–789, 2000.

Midgley, A.R. and Pierce, G.B.: Immunohistochemical localization of human chorionic gonadotropin. J. Exp. Med. **115**:289–297, 1962.

Miller, D., Pelton, R., Deryick, R. and Moses, H.: Transforming growth factor-β. A family of growth regulatory peptides. Ann. N.Y. Acad. Sci. **593**:208–217, 1990.

Miller, R.K. and Thiede, H.A. eds.: Fetal nutrition, metabolism, and immunology. The role of the placenta. Trophoblast Res. **1**:1–387, 1984.

Minot, C.S.: Uterus and embryo. I. Rabbit. II. Man. J. Morphol. **2**:341–460, 1889.

Mitchell, M.D., Trautman, M.S. and Dudley, D.J.: Cytokine networking in the placenta. Placenta **14**:249–275, 1993.

Moe, N.: Deposits of fibrin and plasma proteins in the normal human placenta. Acta Pathol. Microbiol. Scand. **76**:74–88, 1969a.

Moe, N.: Histological and histochemical study of the extracellular deposits in the normal human placenta. Acta Pathol. Microbiol. Scand. **76**:419–431, 1969b.

Moe, N.: The deposits of fibrin and fibrin-like materials in the basal plate of the normal human placenta. Acta Pathol. Microbiol. Scand. **75**:1–17, 1969c.

Moe, N.: Mitotic activity in the syncytiotrophoblast of the human chorionic villi. Amer. J. Obstet. Gynecol. **110**:431, 1971.

Moe, N. and Joergensen, L.: Fibrin deposits on the syncytium of the normal human placenta: evidence of their thrombogenic origin. Acta Pathol. Microbiol. Scand. **72**:519–541, 1968.

Moll, U.M. and Lane, B.L.: Proteolytic activity of first trimester human placenta: localization of interstitial collagenase in villous and extravillous trophoblast. Histochemistry **94**:555–560, 1990.

Morrish, D.W., Bhardwaj, D., Dabbagh, L.K., Marusyk, H. and Siy, O.: Epidermal growth factor induces differentiation and secretion of human chorionic gonadotropin and placental lactogen in normal human placenta. J. Clin. Endocrinol. Metabol. **65**:1282–1290, 1987.

Morrish, D.W., Marusyk, H. and Bhardwaj, D.: Ultrastructural localization of human placental lactogen in distinctive granules in human term placenta: comparison with granules containing human chorionic gonadotropin. J. Histochem. Cytochem. **36**:193–197, 1988.

Morrish, D.W., Bhardwaj, D. and Paras, M.T.: Transforming growth factor b1 inhibits placental differentiation and human chorionic gonadotropin and placental lactogen secretion. Endocrinology **129**:22–26, 1991.

Morrish, D.W., Dakour, J., Li, H., Xiao, J., Miller, R., Sherburne, R., Berdan, R.C. and Guilbert, L.J.: In vitro cultured human term cytotrophoblast: a model for normal primary epithelial cells demonstrating a spontaneous differentiation programme that requires EGF for extensive development of syncytium. Placenta **18**:577–585, 1997.

Morrish, D.W., Dakour, J., and Li, H.S.: Functional regulation of human trophoblast differentiation. J. Reprod. Immunol. **39**:179–195, 1998.

Moskalewski, S., Ptak, W. and Czarnik, Z.: Demonstration of cells with IgG receptor in human placenta. Biol. Neonate **26**:268–273, 1975.

Moussa, M., Mognetti, B., Dubanchet, S., Menu, E., Roques, P., Dormont, D., Barre-Sinoussi, F. and Chaouat, G.: Expression of beta chemokines in explants and trophoblasts from early and term human placentae. Am. J. Reprod. Immunol. **46**:309–317, 2001

Mues, B., Langer, D., Zwadlo, G. and Sorg, C.: Phenotypic characterization of macrophages in human term placenta. Immunology **67**:303–307, 1989.

Mühlhauser, J., Crescimanno, C., Kaufmann, P., Höfler, H., Zaccheo, D. and Castellucci, M.: Differentiation and proliferation patterns in human trophoblast revealed by c-erbB-2 oncogene product and EGF-R. J. Histochem. Cytochem. **41**:165–173, 1993.

Mühlhauser, J., Crescimanno, C., Rajaniemi, H., Parkkila, S., Milovanov, A.P., Castellucci, M. and Kaufmann, P.: Immunohistochemistry of carbonic anhydrase in human placenta and fetal membranes. Histochemistry **101**:91–98, 1994.

Mühlhauser, J., Crescimanno, C., Kasper, M., Zaccheo, D. and Castellucci, C.: Differentiation of human trophoblast populations involves alterations in cytokeratin patterns. J. Histochem. Cytochem. **43**:579–589, 1995.

Mühlhauser, J., Marzioni, D., Morroni, M., Vuckovic, M., Crescimanno, C., and Castellucci, M.: Codistribution of basic fibroblast growth factor and heparan sulfate proteoglycan in the growth zones of the human placenta. Cell Tissue Res. **285**: 101–107, 1996.

Muir, A., Lever, A. and Moffet, A.: Expression of human endogenous retroviral RNA and protein in first trimester trophoblast populations and regulation by steroid hormones. Placenta **24**:A6, 2003.

Müller, H.: Abhandlung über den Bau der Molen. Bonitas-Bauer, Würzburg, 1847.

Murphy, B.E.P.: Cortisol and cortisone in human fetal development. J. Steroid Biochem. **11**:509–513, 1979.

Myatt, L., Brewer, A. and Brockman, D.E.: The action of nitric oxide in the perfused human fetal-placental circulation. Amer. J. Obstet. Gynecol. **164**:687–692, 1991.

Myatt, L., Brockman, D.E., Eis, A.L.W. and Pollock, J.S.: Immunohistochemical localization of nitric oxide synthase in the human placenta. Placenta **14**:487–495, 1993.

Myatt, L., Eis, A.L., Brockman, D.E., Kossenjans, W., Greer, I.A. and Lyall, F.: Differential localization of superoxide dismutase isoforms in placental villous of normotensive, pre-eclamptic, and intrauterine growth-restricted pregnancies. J. Histochem. Cytochem. **45**:1433–1438, 1997.

Myers, R.E. and Fujikura, T.: Placental changes after experimental abruptio placentae and fetal vessel ligation of rhesus monkey placenta. Am. J. Obstet. Gynecol. **100**:846–851, 1968.

Nagy, T., Boros, B. and Benkoe, K.: Elektronenmikroskopische Untersuchungen junger und reifer menschlicher Plazenten. Arch. Gynäkol. **200**:428–440, 1965.

Naito, M., Yamamura, F., Nishikawa, S. and Takahashi, K.: Development, differentiation, and maturation of fetal mouse yolk sac macrophages in cultures. J. Leukocyte Biol. **46**:1–10, 1989.

Nakamura, Y. and Ohta, Y.: Immunohistochemical study of human placental stromal cells. Hum. Pathol. **21**:936–940, 1990.

Nanaev, A.K., Rukosuev, V.S., Shirinsky, V.P., Milovanov, A.P., Domogatsky, S.P., Duance, V.C., Bradbury, F.M., Yarrow, P., Gardiner, L., D'Lacey, C. and Ockleford, C.D.: Confocal and conventional immunofluorescent and immunogold electron microscopic localization of collagen types III and IV in human placenta. Placenta **12**:573–595, 1991.

Nanaev, A.K., Kohnen, G., Milovanov, A.P., Domogatsky, S.P. and Kaufmann, P.: Stromal differentiation and architecture of the human umbilical cord. Placenta **18**:53–64, 1997.

Nelson, D.M.: Apoptotic changes occur in syncytiotrophoblast of human placental villi where fibrin type fibrinoid is deposited at discontinuities in the villous trophoblast. Placenta **17**:387–391, 1996.

Nelson, D.M., Smith, C.H., Enders, A.C. and Donohue, T.M.: The non-uniform distribution of acidic components on the human placental syncytial trophoblast surface membrane: a cytochemical and analytical study. Anat. Rec. **184**:159–182, 1976.

Nelson, D.M., Enders, A.C. and King, B.F.: Galactosyltransferase activity of the microvillous surface of human placental syncytial trophoblast. Gynecol. Invest. **8**:267–281, 1977.

Nelson, D.M., Smith, R.M. and Jarett, L.: Nonuniform distribution and grouping of insulin receptors on the surface of human placental syncytial trophoblast. Diabetes **27**:530–538, 1978.

Nelson, D.M., Meister, R.K., Ortman-Nabi, J., Sparks, S. and Stevens, V.C.: Differentiation and secretory activities of cultured human placental cytotrophoblast. Placenta **7**:1–16, 1986.

Nelson, D.M., Crouch, E.C., Curran, E.M. and Farmer, D.R.: Trophoblast interaction with fibrin matrix. Epithelialization of perivillous fibrin deposits as a mechanism for villous repair in the human placenta. Am. J. Pathol. **136**:855–865, 1990.

Nessmann, C., Huten, Y. and Uzan, M.: Placental correlates of abnormal umbilical Doppler index. Trophoblast Res. **3**:309–323, 1988.

Neumann, J.: Beitrag zur Kenntnis der Blasenmolen und des malignen Deciduoms. Monatsschr. Geburtshilfe Gynäkol. **6**:17–36, 1897.

Nikolov, S.D. and Schiebler, T.H.: Über das fetale Gefäßsystem der reifen menschlichen Placenta. Z. Zellforsch. **139**:333–350, 1973.

Nikolov, S.D. and Schiebler, T.H.: Über Endothelzellen in Zottengefäßen der reifen menschlichen Placenta. Acta Anat. (Basel) **110**:338–344, 1981.

Nishihira, M. and Yagihashi, S.: Immunohistochemical demonstration of somatostatin-containing cells in the human placenta. Tohoku J. Exp. Med. **126**:397, 1978.

Nishihira, M. and Yagihashi, S.: Simultaneous detection of immunoreactive hCG- and somatostatin-containing cells and their gestational changes in the human placental villi and decidua. Acta Histochem. Cytochem. **12**:434–442, 1979.

Nishino, E., Matsuzaki, N., Masuhiro, K., Kameda, T., Taniguchi, T., Tagagi, T., Saji, F. and Tanizawa, O.: Trophoblast-derived interleukin-6 (IL-6) regulates human chorionic gonadotropin release through IL-6 receptor on human trophoblasts. J. Clin. Endocrinol. Metab. **71**:436–441, 1990.

Nissley, P., Kiess, W. and Sklar, M.: Developmental expression of the IGF-II/mannose 6-phosphate receptor. Mol. Reprod. Dev. **35**:408–413, 1993.

Ockleford, C.D.: A three dimensional reconstruction of the polygonal pattern on placental coated vesicle membranes. J. Cell Sci. **21**:83–91, 1976.

Ockleford, C.D. and Menon, G.: Differentiated regions of human placental cell surface associated with exchange of materials between maternal and foetal blood: a new organelle and the binding of iron. J. Cell Sci. **25**:279–291, 1977.

Ockleford, C.D., Wakely, J. and Badley, R.A.: The human placental chorionic villous tree. International SEM Symposium, Nijmegen, The Netherlands, 1981a.

Ockleford, C.D., Wakely, J. and Badley, R.A.: Morphogenesis of human placental chorionic villi: cytoskeletal, syncytioskeletal and extracellular matrix proteins. Proc. R. Soc. Lond. Biol. **212**:305–316, 1981b.

Ockleford, C.D., Wakely, J., Badley, R.A. and Virtanen, I.: Intermediate filament proteins in human placenta. Cell Biol. Int. Rep. **5**:762, 1981c.

Ockleford, C.D., Nevard, C.H.F., Indans, I. and Jones, C.J.P.: Structure and function of the nematosome. J. Cell Sci. **87**:27–44, 1987.

Ohashi, K., Burkart, V., Flohe, S. and Kolb, H.: Cutting edge: heat shock protein 60 is a putative endogenous ligand of the toll-like receptor-4 complex. J. Immunol. **164**:558–561, 2000.

Ohlsson, R.: Growth factors, protooncogenes and human placental development. Cell Differ. Dev. **28**:1–16, 1989.

Ohlsson, R., Holmgren, L., Glaser, A., Szpecht, A. and Pfeifer-Ohlsson, S.: Insulin-like growth factor 2 and short-range stimulatory loops in control of human placental growth. EMBO J. **8**:1993–1999, 1989.

Ohno, M., Martinez-Hernandez, A., Ohno, N. and Kefalides, N.A.: Laminin M is found in placental basement membranes, but not in basement membranes of neoplastic origin. Connect. Tissue Res. **15**:199–207, 1986.

Okamura, Y., Watari, M., Jerud, E.S., Young, D.W., Ishizaka, S.T., Rose, J., Chow, J.C. and Strauss, J.F. 3rd: The extra domain A of fibronectin activates Toll-like receptor 4. J. Biol. Chem. **276**:10229–10233, 2001.

Okudaira, Y. and Hayakawa, K.: Electron microscopic study on the surface coat of the human placental trophoblast. J. Electron Microsc. **24**:279–2281, 1975.

Oliveira, L.H.S., Leandro, S.V., Fonseca, M.E.F. and Dias, L. M.S.: A new technique for the isolation of placental phagocyte cells and a description of their macrophage properties after in vitro culture. Braz. J. Med. Biol. Res. **19**:249–255, 1986.

Ong, P.J. and Burton, G.J.: Thinning of the placental villous membrane during maintenance in hypoxic organ culture: structural adaptation or syncytial degeneration? Eur. J. Obstet. Gynäkol. Reprod. Biol. **39**:103–110, 1991.

O'Reilly, L.A., Harris, A.W., Tarlinton, D.M., Corcoran, L.M. and Strasser, A.: Expression of a bcl-2 transgene reduces proliferation and slows turnover of developing B lymphocytes in vivo. J. Immunol. **159**:2301–2311, 1997.

Orgnero de Gaisan, E., Aoki, A., Heinrich, D. and Metz, J.: Permeability studies of the guinea pig placental labyrinth II. Tracer permeation and freeze fracture of fetal endothelium. Anat. Embryol. **171**:297–304, 1985.

Ortmann, R.: Zur Frage der Zottenanastomosen in der menschlichen Placenta. Z. Anat. Entwicklungsgesch. **111**:173–185, 1941.

Ortmann, R.: Untersuchungen an einer in situ fixierten menschlichen Placenta vom 4.-5. Schwangerschaftsmonat. Arch. Gynäkol. **172**:161–172, 1942.

Oswald, B. and Gerl, D.: Die Mikrofibrinoidablagerungen in der menschlichen Placenta. Acta Histochem. (Jena) **42**:356–359, 1972.

Owens, G.P., Hahn, W.E. and Cohen, J.J.: Identification of mRNAs associated with programmed cell death in immature thymocytes. Mol. Cell Biol. **11**:4177–4188, 1991.

Owens, J.A., Kind, K.L., Carbone, F., Robinson, J.S. and Owens, P.C.: Circulating insulin-like growth factors-I and -II and substrates in fetal sheep following restriction of placental growth. J. Endocrinol. **140**:5–13, 1994.

Panigel, M.: Comparative physiological and pharmacological aspects of placental permeability and hemodynamics in the non-human primate placenta and in the isolated perfused human placenta. Excerpta Med. **170**:13, 1968.

Panigel, M. and Anh, J.N.H.: Ultrastructure des villosites placentaires humains. Pathol. Biol. (Paris) **12**:927–949, 1964.

Panigel, M. and Myers, R.E.: Histological and ultrastructural changes in rhesus monkey placenta following interruption of fetal placental circulation by fetectomy or interplacental umbilical vessels ligation. Acta Anat. (Basel) **81**:481–506, 1972.

Parmley, R.T., Takagi, M. and Denys, F.R.: Ultrastructural local-ization of glycoaminoglycans in human term placenta. Anat. Rec. **210**:477–484, 1984.

Parmley, R.T., Barton, J.C. and Conrad, M.C.: Ultrastructural localization of transferrin, transferrin receptor, and iron-binding sites on human placental and duodenal microvilli. Br. J. Haematol. **60**:81–89, 1985.

Patel, B., Khaliq, A., Jarvisevans, J., Mcleod, D., Mackness, M. and Boulton, M.: Oxygen regulation of TGF-beta 1 mRNA in human hepatoma (HEP G2) cells. Biochem. Mol. Biol. Int. **34**:639–644, 1994.

Pavia, J., Munoz, M., Jimenez, E., Martos, F., Gonzalez-Correa, J.A., De la Cruz, J.P., Garcia, V. and Sanchez de la Cuesta, F.: Pharmacological characterization and distribution of musca-rinic receptors in human placental syncytiotrophoblast brush-border and basal plasma membranes. Eur. J. Pharmacol. **320**:209–214, 1997.

Pescetto, G.: Sulla presenza di elementi granulosi basofili meta-cromatici nella placenta fetale umana. Biol. Lat. (Milan) **2**: 744–757, 1950.

Pescetto, G.: Osservazioni istologiche e istochimiche sulle cellule di Hofbauer del villo coriale umano. Riv. Biol. **44**:231–241, 1952.

Peter, K.: Placenta-Studien. 1. Zotten und Zwischen-Zottenräume zweier Placenten aus den letzten Monaten der Schwangerschaft. Z. Mikrosk. Anat. Forsch. **53**:142–174, 1943.

Peter, K.: Placenta-Studien. 2. Verlauf, Verzweigung und Verankerung der Chorionzottenstämme und ihrer Äste in geborenen Placenten. Z. Mikrosk. Anat. Forsch. **56**:129–172, 1951.

Petraglia, F.: Placental neurohormones: secretion and physio-logical implications. Mol. Cell. Endocrinol. **78**:C109-C112, 1991.

Petraglia, F., Sawchenko, P., Lim, A.T.W., Rivier, J. and Vale, W.: Localization, secretion, and action of inhibin in human pla-centa. Science **237**:187–189, 1987.

Petraglia, F., Calza, L., Giardino, L., Sutton, S., Marrama, P., Rivier, J., Genazzani, A.R. and Vale, W.: Identification of immunoreactive neuropeptide-y in human placenta: localiza-tion, secretion, and binding sites. Endocrinology **124**:2016–2022, 1989.

Petraglia, F., Volpe, A., Genazzani, A.R., Rivier, J., Sawchenko, P.E. and Vale, W.: Neuroendocrinology of the human placenta. Front. Neuroendocrinol. **11**:6–37, 1990.

Petraglia, F., Garuti, G., Calza, L., Roberts, V., Giardino, L., Genazzani, A.R. and Vale, W.: Inhibin subunits in human pla-centa: localization and messenger ribonucleic acid levels during pregnancy. Amer. J. Obstet. Gynecol. **165**:750–758, 1991.

Petraglia, F., Woodruff, T.K., Botticelli, G., Botticelli, A., Genaz-zani, A.R., Mayo, K.E. and Vale, W.: Gonadotropin-releasing hormone, inhibin, and activin in human placenta: evidence for a common cellular localization. J. Clin. Endocrinol. Metab. **74**:1184–1188, 1992.

Pfister, C., Scheuner, G., Bahn, H. and Stiller. D.: Immunhisto-chemischer Nachweis von Fibronectin in der menschlichen Placenta. Acta Histochem. **84**:83–91, 1988.

Pfister, C., Scheuner, G. and Städtler, N.: Fluorescenz- und polar-isationsoptische Untersuchungen zur qualitativen und

quantitativen Erfassung neutraler Carbohydrate in Basal-membranen menschlicher Placenta-Zotten. Acta Histochem. **85**:29–37, 1989.

Pierce, G.B. and Midgley, A.R.: The origin and function of human syncytiotrophoblast giant cells. Amer. J. Pathol. **43**: 153–173, 1963.

Pinto, A., Sorrentino, R., Sorrentino, P., Guerritore, T., Miranda, L., Biondi, A. and Martinelli, P.: Endothelial-derived relaxing factor released by endothelial cells of human umbilical vessels and its impairment in pregnancy-induced hypertension. Amer. J. Obstet. Gynecol. **164**:507–513, 1991.

Piotrowicz, B., Niebroj, T.K. and Sieron, G.: The morphology and histochemistry of the full term placenta in anaemic patients. Folia Histochem. Cytochem. **7**:435–444, 1969.

Piotrowicz, R.S., Orchekowski, D.J., Nugent, D.J., Yamada, K.Y. and Kunicki, T.J.: Glycoprotein lc-lla functions as an activation-independent fibronectin receptor on human platelets. J. Cell Biol. **106**:1359–1364, 1988.

Polin, R.A., Fox, W.W. and Abman, S.H., eds.: Fetal and Neonatal Physiology, 3rd Ed., Vol. I, II. Saunders, Philadelphia, 2004.

Poltorak, A., He, X., Smirnova, I., Liu, M.Y., Van Huffel, C., Du, X., Birdwell, D., Alejos, E., Silva, M., Galanos, C., Freuden-berg, M., Ricciardi-Castagnoli, P., Layton, B. and Beutler, B.: Defective LPS signaling in C3H/HeJ and C57BL/10ScCr mice: mutations in Tlr4 gene. Science **282**:2085–2088, 1998.

Ponferrada, V.G., Mauck, B.S. and Wooley, D.P.: The envelope glycoprotein of human endogenous retrovirus HERV-W induces cellular resistance to spleen necrosis virus. Arch. Virol. **148**:659–675, 2003.

Popovici, R.M., Lu, M., Bhatia, S., Faessen, G.H., Giaccia, A.J. and Giudice, L.C.: Hypoxia regulates insulin-like growth factor-binding protein 1 in human fetal hepatocytes in primary culture: suggestive molecular mechanisms for in utero fetal growth restriction caused by uteroplacental insufficiency. J. Clin. Endocrinol. Metab. **86**:2653–2659, 2001.

Pötgens, A.J.G., Schmitz, U., Bose, P., Versmold, A., Kaufmann, P. and Frank, H.-G.: Mechanisms of syncytial fusion: a review. Placenta **23**, Suppl.A. pp.107–113, 2002.

Pötgens, A.J.G., Kataoka, H., Ferstl, S., Frank, H.G. and Kaufmann, P.: A positive immunoselection method to isolate villous cytotrophoblast cells from first trimester and term placenta to high purity. Placenta **24**:412–423, 2003.

Pötgens, A.J.G., Drewlo, S., Kokozidou, M. and Kaufmann, P.: Syncytin: the major regulator of trophoblast fusion? Recent developments and hypotheses on its action. Human Reprod. Update **10**:487–496, 2004.

Prosdocimi, O.: Richerche istochimiche per la localizzazione delle sostanze gonadotrope nel tessuto coriale normale, nella mola vescicolare e corioepitelioma. Riv. Ostet. Ginecol. **35**:133, 1953.

Rao, C.V., Carman, F.R., Chegini, N. and Schultz, G.S.: Binding sites for epidermal growth factor in human fetal membranes. J. Clin. Endocrinol. Metab. **58**:1034–1042, 1984.

Rao, C.V., Ramani, N., Chegini, N., Stadig, B.K., Carman, F.R. Jr., Woost, P.G., Schultz, G.S. and Cook, C.L.: Topography of human placental receptors for epidermal growth factor. J. Biol. Chem. **260**:1705–1710, 1985.

Rasko, J.E., Battini, J.-L., Gottschalk, R.J., Mazo, I. and Miller, D.: The RD114/simian type D retrovirus receptor is a neutral amino acid transporter. Proc. Natl. Acad. Sci. USA **96**:2129–2134, 1999.

Reale, E. Wang, T., Zaccheo, D., Maganza, C. and Pescetto, G.: Junctions on the maternal blood surface of the human placental syncytium. Placenta **1**:245–258, 1980.

Rhodin, J. and Terzakis, J.: The ultrastructure of the human full-term placenta. J. Ultrastruct. Res. **6**:88–106, 1962.

Richart, R.: Studies of placental morphogenesis. I. Radioautographic studies of human placenta utilizing tritiated thymidine. Proc. Soc. Exp. Biol. Med. **106**:829–831, 1961.

Roberts, L., Sebire, N.J., Fowler, D. and Nicolaides, K.H.: Histomorphological features of chorionic villi at 10–14 weeks of gestation in trisomic and chromosomally normal pregnancies. Placenta **21**:678–683, 2000.

Rock, F.L., Hardiman, G., Timans, J.C., Kastelein, R.A., Bazan, J.F.: A family of human receptors structurally related to Drosophila Toll. Proc. Nat. Acad. Sci. USA **95**:588–593, 1998.

Röckelein, G. and Hey, A.: Ultrastrukturelle Untersuchungen der Vakuolenbildung in arteriellen Choriongefäßen der reifen menschlichen Plazenta. Z. Geburtshilfe Perinatol. **189**:65–68, 1985.

Rodway, H.E. and Marsh, F.: A study of Hofbauer's cells in human placenta. J. Obstet. Gynaecol. Br. Emp. **63**:111–115, 1956.

Rote, N.S., Vogt, E., Devere, G., Obringer, A.R. and Ng, A.K.: The role of placental trophoblast in the pathophysiology of the antiphospholipid antibody syndrome. Amer. J. Reprod. Immunol. **39**:125–136, 1998.

Rote, N.S., Chakrabarti, S. and Stetser, B.P.: The role of human endogenous retroviruses in trophoblast differentiation and placental development. Placenta **25**:673–683, 2004.

Rovasio, R.A. and Monis, B.: Cytochemical changes of a glycocalix of human placenta with maturation. Experientia (Basel) **29**:1115–1118, 1973.

Rukosuev, V.S.: Immunofluorescent localization of collagen types I, III, IV, V, fibronectin, laminin, entactin, and heparan sulphate proteoglycan in human immature placenta. Experientia (Basel) **48**:285–287, 1992.

Runic, R., Lockwood, C.J., Ma, Y., Dipasquale, B. and Guller, S.: Expression of Fas ligand by human cytotrophoblasts: implications in placentation and fetal survival. J. Clin. Endocrinol. Metab. **81**:3119–3122, 1996.

Russel, S.W. and Pace, J.L.: The effects of interferons on macrophages and their precursors. Vet. Immunol. Immunopathol. **15**:129–165, 1987.

Ruzycky, A.L., Jansson, T. and Illsley, N.P.: Differential expression of protein kinase C isoforms in the human placenta. Placenta **17**:461–469, 1996.

Saijonmaa, O., Laatikainen, T. and Wahlström, T.: Corticotrophin-releasing factor in human placenta: localization, concentration and release in vitro. Placenta **9**:373–385, 1988.

Sakakibara, R., Yokoo, Y., Yoshikoshi, K., Tominaga, N., Eida, K. and Ishiguro, M.: Subcellular localization of intracellular form of human chorionic gonadotropin in first trimester placenta. J. Biochem. **102**:993–1001, 1987.

Sakata, M.: The study on the fetal placental circulation. Shikoku Acta Med. **16**:796–812, 1960.

Sakbun, V., Koay, E.S.C. and Bryant-Greenwood, G.D.: Immunocytochemical localization of prolactin and relaxin C-peptide in human decidua and placenta. J. Clin. Endocrinol. Metab. **65**:339–343, 1987.

Sakuragi, N., Matsuo, H., Coukos, G., Furth, E.E., Bronner, M.P., VanArsdale, C.M., Krajewsky, S., Reed, J.C. and Strauss, J.F. III: Differentiation-dependent expression of the Bcl-2 proto-oncogene in the human trophoblast lineage. J. Soc. Gynecol. Invest. **1**:164–172, 1994.

Sala, M.A., Matheus, M. and Valeri, V.: Regional variation in the frequency of fibrinoid degeneration in the human term placenta. Z. Geburtshilfe Perinatol. **186**:80–81, 1982.

Salas, S.P., Power, R.F., Singleton, A., Wharton, J., Polak, J.M. and Brown, J.: Heterogeneous binding sites for a-atrial natriuretic peptide in human umbilical cord and placenta. Am. J. Physiol. **261**:R633–R638, 1991.

Salvaggio, A.T., Nigogosyan, G. and Mack, H.C.: Detection of trophoblast in cord blood and fetal circulation. Amer. J. Obstet. Gynecol. **80**:1013–1021, 1960.

Santiago-Schwarz, F. and Fleit, H.B.: Identification of nonadherent mononuclear cells in human cord blood that differentiate into macrophages. J. Leukocyte Biol. **43**:51–59, 1988.

Scheuner, G.: Über die Verankerung der Nabelschnur an der Plazenta. Morphol. Jahrb. **106**:73–89, 1972.

Scheuner, G.: Zur Morphologie der materno-fetalen Stoffwechselschranke in der menschlichen Plazenta. Zentralbl. Gynäkol. **97**:288–300, 1975.

Scheuner, G. and Hutschenreiter, J.: Strukturanalysen an Basalmembranen. Gefäßwand Blutplasma **IV**:217–218, 1972.

Scheuner, G. and Hutschenreiter, J.: Ergebnisse histophysikalischer Untersuchungen zur submikroskopischen Struktur von Basalmembranen. Anat. Anz. Verh. Anat. Ges. **71**:1213–1216, 1977.

Scheuner, G., Ruckhäberle, K.-E., Flemming, G. and Reissig, D.: Submikroskopischer Nachweis orientierter Proteinfilamente im Plasmoditrophoblasten der menschlichen Plazenta. Anat. Anz. **147**:145–151, 1980.

Schiebler, T.H. and Kaufmann, P.: Über die Gliederung der menschlichen Plazenta. Z. Zellforsch. **102**:242–265, 1969.

Schiebler, T.H. and Kaufmann, P.: Reife Plazenta. In, Die Plazenta des Menschen. V. Becker, T.H. Schiebler and F. Kubli, eds., pp. 51–100. Georg Thieme, Stuttgart, 1981.

Schmidt, W.: Der Feinbau der reifen menschlichen Eihäute. Z. Anat. Entwicklungsgesch. **119**:203–222, 1956.

Schmorl, G.: Pathologisch-anatomische Untersuchungen über puerperale Eklampsie. Vogel-Verlag, Leipzig, 1893.

Schönfelder, G., Graf, R. and Schmidt, H.H.H.W.: A possible regulation of the extravascular contractile system in human placenta by nitric oxide synthase immunoreactive cells. Placenta **14**:A69, 1993.

Schröder, H., Nelson, P. and Power, B.: Fluid shift across the placenta. I. The effect of dextran T40 in the isolated guinea pig placenta. Placenta **3**:327–338, 1982.

Schroeder van der Kolk, J.L.C.: Waarnemigen over het maaksel van de menschljike Placenta. Sulpke, Amsterdam, 1851.

Schuhmann, R.: Plazenton: Begriff, Entstehung, funktionelle Anatomie. In, Die Plazenta des Menschen. V. Becker, T.H. Schiebler and F. Kubli, eds. Thieme Verlag, Stuttgart, pp. 199–207, 1981.

Schweikhart, G. and Kaufmann, P.: Zur Abgrenzung normaler, artefizieller und pathologischer Strukturen in reifen menschlichen Plazentazotten. I. Ultrastruktur des Syncytiotrophoblasten. Arch. Gynäkol. **222**:213–230, 1977.

Scott, S.M., Buenaflor, G.G. and Orth, D.N.: Immunoreactive human epidermal growth factor concentrations in amniotic fluid, umbilical artery and vein serum, and placenta in full-term and preterm infants. Biol. Neonate **56**:246–251, 1989.

Sedmak, D.D., Davis, D.H., Singh, U., van de Winkel, J.G.J. and Anderson, C.L.: Expression of IgG Fc receptor antigens in placenta and on endothelial cells in humans. An immunohistochemical study. Amer. J. Pathol. **138**:175–181, 1991.

Seligman, S.P., Nishiwaki, T., Kadner, S.S., Dancis, J. and Finlay, T.H.: Hypoxia stimulates ecNOS mrna expression by differentiated human trophoblasts. Ann. N.Y. Acad. Sci. **828**:180–187, 1997.

Sen, D.K., Kaufmann, P. and Schweikhart, G.: Classification of human placental villi. II. Morphometry. Cell Tissue Res. **200**:425–434, 1979.

Senaris, R, Garcia-Caballero, T., Casabiell, X., Gallero, R., Castro, R., Considine R.V., Dieguez, C. and Casanueva F.F.: Synthesis of leptin in human placenta. Endocrinology **138**:4501–4504, 1997.

Sgambati, E., Biagiotti, R., Marini, M. and Brizzi, E.: Lectin histochemistry in the human placenta of pregnancies complicated by intrauterine growth retardation based on absent or reversed diastolic flow. Placenta **23**:503–515, 2002.

Siddall, R.S. and Hartman, F.W.: Infarcts of the placenta; study of seven hundred consecutive placentas. Amer. J. Obstet. Gynecol. **12**:683–699, 1926.

Sideri, M., de Virgiliis, G., Rainoldi, R. and Remotti, G.: The ultrastructural basis of the nutritional transfer: evidence of different patterns in the plasma membranes of the multilayered placental barrier. Trophoblast Res. **1**:15–26, 1983.

Simpson, R.A., Mayhew, T.M. and Barnes, P.R.: From 13 weeks to term, the trophoblast of human placenta grows by the continuous recruitment of new proliferative units: a study of nuclear number using the dissector. Placenta **13**:501–512, 1992.

Slamon, D.J., Clark, G.M., Wong, S.G., Levin, W.J., Ullrich, A. and McGuire, R.L.: Human breast cancer: correlation of relapse and survival with amplification of the HER-2/Neu oncogene. Science **235**:177–182, 1987.

Smallwood, A., Papageorghiou, A., Nicolaides, K., Alley, M.K., Alice, J., Nargund, G., Ojha, K., Campbell, S. and Banerjee, S.: Temporal regulation of the expression of syncytin (HERV-W), maternally imprinted PEG10, and SGCE in human placenta. Biol. Reprod. **69**:286–93; 2003.

Smith, C.H., Nelson, D.M., King, B.F., Donohue, T.M., Ruzycki, S.M. and Kelley, L.K.: Characterization of a microvillous membrane preparation from human placental syncytiotrophoblast: a morphologic, biochemical and physiologic study. Amer. J. Obstet. Gynecol. **128**:190–196, 1977.

Smith, S.C., Baker, P.N. and Symonds, E.M.: Placental apoptosis in normal human pregnancy. Amer. J. Obstet. Gynecol. **177**:57–65, 1997a.

Smith, S.C., Baker, P.N. and Symonds, E.M.: Increased placental apoptosis in intrauterine growth restriction. Amer. J. Obstet. Gynecol. **177**:1395–1401, 1997b.

Snoeck, J.: Le Placenta Humain. Masson, Paris, 1958.

Sonnenberg, A., Modderman, P.W. and Hogervorst, F.: Laminin receptor on platelets is the integrin VLA-6. Nature (Lond.) **336**:487–489, 1988.

Sorokin, S.P. and Hoyt, R.F. Jr.: Pure population of nonmonocyte derived macrophages arising in organ cultures of embryonic rat lungs. Anat. Rec. **217**:35–52, 1987.

Sorokin, S.P. and Hoyt, R.F. Jr.: Macrophage development: I. Rationale for using *Griffonia simplicifolia* isolectin B4 as a marker for the line. Anat. Rec. **232**:520–526, 1992.

Sorokin, S.P., Hoyt, R.F. Jr., Blunt, D.G. and McNelly, N.A.: Macrophage development: II. Early ontogeny of macrophage populations in brain, liver, and lungs of rat embryos as revealed by a lectin marker. Anat. Rec. **232**:527–550, 1992a.

Sorokin, S.P., McNelly, N.A., Blunt, D.G. and Hoyt, R.F. Jr.: Macrophage development: III. Transformation of pulmonary macrophages from precursors in fetal lungs and their later maturation in organ culture. Anat. Rec. **232**:551–571, 1992b.

Spanner, R.: Mütterlicher und kindlicher Kreislauf der menschlichen Placenta und seine Strombahnen. Z. Anat, Entwicklungsgesch. **105**:163–242, 1935.

Spanner, R.: Zellinseln und Zottenepithel in der zweiten Hälfte der Schwangerschaft. Morphol. Jahrb. **86**:407–461, 1941.

Sporn, M. and Roberts, A.: The transforming growth factor-betas: past, present and future. Ann. N.Y. Acad. Sci. **593**:1–6, 1990.

Stark, J. and Kaufmann, P.: Protoplasmatische Trophoblastabschnürungen in den mütterlichen Kreislauf bei normaler und pathologischer Schwangerschaft. Arch. Gynäkol. **210**:375–385, 1971.

Stark, J. and Kaufmann, P.: Trophoblastische Plasmapolypen und regressive Veränderungen am Zottentrophoblasten der menschlichen Placenta. Arch. Gynäkol. **212**:51–67, 1972.

Stark, J. and Kaufmann, P.: Infarktgenese in der Placenta. Arch. Gynäkol. **217**:189–208, 1974.

Stengelin, S., Stamenkovic, I. and Seed, B.: Isolation of cDNAs for two distinct human Fc receptors by ligand affinity cloning. EMBO J. **7**:1053–1059, 1988.

Stewart, J.L., Jr., Sano, M.E. and Montgomery, T.L.: Hormone secretion by human placenta grown in tissue culture. J. Clin. Endocrinol. **8**:175–188, 1948.

Stieve, H.: Neue Untersuchungen über die Placenta, besonders über die Entstehung der Placentasepten. Arch. Gynäkol. **161**:160–167, 1936.

Stieve, H.: Das Zottenraumgitter der reifen menschlichen Placenta. Z. Geburtshilfe Gynäkol. **122**:289–316, 1941.

Strauss, L., Goldenberg, N., Hiroto, K. and Okudaira, Y.: Structure of the human placenta; with observations on ultrastructure of the terminal chorionic villus. Birth Defects **1**:13–26, 1965.

Stulc, J.: Extracellular transport pathways in the haemochorial placenta. Placenta **10**:113–119, 1989.

Stulc, J., Friederich, R. and Jiricka, Z.: Estimation of the equivalent pore dimensions in the rabbit placenta. Life Sci. **8**:167–180, 1969.

Sutton, L., Gadd, M., Mason, D.Y. and Redman, C.W.G.: Cells bearing class II MHC antigens in the human placenta and amniochorion. Immunology **58**:23–29, 1986.

Sutton, L.N., Mason, D.Y. and Redman, C.W.G.: Isolation and characterization of human fetal macrophages from placenta. Clin. Exp. Immunol. **78**:437–443, 1989.

Tailor, C.S., Nouri, A., Zhao, Y., Takeuchi, Y. and Kabat, D.: A sodium-dependent neutral amino acid transporter mediates infections of feline and baboon endogenous retroviruses and simian type D retrovirus. J. Virol. **73**:4470–4474, 1999.

Taylor-Papadimitriou, J. and Rozengurt, E.A.: Interferons as regulators of cell growth and differentiation. In, Interferons. Their Impact in Biology and Medicine. J. Taylor-Papadimitriou, ed., pp. 81–98. Oxford University Press, Oxford, 1985.

Teasdale, F. and Jean-Jacques, G.: Morphometry of the microvillous membrane of the human placenta in maternal diabetes mellitus. Placenta **7**:81–88, 1986.

Tedde, G.: Ultrastruttura del villo placentare umano nella seconda meta della gravidanza. Arch. Ital. Anat. Embriol. **75**:101–131, 1970.

Tedde, G. and Tedde-Piras, A.: Mitotic index of the Langhans' cells in the normal human placenta from the early stages of pregnancy to the term. Acta Anat. (Basel) **100**:114–119, 1978.

Tedde, G., Tedde-Piras, A. and Berta, R.: A new structural pattern of the human trophoblast: the syncytial units (abstract 117). In, 11th Rochester Trophoblast Conference, Abstract Booklet, 1988a.

Tedde, G., Tedde-Piras, A. and Fenu, G.: Demonstration of an intercellular pathway of transport in the human trophoblast (abstract 77). In, 11th Rochester Trophoblast Conference, Abstract Booklet, 1988b.

Telfer, J.F., Thomson, A.J., Cameron, I.T., Greer, I.A. and Norman, J.E.: Expression of superoxide dismutase and xanthine oxidase in myometrium, fetal membranes and placenta during normal human pregnancy and parturition. Hum. Reprod. (Oxf.) **12**:2306–2312, 1997.

ten Berge, B.S.: Merkwaardige cellen in chorionvlokken. Med. Thesis, University of Utrecht, 1922.

Tenney, B. and Parker, F.: The placenta in toxemia of pregnancy. Am. J. Obstet. Gynecol. **39**:1000–1005, 1940.

Thomsen, K.: Zur Morphologie und Genese der sogenannten Plazentarinfarkte. Arch. Gynäkol. **185**:221–247, 1954.

Thomsen, K. and Berle, P.: Placentarbefunde bei Rh-Inkompatibilität. Arch. Gynäkol. **192**:628–643, 1960.

Thorn, W., Kaufmann, P. and Müldener, B.: Kohlenhydratumsatz, Energiedefizit und Plasmapolypenbildung in der Placenta nach Vergiftung mit Monojodacetat und NaF. Arch. Gynäkol. **216**:175–183, 1974.

Thorn, W., Kaufmann, P., Müldener, B. and Freese, U.: Einfluß von 2,4-Dinitrophenol, Monojodacetat, Natriumfluorid und Hypoxie auf Plasmapolypenbildung in der Placenta von Meerschweinchen. Arch. Gynäkol. **221**:203–210, 1976.

Thornburg, K. and Faber, J.J.: Transfer of hydrophilic molecules by placenta and yolk sac of the guinea pig. Am. J. Physiol. **233**: C111–C124, 1977.

Thorsby, E.: The role of HLA in T cell activation. Hum. Immunol. **9**:1–7, 1984.

Tominaga, R. and Page, E.W.: Accommodation of the human placenta to hypoxia. Am. J. Obstet. Gynecol. **94**:679–685, 1966.

Toth, F., Paal, M., Nemeth, J. and Doemoetoeri, J.: Histochemical studies of fibrinoid, mucopolysaccharides and chorionic gonadotrophin in the normal and pathologic human placenta. Acta Morphol. Acad. Sci. Hung. **21**:89–104, 1973.

Toth, F.D., Juhl, C., Norskov-Lauritsen, N., Mosborg-Petersen, P. and Ebbesen, P.: Interferon production by cultured human trophoblast induced with double stranded polyribonucleotide. J. Reprod. Immunol. **17**:217–227, 1990.

Toth, F.D., Norskov-Lauritsen, N., Juhl, C. and Ebbesen, P.: Human trophoblast interferon: pattern of response to priming and superinduction of purified term trophoblast and choriocarcinoma cells. J. Reprod. Immunol. **19**:55–67, 1991.

Trudinger, B.J., Giles, W.B., Cook, C.M., Bombardieri, J. and Collins, L.: Uteroplacental blood flow velocity-time waveforms in normal and complicated pregnancy. Br. J. Obstetr. Gynaecol. **92**:23–30, 1985.

Truman, P. and Ford, H.C.: The brush border of the human term placenta. Biochem. Biophys. Acta **779**:139–160, 1984.

Truman, P., Wakerfield, J.St.J. and Ford, H.C.: Microvilli of the human term placenta. Biochem. J. **196**:121–132, 1981.

Tse, W.K., Whitley, G.S. and Cartwright, J.E.: Transforming growth factor-beta1 regulates hepatocyte growth factor-induced trophoblast motility and invasion. Placenta **23**:699–705, 2002.

Uckan, D., Steele, A., Cherry, Wang B.-Y., Chamizo, W., Koutsonikolis, A., Gilbert-Barness, E. and Good, R.A.: Trophoblasts express Fas ligand: a proposed mechanism for immune privilege in placenta and maternal invasion. Mol. Hum. Reprod. **3**:655–662, 1997.

Ulesko-Stroganova, K.: Beitraege zur Lehre vom mikroskopischen Bau der Placenta. Monatsschr. Geburt. Gynäkol. **3**:207, 1896.

Unnikumar, K.R., Wegmann, R. and Panigel, M.: Immunohistochemical profile of the human placenta. Studies on localization of prolactin, human chorionic gonadotropin, human placental lactogen, renin and oxytocin. Cell. Mol. Biol. **34**: 697–710, 1988.

Uren, S. and Boyle, W.: Isolation of macrophages from human placenta. J. Immunol. Methods **78**:25–34, 1985.

Uren, S.J. and Boyle, W.: Class II MCH antigen-positive macrophages from human placentae suppress strong MLR and CML reactions. Cell. Immunol. **125**:235–246, 1990.

Vacek, Z.: Electron microscopic observations on the filaments in the trophoblast of the human placenta. Folia Morphol. (Praha) **17**:382–388, 1969.

Vacek, Z.: Derivation and ultrastructure of the stroma cells of the human chorionic villus. Folia Morphol. (Praha) **18**:1–13, 1970.

Vairo, G., Inner, K.M. and Adams, J.M.: Bcl-2 has a cell cycle inhibitory function separable from its enhancement of cell survival. Oncogene **13**:1511–1519, 1996.

Van Furth, R.: Current view on the mononuclear phagocyte system. Immunobiology **161**:178–185, 1982.

Vanderpuye, O. and Smith, C.H.: Proteins of the apical and basal plasma membranes of the human placental syncytiotrophoblast: immunochemical and electrophoretic studies. Placenta **8**:591–608, 1987.

Velardo, J.T. and Rosa, C.: Female genital system. In, Handbuch der Histochemie, Bd. VII/3. W. Graumann and K. Neumann, eds. Fischer, Stuttgart, 1963.

Verhaeghe, J., Billen, J. and Giudice, L.C.: Insulin-like growth factor-binding protein-1 in umbilical artery and vein of term fetuses with signs suggestive of distress during labor. J. Endocrinol. **170**:585–590, 2001.

Verrijt, C.E., Kroos, M.J., van Noort, W.L., van Eijk, H.G. and van Dijk, J.P.: Binding of human isotransferrin variants to microvillous and basal membrane vesicles from human term placenta. Placenta **18**:71–77, 1997.

Villee, C.A., ed.: The Placenta and Fetal Membranes. Williams & Wilkins, Baltimore, 1960.

Vince, G.S. and Johnson, P.M.: Immunobiology of human utero-placental macrophages-friend and foe? Placenta **17**:191–199, 1996.

Virchow, R.: Die krankhaften Geschwülste, Vol. I. Hirschwald, Berlin, 1863.

Virchow, R.: Cellularpathologie in ihrer Begründung auf physiologische und pathologische Gewebelehre. 4th Ed. Hirschwald, Berlin, 1871.

Virtanen, I., Laitinen, L. and Vartio, T.: Differential expression of the extra domain-containing form of cellular fibronectin in human placentas at different stages of maturation. Histochemistry **90**:25–30, 1988.

Voigt, S., Kaufmann, P. and Schweikhart, G.: Zur Abgrenzung normaler, artefizieller und pathologischer Strukturen in reifen menschlichen Plazentazotten. II. Morphometrische Untersuchungen zum Einfluß des Fixationsmodus. Arch. Gynäkol. **226**:347–362, 1978.

Wachstein, M., Meagher, J.G. and Ortiz, J.: Enzymatic histochemistry of the term human placenta. Am. J. Obstet. Gynecol. **87**:13–26, 1963.

Wada, H.G., Gornicki, S.Z. and Sussman, H.H.: The sialogycoprotein subunits of human placental brush border membranes characterized by two-dimensional electrophoresis. J. Supramol. Struct. **6**:473–484, 1977.

Wada, H.G., Hass, P.E. and Sussman, H.H.: Characterization of antigenic sialoglycoprotein subunits of the placental brush border membranes: comparison with liver and kidney membrane subunits by two-dimensional electrophoresis. J. Supramol. Struct. **10**:287–305, 1979.

Wagner, D.: Trophoblastic cells in the blood stream in normal and abnormal pregnancy. Acta Cytol. **12**:137–139, 1968.

Wagner, D., Schunck, R. and Isebarth, H.: Der Nachweis von Trophoblastzellen im strömenden Blut der Frau bei normaler und gestörter Gravidität. Gynaecologia **158**:175–192, 1964.

Wainwright, S.D. and Holmes, G.H.: Distribution of Fo-g receptors on trophoblast during human placental development: an immunohistochemical and immunoblotting study. Immunology **80**:343–351, 1993.

Wainwright, S.D. and Wainwright, L.K.: Preparation of human placental villous surface membrane. Nature (Lond.) **252**:302–303, 1974.

Wang, T. and Schneider, J.: Cellular junctions on the free surface of human placental syncytium. Arch. Gynecol. **240**:211–216, 1987.

Wang, E., Pfeffer, L.M. and Tamm, I.: Interferon increases the abundance of submembranous microfilaments in HeLa-S3 cells in suspension culture. Proc. Natl. Acad. Sci. U.S.A. **78**: 6281–8285, 1981.

Warren, W.B. and Silverman, A.J.: Cellular localization of corticotrophin releasing hormone in the human placenta, fetal membranes and decidua. Placenta **16**:147–156, 1995.

Wasserman, L., Abramovici, A., Shlesinger, H., Goldman, J.A. and Allalouf, D.: Histochemical localization of acidic glycos-aminoglycans in normal human placentae. Placenta **4**:101–108, 1983a.

Wasserman, L., Shlesinger, H., Goldman, J.A. and Allalouf, D.: Pattern of glycosaminoglycan distribution in tissue and blood vessels of human placenta. Gynecol. Obstet. Invest. **15**:242–250, 1983b.

Watson, A.L., Palmer, M.E., Jauniaux, E. and Burton, G.J.: Variations in expression of copper/zinc superoxide dismutase in villous trophoblast of the human placenta with gestational age. Placenta **18**:295–299, 1997.

Weinberg, P.C., Cameron, I.L., Parmley, T., Jeter, J.R. and Pauerstein, C.J.: Gestational age and placental cellular replication. Obstet. Gynecol. **36**:692–696, 1970.

Werner, C. and Bender, H.G.: Phasenkontrastmikroskopie der Plazenta. In, Neue Erkenntnisse über die Orthologie und Pathologie der Plazenta. H.J. Födisch, ed., pp. 63–71. Enke, Stuttgart, 1977.

Whyte, A.: Lectin binding by microvillous membranes and coated-pit regions of human syncytial trophoblast. Histochem. J. **12**:599–607, 1980.

Wielenga, G. and Willighagen, R.G.J.: The histochemistry of the syncytiotrophoblast and the stroma in the normal full-term placenta. Amer. J. Obstet. Gynecol. **84**:1059–1064, 1962.

Wigglesworth, J.S.: The gross and microscopic pathology of the prematurely delivered placenta. J. Obstet. Gynaecol. Br. Commonw. **69**:934–943, 1962.

Wigglesworth, J.S.: Morphological variations in the insufficient placenta. J. Obstet. Gynaecol. Br. Commonw. **71**:871–884, 1964.

Wilkes, B.M., Mento, P.F., Hollander, A.H., Maita, M.E., Sung, S.Y. and Girardi, E.P.: Endothelin receptors in human placenta: relationship to vascular resistance and thromboxane release. Amer. J. Physiol. **258**:E864-E870, 1990.

Wilkin, P.: Pathologie du Placenta. Masson, Paris, 1965.

Wilson, C.B., Haas, J.E. and Weaver, W.M.: Isolation, purification and characteristics of mononuclear phagocytes from human placentas. J. Immunol. Methods **56**:305–317, 1983.

Winterhager, E.: Dynamik der Zellmembran: Modellstudien während der Implantationsreaktion beim Kaninchen. Med. Thesis, Tech. University of Aachen, 1985.

Wislocki, G.B. and Bennett, H.S.: Histology and cytology of the human and monkey placenta, with special reference to the trophoblast. Am. J. Anat. **73**:335–449, 1943.

Wolfsberg, T.G. and White, J.M.: ADAMs in fertilization and development. Dev. Biol. **180**:389–401, 1996.

Wood, G. and King, G.R., Jr.: Trapping antigen-antibody complexes within the human placenta. Cell Immunol. **69**:347–362, 1982.

Wood, G., Reynard, J., Krishnan, E. and Racela, L.: Immunobiology of the human placenta. I. IgGFc receptors in trophoblastic villi. Cell. Immunol. **35**:191–204, 1978a.

Wood, G., Reynard, J., Krishnan, E. and Racela, L.: Immunobiology of the human placenta. II. Localization of macrophages, in vivo bound IgG and C3. Cell Immunol. **35**:205–216, 1978b.

Wood, G.S., Warner, N.L. and Warnke, R.A.: Anti-Leu-3/T4 antibodies react with cells of monocyte/macrophage and Langerhans lineage. J. Immunol. **131**:212–216, 1983.

Wood, G.S., Turner, R.R., Shiurba, R.A., Eng, L. and Warnke, R.A.: Human dendritic cells and macrophages: in situ immunophenotypic definition of subsets that exhibit specific morphologic and microenvironmental characteristics. Am. J. Pathol. **119**:73–82, 1985.

Wood, G.W.: Mononuclear phagocytes in the human placenta. Placenta **1**:113–123, 1980.

Wright, C., Angus, B., Nicholson, S., Sainsbury, J.R., Cairns, J.C., Gullick, W.J., Kelley, P., Harris, A.L. and Horne, C.H.W.: Expression of *c-erbB*-2 oncoprotein: a prognostic indicator in human breast cancer. Cancer Res. **49**:2087–2090, 1989.

Wright, S.D., Ramos, R.A., Tobias, P.S. and Ulevitch, R.J.: CD 14, a receptor for complexes of lipopolysaccharide (LPS) and LPS binding protein. Science **249**:1431–1433, 1990.

Wynn, R.M.: Derivation and ultrastructure of the so-called Hofbauer cell. Amer. J. Obstet. Gynecol. **97**:235–248, 1967a.

Wynn, R.M.: Fetomaternal cellular relations in the human basal plate: an ultrastructural study of the placenta. Amer. J. Obstet. Gynecol. **97**:832–850, 1967b.

Wynn, R.M.: Fine structure of the placenta. In, Handbook of Physiology, Section 7, Endocrinology. R.O. Greep and E.B. Astwood, eds., pp. 261–276. American Physiological Society, Washington D.C., 1973.

Wynn, R.M.: Fine structure of the placenta. In, The Placenta and its Maternal Supply Line. P. Gruenwald, ed. Medical and Technical Publishing, Lancaster, pp. 56–79, 1975.

Yagami-Hiromasa, T., Sato, T., Kurisaki, T., Kamijo, K., Nabeshima, Y. and Fujisawa-Sehara, A.: A metalloproteinase-disintegrin participating in myoblast fusion. Nature **377**:652–656, 1995.

Yagel, S., Hurwitz, A., Rosenn, B. and Keizer, N.: Progesterone enhancement of prostaglandin E2 production by fetal placental macrophages. Amer. J. Reprod. Immunol. **14**:45–48, 1987.

Yallampalli, C. and Garfield, R.E.: Inhibition of nitric oxide synthesis in rats during pregnancy produces signs similar to those of preeclampsia. Amer. J. Obstet. Gynecol. **169**:1316–1320, 1993.

Yamada, T., Isemura, M., Yamaguchi, Y., Munakata, H., Hayashi, N. and Kyogoku, M.: Immunohistochemical localization of fibronectin in the human placentas at their different stages of maturation. Histochemistry **86**:579–584, 1987.

Yamaguchi, Y., Mann, D.M. and Ruoslahti, E.: Negative regulation of transforming growth factor-b by the proteoglycan decorin. Nature (Lond.) **346**:281–284, 1990.

Yang K.: Placental 11 beta-hydroxysteroid dehydrogenase: barrier to maternal glucocorticoids. Rev. Reprod. **2**:129–132, 1997.

Yasuda, M., Umemura, S., Osamura, Y.R., Kenjo, T. and Tsutsumi, Y.: Apoptotic cells in the human endometrium and placental villi: pitfalls in applying the TUNEL method. Arch. Histol. Cytol. **58**:185–190, 1995.

Yeh, C.-J., Mühlhauser, J., Hsi, B.-I., Castellucci, M. and Kaufmann, P.: The expression of receptors for epidermal growth factor and transferrin on human trophoblast. Placenta **10**:459, 1989.

Yoshiki, N., Kubota, T. and Aso, T.: Expression and localization of heme oxygenase in human placental villi. Biochem. Biophys. Res. Commun. **276**:1136–1142, 2000.

Yu, C., Shen, K., Lin, M., Chen, P., Lin, C., Chang, G.-D. and Chen, H.: GCMa regulates the syncytin-mediated trophoblast fusion. J. Biol. Chem. **277**:50062–50068, 2002.

Yui, J., Garcia-Lloret, M.I., Wegmann, T.G. and Guilbert, L.J.: Cytotoxicity of tumor necrosis factor: alpha- and gamma-interferon against primary human placental trophoblasts. Placenta **5**:819–835, 1994.

Yui, J., Hemmings, D., Garcia-Lloret, M.I. and Guilbert, L.: Expression of the human p55 and p75 tumor necrosis factor receptors in primary villous trophoblasts and their role in cytotoxic signal transduction. Biol. Reprod. **55**:400–409, 1996.

Zaccheo, D., Zicca, A., Cadoni, A., Leprini, A., Castellucci, M. and Kaufmann, P.: Preliminary observations on Hofbauer cells in short-term culture. Bibl. Anat. **22**:63–68, 1982.

Zaccheo, D., Pistoia, V., Castellucci, M. and Martinoli, C.: Isolation and characterization of Hofbauer cells from human placental villi. Arch. Gynecol. **246**:189–200, 1989.

Zhou, G.Q., Baranov, V., Zimmermann, W., Grunert, F., Erhard, B., Minchevanilsson, L., Hammarstrom, S. and Thompson, J. Highly specific monoclonal antibody demonstrates that pregnancy-specific glycoprotein (PSG) is limited to syncytiotrophoblast in human early and term placenta. Placenta **18**:491–501, 1997.

Ziegler-Heitbrock, H.-W.L.: The biology of the monocyte system. Eur. J. Cell Biol. **49**:1–12, 1989.

7
Architecture of Normal Villous Trees

Classification of Villous Types

The ramifications of the villous trees can be subdivided into segments that differ mainly as to caliber, stromal structure, vessel structure, and position within the villous tree (Fig. 7.1). Five villous types have been described (Kaufmann et al., 1979; Sen et al., 1979; Castellucci & Kaufmann, 1982a,b; Kaufmann, 1982; Castellucci et al., 1984, 1990, 2000; Burton, 1987), some of which can be further subdivided. As will be discussed below, all villous types derive from single precursors, the mesenchymal villi, which correspond to the tertiary villi of the early stages of placentation.

The following villous types have been described (Fig. 7.2):

1. Stem villi are characterized by a condensed fibrous stroma, arteries and veins, or arterioles and venules with a media or adventitia identifiable by light microscopy (Fig. 7.2). They comprise the following structures (see Fig. 7.17A):

- The main stems (truncus chorii) of a villous tree, which connect the latter with the chorionic plate;
- Up to four generations of branchings (rami chorii of the first to fourth orders), which are short, thick branches derived from the truncus already in the vicinity of the chorionic plate;
- Two to 30 (mean, 10) more generations of unequal dichotomous branchings (ramuli chorii of the first to tenth orders), which are more slender branches that extend into the periphery of the villous trees;
- A special group of stem villi represented by the anchoring villi; these villi are ramuli chorii, which connect to the basal plate by a cell column. The proliferating trophoblast cells of the latter act as a growth zone for both, the anchoring villus as well as for the basal plate.

2. Immature intermediate villi (Fig. 7.2) are bulbous, peripheral, immature continuations of stem villi. They are in a position comparable to that of the mature intermediate villi, that is, interposed between stem villi and peripheral branches, and they prevail in immature placentas. Normally, this type persists in small groups within the centers of the villous trees (placentones) and represents the immature forerunners of stem villi.

3. Mature intermediate villi (Fig. 7.2) are long, slender, peripheral ramifications characterized by the absence of vessels with a light-microscopically identifiable media and/or adventitia.

4. Terminal villi (Fig. 7.2) are the final, grape-like ramifications of the mature intermediate villi, characterized by their high degree of capillarization and the presence of highly dilated sinusoids. They represent the main sites of fetomaternal exchange.

5. Mesenchymal villi (Fig. 7.2) are the most primitive. They prevail during the first stages of pregnancy, where they are the forerunners of immature intermediate villi. During later stages of pregnancy, these villi are inconspicuous, mostly small, slender structures that can be found along the surfaces of immature intermediate villi or at the tips of mature intermediate villi. At this stage they also act as zones of villous proliferation and further branching.

The principal morphometric data of the various villous types are shown in Chapter 28, Table 28.7, and in Fig. 7.15.

Stem Villi

Trunci chorii, rami chorii, ramuli chorii, and the anchoring villi are summarized as stem villi because they exhibit similar histologic features and differ from each other only in caliber and position within the hierarchy of villous branching (Demir et al., 1997). The calibers vary from

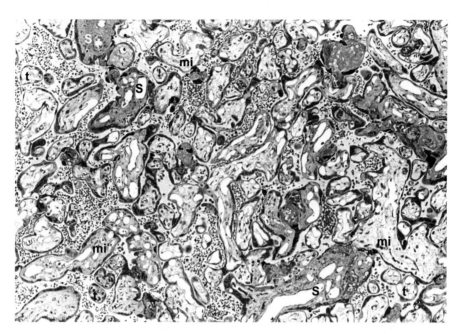

FIGURE 7.1. Semithin section from the 40th week postmenstruation (p.m.) to demonstrate the structural and staining variability of villous cross sections. Such pictures suggest that the villous tree is composed of several villous types that differ from each other regarding size, stromal fibrosis, and density of fetal vascularization. s, stem villi; mi, mature intermediate villi; t, terminal villi. ×140.

about 80 μm (smallest ramuli chorii) to about 3000 μm (some trunci, near the chorionic plate). In the normal mature placenta, they make up 20% to 25% of the total villous volume (see Table 28.7). Because of the typical branching patterns of the villous trees, the volumetric share of the stem villi is the highest in the central subchorionic portion of the villous tree.

The trophoblast cover of stem villi is uniformly thick and lacks epithelial plates. Cytotrophoblastic cells, located below the superficial syncytiotrophoblast, can be found on about 20% of the villous surfaces. In the mature placenta, the trophoblast is often degenerated and largely replaced by perivillous fibrinoid (Figs. 7.3A,B and 7.4). The trophoblastic degeneration is more impressive in stem villi of large caliber than in the small peripheral villi. Moreover, there seems to be a certain positive correlation with intrauterine growth retardation (Ara et al., 1984; Macara et al., 1996).

The stroma is characterized by huge, condensed bundles of collagen fibers that encase occasional fibroblasts and rare macrophages (Fig. 7.3C). Within trunci, rami, and large ramuli, the fetal vessels are composed of arteries and veins that are accompanied by smaller arterioles and venules as well as superficially located paravascular capillaries (Fig. 7.3A). The latter are comparable to vasa vasorum of large-caliber vessels of other organs. In the smaller, more peripheral ramuli, arteries and veins are lacking; rather, the fetal vessels are represented by a few arterioles and venules that typically have thin vessel walls and are accompanied by few paravascular capillaries (Fig.

7.3B). The adventitia of arteries and veins continues without sharp demarcation into the surrounding fibrous stroma of the villous core (Fig. 7.3A). The more centrally located connective tissue cells are myofibroblasts, whereas the more peripheral ones are noncontractile fibroblasts (Demir et al., 1992, 1997; Kohnen et al., 1995, 1996).

The central core of myofibroblasts is arranged around the stem vessels (Fig. 7.5) and has been called the perivascular sheath (Graf et al., 1994, 1995, 1997). In stem villi that are not yet fully mature, an additional superficial rim of reticular stroma, composed of undifferentiated, proliferating connective tissue cells but deficient in fibers, may separate the fibrous stroma from the trophoblastic cover (see Chapter 8, Figs. 8.5 to 8.8). All three layers together represent a differentiation gradient; the most peripheral cells are the proliferating stem cells and the most central cells represent the highest degrees of differentiation. As soon as the trophoblastic cover is replaced by fibrinoid, the stromal stem cells stop proliferation and start differentiation, thus leading to a homogeneously fibrosed stem villus stroma (Demir et al., 1997). These data suggest paracrine interactions between trophoblastic epithelium and the stromal stem cells beneath. Macrophages are evenly distributed throughout the stroma (Demir et al., 1992, 1997). Occasionally mast cells are present in the vascular walls of the stem villi (see Chapter 6).

Function: Stem villi serve to mechanically support the structures of the villous trees. Considering the low degree of fetal capillarization and degenerative changes of the trophoblast, their share in fetomaternal exchange and

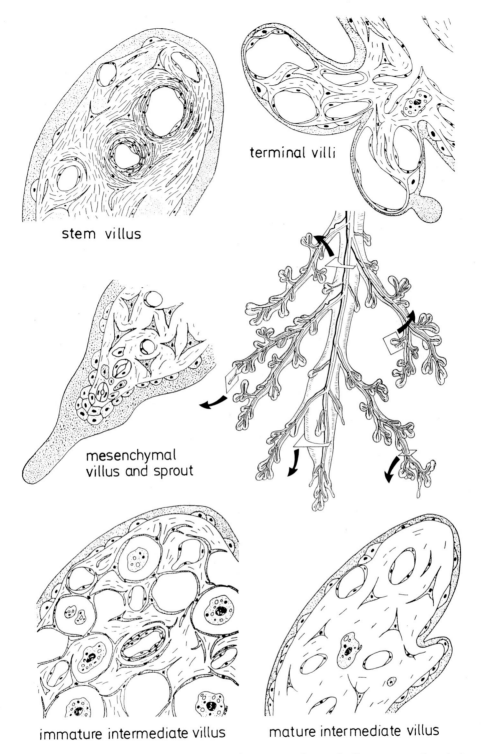

stem villus

terminal villi

mesenchymal villus and sprout

immature intermediate villus

mature intermediate villus

FIGURE 7.2. Simplified representation of the peripheral part of a mature placental villous tree, and typical cross sections of the various villous types. For further details see text. (*Source:* Kaufmann & Scheffen, 1992, with permission.)

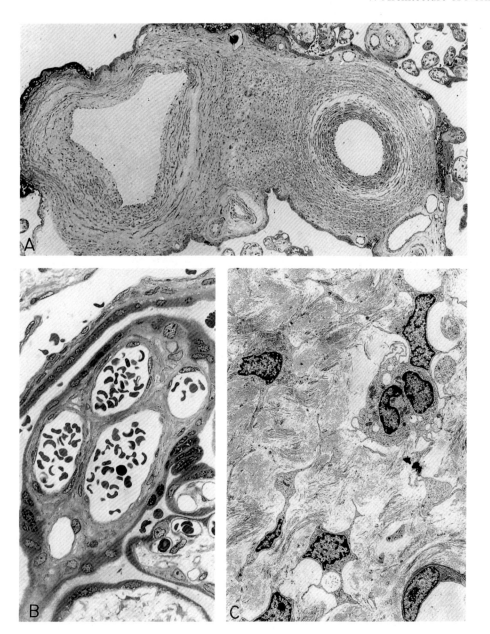

FIGURE 7.3. Structural features of stem villi. A: Semithin cross section of a large stem villus. Note that the adventitias of the artery (right) and vein (left) directly continue into the surrounding dense fibrous stroma of the villus. Superficially, numerous smaller vessels of the paravascular capillary net are seen. As is typical for stem villi of the mature placenta, the trophoblastic covering of this villus has been removed by fibrinoid in many places. ×115. (*Source:* Leiser et al., 1985, with permission.) B: More peripherally positioned stem villi of small caliber can be identified by the condensed fibrous stroma, located between the fetal arterioles and venules (large lumens). Fetal capillaries are rare. ×430. C: Transmission electron micrograph of the fibrous stroma of a stem villus. The interstitial space between the various types of connective tissue cells is mostly occupied by dense bundles of collagen fibers. Residual macrophages (upper right) partly surrounded by sail-like extensions of fibroblasts remind us that fibrous stroma is derived from reticular stroma. ×2400.

endocrine activity is presumably negligible. The presence of the large fetal vessels with thick muscular walls as well as the presence of extravascular myofibroblasts (Demir et al., 1992, 1997; Kohnen et al., 1996) makes their contribution to the autoregulation of the fetoplacental vascular system likely. Moreover, the myofibroblasts that are oriented in parallel to the longitudinal axis of the villous stems, the so-called perivascular sheath (Graf et al., 1994, 1995, 1997), may provide a regulating system for the maternal circulation in the intervillous space (Fig. 7.6). Because many of the larger villous stems are anchoring villi that connect the chorion and basal plate, their longi-

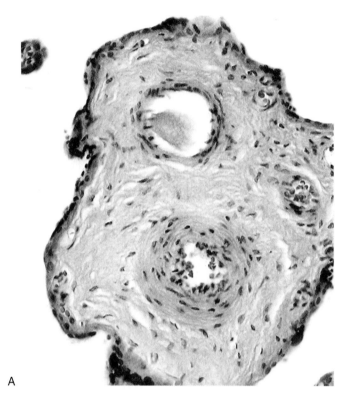

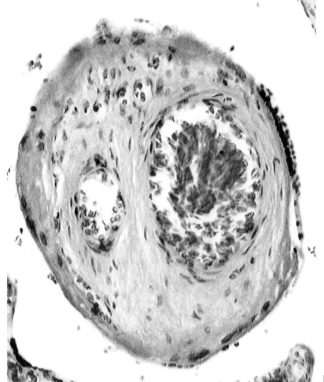

A

B

FIGURE 7.4. Peripheral stem villi. 40 weeks p.m. A: Structural features of a not yet fully matured stem villus from the center of a fetal cotyledon. The trophoblastic surface cover is still largely complete. Below the trophoblastic surface, locally para-vascular capillaries can be seen, which are embedded in highly cellular connective tissue. B: In contrast, in a fully matured stem villus of the same size, derived from the peripheral parts of a fetal cotyledon of the identical placenta, the trophoblast is largely replaced by fibrinoid. The number of subtrophoblastic paravascular capillaries has decreased. Paraffin sections, hematoxylin and eosin (H&E) stain. ×430.

FIGURE 7.5. Mature placental villi immu-nostained with an antibody against γ-smooth muscle actin. This antibody stains both vascular smooth muscle cells and extravascular myofibroblasts. Nuclei counterstained with hematoxylin. Terminal villi and mature intermediate villi are immuno-negative. Only stem villi are immunoreac-tive (brown). Cross sections of small-sized peripheral stem villi (upper and lower left) can be identified by immunoreactive smooth muscle cells concentrically sur-rounding villous arterioles and venules. In the centrally located longitudinally sec-tioned large-caliber stem villus between the immunopositive vessel walls (brown) and villous surface longitudinally sectioned, filiform, immunopositive myofibroblasts can be seen. ×100.

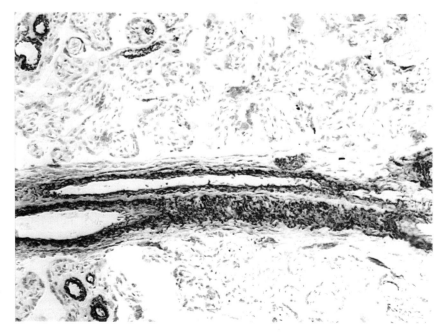

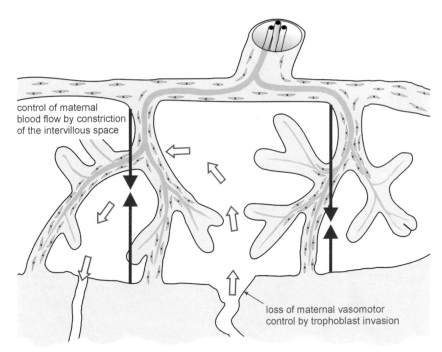

control of maternal
blood flow by constriction
of the intervillous space

loss of maternal vasomotor
control by trophoblast invasion

FIGURE 7.6. Schematic representation of the distribution of villous extravascular myofibroblasts (lilac) in large-caliber stem and anchoring villi. Upon contraction, these cells shorten the length of stem and anchoring villi, thereby reduce the width of the intervillous space, and increase the impedance of maternal intervillous blood flow (red arrows). In this way the fetus is thought to gain control over the maternal blood flow in the placenta, which the mother has lost as a consequence of trophoblast invasion of the uteroplacental arteries.

tudinal contraction decreases intervillous volume (Krantz & Parker, 1963; Kohnen et al., 1996; Demir et al., 1997; Farley et al., 2004) and very likely increases uteroplacental flow impedance. As was discussed in Chapter 6, in this way the fetus gains control over the maternal blood flow in the placenta, which the mother has lost as a consequence of trophoblast invasion of the uteroplacental arteries.

Blood flow and blood pressure control in the intervillous space are important, as has been demonstrated in vitro by Karimu and Burton (1994): pressure increases in the intervillous space reduce the width of the fetoplacental capillaries and thus increase fetoplacental impedance and reduce fetal perfusion of the placenta. Respective malregulation is thought to be a major mechanism in the pathogenesis of intrauterine growth restriction (IUGR) with absent or reversed end-diastolic (ARED) umbilical flow (Kingdom & Kaufmann, 1997; Kingdom et al., 1997a). In conclusion, myofibroblasts may act as an important link adapting maternal and fetal perfusion of the placenta to each other. Increase in fetoplacental blood flow impedance caused by high pressure in the villous surrounding can be downregulated by relaxation of the myofibroblasts (Demir et al., 1997; Kohnen et al., 1995, 1996).

Immature Intermediate Villi

The immature intermediate villi have been known as immature villi or immature terminal villi. We have suggested that the term **immature intermediate** is more appropriate because these villi are not the only immature villous type, nor are they immature forerunners of later terminal villi (Kaufmann et al., 1979; Kaufmann, 1982). Rather, both types of intermediate villi (immature and mature intermediate villi) are differentiated successors of mesenchymal villi:

- The immature intermediate villi result from maturation of mesenchymal villi throughout the first two trimesters. Later they are transformed into stem villi.
- The mature intermediate villi, which derive from mesenchymal precursors during the last trimester, produce the terminal villi.

Thus, both "intermediate" villi are in an intermediate developmental position between mesenchymal and fully mature villi. Moreover, both are in an intermediate topographic position between stem villi and the most peripheral branches.

Histologically, immature intermediate villi have the same uniform, thick trophoblastic cover as stem villi (Figs. 7.2 and 7.7A,B). Epithelial plates are absent. During early pregnancy, Langhans' cells can be found below the syncytium on more than 50% of the villous surfaces. During late pregnancy, their prevalence is reduced to about 20%.

The most characteristic feature of the immature intermediate villi is their reticular stroma, typified by numerous fluid-filled channels that are delimited by large, sail-like processes of the fixed stromal cells (Kaufmann et al., 1977b) (Fig. 7.7A–C). Hofbauer cells are inside the channels (Enders & King, 1970; Castellucci & Kaufmann, 1982a), suspended in some fluid.

Fetal vessels, such as the capillaries, arterioles, and venules, together with scarce bundles of collagen fibers,

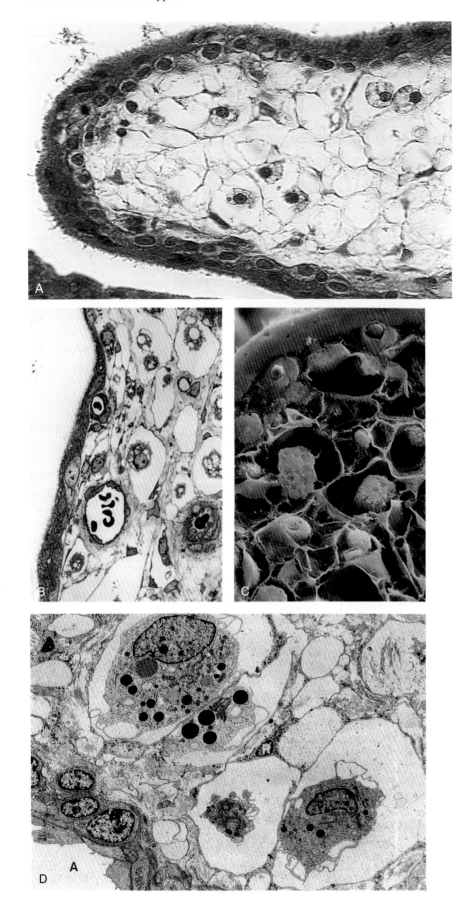

FIGURE 7.7. Typical structure of the immature intermediate villus. A: Paraffin section, 6th week p.m., H&E. staining. Note the reticular appearance of the villous stroma with enmeshed highly vacuolated macrophages. ×400. B: Semithin section of an immature intermediate villus from the 22nd week of pregnancy p.m. with its typical reticular stroma. The rounded, vacuolated macrophages (Hofbauer cells) are located in stromal channels, which are devoid of connective tissue fibers and therefore appear as empty holes. In faintly stained histologic sections, this feature can be misinterpreted as villous edema. ×520. (*Source:* Kaufmann, 1981, with permission.) C: Scanning electron micrograph of a freeze-fractured immature intermediate villus shows the three-dimensional view of the reticular stroma with its characteristic stromal channels. ×1050. (Courtesy of M. Castellucci.) D: Transmission electron micrograph of the reticular stroma of an immature intermediate villus at term. Several stromal channels, each containing a macrophage, can be identified. They are delimited from the surrounding connective tissue fibers by slender, sail-like extensions of fixed connective tissue cells (small reticulum cells, R). A small fetal arteriole (A) is seen in the lower left corner. ×2700. (*Source:* Castellucci & Kaufmann, 1982a, with permission.)

are positioned between the stromal channels. Collagen bundles and vessel walls are separated from the lumina of the channels by the sail-like extensions of the connective tissue cells (Fig. 7.7B,D).

Transformation of immature intermediate villi into stem villi takes place during the first trimester. It is a gradual process that results in numerous intermediate steps. The starting point for the stromal fibrosis is the vascular wall. In the beginning, vessels acquire a distinct media and adventitia. The latter expands in later stages over the entire villous thickness. During this process the intercanalicular bundles of connective tissue fibers increase in diameter and thus compress the neighboring stromal channels. Eventually, they disappear. Residues can be found in all stem villi when one studies the stroma carefully for Hofbauer cells (Fig. 7.3C).

The first immature intermediate villi are formed around the 8th week postmenstruation (p.m.) (compare Figs. 8.2 with 8.3; see Table 8.1). Between the 14th and 20th weeks (Figs. 8.3 to 8.5) they comprise most of the villous cross sections. At term, they may be completely absent; in most cases they can be found in small groups in the centers of the villous trees, the "placentones," where they still act as growth zones and produce new sprouts. At term, a volumetric share of 0% to 5% is normal for immature intermediate villi. This figure is applicable only when all parts of a placentone are equally represented in the histologic section. Sections restricted to the more central parts of a villous tree may show higher values and must thus be interpreted with care.

Function: The immature intermediate villi can be regarded as the growth centers of the villous trees. These produce the true sprouts (see hapter 15), which are transformed into mesenchymal villi as forerunners of all other villous types. Because of the long maternofetal diffusion distances, immature intermediate villi are the principal sites of exchange only during the first two trimesters, so long as other specialized villous types are not yet differentiated.

Immature intermediate villi may cause diagnostic problems, as their reticular stromal core has only a weak affinity for conventional stains because of the lack of collagen. Typical features are depicted in Figs. 7.7A,B and 8.3 through 8.5. The weaker staining, however, often results in the disappearance of the stromal channels so that the resulting histologic picture is that of a seemingly edematous villus that has accumulated much interstitial fluid. Such true edematous villi indeed exist. They are particularly impressive in hydatidiform moles but may also be found in maternal diabetes mellitus and some infections (e.g., syphilis, toxoplasmosis, cytomegalovirus infection). On the other hand, as experienced a pathologist as Harold Fox expressed some doubt when he wrote: "This has long been recognized as one of the characteristic features of placentae from diabetic women and from cases of materno-fetal rhesus incompatibility, though in fact only a proportion of such placentae are edematous." For other cases, he simply stated villous immaturity to be the correct designation (Fox, 1978, 1997). We believe that many villi referred to as "edematous villi" in the literature are in fact normal, immature intermediate villi (e.g., in most cases of rhesus incompatibility) (Pilz et al., 1980; Kaufmann et al., 1987). Naeye et al. (1983) have discussed in much detail the clinical significance of placental villous edema. We cannot exclude, based on their publication, that these changes represent true edematous alterations; however, at least one of the two examples they depicted, their Figure 2, is a normal, immature intermediate villus. They described it as follows: "Villous edema was recognized by the finding of open spaces in the interstitium of the villi," but they pointed to normal stromal channels.

This contradiction does not negate the existence of villous edema. It is probable that true generalized villous edema has functional significance, as it may compress the intervillous space and thus limit maternal blood flow (Alvarez et al., 1972; Fox, 1978); it also increases the maternofetal diffusion distances. Fox (1978) stated that "villous oedema is usually considered to be of no clinical significance," and that "there is, as yet, no clear evidence that villous oedema has, in itself, any effect on fetal growth or nutrition." Perhaps this negative conclusion is based on the interpretation that most cases of "villous edema" are misinterpretations of normal villous structures.

For further details regarding normal structure and function of immature intermediate villi, see the publications by Castellucci and Kaufmann (1982a,b), Castellucci et al. (1984), Highison and Tibbitts (1986), Kaufmann (1982), Kaufmann et al. (1977b, 1979), and Sen et al. (1979).

Mature Intermediate Villi

Mature intermediate villi are long slender villi with diameters of about 60 to 150 mm. As soon as their surfaces bear terminal villi, their shape is characterized by numerous slight bends at points where the terminal villi branch off, resulting in a typical zigzag course (see Fig. 7.10A,D). This pattern is absent when terminal side branches are not present (see Chapter 15), features that may be of diagnostic importance. Mature intermediate villi have roughly the same diameters as terminal villi. Because of their zigzag courses, longitudinal histologic sections are rare. As long as mature intermediate villi do not produce terminal villi, they do not pursue the zigzag course but, rather, remain straight. This appearance, in sections of weeks 32 to 34, is one of groups of cross sections that alternate with bundles of slender longitudinal sections (see Chapter 15, Fig. 15.9).

The trophoblast cover of mature intermediate villi is much thinner than those of stem and immature intermediate villi. Where it covers capillaries, it often is reduced to epithelial plates of less than 1 μm thickness. Also the rare cytotrophoblastic cells are mostly found close to the capillaries.

The stroma of mature intermediate villi is composed of seemingly unoriented, loose bundles of connective tissue fibers and fixed connective tissue cells. In some places it surrounds rudimentary narrow stromal channels that are usually devoid of macrophages (Figs. 7.8 and 7.9).

The vessels comprise numerous capillaries, small terminal arterioles, and collecting venules. The media of the latter is usually too thin for light microscopic identification. Because the terminal villi originate from the surface of the mature intermediate villi, there is a gradual transition. Cross sections are defined as mature intermediate villi, the stroma of which contains fewer than 50% vascular lumens (see Table 28.6). Roughly one fourth of the villous volume in the normal term placenta is composed of this villous type (see Table 28.7).

Function: The mature intermediate villi produce the terminal villi. The high degree of fetal vascularization and the large share in the exchange surface make them important for fetomaternal exchange. When studying the enzyme patterns and the immunolocalization of placental hormones, one gains the impression that they are prominent sites for hormone production. In analogy with the vascular bed of other organs, one may conclude that the presence of terminal arterioles allows participation in vasoregulation and thus intravillous blood distribution (Nikolov & Schiebler, 1973).

Terminal Villi

Terminal villi are the final ramifications of the villous tree during the last trimester. They are grape-like outgrowths of the mature intermediate villi, where they appear as single or poorly branched side branches (Fig. 7.10). The peripheral end of the mature intermediate villus normally branches into a larger aggregate of such terminal villi (Fig. 7.10B). They usually connect to the mature intermediate villi by a narrow neck region (Fig. 7.10C,D; see also Fig. 7.20A). Only an extremely small proportion of the terminal villi are directly connected to stem villi or to immature intermediate villi.

Histologically, the trophoblast cover of terminal villi is thin and forms numerous epithelial plates. Depending on

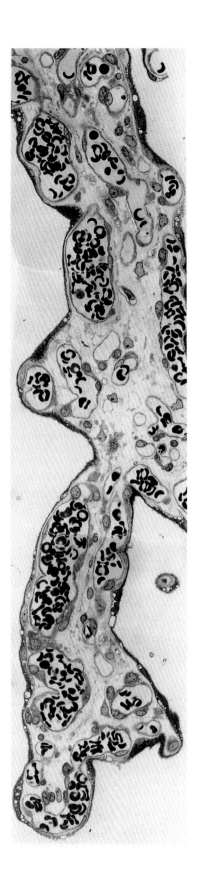

FIGURE 7.8. Semithin section of the richly vascularized peripheral end of a mature intermediate villus (upper half), with a terminal villus (lower half) arising at a narrow neck region (center). The fetal vessels show the typical composition of narrow capillaries and dilated sinusoids. The latter are closely related to the trophoblastic surface, forming thin epithelial plates. ×430. (*Source:* Kaufmann et al., 1979, with permission.)

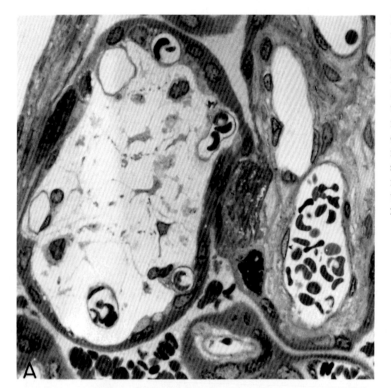

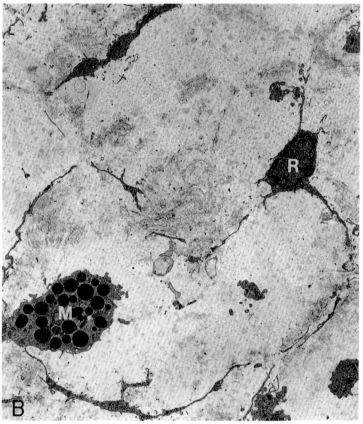

FIGURE 7.9. Typical structure of mature intermediate villi. Semithin cross section of the poorly vascularized, more central portion of a mature intermediate villus. Note the peripheral position of the small fetal capillaries and the ample connective tissue, deficient in cells and fibers. The syncytiotrophoblastic covering of the villus is more uniform in structure than that of the terminal villi. ×730. B: Transmission electron micrograph of the typical loose connective tissue of a mature intermediate villus. The seemingly unoriented mixture of small reticulum cells (R) with long processes, macrophages (M), and loosely arranged connective tissue fibers is highly characteristic for this villous type. ×2150.

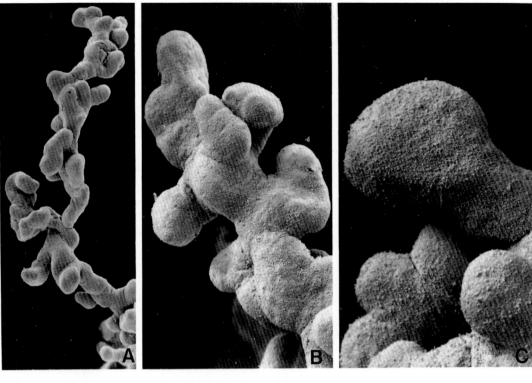

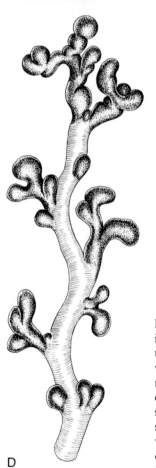

FIGURE 7.10. Scanning electron microscopic appearance of terminal villi. A: A single, long, mature intermediate villus shows the characteristic bends of its longitudinal axis and multiple grape-like terminal villi. Note that the terminal villi largely have the same diameter as the mature intermediate villus from which they branch. ×180. (*Source:* Kaufmann et al., 1979, with permission.) B: Tip of a mature intermediate villus with rich final branching into terminal villi. ×470. (*Source:* Kaufmann et al., 1979, with permission.) C: A group of terminal villi, the central one showing a typical constricted neck region and a dilated final portion. ×500. (*Source:* Kaufmann et al., 1979, with permission.) D: Simplified drawing of a mature intermediate villus (line shaded) and its branching terminal villi (point shading). As is typical, most terminal villi arise from the convex sides of each bend, either directly or with a narrow neck region. They branch repeatedly, particularly at the end of the mature intermediate villus. (*Source:* Kaufmann et al., 1979, with permission.)

the quality of tissue preservation, they amount to 30% to 40% of the villous surface (see Table 28.6 and Fig. 7.20).

Fetal vessels are represented by sinusoidally dilated capillaries. The latter occupy more than 50% of the stromal volume and more than 35% of the villous volume (see Table 28.6) (Figs. 7.8 and 7.11; also see Fig. 7.20) (Kaufmann et al., 1979; Sen et al., 1979). The fetal sinusoids are in intimate contact with the trophoblastic surface and form the epithelial plates.

The remaining connective tissue has scant fibers and cells. Macrophages are rare (Fig. 7.11). The average diameter of terminal villi ranges from 30 to 80 μm. Their histologic appearance differs, depending on where they are sectioned. The slender neck region, containing mostly undilated capillaries, is easily differentiated from the

bulbous tip containing mostly sinusoids and from flat sections across tips (see Fig. 7.20).

It must be pointed out that the light microscopic appearance is heavily influenced by the mode of tissue preservation. Delayed fixation (see Tables 28.6 and 28.9), inappropriate osmolarity of the fixative (see Table 28.10), and time and mode of cord clamping (see Table 28.9) influence the villous structure. In particular, the highly dilated sinusoids respond to postpartal changes of fetal blood pressure. They tend to collapse within minutes, thus dramatically changing the villous proportions (Voigt et al., 1978; Burton & Palmer, 1988). An increase in pressure in the peripheral fetal vessels, as during cord compression (knots, torsion, nuchal cord), leads to congestion in the terminal capillaries and results in seemingly "hyper-

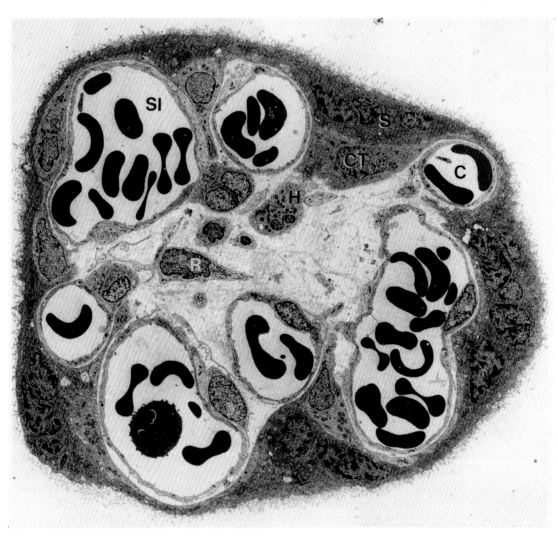

FIGURE 7.11. Survey electron micrograph of a typical, well-fixed terminal villus illustrates the high degree of fetal capillarization, with some of the capillaries (C) being narrow and others dilated, forming sinusoids (SI). The sparse connective tissue is composed of macrophages (H), fibroblasts or small reticulum cells (R), and a loose meshwork of connective tissue fibers. The stroma is surrounded by a structurally highly variable layer of syncytiotrophoblast (S) below which a few cytotrophoblastic cells (CT) can be seen. ×2000. (*Source:* Schiebler & Kaufmann, 1981, with permission.)

capillarized" villi ("chorangiosis"). We found this feature frequently with preterm rupture of membranes, and the correlation is highly significant. There was also an increase in villous blood volume, sometimes of more than 50%. It may be speculated that loss of amnionic fluid predisposes to compression of the umbilical veins and thus inhibits placental venous backflow (Paprocki, 1992).

Function: The high degree of vascularization and minimal mean maternofetal diffusion distance of about 3.7μm (Voigt et al., 1978; Sen et al., 1979; Feneley & Burton, 1991) (see Table 28.6) make this villous type the most appropriate place for diffusional exchange (e.g., transfer of oxygen, carbon dioxide, and water). In the normal mature placenta, the terminal villi comprise nearly 40% of the villous volume. Because of their small diameters, the sum of their surfaces amounts to 50% of the total villous surface. They comprise about 60% of villous cross sections. These figures explain why a remarkable reduction of terminal villi (as in IUGR with ARED umbilical flow) (Macara et al., 1996; Kingdom et al., 1997b) may lead to fetal hypoxia. Also, according to Fox (1978), there is a clear-cut inverse relation between the incidence of villous vasculosyncytial membranes and fetal hypoxia.

Mesenchymal Villi

The term **mesenchymal villi** has been proposed for the first generation of tertiary villi, which are characterized by a seemingly primitive stromal core resembling fetal mesenchyme (Castellucci & Kaufmann, 1982a). From the 5th (onset of villous vascularization) to the 7th week p.m., this is the only vascularized villous type. At later stages, their number continuously decreases. Some of these villi are still found at term, indicating that expansion of the villous trees in normal pregnancies never comes to a standstill.

These villi comprise the first generation of newly formed villi, not only during the first trimester but also at later stages. Differentiation of every new villus starts in the mesenchymal stage. It is derived from trophoblastic sprouts by mesenchymal invasion and vascularization and precedes the formation of new intermediate villi (Figs. 7.12 to 7.14). In accordance with their role as proliferating segments, the mesenchymal villi decrease in number as pregnancy advances. At term, they are primarily found in small numbers on the surfaces of immature intermediate villi. They are located in the centers of the villous trees.

Mesenchymal villi have thick trophoblast surfaces with large numbers of Langhans' cells, which are interposed between syncytium and the trophoblastic basal lamina on 50% to 100% of the villous surfaces (Castellucci et al., 1990, 2000).

The stroma is characterized by loosely arranged collagen fibers that enmesh mesenchymal and some Hofbauer cells (Fig. 7.14). Condensed collagen is sometimes observed.

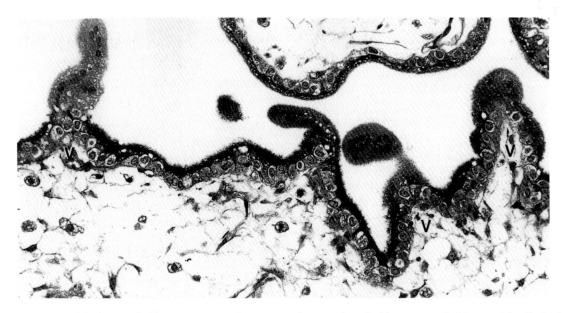

FIGURE 7.12. Structural features of villous sprouts and mesenchymal villi in a methacrylate section of placental villi from the 6th week p.m. From a larger mesenchymal villus (below), several true sprouts protrude into the intervillous space. At their tips, the latter consist merely of syncytiotrophoblast. Nearer the base they are invaded by cytotrophoblast and finally by loose connective tissue (villous sprout, V). The latter is the forerunner of a new mesenchymal villus, which becomes established as soon as the sprout is invaded by fetal vessels. ×390.

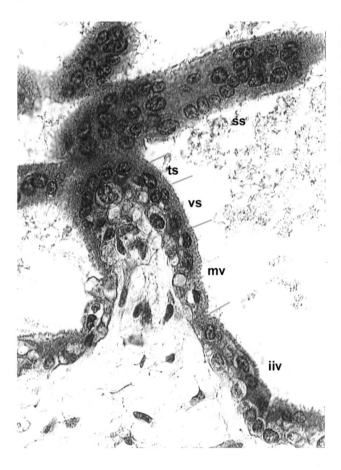

FIGURE 7.13. This longitudinal section of a newly sprouting villus demonstrates the various stages of the sprouting process: as the first step, a group of syncytial sprouts (upper third, ss) is formed; these become invaded by cytotrophoblast (trophoblastic sprout, ts), followed by invasion by dense, avascular cellular stroma (villous sprout, vs). Development of fetal capillaries marks the transition into a mesenchymal villus (mv). The latter branches from an immature intermediate villus (iiv), which was the starting point of the sprouting process. Paraffin section, H&E. staining, ×560.

Fetal capillaries are poorly developed and never show sinusoidal dilatation. Near the villous tips, capillary lumens may still be occluded and are made up of a string of endothelium (Figs. 7.13 and 7.14); several steps in the formation of lumens can be observed.

The still unvascularized tips of mesenchymal villi are referred to as villous sprouts. At their tips, the villous sprouts continue into trophoblastic sprouts (Figs. 7.2, 7.12, and 7.13). In summary, the typical sequence of structures representing the process of villous sprouting is as follows: syncytial sprout, trophoblastic sprout with a central core of cytotrophoblast, villous sprout with some connective tissue, and mesenchymal villus with fetal capillaries (Fig. 7.13).

Function: During the first weeks of pregnancy, mesenchymal villi are not only the places of villous proliferation but also the sites of maternofetal exchange and nearly all endocrine activity. With advancing pregnancy and development of more advanced villous types, their functional importance is reduced to villous growth. At term, their share in total villous volume is far below 1% (Fig. 7.15) (Castellucci et al., 1990, 2000).

Immunohistochemistry of Villous Types

Villous classification is based on two parameters (Kaufmann et al., 1979; Kohnen et al., 1996; see also foregoing text):

- Differences in stromal structure (mesenchymal, reticular, or fibrous);
- Distribution of the various segments of the fetal vessel system: (1) capillaries without media and adventitia; (2) arterioles and venules with thin media and nonfibrous adventitia; or (3) arteries and veins with thick muscular media and fibrous adventitia.

Consequently, immunohistochemistry of cytoskeletal proteins within the villous stroma and the vessel walls provides a useful tool for the identification of various villous types. The above-mentioned differences in stromal structure as well as the differences in vascular wall structure are reflected by different degrees of cytoskeletal differentiation. According to Kohnen et al. (1995, 1996) and Demir et al. (1997), the following mesenchymal derivatives show a highly specific distribution pattern

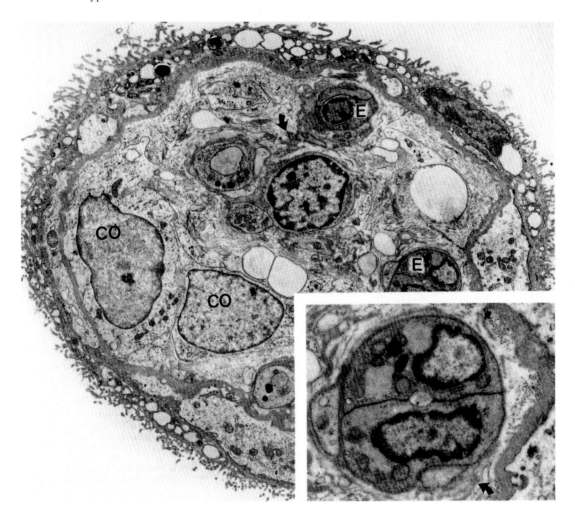

FIGURE 7.14. Transmission electron microscopic cross section of a transitional stage between a villous sprout and a mesenchymal villus from the term placenta. This villus is characterized by large, epithelioid connective tissue cells (CO) and capillary sprouts. The latter consist of densely packed endothelial cells (E) connected to each other by tight junctions, showing no or only minimal lumens (inset), and surrounded by basal laminas. The latter form sometimes thick convolutions (arrow). It is interesting to note that many of the villous sprouts and mesenchymal villi observed exhibit degenerative signs (compare the highly vacuolated syncytiotrophoblast), which can be explained by the fact that not all syncytial sprouts survive, depending on the local circulatory conditions in the intervillous space. By this selection, the shape of the villous tree is adapted to the intervillous hemodynamics. ×5200; inset ×13,000. (*Source:* Demir et al., 1989, with permission.)

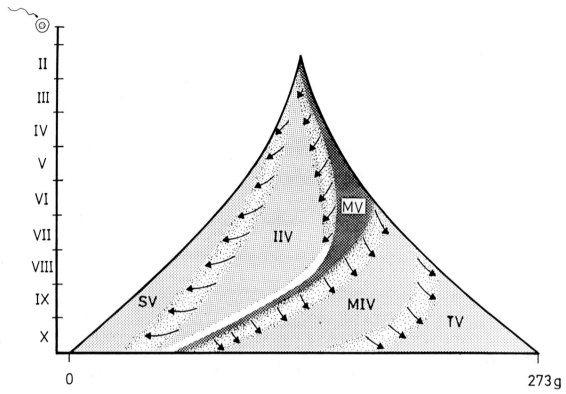

FIGURE 7.15. Development of total villous weight and the weight of the various villous types (in grams), from the 2nd month p.m. until term. Abscissa, villous weight in grams per placenta; ordinate, gestational age p.m. in months. The arrows demonstrate the routes of transformation or formation of villi. The lightly stippled areas around the arrows symbolize transitional stages between closely related villous types. At term, the mean villous weight per placenta amounts to 273 g. After morphometric evaluation of representative histologic sections, this weight can be assigned to the various villous types at term as follows: stem villi (SV), 31 g, 11%; transitional stages to immature intermediate villi, 24 g, 9%; immature intermediate villi (IIV), 9 g, 3%; mesenchymal villi (MV), less than 1%; transitional stages to mature intermediate villi, 3 g, 1%; mature intermediate villi (MIV), 77 g, 28%; transitional stages to terminal villi, 31 g, 11%; terminal villi (TV), 95 g, 35%. Rough data for earlier stages of pregnancy can be deduced from the diagram. It must be pointed out that these data are preliminary, obtained from only a few placentas. There is a considerable local and interindividual variation. It becomes evident that the sum of stem villi (SV) plus immature intermediate villi (IIV) decreases throughout the last 3 months of pregnancy; the decrease can be explained by a massive transformation of stem villi into fibrinoid. (*Source:* Modified from Castellucci et al., 1990, with permission.)

within the various villous types and can be identified immunohistochemically by the expression of the cytoskeletal proteins listed (Table 7.1):

1. Undifferentiated mesenchymal cells express only vimentin (V cells). They are the only fixed connective tissue cells in undifferentiated mesenchymal villi.
2. Fibroblasts express vimentin and desmin (VD cells), and partly even α-smooth muscle actin (VDA cells). Together with the former cell type they make up the stromal core in mesenchymal villi in later pregnancy as well as in mature intermediate and terminal villi.

3. Myofibroblasts in addition to vimentin and desmin are characterized by the expression of α- and γ-smooth muscle actin (VDAG cells). These are the typical representatives of immature intermediate villi.
4. The highest stages of myofibroblast differentiation are characterized by the additional expression of smooth muscle myosin (VDAGM cells). These latter cells share most but not all structural features with smooth muscle cells (see Chapter 6). Their appearance characterizes the transformation of an immature intermediate villus into a stem villus.

TABLE 7.1. Immunohistochemical classification of villous types using monoclonal antibodies directed against various cytoskeletal filaments

Villous type	Stroma	Vimentin	Desmin	α-sm-Actin	γ-sm-Actin	sm-Myosin	Ultrastructure
Undifferentiated mesenchymal villi		+	0	0	0	0	Mesenchymal cells
Differentiated mesenchymal villi		+	+	0	0	0	Mesenchymal and reticulum cells
Immature intermediate villi	Reticular stroma	+	+	0	0	0	Reticulum cells
	Fibrosed surrounding of larger vessels	+	+	+	0	0	Fibroblasts or myofibroblasts
	Inner adventitia of larger vessels	+	+	+	+	0	Myofibroblasts
Stem villi (in general)	Superficial cellular rim	+	+	0	0	0	Reticulum cells or fibroblasts
	Fibrous stroma	+	+	+	0	0	Fibroblasts or Myofibroblasts
	Adventitia of larger vessels	+	+	+	+	Partly +	Myofibroblasts
Type I stem villi (caliber >250 mm)	Adventitia and media of arteries and veins	+	+	+	+ in adventitia and media of arteries and veins	Partly + in adventitia	Myofibroblasts and smooth muscle cells
Type II stem villi (caliber 120–300 mm)	Adventitia and media of arterioles and venules	+	+	+	+ only in media of arterioles and venules	+ in media	Smooth muscle cells
Type III stem villi (caliber <150 mmh)	Adventitia and media of arterioles and venules	+	+	+	+ only in media of arterioles	+ in media	Smooth muscle cells
Mature intermediate villi		+	+	0	0	0	Fibroblasts or reticulum cells
Terminal villi		+	+	0	0	0	Fibroblasts or reticulum cells

Source: Based on findings by Kohnen et al., 1996; Demir et al., 1997. Positive immune reaction (+), no immune reaction (0). For details see text.

Differentiation and Maturation of Villous Types

The mechanisms of villous maturation have attracted little attention, perhaps because they may seem to be unimportant for the understanding of placental pathology. This notion is supported by the experience that, with conventional paraffin histology, it is difficult to identify the various villous types and stages of villous differentiation. Direct structural evidence of villous differentiation and maturation are usually lacking. Only if one compares the villous trees of a mature placenta (see Fig. 8.12) with early villous trees (see Fig. 8.1) does one realize that important developmental steps must have occurred.

Immunohistochemistry and availability of human material from most stages of pregnancy enabled us to consider the mechanism of villous maturation and differentiation in some detail (Kaufmann, 1982; Castellucci et al., 1990, 2000; Kohnen et al., 1996; Demir et al., 1997). Further insights into the dynamics of the growth of the villous trees can be obtained from their topologic analysis of the branching patterns and their later comparison with theoretical branching models (Kosanke et al., 1993). Our insight is still superficial, and our conclusions are accordingly preliminary. We believe, however, that we must discuss this concern because clinical methods (e.g., chorion biopsy and Doppler studies) have caused renewed interest; moreover, our understanding of the pathogenetic mechanisms of IUGR depends on an understanding of villous development.

Development of the Mesenchymal Villi

The first tertiary villi recognizable are represented by mesenchymal villi (Castellucci & Kaufmann, 1982a). They are derived from the following sources (Castellucci et al., 1990, 2000):

- Up to the 6th week p.m., the mesenchymal villi are formed from primary villi via secondary villi (Boyd & Hamilton, 1970). The numerous trophoblastic primary villi are transformed into secondary villi by invagination of extraembryonic mesenchyme. Immediately thereafter, the first capillaries form, giving rise to tertiary villi, the mesenchymal villi considered here.
- Beginning from the 6th week p.m., the supply of primary and secondary villi is exhausted and new mesenchymal villi are henceforth formed by vascularization of trophoblastic sprouts. These structures are trophoblastic outgrowths of the surfaces of mesenchymal and immature intermediate villi and result from trophoblastic proliferation (Figs. 7.12, 7.13, and 7.16).

Not all sprouts (i.e., fungiform outgrowths from the villous surface) are signs of trophoblastic sprouting. Some represent stages of expulsion of apoptotic syncytial nuclei (see Chapters 6 and 15), and others are simply flat sections of villous surfaces (see Chapter 15) (Cantle et al., 1987). The true trophoblastic sprouts correspond to the primary villi of the early stages of placentation; the latter sprouts are invaded by mesenchyme and transformed into villous sprouts. These sprouts then correspond to secondary villi of early development. The first signs of capillary formation mark the transformation into mesenchymal villi.

The concentration of Langhans' cells is greater in mesenchymal villi than in all other villi. In addition, the mitotic index of villous cytotrophoblast, counted from autoradiographs following ^{3}H-thymidine incorporation and from immunohistochemical preparations using the antibodies Ki-67, MIB-1, or proliferating-cell nuclear antigen (PCNA) (Kohnen et al., 1993; Kosanke et al., 1998), considerably exceeds that of all other villi. This fact was not evident in previous publications (Moe, 1971; Tedde & Tedde-Piras, 1978; Kaufmann et al., 1983; Arnholdt et al., 1991) because the authors did not differentiate among the various villous types.

Development and Fate of Immature Intermediate Villi

Beginning between the 7th and 8th weeks p.m., mesenchymal villi transform to immature intermediate villi. This process is characterized by (1) an increase in villous diameter; (2) the formation of the stromal channels (Fig. 7.7) containing numerous macrophages (Enders & King, 1970; Kaufmann et al., 1979; Castellucci & Kaufmann, 1982a,b; Castellucci et al., 1984; King, 1987); (3) the transformation of mesenchymal cells in structurally and immunohistochemically different reticulum cells and fibroblasts (Kohnen et al., 1996); and (4) a decrease in thickness of syncytiotrophoblast and in the number of Langhans' cells.

The reticular stroma is the most characteristic feature of immature intermediate villi. It seems to play an important role during transformation of these villi into fibrosed stem villi. According to G. Petry (personal communication, 1981), the accumulation of connective tissue fibers is preceded by a similar reticular architecture of connective tissue cells during the course of early scar formation in the skin. The significance of this stromal type appears to be defined by the role of macrophages (Hofbauer cells), which are involved in the remodeling of the connective tissue (Scott & Cohn, 1982; Werb, 1983; Castellucci et al., 1984; Takemura & Werb, 1984). There is presently no specific function for the immature intermediate villi, other than being a quickly growing developmental precursor for stem villi (Fig. 7.16).

Development of additional immature intermediate villi from mesenchymal villi gradually ceases at the end of the second trimester (Castellucci et al., 1990, 2000; Bukovsky et al., 1999). Their transformation into stem villi, however, continues to term. Therefore, the number of immature intermediate villi decreases steeply (Fig. 7.15). Sometimes they completely disappear before term. It is common, however, that small numbers persist in the centers of the villous trees and serve as growth zones.

Development of Stem Villi

The development of stem villi is closely related to the formation of the immature intermediate villi. As early as in the 8th week p.m., the central vessels of the proximal segments of immature intermediate villi, near the chorionic plate, commence constructing a compact adventitia. They thus slowly transform into arteries and veins. Centrifugal expansion of the adventitia, paralleled by transformation of reticulum cells and fibroblasts into myofibroblasts, leads to a reduction of the adjacent reticular connective tissue (see Chapter 8, Figs. 8.4 to 8.8).

The transition of immature intermediate villi into stem villi is a gradual process. According to our definition, stem villi are established as soon as the superficial sheet of reticular connective tissue beneath the trophoblast is thinner than the fibrous center surrounding stem vessels (Figs. 8.5, 8.6) (Castellucci et al., 1990, 2000). Stem vessels have then been transformed into arteries and veins or arterioles and venules. The persistence of a small rim of reticular connective tissue beneath the trophoblast in the term placenta can be regarded as a reliable sign of placental immaturity (Kaufmann, 1981).

The formation of additional stem villi depends on the availability of immature intermediate villi. Therefore, the expansion of villous stems gradually ceases during the course of the last trimester, as soon as most of the immature intermediate villi have been transformed and new ones are no longer produced.

Increased stromal fibrosis outside stem villi is considered to be a pathologic phenomenon. Such villi are usually referred to as being fibrotic. Fox (1978) reported several conditions that are commonly associated with fibrotic villi:

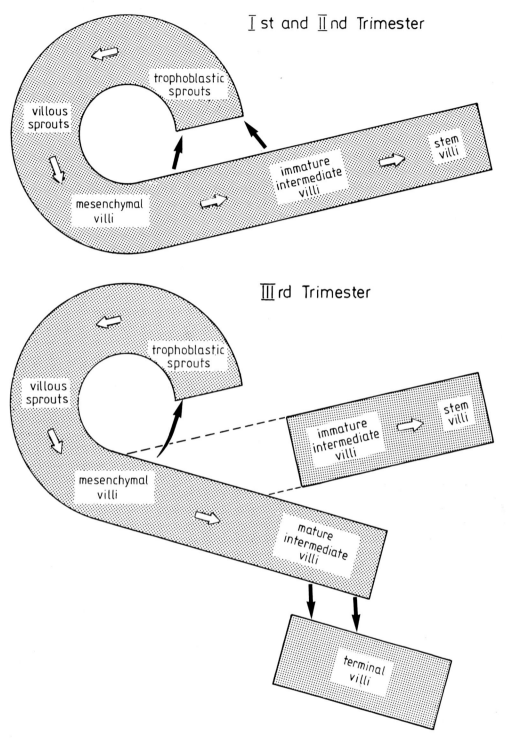

FIGURE 7.16. Routes of villous development during early and late pregnancy. White arrows, transformation of one villous type into another; black arrows, new production of villi or sprouts along the surface of other villi. Upper half: First and second trimester. Trophoblastic sprouts are produced along the surfaces of mesenchymal and immature intermediate villi. Via villous sprouts, they are transformed into mesenchymal villi. The latter differentiate into immature intermediate villi, which produce new sprouts before they are transformed into stem villi. Lower half: Throughout the third trimester, the mesenchymal villi become transformed into mature intermediate villi, which later produce terminal villi along their surfaces. There is no longer transformation of mesenchymal into immature intermediate villi. The remaining immature intermediate villi differentiate into stem villi. Thus, their number steeply decreases toward term. Thus, the base for the formation of new sprouts is also reduced, and the growth capacity of the villous trees gradually slows.

1. Stromal fibrosis is a regular finding of peripheral villi following fetal artery thrombosis.

2. It may also be found in inadequately vascularized villi adjacent to areas of infarction.

3. In placentas from macerated stillbirths, increased numbers of fibrotic villi have also been observed. Fox (1978) concluded that this must be a postmortem change because this feature is absent in placentas from fresh stillbirths. This issue, however, is still debated and probably depends on the causes of fetal demise.

4. A marked increase of fibrosed villi may be found in placentas of prolonged pregnancy.

Contrary to many other reports, Fox (1978) was unable to show an association between villous fibrosis and fetal complications, such as hypoxia or low birth weight. He thus refutes the theory that increased stromal fibrosis is a response to uteroplacental ischemia. In his opinion, it is more likely a result of reduced intravillous blood flow. This situation may result in intravillous hyperoxic conditions as oxygen transfer from the villi to the fetus is impaired (Macara et al., 1996; Kingdom & Kaufmann, 1997; see following).

Development of the Mature Intermediate Villi

One of the most important steps for an understanding of villous development occurs at the beginning of the last trimester. At this time, the transformation of newly formed mesenchymal villi into immature intermediate villi switches to a transformation into mature intermediate villi (Figs. 7.15 and 7.16; also see Figs. 8.7 and 8.8) (Castellucci et al., 1990, 2000). Little is known about the factors causing this switch. The structurally most striking event at this developmental stage (Kaufmann & Kingdom, 2000; Kaufmann et al., 2004) is the switch

- from branching angiogenesis, which is responsible for the development of immature intermediate villi out of mesenchymal ones,
- to nonbranching angiogenesis, which is necessary for the growth of the long, poorly branched capillary loops characteristic for mature intermediate villi developing out of mesenchymal ones.

As will be dealt with later in this chapter, this switch from branching to nonbranching angiogenesis is modulated by a downregulation of vascular endothelial growth factor (VEGF) and an upregulation of placental growth factor (PlGF), as well as by respective changes of their receptors KDR and flt-1 (for review see Kingdom & Kaufmann, 1997; Charnock-Jones et al., 2004; Kaufmann et al., 2004; Mayhew et al., 2004). The factors, however, that trigger this switch in growth factor expression still remain unknown (see below).

Differing in two respects from immature intermediate villi, the mature intermediate villi provide the matrix out of which terminal villi develop, but they do not transform into stem villi.

Development of the Terminal Villi

The first terminal villi, as defined in the past (Kaufmann et al., 1979; Sen et al., 1979), are produced soon after the first mature intermediate villi are formed (Fig. 7.15; see Table 8.1). The formation of terminal villi is closely related to the longitudinal growth of capillaries within the mature intermediate villi (see Figs. 7.19 and 7.23). As soon as longitudinal capillary growth exceeds longitudinal villous growth, the capillaries become coiled and form loops (Kaufmann et al., 1985, 1988). Because of the slender shape of these villi, the loops bulge on the trophoblastic surface and finally protrude as grape-like outgrowths into the intervillous space. This process is not accompanied by trophoblastic proliferation and, therefore, leads to considerable stretching of trophoblast. This process results in numerous vasculosyncytial membranes of terminal villi.

It follows that, in contrast to the development of other villous types, the terminal villi are not active outgrowths induced by proliferation; rather, they represent passive formations caused by capillary coiling. Accordingly, maldevelopment of terminal villi is always an immediate consequence of abnormal fetoplacental angiogenesis.

- Impaired angiogenesis results in deficiency of terminal villi (see Fig. 15.17).
- Overstimulated angiogenesis leads to the development of large conglomerates of terminal villi (see Fig. 15.16).

The slight bends of the mature intermediate villi, at points where terminal villi branch off (see Fig. 7.10A,D), illustrate the mechanical forces that have been active during capillary growth and coiling. Terminal villi, at the surfaces of stem villi and immature intermediate villi and derived from coiling of paravascular capillaries, are the exceptions because these particular capillaries show less impressive longitudinal growth (Leiser et al., 1985).

Angioarchitecture of Villi

Vascular Arrangement in Immature Villi

The first vascular nets formed in early placental villi show no differentiation into arteries, veins, or capillaries (Demir et al., 1989), a picture that changes around the 8th week p.m. (cf. Fig. 7.23, stage III). As a consequence of fusion of locally developed intravillous vascular nets with the fetal vessels that invade the villous trees via the connective stalk (the forerunner of the umbilical cord), the fetoplacental circulation becomes established. Because of pressure gradients between arterial and venous limbs, differently structured vessel walls appear (see Fig. 8.3). Connective tissue cells that aggregate around the endothelial tubes in a circular fashion are the first steps in the formation of the walls of future arteries and veins. Normally, one artery and one vein are formed. The remaining capillary net that surrounds the larger vessels is referred to as the paravascular net. An example of this phenomenon has been illustrated by Boe (1969) (see Fig. 7.18). When he traced single vessels, he found numerous capillaries that formed shortcuts between arteries and veins but also between neighboring arteries (arterioarterial anastomoses). Because of the low blood pressure in the vascular system, effective arteriovenous shunting is unlikely.

The villus depicted by Boe (see Fig. 7.18) is consistent with what we described as an immature intermediate villus. It is an undifferentiated, still growing villous type that can even be found in the mature placenta, although in only small restricted groups. The small branching-off villi described by Boe as "terminal villi" are likely newly formed mesenchymal villi (see Figs. 7.12 and 7.18). As it is typical for newly formed villi, their richly branched capillary nets are connected only with the paravascular net, rather than directly with arteries and veins. Only after further development, as soon as some of their capillaries have been transformed to arterioles and venules, are direct connections to the fetal stem vessel established.

Larger Vessels of Stem Villi

Large stem villi normally contain one artery in a nearly central position. If not constricted or collapsed, the lumen accounts for about one third of the villous caliber (see Fig. 7.3A). The endothelium is surrounded by a few layers of smooth muscle cells. The adventitia is continuous with the surrounding connective tissue without a sharp line of demarcation. The artery is normally accompanied by a corresponding vein. Its luminal width does not much exceed that of the artery in most preparations owing to the collapse occurring after delivery. In addition to the two main vessels, varying numbers of smaller arterioles and venules exist (Leiser et al., 1985; Kaufmann et al., 1988).

The most peripheral generations of stem villi branch or continue into mature intermediate villi and have diameters ranging from 80 to 150 μm (Fig. 7.3B). The stem vessels are represented by arterioles and venules (Fig. 7.17; also see Fig. 7.19) that are surrounded by one or two layers of smooth muscle cells. The inconspicuous venules have one, usually incomplete, layer of muscle cells. Some are surrounded only by pericytes and correspond to the collecting venules of Rhodin (1968), despite their different diameter. Frequently, arterioles and venules of these segments are so similar that they cannot be identified on cross sectioning but only from reconstructions. For quantitative estimations of stem vessels, we refer to a survey by Leiser et al. (1991).

Paravascular Capillary Net of Stem Villi

Beneath the trophoblast, numerous cross sections of capillaries with small calibers appear (Fig. 7.17; also see Figs. 7.19 and 7.24D). They belong to the paravascular net (Boe, 1953). This system is derived from the subtrophoblastic capillary net of the earlier immature villi. Because of vascular obstruction during transformation of the immature intermediate villi into stem villi, a rarefied and poorly branching system of slender capillary loops develops. It can be seen in most stem villi depicted in the literature (Arts, 1961; Thiriot & Panigel, 1978; Habashi et al., 1983; Leiser et al., 1985; Kaufmann et al., 1988). The paravascular capillaries follow a straight course, mostly parallel to the longitudinal axis of the villus. In our material of mature stem villi, net-like connections have been uncommon. We have seen such richly branched and dense paravascular capillary nets as depicted by Burton (1987) only in immature intermediate villi (Fig. 7.18) and in not yet fully matured stem villi. We concede, however, that our impression may be incomplete. The paravascular capillaries are connected to the arteries and veins by short arteriolar and venular segments, measuring up to 100 μm in length.

Only in rare cases do the paravascular capillaries show focal sinusoidal dilatations. If this happens, the dilated and coiling segments bulge on the stem villus surface and form a terminal villus that arises from the stem villus (Kaufmann et al., 1979; Burton, 1987) (Fig. 7.17C, upper half). Such terminal villi are serially intercalated into the paravascular net. According to our experience, this occurrence is rare (less than 5% of all terminal villi), whereas Burton (1987) described it to be a regular finding.

When we traced individual paravascular capillaries from their arteriolar beginnings to their venular ends, we found an average length of 1000 to 2000 μm. Arteriovenous and arterioarterial shortcuts, as described by Boe (1953, 1969) for the earlier stages of development, could no longer be detected in mature stem villi. There is therefore no real basis for speculations that the paravascular net participates in the regulation of fetal blood flow impedance as an arteriovenous shunting system.

The functional relevance of the paravascular capillary net is still uncertain. Thiriot and Panigel (1978) suggested that this was the site for effective fetomaternal exchange. The long diffusion distances in these places make this interpretation implausible. Moreover, the assumption by Arts (1961) that the paravascular net may be of nutritional importance for the stem villi, acting as a kind of vasa vasorum, seems unlikely to us. The concentration of oxygen and most nutrients in the surrounding intervillous space considerably exceeds that in the fetal vessels. Thus, the nutrition by direct diffusion from the maternal blood is probably more effective. This finding is in agreement with those of Zeek and Assali (1950) as well as Fox (1978),

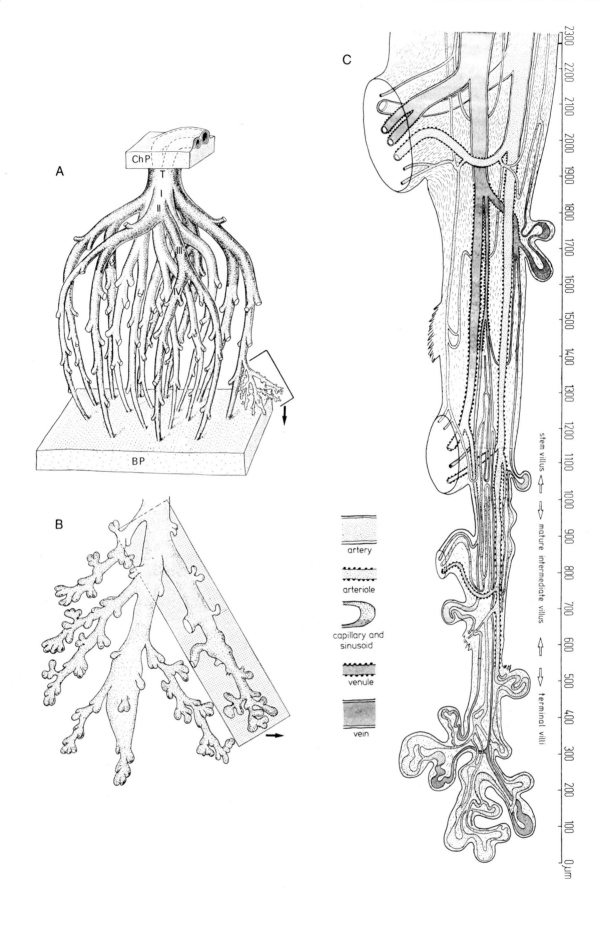

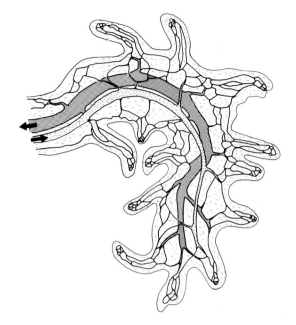

FIGURE 7.18. Classical representation of the villous vascularization by Boe (1969) represents an immature intermediate villus with numerous mesenchymal side branches. The web-like arrangement of the fetal capillaries protruding from the paravascular net of the immature intermediate villus into its sprouting side branches is highly characteristic, not only for early placentas but also for villous sprouting patterns in the term placenta. As depicted in the foregoing pictures, it is normally absent in the mature villous types. (*Source:* Based on findings of Boe, 1969.)

who found not only survival of stroma but also increased fibroblast proliferation and collagen production within stem villi after fetal death.

Boyd and Hamilton (1970) described the paravascular net to be simply a residual indication of better vascularization during early stages of development. Keeping in mind that the developmental forerunners of the stem villi were immature intermediate villi with a well-developed paravascular net (Kaufmann et al., 1988), the respective

capillaries of the mature stem villi probably represent the remains of the immature state where terminal villi with their effective exchange system were absent and the paravascular net had to sustain maternofetal exchange. The development of better-vascularized terminal villi during the course of the last trimester renders the paravascular capillaries largely nonfunctional.

Arrangement of Vessels in Mature Intermediate and Terminal Villi

The mature intermediate villi serve as junctional segments between the most peripheral stem villi and most of the terminal villi. Their vessels are direct continuations of the smallest stem villous vessels (Figs. 7.17C and 7.19). One or two small arterioles, with luminal diameters ranging from 20 to 40 μm, appear histologically as bare endothelial tubes, accompanied by occasional muscle cells. Precapillary sphincters, or comparable narrow segments with complete muscular coats as described for other vascular beds (Rhodin, 1967), have not been identified. Rather, the terminal ends of arterioles continue directly into one or two capillaries by a gradual reduction of their diameters and loss of smooth muscle (Kaufmann et al., 1985; Leiser et al., 1991).

Although the arterioles occupy a more central position in the villous stroma, one or two venules can be found more superficially. Surprisingly, their diameter usually appears to be considerably smaller than that of the arterioles, usually 15 to 20 μm. In agreement with the classification of Rhodin (1968), the term **postcapillary venule** seems to be most appropriate because of the absence of muscle cells and the existence of a nearly complete sheet of pericytes. The most peripheral loops of the paravascular capillaries of the stem villi surround the terminal arterioles and postcapillary venules. They extend to about the middle of the mature intermediate villi (Figs. 7.17C and 7.19).

In the distal half of the mature intermediate villi, the paravascular capillaries are absent. Histologically, the

FIGURE 7.17. Fetal vascularization of term placental villi based on the spatial reconstruction of serial sections. A: Large stem villi of the villous tree. ChP, chorionic plate; BP, basal plate; T, truncus; I, II, III, IV, rami chorii of the first to the fourth order. The more peripheral branches depicted in this drawing are ramuli chorii of the first to the tenth order. The marked peripheral ramulus with its terminal branches refers to part B. B: Higher magnification of peripheral branches of the villous tree. A peripheral stem branches into several mature intermediated villi (slender) and one immature intermediate villus (thick). The shaded rectangular area corresponds to the reconstructed branches depicted in part C. C: Fetal vascular branching patterns of a peripheral stem villus (above), continuing into a

mature intermediate villus, extending into several terminal villi, reconstructed from a series of 2300 semithin sections. Length and caliber of the villi are drawn on the same scale, whereas the diameter of the vessels is reduced to two thirds (necessary because of two-dimensional representation of a three-dimensional system). Occasional spots of fibrinoid necrosis on the villous surface are marked by hatching. Note that the capillary loops of neighboring terminal villi are serially connected. These are normally not continuous with the straight paravascular capillaries of the stem and mature intermediate villi, but form a second independent capillary bed. (*Source:* Modified from Kaufmann et al., 1988, with permission.)

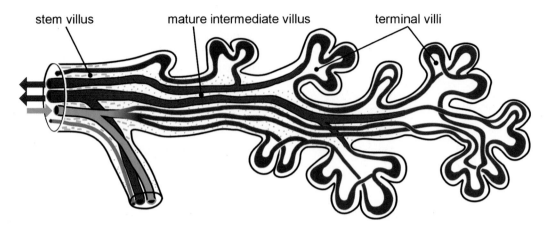

FIGURE 7.19. Arrangement of the fetal vessels in a group of terminal villi (stroma unstained) derived from one mature intermediate villus (green dotted stroma). Based on a three-dimensional reconstruction of the peripheral branches of a mature villous tree. Note the highly complex loop formation of the terminal fetal capillaries. Branching is usually followed shortly later by refusion of the two capillary branches. Such a branching pattern avoids basal shortcuts. Each erythrocyte must pass the terminal capillaries of several terminal villi in their full length. Local dilatations, so-called sinusoids, reduce blood flow impedance. Blue, fetal arteries and arterioles; lilac fetal villous capillaries and sinusoids; red, fetal villous venules and veins.

distal segment can easily be differentiated from the more proximal segments by the absence of larger vessel cross sections and the absence of vessels in the center of the stromal core; most capillaries are located directly beneath the trophoblast. In most cases, the abrupt end of the paravascular "net" causes a sharp line of demarcation between the more proximal segments, which are rich in capillaries, and the distal, less vascularized part (Figs. 7.17C and 7.19).

The terminal capillaries are different from the mostly straight paravascular capillaries and are characterized by the formation of loops and coilings. Focally dilated segments may bulge against the trophoblast and thus form vasculosyncytial membranes, knob-like protrusions, or even terminal villi. As one approaches the peripheral end of the mature intermediate villus, the number and extent of capillary coilings increases and so does the number of terminal outgrowths that cover the surface of the mature intermediate villus (Figs. 7.17, 7.19, and 7.20). At its end, the mature intermediate villus regularly branches into a cluster of terminal villi (Fig. 7.20).

There is no sharp demarcation between mature intermediate and terminal villi. Increased capillary coiling, accompanied by increased sinusoidal dilatation and reduced stromal connective tissue, is responsible for the structural differences. The descriptive name "terminal villus" is used for those villi

1. that contain no vessels other than capillaries and sinusoids, and
2. in which the vascular lumens comprise at least one half of the stromal volume (Kaufmann et al., 1979, 1985).

Depending on the level at which such terminal villi are sectioned, their histologic appearance is highly variable. An example is depicted in Fig. 7.20. The capillary loops of the peripheral terminal villi are direct continuations of terminal arterioles. According to our experience, they show only on occasion cross-connections to peripheral loops of the paravascular capillaries, described as a regular feature by Arts (1961). It is of particular importance to note that the capillary loops of neighboring terminal villi are serially connected to each other (Figs. 7.17C, 7.19, and 7.20A). Fetal blood leaving a terminal arteriole and entering the terminal capillaries normally passes through the capillary loops of three to five terminal villi in series before entering a postcapillary venule. This passage is responsible for the length of terminal capillaries, which we measured as ranging from 3000 to 5000 μm (Kaufmann et al., 1985). Shortcuts at the base of terminal capillary loops are the exception, so that each erythrocyte has to pass the full length of the capillaries. As reported earlier, the paravascular capillary loops measure only 1000 to 2000 μm in length.

When one looks at casts of vessels such as those depicted in Figure 7.20, it seems that the terminal capillary bed is made up of a highly branching network, and it has usually been described as such (Boe, 1953, 1968; Arts, 1961; Boyd & Hamilton, 1970; Thiriot & Panigel, 1978; Habashi et al., 1983; Burton, 1987). In contrast, our reconstructions of terminal vessel beds revealed only a low degree of branching. When discussing this discrepancy, Burton (1987) stated that "the superimposition of SEM [scanning electron microscopy] images can lead to mistaken estimates of the incidence of vessels joining, but it cannot be denied that branching and union

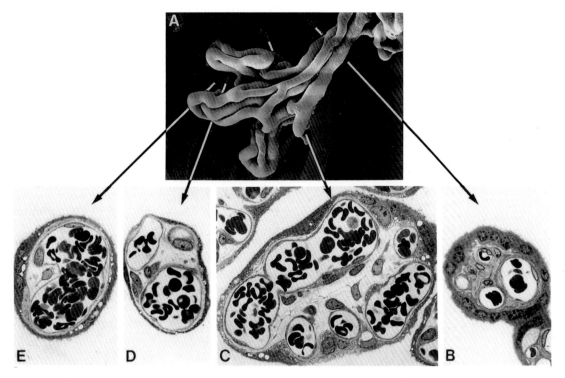

FIGURE 7.20. Fetal vascularization of terminal villi. A: Cast of vessels from a neck region (right) branching into three terminal villi. Comparable to mature intermediate villi, the capillaries of the neck region are strikingly straight and arranged in parallel; however, the diameter of the villus is much smaller. ×520. Corresponding semithin sections of the neck region (B), the basis of the branching terminal villi (C), a single terminal villus near its tip (D), and a flat section of the terminal villous tip (E). The fetal capillaries and the highly dilated sinusoids amount to more than 50% of the stromal volume as long as postpartal collapse can be avoided by early fixation. ×630. (*Source:* From Kaufmann et al., 1988, with permission.)

between capillaries does occur within terminal villi. The problem may be only one of degree. . . ." We admit that our results were obtained from the reconstruction of only a few cases (Kaufmann et al., 1985); it is our opinion, however, that the more likely explanation for the discrepancy is one of definition. Branching, with directly subsequent union, is indeed a frequent feature (Fig. 7.19). It must not be confused with the establishment of true, complex intravillous capillary nets, which offer the possibility of basal shortcuts. The latter arrangement might considerably shorten the individual capillary length. On the other hand, a high degree of coiling with serially intercalated branching and direct fusion has no influence on the mean capillary length. This difference may have physiologic importance for fetal blood flow impedance. Jirkovska and coworkers (1998) have shown that three-dimensional reconstructions of terminal villi using confocal microscopy are a useful approach to solve these questions. This is particularly valid if sophisticated methods of tissue preparation are applied such as dual perfusion fixation (Larsen et al., 1995).

Sinusoids of Terminal Villi

Sinusoids are focal capillary enlargements that attain diameters to about 50 mm (Figs. 7.11 and 7.20). They are thought to be typical features of the mature placenta and are not comparable to the sinusoids of liver, spleen, and bone marrow, as the former possess a continuous endothelium and complete basal lamina. Sinusoids thus differ from conventional capillaries only by their increased diameters.

In semithin sections, the sinusoids are normally positioned near the villous tips. Vascular casts, however, reveal that they are randomly scattered over the full length of the terminal capillaries, rather than dilatations of defined segments (Kaufmann et al., 1985). They may narrow and dilate serially several times (Fig. 7.19). Statistically, they can be found more frequently near the villous tips and along the venous limbs, as well as at points of branching and fusion. The grade of dilatation and the degree of tortuosity of the capillary loops seem to depend on each other.

We have measured the diameters of capillaries and sinusoids in semi-thin sections and compared them to casts of vessels (Kaufmann et al., 1985). The results, obtained with both methods, were largely consistent. The mean diameters of capillaries and sinusoids of the mature placenta varied from 12.2 μm (±0.58 μm) in vessel casts to 14.4 μm (±1.94 μm) in semithin sections. The difference can be explained by different degrees of shrinkage of the resins used for preparation. In our experience, the higher values seem to be more appropriate. The maximum values were 39 μm in casts of vessels and 45 μm in semithin sections. Depending on the method applied, 60% to 80% of the vessel lumens had diameters larger than 10 mm. Our data are largely consistent with those reported by Becker (1962a), Becker and Seifert (1965), and Boyd and Hamilton (1970).

The smaller diameters reported by Habashi et al. (1983) and O'Neill (1983), the latter author giving a range of only 4 to 7 μm, are probably the result of incomplete filling of vessels of their casts and resin shrinkage. Even more contradictory are the physiologic results published by Penfold et al. (1981). These authors perfused capillaries with microspheres of varying diameters and concluded that as many as 25% of capillaries measure less than 4 μm in diameter and virtually no capillary exceeds 11 μm in diameter. Their results were based on the erroneous assumption that narrow and dilated capillary loops are arranged in parallel; their results must be refuted (Habashi et al., 1983). In fact, the capillaries become narrow and dilate serially. Thus, when using microsphere perfusion, the diameter for the narrowest segment of each capillary loop can only be estimated. Even so, the value of 4 mm for 25% of the capillary loops cannot be accepted.

Function: The functional relevance of the sinusoids has caused much speculation. It is evident from the foregoing description that the sinusoidal dilatation cannot be regarded as dilated venous limbs of the capillary loops that allow retarded venous backflow, as was discussed by Nikolov and Schiebler (1973). The localization of most sinusoids near the villous tips supports the conclusion of Arts (1961) that the sinusoids locally decelerate blood flow, thus providing ample opportunity for fetomaternal exchange. This assumption is in agreement with the finding that the sinusoids are regularly situated in contiguity with the epithelial plates (Boyd & Hamilton, 1970; Nikolov & Schiebler, 1973, 1981; Schiebler & Kaufmann, 1981). These plates are thought to represent areas of maximal diffusional exchange (Amstutz, 1960; Kaufmann et al., 1974).

It is still a matter of dispute whether the reduced blood flow velocity facilitates the maternofetal exchange or whether the increased diffusion distance from the center of sinusoids to villous surface negatively influences the diffusion capacity. Another explanation for the existence of sinusoids has been that they serve as functionally specialized segments devoted to specific transport processes. Nikolov and Schiebler (1981) described two types of endothelial cells. These findings, however, cannot serve as arguments for a functional specialization of sinusoids compared to narrow capillaries, as they seem to be evenly distributed in both vessel segments.

We have discussed another explanation for the function of the sinusoids elsewhere (Kaufmann et al., 1985, 1987, 1988). It is remarkable that the sinusoids are pro-duced at the end of pregnancy (Becker, 1981), as soon as the terminal villi achieve the highest degree of branching and twisting and as the terminal capillary loops reach their maximal length of 3000 to 5000 μm. On the other hand, sinusoids are largely absent in the shorter terminal capillary loops of immature placentas and in the shorter paravascular capillaries. Moreover, they are not found in labyrinthine placentas such as those of the guinea pig (Kaufmann & Davidoff, 1977) and chinchilla (Dantzer et al., 1988), both of which are characterized by short fetal capillaries, ranging from 500 to 1000 μm. We have also studied some capybara placentas (Kaufmann, 2004). This species is of the same suborder of caviomorph rodents as the guinea pig and chinchilla but it has a much larger placenta with fetal capillaries of about twice their lengths. Its placenta shows fetal sinusoids. The same is true for the goat placenta, which has long capillary loops comparable to those of the human placenta (Leiser, 1987; Dantzer et al., 1988).

According to the law of Hagen-Poiseuille, blood flow resistance is reduced by the fourth power of the vascular radius. It can be concluded that even limited and focal sinusoidal dilatation of the long terminal capillary loops may considerably decrease blood flow impedance to such a degree that it no longer exceeds that in the shorter paravascular capillaries. In this way, an even blood flow distribution is guaranteed for all capillaries, independent of their length and diameter. In addition, for this low-pressure fetal circulatory system, the perfusion of the huge extracorporeal organ becomes much easier.

Fetoplacental Angiogenesis as the Driving Force for Villous Development

As already noted before, the structural comparison of (1) villous development with (2) vascular development within the villi suggests that both processes depend on each other. This impression is further substantiated by the analysis of normally as compared to abnormally matured terminal villous ramifications:

- More than 95% of terminal villi arise from the surfaces of mature intermediate villi by simple bulging of coiled capillaries (Kaufmann et al., 1985) (Fig. 7.19).
- "Hypermature villi" (Salvatore, 1968; Kaufmann, 1982; Kaufmann et al., 1987), villi in maternal anemia (Kingdom & Kaufmann, 1997; Kosanke et al., 1998), and villi in IUGR with abnormal but still preserved end-diastolic (PED) flow in the umbilical arteries (IUGR with PED) (Todros et al., 1999) show an increased number of highly branched terminal villi, together with highly branched capillary networks (see Fig. 7.23).

- In contrast, placentas from IUGR with ARED umbilical flow exhibit nearly naked, unbranched mature intermediate villi that continue in one single terminal villus (Krebs et al., 1996; Macara et al., 1996; Kingdom et al., 1997a,b). The terminal capillaries are much shorter, and uncoiled, with only a few sinusoidal dilatations (see Fig. 7.23).

We conclude from these observations that the development of terminal villi is influenced by the balance of longitudinal growth of mature intermediate villi with that of their capillary loops. The more capillary growth exceeds the longitudinal villous growth, the more do the capillaries become coiled. The single coils bulge against the surfaces of the mature intermediate villi and thus produce the terminal villi. We interpret the terminal villi as passive outpocketings, rather than the result of trophoblastic proliferation.

Even more simplified, one can say that the placental villous trees are fetoplacental vascular trees covered by a flexible wrapping of trophoblast. The latter does not shape the villi but rather follows the vascular shapes.

General Aspects of Placental Vasculogenesis and Angiogenesis

Because of the obvious importance of formation of vessels for the understanding of decisive steps of villus development, some general principles of vasculogenesis and angiogenesis (Fig. 7.21) as well as the respective findings in the placenta shall be summarized here (for review see also Breier, 2000).

According to Folkman and Shing (1992), Risau and Flamme (1995), and Risau (1997), formation of vessels can be subdivided in two processes that differ regarding mechanisms and control:

- Vasculogenesis involves de novo formation of blood vessels from mesodermally derived precursor cells. Throughout placentation, it takes place during the development of the first villous vessels at the transition from secondary to the tertiary villous stage (from day 18 through about day 35), and later in pregnancy during formation of mesenchymal villi out of immature intermediate ones.
- Angiogenesis is the expansion of a preexisting vessel bed and involves creation of new vessel branches from preexisting ones as well as longitudinal growth of vessels. Throughout placentation it is the principal mechanism for the development of the vascular supply of immature intermediate villi, stem villi, mature intermediate villi, and terminal villi.

Placental angiogenesis must be further subdivided regarding its mechanisms and the geometry of the resulting vascular bed (Kingdom & Kaufmann, 1997; Kaufmann & Kingdom, 2000; Charnock-Jones et al., 2004) into of the following categories:

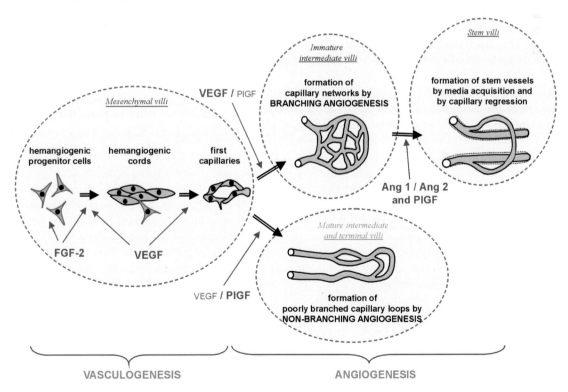

FIGURE 7.21. Diagrammatic survey of basic mechanisms of vasculogenesis and angiogenesis, their attribution to villous development and their presumed paracrine control (red). For details see text.

- **Branching angiogenesis:** This term describes a pattern in which multiple sprouting of microvessels produces a complex, multiply branched capillary web. This is the principal type of angiogenesis from day 32 until about week 24 during development of mesenchymal and immature intermediate villi.
- **Nonbranching angiogenesis:** In this type of angiogenesis branching by sprouting is the exception. Rather, the vascular bed expands by elongation of existing capillary loops. This mode of angiogenesis starts at about week 24 when mesenchymal villi start developing into mature intermediate villi and the latter start producing terminal villi. It lasts until term. Under pathologic conditions it may become the only mode of angiogenesis. Under normal conditions it takes place in combination with branching angiogenesis.

Vasculogenesis 1: Origin of Hemangiogenic Progenitor Cells (Days 15 to 21)

The first generations of placental villi develop by local de novo formation of capillaries (vasculogenesis) rather than protrusion of embryonic vessels via the umbilical cord into the placenta. In the rhesus monkey (gestation 166 days), the onset of vasculogenesis is around day 19 postconception (King, 1987). The few existing respective data in the human (Knoth, 1968; Demir et al., 1989) suggest a slightly later date, at about 21 days postconception, in four-somite embryos. At this stage, the villous trees comprise solid trophoblastic primary villi and secondary villi containing a villous core of loose mesenchymal stroma invading from the exocoelomic cavity.

Hertig (1935) formulated the classic theory that villous mesenchymal cells and hemangioblastic cells are derived from villous cytotrophoblast by in situ delamination. This view has been refuted by all subsequent authors (Dempsey, 1972; Luckett, 1978; King, 1987; Demir et al., 1989), who found that the villous mesenchyme is directly derived from the fetus and invades the villi. The hemangiogenic progenitor cells differentiate locally in the villi from the fetally derived mesenchymal cells. The two cell types are structurally similar.

Using the monoclonal antibody QBend10, which detects the endothelial cell surface marker CD34, the endothelial precursor cells (hemangiogenic progenitor cells) can be demonstrated already from day 15 postconception onwards (Figs. 7.22, 7.23, and 7.24A). Within a short period of time the originally dispersed hemangiogenic progenitor cells form string-like aggregates of polygonal cells (hemangiogenic cords), which differ from their mesenchymal precursors by the absence of cellular extensions and the presence of fewer organelles. The narrow intercellular spaces between these cells are bridged by desmosomes and primitive tight junctions (Fig. 7.22c). Extensions of surrounding mesenchymal cells are often integrated into these clusters.

A variety of angiogenic growth factors are involved in angiogenesis and vasculogenesis (Table 7.2). Basic fibroblast growth factor (FGF-2 or bFGF) and its receptor FGFR are thought to be involved in recruitment of hemangiogenic progenitor cells. Its expression in human placental villi has been described repeatedly (Ferriani et al., 1994; Shams & Ahmed, 1994; Crescimanno et al., 1995) but, due to shortage of respective material, never at this early stage of pregnancy. Vascular endothelial growth factor A (VEGF-A) and its receptor VEGFR-2 (KDR/flk-1), which were found to be responsible for recruitment, growth, and aggregation of the hemangiogenic progenitor cells in other organs, are highly expressed in early placental specimens (Sharkey et al., 1993; Ahmed et al., 1995, 1997; Wheeler et al., 1995; Shore et al., 1997; Vuorela et al., 1997; Demir et al., 2004). In situ hybridization and immunohistochemistry revealed that villous trophoblast and villous stromal macrophages are the main sources of this cytokine (Sharkey et al., 1993; Ahmed et al., 1995; Vuorela et al., 1997; Demir et al., 2004). VEGF-A secretion by human trophoblast was also demonstrated in vitro by Shore et al. (1997). The assumption that macrophages and their cytokines are involved in these first steps of capillary formation is in line with the finding that macrophages differentiate locally in villous stroma even prior to the development of hemangiogenic cords (Demir et al., 1989). Knockout experiments in mice have also highlighted the importance of VEGFR-2 for specification and early differentiation of hemangioblastic precursors of fetoplacental capillaries (Shalaby et al., 1995).

Vasculogenesis 2: Formation of Endothelial Tubes (Days 21 to 32)

Lumen formation within the hemangiogenic cords and thus formation of short segments of endothelial tubes starts at day 21 postconception. This occurs by enlargement of the centrally located intercellular clefts that fuse to become a larger lumen (Fig. 7.22c,d). We have never observed lumen formation by fusion of intraendothelial vacuoles, as this has been described in other organs (Folkman & Haudenschild, 1980; Bär et al., 1984). Rather, the fetoplacental capillary lumen in the human, as in placentas of other mammals, always seems to form by acquisition of a junctionally defined extracellular compartment within the hemangioblastic cords (guinea pig: Davidoff & Schiebler, 1970; rhesus monkey: King, 1987; human: Demir et al., 1989). The acquisition of such still unconnected, isolated segments of capillaries (Fig. 7.23, stage I) defines the transition from secondary to tertiary villi.

pre-vasculogenetic stages (-d 22)

early vasculogenesis (d 22-26th week)

late extension of the vessel bed (angiogenesis) (26th-40th week)

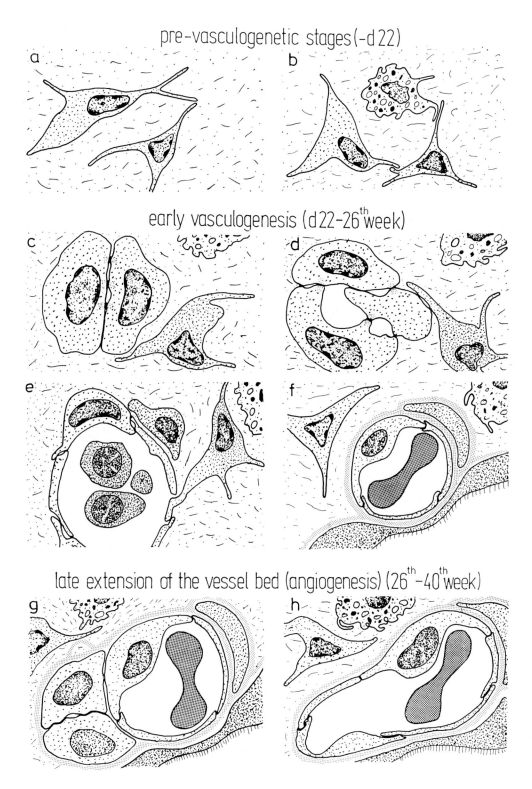

FIGURE 7.22. Vasculogenesis and angiogenesis in early and late placental villi. For further details, see text. (*Source:* Demir et al., 1989, with permission.)

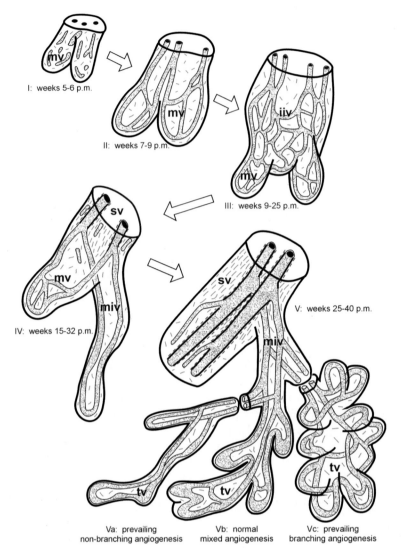

FIGURE 7.23. Villous development in relation to fetal vascular development. Stage I: In the first stage (weeks 5 to 6 p.m.), within mesenchymal villi (mv) fetal capillary segments are formed by vasculogenesis (see Fig. 7.18). Stage II: In weeks 7 to 8 p.m. the primitive vessel segments fuse to form a simple net-like capillary bed. Stage III: During development of immature intermediate villi (iiv) from mesenchymal villi (mv) between weeks 9 and 25 p.m., the preexisting capillary bed enormously expands by branching angiogenesis. This process is likely to be driven predominantly by vascular endothelial growth factor (VEGF). Stage IV: During weeks 15 to 32 p.m., most of the older immature intermediate villi are transformed into highly fibrosed stem villi. In the course of this process, the centrally located capillaries become transformed into stem vessels (arteries and veins), whereas most of the peripheral capillaries undergo regression. In the periphery of these primitive stem villi, mesenchymal villi (mv) are transformed into mature intermediate villi (miv) by nonbranching angiogenesis, resulting in considerable elongation of preexisting capillary loops. The switch from branching angiogenesis toward capillary regression and nonbranching angiogenesis, respectively, is likely to be controlled by increasing levels of placental growth factor (PlGF) and decreasing levels of VEGF. Stage V: Throughout the last trimester (weeks 25 to 40 p.m.), generally increasing levels of angiogenetic growth factors stimulate longitudinal capillary growth within the mature intermediate villi; as a consequence, elongation of capillary loops exceeds elongation of the villi themselves. This difference results in coiling of the capillaries, the coils bulging against the surface, thereby causing the development of terminal villi (tv). Different types of terminal villous development result from varying degrees of imbalance between villous and capillary growth in context with prevalence of branching or nonbranching angiogenesis (compare Fig. 15.5). Prevalence of PlGF is responsible for predominance of non-branching angiogenesis, resulting in long, filiform terminal villi (stage Va), typical for postplacental hypoxia. The prevalence of VEGF stimulates terminal branching angiogenesis, resulting in highly branched convolutes of short and multiply notched terminal villi (stage Vc), typical for preplacental and uteroplacental hypoxia. Well-balanced secretory levels of VEGF and PlGF are responsible for a balance of branching and nonbranching angiogenesis; thus, evenly formed grape-like terminal villi represent the dominating features in normal term pregnancy. Green, collagen fibers; brown, vascular smooth muscle cells; blue, endothelial tubes.

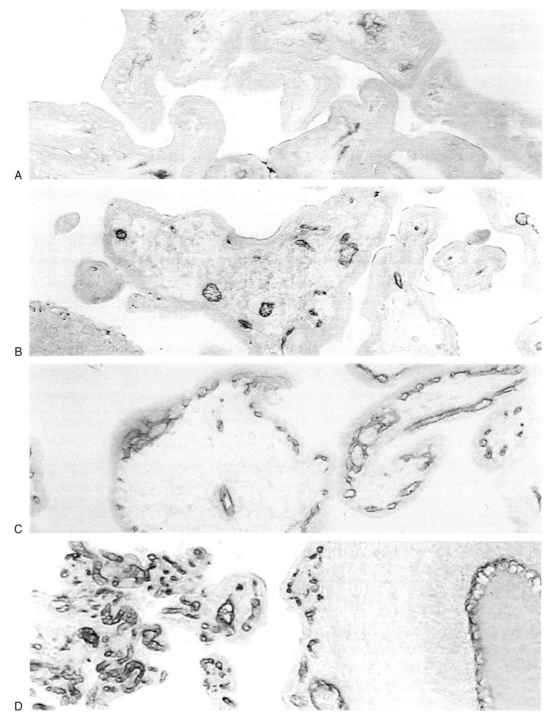

FIGURE 7.24. Stages of villous vasculogenesis and angiogenesis, immunostained with the endothelial marker antibody Qbend10. A: Day 15 to day 20 postconception. The antibody stains weakly hemangiogenic cell cords (light brown). True capillaries are still missing. ×650. (*Source:* From Kaufmann & Kingdom, 2000, with permission). B: Mesenchymal villi in week 7 p.m. The majority of capillary cross sections have developed lumens. The capillaries are still evenly distributed across the villous stroma. ×320. C: Immature intermediate villi at the end of the first trimester. Note the subtrophoblastic localization of richly developed capillary nets. The remaining central vessels are the precursors of arterioles and venules. ×320. D: Terminal and mature intermediate villi (left) and a large-caliber stem villus (right) in week 20 p.m. Note the dense capillarization of the peripheral villous branches, as opposed to the scarce capillarization of the stem villus, largely consisting of superficially located paravascular capillaries. ×320. (*Source:* Kaufmann & Kingdom, 2000, with permission).

TABLE 7.2. Expression of angiogenic growth factors and their receptors in normal and pathologic pregnancies

Growth factors and their receptors	Placental site of expression	Serum levels throughout pregnancy	Data from pathologic pregnancies
VEGF-A	Trophoblast, Hofbauer cells, vascular smooth muscle (1–5)	Moderate increase of total VEGF serum levels throughout pregnancy (including VEGF bound to its antagonist sflt-1) (6,34)	Total is increased in preeclampsia; free VEGF-A may be lower. Placental VEGF-A immunostaining lower (6–10)
VEGF-B	None detected (2)	″	%
VEGF-C	Decidual NK cells (11)	″	%
VEGF-D	None detected	″	%
PlGF	Trophoblast (2,12)	Marked increase of PlGF serum levels throughout pregnancy, peaking at weeks 28–32 (13,15)	Reduced in maternal plasma in preeclampsia (13–15)
VEGFR-1 (flt-1)	Trophoblast, endothelial cells (1,5,10,27)	%	%
VEGFR-2 (kdr)	Villous endothelial cells (1,5,10,28)	%	%
VEGFR-3 (flt-4)	Trophoblast (29 and S. Charnock-Jones, unpublished)	%	%
Soluble VEGFR-1 (sflt-1)	Trophoblast (30–33)	%	Increased in maternal plasma in preeclampsia (10 and S. Charnock-Jones, unpublished)
FGF-1	Trophoblast and vascular smooth muscle (16,17)	%	%
FGF-2	Trophoblast and vascular smooth muscle (16,17)	%	%
Ang-1	(5,19–21)	%	%
Ang-2	Villous trophoblast (5,19–21)	%	%
Tie-2 (Tek)	Villous endothelial cells and trophoblast (5,19–21)	%	%
HGF	Villous core (22–24)	%	Placental HGF mRNA reduced in IUGR; circulating HGF unchanged (25,26)
Met (HGF receptor)	Trophoblast (22–24)	%	No change in mRNA in IUGR (25)

(1) Clark et al., 1996a; (2) Clark et al., 1998c; (3) Sharkey et al., 1993; (4) Shore et al., 1997; (5) Wulff et al., 2002; (6) Sharkey et al., 1996; (7) Lyall et al., 1997; (8) Kupferminc et al., 1997; (9) Baker et al., 1995; (10) Zhou et al., 2002; (11) Li et al., 2001; (12) Khaliq et al., 1996; (13) Torry et al., 1998; (14) Reuvekamp et al., 1999; (15) Chappell et al., 2002; (16) Shams & Ahmed, 1994; (17) Ferriani et al., 1994; (18) Di Blasio et al., 1997; (19) Dunk et al., 2000; (20) Ahmed & Perkins, 2000; (21) Zhang et al., 2001; (22) Clark et al., 1996b; (23) Kilby et al., 1996; (24) Uehara et al., 1995; (25) Somerset et al., 1998; (26) Clark et al., 1998a; (27) Ahmed et al., 1995; (28) Vuckovic et al., 1996; (29) Helske et al., 2001; (30) Banks et al., 1998; (31) Hornig et al., 2000; (32) He et al., 1999; (33) Clark et al., 1998b; (34) Evans et al., 1998.
Ang, angiotensin; FGF, fibroblast growth factor; HGF, hepatocyte growth factor; IUGR, intrauterine growth restriction; PlGF, placental growth factor; VEGF, vascular endothelial growth factor; %, no data available; ″, identical as above.
Extended and modified after Charnock-Jones et al., 2004.

Immunohistochemical studies have found that the receptor VEGFR-1 (flt-1) is expressed on human villous endothelium (Crescimanno et al., 1995; Clark et al., 1996a; Vuckovic et al., 1996; Demir et al., 2004) but also in villous macrophages and trophoblast (Ahmed et al., 1995; Clark et al., 1996a). Analysis of knockout animals by Fong et al. (1995, 1999) has suggested that VEGFR-1 mediates the action of VEGF-A on endothelial precursors. Interestingly, deletion of the tyrosine kinase encoding intracellular portion of the *VEGFR-1* gene has no effect on vascular structures (Hiratsuka et al., 1998), suggesting that it is the extracellular portion of the molecule (i.e., the soluble VEGF antagonist, sflt-1) that is required for placental vascular development.

By day 28 postconception, most villi show clearly defined, long, polygonal capillary lumens with surrounding endothelial cells becoming considerably flattened (Fig. 7.22D,E). Additional mesenchymal cells are integrated by their extensions into both the mesenchymal network and the endothelial tubes (Fig. 7.22E). These "juxta-hemangiogenic" cells are characterized by richly developed rough endoplasmic reticulum and are considered to become pericytes (Dempsey, 1972; King, 1987). Also their inclusion into the endothelial lining has been discussed, since focal extension of these cells may even protrude between endothelial cells (Dempsey, 1972; Challier et al., 1999).

As soon as capillary lumens have been formed, around day 28 postconception, the first hematopoietic stem cells develop by delamination from the primitive vessel walls into the early lumens and start further differentiation (Fig. 7.22E). These cells are not yet circulating since most of the endothelial tubes are still isolated. Also an anatomic connection via the cord to the embryonic circulation does not exist yet. The latter is established a few days later (between days 32 and 35 postconception) by fusion of villous capillaries with each other (Fig. 7.23, stage II) and with the larger, allantoic vessels. The latter are formed by vasculogenesis within the allantois (Downs et al., 1998) and thereafter spread in both embryonic and placental directions and finally establish the connection between intraembryonic and placental vascular beds.

Angiogenesis 1: Branching Angiogenesis (Day 32 to Week 25)

At around day 32 postconception many villous endothelial tubes have created contact among each other (Fig. 7.23, stage II) and with the fetal allantoic vessels in the presumptive umbilical cord. A primitive fetoplacental circulation is established. From this data onward, vasculogenetic de novo formation of capillaries out of mesenchymal precursors is an exception that usually can only be found at the tips of newly sprouting mesenchymal villi. Rather, further expansion of the villous vascular system until term mainly takes place by angiogenesis.

The angiogenic processes from day 32 until term can be divided into three periods that partly overlap:

1. Formation of capillary networks from day 32 to 25 weeks post conception by prevalence of branching angiogenesis (Fig. 7.23, stage III)
2. Regression of peripheral capillary webs and formation of central stem vessels mainly through weeks 15 to 32 postconception (Fig. 7.23, stage IV)
3. Formation of terminal capillary loops by prevalence of nonbranching angiogenesis (25 weeks postconception until term) (Fig. 7.23, stage V)

From day 32 postconception until the end of the first trimester, the endothelial tube segments formed by vasculogenesis are transformed into primitive capillary networks by the interaction of two mechanisms: (1) elongation of preexisting tubes by nonbranching angiogenesis, and (2) ramification of these tubes by lateral sprouting (sprouting angiogenesis; Carmeliet, 2003) and possibly also by intussusceptive microvascular growth (branching of a preexisting vessel by formation of an endothelial pillar along the vessel lumen (Burri & Tarek, 1990).

In the first generation of small-caliber villi (mesenchymal villi), branching angiogenesis is less expressed and the resulting capillary webs are only poorly developed (Fig. 7.23, stage II; Fig. 7.24B). With increasing diameter of the immature intermediate villi differentiating out of the mesenchymal villi, branching angiogenesis is stimulated and results in a dense two-dimensional network which is located just below the villous surface (Fig. 7.23, stage III; Fig. 7.24C).

Around the capillaries differentiation processes occur. The endothelial tubes acquire an incomplete layer of pericytes. First spots of basal lamina material are deposited around the endothelial tubes and around the pericytes from about 6 weeks postconception. Complete wrapping of capillaries by basal lamina has been observed only in the last 10 weeks of pregnancy (Fig. 7.22; Demir et al., 1989).

In vitro experiments on the chorioallantoic membrane of the chicken (Wilting et al., 1995, 1996) have shown that binding of VEGF to both of its receptors (VEGFR-1 and -2) stimulates branching angiogenesis and results in highly branched capillary webs. Expression of VEGF-A and VEGFR-2 are most intense in these early stages of pregnancy. Whether they decline or moderately increase as pregnancy advances is still a matter of controversy (Jackson et al., 1994; Cooper et al., 1996; Sharkey et al., 1996; Shiraishi et al., 1996; Vuckovic et al., 1996; Evans et al., 1998; Kumazaki et al., 2002). By contrast, expression of PlGF and the soluble form of VEGFR-1 (Crescimanno et al., 1995; Clark et al., 1998b,c; He et al., 1999; Kumazaki et al., 2002) have been found steeply to increase toward term when branching angiogenesis is increasingly replaced by nonbranching angiogenic mechanisms. Placental growth factor binds selectively to VEGFR-1 and, in some systems, appears to suppress sprouting angiogenesis (chorioallantoic membrane of the chicken; Wilting, personal communication). However, in other systems (rabbit cornea and mouse skin), PlGF stimulates formation of highly branched capillary networks (Ziche et al., 1997; Odorisio, 2002).

Angiogenesis 2: Formation of Stem Vessels and Regression of Capillaries in Stem Villi (Weeks 15 to 32)

In the third month of pregnancy differentiation of stem villi out of immature intermediate villi is started: some of the centrally located endothelial tubes of immature intermediate villi achieve larger diameters of 100 μm and more. Within a short period of time, they establish thin sheaths of contractile cells expressing α- and γ-smooth (sm) actins in addition to vimentin and desmin. This is followed soon afterward by the expression of sm-myosin (Kohnen et al., 1996; Demir et al., 1997). The surrounding stroma shows concentric, centrifugally spreading fibrosis.

These vessels are forerunners of villous arteries and veins. In larger immature intermediate villi, the adventitia of arteries and veins fuse, thereby forming a fibrosed stromal core within the villus. As soon as more than 50% of the reticular stroma of the former immature intermediate villi is replaced by fibrosed stroma, this type of villus is called a stem villus.

Establishment of the outer parts of vessel walls is thought to be controlled by the balance of angiopoietin-1 (Ang-1), and angiopoietin-2 (Ang-2), interacting at their receptor Tie-2 (Tek) (Hanahan, 1997). Accordingly, Ang-1 and Ang-2 protein and messenger RNA (mRNA) have been detected in perivascular cells of immature intermediate villi (Geva et al., 2002) where differentiation of stem vessels takes place.

In the course of pregnancy, fibrosis of the stroma of the stem villi advances in a centrifugal manner toward the villous trophoblast (Fig. 7.24D). In parallel, the superficial, subtrophoblastic capillary net become rarified into few largely unbranched paravascular capillaries (Fig. 7.23, stage IV) (Arts, 1961; Leiser et al., 1985). The mechanisms by which capillary regression occurs in stem villi are unstudied, nor is it known whether Ang-2 and its receptor Tie-2 (Hanahan, 1997), the lack of VEGF-A, or the increase of PlGF is involved. The latter is under discussion since Cao et al. (1996) and Khaliq et al. (1999) reported that PlGF may antagonize VEGF action and thus suppresses angiogenesis. Interestingly, regression of capillary nets in developing stem villi is contemporaneous with loss of trophoblast at the villous surface and reduction of macrophages in the fibrosing stroma (own data; Demir et al., 1997), both known to be rich sources of VEGF-A (Sharkey et al., 1993, Ahmed et al., 1995, Vuorela et al., 1997).

Angiogenesis 3: Prevailing Nonbranching Angiogenesis (Week 25 to Term)

From about 25 weeks postconception until term, mesenchymal villi transform no longer into immature intermediate villi but rather into a new villous types, the mature intermediate villi. These are slender (80 to 120 μm diameter), elongated villi (>1000 μm long) containing one or two long, poorly branched capillary loops. Differentiation of this new villous type out of mesenchymal precursors becomes possible since the pattern of villous vascular growth switches from prevailing branching angiogenesis (leading to immature intermediate villi) to the prevalence of nonbranching angiogenesis (Kaufmann & Kingdom, 2000).

Analysis of proliferation markers at this stage reveals a relative reduction of trophoblast proliferation and an increase of endothelial proliferation along the entire length of the mature intermediate villi, resulting in nonsprouting angiogenesis by proliferative elongation. An alternative mechanism of capillary elongation would be intercalation (Rafii et al., 2002), that is, by recruitment of circulating endothelial progenitor cells into existing vascular endothelium; but currently there is no evidence to support this.

The final length of these peripheral capillary loops exceeds 4000 μm (Kaufmann et al., 1985, 1988). Most importantly, they grow at a rate that exceeds that of the mature intermediate villi themselves, resulting in coiling of the capillaries (Fig. 7.23, stage V). The looping capillaries bulge toward the trophoblastic surface and thereby contribute to formation of the terminal villi, the number of terminal villi depending on the degree of capillary elongation and the resulting degree of coiling (Fig. 7.23, stage Va–c; Fig. 7.24D). Each of the terminal villi is supplied by one or two capillary coils and is covered by an extremely thin (<2 μm) layer of trophoblast that contributes to the so-called vasculosyncytial membranes. Normally, the capillary loops of five to 10 such terminal villi are connected to each other in series by the slender, elongated capillaries of the central mature intermediate villus (Figs. 7.19 and 7.24D).

Immunohistochemical studies on the expression patterns of VEGF-A, PlGF, and their receptors give hints as to their importance in villous angiogenesis. Expression of VEGF-A and VEGFR-2 are intense early in pregnancy and decline as pregnancy advances (Jackson et al., 1994, Cooper et al., 1996, Shiraishi et al., 1996, Vuckovic et al., 1996; Kumazaki et al., 2002) or at least increase much less than placental weight does (Sharkey et al., 1996; Evans et al., 1998). By contrast, expression of VEGFR-1 and PlGF steeply increase toward term (Crescimanno et al., 1995; Clark et al., 1996a; Kumazaki et al., 2002). Placental growth factor is expressed in both villous syncytiotrophoblast (Shore et al., 1997, Vuorela et al., 1997) and the media of larger stem vessels (Khaliq et al., 1996, 1999). Experiments on the avian chorioallantoic membrane (Wilting et al., 1995, 1996) have shown that binding of VEGF-A to its receptors results in sprouting angiogenesis and a highly branched capillary web. In contrast, PlGF (which binds selectively to VEGFR-1) is reported to suppress angiogenesis (Cao et al., 1996).

As already indicated above, the role of PlGF may be very complex. Initially, it was reported that this factor had little potency in vitro to stimulate endothelial cell proliferation. Therefore, it was suggested that PlGF functioned either as a weak stimulator or, more likely, as an antagonist of the proangiogenic actions of VEGF-A (Cao et al., 1996; Khaliq et al., 1999). However, Lang et al. (2003) showed that PlGF in vivo stimulates proliferation of microvascular endothelial cells in human term placenta, and Ziche et al. (1997) showed that PlGF in vivo is a potent stimulator of angiogenesis. Overexpression of PlGF in mouse skin leads to a substantial increase in vessel growth, and ischemic tissues can revascularize following PlGF treatment (Luttun et al., 2002; Odorisio et al., 2002).

In spite of these contradictions, correlation of growth factor data (Jackson et al., 1994, Cooper et al., 1996, Sharkey et al., 1996; Shiraishi et al., 1996, Vuckovic et al., 1996; Evans et al., 1998; Torry et al., 1998; Chappell et al., 2002; Kumazaki et al., 2002) with development of the villous angioarchitecture (Kaufmann et al., 1985, 1988, Leiser et al., 1985; Kaufmann & Kingdom, 2000) suggests that the final geometry of villous vascular bed is defined, at least to some degree, by the balance of VEGF-A and PlGF together with their receptors.

- Total circulating VEGF is high in early pregnancy (Jackson et al., 1994, Cooper et al., 1996, Sharkey et al., 1996; Shiraishi et al., 1996, Vuckovic et al., 1996; Evans et al., 1998; Kumazaki et al., 2002), whereas circulating PlGF is low (Torry et al., 1998; Chappell et al., 2002). The predominance of VEGF in this period promotes establishment of richly branched, low-resistance capillary beds within mesenchymal and immature intermediate villi, both of which prevail during the first two trimesters of pregnancy.
- By contrast, in the second half of pregnancy VEGF either decreases (Jackson et al., 1994, Cooper et al., 1996; Shiraishi et al., 1996; Vuckovic et al., 1996; Kumazaki et al., 2002) or shows only a moderate further increase (Sharkey et al., 1996; Evans et al., 1998), whereas PlGF levels steeply increase and peak between weeks 28 and 32, the period of the most dramatic nonbranching angiogenesis. The balanced secretion of both cytokines in this period or even the predominance of PlGF and its receptor VEGFR-1 seems to block the development of complex capillary beds to the benefit of poorly branched terminal capillary loops in the last trimester.

Oxygen and Oxygen-Controlled Growth Factors as Regulators of Villous and Vascular Development

Only a little is known concerning the control of villous development. On the other hand, a broad variety of pathologic conditions, such as genetic abnormalities but also such as diabetes mellitus, maternal hypertension, maternal anemia or pregnancy in high altitude, rhesus incompatibility, and smoking during pregnancy, severely affect villous and fetoplacental vascular development. This list suggests that the villous and vascular maturational processes are influenced not only by genes but also by endocrine, metabolic, and environmental parameters. From these, only the role of oxygen has been studied in some more detail.

The Special Role of Oxygen in the Placenta

When discussing effects of oxygen in the placenta, one should be aware of the special role of this gas in the placenta.

First, transplacental oxygen transfer is only one of many villous functions; however, its particular importance becomes evident from the fact that it is nearly the only villous function that, upon disturbance, within a short period of time may cause fetal death. Because of this, it is not surprising that the maternal oxygen supply to the placenta has a stronger impact on villous growth and differentiation than any other known parameter.

Second and even more importantly, in **most organs** the interactions among density of vascularization, tissue oxygenation, and capillary growth follow the same pattern: a low degree of local vascularization results in insufficient oxygen delivery to this tissue. The resulting tissue hypoxia stimulates capillary growth and thus improves capillary density and local tissue oxygenation. On the other hand, optimum capillarization of a tissue under otherwise normal conditions guarantees a high tissue oxygenation and this, in turn, will block further angiogenesis.

By contrast, in **placental villi** tissue oxygenation appears to be inversely related to the numerical density of fetal capillaries since, rather than delivering oxygen to the surrounding tissue, the latter extract it from the villi (Kingdom & Kaufmann, 1997).

- Consequently, a low numerical density of fetal capillaries because of reduced oxygen extraction by the fetal circulation, results in increasing intraplacental oxygen levels (Todros et al., 1999; Sibley et al., 2002), which, in turn, may negatively impact on the already poor vascularization (Charnock-Jones et al, 2004).
- And under otherwise constant conditions, high numerical densities of capillaries, resulting in high oxygen extraction by the fetal circulation, would lower intraplacental oxygen tensions (Todros et al., 1999; Sibley et al., 2002) and thus further stimulate growth of the already well-developed capillary bed (Charnock-Jones et al., 2004).

It is evident that, when exceeding certain limits, both situations are predetermined to develop vicious circles.

Types of Hypoxia and Its Effects on Villous Development

Because of the above-mentioned inverse relationship between the degree of capillarization and the level of tissue oxygenation, the term **hypoxia** in pregnancy often causes confusion. This is particularly true when the hypoxic compartment is not exactly defined. Does the hypoxia relate

FIGURE 7.25. Depending on the origins of fetal hypoxia, placental oxygenation and placental structural reaction patterns to oxygenation are different. In preplacental hypoxia the hypoxic mother (anemia, cyanotic heart disease, high altitude, etc.) causes hypoxia of placenta and fetus. In uteroplacental hypoxia the mother is normoxic, whereas placenta and fetus are hypoxic as the result of uteroplacental malperfusion. In both these conditions, placental hypoxia stimulates angiogenesis and villous proliferation, which may partly compensate for the hypoxic effects. By contrast, in postplacental hypoxia mother and placenta are normoxic and only the fetus is hypoxic from fetoplacental malperfusion; reduced oxygen extraction from the placenta typically results in an intraplacental pO_2 exceeding normal values. This high pO_2 inhibits villous growth and accordingly causes the most severe degrees of intrauterine growth restriction. Red point shading: oxygenation of maternal blood. Blue point shading, oxygenation of fetal blood. Dense point shading, oxygen partial pressure shows normal values for that particular tissue; light point shading, oxygen partial pressure is below normal. (*Source:* Kingdom & Kaufmann, 1997, with permission.)

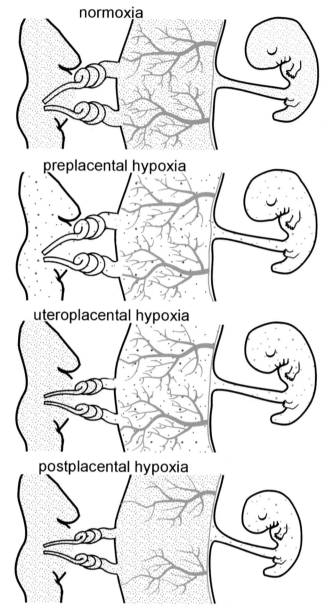

ORIGNS OF FETAL HYPOXIA

• to mother, uterus, placenta, and the fetus, or
• to uterus, placenta, and fetus, or
• only to the fetus?

Based on a respective international symposium 1996 in Banff, the following types of hypoxia in the fetoplacental unit have been defined (Kingdom & Kaufmann, 1997):

1. In **preplacental hypoxia**, the mother, the placenta, and the fetus are hypoxic (Fig. 7.25). Underlying pathologies include pregnancy at high altitude (Jackson et al., 1987; Reshetnikova et al., 1993), maternal anemia (Piotrowicz et al., 1969; Beischer et al., 1970; Kadyrov et al., 1998), and cyanotic maternal cardiac diseases. In this condition, the peripheral placental villi show increased branching angiogenesis with formation of richly branched but shorter terminal capillary loops (Fig. 7.23, stage Vc). These human data are consistent with animal experiments in chronically hypoxic guinea pigs (Scheffen et al., 1990) and chronically hypoxic sheep (Krebs et al., 1997), in which both demonstrated increased branching angiogenesis. Interestingly, in the guinea pig, capillary diameters were reduced under these conditions (Bacon et al., 1984; Scheffen et al., 1990), whereas they were increased in the sheep (Krebs et al., 1997). At the present time, however, we do not understand which factors are responsible for controlling capillary diameter in the human placenta.

2. In **uteroplacental hypoxia** (*e.g.*, preeclampsia with preserved umbilical end-diastolic flow), maternal oxygenation is normal, but because of impaired uteroplacental circulation (Alvarez et al., 1970; for review, see Brosens, 1988), the placenta and fetus are both hypoxic (Fig. 7.25). In this situation, peripheral placental villi similarly show the formation of richly branching capillary networks

(Fig. 7.23, stage Vc), and fetal blood flow impedance is normal or even reduced (Kiserud et al., 1994; Hitschold et al., 1996). Preliminary Western blot data show increased expression of VEGF and reduced PlGF values in placentas of comparable cases (Ahmed et al., 1997), suggesting that placental VEGF expression was upregulated in vivo and caused the changes in angiogenesis.

3. In **postplacental hypoxia** (*e.g.*, IUGR with absent umbilical end-diastolic flow), the fetus is hypoxic whereas the mother is normoxic and the placenta may show even higher pO_2 levels than normal, a situation described as placental hyperoxia (Fig. 7.25) (Macara et al., 1996; Kingdom & Kaufmann, 1997; for commentary, see Ahmed & Kilby, 1997). In this situation, the terminal villus

capillaries are poorly developed, capillary branching is virtually absent (Fig. 7.23, stage Va), and the resulting fetoplacental flow impedance is considerably increased. Perinatal mortality is more than 40% in these circumstances, and survivors of neonatal intensive care are at risk of neurodevelopmental handicap. Similar situations occur in locally restricted parts of the placenta as a consequence of fetoplacental vessel obstruction (Panigel & Myers, 1972; Fox, 1997). Preliminary Western blot data in postplacental hypoxia suggest a pattern of angiogenic growth factor expression in the placenta very different from that of preeclampsia with preserved umbilical end-diastolic flow, namely, a reduction of VEGF expression and relative dominance of PlGF (Ahmed et al., 1997).

Several data support the view that the three variables described above, (1) intraplacental oxygen partial pressure, (2) the balance between VEGF and PlGF expression, and (3) the balance between branching and nonbranching angiogenesis, depend on each other:

- In normal first trimester pregnancy, physiologic intraplacental hypoxia favors VEGF expression and branching angiogenesis.
- In normal third trimester pregnancy, increased intraplacental pO_2 results in a slight prevalence of PlGF expression and dominating but not exclusive nonbranching angiogenesis.
- In several pathologic conditions of third trimester pregnancies, severe intraplacental hypoxia results in prevalence of VEGF expression and marked branching angiogenesis.
- Elevated placental oxygen pressures in severe early-onset IUGR pregnancies (postplacental hypoxia) are combined with the dominance of PlGF expression and complete absence of branching angiogenesis in terminal villi.

Evidence for Oxygen-Controlled Fetoplacental Angiogenesis

Histopathologic and experimental studies have been employed to study the response of fetal villous endothelium to hypoxia (for review, see Kingdom & Kaufmann, 1977).

Histopathology: Complicated pregnancies suffering from intrauterine hypoxia show villous "hypercapillarization" (Hölzl et al., 1974); the same is true for placentas obtained in pregnancies from high altitude (Jackson et al., 1987; Reshetnikova et al., 1993) and those from cases of maternal anemia (Kosanke et al., 1998).

Animal experiments: Experimental chronic hypoxia in pregnant guinea pigs resulted in increased fetal capillarization and in elevated CO_2 diffusion capacity (Bacon et al., 1984). More detailed studies have revealed that this was caused by stimulated sprouting and branching of capillaries; the mean capillary length and the mean capillary diameter were reduced, and the number of parallel capillary loops was considerably increased (Scheffen et al., 1990). As the trophoblastic thickness also decreased, the mean maternofetal diffusion distance was much shorter when compared to normoxic placentas (Bacon et al., 1984). Despite considerable species differences, later repetition of these experiments in sheep revealed a similar reaction pattern (Krebs et al., 1997).

In vitro culture: Using culture of villous explants, the reaction of villous trophoblast to hypoxia was studied in some detail (Tominaga & Page, 1966; Fox, 1970; Amaladoss & Burton, 1985; Ong & Burton, 1991); however, it is difficult to find experimental evidence for an endothelial reactivity in explant culture, because the isolated and unperfused fragments of fetal endothelial tubes tend to disintegrate in culture.

Oxygen-Controlled Angiogenic Growth Factors

The first evidence for the existence of oxygen-controlled endothelial growth factors was obtained from experiments with endothelial cell cultures (Werb, 1983; Ogawa et al., 1991; Shreeniwas et al., 1991). Surprisingly, endothelial cells showed reduced mitotic rates and reduced motility when cultured under hypoxic conditions (Ogawa et al., 1991; Shreeniwas et al., 1991). The addition of conditioned medium obtained from hypoxic macrophages, however, stimulated endothelial proliferation (Ogawa et al., 1991). Moreover, the same authors showed that an increased production of bFGF (FGF-2) by hypoxic macrophages and enhanced expression of bFGF receptor by the hypoxic endothelium were responsible for the enhanced endothelial proliferation.

Since these pilot studies, the list of angiogenic growth factors under discussion to mediate hypoxic signals in the placenta has grown to include

- the platelet-derived growth factor B (PDGF-B) produced by villous cytotrophoblast or by endothelium (Holmgren et al., 1991),
- acidic and basic fibroblast growth factor (FGF-1 and FGF-2) (Ferriani et al., 1994; Shams & Ahmed, 1994; Crescimanno et al., 1995),
- vascular endothelial growth factor (VEGF) (Sharkey et al., 1993; Ahmed et al., 1995, 1997; Wheeler et al., 1995; Shore et al., 1997; Vuorela et al., 1997; for review, see Ahmed et al., 2000), and
- placental growth factor (PlGF) (Khaliq et al., 1996; Ahmed et al., 1997; Shore et al., 1997; Vuorela et al., 1997).

From this list, more recently only VEGF and PlGF and their receptors have been studied in more detail regarding their oxygen dependence

The balance between VEGF-A and PlGF secretion may be regulated by oxygen partial pressures. It has been shown that the expression of VEGF and its receptors in placental and related chorioallantoic tissues is upregulated under conditions of reduced oxygen (Wheeler et al., 1995; Wilting et al., 1995, 1996; Shore et al., 1997; Khaliq et al., 1999), whereas PlGF expression appears to be downregulated under hypoxic conditions (Shore et al., 1997; Khaliq et al., 1999). These findings raise the question of whether or not the switch (from VEGF-A dominance in early pregnancy to PlGF dominance in the second and third trimesters), together with the concomitant changes in vascular geometry, result from increasing intraplacental oxygenation reported by Rodesch et al. (1992).

Throughout the last decade it was shown that oxygen-control of growth factors is mediated by hypoxia-inducible factor (HIF), which transcriptionally regulates the genes of growth factors that are involved in developmental, physiologic, and pathologic responses to hypoxia (Epstein et al., 2001; Semenza, 2001; Pugh & Ratcliffe, 2003). The HIF-1 complex is a heterodimer composed of a constitutively expressed HIF-1β subunit (also known as ARNT, aryl-hydrocarbon receptor nuclear translocator) and the hypoxia-dependent HIF-1α subunit. The level and transcriptional activity of this complex is precisely regulated by the cellular oxygen concentration. In most tissues, the level of the HIF-1α protein is acutely sensitive to cellular oxygen concentration. Under normal oxygen concentrations, the protein is rapidly destroyed, whereas at low oxygen concentrations HIF-1α is stabilized and accumulates within the cell. It then dimerizes with HIF-1β to form an effective transcriptional activator. The HIF-1 dimer binds to specific DNA sequences of the hypoxia-responsive growth factors and activates transcription of the latter.

So far only HIF action in extravillous trophoblast has raised some interest. Relevant data on HIF action in placental villi, however, are scarce. Among the few available data, those by Caniggia et al. (2000) suggest that HIF-1α expression is high in the first trimester, as long as intervillous pO_2 is low and that it decreases thereafter. Unfortunately, the HIF data available at present are not helpful in explaining the oxygen-controlled balance of VEGF and PlGF secretion or the timing mismatch among the increase in placental oxygenation, changes in growth factor expression, and the switch in fetoplacental angiogenesis.

The Timing Mismatch Between Changes in Oxygenation and Morphologic Changes

Throughout pregnancy it is necessary to protect the fetus from the potentially harmful effects of high oxygen tensions (Burton, 1997; Burton & Caniggia, 2001; Hung et al., 2001). Development and remodeling of the fetoplacental vasculature may be part of this protection. As mentioned above, it is tempting to speculate about causal interactions among changes in placental oxygenation, the switch from VEGF-A dominance to PlGF dominance, and the switch from branching to nonbranching angiogenesis. Interestingly, there is a time lag of about 2 months between the rises in intervillous pO_2 levels and perfusion rates (after week 12, Rodesch et al., 1992) and the evidence of morphologic changes (transition from mainly branching to predominantly nonbranching angiogenesis around week 25; Kaufmann & Kingdom, 2000; Mayhew, 2002). The explanation for this time lag may be that the anatomic changes are considerably more protracted than the rapid in vitro effects of altered oxygen tensions on cultured cells. This situation possibly reflects the difference between the acute (short-term and rapid-onset) and chronic (long-term and delayed-onset) responses to oxygen (Semenza, 2001). Sculpting the fetoplacental vascular network takes time and, if the placenta as a whole is to function in a coordinated manner, vascular changes must be integrated with changes in other villous compartments, especially the trophoblast (Mayhew, 2002).

Downregulation of VEGF-A and upregulation of PlGF may occur almost contemporaneously with the oxygen switch, although there is no direct evidence for this at present. The time course of respective vascular adaptation in the placenta is not known, but in the eye and in tumors these events occur within just a few days (Alon et al., 1995; Benjamin & Keshet, 1997). In the placenta stimulated vascularization may take much more time since the interactions between fetoplacental vascularization and villous development are much more complex. Regression of capillaries in immature intermediate villi, together with establishment of a tunica media around maturing vessels in developing stem villi, may begin at about the time of the oxygen switch. The transition from branching angiogenesis (in mesenchymal and immature intermediate villi) to nonbranching angiogenesis (in mature intermediate and terminal villi), however, involves different generations of villi. Only when the key types of villi for nonbranching angiogenesis (mature intermediate villi) are generated, persistently-high pO_2 levels may combine with low VEGF-A and high PlGF levels (and changes in other, as yet unidentified, factors) to facilitate nonbranching angiogenesis.

Intervillous pO_2 values seem to peak during the second trimester (about 60 mm Hg at 16 weeks, Soothill et al., 1986; Rodesch et al., 1992; Jauniaux et al., 2001). This is in seeming contradiction to the assumption that, as pregnancy advances, also the fetal demand for oxygen will rise further. Possibly the final drop to about 45 mm Hg at term (Soothill et al., 1986; Rodesch et al., 1992; Jauniaux et al., 2001) is a consequence of fetoplacental vascular remodeling resulting in increased oxygen extraction from the intervillous space.

Oxygen and Villous Trophoblast

Histopathologic reports unanimously describe that the amount of villous cytotrophoblast is increased in all those pathologic conditions that are thought to be related to intrauterine hypoxia (Fox, 1964, 1970; Piotrowicz et al., 1969; Beischer et al., 1970; Kaufmann et al., 1977a; Kosanke et al., 1998). Arnholdt and coworkers (1991) found evidence that this is the result not only of an increased mitotic index but also of a reduction of the length of the cell cycle. In contrast, unusually good oxygenation of villi reduces the rate of proliferation as well as the quantity of villous cytotrophoblast (Panigel & Myers, 1971, 1972; Myers & Panigel, 1973; Kaufmann et al., 1977a; Macara et al., 1996; for review, see Kingdom & Kaufmann, 1997).

In addition, the villous syncytiotrophoblast is affected by hypoxia as was shown experimentally by Tominaga and Page (1966) and Ong and Burton (1991), and in pathologic specimens (Alvarez et al., 1969, 1970). It is reduced in thickness and simultaneously increased numbers of syncytial knots are produced, the nuclei of which show signs of chromatin clumping and partly of apoptosis. Tominaga and Page interpreted this as a sign of adaptation by reducing diffusion distances. More stringent stereologic studies have suggested, however, that the changes are more likely caused by degenerative processes (Ong & Burton, 1991). Recent experiments by Burton pose the question of whether or not all insults seen after ischemic/hypoxic periods are in fact due to lack of oxygen; the authors found that damage by oxygen radicals in the reoxygenation period may be even more important (Hung et al., 2002a).

Most in vitro studies on the effects of hypoxia have been performed on villous explants rather than on villous cytotrophoblast cultures. For that reason it is still an open question whether cytotrophoblast responds directly to variations of the oxygen partial pressure, or whether this response is mediated by factors released by other hypoxic tissue components such as syncytiotrophoblast or villous macrophages. There are several candidate mediators of hypoxic signals: epidermal growth factor (EGF) may be derived from maternal sources and is additionally produced by syncytiotrophoblast (for review, see Prager et al., 1992); its mitogenic action on trophoblast has been shown by Lysiak and coworkers (1992), and its receptors have been detected on the syncytiotrophoblastic surfaces (Rao et al., 1985) as well as on cytotrophoblastic membranes (Mühlhauser et al., 1993). Transforming growth factor-α (TGF-α) (Lysiak et al., 1992) and tumor necrosis factor-α (TNF-α) (Hung et al., 2002b), the latter produced by macrophages (for review, see Hunt, 1989), and colony-stimulating factor 1 (CSF-1) produced by mesenchymal cells (Jokhi et al., 1992; Shorter et al., 1992) are other candidates. Finally, TGF-β_1 and TGF-β_2, both produced by macrophages (for review, see Hunt, 1989) and by trophoblast (Graham & Lala, 1991), seem to be involved in the regulation of syncytial fusion of the post-proliferative cytotrophoblast to regenerate the hypoxically damaged syncytiotrophoblast. As already mentioned above, oxygen-dependent regulation of most of these cytokines involves HIF as hypoxia-responsive transcriptional factor.

Oxygen and Villous Stroma

It is a common experience in pathologic studies of the placenta that the villous connective tissue responds to variations in the intrauterine oxygen supply. This is nicely illustrated by the low degree of villous fibrosis throughout the first trimester when intervillous pO_2 is low, and the increasing fibrosis, for example, in stem villi at the transition to the second trimester when placental oxygen levels steeply increase. Chronic hypoxia results in minimal fibrosis of the villi (Fox, 1978); in contrast, higher levels of intravillous pO_2 increase villous fibrosis (for example following intrauterine death when intraplacental oxygen partial pressure, because of lacking fetal oxygen extraction, approaches maternal arterial values) (Panigel & Myers, 1971, 1972; Fox, 1978). Related in vitro experiments with placental tissues are still to be done. Possible mediators are macrophage products such as TGF-β, which stimulates collagen-I transcription (Rossi et al., 1988), or interleukin-1, which, among other functions, regulates fibroblast proliferation (Schmidt et al., 1982).

Oxygen and Intervillous Circulation

There are few data concerning hypoxic influences on the maternal vascularization of the placenta. In the guinea pig, volume and surface of maternal blood lacunae are reduced under hypoxic conditions (Bacon et al., 1984). In contrast, in human placentas from patients at high altitude, the intervillous space was described to be increased (Jackson et al., 1987). For the cow placenta, Reynolds and coworkers (1992) have demonstrated maternal endothelial mitogens of endometrial origin.

Numerous experimental data have been provided concerning the influence of oxygen on trophoblast invasion (Genbacev et al., 1996, 1997; Graham & McCrae, 1997; Fitzpatrick & Graham, 1998; Zhou et al., 1998; Caniggia et al., 2000). Trophoblast invasion triggers adaptation of uteroplacental arteries to pregnancy conditions and thus has an important effect on intervillous blood flow. Unfortunately, these data are controversial. Therefore, no actual conclusions can be drawn as to whether hypoxia affects maternal blood flow to the intervillous space, and if so, in which direction.

Hormones as Regulators of Villous Development

Even though it should be expected that villous development is controlled by maternal and fetal hormones, there are only very few relevant clinical indications. Reliable experimental proof is completely missing. Here, we briefly discuss data that look promising for future research.

Ovarian steroids are the most likely group of hormones to be involved in placental development and probably represent the only group of hormones that, in few cases, have been used for the treatment of villous maldevelopment. The following examples may give an idea of how ovarian steroids can influence villous development:

• Placentas from pregnancies complicated by IUGR and combined with decreased or absent end-diastolic blood flow are characterized by very homogeneous features of villous maldevelopment (Macara et al., 1996). These are reduced trophoblastic proliferation rate, reduced numbers of terminal villi, reduced total villous volume, poor branching of terminal villous capillaries, increased terminal villous fibrosis, and increased differentiation of villous myofibroblasts. The functional consequences of these alterations are likely to be responsible for the impaired fetal nutrition, as well as for the increased feto-placental blood flow impedance. Several groups of investigators have found evidence that third trimester treatment with gestagens (allylestre-nol) decreased blood flow impedance and increased fetal birth weight as well as placental weight (Kaneoka et al., 1983; Kurjak & Pal, 1986; Marzolf et al., 1986). The only histologic study of these placentas provided by Papierowski (1981) described a "stimulated development" of villi. As far as we were able to see from Papierowski's data, a numerical increase in immature, proliferating villous types was responsible for the overall increased villous growth rate.
• In contrast, P. Prahalada (personal communication, 1982) found that treatment of rhesus monkeys with higher doses of estrogens during midpregnancy caused reduced placental and fetal growth rates. To our knowledge, these placentas have not been studied histologically.
• The latter findings were supported by experimental data by Yallam-palli and Garfield (1993), Chwalisz et al. (1994), and Garfield et al. (1994). These authors induced symptoms of preeclampsia including IUGR in rats and guinea pigs by blocking nitric oxide synthase by l-NAME, and reversed these effects by treatment with gestagens.

The above data suggest that gestagens and estrogens may have antagonistic effects on villous development and differentiation. Possibly not only the oxygen-controlled balance of VEGF and PlGF (see above) but also both steroid hormones control the switch of mesenchymal villous transformation either into continuously growing immature intermediate villi or into differentiating mature intermediate villi.

Also **insulin** is under discussion regarding its influence on villous development. The prevailing finding in placentas of diabetic mothers is that of an overall increased proliferation rate of villous trophoblast, villous stromal cells, and villous capillaries, resulting in large placentas that are characterized by large-caliber villi with high cellular density (Widmaier, 1970; Werner & Schneiderhan, 1972; Fox, 1978).

So far, all attempts have failed to demonstrate classic insulin effects on the maternal side of the placental barrier, such as stimulation of glucose uptake (Challier et al., 1986), of amino acid transport (Montgomery & Young, 1982), and increase in glycogen levels in trophoblast cells (Schmon et al., 1991). These negative results can be explained by the low levels of insulin receptors on the syncytiotrophoblastic surface during the second half of pregnancy (Jones et al., 1993; Desoye et al., 1994, 1997).

On the other hand, direct growth-promoting effects of insulin (for review, see Strauss, 1984) on the various placental tissues must be considered:

• In the first trimester, insulin receptors available at the maternal/intervillous surface of villous trophoblast are expressed mainly along the surfaces of sprouting segments of the villous trees (true trophoblastic sprouts, mesenchymal villi) (Desoye et al., 1994, 1997). This finding indicates that maternal insulin might be involved in first-trimester villous growth, which is mainly a result of trophoblastic proliferation (Castellucci et al., 1990, 2000).
• In the last trimester, the highest immunoreactivities for insulin receptors are found in fetal villous endothelium (Jones et al., 1993), in particular in segments with capillary sprouting, such as mature intermediate villi and terminal villus necks (Desoye et al., 1994, 1997). In this period, expansion and differentiation of the villous trees are mainly a result of capillary sprouting (Kaufmann et al., 1988; Castellucci et al., 1990, 2000).

A switch in villous growth control from maternal insulin (with insulin receptors along the maternal trophoblastic surface) in early pregnancy to fetal insulin (with endothelial insulin receptors) in late pregnancy would make sense because it would enable the fetus to control villous differentiation in accordance with its own nutritional needs.

Also **thyroid hormones** are candidate regulators of villous development. It is now recognized that in pregnancy, maternal thyroid function is mediated by the placenta (Fisher, 1983). The placenta plays a major role in the synthesis and metabolism of the thyroid hormones: the putative trophoblastic thyrotropin (Hershman, 1972) as well as human chorionic gonadotropin (hCG) (Kennedy & Darne, 1991) stimulate the maternal thyroid hormone production; thyroid-stimulating hormone (TSH), triiodothyronine (T_3), thyroxine (T_4), and thyroglobulin cannot pass the placental barrier, while thyroid-releasing hormone (TRH), iodine, and thyroid-stimulating immunoglobulins can (Cappoen, 1989). Placental tissue as well as the decidua has a high nuclear-binding capacity for T_3. Therefore, Banovac et al. (1986) have suggested the placenta to be a thyroid hormone–dependent tissue. Maruo et al. (1991) have described stimulatory effects of maternal T_3 and T_4 on trophoblastic endocrine functions; moreover, they found that T_3 enhances trophoblastic production of epidermal growth factor (EGF), a potent trophoblastic mitogen, and concluded that thyroid hormone, in synergy with EGF, regulates villous growth (Matsuo et al., 1993).

There are fewer data concerning the correlation of thyroid malfunction with placental function or development. According to experiments in rats (Kumar & Chaudhuri, 1989), the levels of maternal thyroid hormone secretion are positively correlated with fetal growth. Thorpe Beeston et al. (1991) found significantly reduced maternal T_4 levels in small-for-gestational-age fetuses combined with fetal hypoxemia and acidemia.

All these data suggest that maternal thyroid hormones are involved in villous development and thus influence placental transfer functions for nutrients and gases. Relevant clinical data, however, are difficult to interpret. We have seen some placentas of hypothyroid mothers medicated with thyroid hormones. The placentas of all of these cases were characterized by stimulated nonbranching angiogenesis and correspondingly reduced branching of terminal villi; partly, the respective cases comprised persisting villous immaturity with predominance of mature intermediate villi (see Chapter 15, Fig. 15.9) as well as IUGR with ARED flow in the umbilical arteries (Fig. 15.17). We found similar features in two cases of untreated hyperthyroid mothers.

Intervillous Space as Related to the Villous Trees

The human placenta is a hemochorial, villous placental type. After leaving the spiral arteries, the maternal blood circulates through the diffuse intervillous space and flows directly around the villi. The maternal blood is outside the confines of the endothelium of the maternal vascular system.

Width of the Intervillous Space

The anatomical investigations concerning the width of the intervillous space suffer the disadvantage of having been made on delivered placentas, which have lost considerable amount of maternal blood during delivery. They are also usually fixed without the in vivo maternal blood pressure distending the intervillous space. Therefore, the usual appearance of the intervillous space of the delivered placenta is that of a system of **narrow intervillous clefts**. Hörmann (1951, 1953, 1958a,b) and Lemtis (1955) called it the intervillous cleft system. This view was supported by Becker (1962b), who attempted to reestablish in vivo pressure conditions before fixation and found the same narrow clefts. Becker described neighboring villi as clinging closely to one another, the tips of some fitting into notches of others, as in a jigsaw puzzle. Becker interpreted the occasional appearance of a wider intervillous space (in conventional histologic material) as the result of shrinkage. Freese (1966) also failed to demonstrate an intervillous space of larger than capillary dimensions, except for the subchorial lake. Boyd and Hamilton (1970) contradicted these interpretations. According to their experience from in vivo radioangiographs, the rapid filling of the intervillous space is not compatible with a cleft system of capillary dimensions.

Using the data for postpartal intervillous blood volume (23.3% to 37.9% of the placental volume) and for the villous surface (11.0 to 13.3 m²) (see Tables 28.5 and 28.8), we calculate the mean width of the intervillous space (blood volume divided by one half of the villous surface) as ranging from 16.4 to 32 μm. The villous surface must be divided by 2 because it covers the clefts on both sides. Bouw et al. (1976) demonstrated that late cord clamping is responsible for a loss of intervillous volume, probably owing to the decreasing turgor of the villi that border the intervillous space (see Table 28.8). If we calculate the mean width of the intervillous space with their data from term placentas obtained after early cord clamping, it amounts to 31.6 μm. One must bear in mind that there is a considerable subchorial lake, and that wide spaces also exist in the arterial inflow area. Thus, the real "intervillous" volume is likely to be lower and the intervillous clefts narrower. On the other hand, when one adds the considerable loss of maternal blood during labor, we consider that these calculations may be near the truth.

Also recent in vivo studies in various stages of pregnancy using color power Doppler ultrasonography with three-dimensional (3D) option did not answer the question as to the in vivo width of the intervillous space at term (Konje et al., 2003). They suggest, however, that the width of the intervillous space becomes considerably reduced in the course of pregnancy: the 3D reconstruc-

tions (Fig. 7.26B) revealed high maternal blood flow velocities in the maternal inflow and outflow areas on the intervillous space throughout the second and third trimesters of pregnancy. In the second trimester even between peripheral ramifications of the villous trees minor maternal flows could be visualized, suggesting wide intervillous clefts (≫100 μm) with high flow velocities. In the third trimester velocities and width of the intervillous clefts between the peripheral villi were too small for detection.

Organization of Villous Trees

Wigglesworth (1967) studied corrosion casts of fetal vessels and suggested that most villous trees are arranged "as hollow-centered bud-like structures" around a central cavity. When he injected the spiral arteries, Wigglesworth found the injection mass to collect in the loose centers of the villous trees. This finding is in agreement with most descriptions of the maternal arterial inlets as being located near the centers of the villous trees (Schuhmann & Wehler, 1971; Schuhmann, 1981), which direct the bloodstreams into these centers (Panigel & Pascaud, 1968). The 50 to 200 maternal venous outlets of each placenta are thought to be arranged around the periphery of the villous trees. Thus, each fetomaternal circulatory unit is composed of one villous tree with a corresponding, centrifugally perfused portion of the intervillous space (Figs. 4.7, 7.26A, and 7.27A). This unit was called a "placentone" by Schuhmann and Wehler (1971) (for review, see Schuhmann, 1982).

Most placentologists agree that, under in vivo conditions, most of the 40 to 60 placentones are in contact with each other and that they overlap more or less broadly. This supposition is highly probable, as structural borderlines, such as placental septa, are absent (Becker & Jipp, 1963). It is our experience that the peripheral placentones are more clearly separated from each other and thus exhibit typical structural differences between their central and peripheral zones. In the thicker, more central regions of the placenta, most villous trees overlap (Figs. 7.26A and 7.27A), causing less distinct differences between maternal inflow and outflow areas of the placentone.

According to studies of Schuhmann and Wehler (1971), the centers of typical placentones exhibit loosely arranged villi, mostly of the immature intermediate type, and provide a large intervillous space for the maternal arterial inflow, the central arterial inflow area (Figs. 7.26A and 7.27). It is still uncertain if these large, loosely arranged villi regularly delineate a central cavity as described by Wilkin (1965). Schuhmann (1981) suggested that these cavities are pressure-dependent in vivo structures that rapidly collapse after delivery, and his suggestion is borne out by ultrasonographic findings. If one accepts the considerations of Moll (1981), the existence of such a central cavity makes sense because it guarantees the rapid and

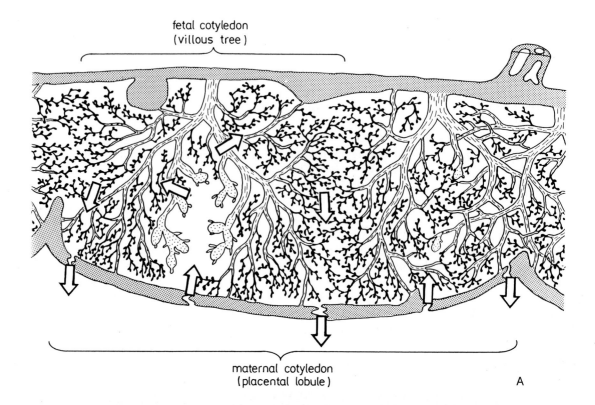

fetal cotyledon
(villous tree)

maternal cotyledon
(placental lobule)

A

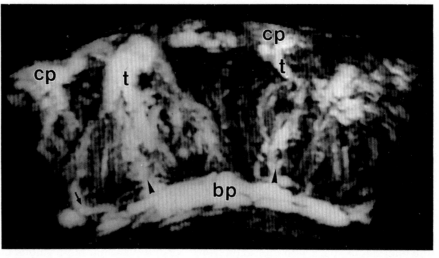

B

FIGURE 7.26. A: Typical spatial relations between villous trees, single villous types, and the maternal bloodstream. According to the placentone theory of Schuhmann (1981), a placentone is one villous tree together with the related part of the intervillous space. In the case of typical placentones (left half of the diagram), which prevail in the periphery of the placenta, the maternal blood (arrows) enters the intervillous space near the center of the villous tree and leaves the intervillous space near the clefts between neighboring villous trees. In the term placenta, the larger stem villi (line shaded), the immature intermediate villi (point shaded), and their tiny branches (unshaded) are concentrated in the centers of the villous trees, surrounding a central cavity as maternal blood inflow area. The mature intermediate villi (black) together with their terminal branches (black, grape-like) make up the periphery of the villous trees, near the venous outflow area. One or few villous trees occupy one placental lobule (see Chapter 2, Fig. 2.2), which is delimited by grooves in the basal surface of the placenta (see Fig. 2.1B). In the central parts of the placenta, the villous trees, because of size and nearby location, may partly overlap (right half of the diagram) so that the zonal arrangement of the placentone disappears. (*Source:* Modified from Kaufmann, 1985, with permission.) B: Corresponding in vivo photograph, generated by power-Doppler ultrasonography with 3D option, shows two villous trees, corresponding to those depicted in part A. The villous trees are derived from villous trunci (t), which are connected to the chorionic plate (cp). As is typical for the power Doppler technique, the picture shows not only the larger vessels in chorionic and basal plates but also the larger stem villi in which the Doppler signals of arteries and veins add to each other. The maternal arterial bloodstreams ("jets") entering the intervillous space (arrowheads), as well as the maternal venous blood (arrow) leaving the intervillous space, are also seen. Since blood flow velocities across the fetal cotyledons are too slow, the remaining parts of the intervillous space are black. Near-term placenta, ×2. (Courtesy of Dr. Justin Konje, Leicester, UK.)

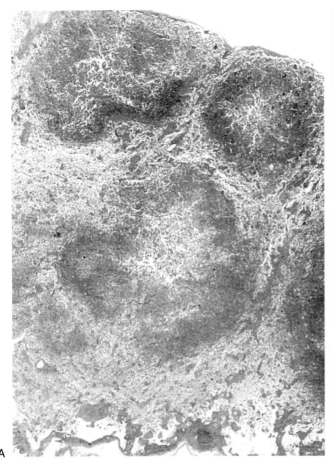

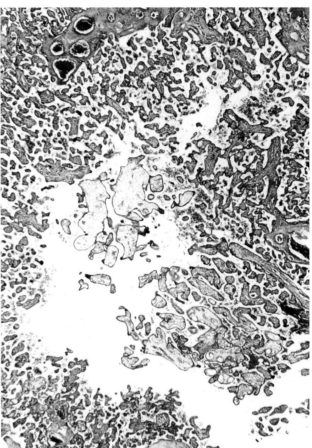

A
B

FIGURE 7.27. Placentone arrangement of villous trees. A: Horizontal paraffin section across the marginal zone of a mature placenta. H&E stain. Note the existence of three ring-shaped placentones (fetal cotyledons), each single one composed of a loose center (arterial inflow area), surrounded by a dense ring of small peripheral villi (exchange area), and finally surrounded by the loosely structured venous outflow area. ×3.6. B: Higher magnification of the placentone center of a fetal cotyledon. Note the large empty appearing arterial inflow area, which is bordered by some immature intermediate villi, easily recognizable by their light staining. This immature center of the cotyledon is surrounded by a densely packed mantle of smaller villi which provide the maternofetal exchange area. ×20.

homogeneous distribution of blood into the surrounding mantle of small, densely packed villi with little loss of pressure.

The surrounding mantle is composed mostly of small villi of the mature intermediate and terminal types and provides the peripheral exchange area. The villi are densely packed. Schmid-Schönbein (1988) described the intervillous space in this zone as a system of randomly shaped and oriented, interconnected clefts, or "connected voids." With respect to their topology, these clefts lack the regular connectivity seen in dichotomously branching vascular beds. The fixed relations of the latter vessels, which orient pressure gradients, are not found in randomly connected voids as in the intervillous space. This feature may be advantageous under normal conditions, but it may also cause hazards to the intervillous circulation.

The most peripheral zone of a placentone, the venous outflow area, is the loosely arranged area that separates neighboring villous trees (Fig. 7.27A) and that, subchorially, is connected to the subchorial lake. It collects the maternal venous blood that has left the high impedance area of the fetomaternal exchange zone of the densely packed terminal villi. Moll (1981) called this the perilobular zone, which is functionally comparable to wide venules of other vascular beds. It allows venous backflow under conditions of low blood flow resistance.

The radioangiographic studies of Ramsey et al. (1963) in rhesus monkey placentas, and those of Borell et al. (1958) in human placentas, are consistent with the placentone concept. They demonstrated rapid filling of the centers of the villous trees and called them "jets," or "spurts." More recent physiologic concepts of intervillous circulation (Moll, 1981; Schmid-Schönbein, 1988) do not agree with these terms, as the actual filling velocities amount to only a few centimeters per second, which might not be enough to describe the driving force of a fountain as implied by the terms **jet** or **spurt**. After passage of the central cavity, a subsequent rather slow centrifugal spreading of the blood toward the subchorial and peripheral zone was observed. Wallenburg et al. (1973) ligated single spiral arteries in rhesus monkeys, which resulted in obliteration of the intervillous space and degeneration of the corresponding villous tree. This experiment demonstrated that each villous tree depends on its own spiral artery. Even though the intervillous space is a widely open, freely communicating system, villous arrangement and pressure gradients are coordinated in such a way that blood perfusion depends strictly on the original flow arrangement. Reversal of the direction is impossible.

If one accepts these considerations, the immature intermediate villi, together with their sprouting mesenchymal side branches (Figs. 7.26A and 7.27B), are concentrated in the placentone center and are thus in the zones of highest pO_2 in the intervillous space. Schuhmann's group found that ^3H-thymidine incorporation, as an index for the mitotic rate, is twice as high in the center of the placentone as at the periphery (Geier et al., 1975). This finding is in seeming contrast to several experimental and histologic findings. The latter authors also suggested that low oxygen concentration serves as a stimulus for trophoblastic proliferation and villous sprouting (Alvarez, 1967; Alvarez et al., 1970; Fox, 1970). The most likely explanation for this discrepancy is that oxygen delivery to the centrally located large villi, those in the central cavity and its close vicinity, is reduced owing to high blood flow velocity and long diffusion distances. The adjacent densely packed zones, although already located nearer the venous pole, probably have a much higher oxygen delivery, as blood flow velocity is reduced in the slender intervillous clefts and diffusion distances are short. This situation results in high mean pO_2 values at the villous surfaces, which is a prerequisite for effective maternofetal oxygen transfer. At the same time, it inhibits villous proliferation and stimulates villous differentiation in the placentone periphery.

These relations may be the basis for regulatory mechanisms. Wide intervillous clefts in the periphery of the villous trees of immature placentas, which lack fine and richly branched terminal villi, result in long diffusion distances and high blood flow velocities—and thus in reduced oxygen delivery. The resulting intravillous pO_2 in this area is low, which stimulates villous sprouting and especially capillary sprouting (Bacon et al., 1984; Scheffen et al., 1990). Increased capillary sprouting is followed by the production of new terminal villi. The latter narrow the intervillous space, reduce blood flow velocity and diffusion distances, and thus increase oxygen delivery. Finally, the elevated pO_2 inhibits further villous branching.

According to this hypothesis, the maternal bloodstream, oxygenation, and villous branching act as limbs of a simple feedback mechanism that regulates growth of the villous trees. As a further consequence, a functional diversity of the placentone is obtained. Whereas the centers act as proliferative zones that guarantee placental growth until term, the periphery is the functionally fully active exchange and secretory area. This situation has also been highlighted by the histochemically and biochemically higher activity of enzymes such as alkaline phosphatase (Schuhmann et al., 1976) and by the higher conversion rate of steroid hormones (Lehmann et al., 1973) in the placentone periphery.

The zonal differences become evident only after the development of mature intermediate villi, at the end of the second trimester. Up to that time, the villous trees are largely homogeneous. In most placentas, the immature placentone centers are present until term, at least in the more peripheral areas of the placenta. Only in cases of preterm maturation of the placenta (hypermaturity, maturitas praecox) do we regularly find mature placentone centers, resulting in a virtually homogeneous structure of the placentones. Thus, such a placenta has lost its capacity to grow, as only the immature intermediate villi and their immediate mesenchymal branches are able to sprout and act as growth zones.

Histopathologic Importance of Inhomogeneity of Villous Trees

For the histopathologist, the inhomogeneity of the villous trees causes considerable problems of interpretation. Because the average diameter of placentone is 1 to 4 cm, histologic sections often do not cover a representative part of the placentone, which would comprise immature growth zones as well as highly differentiated, mature tissue. The prevalence of one or the other tissue may influence the diagnosis. This danger is even greater when one considers that placentones from various locations may show varying degrees of maturation. Thus, even the careful study of several sections from a given placenta may lead to wrong interpretations. This point is of particular importance when performing morphometric evaluations of the placenta. Burton (1987) remarked that "strict attention must be paid to the sampling regimen if meaningful results are to be obtained. Sadly this has not always been taken into consideration in the past, and so many of the published claims must be qualified accordingly."

This problem is greater still when one uses small tissue samples, such as semithin sections for light microscopy or ultrathin sections for electron microscopy. Neither section type allows a diagnosis concerning the degree of maturation upon which one can rely. The same holds true for samples obtained by aspiration from the intact uterus (Alvarez et al., 1964; Aladjem, 1968), the placenta at cesarean section (Schweikhart & Kaufmann, 1977), and chorion villus sampling (CVS). While the latter samples are of greatest value for genetic purposes (Hugentobler et al., 1987), one must be careful with a histologic evaluation of such material (Gerl et al., 1973; Ehrhardt et al., 1974), even during early stages of pregnancy. In these situations one does not have the problem of heterogeneity of the placentones but rather the problem of general heterogeneity.

Fetomaternal Flow Interrelations

The efficiency of diffusional exchange (e.g., oxygen, carbon dioxide, water), among other factors, depends on the arrangement of fetal and maternal blood flows to each other. As early as 1926 Mossman described countercurrent flow conditions in the rabbit placenta; neighboring maternal and fetal bloodstreams were thought to be arranged in parallel but with opposite flow directions.

Later, Mossman (1965) found the same condition to be valid for the human placenta. This finding, however, is not supported by anatomic or physiologic results. Rather, it has been recognized for many years that the anatomic arrangement of placental vascular pathways differs from one species to another. For the human, we have described three major morphologic objections to the existence of countercurrent flow conditions (Kaufmann, 1985):

1. All villi would have to be oriented in the same direction, parallel to the maternal bloodstream. They are, in fact, arranged at varying angles to each other because of the structure of the villous tree.

2. Only one limb of the hairpin-like fetal capillary loops is allowed to have interchange contact with the maternal blood; in fact, both limbs normally exhibit the same structure and the same diffusion distance to the maternal blood.

3. According to the results of Lemtis (1969), one must consider the possibility that considerable amounts of venous maternal blood are recirculated by the arterial "jet" before leaving the intervillous space. Thus, intraplacental circulatory "orbits" are formed.

The anatomic situation and the physiologic effectiveness of the human placenta are much more in agreement with the concept of a multivillous flow arrangement (Bartels & Moll, 1964; Moll, 1981). In this condition, the maternal bloodstream crosses subsequent villi with hairpin-like arranged fetal capillaries. It seems to be of minor importance with which angle the maternal bloodstream crosses the individual villi or whether the vessels of the villi are serially connected to each other or arranged in parallel. The multivillous blood flow is less effective for diffusional transfer (Moll, 1981).

This difference may be the reason why 1 g of human placenta supplies only 6 g of fetus at term, compared to a relation of 1:20 in the guinea pig with a countercurrent flow placenta (see Chapter 4, Table 4.1) (Dantzer et al., 1988). On the other hand, the multivillous arrangement is structurally more flexible. It allows rearrangement and adaptation to changing developmental conditions and the continuous growth to a much greater extent. In this respect, it is worthy of note that the highly effective guinea pig placenta is small (about 5 g) and functions for only 68 days. The capybara (Kaufmann, 2004), which belongs to the same suborder of rodents, has a structurally closely related placenta but a much longer pregnancy (150 days) and a much higher placental weight (150 g), but is less effective than the guinea pig placenta (1 g of placenta at term supplies 10 g of fetus).

References

Ahmed, A. and Kilby, M.: Commentary: Hypoxia or hyperoxia in placental insufficiency? Lancet **350**:826–827, 1997.

Ahmed, A. and Perkins, J.: Angiogenesis and intrauterine growth restriction. Baillieres Best Pract. Res. Clin. Obstet. Gynaecol. **14**:981–988, 2000.

Ahmed, A., Li, X.F., Dunk, C., Whittle, M.J., Rushton, D.I. and Rollason, T.: Colocalisation of vascular endothelial growth factor and its flt-1 receptor in human placenta. Growth Factors **12**:235–243, 1995.

Ahmed, A., Whittle, M.J. and Khaliq, A.: Differential expression of placenta growth factor (PlGF) and vascular endothelial growth factor (VEGF) in abnormal placentation. J. Soc. Gynecol. Invest. **4**:A663, 1997.

Ahmed, A., Dunk, C., Ahmad, S. and Khaliq, A.: Regulation of placental vascular endothelial growth factor (VEGF) and placenta growth factor (PlGF) and soluble Flt-1 by oxygen—a review. Placenta, 21: suppl. A. Troph. Res. **14**:S16–S24, 2000.

Aladjem, S.: Morphopathology of the human placental villi and the fetal outcome. J. Obstet. Gynaecol. Br. Commonw. **75**:1237–1244, 1968.

Alon, T., Hemo, I., Itin, A., Pe'er, J., Stone, J. and Keshet, E.: Vascular endothelial growth factor acts as a survival factor for newly formed retinal vessels and has implications for retinopathy of prematurity. Nature Med. **1**:1024–1028, 1995.

Alvarez, H.: Syncytial proliferation in normal and toxemic pregnancies. Obstet. Gynecol. **29**:637–643, 1967.

Alvarez, H., De Bejar, R. and Aladjem, S.: La placenta human. Aspectos morfologicos y fisio-patologicos. In, 4th Uruguayan Congress for Obstetrics and Gynecology **1**:190–261, 1964.

Alvarez, H., Morel, R.L., Benedetti, W.L. and Scavarelli, M.: Trophoblast hyperplasia and maternal arterial pressure at term. Amer. J. Obstet. Gynecol. **105**:1015–1021, 1969.

Alvarez, H., Benedetti, W.L., Morel. R.L. and Scavarelli, M.: Trophoblast development gradient and its relationship to placental hemodynamics. Amer. J. Obstet. Gynecol. **106**:416–420, 1970.

Alvarez, H., Medrano, C.V., Sala, M.A. and Benedetti, W.L.: Trophoblast development gradient and its relationship to placental hemodynamics. II. Study of fetal cotyledons from the toxemic placenta. Amer. J. Obstet. Gynecol. **114**:873–878, 1972.

Amaladoss, A.S.P. and Burton, G.J.: Organ culture of human placental villi in hypoxic and hyperoxic conditions: a morphometric study. J. Dev. Physiol. **7**:13–118, 1985.

Amstutz, E.: Beobachtungen Über die Reifung der Chorionzotten in der menschlichen Placenta mit besonderer Berücksichtigung der Epithelplatten. Acta Anat. (Basel) **42**:12–30, 1960.

Ara, G., Bari, M.A. and Siddiquey, A.K.: Effects of age, parity and length of pregnancy on the morphology and histology of human placenta. Bangladesh Med. Res. Counc. Bull. **10**:53–58, 1984.

Arnholdt, H., Meisel, F., Fandrey, K. and Löhrs, U.: Proliferation of villous trophoblast of the human placenta in normal and abnormal pregnancies. Virchows Arch. B Cell Pathol. **60**:365–372, 1991.

Arts, N.F.T.: Investigation on the vascular system of the placenta. I. General introduction and the fetal vascular system. Amer. J. Obstet. Gynecol. **82**:147–166, 1961.

Bacon, B.J., Gilbert, R.D., Kaufmann, P., Smith, A.D., Trevino, F.T. and Longo, L.D.: Placental anatomy and diffusing capacity in guinea pigs following long-term maternal hypoxia. Placenta **5**:475–488, 1984.

Baker, P.N., Krasnow, J., Roberts, J.M. and Yeo, K.T.: Elevated serum levels of vascular endothelial growth factor in patients with preeclampsia. Obstet Gynecol **86**:815–821, 1995.

Banks, R.E., Forbes, M.A., Searles, J., Pappin, D., Canas, B., Rahman, D., Kaufmann, S., Walters, C.E., Jackson, A., Eves, P., Linton, G., Keen, J., Walker, J.J. and Selby, P.J.: Evidence for the existence of a novel pregnancy-associated soluble variant of the vascular endothelial growth factor receptor, Flt-1. Mol. Human Reprod. **4**:377–386, 1998.

Banovac, K., Ryan, E.A. and O'Sullivan, M.J.: Triiodothyronine (T3) nuclear binding sites in human placenta and decidua. Placenta **7**:543–549, 1986.

Bär, T., Güldner, F.H. and Wolff, J.R.: "Seamless" endothelial cells of blood capillaries. Cell Tiss. Res. **235**:99–106, 1984.

Bartels, H. and Moll, W.: Passage of inert substances and oxygen in the human placenta. Pfluegers Arch. Gesamte Physiol. **280**:165, 1964.

Becker, V.: Mechanismus der Reifung fetaler Organe. Verh. Dtsch. Ges. Pathol. **46**:309–314, 1962a.

Becker, V.: Funktionelle Morphologie der Plazenta. Arch. Gynäkol. **198**:3–28, 1962b.

Becker, V.: Pathologie der Ausreifung der Plazenta. In, Die Plazenta des Menschen. V. Becker, T.H. Schiebler and F. Kubli, eds., pp. 266–281. Thieme, Stuttgart, 1981.

Becker, V. and Jipp, P.: Über die Trophoblastschale der menschlichen Plazenta. Geburtsh. Frauenheilk. **23**:466–474, 1963.

Becker, V. and Seifert, K.: Die Ultrastruktur der Kapillarwand in der menschlichen Placenta zur Zeit der Schwangerschaftsmitte. Z. Zellforsch. **65**:380–396, 1965.

Beischer, N.A., Sivasamboo, R., Vohra, S., Silpisornkosal, S. and Reid, S.: Placental hypertrophy in severe pregnancy anaemia. J. Obstet. Gynaecol. Br. Commonw. **77**:398–409, 1970.

Benjamin, L.E. and Keshet, E.: Conditional switching of vascular endothelial growth factor (VEGF) expression in tumors: induction of endothelial cell shedding and regression of hemangioblastoma-like vessels by VEGF withdrawal. Proc. Natl. Acad. Sci. USA **94**:8761–8766 1997.

Boe, F.: Studies on the vascularization of the human placenta. Acta Obstet. Gynecol. Scand. (Suppl. 5) **32**:1–92, 1953.

Boe, F.: Studies on the human placenta. II. Gross morphology of the fetal structures in the young placenta. Acta Obstet. Gynecol. Scand. **47**:420–435, 1968.

Boe, F.: Studies on the human placenta. III. Vascularization of the young fetal placenta. A. Vascularization of the chorionic villus. Acta Obstet. Gynecol. Scand. **48**:159–166, 1969.

Borell, U., Fernstroem, I. and Westman, A.: Eine arteriographische Studie des Plazentarkreislaufs. Geburtsh. Frauenheilkd. **18**:1–9, 1958.

Bouw, G.M., Stolte, L.A.M., Baak, J.P.A. and Oort, J.: Quantitative morphology of the placenta. 1. Standardization of sampling. Eur. J. Obstet. Gynecol. Reprod. Biol. **6**:325–331, 1976.

Boyd, J.D. and Hamilton, W.J.: The Human Placenta. Heffer, Cambridge, 1970.

Breier, G.: Angiogenesis in embryonic development—a review. Placenta 21: suppl A. Troph. Res. **14**:S11–S15, 2000.

Brosens, I.A.: The uteroplacental vessels at term-the distribution and extent of physiological changes. Trophoblast Res. **3**:61–67, 1988.

Bukovsky, A., Caudle, M.R., Keenan, J.A., Wimalasena, J. and McKenzie, P.P.: Thy-1 differentiation protein and monocyte-derived cells during regeneration and aging of human placental villi. Amer. J. Reprod. Immunol. **42**:135–152, 1999.

Burri, P. and Tarek, M.R.: A novel mechanism of capillary growth in the rat pulmonary microcirculation. Anat. Rec. **228**:35–45, 1990.

Burton, G.J.: The fine structure of the human placental villus as revealed by scanning electron microscopy. Scanning Electron Microsc. **1**:1811–1828, 1987.

Burton, G.J.: On "Oxygen and placental villous development: origins of fetal hypoxia." Placenta **18**:625–626, 1997.

Burton, G.J. and Caniggia, I.: Hypoxia: implications for implantation to delivery-a workshop report. Placenta **22**: Suppl. A: S63–S65, 2001.

Burton, G.J. and Palmer, M.E.: Eradicating fetomaternal fluid shift during perfusion fixation of the human placenta. Placenta **9**:327–332, 1988.

Caniggia, I., Mostachfi, H., Winter, J., Gassmann, M., Lye, S.J., Kuliszewski, M. and Post, M.: Hypoxia-inducible factor-1 mediates the biological effects of oxygen on human trophoblast differentiation through TGFbeta(3). J. Clin. Invest **105**:577–587, 2000.

Cantle, S.J., Kaufmann, P., Luckhardt, M. and Schweikhart, G.: Interpretation of syncytial sprouts and bridges in the human placenta. Placenta **8**:221–234, 1987.

Cao, Y., Chen, H., Zhou, L., Chiang, M.K., Anand-Apte, B., Weatherbee, J.A., Wang, Y., Fang, F., Flanagan, J.G. and Tsang, M.L.: Heterodimers of placenta growth factor/vascular endothelial growth factor. Endothelial activity, tumor cell expression, and high affinity binding to Flk-1/KDR. J. Biol. Chem. **271**:3154–3162, 1996.

Cappoen, J.P.: Physiology of the thyroid during pregnancy. Various exploratory tests. Rev. Fr. Gynecol. Obstet. **84**:893–897, 1989.

Carmeliet, P.: Angiogenesis in health and disease. Nature Med. **9**:653–660, 2003.

Castellucci, M. and Kaufmann, P.: A three-dimensional study of the normal human placental villous core: II. Stromal architecture. Placenta **3**:269–286, 1982a.

Castellucci, M. and Kaufmann, P.: Evolution of the stroma in human chorionic villi throughout pregnancy. Bibl. Anat. **22**:40–45, 1982b.

Castellucci, M., Schweikhart, G., Kaufmann, P. and Zaccheo, D.: The stromal architecture of the immature intermediate villus of the human placenta. Gynecol. Obstet. Invest. **18**:95–99, 1984.

Castellucci, M., Scheper, M., Scheffen, I., Celona, A. and Kaufmann, P.: The development of the human placental villous tree. Anat. Embryol. (Berl.) **181**:117–128, 1990.

Castellucci, M. and Kaufmann, P.: A three-dimensional study of the normal human placental villous core: II. Stromal architecture. Placenta **3**:269–286, 1982a.

Castellucci, M. and Kaufmann, P.: Evolution of the stroma in human chorionic villi throughout pregnancy. Bibl. Anat. **22**:40–45, 1982b.

Castellucci, M., Schweikhart, G., Kaufmann, P. and Zaccheo, D.: The stromal architecture of the immature intermediate villus of the human placenta. Gynecol. Obstet. Invest. **18**:95–99, 1984.

Castellucci, M., Scheper, M., Scheffen, I., Celona, A. and Kaufmann, P.: The development of the human placental villous tree. Anat. Embryol. (Berl.) **181**:117–128, 1990.

Castellucci, M., Kosanke, G., Verdenelli, F., Huppertz, B., Kaufmann, P.: Villous sprouting: fundamental mechanisms of human placental development. Hum. Reprod. Update **6**:485–494, 2000.

Challier, J.C., Hauguel, S. and Desmaizieres, V.: Effect of insulin on glucose uptake and metabolism in the human placenta. J. Clin. Endocrinol. Metab. **62**:803–807, 1986.

Challier, J.C., Galtier, M., Kacemi, A. and Guillaumin, D.: Pericytes of term human foeto-placental microvessels: Ultrastructure and visualization. Cell Mol. Biol. **45**:89–100, 1999.

Chappell, L.C., Seed, P.T., Briley, A., Kelly, F.J, Hunt, B.J., Charnock-Jones, D.S., Mallet, A.I. and Poston, L.: A longitudinal study of biochemical variables in women at risk of preeclampsia. Amer. J. Obstet. Gynecol. **187**:127–136, 2002.

Charnock-Jones, D.S., Kaufmann, P. and Mayhew, T.M.: Aspects of Human fetoplacental vasculogenesis and angiogenesis. I. Molecular regulation. Placenta **25**:103–113, 2004.

Chwalisz, K., Ciesla, I. and Garfield, R.E.: Inhibition of nitric oxide (NO) synthesis induces preterm parturition and preeclampsia-like conditions in guinea pigs. Presented at the Society for Gynecological Investigation Meeting, Chicago, IL, 1994.

Clark, D.E., Smith, S.K., Sharkey, A.M. and Charnock-Jones, D.S.: Localization of VEGF and expression of its receptors flt and KDR in human placenta throughout pregnancy. Hum. Reprod. (Oxf.) **11**:1090–1098, 1996a.

Clark, D.E., Smith, S.K., Sharkey, A.M., Sowter, H.M. and Charnock-Jones, D.S.: Hepatocyte growth factor scatter factor and its receptor c-met: localization and expression in the human placenta throughout pregnancy. J. Endocrinol. **151**:459–467, 1996b.

Clark, D.E., Salvig, J.D., Smith, S.K. and Charnock-Jones, D.S.: Hepatocyte growth factor levels during normal and intrauterine growth-restricted pregnancies. Placenta **19**:671–673, 1998a.

Clark, D.E., Smith, S.K., He, Y., Day, K.A., Licence, D.R., Corps, A.C., Lammoglia, R. and Charnock-Jones, D.S.: A vascular endothelial growth factor antagonist is produced by the human placenta and released into the maternal circulation. Biol. Reprod. **59**:1540–1548, 1998b.

Clark, D.E., Smith, S.K., Licence, D., Evans, A.L and Charnock-Jones, D.S.: Comparison of expression patterns for placenta growth factor, vascular endothelial growth factor (VEGF), VEGF-B and VEGF-C in the human placenta throughout gestation. J. Endocrinol. **159**:459–467, 1998c.

Cooper, J.C., Sharkey, A.M., Charnock-Jones, D.S., Palmer, C.R. and Smith, S.K.: VEGF mRNA levels in placentae from pregnancies complicated by pre-eclampsia. Br. J. Obstet. Gynaecol. **103**:1191–1196, 1996.

Crescimanno, C., Marzioni, D., Persico, M.G., Vuckovic, M., Mühlhauser, J. and Castellucci, M.: Expression of bFGF, PIGF and their receptors in the human placenta. Placenta **16**:A13, 1995.

Dantzer, V., Leiser, R., Kaufmann, P. and Luckhardt, M.: Comparative morphological aspects of placental vascularization. Trophoblast Res. **3**:235–260, 1988.

Davidoff, M. and Schiebler, T.H.: Über den Feinbau der Meerschweinchenplacenta während der Entwicklung. Z. Anat. Entwicklungsgesch. **130**:234–254, 1970.

Demir, R., Kaufmann, P., Castellucci, M., Erbengi, T. and Kotowski, A.: Fetal vasculogenesis and angiogenesis in human placental villi. Acta Anat. (Basel) **136**:190–203, 1989.

Demir, R., Demir, N., Kohnen, G., Kosanke, G., Mironov, V., Üstünel, I. and Kocamaz, E.: Ultrastructure and distribution of myofibroblast-like cells in human placental stem villi. Electron Microsc. **3**:509–510, 1992.

Demir, R., Kosanke, G., Kohnen, G., Kertschanska, S. and Kaufmann, P.: Classification of human placental stem villi: review of structural and functional aspects. Microsc. Res. Tech. **38**:29–41, 1997.

Demir, R., Kayisli, U.A., Seval, Y., Celik-Ozenci, C., Korgun, E.T., Demir Weusten, A.Y. and Huppertz, B.: Sequential expression of VEGF and its receptors in human placental villi during very early pregnancy: Differences between placental vasculogenesis and angiogenesis. Placenta **25**:560–572, 2004.

Dempsey, E.W.: The development of capillaries in the villi of early human placentas. Am. J. Anat. **134**:221–238, 1972.

Desoye, G., Hartmann, M., Blaschitz, A., Dohr, G., Kohnen, G. and Kaufmann, P.: Insulin receptors in syncytiotrophoblast and fetal endothelium of human placenta. Immunohistochemical evidence for developmental changes in distribution pattern. Histochemistry **101**:277–285, 1994.

Desoye G., Hartmann, M., Jones, C.J.P., Wolf, H.J., Kohnen, G., Kosanke, G. and Kaufmann, P.: Location of insulin receptors in the placenta and its progenitor tissues. Microsc. Res. Tech. **38**:63–75, 1997.

Di Blasio, A.M., Carniti, C., Vigano, P., Florio, P., Petraglia, F. and Vignali, M.: Basic fibroblast growth factor messenger ribonucleic acid levels in human placentas from normal and pathological pregnancies. Mol. Hum. Reprod. **3**:1119–1123, 1997.

Downs, K.M., Gifford, S., Blahnik, M. and Gardner, R.L.: Vascularization in the murine allantois occurs by vasculogenesis without accompanying erythropoiesis. Development **125**:4507–4520, 1998.

Dunk, C., Shams, M., Nijjar, S., Rhaman, M., Qiu, Y., Bussolati, B. and Ahmed, A.: Angiopoietin-1 and angiopoietin-2 activate trophoblast Tie-2 to promote growth and migration during placental development. Amer J Pathol **156**:2185–2199, 2000.

Ehrhardt, G., Gerl, D., Estel, C., Kadner, J. and Günther, M.: Morphologische Auswertbarkeit von in vitro gewonnenen Punktionszylindern der Plazenta. Zentralbl. Gynäkol. **96**:705–711, 1974.

Enders, A.C. and King, B.F.: The cytology of Hofbauer cells. Anat. Rec. **167**:231–252, 1970.

Epstein, A.C., Gleadle, J.M., McNeill, L.A., Hewitson, K.S., O'Rourke, J., Mole, D.R., Mukherji, M., Metzen, E., Wilson, M.I., Dhanda, A., Tian, Y.M., Masson, N., Hamilton, D.L., Jaakkola, P., Barstead, R., Hodgkin, J., Maxwell, P.H., Pugh, C.W., Schofield, C.J. and Ratcliffe, P.J.: C elegans EGL-9 and mammalian homologs define a family of dioxygenases that regulate HIF by prolyl hydroxylation. Cell **107**:43–54, 2001.

Evans, P.W., Wheeler, T., Anthony, F.W. and Osmond, C.: A longitudinal study of maternal serum vascular endothelial growth factor in early pregnancy. Human Reprod. **13**:1057–1062, 1998.

Farley, A.E., Graham, C.H. and Smith, G.N.: Contractile properties of human placental anchoring villi. Amer. J. Physiol. Regul. Integr. Comp. Physiol. **287**:R680–R685, 2004.

Feneley, M.R. and Burton, G.J.: Villous composition and membrane thickness in the human placenta at term: a stereological study using unbiased estimators and optimal fixation techniques. Placenta **12**:131–142, 1991.

Ferriani, R.A., Ahmed, A., Sharkey, A.M. and Smith, S.K.: Colocalization of acidic and basic fibroblast growth factor (FGF) in human placenta and the cellular effects of bFGF in trophoblast cell line JEG-3. Growth Factors **10**:259, 1994.

Fisher, D.A.: Maternal-fetal thyroid function in pregnancy. Clin. Perinatol. **10**:615–626, 1983.

Fitzpatrick, T.E. and Graham, C.H.: Stimulation of plasminogen activator inhibitor-1 expression in immortalized human trophoblast cells cultured under low levels of oxygen. Exp. Cell Res. **245**:155–162, 1998.

Folkman, J. and Haudenschild, C.: Angiogenesis in vitro. Nature (Lond.) **288**:551–556, 1980.

Folkman, J. and Shing, Y.: Angiogenesis. J. Biol. Chem. **267**: 10931–10934, 1992.

Fong, G.-H., Rossant, J., Gertsenstein, M. and Breitman, M.L.: Role of the Flt-1 receptor tyrosine kinase in regulating the assembly of vascular endothelium. Nature (Lond.) **376**:66–70, 1995.

Fong, G.-H., Zhang, L., Bryce, D.M. and Peng, J.: Increased hemangioblast commitment, not vascular disorganization, is the primary defect in flt-1 knock-out mice. Development **126**:3015–3025, 1999.

Fox, H.: The villous cytotrophoblast as an index of placental ischaemia. J. Obstet. Gynaecol. Br. Commonw. **71**:885–893, 1964.

Fox, H.: Effect of hypoxia on trophoblast in organ culture. A morphologic and autoradiographic study. Amer. J. Obstet. Gynecol. **107**:1058–1064, 1970.

Fox, H.: Pathology of the Placenta. 1st Ed. Saunders, London, 1978.

Fox, H.: Pathology of the Placenta. 2nd Ed. Saunders, London, 1997.

Freese, U.E.: The fetal-maternal circulation of the placenta. I. Histomorphologic, plastoid injection, and X-ray cinematographic studies on human placentas. Amer. J. Obstet. Gynecol. **94**:354–360, 1966.

Garfield, R.E., Yallampalli, C., Buhimschi, I. and Chwalisz, K.: Reversal of preeclampsia symptoms induced in rats by nitric oxide inhibition with L-arginine, steroid hormones and an endothelin antagonist. Presented at the Society for Gynecologic Investigation Meeting, 1994.

Geier, G., Schuhmann, R. and Kraus, H.: Regional unterschiedliche Zellproliferation innerhalb der Plazentone reifer menschlicher Plazenten: autoradiographische Untersuchungen. Arch. Gynäkol. **218**:31–37, 1975.

Genbacev, O., Joslin, R., Damsky, C.H., Polliotti, B.M. and Fisher, S.J.: Hypoxia alters early gestation human cytotrophoblast differentiation invasion in vitro and models the placental defects that occur in preeclampsia. J. Clin. Invest. **97**:540–550, 1996.

Genbacev, O., Zhou, Y., Ludlow, J.W. and Fisher, S.J.: Regulation of human placental development by oxygen tension. Science. **277**:1669–1672, 1997.

Gerl, D., Eichhorn, H., Eichhorn, K.-H. and Franke, H.: Quantitative Messungen synzytialer Zellkernkonzentrationen der menschlichen Plazenta bei normalen und pathologischen Schwangerschaften. Zentralbl. Gynäkol. **95**:263–266, 1973.

Geva, E., Ginzinger, D.G., Zaloudek, C.J., Moore, D.H., Byrne, A. and Jaffe, R.B.: Human placental vascular development: vasculogenic and angiogenic (branching and nonbranching) transformation is regulated by vascular endothelial growth factor-A, angiopoietin-1, and angiopoietin-2. J. Clin. Endocrinol. Metab. **87**:4213–4224, 2002.

Graf, R., Langer, J.U., Schönfelder, G., Öney, T., Hartel-Schenk, S., Reutter, W. and Schmidt, H.H.H.W.: The extravascular contractile system in the human placenta. Morphological and immunocytochemical investigations. Anat. Embryol. **190**:541–548, 1994.

Graf, R., Schönfelder, G., Mühlberger, M. and Gutsmann, M.: The perivascular contractile sheath of human placental stem villi; its isolation and characterization. Placenta **16**:57–66, 1995.

Graf, R., Matejevic, D., Schuppan, D., Neudeck, H., Shakibaei, M. and Vetter, K.: Molecular anatomy of the perivascular sheath in human placental stem villi: the contractile apparatus and its association to the extracellular matrix. Cell Tissue Res. **290**:601–607, 1997.

Graham, C.H. and Lala, P.K.: Mechanism of control of trophoblast invasion in situ. J. Cell Physiol. **148**:228–234, 1991.

Graham, C. H. and McCrae, K. R. Hypoxia stimulates expression of the urokinase receptor and invasion of extracellular matrix by trophoblast cells through a heme protein-dependent pathway. Placenta **18**:A24, 1997.

Habashi, S., Burton, G.J. and Steven, D.H.: Morphological study of the fetal vasculature of the human placenta: scanning electron microscopy of corrosion casts. Placenta **4**:41–56, 1983.

Hanahan, D.: Signaling vascular morphogenesis and maintenance. Science **277**:48–50, 1997.

He, Y., Smith, S.K., Day, K.A., Clark, D.E., Licence, D.R. and Charnock-Jones, D.S.: Alternative splicing of vascular endothelial growth factor (VEGF)-R1 (FLT-1) pre-mRNA is important for the regulation of VEGF activity. Mol. Endocrinol. **13**:537–545, 1999.

Helske, S., Vuorela, P., Carpen, O., Hornig, C., Weich, H. and Halmesmaki, E.: Expression of vascular endothelial growth factor receptors 1, 2 and 3 in placentas from normal and complicated pregnancies. Mol. Hum. Reprod. **7**:205–210, 2001.

Hershman, J.M.: Hyperthyroidism induced by trophoblastic thyrotropin. Mayo Clin. Proc. **47**:913–918, 1972.

Hertig, A.T.: Angiogenesis in the early human chorion and in the primary placenta of the macaque monkey. Contrib. Embryol. Carnegie Inst. **25**:37–81, 1935.

Highison, G.J. and Tibbitts, F.D.: Ultrasonic microdissection of immature intermediate human placental villi as studied by scanning electron microscopy. Scanning Electron Microsc. **2**:679–685, 1986.

Hiratsuka, S., Minowa, O., Kuno, J., Noda, T. and Shibuya, M.: Flt-1 lacking the tyrosine kinase domain is sufficient for normal development and angiogenesis in mice. Proc. Natl. Acad. Sci. USA **95**:9349–9354, 1998.

Hitschold, T., Müntefering, H., Ulrich, S. and Berle, P.: Does extremely low fetoplacental impedance as estimated by umbilical artery Doppler velocimetry also indicate fetuses at risk? Ultrasound Gynecol. **8**:39A, 1996.

Holmgren, L., Glaser, A., Pfeifer-Ohlsson, N.S. and Ohlsson, R.: Angiogenesis during human extraembryonic development involves the spatiotemporal control of PDGF ligand and receptor gene expression. Development (Camb.) **113**:749–754, 1991.

Hölzl, M., Lüthje, D. and Seck-Ebersbach, K.: Placentaveränderungen bei EPH-Gestose. Arch. Gynäkol. **217**:315–334, 1974.

Hörmann, G.: Lebenskurven normaler und entwicklungsfähiger Chorionzotten; Ergebnisse systematischer Zottenmessungen. Arch. Gynäkol. **181**:29–43, 1951.

Hörmann, G.: Ein Beitrag zur funktionellen Morphologie der menschlichen Placenta. Arch. Gynäkol. **184**:109–123, 1953.

Hörmann, G.: Versuch einer Systematik plazentarer Entwicklungsstörungen. Geburtsh. Frauenheilkd. **18**:345–349, 1958a.

Hörmann, G.: Zur Systematik einer Pathologie der menschlichen Placenta. Arch. Gynäkol. **191**:297–344, 1958b.

Hornig, C., Barleon, B., Ahmad, S., Vuorela, P., Ahmed, A. and Weich, H.A.: Release and complex formation of soluble VEGFR-1 from endothelial cells and biological fluids. Lab. Invest. **80**:443–454, 2000.

Hugentobler, W., Binkert, F., Haenel, A.F. and Schaetti, D.: Die Chorionzotten-(Plazenta-) Biopsie im II. und III. Trimenon: Neue Perspektiven der Pränataldiagnostik. Geburtsh. Frauenheilkd. **47**:729–732, 1987.

Hung, T.H., Skepper, J.N. and Burton, G.J.: In vitro ischemia-reperfusion injury in term human placenta as a model for oxidative stress in pathological pregnancies. Amer. J. Pathol. **159**:1031–1043, 2001.

Hung, T.H., Skepper, J.N., Charnock-Jones, D.S. and Burton, G.J.: Hypoxia-reoxygenation: a potent inducer of apoptotic changes in the human placenta and possible etiological factor in preeclampsia. Circ. Res. **90**:1274–1281, 2002a.

Hung, T., Charnock-Jones, D. S. and Burton, G. J. Hypoxia/reoxygenation is a potent stimulus for placental production of tumour necrosis factor-alpha. Placenta **23**:Suppl. A, A.9. 2002b.

Hunt, J.S.: Macrophages in human uteroplacental tissues: a review. Amer. J. Reprod. Immunol. **21**:119–122, 1989.

Jackson, M.R., Mayhew, T.M. and Haas, J.D.: Morphometric studies on villi in human term placentae and the effects of altitude, ethnic grouping and sex of newborn. Placenta **8**:487–495, 1987.

Jackson, M.R., Carney, E.W., Lye, S.J. and Ritchie, J.W.K. Localization of two angiogenic growth factors (PDECGF and VEGF) in human placentae throughout gestation. Placenta **15**:341–353, 1994.

Jauniaux, E., Watson, A. and Burton, G.: Evaluation of respiratory gases and acid-base gradients in human fetal fluids and uteroplacental tissue between 7 and 16 weeks gestation. Amer. J. Obstet. Gynecol. **184**:998–1003, 2001.

Jirkovska, M., Kubinova, L., Krekule, I. and Hach, P.: Spatial arrangement of fetal placental capillaries in terminal villi: a study using confocal microscopy. Anat. Embryol. **197**:263–272, 1998.

Jokhi, P., Chumbley, G., King, A., Gardner, L. and Loke, W.: Expression of the colony stimulating factor-1 receptor by cells at the uteroplacental interface. Placenta **13**:A29, 1992.

Jones, C.J.P., Hartmann, M., Blaschitz, A. and Desoye, G.: Ultrastructural localization of insulin receptors in human placenta. Amer. J. Reprod. Immunol. **30**:136–145, 1993.

Kadyrov, M.K., Kosanke, G., Kingdom, J.C.P. and Kaufmann, P. Increased fetoplacental angiogenesis during first trimester in anaemic women. Lancet **352**:1747–1749, 1998.

Kaneoka, T., Taguchi, S., Shimizu, H. and Shirakawa, K.: Prenatal diagnosis and treatment of intrauterine growth retardation. J. Perinat. Med. **11**:204–212, 1983.

Karimu, A.L. and Burton, G.J.: The effects of maternal vascular pressure on the dimensions of the placental capillaries. Br. J. Obstet. Gynaecol. **101**:57–63, 1994.

Kaufmann, P.: Entwicklung der Plazenta. In, Die Plazenta des Menschen. V. Becker, T.H. Schiebler and F. Kubli, eds., pp. 13–50. Thieme Verlag, Stuttgart, 1981.

Kaufmann, P.: Development and differentiation of the human placental villous tree. Bibl. Anat. **22**:29–39, 1982.

Kaufmann, P.: Basic morphology of the fetal and maternal circuits in the human placenta. Contrib. Gynecol. Obstet. **13**:5–17, 1985.

Kaufmann, P.: Capybara. In: Kurt Benirschke: Comparative Placentation. http://medicine.ucsd.edu/cpa/indxfs.html 2004.

Kaufmann, P. and Davidoff, M.: The guinea pig placenta. Adv. Anat. Embryol. Cell Biol. **53**:1–91, 1977.

Kaufmann, P. and Kingdom, J.C.P.: Development of the vascular system in the placenta. In, Morphogenesis of Endothelium. W. Risau and G. M. Rubanyi, pp 255–275. Amsterdam, Harwood Academic Publishers. 2000.

Kaufmann, P. and Scheffen, I.: Placental development. In, Neonatal and Fetal Medicine-Physiology and Pathophysiology, Vol. I. R.A. Polin and W.W. Fox, eds., pp. 47–55. Saunders, Orlando, 1992.

Kaufmann, P., Schiebler, T.H., Ciobotaru, C. and Stark, J.: Enzymhistochemische Untersuchungen an reifen menschlichen Placentazotten. II. Zur Gliederung des Syncytiotrophoblasten. Histochemistry **40**:191–207, 1974.

Kaufmann, P., Gentzen, D.M. and Davidoff, M.: Die Ultrastruktur von Langhanszellen in pathologischen menschlichen Placenten. Arch. Gynaekol **222**:319–332, 1977a.

Kaufmann, P., Stark, J. and Stegner, H.-E.: The villous stroma of the human placenta. I. The ultrastructure of fixed connective tissue cells. Cell Tissue Res. **177**:105–121, 1977b.

Kaufmann, P., Sen, D.K. and Schweikhart, G.: Classification of human placental villi. I. Histology and scanning electron microscopy. Cell Tissue Res. **200**:409–423, 1979.

Kaufmann, P., Nagl, W. and Fuhrmann, B.: Die funktionelle Bedeutung der Langhanszellen der menschlichen Plazenta. Ann. Anat. **77**:435–436, 1983.

Kaufmann, P., Bruns, U., Leiser, R., Luckhardt, M. and Winterhager, E.: The fetal vascularization of term human placental villi. II. Intermediate and terminal villi. Anat. Embryol. (Berl.) **173**:203–214, 1985.

Kaufmann, P., Luckhardt, M., Schweikhart, G. and Cantle, S.J.: Cross-sectional features and three-dimensional structure of human placental villi. Placenta **8**:235–247, 1987.

Kaufmann, P., Luckhardt, M. and Leiser, R.: Three-dimensional representation of the fetal vessel system in the human placenta. Trophoblast Res. **3**:113–137, 1988.

Kaufmann, P., Mayhew, T.M. and Charnock-Jones, D.S.: Aspects of human fetoplacental vasculogenesis and angiogenesis. II. Changes during normal pregnancy. Placenta **25**:114–126, 2004.

Kennedy, R.L. and Darne, J.: The role of hCG in regulation of the thyroid gland in normal and abnormal pregnancy. Obstet. Gynecol. **78**:298–307, 1991.

Khaliq, A., Li, X.F., Shams, M., Sisi, P., Acevedo, C.A., Whittle, M.J., Weich, H. and Ahmed, A.: Localisation of placenta growth factor PlGF in human term placenta. Growth Factors **13**:243–250, 1996.

Khaliq, A., Dunk, C., Jiang, J., Shams, M., Li, X.F., Acevedo, C., Weich, H., Whittle, M. and Ahmed, A.: Hypoxia down-regulates placenta growth factor, whereas fetal growth restriction up-regulates placenta growth factor expression: molecular evidence for "placental hyperoxia" in intrauterine growth restriction. Lab. Invest. **79**:151–170, 1999.

Kilby, M.D., Afford, S., Li, X.F., Strain, A.J., Ahmed, A. and Whittle, M.J.: Localisation of hepatocyte growth factor and its receptor (c-met) protein and mRNA in human term placenta. Growth Factors **13**:133–139, 1996.

King, B.F.: Ultrastructural differentiation of stromal and vascular components in early macaque placental villi. Amer. J. Anat. **178**:30–44, 1987.

Kingdom, J.C.P. and Kaufmann, P.: Oxygen and placental villous development: origins of fetal hypoxia. Placenta **18**:613–621, 1997.

Kingdom, J.C.P., Burrell, S.J. and Kaufmann, P.: Pathology and clinical implications of abnormal umbilical artery Doppler waveforms. Ultrasound Obstet. Gynecol. **9**:271–286, 1997a.

Kingdom, J.C.P., Macara, L.M., Krebs, C., Leiser, R. and Kaufmann, P.: Pathological basis for abnormal umbilical artery Doppler waveforms in pregnancies complicated by intrauterine growth restriction. Trophoblast Res. **10**:291–309, 1997b.

Kiserud, T., Hellevik, L.R., Eik-Nes, S.H., Angelsen, B.A. and Blaas, H.G.: Estimation of the pressure gradient across the fetal ductus venosus based on Doppler velocimetry. Ultrasound Med. Biol. **20**:225–232, 1994.

Knoth, M.: Ultrastructure of chorionic villi from a four-somite human embryo. J. Ultrastruct. Res. **25**:423–440, 1968.

Kohnen, G., Kosanke, G., Korr, H. and Kaufmann, P.: Comparison of various proliferation markers applied to human placental tissue. Placenta **14**:A38, 1993.

Kohnen, G., Castellucci, M., Hsi, B.L., Yeh, C.J.G. and Kaufmann, P.: The monoclonal antibody GB42–a useful marker for the differentiation of myofibroblasts. Cell Tissue Res. **281**:231–242, 1995.

Kohnen, G., Kertschanska, S., Demir, R. and Kaufmann, P.: Placental villous stroma as a model system for myofibroblast differentiation. Histochem. Cell Biol. **101**:415–429, 1996.

Konje, J.C., Huppertz, B., Bell, S.C., Taylor, D. and Kaufmann, P.: 3–dimensional colour power angiography for staging human placental development. Lancet **362**:1199–2101, 2003.

Kosanke, G., Castellucci, M., Kaufmann, P. and Mironov, V.A.: Branching patterns of human placental villous trees: perspectives of topological analysis. Placenta **14**:591–604, 1993.

Kosanke, G., Kadyrov, M., Korr, H. and Kaufmann, P.: Maternal anemia results in increased proliferation in human placental villi. Trophoblast Res. **11**:339–357, 1998.

Krantz, K.E. and Parker, J.C.: Contractile properties of the smooth muscle in the human placenta. Clin. Obstet. Gynecol. **6**:26–38, 1963.

Krebs, C., Macara, L.M., Leiser, R., Bowman, A.W., Greer, I.A. and Kingdom, J.C.P.: Intrauterine growth restriction with absent end-diastolic flow velocity in the umbilical artery is associated with maldevelopment of the placental terminal villous tree. Amer. J. Obstet. Gynecol. **175**:1534–1542, 1996.

Krebs, C., Longo, L.D. and Leiser, R.: Term ovine placental vasculature: comparison of sea level and high altitude conditions by corrosion cast and histomorphometry. Placenta **18**:43–51, 1997.

Kumar, R. and Chaudhuri, B.N.: Altered maternal thyroid function: fetal and neonatal development of rat. Indian J. Physiol. Pharmacol. **33**:233–238, 1989.

Kumazaki, K., Nakayama, M., Suehara, N. and Wada, Y.: Expression of vascular endothelial growth factor, placental growth factor, and their receptors Flt-1 and KDR in human placenta under pathologic conditions. Human Pathol. **33**:1069–1077, 2002.

Kupferminc, M.J., Daniel, Y., Englender, T., Baram, A., Many, A., Jaffa, A.J., Gull, I. and Lessing, J.B.: Vascular endothelial growth factor is increased in patients with preeclampsia. Amer. J. Reprod. Immunol. **38**:302–306, 1997.

Kurjak, A. and Pal, A.: The effect of Gestanon on the fetal and uteroplacental blood flow. Acta Med. Jugosl. **40**:121–131, 1986.

Lang, I., Pabst, M.A., Hiden, U., Blaschitz, A., Dohr, G., Hahn, T. and Desoye, G: Heterogeneity of microvascular endothelial cells isolated from human term placenta and macrovascular umbilical vein endothelial cells. Eur. J. Cell Biol. **82**:163–173, 2003.

Larsen, L.G., Clausen, H.V., Andersen, B. and Graem, N.: A stereologic study of postmature placentas fixed by dual perfusion. Amer. J. Obstet. Gynecol. **172**:500–507, 1995.

Lehmann, W.D., Schuhmann, R. and Kraus, H.: Regionally different steroid biosynthesis within materno-fetal circulation units (placentones) of mature human placentas. J. Perinat. Med. **1**:198–204, 1973.

Leiser, R.: Microvascularisation der Ziegenplazenta dargestellt mit rasterelektronisch untersuchten Gefäßausgüssen. Schweiz. Arch. Tierheilkd. **129**:59–74, 1987.

Leiser, R., Luckhardt, M., Kaufmann, P., Winterhager, E. and Bruns, U.: The fetal vascularisation of term human placental villi. I. Peripheral stem villi. Anat. Embryol. **173**:71–80, 1985.

Leiser, R., Kosanke, G. and Kaufmann, P.: Human placental vascularization. In, Placenta: Basic Research for Clinical Application. H. Soma, ed., pp. 32–45. Karger, Basel, 1991.

Lemtis, H.: Über die Architektonik des Zottengefäßapparates der menschlichen Plazenta. Anat. Anz. **102**:106–133, 1955.

Lemtis, H.: New insights into the maternal circulatory system of the human placenta. In, The Foetoplacental Unit. A. Pecile and D. Finzi, eds. Excerpta Medica, Amsterdam, 1969.

Li, X.F., Charnock-Jones, D.S., Zhang, E., Hiby, S., Malik, S., Day, K., Licence, D., Bowen, J.M., Gardner, L., King, A., Loke, Y.W. and Smith, S.K.: Angiogenic growth factor messenger ribonucleic acids in uterine natural killer cells. J. Clin. Endocrinol. Metab. **86**:1823–1834, 2001.

Luckett, W.P.: Origin and differentiation of the yolk sac and extraembryonic mesoderm in presomite human and rhesus monkey embryos. Amer. J. Anat. **152**:59–97, 1978.

Luttun, A., Tjwa, M., Moons, L., Wu, Y., Angelillo-Scherrer, A., Liao, F., Nagy, J.A., Hooper, A., Priller, J., De Klerck, B., Compernolle, V., Daci, E., Bohlen, P., Dewerchin, M., Herbert, J.M., Fava, R., Matthys, P., Carmeliet, G., Collen, D., Dvorak, H.F., Hicklin, D.J. and Carmeliet, P.: Revascularization of ischemic tissues by PlGF treatment, and inhibition of tumor angiogenesis, arthritis and atherosclerosis by anti-Flt1. Nature Med. **8**:831–840, 2002.

Lyall, F., Greer, I.A., Boswell, F. and Fleming, R.: Suppression of serum vascular endothelial growth factor immunoreactivity in normal pregnancy and in pre-eclampsia. Br. J. Obstet. Gynecol. **104**:223–228, 1997.

Lysiak, J., Khoo, N., Conelly, I., Stettler-Stevenson, W. and Lala, P.: Role of transforming growth factor (TGF) and epidermal growth factor (EGF) on proliferation, invasion, and hCG production by normal and malignant trophoblast. Placenta **13**:A41, 1992.

Macara, L., Kingdom, J.C.P., Kaufmann, P., Kohnen, G., Hair, J., More, I.A.R., Lyall, F. and Greer, I.A.: Structural analysis of placental terminal villi from growth-restricted pregnancies with abnormal umbilical artery Doppler waveforms. Placenta **17**:37–48, 1996.

Maruo, T., Matsuo, H. and Mochizuki, M.: Thyroid hormone as a biological amplifier of differentiated trophoblast function in early pregnancy. Acta Endocrinol. (Copenh.) **125**:58–66, 1991.

Marzolf, G., Lobstein, J.F., Dillmann, J.C., Spizzo, M., Eberst, B. and Gandar, R.: Double blind comparison of the effects of Gestanon versus placebo in intra-uterine growth retardation. Presented at the 4th Asia Oceanic Congress on Perinatology, Tokyo, 1986.

Matsuo, H., Maruo, T., Murata, K. and Mochizuki, M.: Human early placental trophoblasts produce an epidermal growth factor-like substance in synergy with thyroid hormone. Acta Endocrinol. (Copenh.) **128**:225–229, 1993.

Mayhew, T.M.: Fetoplacental angiogenesis during gestation is biphasic, longitudinal and occurs by proliferation and remodeling of vascular endothelial cells. Placenta **23**:742–750, 2002.

Mayhew, T.M., Charnock-Jones, D.S. and Kaufmann, P.: Aspects of human fetoplacental vasculogenesis and angiogenesis. III. Changes in complicated pregnancies. Placenta **25**:127–139, 2004.

Moe, N.: Mitotic activity in the syncytiotrophoblast of the human chorionic villi. Amer. J. Obstet. Gynecol. **110**:431, 1971.

Moll, W.: Physiologie der maternen plazentaren Durchblutung. In, Die Plazenta des Menschen. V. Becker, T.H. Schiebler and F. Kubli, eds., pp. 172–194. Thieme, Stuttgart, 1981.

Montgomery, D. and Young, M.: The uptake of naturally occurring amino acids by the plasma membrane of the human placenta. Placenta **3**:13–20, 1982.

Mossman, H.W.: The rabbit placenta and the problem of placental transmission. Amer. J. Anat. **37**:433–497, 1926.

Mossman, H.W.: The principal interchange vessels of the chorioallantoic placenta of mammals. In, Organogenesis. R.L. DeHann and H. Ursprung, eds., pp. 771–786. Holt Rinehart & Winston, New York, 1965.

Mühlhauser, J., Crescimanno, C., Kaufmann, P., Höfler, H., Zaccheo, D. and Castellucci, M.: Differentiation and proliferation patterns in human trophoblast revealed by c-erbB-2 oncogene product and EGF-R. J. Histochem. Cytochem. **41**:165–173, 1993.

Myers, R.E. and Panigel, M.: Experimental placental detachment in the rhesus monkey: changes in villous ultrastructure. J. Med. Primatol. **2**:170–189, 1973.

Naeye, R.L., Maisels, J., Lorenz, R.P. and Botti, J.J.: The clinical significance of placental villous edema. Pediatrics **71**:588–594, 1983.

Nikolov, S.D. and Schiebler, T.H.: Über das fetale Gefäßsystem der reifen menschlichen Plazenta. Z. Zellforsch. **139**:333–350, 1973.

Nikolov, S.D. and Schiebler, T.H.: Über Endothelzellen in Zottengefäßen der reifen menschlichen Plazenta. Acta Anat. (Basel) **110**:338–344, 1981.

Odorisio, T., Schietroma, C., Zaccaria, M.L., Cianfarani, F., Tiveron, C., Tatangelo, L., Failla, C.M. and Zambruno, G.: Mice overexpressing placenta growth factor exhibit increased vascularization and vessel permeability. J. Cell Sci. **115**:2559–2567, 2002.

Ogawa, S., Leavy, J., Clauss, M., Koga, S., Shreeniwas, R., Joseph-Silverstein, J., Furie, M. and Stern, D.: Modulation of endothelial cell (EC) function in hypoxia: alterations in cell growth and the response to monocyte-derived mitogenic factors. J. Cell. Biochem. Suppl. 15F:213, 1991.

O'Neill, J.E.G.: Vascularizacao da placenta humana. Thesis, Universidade Nova de Lisboa, Portugal, 1983.

Ong, P.J. and Burton, G.J.: Thinning of the placental villous membrane during maintenance in hypoxic organ culture: structural adaptation or syncytial degeneration? Eur. J. Obstet. Gynecol. Reprod. Biol. **39**:103–110, 1991.

Panigel, M. and Myers, R.E.: The effect of fetectomy and ligature of the interplacental fetal vessels on the ultrastructure of placental villosities in Macaca mulatta. C.R. Acad. Sci. Hebd. Seances Acad. Sci. Ser. D **272**:315–318, 1971.

Panigel, M. and Myers, R.E.: Histological and ultrastructural changes in rhesus monkey placenta following interruption of fetal placental circulation by fetectomy or interplacental umbilical vessel ligation. Acta Anat. (Basel) **81**:481–506, 1972.

Panigel, M. and Pascaud, M.: Les orifices artériels d'entrée du sang maternel dans la chambre intervilleuse du placenta humain. Bull. Assoc. Anat. **142**:1287–1298, 1968.

Papierowski, Z.: Effects of selected progestogens used for the protection of high-risk pregnancy on the clinical course, morphological changes and proliferative activity of the trophoblast. Ginekol. Pol. **52**:298–303, 1981.

Paprocki, M.: Morphologie und Morphometrie der Zottengefässe der reifen menschlichen Plazenta nach vorzeitigem Blasensprung. Med. Thesis, University of Technology Aachen, 1992.

Penfold, P., Wootton, R. and Hytten, P.E.: Studies of a single placental cotyledon in vitro. III. The dimensions of the villous capillaries. Placenta **2**:161–168, 1981.

Pilz, I., Schweikhart, G. and Kaufmann, P.: Zur Abgrenzung normaler, artefizieller und pathologischer Strukturen in reifen menschlichen Plazentazotten. III. Morphometrische Untersuchungen bei Rh-Inkompatibilität. Arch. Gynecol. Obstet. **229**:137–154, 1980.

Piotrowicz, B., Niebroj, T.K. and Sieron, G.: The morphology and histochemistry of the full term placenta in anaemic patients. Folia Histochem. Cytochem. **7**:436–444, 1969.

Prager, D., Weber, M.M. and Herman-Bonert, V.: Placental growth factors and releasing/inhibiting peptides. Semin. Reprod. Endocrinol. **10**:83–94, 1992.

Pugh, C.W. and Ratcliffe, P.J.: Regulation of angiogenesis by hypoxia: role of the HIF system. Nature Med. **9**:677–684, 2003.

Rafii, S., Meeus, S., Dias, S., Hattori, K., Heissig, B., Shmelkov, S., Rafii, D. and Lyden, D.: Contribution of marrow-derived progenitors to vascular and cardiac regeneration. Semin. Cell Dev. Biol. **13**:61–67, 2002.

Ramsey, E.M., Corner, G.W. and Donner, M.W.: Serial and cine-radioangiographic visualization of maternal circulation in the primate (hemochorial) placenta. Amer. J. Obstet. Gynecol. **86**:213–225, 1963.

Rao, C.V., Ramani, N., Chegini, N., Stadig, B.K., Carman, F.R., Jr., Woost, P.G., Schultz, G.S. and Cook, C.L.: Topography of human placental receptors for epidermal growth factor. J. Biol. Chem. **260**:1705–1710, 1985.

Reshetnikova, O.S., Burton, G.J. and Milovanov, A.P.: The effects of hypobaric hypoxia on the terminal villi of the human placenta. J. Physiol. **459**:308P, 1993.

Reuvekamp, A., Velsing-Aarts, F.V., Poulina, I.E., Capello, J.J. and Duits, A.J.: Selective deficit of angiogenic growth factors characterises pregnancies complicated by pre-eclampsia. Br. J. Obstet. Gynaecol. **106**:1019–1022, 1999.

Reynolds, L.P., Killilea, S.D. and Redmer, D.A.: Angiogenesis in the female reproductive system. FASEB J. **6**:886–892, 1992.

Rhodin, J.A.G.: The ultrastructure of mammalian arterioles and precapillary sphincters. J. Ultrastruct. Res. **18**:181–223, 1967.

Rhodin, J.A.G.: Ultrastructure of mammalian venous capillaries, venules and small collecting veins. J. Ultrastruct. Res. **25**:452–500, 1968.

Risau, W.: Mechanisms of angiogenesis. Nature **386**:671–674, 1997.

Risau, W. and Flamme, I.: Vasculogenesis. Ann. Rev. Cell Dev. Biol. **11**:73–91, 1995.

Rodesch, F., Simon, P., Donner, C. and Jauniaux, E.: Oxygen measurements in endometrial and trophoblastic tissues during early pregnancy. Obstet. Gynecol. **80**:283–285, 1992.

Rossi, P., Karsenty, G., Roberts, A.B., Roche, N.S., Sporn, M.B. and De Crombrugghe, B.: A nuclear factor 1 binding site mediates the transcriptional activation of a type I collagen promoter by transforming growth factor-β. Cell **52**:405–414, 1988.

Salvatore, C.A.: The placenta in acute toxemia. Amer. J. Obstet. Gynecol. **102**:347–352, 1968.

Scheffen, I., Kaufmann, P., Philippens, L., Leiser, R., Geisen, C. and Mottaghy, K.: Alterations of the fetal capillary bed in the guinea pig placenta following long-term hypoxia. In, Oxygen Transfer to Tissue, XII. J. Piiper, T.K. Goldstick and D. Meyer, eds., pp. 779–790. Plenum Press, New York, 1990.

Schiebler, T.H. and Kaufmann, P.: Reife Plazenta. In, Die Plazenta des Menschen. V. Becker, T.H. Schiebler and F. Kubli, eds., pp. 51–111. Thieme, Stuttgart, 1981.

Schmid-Schönbein, H.: Conceptional proposition for a specific microcirculatory problem: maternal blood flow in hemochorial multivillous placentae as percolation of a "porous medium." Trophoblast Res. **3**:17–38, 1988.

Schmidt, J.A., Mizel, S.B., Cohen, D. and Green, I.: Interleukin 1: a potential regulator of fibroblast proliferation. J. Immunol. **128**:2177–2182, 1982.

Schmon, B., Hartmann, M., Jones, C.J. and Desoye, G.: Insulin and glucose do not affect the glycogen content in isolated and cultured trophoblast cells of human term placenta. J. Clin. Endocrinol. Metab. **73**:888–893, 1991.

Schuhmann, R.: Plazenton: Begriff, Entstehung, funktionelle Anatomie. In, Die Plazenta des Menschen. V. Becker, T.H. Schiebler and F. Kubli, eds., pp. 199–207. Thieme Verlag, Stuttgart, 1981.

Schuhmann, R.A.: Placentone structure of the human placenta. Bibl. Anat. **22**:46–57, 1982.

Schuhmann, R. and Wehler, V.: Histologische Unterschiede an Plazentazotten innerhalb der materno-fetalen Strömungseinheit. Ein Beitrag zur funktionellen Morphologie der Plazenta. Arch. Gynäkol. **210**:425–439, 1971.

Schuhmann, R., Kraus, H., Borst, R. and Geier, G.: Regional unterschiedliche Enzymaktivität innerhalb der Placentone reifer menschlicher Placenten. Histochemische und biochemische Untersuchungen. Arch. Gynäkol. **220**:209–226, 1976.

Schweikhart, G. and Kaufmann, P.: Zur Abgrenzung normaler, artefizieller und pathologischer Strukturen in reifen menschlichen Plazentazotten. I. Ultrastruktur des Syncytiotrophoblasten. Arch. Gynäkol. **222**:213–230, 1977.

Scott, W.A. and Cohn, Z.A.: Secretory products of mononuclear phagocytes. In, Pathobiology of the Endothelial Cell. H.L. Nossel and H.J. Vogel, eds., pp. 240–258. Raven Press, New York, 1982.

Semenza, G.L.: HIF-1, O_2 and the 3 PHDs: How animal cells signal hypoxia to the nucleus. Cell **107**:1–3, 2001.

Sen, D.K., Kaufmann, P. and Schweikhart, G.: Classification of human placental villi. II. Morphometry. Cell Tissue Res. **200**:425–434, 1979.

Shalaby, F., Rossant, J., Yamaguchi, T.P., Gertsenstein, M., Wu, X.-F., Breitman, M. and Schuh, A.C.: Failure of blood island formation and vasculogenesis in Flk-1–deficient mice. Nature (Lond.) **376**:62–66, 1995.

Shams, M. and Ahmed, A.: Localization of mRNA for basic fibroblast growth factor in human placenta. Growth Factors **11**:105–111, 1994.

Sharkey, A.M., Charnock-Jones, D.S., Boocock, C.A., Brown, K.D. and Smith, S.K.: Expression of mRNA for vascular endothelial growth factor in human placenta. J. Reprod. Fertil. **99**:609–615, 1993.

Sharkey, A.M., Cooper, J.C., Balmforth, J.R., McLaren, J., Clark, D.E., Charnock-Jones, D.S., Morris, N.H. and Smith, S.K.: Maternal plasma levels of vascular endothelial growth factor in normotensive pregnancies and in pregnancies complicated by pre-eclampsia. Eur. J. Clin. Invest. **26**:1182–1185, 1996.

Shiraishi, S., Nakagawa, K., Kinukawa, N., Nakano, H. and Sueishi, K.: Immunohistochemical localization of vascular endothelial growth factor in the human placenta. Placenta **17**:111–121, 1996.

Shore, V.H., Wang, T.H., Wang, C.L., Torry, R.J., Caudle, M.R. and Torry, D.S.: Vascular endothelial growth factor, placenta growth factor and their receptors in isolated human trophoblast. Placenta **18**:657–665, 1997.

Shorter, S., Clover, L. and Starkey, P.: Evidence for both an autocrine and paracrine role for the colony-stimulating factors in regulating placental growth and development. Placenta **13**:A58, 1992.

Shreeniwas, R., Ogawa, S., Cozzolino, F., Torcia, G., Braunstein, N., Butura, C., Brett, J., Lieberman, H.B., Furie, M.B. and Joseph-Silverstein, J.: Macrovascular and microvascular endothelium during long-term hypoxia: alterations in cell growth, monolayer permeability, and cell surface coagulant properties. J. Cell. Physiol. **146**:8–17, 1991.

Sibley, C.P., Pardi, G., Cetin, I., Todros, T., Piccoli, E., Kaufmann, P., Huppertz, B., Bulfamente, G., Cribiu, F.M., Ayuk, P., Glazier, J. and Radaelli, T.: Pathogenesis of intrauterine growth restriction (IUGR)—conclusions derived from a European Union Biomed 2 Concerted Action Project 'Importance of Oxygen Supply in Intrauterine Growth Restricted Pregnancies'—A Workshop Report. Placenta 16:S75–S79, 2002.

Somerset, D.A., Li, X.F., Afford, S., Strain, A., Ahmed, A., Sangha, R.K., Whittle, M.J. and Kilby, M.D.: Ontogeny of hepatocyte growth factor (HGF) and its receptor (c-met) in human placenta—reduced HGF expression in intrauterine growth restriction. Amer. J. Pathol. 153:1139–1147, 1998.

Soothill, P.W., Nicolaides, K.H., Rodeck, C.H. and Campbell, S.: Effects of gestational age on fetal and intervillous blood gas and acid-base values in human pregnancy. Fetal Therapy 1:168–175, 1986.

Strauss, D.S.: Growth-stimulatory actions of insulin in vitro and in vivo. Endocr. Rev. 5:356–369, 1984.

Takemura, R. and Werb, Z.: Secretory products of macrophages and their physiological functions. Amer. J. Physiol. 246:C1–C9, 1984.

Tedde, G. and Tedde-Piras, A.: Mitotic index of the Langhans' cells in the normal human placenta from the early stages of pregnancy to the term. Acta Anat. (Basel) 100:114–119, 1978.

Thiriot, M. and Panigel, M.: Microcirculation. La microvascularisation des villosites placentaires humaines. C.R. Acad. Sci. D 287:709–712, 1978.

Thorpe Beeston, J.G., Nicolaides, K.H., Snijders, R.J., Felton, C.V. and McGregor, A.M.: Thyroid function in small for gestational age fetuses. Obstet. Gynecol. 77:701–706, 1991.

Todros, T., Sciarrone, A., Piccoli, E., Guiot, C., Kaufmann, P., and Kingdom, J.: Umbilical Doppler waveforms and placental villous angiogenesis in pregnancies complicated by fetal growth restriction. Obstet. Gynecol. 93:499–503, 1999.

Tominaga, T. and Page, E.W.: Accommodation of the human placenta to hypoxia. Amer. J. Obstet. Gynecol. 94:679–691, 1966.

Torry, D.S., Wang, H.S., Wang, T.H., Caudle, M.R. and Torry, R.J.: Preeclampsia is associated with reduced serum levels of placenta growth factor. Amer. J. Obstet. Gynecol. 179:1539–1544, 1998.

Uehara, Y., Minowa, O., Mori, C., Shiota, K., Kuno, J., Noda, T. and Kitamura, N.: Placental defect and embryonic lethality in mice lacking hepatocyte growth factor/scatter factor. Nature 373:702–705, 1995.

Voigt, S., Kaufmann, P. and Schweikhart, G.: Zur Abgrenzung normaler, artefizieller und pathologischer Strukturen in reifen menschlichen Plazentazotten. II. Morphometrische Untersuchungen zum Einfluss des Fixationsmodus. Arch. Gynäkol. 226:347–362, 1978.

Vuckovic, M., Ponting, J., Terman, B.I., Niketic, V., Seif, M.W. and Kumar, S.: Expression of the vascular endothelial growth factor receptor, KDR, in human placenta. J. Anat. 188:361–366, 1996.

Vuorela, P., Hatva, E., Lymboussaki, A., Kaipainen, A., Joukov, V. and Persico, M.G.: Expression of vascular endothelial growth factor and placenta growth factor in human placenta. Biol. Reprod. 56:489–494, 1997.

Wallenburg, H.C.S., Hutchinson, D.L., Schuler, H.M., Stolte, L.A.M. and Janssens, J.: The pathogenesis of placental infarc-

tion. II. An experimental study in the rhesus monkey. Amer. J. Obstet. Gynecol. 116:841–846, 1973.

Werb, Z.: How the macrophage regulates its extracellular environment. Amer. J. Anat. 166:237–256, 1983.

Werner, C. and Schneiderhan, W.: Plazentamorphologie und Plazentafunktion in Abhängigkeit von der diabetischen Stoffwechselführung. Geburtsh. Frauenheilkd. 32:959–966, 1972.

Wheeler, T., Elcock, C.L. and Anthony, F.W.: Angiogenesis and the placental environment. Placenta 16:289–296, 1995.

Widmaier, G.: Zur Ultrastruktur menschlicher Placentazotten beim Diabetes mellitus. Arch. Gynäkol. 208:396–409, 1970.

Wigglesworth, J.S.: Vascular organization of the human placenta. Nature 216:1120–1121, 1967.

Wilkin, P.: Pathologie du Placenta. Masson, Paris, 1965.

Wilting, J., Birkenhäger, R., Martiny-Baron, G., Marmé, D., Christ, B., Eichmann, A. and Weich, H.A.: Vascular endothelial growth factor (VEGF) and placenta growth factor (PlGF): homologous factors specifically affecting endothelial cells. Ann. Anat. 178:331A, 1995.

Wilting, J., Birkenhäger, R., Eichmann, A., Kurs, H., Martiny-Baron, G., Marme, D., McCarthy, J.E.G., Christ, B. and Weich, H.A.: VEGF(121) induces proliferation of vascular endothelial cells and expression of flk-1 without affecting lymphatic vessels of the chorioallantoic membrane. Dev. Biol. 176:76–85, 1996.

Wulff, C., Wilson, H., Dickson, S.E., Wiegand, S.J. and Fraser, H.M.: Hemochorial placentation in the primate: expression of vascular endothelial growth factor, angiopoietins, and their receptors throughout pregnancy. Biol. Reprod. 66:802–812, 2002.

Yallampalli, C. and Garfield, R.E.: Inhibition of nitric oxide synthesis in rats during pregnancy produces signs similar to those of preeclampsia. Amer. J. Obstet. Gynecol. 169:1316–1320, 1993.

Zeek, P.M. and Assali, N.S.: Vascular changes in the decidua associated with eclamptogenic toxemia of pregnancy. Amer. J. Clin. Pathol. 20:1099–1109, 1950.

Zhang, E.G., Smith, S.K., Baker P.N. and Charnock-Jones, D.S.: The regulation and localization of angiopoietin-1, -2, and their receptor Tie-2 in normal and pathologic human placentae. Mol. Med. 7:624–635, 2001.

Zhou, Y., Genbacev, O., Damsky, C.H. and Fisher, S.J.: Oxygen regulates human cytotrophoblast differentiation and invasion: implications for endovascular invasion in normal pregnancy and in pre-eclampsia. J. Reprod. Immunol. 39:197–213, 1998.

Zhou, Y., McMaster, M., Woo, K., Janatpour, M., Perry, J., Karpanen, T., Alitalo, K., Damsky, C. and Fisher, S.J.: Vascular endothelial growth factor ligands and receptors that regulate cytotrophoblast survival are dysregulated in severe preeclampsia and hemolysis, elevated liver enzymes, and low platelets syndrome. Amer. J. Pathol. 160:1405–1423, 2002.

Ziche, M., Maglione, D., Ribatti, D., Morbidelli, L., Lago, C.T., Battisti, M., Paoletti, I., Barra, A., Tucci, M., Parise, G., Vincenti, V., Granger, H.J., Viglietto, G. and Persico, M.G.: Placenta growth factor-1 is chemotactic, mitogenic, and angiogenic. Lab. Invest. 76:517–531, 1997.

8
Characterization of the Developmental Stages

This chapter is a synopsis and presents brief descriptions of the average data of placenta and membranes throughout the single stages of placental development. Embryologic data concerning embryo and fetus are given only insofar as they are of importance for the definition of the stage. It is not the intention of this chapter to compare data of various sources on a scientific level but rather to present data that are directly applicable to the pathologic and histologic examination of human material. For this purpose, all data have been extrapolated and were standardized where necessary.

The data are based on the following publications: embryonic staging according to O'Rahilly (1973) and Boyd and Hamilton (1970): crown–rump length (CRL), embryonic and fetal weight, mean diameter of the chorionic sac, placental diameter and thickness, placental weight according to Boyd and Hamilton (1970), O'Rahilly (1973), and Kaufmann (1981); placental and uterine thickness in vivo following Johannigmann et al. (1972); length of umbilical cord according to Winckel (1893); villous surfaces, villous volumes, and villous diameters following Hörmann (1951), Knopp (1960), Clavero-Nuñez and Botella-Llusia (1961, 1963), Aherne and Dunnill (1966), Kaufmann (1981), Schiemer (1981), and Gloede (1984); and mean trophoblastic thickness, distribution of villous cytotrophoblast, mean maternofetal diffusion distance according to Kaufmann (1972), Kaufmann and Stegner (1972), Gloede (1984), and Kaufmann (1981). For further details see the summarizing tables in Chapter 28.

Stages of Development

Day 1 p.c. (p.c. = postcoitus)   Carnegie stage 1: one fertilized cell; diameter 0.1 mm.

Day 2 p.c.   Carnegie stage 2a: from 2 to 4 cells; diameter 0.1 to 0.2 mm.

Day 3 p.c.   Carnegie stage 2b: from 4 to about 16 cells; diameter 0.1 to 0.2 mm.

Day 4 p.c.   Carnegie stage 3: free blastocyst, from 16 to about 64 cells; diameter about 0.2 mm.

Day 5 to early day 6 p.c.   Carnegie stage 4: blastocyst attached to the endometrium, from about 128 to about 256 cells; diameter 0.2 to 0.3 mm.

Late day 6 to early day 8 p.c.   Carnegie stage 5a: implantation, prelacunar stage of the trophoblast; the flattened blastocyst measures about $0.3 \times 0.3 \times 0.15$ mm. The blastocyst is partially implanted. The implanted part of the blastocyst wall is considerably thickened, largely consisting of solid syncytiotrophoblast. The still not implanted, thin part of the blastocyst wall consists of a single layer of cytotrophoblast. The embryonic disk measures about 0.1 mm in diameter.

Late day 8 to day 12 p.c.   Lacunar or trabecular stage.
Late day 8 to day 9 p.c.   Carnegie stage 5b: diameter of chorionic sac $0.5 \times 0.5 \times 0.3$ mm; embryonic disk about 0.1 mm. The syncytiotrophoblast at the implantation pole exhibits vacuoles as forerunners of the lacunar system.
Day 10 to day 12 p.c.   Carnegie stage 5c: diameter of chorionic sac $0.9 \times 0.9 \times 0.6$ mm. The vacuoles in the syncytiotrophoblast fuse to form the lacunar system; first lacunae at the antiimplantation pole. First contact of lacunar system with eroded endometrial capillaries. Some maternal erythrocytes may be observed in the lacunae. Around day 11, implantation is complete; the defect in the endometrial epithelium is closed by a blood coagulum and is covered by epithelium on day 12. At the implantation site, the endometrium measures 5 mm in thickness; first signs of decidualization.

Day 13 to day 14 p.c.   Carnegie stage 6, villous stage (first free primary villi).

Day 13 p.c.   The nearly round chorionic sac has a diameter of 1.2 to 1.5 mm; length of embryonic disk is 0.2 mm.

Day 14 p.c.   Diameter of chorionic sac 1.6 to 2.1 mm; length of embryonic disk 0.2 to 0.4 mm. First appearance of primitive streak and of yolk sac.

With the expansion of the lacunar system, the syncytiotrophoblast becomes reduced to radially oriented trophoblastic trabeculae, the forerunners of the stem villi. After invasion of cytotrophoblast into the trabeculae, free trophoblastic outgrowths into the lacunae, the "free primary villi", are formed. The trabeculae are now called villous stems. By definition, from this date onward, the lacunae are transformed into the intervillous space. Cytotrophoblast from the former trabeculae penetrates the trophoblastic shell and invades the endometrium.

Days 15 to 18 p.c.   Villous stage (secondary villi).

Days 15 to 16 p.c.   Carnegie stage 7: diameter of chorionic sac about 5 mm; length of embryonic disk less than 0.9 mm; appearance of notochordal process and primitive node (Hensen).

Day 17 to 18 p.c.   Carnegie stage 8: diameter of embryonic sac less than 8 mm; length of chorionic disk less than 1.3 mm. On the germinal disk, the notochordal and neurenteric canals, and primitive pit can be discerned.

Starting at the implantation pole and continuing all around the circumference to the antiimplantation pole, mesenchyme (derived from the extraembryonic mesoderm in the chorionic cavity) invades the villi, transforming them into secondary villi. The basal feet of the villous stems, connecting the latter with the trophoblastic shell, as well as some villous tips remain free of mesenchyme and thus persist in the primary villous stage (forerunners of the cell columns and cell islands).

Day 19 to 23 p.c.   This is the beginning of the 2nd month postmenstruation (p.m.), villous stage (early tertiary villi).

Day 19 to 21 p.c.   Carnegie stage 9: diameter of chorionic sac less than 12 mm; length of embryonic disk equals the crown–rump length of the embryo, 1.5 to 2.5 mm, 1 to 3 somites. Neural folds appear; first cardiac contractions.

Day 22 to 23 p.c.   Carnegie stage 10: diameter of chorionic sac less than 15 mm; crown–rump length 2.0 to 3.5 mm; 4 to 12 somites. Neural folds start to fuse; two visceral arches.

The villous mesenchyme is characterized by the appearance of the first fetal capillaries (formation of first tertiary villi). The villous diameters are largely homogeneous, presenting two different-sized groups of villi. The larger villous stems and their branches exhibit diameter of 120 to 250 μm. Histologically, the stroma of both is mesenchymal in nature. Along their surfaces, one finds numerous small (diameters 30–60 μm) trophoblastic and villous sprouts.

Days 23 to 29 p.c.   Early tertiary villus stage.

Days 23 to 26 p.c.   Carnegie stage 11: diameter of the chorionic sac less than 18 mm; crown–rump length 2.5 to 4.5 mm; 13 to 20 somites; closure of the rostral neuropore; optic vesicles identifiable.

Days 26 to 29 p.c.   Carnegie stage 12: diameter of chorionic sac less than 21 mm; crown–rump length 3 to 5 mm; 21 to 29 somites; closure of the caudal neuropore; three visceral arches; upper limb buds appear.

The length of villous stems between chorionic plate and trophoblastic shell varies from 1 mm (antiimplantation pole) to 2 mm (implantation pole). The central two thirds are supplied with mesenchyme and capillaries (Fig. 8.1); the peripheral one third remains in the primary villous stage (cell columns). The villous calibers are similar to those described for the previous stage. The amount of trophoblastic and villous sprouts is reduced. Most villi contain loose mesenchyme together with centrally positioned fetal capillaries (mesenchymal villi). Peripherally, they continue via villous sprouts (with unvascularized mesenchymal core) into massive trophoblastic sprouts. In the villous stems, vessels of larger caliber acquire the first signs of a surrounding adventitia (beginning of formation of typical stem villi characterized by fibrous stroma). The villous trophoblastic surface is composed of an outer syncytiotrophoblast and complete inner layer of cytotrophoblast. Together they measure 20 to 30 μm in thickness.

The chorionic plate, consisting of fetal mesenchyme, cytotrophoblast, and syncytiotrophoblast, still lacks fibrinoid. The trophoblastic shell is transformed into the basal plate by intense mixing of decidual and trophoblastic cells. Secretory activities or tissue necrosis of both cell types causes the appearance of the first foci of Nitabuch fibrinoid. The superficial syncytiotrophoblastic layer of the basal plate, bordering the intervillous space, becomes locally replaced by Rohr fibrinoid.

Days 29 to 42 p.c.   Late 2nd month p.m.

Days 29 to 32 p.c.   Carnegie stage 13: diameter of chorionic sac less than 25 mm; crown–rump length 4 to 6 mm; 30 + somites; four limb buds and optic vesicle.

Days 32 to 35 p.c.   Carnegie stage 14: diameter of chorionic sac less than 28 mm; crown–rump length 5 to 8 mm; first appearance of lens pit and optic cup.

Days 35 to 37 p.c.   Carnegie stage 15: diameter of chorionic sac less than 31 mm; crown–rump length 7 to 10 mm; closure of lens vesicle; clear evidence of cerebral vesicles; hand plates.

Days 37 to 42 p.c.   Carnegie stage 16: diameter of chorionic sac less than 34 mm; crown–rump length 8 to 12 mm; embryonic weight about 1.1 g; retinal pigment visible; foot plates.

The net weight of the chorionic sac in stage 16 is about 6 to 10 g; thickness of the chorion at the implantation pole

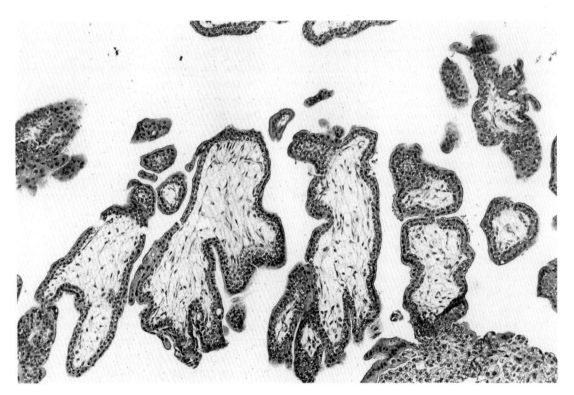

FIGURE 8.1. Placental villi of the 6th week postmenstruation (p.m.). Note the thick trophoblastic covering, consisting of complete layers of cytotrophoblast and syncytiotrophoblast. Fetal capillaries are poorly developed or, in some places, are still lacking. In the lower right corner, an early step of the formation of a cell island can be seen attached to the villous surface. Paraffin section. ×125.

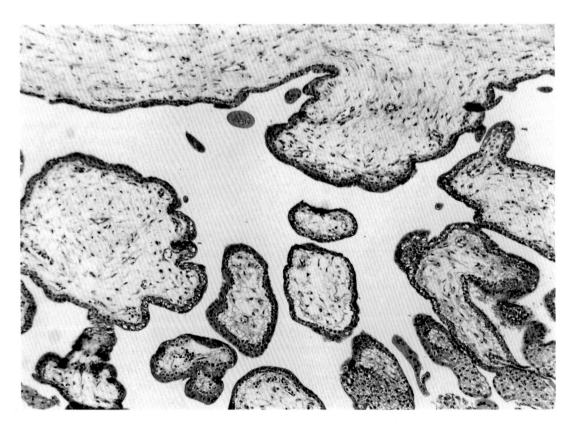

FIGURE 8.2. Placental villi of the 8th week p.m. All villi are vascularized. As can be seen from the diffuse stromal structure, the villi still belong to the mesenchymal type. Paraffin section. ×125. (From Kaufmann, 1981, with permission.)

is about 6 mm and at the antiimplantation pole about 3 mm. The uterine lumen is still open, and parietal and capsular decidua are not yet in contact.

The range of villous calibers changes slightly from the previous stage (Fig. 8.2). The largest stems reach diameters of less than 400 μm. A variety of medium-sized mesenchymal villi is found between the stem villi that measure about 200 μm in diameter and the small sprouts. The mean villous caliber is about 200 μm. The total placental villous surface is about 0.08 m². The connective tissue layer of the chorionic plate is completely fibrosed, the fibrous tissue partly extending in the initial parts of the villous stems. The overwhelming share of the villous stroma is still mesenchymal in nature. The villous cytotrophoblastic layer is incomplete; 85% of the villous surface is double layered (cytotrophoblast plus syncytium). The thickness of the villous trophoblast varies between 10 and 30 μm (mean, 15.4 μm). Near the end of this period, most of the mesenchymal villi show increased numbers of macrophages, as well as the first signs of reticular transformation of their stroma toward immature intermediate villi. Only 2.7% of the villous volume is occupied by fetal vascular lumens. The mean maternofetal diffusion distance is more than 50 μm.

The villous stems are nearly completely occupied by connective tissue; basal segments, persisting in the primary villous stage, are the exception. Those segments now show the typical appearance of cell columns. Short portions of villous side branches, persisting in the primary villus stage and that are positioned somewhere between chorionic and basal plate, may increase in size by continuous cell proliferation with subsequent fibrinoid degeneration; they thus establish the first cell islands.

Third month p.m.   9th to 12th weeks p.m.; days 43 to 70 p.c.

Days 43 to 44 p.c.   Carnegie stage 17: maximum diameter of chorionic sac 38 mm; crown–rump length 10 to 14 mm; finger rays.

Days 44 to 48 p.c.   Carnegie stage 18: maximum diameter of chorionic sac 42 mm; crown–rump length 12 to 16 mm. Elbow region, toe rays, nipples, and eyelids appear.

Days 48 to 51 p.c.   Carnegie stage 19: maximum diameter of chorionic sac 44 mm; crown–rump length 14 to 18 mm.

Days 51 to 53 p.c.   Carnegie stage 20: maximum diameter of chorionic sac 47 mm; crown–rump length 17 to 22 mm. Upper limbs at the elbow region; first signs of finger separation.

Days 53 to 54 p.c.   Carnegie stage 21: maximum diameter of the oval chorionic sac 51 mm; crown–rump length 20 to 24 mm.

Day 54 to 56 p.c.   Carnegie stage 22: maximum diameter of the oval chorionic sac 58 mm; crown–rump length 23 to 28 mm.

Days 56 to 60 p.c.   Carnegie stage 23: maximum diameter of the oval chorionic sac 63 mm; crown–rump length 26 to 31 mm.

Days 61 to 70 p.c.   Maximum diameter of the oval to irregular chorionic sac 68 mm; crown–rump length 26 to 31 mm.

Days 61 to 70 p.c.   Maximum diameter of the oval to irregular chorionic sac 68 mm; crown–rump length 30 to 40 mm.

The embryonic weight increases throughout the 3rd month from 2 g to 17 g and the net weight of the chorionic sac from 10 g to 30 g. The chorionic sac is covered by villi over its surface; it is not yet subdivided into smooth chorion and placenta.

All villi are vascularized. Around the antiimplantation pole, the increased degenerative changes of villi and fibrinoid deposition in the intervillous space indicate that the formation of the smooth chorion will commence soon. Parietal and capsular decidua may come into contact locally, but they remain unfused.

The heterogeneity of villous diameters and villous structures increases. Fibrosis of the villous stems slowly extends into the more peripheral parts of the largest villi (diameters less than 500 μm). During the course of the 3rd month, most of the villi measuring between 100 and 400 μm establish the typical reticular appearance of immature intermediate villi (Fig. 8.3), characterized by numerous macrophages (Hofbauer cells). Small villi with diameters less than 100 μm show mesenchymal stroma. Trophoblastic and villous sprouts are numerous. Total villous surface is about 0.3 m². The trophoblastic thickness varies from 10 to 20 μm. Eighty percent of the villous surfaces are covered by cytotrophoblast. Fetal vessel lumens occupy about 4% of the villous volume. Some of the larger fetal vessels achieve a thick adventitia, consisting of fibrous stroma, which occupies larger parts of the villous stroma. The reticular stroma, as a sign of immaturity of the stem villi, is restricted to the superficial parts of the stroma positioned under the trophoblast.

In the previous stages fibrinoid was restricted to the cell islands and the basal plate, but now spot-like fibrinoid deposition at some of the villous surfaces can be observed. Fibrinoid deposition at the intervillous surface of the chorionic plate is still an exception. The amnionic cavity has extended to such a degree that the amnionic mesoderm comes into contact with the connective tissue layer of the chorionic plate in many places.

Fourth month p.m.   13th to 16th week p.m.; 11th to 14th weeks p.c.

The shape of the chorionic sac becomes more and more irregular because of compression between uterine wall

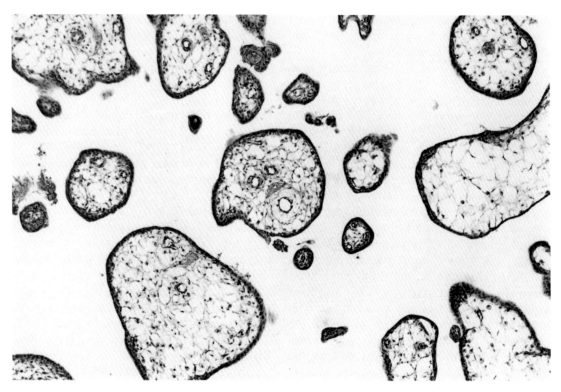

FIGURE 8.3. Placental villi of the 12th week p.m. The larger villi have achieved the reticular stroma of typical immature, intermediate villi. The smaller villi are mesenchymal in structure. The first small fetal arteries and veins can be seen. Paraffin section. ×125.

and fetus. Its maximum diameter increases throughout this period from 68 mm to 80 to 90 mm. The crown–rump length grows from 45 mm to 80 mm, and the fetal weight from 20 g to 70 g. The length of the umbilical cord is between 160 and 200 mm.

The continuous degeneration of placental villi at the antiimplantation pole, which is free of villi from the middle of the 4th month onward, as well as the villous proliferation at the implantation pole, initiates the differentiation of the chorionic sac into smooth chorion and placenta. The placental diameter increases from 50 mm to 75 mm at the end of this month and the placental weight from 30 g to 70 g. The maximal placental thickness in the delivered specimens is 10 to 12 mm. Numerous placental septa become visible. The cell columns become more deeply incorporated into the basal plate by fibrinoid deposition in their surrounding. The chorionic plate is in close contact with the amnion over its entire surface, giving it definite shape and layering. It consists of amnionic epithelium, amnionic mesoderm, chorionic mesoderm, a cytotrophoblast layer, and superficial syncytiotrophoblast.

The distribution of the villous calibers (Fig. 8.4) is similar to that described for the preceding month. The inhomogeneous mixture of villi is composed of stem villi with diameters of 300 to 500 μm, the vascular adventitia of which occupies at least 75% of the villous stroma, and of immature intermediate villi with diameters of 100 to about 300 μm. Mesenchymal villi and sprouts, 40 to 80 μm in diameter, are numerous, but because of their size they occupy only a small proportion of the total villous volume. Because the immature intermediate villi have the most characteristic reticular stroma at this stage and comprise the highest proportion of villi, one observes more villous macrophages (Hofbauer cells) than at all other stages of placental development. The total villous surface was measured to be 0.5 to 0.6 m². The share of fetal vessel lumens is increased to about 6%. Some of the capillaries establish contact with the villous trophoblast. In such places the syncytial nuclei are moved aside, resulting in the first epithelial plates; therefore, the trophoblastic thickness varies between 2 and 12 μm (mean, 9.6 μm). As during the previous month, one observes cytotrophoblast on about 80% of the villous surface. Fibrinoid deposition becomes a usual finding on the villous surfaces.

Fifth month p.m.   17th to 20th week p.m.; 15 to 18th week p.c.

Because of the geometrically irregular outer shape of the fetus, the diameter of the chorionic sac cannot be

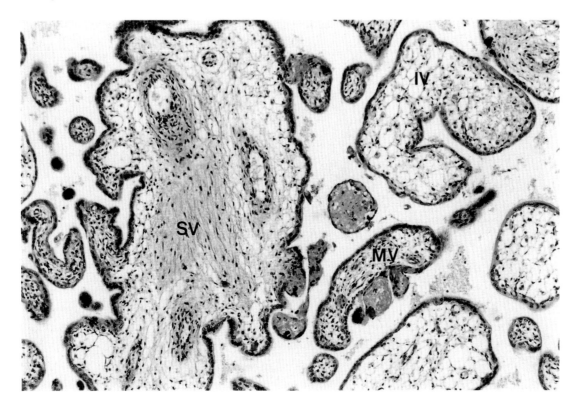

FIGURE 8.4. Placental villi of the 15th week p.m. The larger immature intermediate villi exhibit the first signs of central stromal fibrosis, originating from the larger fetal vessels, thus establishing the first stem villi (SV). Several typical immature intermediate villi (IV) and mesenchymal villi (MV) can be seen. As is typical for mesenchymal villi of the second and third trimester, they are associated with degenerating villi being more or less transformed into intravillous fibrinoid. Paraffin section. ×125.

estimated from this period onward. Over the course of the 5th month the crown–rump length increases from 80 mm to 130 mm and the fetal weight from 70 g to 290 g. The placenta is clearly separated from the smooth chorion. The placental diameter is between 75 mm and 100 mm, and the placental weight increases from 70 g to 120 g. The maximum placental thickness after delivery is about 12 to 15 mm; measured by ultrasonography and in situ, including the uterine wall, it is approximately 28 mm. The length of the umbilical cord varies between 200 and 315 mm.

The structure of the stem villi is nearly the same as in the previous month; however, their number is considerably increased throughout this month (Fig. 8.5). During the 20th week p.m., most of the large caliber villi (those exceeding 300 μm) have achieved the fibrous stroma of stem villi. The number of slender, long mesenchymal villi with diameters around 80 to 100 μm increases. The mean diameter of the remaining immature intermediate villi is slightly reduced to values around 150 μm. The mean villous diameter is 108 μm. The total villous surface is about 1.5 m². Because the amount of villous cytotrophoblast is reduced to about 60% of the villous surface, the extent of thin trophoblastic areas from 1 to 2 μm in thickness increases. Continuous development of fetal capillaries causes the reduction of mean maternofetal diffusion distance to about 22 μm.

Septa and cell islands that originally consisted mainly of accumulations of cells now grow considerably by apposition of fibrinoid. In their centers, cysts are often found.

Sixth month p.m. 21st to 24th week p.m.; 19th to 22nd week p.c.

The fetus grows from 130 mm to 180 mm in crown–rump length. Its weight increases from 290 g to 600 g. The placental diameter is between 100 and 125 mm, and the placental weight increases form 120 g to 190 g. Placental thickness after delivery is 15 to 18 mm, and ultrasonographic measurements in situ, including the uterine wall, indicate a thickness of about 34 mm. The mean length of the cord is between 315 and 360 mm.

The histologic features change considerably. Most of the immature intermediate villi become transformed into stem villi of large caliber. More of the stem villi measure about 200 μm in thickness, some achieving diameters of

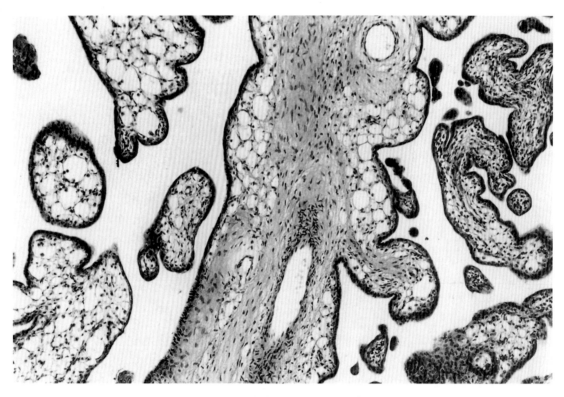

FIGURE 8.5. Placental villi of the 18th week p.m. This picture is comparable to that of the preceding stage. Formation of stem villi with stromal fibrosis is somewhat more expressed. Paraffin section. ×125.

more than 1000 μm. Their fibrous stroma still exhibits a small superficial rim of reticular connective tissue, indicating their immaturity (Fig. 8.6). Different from all earlier stages, increasing numbers of newly formed intermediate villi exhibit small calibers (only 100–150 μm). Some of these villi are reticular in stromal structure, as are their parent villi, whereas others are slender, mature intermediate villi with poorly vascularized and poorly fibrosed, nonreticular stroma (80–120 μm) (Fig. 8.7). At their surfaces, the first richly capillarized terminal villi are formed. They are difficult to identify in the large group of smallest villi, measuring 50 to 80 μm, because the other members of this group, the small mesenchymal villi and villous sprouts, exhibit structural features similar to those of the terminal villi in paraffin sections. The total villous surface amounts to 2.8 m². The mean trophoblastic thickness is reduced to 7.4 μm, and the mean maternofetal diffusion distance is about 22 μm.

Seventh month p.m.   25th to 28th week p.m.; 23rd to 26th week p.c.

When compared to the 6th month, there are only quantitative changes. The crown–rump length increases from 180 mm to 230 mm and the fetal weight from 600 g to 1050 g. The placental diameter is 125 to 150 mm, and the placental weight is increased to 190 to 260 g. The thickness of the

delivered placenta is 18 to 20 mm; by ultrasonography, including the uterine wall, it is 38 mm. The mean length of the umbilical cord increases from 360 to 410 mm.

The total villous surface of the placenta exceeds 4 m². The distribution of structure and caliber of the villi are similar to what was seen during the 6th month. Only 45% of the villous surface is covered by cytotrophoblast. The trophoblastic thickness varies between 0.5 and 8 μm (mean, 6.9 μm). The number of immature intermediate villi decreases in favor of stem villi and mature intermediate and terminal villi. The lumens of fetal vessel amount to 9.1% of the villous volume.

Cell columns are surrounded by increasing amounts of fibrinoid and become deeply invaginated in the basal plate. The syncytiotrophoblastic covering of the chorionic plate begins to degenerate. It becomes replaced by an initially thin layer of fibrinoid that grows in thickness throughout the following weeks and forms the Langhans' stria.

Eighth month p.m.   29th to 32nd week p.m.; 27th to 30th week p.c.

The crown–rump length is 230 to 280 mm, fetal weight is 1050 to 1600 g. The placental diameter normally varies between 150 and 170 mm; the placental weight increases from 260 g to 320 g. The placental thickness after delivery

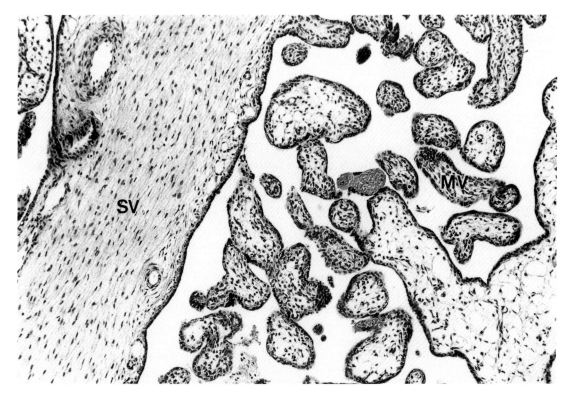

FIGURE 8.6. Placental villi of the 21st week p.m. The stroma of the stem villi (SV) is largely fibrous. Only a discontinuous thin superficial rim of reticular connective tissue is reminiscent of their derivation from immature intermediate villi. Paraffin section. ×125.

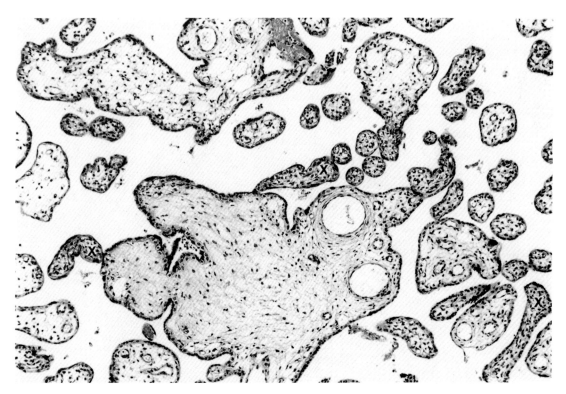

FIGURE 8.7. Placental villi of the 24th week p.m. Compared to the preceding stages, the variability in villous shapes and diameters is sharply increasing. The population of small slender villi (X's at lower left, lower right, and at center), originally referred to as mesenchymal villi, has achieved structural characteristics of mature intermediate villi. Paraffin section. ×125.

is about 20 to 22mm; measured by ultrasonography in situ and including the uterine wall, it is 43mm. The umbilical cord has a mean length between 410 and 455mm.

Steeply increasing numbers of mature intermediate villi and terminal villi, both of which exhibit calibers of 40 to 100μm, are the reason for considerably increased numbers of villous cross sections per square millimeter of histologic sections (Fig. 8.8). The total villous surface is increased to a mean of about 7m². In addition to the villi of small caliber that compose most of the villi, there are mainly stem villi of large caliber. Intermediate calibers of 100 to 200μm are rare, causing a typical gap in the range of calibers. This gap may be evident as early as the second half of the 7th month. The few existing villi of this particular caliber, mostly immature intermediate villi, are grouped together in the centers of the villous trees. Villous cytotrophoblast is reduced to about 35% of the villous surface. As a result of the beginning sinusoidal dilatation of the fetal capillaries in the newly formed terminal villi, the amount of vasculosyncytial membranes (epithelial plates) is increased, and the mean trophoblastic thickness reduced to about 6μm.

Ninth month p.m.   33rd to 36th week p.m.; 31st to 34th week p.c.

The crown–rump length is 280 to 330mm, fetal weight is 1600 to 2400g, placental diameter is 170 to 200mm, and the placental weight is 320 to 400g. The placental thickness postpartum is 22 to 24mm; by ultrasonography in situ, including the uterine wall, it is 45mm. The mean cord length increases from 455 to 495mm.

Histologically, the developmental processes described for the preceding month become even more prominent: The total villous surface of the placenta is increased to about 10m². Capillary growth and continuous sinusoidal dilatation cause the mean maternofetal diffusion distance to decrease to less than 12μm and the mean trophoblastic thickness to about 5μm. Cytotrophoblast is found on only 25% of the villous surfaces. The largest stem villi reach 500 to 1500μm in diameter. The small stromal rim, consisting of reticular connective tissue and indicating their immaturity, has normally disappeared to the credit of fibrous stroma that completely occupies the villous core (Fig. 8.9). The originally reticular superficial zone of the stroma shows an increased number of connective tissue cells for a few weeks, compared to

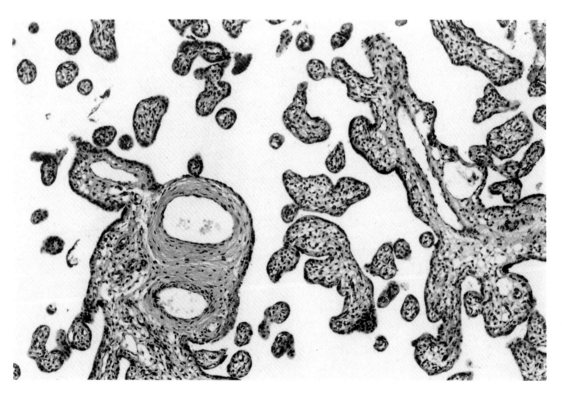

FIGURE 8.8. Placental villi of the 29th week p.m. During this period, the mature intermediate villi and the stem villi (lower left) are the prevailing villous types. Immature intermediate villi with typical reticular stroma (lower right) are less common. Paraffin section. ×125.

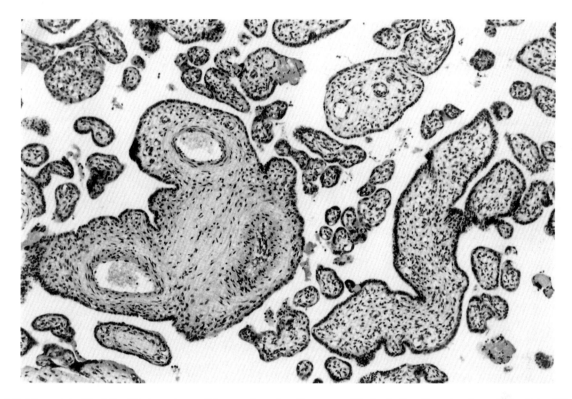

FIGURE 8.9. Placental villi of the 33rd week p.m. The number of immature intermediate villi is further decreasing. Most villi are stem villi and mature intermediate villi; the latter are intermingled with the first few terminal villi, which in paraffin sections (because of their similar diameters) are difficult to differentiate from mature intermediate villi. The stem villi are still not fully fibrosed; rather, they show a thin superficial layer that has few fibers and is rich in connective tissue cells. Paraffin section. ×125.

the more central parts of the stem villi. This difference usually is no longer observed at term. Larger parts of the syncytiotrophoblast of the stem villi are replaced by fibrinoid. Most villi are mature intermediate and terminal villi (Fig. 8.10). Small groups of immature intermediate villi, with calibers of 100 to 200 μm, can regularly be found in the centers of the villous trees, indicating placental growth is still active.

Tenth month p.m.   37th to 40th week p.m.; 35th to 38th week p.c.

The mean crown–rump length is increased from 330 mm to its final value of 380 mm and the mean fetal weight from 2400 to 3400 g. The placental diameter during the last month of pregnancy varies between 200 and 220 mm, and the mean placental weight increases from 400 g to 470 g. There are considerable individual variations. Early clamping of the cord after delivery of the baby may even increase placental weight by as much as 100 g. The final maximal placental thickness postpartum is about 25 mm; measured by ultrasonography in situ, the uterine wall and placenta amount to 45 mm. The mean cord length at term is 495 to 520 mm.

The kind and amount of villous types differ from the foregoing stage in several aspects. There are considerably increased numbers of terminal villi (about 40% of the total villous volume of the placenta) (Fig. 8.11) and a higher degree of capillarization of the latter, mainly because many of the capillary cross sections are dilated sinusoidally to maximally 40 μm. In well-preserved, early-fixed placentas that are not suffering from fetal vessel collapse, the terminal fetal villous capillary lumens amount to 40% or more of the villous volume. About 20% of the villi are stem villi. In the fully matured placenta, the fibrous stroma reaches the trophoblastic or fibrinoid surface of the stem villi everywhere; a superficial reticular rim, or a superficial accumulation of fibroblasts, as during the 9th month, is usually absent at term. If not, it has to be interpreted as a sign of persisting immaturity. The syncytiotrophoblastic cover of the stem villi is degenerated in most places and often it is replaced by fibrinoid (Fig. 8.12). About 30% to 40% of the villous volume is made up of mature intermediate villi, which can be differentiated histologically from the terminal villi by their reduced degree of fetal capillarization, and from the stem villi by the absence of large fetal vessels with media and adventitia identifiable by light microscopy. Maximally, only 10% of the total villous volume is of the immature, intermediate variety; they normally appear as small, loosely arranged groups

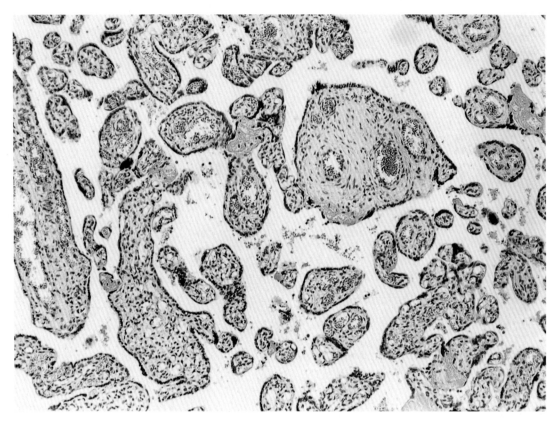

FIGURE 8.10. Placental villi of the 35th week p.m. The distribution of villous types is largely comparable to that demonstrated for the preceding stage. Paraffin section. ×125.

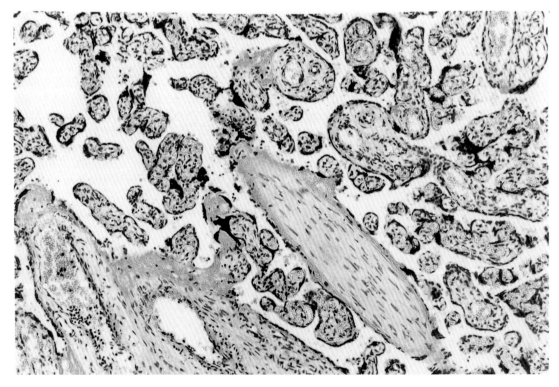

FIGURE 8.11. Placental villi of the 38th week p.m. Dominating villous types are mature intermediate villi and terminal villi, both of small caliber. Several stem villi of varying caliber can be seen in between. As is typical for near-term placentas, the trophoblastic cover of the stem villi is partly replaced by fibrinoid. The stromal core is completely fibrosed. Reticular stroma or cellular connective tissue (which as a typical sign of immaturity was visible below the trophoblast in earlier stages) is absent throughout the last few weeks. Paraffin section. ×125.

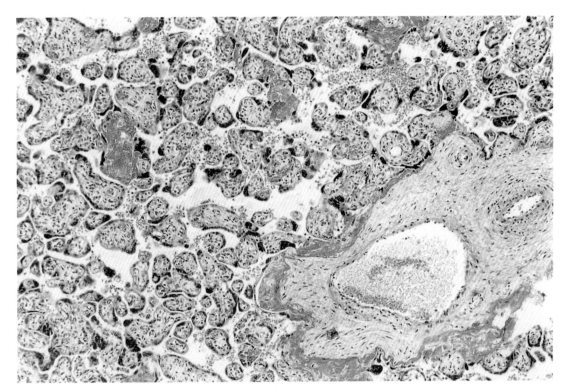

FIGURE 8.12. Placental villi of the 40th week p.m. Caliber distribution is little different from that of the 38th week. Despite this fact, some remarkable changes exist: The fibrinoid deposits (homogeneously gray) around the larger stem villi and the number of terminal villi are considerably increased; also, because of the irregular shapes of terminal villi at term, numerous flat sections of villous surfaces can be seen. Here these structures appear as dark spots of seemingly accumulated nuclei ("trophoblastic knotting"). Paraffin section. ×125.

in the centers of the villous trees, sometimes surrounding a central cavity.

The total villous volume of the placenta is about $12.5 \, m^2$. The mean trophoblastic thickness is reduced to about $4 \mu m$ and the mean maternofetal diffusion distance to less than $5 \mu m$. About 20% of the villous surfaces are double layered, consisting of cytotrophoblast and syncytiotrophoblast; the remaining 80% are only covered by syncytium of highly varying thickness ($0.5–10 \mu m$). The cell bodies of the existing villous cytotrophoblast, however, are so thin at times that they may be difficult to identify; thus, many investigators tend to underestimate their quantity or even deny their existence. The amount of fibrinoid in and around the villi is variable. We have never observed a complete absence of fibrinoid. Amounts exceeding 10% of the total placental villous volume are an exception and likely to be a sign of disease processes. The amount of fibrinoid, inside and at the surfaces of the chorionic and the basal plate, is even more variable.

Table 8.1 summarizes the development of villous types throughout pregnancy.

NUCLEATED RED BLOOD CELLS

There is considerable confusion about the normal numbers of nucleated red blood cells (NRBCs) in neonatal blood and it is for this reason that this information is included here. In the truly normal term pregnancy very few, if any, red blood cells with nuclei are visible in the fetal blood during the microscopic placental examination. When NRBCs are seen in the fetal blood at term (and it is important that they be correctly diagnosed as such), this is a distinctly abnormal finding. The pathologist should endeavor to ascertain the reason for the presence of the NRBCs when they are seen in placental sections (Fig. 8.13). This is most conveniently done by making a blood smear of neonatal blood.

An extensive literature exists on this topic and the findings in these contributions are not always in agreement. They have indeed led to considerable controversy as to how many NRBCs may be found in truly normal neonates. Most studies are based on neonatal blood smears, rather than placental sections. It is difficult to estimate the number accurately by studying placental slides. One reason for the results to be discrepant, especially in the older citations, is that the authors have not always stated the exact age of the neonates they studied. They have also not excluded infants who suffered from any of the many causes of hypoxia. Most reports made no reference to the possible existence of growth retardation and many other factors that are only now becoming known as causing fetal erythropoietin (EPO) release, presumably the main reason for secretion of NRBCs.

One of the earliest contributions to this topic is that by Geissler and Japha (1901), who stated emphatically that "contrary to the dogma,"

Table 8.1. Structural characteristics of the five villous types from the 4th to the 40th week p.m.

Week	Stem villi	Immature intermediate villi	Mesenchymal villi	Mature intermediate villi	Terminal villi
4			Only mesenchymal villi (120–250μm) and trophoblastic sprouts (30–60μm) are present. Large mesenchymal villi (>200μm) may show diffuse, moderate stromal fibrosis.		*Not existing in this stage*
5		*Not existing in this stage*			
6					
7					
8			The first stromal channels appear within the mesenchymal villi.		
9	*Not existing in this stage*	Numerous immature intermediate villi (100–200μm) with reticular stroma; caliber of the largest vessels is 20–30μm.	Numerous short mesenchymal villi (60–100μm), partly continuous with slim trophoblastic sprouts, branch from the surfaces of immature intermediate villi.	*Not existing in this stage*	
10					
11					
12		Increasing amount and size of immature intermediate villi (100–400μm); caliber of stem vessels increased up to 100μm; vessel walls with two to three concentric layers of cells.			
13					
14					
15		Light microscopically apparent bundles of collagen fibers arranged around vessel walls.			
16					
17	About 50% of all villi with calibers >150μm show fusion of the fibrosed adventitial sheaths around the primitive arteries with those of the veins. This is the first step toward formation of the fibrosed stromal core of stem villi.		The numbers of mesenchymal villi and trophoblastic sprouts are slowly decreasing.		
18					
19					

Weeks p.m.	Stem villi	Immature intermediate villi	Mesenchymal villi	Mature intermediate villi	Terminal villi
20–23	First true stem villi appear. Smaller ones (150–300 μm) show centrally fibrosed core with arterial and venous adventitia being fused. Those >300 μm show a largely fibrosed core.	Immature intermediate villi are still the dominating villous type. Those with calibers of 100–150 μm show no stromal fibrosis. The larger ones >300 μm show fibrosis of the walls of larger vessels.	The number of mesenchymal villi with poorly fibrosed and poorly vascularized stroma, rich in cells, increases considerably. They grow in length and in width (calibers 80–150 μm) and show a continuous transition into mature intermediate villi.		
24–25	Caliber >300 μm: completely fibrosed stroma; caliber <300 μm: superficial layer of reticular stroma below the trophoblast.	Number and size of immature intermediate villi are decreasing.			
26–29			Typical mesenchymal villi are rare and mostly located in the surrounding of immature intermediate villi.	Mature intermediate villi with dense stroma, rich in stromal cells and poor in fibers, with calibers of 100–150 μm, comprise the dominating villous type.	Local spot-like groups of first typical terminal villi appear; they show calibers of about 60 μm, about half of their stromal volume being occupied by capillary lumens.
30–34	Caliber >200 μm: completely fibrosed stroma; caliber <200 μm: incomplete superficial rim of reticular stroma.	Only a few evenly distributed immature intermediate villi can be found; the stroma is only partly reticular in nature.			Increasing amount of evenly distributed terminal villi with sinusoidally dilated capillaries and few epithelial plates.
35–37	Usually, all stem villi are void of reticular stroma; however, below the trophoblast still is a less densely fibrosed rim, rich in fibroblasts.	The few remaining immature intermediate villi are no longer evenly dispersed but, rather, concentrated as small groups in the centers of the villous trees lining the central cavities. The extremely loose reticular stroma shows only a few typical stromal channels.	Mesenchymal villi are histologically inconspicuous; the few identifiable ones are usually located around the central cavities.		Terminal villi are the dominating villous type; they amount to about 40% of the total villous volume.
38–40	All stem villi (except a few around the central cavity) are completely fibrosed. The trophoblast of the larger ones often is replaced by fibrinoid.				

Reproduced with permission of Kaufmann and Castellucci (Development and anatomy of the placenta. In: Haines's and Taylor's Textbook of Obstetrical and Gynaecological Pathology. 4th ed. H. Fox and M. Wells (eds). Churchill Livingstone, Edinburgh, 1995).

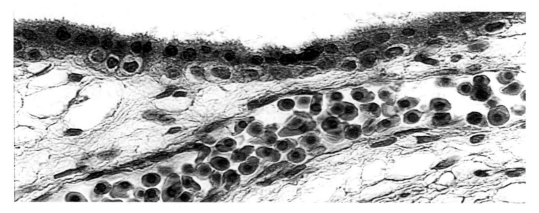

FIGURE 8.13. Immature intermediate villus of the 6th week p.m. The villus is covered by a uniform layer of syncytiotrophoblast lining the intervillous space (above), followed by a nearly complete layer of villous cytotrophoblast directly below. The villous stroma is largely occupied by a fetal vessel containing numerous nucleated red blood cells, as is typical for this stage of pregnancy. Hematoxylin and eosin (H&E) stain. ×800.

NRBCs are not found in young children; it is possible, however, that they occur rarely in prematures. These authors were adamant in their opinion that the presence of NRBCs is to be viewed as "showing disease." As many others, they did not specify the children's ages or clinical conditions of their births. Lippman (1924) enumerated the NRBCs of neonatal blood, followed the children up to 5 days of life, and reviewed all prior literature. Lippman concluded that term neonates have an average of 3.2 NRBCs/100 white blood cells (WBCs). (To express the number of NRBCs per total WBC is a convenient and widely practiced way of enumerating these cells, but an alternate method is referred to below.) The number of NRBCs was found to fall rapidly after birth, and at the age of 5 days there were none left. The condition of the newborns is again not clearly stated in this paper, except that children with congenital syphilis were excluded; however, mothers with preeclampsia were not.

Ryerson and Sanes (1934) undertook one of the more incisive studies of placentally contained NRBCs. They were anxious to ascertain parameters that allowed specifying the age of a gestation by histologic examination of the placenta. They concluded that virtually all NRBCs had disappeared at the end of the third month of pregnancy. They suggested also that, if more than 1% NRBCs are found, this indicated prematurity (Fig. 8.13). Anderson (1941) made the next significant contribution and more or less confirmed the previous findings. He indicated that in approximately 16.5% of term placentas one or two NRBCs could be found among 1000 red blood cells (RBCs); in the remaining 83.5% there were none at term. Stillborns were observed to have greater numbers, and he stated that a "decided increase . . . points to pathologic states." Fox (1967) next published on this phenomenon; he related it to hypoxia or asphyxia. We concur with this interpretation of a relationship to fetal tissue hypoxia, and it is our practice to always take special note of the presence of NRBCs when examining placentas microscopically.

Green and Mimouni (1990) have addressed the question of NRBCs in newborns of diabetic mothers; their observation was that normative data are lacking in the literature. These authors stated the desirability to express NRBCs in absolute numbers, rather than as NRBCs/WBCs, as has been the common practice. One reason for so doing is that elevated WBC counts would lead to artificially low numbers of NRBCs when the usual method of enumeration (NRBC/100 WBCs) is employed. Green and Mimouni also provided rigid criteria for the selection and suggested that "a value greater than 1×10^9/L should be considered as a potential index of intrauterine hypoxia." Normally, there were no NRBCs in term neonates, and the 95th percentile was 1.7 in absolute counts. Diabetic mothers' babies had increased numbers, as did infants with hypoxia and growth-retarded neonates. Shurin (1987) concluded that there are about 200 to 600 NRBCs/mm^3 and 10,000 to 30,000 WBCs; she also stated that the normal infant has 4 to 5 NRBCs/100 WBCs in cord blood samples, which is higher than is our experience. Shurin reflected that this number indicates the erythroid hyperplasia caused by high levels of EPO production.

Erythropoietin, initially made in liver and later in kidneys (Eckardt et al., 1992), is the principal agent in the secretion of NRBCs from the sites of hematopoiesis. It is now being measured with greater frequency in cord blood, and correlations are beginning to be made to perinatal circumstances. Maier et al. (1993) found that elevated levels of EPO in cord blood indicate prolonged fetal hypoxia and advocated that the determination of EPO levels might give the exact time course of events. The EPO levels did not correlate with gestational age, meconium staining, or Apgar scores, but they related to umbilical arterial pH level and were elevated in fetal growth retardation; they also quoted authors who found a relation to fetal death and cerebral palsy. These findings are of great significance to the perinatologist and pathologist with an interest in ascertaining more precisely than now possible the time of possible fetal hypoxia, especially its relation to possible problems during labor. It is hoped that the rapidity (or sluggishness) of the EPO response and the appearance of NRBCs will be further defined in the future so as to allow a better analysis of perinatal hypoxia. Because these phenomena require some significant metabolic steps in fetal performance, one would expect that very many hours must pass from an hypoxic event to significantly elevate the levels of EPO and NRBCs of the fetus; but we do not presently know the exact number of hours. We also do not know whether the fetal response with EPO and numbers of NRBCs secreted to different amounts of acute blood loss is the same or if it is a graded response. There are, however, occasionally specific cases that allow some insight into these questions. They need to be recorded for a better understanding of the response. It is then essential that the precise status of the gestation and the well-being of the fetus be known for accurate assessment. Thus, it would be impossible to compare accurately the levels of NRBCs found after a hemorrhage in a neonate with intrauterine growth restriction (IUGR) and those of a normal neonate; the former may have started at a higher baseline. Experimental observations (presently known only from sheep) are insufficient for the clinical setting. Quantitative and temporal sequences by Shields et al. (1993) have reviewed what is known of this aspect of RBC restoration after experimental hemorrhage in sheep. Despite an initial rise in erythropoietin level, a significant hemorrhage (40%) is not followed by a significant increase in reticulocyte count, nor are the former blood volume and hematocrits restored before birth. Thus, the ovine model may not be adequate to settle these important questions.

Phelan et al. (1993) studied NRBCs in asphyxiated and normal neonates. They found that normal infants do not have NRBCs but that asphyxiated newborns have elevated counts. The most elevated NRBC counts were explicable only by assuming hypoxia to have occurred long before birth. Nicolini et al. (1990) made the observation that IUGR fetuses have elevated NRBC counts in cordocentesis samples.

The following observations may have relevance in this context.

1. A patient at term whom we have known had a major "gush of bright red blood" (later identified as fetal blood from disrupted velamentous vessels) upon insertion of an intrauterine pressure catheter. She was delivered by cesarean section 48 minutes later; the infant was pale but the placenta otherwise entirely normal. The cord arterial pH was 7.05, the fetal hemoglobin 14.6 g, hematocrit 44.8%, WBC 28,000, and platelets 120,000 and falling to 71,000. Three transfusions of packed RBCs were given to the newborn and the hemoglobin level was then only 10.3 g, hematocrit 29.9%. The first enumeration of NRBCs occurred at 1.5 hours as 19 NRBCs/100 WBCs; 6 hours later it was 32 NRBCs/100 WBCs. Thus, there was a continued hematologic response after the delivery of the anemic child, and the initial NRBC response was detectable already within 1 hour. This finding is contrary to the rapid decline of NRBCs postnatally when the hypoxic event has been more remote; under those circumstances most NRBCs are gone on the second day.

2. Another relevant case was a woman who had a car accident while wearing a lap belt and was at 28 weeks' gestation. Approximately 12 (± 1) hours later, the fetus was born with a hematocrit of 25% and an estimated 40 to 50 mL of fetal blood in the maternal circulation; 45 NRBCs/100 WBCs were then found. Moreover, villous edema indicated some degree of early fetal heart failure. This finding may be surprising with a hematocrit of 25% and suggests that final adjustment of blood volume had not yet been made.

3. A 24-year-old gravida 1 was involved in a car accident at 33 weeks. The baby was delivered 12 hours later by cesarean section. There was a large retroplacental hematoma, consistent with age 12 hours. At 0.5 hour later, a complete blood count (CBC) showed 45 NRBCs/100 WBCs and a WBC count of 20,000; hematocrit of 39.7%. Eleven hours later the number of NRBCs was 5/100 WBCs, but packed cells had been given; WBC was then 11,000. The child suffered cerebral palsy.

4. A gravida 1 without toxemia, at 39 weeks and 4 days, with normal pregnancy awoke at 6:45 a.m. with a brief abdominal pain, finding many blood clots in the bed; she ruptured the membranes but stopped bleeding; there was no pain. At 8:12 a.m. she came to the hospital. Findings were fetal heart tone (FHT) 140 to 150; good fetal movements; speculum examination showed blood-tinged fluid in the vagina; no blood from the 1-cm cervix; nontender uterus. At 10:12 a.m. massive bradycardia occurred, followed by emergency cesarean section delivery at 10:37 a.m. Hematocrit was 19%, pH 6.77, PCO_2 125, PO_2 32, base deficit −20; NRBCs 18/100 WBCs; Apgar scores 0/0/0. Despite resuscitation and transfusion with packed cells, the child died the next day having a flat EEG. At autopsy, several myocardial infarcts, brain necroses, and infarcted adrenals, kidneys, spleen, and areas of liver were found. One velamentous vessel had ruptured, of a velamentous cord with bilobed placenta. This happened in bed, and bleeding was presumably stopped because the engaging head compressed the ruptured vessel. The brick-red myocardial necroses and the finding of 18 NRBCs at birth suggest that on admission the damage had already been done.

Through the courtesy of Dr. G. Altshuler, we provide here a more accurate means of assessing the precise number of NRBCs, as it is heavily influenced by WBC counts:

To calculate the absolute NRBC count from NRBCs/WBCs (number/mm³), one first needs to correct the machine-counted WBCs to a CWBC (corrected WBC) by the following formula:

$$CWBC = \frac{WBC_{(machine-counted\ total\ WBC\ count)} \times 100}{100 + (NRBC/100\ WBC)}$$

Then: NRBC = WBC − CWBC, or the total NRBC count = total CWBC × NRBC/100 WBC.

References

Aherne, W. and Dunnill, M.S.: Morphometry of the human placenta. Br. Med. Bull. **22**:5–8, 1966.

Anderson, G.W.: Studies on the nucleated red cell count in the chorionic capillaries and the cord blood of various ages of pregnancy. Amer. J. Obstetr. Gynecol. **42**:1–14, 1941.

Boyd, J.D. and Hamilton, W.J.: The Human Placenta. Heffer, Cambridge, 1970.

Clavero-Nunez, J.A. and Botella-Llusia, J.: Measurement of the villus surface in normal and pathologic placentas. Amer. J. Obstet. Gynecol. **86**:234–240, 1961.

Clavero-Nuñez, J.A. and Botella-Llusia, J.: Ergebnisse von Messungen der Gesamtoberfläche normaler und krankhafter Placenten. Arch. Gynäkol. **198**:56:60, 1963.

Eckardt, K.-U., Ratcliffe, P.J., Tan, C.C., Bauer, C. and Kurtz, A.: Age-dependent expression of the erythropoietin gene in rat liver and kidneys. J. Clin. Invest. **89**:753–760, 1992.

Fox, H. The incidence and significance of nucleated erythrocytes in the foetal vessels of the mature human placenta. J. Obstet. Gynaecol. Br. Commonw. **74**:40–43, 1967.

Geissler, D. and Japha, A.: Beitrag zu den Anämieen junger Kinder. Jahrb. Kinderh. **56**:627–647, 1901.

Gloede, B.: Morphometrische Untersuchungen zur Reifung menschlicher Placentazotten. Medical Thesis, University of Hamburg, 1984.

Green, D.W. and Mimouni, F.: Nucleated erythrocytes in healthy infants and in infants of diabetic mothers. J. Pediatr. **116**:129–131, 1990.

Hörmann, G.: Lebenskurven normaler und entwicklungsfähiger Chorionzotten; Ergebnisse systematischer Zottenmessungen. Arch. Gynäkol. **181**:29–43, 1951.

Johannigmann, J., Zahn, V. and Thieme, V.: Einführung in die Ultraschalluntersuchung mit dem Vidoson. Elektromedica **2**:1–11, 1972.

Kaufmann, P.: Untersuchungen über die Langhanszellen in der menschlichen Placenta. Z. Zellforsch. **128**:283–302, 1972.

Kaufmann, P.: Entwicklung der Plazenta. In, Die Plazenta des Menschen. V. Becker, T.H. Schiebler and F. Kubli, eds., pp. 13–50. Thieme Verlag, Stuttgart, 1981.

Kaufmann, P. and Castellucci, M.: Development and anatomy of the placenta. In, Haines' and Taylor's Textbook of Obstetrical and Gynaecological Pathology, 4th Ed. H. Fox and M. Wells, eds. pp. 1437–1476. Churchill Livingstone, London, 1995.

Kaufmann, P. and Stegner, H.E.: Über die funktionelle Differenzierung des Zottensyncytiums in der menschlichen Placenta. Z. Zellforsch. **135**:361–382, 1972.

Knopp, J.: Das Wachstum der Chorionzotten vom II. bis X.
Monat. Z. Anat. Entwicklungsgesch. **122**:42–59, 1960.

Lippman, H.S.: A morphologic and quantitative study of the
blood corpuscles in the new-born period. Amer. J. Dis. Child.
27:473–536, 1924.

Maier, R.F., Böhme, K., Dudenhausen, J.W. and Obladen, M.:
Cord blood erythropoietin in relation to different markers of
fetal hypoxia. Obstet. Gynecol. **81**:575–580, 1993.

Nicolini, U., Nicolaidis, P., Fisk, N.M., Vaughn, J.I., Fusi, L.,
Gleeson, R. and Rodeck, C.H.: Limited role of fetal blood
sampling in prediction of outcome in intrauterine growth
retardation. Lancet **336**:768–772, 1990.

O'Rahilly, R.: Developmental stages in human embryos.
Part A, Publ. 631. Carnegie Institute, Washington, D.C.,
1973.

Phelan, J.P., Ahn, N.O., Korst, L. and Martin, G.I.: Nucleated red
blood cells: a marker for fetal asphyxia (abstract 49). Amer.
J. Obstet. Gynecol. **170**:286, 1993.

Ryerson, C.S. and Sanes, S.: The age of pregnancy. Histologic
diagnosis from percentage of erythroblasts in chorionic capillaries. Arch. Pathol. **17**:548–651, 1934.

Schiemer, H.G.: Mass und Zahl der Plazenta. In, Die Plazenta
des Menschen. V. Becker, T.H. Schiebler and F. Kubli, eds., pp.
112–122. Thieme Verlag, Stuttgart, 1981.

Shields, L.E., Widness, J.A. and Brace, R.A.: Restoration of fetal
red blood cells and plasma proteins after a moderately severe
hemorrhage in the ovine fetus. Am. J. Obstet. Gynecol.
169:1472–1478, 1993.

Shurin, S.B.: The blood and the hematopoietic system. In,
Neonatal-Perinatal Medicine. A. A. Fanaroff and R.J. Martin,
eds., pp. 826–827. C.V. Mosby, St. Louis, 1987.

Winckel, F.K.L.W.: Lehrbuch der Geburtshilfe. 2nd Ed. Veit,
Leipzig, 1893.

9
Nonvillous Parts and Trophoblast Invasion

H.G. Frank and P. Kaufmann

The nonvillous parts of the placenta include the chorionic plate, cell islands, cell columns, placental septa, basal plate, marginal zone, and fibrinoid deposits in all parts of the organ (Fig. 9.1). In contrast to the villous parts of the placenta, they do not participate in maternofetal exchange since they are never vascularized by both the maternal and fetal circulations, but rather by fetal stem vessels alone (chorionic plate), or maternal stem vessels alone (basal plate), or neither of both (marginal zone, cell islands, cell columns, fibrinoid deposits).

Irrespective of their heterogeneous location and structure, the nonvillous parts of the placenta have the same basic components (Fig. 9.2):

- extravillous trophoblast,
- fibrinoid, and
- in some locations, decidualized endometrial stroma.

These basic tissue components structurally and functionally do not vary from one nonvillous part to another and therefore are considered first.

Extravillous Trophoblast

HISTORICAL ASPECTS AND NOMENCLATURE

Placentologists have known for about 100 years that different cell types exist in the nonvillous parts of the placenta and that they differ markedly in shape and staining patterns. Among those, in particular, the large, intensely basophilic staining cells of all nonvillous parts have raised an enormous interest. Scipiades and Burg (1930) first employed the term **X cells**, the name implying that their origin was in dispute. The search for Barr bodies (sex chromatin, the heterochromatic second X chromosome of females) in X cells gave conflicting results (maternal origin: Klinger & Ludwig, 1957; fetal origin: Zhemkova, 1960). Systematic radioautographic studies on ^{3}H-thymidine incorporation (Kim & Benirschke, 1971), as well as detailed structural (Kaufmann & Stark, 1971) and enzyme histochemical analyses (Stark & Kaufmann, 1971) gave first evidence that X cells are trophoblastic in nature. Final proof for the trophoblastic, fetal origin of the X cells was obtained by Y-specific fluorescence in X cells of placentas from male infants (Faller & Ferenci, 1973; Khudr et al., 1973; Maidman et al., 1973; Steininger, 1978).

Today, normally antibodies against cytokeratin, an epithelial intermediate filament, are used as an easily applicable immunohistochemical marker of these cells (Khong et al., 1986b; Yeh et al., 1988, 1990; Daya & Sabet, 1991; Mühlhauser et al., 1995). This antigen is not trophoblast specific but rather is expressed by all cells of epithelial origin. Because of this, in the nonvillous parts of the placenta, also the amnionic epithelium and residual maternal glandular epithelium are cytokeratin positive; moreover, some smooth muscle cells may express certain isoforms of this cytoskeletal antigen (except cytokeratin 7). In spite of these limitations, cytokeratin antibodies represent the most suitable markers for the distinction of extravillous trophoblast cells from decidual cells (see Fig. 9.4A), since all cells of decidual origin (decidual cells, endometrial stromal cells, macrophages, lymphocytes, natural killer cells) are clearly cytokeratin negative.

Antibodies against different cytokeratin isoforms have been employed to identify special subtypes of trophoblast (Mühlhauser et al., 1995; Pröll et al., 1997a). An antibody against placental protein 19 (PP19) is another immunohistochemical marker that is said to react specifically with extravillous trophoblast (Takayama et al., 1989). The antibody BC-1 (Loke et al., 1992) was shown to differentiate between villous and extravillous trophoblast, binding specifically to the latter.

As soon as the trophoblastic origin of the X cells was proven, new and more appropriate designations were proposed. Among those are extravillous trophoblast, nonvillous trophoblast, intermediate trophoblast. Regrettably, each of these terms has a slightly different definition. In addition, names for trophoblast of special nonvillous localizations have been introduced (e.g., interstitial trophoblast, endovascular trophoblast, intraarterial trophoblast, clear trophoblastic cells, trophoblastic giant cells, trophocytes, and spongiotrophoblast-like cells).

Recently, among placentologists the term **extravillous trophoblast** (EVT) has been generally accepted as general heading for the entire population of trophoblast cells residing outside the villi. This term ideally describes the topographic situation of these trophoblast cells. According to its localization and degree of differentiation, the extravillous trophoblast may be further subdivided. The respective nomenclature is summarized and defined in Figure 9.3.

Among clinicians and pathologists the term **intermediate trophoblast** (Kurman et al., 1984a,b) is still widely applied. Regrettably, this term has never been well defined and it remains open how far, for instance, proliferative extravillous trophoblast and endovascular trophoblast are included. The term intermediate trophoblast was first used for villous trophoblast cells showing a phenotype intermediate between villous cytotrophoblast and syncytiotrophoblast (Tighe et al., 1967). Later it was applied to extravillous trophoblast cells, which were thought to show a similar "intermediate" phenotype (Kurman et al., 1984a,b). Descriptions such as "intermediate trophoblast of the villous sprouts"

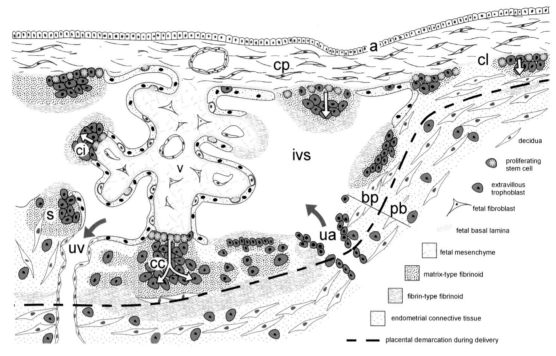

FIGURE 9.1. Schematic drawing of the distribution of the various trophoblast populations (blue) of the human placenta. All those trophoblast cells that rest on the trophoblastic basal lamina of membranes, chorionic plate, villi, cell columns and cell islands, represent the proliferating trophoblastic stem cells (Langhans' cells). Where these are close to the intervillous space (ivs) they differentiate and fuse to form the syncytiotrophoblast. Usually this event takes place in the placental villi (v). Without contact with the intervillous space, the daughter cells of the proliferat-

ing stem cells (marked by asterisks) do not fuse syncytially but rather differentiate and become invasive, forming the extravillous trophoblast cells. Their routes of invasion/migration are symbolized by arrows. Extravillous trophoblast cells can be found in cell columns (c), cell islands (ci), chorionic plate (cp), chorion laeve (cl), septa (s), basal plate (bp), and uteroplacental arteries (ua). Matrix-type fibrinoid: point-shaded; fibrin-type fibrinoid is line-shaded. (*Source:* Modified from Kaufmann and Castellucci, 1997, with permission.)

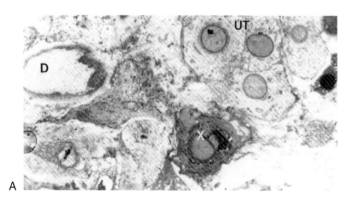

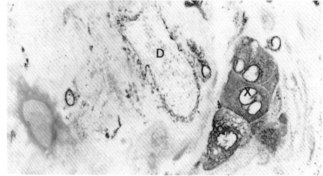

FIGURE 9.2. Semithin sections of the basal plate at term. A: Enzyme histochemical proof of β-glucuronidase to demonstrate the typical mixture of cell types in the basal plate. D, decidua cell with its clearly visible surrounding basal lamina; X, highly differentiated extravillous cytotrophoblast; UT, less differenti- ated, proliferative extravillous cytotrophoblast. ×810. (*Source:*

Stark & Kaufmann, 1973, with permission.) B: Enzyme histo- chemical proof of glucose-6–phosphate dehydrogenase. As is typical for this enzyme, extravillous trophoblast cells (X) exhibit intense reaction patterns, whereas decidua cells (D) stain largely negative, except slight granular staining along their surfaces. ×360.

EXTRAVILLOUS TROPHOBLAST
(all cellular and syncytial
trophoblast outside the villi)

└── **extravillous syncytiotrophoblast**
(syncytiotrophoblast remainders, mostly at the intervillous
surfaces of all nonvillous parts of the placenta)

└── **extravillous cytotrophoblast**
(all mononuclear trophoblast outside the villi)

└── **proliferative phenotype of extravillous trophoblast**
(proliferating stem cells
resting on, or near to the basal lamina facing the villous or chorionic stroma,
= proximal extravillous trophoblast cells)

└── **invasive phenotype of extravillous trophoblast**
(non-proliferative, disseminated daughter cells with invasive phenotype,
= distal extravillous trophoblast cells)

└── **interstitial trophoblast ("intermediate trophoblast")**
(all invasive trophoblast cells
which do not invade uteroplacental vessels)

└── **small spindle-shaped trophoblast cells**
(highly invasive, diploid to tetraploid trophoblast cells,
which prevail in early stages of pregnancy,
from the superficial basal plate until the myometrium)

└── **large polygonal trophoblast cells ("X-cells")[1]**
(polyploid, mononuclear, basophilic cells of low invasiveness,
accumulating preferably in the basal plate;
prevalent extravillous cell type throughout the last trimester)

└── **multinucleated trophoblastic giant cells[1]**
(polyploid multinucleated elements of low invasiveness,
located deep in the invasive zone; probably derived from syncytial
fusion of highly invasive spindle-shaped trophoblast cells)

└── **endovascular trophoblast**
(trophoblast cells invading walls
and lumina of uteroplacental vessels)

└── **intramural trophoblast**
(invasive trophoblast cells infiltrating
the walls of uteroplacental vessels)

└── **intraarterial trophoblast**
(invasive trophoblast cells replacing endothelium and
forming intraluminal plugs in uteroplacental arteries)

[1]The additional widely applied term **placental site giant cells** is a pathologic term for highly differentiated
mono- and multinucleated trophoblastic elements in the maternofetal junctional zone, comprising a degenerative
subset of interstitial trophoblast and multinucleated trophoblastic giant cells.

FIGURE 9.3. Nomenclature of the various subtypes of trophoblast cells residing outside the villous trees (so-called extravillous trophoblast). For developmental relations of these cell types cf. Figure 9.8.

(Pampfer et al., 1992) or "intermediate trophoblast cells at both villous and extravillous sites" (Riley et al., 1992) illustrate how confusing this term can be.

Extravillous Trophoblast Is a Tissue of Its Own

Extravillous trophoblast is derived from the trophoblastic wall of the blastocyst and therefore without doubt is an epithelially derived tissue:

• Extravillous trophoblast reveals its epithelial phenotype by expressing cytokeratins as intermediate filaments. Depending on the stage of differentiation, however, the isoforms pattern may vary (see Immunohistochemical Markers in Chapter 3).

• As in other stratified epithelia, the **proliferation** of extravillous trophoblast is strictly restricted to a population of stem cells resting as a true epithelial layer on a basal lamina. The latter represents the interface between fetoplacental (chorionic) stroma and extravillous trophoblast. Right after leaving the basal lamina, the cells also leave the cell cycle (see next section).

• When leaving the basal lamina, the extravillous trophoblast cells achieve an **interstitial, apolar phenotype** (Fig. 9.1). This process has been analyzed ultrastructurally and immunohistochemically in much detail in the rhesus monkey (Enders, 1995, 1997a,b). Among others, this interstitial phenotype is expressed by the kind and arrangement of extracellular matrix molecules secreted and by the pattern of integrins exposed, binding to this self-produced interstitial extracellular matrix (for review see Kaufmann & Castellucci, 1997) (see below).

- In most cases, this apolar extracellular matrix (ECM) is secreted in the direct vicinity of maternal tissues, namely facing the maternal blood (e.g., cell islands, intervillous surface of the chorionic plate, placental septa) or maternal decidua (basal plate with cell columns, chorion laeve). As a consequence, the maternal tissues add to the formation of the ECM. The maternal ECM additions may be derived from maternal blood (e.g., fibrin) or are secretory products of decidual and endometrial stromal cells. The resulting peritrophoblastic accumulations of extracellular matrix are partly difficult to assign to maternal or fetal origin and are summarized under the summarizing term **fibrinoid** (see below).

- After exiting the cell cycle, the postproliferative daughter cells like typical epithelial cells leave the basal lamina. In a first stage of movement, they are pushed forward by proliferation pressure by the subsequent generations of cells. Only later they start migrating actively in theirself-secreted matrix. In a last step of differentiation, they achieve a **truly invasive phenotype** and pass the maternal host tissue by destroying it (see below).

All of the above features are characteristic for extravillous trophoblast in general. They do not differ in different extravillous locations.

Proliferation Patterns of Extravillous Trophoblast and the Invasive Pathway

When extravillous trophoblast is stained with proliferation markers such as ^{3}H-thymidine, BrdU, Ki-67, MIB-1, or antibodies against proliferating-cell nuclear antigen (PCNA), only those cells are marked that are close to the basal lamina of the neighboring fetal stroma. Extravillous trophoblast cells far from this basal lamina remain unstained (Figs. 9.4 and 9.5) (Bulmer et al., 1988a,c; Mühlhauser et al., 1993; Blankenship & King, 1994a; Kosanke, 1994; Kaufmann & Castellucci, 1997).

The proliferation markers listed above show characteristic differences in their staining patterns, which in the past repeatedly resulted in misinterpretations.

- Nuclei marked by ^{3}**H-thymidine** or by **BrdU** are found only in the basal layer of cells resting directly on the basal lamina; since ^{3}H-thymidine and BrdU are incorporated exclusively during the S-phase of the cell cycle, this pattern indicates that mitosis is restricted to this basal layer of cells.

- **Ki-67** and **MIB-1** are antibodies both directed against the same nuclear antigen (Ki-67 antigen), which is

expressed not only in the S-phase but in all stages of the cell cycle except G_o and G_1. As a result, this marker shows higher staining indices as compared to ^{3}H-thymidine. Normally, with this marker, immunoreactivity is found in two to six proximal layers of columns. Only the deeply invasive and intravascular trophoblast cells are always negative for Ki-67 and MIB-1.

- **Proliferating cell nuclear antigen** is expressed throughout all stages of the cell cycle. It has a half-life of about 20 hours and therefore may even be found in cells that have left the cell cycle already 1 day or more before. For example, PCNA expression was found in intravascular trophoblast (King & Blankenship, 1993), suggesting that these cells were still in the cell cycle. A later study by the same group using Ki-67 made clear that most of the immunoreactivity seen with PCNA did not point to actual mitotic activity but rather was due to the long half-life of the antigen (Blankenship & King, 1994a).

In conclusion, application of the above-mentioned proliferation markers reveals that extravillous trophoblast throughout differentiation passes two subsequent phenotypes (Bulmer et al., 1988a,c; Mühlhauser et al., 1993; Blankenship & King, 1994a; Kosanke, 1994; Kaufmann & Castellucci, 1997):

1. A so-called **proliferative phenotype** of extravillous trophoblast, which according to the ^{3}H-thymidine data is restricted to the basal layer of extravillous trophoblast within the cell columns;

2. A so-called postproliferative, migratory, and invasive phenotype, which starts as early as in the second layer of trophoblast cells of the cell columns (**postproliferative cells**), occupies the distal parts of the cell columns (**migratory trophoblast**), and finally spreads deeply into the maternal tissues (**invasive phenotype**) (for review see Kaufmann & Castellucci, 1997)

Both phenotypes of extravillous trophoblast are generally present in all nonvillous parts of the placenta (Fig. 9.1). This is clearly valid for the first two trimesters of pregnancy. In term pregnancies, extravillous trophoblast shows considerably reduced proliferative activities and locally it may be impossible to find any of the proximal cells still being in the cell cycle. In this case postproliferative cells may be attached to the basal lamina.

We conclude from these findings that the basal layer of trophoblast cells of the cell columns (cells attached to the basal lamina of anchoring villi) represent the **stem cells of the extravillous invasive pathway** (proliferative phenotype), whereas the more distal, nonproliferative extravillous trophoblast cells are the **differentiated, more or less invasive cells**, derived from the nearest proliferative center by migration or invasion (Fig. 9.4A,B). Roughly,

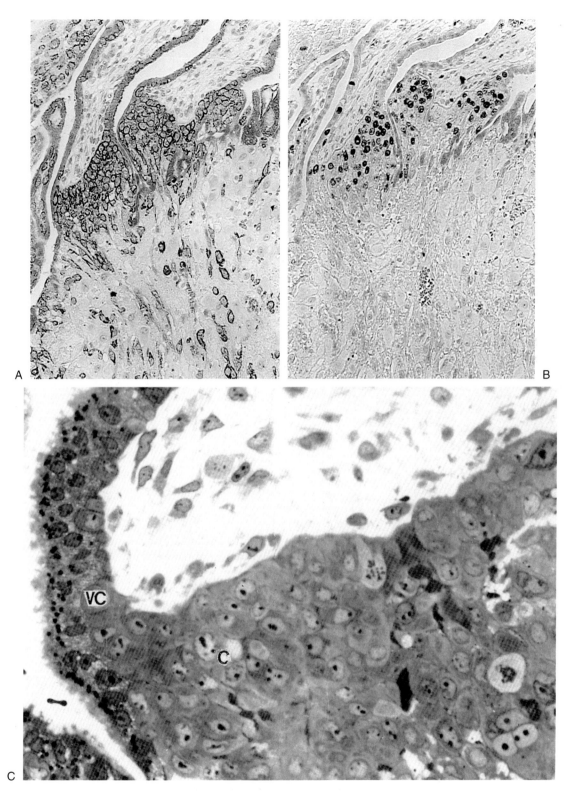

FIGURE 9.4. Serial paraffin sections of two anchoring villi (upper half) attached to the basal plate (below) by cell columns (center), 16th week postmenstruation (p.m.). A: Stained with anticyto-keratin, which binds to all villous and extravillous trophoblast cells. B: Stained with the monoclonal antibody MIB-1, which only stains proliferating cells. Note that the invasive trophoblast cells (lower half) are nonproliferative, whereas those cells facing the basal lamina of the anchoring villus (arrowheads) and villous cytotrophoblast are MIB-1–positive. These cells make up the proliferating stem cells (Langhans' cells). ×100. (Courtesy of Dr. Gaby Kohnen, Aachen, Germany.) C: A 22nd week p.m. semithin section of the transition between the anchoring villus (above) and the cell column (below). The continuity of villous cytotrophoblast (VC) with the proliferating cluster of cytotro-phoblast in the cell column (C) is clearly visible. ×800.

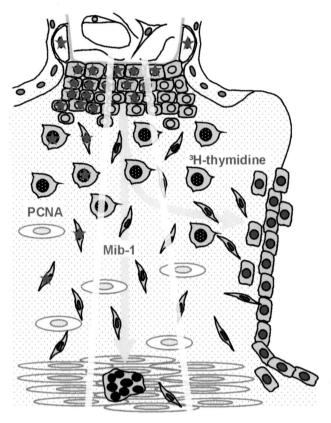

FIGURE 9.5. Schematic drawing of a first trimester anchoring villus (above) attached to the basal plate (center) by a cell column. Extravillous trophoblast cells (blue) derived from the cell column, mix with decidual cells (white) in the depth of the basal plate. The extravillous trophoblast cells are composed of highly invasive spindle-shaped cells and noninvasive large polygonal cells. Depending on the invasion route (interstitial: straight pink arrow; endovascular: curved pink arrow), trophoblast invasion results in the formation of multinucleated giant cells (bottom) or in a cluster of endovascular trophoblast lining uteroplacental arteries (right margin). The red asterisks indicate those trophoblast cells that are marked by the proliferation markers ^{3}H-thymidine, MIB-1/Ki-67, and anti–proliferating-cell nuclear antigen (PCNA). Note that depending on the biologic half-life of the respective antigen and depending on the stage of cell cycle that is identified by the marker, stained cells may even be found deeply invading the basal plate. Truly proliferative cells, marked by ^{3}H-thymidine, can only be found close to the anchoring villus. (*Source:* Modified from Kaufmann & Castellucci, 1997, with permission.)

increasing distance from the underlying basal lamina parallels increasing differentiation.

Stages of Extravillous Trophoblast Differentiation Within the Invasive Pathway

Upon leaving the cell cycle, extravillous trophoblast cells enter a complex differentiation pathway, resulting in various routes of differentiation. Based on the data available, this results in at least seven phenotypes of extravillous trophoblast (Fig. 9.6; also see Fig. 9.12):

Some of these phenotypes are passed subsequently during differentiation of extravillous trophoblast, for example:

- Proliferative stem cells
- Early postproliferative cells (distal compact layer of the cell columns)
- Small spindle-shaped extravillous trophoblast cells.

Others represent alternatives of final differentiation, for example:

- Large polygonal extravillous trophoblast (X-cells)
- Multinucleated trophoblastic giant cells
- Placental site giant cells

- Endovascular trophoblast (including intramural and intraarterial trophoblast).

The various phenotypes shall be defined in some more detail:

Proliferative Stem Cells

These comprise all polar trophoblast cells resting on the basal lamina of cell columns. They are weakly to moderately reactive for cytokeratin 7 (Fig. 9.6A,B). Comparison of data on ^{3}H-thymidine incorporation, as well as Ki-67/MIB-1 and PCNA positivity demonstrate that these are proliferating stem cells but that not all of the cells are actually in the cell cycle (Kosanke et al., 1998). Rather, with advancing gestation the number of cells within the cycle seems to decrease, whereas the number of G_0-cells seems to increase.

The cells of the proliferative layer as well as the postproliferative cells of the next few layers express zona occludens proteins (ZO-1 and occludin) (Marzioni et al., 2001). This suggests the presence of tight junctions in this area. Their function may be to guarantee a tight maternofetal barrier in an area where the syncytiotrophoblast

FIGURE 9.6. Trophoblast cell types in the invasive pathway. av: anchoring villus; cc: cell column; bp: basal plate; pb: placental bed. A: Staining with an antibody against cytokeratin 7 reveals the localization of five different phenotypes of extravillous trophoblast along the invasive pathway, including proliferative and early postproliferative cells (both enlarged in part B), large polygonal cells (enlarged in part C), small spindle-shaped cells (enlarged in part D) and multinucleated giant cells (enlarged in part E). Note the long, filiform profiles of small spindle-shaped EVT, which hardly can be identified as trophoblast cells, in the upper third of part A. They easily can escape the observers' attention. B: The proliferative cells comprise the upper row of cells in direct contact with the basement membrane of anchoring villus. They are followed by a compact cluster of early postproliferative daughter cells. C: A large polygonal trophoblast cell, embedded in ample unstained extracellular matrix (ECM). Note the huge, polyploid nucleus. D: Small spindle-shaped trophoblast cells are surrounded by only little ECM and are in close contact with cytokeratin-negative endometrial cells. The various spot-like cytokeratin reactivities in this picture correspond to cross and oblique sections of the same cell type. E: Multinucleated giant cells are characterized by clusters of nuclei surrounded by ample cytoplasm that only focally shows cytokeratin 7–immunoreactivity. A: ×160; B–D: ×770. (*Source:* From Kemp et al., 2002, with permission.)

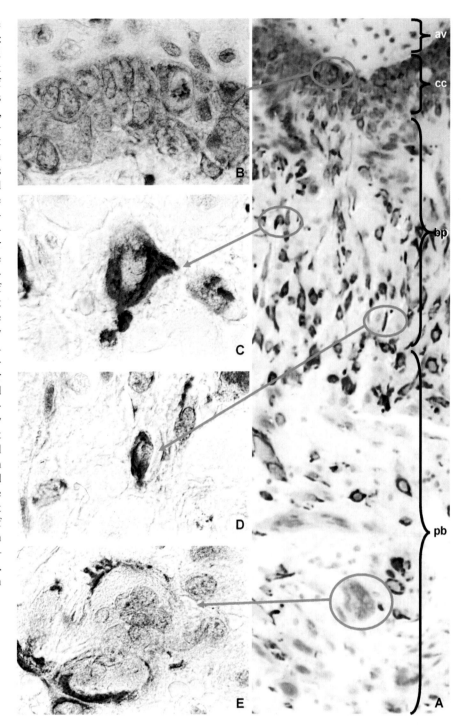

as barrier is interrupted by a cellular epithelium with intercellular clefts.

Early Postproliferative Cells

From the second layer of trophoblast cells distally, the cells very likely have left the cell cycle. There are no indications such as mitotic figures, ^{3}H-thymidine positivity, or BrdU positivity, that after leaving the basal lamina they still stay in the cycle. As described above, positivity for other immunohistochemical proliferation markers (Mib-1 or PCNA, Fig. 9.5) is due to the fact that the respective antigens persist also beyond the cell cycle. It is a question of definition how far peripherally into the invasive pathway cells are subsumed under the heading "early postproliferative cells." According to our definition (Kemp et al., 2002) trophoblast cells belong to this type when they (1) have left the basal lamina; (2) still form a compact cluster of cells, so-called cell columns; and (3) are not separated by light-microscopically visible amounts of extracellular matrix. This differentiation stage, too, is weakly to moderately immunoreactive for cytokeratin 7 (Fig. 9.6A,B).

Small Spindle-Shaped Extravillous Trophoblast Cells

According to distribution, structure, and expression of integrins, ECM, and proteases, these are the truly invasive extravillous trophoblast cells (Kemp et al., 2002). In spite of their moderate to strong immunoreactivity for cytokeratin 7 (Fig. 9.6A,D) these cells are inconspicuous and easily escape the observer's attention. Due to their spindle-shaped to filiform structure they may easily be misinterpreted as tangential sections of larger types of extravillous cells. The cells prevail in the first and second trimester of pregnancy and are only rarely found at term (see Fig. 9.17). Different from all other phenotypes, they do not accumulate in a certain layer of the invasive pathway but rather are homogeneously distributed from the distal parts of cell columns until the first third of the myometrium. Similar to invasive tumor cells (Friedl & Brocker, 2000), their shape reflects invasiveness; movement across their host tissues forces these cells to adapt their morphology and to achieve bipolar, spindle-shaped bodies. Interestingly, those invasive trophoblast cells emerging from villous explants in vitro under the influence of insulin-like growth factor-I (IGF-I) (see Cytokines and Hormones Controlling Differentiation of Extravillous Trophoblast, below) showed the same spindle-shaped phenotype (Aplin et al., 2000). Immunocytochemistry suggests, that they secrete only a little ECM and expose mostly integrins not matching the surrounding ECM (integrin-ECM mismatch) (Kemp et al., 2002). DNA measurements suggest that these cells are diploid to tetraploid (Zybina et al., 2002, 2004).

Large Polygonal Extravillous Trophoblast Cells

This is the structurally most impressive cell type within the population of extravillous trophoblast: large, polygonal, mostly basophilic cell bodies, with large irregular, hyperchromatic nuclei (Fig. 9.6 A,C). Their size and intense staining were the reason that these were the first published extravillous trophoblast cells (X-cells, Scipiades & Burg, 1930). According to Kemp et al. (2002) and Zybina et al. (2002, 2004), they are derived from diploid (spindle-shaped?) extravillous trophoblast cells by polyploidization (Fig. 9.7). Several findings suggest that they are less invasive or noninvasive (Kemp et al., 2002):

- Their number increases with advancing gestation.
- They accumulate usually in the superficial layers of the basal plate and are much less frequent in deeper layers.
- In basal plates of term pregnancies they are by far the dominating trophoblast cell type.
- They embed themselves in large amounts of ECM (laminins, collagen IV, vitronectin, heparan sulfate, fibronectins, vitronectin) and expose the exactly matching integrins along their cell surfaces.
- They can be found deeply in the uterine wall, embedded in large amounts of ECM, even years after the last pregnancy.

Taken together, these findings suggest, that polyploidization and transformation of spindle-shaped trophoblast into large polygonal trophoblast is a mechanism to reduce invasiveness.

Multinucleated Trophoblastic Giant Cells

These are multinucleated trophoblastic elements found in the depth of the basal plate (Fig. 9.6A,E). Often they accumulate in a thin layer close to the endometrial–myometrial border. Their number decreases when pregnancy advances. Attention was first directed to these elements by Kölliker (1861), who called them "Riesenzellen" and "vielkernige Riesenzellen." Similar multinucleated trophoblastic masses have been described in the junctional zone of several mammals. Terms such as **multinuclear giant cells**, **wandering cells**, **migratory cells**, **megalokaryocytes**, and **diplokaryocytes** were employed (for reviews see Mossman, 1937, 1987; Boyd & Hamilton, 1970). Despite the fact that some earlier authors have questioned the fetal origin of these structures (Keiffer, 1928; Park, 1959), there is now agreement concerning their trophoblastic nature based on their immunoreactivity for various cytokeratin isoforms. Unfortunately, they are often negative for cytokeratin 7, the most suitable marker for all uninuclear trophoblast (Fig. 9.6A,E).

There are still some doubts about whether or not multinucleated giant cells can be formed by syncytial fusion of extravillous cytotrophoblast throughout pregnancy. Data by Winterhager et al. (2000) have shown connexin 40 expression by deeply invasive extravillous trophoblast cells as soon as the latter aggregated in clusters (Hellmann et al., 1995). Connexin 40 is a gap junction molecule and formation of gap junctions is a well-studied prerequisite for syncytial fusion (Winterhager et al., 1984). These data in context with the large numbers of multinucleated trophoblastic giant cells in the superficial myometrial parts of the uterine wall (Pijnenborg et al., 1980; 1981) led us to suggest that syncytial fusion takes place preferably at the end of the invasive pathway. The view that multinucleation is a result of syncytial fusion rather than of endomitosis is further supported by the fact that signs of DNA-replication (^{3}H-thymidine incorporation, expres-

FIGURE 9.7. Summarizing overview of changes in the invasive pathway throughout pregnancy. The early postproliferative daughter cells of the cell columns differentiate into highly invasive small spindle-shaped cells. Their invasiveness is limited either by differentiation into ECM-secreting large polygonal EVT, or by syncytial fusion, forming multinucleated giant cells, or by apoptosis. In the first trimester, invasiveness is high since only a few cells undergo polyploidization forming large polygonal cells. In later stages of pregnancy, invasiveness gradually ceases since increasing numbers of spindle-shaped invasive trophoblast leaves the invasive pathway by polyploidization. Syncytial fusion resulting in multinucleated giant cells is a dominant mechanism for the limitation of invasiveness only in early pregnancy. Throughout pregnancy, apoptosis seems to be of marginal importance only. (*Source:* Modified from Kemp et al., 2002, with permission.)

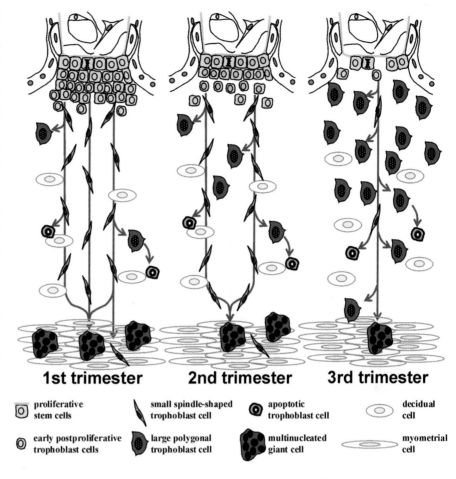

1st trimester   **2nd trimester**   **3rd trimester**

proliferative stem cells	small spindle-shaped trophoblast cell	apoptotic trophoblast cell	decidual cell
early postproliferative trophoblast cells	large polygonal trophoblast cell	multinucleated giant cell	myometrial cell

sion of PCNA or Ki-67 antigen) have never been observed in this deep invasion zone.

Residual extravillous syncytiotrophoblast should not be confused with the multinucleated trophoblastic giant cells. In early pregnancy the nonvillous parts of the placenta (future chorion laeve, primary chorionic plate, and trophoblastic shell) are mostly composed of syncytiotrophoblast; its relative amount in all nonvillous locations is steeply decreasing toward term. In third-trimester pregnancies it is found in only a few locations, all of which face the intervillous space. These comprise largely degenerative syncytial plaques covering small spots of the intervillous surfaces of the chorionic plate, the basal plate, and sometimes even parts of cell columns, cell islands, and septa. In the course of pregnancy, most of this extravillous syncytiotrophoblast degenerates and is replaced by fibrinoid or sometimes even by maternal endothelium evading uteroplacental veins (see below).

Placental Site Giant Cells

This term plays an important role in placental pathology, where these cells are of great diagnostic value for the histopathologist when studying curettings; however, it has never been clearly defined in placental cell biology. The fetal/trophoblastic origin was proven by Khudr et al. (1973), but it remains an open question whether these cells are mononuclear (as extravillous cytotrophoblast) or in part multinucleated cells (Pijnenborg, 1980).

Sauramo (1961) had already characterized these cells from histologic and histochemical studies as cell populations that undergo frequent degeneration and that form, within the extraplacental membranes and placental floor, a separate compartment of cytotrophoblast. Typical placental site giant cells are often vacuolated and sometimes they appear degenerative. They may also be identical with what Yeh et al. (1989) described as a separate extravillous trophoblastic entity, the vacuolated cytotrophoblast. Other historical terms are chorionic giant cells, wandering cells, migratory cells, and megalokaryocytes (for review see Boyd & Hamilton, 1970). Thliveris and Speroff (1977) found an increased amount of fibrinoid deposition around these cells in membranes from preeclamptic women. Wynn (1967a) also noted their frequent or regular association with eosinophilic fibrin-like deposits.

Pathologists are generally reluctant to make the diagnosis of intrauterine pregnancy merely from the presence of extravillous trophoblast cells (X cells) and in the absence of villi. To satisfy this demand for characterization of the placental site, O'Connor and Kurman (1988a,b) used the presence of human placental lactogen (hPL) contained within placental site cells and thus demonstrated in relevant cases that an intrauterine gestation existed in curettings when an ectopic gestation needed to be ruled out.

In our opinion, placental site giant cells are highly differentiated, probably already degenerative extravillous trophoblast cells. This view is further supported by several publications dealing with the placental site trophoblastic tumor (PSTT) (Berger et al., 1984; Young et al., 1988; Duncan & Mazur, 1989; Larsen et al., 1991). This rare variant of trophoblastic disease derives from placental site giant cells and was unequivocally described to be composed of intermediate trophoblast, equivalent to extravillous cytotrophoblast.

Endovascular Trophoblast

This is the summarizing term for all extravillous trophoblast cells found

- within the walls of uteroplacental arteries and veins (**intramural trophoblast**) where it replaces media smooth muscle cells and other vascular wall structures, and
- within the lumens of uteroplacental arteries (**intraarterial trophoblast**) where it either forms a new surface lining replacing maternal endothelium or forms big, multicellular plugs, partly or completely occluding the arterial lumens.

As will discussed later (see Uteroplacental Vessels), endovascular trophoblast is derived from interstitial extravillous trophoblast and represents a side-route of trophoblast invasion (Fig. 9.5).

One Stem Cell Origin for Villous Syncytiotrophoblast and the Extravillous Trophoblast?

Up to now, no obvious differences have been described between the proliferating stem cells of

- the extravillous trophoblast cells that rest on the basal laminas separating anchoring villi and cell columns, and
- villous cytotrophoblast resting on the basal laminas of all other villi.

This refers to all of the following data for expression of receptors and integrins, matrix secretion and endocrine secretion, as well as for major histocompatibility complex I (MHC-I) expression (for review see Kaufmann & Castellucci, 1997). Because of this, it seems justified to speculate that all trophoblast cells resting on the basal lamina separating placental trophoblast and fetoplacental mesenchyme (Fig. 9.1), independent of their location, represent a uniform population of trophoblastic stem cells. This

would apply for the villous cytotrophoblast, the basal layers of proliferating stem cells in cell columns, cell islands, chorionic plate, and chorion laeve.

The future fate of these stem cells, whether they fuse to form syncytiotrophoblast or whether they acquire a migratory or invasive extravillous phenotype very likely depends on surrounding microenvironmental factors (Fig. 9.8), such as

- the presence or absence of contact to maternal blood;
- polar or apolar exposition to extracellular matrix molecules;
- the presence or absence of an intact syncytiotrophoblast covering.

In mouse placental development respective transcription factors directing the cells in the one or other differentiation pathway have been identified (Anson-Cartwright et al., 2000; Cross et al., 2003; Hughes et al., 2004). For human placental development, experimental proof for the one-stem-cell hypothesis is still missing; however, the hypothesis is in agreement with many histologic and experimental findings.

- Peripheral villi, which become embedded in maternal blood clot, transform into cell islands or cell columns, showing degeneration of the covering syncytiotrophoblast and extravillous transformation of the residual cytotrophoblast (see Fibrinoid, below). The same extravillous transformation of trophoblast cells was observed when villous explants were cultivated on or in fibrin, collagens, or matrigel (Castellucci et al., 1990; Genbacev et al., 1991, 1992; Vicovac et al., 1993, 1995a). Interestingly, only first-trimester villi rather than second- or third-trimester villi showed this in vitro behavior.
- In contrast, when cultivating villous explants in tissue culture medium (Castellucci, personal communication) or on agarose (Vicovac et al., 1995b) the trophoblast maintained its villous phenotype.

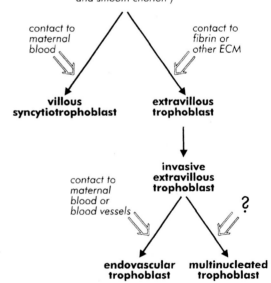

FIGURE 9.8. Factors controlling the various routes of differentiation of trophoblast. (*Source:* Modified from Kaufmann & Castellucci, 1997, with permission.)

Proliferation studies in anchoring villi (Kosanke, 1994) make it very likely that not all daughter cells derived from the proliferative zones of cell columns enter the invasive pathway. Rather, a subset of these cells seems to migrate laterally along the anchoring villi, thus coming into a villous position. These cells finally may be transformed into a syncytiotrophoblast. Accordingly, the stem cells of the cell columns would have a double function, contributing to trophoblast invasion and acting as a growth zone for villous trophoblast of anchoring villi.

Cytokines and Hormones Controlling Differentiation of Extravillous Trophoblast

We focus here on oncogene products, growth factor receptors, and growth factors as well as hormones, which show obvious relations to the various stages of the invasive pathway. Several of those seem to be involved in autocrine loops as well as paracrine loops between extravillous trophoblast and its neighboring tissues. For the discussion of potential interactions between hormones and trophoblast differentiation along the invasive pathway we also refer to the review by Malassine and Cronier (2002). The paper by Islami et al. (2001) specifically addresses the potential influence of human chorionic gonadotropin (hCG) on trophoblast invasion.

EGFR: Epidermal growth factor receptor encoded by the proto-oncogene *c-erbB*-1, is only expressed in those few proximal layers of trophoblastic cell columns that also express proliferation markers (Mühlhauser et al., 1993; Duello et al., 1994; Johki et al., 1994) (Fig. 9.9A). Its best known ligand, epidermal growth factor (EGF), is a potent epithelial mitogen. Moreover, its stimulatory influence on trophoblast invasion has been stressed (Bass et al., 1994). Epidermal growth factor is produced by numerous tissues.

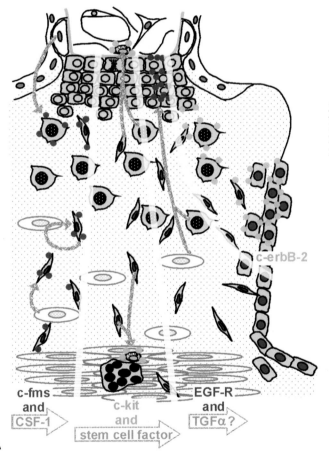

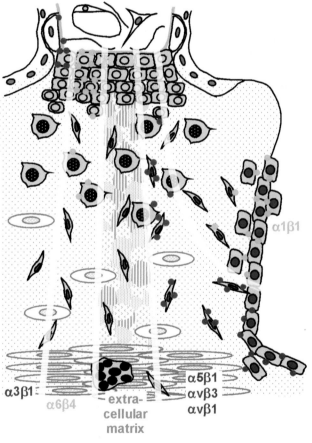

FIGURE 9.9. A: The expression of some growth factor receptors is symbolized by red or yellow dots. Secretion of the respective ligands is indicated by red arrows. These arrows suggest that the invasive pathway of extravillous trophoblast is controlled by autocrine and paracrine regulatory loops. B: Integrin (red and yellow dots) and ECM expression (green) along the invasive pathway. α3β1 and α6β4 integrins are expressed by the proliferative phenotype of extravillous trophoblast. When switching to the invasive phenotype, the above "epithelial" integrins are gradually replaced by "interstitial" integrins such as α5β1, αvβ1, and αvβ3 and finally by α1β1, the latter marking only the deepest cells in the pathway. In the center, the secretion patterns of ECM are depicted. The proliferative phenotype shows polar (basal lamina) or absent secretion of ECM. The invasive trophoblast cells, expressing interstitial integrins, embed themselves in apolarly secreted ECM of different types. (*Source*: Modified from Kaufmann & Castellucci, 1997, with permission.)

Its secretion by extravillous trophoblast has been discussed, suggesting autocrine/paracrine regulatory loops (Hofmann et al., 1992). In contrast, Loke and King (1995) suggested that local secretion at the implantation site is less likely; rather, these authors favor **transforming growth factor-α** (TGF-α) to be the more likely ligand for EGFR. Transforming growth factor is known to have the same mitogenic effects on trophoblast as EGF. It is likely to be secreted by decidual stromal cells as well as by all trophoblast populations (Lysiak et al., 1993).

C-erbB-2: The receptor encoded by the proto-oncogene *c-erbB*-2 is thought to cooperate with other receptors of the *erbB* family in neuregulin/heregulin-mediated signaling (Holmes et al., 1992; Peles et al., 1992; Carraway & Cantley, 1994). This receptor shows a reciprocal expression pattern when compared to EGFR (Fig. 9.9A). It is expressed at the surfaces of all those extravillous trophoblast cells that are negative for EGFR (Mühlhauser et al., 1993; Jokhi et al., 1994). It thus characterizes all differentiated and invasive stages.

HB-EGF: Recent data by Romero's group have shed a new light on the importance of the EGF receptor family in trophoblast differentiation (Leach et al., 2004). The authors have studied the effects of the multifunctional heparin-binding EGF-like growth factor (HB-EGF), which binds to *erbB1* and *erbB4* of the EGF-receptor family. HB-EGF is downregulated in placentas of women with preeclampsia. The addition of HB-EGF during explant culture of first-trimester chorionic villi and during culture of a trophoblast cell line did not alter trophoblast proliferation, but rather enhanced extravillous trophoblast differentiation and invasive activity; expression of α6 integrins decreased to the benefit of α1 integrins. The authors concluded that erbB-mediated autocrine and paracrine signaling by HB-EGF or other EGF family members induces cytotrophoblast differentiation to an invasive phenotype.

C-fms: Also, the expression of the gene product of the oncogene *c-fms*, the receptor for **colony stimulating factor-1** (CSF-1), supports the concept of a differentiation gradient. According to Johki et al. (1993), it is strongly expressed in early invasive stages but weaker during deeper invasion including the endovascular trophoblast (Fig. 9.9A). The corresponding growth factor, CSF-1 can be derived from three different sources (Fig. 9.9A), from villous trophoblast, from endometrial cells (Shorter et al., 1992), and from invasive extravillous trophoblast cells themselves (Hamilton et al., 1995). It is a potent mitogen. Moreover, it is thought to upregulate gelatinase B and tissue inhibitor of metalloproteinase-1 (TIMP-1), both of which are important parameters of invasiveness (Hamilton et al., 1995).

C-kit: Stem cell factor also known as c-kit ligand, another blood cell mitogen, is expressed by invasive extravillous trophoblast cells (Sharkey et al., 1994) (Fig. 9.9A); the receptor for this growth factor, c-kit is expressed by villous macrophages and by the large granular lymphocytes [endometrial natural killer (NK) cells] of the junctional zone (Fig. 9.9A).

TGF-βR: Receptors for transforming growth factor-β have been detected in a variety of cell types at the human implantation site, and the cytokine **TGF-β** itself is abundantly present in decidua, mostly derived from decidual NK cells (Saito et al., 1993a; Loke & King, 1995). Transforming growth factor-β has been implicated as an immunosuppressive factor in decidua by modulating the response of maternal leukocytes to trophoblast (for review see Loke & King, 1995). In contrast to interferon-γ (IFN-γ), TGF-β has been observed to downregulate surface expression of MHC class I antigen (Geiser et al., 1993). The cytokine also restricts trophoblast invasion by downregulation of collagenase secretion and induction of TIMPs (for review, see Loke & King, 1995). The inhibitory effect of TGF-β on trophoblast invasion is mediated by **endoglin**, a member of the TGF-β receptor complex. Transient upregulation of endoglin expression takes place during transition from the proliferative to the invasive phenotype; the addition of endoglin antibodies or of antisense endoglin oligonucleotides to extravillous trophoblast in vitro stimulated the migratory/invasive behavior (Caniggia et al., 1997). Transforming growth factor-β has been reported to enhance the secretion of fibronectins by trophoblast cells in vitro (Feinberg et al., 1994); to upregulate expression of integrins, which make the cells more "adhesive"; to upregulate protease inhibitors such as TIMP-1 and plasminogen activator inhibitor-1 (PAI-1) (for review see Chakraborty et al., 2002); and to upregulate E cadherin expression, which facilitates cell–cell adhesion and impairs cell motility (Karmakar & Das, 2004). Interestingly, TGF-β can be stored extracellularly by binding to **decorin**, an ECM proteoglycan (Xu et al., 2002); the latter has been abundantly found in the decidua (Lysiak et al., 1995). All these observations suggest that TGF-β is a modulator of trophoblast invasion. The secretion of TGF-β seems to be controlled by oxygen via hypoxia-inducible factor-1α (HIF-1α) (Caniggia et al., 2000; Caniggia & Winter, 2002). The same authors suggest that hypoxia via elevated HIF-1α expression leads to TGF-β overexpression, the latter resulting in inhibition of trophoblast differentiation and trophoblast invasion (Caniggia et al., 1999; Caniggia & Winter, 2002). As will be discussed below (see Oxygen-Mediated Regulation of the Invasive Pathway), the interactions between hypoxia and trophoblast invasion are still a matter of controversy.

Transforming growth factor-α, in contrast to TGF-β, appears to be a stimulator of trophoblastic growth in vitro, possibly acting via EGFR (Filla et al., 1993; Lysiak et al., 1993) (see above).

Tumor necrosis factor-α (TNF-α) is a cytotoxic cytokine that according to in vitro data may act to limit trophoblast invasion (Hunt, 1989). The **TNF-receptor I**, which upon ligand binding is able to initiate apoptosis, is expressed by invasive extravillous trophoblast cells (own unpublished observations). Correspondingly, early stages of apoptosis can be found in the same cells (Huppertz et al., 1998a). Even though TNF-α–messenger RNA (mRNA) has been found in a variety of cells at the implantation site, the most likely source for TNF-α protein are decidual macrophages and endometrial NK cells (Vince et al., 1992; Loke & King, 1995; Pijnenborg et al., 1998). Respective cytotoxic effects of macrophages on invasive trophoblast cells are further underlined by the fact that, in preeclampsia, large parts of the spiral arteries are infiltrated by macrophages and do not show trophoblast invasion (Reister et al., 1999). In contrast, in normal pregnancy the utero-placental arteries invaded by trophoblast, and rarely show intramural macrophages. Subsequent in vitro experiments by the same author (Reister et al., 2001) further underlined the notion that activated macrophages induce apoptosis of invasive extravillous trophoblast. Different from earlier assumptions, this is not only a TNF-α effect. Rather, induction of trophoblast apoptosis is a deleterious combination of

• TNF-α/TNF-receptor 1 interaction, with
• local tryptophan depletion by macrophage-secreted indolamine 2,3-dioxygenase (IDO) (see Fig. 9.35).

Interestingly, the preeclampsia-specific increase of macrophages described by Reister et al. (1999) seems to be restricted to the maternal arterial walls, whereas the number of maternal macrophages in the interstitium even seems to be reduced (Burk et al., 2001). (For further details see the sections Macrophages and Uteroplacental Vessels, below.) Tumor necrosis factor-α was shown to be expressed also by invasive extravillous trophoblast cells, the level of expression decreasing with advancing pregnancy and thus correlating with invasiveness of the cells (Pijnenborg et al., 1998). These data suggest that invasive trophoblast cells may exert direct cytotoxic effects during invasion of their host tissue.

HGF: Hepatocyte growth factor is secreted by placental villous stroma (Kauma et al., 1999) and by human decidua (Choy et al., 2004) and acts in a paracrine manner on trophoblast cells that express the HGF receptor **c-met**. In vitro studies by Kauma et al. (1999), Nasu et al. (2000), and Dokras et al. (2001) revealed that HGF significantly increased in vitro invasiveness of trophoblast cell lines. Moreover, in preeclampsia, reduced or absent villous stromal HGF expression was found, whereas expression of the receptor in extravillous trophoblast was unchanged (Nasu et al., 2000). According to Cartwright et al. (1999) the HGF effect on trophoblast invasion is closely linked to invasion, furthering nitric oxide (NO) secretion of extravillous trophoblast.

IGF-I: Insulin-like growth factor-I is secreted among others by villous mesenchyme. In vitro studies by Aplin and coworkers (2000) revealed that serum-free conditioned medium from placental first-trimester fibroblasts stimulated cytotrophoblast to detach from cell columns and to invade the neighboring extracellular matrix. Removal of IGF-I from the conditioned medium decreased the invasive potential, whereas the addition of IGF-I to culture medium increased invasiveness. In contrast, the addition of TGF-β blocked invasiveness completely (see above). These data suggest paracrine interactions between the mesenchyme of anchoring villi and cytotrophoblast in cell columns. A respective paracrine control of trophoblast invasion by stromal cytokines such as IGF-I would be self-limiting because the signal diminishes with increasing invasive depth.

VEGF, PlGF, Ang-2: Finally, angiogenic factors, such as vascular endothelial growth factor (VEGF), placenta growth factor (PlGF), and angiopoietin-2 (Ang-2) are thought to be involved in the regulation of the extravillous pathway. All three factors are expressed by invasive trophoblast (Zhou et al., 2002, 2003a,b). PlGF was found to promote proliferation of extravillous trophoblast but not invasive behavior in vitro (Athanassiades & Lala, 1998). The closely related VEGF is secreted not only by trophoblast but also by decidual cells and decidual macrophages, whereas the VEGF-receptor **flt-1** is expressed by extravillous trophoblast cells (Ahmed et al., 1995). Vascular endothelial growth factor was supposed to be a chemoattractant for the invading trophoblast cells (Lash et al., 1999, 2003). Recent data by Anteby et al. (2004) suggest that VEGF is involved in the control of trophoblastic protease secretion. Moreover, Zhou et al. (2003b) provided in vitro evidence that VEGF, PlGF, and Ang-2 together may be involved in maintenance and turnover of uteroplacental vessels.

Kisspeptin-10, a newly described dekapeptide derived from the translation product of the gene *KISS-1* was recently described to be a potent regulator of trophoblast invasion (Bilban et al., 2004). The *KISS-1* gene is only expressed in villous trophoblast. *KISS-1* receptor was also found in the extravillous trophoblast, suggesting paracrine loops. Kisspeptin-10 inhibited trophoblast migration in vitro in an explant as well as in a transwell assay, but did not affect proliferation. Suppressed motility was paralleled with suppressed gelatinolytic activity suggesting a Kisspeptin-10 effect on matrix metalloproteinase (MMP) secretion.

Interleukins (ILs) are involved at different levels of the control of the invasion process. Their role as proinflammatory (IL-2) or antiinflammatory cytokines (IL-4, -6, -10, and -13), triggering the communication among the various maternal immune cells at the implantation site, is well studied. Less is known about the direct effects on trophoblast cells (for review see Loke & King, 1995;

Bischof et al., 2000a,b). Among others **IL-1** and **IL-6** are secreted by the trophoblast cells themselves and act in an autocrine manner as stimulators of various aspects of extravillous trophoblast differentiation (for review, see Das et al., 2002). Interleukin-1β was found to counteract the effects of TGF-β (see above) by downregulating E-cadherin expression and cell–cell adhesion and thus stimulating cellular invasiveness (Karmakar & Das, 2004a). By contrast, **IL-12** seems to inhibit trophoblast invasion by upregulating MMPs and downregulating TIMPs (see below; Karmakar et al., 2004b).

T$_3$: Triiodothyronine has been known for a long time to play a crucial role in the maintenance of early pregnancy. Moreover, thyroid hormones seem to be involved in maldevelopment of placental villous trees (cf. Hormones as Regulators of Villous Development in Chapter 7). The mechanisms by which thyroid hormones interact with placental development still remain to be elucidated. Recent publications give some hints that an effect of T$_3$ on trophoblast invasion may be the missing link: extravillous trophoblast expresses thyroid hormone receptors (TR) (Barber et al., 2005). T$_3$ in vitro increased the expression of MMPs, fibronectins, and integrin α5β1 (Oki et al., 2004), and it suppressed apoptosis of extravillous trophoblast by a variety of mechanisms (Laoag-Fernandez et al., 2004). All of these findings are consistent with the hypothesis that T$_3$ promotes trophoblast invasion, but they do not clearly prove it yet.

Extracellular Matrix Secretion Along the Invasive Pathway

Extravillous trophoblast cells secrete large amounts of a highly heterogeneous ECM along their invasive pathway. The latter comprises fibronectin isoforms, collagen IV, laminins, vitronectin, and heparan sulfate in a patchy pattern summarized as matrix-type fibrinoid (see Fibrinoid, below). Secretion of ECM by extravillous trophoblast is different from ECM secretion in other epithelia (Frank et al., 1994, 1995; Huppertz et al., 1996, 1998d; Kemp et al., 2002):

- The first layer of still proliferative trophoblast cells behave like epithelial cells and secret ECM in polar fashion as a basal lamina along their basal plasmalemma with collagen IV (Fig. 9.10A) and laminins (Fig. 9.10B) as dominant ECM molecules. Similar to other stratified epithelia, the following layers of early postproliferative cells completely downregulate ECM secretion (Figs. 9.9B and 9.10).
- Different from other stratified epithelia, with advancing differentiation the cells again upregulate ECM secretion, now secreting in an apolar, patchy pattern. The resulting patches of ECM. Deeper in the invasive pathway they increase in number and size, are attached in an apolar pattern to the plasmalemma all around the cell.
- Preliminary data (Kemp et al., 2002) suggest that the highly invasive spindle-shaped trophoblast cells secret only a little ECM, mostly composed of oncofetal fibronectin fibers embedded in a homogeneous matrix of vitronectin and heparan sulfate.
- By contrast, the large, polygonal noninvasive trophoblast cells embed themselves in large amounts of ECM composed of at least three different types of patches: (1) laminins and collagen IV; (2) vitronectin and heparan sulfate; (3) fibronectins, mostly of the non-oncofetal isoforms, embedded in vitronectin and heparan sulfate.

Extracellular Matrix Receptors (Integrins)

The extravillous trophoblast cells embedded in the self-secreted extracellular matrix described above, express the respective ECM receptors (integrins). Depending on the type of cell, the expression and distribution patterns of integrins do not always match with the ECM molecules accumulated around.

Integrins are heterodimeric integral membrane proteins. They act as receptors for ECM molecules (for review, see Humphries, 1990). The functional importance of integrin-binding to ECM molecules has been shown in vitro by blocking them specifically by antibodies which resulted in loss of trophoblast cell adhesion to the ECM (Librach et al., 1991a; Burrows et al., 1995; Irving and Lala, 1995; for review see Burrows et al., 1997).

The following integrins have been described in extravillous trophoblast (for review see Aplin, 1993; Damsky et al., 1993; Kaufmann & Castellucci, 1997):

α3β1 integrin is a receptor for laminin that also localizes to focal contacts in cells cultured on other substrates; it seems to play a role in matrix deposition (DiPersio et al., 1995; Wu et al., 1995). α3β1 is only weakly expressed in villous trophoblast and in few of the most proximal, proliferative trophoblast cells of the cell columns, resting on the basal lamina of anchoring villi (Damsky et al., 1992; Kemp et al., 2002) (Fig. 9.9B).

α6β4 is the dominating integrin of the proliferative and early postproliferative subset of trophoblast (Aplin, 1991a, 1993; Damsky et al., 1992; Burrows et al., 1993a; Kemp et al., 2002). α6β4 integrin is the usual basal lamina receptor. It binds to laminin, which is then linked to collagen IV (Ruoslahti, 1991; Flug & Köpf-Maier, 1995). Its expression in trophoblast, interestingly, is not restricted to the basal trophoblastic surface of the most proximal cells, but rather can be found all around the trophoblast cells of the proximal half of the cell columns of first and second trimester pregnancies (Fig. 9.9B). Most of those are postproliferative cells that

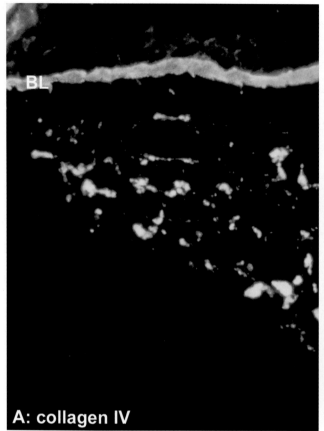

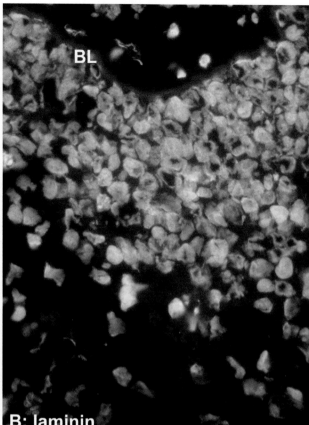

FIGURE 9.10. Immunohistochemistry of extracellular matrix molecules in trophoblastic cell columns. The anchoring villus (above) and the cell column (center and bottom) are separated by a clearly visible basal lamina (BL). A: The collagen IV antibody shows strong immunoreactivity (green) in the basal lamina and a spotwise reaction pattern among the early postprolifera-tive cells and deeper in the invasive pathway. B: The staining pattern of a laminin antibody (red, counterstained with the blue nuclear stain bisbenzimide) is comparable to that of collagen IV. Note the accumulation of spots of laminin in the deeper parts of the invasive pathway (bottom). ×300.

do not express ECM at all. In term pregnancies with reduced proliferative activities of extravillous tropho-blast, also the α6β4 expression is more restrained. In certain mature cell columns (compare Fig. 9.49B) it may completely be lost since only differentiated cells expressing interstitial integrins exist peripherally from the basal lamina.

α5β1, a fibronectin receptor, is upregulated in the same zone where α6β4 expression is downregulated (transition from the compact cluster of early postproliferative cells to loosely arranged, ECM-secreting cells of the invasive phenotype). Its expression is kept constant until the deepest stages of invasion (Fig. 9.9B).

α1β1, a receptor for laminin and collagens I and IV, is turned on slightly later (Fig. 9.9B) (Aplin, 1991a; Fisher et al., 1991; Damsky et al., 1992, 1994; Kemp et al., 2002).

αvβ3 and αvβ5, according to in vitro findings by Irving et al. (1995), are also expressed by the invasive phenotype (Fig. 9.9B).

Integrin Switch

The gradual switch from the basal lamina receptor α6β4 to interstitial receptors such as α5β1, α1β1, and αv integ-rins, in normal intrauterine pregnancies is characteristic of the transition from the proliferative to the invasive phenotype of extravillous trophoblast and has been called the integrin switch. It is still an open question whether in this transitional zone all cells stepwise downregulate α6β4 and upregulate interstitial integrins. The data by Kemp et al. (2002) suggest another possibility. They show that the small spindle-shaped trophoblast cells only express interstitial integrins, independent of the ECM they are attached to. By contrast, the large, polygonal trophoblast cells seem to coexpress all integrins, depend-ing on the matrix they are attached to. If this holds true, the integrin switch would reflect the numerical balance of cells found in the respective area.

The integrin switch has raised considerable interest since it seems to be involved in the regulation of trophoblast invasion in the placental junctional zone (Zhou et al., 1993; Damsky et al., 1993; Lim et al., 1995). Bischof et al. (1995) found α6 expression by extravillous trophoblast to be positively correlated with gelatinase secretion, whereas the secretion ceased as soon as α5 expression was turned on. Cause and effect, however, are not clear. Irving and Lala (1995) stated that blocking of α5β1 by specific antibodies inhibited trophoblast migration in vitro. It is likely, however, that the results of such in vitro studies strongly depend on unknown experimental parameters; thus, Librach et al. (1991a) came to opposite experimental findings. In their in vitro experiments, antibody blocking of the α1β1 integrin impaired trophoblast invasion, whereas antibody blocking of α5β1 even stimulated invasion. Data by Ilic et al. (2001) on the focal adhesion kinase (FAK) underline the importance of integrins for the invasion process; FAK transduces signals from the ECM into the cell. Inhibition of FAK expression reduced invasiveness of cytotrophoblast in to ECM in vitro.

α5β1/α1β1 Balance

These and other findings suggest that the balance of α5β1 and α1β1 expression may be critical for the regulation of trophoblast invasion:

- The importance of this α5/α1 integrin balance is further underlined by recent data concerning the interactions between **antiphospholipid antibodies** and trophoblast invasion. Aminophospholipid antibodies, anticardiolipin antibodies, and antiphospholipid antibodies in lupus anticoagulant were shown to inhibit trophoblast invasion in vitro and in vivo (McIntyre, 2003; Bose et al., 2004). The antibodies primarily seem to affect endovascular trophoblast invasion rather than interstitial invasion (Sebire et al., 2002). Interestingly, antibodies obtained from the same patients decreased α1 integrin expression by cytotrophoblast in vitro, but increased α5 expression (di Simone et al., 2002).
- Also, insulin-like growth factor binding protein-1, **IGFBP-1**, may be involved in the control of integrin expression. Irving and Lala (1994, 1995) have shown that decidua-derived IGFBP-1 binding to α5β1 by means of its arginine-glycin-aspartic acid (RGD)-sequence (and thus blocking the integrin for other ligands?) promoted invasion, an effect that was inhibited by the presence of α5β1 blocking antibodies.
- Tumor necrosis factor-α, **TNFα**, a secretory product of decidual macrophages, upregulates the expression of integrin α1β1 (Defilippi et al., 1992). According to Irving and Lala (1995), **TGF-β** upregulates expression of integrin α5β1 and reduces the migratory effects of invasive trophoblast. Finally, according to the latter group, IGF-II has no obvious effect on integrin expression, but stimulates migration.

Even though partly contradictory, these data suggest that the balance between α5β1 integrin including its ligands and α1β1 including its ligands may be important for regulation of trophoblast invasion. Imbalance may result in insufficient invasion and is discussed as a basic pathogenetic event in preeclampsia (Damsky et al., 1993).

Other Cell Adhesion Molecules and Gap Junction Molecules

E-cadherin is an adhesion molecule that establishes cell-to-cell contacts. Proliferative cells of the proximal cell columns express this adhesion molecule (Fig. 9.11A), whereas it is turned off with increasing invasiveness (MacCalman et al., 1995; Winterhager et al., 1996). In endovascular cytotrophoblast expression it is again upregulated. In tumor pathology, reduction of E-cadherin expression is regarded as an indicator of premalignant changes of epithelial tumors (Pizarro et al., 1995). This notion is further supported by the fact that antiphospholipid antibodies, which decrease trophoblast invasiveness in vitro, at the same time upregulate E-cadherin expression of these cells (di Simone et al., 2002).

N-CAM, the neural cell adhesion molecule, is not only responsible for cell-to-cell contacts but also for matrix adhesion. In early pregnancy, N-CAM–positive extravillous trophoblast cells are abundant in all parts of the basal plate including intraarterial trophoblast cells (Fig. 9.11A); only the intramural trophoblast cells of the arteries stained weaker if at all (King & Blankenship, 1995, findings in the rhesus monkey). With advancing pregnancy, N-CAM expression is restricted to the more proximal, proliferative phenotype. Burrows et al. (1994) confirmed these findings for the human extravillous trophoblast.

Connexin 40 is similarly distributed to E-cadherin. Connexins are gap junction molecules that support cell-to-cell communication and seem to be important for cell proliferation and differentiation. Among the connexins studied so far, only connexin 40 (cx40) has been found in extravillous trophoblast (Winterhager et al., 2000). Its expression is most prominent in the proximal, proliferative parts of the cell columns (Fig. 9.11A) and cell islands where the cells are still in contact with each other (Hellmann et al., 1995; von Ostau et al., 1995; Winterhager et al., 1996). With transition to the invasive phenotype, cx40 is downregulated. Deeply invasive groups of aggregated trophoblast cells again express cx40, whereas endovascular trophoblast cells probably do not (Winterhager et al., 1996). (For further details concerning the role of cell adhesion molecules for the vascular invasion see Trophoblast-Endothelial Adhesion Mechanisms).

CEACAM1 (CD66a, C-CAM, BGP) has raised interest as an adhesion molecule belonging to the carcinoembryonic antigen family. Bamberger et al. (2000)

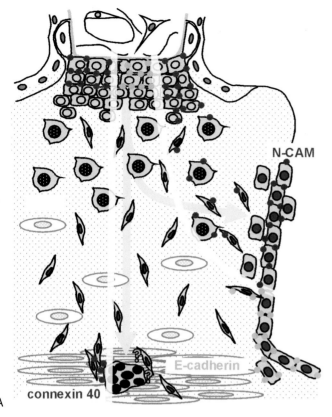
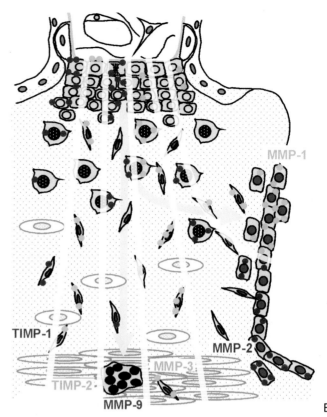

FIGURE 9.11. A: Adhesion molecules. Expression patterns of connexin 40, E-cadherin, and neural cell adhesion molecule (N-CAM) along the invasive pathway. Question marks indicate unclear findings. For details see text. B: Matrix metalloproteinases 1, 2, 3, and 9 and their inhibitors TIMP-1 and TIMP-2 are immunoreactive in extravillous trophoblast cells (red and yellow dots), in decidual cells (not marked) and in the surrounding extracellular matrix (not marked). The distribution patterns depend on the type of trophoblast cell and stage of pregnancy. (*Source:* Modified from Kaufmann & Castellucci, 1997, with permission.)

have shown that CEACAM1 was strongly expressed by the invasive phenotype of extravillous trophoblast as well as by extravillous trophoblast cells with invasive phenotype in vitro. The authors conclude from their data that the molecule is not only a useful marker for invasive trophoblast but also that it might be functionally implicated in mediating trophoblast/endometrial or trophoblast/endothelial interactions during the invasion process.

Proteinases, Activators and Inhibitors Involved in Trophoblast Invasion

Extravillous trophoblast has to fulfill two largely different functions:

- **Invasion of maternal tissues** including infiltration of maternal vessels, supported by lytic activities of proteinases destroying a.o. maternal ECM;
- **Anchorage of the placenta** to the maternal tissues by secretion and continuous turnover of trophoblastic

ECM acting as a kind of glue between cells of maternal and fetal origin (Feinberg et al., 1991b).

Both processes require the secretion of a broad panel of proteases destroying the ECM of the host tissue (for review, see Fisher et al., 1985; Graham & Lala, 1991; Bischof & Martelli, 1992) and providing the turnover of the self-produced trophoblastic ECM. Recent data suggest that these two aspects of extravillous trophoblast function can be attributed to two different subtypes of cells:

- The highly invasive small spindle-shaped trophoblast
- The noninvasive large polygonal trophoblast cells (Kemp et al., 2002)

In accordance with these functions, both cellular subtypes would be expected to express different patterns of proteases. Respective data are, however, still meager.

Among the best studied proteinases are the **matrix metalloproteinases** (MMPs). It has been proven in vitro that they are secreted by trophoblast cells (Bischof et al., 1991). Respective immunoreactivities can be found not only intracellularly but also with increasing invasive depth in the surrounding extracellular matrix.

MMP-1 (interstitial collagenase) degrades various interstitial collagens, among others collagens I and III, which are most abundant in the endometrium. Because of this, it is not surprising that invasive extravillous trophoblast expresses interstitial collagenase (Fig. 9.11B) (Moll & Lane, 1990; Vettraino et al., 1996; Huppertz et al., 1998d). Its expression has also been proven in trophoblast cell culture (Emonard et al., 1990).

MMP-2 (72-kd–type IV collagenase, gelatinase A) degrades mainly collagen IV. Its expression in extravillous trophoblast has been demonstrated by immunohistochemistry and in situ hybridization (Fig. 9.11B) (Autio-Harmainen et al., 1992; Fernandez et al., 1992; Blankenship & King, 1994b; Polette et al., 1994; Huppertz et al., 1998d) as well as by in vitro approaches (Emonard et al., 1990). The mRNA of this proteinase was found only in the invasive phenotype (Polette et al., 1994).

MMP-3 (stromelysin-1) degrades fibronectins, laminin, various collagens, and core proteins of proteoglycans. According to Huppertz et al. (1998d), it is weakly expressed within the proximal proliferating layers, downregulated in early invasive stages, and again upregulated in later invasion (Fig. 9.11B). Most of the extracellular immunoreactivities are linked to the fibronectin fibrils in the ECM.

MMP-7 (matrilysin) is a characteristic product of epithelial cells, cleaving among others proteoglycans, elastin and fibronectins. It was found to be predominantly expressed in the invasive phenotype of trophoblast and decidua; overexpression by the invasive trophoblast was shown in preeclampsia (Vettraino et al., 1996).

MMP-9 (92-kd–type IV collagenase, gelatinase B) mainly degrades collagen IV and in this respect is similar to MMP-2. It is present at both mRNA and protein levels in the proximal, proliferating layers of extravillous trophoblast (Polette et al., 1994). Expression is downregulated in the early invasive stages and then upregulated again in the deeper stages of invasion (Huppertz et al., 1998d) (Fig. 9.11B). An antibody against MMP-9 completely inhibited trophoblast invasion in vitro (Librach et al., 1991b). Expression decreases toward term (Fisher et al., 1989; Librach et al., 1991b; Polette et al., 1994). In vitro findings by Graham et al. (1996) showed reduced active MMP-9 in culture supernatants of trophoblast cells derived from preeclamptic pregnancies.

MMP-11 (stromelysin-3) is a laminin-, collagen IV-, and proteoglycan-degrading proteinase. According to immunohistochemical and in situ hybridization findings by Maquoi et al. (1995, 1997) and Polette et al. (1994), it is expressed only by the invasive phenotype of extravillous trophoblast.

MMPs-14 and **15** (MT-MMPs, membrane-type matrix metalloproteinases) activate MMP-2 and are expressed by proliferating and invasive trophoblast cells in first and third trimesters (Nawrocki et al., 1995, 1996; Hurskainen et al., 1998).

TIMPs, the tissue inhibitors of matrix metalloproteinases, regulate MMPs. In the human placenta **TIMP-1**, an inhibitor of all known MMPs, and **TIMP-2**, which preferentially interacts with MMP-2, have been described as being expressed by both decidual cells and by extravillous trophoblast cells (Fig. 9.11B) (Damsky et al., 1993; Polette et al., 1994; Ruck et al., 1995, 1996, 1997; Marzusch et al., 1996). These data suggest paracrine and autocrine control of MMP action. Moreover, **TIMP-3** an inhibitor of MMP-9 and MT-MMP1, is expressed by invasive trophoblast cells (Bass et al., 1997). The regulatory potential of TIMPs was shown in vitro: TIMP-1 and TIMP-2 completely inhibited human cytotrophoblast invasion in vitro (Librach et al., 1991b).

MMPs and EVT phenotype: There are only a few preliminary data on the expression of MMPs and their inhibitors by the various subtypes of extravillous trophoblast. These suggest that MMP-3 (stromelysin) is preferably expressed by the highly invasive small spindle-shaped trophoblast cells. The fibronectin-degrading activity of this protease would be in agreement with the fact that spindle-shaped trophoblast is mostly embedded in fibronectins rather than in collagens and laminins (Kemp et al., 2002). In contrast, the poorly invasive, large polygonal trophoblast cells throughout pregnancy express all MMP isoforms described so far in extravillous trophoblast (see above). This finding supports the view that MMP expression per se is not an indicator of invasiveness. Rather MMPs such as interstitial collagenase and type IV collagenases may also be required for the turnover of self-secreted ECM by a more or less noninvasive cell. This view is further underlined by recent findings by Huisman et al. (2004), who did not find differences in MMP-2 and MMP-9 activities when comparing placentas with normal trophoblast invasion and those with reduced trophoblast invasion. Also the data by Bauer et al. (2004) suggest that MMP-9 expression does not correlate with invasiveness. Several publications (Bischof et al., 2000a, 2003; Wang et al., 2001; Campbell et al., 2003; Staun-Ram et al., 2004) add further details to this puzzle but do not answer the question as to the role of the various MMPs in invasion and/or anchorage of the placenta by ECM turnover.

Provided that MMPs are involved in the turnover of ECM, acting as "glue" among maternal and fetal tissues, these proteinases may also be related to the initiation of labor and to the separation of the placenta from the uterine wall (for review see Bryant-Greenwood & Yamamoto, 1995; Bryant-Greenwood, 1998). During spontaneous labor, but before delivery, MMP-3 and MMP-9 mRNA levels are significantly increased, whereas after spontaneous delivery tissue-type plasminogen activator (tPA) (see below) and TIMP-1 mRNA levels were increased (Bryant-Greenwood & Yamamoto, 1995).

Leptin seems to regulate MMP expression in extravillous trophoblast. Castellucci and coworkers (2000) found the leptin receptor strongly expressed in the distal, invasive trophoblast of cell columns. In vitro invasiveness of trophoblast cells was stimulated by leptin (Castellucci et al., 2000; Schulz & Widmaier, 2004) and could be blocked by simultaneous administration of MMP inhibitors. Immunohistochemically, the expression of MMP-2 and MMP-9 as well as of oncofetal fibronectin was upregulated by leptin administration in vitro (Castellucci et al., 2000).

Plasminogen activators convert plasminogen to plasmin, which activates other proteinases. Two plasminogen activators are known: urokinase-type plasminogen activator (uPA) and tPA. The expression of uPA by extravillous trophoblast has been shown by Hofmann et al. (1994), and uPA m-RNA has been found in isolated human cytotrophoblast (Eldar Geva et al., 1993). Moreover, uPA receptor is expressed in extravillous trophoblast (Multhaupt et al., 1994; Pierleoni et al., 1998). There are no hints as to the expression of **tPA** by extravillous trophoblast. Also the inhibitors of uPA and tPA (i.e., **PAI-1** and **PAI-2**) have been found in human trophoblast (Astedt et al., 1986; Feinberg et al., 1989). In agreement with the presence of uPA, only PAI-1 is expressed by invasive cytotrophoblast of cell islands and cell columns (Feinberg et al., 1989) and was suggested to control trophoblast invasion (Floridon et al., 2000). Recent data by Chou et al. (2002) suggest that gonadotropin-releasing hormone (GnRH) I and II may facilitate trophoblast invasion by increasing the ratio of uPA/PAI-1 expression via interactions with two distinct GnRH receptors. In contrast, tPA and PAI-2 were found only in villous syncytiotrophoblast where they are thought to regulate fibrinolysis (Feinberg et al., 1989).

Other serine protease inhibitors, such as α_1-antichymotrypsin, α_1-antitrypsin, and inter-α-trypsin inhibitor, have only rarely been studied. None of them was immunoreactive within the extravillous trophoblast; however, the surrounding matrix-type fibrinoid in cell columns and basal plate showed ample reaction product (Castellucci et al., 1994). The authors suggested that the protein is so rapidly exported into the ECM that no intracellular immunoreactivity is detectable.

Nitric Oxide and Trophoblast Invasion

* In lower concentrations, as produced by the endothelial isoform of the enzyme nitric oxide synthase (**eNOS**), NO causes vasodilatation.
* Higher NO levels as produced by the macrophage isoform [macrophage nitric oxide synthase (**mNOS**)/ inducible nitric oxide synthase (**iNOS**)] are said to be cytotoxic.

Nitric oxide synthase immunoreactivities in extravillous trophoblast were described for the first time by Morris et al. (1993). This finding raised little attention.

The potential importance of these results, however, is stressed by experimental findings in rats and guinea pigs; Yallampalli and Garfield (1993), Chwalisz and Garfield (1994), and Garfield et al. (1994) have shown that preeclampsia-like symptoms, including hypertension, proteinuria, and fetal growth restriction, can be induced in rats and guinea pigs by blocking nitric oxide synthase with l-NAME. The experiments were successfully repeated by Osawa et al. (1995) in rats.

These findings led us to study trophoblast invasion in relation to NOS expression by means of immune- and enzyme-histochemistry in guinea pigs (Nanaev et al., 1995). The results indicated that uteroplacental vessel dilatation in this species is related to eNOS expression in periarterial trophoblast cells, the latter corresponding to the interstitial subpopulation of extravillous trophoblast in the human. Invasion and destruction of the vessel walls as well as formation of intraarterial trophoblastic plugs in the guinea pig appeared to be secondary to the NO-mediated arterial dilatation. The question remained open as to whether or not extravillous trophoblast cells in the guinea pig also express mNOS.

These findings obtained in the guinea pig where challenged by Lyall et al. (1999), who did not detect expression of eNOS or iNOS in extravillous trophoblast in human placental bed biopsies from weeks 8 to 19. In contrast, Martin and Conrad (2000), by means of immunohistochemistry and in situ hybridization, found eNOS to be expressed in human interstitial trophoblast. These latter data were further supported by in vitro findings by Cartwright and coworkers (1999): Using a human trophoblast cell line that expressed both the constitutive (eNOS) and the inducible isoforms (iNOS), these authors could demonstrate that also human trophoblast cell motility and invasion strongly depended on trophoblast-derived NO. The effect, however, depended on the contemporaneous availability of hepatocyte growth factor (HGF) (cf. Cytokines and Hormones Controlling Differentiation of Extravillous Trophoblast, above).

Data by Graham's group (Postovit et al., 2001) shed a different light on the role of NO in trophoblast invasion. Their in vitro findings reveal that low concentrations of NO-mimetic drugs (glyceryl trinitrate and sodium nitroprusside) inhibit the ability of trophoblast cells to penetrate through reconstituted ECM (Matrigel). This inhibition was accompanied by a reduced expression of the cell surface urokinase receptor, a molecule important for invasion. The authors conclude that maternal macrophages infiltrating the uteroplacental artery walls in preeclampsia (Reister et al., 1999) might secrete levels of NO high enough to inhibit endovascular trophoblast invasion.

Major Basic Protein

Studies have shown that extravillous trophoblast cells also produce substantial quantities of major basic protein

(MBP) (Wasmoen et al., 1989, 1991). This protein is similar to that contained in the granules of eosinophilic granulocytes. Eosinophil MBP is highly toxic to parasites, as well as to cells (Maddox et al., 1984; Kephart et al., 1988). It was found to circulate in the blood of pregnant women at levels 10 to 20 times higher than in nonpregnant women, in the absence of eosinophilia (Maddox et al., 1983). The concentration of this nonglycosylated protein increases significantly before the onset of labor (Wasmoen et al., 1987). It decreases rapidly after delivery.

Immunohistochemical studies and extraction of placentas, particularly of cyst fluid, showed MBP to be derived from the extravillous trophoblast cells in the placenta (Maddox et al., 1984). Immunoreactivity for the protein was found as early as the sixth week of pregnancy and was confined to trophoblast cells in anchoring villi, septa, basal plate, and placental site giant cells (Fig. 9.12). No immunostaining was observed in villous Langhans' cells, syncytium, fibrinoid, or decidual cells. The trophoblast of ectopic pregnancies and hydatidiform moles stained positively, whereas only one of two choriocarcinomas stained weakly. Immunohistochemistry showed the protein to be present in small granules (Fig. 9.12D) and to be packaged in membranes.

It may be premature to engage in much speculation until more is known about the physiology of this protein. For a complete consideration of all functions of eosinophils, their granules, and related phenomena, the reader is referred to the review by Gleich and Adolphson (1986).

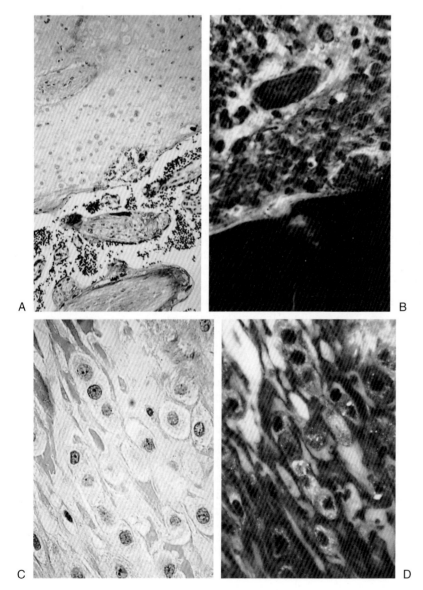

FIGURE 9.12. A,B: Intercotyledonary septum with extravillous trophoblast cells above. There is immunofluorescent localization of major basic proytein (MBP) between septal extravillous trophoblast cells but not in chorionic villi (below). Left: H&E ×100. Right: Anti-eosinophil granule MBP stain. ×100. C,D: Placental septum composed of extravillous trophoblast cells. (Same technique as in A,B.) Note the intense immunofluorescence among and between cells. Left: H&E ×400. Right: Anti-eosinophil granule MBP stain. ×400. (Courtesy of Dr. G. J. Gleich, Mayo Clinic, Rochester, Minnesota.)

Cell Surface Carbohydrates

Carbohydrate epitopes on cell surfaces and on ECM molecules represent an important subgroup of oncofetal antigens. They often have close molecular relations to normal adult blood group antigens, the differences being based either on blockage of the normal synthetic pathways or on unusual synthetic pathways resulting in chain extension or atypical sialylation and fucosylation. Such carbohydrate chains may act as immunologically relevant cell surface markers (blood group antigen "i", Frank et al., 1995). Moreover, they may represent ligands for cell adhesion molecules (sialyl-Lewis[x], King & Loke, 1988; Burrows et al., 1994).

Blood group antigen "i" is the most primitive precursor of the ABO system of blood groups. It is expressed not only by immature red blood cells but also by all stages of invasive extravillous trophoblast (Fig. 9.13) (Frank et al., 1995). Its expression by fetal cells invading the maternal organism raises the question of whether the cell surface expression of an immature blood group antigen that every human organism has expressed throughout embryonic and fetal life prevents immune recognition of extravillous trophoblast cells by the maternal immune system (see Endometrial Large Granular Lymphocytes Endometrial NK Cells, uNK Cells, below). Interestingly, the identical carbohydrate chain "I" was also found extracellularly in the invasive zone bound to trophoblast-secreted fibronectin molecules (Frank et al., 1995; Huppertz et al., 1996). As was shown by Zhu and coworkers, respective glycosylation of ECM molecules decreased their collagen binding and increased their resistance to proteolytic cleavage (Zhu et al., 1984; Zhu & Laine, 1985).

The slightly more mature **blood group antigen "I"** could be detected in human trophoblast only after sialidase pretreatment, thus indicating that not "I" but rather sialyl-"I" is expressed (Frank et al., 1995). Sialyl-"I" immunoreactivity was found on villous syncytiotrophoblast and only in few cases on the surfaces of invasive extravillous trophoblast cells, where it was coexpressed with "i."

Sialyl-Lewis[x], another cell surface carbohydrate, is expressed by intraarterial trophoblast cells (Fig. 9.13) (King & Loke, 1988). It acts as a ligand for the lectins

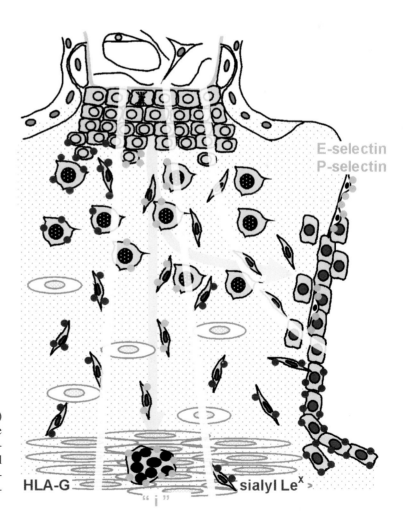

FIGURE 9.13. Human leukocyte antigen G (HLA-G) as well as the glycosyl epitopes "I" and sialyl-Le[x] are expressed only by the invasive phenotype of extravillous trophoblast. The sialyl-Le[x] positive intraarterial trophoblast cells can adhere to the maternal endothelium that expresses the respective receptors, E- and P-selectin only at the implantation site.

E- and **P-selectin** both of which are expressed by maternal endothelium at the implantation site (Fig. 9.13) (Burrows et al., 1994). Usually, both selectins are expressed by endothelium during inflammatory reactions. They enable leukocytes expressing sialyl-Le^x to attach and to leave the vessel wall. These data suggest that at the implantation site, trophoblastic invasion of the arterial walls initiates the respective inflammatory reaction, resulting in selectin expression and intraluminal trophoblast adhesion. Interestingly, the sialyl-Le^x/E-selectin adhesive interaction is also involved in the adhesion of human cancer cells to human umbilical vein endothelial cells in vitro (Takada et al., 1993).

MHC Class I Molecules

Villous cyto- and syncytiotrophoblast separating maternal blood and villous stroma express neither MHC class I nor class II antigens (for review see Loke, 1989). The proliferating stem cells of the cell columns share the MHC negativity with the villous trophoblast. By contrast, the invasive extravillous trophoblast cells express non-classical MHC-I molecules (Schmidt & Orr, 1993; Chumbley et al., 1994a,b; Colbern et al., 1994; McMaster et al., 1995; for review, see Hutter et al., 1996 and Loke et al., 1997).

From the morphologic point of view, the situation becomes even more interesting when one compares the immunohistochemical distribution of MHC-I antigen with the distribution of the class I MHC mRNA (Hunt et al., 1990, 1991). Hunt and coworkers described three different patterns:

- Villous cytotrophoblast (Langhans' cells) contains class I mRNA but does not express the MHC I antigen.
- Villous syncytiotrophoblast neither expresses MHC I antigen nor contains class I mRNA.
- Invasive extravillous cytotrophoblast contains the mRNA message and expresses nonclassical MHC I antigen.

These results are in agreement with findings by Lata et al. (1992), who concluded that MHC-I expression is regulated by posttranscriptional events. Moreover, these findings support the view that the trophoblast cells resting on villous and extravillous basal laminae represent a uniform population of proliferating stem cells for both villous syncytiotrophoblast and extravillous cytotrophoblast (Kaufmann & Castellucci, 1997).

In 1990, these nonclassical, nonpolymorphic MHC-I molecules were identified as **human leukocyte antigen-G (HLA-G)** (Kovats et al., 1990). So far, substantial evidence for the presence of both HLA-G mRNA and protein was found only in extravillous trophoblast (Chumbley et al., 1994a,b; Hutter et al., 1996); in contrast,

HLA-G mRNA was described in various nonplacental tissues (from Loke, 1997; Shukla et al., 1990; Houlihan et al., 1992; Kirszenbaum et al., 1994; Ulbrecht et al., 1994). Detection of the HLA-G protein is difficult, since there seem to be substantial problems in raising antibodies that specifically recognize HLA-G or one of its isoforms. So far HLA-G antibodies have been generated only by using HLA-G transgenic mice (Chumbley et al., 1994a,b). The situation is complicated even more by the fact, that various soluble or membrane-bound HLA-G isoforms exist, probably generated by alternative splicing (from Loke, 1997; Ishitani & Geraghty, 1992; Fuji et al., 1994). Immunohistochemically, HLA-G protein has been detected in the invasive phenotype of extravillous trophoblast (Fig. 9.13), the expression level decreasing toward term in parallel to decreasing invasiveness of the cells (Shorter et al., 1993; McMaster et al., 1995). Also in preeclampsia the HLA-G expression levels in the maternofetal junctional zone were found to be decreased (Colbern et al., 1994); it is still a matter of debate whether this reduction is due to generally reduced numbers of invasive trophoblast cells in this condition.

The functional role of HLA-G is still a matter of investigation. The low degree of polymorphism of its gene locus does not support the hypothesis that HLA-G may have evolved for classical T-cell interaction (Loke et al., 1997). The HLA-G–reactive T cells have never been observed (King et al., 1997). It was proposed that HLA-G acts as a target for decidual NK cells rather than for T cells (King & Loke, 1991; Loke & King, 1991). In this way, extravillous trophoblast may be protected against NK cell attacks, which are to be expected against MHC-I–negative cells. Nevertheless, HLA-G is able to present intracellular nonapeptides like the classical class I molecules (for review, see Hutter et al., 1996), and thus does not necessarily prevent T-cell–mediated immune response. For further discussion of HLA-G functions see Le Bouteiller et al. (2003).

Substantial evidence has accumulated that also **HLA-C**, which is less polymorphic than HLA-A or HLA-B, is expressed in extravillous trophoblast cells (Grabowska et al., 1990; King et al., 1996; for review see Hutter et al., 1996). Similar to HLA-G, HLA-C can present nonapeptides. At the moment, the functional role of HLA-C at the maternofetal interface is discussed along the same lines as for HLA-G, including the interactions with decidual NK cells (Loke & King, 1995).

In addition, **HLA-E**, another nonpolymorphic MHC molecule, is expressed by extravillous trophoblast. Different from the other non- or minimally polymorphic HLA molecules, HLA-E is ubiquitously expressed by a wide variety of cell types. Only HLA-E molecules that present nonamer peptides derived from the signal sequences of other HLA class I molecules, are expressed at the cell surfaces and are recognized by the dimeric receptor

CD94/NKG2A (Borrego et al., 1998; Lee et al., 1998). Binding of HLA-E to this receptor prevents NK cell-mediated lysis of the target cells.

The data on HLA-E raise the question of whether expression of HLA-G or HLA-C alone is sufficient to prevent NK cell attacks or whether coexpression with HLA-E is required, the latter presenting nonapeptides of the former nonclassical MHC molecules (Llano et al., 1998).

Meanwhile there is sufficient evidence, that uterine natural killer cells (uNK cells) in fact sense extravillous trophoblastic HLA-C, HLA-G, and HLA-E molecules and react with an altered NK cell cytokine profile, which modulates the invasive properties of extravillous trophoblast (King et al., 2000).

Normal Extravillous Trophoblast Cells Are Never Proliferative and Invasive at One Time

Taken together, different from tumor cells, normal extravillous trophoblast leaves the cell cycle before becoming invasive. Accordingly, the various stages of differentiation within the invasive pathway have been subdivided in two phenotypes: a proliferative and an invasive one (for review, see Fisher & Damsky, 1993; Kaufmann & Castellucci, 1997). In the light of recent findings, this classification probably is too simple and the following might be closer to the truth:

The **proliferative and early postproliferative phenotype** is characterized by

- the location of the cells on or close to the fetal stromal basal lamina, forming a compact cluster of cells attached to each other by intercellular junctions;
- immunopositivity for the proliferation markers MIB-1/Ki-67 and expression of EGFR (*c-erbB*-1);
- expression of epithelial integrins α6β4, and partly α3β1;
- polar secretion of ECM as a basal lamina (only proximal layer of cells) or absence of visible matrix secretion (all following layers of cells);
- cells either resting on a basal lamina or moving away from the basal lamina by proliferation and proliferation pressure of parent cells, but the absence of the cell's own active migratory or even invasive behavior.

After switching to the **invasive phenotype** (spindle-shaped trophoblast) the trophoblast cells

- have left the basal lamina and have invaded deeper layers of the maternofetal junctional zone;
- have irreversibly left the cell cycle and express the proto-oncogene *c-erbB*-2 rather than *c-erbB*-1;
- express interstitial integrins such as α5β1, α1β1, αvβ3, and αvβ5 either alone or in addition to the epithelial integrin α6β4;
- show different degrees of apolar secretion of extracellular matrix,

- upregulate certain matrix metalloproteinases (MMP-2, MMP-11);
- show active migratory behavior (across their self-secreted ECM) or true invasive behavior (across the maternal host tissue, partially destroying the latter).

The final stage of differentiation is downregulation of invasion

- by polyploidization (large polygonal trophoblast)
- or syncytial fusion (multinucleated giant cells).

These data have prompted placentologists to assume that during normal placentation proliferation and invasion do not coexist in one and the same cell. The switch from the proliferative to the invasive phenotype was thought to comprise synchronous switching of all other parameters belonging to the same phenotype, as defined above. From these conclusions it was deduced that

- **temporal and spatial separation of proliferation and invasiveness** along the normal invasive pathway of extravillous trophoblast limits the depth of trophoblast invasion to the lifespan of the individual trophoblast cell;
- **temporal and spatial coincidence of proliferation and invasion** in "malignant" invasion in tumors increase invasiveness and enable unlimited invasive depth.

These features were thought to embody the major difference between "normal" trophoblast invasion in pregnancy as compared to tumor invasion; however, this view may still be too simple. The clearly defined switch of phenotypes was questioned by earlier in vitro data from the Lala group (for review, see Irving et al., 1995) who immunoselected α5-integrin–positive cells and found them to be still proliferative. Also observations in tubal pregnancies (Kertschanska et al., 1998; Kemp et al., 1999, 2002) revealed proliferation in deeply invasive extravillous trophoblast cells that had undergone the integrin switch from α6β4 to α5β1 and showed apolar matrix secretion. Biologically, the extravillous trophoblast in extrauterine pregnancies is expected to be normal trophoblast, the only difference being the abnormal implantation site.

These data suggest that also in the case of normal extravillous trophoblast, proliferation and invasion do not necessarily exclude each other. More likely, proliferation is downregulated by local factors, an event that in the intrauterine milieu, but not in the fallopian tube, coincides with the integrin switch and the onset of invasion. Partial overlap of proliferation with invasiveness may explain the enhanced invasiveness in tubal pregnancies. Additional factors include missing limitation of invasiveness, for example, by missing polyploidization of spindle-shaped trophoblast (Kemp et al., 2002), by missing syncytial fusion into multinucleated trophoblastic giant cells (Kemp et al., 2002), and by reduced trophoblast apoptosis (von Rango et al., 2003).

Similarly aberrant switching of phenotypes may take place during trophoblast invasion in accreta and percreta intrauterine placentation. Both tubal pregnancy and placenta accreta/percreta have in common locally deficient decidualization. Therefore, decidual factors should be investigated to determine if they are involved in the temporal and spatial coordination of trophoblast proliferation and invasion.

Oxygen-Mediated Regulation of the Invasive Pathway

The **oxygen partial pressure** at the fetomaternal interface varies with gestational age. Studies with oxygen electrodes (Rodesch et al., 1992) have shown that the oxygen pressure in the intervillous space rises at around week 12 of gestation as a result of increased intervillous perfusion (see Uteroplacental Vessels), but is very low throughout the early stages of pregnancy. In the first trimester the following oxygen values were reported (for review, see Lyall & Kaufmann, 2000):

- Intervillous oxygen pressure was measured to be only about 18 mm Hg.
- Maternal intraarterial pO_2 is about 95 to 100 mm Hg.
- Endometrial and myometrial pO_2 are expected to be between both the above values.

Thus, there is a steeply rising pO_2 gradient from the proximal layers of the cell columns (close to the intervillous space) toward the myometrium and even steeper toward the uteroplacental arteries, both representing the two end points of the invasive pathway. The question was raised whether this gradient may be a driving force for trophoblast proliferation, differentiation, and invasion (for review, see Lash et al., 2002), the effects being mediated by oxygen-controlled cytokines (Kourembanas et al., 1991; Shweiki et al., 1992; for review, see Lyall & Kaufmann, 2000).

Hypoxia stimulates trophoblast proliferation: The effects of oxygen concentration on proliferation of trophoblast in vitro were tested by Genbacev et al. (1996, 1997). These authors have shown that hypoxic conditions increase the overall proliferative capacity of isolated trophoblast cells. By contrast, in normoxic conditions, in vitro proliferation was reduced. This in vitro behavior of human trophoblast is in agreement with in vivo data obtained from severely anemic mothers (Kosanke et al., 1997; Kadyrov et al., 2003).

Does hypoxia reduce trophoblast invasiveness? In the same series of in vitro experiments Genbacev et al. (1996, 1997) found evidence that hypoxia did not only stimulate proliferation of isolated trophoblast cells but also inhibited their invasiveness, whereas normoxic conditions enhanced in vitro invasiveness. These data were supported by Kilburn et al. (2000), who found α6-integrin expression increased and α1-integrin expression downregulated under hypoxic conditions.

Genbacev's group explained the reciprocal dependence of proliferation and invasiveness on local oxygen levels by studying the expression of the von Hippel-Lindau tumor-suppressor protein, which regulates the stability of HIF1α and HIF2α (Genbacev et al., 2001). Hypoxia inducible factor transcriptionally regulates the genes of growth factors that are involved in developmental, physiologic, and pathologic responses to hypoxia. The level and transcriptional activity of this complex is precisely regulated by the cellular oxygen concentration (for review see Caniggia & Winter, 2002; for further details see Oxygen-Controlled Angiogenic Growth Factors in Chapter 7). The authors found the von Hippel-Lindau tumor-suppressor protein highly expressed in proliferative trophoblast, but downregulated in the invasive phenotype.

Or does hypoxia stimulate trophoblast invasiveness? The finding of hypoxia-dependent reduction of trophoblast invasiveness was used to explain reduced interstitial trophoblast invasion (e.g., in preeclampsia). As became evident from the data by Kadyrov et al. (2003), trophoblast invasion in preeclampsia is in fact numerically reduced. However, in severe anemia, which provides a clearly hypoxic environment in the uterine wall, the same authors found increased invasiveness of trophoblast (Kadyrov et al., 2003). Therefore the question must be posed whether preeclampsia is really a good in vivo model for hypoxia in the uterine wall. One may argue that intrauterine hypoxia in this entity is not inducing malinvasion of trophoblast but rather that malinvasion of trophoblast induced by other factors is causal for the maladaptation of uteroplacental arteries and thus for intrauterine hypoxia.

Several data underline the notion that hypoxia does not simply impair invasiveness of trophoblast but possibly even stimulates it, as suggested by the in vivo data obtained in anemia:

- The expression of oxygen-controlled genes in trophoblast cells in vitro was studied by various approaches (Pak et al., 1998).
- Fitzpatrick and Graham (1998) could demonstrate increased expression of PAI-1 in immortalized trophoblast cells cultured under low oxygen levels. Plasminogen activator inhibitor-1 is the inhibitor of uPA and is expressed by extravillous trophoblast cells (Feinberg et al., 1989).
- Graham's group (1998) provided evidence that reduced oxygen levels increased in vitro invasiveness of cytotrophoblast, an effect linked to elevated expression of the cell surface receptor for uPA.
- The same conditions resulted in reduced expression of α5 integrin and reduced adhesion to vitronectin and fibronectin (Lash et al., 2001).
- Also, the secretion of MMPs, important tools for cellular invasion, seems to be regulated by oxygen. Whereas hypoxia in vitro upregulates MMP secretion by trophoblast cells, it downregulates at the same

time the secretion of its inhibitors (TIMPs) (Canning et al., 2001).

Data by Campbell et al. (2004) suggest that in vitro experiments with trophoblast generally must be interpreted with care since the experimental design may influence the outcome. These authors found that hypoxia increased trophoblast migration on semipermeable membranes when cultured alone, but not in coculture with decidual endothelial cells due to increased adhesion between the two cell types.

In conclusion, all these data suggest an important role for oxygen in the regulation of cellular invasion (Graham et al., 2000; Lash et al., 2002), a role that more likely points to stimulating effects of hypoxia on invasiveness than to impairing effects.

Extracellular pH as Trigger of Trophoblast Invasion

As discussed above, non-oncofetal cellular fibronectin can universally be found in all extracellular compartments of the placenta. In contrast, oncofetal fibronectins containing the ED-B and III-CS domains are almost exclusively secreted by extravillous trophoblast; the amount of oncofetal fibronectins accumulating around the extravillous trophoblast cells increases along the invasive pathway from early postproliferative to deeply invasive cells (Frank et al., 1994, 1995; Huppertz et al., 1996, 1998b,d; Kaufmann & Castellucci, 1997). Factors affecting the secretion patterns of oncofetal fibronectins, therefore, may be discussed as regulators of differentiation of extravillous trophoblast and of trophoblast invasion.

In a recent study (Gaus et al., 2001) we have shown interesting interactions between pH and trophoblast invasion:

- The peripheral ends of anchoring villi and the attached proliferative zone of cell columns show the strongest tissue acidity (pK about 3.9) measurable within the placenta in vivo; this area is the starting point of trophoblast invasion.
- Acidic extracellular pH stimulates secretion of fibronectins by extravillous trophoblast cell lines in vitro and shifts their isoform pattern toward oncofetal splice variants; this secretory pattern is preserved even following pH normalization.
- This behavior seems to be characteristic for extravillous trophoblast, since choriocarcinoma cells and mesenchymal cells under identical experimental conditions did not show a shift toward the secretion of oncofetal fibronectins, though at least the latter are generally responsive to changes in tissue acidity (Borsi et al., 1996).

Similar data have been reported for pH-dependent alternative splicing of tenascin (Borsi et al., 1996). Taken together, these data suggest that local tissue acidity besides oxygen and various cytokines must be considered as another factor triggering the secretion of ECM proteins along the invasive pathway, and possibly even triggering the transition into the invasive phenotype.

Trophoblastic Mechanisms Limiting Trophoblast Invasion

A variety of mechanisms is under discussion to limit trophoblast invasion. These include

- apoptosis (DiFederico et al., 1999; Genbacev et al., 1999; Reister et al., 1999, 2001),
- polyploidization (Kemp et al., 2002; Zybina et al., 2002, 2004), and
- syncytial fusion (Kemp et al., 2002) of the invasive trophoblast cells (Fig. 9.7).

Apoptosis: It has been shown that both villous and extravillous trophoblast express the molecular machinery of apoptosis (Huppertz et al., 1998a–c). Trophoblast apoptosis was shown to prevent interstitial extravillous trophoblast from invading uteroplacental arterial walls in preeclampsia (Reister et al., 1999, 2001). Moreover, DiFederico et al. (1999) and Genbacev et al. (1999) in two articles derived from the same project, have reported that in preeclampsia 15% to 50% of the extravillous trophoblast cells in "the uterine wall to which the placenta attaches" were TUNEL positive and thus destined to undergo apoptosis. Based on these data the authors suggested that increased trophoblast apoptosis is responsible for reduced interstitial trophoblast invasion in preeclampsia.

In a later study, Kadyrov and coworkers (2003) found much lower apoptosis indices of extravillous trophoblast in the placental bed, ranging from 4.4% (preeclampsia) to 7.2% (normal term placenta). Percentages of up to 50% TUNEL positivity of extravillous trophoblast, as reported by DiFederico, would lead to complete loss of this cell population within few days. Based on the photographs published in DiFederico's paper, it seems likely that the authors did not study placental bed biopsies as claimed but rather basal plate specimens from the delivered placenta.[1] Therefore, it has been suggested

---

[1] At this point, the importance of true placental bed studies must be emphasized: Important pregnancy problems, such as preeclampsia, fetal growth restriction, and spontaneous miscarriage have all been linked to abnormalities in trophoblast invasion into the placental bed. Unfortunately, most of the respective basic research to understand the pathogenetic mechanisms is done either on the more easily available basal plate or on *in vitro* models. In a recent review by Lyall (2002) the various studies that have attempted to sample the placental bed together with the difficulties in obtaining "true" placental bed biopsies have been impressively reviewed.

that DiFederico's unusually high apoptosis indices reflect local tissue degeneration along the demarcation zone between placental basal plate and placental bed, rather than the in vivo situation in the invasive pathway and a true effect of preeclampsia (Kadyrov et al., 2003).

According to von Rango et al. (2003) trophoblast apoptosis is confined to the decidua basalis, the incidence declining with advancing gestation. Interstitial apoptotic trophoblast cells were always closely colocalized with CD56[+] NK cells and the overall number of uNK cells declined parallel to the reduction of trophoblast apoptosis when pregnancy advances. Interestingly, in tubal pregnancies, in which uNK cells were completely missing, the incidence of trophoblast apoptosis was lowest. The authors, therefore, suggest an interaction between uNK cells and trophoblast apoptosis.

The data presented by Kadyrov et al. (2003) and von Rango et al. (2003) support the view that some of the extravillous trophoblast cells may be eliminated by apoptotic death along the invasive pathway, but the same data make it unlikely that apoptosis is the limiting factor for trophoblast invasion. The data obtained from analysis of complete placental bed/uterine wall samples revealed that trophoblast invasion in normal pregnancies clearly exceeded trophoblast invasion in preeclampsia regarding both numerical density of invading trophoblast and invasive depth. But interestingly the incidence of apoptotic death (percentage of total extravillous trophoblast in the invasive pathway) was also higher in normal pregnancy as compared to preeclampsia, suggesting that increased apoptosis cannot be made responsible for the poor and shallow invasion in preeclampsia.

Syncytial fusion: It is generally thought that the multinucleated trophoblastic giant cells of the placental bed are formed by syncytial fusion (Kemp et al., 2002), though respective fusion stages have not been observed yet. Endomitosis as alternative mechanism is very unlikely since MIB-1 reactivity has never been shown in these cells or in neighboring trophoblast cells that may be considered precursors.

Interestingly, the multinucleated trophoblastic giant cells accumulate usually in one layer close to the endometrial-myometrial border. The concentration of giant cells within one layer renders it quite unlikely, that they are mobile or even invasive. Rather, the presence of this layer together with the fact that the uninucleated interstitial trophoblast cells may be found above (toward the placenta) and partly also below this layer, suggest that the multinucleated giant cell layer acts as a kind of net, trapping many of those uninucleated invasive trophoblast cells by fusion that try to pass into deeper layers (Kemp et al., 2002).

Polyploidization: As discussed above, the uninucleated population of interstitial extravillous trophoblast cells is composed of two different phenotypes (Kemp et al., 2002):

- **Small spindle-shaped trophoblast cells,** which express "interstitial integrins" ($\alpha5\beta1$, $\alpha1\beta1$, and αv-integrins) and secrete minor amounts of oncofetal fibronectins. This pattern has for a long time been discussed as an essential mechanism of invasiveness (Fisher & Damsky, 1993; Akiyama et al., 1995; Huppertz et al., 1996; Menzin et al., 1998). Aplin et al., (1999) have provided experimental evidence that the interaction between $\alpha5\beta1$ integrins and fibronectins is crucial for trophoblast invasion. These spindle-shaped trophoblast cells are diploid to tetraploid (Zybina et al., 2002).
- **Large polygonal extravillous trophoblast cells** (the former X cells), which express epithelial ($\alpha6\beta4$) and interstitial integrins and embed themselves in large amounts of self-secreted extracellular matrix (laminins, collagen IV, vitronectin, heparan sulfate, fibronectins). These cells are rare in the depth of the invasive pathway but rather accumulate in the basal plate. Moreover, they are the dominating cell type in the late, less invasive stages of pregnancy. The ample ECM accumulated by these cells possibly acts as a kind of trophoblast-endometrial glue (Feinberg et al., 1991) anchoring not only the cells but also the placenta to its implantation site. These cells are generally polyploid (Zybina et al., 2002). Also in rodents, insectivores, and certain carnivores trophoblastic giant cells accumulate as a compact layer of noninvasive trophoblast and show high degrees of polyploidization (Zybina & Zybina, 1996; Klisch et al., 1999a,b; Zybina et al., 2001).

According to the data by Kemp et al. (2002) and Zybina et al. (2002, 2004), the large polygonal trophoblast cells represent not a separate line of differentiation but rather a final step of differentiation of small spindle-shaped trophoblast cells that polyploidize and thereby differentiate into an ECM-secreting, noninvasive phenotype.

The degree is still open to which all three mechanisms (apoptotic death, syncytial fusion, and polyploidization) contribute to the limitation of trophoblast invasion in normal and various pathologic settings. A high incidence of multinucleated trophoblastic giant cells in the first and second trimester and of mononucleated large polygonal trophoblast cells (X cells) in term pregnancies suggests that the mechanisms vary in the course of pregnancy.

Endocrine Activities of Extravillous Trophoblast

There are few data available on endocrine activities of extravillous trophoblast. Generally, all endocrine activities detectable within the extravillous trophoblast have been found also (mostly with higher activities) in villous trophoblast. Therefore, the question arises of whether endocrine activities of extravillous trophoblast play specific functional roles or whether they are simply due to the fact that all trophoblast, whether villous or extravillous, is derived from the same source and therefore shows similar profiles of gene expression.

TABLE 9.1. Approximate localization of placental proteins in various trophoblastic cells as identified by immunocytochemistry

Trophoblast type	First Trimester			Second Trimester			Third Trimester		
	hCG	hPL	SP$_1$	hCG	hPL	SP$_1$	hCG	hPL	SP$_1$
Cytotrophoblast	–	–	–	–	–	–	–	–	–
X cells ("intermediate")	+	+	+/–	+/–	+	+	–	+	+/–
Syncytiotrophoblast	+	+	+	+	+	+	+	+	+
Syncytial giant cells	+	+	+/–	–	+	+/–	–	+	+/–
Syncytial knots	+	+	+	+	+	+	+	+	+
Placental site trophoblast	+/–	+	+/–	–	+	+/–	–	+	+/–
Membranous trophoblast	+	+		–	+	+	–	+	+/–
Endovascular trophoblast	–	+	+/–	–	+	+/–	–	+	+/–

Source: Modified from Kurman et al. 1984a.

Kurman et al. (1984a,b) has provided information on immunoreactivities of **hCG**, **hPL**, and **SP1** (pregnancy-specific β_1-glycoprotein) in the various forms of trophoblast. The findings are summarized in Table 9.1. Gosseye and Fox (1984) found that the villous syncytiotrophoblast was the principal source of hCG, hPL, PAPP-A, PP5, and SP1; in the invasive extravillous trophoblast, only hPL was present. The intensity of cellular hPL staining increased progressively with deeper penetration of the extravillous trophoblast. SP1 and hPL were also detected in some cell populations of trophoblastic tumors (Kurman et al., 1984b; Manivel et al., 1987). The results concerning hPL and hCG immunoreactivities were largely corroborated by other investigators (Sasagawa et al., 1987; Zeng & Fu, 1991); however, Sakbun and coworkers (1990b) who measured mRNA concentrations of hPL, pointed out that villous trophoblast is the major source and that the extravillous trophoblast adds only minor amounts to total placental hPL production.

Prostaglandin metabolism in extravillous trophoblast cells has been discussed as being involved in control of labor: 15-hydroxy prostaglandin dehydrogenase (type I PGDH) was found not only in villous syncytiotrophoblast but also in invasive extravillous trophoblast (Cheung et al., 1990, 1992), where it is ideally located to metabolize and to maintain low concentrations of prostaglandins, in particular in close vicinity of the myometrium.

Pregnancy-associated prostaglandin synthetase inhibitor (PAPSI) was detected in amnionic epithelium, in villous macrophages, and in trophoblast throughout pregnancy (Mortimer et al., 1989). Its importance for the maintenance of pregnancy and for the control of the onset of parturition was discussed by the authors.

Corticotropin-releasing hormone has been described as being present not only in villous cytotrophoblast (Petraglia et al., 1987; Saijonmaa et al., 1988) but also in extravillous trophoblast of the basal plate (Riley et al., 1991) and membranes (Warren & Silverman, 1995). The authors suggested that this releasing hormone locally affects paracrine/autocrine interactions and that it may be involved in the maturation of the fetal hypothalamic-pituitary-adrenal axis.

Does Extravillous Trophoblast Differ from One Nonvillous Part to the Other?

Most of the above data on extravillous trophoblast were obtained from studying cell columns; only a few data are available on extravillous trophoblast of cell islands, the chorionic plate, and chorion laeve (for details, we refer to the respective chapters; see below). This raises the question as to the homogeneity of extravillous trophoblast population throughout placenta and fetal membranes.

When we compared differentiation patterns of extravillous trophoblast derived from cell columns with those from other sites, largely consistent data were found (Castellucci et al., 1991; Mühlhauser et al., 1993; Nanaev et al., 1993a,b; Frank et al., 1994). In all cases, the basal cells resting on the basal lamina or located close to it represent the proliferative subset (Fig. 9.1) and express epithelial integrins (e.g., $\alpha6\beta4$). Those cells that have left the basal lamina stop proliferating, achieve a migratory/invasive phenotype, express interstitial integrins (e.g., $\alpha5\beta1$ and $\alpha1\beta1$), and start apolar ECM secretion. This is in agreement with the findings of Aplin and Campbell (1985) and Malak et al. (1993), who described the distribution patterns of various ECM molecules around the extravillous trophoblast cells of the chorion laeve. Finally, Genbacev et al. (1993c) cultured explants of cell islands and found no differences when comparing them to cell columns. They concluded that cell islands represent free-floating cell columns. All these findings make it very likely that extravillous trophoblast of all intraplacental sites represents one homogeneous population of cells that differ only regarding their stage of differentiation and their degree of invasiveness.

It has been objected that in term chorion laeve the extravillous trophoblast cells resting on the basal lamina are no longer proliferative and do express interstitial integrins (Aplin, 1993). This behavior, however, is confusing only when comparing term chorion laeve with first trimester cell columns. In third trimester cell columns, as is typical for all third trimester locations of extravillous trophoblast, the proliferative activity is downregulated (Kaufmann & Castellucci, 1997), leading to a "burned out" aspect with the invasive phenotype prevailing.

In conclusion, at the moment there is no convincing evidence for the existence of different populations of extravillous trophoblast residing in different nonvillous parts of the placenta.

Decidua

Composition of Decidua

The changes that occur in the human or animal endometrium in response to physiologic stimuli like blastocyst implantation are called decidualization. If the morphogenetic stimulus was a physiologic one, the resulting tissue is the decidua; the tissue resulting from an experimental or artificial stimulus is called a pseudodecidua or, occasionally, a deciduoma.

There is a long history of confusion regarding the nomenclature. This is due to the fact that the tissue **decidua** is composed of cells of different type and origin:

- Decidualized endometrial stromal cells, the so-called **decidual cells**; and
- Considerable numbers and various types of **maternal leukocytes** invading from the bone marrow via the maternal blood; the latter belong to the decidua and inaccurately are sometimes subsumed under the heading "decidual cells."

From all these cells involved in decidualization, only the transformed endometrial stromal cell should properly be called a decidual cell.

Padykula and Driscoll (1978) described the leukocyte infiltration to occur specifically from the 6th to 11th weeks of pregnancy. Bone marrow–derived cells comprise macrophages, T lymphocytes, few granulocytes, and considerable numbers of large granular lymphocytes (uNK cells, the former "endometrial granular cells" or "K cells") (Enders, 1991; Khan et al., 1991; Dietl et al., 1992; Haller et al., 1993).

According to Marzusch and Dietl (1994), Loke and King (1995), and Loke et al. (1995), the decidual cell population is composed as follows:

Cell designation	First trimester	Term pregnancy
Decidual cells and endometrial stromal cells	30%	30–55%
Large granular lymphocytes (uNK cells)	40%	4–9%
T cells	8–10%	8–17%
B cells and plasma cells	<1%	<1%
Macrophages	20%	20–40%
Granulocytes	2%	3–4%

At term, considerably increased numbers of granulocytes can be found at the separation zone of the placenta and at the maternal surface of the delivered placenta. They are thought to represent an inflammatory response to the mechanisms preceding separation of the placenta.

Endometrial Stromal Cells and Decidual Cells

Under the influence of progesterone, the endometrium is changed into decidua, a structurally different tissue. Faint signs of decidualization first become visible on day 23 of the endometrial cycle. They commence around the spiral arteries from where they spread throughout the tissue.

The youngest human implantation stage [Carnegie stage 5a, late day 6 to early day 8 postcoitus (p.c.); see Chapter 8] does not show decidualization (Enders, 1991); within the following 2 or 3 days it is barely beginning (Carnegie stage 5b). Electron microscopic studies have not been performed on these early human cases from the first 2 weeks of pregnancy, so that the exact starting point of decidualization in the human is difficult to describe.

Structure of Decidual Cells

Decidualization is characterized by the enlargement of endometrial stromal cells that eventually assume an epithelioid appearance. This process has been described in detail by Kaiser (1960), Schmidt-Matthiesen (1963), Stegner et al. (1971), Dallenbach-Hellweg and Sievers (1975), Iwanaga (1983), as well as Welsh and Enders (1985). The final result includes cellular hypertrophy and an increase in number and complexity of cytoplasmic organelles, including the rough endoplasmic reticulum and Golgi complexes; it indicates an increase in synthetic and secretory activities. The cells accumulate glycogen as well as sometimes lipids and large areas with perinuclear bundles of intermediate filaments that are immunohistochemically positive for vimentin. Both together, typical morphology and immunoreactivity for vimentin can be used to identify decidual cells (Fig. 9.14A,C; also see Chapter 3, Figs. 3.2L and 3.4B). One to three euchromatic nuclei with prominent nucleoli can occur. The localization of a variety of enzymes in the decidua was summarized by Kearns and Lala (1983) and Lapan and Friedman (1965). Detailed ultrastructural descriptions have been provided by Wynn (1967b, 1974), Enders (1968), Lawn et al. (1971), and Spornitz and Ludwig (1984). Gap junctions were found by several groups (Lawn et al., 1971; Wadsworth et al., 1980; Ono et al., 1989) and it was then discussed whether these synchronize decidual development or decidual function.

One of the most characteristic features of the mature decidual cells is the presence of club-shaped processes that extend into the surrounding external fibrillar lamina. The tips of these processes contain dense granular bodies of about 0.5 μm diameter (Wynn, 1965; Lawn et al., 1971; Stark & Kaufmann, 1973; Kisalus & Herr, 1988). The granules were identified to contain heparan sulfate proteoglycan, which was also released into the surrounding fibrinoid (Kisalus & Herr, 1988). There, it contributes to the acquisition of a pericellular lamina composed of argyrophilic, fibrillar material (Lawn et al., 1971; Wewer et al., 1985) that also stains with cresyl echt, aldehyde fuchsin, and other dyes (Waidl, 1963) and that resembles the basal lamina of epithelia.

The epithelial appearance of decidual cells is evident from histologic sections (Fig. 9.14C; also see Figs. 3.1K and 3.2L). The cells have often been described as rounded

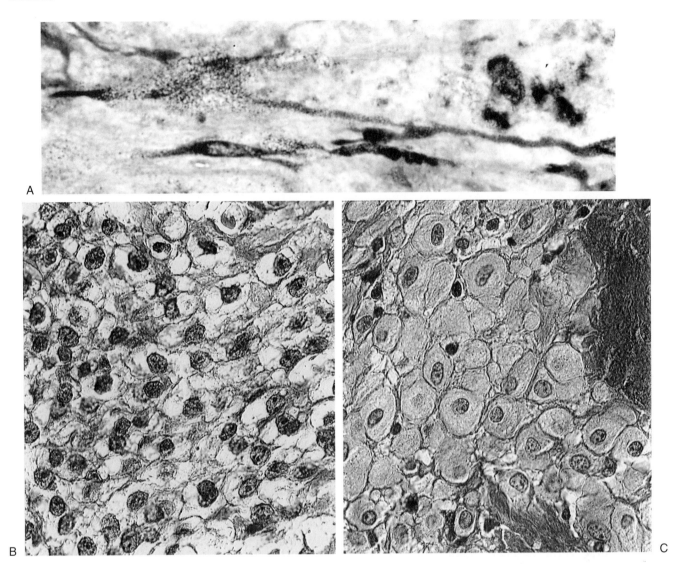

FIGURE 9.14. Comparison of decidua cells with trophoblast cells. A: A 40-μm plastic section of the basal plate. Enzyme histo-chemical proof of isocitrate dehydrogenase. The positively stained cells are decidua cells. In such thick sections the real structure of the elongated cells with extremely long, poorly branched cytoplasmic extensions is revealed. ×520. (*Source:* From Stark & Kaufmann, 1973, with permission.) B: Paraffin section of a cluster of extravillous trophoblast cells at the peripheral end of a cell column. Note the uniformity of cellular shapes and the fact that most cellular profiles contain nuclei. C: Comparable paraffin section of a cluster of decidua cells. Note that the cellular profiles vary very much in diameter and that the numerous small profiles do not contain nuclei. This is due to the fact that most cross sections across the long cellular bodies of decidua cells (cf. part A) do not hit the nucleus. B,C: H&E ×300.

to polygonal (Kisalus & Herr, 1988; Enders, 1991), but according to our experience this impression is incorrect. When we studied decidual cells in thick plastic sections (20 to 50μm), we found large, branched cells (Fig. 9.14A) that resembled hypertrophied connective tissue cells. The length was 100 to 200μm. Thus, the epithelioid appear-ance is the result of cross-sectioning. The low number of nuclear profiles, as compared to the number of cellular cross sections, is one of the easiest available parameters to distinguish decidual from trophoblastic cells (Fig. 9.14B,C; also see Fig. 3.1K).

Control of Decidualization

Few factors have been described that regulate decidual-ization. Progesterone is the most potent stimulator of this differentiation process. Insulin-like growth factor (IGF) is also under discussion in the promotion of decidualiza-tion; its binding protein (IGF-BP) is expressed by decid-ual cells (Bell, 1989; Fazleabas et al., 1989; Rutanen et al., 1991) and appears to be involved in mitosis of endome-trial stromal cells and their later differentiation into decidual cells.

Bone Marrow Derivation of Decidual Cells

Kearns and Lala (1983) and Lala et al. (1984) deduced from experimenting with chimeric mice that the bone marrow was the "ultimate origin" of the decidual cells. According to these authors, the bone marrow derivation is not only valid for decidual macrophages, endometrial NK cells, accidental granulocytes, and T cells, but also for the precursors of the decidualized stromal cells. This special origin could explain why only the intrauterine stromal cells, but not, for example, tubal stromal cells, decidualize under the endocrine and paracrine stimuli of pregnancy. Moreover, it would explain why endometrial stroma once locally removed by uterine connective tissue, for example, in C-section scars and following enforced curettings, does not decidualize in subsequent pregnancies.

Endocrine and Paracrine Aspects of Decidua

Numerous studies have been performed concerning the functional importance of the decidua, and much speculation has been entertained. Even the more commonly suggested functions, such as limiting trophoblastic invasion and providing nourishment for the conceptus, still lack adequate supportive evidence (Enders, 1991). Despite this disillusioning statement, we will try to summarize some interesting findings that may stimulate further discussion.

Relaxin: Several publications ascribe relaxin secretion to decidual tissue (Bigazzi et al., 1982; Bryant-Greenwood et al., 1987; Hansell et al., 1991). Based on old immunohistochemical findings of Dallenbach and Dallenbach-Hellweg (1964), the endometrial granular cells had originally been favored as the origin. But as their identity as large granular lymphocytes has now been settled (see below), relaxin secretory activities are less likely and it is somewhat probable that decidual cells themselves represent the source at the maternofetal interface (Sakbun et al., 1990a; Bogic et al., 1995). On the other hand, relaxin is expressed in villous trophoblast of the human placenta as well as in trophoblast of several other species (Klonisch, personal communication). This suggests the need for reevaluation of the identity of relaxin-expressing cells at the maternofetal interface. In vitro studies of Qin et al. (1997a,b) have shown that trophoblast cells respond to exogenous relaxin with increased expression and activation of various proteinases such as stromelysin-1 (MMP-3), interstitial collagenase (MMP-1), and tPA. The authors suggested a role of decidual relaxin on regulation of ECM degradation in preparation of labor.

hPL: Older publications have favored a decidual production of hPL; however, the decidua was taken from the membranes and placental floor for most of these studies.

It was thus likely to be contaminated by extravillous trophoblast. Kurman et al. (1984a) immunostained specifically for hPL and other hormones in the basal plate, villous tissue, and membranes. They found that hPL was the principal product of what they chose to call the "intermediate trophoblast," the extravillous trophoblast cells. Another possible explanation for the immunoreactivity of decidual cells for hPL is the fact that hPL and prolactin show considerable homology in their amino acid sequence. Correspondingly, in the early period of immunohistochemistry many antibodies were unsuitable to distinguish among both hormones, and, as will be discussed next, there is now convincing evidence that prolactin is a decidual product whereas hPL in the human is exclusively secreted by trophoblast cells.

Prolactin: Proof of the decidual origin of prolactin was obtained by immunohistochemistry (Golander et al., 1979; Rosenberg et al., 1980; Riddick & Daly, 1982; Andersen et al., 1987; Bryant-Greenwood et al., 1987). In vitro studies with isolated cells or tissues (Fukamatsu et al., 1984; Hamaguchi et al., 1990; Daly et al., 1983) and in situ hybridization studies (Wu et al., 1991) confirmed these results. It was noted that prolactin production in various stages of pregnancy was closely related to prolactin concentrations in the amnionic fluid and concluded that prolactin is elaborated by decidual cells contained within the membranes and transported internally, a suggestion made by many investigators. Peak prolactin release into the amnionic fluid is in the 24th week of pregnancy (Neuberg, 1992). The most important functions of decidual prolactin comprised regulatory effects on water and electrolyte transfer across the membranes, thus controlling the fetal water balance. This effect has been observed in vitro when using amnionic fluid prolactin; however, it was absent with human pituitary prolactin (de Bakker-Theunissen et al., 1988). Moreover, it was said to affect the synthesis of fetal surfactant and to influence calcium absorption in the fetal gut (for references, see Neuberg, 1992).

Prostaglandins: The decidual production of prostaglandin E_2 (PGE_2) has been discussed in context with the immunology of gestation; PGE_2 secretion is said to block activation of decidual leukocytes with potential antitrophoblastic killer function, by inhibiting IL-2 receptor generation and IL-2 production (Parhar et al., 1989). Prostaglandins E_2 and $F_{2\alpha}$ have also been discussed in another context: During labor, the production and release of these substances seems to be considerably increased in decidual cells (Khan et al., 1992); the authors discussed the functional relations to labor. The role of PGE_2 is still open, but it may play a role in prepartal ripening of the cervix, whereas $PGF_{2\alpha}$ is essential for the stimulation of uterine muscle during labor (Fuchs & Fuchs, 1984). Casey et al. (1989) proposed that prostaglandin dehydrogenase, resident in the decidua capsularis, regulates levels of prostaglandin therein as well as in amnionic fluid, uterus, and blood. Finally, endothelin-1, a potent vasoconstrictor and its receptors are expressed in human decidual cells (Kubota et al., 1992). Their function during pregnancy and labor is still an open question.

Paracrine regulatory loops: Several such loops between decidual cells and invasive extravillous trophoblast cells are under discussion. Among others, mutual effects of hCG and EGF have been described. Human chorionic gonadotropin is a secretory product not only of villous but also of extravillous trophoblast (Kurman et al., 1984a), whereas EGF is secreted by villous trophoblast (Hofmann et al., 1992; Ladines Llave et al., 1993; Matsuo et al., 1993) but also may be of maternal origin (Fisher et al., 1992). Epidermal growth factor stimulates decidual cell proliferation but inhibits prolactin secretion of decidual cells in culture (Saji et al., 1990). Decidua produces a protein that inhibits hCG release from human trophoblast (Ren & Braunstein, 1991); according to other studies it is likely that prolactin inhibits hCG production (Yuen et al., 1986). On the other hand, decidual cells not only express hCG receptors (Reshef et al., 1990), but hCG (Rosenberg & Bhatnagar, 1984), and in particular αhCG (Blithe et al., 1991) stimulates decidual prolactin production in vitro. Moreover, TNF-α, a secretory product preferentially of decidual macrophages, inhibits trophoblast cell growth (for review, see Briese & Müller, 1992) and promotes trophoblastic apoptosis (Reister et al., 1999, 2001). According to McWey et al. (1982) decidual cells express hPL receptors and may thus be a target for trophoblastic hPL. Finally, decidual large granular lymphocytes (NK cells) are a rich source of TGF-β (Loke & King, 1995), which inhibits trophoblast invasion (Graham et al., 1992; Irving et al., 1995; Lysiak et al., 1995). Respective mechanisms comprise modulation of integrin expression, down-regulation of MMP secretion and induction of TIMPs (Irving et al., 1995; for review see Loke & King, 1995).

Functional Considerations of Decidualization

All of the above studies provide only a little evidence concerning the specific functional activities of the decidua. One must bear in mind that decidualization is not a general phenomenon related to placentation. Rather, it is found in hemochorial placentation, which, unavoidably, is related to invasive processes. In spite of this coincidence, however, it is not the invasive trophoblast itself that stimulates decidualization of endometrial stromal cells; rather, this is very likely to be principally a progesterone effect (see Endometrial Stroma Cells and Decidua Cells, above). In spite of this knowledge, most theories regarding decidual function discuss the decidua in the light of trophoblastic invasion, and the classical descrip-

tions see the decidual cells as being stuffed with glycogen and lipids, to serve as nutrients for the invading trophoblast.

Consequently, a series of studies focused on the interactions between decidualization and trophoblastic invasion (for review, see Bell, 1989). During the menstrual cycle, insulin-like growth factor binding protein (**IGF-BP**) appears to be associated with the stromal fibroblasts (Bell, 1989; Fazleabas et al., 1989; Rutanen et al., 1991; Giudice et al., 1998). It was proposed that IGF-BP is involved in proliferation, inhibition of apoptosis, and decidualization of these cells. Possibly trophoblast cells stimulate the decidual stroma to produce IGF-BP-1 (Lee et al., 1997). Moreover, the RGD tripeptide (Arg-Gly-Asp), which is known to be the recognition site in several adhesive matrix proteins for a range of cell receptors and which is part of the sequence of IGF-BP, has been shown to inhibit tumor cell invasion (Ruoslahti & Pierschbacher, 1987). Therefore, IGF-BP can be interpreted to be part of a paracrine loop by which the decidual cell and decidualization may regulate local proliferation and invasion of trophoblast cells (Bell et al., 1988).

Ruck et al. (1994) have studied the distribution of cell **adhesion molecules** in the decidua throughout pregnancy. The wide variety of cell adhesion molecules found in the various decidual cell populations are likely to allow interactions among all these cells as well interactions between invading trophoblast cells and cells of the decidua.

An interesting publication deals with the secretion of **α₂-macroglobulin** by the rat decidua (Gu et al., 1992). This potent protease inhibitor is specifically expressed by the mesometrial decidua, the site of trophoblastic invasion in the rat. Its expression is regulated in an autocrine loop by prolactin (Gu et al., 1992). On the other hand, the α_2-macroglobulin receptor is expressed by extravillous trophoblast cells (Coukos et al., 1994). Both groups of investigators have speculated that this protease inhibitor may limit tissue damage to decidual cells during extratrophoblastic protease secretion and invasion.

In accordance with all these findings, decidualization may be the answer of the endometrium to trophoblastic invasion, regulating the latter and solving problems posed by hemochorial placentation (Bell, 1989). On the other hand, trophoblast invasion in the human does not induce decidualization in every instance. Pregnancy pathologies that do not show decidualization comprise the following (see Endometrial Stromal Cells and Decidual Cells, above):

• **Tubal pregnancies:** The tubal mucosa does not exhibit any decidual stromal reaction upon implantation and trophoblast invasion; decidua-like cells of the tubal implantation site have been identified by electron microscopy to be invasive trophoblast cells (Spornitz,

1993). Moreover, these tubal implantation sites, in contrast to intrauterine implantation, are largely devoid of large granular lymphocytes (see below) (Vassiliadou & Bulmer, 1998) and of macrophages (own unpublished findings). By contrast, distribution patterns of T cells and B cells are similar in intrauterine and extrauterine implantation sites (von Rango et al., 2001). Trophoblast invasion in this situation is excessive (Kemp et al., 1999).

- **Placenta accreta, increta, and percreta:** Also in these clinical settings, excessive trophoblast invasion is combined with deficient decidualization. Data on leukocyte populations at the implantation site in these cases are not available, to the best of our knowledge.

These data suggest that decidualization is a prerequisite for proper control of trophoblast invasion. It is, however, still an open question whether decidual stromal cells themselves or decidual leukocytes exert this control (see below).

B Cells and T Cells

B cells and plasma cells are virtually absent from normal decidua and are considered to be irrelevant for trophoblast-decidua interactions (Loke & King, 1995). T cells form a minor portion of the decidual lymphocytes (about 10% of all cells in the decidua; see Composition of Decidua, above) (Marzusch & Dietl, 1994; Loke & King, 1995; King & Loke, 1997). The absence of B cells and scarcity of T cells indicate that there is no important influx of cells of the specific adaptive immune system (Loke & King, 1995).

Overall, decidual T cells show a phenotype that would be in agreement with memory cells or activated T cells (Saito et al., 1994; Loke & King, 1995); it is still an open question whether this activated phenotype is specific for pregnancy or already present during the menstrual cycle. Interestingly, however, according to some earlier studies, decidual T cells do express only low levels of T-cell receptor or none at all, the latter being responsible for recognition of MHC-I molecules (Dietl et al., 1990; Marzusch et al., 1991; Chernyshov et al., 1993; for review see Loke & King, 1995). Recent data question the validity of these findings (Ruck & Marzusch, personal communication). This question is of particular importance since paternal peptides presented by trophoblastic HLA-G and HLA-C molecules, upon binding to T-cell receptors are likely to stimulate T-killer-cell–mediated lysis of the invading trophoblast cells.

The relatively low number of T cells in context with the absence of B cells at the site of implantation renders a classical allorecognition reaction of the trophoblast unlikely. This view is in agreement with the fact that the invasive trophoblast cells do not express classical polymorphic MHC I-molecules (see MHC Class I Molecules, above).

It is still a matter of debate why the number of T cells is reduced and B cells are completely absent from the implantation site:

- Inhibition of lymphocyte proliferation by macrophage-derived PGE_2 is one possible explanation (for review see Hunt, 1998).
- An additional attractive hypothesis has been presented by Munn et al. (1998): Indoleamine 2,3-dioxygenase (IDO) secreted by extravillous trophoblast catabolizes extracellularly tryptophan in the maternofetal junctional zone. Local microenvironments with reduced extracellular tryptophan concentration preclude lymphocyte proliferation and thus may protect the invading trophoblast cells from T-cell–mediated lysis. In accordance with this hypothesis, inhibition of tryptophan catabolism in pregnant mice resulted in rejection of the fetuses.
- Another possible mechanism to locally reduce the number of lymphocytes was published by Hammer and coworkers: Invasive extravillous trophoblast cells secrete Fas ligand (Hammer & Dohr, 2000; Murakoshi et al., 2003) and are thus able to stimulate apoptosis of lymphocytes expressing the Fas receptor. Respective clusters of apoptotic leukocytes were found in the implantation site (Hammer & Dohr, 1999; Hammer et al., 1999).
- Kruse et al. (1999) have analyzed the leukocyte homing events in the decidua basalis, in particular the expression of selectins in the decidual vessels. Their data suggest that selective expression patterns in decidual endothelium associated with microdomain specialization within the decidua basalis may be responsible for the selective access of leucocytes to the implantation site. For further review see Zhou et al. (2003a).

In spite of these local mechanisms to reduce the number of maternal lymphocytes in the implantation site, a considerable number of T cells, capable of attaching the invading trophoblast cells, locally persist throughout pregnancy. The functional role of such T cells at the implantation site in many aspects is still a mystery. Among other aspects, their paracrine activities have raised increasing interest (for review, see Hunt, 1998). The balance of two groups of T-helper-cell–derived cytokines is thought to control the maternal immune response against the fetal semiallograft (for review, see Robertson et al., 1994; Mosmann & Sad, 1996):

- T-helper type 1 proinflammatory cytokines (Th1-type cytokines) comprise IFN-γ, IL-2, lymphotoxin, and TNF-α. They are known to activate cytotoxic T cells and are thought to exert adverse effects on trophoblast invasion.
- T-helper type 2 antiinflammatory cytokines (Th2-type cytokines) comprise IL-4, -6, -10, and -13. They are

known to stimulate antibody production by B cells and to support the differentiation of endometrial NK cells (see below), and they are thought to further tropho-blast invasion.

Secretion of these cytokines is not specific for T-helper cells. Rather, macrophages also secrete TNF-α and uNK cells, as well as IFN-γ. These data indicate that a complex cytokine network regulates the interaction of the immune cells at the implantation site (Marzusch et al., 1997). During normal pregnancy, the Th2-cytokines predominate. Their expression is stimulated by progesterone; by contrast, this hormone inhibits macrophage activation and TNF-α secretion. The action of Th1- and Th2-cytokines on trophoblast invasion is further controlled by endometrial NK cells (Hunt, 1998). Interestingly, invasive trophoblast cells share this type of immune response with invasive tumor cells (Mullen et al., 1998).

It is of particular interest that the course of autoimmune diseases often ameliorates throughout pregnancy but relapses after delivery (Beagley & Gockel, 2003). This raises the question as to the activation of general immunosuppressive mechanisms. As one such possibility Aluvihare et al. (2004) found an increase of regulatory T cells in pregnant mice. Regulatory T cells (CD4+CD25+ cells) inhibit inappropriate activation of T- and B-cell responses. In mice the number of regulatory T cells increased generally from 3% to 5% of the T cell pool (nonpregnant) to 9% to 17% (pregnancy), and in the pregnant uterus even to 30%.

Endometrial Large Granular Lymphocytes (Endometrial NK Cells and uNK Cells)

These cells have been well known for many years to occur at the implantation site and they were called "Körnchenzellen," K cells, or granular cells (Hamperl, 1954; Hellweg, 1957; Dallenbach & Dallenbach-Hellweg, 1964; Dallenbach-Hellweg, 1971). Today they are mostly called endometrial NK cells or uNK cells.

Definition: From a comparative point of view, uNK cells are equivalent to the granular metrial gland cells of rodents for which an abundant literature exists (Bulmer & Peel, 1977; Peel & Bulmer, 1977; Bulmer, 1983; Bulmer et al., 1983; Tarachand, 1985, 1986). The human endometrial large granular lymphocytes (LGLs) are regular constituents of all uterine implantation sites (Durst-Zivkovic, 1978) where they amount to about 40% in the first trimester (see Composition of Decidua. above). They are derived from the bone marrow and are closely related to NK cells (endometrial NK cells, uterine NK cells, uNK cells) (Pijnenborg et al., 1980; Bulmer & Sunderland, 1983; Dietl et al., 1992; Marzusch et al., 1993; for reviews, see Enders, 1991; Spornitz, 1992; Loke & King 1995; Whitelaw & Croy, 1996).

Histologically, they are rounded mononuclear cells of approximately 10 μm diameter, with an eccentric, kidney-shaped nucleus. Their typical granular inclusions stain characteristically with phloxine-tartrazine (Pijnenborg

et al., 1980). Sengel and Stöbner (1972) gave a detailed ultrastructural account of these cells. Their appearance within the decidua does not depend on trophoblast invasion but rather is associated with the hormonal conditions of decidualization (Bogaert, 1975; Bulmer et al., 1988a; Pace et al., 1989; Sengupta et al., 1990). Correspondingly, the cells are also present in late proliferative and secretory endometrium.

Surface markers: The LGLs express CD56, a marker molecule of NK cells, but they differ from the majority of NK cells in peripheral blood by the absence of CD57 and CD16. Only 1% to 4% of the NK cells in peripheral blood show this CD56-positive, but CD57- and CD16-negative, phenotype, which is presented by virtually all endometrial large granular lymphocytes (Marzusch et al., 1995; King & Loke, 1997). This distribution has raised the question of which factors are responsible for the specific homing of uNK cells to the decidua. Hanna et al. (2003) have analyzed the chemokine receptor repertoire on various NK cell populations and found the receptors CXCR3 and CXCR4 preferentially expressed on CD16-negative NK cells. Moreover, they found the ligand of CXCR4, CXCL12, to be expressed by the invasive phenotype of extravillous trophoblast. These ligand-receptor interactions were suggested to be responsible for specific accumulation of uNK cells in the invasion zone. The fact, however, that in tubal implantation sites, despite the presence of invasive trophoblast cells, uNK cells do not accumulate (von Rango et al., 2001) suggests that CXCR4/CXCL12 interactions alone cannot be made responsible for specific decidual homing of uNK cells.

Functional aspects: Different from NK cells of the peripheral blood, endometrial NK cells (LGLs) show only moderate in vitro cytotoxicity against the NK cell–sensitive cell line K562 (Ferry et al., 1990). Accordingly, there has been considerable discussion about whether or not they represent NK cells (Watanabe, 1987; Manaseki & Searle, 1989; King & Loke, 1991; Dietl et al., 1992; Saito et al., 1993b; Welsh & Enders, 1993). Their denomination as uterine or endometrial NK cells reflects these differences. Also, the derivation of endometrial NK cells is not yet completely clear. Loke and King (1995) discussed their origin from a common progenitor cell giving rise to both T-cell and NK-cell differentiation.

The mRNA of a number of cytokines was detected in the endometrial NK cells, namely granulocyte CSF (G-CSF), granulocyte-macrophage CSF (GM-CSF), CSF-1, TNF-α, TGF-β, leukemia inhibitory factor (LIF), IL-8, and IFN-γ (Saito et al., 1993b, 1994; Jokhi et al., 1994d; Loke & King, 1995). Also, the presence of the proteins was confirmed for many of these cytokines (Saito et al., 1993b; Jokhi, 1994; for review, see Loke & King, 1995; Whitelaw & Croy, 1996).

Interactions of endometrial NK cells with invading trophoblast cells: The trophoblastic expression of the nonclassical, nonpolymorphic MHC molecules HLA-G and HLA-E, and of the less polymorphic HLA-C (see MHC Class I Molecules, above) is of special importance:

- Trophoblastic expression of the classical polymorphic MHC-I molecules (HLA-A, HLA-B) would trigger a T-cell–mediated immune response against the allohaploid invading trophoblast cells.
- On the other hand, nonexpression of HLA molecules would cause NK-cell attacks. Generally, surface expression of MHC-I molecules prevents NK-cell–mediated lysis of the respective cell (Ljunggren & Kärre, 1990).
- Thus, expression of minimal polymorphic (without individual specificity) HLA molecules by extravillous trophoblast is expected to prevent both T-cell–mediated classical host-versus-graft rejection (for review, see King et al., 1997) as well as susceptibility to decidual NK cell lysis. Indeed, Chumbley et al. (1994a,b) have shown reduction of NK cell–mediated lysis after HLA-G transfection into HLA-G deficient cell lines.

Endometrial NK cells not only recognize the presence or absence of class I molecules but also appear to be able to recognize some basic polymorphism in class I molecules, although they do not detect fine-polymorphic, individual specific differences like T cells (Loke & King, 1995; King & Loke, 1997). The NK cell receptors do also sense nonpolymorphic HLA molecules. These receptors belong to the p58 family of receptors and are now designated as killer cell inhibitory (or activating) receptors (KIR; KAR) (Gumperz & Parham, 1995; for review, see King & Loke, 1997). Human leukocyte antigen-G binding to KIR is thought to inhibit endometrial NK-cell action, whereas binding to KAR activates the endometrial NK cells. Recently it has been shown that prevention of uNK cell–mediated lysis of invasive trophoblast cells requires much more complex interactions than simply HLA-G or HLA-C expression. In addition to the latter two molecules, invasive trophoblast cells express the nonpolymorphic HLA-E; however, only those HLA-E molecules are exposed at the cell surface, which have bound a nonapeptide derived from the signal sequences of HLA-G or HLA-C. Lytic action of uNK dells against their target cell is only prevented by binding of this HLA-E complex to a dimeric uNK cell receptor (CD94/NKG2) (Borrego et al., 1998; Lee et al., 1998; Llano et al., 1998).

In contrast to the classical intramolecular variability of T-cell receptors, the cell-recognition repertoire of NK cells is defined by varying coexpression patterns of KIR- and KAR-like receptors on one and the same NK cell. In addition, besides HLA-G/C/E binding to uNK receptors, trophoblastic surface carbohydrates are thought to be recognized by additional NK-cell receptors (Yokoyama, 1995; for review, see King & Loke, 1997). The coexpres-

sion of nonpolymorphic HLA molecules jointly with cell surface carbohydrates may be responsible for inhibition or activation of NK cells and thus provides a mechanism for the control of trophoblast invasion. As discussed above, invasive extravillous trophoblast cells express respective cell surface carbohydrates, such as sialyl Le^x and blood group antigen "i" (King & Loke, 1988; Frank et al., 1995; Huppertz et al., 1996).

With these findings taken together, evidence is accumulating that there is maternal allorecognition of the fetus by endometrial NK cells, ensuring immunologic protection but also control of the fetal allohaploid transplant (for review, see King et al., 2000). This trophoblast-related allorecognition is thus completely different from both the classical lytic NK-cell action and the T-cell–mediated host-versus-graft reaction. Activated endometrial NK cells are likely to exert paracrine actions on B and T cells as well as on macrophages, the latter again controlling the uNK cells. Such paracrine activities may provide the basis for yet unexplained phenomena such as

- the presence of T cells with an activated phenotype, but paucity of T cell receptors;
- the remarkably low number of B cells and plasma cells at the implantation site; and
- the absence of a significant local humoral response to secreted trophoblastic proteins.

Macrophages

Maternal macrophages are regular constituents of each implantation site and can be demonstrated for instance immunohistochemically by antibodies to CD14 or CD68 (Bulmer & Johnson, 1984; Bulmer et al., 1988b; Vince & Johnson, 1996; Reister et al., 1999; see also Hofbauer Cells in Chapter 6). In spite of their regular presence in the implantation site, only a little is known about the role of macrophages in maternofetal interaction. The recent years have seen a concerted research effort toward the characterization of uNK cells, whereas decidual macrophages have attracted only a little attention.

Macrophages are capable of phagocytosing cellular detritus in the maternofetal battlefield and of clearing immune complexes. Moreover, they are known to be involved in many ontogenetic processes, preferably by paracrine interactions (Werb, 1983). Greater numbers of macrophages are found in the decidua basalis as compared to the decidua parietalis, where trophoblast invasion is limited. This may serve as a hint to so far uncharacterized interactions of trophoblast and macrophages (Oksenberg et al., 1986; Loke & King, 1995).

Cytokines: Generally, decidual macrophages produce and respond to a wide range of cytokines and thus may be involved in paracrine networks of the decidua, either limiting or supporting trophoblast invasion (for review, see Hunt, 1990; Robertson et al., 1994; Loke & King, 1995; Kaufmann & Castellucci, 1997). They may be involved in infection-associated preterm labor (Hunt, 1989); when activated during inflammation, they produce high levels of PGE$_2$ and TNF, both of which can induce myometrial contractions. Moreover, PGE$_2$ has a profound inhibitory effect on lymphocyte proliferation (for review, see Hunt, 1998). Triggering of macrophage cytotoxin production has been shown to mediate early embryo loss in murine pregnancy (Baines et al., 1997). In vitro, macrophages have been shown to stimulate IFN-γ secretion by uNK cells (Marzusch et al., 1997). Further, macrophage cytokines comprise stem cell factor, which is secreted by invading trophoblast cells. The corresponding receptor (c-kit) is expressed by decidual macrophages (Fig. 9.9A). This pattern raises the question of whether macrophages are attracted and activated by the invasive trophoblast (Sharkey et al., 1992, 1994). Another paracrine loop may be provided by the macrophage-derived VEGF; its receptor (flt-1) is expressed by extravillous trophoblast cells (Sharkey et al., 1993).

Induction of trophoblast apoptosis: Also, TNF-α is secreted by macrophages (Hunt, 1989; Todt et al., 1996; Pijnenborg et al., 1998). Its receptor (TNF-R1) is expressed by trophoblast cells (Yui et al., 1996). Interaction between TNF-α and the R1-receptor have been shown to induce trophoblast apoptosis in vitro (Yui et al., 1994). Similar data have been obtained when studying immortalized extravillous trophoblast (EVT) cells in vitro. These EVT cell lines express TNF-R1 (Reister et al., 2001).

We have demonstrated an inverse relation between the number of trophoblast cells in the wall of spiral arteries and the number of macrophages within the vessel wall (Reister et al., 1999):

- In normal pregnancy, the walls of spiral arteries are largely devoid of macrophages and become invaded by trophoblast cells.

- In preeclampsia, deficient arterial trophoblast invasion and increased numbers of apoptotic trophoblast cells around the uteroplacental arteries correlate with large numbers of macrophages in the arterial media. By contrast, in preeclampsia, the number of macrophages in the surrounding interstitium seems to be reduced (Burk et al., 2001).

The positive correlation between activated macrophages and apoptotic trophoblast cells is generally accepted; however, it is still a matter of discussion whether activated macrophages induce trophoblast apoptosis or whether, vice versa, trophoblast apoptosis provides chemotactic signaling for the attraction of macrophages. A later study by Reister et al. (2001) showed that activated macrophages induce apoptosis of invasive extravillous trophoblast. This effect can only partly be abolished by the simultaneous administration of TNF-R1 antibodies. It therefore cannot exclusively be based on TNF-α/TNF-R1 interaction. Rather, induction of trophoblast apoptosis is a deleterious combination of (1) a TNF-α effect with (2) local tryptophan depletion by macrophage-secreted IDO (see Fig. 9.35).

Macrophage function is inhibited by high doses of progesterone. In particular, expression of iNOS and TNF are reduced (Miller et al., 1996; for review, see Hunt, 1998). This explains why progesterone is one of the many factors that supports trophoblast invasion.

Glandular Residues

During decidualization, the endometrial glands initially enlarge and they can often be observed in the decidua of first trimester specimens (Fig. 9.15; also see Chapter 3, Fig. 3.1M). Their epithelium actively secretes material that is discharged into the lumen ("uterine milk"). When pregnancy ensues, the epithelial cell nuclei undergo endomitosis, become polyploid, and acquire the feature known as the Arias-Stella (1973) change. Ultimately, the glands atrophy although their remains can still be found in the basal plate and in the placental bed. Their regressive nature in these stages of pregnancy is also underlined by the absence of immunoreactivity for EGF (Hofmann et al., 1991). Due to the atypical structures of these residues they can usually be identified only by staining with immunohistochemical epithelial markers, such as cytokeratin (Bulmer et al., 1986) (see Chapter 3). However, it should be noted that disintegrating residual glands easily can be mixed up with uterine vessels as soon as the latter are invaded by trophoblast cells and their lumen is lined by cytokeratin-positive intraarterial trophoblast.

Decidual Extracellular Matrix

Extracellular fibrillar material is characteristic of the decidual reaction. It is rich in laminins, collagens, heparan sulfate proteoglycan, and fibronectins (Wewer et al., 1985; Abrahamsohn & Zorn, 1993; Korhonen & Virtanen, 1997). Decidual cells are embedded in a network of type I and III collagens, and enmeshed with collagen V and fibronectins, all of which are produced by the decidual cells and their endometrial stromal precursors. Type IV collagen and laminin prevail in the immediate surrounding of decidual cells. Interestingly, the isoform pattern of laminins changes throughout differentiation; whereas undifferentiated stromal cells secrete preferably laminin 1, following decidualization the newly formed pericellular basal lamina is composed preferentially of laminins 2 and 4 (Church et al., 1996). Antibodies directed against

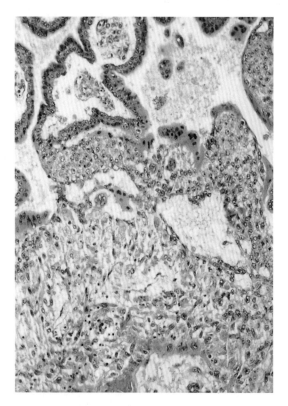

FIGURE 9.15. Early physiologic change in a spiral artery (bottom) in the placental floor of a normal 33-day twin pregnancy. Little of the Nitabuch's and Rohr's fibrin striae are present as yet. Anchoring villi attach with columns, and the intervillous space is lined mostly with syncytium. The basal plate decidua (pale cells) is densely infiltrated with extravillous trophoblast cells, and the arterial wall (bottom) has undergone fibrinoid necrosis. H&E ×100.

osteonectin have shown that the surfaces of mature decidual cells stain heavily with this antibody and that young cells have this protein in their cytoplasm (Wewer et al., 1986).

Kisalus et al. (1987) showed club-shaped processes and secretory bodies on the cellular surfaces of decidual cells containing heparan sulfate that were exocytosed in a merocrine secretory fashion. From our own data we conclude that the ECM surrounding decidual cells is in many places similar in ultrastructure and in immunohistochemical composition to the ECM embedding the extravillous trophoblast cells, the matrix-type fibrinoid (see Fibrinoid, below). Both seem to represent accumulated, modified basal lamina material that is secreted in an unpolarized fashion (Frank et al., 1994; Huppertz et al., 1996). Interestingly, oncofetal fibronectins are found only in decidua that is invaded by extravillous trophoblast (Korhonen & Virtanen, 1997). This raises the question of whether expression of these isoforms reflects a decidual response to invasion or whether

their presence simply points to an admixture of trophoblastic ECM.

In spite of several specific features of both collagen V expression by decidual cells and i-glycosylated oncofetal fibronectins in extravillous trophoblastic ECM, it is still impossible to define the decidual or trophoblastic origin of every matrix component in the junctional zone where matrices derived from both sources intensely mix.

Fibrinoid

DEFINITION AND HISTORICAL REMARKS

Fibrinoid, first described by Langhans (1877), is one of the most prominent components of the human placenta. Accordingly, it has always played a remarkable role in placental pathology. It can be easily identified histologically (Figs. 9.16 and 9.17A). According to Grosser (1925, 1927) all placental material of solid consistency and not composed of cells, syncytium, or connective tissue that shows special affinity to acid stains represents fibrinoid (see Chapter 3, Fig. 3.2C,F,H,I). Its light microscopic appearance changes from glossy and homogeneous to lamellar, fibrous, or reticular. In paraffin sections, using hematoxylin and eosin (H&E), and depending on localization and staining conditions, the color of fibrinoid varies from slightly pink to intense red. When Mallory's connective tissue technique is used, the color is (ideally) a light blue but may vary from dark blue to lilac or even red.

The first attempt to clearly differentiate between "fibrin" and "fibrinoid" and to define the latter was made by Grosser (1925). He proposed that the term fibrin be used only for the precipitates of fibrinogen in blood and tissue fluids. Nonfibrous, noncellular, more or less homogeneous products in the placenta, derived from heterogeneous sources such as cellular secretion and cellular degeneration or of unknown origin, were to be described as being fibrin-like, that is, fibrinoid. Because blood clot and secretory products are usually deposited close together and cannot be easily discriminated with every histologic stain, we propose the more general term fibrinoid as appropriate for placental histology. The general use of the term fibrin is not justified.

The following typical localizations of fibrinoid have been described:

1. Fibrinoid at the intervillous surface of the chorionic plate (subchorial fibrinoid, **Langhans' stria**) (Fig. 9.1; also see Fig. 9.23)
2. **Perivillous fibrinoid** (Fig. 3.2H)
3. **Intravillous fibrinoid** (Fig. 3.2F)
4. Fibrinoid deposits in placental septa (Fig. 3.2K)
5. Fibrinoid of cell islands (Fig. 9.17; also see Chapter 3, Figs. 3.1G and 3.2J)
6. Superficial fibrinoid of the basal plate, facing the intervillous space (**Rohr's stria**) (Figs. 3.2I, 9.16)
7. Fibrinoid of cell columns (Figs. 3.2I and 3.4C,D)
8. Uteroplacental fibrinoid in the depth of the basal plate, where maternal and fetal cells come in close contact to each other (uteroplacental fibrinoid, **Nitabuch's stria**) (Fig. 3.2L)
9. **Intramural fibrinoid** of uteroplacental arteries and veins (Fig. 3.1L)
10. Fibrinoid in the membranes (chorion laeve) (Chapter 11, Fig. 11.1)

Unfortunately, most detailed histochemical, biochemical, immunohistochemical, and experimental studies have been performed at only one of these sites of fibrinoid localization. This selection may explain the considerable discrepancies concerning composition, proposed derivation, and functional interpretation. Immunohistochemical, biochemical,

FIGURE 9.16. Basal plate of mature placenta. Above is the intervillous space. The decidua is covered with Rohr's fibrin stria and "placental site giant cells"; basophilic extravillous trophoblast cells are diffusely scattered throughout the paler decidual cells. Atrophied glandular spaces and small maternal vessels are also present. H&E ×100.

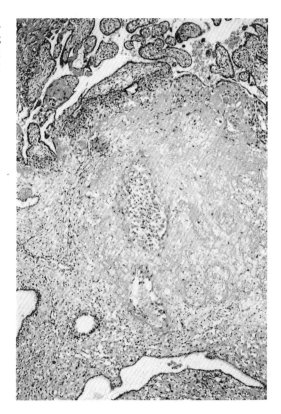

lectin histochemical, and ultrastructural studies have revealed that fibrinoid is composed of two subtypes that differ regarding genesis and composition (Frank et al., 1994; Lang et al., 1994; Huppertz et al., 1996; for review, see Kaufmann et al., 1996):

• Fibrin-type fibrinoid, which is derived from the coagulation cascade and mainly composed of fibrin;
• Matrix-type fibrinoid, which is a secretory product of extravillous trophoblast cells and mainly composed of collagen IV and glycoproteins of the extracellular matrix.

Generally, both subtypes can be found in all of the above-listed localizations, the only differences being varying proportions.

Types of Fibrinoid

Fibrin-type fibrinoid histologically is a densely stained, partly fibrillar, partly net-like matrix (Fig. 9.17A). Ultrastructurally it is characterized by the presence of a dense meshwork of fibers measuring less than 10 nm in thickness, with the characteristic cross striation of fibrin filaments with an approximately 20 nm periodicity (Fig. 9.18). It never contains extravillous trophoblast cells. Immunohistochemically it shows intense reactivity with fibrin antibodies (Figs. 3.4C and 9.17B) that do not cross-react with fibrinogen (e.g., Immunotech fibrin antibody clone E8, directed against the β-peptide; Hui et al., 1983). Moreover, it contains plasma fibronectins. Typically, basal lamina molecules and interstitial matrix molecules such as cellular fibronectins, collagens, laminins are absent. For further details see Frank et al. (1994). Furthermore, fibrin-type fibrinoid can be characterized by binding of Ulex Europaeus lectin (UEA-I), indicating a reaction with encased and disintegrated remnants of endothelial and blood cells that usually bind this lectin (Lang et al., 1994); Bandeiraea simplicifolia lectin (BS-I) and Lycopersicon esculentum lectin (LEA) do not stain this type of fibrinoid.

Matrix-type fibrinoid is characterized by the presence of single or clustered extravillous trophoblast cells (Fig. 9.17), surrounded by ample glossy extracellular matrix. It never stains with fibrin-specific antibodies (Fig. 9.17B), but it contains immunohistochemically detectable traces of fibrinogen. The most characteristic finding for matrix-type fibrinoid is its immunoreactivity for the basal lamina molecules collagen IV and laminin, as well as for cellular fibronectins, especially the oncofetal isoforms (antibodies BC-1 and FDC-6) (Fig. 9.17C) (Frank et al., 1994). Moreover, admixtures of merosin, a laminin-related protein (Leivo et al., 1989; Ehrig et al., 1990; Damsky et al., 1992), heparan sulfate and vitronectin (Castellucci et al., 1993; Huppertz et al., 1996), as well as of fibrillin (King & Blankenship, 1997) have been found. The presence of oncofetal fibronectins in the surrounding of extravillous trophoblast cells has already been reported before (Feinberg et al., 1991b; Feinberg & Kliman, 1993).

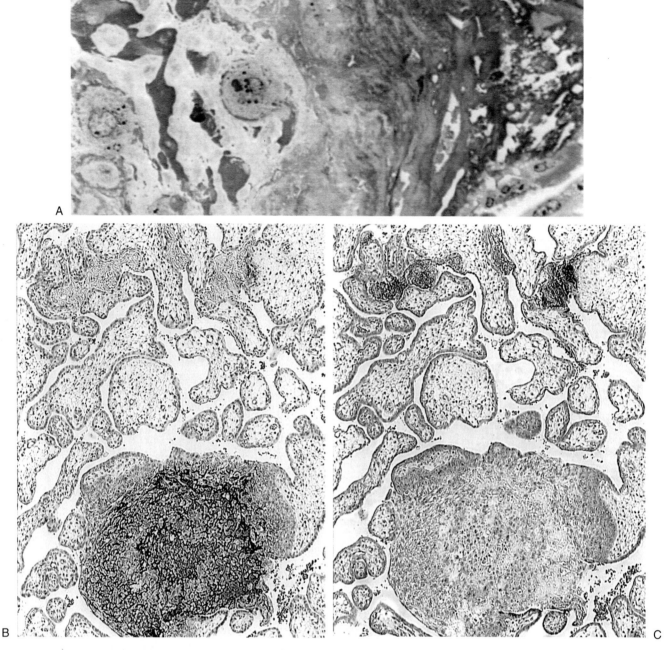

FIGURE 9.17. A: Semithin plastic section of a fibrinoid plaque attached to a cell island; toluidine blue staining. The right half of the picture shows the intensely staining, heterogeneous, partly filamentous structure of fibrin-type fibrinoid. To the left this is continuous with the mosaic pattern of partly densely stained, partly glossy matrix-type fibrinoid, embedding several extravillous trophoblast cells. Term placenta, ×400. B,C: Serial cryostat sections of placental villi and of a cell island (below), 16th week p.m. B: Stained with an antibody directed against oncofetal fibronectin; this matrix molecule can be found specifically in matrix-type fibrinoid that encases the extravillous trophoblast cells of the cell island (brown staining, lower half), but is largely missing in fibrin-type fibrinoid (light brown staining in the upper half). C: Stained with an antibody that detects fibrin but not fibrinogen; fibrin-type fibrinoid in a perivillous position is specifically stained (brown staining), but not the matrix-type fibrinoid of the cell island. ×50.

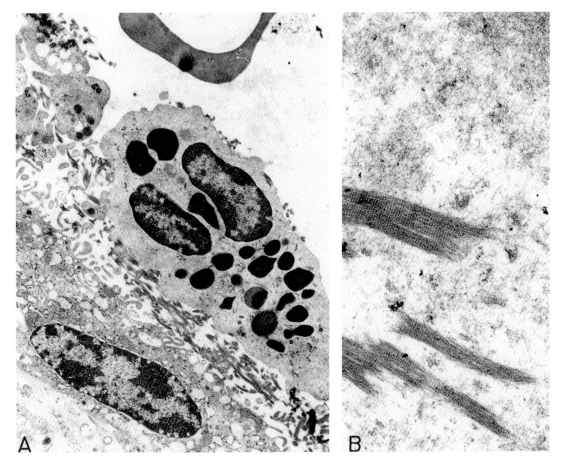

FIGURE 9.18. A: Perivillous fibrin deposition on the trophoblastic surface of an obviously damaged villus (below). A maternal granulocyte (center) as well as several platelets (upper left corner) are attached to the bundles of fibrin. ×9200. B: Higher magnification of fibrin-type fibrinoid from Nitabuch stria from the basal plate. The mixture of granular to fine filamentous material with larger bundles showing typical cross-striation is highly characteristic. ×35,000.

According to the lectin binding studies of Lang et al. (1994), matrix-type fibrinoid is further characterized by the presence of binding with LEA and BS-I, whereas UEA-I does not bind.

Ultrastructurally, matrix-type fibrinoid shows a microheterogeneity (Fig. 9.17A). Three different patches of matrix are arranged around the cells in a mosaic-like pattern. These patches are characterized by the following matrix molecules (Huppertz et al., 1996, 1998d):

- Homogeneous, glossy patches are composed of heparan sulfate and vitronectin.
- Fibrillar patches are composed of various fibronectins embedded in heparan sulfate and vitronectin.
- Granular patches are composed of collagen IV and laminins.

Interestingly, in the more proximal invasive zone every large polygonal extravillous trophoblast cell, the main producers of matrix-type fibrinoid, has contact with any of these patches, the integrin distribution in its plasmalemma matching the extracellular distribution of matrix ligands [see Extracellular Matrix Receptors (Integrins), above]:

- α6ß4 integrins are alwayss in contact with collagen IV and laminin patches.
- α5ß1 integrins are expressed where the fibronectin patches face the plasmalemma.
- αv integrins prevail where the glossy matrix composed of vitronectins and heparan sulfate is apposed (Kertschanska et al., 1997). In the deeper invasive zones where small spindle-shaped trophoblast cells prevail, the integrin distribution within the plasmalemma does not necessarily match the distribution of the surrounding ECM molecules.

Colocalization of integrins and their respective matrix ligands seems to inversely correlate with the invasiveness of the trophoblast; missing colocalization in spindle-shaped trophoblast obviously reflects increasing invasive potential.

Localisation of fibrinoid subtypes: The quantitative proportions of matrix- and fibrin-type fibrinoids vary typically between the different locations:

Fibrinoid at the intervillous surface of the chorionic plate (subchorial fibrinoid, Langhans' stria)	Compact layer, facing the chorionic mesenchyme: matrix-type fibrinoid; reticular layer, facing the intervillous space: fibrin-type fibrinoid
Perivillous fibrinoid	Mostly fibrin-type fibrinoid
Intravillous fibrinoid	Highly variable mixture of both fibrinoid types
Fibrinoid deposits in placental septa	Variable mixture of both subtypes
Fibrinoid of cell islands	Superficially thin layers of fibrin-type fibrinoid; centrally around the extravillous trophoblast cells: matrix-type fibrinoid
Superficial fibrinoid of the basal plate, facing the intervillous space (Rohr's stria)	Fibrin-type fibrinoid
Fibrinoid of cell columns	Superficially, facing the intervillous space: fibrin-type fibrinoid; centrally, embedding the invasive trophoblast cells: matrix-type fibrinoid
Uteroplacental fibrinoid in the depth of the basal plate (uteroplacental fibrinoid, Nitabuch's stria)	Highly variable mixture of both subtypes with predominance of fibrin-type fibrinoid close to the separation zone
Intramural fibrinoid of uteroplacental arteries and veins	Mostly fibrin-type fibrinoid
Fibrinoid of the membranes (chorion laeve)	Within the trophoblast layer: matrix-type fibrinoid; at the trophoblast-decidual junction: fibrin-type fibrinoid

As a general rule, fibrin-type fibrinoid, derived from polymerization of blood fibrinogen, lines the intervillous space in all those locations where the syncytiotrophoblast layer is interrupted; moreover, it prevails in zones of contact between invasive trophoblast and decidua. It is always interposed between matrix-type fibrinoid and maternal blood. Matrix-type fibrinoid, a secretory product of extravillous trophoblast, embeds the postproliferative extravillous trophoblast cells and accordingly can only be found were trophoblast migration/invasion takes place.

Origin of Fibrinoids

Fibrinoid has been shown to react with anti-fibrinogen antibodies in a variety of placental sites (Moe, 1969a,b,c; Gille et al., 1974; Faulk et al., 1975; Johnson & Faulk, 1978), a finding supported by the biochemical findings of Sutcliffe et al. (1982). According to our own experience with anti-fibrinogen binding, it is quite likely that most of the fibrinogen-positive deposits represented **fibrin-type fibrinoid**, even though some immunoreaction for fibrinogen can be found also in matrix-type fibrinoid.

There is no doubt as to the importance of fibrinogen for the formation of fibrin-type fibrinoid. According to Sutcliffe et al. (1982), local, extrahepatic synthesis of fibrinogen is unlikely. Rather, local activation of blood clotting factors must be considered. Indeed, some authors have found enzymes in human trophoblast and uterine cells that were antigenically similar to the blood clotting factor XIII and that were able to polymerize fibrinogen (Chung, 1972; Bohn, 1978).

The typical distribution of fibrin-type fibrinoid lining the intervillous space suggests its origin from maternal blood; however, one cannot exclude that fibrinogen derived from fetal plasma contributes to fibrinoid formation. In particular, in the villous tree, matrix-type fibrinoid is often encapsulated with fibrin from both the intervillous and stromal side, thus suggesting a derivation from both maternal and fetal fibrinogen.

The extracellular matrix molecules found in **matrix-type fibrinoid** are known to be secretory products of epithelial cells (Carnemolla et al., 1987). Castellucci et al. (1993), Hohn et al. (1993), Feinberg and Kliman (1993), and Frank et al. (2000) have provided evidence that also trophoblast cells secrete these matrix molecules. The oncofetal isoforms of fibronectin, containing the ED-B domain, are suitable marker molecules for matrix-type fibrinoid (Frank et al., 1994, 1995). The ED-B domain, which is detected by the antibody BC-1, is not present in plasma fibronectins (Carnemolla et al., 1989). Rather, it is expressed only in oncofetal fibronectins, which are secreted by some fetal and malignant cells, but usually not by normal adult epithelial cells (Carnemolla et al., 1989).

Collagen IV, laminin, heparan sulfate, and cellular fibronectin are secreted also by villous cytotrophoblast together with collagen VI in a polarized manner at their basal surface, constituting the basement membrane (Rukosuev et al., 1990; Castellucci et al., 1993; Nanaev et al., 1993a,b). As a consequence of highly active trophoblastic proliferation in cell columns and cell islands, some of the daughter cells lose the contact with the trophoblastic basal lamina. These extravillous trophoblast cells temporarily stop secretion of detectable amounts of matrix molecules (Castellucci et al., 1993). As soon as the cells are located three or more layers distal to the basal lamina, they start secreting ECM molecules anew, but in a nonpolarized manner. At the same time they change their secretory pattern by replacing collagen VI with oncofetal fibronectins (Frank et al., 1994). The matrix molecules accumulate extracellularly as matrix-type fibrinoid, thereby embedding and separating the extravillous trophoblast cells (Figs. 9.4A and 9.9B).

Decidual cells secrete an ECM showing considerable similarities (see below). They have been shown to express various laminins (Church et al., 1996, 1997) and collagen IV (Mylona et al., 1995); moreover, secretion of heparan sulfate proteoglycan by decidual cells into the surrounding fibrinoid has been described by Kisalus and Herr (1988). These findings raise the question of whether extravillous trophoblast is the only source of matrix-type fibrinoid or whether decidual cells also may contribute to it.

Interactions Between Matrix-Type and Fibrin-Type Fibrinoid

Matrix-type fibrinoid virtually never directly faces the intervillous space; rather, it is always covered by highly variable amounts of fibrin-type fibrinoid. On the other hand, fibrin-type fibrinoid, in our experience, never directly is in contact with cytotrophoblast but rather is separated from the latter by matrix-type fibrinoid. This typical colocalization of both types of fibrinoid suggests that the processes leading to their deposition are linked to each other.

The interactions between fibrin deposition and secretion of matrix-type fibrinoid become particularly obvious in the case of perivillous fibrinoid. It is a common histopathologic finding that villous cytotrophoblast acquires an extravillous phenotype as soon as the covering syncytiotrophoblast is interrupted (Stark & Kaufmann, 1974). Detailed investigation of such areas has revealed that these denuded villous trophoblast cells rarely directly face the maternal blood. Rather, they encapsulate themselves in matrix-type fibrinoid, which is separated from the maternal blood by fibrin-type fibrinoid. The question remains open, whether fibrin deposition as a consequence of syncytiotrophoblast damage induces the extravillous phenotype with subsequent secretion of matrix-type fibrinoid or whether loss of syncytiotrophoblast causes extravillous transformation of the cytotrophoblast with subsequent apolar matrix secretion and induction of the coagulation cascade.

The presence of collagens, laminin, and fibronectins in matrix-type fibrinoid may represent a possible tie between the formation of both types of fibrinoid. Collagens (Kunicki et al., 1988), fibronectins (Piotrowicz et al., 1988), and laminin (Sonnenberg et al., 1988) are known to initiate coagulation by interaction with platelets (Coleman et al., 1987). Platelet antigens have been described in fibrinoid (for review, see Coleman et al., 1987; Faulk, 1989). Thus, it is likely that matrix-type fibrinoid, once secreted by cytotrophoblast, initiates the coagulation cascade and the formation of fibrin-type fibrinoid in all those positions where it is in contact with maternal or fetal blood. In addition, it cannot be excluded that proteases secreted together with the trophoblast-derived ECM directly initiate fibrinogen cleavage with subsequent fibrin deposition. Such atypical pathways of fibrin formation do not involve the coagulation cascade (for review, see Frank et al., 1994).

Functions of Fibrinoid

It is no longer justified to classify fibrinoid merely as the result of degenerative processes caused by placental aging or altered blood flow and nutrition. Rather, most authors consider fibrinoid as an unavoidable constituent of the normal placenta (for review, see Fox, 1997). Several functional aspects are under discussion.

- Hörmann (1965) and Kretschmann (1967a,b) pointed to the mechanical importance of the **constructive principle**. Even though we believe that this aspect has never been studied in detail, it appears reasonable that perivillous fibrin, deposited on the stem villi, may increase their mechanical stability. In the same way, mechanically supportive effects can be attributed to fibrinoid deposits lining the chorionic and the basal plates.

- For matrix-type fibrinoid it has been suggested that it represents the "glue" that guarantees **adhesiveness** of the placenta to the uterine wall (Feinberg et al., 1991b; Frank et al., 1994, 1995). This type of fibrinoid occupies most of the interstitium between extravillous trophoblast and decidual cells; it contains several ECM molecules (e.g., fibronectins, laminins, collagens) (Frank et al., 1994; Huppertz et al., 1996) the cellular receptors of which (integrins) have been found in both the maternal and the fetal cells of the junctional zone (Korhonen et al., 1991; Damsky et al., 1992; Aplin, 1993). Matrix-type fibrinoid, which has a protein composition similar to that of basal laminas (pseudo-basement membrane, Aplin & Campbell, 1985; basement membrane-like layer, King & Blankenship, 1994b), may constitute a three-dimensionally arranged giant basal lamina to which all extravillous trophoblast cells and decidual cells of the maternofetal junctional zone are connected. Jackson and coworkers (1993) have added a partly contrasting view. They found that the production of oncofetal fibronectins by trophoblast cells in vitro was stimulated by inflammatory products (endotoxin, lipopolysaccharide) and by inflammatory mediators (IL-1β). These substances are known to mediate labor by stimulation of prostaglandin secretion. The authors discussed secretion and metabolism of oncofetal fibronectin in relation to the initiation of preterm labor.

- Additional importance may be attributed to fibrin-type fibrinoid as the **regulator of the intervillous circulation** (Stark & Kaufmann, 1974; Becker, 1981; Kaufmann, 1981b). The intervillous space is an open, cleft-like communicating and continuously growing system. In the absence of a clearly defined vascular bed, problems in perfusion are to be expected during the establishment of its maternal circulation. One possibility for continuously adapting the shape of the intervillous space to the maternal blood flow is to obstruct all poorly perfused areas by clotting of blood and fibrinoid deposition. If one were to accept this mechanism, it is then only of secondary importance whether this is achieved by hemostasis with subsequent coagulation or by trophoblastic malnutrition with subsequent syncytial degeneration and induction of fibrinoid deposition.

- The occurrence of fibrinoid at the maternofetal junction correlates with invasive placentation (Pijnenborg et al., 1981). This consideration has prompted several authors to discuss a functional role of fibrinoid as a **barrier to trophoblastic invasion**. The nature of this influence remains an open question. Badarau and Gavrilita (1967), Wynn (1967a), and Moe (1969a,b,c), have suggested that fibrinoid plays a role as a barrier to limit the invasiveness of the trophoblast. This was supported by findings from tubal pregnancies (Kawagoe et al., 1981). For a long time, one had to counter by suggesting that this conclusion is not in agreement with histologic findings: Considerable numbers of trophoblast cells can be found inside fibrinoid or even below Nitabuch's stria, sometimes even in the myometrium. Our recent findings, however, substantiate that the presence of trophoblast cells is related to only one subtype of fibrinoid, the matrix type. In contrast, the fibrin type is never invaded by extravillous cytotrophoblast (Frank et al., 1994) and may thus have the same barrier function against trophoblastic invasion that Dvorak et al. (1983) have suggested to exist for fibrin against tumor invasion.

- Aplin and Foden (1982) described a placental extract, called the "cell spreading factor," that contains fibronectin and fibrinogen. They speculated about its presence in the uteroplacental fibrinoid to restrict or perhaps even promote trophoblast migration and invasion. This was one of the first suggestions for the presence of **invasiveness-promoting activities**. Later this hypothesis has been further substantiated: Oncofetal fibronectins containing the ED-B domain are known to be present in both, the ECMs of malignant tumors (Carnemolla et al., 1989) and in matrix-type fibrinoid (Frank et al., 1994). This suggests interrelations of extravillous trophoblastic invasiveness with matrix-type fibrinoid. In cell columns, the invasive phenotype of the extravillous trophoblast correlates well with increasing amounts of matrix-type fibrinoid. Whereas fibrin-containing matrices have been discussed as acting as barrier against cellular invasion (Dvorak et al., 1983), the self-secreted matrix-type fibrinoid may provide the appropriate microenvironment for extravillous trophoblastic invasion. This assumption is supported by in vitro data: villous trophoblast explanted on ECMs (Matrigel) comparable to matrix-type fibrinoid achieve an extravillous phenotype and easily invade this matrix (Genbacev et al., 1993a,b,c; 1994; Vicovac et al., 1995a,b). The contrasting functions of matrix-type and fibrin-type fibrinoid described above may interact with each other. One example of this is

the morphogenesis of the basal plate, where a barrier of fibrin-type fibrinoid is deposited continuously at the fetal surface. It possibly controls the invasion of trophoblast cells, which themselves secrete matrix-type fibrinoid as a supporting matrix along their invasive pathway.

- Perivillous fibrinoid is discussed as being a **barrier to maternofetal transport processes**. The integrity and completeness of the syncytiotrophoblastic surface of the villi is not perfect. Where the syncytiotrophoblast is interrupted by degeneration or by mechanical forces, the gap is immediately filled by perivillous fibrin (fibrin-type fibrinoid) resulting from the coagulation cascade. Corresponding fibrinoid spots are regular findings in every placenta. Such areas may serve as paratrophoblastic routes for maternofetal macromolecule transfer bypassing the syncytiotrophoblast: Horseradish peroxidase (48,000 d; 3.0-nm molecular radius) was shown to pass through the fibrinoid foci from the maternal circulation into the fetal stroma (Edwards et al., 1991). According to Nelson et al. (1990), these foci of perivillous fibrinoid account for about 7% of the villous surface of the normal human term placenta. They thus possibly provide an effective transfer route for macromolecules amounting to about $1\,m^2$ of villous surface.

- Matrix-type fibrinoid as well as connective tissue related to both types of fibrinoid shows varying degrees of immunoreactivity for tenascin (Castellucci et al., 1991; Frank et al., 1994). Tenascin is a mesenchymal glycoprotein that facilitates epithelial cell migration during development and is thus involved in many embryonic formative processes (Chiquet-Ehrismann et al., 1986; Aufderheide & Ekblom, 1988). Its presence suggests a **morphogenetic function** of fibrinoids during placental development. Nelson et al. (1990) found evidence that trophoblast-fibrinoid interactions modulate trophoblastic differentiation and proliferation and may be involved in reepithelialization of damaged villous surfaces.

- Most of the classical discussion regarding the functional importance of fibrinoid is related to its possible **immunologic significance**, with many authors discussing an immunologically protective function (Bardawil & Toy, 1959; Kirby et al., 1964; Currie & Bagshawe, 1967; McCormick et al., 1971; Azab et al., 1972; Faulk et al., 1975; Wynn, 1975). A particular immunoprotective role of sialic acid as normal constituent of fibrinoid has been stressed by Currie and Bagshawe (1967). This molecule may mask fetal antigens and thus prevent their recognition by maternal cells; moreover, it is thought to protect fetal cells from already sensitized maternal lymphocytes. It is known from several publications that experimental desialation of tumors by in vitro treatment with neuraminidase significantly increases their immunogenicity (for review see

Bagshawe & Lawler, 1975). Also, heparan sulfate proteoglycan, secreted by decidual and extravillous trophoblast cells into the surrounding uteroplacental fibrinoid (Kisalus & Herr, 1988; Huppertz et al., 1996, 1998d), has been suggested as a molecule that provides immunoprotection. A few publications have defined another immunoprotective function of fibrinoid, that is, its action as an immunoabsorptive sponge. This idea was first put forward by Swinburne (1970). He proposed that the fibrinoid expresses target antigens that bind circulating maternal antibodies, and the resulting immune complexes are then thought to contribute to the deposition of fibrinoid. The same concept was later favored by Chaouat et al. (1983) and by Hunziker and Wegmann (1986). Raghupathy et al. (1981, 1984) added two other findings that may be of interest in this context. They found that fibrinoid-bound antibodies are internalized and degraded within 4 to 6 hours and that the capacity of the antigen sponge is regenerated within 48 hours. Also, Montemagno (1967) opined that parts of the fibrinoid derives from antifetal antibodies. Further insight in this subject has been gained through the studies of Redline and Lu (1988). These authors showed that some of the molecules contained within the basal fibrinoid prevent macrophage movement, a subject that is fully discussed in the context of listeriosis (see Chapter 20).

Trophoblast Invasion as a Result of Deciduo-Trophoblastic Interactions

Trophoblast invasion in normal intrauterine pregnancies is a tightly controlled process so that trophoblast cells normally do not penetrate beyond the inner third of the myometrium. The control mechanisms, however, are still poorly understood. It is tempting to speculate that controlled invasion is the well-balanced result of trophoblastic invasiveness and decidual defense mechanisms. This view is supported by pathologic findings: local deficiency of decidualization in tubal pregnancies as well as in placenta accreta and percreta usually coincides with enhanced trophoblast invasion. More recent analysis of the decidua-trophoblastic interactions, however, have revealed a much more complex situation characterized by mechanisms supporting and inhibiting invasion provided from both the trophoblastic and the endometrial side.

We have dealt with the various mechanisms separately for extravillous trophoblast, decidua, and ECM (fibrinoids) in the previous chapters. This chapter briefly summarizes the most important interactions between the various tissue components in the light of trophoblastic invasiveness (Fig. 9.19).

The following **trophoblastic features further its invasiveness:**

- Trophoblast cells leaving the basal lamina achieve an interstitial, apolar phenotype that enables the cells to become invasive.
- The invasive phenotype of extravillous trophoblast cells expresses fewer polymorphic (HLA-C) or non-polymorphic (HLA-G, HLA-E) MHC-I molecules, which enable the cells to escape lytic action of T cells and uNK cells.
- The early invasive extravillous trophoblast shows an apolar extracellular deposition of ECM just matching the distribution of integrins along its plasmalemma; this coordinated colocalization is thought to promote migration of the cells.
- Extravillous trophoblast cells are potential sources of relaxin, which is known to stimulate secretion and activation of MMPs by extravillous trophoblast, and to block the MMP inhibitors (TIMPs).
- Invasive trophoblast cells express a broad pattern of MMPs, which enable the cells to degrade the surrounding ECM.
- The ECM secreted by invasive trophoblast cells is partly "i"-glycosylated and thus less susceptible to degradation by proteolytic enzymes than unglycosylated endometrial matrices.
- Invasive trophoblast cells secrete IDO, which catabolizes and reduces extracellular tryptophan; since adequate microenvironmental concentrations of the latter amino acid are required for T-cell proliferation, T-cell–mediated lysis of invasive trophoblast is reduced.

The following **decidual activities promote trophoblast invasion:**

- Decidua cells are a likely source of relaxin, which is known to further MMP action (see above).
- Transforming growth factor-α (TGF-α) secreted by decidua cells promotes proliferation of the stem cells of the extravillous trophoblast, which express the respective EGFR.
- Endometrial NK cells (uNK cells) have developed receptors (KIRs and the dimer CD94/NKG2) that upon binding to trophoblastic HLA-G, HLA-C, and HLA-E inhibit NK-cell–mediated lysis of the target cells.
- Different from other tissues, T cells at the implantation site possibly express reduced numbers of T-cell receptors (TCRs), which, in other tissues, are used for the host-versus-graft reaction. This reduction may help to avoid lytic action of T cells against extravillous trophoblast cells presenting paternal peptides bound to HLA-G and HLA-C.

The following **trophoblastic mechanisms limit its own invasiveness:**

- Invasive trophoblast cells secrete TIMPs, controlling activation of their self-secreted MMPs.

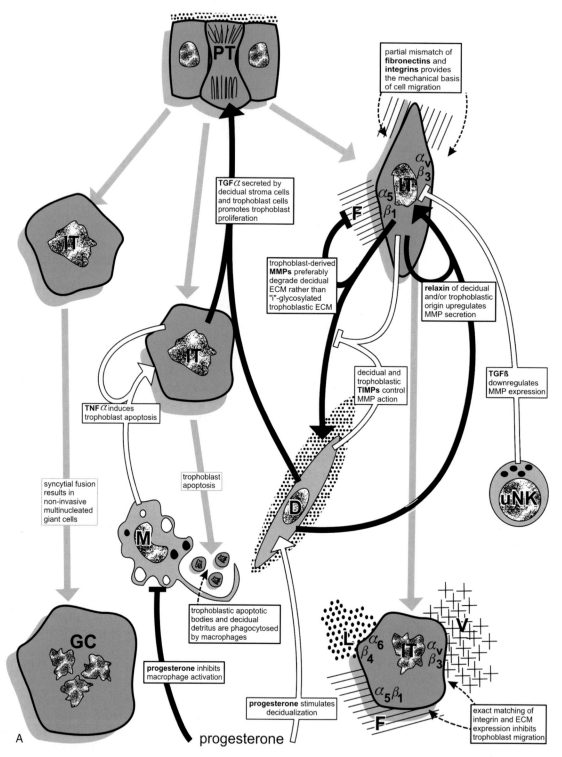

FIGURE 9.19. A,B: Schematic overview of some mechanisms controlling trophoblast invasion. Gray arrows: routes of trophoblast invasion; black arrows: interactions that are thought to exert a promoting net effect on trophoblast invasion; white arrows: interactions that are thought to have an inhibitory net effect on trophoblast invasion. Blue: trophoblast cells; pink: maternal cells; PT, proliferative phenotype of extravillous trophoblast; IT, invasive phenotype of extravillous trophoblast; GC. multinucleated giant cell; D, decidual cell; uNK, uterine natural killer cell; M, macrophage; T, T cell; B, B cell; L, laminins and collagen IV; F, fibronectins; V, vitronectin and heparan sulfate. A: Three different possibilities to limit trophoblast invasion are depicted. Left route: reduction of invasiveness by syncytial fusion resulting in multinucleated giant cells. Central route: elimination of invasive trophoblast by apoptosis, induced either by endogenous mechanisms or by decidual macrophages. Right route: reduction of invasiveness by polyploidization and associated alterations of integrin/ECM interactions. B: Roughly simplified examples of interaction of maternal immune cells (pink) with trophoblast cells (blue) in the implantation site and their effects on trophoblast invasion. Abbreviations and symbols as in part A. For details see text.

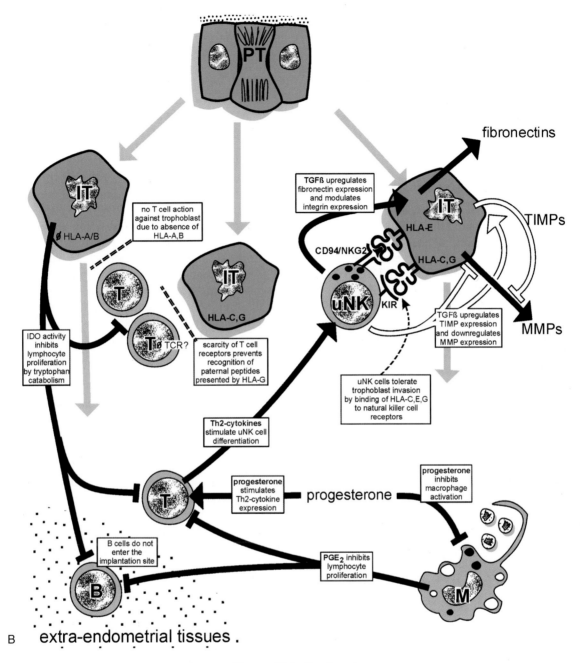

FIGURE 9.19. *Continued*

- With advancing pregnancy, increasing numbers of highly invasive spindle-shaped extravillous trophoblast cells polyploidize and transform into noninvasive large polygonal trophoblast cells.
- Deeply invasive trophoblast cells tend to aggregate and to fuse syncytially; the resulting multinucleated trophoblastic giant cells are thought to be noninvasive.

The following **decidual activities inhibit trophoblast invasion:**

- uNK cells deliver TGF-ß, which downregulates MMP secretion but induces TIMP secretion.

- A subset of invasive trophoblast cells undergoes apoptosis, induced by macrophage-derived TNF-α and by macrophage-induced tryptophan depletion.
- Decidual cells express TIMPs, which inhibit activation of trophoblastic MMPs.

The above very incomplete list of parameters involved in the regulation of trophoblast invasion reveals that promotion and inhibition of invasiveness cannot be allocated to the fetal and maternal tissues, respectively. Rather, every cell type in the maternofetal junctional zone has developed both mechanisms supporting and inhibiting invasion, resulting in an extremely complex but well-balanced control system. It is of particular interest to note that the immune response to malignant tumors shares many similarities with that to normal trophoblast invasion (Mullen et al., 1998). These similarities suggest that tumor invasion makes use of a kind of "immunologic window" that evolved during phylogeny of mammals in order to avoid host-versus-graft rejection of the allohaploid fetal tissues.

Calcification

The basal plate of the mature placenta often has finely divided deposits of calcium salts. They appear yellow and stippled and occur in irregular quantities. They may be detected by ultrasonography, and placental grading was popular in prenatal sonographic studies. In rhesus monkeys, the degree of calcification seems to be generally related to the stage of pregnancy (Bunton, 1986). Also in the human, immature placentas rarely have any significant amount of grossly visible calcification, whereas postmature placentas often have a gritty sensation when the knife passes through the floor of the placenta. It is not a reliable sign of postmaturity, however, and sonographers have largely abandoned its grading. These calcium deposits occur not only in the placental floor but also within the internal structure of the placenta, generally accompanying the septa. Calcium deposits are blue in H&E preparations and, as seen in Figures 9.20 to 9.22, the calcium deposits occur principally within accumulations of fibrin/fibrinoid. Occasionally, one finds calcifications in degenerated villi (see Chapter 15). We have also seen a marked increase in calcification in immature placentas in patients with parathyroid adenomas.

The quantity of placental calcium has been studied chemically by Jeacock et al. (1963), who also reviewed the older literature. These authors found the following calcium concentration in placentas:

Weeks of pregnancy	Mean concentration (mg/g dry tissue)
6–17	4.00
28–36	3.65
37–42	10.26
43–44	10.58

The increment found with postmaturity was small. Binovular twins did not always have the same concentrations. Patients with severe toxemia had higher values when they delivered prematurely but not at term. Stillbirth had no effect and infarcts did not have a high calcium content. Rather than the calcium deposits reflecting placental "aging," Jeacock et al. (1963) suggested that they serve fetal needs.

Fujikura (1963a,b) found that some 15% of placentas had moderate to marked calcification and that it tended to decrease with maternal age; it was most common (in the United States) in placentas delivered between November and February. Fox (1964), who found a significant relation to primigravidity, classified 25% of the placentas as calcified and saw no relation to postmaturity. He emphatically stated that calcification is in no way related to degenerative changes, but that fetal distress and neonatal asphyxia were more common with calcified placentas.

Brown et al. (1988) found by ultrasonographic studies that increased calcification of the placenta occurred in smoking mothers, irrespective of possible fetal weight reduction. When the placenta was studied by radiographic photography, 44% had slight, 30% moderate, and 2% severe calcification (Tindall & Scott, 1965). The manner of deposition varies (see also Hassler, 1969). The findings

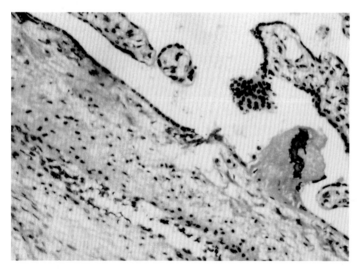

FIGURE 9.20. Focal fibrin deposit on the villous surface (with central calcification: dark) covers trophoblast defect on the villous surface. Note that such lesions in the placenta never have any fibrous ingrowth; they do not "organize" in the sense used by pathologists. H&E ×200.

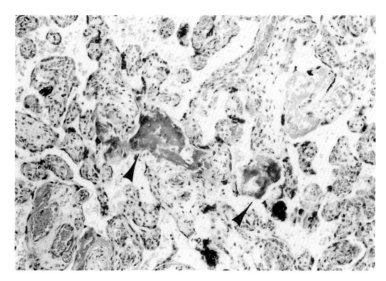

FIGURE 9.21. Irregular calcium salt deposits (dark black) in mature placenta. The dark areas are syncytial buds (knots); the light gray areas (arrowheads) represent fibrin in the intervillous space. H&E ×160.

of Tindall and Scott indicate that calcium deposits increase steadily from 29 to 43 weeks and that the amounts are related to placental and fetal weights. Placentas of stillbirths had generally less calcification. In contrast to the observations of Fujikura (United States), the placentas of Tindall and Scott (England) had more calcification when delivered from June to October. These authors made reference to possible physiologic mechanisms that regulate calcium deposition and did not consider the process to be a pathologic event. Russell (1969) found calcium deposits most commonly in the spring and fall and in younger mothers; interestingly, prosperous women also had more calcium deposits in their placentas. The overall incidence, based on radiographic findings, was 18% of placentas

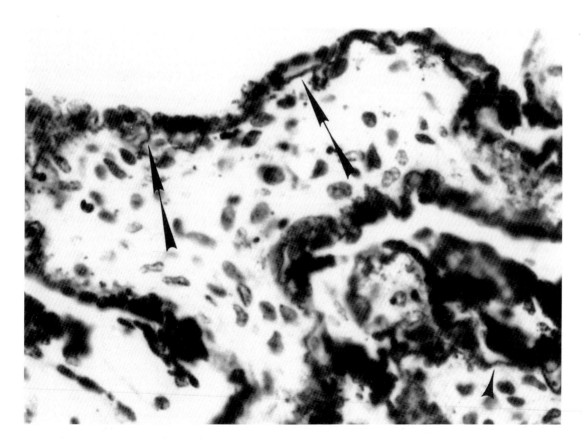

FIGURE 9.22. Mineral salt deposits (arrows) in basement membrane of immature placenta from stillborn fetus. H&E ×640.

after 38 weeks. Al-Zuhair et al. (1984) produced excellent scanning electron micrographs of irregular electron-dense attachments to the villous microvillous projections, but the inference that they are calcium deposits needs further proof.

In addition to the typical calcification that is grossly perceptible, the histopathologist often finds granular, purple deposits on the basement membrane of villous surfaces (Fig. 9.22). They have been described by Avery and Aterman (1971) and they are most common in abortions. We are uncertain that the purple granules that they found also in fibrotic villi truly represent calcium. Pathologists have a tendency to assume something to be calcium when it is amorphous, purple, and stains with the von Kossa reaction. The fact is, however, that there is no specific stain for calcium; phosphorus and carbonate salts of all sorts stain with the von Kossa reaction. The murexide stain may be an exception; it may stain calcium more specifically (Kaufman & Adams, 1957).

That such "calcified" basement membranes may represent largely iron deposits has been shown by Birkenfeld et al. (1989) in a patient with ß-thalassemia major whose pregnancy came to term. Krohn et al. (1967) addressed the relevance of these deposits when they showed that pregnancies complicated by hydramnios had an unusually high (67%) deposition rate of "calcium" at the trophoblastic border. Iron and phosphates are intermixed and not readily separated by the usual methods. McKay et al. (1958) found it to be a feature of second-trimester placentas.

From chemical analysis, Einbrodt et al. (1973) ascertained that, in a large city, the **lead** contamination of calcium in the placentas had increased from 45% to 65% between 1956 and 1961. In addition to these deposits of minerals, **melanin** has been demonstrated in the basement membranes of villi and in Hofbauer cells (Ishizaki & Belter, 1960). With special stains, these authors identified melanin in 85% of the placentas they examined. It was present as often in Caucasians as in African Americans. They suggested that these deposits occur more frequently in association with chronic skin lesions and called the condition "dermatopathic melanosis of placenta." Melanin-containing macrophages in amnion have also been found in cases of prolonged amnion rupture (Bendon & Ray, 1986). Parmley et al. (1981) demonstrated the "aging pigment" **lipofuscin** in placentas beyond 32 weeks. They used fluorescence microscopy for its demonstration and saw it routinely in the trophoblast. In a discussion of that paper, Wynn remarked that one should not necessarily construe this finding as "aging." We agree with him and the many authors who believe that only maturation, not aging, occurs during normal gestation in placental tissue.

We have earlier stated that sonographers have used the presence of calcium and other structural features to "grade" the placenta before birth (Hobbins & Winsberg, 1977). Their grades I to III have been correlated with fetal maturity, as judged by the sphingomyelin/lecithin (L/S) ratios (Grannum et al., 1979). These studies have often shown that placental grading is not accurate enough to diagnose pulmonary maturity without the determination of the L/S ratio (Harman et al., 1982; Petrucha & Platt, 1982). They are also not useful for delineating and monitoring postmature pregnancies (Hill et al., 1983; Monaghan et al., 1987) and have generally been given up. There has been a suggestion, however, that they may be useful to predict intrauterine growth restriction (IUGR) (Kazzi et al., 1983).

This chapter is not the place for a detailed review of maternal/fetal calcium relations. Thoughtful reviews have been provided by Pitkin (1975) and Tsang et al. (1976). It has been said that pregnancy induces a maternal "physiological hyperparathyroidism" (Pitkin et al., 1979). High maternal calcitonin levels of pregnancy protect the mother against bone loss (Garel & Barlet, 1978). During the third trimester the fetus requires 100 to 150 mg calcium/kg fetal weight/day for bone apposition (Tsang et al., 1976), and there is also evidence of placental production of vitamin D (Reddy et al., 1983). The paradox of higher serum levels of ionized calcium in the fetus than in the mother may relate to this finding. Despite many safeguards, abnormalities occur. Neonatal tetanus is not rare, particularly in premature infants, and may reflect secondary vitamin D deficiency (Rosen et al., 1974).

Although numerous investigations have been undertaken to clarify transplacental calcium/phosphorus transfer, none can be found that takes into consideration the simultaneous degree of placental calcium deposits. Are they related to homeostasis, or are they merely a reflection of dystrophic mineral deposits in extracellular matrix? Einbrodt and Schmid (1965) did not think that the excessive calcium deposits they found were the cause of an infant's death. They described two successive pregnancies with massive calcification of the placenta (20% to 30% in excess of the normal) in a woman with latent pregnancy tetany. The first pregnancy had been medicated to alleviate these symptoms; the second pregnancy was not treated, yet excessive amounts of placental calcium accumulated. It is not clear that this was the result of the disturbance in maternal calcium homeostasis. The authors cited another case from the literature with similar pathology but without tetany. They identified the placental mineral deposits as hydroxyapatite, not carbonate. The authors made the point that the excessive calcification was not due to mere fibrin absorption of calcium. At present, then, we do not understand the normal mechanisms that lead to calcification of the placenta, let alone when it attains seemingly pathologic quantities.

Chorionic Plate

DEVELOPMENT

The development of the chorionic plate begins with the formation of the primary chorionic plate. This process starts as soon as the first lacunae appear in the syncytiotrophoblast of the implanting blastocyst on day 8 p.c. (see Chapter 5). Initially, this layer is composed only of syncytiotrophoblast and cytotrophoblast. It separates the early lacunar system from the blastocyst cavity (see Chapter 5, Fig. 5.1C,D). As soon as the extraembryonic mesenchyme develops and spreads around the cytotrophoblastic surface of the blastocyst cavity (Fig. 5.1D), the primary chorionic plate becomes triple-layered, consisting of mesenchyme, cytotrophoblast, and syncytiotrophoblast. At the same time, the trophoblastic trabeculae that separate the lacunae start proliferating and form the first villous outgrowths into the continuously expanding lacunar system (Fig. 5.1D,E). The trabeculae are henceforth called the villous stems; the lacunar system is transformed into the intervillous space. From this stage onward, the chorionic plate represents the "lid" of the intervillous space and at the same time serves as the base from which the villous trees are suspended into the intervillous space.

The layering of the primary chorionic plate described above is maintained until term (Kaufmann, 1981a). Multifocal tissue degeneration with subsequent fibrinoid deposition, however, may considerably disturb its architecture. Fibrinoid deposits within and along the surface of the chorionic plate are called **Langhans' fibrinoid** (Langhans, 1877; Bourne, 1962). Those parts of the fibrinoid that replace tissues of the chorionic plate are usually compact and largely homogeneous in appearance. Toward the intervillous space, it becomes mostly covered by an inhomogeneous material, fibrin-type fibrinoid that is arranged in more or less net-like fashion. It is thought to be derived from blood clotting in the intervillous space (Bourne, 1962). The syncytiotrophoblastic cover of the chorionic plate is usually replaced by Langhans' fibrinoid, which occurs early in pregnancy.

In some places, the cytotrophoblastic layer also degenerates, whereas in other places it proliferates, resulting in multilayered plaques. These plaques consist of either compact **extravillous cytotrophoblast** or scattered trophoblastic cells surrounded by fibrinoid. The basal layer of cytotrophoblast, which rests on the chorionic mesenchyme, retains the characteristics of a proliferating layer of stem cells. Their highly differentiated, nonproliferative daughter cells (extravillous trophoblast cells) lose contact with the mesenchymal layer and migrate into the neighboring matrix-type fibrinoid. Here they grow in size and achieve the histochemical (Weser & Kaufmann, 1978) and ultrastructural (Wiese, 1975) characteristics of specialized, metabolically highly active cells. They are thus largely comparable to the invasive phenotype of extravillous trophoblast cells in other locations (Kaufmann & Castellucci, 1997).

With advancing gestation, numerous small and large **villi become attached** to the fibrinoid. Through coagulation of blood in their surrounding, and with subsequent transformation into fibrinoid, they may become deeply incorporated into the Langhans' fibrinoid layer. The original Langhans' cells of the incorporated villi commence proliferation following degeneration of their syncytial layer. They then transform into extravillous trophoblast cells, and migrate into the fibrinoid. In places that are devoid of such incorporated villi, the thickness of the chorionic plate rarely exceeds 200 μm, whereas conglomerates of encased villi, together with their derivatives, may measure up to several millimeters in thickness.

The extraembryonic **mesenchyme** that has formed after day 9 p.c. initially completely occupies the blastocyst cavity (see Chapter 12, Fig. 12.1, day 13). During the course of the 3rd week p.c., the exocoelomic cavity is formed, reducing the extraembryonic mesenchyme to thin layers that cover the early embryo as well as the chorionic plate (Fig. 12.18, day 18). In the latter position it establishes the chorionic mesoderm. Toward the exocoelomic cavity, the mesoderm is lined by a single layer of flat mesothelium.

During the course of the 2nd month postmenstruation (p.m.), **fetal blood vessels** derive from the allantois via the connecting stalk and establish contact with the chorionic plate (Fig. 12.1; days 28 and 40). There they spread across the chorionic mesoderm and soon enter the early stem villi (Figs. 5.1F, 5.2, and 12.1). The vessels come into contact with locally formed fetal villous capillaries, resulting in the completed fetoplacental circulatory system. The chorionic fetal vessels soon enlarge to form arteries and veins. It must be pointed out that all these vessels pass the chorionic plate and thus connect the villous trees with the umbilical cord. Capillaries for the nutrition of the various tissues of the chorionic plate are a rare and locally very restricted exception.

At 17 weeks p.m. the amnionic vesicle has become so large that it comes into close contact with the chorionic plate (Grosser, 1927). At this time, the **amnion** is composed of an inner epithelial layer (amnionic epithelium) and an intermediate layer of amnionic mesoderm that, on its outer surface, is lined by amnionic mesothelium (see Chapter 11). Where amnion and chorion closely appose each other, their mesothelial layers slowly regress, resulting in mesodermal fusion. As in the membranes, this fusion is never perfect. Rather, it is a focal attachment, with the formation of net-like bridges between the layers (spongy layer). This structure establishes contact that allows easy gliding of the layers against each other. Attachment of the amnion to the primary chorionic plate transforms the latter into the definitive chorionic plate. Ample folding of the amnionic cover on the chorionic plate is a usual histologic finding (Fig. 9.23A). It is difficult to decide from histologic preparations how far they reflect the in vivo situation and how much is a consequence of the collapse of the amnionic vesicle after delivery because of the easy gliding of the amnion.

Structure at Term

Only a few publications deal with the structure of the chorionic plate (Langhans, 1877; Grosser, 1927; Singer & Wislocki, 1948; Bourne, 1962; Boyd & Hamilton, 1970; Wiese, 1975; Weser & Kaufmann, 1978; Schiebler & Kaufmann, 1981). Studies that are especially devoted to the chorionic plate concern the cord insertion (Scheuner, 1964), the subchorial Langhans' fibrinoid layer (Geller, 1959), and the chorionic vessels (Nikolov & Schiebler, 1973). Aspects of its cellular composition have been studied twice, on the electron microscopic level by Wiese (1975) and histologically, including enzyme histochemistry, by Weser and Kaufmann (1978).

The layering of the term chorionic plate is consistent with that described during development. The following layers must be distinguished (Fig. 9.24) and are described in greater detail in the following sections:

- Amnionic epithelium
- Compact layer
- Amnionic mesoderm
- Spongy layer, separating amnion and chorion
- Chorionic mesoderm
- Proliferating cytotrophoblast
- Langhans' fibrinoid layer encasing the extravillous cytotrophoblast

Amnion

The three layers of the amnion, that is, amnionic epithelium, compact layer, and amnionic mesoderm, are struc-

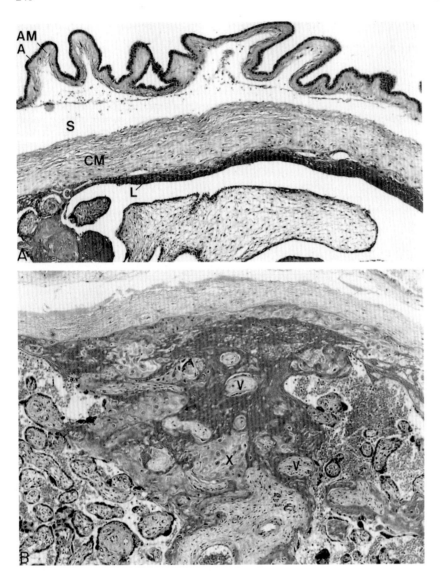

FIGURE 9.23. Paraffin sections prepared to compare the chorionic plate in earlier stages and later stages of pregnancy. A: At the 21st week p.m. B: At the 40th week p.m. The typical layering of the chorionic plate with amnionic epithelium (A), amnionic mesenchyme (AM), spongy layer (S), chorionic mesenchyme (CM), chorionic (extravillous) cytotrophoblast (C), and Langhans' fibrinoid (L) is evident at both time points. The main difference between the two developmental stages is the increased deposition of Langhans' fibrinoid below the chorionic plate near term. Clusters of extravillous trophoblast cells (X) and residues of buried villi (V) are typically incorporated in the mature Langhans' fibrinoid. ×85.

turally largely identical with the respective layers described in Chapter 11. Bourne (1962) has given the most detailed review of these layers. Plaques of squamous metaplasia are common findings, especially surrounding the cord insertion. The usually columnar epithelium is here replaced by a squamous, keratinizing type. Sinha (1971) has dealt with this subject in more detail.

Wiese (1975) studied the arrangement of fibers in both connective tissue layers of the amnion by electron microscopy. The compact layer, devoid of cells, is composed of a condensed three-dimensional lattice of collagen fibers. The neighboring amnionic mesoderm differs in two aspects: vertical collagen fibers are lacking, and the remaining two-dimensional loose network is composed only of fibers that are arranged parallel to the amnionic epithelium. Three to four thin layers of filaments alternate with layers of loosely arranged fibroblasts, thus forming an incomplete irregular network. Kratzsch and Grygiel (1972) have histochemically demonstrated the existence

of diphosphoglucose dehydrogenase in these cells, an enzyme that is involved in the production of matrix proteoglycans. For further details see Chapter 11.

Spongy Layer

The spongy layer (Bourne, 1962) has also been called the intermediate layer (Petry, 1954a,b), jelly layer (Dohrn, 1865), or stratum intermedium (Bautzmann & Schröder, 1955). The layer is structurally similar to the corresponding layer of the free membranes (Chapter 11). It is easier to study at the chorionic plate, however, because here it is less often dislocated by the forces of labor. The spongy clefts that separate amnion and chorion are normally less impressive. The clefts are partially lined by small, rounded cells, which, based on immunohistochemical studies, are likely to be residues of the former amnionic and chorionic mesothelium (Ockleford et al., 1993, 1994; Malak et al., 1993); the latter once lined the exocoelomic cavity

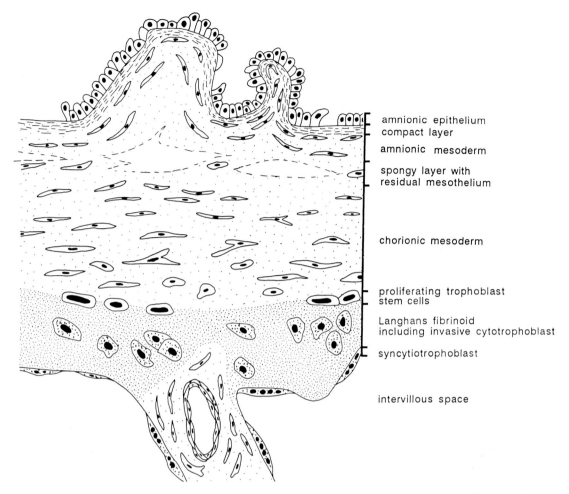

FIGURE 9.24. Layering and cellular composition of mature chorionic plate.

as the so-called Heuser's membrane, prior to fusion of amnionic and chorionic mesoderms.

Chorionic Mesoderm

The chorionic mesoderm of the chorionic plate presents some peculiarities that have not been described in detail for the chorionic mesoderm of the membranes. Several authors (Scheuner, 1964; Wiese, 1975; Weser & Kaufmann, 1978) have described distinct layers, ranging from "oriented" connective tissue facing the spongy layer to "unoriented" connective tissue near the fibrinoid. In the unoriented layers, the collagen fibers seem to be irregularly arranged, with large polymorphic fibroblasts in between. The oriented layers, on the other hand, consist of thin strata with collagen fibers that are oriented in parallel. The layers are separated by small fibroblasts with long extensions and condensed nuclei. These authors suggested that the unoriented layers are the primitive precursors of the oriented layers, a suggestion that is sup-

ported by the fact that during early pregnancy the unoriented layers are more prominent (Fig. 9.23A).

Bertolini et al. (1969) reported the existence of smooth muscle cells within these layers, in agreement with results of Spanner (1935). Later studies, in particular the detailed electron microscopic investigation by Wiese (1975), did not support this finding. Many of the cells, however, display typical immunohistochemical features of myofibroblasts (see Chorionic Mesoderm in Chapter 11).

The oriented layers of the mesoderm comprise the site of the chorionic vessels, which originate by branching from the umbilical vessels. These vessels have been described in greater detail in Chapter 12 (see Placental Surface Vessels).

Extravillous Cytotrophoblast

The chorionic mesoderm is followed by an incomplete basal lamina. A layer of extravillous cytotrophoblast is found on its other side. In the central parts of the pla-

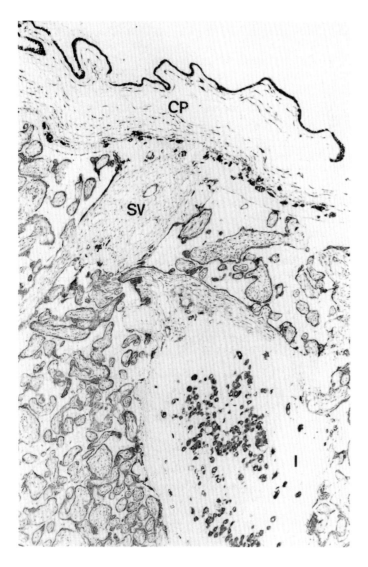

FIGURE 9.25. Cryostat survey picture at the 40th week p.m. showing the chorionic plate (CP) with a branching-off stem villus (SV), numerous small villous branches, and a cell island (I). Because of the histochemical reaction for malate dehydrogenase applied to this section, amnionic epithelium, cytotrophoblast, and syncytiotrophoblast show intense staining, whereas connective tissue cells are only weakly stained. Note the immediate relation of the cell island to a large stem villus. ×115. (*Source:* From Schiebler & Kaufmann, 1981, with permission.)

centa, it is a discontinuous layer of small groups of cells (Figs. 9.24 and 9.25). Near the placental margin, it becomes continuous and is finally multilayered. The location at the exact mesodermal–fibrinoid interface is characteristic for these cells. Where several cells lie close together, their cell membranes show intense interdigitations. They are fixed to each other by desmosomes. Foot-like extensions, equipped with hemidesmosomes, connect the cells to the basal lamina. The latter is absent where the chorionic mesoderm directly faces the Langhans' fibrinoid without interposed cytotrophoblast. The basal ones of these cells present the germinative layer; still, at term, some of these cells can be stained by immunohistochemical proliferation markers (MIB-1, PCNA). Accumulations of proliferating cells up to multilayered groups in the marginal zone of the placenta (Arnold, 1975a,b) account for particular growth activities at the placental margin.

The chorionic plate trophoblast cells lining the chorionic mesoderm were thought in earlier publications to represent a source for the differentiation of chorionic mesoderm (Hertig, 1935; Wislocki & Streeter, 1938). The histologic studies by Luckett (1978) and experimental findings in chimeric mice (Rossant & Croy, 1985), however, have clearly ruled out this possibility. All placental mesoderm is of fetal origin and invades the chorion.

Langhans' Fibrinoid Layer

Langhans' fibrinoid layer is a rather constant feature, with a thickness and structure that increase continuously throughout pregnancy. In its early stages, the intervillous surface of Langhans' layer is still mostly covered by syncytiotrophoblast, which becomes completely replaced by additional fibrinoid during later pregnancy.

Abundant scattered or aggregated **extravillous trophoblast cells** can be seen in the fibrinoid. Ultrastructurally (Wiese, 1975), enzyme-histochemically (Weser & Kaufmann, 1978), and immunohistochemically the cells are comparable to the invasive stages of extravillous tro-phoblast cells of other origin. The assumption by Bertolini and Klinger (1966) that these cells are decidual cells is no longer tenable but it has to be pointed out that sometimes decidual cells may be present in the chorionic plate, in particular near the placental margin (see below). They are the result of folding of basal plate tissue into chorionic plate tissue and can be interpreted as mild transitional stages toward placental circumvallation (see Chapter 13).

Nearly all earlier authors described the fibrinoid of the chorionic plate as normally composed of two distinct layers that differ in structure: a deep compact layer that, in the mature placenta, is nearly continuous and follows the chorionic connective tissue; and, where present, the chorionic cytotrophoblastic layer (Fig. 9.23). This compact fibrinoid represents **matrix-type fibrinoid** (Frank et al., 1994; Lang et al., 1994). It encases the extravillous tro-phoblast cells of the chorionic plate, which contribute to its growth by secretion.

This layer is usually covered by a second fibrinoid layer of more reticulated fibrinoid that corresponds immuno-histochemically to **fibrin-type fibrinoid** (Fig. 9.23B) (Frank et al., 1994; Lang et al., 1994). The latter had been described as canalized fibrin by Langhans (1877).

The amount of subchorial fibrinoid at term varies considerably. According to our anatomic experience, it is impossible to define the amount that is compatible with normal pregnancy. Note, however, that the most impres-sive cases of subchorial fibrinoid deposition we have observed occurred in cases of Rh incompatibility. Here the Langhans' stria extended without identifiable demarca-tion into ample perivillous fibrinoid and numerous sub-chorial cell islands, occupying up to one half of the placental volume. The subchorial fibrinoid is the basis for the bosse-lations and the laminated subchorial plaques that vary so much from one placenta to another. The latter are deposits resulting from eddying in the places where the intervillous blood is turned back toward the basal plate.

At times, large **laminated hematomas** are found under-neath the Langhans' fibrinoid. Such cases have been reported by Torpin (1960), Shanklin and Scott (1975), and Oláh et al. (1987), with the latter authors diagnosing it even during ultrasonographic examination. The 25 weeks pregnant patient they described suffered a falling hemo-globin level and a rapidly enlarging abdomen. A fatally ill premature infant was delivered by cesarean section. The circumvallate placenta weighed 700 g (28 weeks) and had a 15 × 5 cm laminated thrombus under the chorionic plate. This case is not unlike the classical Breus' mole (tuberous subchorionic hematoma) of earlier abortions, except for the sacculations that Breus delineated (1892). Although Breus thought that these sacculations devel-oped after fetal death, Oláh et al. (1987) cited evidence that the hematoma may be primary, albeit a rare event. A somewhat similar condition was reported by Howorka

and Kapczynski (1971). In their patient, the hematoma was circumferential. It had disrupted the chorion laeve, much as in acute circumvallation. The authors included an interesting diagram that depicts their operative obser-vations. It suggested to them that separate contractions, within sacculations of the uterine fundus were the basis for the detachment. More extensive consideration is given to these "thrombohematomas" in Chapter 11 (see Cysts, Tumors, and Hemorrhage).

Marginal Zone

The marginal zone is not precisely defined. It consists of the transitional zone of the chorionic plate, the basal plate, and the membranes, and it has characteristics of all three regions. The internal margin, separating it by defini-tion from the chorionic plate (Bühler, 1964), is the line connecting those points where the most peripheral branches of the chorionic plate vessels make their verti-cal bend to enter the most peripheral villous trees. The outer margin that separates it from the membranes rep-resents the macroscopically visible transition from pla-centa to membranes (Bühler, 1964). It is largely identical with that line where the intervillous space is occluded by fusion of the chorionic plate with the basal plate.

Subchorial Closing Ring

Macroscopically, the marginal zone is often represented by a slightly prominent opaque ring which is about 1 cm in width, the subchorial closing ring (Boyd & Hamilton, 1970). An increase in thickness of the marginal zone is represented by the designation "placenta marginata" (Kölliker, 1879). The transposition of the subchorial closing ring nearer to the cord, with origination of the membranes from the chorionic surface of the placenta rather than from the margin, is referred to as "placenta circumvallata" (see Chapter 13). In circumvallate placen-tas, the intervillous space, together with smaller villous trees peripherally, exceeds the marginal zone. A com-plete, macroscopically identifiable subchorial closing ring was described by Bühler (1964) in 71% of placentas studied; in 21% it was incomplete, in 8% it was absent.

The structures of the marginal amnion and the mar-ginal chorionic mesoderm are comparable to those of the neighboring zones: chorionic plate and membranes (Arnold, 1975a,b). The structural basis for the promi-nence and the opaque appearance of the subchorial closing ring is the presence of both an increased number of extravillous trophoblast cells in the Langhans' fibri-noid and local accumulations of decidua cells (Arnold, 1975a,b). The latter usually form a hook-like extension of the basal decidua, which laterally surrounds the placental margin and protrudes into the Langhans' layer.

Trabeculae

In histologic preparations of the marginal zone, rounded or elongated plaques of connective tissue or trabeculae become apparent. They are nearly uniformly scattered over the Langhans' fibrinoid and extravillous trophoblast layer. They must not be confused with the trabeculae of the early stages of previllous development. Krafft (1973) studied these structures in serial sections and was able to demonstrate convincingly that they are continuous on the one side with encased branches of the most peripheral villous trees. Their peripheral ends extend far into the membranes, where they end blindly at the decidual layer. According to Krafft (1973), they are residues of villous branches that have been incorporated into the marginal zone during regression of the chorion frondosum. They are thought to be important for the mechanical stability of the marginal zone and for anchoring the membranes to the placenta.

Marginal Sinus

Large maternal veins exist near the placental margin that open into the intervillous space. This coincidence has caused intense speculation regarding the intervillous circulation of blood. Spanner (1935, 1941) described this as the "marginal sinus" and concluded that this sinus drains more or less all of the maternal intervillous blood into the uterine veins. Ramsey (1956) and Arts (1961) called it the "marginal lake." The beautiful studies of Ramsey (1956), Ramsey and Harris (1966), Ramsey et al. (1966), and Ramsey and Donner (1980) showed that this is indeed a prominent area of venous outflow, but also that it does not have the exclusive characteristics attributed to it by Spanner (1935, 1941). Numerous venous openings, scattered over the entire surface of the basal plate, offer sufficient venous drainage at the base of the placenta.

The wall of the initial part of the marginal uteroplacental veins is largely replaced by fibrinoid; in addition, numerous signs of cellular degeneration can be observed in the surrounding tissues (Arnold, 1975a,b). It has been speculated that it is the structural basis for the so-called marginal sinus hemorrhage (Schultze, 1953, 1968), as the peripheral decidual cover is very thin.

In the marginal zone of the placenta, the border between maternal veins and intervillous space is difficult to define for two reasons: First, maternal endothelial cells spread from the venous lumina deeply into the placenta, and there they usually line the intervillous surfaces of the basal and chorionic plates in the entire marginal zone (Nanaev et al., 2000a; see also Lang et al., 1993). Second, the smooth muscle cells of the venous media extend far into the placenta, forming a loosely arranged muscular ring around the placental margin (Nanaev et al., 2000a). This ring has an average width of some centimeters and extends into both the basal plate and the chorionic plate. The functional meaning of this circumplacental muscular ring is still an open question. Based on the coexistence of maternal endothelium and vascular smooth muscle cells, one may argue that the intervillous space of the marginal zone ("marginal sinus") represents dilated venous openings. This view is in agreement with the finding by Craven et al. (1997) that lateral placental growth takes place by villous "invasion" into the marginal veins with subsequent widening of the maternal venous openings.

Basal Plate

TROPHOBLASTIC SHELL AND DEVELOPMENT OF THE BASAL PLATE

The basal plate is defined as the maternal aspect of the intervillous space. It is the most intimate and most important contact zone of maternal and fetal tissues (see Figs. 4.7 and 5.1F). The definitive basal plate is a highly complex structure. It is composed of various tissues, for example, extravillous trophoblast, endometrial stroma with its pregnancy-specific specialization, fibrinoid, residues of degenerating villi, and maternal vessels. General information concerning all of these tissues has been provided separately at the beginning of this chapter.

The early precursor of the basal plate is the **trophoblastic shell** (Fig. 9.26), a particular trophoblastic layer that, in the implanting blastocyst, separates the lacunar system from the endometrial tissues (Fig. 5.1C,D). Its development has been analyzed in detail in the rhesus monkey (Enders, 1995). Because of the intimate relationship between trophoblastic shell and the surrounding endometrium, the first steps in

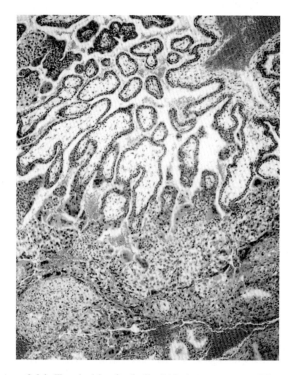

FIGURE 9.26. Trophoblastic shell of 13-day pregnancy. The cytotrophoblastic columns are covered with syncytium. Placental site giant cells are intermingled with decidua (right). H&E ×300.

the formation of the basal plate are coupled with the mechanisms of implantation (see Chapter 5).

Representing the invasive front of the blastocyst, the trophoblastic shell has an irregular surface that interdigitates intensively with the endometrial connective tissue. During early implantation the trophoblastic shell consists merely of syncytiotrophoblast. On day 13 p.c., cytotrophoblast reaches the shell via the trabeculae and splits the syncytiotrophoblast (Fig. 5.1D,E). Because of this, increasing amounts of cytotrophoblast come into contact with the endometrium. As typical sign of their invasive activity, these cells relinquish their closed epithelial formation and commence to invade the stroma as single cells or in small groups (Figs. 9.27 to 9.29; also see Fig. 5.1E,F). It is the first time at which an exact border—one separating the trophoblastic shell and the endometrium—can no longer be defined. An exactly dated, 22-day-old human specimen, described in detail by Larsen and Knoth (1971), illustrated this situation. From this date onward, the term trophoblastic shell is usually replaced by the term **basal plate**, a term that includes the base of the intervillous space together with all placental and maternal tissues that adhere to it after parturition.

The deeper tissue layers of the placental site, which remain in utero and are later discharged as lochia, show a similar admixture of maternal and placental tissues, the **placental bed**. In situ, the placental bed and basal plate cannot be delimited from each other because the demarcation zone becomes visible only shortly before delivery. Therefore, they together composed the **junctional zone** for in situ specimens. They encompass all regions of admixed maternal and fetal composition that lie basal to the intervillous space (Fig. 5.1F). Note that the term basal plate is applicable only to the delivered placenta.

During the first stages of pregnancy, **residual endometrial glands** are still visible in the deep parts of the decidua of the implantation site (see Chapter 3, Fig. 3.1M). So long as these remnants exist, trophoblastic invasion is largely limited to those parts of the compact and spongy layers of the decidua that overlie the glands (Pijnenborg et al., 1980). Only scattered trophoblast cells are found amidst the glands and they are only occasionally closely related to them. During the 15th to 18th weeks p.m., only occasional, isolated fragments of the glands are seen. Most are located in the lateral parts of the placental site, whereas in the central areas the glandular tissue is completely lost. The trophoblast invades the entire thickness of the decidua, down to the myometrium where glands are absent. One may speculate whether the existence of glands prevents trophoblastic invasion or the invasive activities of the trophoblast contribute to the destruction of the glands. We believe the latter to be more likely. Moreover, the prolonged presence of progesterone causes atrophy of the glandular epithelium during advancing gestation.

Much tissue necrosis occurs where maternal and fetal cells come close together. This degeneration has been interpreted as the consequence of proteolytic activity of the invading trophoblast. Large necrotic foci of the decidua in this region may also be a consequence of obstruction of spiral arteries. The necrotic residues of decidua and trophoblast are transformed into fibrinoid with a considerable admixture of fibrin being probable. Two layers of fibrinoid exist. **Rohr's fibrinoid** is a superficial, multiply interrupted, more or less focal layer. It faces the intervillous space (Figs. 5.1F and 9.27B), where it replaces the superficial layer of basal plate syncytiotrophoblast. By contrast, **Nitabuch's fibrinoid** is a layer of uteroplacental fibrinoid. As is expressed by its name, this layer is believed to mark the border of the placental and maternal tissues (Fig. 5.1F) and thus represents the immediate "battle-field" of the tissues (Kaufmann & Stark, 1971). Nitabuch's fibrinoid separates a superficial trophoblastic layer from a deeper decidual layer exactly in only few areas (Figs. 3.2L and 9.27B; also see Fig. 9.31). In other places, the cell types may be intensely intermixed on one or both sides of the Nitabuch layer. Finally, the order of layers can be inverted in exceptional cases, with the decidua nearer the intervillous space and the extravillous trophoblast cells making up the base of the basal plate.

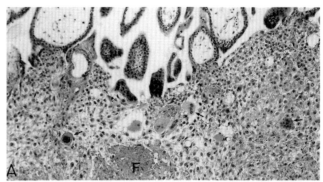

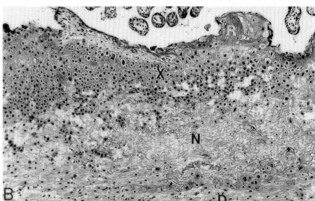

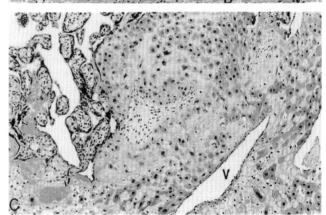

FIGURE 9.27. Developmental stages of the basal plate, paraffin sections. A: At the 8th week p.m. The basal plate is composed of a dense mixture of extravillous trophoblastic and decidual cells, intermingled with a few trophoblastic giant cells (arrows). There is little fibrinoid (F). ×75. B: At the 23rd week of gestation. The typical layering of the basal plate is evident. Facing the intervillous space, it is covered by an interrupted layer of Rohr's fibrinoid (R), followed by a nearly complete layer of extravillous cytotrophoblast (X). The latter is largely separated from the decidua cells (D) by a loose layer of Nitabuch's fibrinoid (N). ×85. C: At the 37th week p.m. During the last trimester of pregnancy the typical layering of the basal plate is again abolished by trophoblastic cells and decidual cells penetrate the originally separating Nitabuch's layer in both directions. The result is a colorful mixture of fibrinoid and cells of maternal and fetal origin. A few cross sections of a fetal vein (V), lined by innocuous endothelium, can be seen. ×85.

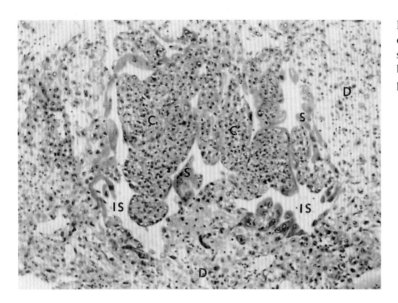

FIGURE 9.28. Implantation site of a 13–day human ovum to show the cytotrophoblastic cell columns (C), syncytium (S), intervillous space (IS) without maternal blood as yet and the decidua (D) with infiltrating trophoblastic elements. H&E ×260.

Growth of the basal plate, laterally as well as in thickness, is largely a consequence of extravillous cytotrophoblast proliferation originating from cell columns. The migration of their daughter cells into tissues of the basal plate can readily be demonstrated (for review, see Extravillous Trophoblast, above). The lateral growth of the basal plate probably is not always accompanied by a corresponding degree of local distention of the uterine wall. This lack may cause a lateral movement and enhance the folding of the basal plate and the uterine wall over each other. Such folding processes result in the dislocation of basal plate tissues into the intervillous space, including all of its normal constituents. The placental septa are thus formed. Detached parts of the septa that are connected to the villous trees only by some interposed fibrinoid make up a subpopulation of the cell islands.

Layers of the Basal Plate at Term

The mature basal plate is of variable thickness, ranging from 100 μm to 1.5 mm. In most places it has lost its typical earlier layering (Fig. 9.27C; also see Fig. 9.31). Only rarely can all of the following layers be identified in an undisturbed order (Hein, 1971; Kaufmann & Stark, 1971):

Basal plate syncytiotrophoblast: The inner surface of the basal plate, which faces the intervillous space, shows residues of the former syncytiotrophoblastic lining in only very few places. These areas are small patches of largely degenerative syncytium and an underlying cytotrophoblast is normally absent. Wanner (1966) reported the existence of **maternal endothelial cells** in the same location that were thought to be derived from the ostia of the uteroplacental veins. According to recent immunohistochemical studies, maternal endothelium lines not only large parts of the intervillous surface of the basal plate (Fig. 9.30; also see Fig. 9.37C,D) but also parts of the septa and of the marginal zone (Lang et al., 1993; Nanaev et al., 2000a). Where syncytiotrophoblast and maternal endothelium are absent, the basal plate is superficially covered by Rohr's fibrinoid.

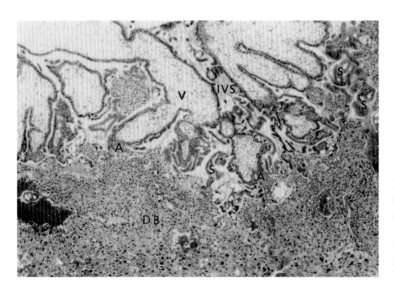

FIGURE 9.29. Very young placental floor with villi (V) containing connective tissue but no fetal vessels as yet, syncytium (S), intervillous space (IVS) with maternal blood, and the confusing intermixed population of cells in the decidua basalis (DB). The placental site giant cells are largely mononuclear but dark, in contrast to the lighter decidual cells. H&E ×40.

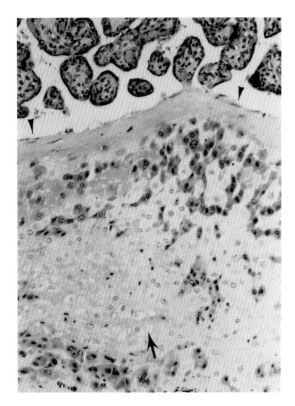

FIGURE 9.30. Extravillous trophoblast cells (dark cells) in decidua basalis of a near-term placenta. The arrow indicates a decidual stromal cell. The endothelial cells that are believed to line the basal portion of the intervillous space, above Rohr's fibrin layer, are indicated by arrowheads. H&E ×240.

Rohr's stria: The superficial fibrinoid layer of the basal plate, Rohr's stria was first described in 1888 by Wolska as superficially located, homogeneous or lamellar material in the basal plate (Fig. 9.27B) that shows structural similarities to a deeper layer characterized 1 year earlier by Nitabuch (1887). A year later, Rohr (1889) dealt with this superficial fibrinoid in some greater detail, pointing particularly to the fact that the superficial fibrinoid layer is less complete and more irregularly structured. His name was later attached to this layer. Rohr's stria is basically similar to Langhans' stria of the chorionic plate. Where villi are attached, it is continuous with perivillous fibrin, engulfing these villi. In most places, Rohr's fibrinoid shows immunohistochemical characteristics of fibrin-type fibrinoid (Frank et al., 1994). Only where Rohr's fibrinoid encases extravillous trophoblast cells, usually in the neighborhood of cell columns, patches of matrix-type fibrinoid can be found that are free of fibrin and rich in other ECM molecules.

Extravillous trophoblast layer: The principal layer of the basal plate is highly variable in composition and thickness, measuring 50μm to 1mm in thickness. It is composed of **extravillous cytotrophoblast**, patches of **fibrinoid**, loosely arranged **connective tissue**, admixed **decidual cells**, remnants of encased anchoring villi, and

"buried" cell columns. Most of the connective tissue of this region is of maternal origin. It is composed of endometrial stromal cells, small, highly branched fibroblast-like cells, and some macrophages. Because of the presence of maternal connective tissue in this layer, decidualization may also be present. Locally, there may be an admixture of fetal connective tissue cells that are derived from the stroma of encased and degenerating anchoring villi. Both lines of connective tissue cells can easily be distinguished by the application of the enzymatic histochemical reaction for leucine aminopeptidase. It results in positive staining of only the fetally derived connective tissue (Stark & Kaufmann, 1971).

A vast traditional descriptive literature deals in much detail with the structural, ultrastructural, histochemical, and functional aspects of the extravillous trophoblast cells of the basal plate (Wislocki, 1951; Ortmann, 1955; McKay et al., 1958; Thomsen & Willemsen, 1959; Weber, 1961; Dallenbach-Hellweg & Nette, 1963a,b, 1964; Wachstein et al., 1963; Hein, 1971; Kaufmann & Stark, 1971; Stark & Kaufmann, 1971). It has now become clear that these cells represent the largely nonproliferative, invasive portion of the extravillous trophoblast cells emanating from the cell columns (Schindler et al., 1984; Eidelman et al., 1989; Feinberg et al., 1989, 1991a; Loke et al., 1989, 1992a; Wakuda & Yoshida, 1990, 1992; Castellucci et al., 1991; Librach et al., 1991a,b; Damsky et al., 1992; Burrows et al., 1993; Fisher & Damsky, 1993; Mühlhauser et al., 1993; for review see Kaufmann & Castellucci, 1997). We refer the reader to the earlier section on Extravillous Trophoblast in this chapter.

The number of decidual cells present in this layer varies greatly. These cells may be absent or they can represent the majority of cells. For structural features of the decidual cells, see the section on Decidua. Cytotrophoblast and decidual cells may be intensively admixed (Figs. 9.2A and 9.28). According to Wynn (1967a), these cell types never establish direct intercellular contacts; rather, they are separated by fibrillar networks (external lamina of the decidual cells) (Kisalus & Herr, 1988), fibrinoid, or both. This finding is in partial disagreement with the results published by Hein (1971), who found the two types to be in intimate contact. The possibility of such contacts, even though established only occasionally in the human, is supported by findings in rats and mice (Martinek, 1970, 1971).

Nitabuch fibrinoid layer: The next layer of the basal plate is a fibrinoid layer (**uteroplacental fibrinoid**), which is a net-like to lamellar structure that is variably interrupted (Figs. 5.1 and 9.27B). It is located in the immediate maternofetal "battlefield" of the junctional zone (see Fig. 5.1). Because of this location, it has commonly been regarded as the site of immunologic processes.

This fibrinoid stria, first described by Nitabuch in 1887, is a rather consistent, more or less uninterrupted layer that is 20μm to more than 100μm in thickness. In many places, the layer may split and rejoin, with trophoblastic and decidual cells or endometrial connective tissue interposed. In its most ideal, but rarely executed situation, Nitabuch's fibrinoid separates superficially positioned trophoblastic cells from more basally located decidual cells (Figs. 5.1 and 9.27B). In these cases, it marks the exact maternofetal border (Wynn, 1967a). Usually, however, the arrangement of maternal and fetal cells is more irregular. Mixed populations of the two cell types on one or both sides of the stria are the commonest finding (Fig. 9.31).

Electron-microscopically and immunohistochemically, Nitabuch's fibrinoid represents a mixture of both, matrix-type fibrinoid and fibrin-type fibrinoid (Frank et al., 1994; Lang et al., 1994; Huppertz et al., 1996, 1998d). Its biochemical analysis by Sutcliffe et al. (1982) showed a prevailing composition of proteins of 48,000 and 105,000 d, thus corresponding to components of blood fibrin.

Whether other minor protein bands were of serum or local tissue origin remained an open question. In addition, Kisalus and Herr (1988) found immunocytochemical proof for a decidual secretion of heparan sulfate proteoglycan into the surrounding fibrinoid, and Frank et al. (1994, 1995) as well as Huppertz et al. (1996, 1998d) reported trophoblastic secretion of ECM molecules into it. According to the latter studies, those parts that encase extravillous trophoblast or decidual cells represent largely pure matrix-type fibrinoid. Cell free areas and in particular those layers that cover the basal surface of the delivered placenta are usually composed of fibrin-type fibrinoid. This explains why Sutcliffe et al. (1982) biochemically detected mostly blood clotting products because their material was derived from the basal surface.

Kirby et al. (1964) pointed to the interesting finding that large genetic differences between mother and fetus result in increasing amounts of uteroplacental fibrinoid.

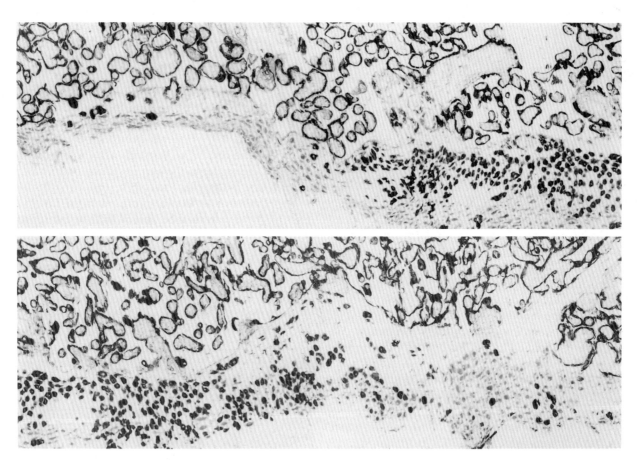

FIGURE 9.31. Cryostat survey section of the basal plate. Enzyme histochemical proof of glucose-6–phosphate dehydrogenase. **The right half of the upper picture is a continuation of the left half of the lower picture**. **At the upper side** of each picture one can see the intervillous space with numerous villi. The ability of the glucose-6-phosphate-dehydrogenase reaction to discriminate between extravillous trophoblast and decidua is used to illustrate the distribution of both cell types in the basal plate. The extravillous cytotrophoblast cells can be identified as darkly stained polygonal cells, whereas the decidua is composed of slender, faintly stained cell bodies. Note that there are segments of the basal plate with perfect layering (upper **right**) but also segments consisting merely of decidua (upper **middle**) or extravillous trophoblast cells (lower **left**). A colorful mixture of the two cell types is the most usual feature. ×65. (From Stark & Kaufmann, 1971, with permission.)

Consequently, a functionally protective immunological mechanism was proposed. Bardawil and Toy (1959), Kirby et al. (1964), Currie and Bagshawe (1967), Azab et al., (1972), Wynn (1975), and Sutcliffe et al. (1982) suggested a barrier function that protects fetal antigens against identification by maternal cells so as to avoid direct contact of fetal tissues with sensitized maternal lymphocytes. In the same context, Sutcliffe et al. (1982) have pointed to the ample uteroplacental fibrinoid present in human and rodent placentas with invasive implantation, in contrast to the relative lack in artiodactyls and perissodactyls that are characterized by noninvasive implantation with largely intact maternal and fetal epithelial surfaces facing each other.

Separation zone: Demarcation and separation of the placenta from the placental bed usually does not take place within Nitabuch's stria, but rather in most cases somewhat deeper. Therefore, some additional tissues may be attached to the placental floor and form the deepest layer of the basal plate. Most cells in this layer are decidual cells and other components of the endometrial stroma, and a certain admixture of trophoblastic elements is a regular finding.

With increasing distance from the intervillous space, the number of multinucleated giant cells (Kölliker, 1861; Boyd & Hamilton, 1960; Hein, 1971; Pijnenborg et al., 1980) increases. These cells are large, highly differentiated, multinucleated elements with diameters up to 100 μm. With the use of serial sections, they appear as slender, branching streamers with syncytial character (Boyd & Hamilton, 1960; Uhlendorf & Kaufmann, 1979).

This layer is the site of placental separation, a mechanism that is not fully understood. Even when separation is a rapid process, taking place within a few minutes, it must be assumed that tissue changes precede its occurrence. From clinical findings it seems likely that placental separation depends on the existence of decidua at the placental site. Where a decidual layer is lacking, as with an extrauterine pregnancy or placenta accreta, the placenta cannot separate spontaneously. We believe that placental separation occurs primarily on a mechanical basis, the contracting uterus shearing off the turgid placenta at the site of degeneration: In specimens of delivered human placentas as well as of remaining placental beds, decidual changes can be observed morphologically in the future zone of separation. These changes comprise a reduction of collagen fibers, an accumulation of interstitial fluid, and many degenerative changes. Kaiser (1960) reported the preterm reduction in the thickness of the decidual spongy zone from an original 4 mm to 0.2 mm. After placental separation, both surfaces, those of the placental bed and the basal plate are covered by a thin layer of fibrin (Ludwig & Metzger, 1971). This was interpreted by these authors as being a peripartal or perhaps even postpartal phenomenon.

Uteroplacental Vessels

Development

The basal plate is traversed by maternal uteroplacental vessels. The uteroplacental arteries are branches or direct continuations of myometrial arteries. As soon as they enter the decidua and the basal plate, they are also called spiral arteries or spiral arterioles because of their spiral course (Fig. 9.32A). Some authors restrict the term spiral artery to the nonpregnant endometrium and rename the vessel after a placenta is established as the uteroplacental artery. In most publications the terms are used synonymously.

The first contacts between maternal endometrial vessels and the intraplacental lacunar system become established around days 11 to 12 p.c. (Boyd & Hamilton, 1970). At this time, the first maternal erythrocytes leave the eroded capillaries and enter the trophoblastic lacunae. For the human there is some doubt whether it results in an effective uteroplacental circulation. Boyd and Hamilton (1970) failed to find openings of spiral arteries into the intervillous space, even in the case of an embryo with 28 somites, which corresponds to the 28th to 29th day p.c. Their earliest specimen with such openings was around 40 days old (10 mm crown–rump length), while Harris and Ramsey (1966) have reported this situation to exist as early as day 30 p.c. (5 mm crown–rump length). Further classical studies concerning this crucial question are summarized in the large study of Harris and Ramsey (1966).

Doppler studies of the uteroplacental circulation have again stimulated the discussion. A provocative and challenging study with ultrasonography, histology, and barium injection of the maternal plate came from Hustin and Schaaps (1987), Hustin et al. (1988), and Schaaps and Hustin (1988). They had earlier observed that chorionic villous sampling (CVS) biopsies are always bloodless. They also found no echogenic evidence of intervillous blood flow before 13 weeks' gestation. Moreover, when they were able to observe the placenta in vivo during the first trimester it was pale, and barium could not be forced into the intervillous space. Furthermore, few maternal blood cells were ever observed histologically in this area. Hustin and Schaaps suggested that the intraarterial trophoblast so much obstructs the arterial lumen (Fig. 9.33) that only filtered plasma reaches the intervillous space before 12 weeks' gestation. Careful inspection of sections from such immature placentas (Figs. 9.12, 9.15, 9.16, and 9.33) shows indeed in many cases the lack of red blood cells in our cases as well.

This **hypothesis of delayed onset of an uteroplacental circulation** has raised a highly controversial debate (Moll, 1995; Hustin, 1995; Jauniaux, 1996; Carter, 1997) and stimulated new, more detailed studies. Enders and Blankenship (1997) showed patent uteroplacental artery lumina in the macaque placenta already in the first month of gestation, even though some arteries may become temporarily blocked; and in the same species, Simpson and coworkers (1997) noted maternal intervillous blood flow from day 20 of gestation onward. When reevaluating human first trimester hysterectomy specimens, Meekins et al. (1997) found maternal blood in the villous space in all stages; moreover, according to their data, total plugging of uteroplacental arteries is a rare event. Also, these authors concluded that uteroplacental circulation is not interrupted in the first trimester.

In the fall of 1997, on the occasion of the European Placenta Group Meeting the authors mentioned in the foregoing paragraph met in Vigsoe/Danmark and discussed their data obtained in human and monkey pregnancies. The members of this workshop reached agreement that the maternal circulation throughout the first trimester may be reduced by

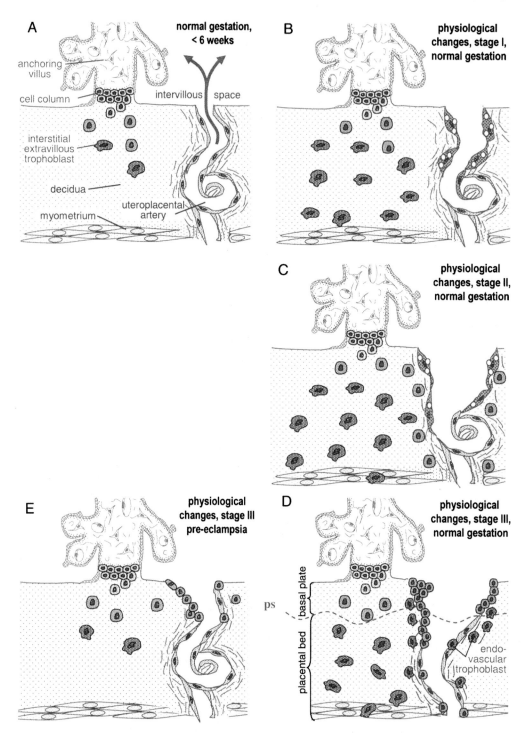

FIGURE 9.32. Schematic representation of interstitial and endovascular trophoblast invasion in human pregnancy. A: Before week 6 of gestation, the uteroplacental arteries are unaltered. B: Stage 1 of the pregnancy-induced physiologic changes of arteries is characterized by generalized endothelial basophilia, endothelial vacuolization, muscular disorganization, and slight lumen dilation. C: After appearance of trophoblast cells in the vascular surrounding, but prior to trophoblast invasion of the vascular walls, in stage 2 of vascular changes, maximum arterial dilatation occurs. D: Only in the final stage of pregnancy-induced changes of uteroplacental arteries, smooth muscle cells and endothelium of the already maximally dilated arteries are replaced by trophoblast. E: Note that failure of endovascular trophoblast invasion in intrauterine growth restriction (IUGR) and preeclampsia is restricted to the placental bed and does not affect segments of the uteroplacental arteries in the later basal plate of the placenta. Blue, fetal tissues; red, Maternal tissues; ps, zone of placental separation where the basal plate (above, attached to the placenta) separates from the placental bed (remaining in the uterus after delivery). (*Source:* Modified and extended from Kaufmann et al., 2003, with permission.)

FIGURE 9.33. Arteries in the basal plate in the same placenta as in Figure 9.15. Note the fibrin in the wall, whose muscular coat is destroyed; the vessels are surrounded and thoroughly infiltrated by extravillous trophoblast cells. The paler cells at the bottom are decidual stromal cells; endometrial glands are at bottom right. H&E ×160.

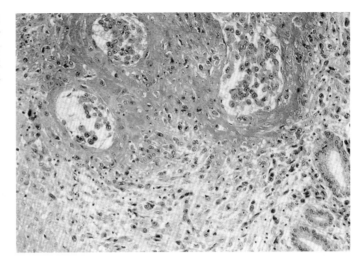

partial plugging of the arteries but that it never is completely interrupted. This consensus is in agreement with the low oxygen partial pressures measured in the intervillous space throughout the first trimester; only from week 13 p.m. onward the pO$_2$ values were raised (Rodesch et al., 1992). These data have interesting implications; for instance, is relative hypoxia an important modulator of trophoblast behavior controlling the balance between proliferation and invasion (Genbacev et al., 1996, 1997)? (See Oxygen-Mediated Regulation of the Invasive Pathway, above.)

The uteroplacental arteries cross the uterine wall almost perpendicularly up to the 8th week p.m. (Pijnenborg et al., 1980). With advancing gestation, as the placental area enlarges, the course of the peripheral arteries becomes more oblique, so that by 10 weeks distal segments are almost parallel to the basal plate. Invading trophoblast breaches these horizontal segments to form new openings into the intervillous space (Harris & Ramsey, 1966). Alteration of the blood flow, which is caused by these new openings, was thought to be the consequence in the most distal segments. Degeneration of the latter can be followed by necrosis of the surrounding decidua. This finding is common in the periphery of the placental site between 8 and 14 weeks of pregnancy. In most instances, obliterated arterial segments can be found within the areas of necrosis. Trophoblastic invasion of the necrotic areas is reduced (Pijnenborg et al., 1980).

The number of spiral arterial turns appears to decrease throughout pregnancy. Intense spiraling, with formation of large loops directly beneath the basal plate, may result in up to seven openings, one after the other, in consecutive loops of one and the same spiral artery. On the other hand, multiple openings of one artery can also be produced by branching in the superficial layers of the basal plate. Both are common findings in early placentas. Near term, most of these additional openings and branches are apparently obstructed by blood clots, resulting in the final finding of one opening per artery. Some smaller branches, arterioles, and venules, may branch off in the deeper layers of the junctional zone and in the superficial myometrial layers. They are nutritional vessels that result in only poorly developed capillary nets.

Number and Position of the Uteroplacental Vessels

Comparative studies of the maternal circulations of rhesus monkey and human placentas have shown that they are similar. Thus, appropriate deductions can be made from observations in monkeys (Freese, 1968). It is remarkable that, after all these studies, we still do not know the **number of spiral arteries** that perfuse the placenta. Panigel and Pascaud (1968) reviewed the topic; they wrote that in 1890 Klein found 53 arteries and 31 veins, whereas Spanner in 1934 and 1935 counted 80 to 90 arteries with 488 openings! Franken (1954) described 263 arterial and 79 venous openings. Marais (1962) counted 105 arterial ostia, Reynolds (1966) 40 to 50, and Boyd (1956) 102 to 156 at the end of the first trimester, and about 180 to 320 at term. Brosens (1988) reported 120 spiral arteries for the term placenta, each with a single opening. In contrast to Boyd's observations, Harris and Ramsey (1966) found decreasing numbers of arterial inlets during the course of pregnancy. The final density of arterial openings at term was reported to be one per square centimeter of basal plate surface (Harris & Ramsey, 1966) or 0.5 per square centimeter (Brosens, 1964). Haller (1968) found some 200 to 300 vascular openings in the floor of the delivered placenta; he described their morphology and stated that it was difficult to differentiate between arteries and veins. These conflicting data reflect the methodologic problems when identifying and counting such highly coiled and branched structures. Fewer figures have been given for the **number of venous openings**. Most authors agree that their number is considerably lower than that of the arterial ostia (Franken, 1954; Gruenwald, 1966; Boyd & Hamilton, 1970). All these numbers are in disagreement with those of Borell et al. (1965), who, in cineradiographic studies of pregnant women, observed 25 arteries at term. These authors cautioned that erroneous enumeration of placental lobules causes false numbers of arteries.

Regarding the **position of uteroplacental vessels**, many authors now agree that a single decidual spiral artery delivers its blood into the center of a cotyledon, and on occasion lateral vessels add to the supply. This fact has been amply demonstrated by the injection studies of Freese (1968), Freese and Maciolek (1969), Wigglesworth (1969), Panigel and Pascaud (1968), Schuhmann and Wehler (1971), and Schuhmann (1981). Only Gruenwald (1966), Nikolov and Schiebler (1973), and Brosens (1988) came to different conclusions. The latter authors found the arteries to open in the periphery of the cotyledons, at the base, or in the lower one third of the septa. The venous openings are thought to be in a more peripheral position of the cotyledons, which is in contrast to the views presented by Spanner (1934, 1935), who concluded that the intervillous venous blood is mainly drained via the marginal venous sinus. This opinion, in turn, has been contradicted by Arts (1961), who found the venous openings more evenly distributed over the basal plate.

It must be pointed out that the idealized arrangement, with one artery opening near the center of a villous tree (see Intervillous Space as Related to the Villous Trees in Chapter 7), is rare. It is seen only at the placental periphery, where the average diameter of the cotyledons or lobules is small. Here the numerical relation of villous trees to basally visible lobes is 1:1 (see Chapter 2, Fig. 2.2). Larger lobules, in particular those of the more central parts of the organ, normally contain two to four villous trees that usually overlap partially at the margin (see Figs. 2.2 and 7.26). Here the position of vascular openings, as they relate to the villous trees, is more confusing, and this fact may have contributed to the above controversy.

The villous tissue within the central cotyledonary region, where the maternal "jet" enters, is usually composed of larger, more immature appearing villous types. Here they are separated by wider intervillous clefts (Schuhmann & Wehler, 1971; Schuhmann, 1981; Kaufmann, 1985) (see Fig. 7.26). This can be easily seen when a fresh placenta is sectioned. The area shows apparently empty spaces—the central cavities (Ramsey, 1962; Ramsey et al., 1963, 1966; Gruenwald, 1966, 1971, 1973; Freese, 1968). Wigglesworth (1969) considered this area to be the site where intervillous thrombi most commonly occur, and we agree. Most intervillous thrombi are fresh and apparently result from local stasis of blood flow during labor. At times one can see that their triangular shape originates from vessels in the placental floor. The villous architecture is draped around these central cavities. Serial roentgenographic studies, with injection of radiopaque dyes, demonstrate them adequately. After these spaces are filled, the radiopaque material is dissipated peripherally, producing the familiar and oft-mentioned "smoke rings" (Freese, 1968).

Importance of Physiologic Changes of Uteroplacental Arteries

The trophoblastic invasion of the uteroplacental arteries and the subsequent alterations have been designated as physiologic changes to distinguish them from the pathologic changes seen in the placental bed vessels of patients with IUGR and preeclampsia (Brosens et al., 1967). The process has been succinctly reviewed by Ramsey (1981), Brosens (1988), and Sheppard and Bonnar (1988).

Trophoblast invasion of uteroplacental arteries with respective physiologic changes is seen in many other species with invasive placentation and is considered to have important ramifications for ensuring placental perfusion. In the course of this process, the spiral arteries are remodeled into low-resistance vessels that are unable to constrict. Because of the absence of local regulatory mechanisms in uteroplacental vessels, the mother cannot reduce the nutrient supply to the placenta without reducing nutrient supply to her own tissues (Haig, 1993).

The physiologic changes according to Brosens et al. (1967) include (1) apparent replacement of endothelium and media smooth muscle cells by invasive trophoblast; (2) loss of elasticity; (3) dilatation to wide, incontractile tubes; and (4) loss of vasomotor control (Fig. 9.32A–D).

The purposes of pregnancy-specific spiral artery remodeling are threefold:

- Maternal blood flow resistance is reduced and uteroplacental perfusion is increased to meet the increasing nutritional requirements of the fetus.
- The loss of contractility and loss of maternal vasomotor control guarantees maximum maternal blood supply to the placenta, irrespective of maternal attempts to regulate the blood distribution within her own body (Moll et al., 1988).
- As already described earlier (see Myofibroblasts in Chapter 6), local loss of maternal vasomotor control enables the fetus to gain control over maternal blood flow resistance and blood flow distribution within the intervillous space.

Deficiency of physiologic changes of the spiral arteries (Fig. 9.32E) has been demonstrated to be abnormal (Feinberg et al., 1991a). It represents a significant characteristic of preeclampsia and of hypertension during pregnancy; it is also typically associated with fetal growth retardation (Brosens et al., 1972, 1977; Sheppard & Bonnar, 1976; deWolf et al., 1980; Brosens, 1988). Khong et al. (1986a) and Sheppard and Bonnar (1988) have even reported complete absence of such physiologic change throughout the length of some of the spiral arteries in cases of preeclampsia and IUGR.

Stages of Physiologic Changes in Uteroplacental Arteries

Different from earlier views, it is important to note that trophoblast invasion of the arteries is not the primary event, which is responsible for all other pregnancy-specific alterations of the arteries; rather, most of the changes happen already prior to or concomitant with trophoblast infiltration. Trophoblast cells invade already severely altered, physiologically changed arteries. According to structural criteria, physiologic changes of uteroplacental arteries can be subdivided into three subsequent stages:

Stage 1: Vascular changes preceding trophoblast invasion (Fig. 9.32B): The initial arterial changes involve a generalized endothelial basophilia and vacuolation, disorganization of vascular smooth muscle, and lumen dilation (Craven et al., 1998). These changes are independent from direct trophoblast invasion and are considered to involve maternal activation of local decidual artery renin-angiotensin systems (Craven et al., 1998). The same authors demonstrated that during intrauterine pregnancies spiral arteries from both implantation and nonimplantation regions display these physiologic changes. Last but not least, in ectopic pregnancies endometrial spiral arteries undergo the same physiologic vascular modifications.

Stage 2: Vascular remodeling induced by perivascularly located extravillous trophoblast (Fig. 9.32C): Only after the appearance of the trophoblast invasion-independent changes, the uteroplacental arteries within the implantation region are invaded by extravillous trophoblast cells. As soon as extravillous trophoblast cells approach the uteroplacental arteries, further vascular remodeling starts. This has been analyzed in detail in the guinea pig (Hees et al., 1987; Moll et al., 1988; Nanaev et al., 1995). This second set of changes comprise reduction of media smooth muscle cells and deposition of fibrinoid material prior to infiltration of the media by trophoblast. The question came up as to the mechanisms that drive this second group of changes. Nanaev et al. (1995) analyzed arterial trophoblast invasion in the guinea pig and described arterial dilatation already prior to trophoblastic infiltration of the wall. They found indications for nitric oxide secretion of periarterial trophoblast cells, resulting in maximum arterial dilatation (for further discussion of the role of nitric oxide, see Nitric Oxide and Trophoblast Invasion, above).

Stage 3: Trophoblast infiltration of vessel walls (Fig. 9.32D): Only the third and last stage of uteroplacental vascular remodeling is characterized by infiltration of the arterial wall by endovascular trophoblast:

- The uteroplacental arteries undergo further **dilatation** up to several times the original diameter of the lumen (Brosens et al., 1967; Hirano et al., 2002). The increase in luminal width is particularly impressive near the intervillous space, where the spiral arteries may finally reach as much as five times their original luminal diameter. Panigel and Pascaud (1968), Boyd and Hamilton (1970), and Sheppard and Bonnar (1974a,b) reported arterial luminal diameters of about $200\,\mu m$ in the myometrial segments, compared to 500 to $1000\,\mu m$ near their opening into the intervillous space. The diameter of the arterial ostia may be as much as $2000\,\mu m$. A terminal constriction of the lumens, and in particular a flow-regulating sphincter, as described by Spanner (1935) and Debiasi et al. (1963), have later been refuted by all subsequent authors.

- The trophoblastic infiltration of the arterial media coincides with **loss of elastic fibers** (Robertson, 1976; Robertson & Manning, 1974). The latter authors suggested that even more elastic fibers develop in these vessels throughout gestation; but because of invasion-related degenerative processes, most of these fibers seem to be lost again later. Destruction of elastic fibers usually is attributed to proteolytic activities of the invasive endovascular trophoblast cells. The process has been mimicked in vitro by Aplin (personal communication). Accordingly, the expression of proteases such as interstitial collagenase (MMP-1), gelatinase A (MMP-2), stromelysin 1 (MMP-3), and gelatinase B (MMP-9) was shown (Moll & Lane, 1990; Blankenship & Enders, 1997; Kaufmann & Castellucci, 1997). In this context it is, however, of interest that the two proteinase inhibitors α_1-antitrypsin and α_1-antichymotrypsin were found to be expressed only in the intraarterial trophoblast cells, whereas the interstitial subpopulation of invasive extravillous trophoblast cells was negative for both inhibitors (Earl et al., 1989).

- According to Brosens et al. (1967), the trophoblast invasion is paralleled by an increase in **intramural fibrinoid masses**, which cause transformation of the originally flexible vessels into rigid channels.

- Regarding the **media smooth muscle cells**, the original view was that smooth muscle cells are destroyed by invasive trophoblast and become replaced by endovascular trophoblast (Ramsey & Harris, 1966; Brosens et al., 1967; Boyd & Hamilton, 1970; Nikolov & Schiebler, 1973). In fact, Aplin (personal communication) has shown that invasive trophoblast cells in vitro when invading isolated arterial segments, induced apoptosis of vascular smooth muscle cells. In the older literature the vessels were described as being finally more or less devoid of smooth muscle cells (Wilkin, 1958; Brettner, 1964; Panigel & Pascaud, 1969), the loss being less impressive in the decidual portion than at the more superficial levels (deWolf et al., 1973; Nikolov & Schiebler, 1973; Sheppard & Bonnar, 1974b; Brosens, 1988). More recently, it was shown in the guinea pig that at least the majority of smooth muscle cells under the influence of trophoblast cells does not degenerate but rather dedifferentiates to myoblasts (Nanaev et al., 1995). The resulting myoblasts, which are phenotypically similar to trophoblast cells, are the basis for postpartal arterial reconstitution (Nanaev et al., 2000b). The trophoblast cells, in this species only in a secondary step, infiltrated the already maximally dilated and dedifferentiated vessel wall. The data support earlier reports in the same species, which showed vascular changes preceding trophoblastic infiltration (Hees et al., 1987; Moll et al., 1988). Also for the human it was immunohistochemically shown, that α-smooth muscle actin is still present in segments of uteroplacental arteries that are phenotypically void of smooth muscle cells (Craven & Ward, 1996).

- The **endothelial cells** in the peripheral parts of uteroplacental arteries are largely replaced by a mono-to polylayer of cytotrophoblast (intraarterial trophoblast). The latter partly even form large **trophoblastic plugs**, which locally may obstruct the lumen. It is still an open question whether such trophoblastic plugs may completely block blood flow in certain arteries thus resulting in reduced or even absent perfusion of the intervillous space (Hustin, 1995; Moll, 1995; Jauniaux, 1996; Carter, 1997). One should bear in mind that uteroplacental arteries show final branching before entering the intervillous space (see Number and Position of the Uteroplacental Vessels, above) and that obstruction of single side-branches must not influence intervillous blood flow.

The discrimination between intraarterial trophoblast cells and maternal endothelial cells is not always easy since trophoblast cells, when replacing the endothelium, may achieve an endothelial phenotype. By contrast, also maternal endothelium may contribute to the formation of the intraarterial plugs: When the placental bed was examined with antibodies directed against hCG and factor VIII–related antigens, Tuttle et al. (1985) found that many large endovascular cells had factor VIII activity but no hCG-immunoreactivity, which suggested that they are endothelium, rather than trophoblast.

These problems underline the usefulness of antibodies specifically directed against endovascular trophoblast, such as anti–cytokeratin 17 (Pröll et al., 1997a) or GZ 112 (Hartmann et al., 1997). Application of such antibodies reveals that the majority of cells lining the lumina of the endometrial segments of uteroplacental arteries, and of those parts passing the luminal third of the myometrium, represent intraarterial trophoblast. This is quite different from uteroplacental veins (see below), the maternal endothelium of which becomes replaced only in extremely rare cases by trophoblast.

Sites and Routes of Endovascular Trophoblast Invasion

Endovascular trophoblast invasion is not a homogeneous process. The density of extravillous trophoblast and the depth of invasion of uteroplacental arteries are most pronounced in the central region of the placental bed. The density and depth of invasion of extravillous trophoblast as well as the degree of invasion of spiral arteries diminish toward the placental margin (Brosens, 1988). Central-region placental bed specimens obtained from normal pregnancies reveal endovascular trophoblast that invaded and dilated uteroplacental arteries up to the first third of the myometrium—a depth similar to interstitial trophoblast invasion in this region.

The anatomic pathways taken by the endovascular trophoblast have been a matter of controversy. Two different

models, the extravasation and the intravasation model, are under discussion.

Extravasation: Based on detailed studies on the rhesus monkey, Blankenship and coworkers (1993a) concluded that endovascular trophoblast derived from an unknown source gained access to the arterial lumens via or close to their point of confluence with the intervillous space. Thereafter the cells migrate along the arterial lumens retrograde to blood flow by adhering to the endothelium and replacing it (Fig. 9.34A). Finally a certain number of these cells were thought to leave the lumen (extravasate) and centrifugally invade media and adventitia. This view would imply that endovascular trophoblast cells have a different origin from the interstitial route of trophoblast invasion. And indeed, immunohistochemical markers have been described that allow discrimination of endovascular trophoblast from interstitial extravillous trophoblast (Hartmann et al., 1997; Pröll et al., 1997a).

Intravasation: Based on studies in the human, the majority of researchers favor the contrasting concept of intravasation (Pijnenborg et al., 1983; Kurman et al., 1984a; Damsky et al., 1992, 1993; Loke et al., 1992; Fisher & Damsky, 1993; Kaufmann & Castellucci, 1997; Redman, 1997) (Fig. 9.34B). Structural criteria (Pijnenborg et al., 1983) and immunohistochemical data (Damsky et al., 1992; Fisher & Damsky, 1993) suggested that endovascular trophoblast represents an end stage of differentiation of interstitial trophoblast derived from the cell columns. As a sidestep, a subpopulation of extravillous trophoblast cells invade the arterial walls from the surrounding junctional zone and finally enter the arterial lumens. Whether or not the intravasated cells then migrate inside the arterial lumens and even locally may extravasate remains an open question.

A combination of both hypotheses was suggested by Loke's group (Kam et al., 1999). These authors described infiltration and replacement of arterial media and adventitia by interstitial trophoblast, followed by the replacement of endothelium by a separate population of endovascular trophoblast, the derivation of which was not described.

The answer to the question whether extra- or intravasation takes place in uteroplacental arteries is crucial for the understanding of the various hypotheses below. Here it is important to recognize that extravasation was described in the rhesus monkey, a species with a nearly complete trophoblastic shell separating the intervillous space and maternofetal junctional zone. This trophoblastic shell may be a source for intraluminal trophoblast migration. In contrast, the trophoblastic shell of the very early gestation human placenta becomes rarefied to widely spread cell columns not in contact with the terminal structures of the maternal arteries.

In agreement with the extravasation theory, the endovascular trophoblast in the rhesus monkey has been described by King and Blankenship (1993) to maintain proliferation based on PCNA immunohistochemistry (proliferative cell nuclear antigen; antibody PC10). The PCNA displays a long half-life (20+ hours) (Bravo & Macdonald-Bravo, 1987); therefore, cells may remain immunopositive for days after leaving the cell cycle. Human endovascular trophoblast has not been observed to proliferate according to Ki-67 immunohistochemistry, ^{3}H-thymidine incorporation

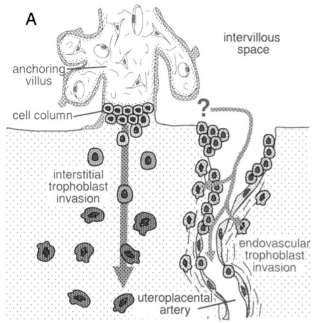

Endovascular trophoblast invasion by extravasation

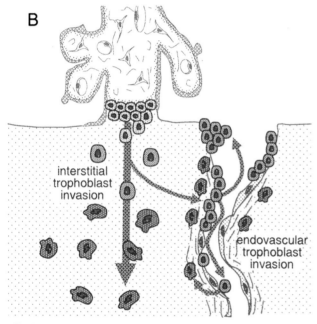

Endovascular trophoblast invasion by intravasation

FIGURE 9.34. Hypothetical routes of endovascular trophoblast invasion. Blue: fetal tissues including interstitial trophoblast and its "intravasating" derivatives. Green: extravasation route of endovascular trophoblast. Red: Maternal tissues. Note that in the hypothetical case of "extravasation" (A) the endovascular trophoblast cells invade via the arterial lumen and are derived from an unknown origin. By contrast, in the more likely case of "intravasation" (B), endovascular trophoblast is derived from cell columns via the interstitial invasion route. (*Source:* Modified from Kaufmann et al., 2003, with permission.)

studies, or assessment of mitotic figures. Proliferation of human extravillous trophoblast has been observed exclusively in trophoblast resting on the basal lamina of cell columns (Kaufmann & Castellucci, 1997).

We conclude from these data that extravillous trophoblast emanating from the cell columns, provides cells for the interstitial route of trophoblast invasion. Cells from the latter route invade (intravasate) uteroplacental arteries and contribute to the remodeling process by replacing arterial media and endothelium (Fig. 9.34B). It may, however, happen that these cells enter the vessel lumina quite early, close to the intervillous space, then migrating along the endothelium against the blood flow to more central portions of the arteries (Enders et al., 1996). In the latter position they may even extravasate again. A similar situation has been observed in guinea pig placentation (Nanaev et al., 1995).

Trophoblast-Endothelial Adhesion Mechanisms

To understand the pathogenetic mechanisms of IUGR and preeclampsia, there as been increasing interest in the molecular mechanisms behind endovascular trophoblast invasion and concomitant vascular changes. Most of these studies have focused on adhesion mechanisms, which enable the trophoblast to enter the arterial walls and to replace the endothelial lining by a new trophoblastic lining. The expression of cell adhesion molecules is necessary for trophoblast invasion as these molecules enable trophoblast to adhere to the ECM, form colonies, and target cells in the vessel wall. Numerous studies reported that (1) proliferative and early postproliferative cells within the proximal invasive pathway (immunoreactive with proliferation marker MIB-1) express epithelial adhesion molecules, and (2) nonproliferative trophoblast of the distal invasive pathway (immunonegative with MIB-1) acquire an invasive phenotype by switching their repertoire of adhesion molecules to one resembling that of mesenchymal derivatives as, for example, endothelial cells (Vicovac & Aplin, 1996; Merviel et al., 2001).

Selectins: The first respective studies on trophoblast-endothelial interactions were performed by the Loke group in Cambridge. These authors found that intra-arterial trophoblast cells express **sialyl-Lewis**[x] (King & Loke, 1988). Expression of this cell surface carbohydrate was already known from various leukocytes. It is the ligand of the lectins **E-** and **P-selectin**, both of which are expressed by endothelium during inflammatory reactions. Interactions between sialyl-Le[x] and selectins enable the leukocytes to attach to the endothelium and subsequently to pass the vessel wall. Interestingly, both selectins were found to be expressed also by maternal endothelium during pregnancy exclusively at the implantation site (Burrows et al., 1994). The authors suggest that sialyl-Le[x]/selectin interaction is used for trophoblast attachment to the arterial endothelium and for trophoblast migration along the vessels lumina. The sialyl-Le^x–E-selectin interaction is also involved in adhesion of cancer cell lines to human umbilical vein endothelial cells in vitro (Takada et al., 1993).

N-CAM: Also the **neural cell adhesion molecule** (N-CAM, CD56) is thought to be involved in the process of vascular invasion. It is a homophilic cell–cell adhesion molecule and permits cells to adhere to ECMs. It is expressed by extravillous trophoblast in nearly all stages of its development (Pröll et al., 1997b; for review, see Kaufmann & Castellucci, 1997). According to data obtained in the rhesus monkey, also intraarterial trophoblast cells are distinctly N-CAM–positive, whereas intramural trophoblast cells and maternal endothelium reveal reduced or no immunoreactivity (Blankenship & King, 1996). The latter authors assign this adhesion molecule a special role of trophoblast/trophoblast adhesion during formation of intraluminal plugs.

ICAM-1: According to Ruck et al. (1994), intercellular adhesion molecule-1 (ICAM-1) is expressed by the maternal endothelium at the implantation site. Burrows et al. (1994) found this adhesion molecule not only to be expressed by all maternal endothelial cells, large granular lymphocytes, macrophages, but also by perivascular interstitial trophoblast and endovascular trophoblast. The ligand for ICAM-1 is the β2 integrin heterodimer CD11a/18 (Springer, 1990), which is expressed by large granular lymphocytes/uNK cells (Burrows et al., 1993b) but not by trophoblast cells. These data are partly in contrast to those of Labarrere and Page Faulk (1995), who detected ICAM-1 only in endovascular trophoblast from abnormal pregnancies characterized by arterial malinvasion (IUGR and preeclampsia), whereas endovascular trophoblast from normal pregnancies was immunonegative. It is speculated that expression of ICAM-1 at the implantation site is unimportant for vascular trophoblast invasion itself but rather for local adhesion and subsequent migration of endometrial NK cells (CD56$^+$ lymphocytes, uNK cells) from the peripheral blood into the decidua.

Arguments for endothelial mimicry: Susan Fisher's group (Zhou et al., 1997a,b) introduced the hypothesis that impaired invasion of uteroplacental arteries is due to trophoblastic failure to acquire the vascular repertoire of adhesion molecules. In normal pregnancies these authors reported a generally reduced expression of E-cadherin in extravillous trophoblast, but an upregulation of expression of **VE-cadherin** (endothelial cadherin), **PECAM-1** (platelet-endothelial adhesion molecule-1), **VECAM-1** (vascular endothelial adhesion molecule-1), and **α4 integrins** (Zhou et al., 1997a). Endovascular trophoblast continues to express these receptors and, like activated endothelial cells, acquires αvβ3 (Zhou et al., 1997b). In the latter publication, this group reported that extravillous trophoblast in preeclampsia failed to express most of these endothelial markers and hypothesized that

expression of a vascular phenotype by the trophoblast is required for successful endovascular invasion.

Arguments against endothelial mimicry: The trophoblast-endothelial mimicry model has not been supported by other investigators. For example, Lyall and co-workers (2001) studied human placental bed biopsies and found that PECAM-1 expression was not detected in extravillous trophoblast but rather observed only in endothelial cells. Moreover, no differences in cell-type patterns of PECAM-1 expression were observed among normal pregnancy, preeclampsia, and IUGR. Also regarding integrins, the patterns found in normal pregnancies were comparable to those in preeclampsia (Divers et al., 1995). The downregulation of E-cadherin during trophoblast invasion, described by Zhou et al. (1997a,b), was not supported by Floridon et al. (2000). Finally, Jaakkola and coworkers (2000), after studying a broad panel of leukocyte-endothelium adhesion or lymphocyte homing-associated antigens including ICAM-1, ICAM-2, VCAM, P-selectin, E-selectin, L-selectin, CLA-1, CD73, and VAP-1 in the invasion area, concluded that there is no major change in the adhesive properties of the endothelium of the placental bed in preeclampsia.

Induction of endothelial apoptosis: Different from the above models, the in vitro data of Ashton et al. (2005) do not require trophoblast-endothelial adhesion, with or without endothelial mimicry, as prerequisites for intra-arterial trophoblast invasion. Rather, based on their data, these authors concluded that trophoblast by means of FasL secretion forces Fas-positive maternal arterial endothelium into apoptosis and thereafter replaces it.

The Role of Macrophages in the Control of Endovascular Trophoblast Invasion

Maternal macrophages are normal constituents of the placental implantation site and can be demonstrated by antibodies to CD14 or CD68 (Bulmer et al., 1984; Reister et al., 1999). Greater numbers of macrophages are found in the decidua basalis as compared to the decidua parietalis, where trophoblast invasion is limited. This may hint at interactions between trophoblast invasion and macrophages (Loke & King, 1995). Macrophages produce and respond to a wide range of cytokines and may well be involved in local paracrine networks regulating trophoblast invasion (for review, see Hunt, 1989, 1990). Among others, activated macrophages produce high levels of TNF-α (Hunt, 1989). Its receptor TNF-R1 is expressed by trophoblast cells (Yui et al., 1996; Reister et al., 2001). Interactions between TNF-α and TNF-R1 were described as inducing trophoblast apoptosis in vitro (Yui et al., 1994; Reister et al., 2001).

As already dealt with above, in preeclampsia, segments of the spiral arteries located in the inner third of the myometrium and in the deep endometrium are infiltrated by macrophages and do not show any trophoblast

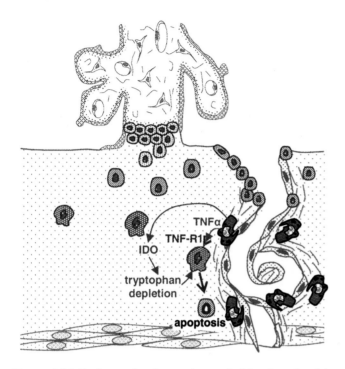

FIGURE 9.35. Defense of endovascular trophoblast invasion (via intravasation) by activated maternal macrophages of the arterial walls in preeclampsia or IUGR. These macrophages force approaching trophoblast cells into apoptosis by secretion of tumor necrosis factor-α (TNF-α) and indolamine 2,3-dioxygenase (IDO), the latter causing local tryptophan depletion. Blue: fetal tissues including trophoblast. Red: maternal tissues. Lilac: Activated maternal macrophages. Note that in the case of preeclampsia activated maternal macrophages accumulate in the proximal parts of the uteroplacental arteries located in the deeper zones of the placental bed. There they prevent perivascular and endovascular trophoblast invasion and thereby block the physiologic changes of arteries. (*Source:* Modified from Kaufmann et al., 2003, with permission.)

invasion (Reister et al., 1999). In normal pregnancy, the respective segments are invaded by trophoblast, but rarely show intramural macrophages. Interestingly, the preeclampsia-specific increase of macrophages seems to be restricted to the maternal arterial walls. By contrast, the number of maternal macrophages in the interstitium even was described as being reduced in preeclampsia (Burk et al., 2001).

To analyze the inverse relation between invasive trophoblast cells and maternal macrophages, Reister et al. (2001) have performed in vitro experiments using an immortalized extravillous trophoblast cell line and primary macrophages. The experiments revealed that activated macrophages induce trophoblast apoptosis by the concerted action of two mechanisms (Fig. 9.35):

- By secretion of TNF-α, which binds to the trophoblastic TNF-R1;
- By secretion of IDO, which catabolizes and depletes local levels of tryptophan.

These data explain the immunohistochemically evident inverse relation between the number of endovascular trophoblast and macrophages in the wall of uteroplacental arteries (Reister et al., 1999). The fact that macrophages induce trophoblast apoptosis in vitro renders it unlikely that the increased macrophage population in the arterial walls in preeclampsia is simply due to apoptotic attraction of macrophages. However, combining both possible interactions between macrophages and trophoblast, it could be hypothesized that macrophage-induced trophoblast apoptosis attracts and activates more macrophages leading to a vicious cycle.

Incompetent Trophoblast Invasion or Exaggerated Maternal Defense as Causes for Maladaptation of Uteroplacental Arteries

Several authors suggest that shallow interstitial trophoblastic invasion results in impaired endovascular trophoblast invasion and leads to maladaptation of uteroplacental arteries. This view is expressed by statements such as "pre-eclampsia is associated with abnormally shallow placentation" (Zhou et al., 1998); "hypoinvasive placental phenotype characteristic of pre-eclampsia" (Caniggia et al., 1999); "shallow trophoblast invasion ... predisposing the pregnancy to pre-eclampsia" (Caniggia et al., 2000). In agreement with this view, it is often believed that IUGR and preeclampsia are associated with a generalized impairment of trophoblast invasion that includes both reduced interstitial and reduced endovascular trophoblast invasion.

Recent quantitative studies on interstitial trophoblast invasion in hysterectomized uteri from patients with preeclampsia have revealed in fact that both invasive depth and numerical density of interstitial extravillous trophoblast in this entity are significantly reduced compared to normal (Kadyrov et al., 2003). However, in contrast to previous studies on basal plates from delivered placentas (DiFederico et al., 1999) interstitial trophoblast apoptosis within the placental bed was not increased but rather reduced in preeclampsia (Kadyrov et al., 2003), while endovascular trophoblast apoptosis was increased (Reister et al., 1999).

These contrasting apoptosis features led us to doubt that shallow trophoblast invasion or increased trophoblast apoptosis per se are the cause of impaired endovascular invasion. Mere intrinsic trophoblastic phenomena, such as missing expression of a vascular phenotype, reduced NO secretion by the trophoblast, and altered trophoblast behavior caused by deficient oxygenation (Zhou et al., 1998; Caniggia et al., 2000) are unlikely to be the exclusive causes of malinvasion of uteroplacental arteries with subsequent IUGR or preeclampsia.

Rather, the clinical and basic research data discussed above suggest that maladaptation and malinvasion of uteroplacental arteries characteristic of IUGR and preeclampsia result from a variety of factors interacting with each other in a cascade of events:

- intrinsic factors, namely abnormal biology of the extravillous trophoblast, acting in concert with
- extrinsic, maternal uterine factors operating around the uteroplacental arteries, which might include a.o.
- impaired decidual remodeling (Aplin 1991b; Brosens et al., 2002),
- macrophage-based defense mechanisms (Reister et al., 1999; 2001),
- impaired function of uterine NK cells (Ashkar et al., 2000), and
- maternal endothelial failure to express selectins (King & Loke, 1988; Burrows et al., 1994).

Structure of Uteroplacental Veins

The structure of the uteroplacental veins differs in some minor aspects from that of the spiral arteries. The muscular coat is even more reduced than that of the arteries, and smooth muscle cells are usually absent near the venous openings (Nikolov & Schiebler, 1973). The discontinuous endothelium is surrounded by some connec-

tive tissue. Trophoblast cells may be locally absent from the vessel walls (Fig. 9.36A) or may show a low degree of infiltration. In the rhesus monkey, trophoblast cells sometimes have been observed even intraluminally to replace the endothelium in venous segments near the intervillous space (Blankenship et al., 1993b).

Wanner (1966) described that maternal endothelium may leave the venous lumina and cover the surrounding parts of the basal plate. This finding has been supported immunohistochemically by applying a panel of endothelium-specific antibodies (Lang et al., 1993). Using an antibody directed against the factor VIII–related antigen we found maternal endothelium not only in the vicinity of the venous openings (Fig. 9.37) but also covering other parts of the basal plate (see Chapter 3, Fig. 3.3C), parts of septa, cell islands, and sometimes even perivillous fibrinoid deposits.

The maternal endothelial lining of the intervillous space is particularly impressive in the marginal zone of the placenta. In this area, maternal veins show funnel-like terminal dilatations that, without clear border, continue into

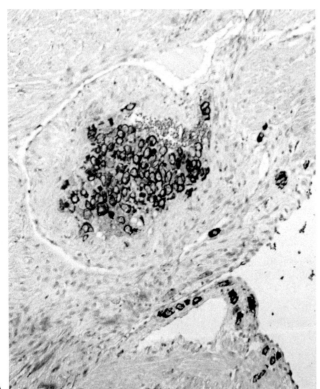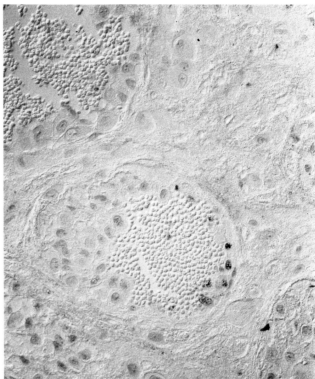

FIGURE 9.36. Uteroplacental vessels, paraffin sections, 16th week p.m. A: Stained with an anticytokeratin antibody that detects extravillous trophoblast cells (brown). The spiral artery (center) is largely occluded by a plug of intraarterial trophoblast cells. The uteroplacental vein beneath (lower third) shows only few intramural trophoblast cells. ×100. B: Stained with MIB-1, which binds to the nuclei of proliferating cells. The tro-

phoblastic plug protruding into the arterial lumen is obviously nonproliferative as are the trophoblast cells lining the upper vessel. The trophoblastic nature of these cells has been proven by anticytokeratin staining of a parallel section. The only positive (proliferating) nuclei (brown) belong to cytokeratin-negative (endothelial) cells. ×250. (Courtesy of Dr. Gaby Kohnen, Aachen, Germany.)

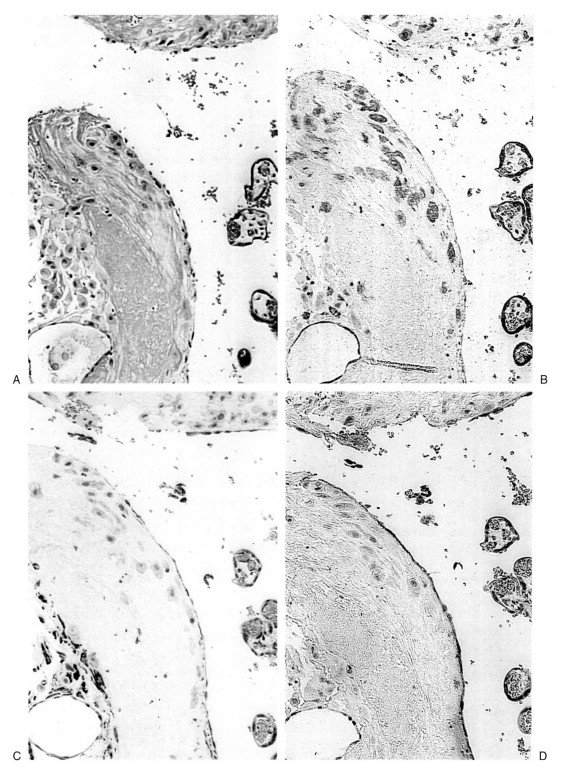

FIGURE 9.37. Cryostat serial sections of the basal plate of the mature placenta with a cross section of a spiral artery (lower left); moreover, the basal plate is passed in full thickness by a uteroplacental vein (upper left). A: Stained with H&E, which does not allow one to identify the various cellular components. B: Stained with anticytokeratin, which binds to syncytiotrophoblast of placental villi (right margin), extravillous trophoblast (oval brownish cells in the center) and to the trophoblastic lining of the spiral artery (lower left). C: Stained with antivimentin, a marker for mesenchymal derivatives. It stains decidual cells (above the spiral artery, lower left) and maternal endothelium lining the venous opening and spreading over the surface of the basal plate (center). D: Stained with anti–factor VIII–related antigen, a specific endothelial marker. Note the absence of staining from the wall of the spiral artery (lower left), but the presence of maternal endothelium at the basal plate surface (center). ×95. All sections are counterstained with hematoxylin so that all nuclei appear dark. (Courtesy of Dr. Sonya Kertschanska, Aachen, Germany.)

the chorionic and basal plates. These observations have prompted Craven and coworkers (2000) to study the interactions between lateral uteroplacental veins and placental villi in more detail. They found very often peripheral villi expanding deeply into the openings of maternal placental veins. Some of the villi were attached to venous walls in places were venous endothelial cells expressed vascular cell adhesion molecule (VCAM). And mononuclear trophoblast cells that were integrin β4 positive and β1 negative evaded the villi and started invading the surrounding decidual stroma. Oncofetal fibronectin was present at sites of trophoblast invasion. The authors concluded that the combination of three findings suggests that placental surface expansion throughout pregnancy is at least partly due to **lateral expansion of the placenta** by transformation of marginal veins into intervillous space:

- Dilation of lateral placental veins with transformation into marginal parts of the intervillous space is strongly supported by the fact that marginal parts of the intervillous space are lined by maternal endothelium with smooth muscle cells underneath (cf. Nanaev et al., 2000a).
- Branches of marginal villous trees develop into these newly developed parts of the intervillous trees.
- There they form anchoring villi and cell columns, which are starting points of trophoblast invasion and thus guarantee that also the junctional zone spreads in accord with placental expansion.

On the other hand, not every villous cross section observed in uteroplacental veins is an indication of villous anchorage and points to lateral expansion of the placenta. Rather, peripheral villi may segregate from the villous trees and may be deported with the maternal blood flow into myometrial segments of uteroplacental veins (Fig. 9.38) or even deeper (Fujikura, 2005).

Intramural Fibrinoid of Uteroplacental Arteries and Veins

Fibrinoid of the uteroplacental arteries is very likely to be composed mainly of fibrin-type fibrinoid. At present, there is no evidence for the secretion of matrix-type fibrinoid by endovascular trophoblast cells. Rather, Sheppard and Bonnar (1974b, 1988) and Bonnar and Sheppard (1977) described typical fibrin with a 200-Å cross-striation in all layers of these vessel walls. They observed intraluminal fibrin thrombi attached to the intimal lining and noted that muscular and elastic components of the vessel walls may be replaced by fibrin.

Whether the deposition is caused by increased fibrin polymerization or by decreased fibrinolytic activity is a matter of dispute. Endothelium is well known to have fibrinolytic activity. The endothelium of the uteroplacental arteries, however, becomes largely replaced by trophoblast during pregnancy. According to Sheppard and Bonnar (1974a), also trophoblast is discussed as being a potent source of antifibrinolytic activity. The latter is said to prevent the enzymatic digestion of fibrin (Kawano et al., 1968).

Functional Aspects of Uteroplacental Vessels

During the course of pregnancy, uteroplacental flow resistance is decreased by structural widening of the lumens of the uterine and terminal spiral arteries, so that maternal blood supply to the placenta is adjusted to fetal growth. When comparing parameters such as blood flow velocity, arterial widening, and timing of trophoblast invasion in rats and guinea pigs, it was found that the vascular changes proceed normally, even under conditions of reduced blood flow (Moll et al., 1988). They appeared earlier than the

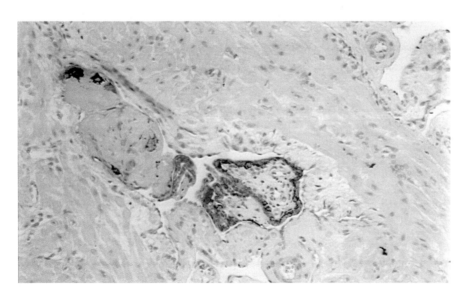

FIGURE 9.38. Paraffin section of a myometrial vein from a 16th week pregnant uterus. The vein is blocked by two placental villi (center), which are lined by trophoblast (dark brown anticytokeratin staining), and by a big fibrinoid conglomerate (left), which contains several cytokeratin-positive (brown) extravillous trophoblast cells. ×80. (Courtesy of Dr. Gaby Kohnen, Aachen, Germany).

trophoblastic invasion and could be induced by long-term estradiol treatment. Moll et al. (1988) concluded that the changes in luminal width are not induced by the intraarterial trophoblast invasion but rather by endocrine/paracrine factors. Later studies of vascular trophoblast invasion in the guinea pig (Nanaev et al., 1995) and in the human (Craven et al., 1998) have supported this view.

The increased arterial diameters are thought to guarantee sufficient uteroplacental blood flow volumes and to prevent excessively high blood pressures in the intervillous space. Only a balance between the intervillous maternal blood pressure and the intravillous fetal blood pressure keeps the fetal vessels open and allows intravillous fetal blood flow (Karimu & Burton, 1994a,b). As is known from experimental studies in the guinea pig (Kaufmann et al., 1982) and in the isolated, dually perfused human cotyledon (Kaufmann, 1985), corresponding elevation of the fetal blood pressure would be an inadequate answer to intervillous pressure increases. Elevation of fetal blood pressure results in filtration through fetal vessels and finally in villous edema. Thus, the only realistic consequence is a reduction of the intervillous blood pressure to that of the fetus. All pregnancy-induced physiologic changes of the spiral arteries must be seen in the light of such considerations.

Failure of physiologic dilatation of uteroplacental arteries due to deficient arterial trophoblast invasion is generally accepted as underlying pathogenetic mechanism in preeclampsia and fetal IUGR (for review, see Brosens, 1988). As discussed above, absent dilation will result in increased maternal flow impedance. From a theoretical point of view, the maternal organism has two different options to adjust to this situation:

- If the maternal blood pressure is kept constant, the increased impedance will cause reduced intervillous perfusion. This directly will impair delivery of oxygen and nutrients into the placenta and into the fetal circulation. The placenta and the fetus become hypoxic (uteroplacental hypoxia, see Types of Hypoxia and Its Effects on Villous Development in Chapter 7).
- If the maternal blood pressure is increased, maternal perfusion of the placenta as well as delivery of oxygen and nutrients into the placenta may be kept constant. This situation, however, will result in increased intervillous blood pressure, which results in compression of the villi, increased fetoplacental impedance, reduced fetoplacental circulation, and reduced oxygen and nutrient transfer to the fetus. The fetus is hypoxic, whereas the placenta may show oxygen partial pressures higher than normal (postplacental hypoxia, see Types of Hypoxia and Its Effects on Villous Development in Chapter 7).

As a consequence, depending on the maternal response to deficient vascular trophoblast invasion, different clinical features may result such as IUGR with preserved end-diastolic (PED) flow in the umbilical arteries or IUGR with absent or reversed end-diastolic (ARED) flow in the umbilical arteries. Whether or not IUGR is further complicated by preeclampsia very likely depends on the way in which villous trophoblast turnover responds to these changes (see Chapter 15).

Septa, Cell Islands, and Cell Columns

Septa

Placental septa are irregular protrusions of the basal plate that are composed of fibrinoid and various cell types (Figs. 9.12 and 9.39). Boyd and Hamilton (1966) gave a detailed historical and analytical description of these structures. As early as in the 6th week p.m. we observed short basal plate protrusions into the intervillous space that were composed of cytotrophoblastic cells, likely precursors of future septa. The septum depicted in Figure 9.40 was found in a placenta from the 8th week p.m.

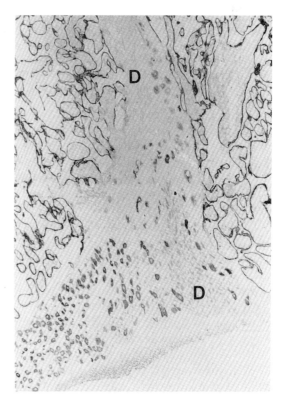

FIGURE 9.39. Cryostat section of a placental septum (center and above) resting on the basal plate (below). Glucose-6-phosphate dehydrogenase reaction. It becomes evident from this enzyme reaction that the faintly stained decidual cells (D) extend from the basal plate into the septum. Ample numbers of anchoring villi are attached to the septum. These similarities of basal plate and septum support the theory that the septa are results of folding of the basal plate. 40th week p.m. ×65.

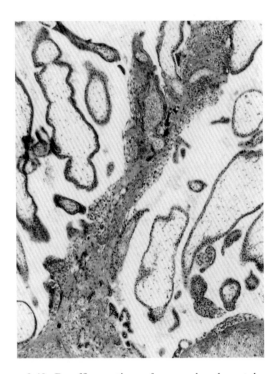

FIGURE 9.40. Paraffin section of an early placental septum (middle) during the 8th week p.m. In this stage the septa have a cellular composition similar to that of the early basal plate (see Fig. 9.27). As in the latter, they are largely devoid of fibrinoid and can be interpreted as being extensions and folds of the early basal plate. ×90.

Septa can be found in nearly every mature placenta. Absence of septa is a rare event in mature placentas that is usually linked to pathologic conditions (Fig. 9.41). The fetus of the placenta shown in Figure 9.41 had hygroma and X monosomy. True septa are also absent from abdominal pregnancies.

The **shape of septa** is one of irregular plates, or pillars, that partially subdivide the intervillous space. Their position normally corresponds to that of the grooves that are visible at the basal surface of the delivered placenta (Wilkin, 1958) (Fig. 9.42; also see Fig. 2.1)—hence their designation as "intercotyledonary septa." Many observers, such as Spanner (1935), Stieve (1940), and Stieve and von der Heide (1941), have suggested that septa partly serve as subdivisions of intervillous blood flow. The famous drawings of Spanner and Stieve depicted chamber-like compartments of the intervillous space. In contrast, Becker (1962; Becker & Jipp, 1963) found that septa never subdivide truly functional units of placental tissue. Most often they were found to be rather shallow "vela," measuring between 12 and 18 mm in height, originating from the floor of the placenta, and rarely reaching the fetal surface. They represent furrows or folds in the maternal surface or basal decidua, rather than complete septations of the villous tissue.

Concerning the **development of septa**, Boyd and Hamilton (1966) suggested that they probably result from buckling of the basal decidua. They envisaged this buckling to be induced by the pressures of expanding villous lobules and found further support for this idea from the relative paucity of villous attachments on only one side of the septa. When the septa are dissected, this side is found to be much smoother than the other. When we studied early specimens from the 6th to 8th weeks p.m. that showed the first signs of formation of septa (Fig. 9.40), we found them to be composed of cytotrophoblast. Anchoring villi can often be observed near their tips (Fig. 9.40). We concluded, therefore, that one of the initial causes of septum formation is traction of these anchoring villi combined with excessive proliferation of their cytotrophoblastic feet. Only later, a considerable admixture of decidua can be found (Figs. 9.39 and 9.42).

As was already discussed, it is likely that the combination of septa with groves in the basal plate (Fig. 9.42) is a consequence of secondary folding of the basal plate along those points where the cytotrophoblastic septal precursors originate. This process can be induced by lateral movements between uterine wall and basal plate and is due to placental growth.

According to this concept of their genesis, it is understandable that the **composition of septa** resembles that of the basal plate. They are composed of both decidual cells and extravillous trophoblast cells embedded in matrix-type fibrinoid, and partly surrounded by fibrin-type fibrinoid. Anchoring villi are attached to the septa by means of cell columns, the latter representing the foci of extravillous trophoblastic proliferation. In addition, the septa may contain all other basal plate constituents like

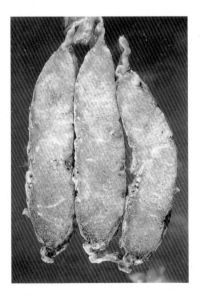

FIGURE 9.41. Third trimester placenta without septa or folds of the maternal floor. This placenta comes from an 45,X fetus with hygroma.

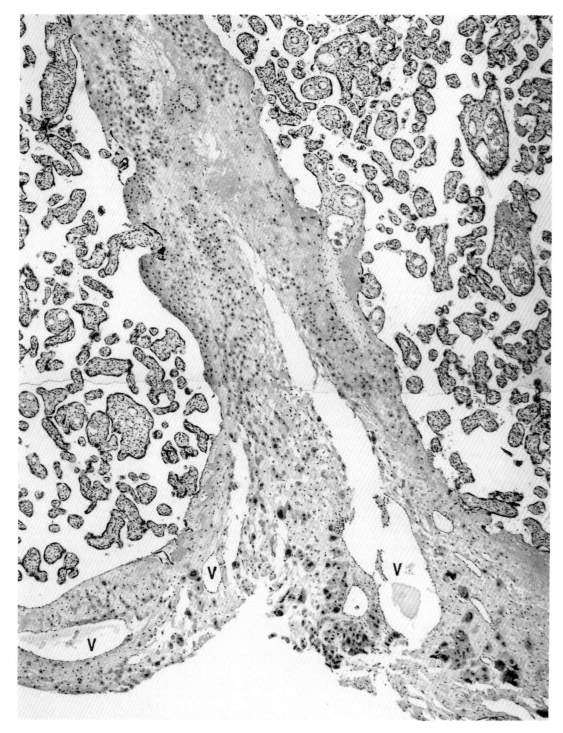

FIGURE 9.42. Paraffin section of a placental septum, 37th week p.m. Note the numerous anchoring villi inserting at the septum. In its base several vessel cross sections (V) represent uteroplacental veins. ×65.

glands (Fig. 9.42) and vessels. Brosens (1988) interpreted the latter to be predominantly spiral arteries, which is in disagreement with current views. Also, the vessels depicted in the septal base of Figure 9.42 are more likely veins. The ultrastructure of septa has been described in much detail by Glienke (1974). Another ultrastructural

study of septa by Demir and Erbengi (1984) distinguished five cell types but does not draw conclusions as to their origin. Whereas in the early stages of pregnancy (Fig. 9.40) the septa are composed mostly of cells, with advancing gestation trophoblast-derived matrix-type fibrinoid is accumulated and embeds the extravillous

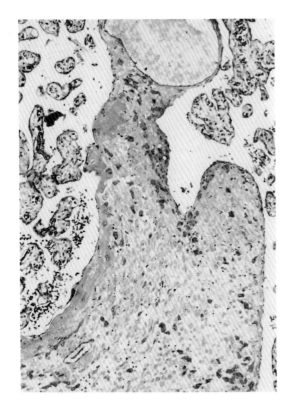

FIGURE 9.43. Intercotyledonary septum with cyst at its tip (top center). The darker cells are extravillous trophoblast cells, which are intermingled with a larger number of decidua cells. Note that Rohr's fibrin stria (at left) follows the outline of the septum. H&E ×80.

trophoblast cells. From the intervillous space, fibrin-type fibrinoid is added. At term, both type of fibrinoid are the predominant elements of septa.

Septa are a frequent site of **placental cysts** (Figs. 9.43 and 9.44). Macroscopically identifiable cysts are less

common, but microscopically one finds septal cysts in nearly every placenta. Wieloch (1923) described such cysts as artifacts. Stieve and von der Heide (1941) identified trophoblastic necrosis in the walls of septa and concluded that it is the causal mechanism of cysts. Hörmann (1966) came to similar conclusions. In his studies of what he called "pseudocysts," however, the degenerating cell population is decidua. Also, Schwartz et al. (1973) described the cysts to be the result of cellular necrosis and liquefaction. In many cases, particularly near the base, we found irregular clefts (Fig. 9.42) that can be interpreted to have resulted from laceration of intercellular debris and fibrinoid during labor. On the other hand, cysts with well-developed cellular walls and similar to the cysts of the cell islands (see Fig. 9.47B) are not mechanically induced artifacts.

Cell Islands

Cell islands are macroscopically round or irregularly shaped white structures connected to either the villous tree or the chorionic plate. Their diameter varies between several hundred micrometers and 3mm. As the term implies, they are composed primarily of extravillous trophoblast cells (Fig. 9.45) that, with advancing gestation, are encased in increasing amounts of fibrinoid (Fig. 9.46). Fetal or maternal vessels are absent. They resemble septa in structure and composition. When one uses histologic sections, it cannot be excluded that apparent cell islands are, in fact, tangential or cross sections of septa.

The **development of cell islands** never caused much controversy. Most authors agree that cell islands are derived from trophoblast, without an admixture of decidual cells (Spanner, 1935, 1941; Stieve, 1936; Ortmann,

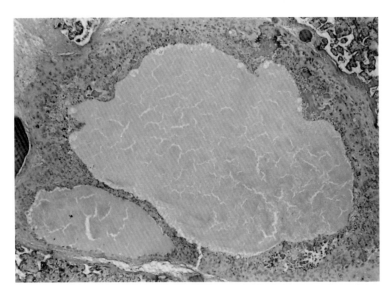

FIGURE 9.44. Septum with cystic centers. H&E ×40.

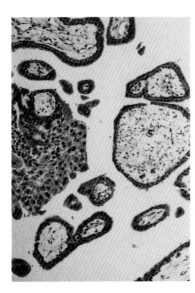

FIGURE 9.45. Placenta from tubal ectopic pregnancy at 5 weeks' gestation. A cluster of extravillous trophoblast cells forming an early cell island is shown above, attached to villi and interspersed with syncytiotrophoblast. No interstitial "fibrinoid" is present as yet. H&E ×240.

1955, 1960). Steininger (1978) described a very small number of cell islands in which both decidual and trophoblast cells were present. It is likely that these represent either cross-sectioned tips of septa or former portions of septa that during placental development by traction of anchoring villi have been be detached from the septum. Boe (1967) studied trophoblast proliferation in cell

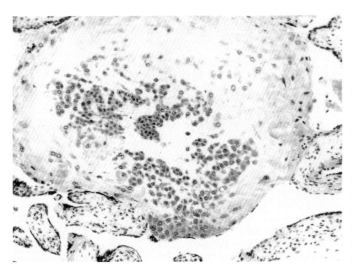

FIGURE 9.46. Cell island at 20 weeks' gestation. The mononuclear cells with dark cytoplasm in the center are the extravillous trophoblast cells. They are surrounded by "fibrinoid." Note that there is no differentiation to syncytium among the extravillous trophoblast cells. H&E ×160.

islands in placentas from therapeutic abortions. His view was that the extravillous trophoblast cells derive from the aggregation of "erupted" proliferative masses of cytotrophoblast originating in villous tips. According to Boe's data, cell islands correspond to persistent primary villi that have not been occupied by villous stroma. They are comparable to the basal ends of the anchoring villi, the "cell columns."

This view has been supported by several cell biologic and in vitro studies (e.g., Castellucci et al., 1991; Genbacev et al., 1993c; Mühlhauser et al., 1993). All these studies arrived at the conclusion that the major difference between a cell island and a cell column is the topographical relation: cell islands are freely floating cell columns, and cell columns in the narrow sense are anchored to the basal plate or to septa. A further immunologic difference may be derived from the fact that the extravillous trophoblast of cell columns invades decidual tissues, whereas that of the cell islands only migrates within its own ECM and finally degenerates under formation of cysts (Fig. 9.47).

Krönicher (1975) presented a detailed **ultrastructural description** of the cell islands from early to late pregnancy. He reported different stages of cytotrophoblastic differentiation in the trophoblastic islands. In particular, when studying cell islands from the second and third months, one does not get the impression that they are degenerative or useless groups of cells. Arnholdt and Löhrs (1989, 1991) demonstrated a high mitotic rate in the cells.

The basophilia of the extravillous trophoblast cells, an expression of a richly developed rough endoplasmic reticulum, led investigators to believe that these cells are a potent source of protein hormones, such as hCG (Ortmann, 1955, 1960; Bargmann, 1957; Boyd & Hamilton; 1970). Also, in this respect they are fully comparable to extravillous trophoblast cells of other origin.

Cell Columns

Cell columns are the massive trophoblastic connections between anchoring villi and basal plate or placental septa. The **development of cell columns** starts around day 15 p.c. when the primary villi become invaded by extraembryonic mesenchyme (see Chapter 5, Fig. 5.1E,F). This process is followed by capillarization of the newly formed villous stroma, which then results in formation of the tertiary villi. Both processes spread from the chorionic plate peripherally but do not reach the basal plate. Rather, the basal parts of the villous stems that connect the latter with the basal plate persist in the primary villous stage. These massive trophoblastic segments of the anchoring villi are called the cell columns. These developmental events are identical to those at some free-floating villous tips, leading to the formation of cell islands.

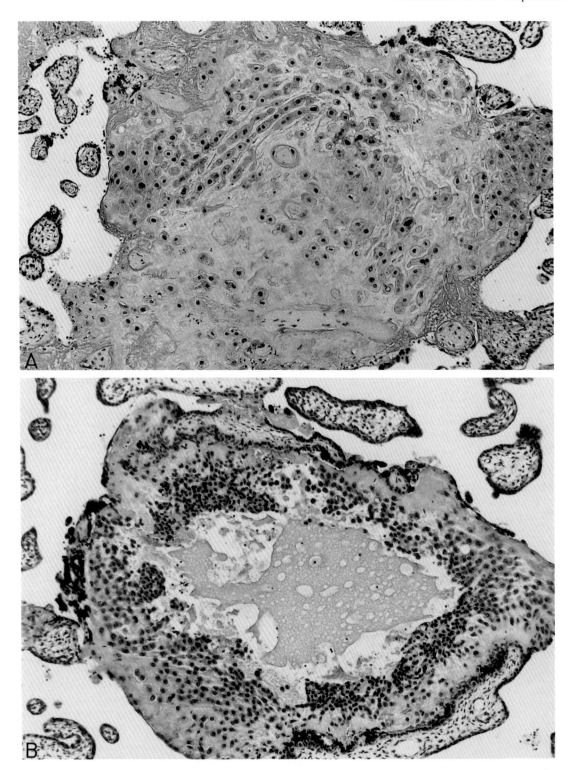

FIGURE 9.47. Paraffin sections of cell islands. A: At the 37th week p.m., the cell island is largely composed of a fibrinoid matrix in which strings of proliferating cytotrophoblastic cells are embedded. Incorporated decidual cells are rare findings. The surrounding placental villi may be attached to the surface; sometimes they are incorporated into the fibrinoid. Note the heterogeneous structure of the darker superficial patches of fibrin-type fibrinoid as compared to the glossy, lighter matrix-type fibrinoid that makes up the center of the cell island. ×110. B: At the 19th week p.m. In the centers of large cell islands central cavities, or "cysts" are found. They must be considered to be a result of degeneration with subsequent liquefaction. Note two "anchoring villi" attached to this island (above and bottom right). The trophoblast cells lining the border from cell island to anchoring villus represent the proliferating subpopulation, comparable to cell columns. ×120. (*Source:* From Kaufmann, 1981a, with permission.)

The cell columns have been the topic of electron microscopic (Enders, 1968; Larsen & Knoth, 1971; Okudaira et al.,1971,1991),enzyme-histochemical (Stark & Kaufmann, 1971), immunohistochemical (Okudaira et al., 1971; Feinberg et al., 1989, 1991b; Castellucci et al., 1991, 1993; Librach et al., 1991a,b; Damsky et al., 1992; Fisher & Damsky, 1993; Mühlhauser et al., 1993; Zhou et al., 1993), and numerous in vitro studies, for example by Genbacev et al. (1992, 1993a,b). This particular interest is because they represent the most impressive proliferation zones of extravillous trophoblast, and that the various steps from trophoblastic proliferation via differentiation to invasion cannot be so easily studied anywhere else. All respective data were discussed earlier (see Extravillous Trophoblast). In this context we only briefly discuss some additional **structural features**. Cell columns are composed of a multilayered core of cytotrophoblast surrounded by an incomplete sleeve of syncytiotrophoblast (see Figs. 3.1I and 11.40) (Enders, 1968; Boyd & Hamilton, 1970; Larsen & Knoth, 1971; Okudaira et al., 1971). As soon as cell columns are surrounded by fibrinoid and thus buried in the basal plate, their syncytiotrophoblastic cover becomes replaced by fibrin-type fibrinoid (Fig. 9.48B) (Stark & Kaufmann, 1971). The cytotrophoblastic core continues without sharp demarcation into the Langhans' layer of the anchoring villus at one side (see Fig. 9.4C); on the opposite side, it is connected to loose streamers of invasive extravillous trophoblast.

The border between cell columns and stroma of the anchoring villus is represented by a basal lamina (Fig. 9.4C) (Enders, 1968; Okudaira et al., 1971). It represents the indispensable pad for trophoblast proliferation, and all extravillous trophoblast cells invading the basal plate and the placental bed are derived from this stem cell population (see Fig. 9.1) (Arnholdt et al., 1991; Castellucci et al., 1993; Mühlhauser et al., 1993; Kaufmann & Castellucci, 1997).

As has already been discussed above (see Fig. 9.5), the cell columns function as growth zones for both the basal plate and the anchoring villi. Postmitotic cells derived from the proliferative stem cell population migrate laterally into the villous trophoblastic epithelium as well as basally into the basal plate. With advancing gestation, the cellular layer of the cell columns is reduced by decreasing proliferative activity but continuous migration of the trophoblast (Fig. 9.48). Sometimes there are almost no trophoblast cells left so that anchoring villous stroma and the nearly naked basal lamina directly face basal plate fibrinoid (Figs. 9.48 and 9.49; also see Fig. 3.2I). Because of this situation, Baker et al. (1944) and Ortmann (1960) reported that the cell columns disappear at the end of the third month of pregnancy. But this is certainly incorrect, and with some care one still can find largely intact cell columns even in term placentas.

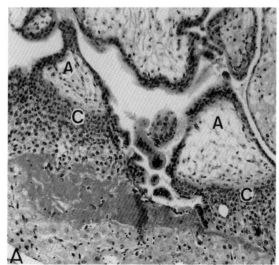
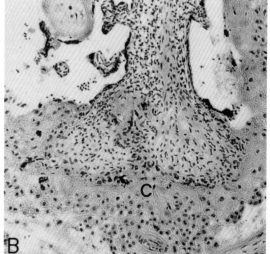

FIGURE 9.48. Paraffin histology of cell columns. A: At the 15th week p.m. During early stages of pregnancy the anchoring villi (A) are connected to the basal plate (below) by broad orv slender feet consisting of cytotrophoblast, the so-called cell columns (C). They are proliferative zones for the villous trophoblast as well as for the trophoblast of the basal plate. ×95. B: At the 28th week p.m. During later stages of pregnancy the cell columns are deeply incorporated into the basal plate by surrounding fibrinoid deposition. Also, its cytotrophoblast is progressively replaced by fibrinoid, indicating reduced proliferative activity of these growth zones. A final stage of this process is depicted in Figure 9.49B. ×95. (From Kaufmann, 1981a, with permission.)

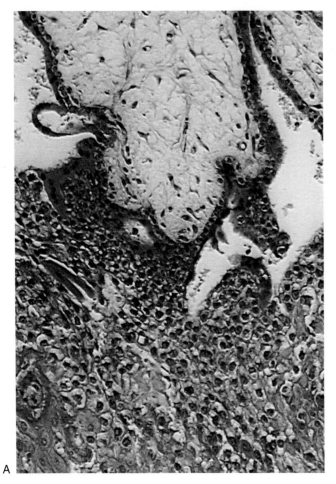

FIGURE 9.49. Comparison of a cell column from the 6th week of pregnancy (A) with a cell column from the 40th week (B). Note the big cluster of early postproliferative and invasive trophoblast cells emanating from the cell column in early pregnancy, as compared to the term anchoring villus, which is connected to the basal plate by fibrinoid, which contains few barely visible trophoblast cells as remainders of the former cell column. As is typical for this stage of pregnancy, this cell column is "burned out." H&E, ×300.

Pathology of Trophoblast Invasion

Placenta Accreta

Placenta accreta is an important condition clinically. It may be life threatening (Manyonda & Varma, 1991). In placenta accreta the villous tissue is in direct contact with the myometrium, and the placental villi are anchored to muscle fibers rather than to intervening decidual cells. The deficiency of decidua prevents normal separation of the placenta after delivery. Normally, the placenta separates from the uterine musculature in a plane just peripheral to Nitabuch's fibrin layer. It is accomplished by the shearing action of contracting myometrium against the stationary, noncontracting placenta and occurs in irregular planes of friable decidual cells. Thus, either the entire placenta is retained, or when the focus of adherence is small, only a portion of placenta is retained. These adherent areas tend to bleed; fibrin and clot continue to accumulate around such retained placental tissue and, over time, a placental polyp develops that may necessitate operative removal. Lester et al. (1956) found placental fragments to be an unimportant feature of immediate postpartum hemorrhage (4.5%). When hemorrhage occurred in a later stage of the puerperium, however, placental polyp was the cause in 44.4% of affected mothers (see Chapter 10).

Placenta accreta cannot easily be diagnosed from the delivered placenta, but it has been shown that it is often (in 45%) associated with elevated maternal serum α-fetoprotein levels (Zelop et al., 1992; Kupferminc et al., 1993). The placenta may be disrupted during the delivery because of the accretion, and there may thus be missing cotyledons. Occasionally, one can palpate these retained cotyledons by manual exploration in the postpartum uterus. When histologic sections of such a placenta are made, however, the deficiency of endometrium that underlies placenta accreta is not evident. For such a diagnosis one needs to examine the entire uterus or curettings that include the myometrium. Even then it may be difficult to orient the lesion, and a firm diagnosis may be difficult to render. It is more easily done when whole specimens are available, but this is the less acceptable outcome for the patient. Nevertheless, hysterectomy is a frequent sequel when large areas of placenta accreta exist. If the site of attachment is fixed before trimming the tissues for histology, the lesion is easily diagnosed microscopically (Fig. 9.50). Pathologists must be aware of the difficulties existing in distinguishing the populations of cells that make up the placental floor, especially when they do not examine many placentas. In this differential diagnosis the pathologist must distinguish between the basal decidual cells and the unicellular trophoblast (extravillous trophoblast), cells that are abundant at the site of placenta previa implantation. There is usually an abundance of basal fibrin, and the maternal vessels show the focally deficient physiologic change described by Khong and Robertson (1987). It should also be mentioned that there is a poorly understood increased fetal mortality after 34 weeks' gestation when a prior section had been done (Lumley, 2003; Smith et al., 2003). The increased neonatal problems that are associated with uterine rupture are perhaps more easily understood (Bujold & Gauthier, 2002).

It may be of parenthetical interest here to mention that successful treatment with methotrexate has been undertaken in cervical accretas to destroy trophoblastic cells

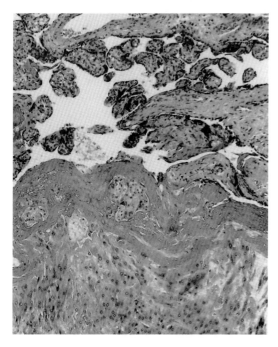

FIGURE 9.50. Placenta accreta at term. Villi are attached to myometrium, and the cellular layer at the bottom is composed of only cellular trophoblast (X cells). There is still a large amount of Nitabuch's fibrin layer. H&E ×125.

(Oyer et al., 1988; Palti et al., 1989; Bakri et al., 1993). Also, microembolization through the internal iliac artery (Kivikoski et al., 1988) has been used to treat these abnormal implantation sites.

Various antecedents to placenta accreta have been described, such as constitutional endometrial defect, scars, diverticula, cornual implantation, leiomyoma (Fig. 9.51), antecedent cesarean section with placenta previa, and previous curettage (Sumawong et al., 1966). The classic article on placenta accreta is by Irving and Hertig (1937), who studied 18 cases of this condition and reviewed 80 cases from the literature. Their incidence was 1 in 1956 deliveries. Deficiency of endometrium as it was formerly induced by endometrial cautery (e.g., by steam), is no longer a problem, but endometrial defects caused by curettage and by cesarean section have become very prevalent. A familial occurrence was once described to exist in Eskimos, but it has not been confirmed (Schaefer, 1960). Patients successfully treated for Asherman's syndrome (intrauterine adhesions) often develop accretas and other complications (Friedman et al., 1986).

Fox (1972) presented a comprehensive review of this relatively frequent condition and chose to combine all stages of accretion, including increta and percreta. He reiterated that it is a condition of elderly multigravidas, many of whom have uterine malformations (septa) or other complications listed earlier. Of the 622 reported cases covered by his 25-year review, 213 were associated with placenta previa (34%) and seven were placentas membranaceas (vide infra); in only 43 cases were there no predisposing factors. The fact that 57 maternal deaths occurred in these women (9.2%) with 9.6% fetal deaths, attests to the gravity of the condition. Another review of the antecedents to placenta accreta comes from Gielchinsky et al. (2002), whose incidence is higher than usually quoted—0.9% of all deliveries. They affirmed frequent multigravid status, prior section (12%), and placenta previa (10%), but excluded myomas from their review. In their experience, hysterectomy was needed in 3.5% and they had one maternal death. Amazingly, 16% of their patients with accreta had a prior placenta accreta. The rate of maternal complications was higher in the experience of Armstrong et al. (2004), who did hysterectomy in 91%. Similarly, Landon et al. (2004) have evaluated the risk of a trial of labor following prior cesarean section and they enumerate the frequency of maternal and fetal outcomes. The American College of Obstetricians and Gynecologists (ACOG) committee opinion has suggested that there is a 10-fold increase of placenta accreta in the last 50 years (ACOG, 2002) and occurs now with a frequency of 1 in 2500 deliveries.

The frequent antecedent of cesarean section was also stressed by Breen et al. (1977), who reviewed the literature and found an overall incidence of 1 in 7000 pregnancies. This figure is only a rough estimate, however; the higher

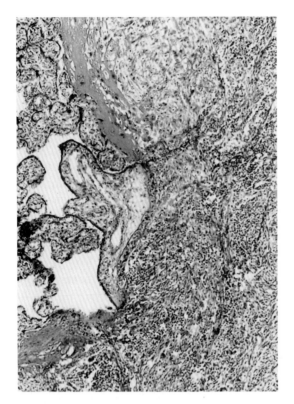

FIGURE 9.51. Placenta accreta over a leiomyoma. The leiomyoma (right) was delivered with the placenta at term (see also Cramer, 1987). H&E ×100. (Courtesy of Dr. Ralph Richart, New York, New York.)

frequency reported from Thailand (1:540) by Sumawong et al. (1966) was speculated to relate possibly to the higher incidence there of proliferative trophoblastic disease. This argument is unjustified, we believe, as there is no evidence that accretas are the result of an overly aggressive trophoblast. Conversely, all correlations point to a defective uterus. To and Leung (1995) also noted the higher prior section frequency of previas and saw an incidence of 1.18% accreta with placenta previa. Another comprehensive study of placenta accreta comes from Millar (1959), and an overview of the risks were elaborated by Windrim (2005). Millar reviewed not only the morphology of this condition but also its etiology. The decidua was always absent at the attachment site, and it was frequently deficient elsewhere in the uterus, and Comstock et al. (2004) indicated that placenta accreta after prior section can be detected sonographically as early as 15 to 20 weeks' gestation. Fox (1972) pointed out correctly that there is usually a deficiency of placental septum formation with placenta accreta. When septa are present in a placenta accreta, they are composed of uterine muscle. He considered that there may be an endocrine deficiency that fails to support normal endometrial growth. Fox also reported some early cases in which decidua was already lacking. One very young placenta accreta was also found accidentally at hysterec-

tomy by Begneaud et al. (1965). The histologic features were identical to those of other accretas. An interesting observation was recorded by Cramer (1987). He observed a placenta increta in a patient who had previously needed to be curetted for a placenta accreta. Cramer did not give the patient's prior history and deduced, incorrectly we think, that some placenta have greater invasive qualities than others and do not respect the decidual limitation because of innate qualities.

It has been suggested that the clinical picture associated with placenta previa has been changing (Read et al., 1980); certainly, associated fetal mortality figures have improved. Weckstein et al. (1987) reported a case of placenta percreta and stated their belief that this condition is increasing in frequency because of increased cesarean section rates, which is our observation as well. Importantly, placenta previa can now be diagnosed with some accuracy by sonography, especially with transvaginal probe (Timor-Tritsch & Yunis, 1993; Timor-Tritsch & Monteagudo, 1993). In addition to the diagnosis of the abnormal location, sonography of placenta accreta often displays irregular lucencies in the villous tissue (Finberg & Williams, 1992; Bromley et al., 1995). These "lakes" presumably derive from an abnormal disposition of maternal spiral arterioles to the intervillous space. Their appearance and turbulence within was much enhanced by power amplitude ultrasonographic angiography in a case of placenta previa increta described by Chou and Ho (1997) and reflect the "lacunae" described macroscopically by earlier observers (see above). These authors made a cogent argument for the employment of this methodology for preoperative diagnosis so as to much improve the outcome. The use of magnetic resonance imaging (MRI) has been advocated by Thorp et al. (1998), who were able to make an accurate diagnosis of placenta previa percreta in the first trimester of pregnancy. Fujikura and Sho (1997) studied the occurrence of what they called "cavities" but which correspond to the lacunae of other observers. They found them to be increased primarily in thicker, more voluminous placenta.

Considering the above findings, placenta accreta is a nice example of the importance of endometrial decidualization for proper control of trophoblast invasion. This correlation is further underlined by the fact that the absence of decidualization also in tubal pregnancy coincides with increased trophoblastic invasiveness (see below). At present, the decidual parameters responsible for missing control of invasiveness are still unknown (see Subchapter on Decidua). Several factors are under discussion: deficient decidualization of endometrial stromal cells, absence of endometrial NK cells, paucity of decidual macrophages, presence of B cells, increased numbers of T cells, or a concerted action of all these factors (see Trophoblast Invasion as a Result of Deciduo-Trophoblastic Interactions, below).

Placenta Increta and Percreta

Many authors, Fox (1972) for instance, do not distinguish accretas from incretas and percretas, and Luke et al. (1966) criticized terms that have become fairly accepted in the medical nomenclature when they recalled 427 cases from the literature of accretas, incretas, and percretas. And we have to admit that the underlying pathogenetic mechanisms are likely to be the same, the only difference being a quantitative one that may be of considerable clinical importance.

In contrast to placenta accreta, in incretas the myometrium is apparently "invaded" by the placental villous tissue, whereas in percretas the villi penetrate the entire wall and the uterus may rupture. This may then become an acutely life-threatening condition. In general, the causes of such "invasive" placentas are similar to those of the placenta accreta vera. These conditions are nearly always present when tubal ectopic pregnancies rupture. Placenta percreta has also been reported to follow tubal reconstructive surgery at the uterine fundus (Stromme, 1963), in septate uteri (Ries & Middleton, 1972), complicating therapy for "missed abortion" (Harden et al., 1990), and through former Cesarean section sites (Berchuck & Sokol, 1983). The "invading" placenta may be intramural in position (Cava & Russell, 1978; Fait et al., 1987), perhaps its rarest site. Although adenomyosis is an attractive and often proposed cause of such unusual cases, it has rarely been found. McGowan (1965) proposed previous instrumental injury as a possibility because he saw two cases that were interpreted to have resulted from curettage. Ayers et al. (1971) have even reported the presence of fetal tissues within placenta increta sites of women who had previously suffered abortion. Dessouky (1980) found viable abdominal villi in the omentum following an instrumental abortion; the patient recovered after resection. Similarly, Davis and Cruz (1996) reported a case of persistent villi in myometrium (placenta increta) following earlier section and tubal ligation.

The most demonstrative pictures of placenta accreta and percreta were produced by Morison (1978). Among a population of 645,000 deliveries from his institution, he found 67 uteri thus affected. Of them, 31 were accretas (14 focal, 17 partial), three were incretas, and three were percretas; 17 were placentas previa accreta, 11 were placenta previa increta, and two were placenta previa percreta. In most of these cases, there was massive hemorrhage. Maternal death (only twice in his series) is a possible outcome; we have seen this also when the accreta had been incompletely removed and subsequent bacterial invasion led to sepsis. The fetus also often dies, but Gribble and Fitzsimmons (1985) described fetal survival (890 g) with such a complication.

Placenta accreta (vera) is usually detected after delivery when the placenta fails to separate or is incompletely delivered. Incretas and percretas more frequently manifest during earlier gestation because of hemorrhage or uterine rupture. They are now often diagnosed by ultrasonography (Cox et al., 1988; Finberg & Williams, 1992; Hoffman-Tretin et al., 1992; Shapiro et al., 1992). Cox diagnosed the event at 16 weeks, closed the disrupted uterus, and allowed the pregnancy to continue for another 8 weeks. The infant was then delivered by cesarean section. After a stormy course over 2 months, the malformed neonate died. Five other conservatively managed cases were reviewed by Cox et al. as well. Other instances of young percretas have been described at 19 weeks' gestation (deWane & McCubbin, 1981) and 22 weeks' gestation (Bateman, 1967). The etiology of percreta, however, was not always clearly documented. On the other hand, Hassim et al. (1968) treated a mother with uterine rupture that occurred at 26 weeks. The patient expired. Another case involved rupture through a cesarean section scar at 37 weeks' gestation. Percreta with hemorrhage was documented by Hornstein et al. (1984) as occurring during elective termination of a 16-week pregnancy. The mother was 40 years of age and had leiomyomas but no other known risk factor. Rupture of the uterus is sometimes associated with the presence of an intrauterine device (Axelsson & Winblad, 1976), and it has occurred with pregnancy in bicornuate uteri (Zabrieskie, 1962). Zabrieskie reviewed the outcome of pregnancy in 92 patients with malformed uteri; he found that retained placentas occurred in 15% of patients, and that rupture occurred in four. Placenta percreta that invades the bladder and causes hematuria or massive hemorrhage has also been described and it is now seen more frequently with sonography or MRI (Taefi et al., 1970; Silber et al., 1973; Thorp et al., 1992; Leaphart et al., 1997). Nagy (1989) described a primigravida with placenta percreta at 23 weeks' gestation. The placenta had implanted at the fundus and it had spontaneously penetrated. He believed that percretas in primigravidae, at this stage of gestation, are exceptionally rare events.

Two cases of percreta are shown in Figure 9.52. The first was a patient whose erythroblastotic placenta would not separate after delivery. Hemorrhage necessitated hysterectomy. The mother's obstetrical history included five previous cesarean sections. The bulging placenta can readily be seen in Figure 9.52A at the arrows. In this case, only the peritoneum separated the villous tissue from the cul-de-sac. The specimen was much disrupted during the traumatic event. The "invasive" nature of the placenta into the lower uterine segment is seen in Figure 9.52B, it was actually a placenta increta. The placenta shown later in Figure 9.54A, on the other hand, came from what was thought to be an abdominal pregnancy near term with a surviving infant. Most of the placenta had an abdominal position and was attached to a defect in the uterus. The placenta had more or less herniated through a uterine

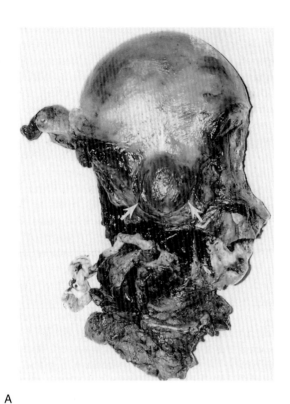

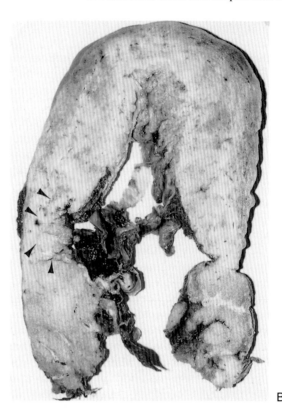

A   B

FIGURE 9.52. A: Placenta increta-near-percreta. The patient bled during delivery, and the placenta would not separate, so a hysterectomy was done. At the posterior aspect of the lower uterine segment, one can see the nodular protrusion (arrows) of peritoneum-covered placenta. B: Same specimen as in part A after fixation and sagittal sectioning. Placental outline is indicated by arrows where it is invasive. The blood overlying this area is visible. Also seen are the scars from preceding cesarean sections in the anterior wall (right).

defect. It was covered with old blood and hemosiderin. There was no basal decidua, and there were virtually no free membranes. This case then represented nearly a placenta membranacea with the final implantation on the peritoneum (see Fig. 9.54B); there was significant salpingitis present also. In another nearly fatal case of placenta previa, the pregnancy had followed curettage and therapy for postabortal endometritis. Because such cases usually require hysterectomy, it is not common that one can evaluate possible future reproductive events. We had the opportunity to examine material from a first-trimester percreta that nearly led to fatal hemorrhage. The tissue was excised, and the patient had a successful second pregnancy. In her third pregnancy, however, another percreta developed at 14 weeks, necessitating hysterectomy. Despite careful search, we were unable to identify adenomyosis or other predisposing factors (W.J. Mulligan, personal communication, 1962). Following rupture and hemoperitoneum the α-fetoprotein levels may be increased (McDuffie et al., 1994). Because of the serious nature of this pregnancy complication, various therapeutic modalities have been advocated for placenta percreta and are reviewed in contributions by Legro et al. (1994), O'Brien et al. (1996), and Dubois et al. (1997). Sono-

graphic diagnosis of this now so much more frequent entity is feasible (Bromley et al., 1995).

The reason why placenta percreta is now so common undoubtedly relates to the greater frequency of cesarean sections. But what is it that causes the percretion? In our view it is the manner in which the uterus is repaired and reconstituted after section. After all, when the section site is closed, the uterus commences a rapid involutionary stage; little regeneration of myometrium can then be expected anyway. Moreover, there is probably little if any myometrial growth after incision, and reconstitution of a normal uterine wall is impossible, we believe. Therefore, when the next pregnancy occurs, the expanding uterus often dehisces at the former section site, and it is not unusual for the obstetrician to witness such dehiscence at repeat cesarean section (Fig. 9.53). Alternatively, when the placenta implants over this previous scar, there is no underlying endomyometrium and, with uterine expansion, the placenta comes to implant on very thin scar tissue and/or peritoneum. Such a condition is seen in Figure 9.54. In this case and others we have witnessed, much distortion of the intervillous space had occurred (lacunae) and there was marked chronic villitis with plasma cells, at this site only. Additionally it needs to be

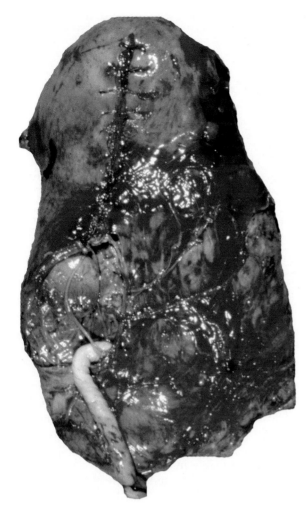

FIGURE 9.53. Placenta precreta in the region of a former cesarean section scar. It necessitated total hysterectomy.

considered that, in the past, closure after cesarean section was accomplished with silk sutures, a practice that has more recently been abandoned, perhaps with dire consequences. The microscopic appearance typical of the placenta accreta in such cases is shown in Figure 9.55.

Uterine Rupture

The uterus may rupture and expel its contents into the peritoneal cavity, there may massive hemorrhage, or it may be "sealed" by the fetal membranes. Such a case was eloquently illustrated by Murta and Nomelini (2004), in which the former cesarean section scar had dehisced and the amnionic membrane protruded through the separated uterine wall. These authors cited a number of relevant publications, of which there are many in the obstetrical literature. Only a few are cited here. Aboulafia et al. (1994) found rupture and abdominal hemorrhage in the second trimester and sutured the myometrial defect through which the placenta protruded. They advocated

conservative treatment because they obtained a viable neonate. Endres and Barnhart (2000) were not so fortunate. In their patient a hysterectomy was necessary at 15 weeks' gestation. Bujold et al. (2002a) examined the rate of rupture after prior transverse cesarean section. When single-layer suture had been performed, rupture in the next pregnancy occurred in 5.6% of cases if the pregnancy took place less than 2 years after prior section; the rate

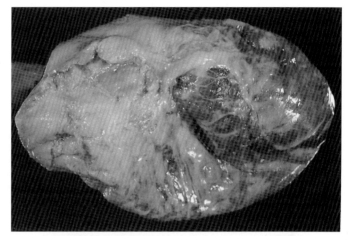

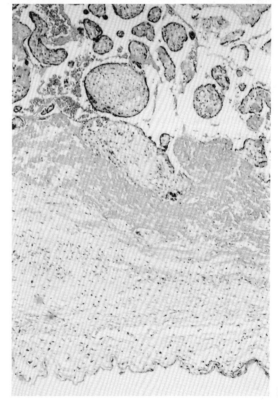

FIGURE 9.54. A: Placental percreta from the maternal side with much old blood covering the protruding tissue. (Courtesy of Dr. J. Carey, San Diego.) B: Same specimen as in part A, showing peritoneal implantation. The villi are anchored by a broad band of fibrin to the connective tissue of the peritoneum (below). H&E. ×60.

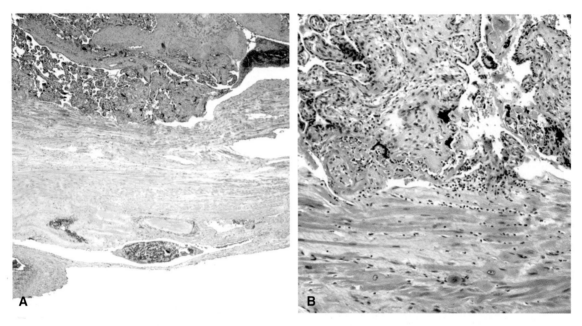

FIGURE 9.55. Placenta accreta in patient with prior cesarean section. Note the absence of decidua basalis. Also, in a large vein to the right a portion of villous tissue has "herniated." There is minimal inflammation at the site of adherence. A: H&E ×160. B: ×260.

was lower after a longer interval. LeMaire et al. (2001) described fundal rupture necessitating hysterectomy at 16 weeks in a pregnancy in which the uterus had no prior injury or section, although the patient had two previous pregnancies. This and a similar case reported by Caglar and Sezik (2003) must be most unusual events and were considered to be due to a "spontaneous" placenta percreta in an unscarred uterus (Fig. 9.56). Chauhan and colleagues (2003) searched a large database (142,075 patients) and found that 6.2 per 1000 trials of labor after cesarean section led to rupture, and Lin and Raynor (2004) reported

that induction of labor with oxytocin and/or misoprostol was followed by an approximately 1% uterine rupture.

This literature also considers the possible reason for the apparent increase in placenta percreta and uterine rupture. One possibly important aspect as precursor to percretas has been examined by Durnwald and Mercer (2003), for instance. They studied the relationship of single- vs. double-layered suture at hysterectomy. Of 768 women studied, 267 had a single-layer closure, while 501 had a double layer closure of the cesarean section site. The single layered closure was associated with shorter

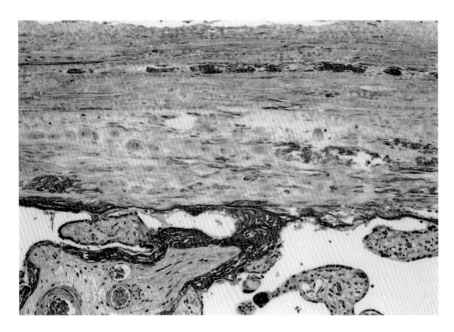

FIGURE 9.56. Placental site of placenta "percreta." This was a thin square fibrous scar at the location of previous cesarean section. The placenta was a total previa with expansion from mid-anterior uterus to low-posterior uterus, spanning over the internal cervical os. Focal villitis was present in anchoring villi. H&E. ×160.

operative time, slightly less blood loss, less endometritis, and shorter postoperative hospitalization. Importantly, it was not associated with uterine rupture, but there was an increase of what they called "uterine windows," which is the same as is commonly referred to as placenta percreta (see Fig. 9.53). Bujold et al. (2002b) had found a four-fold increase of uterine rupture after single-stitch repair; however, the ensuing discussion following this paper (Joura et al., 2003; Shipp & Lieberman, 2003; Vidaeff & Lucas, 2003) that discusses the nature of suture material and other controversies should be read to gain full understanding of these issues. Single- *vs.* double-stitch methods and their history are adequately reviewed by Cohain (2004). That summary recommends sonographic study after a prior cesarean section and the usage of Vicryl as suture material.

Perhaps the most important question for the pathologist is whether there has to be a prior uterine injury for a placenta percreta to occur or whether the placenta can march through the uterus spontaneously. This question is posed because of the enormous number of pregnancies that occur and the real scarcity of reports on spontaneous percretas (uterine rupture from other causes such as abnormal fetal position and arrested labor aside; they are covered by Ofir et al., 2004). We consider that this must be extremely uncommon and at least on occasion explicable by the reduced uterine collagen content in a woman with osteogenesis imperfecta type IA, as demonstrated by Di Lieto et al. (2003).

Placenta in Ectopic (Tubal) Pregnancy

This topic is relevant here because ectopic pregnancies in many cases are also placentas accreta and percreta, and Fylstra et al. (2002) have even described a case of gestation within a uterine section scar. Additionally, the obstetrician faces interesting issues. For instance, Kemp et al. (1997) reported Doppler sonographic criteria for the viability of (as yet) symptomless tubal pregnancies. They saw two different types: (1) Viable pregnancies characterized by signal-intensive rings of maternal vessels around the gestational sac; these were likely to be followed by rupture if not treated surgically. These are implanted generally on the mesosalpingeal portion of the tubal circumference. (2) Nonviable tubal pregnancies implant on the other side, lack a highly vascularized ring, show little or no trophoblast invasion, and do not require surgical intervention. The authors concluded that differences in maternal vascularization within the tubal wall account for the differences in fate of ectopic pregnancies.

Trophoblast invasion on the mesosalpingeal side of tubal pregnancy is excessive and usually completely penetrates the tubal wall and deeply invades the tubal mesenterium (Kemp et al., 1997, 2002). This invasion behavior is made responsible for the high risk of tubal rupture.

There are no hints that differences in trophob–last biology can be made responsible for this excessive invasiveness. As was already discussed above (see Decidua) the more likely explanation are differences in the tubal host tissue, which largely lacks decidualization, contains only few macrophages, and is completely void of uNK cells (von Rango et al., 2001, 2003; Kemp et al., 2002).

Virtually all mesosalpingeally implanted tubal pregnancies are at least placentas accreta. When they rupture, they do so because the placenta almost always has become a placenta percreta. Overdistention of the tube is not the primary cause of tubal rupture in ectopic pregnancy, which is somewhat in contrast to what has been reported by Philippe et al. (1970). In a review of 112 tubal pregnancies, these authors observed that ectopic implantation is often superficial and that it leads to bleeding at the site of attachment. They did not specifically discuss the rupture. Numerous case reports of viable term fetuses from tubal pregnancies testify to tubal expansibility, and a relevant case is shown in Figure 9.57. McElin and Randall (1951) established criteria for this entity and collected 45 cases from the literature. The placenta they reported was clearly an accreta and was difficult to separate at operation. The fetal mortality in the literature was 75%, and the maternal mortality 10%. Frachtman (1953) also reviewed this topic extensively. He found at least 75 reported cases, to which he added his own. His case had a thin placenta. Large infarcts were found in O'Connell's case (1952). Sunde (1965) emphasized the need to attempt complete removal of the placenta. Augensen (1983) found the placenta to possess a short cord (22 cm) and observed extensive decidualization of the sac's wall, as well as many placental infarcts. One wonders if the "decidualization" was truly endometrium or whether it could have been extravillous trophoblast cells. Short cords are expected because of the reduced inability of the fetus to move. Thus, Willemen et al. (1965) recorded 31 cm for the cord's length, and a case described by Chokroverty et al. (1986) had a 38 cm long cord with a macerated fetus. Many areas of placental degeneration were found as well.

The report by Gustafson et al. (1953) included a color picture of a placenta with velamentous cord insertion. It described a decidual reaction, but it actually depicted a typical placenta accreta with many extravillous trophoblast cells. We believe that, as is not uncommon, these cells were mistakenly interpreted to be decidua. This consideration is an important one that was once specifically studied by Moritz and Douglass (1928). These authors claimed that they regularly found decidua in tubal pregnancies at the villous attachment site "if the chorionic villi are intact." This finding is contrary to our experience. True decidual transformation is rare in the tubal mucosa and all tubal pregnancies in our patients have been accretas. The connection to the tubal musculature is afforded by extravillous trophoblast cells, or the placental site cells.

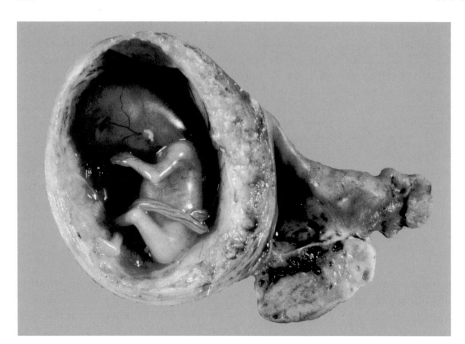

FIGURE 9.57. Large ectopic, interstitial pregnancy with placenta accreta.

They often have a superficial resemblance to decidual cells but are of trophoblastic origin. It was for this reason that they were referred to as X cells in the first place, because of the difficulties in differentiating them from maternal tissue elements. Silver stains would quickly delineate the characteristically crisp borders of decidual stromal cells, while cytokeratin stain is useful to distinguish extravillous trophoblast cells.

It is also surprising to find striking contradictions in a study of 90 placentas (young abortions) of tubal pregnancies by Laufer et al. (1962). In their introduction, these authors wrote that decidua was lacking in the tube, but in their summary they stated that, aside from the hydropic degeneration and placental infarcts that are expected, decidua was found in all cases. Not only are tubal ectopic pregnancies accretas, when they rupture (as is commonly the case) they do so because the placenta becomes a placenta percreta with blood issuing from the intervillous space into the peritoneal cavity.

Reports of intraligamentary pregnancy (Vierhout & Wallenburg, 1985) merge with the next topic, abdominal pregnancy. The patient Vierhout and Wallenburg described was presumed to have developed interstitial placentation from rupture of a tubal implantation; the patient suffered severe toxemia, and the placenta was left behind and resorbed spontaneously. Interstitial implantation also occurred in the case described by Schmitt and Dittrich (1973), probably secondary to an abdominal pregnancy. As in so many other abdominal pregnancies, there was no amnionic fluid, and the child had deformations. The placenta had succenturiate lobes, many infarcts and intervillous thrombi. It was small and had unusually thick membranes. Similar cases of "interstitial" tubal pregnancy, related to previous tubal surgery, were recorded by Kalchman and Meltzer (1966), and Woolam et al. (1967); these authors reviewed the literature and provided good illustrations.

Placenta in Abdominal Pregnancy

Implantation in the abdominal cavity, particularly when associated with term fetuses, has long been a topic of heated discussion. It may be associated with tubal disease and contraceptive devices, as in the case described by Tisdall et al. (1970), and Ross et al. (1997) described massive sanguineous ascites in association with it. Early diagnosis is a matter of concern, as it is difficult (Atrash et al., 1987). Ultrasonography and magnetic resonance studies have been advocated (Spanta et al., 1987). This complication of pregnancy is estimated to occur once in 3000 to 8000 births, according to the review of Martin et al. (1988). It also is associated with high fetal (83%) and some maternal mortality, according to these authors. They described nine cases of early and six cases of advanced abdominal pregnancy, and also provided an excellent review of current management. Abdominal pregnancy occurring after gonadotropin-induced pregnancy was reported by Cheng et al. (1994). The young pregnancy was located in the cul-de-sac and easily removed. When both intra- and extrauterine pregnancies exist, we speak of heterotopic gestations, very rare occurrences. Crabtree et al. (1994) reported such a case, a woman who remained pregnant after preterm delivery. After several irrelevant treatments, sonography showed the presence of an abdominal fetus. It was delivered by section; the placenta had an implantation on top of the uterus and was left behind.

Abdominal pregnancy also causes concern because of the unanswered question of how to deliver the placenta (Hreshchyshyn et al., 1961), as it does not deliver spontaneously because it is invariably a placenta accreta. There is extraordinary local vascular development in response to implantation. When that tissue is dislodged, exsanguinating hemorrhage may occur. These authors analyzed 101 such cases and found that attempted placental removal was the commonest practice; they also advocated it when it is surgically feasible. They found a high morbidity when the placenta was retained; for example, Caruso et al. (1963) reported a patient who had subsequent bowel perforation.

StClair et al. (1969) intentionally left the placenta in the abdomen and perfused the umbilical vessels with methotrexate. They undertook this measure because methotrexate is highly toxic to trophoblast. The placenta involuted rapidly and the gonadotropin titers fell. They believed that this therapy may have improved the involution, which is otherwise considered to take as long as 50 days. Rahman et al. (1982) have also reported the use of this agent, but they were less enthusiastic about its benefit. These authors reported that 10 cases occurred among 102,000 deliveries. Somewhat similar figures were obtained in other large series dealing with ectopic pregnancy (Hallatt & Grove, 1985). Jaffe et al. (1994), who also left a placenta percreta behind, ineffectively treated the patient with methotrexate, only to have to remove the bleeding tissue 7 weeks after initial surgery.

Many abdominal pregnancies are secondary to tubal abortion; Hallatt and Grove depicted the typical accreta on uterine muscle and provided a distribution of the major implantation sites. The first successful removal of the gestational sac and most of the placenta by laparoscopy was reported by Dover and Powell (1995).

The placenta in abdominal pregnancy is rarely described in detail. It has been mentioned that the placental floor lacks decidua, that a large vascular supply supports the intervillous space, and that the placenta may develop on many maternal organs. Holzer and Pickel (1976) found such a case to have a large succenturiate lobe and a velamentous cord insertion. A remarkable vascular attachment to the mother was described by Norén and Lindblom (1986). Their normal term infant had a thickened placental sac over which many islands of placenta were distributed. The only connection to the mother was a 2 cm wide and 3 cm long vascular pedicle that connected the placenta to the uterine fundus. It was easily ligated. The placenta membranacea had many intervillous thrombi and infarcts. Fetal growth restriction (Shott et al., 1973), anomalies and deformations (Paintin, 1970; Guha-Ray & Hamblin, 1977), and occasionally fetal pulmonary hypoplasia (Cartwright et al., 1986) are often described. Several publications of abdominal pregnancy have appeared in which the condition occurred after hysterectomy (Kornb-

latt, 1968; Niebyl, 1974; Nehra & Loginsky, 1984). The latter authors collected 30 such cases from the literature.

The fate of the retained placenta is also rarely described in detail. When complications such as perforations and adhesions necessitate reoperation, the placental tissue is usually not described. Only sonographic studies of the atrophy are available (Belfar et al., 1986). An interesting report comes from Spinnato et al. (1987), who saw a cyst develop 3 weeks after the term delivery of a normal infant from an abdominal pregnancy. The umbilical cord was tied near its base and the chorion laeve was not removed or closed. Despite the absence of a fetus, the membranes reaccumulated a large amount of fluid. When the mass was finally excised, the fluid was brown and thick. It contained much necrotic debris and the remains of a macerating umbilical cord with its ligature, which were clearly depicted. Regrettably, no histology is available.

Ovarian pregnancies usually abort. The definition of ovarian pregnancy generally follows the strict criteria set in the past. These criteria are often attributed to Spiegelberg (1878), but they were actually delineated by Cohnstein the year before. A term pregnancy has rarely been reported in the ovary, although Williams et al. (1982) described such a case. As expected, the umbilical cord was very short (22 cm), but the placenta was unusually large (1500 g). When sections are made of the implantation site of ovarian pregnancies, the placental villi often insert on the cells of the corpus luteum. The cellular component of the placental floor is the extravillous trophoblast cell, frequently mistakenly identified (Yu et al., 1984). The English-language literature of ovarian pregnancy was reviewed by Boronow et al. (1965), who found 62 cases in 13 years. In other words, it is not a really uncommon entity. They noted that the usual antecedents of ectopic pregnancy (pelvic and tubal inflammation, sterility, and endometriosis) are not important in this disease. The site of implantation often contains much hemorrhage and only some trophoblastic giant cells. True placental tissue is frequently absent, except for some degenerating villi.

Cysts and Breus' Mole

Placental cysts occur in many normal placentas. They may be found in the placental septa, in cell islands, and under the fetal surface. In addition, there are cystic structures in placental villi. The latter have a completely different pathogenesis and are largely ignored in this context and further considered in Chapters 21 and 22.

Also present and having a somewhat overlapping quality are liquefying hematomas ("Breus' mole"), which may occur in the subchorionic space of the placenta. They are included for discussion here merely for convenience, as they are not related to the common cysts of the mature placenta. A detailed chemical analysis was undertaken of cyst fluid from a large (4 cm) prenatally diagnosed subchorionic cyst by Shipley and Nelson (1993). They compared the content of many components with those of amnionic fluid, cord, and maternal serum. Unusually high concentrations of iron, aspartate- and alanine aminotransferase, and lactic dehydrogenase were found in the fluid.

Placental cysts may be numerous and large (Fig. 9.58). Although the cysts probably have no clinical significance—at least none is recognized as yet—their origin is interesting and has been a matter of controversy. The cells that produce the cysts have also had a varied nomenclature, as they were often mistaken for decidual cells. The cells that produce the cysts and the biochemical features of their viscid, mucin-like product have now been examined more closely. Grosser (1927) considered placental cysts to represent a special form of trophoblastic degeneration. He equated cyst formation with a process of fibrinoid degeneration. Bret et al. (1960) beautifully illustrated these structures in a study of 589 placental cysts and provided an extensive literature review. Cysts have been as large as a fetal head on rare occasion. Sanguineous material is often included and mixed with the normally "serous" content of cysts.

There are thus three principal types of cysts in the placenta. One is a **cystic "degeneration" of villi**. In this form (Fig. 9.59) some villi distend remarkably with fluid. More commonly, however, the villous edema involves scattered areas of the placenta, and the process is related to the hydatidiform mole. It is commonly found in triploid conceptuses and is then referred to as a "partial" mole. Partial moles are considered in Chapter 22.

Next, **cystic "degeneration" of subchorionic intervillous thrombi** occurs. Laminated thrombi form, almost regularly and in small quantities, in the subchorionic space. It is this site where the intervillous (maternal)

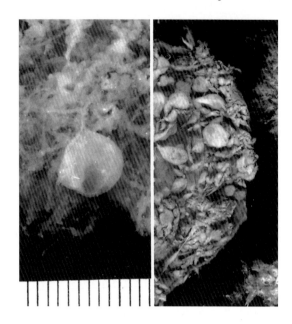

FIGURE 9.59. Two variants of villous "cysts," actually hydropic changes of villi. All are triploid conceptuses at different stages of gestation. The cysts are actually within villous tissue.

blood is deflected backward. Most likely, eddying of intervillous blood accounts for the deposition of the small amounts of fibrin that normally accumulate here. This process leads to the formation of some white patches of subchorionic fibrin and to the "bosselation" ("tessellation") of the fetal surface of the placenta. The fibrin accumulations increase with maturation, and much more thrombotic material accumulates underneath the chorion in some abnormal placentas.

It is more often found when maternal circulatory disorders exist; we have seen it repeatedly, for instance, in mothers with complex heart disease. These large patches of subchorionic coagulation may protrude on the fetal surface; and when they contract, fluid may be extruded from the clot. In this way, cysts can develop that contain old blood clot (Fig. 9.60). Some of these subchorionic cystic hematomas have been so large that they were diagnosed antenatally by sonography (Kirkinen & Jouppila, 1986). In one of the cases reported by Kirkinen and Jouppila, Doppler velocimetry of blood flow in the umbilical cord identified that the hematoma, having dissected into the base of the cord, caused a venous obstruction to blood flow. It was also the cause of furcate cord insertion. Occasional association with circumvallate placentas has been noted.

On rare occasions, cysts with this macroscopic appearance associate with a fetus papyraceus. This type of cyst is akin to the "**Breus mole**" (Fig. 9.61). Breus (1892) had described these lesions in five cases of missed abortions. He interpreted them as sacculations ("diverticula") produced by the continued intervillous blood pressure against a decreased amnionic sac pressure. He believed that the

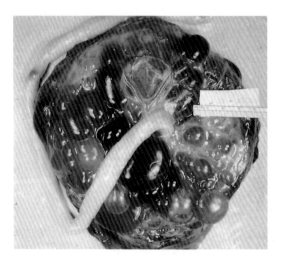

FIGURE 9.58. Multiple subchorionic cysts in a near-term placenta. Many cysts were discolored (red, brown, green) due to prior hemorrhage. The placenta had typical "maternal floor infarction" and was the fifth so affected pregnancy of this patient.

FIGURE 9.60. Term placenta with a large subchorionic intervillous thrombus that had liquefied and produced a protruding cyst. When the cyst was opened, it contained clot, contiguous with the intervillous space.

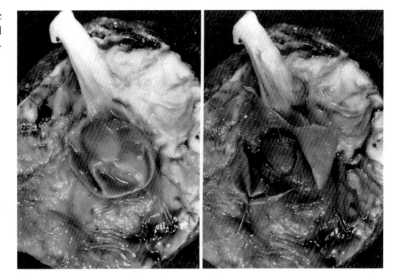

membranous cover continues to grow after fetal death, and he called the lesion "subchorionic tuberous hematoma," wanting to differentiate this condition from hydatidiform moles.

The term Breus mole, however, is confusing. It has to do with "mass" rather than the process of molar "degeneration" as seen in hydatidiform moles. Torpin (1960, 1966) referred to these coagula as "hematoma moles" and also related them to circumvallate placentas. He suggested that abnormally deep implantation is their cause. Linthwaite (1963) conjectured that this placental abnormality precedes fetal demise. This view and "excessive implantation" were upheld by Thomas (1964). He cited authors who disagreed with Breus' opinion, an aspect that was comprehensively discussed in the report by Shanklin and Scott (1975), who studied 10 cases past 25 weeks' gestation. Seven infants were liveborn, but only three survived the neonatal period. These findings argue strongly against the view that fetal death is primary in the development of the tuberous subchorionic hematoma. The authors also reviewed case reports that supported their opinion. Their incidence was 1:1200 placentas. Many of their patients had various diseases, including diabetes and hypertension. Despite these observations and their meticulous illustrations, no unified etiology for subchorionic tuberous hematomas emerged from this study.

Breus mole apparently is more commonly associated with monosomy X (45,X, Turner syndrome; Fig. 9.61) (see also Perrin, 1984). It is always a benign condition, and although it correlates with missed abortion, it is not limited to it, as Breus had suggested.

Finally, there are **true cysts** (Figs. 9.62 and 9.63), which are the principal focus of this discussion. These cysts are often blood-tinged, frequently multiple, and most often

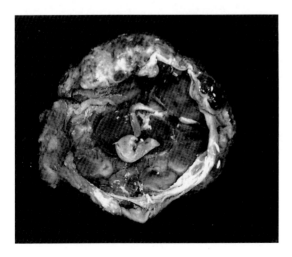

FIGURE 9.61. Breus' mole (subchorionic tuberous hematoma) in an immature placenta from a "missed abortion." Note the numerous blood-filled protrusions on the surface.

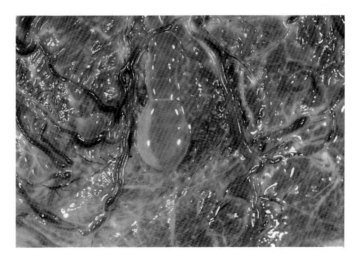

FIGURE 9.62. Multicameral subchorionic cysts issuing from subchorionic deposits of extravillous trophoblast cells in a mature placenta.

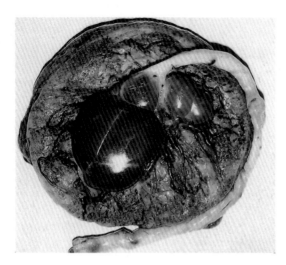

FIGURE 9.63. Large subchorial cysts, some discolored by blood, in mature placenta. Note that one of the cysts dissects into the base of the umbilical cord. They may cause compression of vessels.

found in mature placentas. Their frequency is more difficult to ascertain. In our experience, about 5% of mature placentas have surface cysts of varying size. We find a much higher percentage of septal and cell island cysts, provided the placentas are sliced at thin intervals. Paddock and Greer (1927) found 14% in a macroscopic study of 1965 placentas; Carter et al. (1963) found 7% subchorial and 17% septal cysts in 400 mature placentas that they examined for vascular lesions. Cysts may originate below chorial vessels and elevate them much above the rest of the fetal surface. There is no evidence, however, that this compromises the fetal circulation (Bret et al., 1960).

Subchorial cysts are rarely encountered at the margin of the placenta (Fig. 9.64) and they have not been recorded to occur on the extraplacental membranes. These cysts arise from the same extravillous trophoblast cells at the margin of the placenta that surrounds the entire membranous sac.

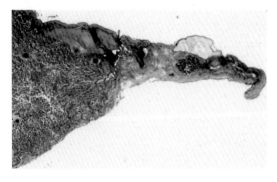

FIGURE 9.64. Subchorial cyst on membranes near the edge of the placental disk. It overlies an area of placental atrophy. H&E ×2.

Cysts are most commonly found in placental septa (Figs. 9.43, 9.44, and 9.65 to 9.67) and in the cell islands (Fig. 9.47B) of mature placentas. They contain a colorless, thin fluid that is frequently slightly mucinous in character. Real mucin, however, is not found. The fluid is a rich source of major basic protein (MBP). The rich protein content of these cysts is evident by the precipitate found in histologic sections (Fig. 9.68). Paddock and Greer (1927) likened the content of cysts to colloid, while Grosser (1927) wrote of "colliquation necrosis" as the origin of the cystic fluid. It has been the experience of many writers that X-cell cysts are particularly often found in placentas that have fibrinoid degeneration. Thus, in maternal floor infarction, an unusual condition to be discussed later in this chapter, an excessive number of cysts surrounded by extravillous trophoblast are typical (Figs. 9.58 and 9.68). Their lining is irregular and ragged. Spaces develop between the extravillous trophoblast cells during their expansion, and they ultimately coalesce to make cysts.

According to Soma et al. (1991) increased numbers of X-cell cysts can be found in placentas from high altitude (Tibet and Nepal). This finding supports the view that cyst formation is a result of degenerative processes due to malnutrition and hypoxia in the centers of large accumulations of extravillous trophoblast. Further support is derived from the fact that cysts are formed within the

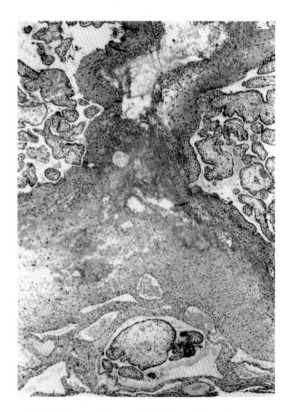

FIGURE 9.65. Placental floor with the origin of a septum of a near-term placenta. The septum shows cystic cavitation in extravillous trophoblast cell deposits. H&E ×60.

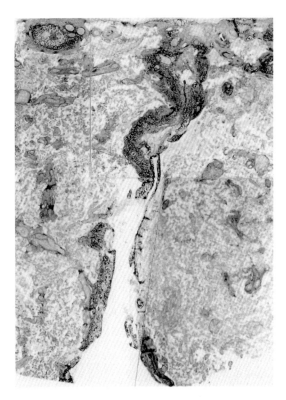

FIGURE 9.66. Placental septum that reaches the chorionic surface (top). The intercellular substance has been stained dark (purple) with aldehyde-fuchsin (Waidl, 1963). At top left and in the top portion of the septum are small cysts developing in subchorial deposits of extravillous trophoblast cells. Aldehyde-fuchsin ×8; Montage.

extravillous trophoblast of the chorionic plate, the septa, and the cell islands rather than in those of the basal plate, the difference being that in the basal plate the extravillous trophoblast cells are intermingled with macrophages. These macrophages might easily remove degenerative products by phagocytosis and thus avoid liquefaction of degenerative masses.

Maternal Floor Infarction

In maternal floor infarction (MFI), the floor of the placenta is thick, stiffened, and often yellow. The maternal surface has a corrugated appearance, and the placental septa are prominent (Fig. 9.69). Often, the lesion is associated with excessive proliferation of extravillous trophoblast cells and cyst formation (Fig. 9.70). Frequently, but not always, there is a massive "net-like" fibrin deposition throughout the placental tissue as well, occasionally referred to as Gitterinfarkt or Netzinfarkt in the German literature (Figs. 9.71 and 9.72) (Becker, 1981). The same features occur also in association with villitis of unknown etiology (VUE) (see Chapter 20). The placenta in MFI is often small and firm, and no other major pathologic lesions exist when it is sectioned. Maternal floor infarction is not associated with abruption, but fetal growth retardation is often a sequela. Most importantly, the condition may lead to fetal death, and it recurs frequently in subsequent pregnancies.

One patient seen by us had nine consecutive losses due to MFI. With other patients in whom the lesion had previously occurred, the anticipation of its recurrence has led to intense fetal monitoring, including an evaluation of estriol excretion. Twice, when fetal activity declined, Clewell and Manchester (1983) were able to obtain a living fetus by cesarean section. The placenta had the same changes as those of the original descriptions of MFI (Benirschke, 1961; Benirschke & Driscoll, 1967). This strongly argues against the notion, expressed by Fox (1978), that MFI is a postmortem change of the placenta of stillborns. Likewise, Katz and colleagues (1987) found typical MFI in a patient whose baby survived and did well. That patient had previously had three abortions and one abruptio placentae with stillbirth. All of her placentas had excessive fibrin deposits. The patient had chronic hypertension, and during the last pregnancy there was growth retardation, and a 7.2-fold elevation of α-fetopro-

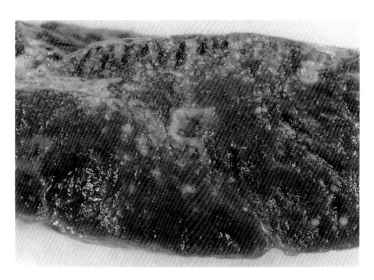

FIGURE 9.67. Typical septal cyst. Note that it is in the center of the placenta, at the tip of the partial septum.

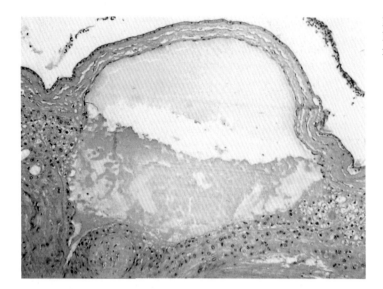

FIGURE 9.68. Subchorionic "X cell" cyst of the placenta. Note that the cyst contains precipitated protein. H&E ×40.

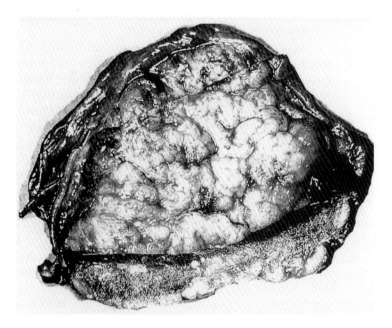

FIGURE 9.69. Maternal floor with maternal floor infarction. The entire decidual floor is thickened, yellowish, and infiltrated with fibrin. The cut section (below) shows the relatively shallow depth of fibrin infiltration.

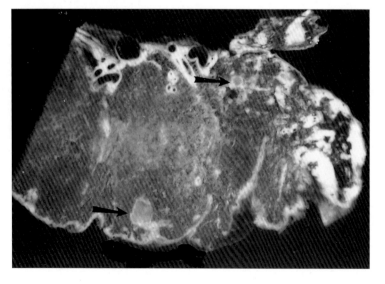

FIGURE 9.70. Typical maternal floor infarction (MFI) in the placenta of a premature infant who died with hyaline membrane disease. The infant had been reported to "never be active" in utero. The floor and septa have increased fibrin infiltrates, and there are two septal cysts (arrows) in this section. The entire placenta had a firm appearance.

FIGURE 9.71. Massive intervillous fibrin deposition: "Gitterinfarkt." It was a 34 weeks' gestation placenta of a growth-retarded infant who did well. The previous pregnancy had also resulted in an infant with growth restriction.

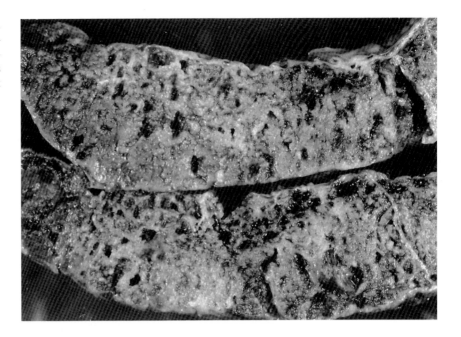

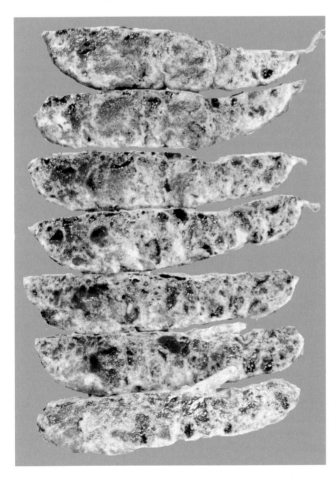

FIGURE 9.72. Case similar to that in Figure 9.71: massive diffuse fibrin encasement of villous tissue in MFI with "Gitterinfarkt." It was the third stillborn of a healthy mother; the maternal serum MBP levels were markedly elevated.

tein (AFP) was detected from 17 weeks on. She delivered at 34 weeks and the growth-retarded infant eventually did well. The elevated AFP levels were interpreted to result from a disruption at the maternal–fetal interface and at least once a fetal hemorrhage of 4 mL was detected by Kleihauer test. The MBP levels in maternal serum were significantly elevated in one of our patients with MFI, which was established by elevated maternal serum AFP levels; the patient had had two previous stillbirths (G.J. Gleich, personal communication, 1989).

Subsequent evaluation of the possible utility of MBP levels in maternal serum for the anticipation of MFI was not productive (Vernof et al., 1992). Robinson et al. (1989) found a strong correlation between elevated AFP levels and poor pregnancy outcome, even when congenital anomalies and twins were excluded. Thus, MFI and its variants must be entertained in the differential diagnosis of an unexplained elevation of AFP during pregnancy. Mandsager et al. (1993) established ultrasonographic criteria for the diagnosis of MFI and found them useful in anticipating the disease.

It is true that when a placenta has been retained for a long time after fetal death the organ accumulates fibrin and becomes firm. It is not the case, however, with most stillborns. Their placentas usually show no increased fibrin imbibition. Nor have the fetuses of some of the placentas with MFI been dead for especially long periods. As indicated earlier, this condition occurs with liveborn infants as well, especially with growth-restricted infants. Although MFI is a specific entity, it is not always completely expressed; that is, in some placentas, the characteristic fibrin deposition does not involve the entire floor. This variability occasionally makes the diagnosis difficult.

One atypical case has been described in which the fetus ultimately developed microcephaly (Pfeiffer, 1974).

The histologic findings of MFI include a marked increase in fibrinoid deposits of the decidual floor with encasement of many villous tips. Those villi then are sclerotic and avascular. The fibrinoid stains faintly with Congo red, but it is not amyloid by electron microscopic study. There is an increase of extravillous trophoblast (X cells) and septal cyst formation. Occasionally, many subchorionic cysts are found in this condition. Inflammation is usually not present, and the trophoblast in uninvolved areas is normal. The Gitterinfarkt features are shown in Figures 9.71 and 9.72. Villi are encased in masses of fibrinoid and appear to have been strangled, whereas adjacent villi are normal (Figs. 9.73 and 9.74). There is usually no inflammation. In some specimens of MFI, however, there is a moderate degree of lymphoid cell infiltration around the necrotic villi (Fig. 9.75). Plasma cells are absent, and there is usually no villitis. These placentas are also not associated with the decidual vasculopathy (atherosis) of preeclampsia.

It must be emphasized that MFI is macroscopically and microscopically different from common infarcts. No large areas of villous infarction are present; the lesion is usually confined to the floor of the placenta, and the deposition of fibrinoid is an outstanding feature of this entity. Therefore, when studies of the nature and frequency of infarcts are made (e.g., Fox, 1967), this lesion is not encompassed. In considerations of the placenta in placental insufficiency, however, there is more often mention of fibrin-encasement, lesions that apparently represent similar pathologic features. Thus, Wigglesworth (1964) found among the normotensive cases in his study that "the most extensive placental infarction was seen in cases of unexplained stillbirth. The lesions in those placentas were not always pure infarcts but consisted of true infarction and massive arborescent fibrin deposits."

Kubli (1968), in a consideration of chronic placental insufficiency, mentioned that the lesions are variable and comprise cases with "disseminated ischemic necroses with fibrinoid degeneration ('essential' placental insufficiency, prolonged pregnancy)." Ermocilla and Altshuler (1973) found similar lesions, particularly prominent proliferation of extravillous trophoblast cells (X cells) in three growth-retarded infants. They suggested that it would be better if we devoted our efforts to determining the function of X cells than be concerned with their origin. Davies et al. (1984), although not referring directly to MFI, also found an increased amount of fibrin in the placentas of growth-restricted infants.

The only author who has paid more attention to this lesion is Naeye (1985). He attempted to ascertain the incidence of MFI and its significance from the 39,215 placentas examined in the Collaborative Perinatal Study. He found that MFI was reported in 1 of 200 placentas. That figure is much higher than is our experience and

may be related to the variability of observers. The fetuses were stillborn in 17%, and 50% of the patients had had previous stillbirths or abortions (27% of controls had such). He also found chorioamnionitis and twice the expected frequency of fetal growth retardation. His experience of an increased incidence of preeclamptic decidual lesions is not supported by our cases. Smoking had no influence, but women with MFI had higher hemoglobin values. Nickel (1988) also described a case and discussed the recurrence and related diseases.

The etiology of MFI is unknown. We are convinced, partly because of its frequently recurrent nature, that MFI is a specific entity. Naeye (1985), on the other hand, believed that it represents the "final common pathway for a number of disorders, some of which are the result of damage to the decidua." He favored a relation to infection, with which we disagree. It is true that MFI and especially "Gitterinfarkt" are seen in some cases of chronic villitis, but not all MFI placentas have villitis. We have suggested that MFI relates to an abnormal host/placental interaction but not necessarily an immunologic one. Because the lesion has generally been poorly recognized, no further support has been forthcoming for this notion. Be that as it may, it is important for the obstetrician to know of its existence because, as the case reported by Clewell and Manchester (1983) clearly showed, subsequent pregnancies may be salvaged when the disease is recognized to have caused stillbirth or abortion.

We know nothing of the pathogenesis of MFI. The excessive fibrinoid (and perhaps extracellular substances, such as fibronectin) deposits may reduce the flow into the intervillous space and thus be responsible for fetal malnutrition. We have not observed any specific maternal vascular disease in these patients, and lupus anticoagulants have not been present in the mothers. The few clinical correlations and histologic observations have suggested that the fibrinoid deposition occurs relatively quickly. Usually, this situation is the case during the second and third trimesters. With the exception of occasional diabetic patients, the mothers have been clinically normal.

One promising avenue for future study is based on the findings of Robb et al. (1986a,b). Using an immunohistochemical technique, these investigators located what was interpreted as herpes virus antigen in the floor of most specimens diagnosed as having MFI. They suggested that this deposition of antigen may represent a manifestation of latent herpes simplex virus infection. The problematic associated with demonstrating conclusively HSV antigen by immunoperoxidase staining, however, is significant and taints these efforts.

Decidual Degeneration

Degenerative changes and hemorrhages are frequent features of the decidua in the basal plate and the membranes. The slowly progressive necrosis of the decidua

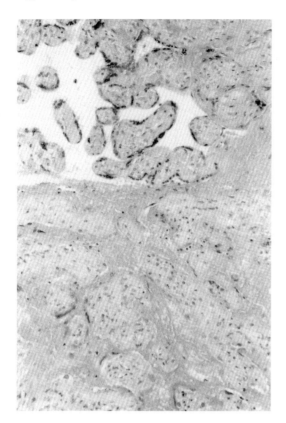

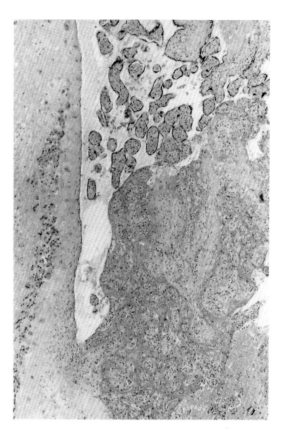

FIGURE 9.73. Histologic features of Gitterinfarkt. Villi are encased in masses of pale eosinophilic fibrin-like material. Adjacent villi are normal. The encasement usually begins, and is most severe, at the anchoring tips of the villi. H&E ×160.

FIGURE 9.74. Case similar to that in Figure 9.73. Fibrin-engulfed clusters of mature villi exist adjacent to normally preserved villi. H&E ×60.

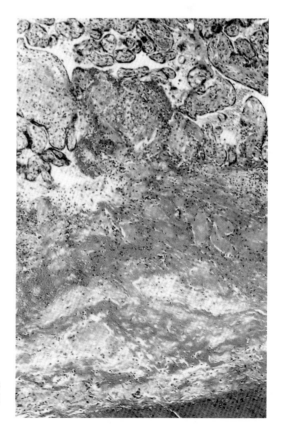

FIGURE 9.75. Histologic appearance of a maternal floor infarction. There is an excessive amount of fibrin in the decidua. Many basal villi are dead and are surrounded by chronic inflammatory cells. H&E ×100.

capsularis was believed to be the result of progressively decreasing vascularization (Grosser, 1927). The more likely explanation is endocrinologic. One may presume that reduced concentrations of those steroid hormones that induced decidualization occur locally. It may be so because with increasing distance from the placenta decidual degeneration increases (Dallenbach-Hellweg & Sievers, 1975). This view has been supported by the findings of Welsh and Enders (1985), who found decidual involution at the mesometrial side of rodent uteri, opposite the placental site.

Decidual necrosis is often combined with local hemorrhages and may result in prenatal bleeding. McCombs and Craig (1964) reviewed the basal plates of 34 uteri from therapeutic hysterectomies and found decidual necrosis in 81%. In 52% the necrosis was present at some distance from the implantation site. They regarded it to be a normal phenomenon, which is also our opinion. At early implantation sites, hemorrhages of the decidua are normal, although it may be a different matter when they become clinically evident by vaginal bleeding. The latter may be a sign of "decidual angiomatosis," according to Bittencourt and Sadigursky (1977). Their finding, however, may merely represent exaggerated dilatation of basal plate vessels with thrombosis.

In the delivered placenta, one often finds small retromembranous hematomas. They appear as patches of adherent brown-yellow clot, which when they are old, look as though they are composed of fibrous tissue (Fig. 9.76). Occasionally, this situation ensues after amniocentesis (Fig. 9.77). Moreover, when an intrauterine device (IUD) remains into pregnancy, it is frequently locally associated with old hemorrhages (see Chapter 1, Figs. 1.4 and 1.5). These IUDs also lead to frequent placental "wandering" (trophotropism) with marginal or velamentous insertions of the umbilical cord.

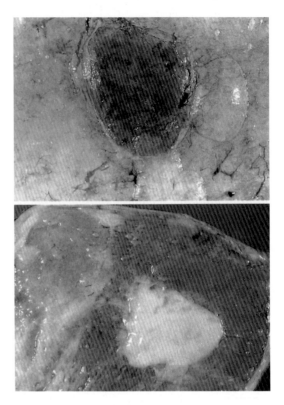

FIGURE 9.76. Localized retromembranous hematomas in uncomplicated pregnancy. Top: Note the brown patch of old blood in the decidua capsularis. Bottom: There is an old, white retromembranous hematoma in an otherwise uncomplicated pregnancy at term.

Massive hemorrhage during early pregnancy has once been reported to break into the amnionic sac, producing a sonographically apparent umbilical cord mass (Witter & Sanders, 1986). Retromembranous bleeding from venous lakes has also been described to occur, according

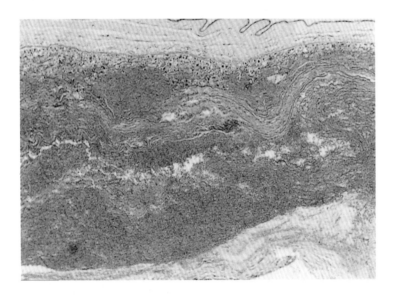

FIGURE 9.77. Retromembranous hematoma 4 weeks after amniocentesis. Note the vacuolated trophoblast beneath chorion and the degenerating clot in dead decidua capsularis (below). H&E ×64.

to Pozniak et al. (1988), following chorionic villus sampling. They found venous lakes to be uncommon in first trimester uteri and cautioned that they must be avoided in chorionic villus sampling (CVS).

Decidual necrosis and local hemorrhages have been linked to potential adverse effects on embryonic development. Ornoy et al. (1976) found an increase in severe congenital anomalies when prenatal bleeding had occurred, whereas Mau and Netter (1974), in their paired prospective analysis of 5257 pregnancies, found no statistical difference of anomalies occurring in infants of mothers who bled and those who did not. Rutherford (1942) had suggested that prenatal bleeding was an ominous feature. That opinion paved the way for future experimental decidual support with hormone replacement. Javert (1955), who observed that the expansion of the placenta lends itself to decidual bleeding, found administration of vitamin C to be helpful.

References

Aboulafia, Y., Lavie, O., Granovsky-Grisaru, Shen, O. and Diamant, Y.Z.: Conservative surgical management of acute abdomen caused by placenta percreta in the second trimester. Amer. J. Obstet. Gynecol. **170**:1388–1389, 1994.

Abrahamsohn, P.A. and Zorn, T.M.: Implantation and decidualization in rodents. J. Exp. Zool. **266**:603–628, 1993.

ACOG: ACOG committee opinion. Placenta accreta. Number 266, January 2002. American College of Obstetricians and Gynecologists. Intern. J. Gynaecol. Obstet. **77**:77–78, 2002.

Ahmed, A., Li, X.F., Dunk, C., Whittle, M.J., Rushton, D.I. and Rollason, T.: Colocalisation of vascular endothelial growth factor and its flt-1 receptor in human placenta. Growth Factors **12**:235–243, 1995.

Akiyama, S.K., Olden, K. and Yamada, K.M.: Fibronectin and integrins in invasion and metastasis. Cancer Metastasis Rev. **14**:173–189, 1995.

Aluvihare, V.R., Kallikourdis, M. and Betz, A.G.: Regulatory T cells mediate maternal tolerance to the fetus. Nature Immunology **5**:266–271, 2004.

Al-Zuhair, A.G.H., Ibrahim, M.E.A. and Mughal, S.: Calcium deposition on the maternal surface of the human placenta: a scanning electron microscopic study. Arch. Gynecol. **234**:167–172, 1984.

Andersen, J.R., Borggaard, B., Olsen, E.B, Stimpel, H., Nyholm, H.C. and Schroeder, E.: Decidual prolactin content and secretion at term: correlations with the clinical data. Acta Obstet. Gynecol. Scand. **66**:591–596, 1987.

Anson-Cartwright, L., Dawson, K., Holmyard, D., Fisher, S.J., Lazzarini, R.A. and Cross, J.C.: The glial cells missing-1 protein is essential for branching morphogenesis in the chorioallantoic placenta [see comments]. Nature Genet. **25**:311–314, 2000.

Anteby, E.Y., Greenfield, C., Natanson-Yaron, S., Goldman-Wohl, D., Hamani, Y., Khudyak, V., Ariel, I. and Yagel, S.: Vascular endothelial growth factor, epidermal growth factor and fibroblast growth factor-4 and -10 stimulate trophoblast

plasminogen activator system and metalloproteinase-9. Mol. Hum. Reprod. **10**:229–235, 2004.

Aplin, J.D.: Loss of integrin alpha-6–beta-4 from extravillous trophoblast. Placenta **12**:366, 1991a.

Aplin, J.D.: Implantation, trophoblast differentiation and haemochorial placentation: mechanistic evidence in vivo and in vitro. J. Cell Sci. **99**:681–692, 1991b.

Aplin, J.D.: Expression of integrin alpha 6 beta 4 in human trophoblast and its loss from extravillous cells. Placenta **14**:203–215, 1993.

Aplin, J.D. and Campbell, S.: An immunofluorescence study of extracellular matrix associated with cytotrophoblast of the chorion laeve. Placenta **6**:469–479, 1985.

Aplin, J.D. and Foden, L.J.: A cell spreading factor, abundant in human placenta, contains fibronectin and fibrinogen. J. Cell Sci. **58**:287–302, 1982.

Aplin, J.D., Haigh, T., Jones, C.J., Church, H.J. and Vicovac, L.: Development of cytotrophoblast columns from explanted first-trimester human placental villi: role of fibronectin and integrin alpha5beta1. Biol. Reprod. **60**:828–838, 1999.

Aplin, J.D., Lacey, H., Haigh, T., Jones, C.J, Chen, C.P. and Westwood, M.: Growth factor-extracellular matrix synergy in the control of trophoblast invasion. Biochem. Soc. Trans. **28**:199–202, 2000.

Arias-Stella, J.: Gestational endometrium. In, The Uterus. H.J. Norris, A.T. Hertig, A.T. and M.R. Abel, eds., pp. 183–212. Williams and Wilkins, Baltimore, 1973.

Armstrong, C.A., Harding, S., Matthews, T. and Dickinson, J.E.: Is placenta accreta catching up with us? Austral. New Zeal. J. Obstet. Gynaecol. **44**:210–213, 2004.

Arnholdt, H. and Löhrs, U.: Proliferation and differentiation of Langhans' cells. Placenta **10**:458, 1989.

Arnholdt, H., Meisel, F., Fandrey, K. and Löhrs, U.: Proliferation of villous trophoblast of the human placenta in normal and abnormal pregnancies. Virchows Arch. B. Cell Pathol. **60**:365–372, 1991.

Arnold, J.: Über die Randzone der reifen menschlichen Plazenta. Inaugural Dissertation, Würzburg, 1975a.

Arnold, J.: Über den Schlussring reifer menschlicher Plazenten. Verh. Anat. Ges. **69**:303–306, 1975b.

Arts, N.F.T.: Investigations on the vascular system of the placenta. Amer. J. Obstet. Gynecol. **82**:147–166, 1961.

Ashkar, A.A., Di Santo, J.P. and Croy B.A.: Interferon gamma contributes to initiation of uterine vascular modification, decidual integrity, and uterine natural killer cell maturation during normal murine pregnancy. J. Exp. Med. **192**:259–270, 2000.

Ashton, S.V., Whitley, G.S., Dash, P.R., Wareing, M., Crocker, I.P., Baker, P.N. and Cartwright, J.E.: Uterine Spiral Artery Remodeling Involves Endothelial Apoptosis Induced by Extravillous Trophoblasts Through Fas/FasL Interactions. Arterioscler. Thromb. Vasc. Biol. **25**:102–108, 2005.

Astedt, B., Hagerstrand, I. and Lecander, I.: Cellular localisation in placenta of placental type plasminogen activator inhibitor. Thromb. Haemost. **56**:63–65, 1986.

Athanassiades, A. and Lala, P.K.: Role of placenta growth factor (PlGF) in human extravillous trophoblast proliferation, migration and invasiveness. Placenta **19**:465–473, 1998.

Atrash, H.K., Friede, A. and Hogue, C.J.R.: Abdominal pregnancy in the United States: frequency and maternal mortality. Obstet. Gynecol. **69**:333–337, 1987.

Aufderheide, E. and Ekblom, P.: Tenascin during gut development: appearance in the mesenchyme, shift in molecular forms, and dependence on epithelial-mesenchymal interactions. J. Cell Biol. **107**:2341–2349, 1988.

Augensen, K.: Unruptured tubal pregnancy at term with survival of mother and child. Obstet. Gynecol. **61**:259–261, 1983.

Autio Harmainen, H., Hurskainen, T., Niskasaari, K., Hoyhtya, M. and Tryggvason, K.: Simultaneous expression of 70 kilodalton type IV collagenase and type IV collagen alpha 1 (IV) chain genes by cells of early human placenta and gestational endometrium. Lab. Invest. **67**:191–200, 1992.

Avery, C.R. and Aterman, K.: Calcification of the basement-membrane of placental villi. J. Pathol. **103**:199–200, 1971.

Axelsson, H. and Winblad, B.: Dislocated IUD and intrauterine ectopic pregnancy with uterine rupture. Obstet. Gynecol. **47**:365–366, 1976.

Ayers, L.R., Drosman, S. and Saltzstein, S.L.: Iatrogenic paracervical implantation of fetal tissue during therapeutic abortion: a case report. Obstet. Gynecol. **37**:755–760, 1971.

Azab, I., Okamura, H. and Beer, A.: Decidual cell production of human placental fibrinoid. Obstet. Gynecol. **40**:186–193, 1972.

Badarau, L. and Gavrilita, L.: Intervillous fibrin deposition, the Rohr, Nitabuch and Langhans striae. Amer. J. Obstetr. Gynecol. **98**:252–260, 1967.

Bagshawe, K. and Lawler, S.: The immunogenicity of the placenta and trophoblast. In, Immunobiology of Trophoblast. R.G. Edwards, C.W.S. Howe and M.H. Johnson, eds., pp. 171–182. Cambridge University Press, London, 1975.

Baines, M.G., Duclos, A.J., Antecka, E. and Haddad, E.K.: Decidual infiltration and activation of macrophages leads to early embryo loss. Amer. J. Reprod. Immunol. **37**:471–477, 1997.

Baker, B.L., Hook, J. and Severinghaus, A.E.: The cytological structure of the human chorionic villus and decidua parietalis. Amer. J. Anat. **74**:291–325, 1944.

Bakri, Y.N., Rifai, A. and Legarth, J.: Placenta previa-percreta: Magnetic resonance imaging findings and methotrexate therapy after hysterectomy. Amer. J. Obstet. Gynecol. **169**:213–214, 1993.

Bamberger, A.M., Sudahl, S., Loning, T., Wagener, C., Bamberger, C.M., Drakakis, P., Coutifaris, C. and Makrigiannakis, A.: The adhesion molecule CEACAM1 (CD66a, C-CAM, BGP) is specifically expressed by the extravillous intermediate trophoblast. Amer. J. Pathol. **156**:1165–1170, 2000.

Barber, K., Franklyn, J., McCabe, C., Khanim, F., Bulmer, J., Whitley, G.S., Franklyn, J. and Kilby, M: The in vitro effects of tri-iodothyronine on epidermal growth factor-induced trophoblast function. J. Clin. Endocrinol. Metab. 2005 (in press).

Bardawil, W.A. and Toy, B.L.: The natural history of choriocarcinoma: Problems of immunity and spontaneous regression. Ann. N.Y. Acad. Sci. **80**:197–261, 1959.

Bargmann, W.: Über den Bildungsort der Choriongonadotropine und Plazentarsteroide. Geburtshilfe Frauenheilk. **17**:865–875, 1957.

Bass, K.E., Morrish, D.W., Roth, I., Bhardway, D., Taylor, R. Zhou, Y. and Fisher, S.J.: Human cytotrophoblast invasion is

up-regulated by epidermal growth factor: Evidence that paracrine factors modify this process. Dev. Biol. **164**:550–561, 1994.

Bass, K.E., Li, H., Hawkes, S.P., Howard, E., Bullen, E., Vu, T.-K.H., McMaster, M., Janatpour, M. and Fisher S.J.: Tissue inhibitor of metalloproteinase-3 expression is upregulated during human cytotrophoblast invasion in vitro. Dev. Genetics **21**:61–67, 1997.

Bateman, D.E.R.: Spontaneous rupture of uterus at 22 weeks' pregnancy. Brit. Med. J. **2**:844, 1967.

Bauer, S., Pollheimer, J., Hartmann, J., Husslein, P., Aplin, J.D. and Knofler, M.: Tumor necrosis factor-alpha inhibits trophoblast migration through elevation of plasminogen activator inhibitor-1 in first-trimester villous explant cultures. J. Clin. Endocrinol. Metab. **89**:812–822, 2004.

Bautzmann, H. and Schröder, R.: Vergleichende Studien über Bau und Funktion des Amnions. Neue Befunde am menschlichen Amnion mit Einschluss seiner freien Bindegewebs-oder sog. Hofbauerzellen. Z. Anat. **119**:7–22, 1955.

Beagley, K.W. and Gockel, C.M.: Regulation of innate and adaptive immunity by the female sex hormones oestradiol and progesterone. FEMS Immunol. Med. Microbiol. **38**:13–22, 2003.

Becker, V.: Funktionelle Morphologie der Placenta. Arch. Gynäkol. **198**:3–28, 1962.

Becker, V.: Gefäße der Chorionplatte und Stammzotten. In, Die Plazenta des Menschen. V. Becker, Th.H. Schiebler and F. Kubli, eds. Thieme Verlag, Stuttgart, pp. 311–313, 1981.

Becker, V. and Jipp, P.: Über die Trophoblastschale der menschlichen Plazenta. Geburtshilfe Frauenheilk. **23**:466–474, 1963.

Begneaud, W., Dougherty, C.M. and Mickal, A.: Placenta accreta in early gestation; report of 2 cases. Amer. J. Obstet. Gynecol. **92**:267–268, 1965.

Belfar, H.L., Kurtz, A.B. and Wagner, R.J.: Long-term follow-up after removal of an abdominal pregnancy. J. Ultrasound Med. **5**:521–523, 1986.

Bell, S.C.: Decidualization and insulin-like growth factor (IGF) binding protein: implications for its role in stromal cell differentiation and the decidual cell in haemochorial placentation. Human Reprod. **4**:125–130, 1989.

Bell, S.C., Patel, S.R., Jackson, J.A. and Waites, G.T.: Major secretory protein of human decidualized endometrium in pregnancy is an insulin-like growth factor binding protein. J. Endocrinol. **118**:317–328, 1988.

Bendon, R.W. and Ray, M.B.: The pathologic findings of the fetal membranes in very prolonged amniotic fluid leakage. Arch. Pathol. Lab. Med. **110**:47–50, 1986.

Benirschke, K.: Examination of the placenta. Obstet. Gynecol. **18**:309–333, 1961.

Benirschke, K. and Driscoll, S.G.: The Pathology of the Human Placenta. Springer-Verlag, New York, 1967.

Berchuck, A. and Sokol, R.J.: Previous cesarean section, placenta increta, and uterine rupture in second-trimester abortion. Amer. J. Obstet. Gynecol. **145**:766–767, 1983.

Berger, G., Verbaere, J. and Feroldi, J.: Placental site trophoblastic tumor of the uterus: an ultrastructural and immunohistochemical study. Ultrastruct. Pathol. **6**:319–329, 1984.

Bertolini, R. and Klinger, M.: Über deziduaähnliche Zellnester in der Chorionplatte von geburtsreifen menschlichen Plazenten. Zentralbl. Gynäkol. **17**:521–524, 1966.

Bertolini, R., Reissig, D. and Schippel, K.: Elektronenmikroskopische Befunde an den Zellen in der Chorionplatte der reifen menschlichen Plazenta. Z. Mikrosk. Anat. Forsch. **80**:358–368, 1969.

Bigazzi, M., Bruni, P., Nardi, E., Petrucci, F., Pollicino, G., Franchini, M., Scarselli, G. and Farnararo, M.: Human decidual relaxin. Ann. N.Y. Acad. Sci. **380**:87–99, 1982.

Bilban, M., Ghaffari-Tabrizi, N., Hintermann, E., Bauer, S., Molzer, S., Zoratti, C., Malli, R., Sharabi, A., Hiden, U., Graier, W., Knofler, M., Andreae, F., Wagner, O., Quaranta, V. and Desoye, G.: Kisspeptin-10, a KiSS-1/metastin-derived decapeptide, is a physiological invasion inhibitor of primary human trophoblasts. J. Cell Sci. **117**:1319–1328, 2004.

Birkenfeld, A., Mordel, N. and Okon, E.: Direct demonstration of iron in a term placenta in a case of β-thalassemia major. Amer. J. Obstet. Gynecol. **160**:562–563, 1989.

Bischof, P. and Martelli, M.: Current topic: proteolysis in the penetration phase of the implantation process. Placenta **13**:17–24, 1992.

Bischof, P., Friedli, E., Martelli, M. and Campana, A.: Expression of extracellular matrix-degrading metalloproteinases by cultured human cytotrophoblast cells: effects of cell adhesion and immunopurification. Amer. J. Obstet. Gynecol. **165**:1791–1801, 1991.

Bischof, P., Haenggeli, L. and Campana, A.: Gelatinase and oncofetal fibronectin secretion is dependent on integrin expression on human cytotrophoblasts. Hum. Reprod. **10**:734–743, 1995.

Bischof, P., Meisser, A. and Campana, A.: Mechanisms of endometrial control of trophoblast invasion. J. Reprod. Fertil. Suppl. **55**:65–71, 2000a.

Bischof, P., Meisser, A. and Campana, A.: Paracrine and autocrine regulators of trophoblast invasion—a review. Placenta. **21** (Suppl A):S55–60, 2000b.

Bischof, P., Truong, K. and Campana, A.: Regulation of trophoblastic gelatinases by proto-oncogenes. Placenta. **24**:155–163, 2003.

Bittencourt, A.L. and Sadigursky, M.: Decidual angiomatosis with abortion. Patologia (Mexico) **15**:45–47, 1977.

Blankenship, T.N. and King, B.F.: Developmental expression of Ki-67 antigen and proliferating cell nuclear antigen in macaque placentas. Develop. Dynam. **201**:324–333, 1994a.

Blankenship, T.N. and King, B.F.: Identification of 72–Kilodalton Type-IV collagenase at sites of trophoblastic invasion of macaque spiral arteries. Placenta **15**:177–187, 1994b.

Blankenship, T.N. and King, B.F.: Macaque intra-arterial trophoblast and extravillous trophoblast of the cell columns and cytotrophoblastic shell express neural cell adhesion molecule (NCAM). Anat. Rec. **245**:525–531, 1996.

Blankenship, T.N. and Enders, A.C.: Trophoblast cell-mediated modifications to uterine spiral arteries during early gestation in the macaque. Acta Anat. **158**:227–236, 1997.

Blankenship, T.N., Enders, A.C. and King, B.F.: Trophoblastic invasion and the development of uteroplacental arteries in the macaque: immunohistochemical localization of cytokeratins, desmin, type IV collagen, laminin, and fibronectin. Cell Tissue Res. **272**:227–236, 1993a.

Blankenship, T.N., Enders, A.C. and King, B.F.: Trophoblastic invasion and the development of uteroplacental arteries in the macaque—immunohistochemical localization of cytokeratins, desmin, type-IV collagen, laminin, and fibronectin. Cell Tissue Res. **272**:227–236, 1993b.

Blithe, D.L., Richards, R.G. and Skarulis, M.C.: Free alpha molecules from pregnancy stimulate secretion of prolactin from human decidual cells: a novel function for free alpha in pregnancy. Endocrinology **129**:2257–2259, 1991.

Boe, F.: Studies on the human placenta. I. The cell islands in the young placenta. Acta Obstet. Gynecol. Scand. **46**:591–603, 1967.

Bogaert, L.J.: Endometrial granulocytes in proliferative endometrium. Brit. J. Obstet. Gynaecol. **82**:995–998, 1975.

Bogic, L.V., Mandel, M. and Bryant-Greenwood, G.D.: Relaxin gene expression in human reproductive tissues by in situ hybridization. J. Clin. Endocrinol. Metab. **80**:130–137, 1995.

Bohn, H.: The human fibrin-stabilizing factors. Mol. Cell. Biochem. **20**:67–75, 1978.

Bonnar, J. and Sheppard, B.L.: Treatment of poor intrauterine fetal growth with heparin and dipyridamole. In, Poor Intrauterine Fetal Growth. B. Salvadori and B. Modena, eds. Minerva Med. 465–468, 1977.

Borell, U., Fernstroem, I., Ohlson, L. and Wiqvist, N.: Effect of uterine contractions on the uteroplacental blood flow at term. Amer. J. Obstet. Gynecol. **93**:44–57, 1965.

Boronow, R.C., McElin, T.W., West, R.H. and Buckingham, J.C.: Ovarian pregnancy: report of four cases and a thirteen-year survey of the English literature. Amer. J. Obstet. Gynecol. **91**:1095–1106, 1965.

Borrego, F., Ulbrecht, M., Weiss, E.H., Coligan, J.E. and Brooks, A.G.: Recognition of human histocompatibility leukocyte antigen (HLA)-E complexed with HLA class I signal sequence-derived peptides by CD94/NKG2 confers protection from natural killer cell-mediated lysis. J. Exp. Med. **187**:813–818, 1998.

Bose, P., Black, S., Kadyrov, M., Bartz, C., Shlebak, A., Regan, L. and Huppertz, B.: Adverse effects of lupus anticoagulant positive blood sera on placental viability can be prevented by heparin in vitro. Amer. J. Obstet. Gynecol. **191**:2125–2131, 2004.

Bourne, G. L.: The Human Amnion and Chorion. Lloyd-Luke, London, 1962.

Boyd, J.D.: Morphology and physiology of the utero-placental circulation. In, Gestation. C.A. Villee, ed., pp. 132–194, Macy, New York, 1956.

Boyd, J.D. and Hamilton, W.J.: The giant cells of the pregnant human uterus. J. Obstet. Gynaecol. Brit. Emp. **67**:208–218, 1960.

Boyd, J.D. and Hamilton, W.J.: Placental septa. Z. Zellf. **69**:613–634, 1966.

Boyd, J.D. and Hamilton, W.J.: The Human Placenta. Heffer & Sons, Cambridge, 1970.

Bravo, R. and Macdonald-Bravo, H.: Existence of two populations of cyclin/proliferating cell nuclear antigen during the cell cycle: Associated with DNA replication sites. J. Cell Biol. **105**:1549–1554, 1987.

Breen, J.L., Neubecker, R., Gregori, C.A. and Franklin, J.E.: Placenta accreta, increta, and percreta: a survey of 40 cases. Obstet. Gynecol. **49**:43–47, 1977.

Bret, A.-J., Legros, R. and Toyoda, S.: Les kystes placentaires. Press Méd. **68**:1552–1555, 1960.

Brettner, A.: Zum Verhalten der sekundären Wand der Utero-Plazentargefässe bei der decidualen Reaktion. Acta Anat. (Basel) **57**:367–376, 1964.

Breus, C.: Das Tuberöse Subchoriale Hämatom der Decidua. Eine typische Form der Molenschwangerschaft. F. Deuticke, Leipzig, 1892.

Briese, V. and Muller, H.: Fetomaternal signal transduction by growth factors. Zentralbl. Gynäkol. **114**:219–223, 1992.

Bromley, B., Pitcher, B.L., Klapholz, H., Lichter, E. and Benacerraf, B.R.: Sonographic appearance of uterine scar dehiscence. Intern. J. Gynecol. Obstet. **51**:53–56, 1995.

Brosens, I.: A study of the spiral arteries of the decidua basalis in normotensive and hypertensive pregnancies. J. Obstet. Gynaecol. Brit. Commonw. **71**:222–230, 1964.

Brosens, I.: The utero-placental vessels at term—the distribution and extent of physiological changes. Trophoblast Res. **3**:61–68, 1988.

Brosens, I., Robertson, W.B. and Dixon, H.G.: The physiological response of the vessels of the placental bed to normal pregnancy. J. Pathol. Bacteriol. **93**:569–579, 1967.

Brosens, I., Robertson, W.B. and Dixon, H.G.: The role of the spiral arteries in the pathogenesis of preeclampsia. Obstet. Gynecol. Ann. **1**:177–191, 1972.

Brosens, I., Dixon, H.G. and Robertson, W.B.: Fetal growth retardation and the arteries of the placental bed. Brit. J. Obstet. Gynaecol. **84**:656–663, 1977.

Brosens, J.J., Pijnenborg, R. and Brosens, I.A.: The myometrial junctional zone spiral arteries in normal and abnormal pregnancies: a review of the literature. Amer. J. Obstet. Gynecol. **187**:1416–1423, 2002.

Brown, H.L., Miller, J.M., Khawli, O. and Gabert, H.A.: Premature placental calcification in maternal cigarette smokers. Obstet. Gynecol. **71**:914–917, 1988.

Bryant-Greenwood, G.D., Rees, M.C.P. and Turnbull, A.C.: Immunohistochemical localization of relaxin, prolactin and prostaglandin synthase in human amnion, chorion and decidua. J. Endocr. **114**:491–496, 1987.

Bryant-Greenwood, G.D.: The extracellular matrix of the human fetal membranes: structure and function. Placenta **19**:1–11, 1998.

Bryant-Greenwood, G.D. and Yamamoto, S.Y.: Control of peripartal collagenolysis in the human chorion-decidua. Amer. J. Obstet. Gynecol. **172**:63–70, 1995.

Bühler, F.R.: Randbildungen der menschlichen Placenta. Acta Anat. (Basel) **59**:47–76, 1964.

Bujold, E. and Gauthier, R.J.: Neonatal morbidity associated with uterine rupture: What are the risk factors? Amer. J. Obstet. Gynecol. **186**:311–314, 2002.

Bujold, E., Bujold, C., Hamilton, E.F., Harel, F. and Gauthier, R.J.: The impact of a single-layer or double-layer closure on uterine rupture. Amer. J. Obstet. Gynecol. **186**:1326–1330, 2002a.

Bujold, E., Mehta, S.H., Bujold, C. and Gauthier, R.J.: Inter-delivery interval and uterine rupture. Amer. J. Obstet. Gynecol. **187**:1199–1202, 2002b.

Bulmer, D.: The metrial gland and endometrial granulocytes. J. Anat. **137**:787–826, 1983.

Bulmer, D. and Peel, S.: The demonstration of immunoglobulin in the metrial gland cells of the rat placenta. J. Reprod. Fertil. **49**:143–145, 1977.

Bulmer, D., Stewart, I. and Peel, S.: Endometrial granulocytes of the pregnant hamster. J. Anat. **136**:329–337, 1983.

Bulmer, J.N. and Johnson, P.M.: Macrophage populations in the human placenta and amniochorion. Clin. Exp. Immunol. **57**:393–403, 1984.

Bulmer, J.N. and Sunderland, C.A.: Bone-marrow origin of endometrial granulocytes in the early human placental bed. J. Reprod. Immunol. **5**:383–387, 1983.

Bulmer, J.N., Wells, M., Bhabra, K. and Johnson, P.M.: Immuno-histological characterization of endometrial gland epithelium and extravillous fetal trophoblast in third trimester human placental bed tissues. Brit. J. Obstet. Gynaecol. **93**:823–832, 1986.

Bulmer, J.N., Johnson, P.M., Sasagawa, M. and Takeuchi, S.: Immunohistochemical studies of fetal trophoblast and maternal decidua in hydatidiform mole and choriocarcinoma. Placenta **9**:183–200, 1988a.

Bulmer, J.N., Morrison, L. and Smith, J.C.: Expression of class II MHC gene products by macrophages in human uteroplacental tissue. Immunology **63**:707–714, 1988b.

Bulmer, J.N., Smith, J., Morrison, L. and Wells, M.: Maternal and fetal cellular relationships in the human placental basal plate. Placenta **9**:237–246, 1988c.

Bunton, T.E.: Incidental lesions in nonhuman primate placentae. Vet. Pathol. **23**:431–438, 1986.

Burk, M.R., Troeger, C., Brinkhaus, R., Holzgreve, W. and Hahn, S.: Severely reduced presence of tissue macrophages in the basal plate of pre-eclamptic placentae. Placenta **22**:309–316, 2001.

Burrows, T.D., King, A. and Loke, Y.W.: Expression of integrins by human trophoblast and differential adhesion to laminin or fibronectin. Hum. Reprod. **8**:475–484, 1993a.

Burrows, T.D., King, A. and Loke, Y.W.: Expression of adhesion molecules by human decidual large granular lymphocytes. Cell Immunol. **147**:81–94, 1993b.

Burrows, T.D., King, A. and Loke, Y.W.: Expression of adhesion molecules by endovascular trophoblast and decidual endothelial cells—implications for vascular invasion during implantation. Placenta **15**:21–33, 1994.

Burrows, T.D., King, A. and Loke, Y.W.: Trophoblast–matrix interactions and integrin-mediated signal transduction in vitro. Placenta **16**:A9, 1995.

Burrows, T.D., King, A., Smith, S.K. and Loke Y.W.: Trophoblast-matrix interactions in human implantation. A review. Trophoblast Res. **10**:163–172, 1997.

Caglar, G.S. and Sezik, M.: Repair of an extensive tear of the unscarred uterus resulting from spontaneous rupture. Ann. Saudi Med. **23**:196–197, 2003.

Campbell, S., Rowe, J., Jackson, C.J. and Gallery, E.D.: In vitro migration of cytotrophoblasts through a decidual endothelial cell monolayer: the role of matrix metalloproteinases. Placenta **24**:306–315, 2003.

Campbell, S., Rowe, J., Jackson, C.J. and Gallery, E.D.: Interaction of cocultured decidual endothelial cells and cytotrophoblasts in preeclampsia. Biol. Reprod. **71**:244–252, 2004.

Caniggia, I. and Winter, J.L.: Hypoxia inducible factor-1: oxygen regulation of trophoblast differentiation in normal and pre-eclamptic pregnancies—a review. Placenta **23**(Suppl A):S47–57, 2000.

Caniggia, I., Taylor, C.V., Knox Ritchie, J.W., Lye, S.J. and Letarte, M.: Endoglin regulates trophoblast differentiation along the invasive pathway in human placental villous explants. Endocrinology **138**:4977–4988, 1997.

Caniggia, I., Grisaru-Gravnosky, S., Kuliszewsky, M., Post, M. and Lye, S.J.: Inhibition of TGF-beta (3) restores the invasive capability of extravillous trophoblasts in preeclamptic pregnancies. J. Clin. Invest. **103**:1641–1650, 1999.

Caniggia, I., Winter, J., Lye, S.J. and Post, M.: Oxygen and placental development during the first trimester: implications for the pathophysiology of pre-eclampsia. Placenta **21**(suppl A): S25–30, 2000.

Canning, M.T., Postovit, L.M., Clarke, S.H. and Graham, C.H.: Oxygen-mediated regulation of gelatinase and tissue inhibitor of metalloproteinases-1 expression by invasive cells. Exp. Cell Res. **267**:88–94, 2001.

Carnemolla, B., Borsi, L., Zardi, L., Owens, R.J. and Baralle, F.E.: Localization of the cellular-fibronectin-specific epitope recognized by the monoclonal antibody IST-9 using fusion proteins expressed in E. coli. FEBS Lett. **215**:269–73, 1987.

Carnemolla, B., Balza, E., Siri, A., Zardi, L., Nicotra, M.R., Bigotti, A. and Natali, P.G.: A tumor associated fibronectin isoform generated by alternative splicing of messenger RNA precursors. J. Cell Biol. **108**:1139–48, 1989.

Carraway, K.L. and Cantley, L.C.: A new acquaintance for erbB3 and erbB4: A role for receptor heterodimerization in growth signaling. Cell **78**:5–8, 1994.

Carter, A.M.: When is the maternal placental circulation established in man? Placenta **18**:83–87, 1997.

Carter, J.E., Vellios, F. and Huber, C.P.: Histologic classification and incidence of circulatory lesions of the human placenta, with a review of the literature. Amer. J. Clin. Pathol. **40**:374–378, 1963.

Cartwright, J.E., Holden, D.P. and Whitley, G.S.: Hepatocyte growth factor regulates human trophoblast motility and invasion: a role for nitric oxide. Br. J. Pharmacol. **128**:181–189, 1999.

Cartwright, P.S., Brown, J.E., Davis, R.J., Thieme, G.A. and Boehm, F.H.: Advanced abdominal pregnancy associated with fetal pulmonary hypoplasia: report of a case. Amer. J. Obstet. Gynecol. **155**:396–397, 1986.

Caruso, L.J., Liegner, B. and Tamis, A.B.: Advanced abdominal pregnancy: report of a case. Obstet. Gynecol. **22**:795–797, 1963.

Casey, M.L., Delgadillo, M., Cox, K.A., Nisert, S. and MacDonald, P.C.: Inactivation of prostaglandins in human decidua vera (parietalis) tissue: substrate specificity of prostaglandin dehydrogenase. Amer. J. Obstet. Gynecol. **160**:3–7, 1989.

Castellucci, M., Kaufmann, P. and Bischof, P.: Extracellular matrix influences hormone and protein production by human chorionic villi. Cell Tissue Res. **262**:135–142, 1990.

Castellucci, M., Classen-Linke, I., Mühlhauser, J., Kaufmann, P. and Zardi, L.: The human placenta: a model for tenascin expression. Histochemistry **95**:449–458, 1991.

Castellucci, M., Crescimanno, C., Schröter, C.A., Kaufmann, P. and Mühlhauser, J.: Extravillous trophoblast: immunohistochemical localization of extracellular matrix molecules. In, Frontiers in Gynecologic and Obstetric Investigation. A.R. Genazzani, F. Petraglia, A.D. Genazzani, eds. Parthenon Publishing Group, New York, pp. 19–25, 1993.

Castellucci, M., Theelen, T., Pompili, E., Fumagalli, L., De Renzis, G. and Mühlhauser, J.: Immunohistochemical localization of serine-protease inhibitors in the human placenta. Cell Tissue Res. **278**:283–289, 1994.

Castellucci, M., De Matteis, R., Meisser, A., Cancello, R., Monsurro, V., Islami, D., Sarzani, R., Marzioni, D., Cinti, S. and Bischof, P.: Leptin modulates extracellular matrix molecules and metalloproteinases: possible implications for trophoblast invasion. Mol. Hum. Reprod. **6**:951–958, 2000.

Cava, E.F. and Russell, W.M.: Intramural pregnancy with uterine rupture. A case report. Amer. J. Obstet. Gynecol. **131**:214–216, 1978.

Chakraborty, C., Gleeson, L.M., McKinnon, T. and Lala, P.K.: Regulation of human trophoblast migration and invasiveness. Can. J. Physiol. Pharmacol. **80**:116–124, 2002.

Chaouat, G., Kolb, J.P. and Wegmann, T.G.: The murine placenta as an immunological barrier between the mother and the fetus. Immunol. Rev. **75**:31–60, 1983.

Chaouat, G., Tranchot Diallo, J., Volumenie, J.L., Menu, E., Gras, G., Delage, G. and Mognetti, B.: Immune suppression and Th1/Th2 balance in pregnancy revisited: a (very) personal tribute to Tom Wegmann. Amer. J. Reprod. Immun. **37**:427–434, 1997.

Chauhan, S.P., Martin, J.N., Henrichs, C.E., Morrison, J.C. and Magann, E.F.: Maternal and perinatal complications with uterine rupture in 142,075 patients who attempted vaginal birth after cesarean delivery: A review of the literature. Amer. J. Obstet. Gynecol. **189**:408–417, 2003.

Cheng, W.F., Ho, H.N., Yang, Y.S. and Huang, S.C.: Abdominal pregnancy after gonadotropin superovulation and intrauterine insemination: A case report. Amer. J. Obstet. Gynecol. **171**:1394–1395, 1994.

Chernyshov, V.P., Slukvin, I.I. and Bondarenko, G.I.: Phenotypic characterization of CD7+, CD3+, and Cd8+ lymphocytes from first trimester human decidua using two-color flow cytometry. Amer. J. Reprod. Immunol. **29**:5–16, 1993.

Cheung, P.Y., Walton, J.C., Tai, H.H., Riley, S.C. and Challis, J.R.: Immunocytochemical distribution and localization of 15–hydroxyprostaglandin dehydrogenase in human fetal membranes, decidua, and placenta. Amer. J. Obstet. Gynecol. **163**:1445–1449, 1990.

Cheung, P.Y., Walton, J.C., Tai, H.H., Riley, S.C. and Challis, J.R.: Localization of 15–hydroxy prostaglandin dehydrogenase in human fetal membranes, decidua, and placenta during pregnancy. Gynecol. Obstet. Invest. **33**:142–146, 1992.

Chiquet-Ehrismann, R., Mackie, E.J., Pearson, C.A. and Sakakura, T.: Tenascin: an extracellular matrix protein involved in tissue interactions during fetal development and oncogenesis. Cell **47**:131–139, 1986.

Chokroverty, M., Caballes, R.L. and Gear, P.E.: An unruptured tubal pregnancy at term. Arch. Pathol. Lab. Med. **110**:250–251, 1986.

Chou, M.M. and Ho, E.S.C.: Prenatal diagnosis of placenta previa accreta with power amplitude ultrasonic angiography. Amer. J. Obstet. Gynecol. **177**:1523–1525, 1997.

Chou, C.S., Zhu, H., Shalev, E., MacCalman, C.D. and Leung, P.C.: The effects of gonadotropin-releasing hormone (GnRH) I and GnRH II on the urokinase-type plasminogen activator/plasminogen activator inhibitor system in human extravillous cytotrophoblasts in vitro. J. Clin. Endocrinol. Metab. **87**:5594–5603, 2002.

Choy, M.Y., Siu, S.S., Leung, T.N. and Lau, T.K.: Human decidual production of hepatocyte-growth factor is not influenced by trophoblastic invasion in vivo. Fertil. Steril. **82** Suppl. 3:1220–1225, 2004.

Chumbley, G., King, A., Gardner, L., Howlett, S., Holmes, N. and Loke, Y.W.: Generation of an antibody to HLA-G in transgenic mice and demonstration of the tissue reactivity of this antibody. J. Reprod. Immunol. **27**:173–186, 1994a.

Chumbley, G., King, A., Robertson, K., Holmes, N. and Loke, Y.W.: Resistance of HLA-G and HLA-A2 transfectants to lysis by decidual NK cells. Cell Immunol. **155**:312–322, 1994b.

Chung, S.I.: Comparative studies on tissue transglutaminase and factor XIII. Ann. N.Y. Acad. Sci. **202**:240–255, 1972.

Church, H.J., Vicovac, L.M. Williams, J.D., Hey, N.A. and Aplin, J.D.: Laminins 2 and 4 are expressed by human decidual cells. Lab. Invest. **74**:21–32, 1996.

Church, H.J., Richards, A.J. and Aplin, J.D.: Laminins in decidua, placenta and choriocarcinoma cells. Trophoblast Res. **10**:143–162, 1997.

Chwalisz, K. and Garfield, R.: Role of progesterone during pregnancy: models of parturition and preeclampsia. Geburtsh. Perinatol. **198**:170–180, 1994.

Clewell, W.H. and Manchester, D.K.: Recurrent maternal floor infarction: a preventable cause of fetal death. Amer. J. Obstet. Gynecol. **147**:346–347, 1983.

Cohain, J.S.: The many ways to sew up a uterus. "Single-layer" vs. "double-layer" cesarean repair: what's best? Midwifery Today Int. Midwife **70**:32–34, 2004.

Colbern, G.T., Chiang, M.H. and Main, E.K.: Expression of the nonclassic histocompatibility antigen HLA-G by preeclamptic placenta. Amer. J. Obstet. Gynecol. **170**:1244–1250, 1994.

Coleman, R.W., Marder, V.J., Salzman, E.W. and Hirsh, J.: Overview of hemostasis. In: Coleman, R.W., Hirsh, J., Marder, V.J. and Salzman, E.W. (eds.) Hemostasis and Thrombosis (2nd edition). J.P. Lippincott, Philadelphia pp. 3–17, 1987.

Comstock, C.H., Love, J.J., Bronsteen, R.A., Lee, W., Vettraino, I.M., Huang, R.R. and Lorenz, R.P.: Sonographic detection of placenta accrete in the second and third trimesters of pregnancy. Amer. J. Obstet. Gynecol. **190**:1135–1140, 2004.

Corsi, L., Allemanni, G., Gaggero, B. and Zardi, L.: Extracellular pH controls pre-mRNA alternative splicing of tenascin-C in normal, but not malignantly transformed cells. Int. J. Cancer **66**:632–635, 1996.

Coukos, G., Gafvelsa, M.E., Wisel, S., Ruelaz, E.A., Strickland, D.K., Strauss, J.F. and Coutifaris, C.: Expression of alpha 2–macroglobulin receptor/low density lipoprotein receptor-related protein and the 39–kd receptor-associated protein in human trophoblasts. Amer. J. Pathol. **144**:383–392, 1994.

Cox, S.M., Carpenter, R.J. and Cotton, D.B.: Placenta percreta: ultrasound diagnosis and conservative surgical management. Obstet. Gynecol. **71**:454–456, 1988.

Crabtree, K.E., Collet, B. and Kilpatrick, S.J.: Puerperal presentation of a living abdominal pregnancy. Obstet. Gynecol. **84**:646–648, 1994.

Cramer, S.F.: Letter to the Editor. Pediatr. Pathol. **7**:473–447, 1987.

Craven, C.M. and Ward, K.: Alpha smooth muscle actin is preserved in arteries showing physiologic change. Placenta **17**:A17, 1996.

Craven, C., Zhao, L. and Ward, K.: Trophoblast $\beta1$ & $\beta4$ integrin switching in villous invasion of decidual veins, a mechanism of lateral placental growth. Placenta **18**:A18, 1997.

Craven, C.M., Morgan, T. and Ward, K.: Decidual spiral artery remodelling begins before cellular interaction with cytotrophoblasts. Placenta **19**:241–252, 1998.

Craven, C.M., Zhao, L. and Ward, K.: Lateral placental growth occurs by trophoblast cell invasion of decidual veins. Placenta **21**:160–169, 2000.

Cross, J.C., Baczyk, D., Dobric, N., Hemberger, M., Hughes, M. and Simmons, D.G.: Genes, development and evolution of the placenta. Placenta **24**:123–130, 2003.

Currie, C.A. and Bagshawe, K.D.: The masking of antigens on trophoblast and cancer cells. Lancet **1**:708–710, 1967.

Dallenbach, F.D. and Dallenbach-Hellweg, G.: Immunohistologische Untersuchungen zur Lokalisation des Relaxins in menschlicher Placenta und Decidua. Virchows Arch. [Pathol. Anat.] **337**:301–316, 1964.

Dallenbach-Hellweg, G.: Histopathology of the Endometrium. pp. 24–27. Springer-Verlag, Berlin, 1971.

Dallenbach-Hellweg, G. and Nette, G.: Über Proteineinschlüsse in basalen Trophoblastzellen der reifen menschlichen Plazenta. Virchows Arch. [Pathol. Anat.] **336**:528–543, 1963a.

Dallenbach-Hellweg, G. and Nette, G.: Über Glykoproteideinschlüsse in den Trophoblastzellen der menschlichen Plazenta und die Frage ihres Zusammenhangs mit der Bildung von Gonadotropin. Z. Zellforsch. **61**:145–158, 1963b.

Dallenbach-Hellweg, G. and Nette, G.: Morphological and histochemical observations on trophoblast and decidua of the basal plate of the human placenta at term. Amer. J. Anat. **115**:309–326, 1964.

Dallenbach-Hellweg, G. and Sievers, S.: Die histologische Reaktion des Endometrium auf lokal applizierte Gestagene. Virchows Arch. Pathol. Anat. **368**:289–298, 1975.

Daly, D.C., Maslar, I.A. and Riddick, D.H.: Prolactin production during in vitro decidualization of proliferative endometrium. Amer. J. Obstet. Gynecol. **145**:672–678, 1983.

Damsky, C.H., Fitzgerald, M.L. and Fisher, S.J.: Distribution patterns of extracellular matrix components and adhesion receptors are intricately modulated during first trimester cytotrophoblast differentiation along the invasive pathway, in vivo. J. Clin. Invest. **89**:210–222, 1992.

Damsky, C., Sutherland, A. and Fisher, S.: Extracellular matrix 5: Adhesive interactions in early mammalian embryogenesis, implantation, and placentation. FASEB J. **7**:1320–1329, 1993.

Damsky, C.H., Librach, D., Lim, K.H., Fitzgerald, M.L., McMaster, M.T., Janatpour, M., Zhou, Y., Logan, S.K. and Fisher, S.J.: Integrin switching regulates normal trophoblast invasion. Development **120**:3657–3666, 1994.

Davies, B.R., Casanueva, E. and Arroyo, P.: Placentas of small-for-dates infants: a small controlled series from Mexico City, Mexico. Amer. J. Obstet. Gynecol. **149**:731–736, 1984.

Davis, J.D. and Cruz, A.: Persistent placenta increta: A complication of conservative management of presumed placenta accreta. Obstet. Gynecol. **88**:653–654, 1996.

Daya, D. and Sabet, L.: The use of cytokeratin as a sensitive and reliable marker for trophoblastic tissue. Amer. J. Clin. Pathol. **95**:137–141, 1991.

de Bakker-Theunissen, O.J.G.B., Arts, N.F.T. and Mulder, G.H.: Fluid transport across human fetal membranes affected by human amniotic fluid prolactin: an in vitro study. Placenta **9**:533–545, 1988.

Debiasi, E., Damiani, N. and Capodacqua, R.: Contributo allo studio della circolazione utero-placentare nelle donna. Minerva Ginecol. **15**:539–545, 1963.

Defilippi, P., Silengo, L. and Tarone, G.: Alpha 6 beta 1 integrin (laminin receptor) is down regulated by tumor necrosis factor alpha and interleukin 1 beta in human endothelial cells. J. Biol. Chem. **267**:18303–18307, 1992.

Demir, R. and Erbengi, T.: The cells of the intercotyledonary septae in full-term placenta. In, Proceedings of the 8th European Congress of Electron Microscopy. **3**:2017–2018, 1984.

Dessouky, D.A.: Ectopic trophoblast as a complication of first-trimester induced abortion. Amer. J. Obstet. Gynecol. **136**:407–408, 1980.

DeWane, J.C. and McCubbin, J.H.: Spontaneous rupture of an unscarred uterus at 19 weeks' gestation. Amer. J. Obstet. Gynecol. **141**:222–223, 1981.

DeWolf, F., DeWolf-Peeters, C. and Brosens, I.: Ultrastructure of the spiral arteries in the human placental bed at the end of normal pregnancy. Amer. J. Obstet. Gynecol. **117**:833–848, 1973.

DeWolf, F., Brosens, I. and Renaer, M.: Fetal growth retardation and the maternal arterial supply of the human placenta in the absence of sustained hypertension. Brit. J. Obstet. Gynaecol. **87**:678–685, 1980.

Dietl, J., Horny, H.-P., Ruck, P., Marzusch, K., Kaiserling, E., Griesser, H. and Kabelitz, D.: Intradecidual T-lymphocytes lack immunohistochemically detectable T-Cell receptors. Amer. J. Reprod. Immunol. **24**:33–36, 1990.

Dietl, J., Ruck, P., Horny, H.P., Handgretinger, R., Marzusch, K., Ruck, M., Kaiserling, E., Griesser, H. and Kabelitz, D.: The decidua of early human pregnancy—immunohistochemistry and function of immunocompetent cells. Gynecol. Obstet. Invest. **33**:197–204, 1992.

DiFederico, E., Genbacev, O. and Fisher, S.J.: Preeclampsia is associated with widespread apoptosis of placental cytotrophoblasts within the uterine wall. Amer. J. Pathol. **155**:293–301, 1999.

DiPersio, C.M., Shah, S. and Hynes, R.O.: α3β1 integrin localizes to focal contacts in response to diverse extracellular matrix proteins. J. Cell Sci. **108**:2321–2336, 1995.

Di Simone, N., Castellani, R., Caliandro, D. and Caruso, A.: Antiphospholipid antibodies regulate the expression of trophoblast cell adhesion molecules. Fertil. Steril. **77**:805–811, 2002.

Divers, M.J., Bulmer, J.N., Miller, D. and Lilford, R.F.: Beta 1 integrins in third trimester human placentae: no differential expression in pathological pregnancy. Placenta **16**:245–260, 1995.

Dohrn, M.: Ein Beitrag zur mikroskopischen Anatomie der reifen menschlichen Eihüllen. Monatsschr. Geburtshilfe Frauenkr. **26**:114–127, 1865.

Dokras, A., Gardner, L.M., Seftor, E.A. and Hendrix, M.J.: Regulation of human cytotrophoblast morphogenesis by hepatocyte growth factor/scatter factor. Biol. Reprod. **65**:1278–1288 2001.

Dover, R.W. and Powell, M.C.: Management of a primary abdominal pregnancy. Amer. J. Obstet. Gynecol. **172**:1603–1604, 1995.

Dubois, J., Garel, L., Grignon, A., Lemay, M. and Leduc, L.: Placenta percreta: Balloon occlusion and embolization of the iliac arteries to reduce intraoperative blood loss. Amer. J. Obstet. Gynecol. **176**:723–726, 1997.

Duello, T.M., Bertics, P.J., Fulgham, D.L. and Vaness, P.: Localization of epidermal growth factor receptors in first- and third-trimester human placentas. J. Histochem. Cytochem. **42**:907–915, 1994.

Duncan, D.A. and Mazur, M.T.: Trophoblastic tumors: ultrastructural comparison of choriocarcinoma and placental-site trophoblastic tumor. Hum. Pathol. **20**:370–381, 1989.

Durnwald, C. and Mercer, B.: Uterine rupture, perioperative and perinatal morbidity after single-layer and double-layer closure at cesarean delivery. Amer. J. Obstet. Gynecol. **189**:925–929, 2003.

Durst-Zivkovic, B.: Endometrial granular cells in fetal membranes. Anat. Anz. **143**:258–261, 1978.

Dvorak, H.F., Senger, D.R. and Dvorak, A.M.: Fibrin as a component of the tumor stroma: origins and biological significance. Cancer Metastasis Rev. **2**:41–73, 1983.

Earl, U.M., Bulmer, J.N. and Briones, A.: Placenta accreta: an immunohistological study of trophoblast populations. Placenta **8**:273–282, 1987.

Earl, U., Morrison, L., Gray, C. and Bulmer, J.N.: Proteinase and proteinase inhibitor localization in the human placenta. Int. J. Gynecol. Pathol. **8**:114–124, 1989.

Edwards, D., Jones, C.J.P., Sibley, C.P., Farmer, D.R. and Nelson, D.M.: Areas of syncytial denudation may provide routes for paracellular diffusion across the human placenta. Placenta **12**:383 (abstract), 1991.

Ehrig, K., Leivo, I., Argraves, W.S., Ruoslahti, E. and Engvall, E.: Merosin, a tissue-specific basement membrane protein, is a laminin-like protein. Proc. Natl. Acad. Sci. U.S.A. **87**:3264–3268, 1990.

Eidelman, S., Damsky, C.H., Wheelock, M.J. and Damjanov, I.: Expression of the cell-cell adhesion glycoprotein cell-CAM 120/80 in normal human tissues and tumors. Amer. J. Pathol. **135**:101–110, 1989.

Einbrodt, H.J. and Schmid, K.O.: Über abnorme Verkalkungen der menschlichen Placenta bei Maternitätstetanie. Arch. Gynäkol. **200**:327–339, 1965.

Einbrodt, H.J., Schiereck, F.W. and Kinny, H.: Über die Ablagerung von Blei in den Verkalkungen der menschlichen Placenta. Arch. Gynäkol. **213**:303–306, 1973.

Eldar Geva, T., Rachmilewitz, J., De Groot, N. and Hochberg, A.A.: Interaction between choriocarcinoma cell line (JAr) and human cytotrophoblasts in vitro. Placenta **14**:217–223, 1993.

Emonard, H., Christiane, Y., Smet, M., Grimaud, J.A. and Foidart, J.M.: Type IV and interstitial collagenolytic activities in normal and malignant trophoblast cells are specifically regulated by the extracellular matrix. Invasion Metastasis **10**:170–177, 1990.

Enders, A.C.: Fine structure of anchoring villi of the human placenta. Amer. J. Anat. **122**:419–452, 1968.

Enders, A.C.: Current topic: structural responses of the primate endometrium to implantation. Placenta **12**:309–325, 1991.

Enders, A.C.: Transition from lacunar to villous stage of implantation in the macaque, including establishment of the trophoblastic shell. Acta Anat. **152**:151–169, 1995.

Enders, A.C.: Cytodifferentiation of trophoblast in the anchoring villi and trophoblastic shell in the first half of gestation in the macaque. Microsc. Res. Tech. **38**:3–20, 1997a.

Enders, A.C.: Cytotrophoblast invasion of the endometrium in the human and macaque early villous stage of implantation. Trophoblast Res. **10**:83–95, 1997b.

Enders, A.C. and Blankenship, T.N.: Modification of endometrial arteries during invasion by cytotrophoblast cells in the pregnant macaque. Acta Anat. **159**:169–193, 1997.

Enders, A.C., Lantz, K.C. and Schlafke, S.: Preference of invasive cytotrophoblast for maternal Vessels in early implantation in the macaque. Acta Anat. **155**:145–162, 1996.

Endres, L.K. and Barnhart, K.: Spontaneous second trimester uterine rupture after classical cesarean. Obstet. Gynecol. **96**:806–808, 2000.

Ermocilla, R. and Altshuler, G.: The origin of "X cells" of the human placenta and their possible relationship to intrauterine growth retardation: An enigma. Amer. J. Obstet. Gynecol. **117**:1137–1140, 1973.

Fait, G., Goyert, G., Sundareson, A. and Pickens, A.: Intramural pregnancy with fetal survival: case history and discussion of etiologic factors. Obstet. Gynecol. **70**:472–474, 1987.

Faller, T. and Ferenci, P.: Der Aufbau der Placenta-Septen: Untersuchungen mit Hilfe der Quinacrinfluorescenzfärbung des Y-Chromatins. Z. Anat. Entwicklungsgesch. **142**:207–217, 1973.

Faulk, P., Trenchev, P., Dorling, J. and Holborow, J.: Antigens on post-implantation placentae. In, Immunobiology of Trophoblast. R.G. Edwards, C.W.S. Howe and M.H. Johnson, eds. Cambridge University Press, Cambridge, pp. 113–130, 1975.

Faulk, W.P.: Placental fibrin. Amer. J. Reprod. Immunol. **19**:132–135, 1989.

Fazleabas, A.T., Verhage, H.G., Waites, G. and Bell, S.C.: Characterization of an insulin-like growth factor binding protein, analogous to human pregnancy-associated secreted endometrial alpha 1–globulin, in decidua of the baboon (Papio anubis) placenta. Biol. Reprod. **40**:873–885, 1989.

Feinberg, R.F. and Kliman, H.J.: Tropho-uteronectin (TUN): A unique oncofetal fibronectin deposited in the extracellular matrix of the tropho-uterine junction and regulated in vitro by cultured human trophoblast cells. Trophoblast Res. **7**:167–181, 1993.

Feinberg, R.F., Kao, L.C., Haimowitz, J.E., Queenan, J.T., Jr., Wun, T.C., Strauss, J.F. and Kliman, H.J.: Plasminogen activator inhibitor types 1 and 2 in human trophoblasts. PAI-1 is an immunocytochemical marker of invading trophoblasts. Lab. Invest. **61**:20–26, 1989.

Feinberg, R.F., Kliman, H.J. and Cohen, A.W.: Preeclampsia, trisomy 13, and the placental bed. Obstet. Gynecol. **78**:505–508, 1991a.

Feinberg, R.F., Kliman, H.J. and Lockwood, C.J.: Is oncofetal fibronectin a trophoblast glue for human implantation? Amer. J. Pathol. **138**:537–543, 1991b.

Feinberg, R.F., Kliman, H.J. and Wang, C.-L.: Transforming growth factor-beta stimulates trophoblast oncofetal fibronectin synthesis in vitro: implications for trophoblast implantation in vivo. J. Clin. Endocrinol. Metab. **78**:1241–1248, 1994.

Fernandez, P.L., Merino, M.J., Nogales, F.F., Charonis, A.S., Stetler Stevenson, W.G. and Liotta, L.: Immunohistochemical profile of basement membrane proteins and 72 kilodalton type-IV collagenase in the implantation placental site—an integrated view. Lab. Invest. **66**:572–579. 1992.

Ferry, B.L., Starkey, P.M., Sargent, I.L., Watt, G.M.O., Jackson, M., and Redman, C.W.G.: Cell populations in the human early pregnancy decidua: natural killer activity and response to interleukin-2 of CD56–positive large granular lymphocytes. Immunology **70**:446–452, 1990.

Filla, M.S., Zhang, C.X. and Kaul, K.L.: A potential transforming growth factor alpha/epidermal growth factor receptor autocrine circuit in placental cytotrophoblasts. Cell Growth and Differentiation **4**:387–393, 1993.

Finberg, H.J. and Williams, J.W.: Placenta accreta: Prospective sonographic diagnosis in patients with placenta previa and prior cesarean section. J. Ultrasound Med. **11**:333–343, 1992.

Fisher, S.J. and Damsky, C.H.: Human cytotrophoblast invasion. Semin. Cell Biol. **4**:183–188, 1993.

Fisher, S.J., Leitch, M.S., Kantor, M.S., Basbaum, C.B. and Kramer, R.H.: Degradation of extracellular matrix by the trophoblastic cells of first-trimester human placentas. J. Cell Biochem. **27**:31–41, 1985.

Fisher, S.J., Cui, T.Y., Zhang, L., Hartman, L., Grahl, K., Guo-Yang, Z., Tarpey, J. and Damsky, C.H.: Adhesive and degradative properties of human placental cytotrophoblast cells in vitro. J. Cell Biol. **109**:891–902, 1989.

Fisher, S.J., Librach, D.L., Fitzgerald, M.L. and Damsky, C.H.: Human cytotrophoblast invasion is mediated by metalloproteinases and α1 integrins and is accompanied by changes in the expression of adhesion molecules and HLA-G. Placenta **12**:387–388, 1991.

Fisher, S.J., Librach, C., Zhou, Y., Dao, D., Kosten, K., Roth, I., Bass, K. and Damsky, C.H.: Regulation of human cytotrophoblast invasion. Placenta **13**:A.17, 1992.

Fitzpatrick, T.E. and Graham, C.H.: Stimulation of plasminogen activator inhibitor-1 expression in immortalized human trophoblast cells cultured under low levels of oxygen. Exp. Cell Res. **245**:155–162, 1998.

Floridon, C., Nielsen, O., Holund, B., Sunde, L., Westergaard, J.G., Thomsen, S.G. and Teisner, B.: Localization of E-cadherin in villous, extravillous and vascular trophoblasts during intrauterine, ectopic and molar pregnancy. Mol. Hum. Reprod. **6**:943–950, 2000.

Flug, M. and Köpf-Maier, P.: The basement membrane and its involvement in carcinoma cell invasion. Acta Anat. **152**:69–84, 1995.

Fox, H.: Calcification of the placenta. J. Obstet. Gynaecol. Brit. Commonw. **71**:759–765, 1964.

Fox, H.: The significance of placental infarction in perinatal morbidity and mortality. Biol. Neonat. **11**:87–105, 1967.

Fox, H.: Placenta accreta, 1945–1969. Obstet. Gynecol. Surv. **27**:475–490, 1972.

Fox, H.: Pathology of the Placenta. 1st edition, Saunders, London, 1978.

Fox, H.: Pathology of the Placenta. 2nd edition, Saunders, London, 1997.

Frachtman, K.G.: Unruptured tubal term pregnancy. Amer. J. Surg. **86**:161–168, 1953.

Frank, H.G., Malekzadeh, F., Kertschanska, S., Crescimanno, C., Castellucci, M., Lang, I., Desoye, G. and Kaufmann, P.: Immunohistochemistry of two different types of placental fibrinoid. Acta Anat. **150**:55–68, 1994.

Frank, H.G., Huppertz, B., Kertschanska, S., Blanchard, D., Roelcke, D. and Kaufmann, P.: Anti-adhesive glycosylation of fibronectin-like molecules in human placental matrix-type fibrinoid. Histochem. Cell Biol. **104**:317–329, 1995.

Frank, H.G., Gunawan, B., Ebeling-Stark, I., Schulten, H.J., Funayama, H., Cremer, U., Huppertz, B., Gaus, G., Kaufmann, P. and Füzesi, L.: Cytogenetic and DNA-fingerprint characterization of choriocarcinoma cell lines and a trophoblast/choriocarcinoma cell hybrid. Cancer Gen. Cytogen. **116**:16–22, 2000.

Franken, H.: Beitrag zur Veranschaulichung von Struktur und Funktion der Plazenta. Zentralbl. Gynäkol. **76**:729–745, 1954.

Freese, U.E.: The uteroplacental vascular relationship in the human. Amer. J. Obstet. Gynecol. **101**:8–16, 1968.

Freese, U.E. and Maciolek, B.J.: Plastoid injection studies of the uteroplacental vascular relationship in the human. Obstet. Gynecol. **33**:160–169, 1969.

Friedl, P. and Brocker, E.B.: The biology of cell locomotion within three-dimensional extracellular matrix. Cell Mol. Life Sci. **57**:41–64, 2000.

Friedman, A., deFazio, J. and deCherney, A.: Severe obstetric complications after aggressive treatment of Asherman syndrome. Obstet. Gynecol. **67**:864–867, 1986.

Fuchs, A.R. and Fuchs, F.: Endocrinology of human parturition: a review. Brit. J. Obstet. Gynaecol. **91**:948–967, 1984.

Fujii, T., Ishitani, A. and Geraghty, D.E.: A soluble form of the HLA-G antigen is encoded by a messenger ribonucleic acid containing intron 4. J. Immunol. **153**:5516–5524, 1994.

Fujikura, T.: Placental calcification and maternal age. Amer. J. Obstet. Gynecol. **87**:41–45, 1963a.

Fujikura, T.: Placental calcification and seasonal difference. Amer. J. Obstet. Gynecol. **87**:46–47, 1963b.

Fujikura, T.: The openings of uteroplacental vessels with villous infiltration at different gestational ages. Arch. Pathol. Lab. Med. **129**:382–385, 2005.

Fujikura, T. and Sho, S.: Placental cavities. Obstet. Gynecol. **90**:112–116, 1997.

Fukamatsu, Y., Tomita, K. and Fukuta, T.: Further evidence of prolactin production from human decidua and its transport across fetal membrane. Gynecol. Obstet. Invest. **17**:309–316, 1984.

Fylstra, D.L., Pound-Chang, T., Miller, G., Cooper, A. and Miller, K.M.: Ectopic pregnancy within a cesarean section delivery scar: A case report. Amer. J. Obstet. Gynecol. **187**:302–304, 2002.

Garel, J.-M. and Barlet, J.-P.: Calcitonin in the mother, fetus and newborn. Ann. Biol. Anim. Biochem. Biophys. **18**:53–68, 1978.

Garfield, R.E., Yallampalli, C., Buhimschi, I. and Chwalisz, K.: Reversal of preeclampsia symptoms induced in rats by nitric oxide inhibition with L-arginine, steroid hormones and an endothelin antagonist. Soc. Gynecol. Invest., Chicago (III) Abstract No. 384, 1994.

Geiser, A.G., Letterio, J.J., Kulkarni, A.B. Karlsson, S., Roberts, A.B. and Sporn, M.B.: Transforming growth factor beta 1 (TGF-beta 1) controls expression of major histocompatibility genes in the postnatal mouse: aberrant histocompatibility antigen expression in the pathogenesis of the TGF-beta null

mouse phenotype. Proceedings of the National Academy of Sciences USA **90**:9944–9948, 1993.

Geller, H.F.: Über die Bedeutung des subchorialen Fibrinstreifens in der menschlichen Plazenta. Arch. Gynäkol. **192**:1–6, 1959.

Genbacev, O., Papic, N., Cuperlovic, M., Vicovac, L., Vuckovic, M. and Miller, R.K.: First trimester chorionic villous explants in culture as a model to study the origin and characteristics of extravillous cytotrophoblast. Placenta **12**:389 (abstract), 1991.

Genbacev, O., Schubach, S.A. and Miller, R.K.: Villous culture of first trimester human placenta—model to study extravillous trophoblast EVT) differentiation. Placenta **13**:439–461, 1992.

Genbacev, O., White, T.E.K., Gavin, C.E. and Miller, R.K.: Human trophoblast cultures: models for implantation and peri-implantation toxicology. Reproduct. Toxicol. **7**:75–94, 1993a.

Genbacev, O., DeMesey Jensen, K., Schubach Powlin, S. and Miller, R.K.: In vitro differentiation and ultrastructure of human extravillous trophoblast (EVT) cells. Placenta **14**:463–475, 1993b.

Genbacev, O., Gerdner, K. and Miller, R.K.: Human cytotrophoblastic cell islands from first trimester placentae—proliferative and functional activity in vitro. Placenta **14**:A.25, 1993c.

Genbacev, O., Powlin, S.S. and Miller, R.K.: Regulation of human extravillous trophoblast (EVT) cell differentiation and proliferation in vitro—role of epidermal growth factor (EGF). Trophoblast Res. **8**:427–442, 1994.

Genbacev, O., Joslin, R., Damsky, C.H., Polliotti, B.M. and Fisher, S.J.: Hypoxia alters early gestation human cytotrophoblast differentiation/invasion in vitro and models the placental defects that occur in preeclampsia. J. Clin. Invest. **97**:540–550, 1996.

Genbacev, O., Zhou, Y., Ludlow, J.W. and Fisher S.J.: Regulation of human placental development by oxygen tension. Science **277**:1669–1672, 1997.

Genbacev, O., DiFederico, E., McMaster, M. and Fisher, S.J. Invasive cytotrophoblast apoptosis in pre-eclampsia. Hum. Reprod. **14**:59–66, 1999.

Genbacev, O., Krtolica, A., Kaelin, W. and Fisher, S.J.: Human cytotrophoblast expression of the von Hippel-Lindau protein is downregulated during uterine invasion in situ and upregulated by hypoxia in vitro. Dev. Biol. **233**:526–536, 2001.

Gielchinsky, Y., Rojansky, N., Fasouliotis, S.J. and Ezra, Y.: Placenta accreta—summary of 10 years: a survey of 310 cases. Placenta **23**:210–214, 2002.

Gille, J., Börner, P., Reinecke, J., Krause, P.-H. and Deicher, H.: Über die Fibrinoidablagerungen in den Endzotten der menschlichen Placenta. Arch. Gynäkol. **217**:263–271, 1974.

Giudice, L.C., Mark S.P. and Irwin, J.C.: Paracrine actions of insulin-like growth factors and IGF binding protein-1 in non-pregnant human endometrium and at the decidual-trophoblast interface. J. Reprod. Immunol. **39**:133–148, 1998.

Gleich, G.J. and Adolphson, C.R.: The eosinophilic leukocyte: Structure and function. Adv. in Immunol. **39**:177–253, 1986.

Glienke, W.: Zur Ultrastruktur der Septen der menschlichen Plazenta. Z. Mikrosk. Anat. Forsch. **88**:111–147, 1974.

Golander, A., Hurley, T.W., Barret, J. and Handwerger, S.: Synthesis of prolactin by human decidua in vitro. J. Endocrinol. **82**:263–267, 1979.

Gosseye, S. and Fox, H.: An immunohistological comparison of the secretory capacity of villous and extravillous trophoblast in the human placenta. Placenta 5:329–348, 1984.

Grabowska, A., Chumbley, G., Carter, N. and Loke, Y.W.: Human trophoblast cells in culture express an unusual major histocompatibility complex class I-like antigen. Amer. J. Reprod. Immun. 23:10–18, 1990.

Graham, C.H. and Lala, P.K.: Mechanism of control of trophoblast invasion in situ. J. Cellular Physiol. 148:228–234, 1991.

Graham, C.H. and McCrae, K.R.: Altered expression of gelatinase and surface-associated plasminogen activator activity by trophoblast cells isolated from placentas of preeclamptic patients. Amer. J. Obstet. Gynecol. 175:555–562, 1996.

Graham, C.H., Lysiak, J.J., McCrae, K.R. and Lala, P.K.: Localization of transforming growth factor-beta at the human fetal-maternal interface: role in trophoblast growth and differentiation. Biol. Reprod. 46:561–572, 1992.

Graham, C.H., Fitzpatrick, T.E. and McCrae, K.R.: Hypoxia stimulates urokinase receptor expression through a heme-protein-dependent pathway. Blood 91:3300–3307, 1998.

Graham, C.H., Postovit, L.M., Park, H., Canning, M.T. and Fitzpatrick, T.E.: Role of oxygen in the regulation of trophoblast gene expression and invasion. Placenta 21:443–450, 2000.

Grannum, P.A.T., Berkowitz, R.L. and Hobbins, J.C.: The ultrasonic changes in the maturing placenta and their relation to fetal pulmonic maturity. Amer. J. Obstet. Gynecol. 133:915–922, 1979.

Gribble, R.K. and Fitzsimmons, J.M.: Placenta previa percreta with fetal survival. Amer. J. Obstet. Gynecol. 153:314–316, 1985.

Grosser, O.: Über Fibrin und Fibrinoid in der Placenta. Z. Anat. Entwicklungsgesch. 76:304–314, 1925.

Grosser, O.: Frühentwicklung, Eihautbildung und Placentation des Menschen und der Säugetiere. J.F. Bergmann, München, 1927.

Grünwald, P.: The lobular architecture of the human placenta. Bull. Johns Hopkins Hosp. 119:172–190, 1966.

Grünwald, P.: Fetal deprivation and placental insufficiency. Obstet. Gynecol. 37:906–908, 1971.

Grünwald, P.: Lobular structure of hemochorial primate placentas and its relation to maternal vessels. Amer. J. Anat. 136:133–151, 1973.

Gu, Y., Jayatilak, P.G., Parmer, T.G., Gauldie, J., Fey, G.H. and Gibori, G.: Alpha 2–macroglobulin expression in the mesometrial decidua and its regulation by decidual luteotropin and prolactin. Endocrinology 131:1321–1328, 1992.

Guha-Ray, D.K. and Hamblin, M.H.: Arthrogryposis multiplex congenita in an abdominal pregnancy. J. Reprod. Med. 18:109–112, 1977.

Gumperz, J.E. and Parham, P.: The enigma of the natural killer cell. Nature, 378:245–248, 1995.

Gustafson, G.W., Bowman, H.E. and Stout, F.E.: Extrauterine pregnancy at term. Obstet. Gynecol. 2:17–21, 1953.

Gustavii, B.: Release of lysosomal acid phosphatase into the cytoplasm of decidual cells before the onset of labour in humans. Brit. J. Obstet. Gynaecol. 82:177–181, 1975.

Haig, D.: Genetic conflicts in human pregnancy. The Quarterly Review of Biology 68:495–532, 1993.

Hallatt, J.G. and Grove, J.A.: Abdominal pregnancy: a study of twenty-one consecutive cases. Amer. J. Obstet. Gynecol. 152:444–449, 1985.

Haller, U.: Beitrag zur Morphologie der Utero-Placentargefäße. Arch. Gynäkol. 205:185–202, 1968.

Haller, H., Radillo, O., Rukavina, D., Tedesco, F., Candussi, G., Petrovic, O. and Randic, L.: An immunohistochemical study of leucocytes in human endometrium, first and third trimester basal decidua. J. Reprod. Immunol. 23:41–49, 1993.

Hamaguchi, M., Yamamoto, T. and Sugiyama, Y.: Production of prolactin by cultures of isolated cells from human first-trimester decidua. Obstet. Gynecol. 76:783–787, 1990.

Hamilton, G.S., Lysiak, J.J., Watson, A.J. and Lala, P.K.: Colony-stimulating factor-1 provides an autocrine signal for first trimester extravillous trophoblast cell proliferation. Placenta 16:A24, 1995.

Hammer, A. and Dohr, G.: Apoptotic nuclei within the uterine decidua of first trimester pregnancy arise from CD45 positive leukocytes. Amer. J. Immunol. 42:88–94, 1999.

Hammer, A. and Dohr, G.: Expression of Fas-ligand in first trimester and term human placental villi. J. Reprod. Immunol. 46:83–90, 2000.

Hammer, A., Blaschitz, A., Daxboeck, C., Walcher, W. and Dohr, G.: Fas and fas-ligand are expressed in the uteroplacental unit of first-trimester pregnancy. Amer. J. Reprod. Immunol. 41:41–51, 1999.

Hamperl, H.: Über die endometrialen Granulozyten (endometriale Körnchenzellen). Klin. Wochenschr. 32:665–668, 1954.

Hanna, J., Wald, O., Goldman-Wohl, D., Prus, D., Markel, G., Gazit, R., Katz, G., Haimov-Kochman, R., Fujii, N., Yagel, S., Peled, A. and Mandelboim, O.: CXCL12 expression by invasive trophoblasts induces the specific migration of CD16– human natural killer cells. Blood 102:1569–1577, 2003.

Hansell, D.J., Bryant Greenwood, G.D. and Greenwood, F.C.: Expression of the human relaxin H1 gene in the decidua, trophoblast, and prostate. J. Clin. Endocrinol. Metab. 72:899–904, 1991.

Harden, M.A., Walters, M.D. and Valente, P.T.: Postabortal hemorrhage due to placenta increta: a case report. Obstet. Gynecol. 75:523–526, 1990.

Harman, C.R., Manning, F.A., Stearms, E. and Morrison, I.: The correlation of ultrasonic placental grading and fetal pulmonary maturation in five hundred sixty-three pregnancies. Amer. J. Obstetr. Gynecol. 143:941–943, 1982.

Harris, J.W.S. and Ramsey, E.M.: The morphology of human uteroplacental vasculature. Carnegie Inst. Contrib. Embryol. 38:43–58, 1966.

Hartmann, M., Blaschitz, A., Hammer, A., Haidacher, S., Mahnert, W., Walcher, W. and Dohr, G.: Immunohistochemical examination of trophoblast populations in human first trimester and term placentae and of first trimester spiral arteries with the monoclonal antibody GZ 112. Placenta 18:481–489, 1997.

Hassim, A.M., Lucas, C. and Elkabbani, S.A.M.: Spontaneous uterine rupture caused by placenta percreta. Brit. Med. J. 2:97–98, 1968.

Hassler, O.: Placental calcifications. Amer. J. Obstet. Gynecol. 103:348–353, 1969.

Hees, H., Moll, W., Wrobel, K.H. and Hees, I.: Pregnancy-induced structural changes and trophoblastic invasion in the segmental mesometrial arteries of the guinea pig (Cavia porcellus L.) Placenta **8**:609–626, 1987.

Hein, K.: Licht-und elektronenmikroskopische Untersuchungen an der Basalplatte der reifen menschlichen Plazenta. Z. Zellforsch. **122**:323–349, 1971.

Hellmann, P., von Ostau, C., Grümmer, R. and Winterhager, E.: Connexin-40 expression in the human trophoblast: implicator for proliferation and invasion properties. Placenta **16**:A26, 1995.

Hellweg, G.: Über Auftreten und Verhalten der endometrialen Körnchenzellen im Verlauf der Schwangerschaft, im krankhaft veränderten Endometrium und außerhalb des Corpus Uteri. Virchows Arch. [Pathol. Anat.] **330**:658–680, 1957.

Hertig, A.T.: Angiogenesis in the early human chorion and in the primary placenta of the macaque monkey. Contrib. Embryol. Carnegie Inst. **25**:37–81, 1935.

Hill, L.M., Breckle, R., Ragozzino, M.W., Wolfgram, K.R. and O'Brien, P.C.: Grade 3 placentation: Incidence and neonatal outcome. Obstet. Gynecol. **61**:728–732, 1983.

Hirano, H., Imai, Y. and Ito, H.: Spiral artery of placenta: development and pathology—immunohistochemical, microscopical, and electron-microscopic study. Kobe J. Med. Sci. **48**:13–23, 2002.

Hobbins, J.C. and Winsberg, F.: Ultrasonography in Obstetrics and Gynecology. Williams & Wilkins, Baltimore, 1977.

Hoffman-Tretin, J.C., Koenigsberg, M., Rabin, A. and Anyaegbunam, A.: Placenta accreta: Additional sonographic observations. J. Ultrasound Med. **11**:29–34, 1992.

Hofmann, G.E., Scott, R.T., Jr., Bergh, P.A. and Deligdisch, L.: Immunohistochemical localization of epidermal growth factor in human endometrium, decidua, and placenta. J. Clin. Endocrinol. Metab. **73**:882–887, 1991.

Hofmann, G.E., Drews, M.R., Scott, R.T., Jr., Navot, D., Heller, D. and Deligdisch, L.: Epidermal growth factor and its receptor in human implantation trophoblast: immunohistochemical evidence for autocrine/paracrine function. J. Clin. Endocrinol. Metab. **74**:981–988, 1992.

Hofmann, G.E., Glatstein, I., Schatz, F., Heller, D. and Deligdisch, L.: Immunohistochemical localization of urokinase-type plasminogen activator and the plasminogen activator inhibitors 1 and 2 in early human implantation sites. Amer. J. Obstet. Gynecol. **170**:671–676, 1994.

Hohn, H.P., Boots, L.R., Denker, H.W. and Höök, M.: Differentiation of human trophoblast cells in vitro stimulated by extracellular matrix. Trophoblast Res. **7**:181–201, 1993.

Holmes, W.E., Sliwkowski, M.X., Akita, R.W., Henzel, W.J., Lee, J., Park, J.W., Yanssura, D., Abardi, N., Raab, H., Lewis, G.D., Shepard, H.M., Kuang, W.-J., Wood, W.I., Goeddel, D.V. and Vandlen, R.L.: Identification of heregulin, a specific activator of p185 erbB2. Science **256**:1205–1210, 1992.

Holzer, E. and Pickel, H.: Ausgetragene ektopische Schwangerschaft mit lebendem Kind. Zentralbl. Gynäkol. **98**:52–55, 1976.

Hörmann, G.: Die Fibrinoidisierung des Chorionepithels als Konstruktionsprinzip der menschlichen Plazenta. Z. Geburtshilfe Gynäkol. **164**:263–269, 1965.

Hörmann, G.: Über die sogenannten Septen, Inseln, Zysten, Furchen und die Randzone der menschlichen Plazenta. Z. Geburtshilfe Gynäkol. **165**:125–134, 1966.

Hornstein, M.D., Niloff, J.M., Snyder, P.F. and Frigoletto, F.D.: Placenta percreta associated with a second-trimester pregnancy termination. Amer. J. Obstet. Gynecol. **150**:1002–1003, 1984.

Hoshina, M., Boothby, M., Hussa, R., Pattillo, R., Camel, H.M. and Boime, I.: Linkage of human chorionic gonadotrophin and placental lactogen biosynthesis to trophoblast differentiation and tumorigenesis. Placenta **6**:163–172, 1983.

Houlihan, J.M., Biro, P.A., Fergar-Payne, A., Simpson, K.L. and Holmes, C.H.: Evidence for the expression of non-HLA-A, -B, -C class I genes in the human fetal livers. J. Immunol. **149**:668–675, 1992.

Howorka, E. and Kapczynski, W.: Marginal circular haematoma disrupting the chorionic plate of the placenta. J. Obstet. Gynaecol. Brit. Commonw. **78**:280–282, 1971.

Hreshchyshyn, M.M., Bogen, B. and Loughran, C.H.: What is the actual present-day management of the placenta in late abdominal pregnancy? Amer. J. Obstet. Gynecol. **81**:302–317, 1961.

Hughes, M., Dobric, N., Scott, I.C., Su, L., Starovic, M., St-Pierre, B., Egan, S.E., Kingdom, J.C.P. and Cross, J.C.: The Hand1, Stra13 and Gcm1 transcription factors override FGF signaling to promote terminal differentiation of trophoblast stem cells. Dev. Biol. **271**:26–37, 2004.

Hui, K.Y., Haber, E. and Matsueda, G.R.: Monoclonal antibodies to a synthetic fibrin-like peptide bind to human fibrin but not to fibrinogen. Science **222**:1129–1132, 1993.

Huisman, M.A., Timmer, A., Zeinstra, M., Serlier, E.K., Hanemaaijer, R., Goor, H. and Erwich, J.J.: Matrix-metalloproteinase activity in first trimester placental bed biopsies in further complicated and uncomplicated pregnancies. Placenta **25**:253–258, 2004.

Humphries, M.J.: The molecular basis and specificity of integrin-ligand interactions. J. Cell Science **97**:585–592, 1990.

Hunt, J.S.: Cytokine networks, in the uteroplacental unit: macrophages as pivotal regulatory cells. J. Reprod. Immun. **16**:1–17, 1989.

Hunt, J.S.: Current topic: The role of macrophages in the uterine response to pregnancy. Placenta **11**:467–475, 1990.

Hunt, J.S.: Immunobiology of the maternal-fetal interface. Prenat. Neonat. Med. **3**:72–75, 1998.

Hunt, J.S., Fishback, J.L., Chumbley, G. and Loke, Y.W.: Identification of class I MHC mRNA in human first trimester trophoblast cells by in situ hybridization. J. Immunol. **144**:4420–4425, 1990.

Hunt, J.S., Hsi, B.L., King, C.R. and Fishback, J.L.: Detection of class I MHC mRNA in subpopulations of first trimester cytotrophoblast cells by in situ hybridization. J. Reprod. Immunol. **19**:315–323, 1991.

Hunziker, R.D. and Wegmann, T.G.: Placental immunoregulation. Crit. Rev. Immunol. **613**:245–285, 1986.

Huppertz, B., Kertschanska, S., Frank, H.G., Gaus, G. Funayama, H. and Kaufmann, P.: Extracellular matrix components of the placental extravillous trophoblast: Immunocytochemistry and ultrastructural distribution. Histochem. Cell Biol. **106**:291–301, 1996.

Huppertz, B., Frank, H.G. and Kaufmann, P.: Apoptosis along the invasive trophoblastic pathway. Placenta, **19**, A34, 1998a.

Huppertz, B., Kertschanska, S. and Kaufmann, P.: Changes in cell-matrix-interactions of invasive trophoblast lead to apoptosis. Placenta 19:A20, 1998b.

Huppertz, B., Frank, H.G., Kingdom, J.C.P., Reister, F. and Kaufmann, P.: Villous cytotrophoblast regulation of the syncytial apoptotic cascade in the human placenta. Histochem. Cell Biol. 110:495–508, 1998c.

Huppertz, B., Kertschanska, S., Demir, A.Y., Frank, H.G. and Kaufmann, P.: Immunohistochemistry of matrix metalloproteinases (MMP), their substrates, and their inhibitors (TIMP) during trophoblast invasion in the human placenta. Cell Tissue Res. 291:133–148, 1998d.

Hurskainen, T., Seiki, M., Apte, S.S., Syrjäkallio-Ylitalo, M., Sorsa, T., Oikarinen, A. and Autio-Harmainen, H.: Production of membrane-type matrix metalloproteinase-1 (MT-MMP-1) in early human placenta: A possible role in placental implantation? J. Histochem. Cytochem. 46:221–229, 1998.

Hustin, J.: Blood flow in the intervillous space in the first trimester (Letter to the Editors). Placenta 16:659–660, 1995.

Hustin, J. and Schaaps, J.-P.: Echocardiographic and anatomic studies of the maternotrophoblastic border during the first trimester of pregnancy. Amer. J. Obstet. Gynecol. 157:162–168, 1987.

Hustin, J., Schaaps, J.-P. and Lambotte, R.: Anatomical studies of the utero-placental vascularization in the first trimester of pregnancy. Trophoblast Res. 3:49–60, 1988.

Hutter, H., Hammer, A., Blaschitz, A., Hartmann, M. Ebbesen, P., Dohr, G., Ziegler, A. and Uchanska-Ziegler, B.: Expression of HLA class I molecules in human first trimester and term placenta trophoblast. Cell Tissue Res. 286:439–447, 1996.

Irving, F.C. and Hertig, A.T.: A study of placenta accreta. Surg. Gynecol. Obstet. 64:178–200, 1937.

Irving, J.A. and Lala, P.K.: Decidua-derived IGFBP-1 stimulates human intermediate trophoblast migration by binding to the alpha5/beta1 integrin subunits. Placenta 15:A31, 1994.

Irving, J.A. and Lala, P.K.: Functional role of cell surface integrins on human trophoblast cell migration: regulation by TGF-beta, IGF-II, and IGFBP-1. Exp. Cell Res. 217:419–427, 1995.

Irving, J.A., Lysiak, J.J., Graham, C.H., Hearn, S., Han, V.K.M. and Lala, P.K.: Characteristics of trophoblast cells migrating from first trimester chorionic villous explants and propagated in culture. Placenta 16:413–433, 1995.

Ishitani, A. and Geraghty, D.E.: Alternative splicing of HLA-G transcripts yields proteins with primary structures resembling both class I and class II antigens. Proc. Natl. Acad. Sci. USA 89:1–5, 1992.

Ishizaki, Y. and Belter, L.F.: Melanin deposition in the placenta as a result of skin lesions (dermatopathic melanosis of placenta). Amer. J. Obstet. Gynecol. 79:1074–1077, 1960.

Islami, D., Mock, P. and Bischof, P.: Effects of human chorionic gonadotropin on trophoblast invasion. Semin. Reprod. Med. 19:49–53, 2001.

Iwanaga, S.: Ultrastructural observations on human endometrial stromal cells during the normal menstrual cycle—with special reference to so-called "predecidual cells". Nippon. Sanka. Fujinka. Gakkai. Zasshi. 35:177–182, 1983.

Jaakkola, K., Jokimaa, V., Kallajoki, M., Jalkanen, S. and Ekholm, E.: Pre-eclampsia does not change the adhesion molecule status in the placental bed. Placenta. 21:133–141, 2000.

Jackson, G.M., Edwin, S.S., Varer, M.W., Casal, D. and Mitchell, M.D.: Regulation of fetal fibronectin production in human chorion cells. Amer. J. Obstet. Gynecol. 169:1431–1435, 1993.

Jaffe, R., DuBeshter, B., Sherer, D.M., Thompson, E.A. and Woods, J.R.: Failure of methotrexate treatment for term placenta previa. Amer. J. Obstet. Gynecol. 171:558–559, 1994.

Jauniaux, E.: Intervillous circulation in the first trimester: the phantom of the color Doppler obstetric opera. Ultrasound Obstet. Gynecol. 8:73–76, 1996.

Javert, C.T.: Decidual bleeding in pregnancy. Ann. N.Y. Acad. Sci. 61:700–712, 1955.

Jeacock, M.K., Scott, J. and Plester, J.A.: Calcium content of the human placenta. Amer. J. Obstet. Gynecol. 87:34–40, 1963.

Johnson, P.M. and Faulk, W.P.: Immunological studies of human placenta: identification and distribution of proteins in immature chorionic villi. Immunology 34:1027–1036, 1978.

Jokhi, P.P., Chumbley, G., King, A., Gardner, L. and Loke, Y.W.: Expression of the colony stimulating factor-1 receptor (c-fms product) by cells at the human uteroplacental interface. Lab. Invest. 68:308–320, 1993.

Jokhi, P.P., King, A. and Loke, Y.W.: Reciprocal expression of epidermal growth factor receptor (EGF-R) and c-erbB2 by non-invasive and invasive human trophoblast populations. Cytokine 6:433–442, 1994a.

Jokhi, P.P., King, A., Sharkey, A.M. Smith, S.K. and Loke, Y.W.: Screening for cytokine mRNAs in purified human decidual lymphocyte populations by the reverse-transcriptase polymerase chain reaction (RT-PCR). J. Immunol. 153:4427–4435, 1994b.

Joura, E.A., Nather, A., Hohlagschwandtner, M. and Husslein, P.: The impact of single- or double-layer closure on uterine rupture. Amer. J. Obstet. Gynecol. 188:895–896, 2002.

Kadyrov, M., Schmitz, C., Black, S., Kaufmann, P. and Huppertz, B.: Pre-eclampsia and maternal anaemia display reduced apoptosis and opposite invasive phenotypes of extravillous trophoblast. Placenta 24:540–548, 2003.

Kaiser, R.: Über Rückbildungsvorgaenge in der Dezidua während der Schwangerschaft. Arch. Gynäkol. 192:209–220, 1960.

Kalchman, G.G. and Meltzer, R.M.: Interstitial pregnancy following homolateral salpingectomy. Amer. J. Obstet. Gynecol. 96:1139–1143, 1966.

Kam, E.P.Y., Gardner, L., Loke, Y.W. and King, A.: The role of trophoblast in the physiological change in decidual spiral arteries. Hum. Reprod. 14:2131–2138, 1999.

Karimu, A.L. and Burton, G.J.: Significance of changes in fetal perfusion pressure to factors controlling angiogenesis in the human term placenta. J. Reprod. Fertil. 102:447–450, 1994a.

Karimu, A.L. and Burton, G.J.: The effects of maternal vascular pressure on the dimensions of the placental capillaries. Brit. J. Obstet. Gynaecol. 101:57–63, 1994b.

Karmakar, S. and Das, C.: Modulation of ezrin and E-cadherin expression by IL-1beta and TGF-beta1 in human trophoblasts. J. Reprod. Immunol. 64:9–29, 2004a.

Karmakar, S., Dhar, R. and Das, C.: Inhibition of cytotrophoblastic (JEG-3) cell invasion by IL-12 involves an interferon gamma mediated pathway. J. Biol. Chem. 279:55297–55307, 2004b.

Katz, V.L., Bowes, W.A. and Sierkh, A.E.: Maternal floor infarction of the placenta associated with elevated second trimester serum alpha-fetoprotein. Amer. J. Perinatol. 4:225–228, 1987.

Kaufman, H. and Adams, E.: Murexide, another approach to the histochemical staining of calcium. Lab. Invest. **6**:275–280, 1957.

Kaufmann, P.: Entwicklung der Plazenta. In, Die Plazenta des Menschen. V. Becker, Th.H. Schiebler and F. Kubli, eds. Thieme, Stuttgart, 1981a.

Kaufmann, P.: Fibrinoid. In, Die Plazenta des Menschen. V. Becker, Th.H. Schiebler and F. Kubli, eds. Thieme, Stuttgart, 1981b.

Kaufmann, P.: Basic morphology of the fetal and maternal circuits in the human placenta. Contrib. Gynecol. Obstet. **13**:5–17, 1985.

Kaufmann, P. and Castellucci, M.: Extravillous Trophoblast in the Human Placenta. Trophoblast Res. **10**:21–65, 1997.

Kaufmann, P. and Stark, J.: Die Basalplatte der reifen menschlichen Placenta. I. Semidünnschnitt-Histologie. Z. Anat. Entwicklungsgesch. **135**:1–19, 1971.

Kaufmann, P., Schröder, H. and Leichtweiss, H.-P.: Fluid shift across the placenta: II. Fetomaternal transfer of horseradish peroxidase in the guinea pig. Placenta **3**:339–348, 1982.

Kaufmann, P., Huppertz, B. and Frank, H.G.: The fibrinoids of the human placenta: origin, composition and functional relevance. Ann. Anat. **178**:485–501, 1996.

Kaufmann, P., Black, S. and Huppertz, B.: Endovascular trophoblast invasion: implications for the pathogenesis of intrauterine growth retardation and preeclampsia. Biol. Reprod. **69**:1–7, 2003.

Kauma, S.W., Bae-Jump, V. and Walsh, S.W.: Hepatocyte growth factor stimulates trophoblast invasion: a potential mechanism for abnormal placentation in preeclampsia. J. Clin. Endocrinol. Metab. **84**:4092–4096 1999.

Kawagoe, K., Kawana, T. and Sakamoto, S.: Ultrastructure of the nidatory site in tubal pregnancy. Acta Obstet. Gynaecol. Jpn. **33**:403–410, 1981.

Kawano, T., Morimoto, K. and Uemura, Y.: Urokinase inhibitor in human placenta. Nature **217**:253–254, 1968.

Kazzi, G.M., Gross, T.L. and Sokol, R.J.: Fetal biparietal diameter and placental grade: Predictors of intrauterine growth retardation. Obstet. Gynecol. **62**:755–759, 1983.

Kearns, M. and Lala, P.K.: Life history of decidual cells: a review. Amer. J. Reprod. Immunol. **3**:78–82, 1983.

Keiffer, H.: Le placenta myometrial humain; le mechanisme de sa secretion, excretion et absorption. Arch. Biol. **38**:93–108, 1928.

Kemp, B., Funk, A., Hauptmann, S. and Rath, W.: Doppler sonographic criteria for viability in symptomless ectopic pregnancies. Lancet **349**:1220–1221, 1997.

Kemp, B., Kertschanska, S., Handt, S., Funk, A., Kaufmann, P. and Rath, W.: Different placentation patterns in viable as compared to non-viable tubal pregnancy suggest a divergent clinical management. Amer. J. Obstet. Gynecol. **181**:615–620, 1999.

Kemp, B., Kertschanska, S., Kadyrov, M., Rath, W., Kaufmann, P. and Huppertz, B.: Invasive depth of extravillous trophoblast correlates with cellular phenotype—a comparison of intra- and extrauterine implantation sites. Histochem. Cell Biol. **117**:401–414, 2002.

Kephart, G.M., Andrade, Z.A. and Gleich, G.J.: Localization of eosinophil major basic protein onto eggs of Schistosoma mansoni in human pathologic tissue. Amer. J. Pathol. **133**:389–396, 1988.

Kertschanska, S., Frank, H.G., Huppertz, B. and Kaufmann, P.: Coexpression of integrins and their ligands in extravillous trophoblast and matrix-type fibrinoid of the human placenta. Placenta **18**:A32, 1997.

Kertschanska, S., Kemp, B., Kosanke, G. and Kaufmann, P.: Die vitale Tubargravidität beim Menschen—ein Modell für gesteigerte Invasivität des Trophoblasten. Ann. Anat. **180**:6, 1998.

Khan, H., Ishihara, O., Elder, M.G. and Sullivan, M.H.: A comparison of two populations of decidual cells by immunocytochemistry and prostaglandin production. Histochemistry **96**:149–152, 1991.

Khan, H., Ishihara, O., Sullivan, M.H. and Elder, M.G.: Changes in decidual stromal cell function associated with labour. Brit. J. Obstet. Gynaecol. **99**:10–12, 1992.

Khong, T.Y. and Robertson, W.B. Placenta creta and placenta praevia creta. Placenta **8**:399–409, 1987.

Khong, T.Y., DeWolf, F., Robertson, W.B. and Brosens, I.: Inadequate maternal vascular response to placentation in preeclampsia and intrauterine fetal growth retardation. Brit. J. Obstet. Gynaecol. **93**:1049–1059, 1986a.

Khong, T.Y., Lane, E.B. and Robertson, W.B.: An immunocytochemical study of fetal cells at the maternal-placental interface using monoclonal antibodies to keratins, vimentin and desmin. Cell Tissue Res. **246**:189–195, 1986b.

Khudr, G., Soma, H. and Benirschke, K.: Trophoblastic origin of the X-cell and the placental giant cell. Amer. J. Obstet. Gynecol. **115**:530–533, 1973.

Kilburn, B.A., Wang, J., Duniec-Dmuchowski, Z.M., Leach, R. E., Romero, R. and Armant, D.R.: Extracellular matrix composition and hypoxia regulate the expression of HLA-G and integrins in a human trophoblast cell line. Biol. Reprod. **62**:739–747, 2000.

Kim, C.K. and Benirschke, K.: Autoradiographic study of the "X-cells" in the human placenta. Amer. J. Obstet. Gynecol. **109**:96–102, 1971.

King, A. and Loke, Y.W.: Differential expression of blood-group-related carbohydrate antigens by trophoblast subpopulations. Placenta **9**:513–521, 1988.

King, A. and Loke, Y.W.: Uterine large granular lymphocytes: a possible role in embryo implantation? Amer. J. Obstet. Gynecol. **162**:308–310, 1990.

King, A. and Loke, Y.W.: On the nature and function of human uterine granular lymphocytes. Immunol. Today **12**:432–435, 1991.

King, A. and Loke, Y.W.: Trophoblast Interaction with Decidual NK cells in Human Implantation. Trophoblast Res. **10**:173–180, 1997.

King, A., Jokhi, P.P., Burrows, T.D., Gardner, L., Sharkey, A.M. and Loke, Y.W.: Functions of human decidual NK cells. Amer. J. Reprod. Immunol. **35**:258–260, 1996.

King, A., Hilby, S.E., Verma, S., Burrows, T., Gardner, L. and Loke, Y.W.: Uterine NK Cells and Trophoblast HLA Class I Molecules. Amer. J. Reprod. Immunol. **37**:459–462, 1997.

King, A., Hilby, S.E., Gardner, L., Joseph, S., Bowen, J.M., Verma, S., Burrows, T.D. and Loke, Y.W.: Recognition of trophoblast call I molecules by decidual NK cell receptors—a review. Placenta **21**:S81–S85, 2000.

King, B.F. and Blankenship, T.N.: Expression of proliferating cell nuclear antigen (PCNA) in developing macaque placentas. Placenta **14**:A36, 1993.

King, B.F. and Blankenship, T.N.: Ultrastructure and development of a thick basement membrane-like layer in the anchoring villi of macaque placentas. Anat. Res. **238**:498–506. 1994.

King, B.F. and Blankenship, T.N.: Immunohistochemical localization of fibrillin in developing macaque and term human placentas and fetal membranes. Micr. Res. Techn. **38**:42–51, 1997.

Kirby, D.R.S., Billington, W.D., Bradbury, S. and Goldstein, D.J.: Antigen barrier of mouse placenta. Nature **204**:548–549, 1964.

Kirkinen, P. and Jouppila, P.: Intrauterine membranous cyst: a report of antenatal diagnosis and obstetric aspects in two cases. Obstet. Gynecol. **67**:26S–30S, 1986.

Kirszenbaum, M., Moreau, P., Gluckman, E., Dausset, J. and Carosella, E.: An alternatively spliced form of HLA-G mRNA in human trophoblasts and evidence for the presence of HLA-G transcript in adult lymphocytes. Proc. Natl. Acad. Sci. USA **91**:4209–4213, 1994.

Kisalus, L.L. and Herr, J.C.: Immunocytochemical localization of heparan sulfate proteoglycan in human decidual cell secretory bodies and placental fibrinoid. Biol. Reprod. **39**:419–430, 1988.

Kisalus, L.L., Herr, J.C. and Little, C.D.: Immunolocalization of extracellular matrix proteins and collagen synthesis in first trimester human decidua. Anat. Rec. **218**:402–415, 1987.

Kivikoski, A.I., Martin, C., Weyman, P., Picus, D. and Giudice, L.: Angiographic arterial embolization to control hemorrhage in abdominal pregnancy: a case report. Obstet. Gynecol. **71**:456–457, 1988.

Klein, G.: Makroskopisches Verhalten der UteroPlacentargefässe. In, Die menschliche Placenta. Beiträge zur normalen und pathologischen Anatomie derselben. Hofmeier, ed., pp. 72–87. Bergmann, Wiesbaden 1890.

Klinger, H.P. and Ludwig, K.S.: Sind die Septen und die grosszelligen Inseln der Placenta aus mütterlichem oder kindlichem Gewebe aufgebaut? Z. Anat. Entwicklungsgesch. **120**:95–100, 1957.

Klisch, K., Hecht, W., Pfarrer, C., Schuler, G., Hoffmann, B. and Leiser, R.: DNA content and ploidy level of bovine placentomal trophoblast giant cells. Placenta **20**:451–458, 1999a.

Klisch, K., Pfarrer, C., Schuler, G., Hoffmann, B., Leiser, R.: Tripolar acytokinetic mitosis and formation of feto-maternal syncytia in the bovine placentome: different modes of the generation of multinuclear cells. Anat. Embryol. **200**:229–237, 1999b.

Kölliker, A.: Entwicklungsgeschichte des Menschen und der höheren Thiere. 1st ed., Engelmann, Leipzig, 1861.

Kölliker, A.: Entwicklungsgeschichte des Menschen und der höheren Thiere. 2nd ed., Engelmann, Leipzig, 1879.

Korhonen, M. and Virtanen, I.: The distribution of laminins and fibronectins is modulated during extravillous trophoblastic cell differentiation and decidual cell response to invasion in the human placenta. J. Histochem. Cytochem. **45**:569–581, 1997.

Korhonen, M., Ylanne, J., Laitinen, L., Cooper, H.M., Quaranta, V. and Virtanen, I.: Distribution of the alpha 1–alpha 6 integrin subunits in human developing and term placenta. Lab. Invest. **65**:347–356, 1991.

Kornblatt, M.B.: Abdominal pregnancy following a total hysterectomy. Report of a case. Obstet. Gynecol. **32**:488–489, 1968.

Kosanke, G.: Proliferation, Wachstum und Differenzierung der Zottenbäume der menschlichen Placenta. Shaker Publishers, Aachen, Germany, 1994.

Kosanke, G., Kadyrov, M., Korr, H. and Kaufmann P.: Maternal anemia results in increased proliferation in human placental villi. Trophoblast Res. **11**:339–357, 1998.

Kourembanas, S., Marsden, P., McQuillan, L. and Faller D.: Hypoxia induces endothelin gene expression and secretion in cultured endothelium. J. Clin. Invest. **86**:670–674, 1991.

Kovats, S., Main, E.K., Librach, C., Stubblebine, M., Fisher, S.J. and DeMars, R.: A class I antigen, HLA-G, expressed in human trophoblasts. Science **248**:220–223, 1990.

Krafft, M.-L.: Über den Halte- und Verspannungsapparat der plazentaren Randzone und der Eihäute. (Nach graphischen Rekonstruktionen.) Inaugural Dissertation, Berlin, 1973.

Kratzsch, E. and Grygiel, I.-H.: Über das Vorkommen eines spezifischen Enzyms der Glucuronsäurebildung im menschlichen Amnion. Z. Zellforsch. **123**:566–571, 1972.

Kretschmann, H.-J.: Über Feinstruktur des subchorialen Placentarfibrins im Vergleich mit der des Blutfibrins. I. Orthoskopische Analyse. Acta Anat. (Basel) **66**:339–364, 1967a.

Kretschmann, H.-J.: Über die Feinstruktur des subchorialen Placentarfibrins im Vergleich mit der des Blutfibrins. II. Experimentelle Studie über Veränderungen der Feinstruktur des Blutfibrins. Acta Anat. (Basel) **66**:494–503, 1967b.

Krohn, K., Ljungqvist, A. and Robertson, B.: Trophoblastic and subtrophoblastic mineral salt deposition in hydramnios. Acta Pathol. Microbiol. Scand. **69**:514–520, 1967.

Krönicher, W.D.: Ein Beitrag zur Genese der Inseln in der menschlichen Placenta. Z. Mikrosk. Anat. Forsch. **89**:777–803, 1975.

Kruse, A., Merchant, M.J., Hallmann, R. and Butcher, E.C.: Evidence of specialized leukocyte-vascular homing interactions at the maternal/fetal interface. Eur. J. Immunol. **29**:1116–1126, 1999.

Kubli, F.: Die chronische Placentarinsuffizienz. Gynäkologe **1**:53–60, 1968.

Kubota, T., Kamada, S., Hirata, Y., Eguchi, S., Imai, T., Marumo, F. and Aso, T.: Synthesis and release of endothelin-1 by human decidual cells. J. Clin. Endocrinol. Metab. **75**:1230–1234, 1992.

Kunicki, T.J., Nugent, D.J., Staats, S.J., Orchekowski, R.P., Wayner, E.A. and Carter W.G.: The human fibroblast class II extracellular matrix receptor mediates platelet adhesion to collagen and is identical to the platelet Ia-IIa complex. J. Biol. Chem. **263**:4516–4519, 1988.

Kupferminc, M.J., Tamura, R.K., Wigton, T.R., Glassenberg, R. and Socol, M.L.: Placenta accreta is associated with elevated maternal serum alpha-fetoprotein. Obstet. Gynecol. **82**:266–269, 1993.

Kurman, R.J., Main, C.S. and Chen, H.C.: Intermediate trophoblast: a distinctive form of trophoblast with specific morphological, biochemical and functional features. Placenta **5**:349–369, 1984a.

Kurman, R.J., Young, R.H., Norris, H.J., Main, C.S., Lawrence, W.D. and Scully, R.E.: Immunocytochemical localization of placental lactogen and chorionic gonadotropin in the normal placenta and trophoblastic tumors, with emphasis on intermediate trophoblast and the placental site trophoblastic tumor. Intern. J. Gynecol. Pathol. **3**:101–121, 1984b.

Labarrere, C. and Page Faulk, W.: Intercellular adhesion molecule-1 (ICAM-1) and HLA-DR antigens are expressed on endovascular cytotrophoblasts in abnormal pregnancies. Amer. J. Reprod. Immun. 33:47–53, 1995.

Ladines Llave, C.A., Maruo, T., Manalo, A.M. and Mochizuki, M.: Decreased expression of epidermal growth factor and its receptor in the malignant transformation of trophoblasts. Cancer 71:4118–4123, 1993.

Lala, P.K., Kearns, M. and Colavincenzo, V.: Cells of the fetomaternal interface: their role in the maintenance of viviparous pregnancy. Amer. J. Anat. 170:501–517, 1984.

Landon, M.B., Hauth, J.C., Leveno, K.J., Spong, C.Y., Leindecker, S., Varner, M.W., Moawad, A.H., Caritis, S.N., Harper, M., Wapner, R.J., Sorokin, Y., Miodovnik, M., Carpenter, M., Peaceman, A.M., O'Sullivan, M.J., Sibai, B., Langer, O., Thorp, J.M., Ramin, S.M., Mercer, B.M. and Gabbe, S.G.: Maternal and perinatal outcomes associated with a trial of labor after prior Cesarean delivery. NEJM 351:2581–2589, 2004.

Lang, I., Hartmann, M., Blaschitz, A., Dohr, G., Skofitsch, G. and Desoye, G.: Immunohistochemical evidence for the heterogeneity of maternal and fetal vascular endothelial cells in human full-term placenta. Cell Tissue Res. 274:211–218, 1993.

Lang, I., Hartmann, M., Blaschitz, A., Dohr, G., Kaufmann, P., Frank, H.G., Hahn, T., Skofitsch, G. and Desoye, G.: Differential lectin binding to the fibrinoid of human full term placenta: correlation with a fibrin antibody and the PAF-Halmi method. Acta Anat. 150:170–177, 1994.

Langhans, T.: Untersuchungen über die menschliche Placenta. Arch. Anat. Physiol., Anat. Abt. 188–267, 1877.

Laoag-Fernandez, J.B., Matsuo, H., Murakoshi, H., Hamada, A.L., Tsang, B.K. and Maruo, T.: 3,5,3′-Triiodothyronine down-regulates Fas and Fas ligand expression and suppresses caspase-3 and poly (adenosine 5′-diphosphate-ribose) polymerase cleavage and apoptosis in early placental extravillous trophoblasts in vitro. J. Clin. Endocrinol. Metab. 89:4069–4077, 2004.

Lapan, B. and Friedman, M.M.: Tissue enzymes in gestation: comparative activities in the placenta and fetal membranes. Amer. J. Obstet. Gynecol. 93:1157–1163, 1965.

Larsen, J.F. and Knoth, M.: Ultrastructure of the anchoring villi and trophoblastic shell in the second week of placentation. Acta Obstet. Gynecol. Scand. 50:117–128, 1971.

Larsen, L.G., Theilade, K., Skibsted, L. and Jacobsen, G.K.: Malignant placental site trophoblastic tumor. A case report and a review of the literature. APMIS Suppl. 23:138–145, 1991.

Lash, G.E., Cartwright, J.E., Whitley, G.S., Trew, A.J. and Baker, P.N.: The effects of angiogenic growth factors on extravillous trophoblast invasion and motility. Placenta 20:661–667, 1999.

Lash, G.E., Fitzpatrick, T.E. and Graham, C.H.: Effect of hypoxia on cellular adhesion to vitronectin and fibronectin.: Biochem. Biophys. Res. Commun. 287:622–629, 2001.

Lash, G.E., Postovit, L.M., Matthews, N.E., Chung, E.Y., Canning, M.T., Pross, H., Adams, M.A. and Graham, C.H.: Oxygen as a regulator of cellular phenotypes in pregnancy and cancer. Can. J. Physiol. Pharmacol. 80:103–109, 2002.

Lash, G.E., Warren, A.Y., Underwood, S. and Baker, P.N.: Vascular endothelial growth factor is a chemoattractant for trophoblast cells. Placenta 24:549–556, 2003.

Lata, J.A., Tuan, R.S., Shepley, K.J., Mulligan, M.M., Jackson, L.G. and Smith, J.B.: Localization of major histocompatibility complex class I and II mRNA in human first-trimester chorionic villi by in situ hybridization. J. Exp. Med. 175:1027–1032, 1992.

Laufer, A., Sadovsky, A. and Sadovsky, E.: Histologic appearance of the placenta in ectopic pregnancy. Obstet. Gynecol. 20:350–353, 1962.

Lawn, A.M., Wilson, E.W. and Finn, C.A.: The ultrastructure of human decidual and predecidual cells. J. Reprod. Fertil. 26:85–90, 1971.

Leach, R.E., Kilburn, B., Wang, J., Liu, Z., Romero, R. and Armant, D.R.: Heparin-binding EGF-like growth factor regulates human extravillous cytotrophoblast development during conversion to the invasive phenotype. Dev. Biol. 266:223–237, 2004.

Leaphart, W.L., Schapiro, H., Broome, J., Welander, C.E. and Bernstein, I.M.: Placenta previa percreta with bladder invasion. Obstet. Gynecol. 89:834–835, 1997.

Le Bouteiller, P., Pizzato, N., Barakonyi, A. and Solier, C.: HLA-G, pre-eclampsia, immunity and vascular events. J. Reprod. Immunol. 59:2192–2234, 2003.

Lee, N., Llano, M., Carratero, M., Ishitani, A., Navarro, F., Lopez-Botet, M. and Geraghty, D.E.: HLA-E is a major ligand for the natural killer inhibitory receptor CD94/NKG2A. Proc. Natl. Acad. Sci. USA 95:5199–5204, 1998.

Lee, P.D., Giudice, L.C. Conover, C.A. and Powell, D.R.: Insulin-like growth factor binding protein-1: recent findings and new directions. Proc. Soc. Exp. Biol. Med. 216:319–357, 1997.

Legro, R.S., Price, F.V., Hill, L.M. and Caritis, S.N.: Nonsurgical management of placenta percreta: A case report. Obstet. Gynecol. 83:847–849, 1994.

Leivo, I., Laurila, P., Wahlstrom, T. and Engvall, E.: Expression of merosin, a tissue-specific basement membrane protein, in the intermediate trophoblast cells of choriocarcinoma and placenta. Lab. Invest. 60:783–790, 1989.

LeMaire, W.J., Louisy, C., Dalessandri, K. and Muschenheim, F.: Placenta percreta with spontaneous rupture of an unscarred uterus in the second trimester. Obstet. Gynecol. 98:927–929, 2001.

Lester, W.M., Bartholomew, R.A., Colvin, E.D., Grimes, W.H., Fish, J.S. and Galloway, W.H.: Role of retained placental fragments in immediate and delayed postpartum hemorrhage. Amer. J. Obstet. Gynecol. 72:1214–1226, 1956.

Librach, C.L., Fisher, S.J., Fitzgerald, M.L. and Damsky, C.H.: Cytotrophoblast-fibronectin and cytotrophoblast-laminin interactions have distinct roles in cytotrophoblast invasion. J. Cell Biol. 115:6a, 1991a.

Librach, C.L., Werb, Z., Fitzgerald, M.L., Chiu, K., Corwin, N.M., Esteves, R.A., Grobelny, D., Galardy, R., Damsky, C.H. and Fisher, S.J.: 92–kD type IV collagenase mediates invasion of human cytotrophoblasts. J. Cell Biol. 113:437–449, 1991b.

Lieto, A.Di, Pollio, F., Falco, M.De, Iannotti, F., Mascolo, M., Somma, P. and Staibano, S.: Collagen content and growth factor immunoexpression in uterine lower segment of type IA osteogenesis imperfecta: Relationship with recurrent uterine rupture in pregnancy. Amer. J. Obstet. Gynecol. 189:584–600, 2003.

Lim, K.H., Damsky, C.H. and Fisher, S.J.: Basic fibroblast growth factor and heparin stimulate integrin-alpha-1 expression by cytotrophoblasts. J. Soc. Gynecol. Invest. 2:287, 1995.

Lin, C. and Raynor, D.: Risk of uterine rupture in labor induction of patients with prior cesarean section: An inner city hospital experience. Amer. J. Obstet. Gynecol. **190**:1476–1478, 2004.

Linthwaite, R.F.: Subchorial hematoma mole (Breus' mole). JAMA **186**:867–870, 1963.

Ljunggren, H.-G. and Kärre, K.: In search of the 'missing self': MHC molecules and NK cell recognition. Immunology Today **11**:237–244, 1990.

Llano, M., Lee, N., Navarro, F., Garcia, P., Albar, J.P., Geraghty, D.E. and Lopez-Botet, M.: HLA-E bound peptides influence recognition by inhibitory and triggering CD94/NKG2 receptors: preferential response to an HLA-G-derived nonamer. Eur. J. Immunol. **28**:2854–2863, 1998.

Loke, Y.W.: Trophoblast antigen expression. Curr. Opin. Immunol. **1**:1131–1134, 1989.

Loke, Y.W. and King, A.: Recent developments in the human maternal-fetal immune interaction. Curr. Opin. Immunol. **3**:762–766, 1991.

Loke, Y.W. and King, A.: Human Implantation—Cell Biology and Immunology. Cambridge University Press, 1995.

Loke, Y.W., Gardner, L., Burland, K. and King, A.: Laminin in human trophoblast—decidua interaction. Hum. Reprod. **4**:457–463, 1989.

Loke, Y.W., Hsi, B.L., Bulmer, J.N., Grivaux, C., Hawley, S., Gardner, L., King, A. and Carter, N.P.: Evaluation of a monoclonal antibody, BC-1, which identifies an antigen expressed on the surface membrane of human extravillous trophoblast. Amer. J. Reprod. Immunol. **27**:77–81, 1992.

Loke, Y.W., King, A. and Burrows, T.D.: Decidua in human implantation. Hum. Reprod. **10**:14–21, 1995.

Loke, Y.W., King, A., Burrows, T.D., Gardner, L., Bowen, M., Hiby, S., Howlett, S., Holmes, N. and Jacobs, D.: Evaluation of trophoblast HLA-G antigen with a specific monoclonal antibody. Tissue Antigens **50**:135–146, 1997.

Luckett, W.P.: Origin and differentiation of the yolk sac and extraembryonic mesoderm in presomite human and rhesus monkey embryos. Amer. J. Anat. **152**:59–97, 1978.

Ludwig, H. and Metzger, H.: Das uterine Placentarbett post partum im Rasterelektronenmikroskop, zugleich ein Beitrag zur Frage der extravasalen Fibrinbildung. Arch. Gynäkol. **210**:251–266, 1971.

Luke, R.K., Sharpe, J.W. and Greene, R.R.: Placenta accreta: the adherence or invasive placenta. Amer. J. Obstet. Gynecol. **95**:660–668, 1966.

Lumley, J.M.: Unexplained antepartum stillbirth in pregnancies after caesarean delivery. Lancet **362**:1774–1775, 2003.

Lyall, F.: The human placental bed revisited. Placenta **23**:555–562, 2002.

Lyall, F. and Kaufmann, P.: The uteroplacental circulation: Extravillous trophoblast. In: Intrauterine Growth Restriction. P. Baker and J. Kingdom (Eds.), Springer Publ. London, pp 85–130, 2000.

Lyall, F., Bulmer, J.N., Kelly, H., Duffie, E. and Robson, S.C.: Human trophoblast invasion and spiral artery transformation—the role of nitric oxide. Am. J. Pathol. **154**:1105–1114, 1999.

Lyall, F., Bulmer, J.N., Duffie, E., Cousins, F., Theriault, A. and Robson, S.C.: Human trophoblast invasion and spiral artery transformation. The role of PECAM-1 in normal pregnancy, preeclampsia, and fetal growth restriction. Amer. J. Pathol. **158**:1713–1721, 2001.

Lysiak, J.J., Han, V.K. and Lala, P.K.: Localization of transforming growth factor alpha in the human placenta and decidua: role in trophoblast growth. Biol. Reprod. **49**:885–894, 1993.

Lysiak, J.J., Hunt, J., Pringle, G.A. and Lala, P.K.: Localization of transforming growth factor β and its natural inhibitor decorin in the human placenta and decidua throughout gestation. Placenta **16**:221–231, 1995.

MacCalman, C.D., Omigbodun, A., Bronner, M.P. and Strauss, J.F.: Identification of the cadherins present in the human placenta. J. Soc. Gynecol. Invest. **2**:146, 1995.

Maddox, D.E., Butterfield, J.H., Ackerman, S.J., Coulam, C.B. and Gleich, G.J.: Elevated serum levels in human pregnancy of a molecule immunochemically similar to eosinophil granule major basic protein. J. Exp. Med. **158**:1211–1226, 1983.

Maddox, D.E., Kephart, G.M., Coulam, C.B., Butterfield, J.H., Benirschke, K. and Gleich, G.J.: Localization of a molecule immunochemically similar to eosinophil major basic protein in human placenta. J. Exp. Med. **160**:29–41, 1984.

Maidman, J.E., Thorpe, L.W., Harris, J.A. and Wynn, R.M.: Fetal origin of X-cells in human placental septa and basal plate. Obstet. Gynecol. **41**:547–552, 1973.

Malak, T.M., Ockleford, C.D., Bell, S.C., Dalgleish, R., Bright, N. and MacVicar, J.: Confocal immunofluorescence localization of collagen type-I, type-III, type-IV, type-V and type-VI and their ultrastructural organization in term human fetal membranes. Placenta **14**:385–406, 1993.

Malassine, A. and Cronier, L.: Hormones and human trophoblast differentiation: a review. Endocrine **19**:3–11, 2002.

Manaseki, S. and Searle, R.F.: Natural killer (NK) cell activity of first trimester human decidua. Cell Immunol. **121**:166–173, 1989.

Manivel, J.C., Niehans, G., Wick, M.R. and Dehner, L.P.: Intermediate trophoblast in germ cell neoplasms. Amer. J. Surg. Pathol. **11**:693–701, 1987.

Mansager, N., Bendon, R., Rosen, B., Miodovnik, M., Mostello, D. and Siddiqi, T.A.: Maternal floor infarction: Prenatal diagnosis and clinical significance. Amer. J. Obstet. Gynecol. **168**:347 (abstract 170), 1993.

Manyonda, I.T. and Varma, T.R.: Massive obstetric hemorrhage due to placenta previa/accreta with prior cesarean section. Intern. J. Gynecol. Obstet. **34**:183–186, 1991.

Maquoi, E., Polette, M., Nawrocki, B., Bischof, P., Noel, A., Pintiaux, A. Birembaut, P., Basset, P. and Foidart, J.M.: Expression of stromelysin-3 in the human implantation placental site. Placenta **16**:A46, 1995.

Maquoi, E., Polette, M., Nawrocki, B., Bischof, P., Noel, A., Pintiaux, A., Santavicca, M., Schaaps, J.-P., Pijnenborg, R., Birembaut, P. and Foidart, J.-M.: Expression of stromelysin-3 in the human placenta and placental bed. Placenta **18**:277–285, 1997.

Marais, W.D.: Human decidual spiral artery studies. I. Anatomy, circulation and pathology of the placenta. Observations with a colposcope. J. Obstet. Gynaecol. Brit. Commonw. **69**:1–122, 1962.

Martin, D. and Conrad, K.P.: Expression of endothelial nitric oxide synthase by extravillous trophoblast cells in the human placenta. Placenta **21**:23–31, 2000.

Martin, J.N., Sessums, J.K., Martin, R.W., Pryor, J.A. and Morrison, J.C.: Abdominal pregnancy: current concepts of management. Obstet. Gynecol. **71**:549–557, 1988.

Martinek, J.J.: Fibrinoid and the fetal-maternal interface of the rat placenta. Anat. Rec. **166**:587–604, 1970.

Martinek, J.J.: Ultrastructure of the deciduotrophoblastic interface of the mouse placenta. Amer. J. Obstet. Gynecol. **109**:424–431, 1971.

Marzioni, D., Banita, M., Felici, A., Paradinas, F.J., Newlands, E., De Nictolis, M., Muehlhauser, J. and Castellucci, M.: Expression of ZO-1 and occluding in normal human placenta and in hydatiform moles. Mol. Hum. Reprod. **7**:279–285, 2001.

Marzusch, K. and Dietl, J.: Immunologische Aspekte im Rahmen der regelrechten und gestörten Schwangerschaft beim Menschen. Publ.: Universitäts-Frauenklinik Tübingen, Tübingen, 1994.

Marzusch, K., Dietl, J., Horny, H.-P., Ruck, P., Kaiserling, E., Griesser, H. and Kabelitz, D.: Tolerance and the fetal graft. Lancet **337**:52, 1991.

Marzusch, K., Ruck, P., Geiselhart, A., Handgretinger, R., Dietl, J.A., Kaiserling, E., Horny, H.-P., Vince, G. and Redman, C.W.G.: Distribution of cell adhesion molecules on CD56++, CD3–, CD16– large granular lymphocytes and endothelial cells in first-trimester human decidua. Human Reprod. **8**:1203–1208, 1993.

Marzusch, K., Ruck, P., Handgretinger, R., Dietl, J.A., Horny, H.P. and Kaiserling, E.: Zur funktionellen Bedeutung der CD56++ large granular lymphocytes (LGL) in der Dezidua der Frühschwangerschaft beim Menschen. Gynaekol. Geburtsh. Rundsch. **35**:88–92, 1995.

Marzusch, K., Ruck, P., Dietl, J.A., Horny, H.-P. and Kaiserling, E.: Immunohistochemical localization of tissue inhibitor of metalloproteinases-2 (TIMP-2) in first trimester human placental decidua. Europ. J. Obstet. Gynecol. Reprod. Biol. **68**:105–107, 1996.

Marzusch, K., Buchholz, F., Ruck, P., Handgretinger, R., Geiselhart, A., Engelmann, L. and Dietl, J.: Interleukin-12– and interleukin-2–stimulated release of interferon-gamma by uterine CD56++ large granular lymphocytes is amplified by decidual macrophages. Human Reprod. **12**:921–924, 1997.

Matsuo, H., Maruo, T., Murata, K. and Mochizuki, M.: Human early placental trophoblasts produce an epidermal growth factor-like substance in synergy with thyroid hormone. Acta Endocrinol. Copenh. **128**:225–229, 1993.

Mau, G. and Netter, P.: Blutungen in der Frühschwangerschaft: Ein Hinweis auf kindliche Mißbildungen? Z. Kinderheilk. **117**:79–88, 1974.

McCombs, H.L. and Craig, J.M.: Decidual necrosis in normal pregnancy. Obstet. Gynecol. **24**:436–442, 1964.

McCormick, J.N., Faulk, W.P., Fox, H. and Fudenberg, H.H.: Immunohistological and elution studies of the human placenta. J. Exp. Med. **91**:1–13, 1971.

McDuffie, R.S., Harkness, L., McVay, R.M. and Haverkamp, A.D.: Midtrimester hemoperitoneum caused by placenta percreta in association with elevated maternal serum α-fetoprotein level. Amer. J. Obstet. Gynecol. **171**:565–566, 1994.

McElin, T.W. and Randall, L.M.: Intratubal term pregnancy without rupture: review of the literature and presentation of diagnostic criteria. Amer. J. Obstet. Gynecol. **61**:130–137, 1951.

McGowan, L. Intramural pregnancy. JAMA **192**:637–639, 1965.

McIntyre, J.A.: Antiphospholipid antibodies in implantation failures. Amer. J. Reprod. Immunol. **49**:221–229, 2003.

McKay, D.G., Hertig, A.T., Adams, E.C. and Richardson, M.V.: Histochemical observations on the human placenta. Obstet. Gynecol. **12**:1–36, 1958.

McMaster, M.T., Librach, C.L., Zhou, Y., Lim, K.H., Janatpour, M.J., DeMars, R., Kovats, S., Damsky, C.H. and Fisher, S.J.: Human placental HLA-G expression is restricted to differentiated cytotrophoblasts. J. Immunol. **154**:3771–3778, 1995.

McWey, L.A., Singhas, C.A. and Rogol, A.D.: Prolactin binding sites on human chorion-decidua tissue. Amer. J. Obstet. Gynecol. **144**:283–288, 1982.

Meekins, J.W., Luckas, M.J.M., Pijnenborg, R. and McFadyen, I.R.: Histological study of decidual spiral arteries and the presence of maternal erythrocytes in the intervillous space during the first trimester of normal human pregnancy. Placenta **18**:459–464, 1997.

Menzin, A.W., Loret de Mola, J.R., Bilker, W.B., Wheeler, J.E., Rubin, S.C. and Feinberg, R.F.: Identification of oncofetal fibronectin in patients with advanced epithelial ovarian cancer: detection in ascitic fluid and localization to primary sites and metastatic implants. Cancer **82**:152–158, 1998.

Merviel, P., Challier, J.C., Carbillon, L., Foidart, J.M. and Uzan, S.: The role of integrins in human embryo implantation. Fetal Diagn. Ther. **16**:364–371, 2001.

Millar, W.G.: A clinical and pathological study of placenta accreta. J. Obstet. Gynaecol. Brit. Emp. **66**:353–364, 1959.

Miller, L., Alley, E.W., Murphy, W.J., Russel, S.W. and Hunt, J.S.: Progesterone inhibits inducible nitric oxide synthase gene expression and nitric oxide production in murine macrophages. J. Leukoc. Biol., **59**:442–450, 1996.

Moe, N.: Deposits of fibrin and plasma proteins in the normal human placenta. Acta Pathol. Microbiol. Scand. **76**:74–88, 1969a.

Moe, N.: Histological and histochemical study of the extracellular deposits in the normal human placenta. Acta Pathol. Microbiol. Scand. **76**:419–431, 1969b.

Moe, N.: The deposits of fibrin and fibrin-like materials in the basal plate of the normal human placenta. Acta Pathol. Microbiol. Scand. **75**:1–17, 1969c.

Moll, U.M. and Lane, B.L.: Proteolytic activity of first trimester human placenta: localization of interstitial collagenase in villous and extravillous trophoblast. Histochemistry **94**:555–560, 1990.

Moll, W.: Invited Commentary: Absence of intervillous blood flow in the first trimester of human pregnancy. Placenta **16**:333–334, 1995.

Moll, W., Nienartowicz, A., Hees, H., Wrobel, K.-H. and Lenz, A.: Blood flow regulation in the uteroplacental arteries. Trophoblast Res. **3**:83–96, 1988.

Monaghan, J., O'Herlihy, C. and Boylan, P.: Ultrasound placental grading and amniotic fluid quantitation in prolonged pregnancy. Obstet. Gynecol. **70**:349–352, 1987.

Montemagno, U.: La sostanza fibrinoide placentare. Arch. Ostetr. Ginecol. (Napoli) **72**:585–596, 1967.

Morison, J.E.: Placenta accreta: a clinicopathologic review of 67 cases. Obstet. Gynecol. Annual **7**:107–123, 1978.

Moritz, A.R. and Douglass, M.: A study of uterine and tubal decidual reaction in tubal pregnancy. Based on the histological examination of the tubes and endometria of fifty-three cases of ectopic gestation. Surg. Gynecol. Obstet. **47**:785–790, 1928.

Morris, N.H., Eaton, B.M., Sooranna, S.R. and Steer, P.J.: NO synthase activity in placental bed and tissues from normotensive pregnant women. Lancet **342**:679–680, 1993.

Mortimer, G., Mackay, M.M. and Stimson, W.H.: The distribution of pregnancy-associated prostaglandin synthetase inhibitor in the human placenta. J. Pathol. **159**:239–243, 1989.

Mosmann, T.R. and Sad, S.: The expanding universe of T-cell subsets: Th1, Th2 and more. Immunol. Today **17**:138–146, 1996.

Mossman, H.W.: Comparative morphogenesis of the foetal membranes and accessory uterine structures. Contrib. Embryol. Carnegie Inst. **26**:129–246, 1937.

Mossman, H.W.: Vertebrate Fetal Membranes: Comparative Ontogeny and Morphology; Evolution; Phylogenetic Significance; Basic Functions; Research Opportunities. Macmillan, London, 1987.

Mühlhauser, J., Crescimanno, C., Kaufmann, P., Höfler, H., Zaccheo, D. and Castellucci, M.: Differentiation and proliferation patterns in human trophoblast revealed by c-erbB-2 oncogene product and EGF-R. J. Histochem. Cytochem. **41**:165–173, 1993.

Mühlhauser, J., Crescimanno, C., Kasper, M., Zaccheo, D. and Castellucci, M.: Differentiation of human trophoblast populations involves alterations in cytokeratin patterns. J. Histochem. Cytochem. **43**:579–589, 1995.

Mullen, C.A.: Review: analogies between trophoblastic and malignant cells. Amer. J. Reprod. Immunol. **39**:41–49, 1998.

Multhaupt, H.A.B., Mazar, A., Cines, D.B., Warhol, M.J. and McCrae, K.R.: Expression of urokinase receptors by human trophoblast. A histochemical and ultrastructural analysis. Lab. Invest. **71**:392–400, 1994.

Munn, D.H., Zhou, M., Attwood, J.T., Bondarev, I., Conway, S. J., Marshall, B., Brown, C. and Mellor, A.L.: Prevention of allogeneic fetal rejection by tryptophan catabolism. Science **281**:1191–1193, 1998.

Murakoshi, H., Matsuo, H., Laoag-Fernandez, J.B., Samoto, T, and Maruo, T.: Expression of Fas/Fas-ligand, Bcl-2 protein and apoptosis in extravillous trophoblast along invasion to the decidua in human term placenta. Endocr J. **50**:199–207, 2003.

Murta, E.F.C. and Nomelini, R.S.: Is repeated caesarean section a consequence of elective caesarean section? NEJM **364**:649–650, 2004.

Mylona, P., Kielty, C.M. Hoyland, J.A. and Aplin, J.D.: Expression of type VI collagen mRNAs in human endometrium during the menstrual cycle and first trimester of pregnancy. J. Reprod. Fertil. **103**:159–167, 1995.

Naeye, R.L.: Maternal floor infarction. Hum. Pathol. **16**:823–828, 1985.

Nagy, P.S.: Placenta percreta induced uterine rupture and resulted in intraabdominal abortion. Amer. J. Obstet. Gynecol. **161**:1185–1186, 1989.

Nanaev, A.K., Milovanov, A.P. and Domogatsky, S.P.: Immunohistochemical localization of extracellular matrix in various types of fibrinoid of the normal human term placenta. Placenta **14**:A.55, 1993a.

Nanaev, A.K., Milovanov, A.P. and Domogatsky, S.P.: Immunohistochemical localization of extracellular matrix in perivillous fibrinoid of normal human term placenta. Histochemistry **100**:341–346, 1993b.

Nanaev A., Chwalisz, K., Frank, H.-G., Kohnen, G., Hegele-Hartung, C. and Kaufmann, P.: Physiological dilation of uteroplacental arteries in the guinea pig depends on nitric oxide synthase activity of extravillous trophoblast. Cell Tissue Res. **282**:407–421, 1995.

Nanaev, A.K., Kosanke, G., Kemp, B., Frank, H.G., Huppertz, B. and Kaufmann, P.: The human placenta is encircled by a ring of smooth muscle cells. Placenta **21**:122–125, 2000a.

Nanaev, A.K., Kosanke, G., Reister, F., Kemp, B., Frank, H.G. and Kaufmann, P.: Pregnancy-induced de-differentiation of media smooth muscle cells in uteroplacental arteries of the guinea pig is reversible after delivery. Placenta **21**:306–312, 2000b.

Nasu, K., Zhou, Y., McMaster, M.T. and Fisher, S.J.: Upregulation of human cytotrophoblast invasion by hepatocyte growth factor. J. Reprod. Fertil. Suppl. **55**:73–80, 2000.

Nawrocki, B., Polette, M., Marchand, V., Foidart, J.M. and Birembaut, P.: MT-MMP expression in the development of human placenta. Placenta **16**:A52, 1995.

Nawrocki, B., Polette, M. Marchand, V., Maquoi, E., Boerchia, A., Tournier, J.M. Foidart, J.M. and Birembaut, P.: Membrane-type matrix metalloproteinase-1 expression at the site of human placentation. Placenta **17**:565–572, 1996.

Nehra, P.C. and Loginsky, S.J.: Pregnancy after vaginal hysterectomy. Obstet. Gynecol. **64**:735–737, 1984.

Nelson, D.M., Crouch, E.C., Curran, E.M. and Farmer, D.R.: Trophoblast interaction with fibrin matrix. Epithelialization of perivillous fibrin deposits as a mechanism for villous repair in the human placenta. Amer. J. Pathol. **136**:855–865, 1990.

Neuberg, M.: Decidual prolactin. Wiad. Lek. **45**:376–380, 1992.

Nickel, R.E.: Maternal floor infarction: an unusual cause of intrauterine growth retardation. Amer. J. Dis. Child. **142**:1270–1271, 1988.

Niebyl, J.R.: Pregnancy following total hysterectomy. Amer. J. Obstet. Gynecol. **119**:512–515, 1974.

Nikolov, Sp.D. and Schiebler, T.H.: Über die Gefässe der Basalplatte der reifen menschlichen Placenta. Licht- und elektronenmikroskopische Untersuchungen. Z. Zellforsch. **139**:319–332, 1973.

Norén, H. and Lindblom, B.: A unique case of abdominal pregnancy: what are the minimal requirements for placental contact with the maternal vascular bed? Amer. J. Obstet. Gynecol. **155**:394–396, 1986.

O'Brien, J.M., Barton, J.R. and Donaldson, E.S.: The management of placenta percreta: Conservative and operative strategies. Amer. J. Obstet. Gynecol. **175**:1632–1638, 1996.

O'Connell, C.P.: Full-term tubal pregnancy. Amer. J. Obstet. Gynecol. **63**:1305–1311, 1952.

O'Connor, D.M. and Kurman, R.J.: Utilization of intermediate trophoblast in the diagnosis of an in utero gestation in endometrial curettings without chorionic villi. Mod. Pathol. **1**:68A, 1988a.

O'Connor, D.M. and Kurman, R.J.: Intermediate trophoblast in uterine curettings in the diagnosis of ectopic pregnancy. Obstet. Gynecol. **72**:665–670, 1988b.

Ockleford, C.D., Malak, T., Hubbard, A., Bracken, K., Burton, S.A., Bright, N., Blakey, G., Goodliffe, J., Garrod, D. and d'Lacey, C.: Human amniochorion cytoskeletons at term. Placenta **14**:A56, 1993.

Ockleford, C., Bright, N., Hubbard, A., d'Lacey, C., Smith, J., Gardiner, L., Sheikh, T., Albentosa, M. and Turtle, K.: Microtrabeculae, macro-plaques or mini-basement membranes in human term fetal membranes. Phil. Trans. R. Soc. Lond. B **342**:121–136, 1994.

Ofir, K., Sheiner, E., Levy, A., Katz, M. and Mazor, M.: Uterine rupture: Differences between a scarred and an unscarred uterus. Amer. J. Obstet. Gynecol. **191**:425–429, 2004.

Oki, N., Matsuo, H., Nakago, S., Murakoshi, H., Laoag-Fernandez, J.B. and Maruo, T.: Effects of 3,5,3′-triiodothyronine on the invasive potential and the expression of integrins and matrix metalloproteinases in cultured early placental extravillous trophoblasts. J. Clin. Endocrinol. Metab. **89**:5213–5221 2004.

Oksenberg, J.R., Mor-Yosef, S., Persitz, E., Schenker, Y., Mozes, E. and Brautbar, C.: Antigen-presenting cells in human decidual tissue. Amer. J. Reprod. Immunol. **11**:82–88, 1986.

Okudaira, Y., Hashimoto, T., Hamanaka, N. and Yoshinare, S.: Electron microscopic study on the trophoblastic cell column of human placenta. J. Electron Microsc. **20**:93–106, 1971.

Okudaira, Y., Matsui, Y. and Kanoh, H.: Morphological variability of human trophoblasts in normal and neoplastic conditions—an ultrastructural reappraisal. In, Placenta: Basic Research for Clinical Application. H. Soma, ed. Karger, Basel 1991.

Oláh, C.S., Gee, H., Rushton, I. and Fowlie, A.: Massive subchorionic thrombohaematoma presenting as a placental tumour. Case report. Brit. J. Obstet. Gynaecol. **94**:995–997, 1987.

Ono, H., Ide, C. and Nishiya, I.: Electron microscopic study on early decidualization of the endometrium of pregnant mice, with special reference to gap junctions. Placenta **10**:247–261, 1989.

Ornoy, A., Benady, S., Kohen-Raz, R. and Russell, A.: Association between maternal bleeding during gestation and congenital anomalies in the offspring. Amer. J. Obstet. Gynecol. **124**:474–478, 1976.

Ortmann, R.: Histochemische Untersuchungen an menschlicher Plazenta mit besonderer Berücksichtigung der Kernkugeln (Kerneinschlüsse) und der Plasmalipoideinschlüsse. Z. Anat. Entwicklungsgesch. **119**:28–55, 1955.

Ortmann, R.: Morphologie der menschlichen Placenta. Anat. Anz. **106/107**:27–56, 1960.

Osawa, H., Iida, S., Tomioka, Y. and Hirano, M.: The effects of NOS inhibitor on pregnancy. Placenta **16**:A54, 1995.

Oswald, B. and Gerl, D.: Die Mikrofibrinoidablagerungen in der menschlichen Placenta. Acta Histochem. (Jena) **42**:356–359, 1972.

Oyer, R., Tarakjian, D., Lev-Toaff, A., Friedman, A. and Chatwani, A.: Treatment of cervical pregnancy with methotrexate. Obstet. Gynecol. **71**:469–471, 1988.

Pace, D., Morrison, L. and Bulmer, J.N.: Proliferative activity in endometrial stromal granulocytes throughout menstrual cycle and early pregnancy. J. Clin. Pathol. **42**:35–39, 1989.

Paddock, R. and Greer, E.D.: Origin of common cystic structure of human placenta. Amer. J. Obstet. Gynecol. **13**:164–173, 1927.

Padykula, H.A. and Driscoll, S.G.: Decidual cell differentiation in the normal early gestational uterus includes lymphoid infiltration. Anat. Rec. **190**:500–501, 1978.

Paintin, D.B.: Abdominal pregnancy carried to term following the treatment of pelvic tuberculosis. Proc. R. Soc. Med. **63**:54–55, 1970.

Pak, B.J., Park, H., Chang, E.R., Pang, S.C. and Graham, C.H.: Differential display analysis of oxygen-mediated changes in gene expression in first trimester human trophoblast cells. Placenta **19**:483–488, 1998.

Palti, Z., Rosenn, B., Goshen, R., Ben-Chitrit, A. and Yagel, S.: Successful treatment of a viable cervical pregnancy with methotrexate. Amer. J. Obstet. Gynecol. **161**:1147–1148, 1989.

Pampfer, S., Daiter, E., Barad, D. and Pollard, J.W.: Expression of the colony-stimulating factor-1 receptor (c-fms proto-oncogene product) in the human uterus and placenta. Biol. Reprod. **46**:48–57, 1992.

Panigel, M. and Pascaud, M.: Les orifices artériels d'entrée du sang maternel dans la chambre intervilleuse du placenta humain. Bull. Assoc. Anat. 53rd Congres (Tours. No. 142), pp. 1287–1298, 1968.

Parhar, R.S., Yagel, S. and Lala, P.K.: PGE2–mediated immunosuppression by first trimester human decidual cells blocks activation of maternal leukocytes in the decidua with potential anti-trophoblast activity. Cell Immunol. **120**:61–74, 1989.

Park, W.W.: Disorders arising from the human trophoblast. In, Modern Trends in Pathology. D.H. Collins, ed., pp. 180–211, Butterworth, London, 1959.

Parmley, T.H., Gupta, P.K. and Walker, M.A.: "Aging" pigments in term human placenta. Amer. J. Obstet. Gynecol. **139**:760–766, 1981.

Peel, S. and Bulmer, D.: The fine structure of the rat metrial gland in relation to the origin of the granulated cells. J. Anat. **123**:687–969, 1977.

Peles, E., Bacus, S.S., Koski, R.A., Lu, H.S., Wen, D., Ogden, S. G., Ben-Levy, R. and Yarden, Y.: Isolation of the neu/Her-2 stimulatory ligand: a 44kd glycoprotein that induces differentiation of mammary tumor cells. Cell **69**:205–216, 1992.

Perrin, E.V.D.K.: Placenta as a reflection of fetal disease: A brief overview. In, Pathology of the Placenta. E.V.D.K. Perrin, ed. Churchill Livingstone, New York, 1984.

Petraglia, F., Sawchenko, P., Lim, A.T.W., Rivier, J. and Vale, W.: Localization, secretion, and action of inhibin in human placenta. Science **237**:187–189, 1987.

Petrucha, R.A. and Platt, L.D.: Relationship of placental grade to gestational age. Amer. J. Obstet. Gynecol. **144**:733–735, 1982.

Petry, G.: Studien über die morphologischen Grundlagen des Blasensprungs. Zentralbl. Gynäkol. **76**:655–675, 1954a.

Petry, G.: Der Bau der menschlichen Eihaut und seine funktionelle Bedeutung. Klin. Wochenschr. **32**:1020, 1954b.

Pfeiffer, R.A.: Nanisme microcephalique letal: Exemple de pathologie placentaire d'origine genetique? J. Génét. Hum. **22**:259–261, 1974.

Philippe, E., Ritter, J., Lefakis, P., Laedlein-Greilsammer, D., Itten, S. and Foussereau, S.: Grossesse tubaire, ovulation tardive et anomalie de nidation. Gynécol. Obstétr. (Paris) **69**:617–628, 1970.

Pierleoni, C., Samuelsen, G.B., Graem, N., Ronne, E., Nielsen, B.S., Kaufmann, P. and Castellucci, M.: Immunohistochemical identification of the receptor for urokinase plasminogen activator associated with fibrin deposition in normal and ectopic human placenta. Placenta **19**:501–508, 1998.

Pijnenborg, R., Dixon, G., Robertson, W.B. and Brosens, I.: Trophoblastic invasion of human decidua from 8 to 18 weeks of pregnancy. Placenta **1**:3–19, 1980.

Pijnenborg, R., Robertson, W.B., Brosens, I. and Dixon, G.: Trophoblast invasion and the establishment of haemochorial placentation in man and laboratory animals. Placenta **2**:71–92, 1981.

Pijnenborg, R., Bland, J.M., Robertson, W.B. and Brosens, I.: Uteroplacental arterial changes related to interstitial trophoblast migration in early human pregnancy. Placenta **4**:397–414, 1983.

Pijnenborg, R., McLaughlin, P.J., Vercruysse, L., Hanssens, M., Johnson, P.M., Keith, J.C. and Van Assche, F.A.: Immunolocalization of tumour necrosis factor-α (TNF-α) in the placental bed of normotensive and hypertensive human pregnancies. Placenta **19**:231–239, 1998.

Piotrowicz, R.S., Orchekowski, D.J., Nugent, D.J., Yamada, K.Y. and Kunicki T.J.: Glycoprotein Ic-IIa functions as an activation-independent fibronectin receptor on human platelets. J. Cell Biol. **106**:1359–1364, 1988.

Pitkin, R.M.: Calcium metabolism in pregnancy: a review. Amer. J. Obstet. Gynecol. **121**:724–737, 1975.

Pitkin, R.M., Reeynolds, W.A., Williams, G.A. and Hargis, G.K.: Calcium metabolism in normal pregnancy: a longitudinal study. Amer. J. Obstet. Gynecol. **133**:781–790, 1979.

Pizarro, A., Gamallo, C., Benito, N., Palacios, J., Quintanilla, M., Cano, A. and Contreras, F.: Differential patterns of placental and epithelial cadherin expression in basal cell carcinoma and in the epidermis overlying tumours. Brit. J. Cancer **72**:327–332, 1995.

Polette, M., Nawrocki, B., Pintiaux, A., Massenat, C., Maquoi, E., Volders, L., Schaaps, J.P., Birembaut, P. and Foidart, J.M.: Expression of gelatinases A and B and their tissue inhibitors by cells of early and term human placenta and gestational endometrium. Lab. Invest. **71**:838–846, 1994.

Postovit, L.M., Adams, M.A. and Graham, C.H.: Does nitric oxide play a role in the aetiology of pre-eclampsia? Placenta **22** Suppl A:S51–S55, 2001.

Pozniak, M.A., Cullenward, M.J., Zickuhr, D. and Curet, L.B.: Venous lake bleeding: a complication of chorionic villus sampling. J. Ultrasound Med. **7**:297–299, 1988.

Pröll, J., Blaschitz, A., Hartmann, M., Thalhamer, J. and Dohr, G.: Cytokeratin 17 as an immunohistochemical marker for intramural cytotrophoblast in human first trimester uteroplacental arteries. Cell Tissue Res. **288**:335–343, 1997a.

Pröll, J., Blaschitz, A., Hartmann, M., Thalhamer, J. and Dohr, G.: Human first-trimester placenta intra-arterial trophoblast cells express the neural cell adhesion molecule: References. Early Pregnancy: Biology and Medicine **3**:125–126, 1997b.

Qin, X.J., Chua, P.K., Ohira, R.H. and Bryant-Greenwood, G.D.: An autocrine/paracrine role of human decidual relaxin. 2. Stromelysin-1 (MMP-3) and tissue inhibitor of matrix metalloproteinase-1 (TIMP-1). Biol. Reprod. **56**:812–820, 1997a.

Qin, X.J., Garibaytupas, J., Chua, P.K., Cachola, L. and Bryant-Greenwood, G.D.: An autocrine/paracrine role of human decidual relaxin. 1. Interstitial collagenase (matrix metalloproteinase-1) and tissue plasminogen activator. Biol. Reprod. **56**:800–811, 1997b.

Raghupathy, R., Singh, B., Barrington-Leigh, J. and Wegmann, T.G.: The ontogeny and turnover kinetics of paternal H-2 K antigenic determinants on the allogenic murine placenta. J. Immunol. **127**:2074, 1981.

Raghupathy, R., Singh, B. and Wegmann, T.G.: Fate of antipaternal H-2 antibodies bound to the placenta in vivo. Transplantation **37**:296, 1984.

Rahman, M.S., Al-Suleiman, S.A., Rahman, J. and Al-Sibai, M. H.: Advanced abdominal pregnancy-Observations in 10 cases. Obstet. Gynecol. **59**:366–372, 1982.

Ramsey, E.M.: Circulation in the maternal placenta of the rhesus monkey and man, with observations on the marginal lakes. Amer. J. Anat. **98**:159–190, 1956.

Ramsey, E.M.: Circulation in the intervillous space of the primate placenta. Amer. J. Obstet. Gynecol. **84**:1649–1663, 1962.

Ramsey, E.M.: The story of the spiral arteries. J. Reprod. Med. **26**:393–399, 1981.

Ramsey, E.M. and Donner, M.W.: Placental Vasculature and Circulation. Thieme, Stuttgart 1980.

Ramsey, E.M., Corner, G.W., Jr. and Donner, M.W.: Serial and cineradioangiographic visualization of maternal circulation in the primate (hemochorial) placenta. Amer. J. Obstet. Gynecol. **86**:213–225, 1963.

Ramsey, E.M. and Harris, J.W.S.: Comparison of uteroplacental vasculature and circulation in the rhesus monkey and man. Contrib. Embryol. Carnegie Inst. **38**:59–70, 1966.

Ramsey, E.M., Martin Jr., C.B., McGaughey, Jr., H.S., Kaiser, I.H. and Donner, M.W.: Venous drainage of the placenta in rhesus monkeys: radiographic studies. Amer. J. Obstet. Gynecol. **95**:948–955, 1966.

Read, J.A., Cotton, D.B. and Miller, F.C.: Placenta accreta: changing clinical aspects and outcome. Obstet. Gynecol. **56**:31–33, 1980.

Reddy, G.S., Norman, A.W., Willis, D.M., Goltzman, D., Guyda, H., Solomon, S., Philips, D.R., Bishop, J.E. and Mayer, E.: Regulation of vitamin D metabolism in normal human pregnancy. J. Clin. Endocrinol. Metabol. **56**:363–370, 1983.

Redline, R.W. and Lu, C.Y.: Specific defects in the anti-listerial immune response in discrete regions of the murine uterus and placenta account for susceptibility to infection. J. Immunol. **140**:3947–3955, 1988.

Redman, C.W.G.: Cytotrophoblasts: Masters of disguise. Nature Medicine **3**:610–611, 1997.

Reister, F., Frank, H.G., Heyl, W., Kosanke, G., Huppertz, B., Schröder, W., Kaufmann, P. and Rath, W.: The distribution of macrophages in the placental bed in preeclampsia differs from that in healthy patients. Placenta **20**:229–233, 1999.

Reister, F., Frank, H.G., Kingdom, J.C.P., Heyl, W., Kaufmann, P., Rath, W. and Huppertz, B.: Macrophage-induced apoptosis limits endovascular trophoblast invasion in the uterine wall of preeclamptic women. Lab. Invest. **81**:1143–1152, 2001.

Ren, S.G. and Braunstein, G.D.: Decidua produces a protein that inhibits choriogonadotrophin release from human trophoblasts. J. Clin. Invest. **87**:326–330, 1991.

Reshef, E., Lei, Z.M., Rao, C.V., Pridham, D.D., Chegini, N. and Luborsky, J.L.: The presence of gonadotropin receptors in nonpregnant human uterus, human placenta, fetal membranes, and decidua. J. Clin. Endocrinol. Metab. **70**:421–430, 1990.

Reynolds, S.R.M.: Formation of fetal cotyledons in the hemochorial placenta: a theoretical consideration of the functional implication of such an arrangements. Amer. J. Obstet. Gynecol. **94**:425–439, 1966.

Riddick, D.H. and Daly, D.C.: Decidual prolactin production in human gestation. Semin. Perinatol. **6**:229–237, 1982.

Ries, K.J. and Middleton, E.B.: Rupture of septate uterus due to placenta percreta. Obstet. Gynecol. **39**:705–712, 1972.

Riley, S.C., Walton, J.C., Herlick, J.M. and Challis, J.R.: The localization and distribution of corticotropin-releasing hormone in the human placenta and fetal membranes throughout gestation. J. Clin. Endocrinol. Metab. **72**:1001–1007, 1991.

Riley, S.C., Dupont, E., Walton, J.C., Luuthe, V., Labrie, F., Pelletier, G. and Challis, J.R.G.: Immunohistochemical localization of 3β-hydroxy-5-ene-steroid dehydrogenase delta5-delta4 isomerase in human placenta and fetal membranes throughout gestation. J. Clin. Endocrinol. Metab. **75**:956–961, 1992.

Robb, J.A., Benirschke, K. and Barmeyer, R.: Intrauterine latent herpes simplex virus infection. I. Spontaneous abortion. Hum. Pathol. **17**:1196–1209, 1986a.

Robb, J.A., Benirschke, K., Mannino, F. and Voland, J.: Intrauterine latent herpes simplex virus infection. II. Latent neonatal infection. Hum. Pathol. **17**:1210–1217, 1986b.

Robertson, S.A., Seamark, R.F., Guilbert, L.J. and Wegmann, T.G.: The role of cytokines in gestation. Critical Reviews in Immunology **14**:239–292, 1994.

Robertson, W.B. and Manning, P.J.: Elastic tissue in uterine blood vessels. J. Pathol. **112**:237–243, 1974.

Robertson, W.B.: Uteroplacental vasculature. J. Clin. Pathol. [Suppl.] **29**:9–17, 1976. (R. Coll. Pathol.) **10**:9–17, 1976.

Robinson, L., Grau, P. and Crandall, B.F.: Pregnancy outcomes after increasing maternal serum alpha-fetoprotein levels. Obstet. Gynecol. **74**:17–20, 1989.

Rodesch, F., Simon, P., Donner, C. and Jauniaux, E.: Oxygen measurements in endometrial and trophoblastic tissues during early pregnancy. Obstet. Gynecol. **80**:283–285, 1992.

Rosen, J.F., Roginsky, M., Nathenson, G. and Finberg, L.: 25-hydroxyvitamin D: Plasma levels in mothers and their premature infants with neonatal hypocalcemia. Amer. J. Dis. Child. **127**:220–223, 1974.

Rosenberg, S.M., Maslar, I.A. and Riddick, D.H.: Decidual production of prolactin in late gestation: further evidence for a decidual source of amniotic fluid prolactin. Amer. J. Obstet. Gynecol. **138**:681–685, 1980.

Rosenberg, S.M. and Bhatnagar, A.S.: Sex steroid and human chorionic gonadotropin modulation of in vitro prolactin production by human term decidua. Amer. J. Obstet. Gynecol. **148**:461–465, 1984.

Ross, J.A., Hacket, E., Lawton, F. and Jurkovic, D.: Massive ascites due to abdominal pregnancy. Human Reprod. **12**:390–391, 1997.

Rossant, J. and Croy, B.A.: Genetic identification of tissue of origin of cellular populations within the mouse placenta. J. Embryol. Exp. Morphol. **86**:177–189, 1985.

Ruck, P., Marzusch, K., Kaiserling, E., Horny, H.-P., Dietl, J., Geiselhart, A., Handgretinger, R. and Redman, C.W.G.: Distribution of cell adhesion molecules in decidua of early human pregnancy. Lab. Invest. **71**:94–101, 1994.

Ruck, P., Marzusch, K., Horny, H.-P., Dietl, J. and Kaiserling, E.: Distribution of tissue inhibitor of metalloproteinases-2 (TIMP-2) in trophoblast of early human pregnancy. Placenta **16**:A62, 1995.

Ruck, P., Marzusch, K., Horny, H.-P., Dietl, J. and Kaiserling, E.: The distribution of tissue inhibitor of metalloproteinases-2 (TIMP-2) in the human placenta. Placenta **17**:263–266, 1996.

Ruck, P., Marzusch, K., Kröber, S., Horny, H.-P., Dietl, J. and Kaiserling, E.: The Distribution of tissue inhibitor of metalloproteinases-2 (TIMP-2) in decidua and trophoblast of early human pregnancy. Trophoblast Res. **10**:115–121, 1997.

Rukosuev, V.S., Nanaev, A.K. and Milovanov, A.P.: Participation of collagen types I, III, IV, V, and fibronectin in the formation of villi fibrosis in human term placenta. Acta Histochem. (Jena) **89**:11–16, 1990.

Ruoslahti, E.: Integrins as receptors for extracellular matrix. In: Cell Biology of Extracellular Matrix. E.D. Hay, (ed). New York: Plenum Press, Ed. **2**:343–363, 1991.

Ruoslahti, E. and Pierschbacher, M.D.: New perspectives in cell adhesion: RGD and integrins. Science **238**:491–497, 1987.

Russell, J.G.B.: Antenatal diagnosis of placental calcification. J. Obstet. Gynaecol. Brit. Commonw. **76**:813–126, 1969.

Rutanen, E.M., Partanen, S. and Pekonen, F.: Decidual transformation of human extrauterine mesenchymal cells is associated with the appearance of insulin-like growth factor-binding protein-1. J. Clin. Endocrinol. Metab. **72**:27–31, 1991.

Rutherford, R.N.: The significance of bleeding in early pregnancy as evidenced by decidual biopsy. Surg. Gynecol. Obstet. **74**:1139–1153, 1942.

Saijonmaa, O., Laatikainen, T. and Wahlström, T.: Corticotrophin-releasing factor in human placenta: localization, concentration and release in vitro. Placenta **9**:373–385, 1988.

Saito, S., Morii, T., Enomoto, M., Sakakura, S., Nishikawa, K., Narita, N. and Ichijo, M.: The effect of interleukin 2 and transforming growth factor-β2 (TGF-β2) on the proliferation and natural killer activity of decidual CD16-CD56 bright natural killer cells. Cell. Immunol. **152**:605–613, 1993a.

Saito, S., Nishikawa, K., Morii, T., Enomoto, M., Narita, N., Motoyoshi, K. and Ichijo, M.: Cytokine production by CD16-CD56 (bright) natural killer cells in the human early pregnancy decidua. Int. Immunol. **5**:559–563, 1993b.

Saito, S., Nishikawa, K., Morii, T., Narita, N., Enomoto, M., Ito, A. and Ichijo, M.: A study of CD45RO, CD45RA and CD29 antigen expression on human decidual T cells in an early stage of pregnancy. Immunol. Letters **40**:193–197, 1994.

Saji, M., Taga, M. and Minaguchi, H.: Epidermal growth factor stimulate cell proliferation and inhibits prolactin secretion of the human decidual cells in culture. Endocrinol. Jpn. **37**:177–182, 1990.

Sakbun, V., Ali, S.M., Greenwood, F.C. and Bryant Greenwood, G.D.: Human relaxin in the amnion, chorion, decidua parietalis, basal plate, and placental trophoblast by immunocytochemistry and northern analysis. J. Clin. Endocrinol. Metab. **70**:508–514, 1990a.

Sakbun, V., Ali, S.M., Lee, Y.A., Jara, C.S. and Bryant Greenwood, G.D.: Immunocytochemical localization and messenger ribonucleic acid concentrations for human placental lactogen in amnion, chorion, decidua, and placenta. Amer. J. Obstet. Gynecol. **162**:1310–1317, 1990b.

Sasagawa, M., Yamazaki, T., Sudo, Y., Kanazawa, K. and Takeuchi, S.: Immunohistochemical localization of hCG α, hCG β, CTP, hPL and SP1 on villous and extravillous trophoblasts in normal human pregnancy. Nippon. Sanka. Fujinka. Gakkai. Zasshi. **39**:1073–1079, 1987.

Sauramo, H.: Cytotrophoblast of the placenta and foetal membranes in normal and pathological obstetrics. Ann. Med. Exper. Fenn. **39**:7–12, 1961.

Schaaps, J.P. and Hustin, J.: In vivo aspect of the maternal-trophoblastic border during the first trimester of gestation. Trophoblast Res. **3**:39–48, 1988.

Schaefer, O.: Familial occurrence of abnormal placentation and fetal malformations, observed in Baffin Island Eskimos. Canad. Med. Assoc. J. **83**:437–438, 1960.

Scheuner, G.: Über die Verankerung der Nabelschnur an der Plazenta. Morphol. Jahrb. **106**:73–89, 1964.

Schiebler, T.H. and Kaufmann, P.: Reife Plazenta. In, Die Plazenta des Menschen. V. Becker, T.H. Schiebler and F. Kubli, eds. Thieme, Stuttgart, 1981.

Schindler, A.M., Bordignon, P. and Bischof, P.: Immunohistochemical localization of pregnancy-associated plasma protein A in decidua and trophoblast: comparison with human chorionic gonadotrophin and fibrin. Placenta **5**:227–235, 1984.

Schmidt, C.M. and Orr, H.T.: Maternal/fetal interactions—the role of MHC class I molecule HLA-G. Crit. Rev. Immunol. **13**:207–224, 1993.

Schmidt-Matthiesen, H.: Das normale menschliche Endometrium. Thieme, Stuttgart 1963.

Schmitt, R. and Dittrich, A.: Ausgetragene Extrauteringravidität bei lebendem Kind. Zentralbl. Gynäkol. **95**:28–31, 1973.

Schuhmann, R.: Plazenton: Begriff, Entstehung, funktionelle Anatomie. In, Die Plazenta des Menschen. V. Becker, T.H. Schiebler and F. Kubli, eds. pp. 192–207. Thieme, Stuttgart, 1981.

Schuhmann, R. and Wehler, V.: Histologische Unterschiede an Plazentazotten innerhalb der materno-fetalen Strömungseinheit. Ein Beitrag zur funktionellen Morphologie der Plazenta. Arch. Gynäkol. **210**:425–439, 1971.

Schultze, K.W.: Über Randsinusblutungen aus der Plazenta in der Schwangerschaft und unter der Geburt. Geburtshilfl. Frauenheilk. **13**:708–715, 1953.

Schultze, K.W.: Über sog. Plazenta-Randsinusblutungen. Dtsch. Hebammen-Z. **20**:1–4, 1968.

Schulz, L.C. and Widmaier, E.P.: The effect of leptin on mouse trophoblast cell invasion. Biol Reprod. **71**:1963–1967, 2004.

Schwartz, A., Sauer, J., Hradeckky, L. and Pavlik, V.: Die Zysten der menschlichen Plazenta. Zentralbl. Allg. Pathol. **117**:185–190, 1973.

Scipiades, E. and Burg, E.: Über die Morphologie der menschlichen Placenta mit besonderer Rücksicht auf unsere eigenen Studien. Arch. Gynäkol. **141**:577–619, 1930.

Sebire, N.J., Fox, H., Backos, M., Rai, R., Paterson, C. and Regan, L.: Defective endovascular trophoblast invasion in primary antiphospholipid antibody syndrome-associated early pregnancy failure. Hum. Reprod. **17**:1067–1071, 2002.

Sengel, A. and Stöbner, P: Ultrastructure de l'endometre humain normal. III. Les cellules K.Z. Zellforsch. **133**:47–57, 1972.

Sengupta, J., Given, R.L., Talwar, D. and Ghosh, D.: Endometrial response to deciduogenic stimulus in ovariectomized rhesus monkeys treated with oestrogen and progesterone: an ultrastructural study. J. Endocrinol. **124**:53–57, 1990.

Shanklin, D.R. and Scott, J.S.: Massive subchorial thrombohaematoma (Breus' mole). Brit. J. Obstet. Gynaecol. **82**:476–487, 1975.

Shapiro, J.L., Sherer, D.M., Hurley, J.T., Metlay, L.A. and Amstey, M.S.: Postpartum ultrasonographic findings associated with placenta accreta. Amer. J. Obstet. Gynecol. **167**:601–601, 1992.

Sharkey, A.M., Charnock-Jones, D.S., Brown, K.D. and Smith, S. K.: Expression of mRNA for kit ligand in human placenta: localisation by in-situ hybridisation and identification of alternatively spliced variants. Mol. Endocrinol. **6**:1235–1241, 1992.

Sharkey, A.M., Charnock-Jones, D.S., Boocock, C.A., Brown, K.D. and Smith, S.K.: Expression of mRNA for vascular endothelial growth factor in human placenta. J. Reprod. Fertil. **99**:609–615, 1993.

Sharkey, A.M., Jokhi, P.P., King, A., Loke, Y.W., Brown, K.D. and Smith, S.K.: Expression of c-kit and kit ligand at the human maternofetal interface. Cytokine **6**:195–205, 1994.

Sheppard, B.L. and Bonnar, J.: Scanning electron microscopy of the human placenta and decidual spiral arteries in normal pregnancy. J. Obstet. Gynaecol. Brit. Commonw. **81**:17–20, 1974a.

Sheppard, B.L. and Bonnar, J.: The ultrastructure of the arterial supply of the human placenta in early and late pregnancy. J. Obstet. Gynaecol. Brit. Commonw. **81**:497–511, 1974b.

Sheppard, B.L. and Bonnar, J.: The ultrastructure of the arterial supply of the human placenta in pregnancy complicated by fetal growth retardation. Brit. J. Obstet. Gynaecol. **83**:948–959, 1976.

Sheppard, B.L. and Bonnar, J.: The maternal blood supply to the placenta in pregnancy complicated by intrauterine fetal growth retardation. Trophoblast Res. **3**:69–82, 1988.

Shipley, C.F. and Nelson, G.H.: Prenatal diagnosis of a placental cyst: Comparison of postnatal biochemical analyses of cyst fluid, amniotic fluid, cord serum, and maternal serum. Amer. J. Obstet. Gynecol. **168**:211–213, 1993.

Shipp, T.D. and Lieberman, E.: Impact of single- or double-layer closure on uterine rupture. Amer. J. Obstet. Gynecol. **188**:601–603, 2003.

Shorter, S.C., Vince, G.S. and Starkey, P.M.: Production of granulocyte colony-stimulating factor at the materno-fetal interface in human pregnancy. Immunol. **75**:468–474, 1992.

Shorter, S.C., Starkey, P.M., Ferry, B.L., Clover, L.M., Sargent, I.L. and Redman, C.W.G.: Antigenic heterogeneity of human cytotrophoblast and evidence for the transient expression of MHC class I antigens distinct from HLA-G. Placenta **14**:571–582, 1993.

Shott, R.J., Cook, L.N. and Andrews, B.F.: Intra-abdominal pregnancy: an unusual cause of fetal growth retardation. Amer. J. Dis. Child. **126**:361–362, 1973.

Shukla, H., Swaroop, A., Srivastava, R. and Weissman, S.M.: The mRNA of a human class I gene HLA G/GLA 6.0 exhibits a restricted pattern of expression. Nucleic Acids Res. **18**:2189, 1990.

Shweiky, D., Itin, A., Soffer, D. and Keshet, E.: Vascular endothelial growth factor induced by hypoxia may mediate hypoxia-initiated angiogenesis. Nature **359**:843–845, 1992.

Simpson, N.A.B., Nimrod, C., De Vermette, R. and Fournier, J.: Determination of intervillous flow in early pregnancy. Placenta **18**:287–293, 1997.

Silber, S.J., Breakey, B., Campbell, D., Williams, H. and Fellman, S.: Placenta percreta invading bladder. J. Urol. **109**:615–618, 1973.

Singer, M. and Wislocki, G.B.: The affinity of syncytium, fibrin and fibrinoid of the human placenta for acid and basic dyes under controlled conditions of staining. Anat. Rec. 102:175–194, 1948.

Sinha, A.A.: Ultrastructure of human amnion and amniotic plaques of normal pregnancy. Z. Zellforsch. 122:1–14, 1971.

Smith, G.C.S., Pell, J.P. and Dobbie, R.: Caesarean section and risk of unexplained stillbirth in subsequent pregnancy. Lancet 362:1779–1784, 2003.

Soma, H., Satoh, M., Higashi, S., Horikiri, H., Hata, T., Isaka, K. and Malla, D.: Fine structure and biological properties of chorionic cysts. In: Placenta: Basic Research for Clinical Application. Soma, H., ed. pp. 200–208, Karger, Basel, 1991.

Sonnenberg, A., Modderman, P.W. and Hogervorst, F.: Laminin receptor on platelets is the integrin VLA-6. Nature (Lond.) 336:487–489, 1988.

Spanner, R.: Der Kreislauf im intervillösen Raum des Menschen. Untersuchungen an den Uteroplacentargefässen schwangerer Uteri. Anat. Anz. 78:127–129, 1934.

Spanner, R.: Mütterlicher und kindlicher Kreislauf der menschlichen Placenta und seine Strombahnen. Z. Ges. Anat. 105:163–242, 1935.

Spanner, R.: Zellinseln und Zottenepithel in der zweiten Hälfte der Schwangerschaft. Morphol. Jahrb. 86:407–461, 1941.

Spanta, R., Roffman, L.E., Grissom, T.J., Newland, J.R. and McManus, B.M.: Abdominal pregnancy: magnetic resonance identification with ultrasonographic follow-up of placental involution. Amer. J. Obstet. Gynecol. 157:887–889, 1987.

Spiegelberg, O.: Zur Casuistik der Ovarialschwangerschaft. Arch. Gynäkol. 13:73–79, 1878.

Spinnato, J.A., Aksel, S. and Mendenhall, H.W.: Postpartum polyhydramnios: a unique complication of advanced pregnancy. Obstet. Gynecol. 70:490–492, 1987.

Spornitz, U.M.: The functional morphology of the human endometrium and decidua. Adv. Anat. Embryol. Cell Biol. 124:1–99, 1992.

Spornitz, U.M.: Pseudo-decidualization at the site of implantation in tubal pregnancy. Arch. Gynecol. Obstet. 253:85–95, 1993.

Spornitz, U.M. and Ludwig, K.S.: Die Ultrastruktur der menschlichen Deziduazelle. Acta Anat. 120:245, 1984.

Springer, T.A.: Adhesion receptors of the immuno system. Nature 346:425–434, 1990.

Stark, J. and Kaufmann, P.: Die Basalplatte der reifen menschlichen Placenta. II. Gefrierschnitt-Histochemie. Z. Anat. Entwicklungsgesch. 135:185–201, 1971.

Stark, J. and Kaufmann, P.: Die Basalplatte der reifen menschlichen Placenta. III. Bindegewebs- und Deciduazellen. Arch. Gynäkol. 213:399–417, 1973.

Stark, J. und Kaufmann, P.: Infarktgenese in der Placenta. Arch. Gynäkol. 217:189–208, 1974.

Staun-Ram, E., Goldman, S., Gabarin, D. and Shalev, E.: Expression and importance of matrix metalloproteinase 2 and 9 (MMP-2 and -9) in human trophoblast invasion. Reprod. Biol. Endocrinol. 2:59, 2004.

St. Clair, J.T., Wheeler, D.A. and Fish, S.A.: Methotrexate in abdominal pregnancy. JAMA 208:529–531, 1969.

Stegner, H.E., Sachs, H. and Uthmöller, E.: Elektronenmikroskopische Untersuchungen am experimentellen Deziduom der Ratte. Z. Geburtsh. Gynäkol. 174:241–251, 1971.

Steininger, H.: Über die Herkunft von Septen und Inseln der menschlichen Plazenta. Arch. Gynecol. 226:261–275, 1978.

Stieve, H.: Neue Untersuchungen über die Placenta, besonders über die Entstehung der Placentasepten. Arch. Gynäkol. 161:160–167, 1936.

Stieve, H.: Die Entwicklung und der Bau der menschlichen Placenta. I. Zotten, Trophoblastinseln und Scheidewaende in der ersten Hälfte der Schwangerschaft. Z. Mikrosk. Anat. Forsch. 48:287–358, 1940.

Stieve, H. and von der Heide, I.: Über die Entwicklung der Septen in der menschlichen Plazenta. Anat. Anz. 92:1–16, 1941.

Stromme, W.B.: Placenta increta: report of a case with unusual etiology. Obstet. Gynecol. 21:133–135, 1963.

Sumawong, V., Nondasuta, A., Thanapath, S. and Budthimedhee, V.: Placenta accreta: a review of the literature and a summary of 10 cases. Obstet. Gynecol. 27:511–516, 1966.

Sunde, A.: Advanced extrauterine pregnancy. Acta Obstet. Gynecol. Scand. 44:159–162, 1965.

Sutcliffe, R.G., Davies, M., Hunter, J.B., Waters, J.J. and Parry, J.E.: The protein composition of the fibrinoid material at the human uteroplacental interface. Placenta 3:297–308, 1982.

Swinburne, L.M.: Leucocyte antigens and placental sponge. Lancet 2:592–593, 1970.

Taefi, P., Kaiser, T.F., Sheffer, J.B., Courey, N.G. and Hodson, J.M.: Placenta percreta with bladder invasion and massive hemorrhage: report of a case. Obstet. Gynecol. 36:686–687, 1970.

Takada, A., Ohmori, K., Yoneda, T., Tsuyuoka, K., Hasegawa, A., Kiso, M. and Kannagi, R.: Contribution of carbohydrate antigens sialyl Lewis-a and sialyl Lewis-x to adhesion of human cancer cells to vascular endothelium. Cancer Res. 53:354–361, 1993.

Takayama, M., Isaka, K., Suzuki, Y., Funayama, H., Akiya, K. and Bohn, H.: Comparative study of placental protein 19, human chorionic gonadotrophin and pregnancy-specificß1–glycoprotein as immunohistochemical markers for extravillous trophoblast in pregnancy and trophoblastic disease. Histochemistry 93:167–173, 1989.

Tang, B., Guller, S. and Gurpide, E.: Mechanism of human endometrial stromal cells decidualization. Ann. N.Y. Acad. Sci. 734:19–25, 1994.

Tarachand, U.: Morphogenesis and postulated functions of decidual cells. Biol. Res. Pregnancy. Perinatol. 6:187–190, 1985.

Tarachand, U.: Decidualisation: origin and role of associated cells. Biol. Cell 57:9–16, 1986.

Thliveris, J.A. and Speroff, L.: Ultrastructure of the placental villi, chorion laeve, and decidua parietalis in normal and hypertensive pregnant women. Amer. J. Obstet. Gynecol. 129:492–498, 1977.

Thomas, J.B.: Breus' mole. Obstet. Gynecol. 24:794–797, 1964.

Thompson, M.O., Vines, S.K., Aquilina, J., Wathen, N.C. and Harrington, K.: Are placental lakes of any clinical significance? Placenta 23:685–690, 2002.

Thomsen, K. and Willemsen, R.: Histochemische Untersuchungen über die Produktionsorte der Choriongonadotropine. Acta Endocrinol. (Copenh.) 30:161–174, 1959.

Thorp, J.M., Councell, B., Sandridge, D.A. and Wiest, H.H.: Antepartum diagnosis of placenta previa percreta by magnetic resonance imaging. Obstet. Gynecol. 80:506–508, 1992.

Thorp, J.M., Wells, S.R., Wiest, H.H., Jeffries, L. and Lyles, E.: First-trimester diagnosis of placenta previa percreta by magnetic imaging. Amer. J. Obstet. Gynecol. **178**:616–618, 1998.

Tighe, J.R., Garrod, P.R. and Curran, R.C.: The trophoblast of the human chorionic villus. J. Pathol. Bacteriol. **93**:559–567, 1967.

Timor-Tritsch, I.E. and Monteagudo, A.: Diagnosis of placenta previa by transvaginal sonography. Ann. Med. **25**:279–283, 1993.

Timor-Tritsch, I.E. and Yunis, R.A.: Confirming the safety of transvaginal sonography in patients suspected of placenta previa. Obstet. Gynecol. **81**:742–744, 1993.

Tindall, V.R. and Scott, J.S.: Placental calcification: a study of 3,025 singleton and multiple pregnancies. J. Obstet. Gynaecol. Brit. Commonw. **72**:356–373, 1965.

Tisdall, L., Nichols, R.A. and Sicuranza, B.J.: Abdominal pregnancy associated with an intrauterine contraceptive device. Amer. J. Obstet. Gynecol. **106**:937–939, 1970.

To, W.W.K. and Leung, W.C.: Placenta previa and previous cesarean section. Intern. J. Gynecol. Obstet. **51**:25–31, 1995.

Todt, J.C., Yang, Y., Lei, J., Lauria, M.R., Sorokin, Y., Cotton, D.B. and Yelian, F.D.: Effects of tumor necrosis factor-alpha on human trophoblast cell adhesion and motility. Amer. J. Reprod. Immunol. **36**:65–71, 1996.

Topuz, S.: Spontaneous uterine rupture at an unusual site due to placenta percreta in a 21-week twin pregnancy with previous cesarean section. Clin. Exp. Obstet. Gynecol. **31**:239–241, 2004.

Torpin, R.: Subchorial haematoma mole: hypothetical aetiology. J. Obstet. Gynaecol. Brit. Emp. **67**:990, 1960.

Torpin, R.: Breus subchorial hematoma mole at three or four months of pregnancy. Pacific Med. Surg. **74**:226–227, 1966.

Tsang, R.C., Donavan, E.F. and Steichen, J.J.: Calcium physiology and pathology in the neonate. Pediatr. Clin. North Amer. **23**:611–626, 1976.

Tulani, T. and Al-Jaroudi, D.: Nonclosure of peritoneum: A reappraisal. Amer. J. Obstet. Gynecol. **189**:609–612, 2003.

Tuttle, S.E., O'Toole, R.V., O'Shaughnessy, R.W. and Zuspan, F.P.: Immunohistochemical evaluation of human placental implantation: An initial study. Amer. J. Obstet. Gynecol. **153**:239–244, 1985.

Uhlendorf, B. and Kaufmann, P.: Die Entwicklung des Plazentastieles beim Meerschweinchen. Zentralbl. Veterinar. Med. [C] **8**:233–247, 1979.

Ulbrecht, M., Rehberger, B., Strobel, I., Messer, G., Kind, P., Degitz, K., Bieber, T. and Weiss, E.H.: HLA-G: expression in human kertinocytes in vitro and in human skin in vivo. Eur. J. Immunol. **24**:176–180, 1994.

Vasssiliadou, N. and Bulmer, J.N.: Characterization of tubal and decidual leukocyte populations in ectopic pregnancy: evidence that endometrial granulated lymphocytes are absent from the tubal implantation site. Fertil. Steril. **69**:760–767, 1998.

Vernof, K.K., Benirschke, K., Kephart, G.M., Wasmoen, T.L. and Gleich, G.J.: Maternal floor infarction: Relationship to X cells, major basic protein, and adverse perinatal outcome. Amer. J. Obstet. Gynecol. **167**:1355–1963, 1992.

Vettraino, I.M., Roby, J., Tolley, T. and Parks, W.C.: Collagenase-I, stromelysin-I, and matrilysin are expressed within the placenta during multiple stages of human pregnancy. Placenta **17**:557–563, 1996.

Vicovac, L. and Aplin, J.D.: Epithelial-mesenchymal transition during trophoblast differentiation. Acta Anat (Basel) **156**:202–216, 1996.

Vicovac, L., Jones, C.J.P. and Aplin, J.D.: Morphogenesis of human placental anchoring villi in culture. Placenta **14**:A.80, 1993.

Vicovac, L.J., Jones, C.J.P. and Aplin, J.D.: Trophoblast differentiation during formation of anchoring villi in a model of the early human placenta in vitro. Placenta **16**:41–56, 1995a.

Vicovac, L.J., Jones, C.J.P., Church, H.J. and Aplin, J.D.: Factors controlling trophoblast entry into the extravillous lineage. Placenta **16**:A74, 1995b.

Vidaeff, A.C. and Lucas, M.J.: Impact of single- or double-layer closure on uterine rupture. Amer. J. Obstet. Gynecol. **188**:602–603, 2003.

Vierhout, M.E. and Wallenburg, H.C.S.: Intraligamentary pregnancy resulting in a live infant. Amer. J. Obstet. Gynecol. **152**:878–879, 1985.

Vince, G.S. and Johnson, P.M.: Immunobiology of human uteroplacental macrophages-friend and foe? Placenta **17**:191–199, 1996.

Vince, G., Shorter, S., Starkey, P., Humphreys, J., Clover, L., Wilkins, T., Sargent, I. and Redman, C.: Localization of tumour necrosis factor production in cells at the materno/fetal interface in human pregnancy. Clinical Exp. Immunol. **88**:174–180, 1992.

von Ostau, C., Grümmer, R., Kohnen, G., Kaufmann, P. and Winterhager, E.: Expression verschiedener Connexine während der Entwicklung der humanen Plazenta. Ann. Anat. **2**:A102/103, 1995.

von Rango, U., Classen-Linke, I., Kertschanska, S., Kemp, B. and Beier, H.M.: Effects of trophoblast invasion on the distribution of leukocytes in uterine and tubal implantation sites. Fertil. Steril. **76**:116–124, 2001.

von Rango, U., Krusche, C.A., Kertschanska, S., Alfer, J., Kaufmann, P. and Beier, H.M.: Apoptosis of extravillous trophoblast cells limits the trophoblast invasion in uterine but not in tubal pregnancy during first trimester. Placenta **24**:929–940, 2003.

Wachstein, M., Meagher, J.G. and Ortiz, J.: Enzymatic histochemistry of the term human placenta. Amer. J. Obstet. Gynecol. **87**:13–26, 1963.

Wadsworth, P.F., Lewis, D.J. and Heywood, R.: The ultrastructural features of progestagen-induced decidual cells in the rhesus monkey (Macaca mulatta). Contraception **22**:189–198, 1980.

Waidl, E.: Die Entstehung der Septen und Furchen der menschlichen Plazenta. Geburtsh. Frauenheilk. **23**:757–766, 1963.

Wakuda, K. and Yoshida, Y.: Cytofluorometric nuclear DNA analysis and immunohistochemical study on the proliferative activity of the trophoblasts in human early gestation. Nippon. Sanka. Fujinka. Gakkai. Zasshi. **42**:1182–1188, 1990.

Wakuda, K. and Yoshida, Y.: DNA ploidy and proliferative characteristics of human trophoblasts. Acta Obstet. Gynecol. Scand. **71**:12–16, 1992.

Wang, H., Li, Q., Shao, L. and Zhu, C.: Expression of matrix metalloproteinase-2, -9, -14, and tissue inhibitors of metalloproteinase-1, -2, -3 in the endometrium and placenta of rhesus monkey (Macaca mulatta) during early pregnancy. Biol. Reprod. 65:31–40, 2001.

Wanner, A.: Wird bei der Geburtsplacenta des Menschen die Basalplatte von Trophoblastzellen oder Zellen mütterlicher Herkunft überzogen? Acta Anat. (Basel) 63:545–558, 1966.

Warren, W.B. and Silverman, A.J.: Cellular localization of corticotrophin releasing hormone in the human placenta, fetal membranes and decidua. Placenta 16:147–156, 1995.

Wasmoen, T.L., Coulam, C.B., Leiferman, K.M. and Gleich, G. J.: Increase of plasma eosinophil major basic protein levels late in pregnancy predicts onset of labor. Proc. Natl. Acad. Sci. 84:3029–3032, 1987.

Wasmoen, T.I., McKean, D.J., Benirschke, K., Coulam, C.B. and Gleich, G.J: Evidence of eosinophil granule major basic protein in human placenta. J. Exp. Med. 170:2051–2063, 1989.

Wasmoen, T.L., Coulam, C.B., Benirschke, K. and Gleich, G.J.: Association of immunoreactive eosinophil major basic protein with placental septa and cysts. Amer. J. Obstetr. Gynecol. 165:416–420, 1991.

Watanabe, S.: Studies of endometrial granulocytes in early pregnant decidual tissue by means of double immunofluorescent staining and flow cytometry. Nippon. Sanka. Fujinka. Gakkai. Zasshi. 39:972–979, 1987.

Weber, J.: The site of production of gonadotrophin in the placenta at term. Acta Obstet. Gynecol. Scand. 40:139–151, 1961.

Weckstein, L.N., Masserman, J.S.H. and Garite, T.J.: Placenta accreta: a problem of increasing clinical significance. Obstet. Gynecol. 69:480–482, 1987.

Welsh, A.O. and Enders, A.C.: Light and electron microscopic examination of the mature decidual cells of the rat with emphasis on the antimesometrial decidua and its degeneration. Amer. J. Anat. 172:1–29, 1985.

Welsh, A.O. and Enders, A.C.: Chorioallantoic placenta formation in the rat. III. Granulated cells invade the uterine luminal epithelium at the time of epithelial cell death. Biol. Reprod. 49:38–57, 1993.

Werb, Z: How the macrophage regulates its extracellular environment. Amer. J. Anat. 166:237–256, 1983.

Weser, H. and Kaufmann, P.: Lichtmikrosskkopische und histochemische Untersuchungen an der Chorionplatte der reifen menschlichen Placenta. Arch. Gynäkol. 225:15–30, 1978.

Wewer, U.M., Faber, M., Liotta, L.A. and Albrechtsen, R.: Immunochemical and ultrastructural assessment of the nature of pericellular basement membrane of human decidual cells. Lab. Invest. 53:624–633, 1985.

Wewer, U.M., Faber, M., Liotta, L.A. and Albrechtsen, R.: Correspondence: decidual cells. Lab. Invest. 55:120–121, 1986.

Whitelaw, P.F. and Croy, B.A.: Granulated lymphocytes of pregnancy. Placenta 17:533–543, 1996.

Wieloch, J.: Beitrag zur Kenntnis des Baues der Placenta. Arch. Gynäkol. 118:112–119, 1923.

Wiese, K.-H.: Licht- und elektronenmikroskopische Untersuchungen an der Chorionplatte der reifen menschlichen Plazenta. Arch. Gynäkol. 218:243–259, 1975.

Wigglesworth, J.S.: Morphological variations in the insufficient placenta. J. Obstet. Gynaecol. Brit. Commonw. 71:871–884, 1964.

Wigglesworth, J.S.: Vascular anatomy of the human placenta and its significance for placental pathology. J. Obstet. Gynaecol. Brit. Commonw. 76:979–989, 1969.

Wilkin, P.: Morphogenese. In, Le Placenta Humain. J. Snoeck, ed., pp. 23–70, Masson, Paris, 1958.

Willemen, D.F.W., Bol, J.J., Unnik, A.J.M. and Breda, A.T.: Een voldragen tubaire Zwangerschap. Nederl. Tijdschr. Geneesk. 109:2339–2341, 1965.

Williams, P.C., Malvar, T.C. and Kraft, J.R.: Term ovarian pregnancy with delivery of a live female infant. Amer. J. Obstet. Gynecol. 142:589–591, 1982.

Windrim, R.: Vaginal delivery in birth centre after previous cesarean section. Lancet 365:106–107, 2005.

Winkler, F.N.: Zur Kenntnis der menschlichen Plazenta. Arch. Gynäkol. 4:238–265, 1872.

Winterhager, E., Busch, L.C. and Kühnel, W.: Membrane events involved in fusion of uterine epithelial cells in pseudopregnant rabbits. Cell Tissue Res. 235:357–363, 1984.

Winterhager, E., von Ostau, C., Grümmer, R. Kaufmann, P. and Fisher, S.J.: Connexin und E-cadherin Expression während der Differenzierung des humanen Trophoblasten. 91. Versammlung der Anat. Gesellschaft, Jena, März 1996.

Winterhager, E., Kaufmann, P. and Gruemmer, R.: Cell-cell-communication during placental development and possible implications for trophoblast proliferation and differentiation. Placenta 21 Suppl A:S61–S68, 2000.

Wislocki, G.B. and Streeter, G.L.: On the placentation of the macaque (Macaca mulatta) from the time of implantation until the formation of the definitive placenta. Contrib. Embryol. Carnegie Instit. 27:1–66, 1938.

Wislocki, G.B.: The histology and cytochemistry of the basal plate and septa placentae of the normal human placenta delivered at full term. Anat. Rec. 109:359, 1951.

Witter, F.R. and Sanders, R.C.: Maternal hemorrhage into the amniotic sac producing an apparent umbilical cord mass on sonogram. Amer. J. Obstet. Gynecol. 155:649–651, 1986.

Wolska, W.: Über die von Ruge beschriebene Vaskularisation der Serotina. Thesis, Bern, 1888.

Woolam, G.I., Pratt, J.H. and Wilson, R.B.: Uterine rupture following tubal implantation: report of 2 cases. Obstet. Gynecol. 29:415–419, 1967.

Wu, C., Chung, A.E. and McDonald, J.A.: A novel role for $\alpha 3\beta 1$ integrins in extracellular matrix assembly. J. Cell Sci. 108:2511–2523, 1995.

Wu, W.X., Brooks, J., Millar, M.R., Ledger, W.L., Saunders, P.T., Glasier, A.F. and McNeilly, A.S.: Localization of the sites of synthesis and action of prolactin by immunocytochemistry and in-situ hybridization within the human utero-placental unit. J. Mol. Endocrinol. 7: 241–247, 1991.

Wynn, R.M.: Electron microscopy of the developing decidua. Fertil. Steril. 16:16–26, 1965.

Wynn, R.M.: Fetomaternal cellular relations in the human basal plate: an ultrastructural study of the placenta. Amer. J. Obstet. Gynecol. 97:832–850, 1967a.

Wynn, R.M.: Intra-uterine devices: effects on ultrastructure of human endometrium. Science 156:1508–1510, 1967b.

Wynn, R.: Ultrastructural development of the human decidua. Amer. J. Obstet. Gynecol. 118:652–670, 1974.

Wynn, R.M.: Fine structure of the placenta. In, The Placenta and its Maternal Supply Line. P. Gruenwald, ed. Medical Technical Publications, Lancaster, pp. 56–79, 1975.

Xu, G., Guimond, M.J., Chakraborty, C. and Lala, P.K.: Control of proliferation, migration, and invasiveness of human extravillous trophoblast by decorin, a decidual product. Biol. Reprod. **67**:681–689, 2002.

Yallampalli, C. and Garfield, R.E.: Inhibition of nitric oxide synthesis in rats during pregnancy produces signs similar to those of preeclampsia. Amer. J. Obstet. Gynecol. **169**:1316–1320, 1993.

Yeh, I., O'Connor, D.M. and Kurman, R.J.: Further immunocytochemical characterization of intermediate trophoblast. Modern Pathol. **1**:106A, 1988.

Yeh, I., O'Connor, D.M. and Kurman, R.J.: Vacuolated cytotrophoblast: a sub-population of trophoblast in the chorion laeve. Placenta **10**:429–438, 1989.

Yeh, I.T., O'Connor, D.M. and Kurman, R.J.: Intermediate trophoblast: further immunocytochemical characterization. Modern Pathol. **3**:282–287, 1990.

Yokoyama, W.M.: Natural killer cell receptors. Current Opinion in Immunology **7**:110–120, 1995.

Young, R.H., Kurman, R.J. and Scully, R.E.: Proliferations and tumors of intermediate trophoblast of the placental site. Semin. Diagn. Pathol. **5**:223–237, 1988.

Yu, T.J., Iwasaki, I., Teratani, T., Tanaka, T. and Aoki, M.: Primary ovarian pregnancy in a cystic teratoma. Obstet. Gynecol. **64**:52s–54s, 1984.

Yuen, B.H., Moon, Y.S. and Shin, D.H.: Inhibition of human chorionic gonadotropin production by prolactin from term human trophoblast. Amer. J. Obstet. Gynecol. **154**:336–340, 1986.

Yui, J., Garcia Lloret, M.I., Wegmann, T.G. and Guilbert, L.J.: Cytotoxicity of tumour necrosis factor-alpha and gamma-interferon against primary human placental trophoblasts. Placenta **15**:819–835, 1994.

Yui, J., Hemmings, D., Garcia Lloret, M.I. and Guilbert, L.J.: Expression of the human p55 and p75 tumor necrosis factor receptors in primary villous trophoblasts and their role in cytotoxic signal transduction. Biol. Reprod. **55**:400–409, 1996.

Zabrieskie, J.R.: Pregnancy and the malformed uterus. West. J. Surg. Obstet. Gynecol. **70**:293–296, 1962.

Zelop, C., Nadel, A., Frigoletto, F.D., Pauker, S., MacMillan, M. and Benacerraf, B.R.: Placenta accreta/percreta/increta: A cause of elevated maternal serum alpha-fetoprotein. Obstet. Gynecol. **80**:693–694, 1992.

Zeng, C.X. and Fu, X.S.: Immunocytochemical localization of human chorionic gonadotropin and placental lactogen in normal placentae. Chung. Hua. Fu. Chan. Ko. Tsa. Chih. **26**:155–7, 188, 1991.

Zhemkova, Z.P.: Sex chromatin in human placenta. Arkh. Anat. Histol. Embriol. **39**:24–32, 1960.

Zhou, Y., Damsky, C.H., Chiu, K., Roberts, J.M. and Fisher, S.J.: Preeclampsia Is Associated with Abnormal Expression of

Adhesion Molecules by Invasive Cytotrophoblasts. J. Clin. Invest. **91**:950–960, 1993.

Zhou, Y., Fisher, S.J., Janatpour, M., Genbacev, O., Dejana, E. and Wheelock, M.: Human cytotrophoblasts adopt a vascular phenotype as they differentiate. A strategy for successful endovascular invasion? J. Clin. Invest. **99**:2139–2151, 1997a.

Zhou, Y., Damsky, C.H. and Fisher, S.J.: Preeclampsia is associated with failure of human cytotrophoblasts to mimic vascular adhesion phenotype. One cause of defective endovascular invasion in this syndrome? J. Clin. Invest. **99**:2152–2164, 1997b.

Zhou, Y., Genbacev, O., Damsky, C.H. and Fisher, S.J.: Oxygen regulates human cytotrophoblast differentiation and invasion: implications for endovascular invasion in normal pregnancy and in pre-eclampsia. J. Reprod. Immunol. **39**:197–213, 1998.

Zhou, Y., McMaster, M., Woo, K., Janatpour, M., Perry, J., Karpanen, T., Alitalo, K., Damsky, C. and Fisher, S.J.: Vascular endothelial growth factor ligands and receptors that regulate human cytotrophoblast survival are dysregulated in severe preeclampsia and hemolysis, elevated liver enzymes, and low platelets syndrome. Amer. J. Pathol. **160**:1405–1423, 2002.

Zhou, Y., Genbacev, O. and Fisher, S.J.: The human placenta remodels the uterus by using a combination of molecules that govern vasculogenesis or leukocyte extravasation. Ann. N.Y. Acad. Sci. **995**:73–83, 2003a.

Zhou, Y., Bellingard, V., Feng, K.T., McMaster, M. and Fisher, S.J.: Human cytotrophoblasts promote endothelial survival and vascular remodeling through secretion of Ang2, PlGF, and VEGF-C. Dev. Biol. **263**:114–125, 2003b.

Zhu, B.C.R. and Laine, R.A.: Polylactosamine glycosylation on human fetal placental fibronectin weakens the binding affinity of fibronectin to gelatin. J. Biol. Chem. **260**:4041–4045, 1985.

Zhu, B.C.R., Fisher, S.F., Pande, H., Calaycay, J., Shively, J.E. and Laine, R.A.: Human placental (fetal) fibronectin: increased glycosylation and higher protease resistance than plasma fibronectin. J. Biol. Chem. **259**:3962–3970, 1984.

Zybina, E.V. and Zybina, T.G.: Polytene chromosomes in mammalian cells. Int. Rev. Cytol. **165**:53–119, 1996.

Zybina, T.G., Zybina, E.V., Kiknadze, I.I. and Zhelezova, A.I.: Polyploidization in the trophoblast and uterine glandular epithelium of the endotheliochorial placenta of silver fox (Vulpes fulvus Desm.), as revealed by the DNA content. Placenta **22**:490–498, 2001.

Zybina, T.G., Kaufmann, P., Frank, H.G., Freed, J., Kadyrov, M. and Biesterfeld, S.: Genome multiplication of extravillous trophoblast cells in human placenta in the course of differentiation and invasion into endometrium and myometrium. I. Dynamics of polyploidization. Tsitologiia **44**:1058–1067, 2002.

Zybina, T.G., Frank, H.G., Biesterfeld, S. and Kaufmann, P.: Genome multiplication of extravillous trophoblast cells in human placenta in the course of differentiation and invasion into endometrium and myometrium. II. Mechanisms of polyploidization. Tsitologiia **46**:640–648, 2004.

10
Involution of Placental Site: Retained Placenta

Involution of the Placental Site

Pathologists rarely obtain a postpartum uterus to enable a detailed study of the involutional changes that take place at the former site of implantation. Therefore, involution of the normal placental site has been studied by only a few investigators. Normally, the postpartum lochia contains the decidual remnants, including perhaps some of the degenerating remnants of the vasculature that had previously undergone the so-called physiologic changes of pregnancy. Only when significant postpartum hemorrhage occurs and hysterectomy is performed, is the pathologist asked to seek the cause of the bleeding. He or she may then find remains of villi, incompletely thrombosed vessels, placental polyps, and some degree of inflammatory reaction. Frisoli (1981) suggested that retained placental tissue is found in about 50% of such cases at curettage. The curettings and postpartum uteri are difficult tissues to study objectively because most pathologists have little experience with the normal, complex process of placental site involution. Williams (1931), in a classic paper, attempted to rectify this situation. His study should be read before any interpretation of such a postpartum uterus is undertaken. It must also be recognized that in 85% of normal, delivered placentas the decidua basalis shows foci of polymorphonuclear leukocyte infiltration (Schneider, 1970). These cells are part of an apparently normal process of implantation and are not considered an expression of deciduitis or infection. Nevertheless, postpartum hemorrhage and subinvolution are nearly always associated with significant inflammation, if only because the cervix remains open and patulous.

The placenta separates from the uterus in the decidua basalis, deep to Nitabuch's fibrin layer. This fibrin layer is usually present in the floor of the delivered placenta but, contrary to some opinions, it does not serve as the cleavage plane. Placental separation probably occurs largely because of the shearing action of the underlying myome-

trium against the noncontractile placenta. One may speculate that detachment might be easier when the placenta is more turgid and still filled with fetal blood, but it is apparently not the case. Walsh (1968) found that when the cord is clamped early and more fetal blood remains in the placenta, postpartum hemorrhage is significantly more common than when this blood was allowed to drain into the fetus.

Immediately following delivery, the uterine surface becomes covered with fibrin and blood clot; the contraction of the uterus clamps the maternal vessels and this stops uterine bleeding. Ludwig (1971), and Ludwig and Metzger (1971) have made elegant electron-microscopic observations of this area postpartum. In their scanning electron-microscopic study, they speak of a "wallpapering" of the endometrial surface with a delicate meshwork of cross-linked fibrin that includes deformed erythrocytes. They had shown earlier that, with the first contraction after expulsion of the placenta, this fibrin is deposited and that it aids hemostasis. There is pronounced furrowing of the inner surface of the uterus following delivery that is bridged by the "tapestry" of fibrin. Mukaida et al. (1975), who also investigated this topic, came to similar conclusions.

Friedländer (1870) found that most of the endometrium degenerates after birth and that regeneration takes place from the glands and stroma in the spongy layer of the endometrium; this process is largely completed by 4 weeks postpartum, at least in the area away from the implantation site. The endometrium of the implantation site itself is not reformed for several additional weeks after delivery. The controversy over what constitutes physiologic changes after birth did not cease until Williams (1931) published his comprehensive study of normal uteri that had been removed up to 4 months after delivery. He showed that the detachment of the placental site proceeded with little inflammation or necrosis. The cessation of blood flow through the endometrial vessels was largely accomplished by contraction of the uterus itself. In the

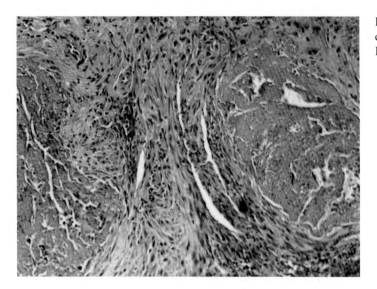

FIGURE 10.1. Poorly thrombosed uterine vessels of the placental site 2 weeks after delivery of a hydatidiform mole. H&E ×160.

absence of contraction, as in cases following former overdistention (e.g., in multiple pregnancy, hydramnios), these vessels may bleed extensively. This uterine atony presents a life-threatening situation that demands emergency attention. Normally then, these vessels are clamped by uterine contraction; they thrombose subsequently (Fig. 10.1), and the vascular placental site eventually becomes a mass of hyaline plaques (Fig. 10.2). The vessels

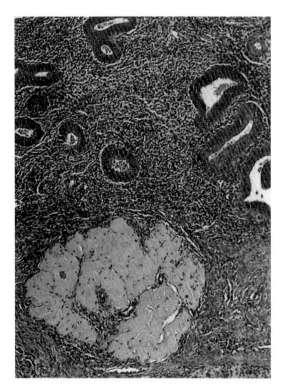

FIGURE 10.2. Agglomeration of hyaline masses from placental site vessels 6 weeks after normal delivery. H&E ×64.

become "organized" by the ingrowth of fibrocytes and endothelium, and they are later recanalized. This process takes many weeks. One can then readily identify former implantation sites by the presence of these unusual hyalinized vessels and by the remains of some placental site giant cells. These residua of implantation have been demonstrated particularly impressively in several monkey species, in which they form macroscopically visible plaques (Bronson et al., 1972). Although the changes in monkeys are, in general, similar, they differ by involving usually both uterine sides, as their placenta is commonly bidiscoid. Moreover, they are much more massive and persist much longer than the approximately 7 weeks considered to be the normal for women. Also, some calcification occurs in the hyaline areas of simian placental site involution, which is not often the case in humans.

The placental site is then "exfoliated," as Williams (1931) called it, rather than being absorbed into the myometrial tissue. At least the portions that are central to the myometrium are undermined. Williams considered that the decidual site is undermined by regrowth and by extension and downgrowth of endometrium that originates from remaining endometrial glands and stroma. He described it to be a "conservative" effort of nature to thus dispose of the thrombosed vessels. It must be borne in mind, however, that it applies only to the decidual portions of the placental site; the myometrial part has a much different regressive curve. One mystery of postpartum uterine involution is the rapidity with which the muscle mass is reduced. The average uterus weighs about 1000 g after term delivery and, largely through the dissolution of cytoplasm, it shrinks to less than 100 g, usually within 2 months. An appreciation of this massive involution of myometrium postpartum is especially important in our understanding of the "healing" of cesarean section incisions. Virtually no myometrium repairs the incisional defect. Only a thin fibrous scar approximates the muscle layers. Thus, in subsequent pregnancies the probability of dehiscence exists (see Chapter 9).

The nature of the vascular changes that take place at the placental site postpartum was the topic of a study by Maher (1959). He observed that the elastic membranes of placental site vessels lose their staining qualities for 25 to 30 days. After that, the elastica is restored, but there is persistence of abnormalities in the pattern of the elastic membrane for a long time. Maher described striking involutional and regenerative changes of the placental site vessels and compared them with the much less prominent effect of pregnancy in those portions of the uterus and fallopian tube that are remote from the implantation site.

Anderson and Davis (1968) made the next major contribution to the study of placental site involution. They believed that vascular constriction and occlusion cause necrosis and sloughing of the former decidua basalis. They confirmed the findings of Sharman (1953), which were made from 626 postpartum biopsies and 11 uteri, removed 1 to 9 months after delivery. Anderson and Davis suggested that the absence of necrosis observed by Williams (1931) was due to his lack of appropriate material from days 4 to 7 postpartum. They corrected this deficiency and measured the placental site. Immediately after birth of the infant, the placental site was 18 cm; after the placenta detached, it measured 9 cm (largely because of uterine contraction), and it was 4 mm in thickness. At 8 days postpartum, the placental site measured only 4.5 cm in diameter, and by 8 weeks it had shrunken to 2 cm. The latest time at which a formerly normal placental site was visible macroscopically was 11 weeks after delivery. In contrast to Williams' opinion, a 6-mm-deep area of necrosis of the placental site, extending onto the myometrium, was observed from 2 to 6 days. A mixed "granulocytic and mononuclear inflammatory infiltrate occurred in the slough and the viable endomyometrium." Anderson and Davis described the "physiologic adenomyosis" that occurs in the superficial myometrium, particularly in the center of the former placental site, and they delineated the development of pleomorphic nucleated cells of the endometrial glands. In their experience, placental site giant cells persisted for several days, were confined to the

superficial layers, and did not extend deeply into the myometrium. Villi were found in four early specimens from apparently uncomplicated pregnancies. None of these elements normally persisted past 4 weeks. Vessels were described as thrombosed and showing "endophlebitis." Endothelial proliferation was a particularly prominent feature in the veins. Toward the end of the first week, the veins showed the beginning of organization of clots; arterial thrombosis was not a prominent feature. Because these normal changes are often misinterpreted as possibly being pathologic, a summary of the features of these sequential events is presented in Table 10.1.

Anderson and Davis (1968) were unable to resolve the nature of the placental site giant cells but favored a trophoblastic origin for these cellular elements. They stated emphatically that involution of the placental site does not lead to fibrosis of the uterus. They insisted that the term **subinvolution** must be understood within the framework of these normal involutional processes.

Sharman (1953) found that mitoses of the endometrium first occurred 8 days after delivery. By 16 days, the endometrium was structurally intact again. He also observed an "appreciable number" of plasma cells to be present 6 weeks after birth in 50% of his cases (37% had plasma cells at 3 to 4 months postpartum). This result is surprising, as it implies infection in one half of postpartum patients. It must be reiterated, however, that the inflammatory reaction of the normal placental site involutional process is usually sparse, and in most women it is confined to the first few days. Moreover, this infiltrate is made up of granulocytes and macrophages; plasma cells appear only late in this process.

In step with the involution of placental bed trophoblast are the endocrine signals of pregnancy. Human chorionic gonadotropin (hCG) disappears within 2 weeks from the maternal serum completely, regulated largely by its half-life of 9 to 37 hours (Midgley & Jaffe, 1968; Jaffe et al., 1969). Human placental lactogen (hPL), on the other hand, having a shorter half-life of up to 30 minutes, disappears within a day (Geiger, 1973). The disappearance of other pregnancy markers is less well defined (Tulchinsky & Ryan, 1980). Korhonen et al. (1997) studied the hCG decline in some detail in six women following

TABLE 10.1. Structural alterations in the postpartum placental site

Time	Size (cm)	Slough	Glands	Decidua	Veins	Arteries
Term	9	Hemorrhage	Present	Viable	Hyaline	Fibrinoid
1–3 d	7–8	Early necrosis	Prominent	Necrosis	Thrombosis	Obliterated
3–5 d	6	With reaction	Atypia	Necrosis	Organization	Hyalinized
5–8 d	4.5	Demarcated	Increased	Regression	Organization	Hyalinized
4–20 w	2	Hemosiderin	Inactive	Absent	Recanalized	Remnants of hyaline

Source: From Anderson and Davis (1968), with permission.

normal delivery. From levels of around 35,000 IU/mL at the end of pregnancy, rapid decline leads to virtual elimination (5 IU/mL) by 21 days after delivery, α-hCG having a much more rapid decline than β-hCG. Inasmuch as one may see extravillous trophoblast (X cells) for some time following delivery in the hyalinizing placental site, however, it is likely that some of the large quantity of major basic protein (MBP) that exists during gestation can be detected for longer periods, but measurements have not been made.

Subinvolution

At times the uterus does not involute properly, and the clinical diagnosis of "uterine subinvolution" is entertained. What are the pathologic equivalents of this condition? Khong and Khong (1993) are the most recent authors to have examined this phenomenon, with the evaluation of 169 specimens from "delayed postpartum hemorrhage" that followed a singleton delivery. They provided some reason why such studies should be divided into periods before and after 6 weeks postpartum, not an important issue for pathologists, we believe. Retained placental tissue was most common (45 cases), to be followed by "subinvolution," that is, widely patent uteroplacental arteries in 30 patients. Endometritis (seven patients) was uncommon and most of the other patients had essentially normal histologic findings. Placental tissue may have been retained because it resulted from placenta accreta, or because the fragmentation of a manually removed placenta was not appreciated at delivery, and a portion of a cotyledon was left behind.

Normally, the uterus shrinks rapidly, with dissolution of the myometrium. Within 2 weeks, its size reduces from about 1000 g to nearly 100 g, and the endometrium and placental site are cast off. With subinvolution this regression is delayed; the uterus remains boggy and edematous and may actually be retroflexed and congested. Often there is bleeding and some remaining placental tissue ("placental polyp"), or an infection may cause uterine subinvolution. Thorsteinsson and Kempers (1970) studied the records of 148 patients with delayed postpartum bleeding, occuring in 1% of deliveries. They found the bleeding most commonly resulted from subinvolution of the placental site. Curettage was done in 94 patients, and 78 were found to harbor microscopic fragments of placental tissue; seven additional patients had grossly visible placental remains. Curettage cured most patients. It is interesting to note here also that most of the patients (135) were said to have had normal placentas at delivery.

According to Stamm (1961), incompletely removed placentas have been the cause of litigation. For that reason, others had suggested that placentas be injected for completeness. Stamm, however, believed that the evaluation for completeness of the placenta through the injection of milk is inaccurate, and that it should not become a routine procedure. Tears in the placenta often occur, which makes it difficult to ascertain with certainty that removal was complete. Stamm suggested that manual exploration of the uterus is necessary when one is uncertain whether a placenta has been removed completely.

Placental Polyps

Placental polyps were described in three patients by Hoberman and his colleagues (1963), who also reviewed the sparse English-language literature on this topic. Placental polyps are usually made up of remnants of villous tissue that have become encased in layered clot. At times, one finds that the villi are directly attached to the myometrium; they are thus focal placentas accretas, but because of degenerative changes this diagnosis is often impossible to verify.

When these "polyps" are removed, the symptoms usually abate. If they are not removed, life-threatening bleeding may occur. This possibility was emphasized in the study of placental polyps undertaken by Dyer and Bradburn (1971). They decried that this important complication of the puerperium is rarely mentioned in modern textbooks. Dyer and Bradburn described the "immediate type" of polyp, which occurs during the first month after delivery, and the "delayed type," where the tissue may be discovered months or even years later. They acknowledged that accretas may be part of the problem but believed that other, unrecognized factors play a role as well. Finally, they speculated that such retained fragments are the possible sites of future trophoblastic tumors. In our opinion, there is little evidence for the latter speculation, even though the placental site trophoblastic tumor has become a delineated entity (see Chapter 23). It is true, however, that an exaggerated placental site may pose as tumor and the differential diagnosis is not always easy (Benirschke, 1997). Philippe et al. (1968) claimed that a deficient arterial occlusion at the site of involution is a probable cause of postpartum hemorrhage. After studying and depicting the normal vascular occlusions, these authors showed hugely distended vessels with poorly organized thrombi, as well as increased hyaline masses, to be a cause of the bleeding that may take place later, when early postpartum hemorrhage has occurred. Philippe and his colleagues speculated that these vascular changes may result from inadequate hormonal effects on these vessels during the immediate postpartum period. They also suggested that therapy with 17-hydroxyprogesterone caproate may resolve the condition and that hysterectomy is not always indicated. Rutherford and Hertig (1945) showed placental polyps in three postpartum patients who had neither placental remains nor inflammation, but had hugely dilated, improperly occluded, placental site blood vessels. Perhaps this situation constitutes the "true" subinvolution, a process whose etiology is yet to be clarified. Most recently, late bleeding has been associated with the discovery of hyalinized masses (placental-site nodules); when stained with antibodies to hPL, these masses were found to contain positively staining placental-site giant cells (Young et al., 1990) (see Chapter 23). The authors cautioned that these masses are benign remnants of placentation that must not be mistaken for tumor. Suffice it to say, retained placental villi are not always present in patients who experience postpartum hemorrhage. Incomplete occlusion of vessels alone may be the cause of subinvolution, as also may be an idiopathic failure of trophoblastic placental site cells to involute.

In addition to these features of subinvolution, there is the postpartum endometritis, "puerperal fever," an infection caused by a variety of microorganisms. Its prototype, however, is caused by group A streptococci. The histologic features may be similar to those seen with other subinvolutional events, although there are additionally pronounced acute inflammation, infiltration with plasma cells, phlebothrombosis, and often colonies of bacterial organisms. All are life-threatening processes that may also lead to pulmonary embolism. Various aspects of a placental polyp, symptomatic 9 years after abortion of the last known pregnancy, were reported by Lawrence et al. (1988). At that time the patient had undergone sterilization. The polyp was composed mostly of "necrotic and hyalinized villi, without identifiable trophoblast." A few syncytial cells exhibited hCG immunohistochemically, and abundant X cells were present with the hPL reaction. Regrettably, the authors did not report on the status of the ovaries so as to rule out a possible recent pregnancy. They also reviewed the few case reports and case series

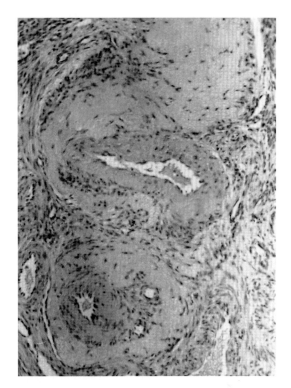

FIGURE 10.3. Myometrial remnants of a former placental site with hyalinization, 2 years after normal delivery and death for unrelated reasons. H&E ×160.

from the literature, which included a placental polyp 21 years after pregnancy.

In our experience, the hyaline scars of former placental sites may persist in the uterus for much longer than has been indicated in most of the literature cited here, much as the corpus albicans persists for years in the ovary. The myometrial remnants of former placental site vessels are shown in Figures 10.3 and 10.4, assuredly 2 years after the

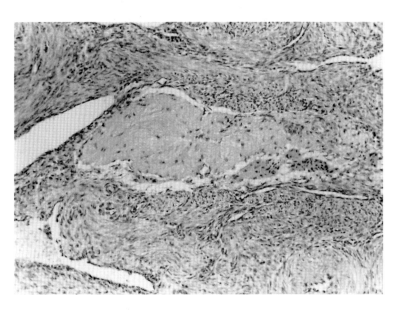

FIGURE 10.4. Finding similar to that in Figure 10.3 but deeper in the myometrium. H&E ×160.

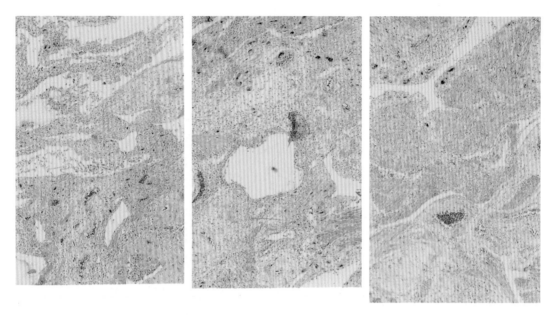

FIGURE 10.5. Composite of implantation site with endometrium above. This patient had retained placental tissue for 16 weeks (see Fig. 10.6), and many of the placental site giant cells (dark) persist deep in the myometrium. No vascular thrombosis had occurred. H&E ×16.

last pregnancy. Figure 10.5 shows the uterus of a patient with retained placental tissue who died 16 weeks postpartum. Numerous trophoblastic cells can be seen throughout the myometrium of the placental site. Most, but not all, villi were completely necrotic in this patient (Fig. 10.6).

Somewhat related to these rare pathological findings are the observations made by Craven and Ward (1997)

on placental bed biopsy. This was done after cesarean section delivery of a multiparous patient for a study of preeclampsia. Microscopically, squamous epithelial masses, undoubtedly of vernix origin, were embedded in endomyometrium and maternal vessels. There was intense inflammation also present, and the authors considered this to be the result of membrane rupture.

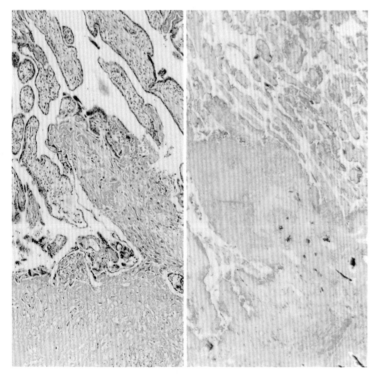

FIGURE 10.6. Live and necrotic villi forming the placental polyp of the uterus shown in Figure 10.5, 16 weeks after delivery. H&E ×64.

Involution of a Remaining Placenta

Involution of a remaining placenta is conveniently dealt with at this point because some of its features resemble the findings of retained placental tissue and placental polyps. When fetectomy had been performed in rhesus monkeys between the 10th and 23rd weeks of pregnancy, it was alleged that the placenta was later delivered "on time" (Van Wagenen & Newton, 1943), that is, at term for this species. Lewis and Hertz (1966) found that most of the monkeys developed degenerated placentas when fetectomy was done between the 14th and 35th days of gestation. They had expected to find hydatid swelling, perhaps molar transformation, but it did not occur. In similar, larger experiments, Panigel and Myers (1972) also did not find hydatid changes following either fetectomy or ligation of the vessels that extend to the monkey's second placental disk (the "bridging vessels"). They observed that some villi remained structurally normal for several weeks, although their fetal capillaries and red blood cells soon disintegrated. The maintenance of some fine structural detail in these surviving villi is indeed remarkable. The villi become usually more compacted, rather than hydropic. Detaching a disk of the placenta and thereby interrupting the maternal perfusion in monkeys, however, led to placental infarction (Myers & Panigel, 1973). In many ways the villous changes found after prolonged retention of the placenta resemble those encountered following fetal demise (Fox, 1968). They are initiated by syncytial knotting, stromal fibrosis with loss of capillaries, and fibrosis of major stem vessels. Calcification and complete villous hyalinization are end stages.

When investigation of the factors that initiate labor required reexamination of the role of fetectomy, specifically as it relates to the role played by the fetal adrenal and pituitary glands, Lanman et al. (1975) restudied the placental changes following fetectomy in the rhesus monkey. In the 13 animals examined by these authors, fetectomy was performed between 65 and 143 days, term being 168 days. Nine of the placentas remained in situ beyond the expected date of delivery, two delivered near term, and two delivered prematurely. Histologic study revealed empty vessels, stromal fibrosis of villi, hyalinization, and calcification 17 to 108 days after fetectomy. X-cell hyperplasia was prominent in two placentas. The placental weights were similar to what was expected at the time of fetectomy, but they were much smaller than expected for the gestational age of the placenta. Somewhat different results were obtained by Nathanielsz et al. (1992). These authors were unable to obtain the placentas for dissection but, from the endocrine changes that occurred after fetectomy, they decided that a functional fetal circulation in necessary for normal gestational control.

The anatomic results just reviewed have also been the experience with retained placentas in women whose fetus has died or when only one fetus of twins survives. The placental tissue remains structurally intact for a long time. It first loses its fetal vasculature and undergoes fibrosis, and much fibrin accumulates, particularly in the intervillous space. The trophoblast continues to be perfused by the maternal circulation and so survives longer. The placenta eventually atrophies and comes to resemble an infarct. The result is not a true infarct, because an infarct occurs only after interruption of the maternal intervillous circulation.

References

Anderson, W.R. and Davis, J.: Placental site involution. Amer. J. Obstet. Gynecol. **102**:23–33, 1968.

Benirschke, K.: Critical commentary to: Placental site trophoblastic tumor (PSTT) initially misdiagnosed as cervical carcinoma (by L.C. Horn, et al.) Pathol. Res. Pract. **193**:233–234, 1997.

Bronson, R., Volk, T.L. and Ruebner, B.H.: Involution of placental site and corpus luteum in the monkey. Amer. J. Obstet. Gynecol. **113**:70–75, 1972.

Craven, C.M. and Ward, K.: Premature rupture of the amniotic membranes diagnosed by placental bed biopsy. Arch. Pathol. Lab. Med. **121**:167–168, 1997.

Dyer, I. and Bradburn, D.M.: An inquiry into the etiology of placental polyps. Amer. J. Obstet. Gynecol. **109**:858–867, 1971.

Fox, H.: Morphological changes in the human placenta following fetal death. J. Obstetr. Gynaecol. Brit. Cwlth. **75**:839–843, 1968.

Friedländer, C.: Physiologisch-anatomische Untersuchungen über den Uterus. Simmel and Co., Leipzig, 1870.

Frisoli, G.: Physiology and Pathology of the Puerperium. Chapter 93 in, Principles and Practice of Obstetrics & Perinatology. L. Iffy and H.A. Kaminetzky, eds. John Wiley, New York, 1981.

Geiger, W.: Radioimmunological determination of human chorionic gonadotropin, human placental lactogen, growth hormone and thyrotropin in the serum of mother and child during the early puerperium. Horm. Metab. Res. **5**:342–346, 1973.

Hoberman, L.K., Hawkinson, J.A. and Beecham, C.T.: Placental polyp: report of 3 cases. Obstet. Gynecol. **22**:25–29, 1963.

Jaffe, R.B., Lee, P.A. and Midgley, A.R.: Serum gonadotropins before, at the inception of, and following human pregnancy. J. Clin. Endocrinol. Metabol. **29**:1281–1283, 1969.

Khong, T.Y. and Khong, T.K.: Delayed postpartum hemorrhage: a morphologic study of causes and their relation to other pregnancy disorders. Obstet. Gynecol. **82**:17–22, 1993.

Korhonen, J., Alfthan, H., Ylöstalo, P., Veldhuis, J. and Stenman, U.-H.: Disappearance of human chorionic gonadotropin and its α- and β-subunits after term pregnancy. Clin. Chem. **43**:2155–2163, 1997.

Lanman, J.T., Mitsudo, S.M., Brinson, A.O. and Thau, R.B.: Fetectomy in monkeys (Macaca mulatta); retention of the placenta past term. Biol. Reprod. **12**:522–525, 1975.

Lawrence, W.D., Qureshi, F. and Bonakdar, M.I.: "Placental polyp": light microscopic and immunohistochemical observations. Hum. Pathol. **19**:1467–1470, 1988.

Lewis, J. and Hertz, R.: Effects of early embryectomy and hormonal therapy on the fate of the placenta in pregnant rhesus monkeys. Proc. Soc. Exp. Biol. Med. **123**:805–809, 1966.

Ludwig, H.: Surface structure of the human term placenta and of the uterine wall post partum in the screen scan electron microscope. Amer. J. Obstet. Gynecol. **111**:328–344, 1971.

Ludwig, H. and Metzger, H.: Das uterine Placentarbett post partum im Rasterelektronenmikroskop, zugleich ein Beitrag der extravasalen Fibrinbildung. Arch. Gynäkol. **210**:251–266, 1971.

Maher, J.A.: Morphologic and histochemical changes in postpartum uterine blood vessels. AMA Arch. Pathol. **67**:175–180, 1959.

Midgley, A.R. and Jaffe, R.B.: Regulation of human gonadotropins. II. Disappearance of human hCG following delivery. J. Clin. Endocrinol. Metabol. **28**:1712–1718, 1968.

Mukaida, T., Yoshida, K. and Soma, H.: A surface ultrastructural study of the placental separation site. J. Clin. Electron Microsc. **8**:5–6, 1975.

Myers, R.E. and Panigel, M.: Experimental placental detachment in the rhesus monkey: Changes in villous ultrastructure. J. Med. Primatol. **2**:170–189, 1973.

Nathanielsz, P.W., Figueroa, J.P. and Honnebier, M.B.O.M.: In the rhesus monkey placental retention after fetectomy at 121 to 130 days' gestation outlasts the normal duration of pregnancy. Amer. J. Obstet. Gynecol. **166**:1529–1535, 1992.

Panigel, M. and Myers, R.E.: Histological and ultrastructural changes in rhesus monkey placenta following interruption of fetal placental circulation by fetectomy or interplacental umbilical vessel ligation. Acta Anat. (Basel) **81**:481–506, 1972.

Philippe, E., Ritter, J., Renaud, R., Dellenbach, P., Fonck-Cussac, Y. and Gandar, R.: Les métrorrhagies tardives du post-partum par anomalie d'involution des artères utéro-placentaires. Rev. Fr. Gynécol. **63**:255–262, 1968.

Rutherford, R.N. and Hertig, A.T.: Noninvolution of the placental site. Amer. J. Obstet. Gynecol. **49**:378–384, 1945.

Schneider, L.: Über Vorkommen und Bedeutung leukocytärer Infiltrate im Ablösungsbereich der spontan geborenen Placenta. Arch. Gynäkol. **208**:247–254, 1970.

Sharman, A.: Post-partum regeneration of the human endometrium. J. Anat. **87**:1–10, 1953.

Stamm, H.: Alte und neue Probleme bei Plazentarpolypen. Gynaecologia **151**:252–260, 1961.

Thorsteinsson, V.T. and Kempers, R.D.: Delayed postpartum bleeding. Amer. J. Obstet. Gynecol. **107**:565–571, 1970.

Tulchinsky, D. and Ryan, K.J.: Maternal-Fetal Endocrinology. W.B. Saunders, Philadelphia, 1980.

van Wagenen, G. and Newton, W.H.: Pregnancy in the monkey after removal of the fetus. Surg. Gynecol. Obstet. **77**:539–549, 1943.

Walsh, S.Z.: Maternal effects of early and late clamping of the umbilical cord. Lancet **1**:996–997, 1968.

Williams, J.W.: Regeneration of the uterine mucosa after delivery, with especial reference to the placental site. Amer. J. Obstet. Gynecol. **22**:664–696, 793–796, 1931.

Young, R.H., Kurman, R.J. and Scully, R.E.: Placental site nodules and plaques. An analysis of 20 cases. Amer. J. Surg. Pathol. **14**:1001–1009, 1990.

11
Anatomy and Pathology of the Placental Membranes

Overview

The term **membranes** is usually taken to be synonymous with the amnion and the chorion laeve. The membranes represent the "bag of waters" that encloses the fetus. The membranes are distinct from the chorion frondosum, which is the actual placental tissue and forms a specialized, thickened part of the membranes. In other usage, placental membranes is occasionally also used as denominating the entire afterbirth. The true membranes normally insert at the edge of the placenta and contain the amnionic fluid and fetus. Membranes rupture during delivery owing to stretching or because of the mechanical force of the accoucheur. Several distinct layers are present in the membranes, and the structure and function of the membranes have received considerable attention primarily because of an interest in the turnover of the water they contain. Enzymatic activity of the membranes during the initiation of labor has been of additional interest. Most recently, the composition of the various extracellular connective tissue components has come under scrutiny (for review, see Bryant-Greenwood, 1998). Comprehensive surveys of many of these aspects, particularly the structural nature of the membranes, are found in Bourne's (1962) and Schmidt's (1992) books on the topic. Millar et al. (2000) measured the surface of the entire membranes in preterm and term placentas sonographically. It was 1037 cm² between 25 and 29 weeks; 1376 cm² from 30 to 34 weeks, and 1876 cm² at term. The measured surface area of expelled membranes, however, was only 737 cm², 855 cm², and 1115 cm², respectively, from which they deduced that the membranes are stretched in utero. The structural basis for premature rupture of the membranes was reviewed by Malak and Bell (1996). Amnionic fluid dynamics were reviewed comprehensively by Barnes and Seeds (1972), and they have been modeled by Mann et al. (1996). The turnover of amnionic fluid has also been reexamined by Gilbert et al. (1997) in rhesus monkeys undergoing chronic catheterization. The absorption of technetium-99 m from the fluid led these authors to conclude that much fluid turnover occurs through the placental membranes. Measurements of tensile strength with determination of gene regulation of membrane rupture were provided by Nemeth et al. (2000a,b), who constructed a special apparatus for the purpose. They found upregulation of interleukin-8 and pre–B-cell colony-enhancing factor by distention.

There are three distinct layers of the membranes. Their origin and interdependence must be understood if one wishes to comprehend their complexity (Fig. 11.1; also see Fig. 11.6. The inner layer is the **amnion**. A thin, avascular layer of epithelial cells and connective tissue, it is derived from the fetal ectoderm by cavitation within the embryonic knot (Luckett, 1973) and is contiguous, over the umbilical cord, with the fetal skin. Confirmation of its epidermal origin has come from the studies of Nanbu et al. (1989), who demonstrated the fetal differentiation antigen CA 125 in the fetal periderm (outer layer of epidermis) and the amnionic epithelium.

The amnion is passively attached to the next layer, the **chorion laeve**, by the internal pressures of amnionic fluid. The chorion laeve, a much more complex tissue, is composed of connective tissue within which there are the fetal (chorioallantoic) blood vessels. The villi of the chorion frondosum originate from the chorion. At the parietal, free surface of the membranes, one finds their atrophied remains, even in term pregnancy specimens. These former villi then are round balls of connective tissue, usually lacking trophoblastic cover and possessing no vessels. On the outer surface of the chorion rest also the remains of the cytotrophoblastic cells of the trophoblastic shell. They undergo much change with advancing gestation; they are somewhat vesicular and often atrophy. Small cysts are often found in these cell collections that are similar to the X-cell cysts in the placental tissue (see Fig. 11.13).

These cells, as the remaining villi, are intimately intermingled with the outermost layer, the **decidua capsularis**.

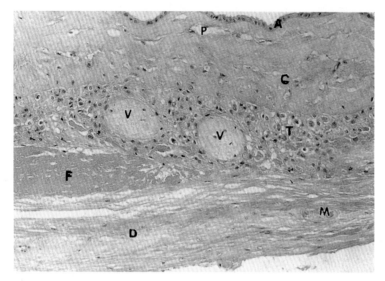

FIGURE 11.1. Microscopic appearance of normal "membranes." Amnion epithelium (A) sits on a thin layer of connective tissue that is separable from chorionic connective tissue (C) in an ill-defined plane (P) representing the so-called spongy layer (see Fig. 9.20). The following layer of extravillous trophoblast cells (T) is irregularly studded with atrophic "ghost villi" (V). At the periphery one finds the decidua capsularis (D) with maternal vessels (M) and frequent fibrinoid (F) deposits. H&E ×16.

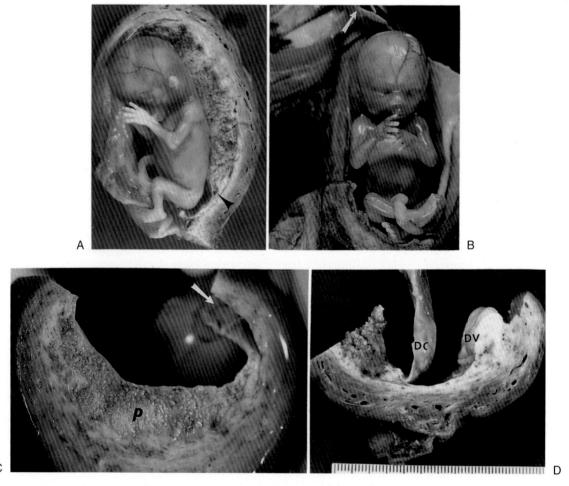

FIGURE 11.2. A–C: Uterus of a first trimester pregnancy with a 7.5-cm fetus in situ that was removed because of carcinoma of the cervix. Note the large myometrial vessels and the distance of the implanted placenta from the endocervix. The arrows point to the "marginal sinus." P, placenta. D: The membranes have been elevated from the decidua vera (DV) to show the fact that the decidua vera and decidua capsularis (DC) do not "grow together." The cervix has been removed.

The decidua, representing modified endometrium, is the only maternal component of the membranes. A variety of trophoblastic cells are present within this area, and it is essentially impossible to obtain "clean" decidual cells from this tissue for experimental work. The decidua capsularis also normally contains a few maternal blood vessels, some phagocytes, and other inflammatory cells. At the placental margin, this decidua capsularis is contiguous with the decidua basalis and here delimits the marginal sinus. The tissue at the base of the actual placenta, to which the normal villous tissue is anchored, is the maternal floor. One often finds degenerative processes and inflammation at this location, and hemorrhages are also frequent at this site. They have been referred to as being the result of a marginal sinus thrombosis, a term that is no longer defensible. When one stretches the edge of the membranes away from the placenta, one can see the friable tissue that constitutes this marginal decidua. When it is disrupted, one enters the intervillous blood space, the marginal sinus. In Figure 11.2, the margin of the placental membrane attachment is seen in situ. The uterus depicted also clearly shows a lack of fusion between the decidua capsularis and the decidua vera (or parietal decidua), as is similarly shown in Figure 11.3.

For the purposes of this presentation, we start with a brief summary of the development of the membranes. In the following sections we discuss each layer separately and identify the associated pathologic processes. This organization of material is not meant to suggest that these structures are independent; often they have substantial interactions. There is, however, much misunderstanding of the perceived unity of the membranes, particularly in biochemical studies. It is thus important that one clearly distinguishes between these different structures.

DEVELOPMENT

The trophoblast of the implanting blastocyst can be subdivided into one early implanting half (the cells surrounding the implantation pole or the

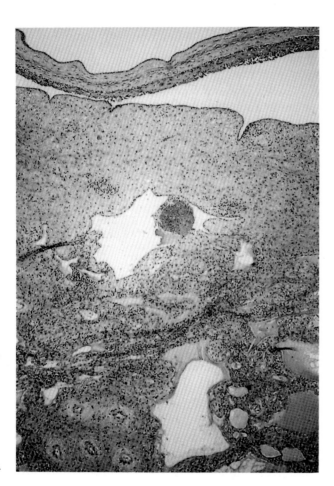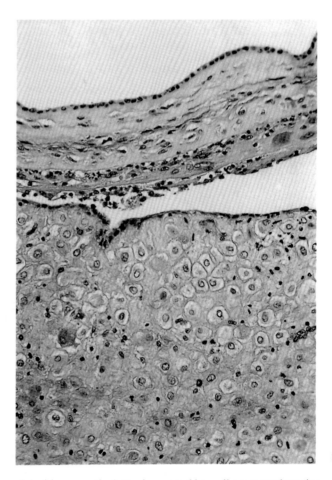

FIGURE 11.3. Membranes and decidua vera at term. The membranes of this placenta had a "plaque" attached to their external surface that was a portion of the decidua vera from the opposite side of the uterus. There is a space between decidua capsularis and decidua vera; the latter is covered by well-preserved uterine epithelium. True "fusion" between the two deciduas has not occurred. H&E. A ×10; B ×240.

basal chorion) and one later implanting half (that surrounding the anti-implantation pole or the capsular chorion) (see Figs. 4.1B,C and 12.1). The developmental processes, described in Chapter 5, are valid for the basal chorion. With the appearance of the first villi, the basal chorion becomes the chorion frondosum, the forerunner of the later placenta (Fig. 11.4). The capsular chorion, which implants a few days later (see Fig. 5.1B,C), initially undergoes a corresponding although delayed development. It proceeds with the identical processes of lacuna formation and consecutive transformation of the trabeculae into small villous trees, as those that take place at the implantation pole. At this stage, it is called the **capsular chorion frondosum**. Within a few days, however, beginning at the end of the 3rd week postcoitus (p.c.), the first degenerative changes at the antiimplantation pole can be observed. These result in the regression of newly formed villi, a process that slowly spreads laterally over the blastocyst surface (Hamilton & Boyd, 1960). As soon as the villi degenerate, the surrounding intervillous space obliterates. Finally, the primary chorionic plate of the respective region, the obliterated intervillous space together with its villous remnants, and the trophoblastic shell fuse (see Fig. 12.1), forming a multilayered compact lamella, the **smooth chorion (chorion laeve)** (Fig. 11.4). The first patches of the smooth chorion are formed roughly opposite the implantation pole. From there they gradually spread over about 70% of the surface of the chorionic sac. This process continues until the fourth lunar month, when it slowly comes to a halt (Wynn, 1968; Boyd & Hamilton, 1970).

The differentiation process into chorion frondosum and chorion laeve is paralleled by changes in the surrounding maternal tissues. The superficial layer of the endometrium, which is characterized throughout implantation by the transformation of endometrial stromal cells into decidual cells, is henceforth called the decidua. Depending on its spatial relation to the implanting chorionic sac, the decidua is subdivided into several segments (Fig. 11.4). The decidua below and lateral to the blastocyst or, later, that below the placenta, is called the **basal decidua (decidua basalis)**. With complete interstitial implantation, the decidua closes over the blastocyst. This protruding layer is called the **capsular decidua (decidua capsularis)**. All those parts of the decidua that line the uterine cavity without being in contact with the blastocyst (i.e., at the opposing uterine wall) are called the **parietal decidua (decidua vera)**. With increasing diameter of the chorionic sac, the capsular decidua focally degenerates, so that in such places the external surface of the smooth chorion (trophoblast cells) borders the uterine cavity (Fig. 11.4C). This surface finally touches the parietal decidua (Fig. 11.4B,C). Between the 15th and 20th weeks p.c., the smooth chorion, together with its attached residual capsular decidua, locally fuses with the parietal decidua, thereby largely obliterating the uterine cavity (Fig. 11.4C). From this date onward, the smooth chorion has contact with the decidual surface of the uterine wall over nearly its entire surface and may function as a paraplacental exchange organ. The efficiency of this exchange, however, is limited by the absence of fetal vessels within the smooth chorion.

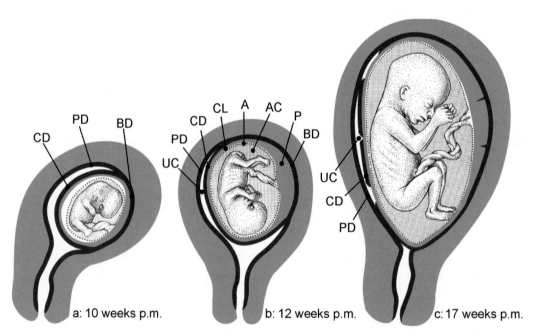

FIGURE 11.4. Late stages of the development of the fetal membranes. Fetus and amnion: black. Trophoblast: blue. Decidua: red. Myometrium: brown. A: Until 10 weeks postmenstruation (p.m.), the embryo is surrounded by a unit of chorion frondosum (blue); its later specialization into chorion leave and the placenta is indicated by a slight increase in thickness only. The capsular part of the chorion frondosum is covered by the capsular decidua (CD), which is continuous with basal decidua (BD) at the placental site, and with the parietal decidua (PD), which lines the uterine cavity. The amnion (black dotted line) is not fused in most places with the chorion frondosum. B: Two weeks later (12th week p.m.), the original chorion frondosum

has differentiated into the thick placenta (P) and the thinner fetal membranes that surround the inner amnionic cavity (AC). At this stage, the membranes are three-layered, composed of inner amnion (A), intermediate chorion laeve (CL), and outer capsular decidua (CD). Because of the embryo's small size, the uterine cavity (UC) is largely open. C: From 17 weeks on, the membranes come into close contact with the uterine wall. The remainder of the capsular decidua (CD) fuses with the parietal decidua (PD) and largely closes the uterine cavity (UC). From then on, the chorion laeve contacts the parietal decidua. (*Source:* Modified from Kaufmann, 1981.)

A third tissue, the amnion, contributes to the development of the membranes. During the first steps of implantation, an enlarged intercellular space between embryoblast and neighboring trophoblastic cells can be observed. Some small cells that line the inner surface of the trophoblast in this particular region have been named the amniogenic cells. They are the forerunners of the **amnionic epithelium**; the cleft separating them from the embryoblast is the early **amnionic cavity** (Hertig & Rock, 1941; Starck, 1975; Hinrichsen, 1990) (see Fig. 12.1). Because of its continuous expansion, the amnionic cavity slowly surrounds the embryo from all sides and finally covers the umbilical cord. In addition, through fetal growth and the production of **amnionic fluid**, the amnionic cavity is expanded.

Extraembryonic mesoblast, formed in the lacunar stage (see Chapter 5; Fig. 5.1D), not only lines the inner surface of the blastocyst cavity but also covers the external surface of the amnionic epithelium, thus giving rise to the **amnionic mesoderm**. Amnionic mesoderm and the extraembryonic mesoblast covering the trophoblast (**chorionic mesoderm**) are separated by a cavity called the exocoel (see Fig. 12.1) (Hertig, 1945, 1968). Those mesoblast cells that line the cavity are transformed into a mesothelium (Heuser's membrane). Fluid accumulation within the amnionic cavity causes its expansion so that it slowly compresses the exocoel. During the 6th to 7th week p.c., the amnionic vesicle has become so large that its mesoderm locally fuses with the chorionic mesoderm (see Fig. 12.1). This process starts in the areas surrounding the cord insertion at the chorionic plate and is largely completed after another 5 weeks (until the 12th week p.c.). The amnionic vesicle then completely occupies the exocoel (see Fig. 11.4) (Boyd & Hamilton, 1970). Only cleft-like remnants of the latter may be detectable in later stages of pregnancy, although one can always detach the amnion from the chorion. There is some sonographic indication that complete fusion may be delayed in pregnancies with trisomy 21 (Down syndrome) (Appelman et al., 1998). According to Grosser (1927), the mesothelium of both mesoderm layers disappears as soon as they come into contact with each other or even fuse. Fusion is never perfect, and amnion and chorion can always easily slide against each other. There are numerous clinical descriptions of "double sacs", that is, the presence of more fluid than expected between the amnion and chorion (e.g., Borlum, 1989). Generally, they have no relevance and are not pathologic. Histologically, they even seem to be separated by a system of slender, fluid-filled clefts (see Intermediate Zone of Chorion, below). Bundles of connective tissue fibers exist, crossing from one to the other layer; however, they are locally restricted and are laterally surrounded by these clefts. Differing from the situation in the membranes, the expanding amnion not only becomes closely attached to the surface of the cord but firmly fuses with it. It cannot be dislodged from the cord.

As soon as the amnion is attached to the surfaces of the placenta, umbilical cord, and the chorion laeve, its nomenclature becomes specified. The terms **placental amnion**, **umbilical amnion**, and **reflected amnion** are widely used. Although histologically the reflected amnion and chorion laeve are evidently separate structures, macroscopically they are summarized under the term **membranes**.

In spite of the considerable expansion of the amnionic cavity (Fig. 11.5), the structure of the membranes generally remains constant from the 4th month until term (Petry, 1962; Schmidt, 1992). Their mean thickness after separation from the uterine wall during labor is from about 200 to 300 mm, with a slight tendency to increase closer to the placenta. Because of local edematous swelling of the amnionic mesoderm, considerably thicker membranes are sometimes observed (Bourne, 1962). After birth, the following layers can be seen histologically (Fig. 11.6):

1. Amnionic epithelium and basal lamina (20–30 μm in thickness)
2. Amnionic mesoderm (about 15–30 μm in thickness)
3. Intermediate zone (highly variable in thickness)
4. Chorionic mesoderm (15–20 μm in thickness)
5. Trophoblast (10–50 μm in thickness)
6. Decidua (up to 50 μm in thickness)

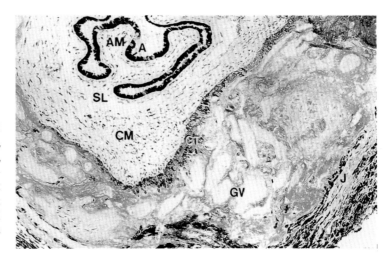

Figure 11.5. Membranes near their lateral placental attachment, showing lactate dehydrogenase activity. A, amnion epithelium; AM, amnionic mesenchyme; SL, spongy (intermediate) layer; CM, chorionic mesenchyme; CT, cytotrophoblast; GV, degenerative ghost villi; J, junctional zone, consisting of basal trophoblast and decidua. Ghost villi are frequent at the placental margin; further peripherally, the trophoblastic layers will fuse. Cryostat section. ×75.

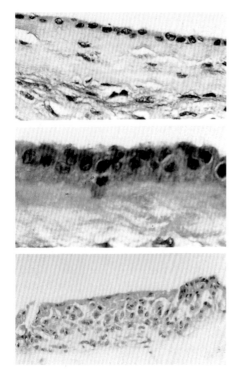

FIGURE 11.6. Different thicknesses of amnionic epithelium from three normal pregnancies. H&E ×160.

Amnion

The amnion is composed of an inner layer of epithelial cells, planted on a basement membrane that, in turn, is connected to a thin connective tissue layer by filamentous strands (Danforth & Hull, 1958). When the membrane is allowed to fix while stretched, the surface appears flat; when it is allowed to contract, many folds appear. It is a translucent structure that is frequently detached from the rest of the membranes by the forces of labor. It can almost always be easily separated from the underlying chorion, with which it never truly fuses, cellularly speaking.

As mentioned, this "fusion" of amnion and chorion completes around the 12th week of development (Boyd & Hamilton, 1970). Before that time, the amnion forms a separate bubble within the chorionic sac; it is surrounded and separated from the chorion by chorionic fluid, the magma reticulare, a viscous and thixotropic gel within which some stellate cells are dispersed (Fig. 11.7). It is important to recognize that the amnion does not possess its own blood vessels, in contrast to the opinion expressed by Donskikh (1957), who believed them to be present in early embryos. His drawings, however, are not convincing.

The amnion obtains its nutrition and oxygen from the surrounding chorionic fluid, the amnionic fluid, and the fetal surface vessels and, during early gestation, from the magma reticulare. It is of parenthetical interest here to note that magma reticulare–like differentiation has been described in yolk sac tumors, and that these elements stain positively with antibodies to vimentin and cytokeratin, thus displaying both mesenchymal and epi-

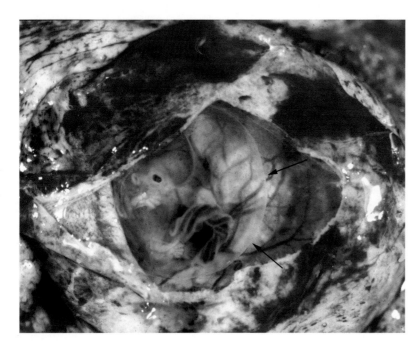

FIGURE 11.7. Intact placenta and fetus at 8 weeks of pregnancy, the chorion laeve having been opened. The arrows point to the amnionic bubble within the magma reticulare. Note also the early spiraling of the umbilical cord.

thelial characteristics (Michael et al., 1988). The latter is valid also for the amnionic epithelium. Despite its clearly epidermal origin, the cells not only express epidermal markers such as CA 125 (Nanbu et al., 1989) and such general epithelial markers as cytokeratins (Beham et al., 1988), but also vimentin staining is observed (Beham et al., 1988; Wolf et al., 1991). The latter is thought to be a marker for mesenchymally derived cells.

It is of historical interest also to note that Cane (1888) considered the amnion to secrete the amnionic fluid, which then was said to mold the early amnionic membrane. He also considered that it was responsible for the supply of oxygen by its rhythmic contractions, deemed to be analogous to the condition prevailing in birds. These hypotheses can now be laid aside.

Amnionic Epithelium: Different Cell Types or Cell Degeneration

The amnionic epithelium is a highly variable tissue, composed of a single layer of flat, cuboidal to columnar cells (Bautzmann & Schröder, 1955; Hempel, 1972; Schmidt, 1992). Columnar cells normally have been observed near the insertion of the membranes at the placental margin (Bou-Resli et al., 1981), whereas the cells generally flatten further in the periphery. Despite the diversity in shape, there appears to be only one single, uniform cell type (Sinha, 1971; Hempel, 1972; King, 1980). Previous findings by Thomas (1965), Armstrong et al. (1968), and Wynn and French (1968) resulted in the suggestion of the existence of different cell types, such as Golgi and fibrillar cells, or light and dark cells. These types could not be verified, however, in later studies.

According to Hoyes (1972), an artifactual genesis of the previous findings (due to inappropriate fixation and inappropriate osmolarity of the fixative) may be the explanation. The differences in nomenclature may also result from different amounts of fluid content. Thus, Hebertson et al. (1986) noted in their electron microscopic study of the epithelium that the normal thickness was much increased (to 18–56 μm) in diabetic pregnancies, channels (see following) were reduced in hydramnios, and other changes could be correlated with oligo- and polyhydramnios. Moreover, as discussed by Wynn and French (1968), a certain structural diversity of the cells may result from degenerative processes. These authors suggested that the often-present vesicles may reflect pinocytotic events. Histologic examination of the amnionic epithelium shows it to exhibit many different appearances. Often it is tall and columnar, whereas in other specimens it is flat and more squamous (Fig. 11.5). The varied appearance of the epithelial cells may be the result of different methods of fixation during preparation for

microscopy, and it may also result from different amounts of fluid content. Numerous gaps in the amnionic epithelium may be signs of such an expulsion of dying cells from the epithelium into the amnionic fluid, resulting in frequent defects of the epithelial layer. The remains may be the channels that Bourne and Lacy (1960) interpreted to be channels for preferred fluid exchange. Similar channels and complex cellular arrangements of the amnionic epithelium have been identified in the surface by the electron-microscopic studies of King (1982). This investigator also drew attention to the significant differences in the epithelial structure of the amnion when it is obtained from the free membranes or represents that of the cord. The development of micro-"blebs," frequent cell shedding, and the importance of the basal membrane for the maintenance of the integrity of the sac have been emphasized in the studies of Herendael et al. (1978). The influence of labor on the structure of the amnionic epithelium has been studied by Sonek et al. (1991).

Cytologic and Functional Aspects of the Amnionic Epithelium

During early pregnancy the bulging apical surfaces of the cells are covered by loosely scattered microvilli (Hoyes, 1968a; Lister, 1968; Ludwig et al., 1974). The number of microvilli increases later in pregnancy. The microvillous surface is characterized by a densely packed glycocalix with a high concentration of anionic binding sites (King, 1982). Intracellularly, a pronounced rough endoplasmic reticulum, numerous lipid droplets, and glycogen stores are evident. The ultrastructural findings are thought to favor intraamnionic lipid synthesis, rather than a degenerative origin of the droplets (Armstrong et al., 1968; van Bogaert et al., 1978; King, 1980). So far, however, there is no explanation for such a possible secretion. According to Benedetti et al. (1973), the lipids cannot be explained as the result of absorption from the amnionic fluid because the respective hydrolytic enzymes are absent. Most authors favor the view that the lipids are derived from the maternal circulation and, after some chemical changes, are secreted into the amnionic fluid (Polano, 1922; Szendi, 1940; Schmidt, 1965a,b, 1967; Armstrong et al., 1968; Pomerance et al., 1971; Schmidt et al., 1971). It is, however, difficult to understand how such quantities of maternally derived lipids should pass all layers of the membranes, and accordingly not all findings are in agreement with this concept. Some point to a fetal origin of the lipids and thus to their resorption from the amnionic fluid. According to Polishuk et al. (1965) and Pritchard et al. (1968), the intraamnionic lipids are chemically similar to those of the vernix. Vernix caseosa is derived from fetal sources, that is, secretory products of the fetal skin mixed with desquamated skin cells (Brusis et al., 1975). Even the degenerative character of the lipid droplets is still under discussion, although there is no ultrastructural evidence to support degeneration. The amount of lipid droplets increases throughout pregnancy (Yoshimura et al., 1980); maximum amounts have been reported following fetal hypoxia (Bourne, 1962; Bartman & Blanc, 1970) and fetal death (Yoshimura et al., 1980).

Substantial evidence exists to suggest a significant role for prostaglandins in the initiation and maintenance of uterine contractions (Smieja et al., 1993). Among the sources of prostaglandins for parturition, the amnionic epithelium seems to play a pivotal role because of its strategic anatomic location, with its close relation to amnionic fluid, myometrium, and uterine cervix. With the onset of labor, production of prostaglandins increases (Olson et al., 1983; Kinoshita et al., 1984; Skinner & Challis, 1985; Lopez Bernal et al., 1989; Mitchell, 1988). Moreover, amnionic epithelium is the nearly exclusive source for prostaglandin E_2 (PGE$_2$) (Okazaki et al., 1981a). The release of the latter hormone is regulated by intrinsic stimulatory properties of the membranes, but not of the villous chorion (McCoshen et al., 1986).

In this context, several questions arise: Do the membranes have the lipid precursors (arachidonic acid) for the synthesis of prostaglandins, and where are these metabolites manufactured and located? Foster and Das (1984) have contributed relevant studies. They separated amnion from chorion of normal membranes that they obtained following the normal onset of labor and analyzed the lipid content. This investigation contrasts with earlier studies that used combined membranes. It must be mentioned that the chorion was not freed from its decidual investment and that inferences drawn with respect to the precise localization of prostaglandin precursors cannot be made from this study alone. Nevertheless, the chorion had considerably more lipid (in milligram per deciliter) than the amnion, as can be seen in the following summary of their findings:

Lipid components	Amnion (mg/dL)	Chorion (mg/dL)
Total lipid	470	1530
Nonpolar lipids	319	1042
Cholesterol esters	44	263
Cholesterol	71	210
Triglycerides	160	416
Free fatty acids	44	153
Phospholipids	150	488

Olson and Smieja (1988) studied the incorporation of arachidonic acid into amnion and found that there was no difference, regardless of whether labor had preceded.

Enzymes involved in prostaglandin biosynthesis include phospholipases, prostaglandin synthase, and prostaglandin endoperoxide synthase (or cycloxygenase). They have been found in human amnion (Okazaki et al., 1981b; Bryant-Greenwood et al., 1987; Smieja et al., 1993; Toth et al., 1993; Toth & Rao, 1992). Interestingly, the enzymes are regulated by human chorionic gonadotropin (hCG) (Toth & Rao, 1992), the receptors of which are found on the amnionic epithelium (Rao & Lei, 1989; Reshef et al., 1990; Toth et al., 1993). The complexity of the intraamnionic regulatory mechanisms is increased by some additional findings: corticotropin-releasing hormone (CRH) (Jones & Challis, 1989) and glucocorticoids (Gibb & Lavoie, 1990) modulate prostaglandin production; CRH messenger RNA (mRNA) was demonstrated in the amnion of term pregnancies (Okamoto et al., 1990). Its production is modulated by glucocorticoids and progesterone (Jones et al., 1989).

Interleukins also are well known to regulate prostaglandin biosynthesis. According to the in situ hybridization and polymerase chain reaction studies by Rote et al. (1993), explants of normal amnion and chorion laeve produce interleukin-1β in vitro; the application of endotoxin induced additional expression of interleukin-6. In conclusion, the authors speculated that intraamnionic infections induce production of interleukins that increase prostaglandin production. Much additional investigation relates to prostaglandin initiation during the process of chorioamnionitis and is covered in Chapter 20. 15-Hydoxyprostaglandin dehydrogenase as a prostaglandin-metabolizing and -inactivating enzyme was found in membranes and villous trophoblast (Cheung et al., 1990). Casey et al. (1989) found prostaglandin dehydrogenase in the decidua capsularis and proposed that it regulates levels of prostaglandin therein as well as in the amnionic fluid, uterus, and blood.

The interactions between prostaglandins and oxytocin in the regulation of uterine contractions are only poorly understood. In humans, oxytocin acts as the myometrial contraction stimulator, but only when it is combined with increased levels of PGF$_{2\alpha}$ (Fuchs et al., 1982). The production of the latter is stimulated by oxytocin through a receptor-mediated process (Roberts et al., 1976). Benedetto et al. (1990) were able to demonstrate the oxytocin receptors in the amnion as well as in the chorion laeve. Finally, leukotrienes, another cytokine group derived from arachidonic acid, are produced by the amnion (Rees et al., 1988). The authors stated that these cytokines may affect uterine contractility besides their function as mediators of immune reaction and vasodilation.

From a functional perspective, perhaps more interesting are some findings concerning the intercellular junctions and the basal lamina of the amnion. The amnionic cells are connected to each other by numerous desmosomes that focally bridge the long, winding lateral intercellular spaces; some additional gap junctions have been observed in the laterobasal region (King, 1982; Bartels & Wang, 1983; Wang, 1984). Tight junctions occluding the lateral intercellular spaces, and thus limiting paracellular transport, could not be observed between the cells, with the exception of a few during the first months of pregnancy (King, 1982; Bartels & Wang, 1983). Consequently, the intercellular clefts may represent an effective route for paracellular transfer, as has been demonstrated by tracer studies (King, 1982; Matsubara & Tamada, 1991). This point is of particular importance, as there are no hints of an effective transcellular pathway for macromolecules.

There are, however, some findings concerning the basal lamina that restrict the relevance of these interpretations. The amnionic cells have a highly folded basal surface that interdigitates intensely with the basal lamina to which they are fixed by numerous hemidesmosomes (Danforth & Hull, 1958; Verbeek et al., 1967; King, 1980, 1982; Bartels & Wang, 1983; Wang, 1984). According to the histochemical studies of King (1985), the basal lamina contains large quantities of proteoglycans, rich in heparan sulfate. The latter substance may serve as a permeability barrier to anionic macromolecules. Also, Klima et al. (1991), Wolf and Schmidt (1991), and Singhas (1992) have described by means of lectin-binding studies the presence of glycoconjugates in the amnion and discussed the influence of these substances on amnionic fluid transfer. These findings are in agreement with two other studies. Liotta et al. (1980) observed restricted permeability of an isolated basal lamina preparation of human amnion to a 60,000-dalton protein, and Sutcliffe (1975) reported that the amnionic fluid contains a much smaller amount of protein than is found in fetal and maternal serum. Thus, the amnionic basal lamina must also be considered to participate in the barrier function (King, 1985).

Concerning the regulation of transamnionic fluid transfer, Beham et al. (1988), Wolf et al. (1991), and Ockleford et al. (1993) have studied the distribution of cytoskeletal filaments within the amnionic epithelium. Actin, α-actinin, spectrin, ezrin, cytokeratins, vimentin, and desmoplakin have all been found. The specialized arrangement of this intracellular filament system indicates a role in the structural integrity and modulation of cell shape as well as in junctional permeability (Wolf et al., 1991). Casey et al. (1991) demonstrated that amnionic epithelial cells produce endothelin-1 and are thus one of the potential sources for endothelin in the amnionic fluid where it appears in concentrations exceeding those of the blood plasma by 10- to 100 fold. Epidermal growth factor, interleukin-1, and tumor necrosis factor-α (TNF-α) increased amnionic endothelin production. Amnionic endothelin may be involved in the regulation of amnionic fluid homeostasis as it is known to promote water transfer across the epithelia of other organs.

The amnion is involved in the turnover of the amnionic fluid. There is great immunohistochemical activity of carbonic anhydrase isoenzymes CA-1 and CA-2 (Crescimanno et al., 1993; Mühlhauser et al., 1994); this enzyme is involved in bicarbonate-carbon dioxide exchange. This fact makes it likely that the epithelium is responsible for regulating the pH of the amnionic fluid, keeping it constant at about pH 7.10. In doing so, the amnionic epithelium is at least partly involved in fetal pH regulation because the fetus delivers considerable amounts of protons and bicarbonate via his or her kidneys into the amnionic fluid. In addition, aquaporins may be involved in fluid balance, as they are found in amnion and chorion of the human placenta (Mann et al., 2002). These authors suggested that the presence of aquaporin may be responsible for the rapid water turnover from amnionic fluid to the fetal circulation (400 mL/day).

Amnionic epithelium participates not only in fetal CO_2 clearance but also in the clearance of fetal vasopressin, for instance, which is excreted via the fetal urine. It is removed from the amnionic fluid by diffusion- and swallowing-independent mechanisms (Uyehara & Claybaugh, 1988). It is likely that the degrading peptidases are active in the amnionic epithelium as well as in the amnionic fluid. In this context it may be of interest that Gossrau et al. (1987) described dipeptidylpeptidase IV activities in the amnionic epithelium and speculated about its hydrolytic action, both intracellularly as well as in the amnionic fluid.

Epithelial participation in the secretion of amnionic fluid and in its resorption has long been under discussion (Bourne, 1962; Armstrong et al., 1968; Kratzsch & Grygiel, 1972; Smadja et al., 1974; Weser & Kaufmann, 1978), but until now this secretory activity has been speculative. It is generally accepted that the sources of the amnionic fluid are multiple and that the role of the amnion in maintaining its composition is still uncertain. The general functional description of the amnion as an epithelial lining that is contributing to the homeostasis of the amnionic fluid is supported by many clinical findings (see following), but they add little to the resolution of the precise interactions. Several groups of investigators have detected, by immunohistochemical means, hormones such as hCG and somatotropin (hCS) in the amnionic cells (Thiede & Choate, 1963; Kim et al., 1971; de Ikonicoff & Cedard, 1973). It is likely, however, that these hormones are the result of resorption from the amnionic fluid with subsequent degradation, rather than reflecting any local hormone synthesis.

The structural studies support the view that the amnionic epithelium is metabolically highly active throughout gestation. This point is also supported by the histochemical proof of high activity of various enzymes (Weser & Kaufmann, 1978). The histochemical study of enzymes related to energy metabolism suggested a predominating anaerobic glycolysis caused by restricted oxygen supply (Benedetti et al., 1973). The absence of vessels in the mesenchymal layers of the amnion raises the question concerning the source of its nutrients and oxygen. They may be supplied by diffusion from the deeper layers of the uterine wall or via the amnionic fluid from the fetus. Wolf and Desoye (1993) have described the presence of glucose transporter protein-1 and -3 predominantly at the apical surface of amnionic epithelial cells, whereas glucose transporter protein-4 and insulin receptor could not be detected. Thus, it is quite likely that these cells cover their glucose requirements from the amnionic fluid with an insulin-independent mechanism. Furthermore, Bourne (1962) reported a monochorionic, diamnionic twin pregnancy in which the ipsilateral amnion in the "dividing membrane" degenerated following the death of one fetus. This finding can be explained in different ways; it simply may be an indicator that the fetus is important for supplying the amnion with nutrients and gases or, alternatively, the degenerating fetal tissues may affect adversely the epithelium.

The question of possible repair mechanisms of amnion epithelium and the mesenchymal cells after mechanical injury was studied in vitro by Bilic et al. (2004). They produced monolayers of epithelial and mesenchymal cells and then injured them. Repair of the epithelium was generally complete within 40 hours but less efficiently so in mesenchymal cells, although it was more extensive in preterm than term tissues. The addition of platelet-derived growth factor (PDGF) and TNF-α had no beneficial effect on cell proliferation.

AMNIONIC FLUID

It is commonly accepted that the amnionic fluid is derived from multiple sources: (1) possible secretory processes of the amnionic epithelium; (2) filtration of fluid from maternal vessels via the parietal decidua and the chorion laeve; (3) filtration from the fetal vessels via the chorionic plate and via the umbilical cord; (4) urination by the fetus; and (5) during earlier stages of pregnancy, by filtration from intracorporeal fetal vessels via the fetal skin. Its composition is influenced by continuous resorptive processes by the fetal digestive tract and the amnion and by pressure-dependent fetomaternal filtration across the membranes. The volume of the fluid is not static, varying among the stages of pregnancy as well as among individuals. A careful determination of the development of amnionic fluid volumes throughout pregnancy by a dilution method during amniocentesis has been presented by Queenan et al. (1972) (Fig. 11.8). The results showed a wide range of volumes, with a mean of 239 mL at 15 to 16 weeks postmenstruation (p.m.), a maximum mean of 984 mL at 33 to 34 weeks p.m., and a slight final decrease to term (836 mL). After term (41 to 42 weeks p.m.), the mean volume was reduced to 544 mL.

The composition of the amnionic fluid has been described in detail by Schmidt (1992) and is reviewed only briefly here. The pH is usually 7.10, with maximum values of 7.40; the osmotic pressure is about 255 mOsm. Further constituents include:

- Glucose (5–20 mg/100 mL)
- Amino acids

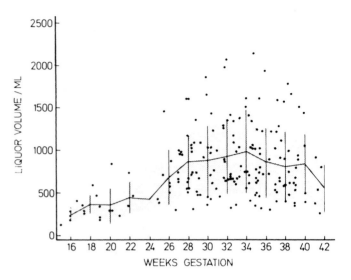

FIGURE 11.8. Volume of amnionic fluid during gestation in 187 determinations. Mean values ±1 SD. There is a wide range, with a final decrease during the last 4 weeks of gestation. (*Source:* Modified from Queenan et al., 1972.)

- Proteins (280–780 mg/100 mL) (α_1-albumin; α_2-albumin; β-globulin; γ-globulins: immunoglobulins IgA, IgG, IgM; α_1-fetoprotein; lipoproteins); the recent identification of elevated S100B protein levels by Florio et al. (2004) was used to anticipate fetal demise at mid-gestation; similarly, elevated maternal α-fetoprotein levels anticipated sudden fetal demise (Smith et al., 2004).
- Lipids (40 mg/100 mL), largely as lipid droplets measuring 1 to 30 mm in diameter, composed of cholesterol, triglycerides, diglycerides, free fatty acids, phospholipids (among the latter, the ratio of lecithin to sphingomyelin (L/S ratio) as performed during prenatal diagnosis is thought to be a reliable parameter in determining pulmonary maturity; it has also been suggested that surfactant may stabilize the amnionic sac) (Hills, 1994); Longo et al. (1996) found no lecithin/sphingomyelin but a substance with similar migratory pattern and may thus be confusing.
- Urea (20–40 mg/100 mL)
- Uric acid
- Creatinine
- Bilirubin

In addition, a broad variety of hormones has been found in the amnionic fluid (Schindler, 1982):

- Progesterone, estradiol, estriol, testosterone, aldosterone, cortisol
- Luteinizing hormone (LH), follicle-stimulating hormone (FSH), hCG, human placental lactogen (hPL), prolactin, adrenocorticotropic hormone (ACTH), human growth hormone (hGH), somatomedin, thyrotropin (thyroid-stimulating hormone, TSH)
- Thyroid hormones, parathyroid hormone, oxytocin, glucagon, insulin, hypothalamic-releasing hormones, neurophysin. We have had an interest in the presence of endorphin in amnionic fluid (Gautray et al. (1977)). This central nervous system (CNS)- or pituitary-derived hormone was present late in gestation, has its source in fetal urine, and was elevated in amnionic fluid of gestations with gastroschisis (Akgur & Olguner, 2004; Mahieu-Caputo et al., 2004). We speculate that variations in levels may indicate different levels of response to pain by the fetus, as for instance in osteogenesis imperfecta.

Numerous enzymes have been found, most of which, according to Schmidt (1992), are thought to be derived from the membranes by secretion or by cell shedding. Among the activators and inhibitors of proteases are tissue-type plasminogen activator (tPA) and urokinase-type plasminogen activator (uPA), as well as their respective inhibitors PAI-1 and PAI-2 (Kjaeldgaard et al., 1989). They regulate the fibrinolytic and proteolytic activities of amnionic fluid plasminogen, which is considered to be involved in the etiology of membrane rupture (Jenkins et al., 1983) (see following).

After staining with Nile blue (Nieland et al., 1970), hematoxylin and eosin (H&E), Giemsa, or Papanicolaou stains, a variety of amnionic fluid cells can be observed, their number steadily increasing throughout pregnancy and reaching values at term to 80 cells/mm^3. Their origin has not been satisfactorily determined in every case because, after exfoliation from their tissue of origin, they usually undergo structural changes (Schmidt, 1992). The following cell types have been classified by Schmidt (1992):

- Large anuclear flat cells (diameter 40–50 mm), probably exfoliated keratinocytes
- Nucleated squamous epithelial cells (diameter 30–50 mm): type b originating from the oral mucous membrane, type c possibly originating from the amnionic epithelium of the cord, type d derived from the fetal vulva and vagina
- Small round to oval cells (diameter 18–25 mm), originating from the fetal urinary tract
- In addition, a variety of special cell forms such as polynuclear cells from the urinary tract (transitional epithelium) and others have been found. This has included neurogenic cells (Prusa et al., 2004) whose origin may be the fetal hair follicles (Sieber-Blum & Grim, 2004).

CHROMOSOMAL DETERMINATIONS

Bautzmann et al. (1960) and other students of the amnionic membrane have often made flat membrane preparations for investigation. These preparations allow one to see more clearly the squamous nature of the epithelium and to demonstrate its occasional defects. These preparations also lend themselves to observing the lipid droplets in the epithelium whose numbers increase with maturation (Bautzmann & Hertenstein, 1957; Danforth & Hull, 1958; Schmidt, 1963). Occasional giant cells ("colossal cells") with large vacuoles are seen to include large vacuoles. Such preparations also show relatively frequent polyploid nuclei. The epithelial cells, however, divide under normal conditions by regular mitosis (Schwarzacher & Klinger, 1963). Multinucleated cells, particularly binucleated cells, are most commonly found in newborns. Mitoses become rare after the sixth gestational month. In cytophotometric measurements, Schindler (1961) showed, in specimens from early gestation, that the polyploid cells are tetraploid and octoploid, with a concomitant increase in their cytoplasm. These observations have assumed greater significance as the use of amniocentesis for chromosomal determination of the fetus has been more widely practiced. The finding of mixed cell populations (mosaicism) is here of concern; it demands an explanation (Kalousek & Dill, 1983). These authors studied 117 specimens and concluded that the mosaic (aneuploid) cell populations they found invariably came from the membranes. Aneuploid cells were not found in fetal lymphocytes when these were studied after birth. They had only 47 completely successful cultures with two aneuploid admixtures, but it is not clear that they grew amnion epithelium, as opposed to chorionic fibroblasts. Nevertheless, they reviewed other reports of mosaicism of cell lines from amnionic fluid culture (origin of these cells also unknown), where the fetus was eventually found to be normal.

Similarly perplexing mosaicism has been detected in chorionic villus sampling (CVS) biopsy by a number of investigators. Linton and Lilford (1986), for instance, found complex XY/XYY mosaicism, and all 14 metaphases contained an extra chromosome 16q-. It was associated with a karyotypically normal fetus in a case described by Breed et al.

(1986). In parallel cultures of amnionic fluid cells and samples from CVS, Verjaal et al. (1987) also found discrepancies and warned that great care must be taken when interpreting such abnormalities. Their findings supported the view of Hogge et al. (1985) that such errors occur as often as in 2% of CVS. Schulze et al. (1987) had experience with two aneuploid mosaics (46,XX/47,XX + 3; 46,XX/47,XX + 15) and normal 46,XX newborns. Crane and Cheung (1988) suggested that postzygotic nondisjunction of chromosomes in the cytotrophoblast is the most likely cause of such mosaicism. They described 15 cases of mosaicism in CVS, identified in direct preparations from the biopsy, thus ruling out an artifact of tissue culture. They suggested that the processing of multiple individual fragments of tissue might avoid mistaken diagnosis. Further consideration of confined placental mosaicism is to be found in Chapter 21. The most recent methodology for the evaluation of the fetal genotype and for the study of differences in the genetic contributions of fetus versus placenta involves a molecular analysis of the DNA extracted from both tissues. Butler et al. (1988) studied 50 paired samples from these sources and found differences in the hypervariable regions of repetitive DNA in four pairs, whereas they were alike in the others. This finding may indicate that mitotic crossing-over or other mechanisms of chromosomal segregation occur. These points must be considered for a meaningful interpretation of cytogenetic studies from placenta and amniotic fluid. Furthermore, mitotic errors in the delicate amnionic membrane of early gestation might be one mechanism that leads to defects in its structure and thus to the future amnionic band development. Additional discussion of this important topic is found in Chapter 21, on abortion.

Another still poorly understood feature of the developing membranes is that the X inactivation ("lyonization") of its cells appears to be non-random. Ropers et al. (1978) reviewed the studies on this topic and analyzed the glucose-6-phosphate dehydrogenase (G-6-PD) activity of heterozygotic females. Preferential activity of the maternal X chromosome–derived isozyme activity was found in the membranes of the placenta, analogous to earlier observations made in rodents (Frels et al., 1979; Rastan et al., 1980). Confirmation of these results has come from the study by Harrison and Warburton (1986). They also used the variants of G-6-PD as markers for "lyonization," but the mechanism (DNA methylation) leading to this preferential expression of the maternal allele ("imprinting") and the possible reasons for it are unknown at present.

Cellular Metaplasia and Glycogen

Metaplastic processes are frequent in the amnionic epithelium. They are present in at least one fourth of mature placentas, most prominently around the umbilical cord; they must not be confused with amnion nodosum. We refer to them as "squamous metaplasia," a misnomer, as Bourne (1960) noted. The amnion is squamous, and these areas of metaplasia do not form in response to some chronic irritation or inflammation, as for instance in the bronchus of smokers. They merely betray maturity and are not found in immature placentas. This so-called squamous metaplasia of the amnion is actually only the focal keratinization of the epithelium (Figs. 11.9 and 11.10). It is a regular feature of the amnion in many other species, such as whales and sheep, in which nodules of keratin stud the cord and amnion. Some species even have melanin pigment in these structures. In the term human placenta these areas of squamous metaplasia are visible

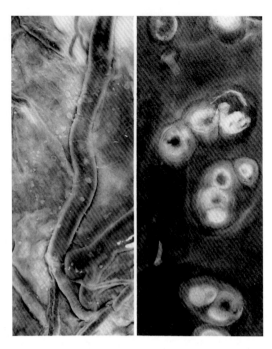

FIGURE 11.9. Squamous metaplasia of the amnion. At left is a surface view showing the concentric layers of keratin. At right one sees the tiny nodules of keratin irregularly present over vessels and chorion, different from amnion nodosum.

as hydrophobic foci of tiny, concentric elevations. They are most commonly found in the vicinity of the cord insertion. Squamous metaplasia occurs in up to 60% of term placentas. Sinha (1971) and Nieland et al. (1970) provided a detailed electron-microscopic study of squamous metaplasia. In animals, these plaques (occasionally referred to as pustules) may be 15 cells thick. They may have no similarity to amnion cells but more resemble the epidermis and usually include keratohyaline granules and melanin. In this context, one must recall the developmental and structural continuity (see Fig. 12.1) of amnionic epithelium and the squamous fetal skin.

An interesting consideration is whether, in cases of ichthyosis congenita, the amnion participates in the excessive keratinization that is seen in the epidermis. One report of marked plaque formation in ichthyosis has come from Coston (1908). He observed a large placenta whose cord and amnion were covered with ichthyotic patches. This finding has not been our experience. The placenta of the X-linked type of ichthyosis (the commonest form of this disease) is structurally normal. A biochemical study by Bedin et al. (1981) of the steroid sulfatase in placentas from heterozygous women has shown that the locus (localized at Xp22.3) determining this critical enzyme for the disease is not inactivated by lyonization. It can now be identified by fluorescent in situ hybridization, and deficiency should be suspected when abnormally low estriol values are found in pregnancy

(Ahmed et al., 1998). Garcia et al. (1977) observed the concurrence of amnion nodosum and congenital ichthyosis in four cases. Amnionic plaques of the membranes were correctly interpreted to result from oligohydramnios, rather than from excessive squamous metaplasia. Our conclusion is that the amnion, although ectodermal in origin, does not have the capacity to exhibit the lesion of ichthyosis congenita. In a case of severe, fatal lamellar ichthyosis seen by us, the amnion was attached to the fetal skin because of oligohydramnios, but its remnants, located around the cord insertion, were free from keratinization. There was some excessive squamous metaplasia on the cord surface, with prominent desmosomes but lacking keratohyaline granules and true keratin. Moreover, no macroscopic plaques were present despite severe fetal skin involvement. A case of harlequin (lamellar, collodion) ichthyosis was described in detail by Shareef et al. (2000), but the placental findings were not noted. Interestingly, after adequate neonatal care of this severely affected neonate, its skin was normal at 2-month follow-up. An unresolved question is the cause of the common oligohydramnios in these pregnancies and the concomitant fetal deformities. The latter are frequently much in excess of those found with Potter's syndrome and are presumably a part of the genetic abnormality ichthyosis. Moirot and colleagues (1990), on the other hand, suggested that polyhydramnios is frequent in lamellar ichthyosis cases. They also found no typical changes in

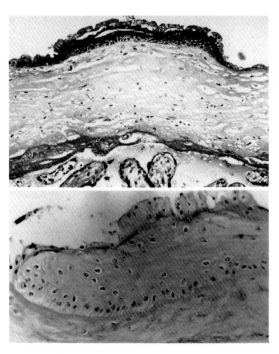

FIGURE 11.10. Squamous metaplasia, typical of mature placenta (top), and amnion epithelium (bottom). H&E. Top ×160; bottom ×250.

FIGURE 11.11. Ballooning degeneration of amnionic epithelium in a 20–week abortus after 3 weeks of bleeding. H&E ×400.

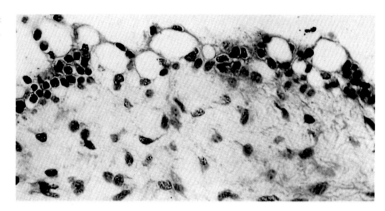

amnion, only keratinization. The fluid was found to be yellow and "flocculent," and the placenta edematous. Keratinization was also found to be absent in the rare harlequin fetuses of the Neu-Laxova syndrome (Karimi-Nejad et al., 1987), in which hyperkeratosis is a prominent feature of the infant's skin.

During early pregnancy, the amnionic epithelium contains cytoplasmic glycogen, and it is not significantly increased in the placentas of women with diabetes. Increased amounts of glycogen in the placentas of diabetics have been found to occur only around the major fetal vessels (Robb & Hytten, 1976). Other vacuoles are frequently present in the epithelial cells; they may be engaged in transport activity (Fig. 11.11). In cases of fetal death, the epithelium shows extensive degeneration, particularly when studied by electron microscopy (Mukaida et al., 1977). For a consideration of the vacuolization of amnionic epithelium, see the following section.

Amnionic Mesoderm

The amnionic epithelium rests on a basal lamina that is mainly composed of collagen IV fibrils (Yurchenco & Ruben, 1994), laminin (Aplin et al., 1985), and heparan sulfate proteoglycan (Foltz et al., 1982). It is associated with the basal cell surface by means of fibronectins. Its functional influence on transamnionic transfer has been discussed earlier. The lamina is fixed to the neighboring stroma by anchoring plaques containing collagen IV, which are attached to anchoring fibrils in the surrounding tissues that contain collagen VII (Keene et al., 1987). In addition, collagen V appears in the area immediately surrounding the basal lamina (Modesti et al., 1984). Proteoglycans embedding the collagen fibers can imbibe water and swell, leading to sliding of the amnion over the chorion; this might provide a short-term sealing mechanism of ruptured membranes (Behzad et al., 1994; Bryant-Greenwood, 1998).

The following layer, the compact stromal layer, has a varying thickness. It contains collagen types I and III (Madri et al., 1983) and fibronectins (Linnala et al., 1993) that are largely secreted by the amnionic epithelial cells. The distribution of the different collagen types in the various mesenchymal layers of the amnion has been described in detail by Malak et al. (1993). The compact stroma is composed of bundles of 50-nm collagen fibrils that are intermingled with 18-nm fibrils (Aplin & Allen, 1985). The three-dimensional structure of these fibrils and their association with the basal lamina as well as with the basal surface of amnionic epithelium has been beautifully illustrated by Campbell et al. (1989). The two types of fibers together form a coarse meshwork of bundles, in which, according to Bourne (1962), some elastic fibers can also be integrated. The latter finding has been contested by Aplin and Allen (1985), so that it remains an open question whether the well-known elasticity of the amnion results from the presence of elastic material or the arrangement of the collagenous bundles.

A characteristic layering of the amnionic mesoderm, as it has been described for the amnion of the **chorionic plate** (Bourne, 1962), is less pronounced in the **amnionic membrane**. The ability to identify several distinct layers of connective tissue probably depends to some degree on the state of its contraction and fixation, as well as on one's imagination. It is evident, however, that the compact, collagenous layer nearer to the epithelium is largely devoid of connective tissue cells. Ockleford et al. (1993), based on immunohistochemical studies, have suggested that it represents a giant lamina reticularis making up the inner part of a basal membrane and thus belongs to the amnionic basal lamina.

The deeper part of the amnionic mesenchyme, also called the fibroblast layer (Bou-Resli et al., 1981), contains a more or less dense network of branched fibroblasts. Bartels and Wang (1983) failed to observe intercellular junctions connecting these cells. Additionally, some macrophages can be observed as early as in the

7th week of gestation (5- to 6-mm embryo). Schwarzacher (1960) likened them to Hofbauer cells. In electron microscopic studies of the amnion, Hoyes (1968b) suggested that these macrophages derive from the epithelium and that they decrease in number toward term. In light of the modern findings regarding the biology of placental macrophages (see Chapter 6), however, there are no longer arguments regarding an epithelial derivation. The bundles of collagen fibers are arranged in clearly separated layers of varying fiber orientation (Bou-Resli et al., 1981). Aplin and Allen (1985) described the synthesis of collagens I, III, and IV, as well as of laminin and fibronectin, by amnionic epithelial cells in culture. From these findings, they concluded that the epithelium not only produces the basal lamina but is also involved in the synthesis of the stromal fibers, at least of the compact layer, which is largely devoid of fibroblasts.

A MEDLEY OF THEMES

The sex chromatin (Barr body) of amnionic epithelial cells and of the underlying connective tissue is easily observed. Using this marker, Klinger & Schwarzacher (1962) demonstrated in a fetus with XY/XXY mosaicism that the amnion was also mosaic. Some areas were sex chromatin–positive and others were sex chromatin–negative. Moreover, they showed clearly that the connective tissue underlying one type of epithelium occasionally had a different karyotype. This observation proved, once and for all, that these tissues have different embryologic origins. We indicated earlier that we believe the peripheral connective tissue of the amnion is a condensation of the cellular elements that are dispersed in the magma reticulare of the primitive chorionic sac. Parenthetically, it may be noted that an improved method for the histologic detection of sex chromatin in formalin-fixed tissues has been described (Davis & Penny, 1981); it employs pronase and acid hydrolysis before quinacrine staining. Perhaps the earliest time sex chromatin can be observed in human embryos is on day 13. Thorburn (1964) identified the Barr bodies readily in trophoblast. The sex chromatin in membranes

and trophoblast has also been described by Bohle and Hienz (1956) and Verma and Ghai (1971).

Efforts to study the possible existence of smooth musculature in human amnions have usually employed flat, surface preparations of membranes. From studies in chicken and reptiles it is known that an orderly arrangement of a smooth muscle plexus in the amnion produces regular contractions, possibly to ensure mixing of fluid and rocking of the embryo (Bautzmann & Schröder, 1953; Bautzmann, 1956). Such structures have not been found in mammals. In early human amnions, only net-like fibrocytic cell arrangements are identifiable in the connective tissue of the amnion; muscle is absent.

There are also no nerves, lymphatics, or blood vessels in the amnion. Because the amnion is avascular, it must subsist on the nutrients and gaseous exchange of surrounding fluids and structures. As mentioned earlier, this point is particularly well demonstrated by the large portions of amnion that are apposed as the "dividing membranes" in diamnionic monochorionic twins. Here the large stretches of amnion are kept alive by the amnionic fluid surrounding them. Consequently, when one fetus dies, that portion of its amnionic surface dies as well. The epithelial cells undergo necrosis, as shown in Figure 11.12A (see also Bourne, 1962). It is surprising that the living amnion from the opposing twin's side is not able to sustain this portion of membrane, as the dividing membranes are so thin and delicate. Although it is also possible that the death of the amnionic epithelium in these circumstances comes about by the liberation of noxious substances from a macerating fetus, it is unlikely. The amnion overlying the placenta proper takes much longer to die; it is obviously being kept alive by the oxygen gradients from the persisting intervillous circulation.

CLINICAL AND RESEARCH APPLICATIONS

Because the amnion can be so readily separated from the chorion, and because it is so widely available, it has often been used as dressing for burns and other wounds (Editorial, 1984; Redmond, 1984). This practice appears to have special merits in that the epithelium does not possess human leukocyte antigen (HLA)-type antigens and even fails to elicit an immunologic reaction when transplanted (Akle et al., 1981). Moreover, antibacterial properties of the amnion are well documented. The antimicrobial effect is thought to be related to the close adherence of the membrane to the wound surface (Talmi et al., 1981).

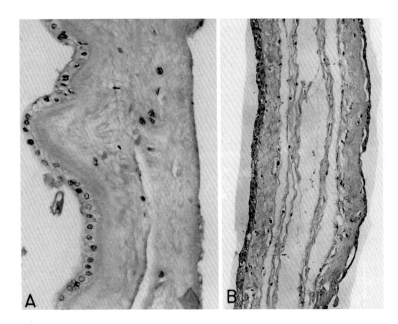

FIGURE 11.12. Two sets of "dividing membranes" (A,B) of diamnionic, monochorionic twins with one twin having died days before birth. Note the necrosis of the epithelium on the right sides at various stages of degeneration. H&E. A ×160; B ×250.

Amnion has also been a favorite cellular material for virologists in that it can readily be established in culture, particularly when it is obtained from young pregnancies and from patients with toxemia of pregnancy (Jonas & Caunt, 1965). When such cultures are treated with cortisone, profound changes occur in the membranous surface of the amnionic epithelial cells (Polet, 1966). It is also worthy of note that the injection of transformed human amnion cells into cortisone-treated mice induces tumor growth with cartilage and bone formation, presumably by stimulating host cells to undergo this differentiation (Anderson et al., 1964). In other studies, the amnion has been used to serve as a substratum for axons in tissue culture (Davis et al., 1987) and for the cultivation of trophoblast; after removal of the epithelial cells, the remaining connective tissue matrix, together with the epithelial basal lamina, serves as an excellent substratum for the monolayer culture of cytotrophoblast, even allowing syncytial fusion of the latter (Bullen et al., 1990).

Chorion Laeve

The chorionic membrane is a tough fibrous tissue layer that carries the fetal blood vessels. The villi arise from its outer surface; on the inside of the chorion is the amnion, which is only loosely attached. It has been convenient for many authors to speak of the "placental chorion," the membrane that covers the placental disk proper. In agreement with the anatomic literature, we call it the chorionic plate. On the other hand, the "reflected chorion" is the chorion laeve or extraplacental membrane (Bourne, 1962), which is the tissue that we discuss in greater detail in this chapter.

Intermediate (Spongy) Layer

When studying the membranes after birth, one realizes that the reflected amnion and chorion can easily slide, separating the two membranes from each other. This phenomenon is due to the existence of the spongy layer, which results from incomplete fusion of amnionic and chorionic mesoderm during early pregnancy. This intermediate layer is composed of loosely arranged bundles of collagen fibers with a few scattered fibroblasts, separated by a communicating system of clefts (Schmidt, 1956; Petry, 1962; Bou-Resli et al., 1981). The clefts are remainders of the formerly existing and now largely obstructed exocoel (see Fig. 12.1). This view has been corroborated by immunohistochemical/confocal laser studies by Ockleford et al. (1993).

It is difficult to decide whether accidental cells lining these clefts are also fibroblasts or whether they are the remainder of the original amnionic and chorionic mesothelium. The presence of collagen type IV in this zone (Malak et al., 1993; Ockleford et al., 1993), which is a typical basal lamina molecule, means that a mesothelial origin of these cells is quite likely (Ockleford et al., 1993). In addition, macrophages have been observed (Schmidt, 1956).

Chorionic Mesoderm

The spongy layer continues without sharp demarcation into the next connective tissue layer, already belonging to the chorion laeve.

This connective tissue is derived from the embryo (Luckett, 1971). When restudying human and rhesus monkey embryonic material, Luckett found that the extraembryonic mesoderm comes from the primitive streak. It develops on day 12 from the caudal pole of the embryonic shield and differentiates in human embryos on about day 14. He interpreted this to mean that the cells of the primitive streak move peripherally; there they form the cores of the primitive villi. Luckett did not totally exclude the idea that there may be some minor contribution derived from trophoblast, but in our view this is unlikely. For example, even well-differentiated choriocarcinomas never produce connective tissue, which would be expected at least occasionally; as such behavior is seen with virtually all other neoplasms. The meticulous study by Enders and King (1988) referred to below clearly shows now that the connective tissue of the placenta derives ultimately from the "epiblast."

Another reason for asserting that chorionic connective tissue has an embryonic origin comes from the embryologic studies on reconstituted mouse embryos (Rossant & Croy, 1985). Rossant and Croy took inner cell masses of mice with distinct isoenzymes and in situ genetic markers and placed them into different trophoblastic shells. They then followed the placental development and deduced that only 4% of the mouse placenta was derived from the embryo. This portion was composed primarily of fetal capillaries. Mouse placental tissue has generally little connective tissue.

The formation of the extraembryonic mesenchyme has been studied in exquisitely prepared electron micrographs from early rhesus monkey ova from days 19 to 60 (Enders & King, 1988). This is an important topic as inferences made from various divergent cytogenetic procedures (CVS, amnionic fluid study, fetal biopsy) have often yielded findings that are difficult to interpret unless this is understood. These authors found that the first evidence of mesenchyme was peripheral to the primitive endoderm, the "hypoblast." They showed convincing evidence that the rough endoplasmic reticulum of this mesenchyme has intracisternal densities that are not shared by other connective tissue. This feature allows one also to determine its origin. It could be followed into the early villous structures on day 13. Also arguing against a trophoblastic origin of villous mesenchyme is the finding that there is always a complete basal lamina underlying the trophoblast. The meticulous study of Enders and King showed that the earliest blood vessel formation comes from this villous mesenchyme, which differentiates focally into endothelium as early as on day 13 but more actively later.

The composition of the chorionic mesoderm is similar to that of the fibroblast layer of the amnion, consisting of a coarse network of collagen bundles intermingled with finer argyrophilic fibrils. The distribution of the various collagen types I, III, IV, V, and VI has been detailed by Malak et al. (1993). Hessle and Engvall (1984) and Hessle et al. (1984) focused on the distribution of collagen VI. Fibroblasts and macrophages are regular findings. According to Wang and Schneider (1982) and Bartels and Wang (1983), many of the fibroblasts are likely to represent myofibroblasts. They are connected to each other by gap junctions, which allow intercellular coupling. McParland et al. (2003) found thickening and expression of smooth muscle actin in the region overlying the internal os. Most of the studies that concern collagen composition and tensile properties of the membranes (Aplin et al., 1986; Teodoro et al., 1990; Manabe et al., 1991; Malak et al., 1993) consider both the mesenchyme of the amnion and that of the chorion. For details we refer the reader to these papers. It is very likely that both layers equally contribute to the mechanical stability of the membranes. Meirowitz et al. (2002) found an increase of collagen I/XIV mRNA ratios in premature rupture of membranes that was not associated with infection.

The structure of the chorion laeve has been extensively studied by Hoyes (1970, 1971). His earlier contribution, although specifically dealing with the mesenchyme of the amnion, has two important features. Hoyes stated that, before the attachment of amnion to chorion, the mesenchymal cells have a continuous configuration with highly developed endoplasmic reticulum. Later, these cells disintegrate into dispersed elements. Hoyes believed that the Hofbauer cells found during later development resulted from degenerating connective tissue elements, a notion that is no longer in agreement with the modern views regarding the derivation of the placental macrophages (see Chapter 6). It appears to us more likely that these cells take their origin from the fetal vascular compartment. Santiago-Schwarz and Fleit (1988) described a population of cells in cord blood that, upon culturing, developed into macrophages. In a later paper, Hoyes (1971) described the mesenchymal elements. He considered them to be similar to those of the amnion.

The connective tissue is followed by a basal lamina that is highly variable in terms of thickness and structure. It is composed of laminin and collagen IV and shows accumulations of fibronectin and collagen III in its immediate surrounding (Aplin & Campbell, 1985). Near the basal lamina, increased amounts of extracellular debris can be observed (Lister, 1968). Fetal vessels exist up to the 6th month; they are branches of the umbilical vessels, extending via the chorionic plate into the mesoderm of the former chorion frondosum. During the last trimester, these vessels are usually absent (Hoyes, 1971). Band-like groups of cells that are rich in lipid droplets and glycogen stores (found between the collagen bundles) have been discussed to be residues of the former capillary endothelium (Hoyes, 1971). This author traced the development of those capillaries that are present up to the 3rd month; they thrombose and gradually disappear. Lister (1968) claimed to have found some capillaries in abnormal placentas near term, but this observation was shared by neither Hoyes (1971) nor us.

From histochemical studies of fetal membranes, largely periodic acid-Schiff (PAS) and similar reactions, Sala and Matheus (1984) concluded that the membranes are not merely a container for the fetus, but that because of their polysaccharide content they participate in the exchange of water and electrolytes. They found that more neutral polysaccharides were present in the trophoblastic shell of term placental membranes and decidua than elsewhere; the acid mucopolysaccharides were most prominent in the connective tissue layers and decidua.

Trophoblast Layer

A highly variable layer of trophoblast cells persists until term. These cells are the only residues of the former villi of the chorion frondosum, intermingled with the trophoblastic residues of the primary chorionic plate and the trophoblastic shell.

The trophoblast is separated from the chorionic mesoderm by this basal lamina, on which it rests as a more or less uninterrupted, mostly even, multilayered stratum. Toward the uterine wall, the trophoblast interdigitates intensely with the decidua. Near the placental margin, the trophoblast splits into two layers, flanking an intermediate fibrinoid lamella of increasing thickness. Ghost villi may be encased in the fibrinoid, which consist of clearly identifiable villous stroma surrounded by fibrinoid with some scattered trophoblast cells (see Figs. 11.1 and 11.6). At the placental margin, transition of the ghost villi into intact villi, surrounded by maternal blood, may lead smoothly to the placenta (Bühler, 1964). In other cases, abrupt changes from placental margin into a uniform trophoblast layer of the chorion laeve are observed.

The trophoblast cells of the membranes, together with all the other cytotrophoblast residing outside the placental villi, are now subsumed under the term **extravillous cytotrophoblast**. This summarizing term is justified because all these cells show the same behavior despite their different locations (chorionic plate, basal plate, cell columns, cell islands, septa, membranes). The structure of the trophoblast cells of the membranes is variable (Bou-Resli et al., 1981), as it is in all other extravillous trophoblast populations. Several stages of differentiation can be found, including proliferating, undifferentiated rounded cells with large, oval nuclei and scarce organelles resting on the basal lamina that incorporate ^{3}H-thymidine (Kaltenbach & Sachs, 1979) and nonproliferating, differentiated, large polygonal cells with highly irregular, invaginated nuclei and condensed cytoplasm, with ample rough endoplasmic reticulum, lipid droplets, and glycogen. These cells have a highly active energy metabolism and express alkaline phosphatase (Petry, 1962). Some of the latter cells that are located nearer the decidua are obviously degenerative in nature. Foci of matrix-type fibrinoid can be observed between the cells. It is probably identical with the amorphous material described by Bou-Resli et al. (1981).

The trophoblast cells are separated from each other by a system of partly dilated intercellular clefts, bordered by a few microvilli and irregular cytoplasmic processes. The clefts are filled with a largely amorphous material

(Bou-Resli et al., 1981), with some loosely arranged collagen fibers, and with bundles of a fine fibrillar material. Immunohistochemically, this material contains laminin, collagen IV, and heparan sulfate proteoglycan, all three known to be usual basal lamina constituents; in addition, oncofetal fibronectin but no fibrin is present. Thus, the area corresponds to the matrix-type fibrinoid described by Frank et al. (1994) and Huppertz et al. (1996), which is a secretory product of trophoblast rather than a blood-clotting product as postulated for fibrin. These secretions are frequently found in small cysts that correspond to the cysts in the placenta, the so-called X-cell cysts (Fig. 11.13). The content is, in part, major basic protein. The presence of fibronectin in this trophoblastic layer has also been described by Yamaguchi et al. (1985) and that of collagen IV and laminin by Aplin and Campbell (1985), Malak et al. (1993), and Ockleford et al. (1993); the latter authors pointed to the similarity with basal lamina material.

The trophoblast cells are connected to each other by desmosomes (Bourne, 1962; Lister, 1968; Bou-Resli et al., 1981; Bartels & Wang, 1983; Wang & Schneider, 1987). In addition, occluding junctions and gap junctions have been described (Bartels & Wang, 1983). The function of the occluding junctions is still open to question. As concluded from their focal arrangement and from physiologic studies

(Battaglia et al., 1968; Lloyd et al., 1969; Chez et al., 1970; Seeds et al., 1977), the junctions cannot limit the permeability of the chorion laeve; physiologically, this layer must be regarded as a leaky membrane. The extracellular matrix may be involved in the permeability properties (Bartels & Wang, 1983), as discussed for the amnionic epithelium. This assumption, however, also cannot explain why the layer seems to be permeable for placental lactogen with a molecular weight of about 22,000 daltons (Chez et al., 1970), whereas it was found to be impermeable to the much smaller inulin molecule (5500 daltons) (Battaglia et al., 1962).

Another interesting view has been stressed by Bartels and Wang (1983). The existence of gap junctions between the trophoblast cells suggests that these cells are coupled metabolically. Gap junctions could not be detected between the individual cells of the villous cytotrophoblast or between villous cytotrophoblast and syncytiotrophoblast (Metz et al., 1979; Reale et al., 1980). Large amounts of renin have been detected immunohistochemically within the cytotrophoblast of the chorion laeve (Symonds et al., 1970; Poisner et al., 1981), and it has been demonstrated in other tissues that renin-producing cells are coupled by gap junctions (Boll et al., 1975; Forssmann & Taugner, 1977). The probable renin synthesis attributed to these cells is the only concrete functional finding, although there are some vague histochemical hints that the trophoblast of the smooth chorion is also involved in steroid biosynthesis (Benedetti et al., 1973) and that some cells at the trophoblastic decidual interface express hPL (Sakbun et al., 1990b). Another finding makes it likely that the trophoblast cells of this site are more than mere residual or even degenerating elements, as they bind epidermal growth factor to such an extent that they must be designated a real target tissue of this growth-stimulating and growth-regulating molecule (Rao et al., 1984).

Trophoblast cells of the membranes are an easily available source for the isolation of extravillous trophoblast cells for in vitro purposes because extravillous trophoblast cells are the only cells of epithelial origin within the membranes after stripping off the amnion (Lewis et al., 1996; Gaus et al., 1997).

Decidua

The decidual layer that is attached to the membranes after birth is largely derived from the parietal decidua (see Fig. 11.4), with some additional residual elements of the capsular decidua. Whether the individual cells are derived from one or the other layer cannot be distinguished. Because the capsular decidua usually undergoes degeneration early and becomes discontinuous (Fig. 11.4C; compare Fig. 11.3), it is likely that the remaining cells are mostly of parietal origin.

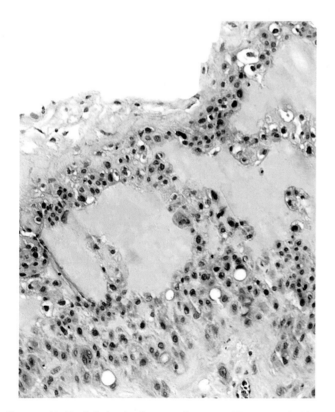

FIGURE 11.13. Subchorionic cysts in extravillous trophoblast. H&E ×250.

In most morphologic descriptions of the membranes, the decidua is only peripherally discussed or is not mentioned at all. Therefore, it is difficult to decide if it is structurally different from the basal decidua, which has been the subject of numerous studies. The only modern description of the parietal decidua is based on rhesus monkey membranes (King, 1981). As far as can be determined from the early descriptions by Petry (1962) and Bourne (1962), the results can be extrapolated to humans. The cells of this layer obviously do not comprise a uniform population. They all have elongated cell bodies surrounded by more or less prominent and partly condensed meshworks of fine fibrils. Most of the cells have well-developed granular endoplasmic reticulum, numerous mitochondria, and a prominent Golgi apparatus. The cell surfaces of many cells are characterized by stalk-like cytoplasmic processes that contain secretory granules, which are also well known in the decidua basalis (Wynn, 1974; Kisalus & Herr, 1988).

The cells are surrounded by a basal membrane–like material that contains various collagens (Wewer et al., 1985; Malak et al., 1993), heparan sulfate proteoglycan (Kisalus & Herr, 1988), and laminin. Charpin et al. (1985) studied laminin distribution. They considered laminin to be the protein that was demonstrated around decidual cells by Wynn (1974). Because laminin has never been found in nondecidualized endometrium, they suggested that it is deposited under hormonal control. The same is probably valid for the other basal lamina molecules. Because laminin has an adhesive quality, they proposed that it may be involved in the attachment and nesting of the blastocyst.

In their delineation of placental villi with immunofluorescent antibodies directed against complement C3 breakdown products (C3d), Leivo and Engvall (1986) observed a strong localization in the trophoblastic basement membrane and decidua but none in the basement membranes of villous capillaries. They considered it possible that the complement originates from maternal plasma, as none was found in fetal capillaries, and it was also not produced by trophoblast. Because C3d has been found in glomeruli, its immunologic relation to placenta, amply demonstrated in studies of the past, may have a new explanation. Laminin has a strong affinity for C3d, and it may be for this reason that it is bound at these sites. Some of the decidual cells have been shown to express relaxin, a hormone, however, that is secreted also by cyto- and syncytiotrophoblast of different origin (Sakbun et al., 1990a).

The deeper layers of the parietal decidua, which remain in utero, are richly supplied with maternal blood vessels (Arts, 1961). In the superficial parts of the decidua that are attached to the membranes after birth, maternal vessels are the exception. If there are any vessels here, only some capillaries, smaller arterioles, and venules can be identified.

Tensile Properties of the Membranes

Some investigators have wondered why the relatively thin amnion withstands pressures so readily, and many have conducted measurements of its tensile strength. Independently, Polishuk et al. (1962, 1964), Laufer et al. (1966), and MacLachlan (1965) developed an apparatus to measure the tensile strengths of amnion and whole membranes. The tensile strength of amnion is greater than that of chorion. According to Klima et al. (1989), it is the amount and arrangement of fibers of the compact layer of amnionic mesenchyme that are primarily responsible for the tensile properties. The tensile strength of the amnion was estimated to be even greater than would be needed for a successful gestation, and they found that the strength is greater still during early gestation than near term (see also Wyatt-Ashmead and Ashmead, 2004).

The average thickness of the membranes is 0.56mm, the amnion making up one third. The average tensile strength is 205g/cm (50–500g/cm) (Lavery et al., 1980). More recent studies have pointed out that the membranes have a great ability to withstand trauma. They can expand to twice normal size during pregnancy and labor; their physical properties are both viscous and elastic, and these properties are believed to explain the various unusual physical features (Lavery & Miller, 1977). Kanayama et al. (1985) were unable to demonstrate the presence of elastins in any membranes, a finding that was contradicted by the results of Malak and Bell (1994a) and Hieber et al. (1997).

Pathology of the Membranes

Preterm Rupture of the Membranes

Studies of details in membrane strength in prematurely ruptured sacs have supported earlier findings (Danforth et al., 1953). They pointed out that the membranes thin out appreciably at the site of rupture, but that their possibly reduced strength is not the explanation for rupture (Artal et al., 1976). Surprisingly, amnions from pregnancies with premature rupture of membranes had even higher tensile strengths than those with timely membrane rupture (Lavery et al., 1980).

It is not logical to deduce from a study of the membranes in general what the nature of the membranes may be at the site of rupture. It seems that it is not so much the general membrane strength that is important but rather that a local alteration occurs near the site of the membranes overlying the endocervix in the process that leads to their rupture. Malak and Bell (1994b, 1996) have reported local reduction of trophoblast, absence of decidua, and edematous swelling of connective tissue ("zone of altered morphology") as well as local activation of a variety of proteinases (see following). Moreover, Lei et al. (1996) have shown in the rat placenta that the amnionic epithelium undergoes apoptotic cell death followed by degradation of collagen I before the onset of labor. In contrast, older morphologic studies indicated that widespread apoptosis and degeneration do not occur in humans (Aplin et al., 1985). Nonetheless, the latter group did not exclude that weakening of the membranes may result from more localized changes in the tissue (Streuli & Aplin, 1996).

Amnionic epithelium and the few neighboring fibroblasts continue to synthesize and to depose basal lamina and interstitial collagens and other matrix molecules until term, depending on the presence of vitamin C (Aplin et al., 1986). When collagen content of amnionic membranes was quantified, it was found to decrease significantly during the last 8 weeks of pregnancy; it may be reduced in membranes from prematurely ruptured sacs (Skinner et al., 1981). According to Teodoro et al. (1990), the membranes of patients with premature rupture have 44% less collagen than is normal. In contrast, Evaldson et al. (1987) and Al-Zaid and colleagues (1980) found no decrease but rather a dissolution of fibers near the site of membrane rupture. This change was examined electron microscopically by Ibrahim et al. (1983). From samples taken at cesarean section at the cervical and opposite sides of membranes, they showed that disruption of the collagen fibrils occurs near the site of membrane rupture. In spite of these contradictions, the role of connective tissue fibers in the pathogenesis of premature rupture is illustrated by the Ehlers-Danlos syndrome. Infants affected with this inherited, generalized disorder of the connective tissue have a greatly increased incidence of preterm prelabor membrane rupture (Barabas, 1996).

It must be said that the crucial point is not the overall content of collagens, but rather the distribution of isoforms, their cross-linkage, and the availability and activity of the respective cleaving enzymes. Several publications underscore this view. Kanayama and colleagues (1985) analyzed the collagen isoforms of normal and prematurely ruptured membranes. They recognized types I, III, and V in these extracts and found altered ratios between the types in specimens from prematurely ruptured membrane cases. There was a particular reduction in collagen type III, and they deduced from their analysis that it related to an increase in trypsin content and a decrease in α_1-antitrypsin. The findings were generally supported by Keene et al. (1987), Malak et al. (1993), and Bryant-Greenwood (1998), who concluded that collagens I and II together with smaller amounts of collagens V, VI, and VII are involved in the tensile properties.

Not only is the presence of the various types of collagen fibers critical for the mechanical properties but so is their cross-linkage. Availability of copper ions is required to cross-link collagen fibers. King et al. (1997) have shown that amnionic expression of metallothioneins and amnionic fluid levels of this Cu^{2+}-binding peptide are increased in smokers. These data suggest a reduced availability of copper for cross-linking of collagens and may help explain the increased incidence of premature rupture of membranes in smokers. Shimizu et al. (1992) provided an additional, closely related explanation for the obvious correlation between smoking and preterm membrane rupture: fibronectins are also involved in the tensile properties of connective tissues by cross-connecting collagen filaments. These authors found inhibition of fibronectin expression in smokers.

Lower collagen/hexosamine ratios reduce tensile strength. Meudt (1966) found that meconium exposure had the same effect but offered no quantitative data. Lavery et al. (1980) provided such data and noted that although tensile strength is reduced, the presence of meconium does not correlate with premature rupture of membranes. In an attempt to explain why the membrane rupture occurs frequently away from the internal uterine os, Lavery et al. (1982) constructed a complex rheologic model. From it they suggested that local flaws develop under the stress of Braxton-Hicks contractions and with labor. Opitz and Bernoth (1962) examined the site of rupture with polarizing optics; they observed the development of parallel "rupture lines" of collagen. The ability of the amnion to slide over the chorion is probably partly responsible for the variations in membrane rupture. This is enhanced, as Schwarzacher (1960) pointed out, by residues of magma reticulare [see Intermediate (Spongy) Layer, above] between amnion and chorion that exist to term. This remnant of extraamnionic fluid is presumably also responsible for the sonographic "tenting" of some amnions seen after failed amniocentesis (Platt et al., 1982). It is also possibly the reason why, with repeated amniocentesis, the amnion often detaches from the chorion and thus allows the collection of amnionic fluid underneath. This mechanism probably led to the retained chorion of the patient reported by Stempel and Nelson (1982). The studies by Wynn et al. (1967) with pig amnion suggested that "healing" of earlier defects may result from the regenerative processes in the amnion. They may also explain cessation of fluid leakage in such pregnancies. These authors are the only ones who clearly stated their opinion that the amnion is nourished by amnionic fluid.

Studies of active and latent collagenases (matrix metalloproteinases) have shown that during labor the placenta, cervix, and maternal serum contain high levels of the active enzymes whereas the levels in the umbilical cord are markedly lower (Rajabi et al., 1990). By incubating membranes in "pseudoamnionic fluid" and studying the biomechanical properties with and without the addition of enzyme inhibitors, Artal et al. (1979) suggested that membrane rupture is perhaps regulated by enzymes.

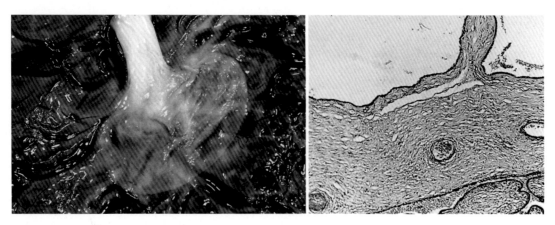

FIGURE 11.14. Amnionic cyst surrounding the umbilical cord. The cyst (left) contained 5 mL of clear fluid. There was no evidence of a vanished twin. H&E ×160.

According to Jenkins et al. (1983), amnionic fluid plasminogen must also be considered as an etiologic factor in preterm rupture. Its proteolytic activity is regulated by tPA and uPA and their respective inhibitors (PAI-1 and PAI-2) (see earlier discussion). Plasminogen as well as its activators and inhibitors were detected in amnionic fluid (Kjaeldgaard et al., 1989). Other studies showed that proteases, presumably released from bacteria, reduce the strength and elasticity of membranes (McGregor et al., 1987). This finding is relevant because of the well-known fact that premature rupture occurs with chorioamnionitis (Naeye, 1982) (see Chapter 20).

The studies and reviews by Vadillo-Ortega et al. (1995, 1996), Fortunato et al. (1997), and Bryant-Greenwood (1998) attributed a special role to the broad variety of matrix metalloproteinases (MMPs) and their inhibitors (tissue inhibitors of metalloproteinases, TIMPs) within the membranes. Furthermore, Bryant-Greenwood (1998) reported that activation of MMPs by relaxin decreased the tensile strength of the membranes. For the first time, these data point to the existence of a local autocrine-paracrine signaling system coordinating the local events during membrane rupture.

Cysts, Tumors, and Hemorrhage

Localized edema with resultant cyst formation is occasionally seen on the amnionic surface. It is not usually associated with clinical problems (Fig. 11.14). Occasionally, such cysts are amnionic epithelial inclusions. No real tumors have been described to develop in the amnion. To be sure, rare nests of cartilage, skin, or bone may be found underneath the amnionic epithelium (Fig. 11.15), but they are not generally neoplastic. Some of these structures may represent the remains of aborted ("vanished") twins. This possibility is unlikely because vanished twins (discussed in Chapter 25) have usually a different microscopic appearance. An unusual case of an epidermoid cyst

is seen in Figure 11.16. Other investigators have described teratomas in the membranes (e.g., Fox & Butler-Manuel, 1964; Joseph & Vogt, 1973; Nickell & Stocker, 1987). These "tumors" have usually had the appearance of acardiac twins, also discussed in greater detail in Chapter 25. Although these authors stated emphatically that no umbilical cord attached them to the membranes, a feature

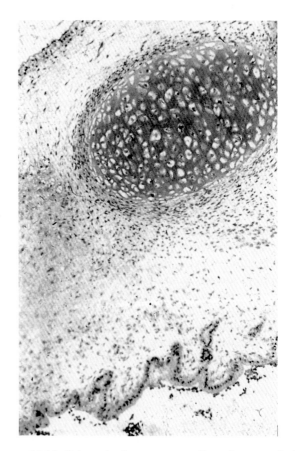

FIGURE 11.15. Subamnionic mature cartilage in normal placenta. H&E ×100.

FIGURE 11.16. Subamnionic squamous epithelium-lined cyst with keratinization in normal placenta. H&E ×160.

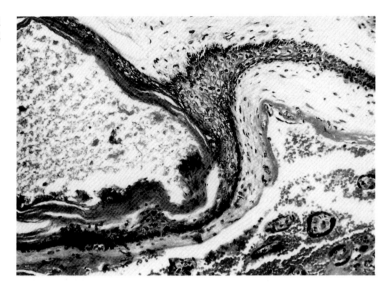

that is usually held to be a sine qua non for acardiac twins, the appearance of the lesions described is that of acardiacs. Smith and Pounder (1982) came to the same conclusion. They described a 3.0 × 2.0 × 1.5 cm mass at the edge of a placenta, covered with skin, and broadly attached to the chorion (not decidua, as they stated). It also contained glia, intestine, cartilage, and fat. They referred to other, similar cases that were originally described by Küster (1928) and suggested that the lesion was most similar to an amorphous acardiac twin, under which heading this topic is further developed (see Chapter 25). Despite the lack of organization of such "teratomas," a feature that is also found in some bona fide acardiacs, some recognizable structures are depicted in most of the foregoing descriptions. The difficult decision as to whether such a lesion represents a teratoma or an acardiac twin has been pursued since Küster (1928) described a walnut-sized lesion composed of external skin, bone, cartilage, connective tissue, nerves, fat, glands, and smooth muscle; she leaned toward a diagnosis of teratoma. Unger (1989) has reconsidered this problem, but there is no resolution. To invoke their origin from aberrant germ cells seems unwarranted without further supportive evidence. Other teratomas of the placenta fall into the same category. See further details in Acardiac Twins in Chapter 25 on multiple pregnancy.

Hemorrhage into areas underneath the amnion most commonly originates from chorionic vessels. It is seen in many placentas when they are examined by the pathologist because the attendants in the delivery room have collected blood for the determination of fetal pH and blood groups and to undertake other laboratory tests. Rarely is such subamnionic blood of prenatal origin, and the age-old question of whether the placental surface can be damaged by the fetus (scratching) has remained unresolved. Shanklin and Scott (1975) found subamnionic

hemorrhages in 1 of 400 placentas. They preferred to call them hematomas and indicated that inappropriate traction on the umbilical cord by the accoucheur to be the common cause of this hemorrhage. There are, however, ultrasonographic observations before birth that suggest the occurrence of subamnionic and, certainly more frequently, **subchorionic** hematomas, representing intervillous thromboses. It is normal to find small laminated fibrin deposits beneath the chorionic plate at term, presumably accumulating from eddying in the intervillous circulation. These deposits may acquire major proportions, however, and they then represent a pathologic feature. Sonographers have been much interested in this topic, as it is readily demonstrable with their equipment. It must be cautioned, however, that so-called subchorionic hematomas, seen sonographically as often as in 60% of pregnancies, may represent merely some blood eddying rather than representing the typical "thrombohematomas." The differentiation may not be easy and the consequences may differ materially. Nyberg et al. (1990) found that marginal abruptios "tend to dissect beneath the placental membranes," resulting in subchorionic hematomas. This site is by far the most common type of abruptio seen by sonography (91% before 20 weeks) and may mimic other placental sonographic masses, such as angiomas. In addition, these authors recognized what they termed "preplacental hematomas," deposits between placenta and amnionic fluid. They are considered to be subchorial or subamnionic in location; some authors believed that they may originate from ruptured vessels (DeSa, 1971) and large ones possibly correspond to the Breus' mole (Shanklin & Scott, 1975).

Anechoic placental "lakes" beneath the chorionic plate are common and probably of no significance, as most disappear with delivery. It was found that 80% of the subchorial hematomas that were recognized before 20 weeks result in normal term delivery and that their size is the most important prognostic determinant. Thus, Abu-Yousef (1987) found significantly large hematomas to have a grave prognosis, and also that they always extend to the placental margin. Pearlstone and Baxi (1993) reviewed 14 studies and found that these lesions are common (occurring as often as in 4% to 48% of pregnancies), that their etiology was still undetermined, and that a risk for premature delivery exists with large thrombi. One such large thrombus was shown in an early publication by Cooperberg et al. (1979). Oláh et al. (1987) delivered a normally grown fetus at 28 weeks with a huge subchorionic "thrombohematoma" that appeared sonographically as a placental tumor. The neonate succumbed at 5 days of age. The placenta weighed 700 g (!) and was circumvallate; the hematoma was 15 × 5 cm. Conversely, Pedersen and Mantoni (1990), while also finding subchorionic hematomas with great frequency among threatened abortions that had vaginal bleeding (18%), stated that their presence did not enhance the frequency of abortion. Large preplacental hematomas (Pedersen and Mantoni observed hematomas of 2 to 150 mL) may produce clinical symptomatology similar to abruptios, and fetal demise can occur when the hematoma is large enough. Some authors believe they can compress the umbilical cord. The various controversies about this entity were discussed by Spirt et al. (1993). Dickey et al. (1992) also found these hematomas commonly by sonography and related adverse outcomes only to cases with vaginal bleeding. Fleischer et al. (1988) found a correlation with elevated α-fetoprotein levels, as did Bernstein et al. (1992). Because of the presence of antinuclear antibodies in three of five patients with subchorionic hematomas, Baxi and Pearlstone (1991) recommended that these patients be screened for such antibodies, irrespective of the obstetric history. We have seen a number of such hematomas among midtrimester losses. They differ from Breus' moles in that they are not focal and the chorionic plate is uniformly elevated rather than, as in Breus' moles, in pockets. When fetuses survive, they often become growth retarded. Al-Nuaim et al. (1996) found an 8.5% incidence of sonographically diagnosed subchorionic hematomas in patients with bleeding in early pregnancy, with a 20.7% abortion rate, a frequency similar to that of other studies.

True amnionic cysts are rarely present on the placental surface. The most common cysts found here are located underneath the chorion; they take their origin from extravillous trophoblast cell deposits in which central liquefaction has occurred. Bleeding into such cysts may occur, and the cysts may also be large and multiple. The associated fetus or newborn may be normal or small for gestational age; growth restriction occurs occasionally because extravillous trophoblast cells are especially prevalent in placentas with severe, extensive ischemic degeneration. These features are discussed further in Chapter 9.

Many term placentas exhibit the remnants of yolk sac as small yellow-white, calcific plaques beneath the amnion (Fig. 11.17) and there may even be on very rare occasions the remains of an omphalo-mesenteric duct present (Fig. 11.18).

Amnionic Fluid Embolism

Vernix Dissection

Vernix caseosa often dissects underneath the amnion. Indeed, the occasional rupture of only the amnionic sac

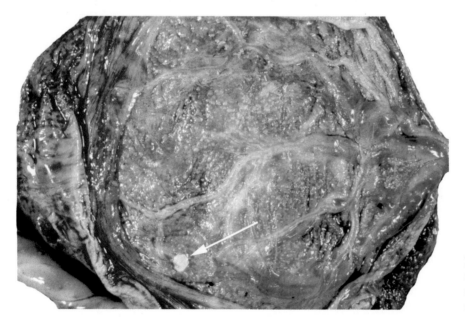

FIGURE 11.17. Placental surface with remnant of yolk sac beneath amnion at arrow. There is also extensive amnion nodosum.

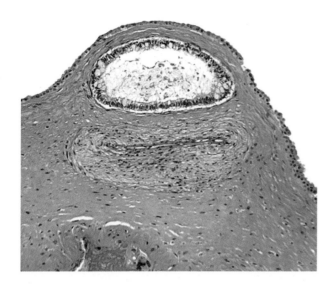

FIGURE 11.18. Subamnionic remnant of omphalo-mesenteric (vitelline) duct. H&E ×160.

can lead to the formation of "double sacs," a condition seen also in patients with "high leaks." Such accumulations of vernix also occur occasionally in large patches of greasy material that may be mistaken for a vanished twin (Fig. 11.19). Jacques and Qureshi (1994) summarized 18 cases of subamnionic vernix collection and emphasized that no cellular reaction to this material had taken place. There were also no clinical events that suggested a mechanism leading to this benign subamnionic vernix accumulation. Spontaneous amnionic membrane rupture seems

to have occurred as the initiating mechanism, as was observed by Yang (1990) in his study of amnionic bands. In placental bed biopsies, vernix has also been observed; indeed, vernix can then lead to an inflammatory reaction, as shown by Craven and Ward (1997). They found vernix with neutrophilic reaction in the myometrium and decidual bed at incidental placental bed biopsy. It was also found in uterine veins, associated with thrombi in this postpartum patient. Patients who have had clinical fluid discharge and in whom later intact membranes were observed have similar membrane ruptures. Reisfield (1958) considered it to result from a congenital defect, but this conclusion is probably not valid. This rupture may occur before delivery, presumably when the amnion breaks before the chorion does. Amnionic fluid with cellular debris (squames, fat, hair) can then be pushed underneath the amnion (Fig. 11.20), at times in impressive amounts. This material appears as white flakes that can be moved back and forth under the amnion. In general, this finding has no significance whatsoever; earlier students of the matter, however (Leary & Hertig, 1950), considered that such subamnionic vernix may gain access to the maternal vascular space and thus initiate the clinical spectrum of amnionic fluid embolism. Indeed, some of their pictures showed squamous cells in the intervillous space and within the decidual sinusoids. Whether the vernix got there by dissection from the subamnionic space is a matter of conjecture. This separation between amnion and chorion can also occur spontaneously before birth, and amnionic fluid may then enter this space, a feature that is sometimes recognized sonographically

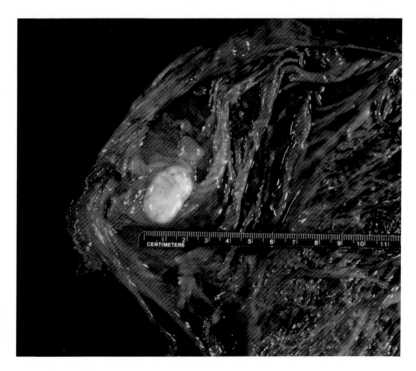

FIGURE 11.19. Large, white accumulation of pasty vernix caseosa beneath (dissected) amnion. It is much larger than a yolk sac remnant and must not be mistaken for a fetus papyraceus.

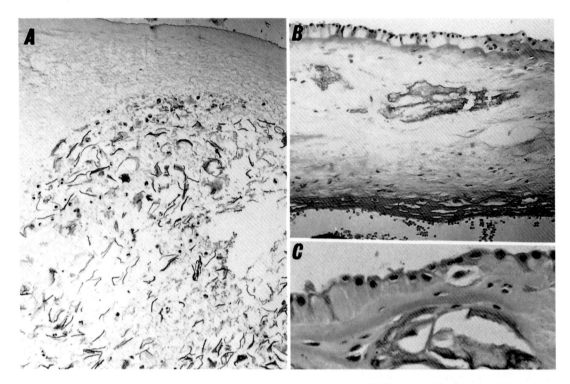

FIGURE 11.20. Dissection of vernix underneath the amnion. H&E. A ×64; B ×125; C ×400.

(Borlum, 1989). Borlum emphasized that such "chorio-amniotic separation" is not a contraindication to amniocentesis.

Amnionic fluid embolism has been recognized as an important cause of maternal deaths. It occurs most commonly after tumultuous labor, occasionally during cesarean section, and rarely after amnioinfusion for the treatment of thick meconium (Maher et al., 1994). Steiner and Lushbaugh (1941) first reported this entity. It occurred in 70% of cases during labor, in 11% after vaginal delivery, and during cesarean section in 19% (Clark et al., 1995). Clinical features include severe dyspnea, shock,

and afibrinogenemia. Amnionic fluid embolism may lead to death; indeed, Clark et al. (1995) found it to have a 61% mortality. At autopsy one finds fragments of vernix caseosa, fat, squames, and fetal hair, as well as thrombotic material in the pulmonary capillaries (Fig. 11.21). The problem is well illustrated in an authoritative study by Landing (1950b). Although the diagnosis of amnionic fluid embolism is often suspected, it is only occasionally diagnosed with accuracy during life (Resnik et al., 1976; Haddad, 1985). The pathologic interpretation of vernix in pulmonary capillaries is frequently difficult, particularly when it is attempted from blood smears of living patients.

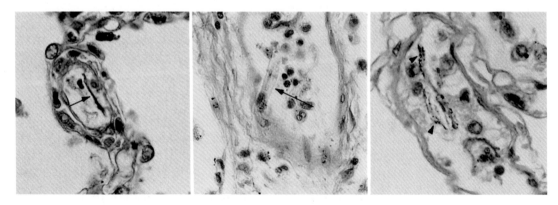

FIGURE 11.21. Pulmonary blood vessels containing various elements of vernix in a fatal amnionic fluid embolism. On the left is a squame (arrow), in the middle a hair (arrow), and on the right squames with meconium pigment (arrow heads). H&E ×240.

It must be realized that the embolization is probably a relatively brief event, wherein circulating vernix is quickly filtered out in the periphery and lung. Contamination of specimens by dandruff (during handling or staining) simulates the microscopic appearance closely. Squames are often contained in the histologic staining solutions and so simulate the true vernix that one must make a positive interpretation with great circumspection. The finding of vernix in blood smears, however, is absolutely diagnostic. It seems unlikely that vernix enters maternal vessels by dissection of the amnion. It probably enters large veins that are opened during cesarean section or tumultuous labor, and in patients with placenta previa accreta. Similarly opened uterine vessels were considered by Landing (1950b) to be sites of entry. Bendon and Ray (1986) reported five cases of prolonged amnionic fluid leakage; they believed that the squames they found in and underneath the chorion represented vernix. In one, it had elicited a foreign-body giant cell reaction. Although it was certainly not the cause of the chorioamnionitis in that case, their Figure 2 clearly showed that the squames had access to the maternal intervillous space.

Amnionic fluid embolism is fatal in more than 60% of cases. The clinical diagnosis is thus of considerable importance (Tuller, 1957; Philippe et al., 1961; Guidotti et al., 1981). Cases have been reported after repeated amniocentesis (Paterson et al., 1977) and even in undelivered patients with cord entanglement that had led to abruption of the placental margin (Corridan et al., 1980). Amnionic fluid embolism causes not only pulmonary hypertension when the lung capillaries are plugged but also shock, hypotension, and uncontrolled bleeding. The "consumption coagulopathy" that follows the disseminated intravascular coagulation event has been thought to result from the thromboplastin-containing liquor. Many coagulation studies on amnionic fluid have been published (Beller et al., 1963). The principal coagulative protein in amnionic fluid appears to be tissue factor (Lockwood et al., 1991). It must be cautioned again, however, that the accurate diagnosis of embolism may be difficult during life; afibrinogenemia more often results from abruption, the dead fetus syndrome, and other complications of pregnancy than from embolism with liquor. Moreover, it must be appreciated that several studies have supported earlier notions of the possible involvement of arachidonic acid and leukotrienes in the catastrophic process that follows amnionic fluid embolism (Clark, 1985, 1988; Azegami & Mori, 1986). Although a central focus of past considerations has been the presumed pulmonary hypertension in this condition, Clark et al. (1988) have shown convincingly that left-sided heart failure is the principal cause of death in this devastating disorder. Clark et al. (1995) later reviewed data from a National Registry with 46 cases and found that the disease simulates the clinical picture of septic shock. Many

patients in their review had histories of allergic reactions and atopy. For all these reasons, they suggested that anaphylactic shock may be an important underlying mechanism. Importantly, during the lengthy discussion of this presentation, Clark et al. indicated that, as the clinical picture is not of the nature of an embolic event, the identification of fetal squames may not be a reliable indicator of the amnionic fluid embolism. Benson and Lindberg (1996) reviewed suggestions that amnionic fluid embolism initiates anaphylaxis in the patient. Because tryptase is a reliable indicator of mast cell degranulation, they suggested that it be measured in future embolic events to obtain more insight into the disease.

Even greater care must be exercised in the diagnosis of amnionic fluid embolism during early pregnancy. The overwhelming evidence suggests that the fluid before 20 weeks is unable to cause coagulation. Vernix is not found in any quantity before the third trimester, certainly not at times of genetic amniocentesis. Also, Clark et al. (1986) made the point that blood obtained from pulmonary arteries of pregnant and nonpregnant patients often contain squamous cells. They assumed that this cellular material originates from venous puncture, rather than from amnionic fluid. Although this statement may be true, it is our opinion that these cells usually derive from contamination with debris contained in fixing or staining solutions and, most commonly, from dandruff of technicians.

Meconium

Meconium is the bile-stained intestinal content of the fetus. It is often admixed with mucus. Meconium is present in the small bowel of fetuses long before mid-gestation but is usually not eliminated until after birth. Its chemical composition has been partially determined by the early studies of Rapoport and Buchanan (1950). These investigators found it to contain mucopolysaccharides, blood group antigens and some small amount of protein. In infants with cystic fibrosis, there is more protein (nitrogen) than in normal infants, presumably because of the absence of trypsin digestion. When meconium is discharged before parturition, the baby and placenta may be meconium stained and deeply green. It is a common event. In consecutive placental examinations, we have found in San Diego that macroscopic meconium staining occurred in 17.81% of 12,951 placentas, whereas Nathan et al. (1994) found it in 19%. In addition, in our material there were 130 hemosiderin-stained placentas (1%); thus there was a total of 5% hemosiderin staining of the stained placentas overall. Fujikura and Klionsky (1975) reviewed the 42,000 placenta examinations of liveborn infants that were enrolled in the oft-cited large, prospective Collaborative Perinatal Study that was conducted in the 1960s. These authors identified staining in 10.3%, and

18.1% of neonatal deaths had meconium-stained placentas. Their case material, however, contained many instances of erythroblastosis, a condition that is now rarely encountered. Therefore, many of the placentas may well have been stained with hemolyzed blood pigments rather than with meconium. Kallakury et al. (1993) found that 19 of 23 discolored placentas (of 100 consecutive organs examined) contained meconium and even more contained iron pigment. They concluded that no relation to fetal well-being could be identified. This result is contrary to the opinions published by Spinillo et al. (1997), who correlated "meconium-stained amniotic fluid" with cerebral palsy in infants born from 24 to 33 weeks. Regrettably, it is impossible to ascertain whether truly meconium rather than hematoidin or hemosiderin discolored the fluid. As we will see, this is an important and occasionally difficult differential diagnosis.

The reason for the discharge of meconium is complex and has been reviewed in some detail in the past (Benirschke, 2001). One early review of this intestinal content of the fetus comes from Antonowicz and Schwachman (1979) when intestinal functions in patients with cystic fibrosis were dominant. When intestinal function was studied sonographically in fetuses between 15 and 41 weeks of gestation, Cajal and Martinez (2003) concluded that all passed material through a dilating anus at one time or another and considered discharge to be physiologic. When it occurs, it usually takes place during the last month of pregnancy and with an even greater frequency in postterm pregnancies. It may be of some importance to differentiate various types of meconium staining of the fetal surface of the placenta. Such differentiation is represented in a simplified fashion as follows:

Gross features	Clinical outcome
Acute meconium staining: blue-green, glistening placenta, covered with green, slimy meconium	Typically normal
Subacute meconium staining: slippery, edematous membranes with dark discoloration	High risk of association with asphyxia and cerebral palsy; meconium aspiration syndrome
Chronic meconium staining: dull and diffuse, muddy, cord sometimes stained throughout	Some of the infants with brown-green discoloration later manifest placental and membranes damage, assumed to be secondary to prenatal hypoxia sometimes later manifest

In a study conducted by Usher et al. (1988) of 5915 pregnancies 1 week before term, 1408 pregnancies lasting 1 to 2 weeks past term, and 340 pregnancies lasting more than 42 weeks, meconium staining was observed in 15.3%, 27%, and 31.5%, respectively. Although meconium discharge was also positively correlated with fetal distress, meconium staining occurred without fetal distress in 10.9%, 18.8%, and 16.2% in the respective groups. Similarly, Rogers et al. (1990) found no good correlation between meconium discharge and neonatal blood pH determinations. Trimmer and Gilstrap (1991) unsuccessfully attempted to correlate the thickness (the "meconiumcrit" of Weitzner et al., 1990) of meconium-stained fluid with outcome. Despite these findings, meconium has assumed great importance in medicolegal pursuits (see Chapter 26 and below).

Meconium is moved in the intestinal lumen by contractions of the intestine's muscular wall. This movement is regulated by a variety of hormones. Because of the difficulty of passage in Hirschsprung's disease, various neurogenic factors have been implicated. These are reviewed by Acosta et al. (2005), who studied the cholinergic influences and electromechanical aspects in sheep. Others have suggested that muscarinic acid receptors may be playing a role in fetal intestinal transport. Yet another motility factor is motilin, a 22-amino-acid polypeptide. Motilin is released during the fasting period and induces movement of the "activity front" of the small intestine. In a variety of experimental animals and in human volunteers, the infusion of this polypeptide caused intestinal motor activity that can be interrupted by high doses of gastrin and insulin (Vantrappen et al., 1979). When motilin was measured in the umbilical cord blood of neonates, it was found that those with fetal distress had levels elevated above the normal 32 to 127 pmol/L (Lucas et al., 1979a). Lucas et al. suggested that meconium discharge was the result of elevated motilin levels, which in turn were induced by fetal distress. In subsequent studies (Lucas et al., 1979b), it was found that six of eight gastrointestinal hormones were also elevated in cases complicated by fetal distress. This finding suggested to these investigators that these hormones may be powerful mediators in the many complications that follow fetal distress.

Immature fetuses had significantly lower levels of motilin than did mature infants. This conclusion, however, has been challenged by the report on motilin levels by Kowalewska-Kantecka (1995). She found only small and statistically nonsignificant lower values in premature infants. Our own studies of motilin levels in mature infants with and without meconium discharge are also somewhat different (Mahmoud et al., 1988). In part, the different findings may have occurred because we used different antibodies. We found that motilin levels of infants who had passed meconium were 177 pmol/L of cord blood, whereas those who did not pass meconium had only 111 pmol/L. No relation to fetal distress was found in this study. Because of the underdeveloped production of motilin in immature fetuses, it may be easily understood that meconium discharge is rare in premature infants, whereas it is common in postmature infants. Whether fetal distress is a primary signal for an increase in motilin and for meconium discharge is still uncertain. It is certainly true that many term stillbirths never have discharged meconium despite prolonged periods of distress that eventually lead to their demise.

Putative meconium presence in greenish amnionic fluid of very premature infants often results from hematoidin and other blood-derived pigments that have the same spectral absorbance when amnionic fluid is studied. It must be said that it then may be very difficult to properly define meconium staining of amnionic fluid. For instance, Falciglia et al. (1993) described a 610-g infant with intrauterine meconium aspiration syndrome and pigmented material in the lung at autopsy. It is not clear to us that this green-stained fluid and the yellow pigment of the lung truly represented discharged meconium, as other pigments have similar spectral characteristics. In fact, we have never seen meconium discharge at that young gestational age. However, Kearney (1999), Scott et al. (2001), and others have reported meconium discharge to occur in immature gestations. In fact, the worst effect on the umbilical cord I have ever seen occurred in a 34-week premature infant and is shown in Figure 11.22. There were numerous meconium macrophages in cord and membranes, and part of the Wharton's jelly had disintegrated to allow the fetal vessels to lie free. Remarkably, the neonate did well. We may need to have a better definition for the material in the amnionic fluid and lungs. For each of the cases of midtrimester amniocenteses with meconium-stained liquor, Karp and Schiller (1977) suggested that a reason for fetal distress could be envisaged. Three times it had been caused by significant prenatal bleeding, once there was marked hypertensive disease in the mother, and twice unsuccessful amniocenteses had preceded it. These investigators did spectrophotometric studies and found absorbance peaks at 405 nm, which is usually considered to be diagnostic of meconium but can be mimicked by other bile pigments. Their fetuses did well, and the pigment may have been hematoidin.

Golbus and Stephens (1979) did similar spectrophotometric studies on fluid obtained from genetic amniocentesis. Discolored fluid had a large 405- to 415-nm peak, shared with meconium and oxyhemoglobin, as well as peaks at 540 and 575 nm. The latter peaks were the result of blood pigments, believed to derive from disintegrating old blood. Allen (1985) found a 1.67% incidence of "meconium"-stained fluid among 4709 midtrimester amniocenteses, with a 5.06% fetal mortality. He excluded fetuses with brownish amnionic fluid from the analysis. In the discussion that followed his paper, various data were summarized and a consideration of the difficulty with the use of spectrophotometry as a sole determinant of meconium was given. In studies of brown and green fluids from amniocenteses, Hankins et al. (1984) found that brown and green fluids had similar absorption spectra; the authors concluded that the staining at mid-gestation is more likely secondary to hemolysis than to meconium discharge. We concur with that assessment. We have seen only one case of meconium discharge before 30 weeks (courtesy of Dr. C. Kaplan); this occurred in a 29-week gestation stillbirth in a mother with uncontrollable hyperthyroidism, allergy to propylthiouracil, and thyroidectomy during the second trimester. The fetus had 242 nucleated red blood cells (NRBCs)/100 white blood cells (WBCs) and the membranes had a massive meconium macrophage population; iron stains were negative. Moreover, the umbilical arterial walls were focally necrotic and had mural thrombosis. One may assume that the maternal hyperthyroidism stimulated fetal motilin production, but that remains speculative, although meconium discharge is more frequent in maternal hyperthyroidism. Legge (1981) detected the presence of hemoglobin in brownish fluids by chemical means. Alger et al. (1984)

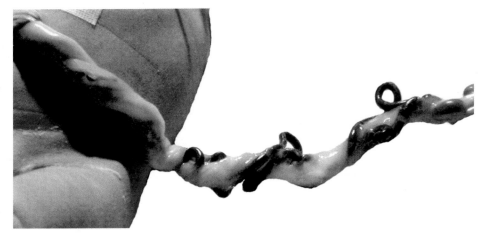

FIGURE 11.22. Umbilical cord of a 34-week fetus. The 24-year-old mother had been "hyperthyroid" and was treated with radioactive iodine and was on Synthroid medication. The neonate did well. The dissolution of Wharton's jelly and isolation of fetal vessels is remarkable. (Courtesy of Dr. S.L. Pedron, Tucson, Arizona.)

made a determined effort to differentiate among the pigments of second-trimester "meconium-like" substances. They studied 123 fluids, irrespective of their gross discoloration, finding that 91% of the clear fluids had an absorption peak at 405 nm, which is that of a pigment generally absent at term. The presence of this peak was not correlated with fetal outcome but it had a higher frequency in the presence of circumvallate placentas and in those with abruptio placentae. The substance was identified as methemoglobin. The authors emphatically denied the ability of a fetus to be able to discharge meconium before 20 weeks; they reviewed what is known of early fetal intestinal motility and anal innervation. Abramovich and Gray (1982), on the other hand, went so far as to suggest that the fetus routinely defecates until 16 weeks but ceases to do so by 18 to 20 weeks.

Boué et al. (1988) found the appearance of intestinal "microvillar enzymes" in amnionic fluid as early as at 12 to 13 weeks' gestation and suggested that this occurred as the anal membrane ruptured. When fetal anal sphincter control is established (18 weeks), however, the enzyme disappears quickly. Whether this evidence should be considered as "defecation" is moot. Ostrea and Naqvi (1982) found that the passage of meconium was strongly dependent on gestational age. Eighty percent of their premature neonates with meconium staining were older than 34 weeks' gestation, even when they had presented as breeches. Their overall incidence was only 6.5%. Recall that although the tensile strength of meconium-stained membranes is reduced, the frequency of premature rupture of membranes is not increased with meconium staining (Lavery et al., 1980). Franqoual et al. (1986) identified coproporphyrin and hemoglobin chemically in stained fluids. Zorn et al. (1986) also studied midtrimester staining to rule out the presence of true meconium. Bilirubin staining of amnionic fluid has been associated with intestinal obstruction and hydramnios (Grimes & Cassady, 1970); these authors suggested that the pigment may derive from disturbed placental exchange. Could it not equally well derive from prenatal vomiting of bile-stained gastrointestinal content? This situation certainly occurred in two of our cases with duodenal or jejunal obstruction, which was complicated by hydramnios. The fetal surfaces of the placentas were diffusely yellow, rather than green as in meconium discharge. Griffiths and Burge (1988) found three similar cases with intestinal obstruction and bile vomiting in utero. Yellow fetal surfaces, especially in the loose connective tissue next to the fetal vessels, are often caused by hematoidin (bilirubin) from hemolysis, as in rhesus incompatibility. We have also seen it complicating Bart's hemoglobinopathy (α-thalassemia) and associated with an abnormal hemoglobin.

The conclusion that can be reached from all these investigations is that meconium discharge of immature pregnancies is rare and that it is unreliably assessed by current technology. The reason is that hemoglobin is the common precursor of all these pigments. It may be more useful to determine if hemosiderin is present as iron-containing crystals in histologic preparations of the discolored placental surface. This test would be a more reliable indicator of decomposed blood. The formation of pigments in vivo has been a long-standing investigative challenge for pathologists. In particular, it has been questioned whether extracellular formation of hemosiderin and hematoidin is possible. This topic was fully reviewed by Muir and Niven (1935), who experimented with the injection of red blood cells and hemolyzed blood into rodents and rabbits. Generally speaking, hemosiderin was formed within cells only after about 24 hours; hematoidin, in crystal form, followed in about 7 days. Muir and Niven did not find it in extracellular sites. They assumed that it derives intracellularly from hemosiderin after removal of the iron. This moiety is the same as the bilirubin of meconium. We believe that hematoidin and bilirubin cannot be reliably distinguished from each other at present by either light microscopy or spectrophotometry.

For some reason, meconium has become the "red flag" for obstetricians and for the law profession as well (Sepkowitz, 1987). Meconium, so it is often portrayed, is the result of preceding fetal distress and hypoxia (Mitchell et al., 1985; Zorn et al., 1986). Numerous studies, on the other hand, indicate that correlations between meconium discharge and fetal pH or with tocograms are poor (Steer et al., 1989; Richey et al., 1995), although elevated erythropoietin levels are recorded (Manchanda et al., 1999; Jazayeri et al., 2000). The finding of meconium during labor is in fact a complex topic. The amount of gastrointestinal hormone accumulating in the fetus may reach an optimal quantity at the normal 40 weeks' gestation; when gestation continues beyond that time, meconium discharge becomes increasingly likely. Meconium is thus perhaps correlated with postmaturity (or "postdatism") more closely than with distress (Ostrea & Naqvi, 1982). This is not to say that postmature babies infrequently suffer some distress. Their discharge of meconium, however, may merely reflect the maturation of the system (see also Usher et al., 1988). As mentioned earlier, many term stillbirths never have discharged meconium, despite prolonged periods of distress that eventually lead to their demise. Yeomans and colleagues (1989) correlated meconium in amnionic fluid with fetal acid-base status. They concluded that "meconium-stained amnionic fluid correlates poorly with infant condition at birth as reflected by umbilical cord acid-base measurements." Their report also provided a valuable review of the views, pro and con, that meconium relates to fetal hypoxia. It must be appreciated that the mere presence of meconium at the time of birth may be irrelevant, while the prolonged presence in utero with staining of membranes and cord may signal significant problems to have existed. The important question is, How are we to separate what is meaningful meconium staining from its accidental presence? Some answers have been provided by Phelan et al. (1994, 1999), Redline and O'Riordan (2000), Kaspar et al. (2000), and Spinillo et al. (1998) that suggested a relationship to neonatal impairment and the presence of meconium at birth. Further, the experimental studies performed by Blackwell et al. (2004) found minor CNS learning deficiencies in rats that had been exposed in uteri to meconium late in gestation. None of these studies, however, is designed to show that fetal hypoxia is the cause of meconium discharge; it could as well be its consequence.

Meconium has deleterious sequelae when it is aspirated by the fetus (Byrne & Gau, 1987) and on the amnion and umbilical cord as well. A deleterious effect on the conversion of surfactants has been demonstrated by Kakinuma et al. (2002). Nathan et al. (1994) reviewed the impact of meconium-stained fluid in a very large sample and concluded that the impact on fetal morbidity and mortality is small and primarily related to the meconium aspiration syndrome. An increased viscosity of the meconium-stained amnionic fluid also was not apparently related to a worse outcome. At times, the meconium is quickly expectorated when aspirated and has then no untoward consequence, whereas at other times it leads to fatal pulmonary complications despite proper airway management (Davis et al., 1985). Thureen et al. (1997) found that much of the pulmonary damage had usually a prenatal onset and that significant placental abnormalities were frequent. Dooley et al. (1985) studied outcome in infants who had meconium present below the vocal cords and related its discharge to intrapartum events; they found that no change in therapeutic maneuvers would have saved the infants (see, however, Falciglia, 1988). The quality of meconium differs from case to case. In some infants, mucinous material may be present that the newborn's respiratory tract finds more difficult to eliminate. Likewise, it must be appreciated that not all babies born from a meconium-containing amnionic environment suffer meconium aspiration. They may have ceased to breathe in utero as a result of chronic distress (Kaplan, 1983). Thus, the problem is complicated and must be evaluated on individual merits. One must also consider the possibility that aspirated meconium causes degenerative changes in the alveolar epithelium similar to those seen in the amnionic epithelium. Thus, the meconium aspiration syndrome may represent a form of chemical pneumonitis with acute respiratory distress syndrome. Others (Katz & Bowes, 1992) have suggested that the deleterious pulmonary effect of meconium aspiration may be initiated by asphyxia. Kearney (1999) impressively demonstrated the production of subpleural plaques and infarcts with inspissated meconium, and later (2000) found eight "unequivocal intrauterine meconium aspirations" in midtrimester fetuses. How controversial the

topic is may be learned from the study of Ghidini and Spong (2001), who concluded that most so-called meconium aspiration syndromes are the result of prenatal asphyxial and infectious problems. Many experimental studies have been conducted with meconium inhalation before and after birth; some have yielded conflicting results. Goodlin (1968), for instance, found that there was little difference between saline and meconium in his rabbit experiments. Wiswell et al. (1992) observed the changes in piglets, and Goetzman (1992) summarized all aspects of the meconium aspiration syndrome. Yoder (1994) reviewed treatment regimes and reemphasized that not all meconium is equal. Of what element exactly the noxious quality of meconium consists, however, is unknown. It is possible that bile acids constitute the toxic material, as reported in maternal sclerosing cholangitis (Nolan et al., 1994) and in the cholestasis of pregnancy (Sepulveda et al., 1991). It should be noted, however, that experimental infusion of cholic acid during gestation into fetal lambs did not appear to be toxic (Campos et al., 1986). Alternatively, perhaps it is trypsin that causes the toxicity. Thus, Maradny (1994) showed that fetal urine and amnionic fluid contain urinary trypsin inhibitor-related (UTI-R) substance, that it can be demonstrated immunochemically in amnion epithelium, and speculated that it may have a stabilizing effect on intracellular calcium. Resolution of this question is desirable as it may lead to effective therapeutic measures for the meconium aspiration syndrome. The investigations by Uotila and Kääpä (1998) showed that meconium dose-dependently stimulates the expression of cyclooxygenase-2 in monocytes. These authors suggested that, if a similar stimulation of alveolar macrophages occurs in response to meconium exposure, perhaps their production of prostaglandins participates in the creation of the meconium aspiration syndrome.

Meconium is noxious in other ways (Rubovits et al., 1938). When meconium has been present in the amnionic cavity for many hours, the amnionic epithelium begins to show degenerative changes. Vacuolation, heaping up, loss of cells, and eventually necrosis are seen (Fig. 11.23). Moreover, muscle cells of the umbilical vessels of the umbilical cord, and their ramifications on the placental surface may degenerate when meconium presence has been long-standing (Figs. 11.22 and 11.24). This change was first described by Altshuler and Hyde (1989), who also provided evidence that damage to the fetal vascular tissue may exacerbate fetal cerebral hypoperfusion and thereby augment possibly existing fetal hypoxia. When they experimentally exposed segments of umbilical veins obtained from cesarean sections to meconium solutions, the muscular wall contracted markedly and rapidly. In addition, necrosis of vascular walls was believed to be a consequence of meconium exposure. Exactly how long this exposure must have existed before visual vascular

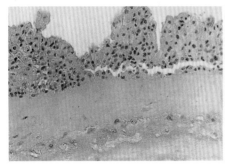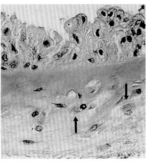

FIGURE 11.23. Heaping and degeneration of amnionic epithelium with meconium macrophage (arrows) after 20 hours of exposure (right) to meconium. H&E. Left ×160; right ×400.

alterations occur is not known, but we estimate that it is many hours. In subsequent studies, Altshuler et al. (1992) examined 1100 meconium-stained placentas among which they found 10 with vascular necrosis; two placentas had ulcerated cords. It is also common that the fetal surface blood vessels suffer damage and may contain mural thrombi. Holcberg et al. (1999) confirmed the vasoconstrictive result by injecting variable concentrations into isolated placenta cotyledons and found a concentration-dependent effect. Moreover, when they dialyzed the meconium-containing amnionic fluid, the constrictive effect vanished. Sienko and Altshuler (1999) found interleukin-1β in the meconium-containing macrophages, and specifically ruled out inflammatory reactions of the placentas studied. Hsieh et al. (1998) found no relation of meconium discharge and interleukin levels but detected interleukin-1β in meconium. The degenerative effect of meconium on cord smooth muscle was studied in vitro by Lembel et al. (2000) and essentially confirmed. This topic is further discussed in Chapter 12.

It is incorrect to assert, however, that meconium causes chorioamnionitis (Dominguez et al., 1960; see also Lauweryns et al., 1973) although, when it is present simultaneously, the neonatal outcome is poorer (Rao et al., 2001). To be sure, when degenerative changes in the surface do occur, they are sometimes followed by inflammation, but the amnionic sac infection syndrome is not caused

by meconium. We believe this to be true despite the observations by Beaufort et al. (1998) that meconium contains interleukin-8 and also demonstrated some leukotactic activity. Bacterial cultures from meconium-stained fluid, however, are more frequently positive than those from controls (Romero et al., 1991; Mazor et al., 1995). Meconium additionally inhibits neutrophil performance (Clark & Duff, 1995), thus further decreasing fetal defense. In the retrospective study undertaken by Burgess and Hutchins (1994), the authors thought not only that meconium induces the typical arterial necrosis of the cord but also that inflammation may result in membranes and fetal lung from meconium. Their inflammation of the membranes was less severe than that usually seen in chorioamnionitis. We often see deeply meconium-stained placentas, obviously having been exposed to meconium for many hours that do not have any inflammation. A study by Novak and Kokomoor (1988) found meconium in about 13% of 1024 consecutive placentas, 30 of which came from prematures. The latter had 53% "chronic staining" in contrast to 17% in the term placentas. Also, 60% of the premature infants had inflammation with the staining; it occurred in only 26% of the mature neonates. Villous edema was also more common in the prematurely delivered infants' placentas, and the authors concluded that meconium-stained placentas come from populations with different characteristics. It is likely

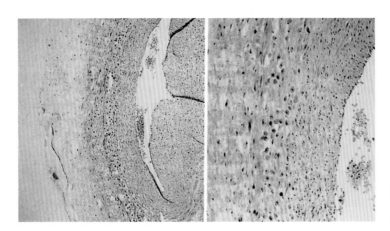

FIGURE 11.24. Degenerating muscle of umbilical cord blood vessel after chronic meconium exposure. H&E. Left ×64; right ×160. (Courtesy of Dr. G. Altshuler.)

FIGURE 11.25. Viscous, mucinous fluid beneath the amnion is a frequent feature of prolonged meconium exposure. Note the heaped, dissociated amnionic epithelium. H&E ×250.

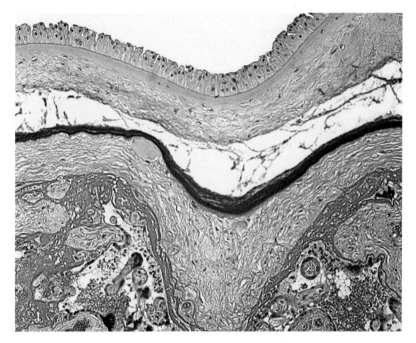

that the more immature babies had chorioamnionitis independent of the meconium discharge because inflammation is much more common in prematures in any event.

It has been our experience that, after meconium has been present on the placental surface for some time, it leads to an accumulation of a viscous fluid between amnion and chorion. It is readily apparent histologically (Fig. 11.25)

The pigment of meconium can be seen in cells of the membranes. It is not only the pigment that is found; phagolysosomes are full of debris when examined ultrastructurally (Fig. 11.26). For routine purposes, it suffices to make light microscopic observations. When hemosiderin is to be ruled out, a Prussian blue stain quickly differentiates between these two pigments. Meconium-laden macrophages are large, ovoid, or round cells in amnion and later in the chorion that have a yellow-brown-green

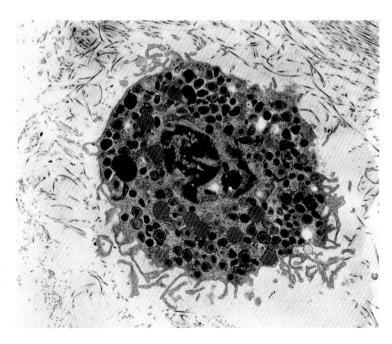

FIGURE 11.26. Meconium macrophage filled with lipid and lysosomes in a patient also having gastroschisis. Some lysosomes contain membranous debris and other heterogeneous material. Transmission electron micrograph. ×15,200. (Courtesy of Dr. M. Grafe.)

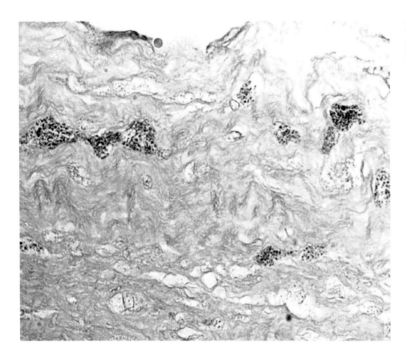

FIGURE 11.27. Numerous meconium-laden macro-phages in amnion and chorion. Iron stains were negative. H&E ×280.

content (Fig. 11.27). They are often vacuolated (Fig. 11.28). It is our opinion that these macrophages usually "lie in waiting" in amnion and in chorion, and that they are normally inactive and unoccupied. When meconium or other substances come by, they spring into functional activity. Although iron stains (Prussian blue) readily differentiate hemosiderin, the only other significant pigmentation, the bile in meconium is not readily confirmed positively. Its association with fine vacuoles helps, but a Luna-Ishak stain (Luna, 1968) may be necessary to

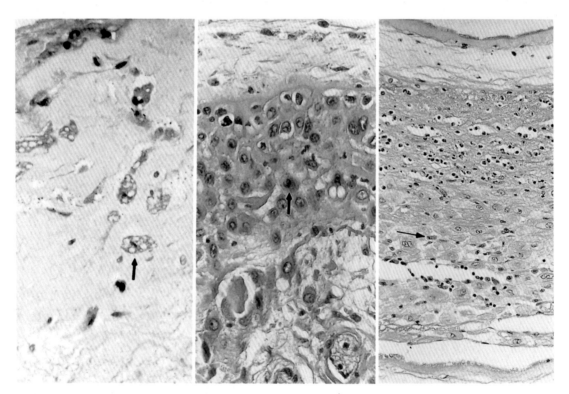

FIGURE 11.28. Different types of meconium macrophages in membranes after prolonged exposure. Note that the amnion is degenerated in all sections, and only the right membranes show minimal inflammation. Left: Vacuolated cells with pigment. Middle: Finely pigmented cells penetrating into trophoblast layer. Right: Degenerating decidua with macrophages at arrow. H&E. Left, middle ×400; right ×200.

confirm the pigment on occasion; it stains the bile a greenish color. The stain is not always easily performed. Bourne (1962) showed some photographs suggesting that meconium may stream through passageways of the epithelium, but it is more likely that these areas represent already damaged epithelium. In detailed studies of the ultrastructure of placenta and membranes, Lister (1968) concluded that the meconium appears as electron-dense granules that are associated with debris and frequent cellular degeneration. There are, however, also rare circumstances in which the membranes definitely do not have green meconium staining and histologically have pigmented macrophages that do not stain with iron stains. This finding was prominent in a placenta of a case of characteristic α-thalassemia that we saw. Hemolysis was not clinically observed and the nature of the pigment was not determined. One can always speculate that meconium had been discharged days earlier, but there was no evidence for this. Further, in a child with anal atresia and rectourinary fistula we saw meconium staining because of meconuria. In other cases, bile vomiting may be the cause of such pigmented macrophages (Vijayakumar & Koh, 2001). Not only that, Ohyama et al. (1999, 2000) described a number of newborns with ulcers of umbilical cords in which there was atresia of the intestines below the papilla of Vater. They concluded that this results from vomiting of the upper intestinal content.

When meconium is discharged a short time before birth, it may be wiped or washed off the surface without leaving a stain. Later, it stains the amnion, and thereafter the chorion stains permanently. When studies were done to estimate the time interval for the staining to become permanent, it was found that one may find histologic meconium-stained macrophages in the amnion within 1 hour of exposure; staining of the chorion occurred after 3 hours (Miller et al., 1985). Poggi et al. (2003), however, deduced from their experiments that it takes much longer (~12 hours) for the staining to take place. When it has been present for longer times, it cannot be dated reliably. From their review of the literature, Fujikura and Klionsky (1975) estimated 4 to 6 hours before meconium reaches the chorion. These figures are estimates only, because it is difficult to undertake such observations prospectively in vivo. Similar timetables have been established for the staining of fingernails and vernix. Desmond et al. (1956) found that it took 4 to 6 hours of bathing the toes of neonates in meconium-containing fluid before the nails were stained, and 12 to 14 hours for the vernix to be stained. The further progression of meconium staining of the membranes is the following: Bile pigment stains the center of the umbilical cord, usually without being contained in many macrophages, and the amnionic epithelium degenerates. The meconium is then handed to macrophages that reside within the decidua. With very long-standing meconium exposure and when the rare uterus with attached placenta becomes available for study, one may even observe meconium-stained macrophages within the myometrium. It is possible that some meconium is ultimately completely removed by this exchange, by swallowing, and by in utero inhalation of the material. It is also conceivable that, in some instances, fetuses discharge meconium repeatedly. This fact further complicates our ability to assign firm time sequences of placental meconium staining. It must also be remembered that the staining quality of meconium is reduced or eliminated when slides that contain meconium macrophages are exposed to light for longer periods of time (Morhaime et al., 2003). This is similar to the effect of exposure of jaundiced neonates to ultraviolet (UV) light. The frequent meconium discharge in postterm fetuses and its effect on the fetus is complicated by the increasing incidence of oligohydramnios after term. The volume of amnionic fluid decreases significantly near term and thereafter (Clement et al., 1987). Suggestions that indomethacin induces both (Itskovitz et at., 1980) have not yet been confirmed. Prophylactic amnioinfusion with saline in thick meconium discharge has sometimes been beneficial in the ultimate outcome (Macri et al., 1992; Uhing et al., 1993). The overall benefit of this procedure, however, is still controversial (Dye et al., 1994; Usta et al., 1995). Importantly also, several cases of maternal amnionic fluid embolism have been reported following this procedure (Maher et al., 1994). Many of the outstanding questions regarding meconium have been addressed in a searching contemporary contribution (Benirschke, 1994).

It is essential that hemosiderin be differentiated from meconium. It derives from hemolyzed red blood cells and is commonly found in association with circumvallate placentas, in the placentas of erythroblastotic infants, with abruptio placentae, and with thromboses and other circumstances wherein bleeding has occurred. Although such placentas often have a brownish tint, they may be green and simulate meconium macroscopically, except that the membranes are not then slimy. Clayton et al. (1969) spectrophotometrically studied the fluid pigments of hydropic fetuses and those with hemolyzed blood; they emphasized the difficulties of differentiating these moieties. Hemosiderin is composed of granular particles, and it has a characteristic sheen (refringence) when the focus of the light microscope, or its substage, is changed (Figs. 11.29 and 11.30). Hemosiderin is strongly positive with iron stains but, as mentioned earlier in this chapter, hematoidin cannot be reliably distinguished from the bilirubin of meconium. Finally, one should be aware that the bilirubin that stains the macrophages laden with meconium bleaches when it is exposed to the light of the laboratory.

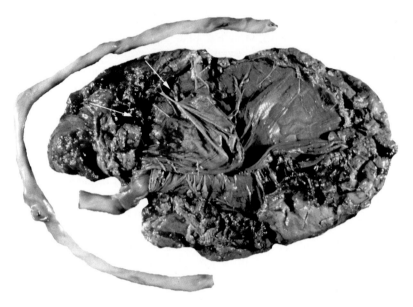

FIGURE 11.29. Circumvallate placenta with extensive hemosiderin staining. Although it looks green, it is all hemosiderin, not meconium. Disrupted fetal vessels are shown at white arrows.

GASTROSCHISIS

The amnionic epithelial cells in gastroschisis have a characteristic fine, uniform, extensive vacuolation (Ariel & Landing, 1985) (Figs. 11.31 and 11.32). Although this association was startling when first found, it is now known to be regularly present, is virtually diagnostic of gastroschisis, and is not found in fetuses with omphalocele. The fine vacuoles of amnion in gastroschisis contain lipid when examined by electron microscopy (Grafe & Benirschke, 1990), but the origin of the lipid is still obscure. When young pregnancies (>20 weeks) are studied, the vacuolization of the epithelium is not yet present; only later in gestational age does it accumulate, and the lipids then stain intensely with oil red O and other lipid stains. It is possible that the lipid comes from the opened abdominal cavity of the fetus, but that possibility should be ascertained by future studies. This assumption is somewhat contradicted by the finding that the fibrin/fibrous coating of intestines in this condition apparently contains no lipid (Tibboel et al., 1986). As was summarized earlier in this chapter, lipid has been found in small quantities by histochemical staining of the amnionic epithelium during early pregnancy, but particularly in specimens from term pregnancies. Moreover, the quantity of cellular lipid content in amnionic fluid cells was formerly used reasonably successfully to estimate the length of gestation (van Bogaert et al., 1978). Schmidt (1963) studied lipid removal from the amnionic sac in the chick embryo and concluded that lipid injected into the extraembryonic coelom of the chick is absorbed by amnionic epithelium. Later, lipid in amnionic cells again becomes a component of the amnionic fluid, from where it reaches the fetal intestine. Schmidt considered similar pathways for the human embryo. Pritchard et al. (1968) found the composition of the lipid in amnionic cells to be similar to that of the amnionic fluid and to vernix; they suggested that most of the lipid in vernix is produced by amnionic epithelium. We believe that the reverse occurs, and that vernix is derived from fetal sebum, which becomes incorporated into amnionic epithelium. The difference of normal versus gastroschisis amnionic epithelial vacuolation is evident in the dividing membranes of discordant dichorionic twins (Fig. 11.32).

EPIDERMOLYSIS BULLOSA

Epidermolysis bullosa, a rare condition, has been associated with amnionic lesions. Faulk et al. (1988) reported that a term newborn with

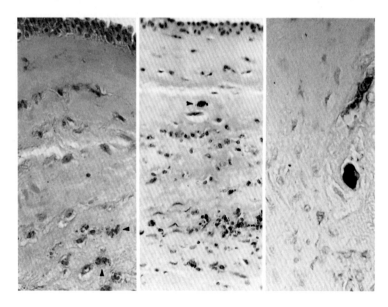

FIGURE 11.30. Hemosiderin macrophages (arrowheads) in circumvallate placentas of the second trimester. Left: H&E ×160. Middle: H&E ×100. Right: Prussian blue ×400.

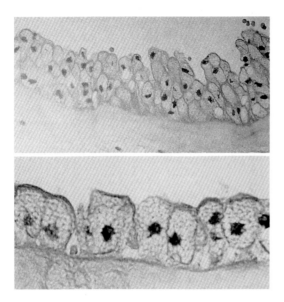

FIGURE 11.31. Characteristically vacuolated amnionic epithelium in two cases of gastroschisis. H&E. Top ×400; bottom ×640.

this disease had an amnionic surface with multiple polypoid protrusions that were covered by epithelial cells. We saw a 26-week premature infant with this disease and with duodenal atresia. Its amnion also had lesions similar to those described by Faulk et al. (1988). There were apparent protrusions of the connective tissue through epithelial defects. Thus, polyp-like excrescences were produced that were partially covered by amnionic epithelium (Fig. 11.33). There was no inflammation but many pigmented macrophages existed in the connective tissue of the

membranes. Thus, it would appear that the amnion shares the immunologic features of this disease with the skin.

Amnion Nodosum

Amnion nodosum, a relatively common condition, was first so named by Landing (1950a) when he observed small granules on the placental surfaces from pregnancies that were complicated by severe oligohydramnios. The lesion had been known since Pilgram (1889) and was described in the German literature as *Amnionknötchen*, so termed by Franqué (1897). Blanc (1961) assigned the term **vernix granulomas** to it and expanded on the pathology of associated fetal lesions in a later contribution (Blanc et al., 1962). The term **vernix granuloma,** although denoting its relation to vernix, was not adopted because the lesions are clearly not granulomas.

Amnion nodosum is most commonly found in the placentas of fetuses with renal agenesis or following premature and prolonged amniorrhea, in the placenta of the donor twin of the twin transfusion syndrome (the "stuck twin"), in diamnionic acardiac twins, characteristically in sirenomelia, and with some other disturbances that lead to prolonged oligohydramnios. It is clearly the result of deficient amnionic fluid over a prolonged period of time. The nodules are most pronounced on the placental surface, but they may rarely extend onto the membranes as well. They are only very rarely found on the umbilical cord surface. Most cases of amnion nodosum show fine

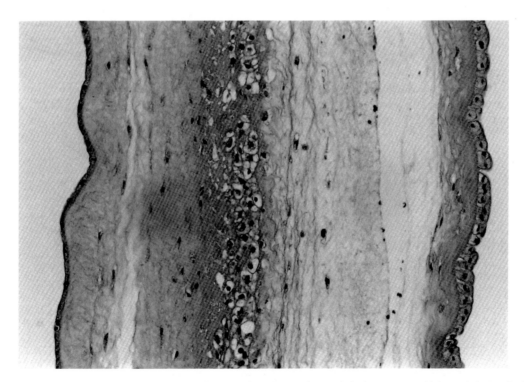

FIGURE 11.32. Dividing membranes of diamnionic, dichorionic twins. Twin on right has gastroschisis and the typical cytoplasmic vacuolation. H&E ×160. (Courtesy of Dr. C. Kaplan, New York, New York.)

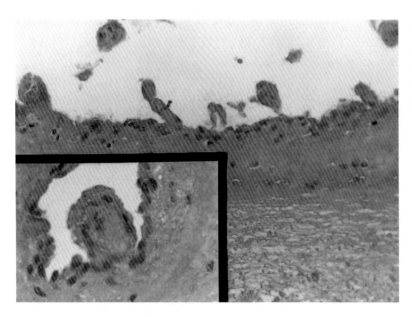

FIGURE 11.33. Amnion in a case of congenital epidermolysis bullosa and duodenal atresia. The child was delivered at 26 weeks' gestation and had numerous bullae. The amnion has polypoid expansions that were produced by apparent "herniation" of connective tissue through superficial defects. These protrusions were covered by degenerating amnionic epithelium. H&E ×256; inset ×400.

granules that are best seen in oblique light (Fig. 11.34). They are quite different from the granules of squamous metaplasia, which is typically more plaque like, patchy, and hydrophobic. Amnion nodosum is frequently brown-yellow and not shiny. The nodules are composed of squames and hair intermixed with sebum. They are from vernix that has been "rubbed" into defects of the amnionic surface. Probably the first event is that the amnionic epithelium becomes defective because of absent fluid; this then allows vernix to attach to the defect (Figs. 11.35 and 11.36). There is no inflammatory or other tissue reaction of the amnion to the presence of the vernix. At times, the edges of the granules become covered with regenerating amnionic epithelial cells.

Electron-microscopic studies have shown that most of the nodules are composed of acellular debris, degenerating cellular walls, hair fragments, and squamous cells. Bartman abd Driscoll (1968) discussed the possibility, originally suggested by Bourne (1960), that the nodules originate from the amnionic epithelium, but Salazar et al. (1974) clearly demonstrated their origin from vernix. The later authors described many cell types present within the nodules; these also contain remnants of cells, old cell walls, and fibrillar material. The centers of amnion nodosum are positive with PAS and Alcian blue stains. Salazar et al. (1974) laid to rest the notion of the cellular origin from squamous hyperplasia and metaplasia. Surprisingly, they saw some nodules covered by thin, symplastic amnionic epithelium that they considered as possibly having regenerated.

Amnion nodosum develops during late fetal life. There is not enough vernix during early pregnancy to produce this lesion. Although oligohydramnios has been verified as early as at 16 weeks in the case of urethral obstruction reported by Wagner and Tygstrup (1963), the amnion was still normal. Alternatively, as shown in Figure 11.35, in such gestations the amnion shows only minute foci of cellular

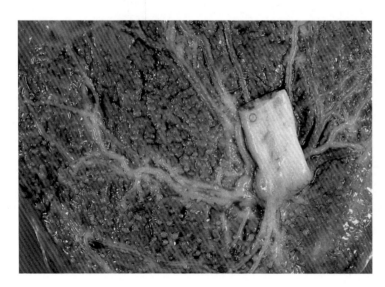

FIGURE 11.34. Macroscopic appearance of amnion nodosum in a child with renal agenesis. Note the uniform presence of fine granules, mostly sparing the vessel surfaces and not present on the cord.

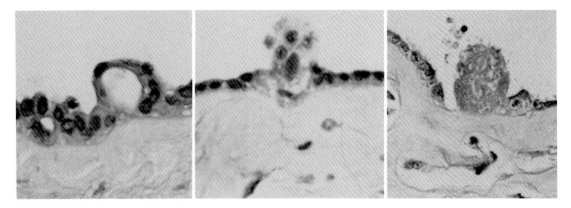

FIGURE 11.35. Early stages in the development of amnion nodosum. Focal ballooning, necrosis, and apposition of debris are present in therapeutic abortions performed for recognized oligohydramnios caused by renal agenesis or renal cystic disease. H&E ×400.

degeneration. When renal anomalies exist in only one of monoamnionic twins, as in the sirenomelia described by Kohler (1972) and substantiated by many subsequent cases, there is no amnion nodosum. Not only does amnion nodosum not develop in such monoamnionic twins, but the pulmonary hypoplasia that is so characteristic of newborns associated with severe oligohydramnios is also prevented. Brown et al. (1978) described two cases of oligohydramnios secondary to amniorrhea, similar to that originally delineated by Bain et al. (1964). In Brown et al.'s two cases, amnion nodosum was present in only one, a fetus of 1000 g; the other, weighing 600 g at 27 weeks, lacked amnion nodosum. The explanation for such apparent discrepancies is that at that early age little vernix exists to allow amnion nodules to develop. It needs not be hypothesized, as did Bain and colleagues, that the vernix had drained out with the amniorrhea, or that real "trauma" or very close contact with the fetal surface is necessary to produce the nodules, as has been suggested. The nodules are much too finely distributed to have derived from trauma of scratching or from close fetal contact with the amnion. We believe that it forms by apposition of vernix debris to foci of dying amnion epithelium-areas of epithelium that are no longer sup-

ported by the nutrition and oxygen normally contained in amnionic fluid. If the amnion had ruptured earlier, as in cases with amnionic bands, similar nodules may develop on the chorionic surface, something we have termed "chorion nodosum" in a case of congenital high airway obstruction syndrome (CHAOS) (Welsh et al., 2000).

There are numerous other reports of amnion nodosum, itemized in the contributions of Thompson (1960), Masson et al. (1966), Fitch and Lachance (1972), and Wentworth and Turnbull (1969). A comprehensive study of 100 cases of oligohydramnios may be found in the poorly accessible thesis of Déglon (1978). These studies also considered the pathogenesis of pulmonary hypoplasia and the fetal deformities associated with oligohydramnios. The dispute here is whether pulmonary hypoplasia follows the inability of the lung to inhale normal amounts of liquor, or whether it is a phenomenon caused by compression from life in a too-tight uterus. Breathing motions alone do not determine the future of lung development; it is the availability of amnionic fluid that is a prerequisite for useful breathing expansion of the lung (Wigglesworth & Desai, 1982; Kilbride et al., 1988). This claim is supported by experimental studies of fluid withdrawal from the amnion

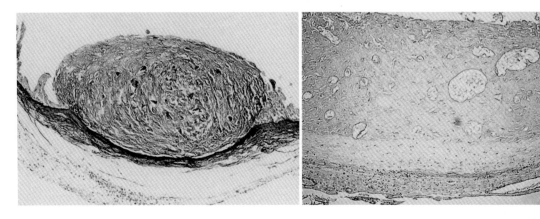

FIGURE 11.36. Late stages of amnion nodosum. Left: One nodule. Phosphotungstic acid hematoxylin (PTAH). Right: A larger plaque. Both contain squames, fat, and hair. Left: PTAH ×1160. Right: H&E ×200.

of rats (Symchych & Winchester, 1978). Lung fluid production may be another important facet, as derives from rare and complex anomalies.

The poor prognosis of fetuses associated with oligohydramnios and identified sonographically during the second trimester has been the topic of articles by Barss et al. (1984) and Mercer and Brown (1986). Wong and colleagues (1985) criticized this mode of detection if it is not followed up by confirmation through amnioscopy or amniocentesis. An additional consideration regarding pulmonary development is the secretion of fluid by the respiratory tract. When laryngeal atresia exists, the fetal lung may overexpand owing to this secretion, with hydramnios ensuing from obstruction to venous return (Silver et al., 1988).

Amnionic Bands

The existence of amnionic bands as a cause of amputations and other fetal debilities can hardly be disputed, although such doubts are expressed in the literature with regularity. These doubts began with Streeter (1930), who believed the defects to be of "germ plasm" origin. Others have shared this doubt in the primacy of amnion disruption (Patterson, 1962; Woolnough, 1987; Lockwood et al., 1989). Doubt has been expressed particularly with cases involving major congenital anomalies, such as exencephaly, ectopia cordis, and spinal disruptions (Chaurasia, 1978). These cases are frequently associated with broad amnionic adhesions. Several reviews of these cases have suggested that we may be faced with two or three distinct entities: (1) amnionic bands (with constriction possible of fingers, extremities, or umbilical cord but a generally normally formed fetus); (2) amnionic sheets (usually attached broadly to the skull and often the facies); and (3) the limb-body wall complex (with amnionic sheets and gross disruptions). The last word has not been spoken on this complicated issue, especially as to etiology and pathogenesis. Two considerations in the literature have suggested that amnionic bands and the limb-body wall complex are two distinct entities (Martinez-Frias, 1997a,b). It is also clear that the amnionic sheets are very frequently associated with many other fetal anomalies [e.g., exencephaly, meningocele, bony defects, single umbilical artery (SUA)], which is not the case with the typical bands that entangle the fingers. There may be overlaps, as also suggested by Moerman et al. (1992). These authors provided a useful differentiation between these features and suggested that the latter two categories are associated with disturbances of early embryogenesis, thus leaving the amnion attached to the forehead in a broad sheet. Numerous cases of constriction of umbilical cord, limbs, and fingers have been presented that leave little doubt, however, that true bands from disruption of the amnionic sac do occur, that these can cause amputations, even fusion of fingers and toes, and that they may cause fetal death by encircling the

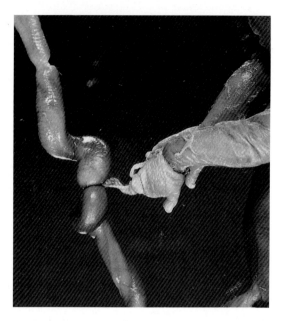

FIGURE 11.37. Spontaneous abortion at 15 weeks with amnionic bands encircling a constricting umbilical cord and tips of fingers.

cord (Hong & Simon, 1963; Ashkenazy et al., 1982). Baker and Rudolph (1971), who reported on 13 cases, believed that bands occurred only rarely, once in 10,000 births. Bands can be a cause of spontaneous abortion with macerated fetuses, which must be carefully inspected to arrive at the correct diagnosis (Figs. 11.37 to 11.39). Kalousek

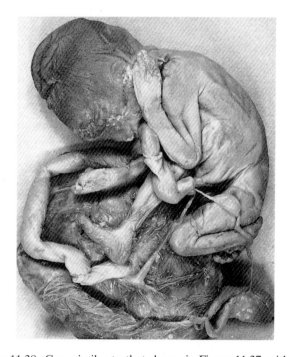

FIGURE 11.38. Case similar to that shown in Figure 11.37, with encircling of extremities and cord. Aborted fetus. (Courtesy of Dr. G. Altshuler. *Source:* Altshuler & McAdams, 1972, with permission.)

FIGURE 11.39. Surface of the placenta of a term fetus with an amnionic remnant issuing from the base of the cord. The band had encircled the leg and nearly amputated it (see Fig. 11.41). Note the opacity of the membranes.

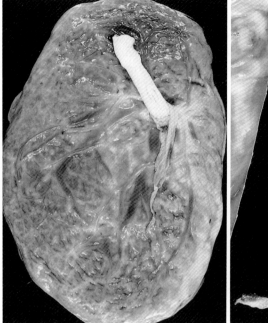
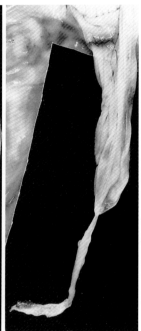

(1987; Kalousek & Bamforth, 1988) found amnionic bands much more frequently. They occurred as often as 1 per 53 previable fetuses compared to 1 per 2500 to 10,000 liveborns.

At times, it has even been witnessed that a smaller limb is delivered with a fetus. We have seen a newborn with foot amputation whose placenta was accompanied by one small macerated foot. The gestational age of the foot was estimated (from its length) to be 20 weeks. The term neonate suffered osteomyelitis later in the amputated stump. These findings indicated to us that amputation had occurred at an earlier fetal age. Such was also the case in the patient reported by Torpin and Faulkner (1966). Shipp et al. (1996) observed fetal decapitation caused by amni-

onic bands. Remarkably, the fetus continued to grow for 7 weeks after decapitation. The fetus also had clubbed feet and hepatic calcifications, presumably from hypoxia. Doubtless, the fetus moves and becomes entangled in these remnants of amnion; because the fingers move most actively it is probable that amputation of fingertips is the most common sequel in amnionic bands. Most fetuses with amputations caused by amnionic bands are otherwise normal, and the placental surface is usually completely devoid of amnion. In such cases, one usually finds remnants of amnion only around the umbilical cord. A small sac is often found at the placental end of the cord whence the bands originate (Figs. 11.39 and 11.40) (Patterson, 1962). The amnion is so firmly attached to the cord

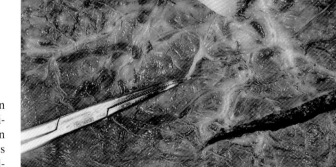

FIGURE 11.40. Placental surface of an infant with an amputated arm. The tiny remnants (clamp) of amnionic bands were initially not recognized at inspection after delivery. The importance of recognizing bands cannot be overemphasized if proper clinical counseling is to occur.

surface that it does not detach from it and is not capable of disruption with band formation. The placental surface is usually somewhat opaque owing to infiltration with enlarged macrophages. This situation is particularly true when the amnion has been missing for long periods (Fig. 11.39). The entire topic of amnionic disruption and bands has been exhaustively treated by Torpin (1968) in a book that has innumerable references and illustrations. Not only did Torpin collect more than 400 cases from the literature, he also gave a detailed account of the many cases he had himself encountered. This volume should be consulted with respect to the history and other aspects of this relatively common cause of fetal anomalies. Moreover, it was Torpin who first contradicted the theories of Streeter and assigned a later amnion rupture as the etiologic event. Constriction of extremities is perhaps the most common or best known feature (Fig. 11.41). We believe that the mobility of hands and feet is responsible for this. It should be cautioned, however, that not every case of amnionic rupture necessarily leads to entangling and constrictions.

Another comprehensive review of most aspects of amnionic bands is that of Seidman et al. (1989). These authors bemoan that the syndrome is surely underdiagnosed and emphasize that no two cases are alike. This is especially so when one includes the limb–body wall complex. Single umbilical artery and short umbilical cords were found to be common associations. The karyotype of associated fetuses has almost always been normal, and the etiology is still disputed. This other type of amnionic disruption leads to very different fetal deformities. These have been assumed to be associated with **early** amnion rupture, although different interpretations exist. Indeed, the sheets are so large and often so well shown in sonography (they are contiguous with the ectoderm of the face and other parts of the body) that one should question the association with amniotic disruption. The anomalies are characterized by more profound defects commonly involving the face, skull, and abdomen. Often exencephaly, clubbed feet, and a variety of other features are observed. Although these disruptive events were once also held to be sequelae of amnion rupture, the mechanism that produces them is surely different from the typical bands. Yang (1990) has reviewed the topic well, added a number of band cases and sheets to the literature, and believed that amnionic bands were doubtless the result of early amnion rupture. He also highlighted the fact that not all ruptures lead to band constrictions and that vernix is often incorporated into the membranes after rupture. Shephard et al. (1988) conjectured that the frequent facial disruption of these fetuses may result from the "stickiness" of these areas in early embryos. This is highly unlikely. Stickiness would not produce the large variety of other anomalies, nor would it be associated with a sheet of amnion whose epithelium is contiguous with the facial ectoderm. Incomplete embryonic folding and neural tube closure are more likely the mechanism. Because of fetal growth retardation and hydramnios, these "limb–body wall complexes" (Patten et al., 1986) are often recognized antenatally. Pysher (1980) described such a case that affected only one of monozygotic twins, and Woolnough (1987) described it in a dizygotic twin. We have seen it in one of presumably monozygotic but dichorionic twins. It had broad amnionic adhesions and many other anomalies (truncus, short bowel, ureteromegaly).

In observations of amnionic bands described by Lockwood et al. (1989) and their review of the literature, emphasis was laid on the fact that only one of monozygotic (rarely a dizygotic) twins may be affected, thus making an external cause such as infection unlikely. Hartwig et al. (1989) reviewed this limb–body wall mal-

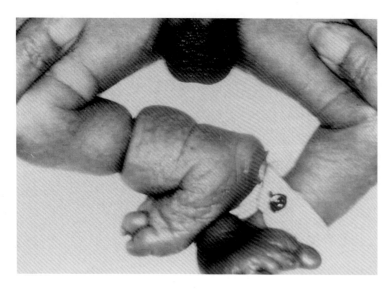

FIGURE 11.41. Note the extreme constriction of the right foreleg by the amnionic bands shown in Figure 11.39. The infant also had several amputated toes.

formation complex more completely and concluded that only some cases have broad amnionic adhesions and that others cannot be explained by this mechanism. They favored other, more complex disturbances of early embryogenesis as their etiology. It was especially deemed to be so because apparently unrelated anomalies (e.g., truncus arteriosus) were sometimes encountered in such fetuses. It must be cautioned, however, that delivery often disrupts the areas of amnionic adhesion, and reconstruction may be difficult. Characteristic of the limb–body wall complex is that the amnion is contiguous with some portion of the body wall, often either the abdomen or the skull (Fig. 11.42). This interesting spectrum of anomalies has therefore received attention since the beginning of the 20th century (e.g., Ballantyne, 1904; Woyton, 1961; Torpin, 1968; Chaurasia, 1978; Higginbottom et al., 1979; Bieber et al., 1984; Seidman et al., 1989). Most commonly it has been assumed that these gross malformations result from an "early amnion rupture" but truthfully the exact differences of etiology between it and the more classical amnionic band syndrome are not known. We prefer to see them as a different entity and consider amnionic sheets separately from true bands.

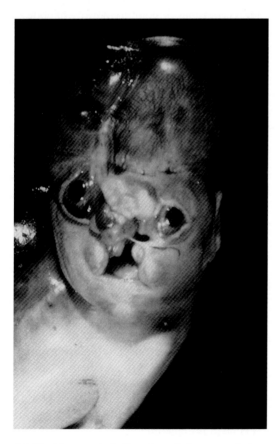

Figure 11.42. Abnormal skull and partial exencephaly secondary to broad amnionic adhesions. (Courtesy of Dr. Cynthia Kaplan. *Source:* Kaplan, 1980, with permission.)

For these reasons and because "amnionic intrusion" (Fort, 1971) (i.e., the prenatal intraamnionic invasion by perinatologists) is now so common, many investigators have attempted to understand these features by experimental reduction of amnionic fluid and disruption of the fetal sacs. After doing this in mice, Trasler et al. (1956) found a high incidence of cleft palate, which is also a common feature of this syndrome in humans. De Myer and Baird (1969) found similar defects and skeletal abnormalities in rat fetuses when amniocentesis was done between days 14 and 16; Kino (1972), Singh and Singh (1978), and Houben and Huygens (1987) observed that limb defects follow focal hemorrhages in the limbs after amniocentesis in rats. None of these experiments, however, produced adhesions. Whether they bear any relation to the massive anomalies seen in the limb–body wall complex is doubtful. Lockwood et al. (1989) suggested that these hemorrhages are a primary agency in the formation of amputations and the band syndrome in general. Among the 2300 amniocenteses reported by Porreco et al. (1982), adverse outcomes usually related to complications from anterior placentas; amnionic adhesions were not recorded (see following). In at least one case that we have seen with many amputations, cleft face, and skull adhesion, the mother had been a heavy user of intoxicating drugs. She had fallen onto her abdomen from a second-story window during her second month of gestation. Whether this was the cause of amnionic rupture remains speculative but should stimulate the detailed review of patients' histories. Moreover, it instills doubt into the hypothesis that these conditions (amnionic bands and facial disruptions) are etiologically different.

It has been noted that pregnancies complicated by apparent bands as identified with ultrasonographic techniques often have a benign outcome, without fetal adhesions present; at birth, no amnionic bands can be found (Wehbeh et al., 1993). The discrepancy was first noted by Mahony et al. (1985) and further elaborated on by Randel et al. (1988) in their sonographic study of 17 patients. In the patients with this condition, the membranes were intact, and the apparent bands represented indentations of the free membranes by endometrial synechiae or were the sequelae of former endometrial trauma. In most patients there is a history of repeated therapeutic abortion, myomectomy, or infection. Presumably, such history has led to the formation of endometrial synechiae, around which the amnion expands; sonographically it appears as bands. In two cesarean sections of patients with amnionic sheets, however, no uterine anomalies were identified. Such a case is shown in Figure 11.43. During sonography, a peculiar "stalk" was seen near term. This 36-year-old patient had a transverse lie with primary cesarean section. Although she was multiparous, no other risk factors were ascertained. The decidual adhesive band is clearly visible. There were no other pathologic findings or complications.

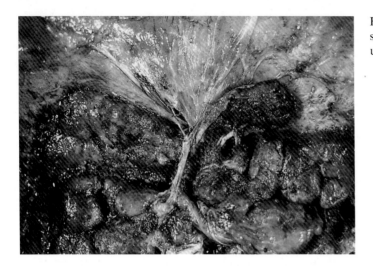

FIGURE 11.43. "Amnionic sheet." This stalk was identified sonographically as a stalk. It represents an adhesion in the uterine cavity.

Future studies are needed to clarify this condition. For clinical purposes, it is important to distinguish it from true amnionic bands. These uterine adhesions have also been termed amniotic sheets, but they are different from the sheets discussed earlier in the limb–body wall complex. It is unfortunate that the two names have been used for quite different conditions. It has occasionally been questioned whether ruptured amnion may heal or if it always must lead to defects and bands. Behzad et al. (1994) have attempted to answer this by causing laser-induced amnionic defects and immediately fixing the tissues in a controlled manner. They observed that the amnion tends to slide in its spongy layer over the chorion, thus possibly sealing the defect. We have also observed that typical constriction of a limb, undoubtedly formed by a band, can be associated with an apparently normal placenta. In such a case the amnionic surface of the chorion frondosum was entirely normal but, over the chorion laeve, the amnion was necrotic over long distances, amnion nodosum existed, and, most challenging, there was extensive vernix caseosa in the decidua capsularis. Undoubtedly a focal rupture had occurred, vernix and a limb had extruded, and thus the band-like constriction took place.

When sections are made of amnionic bands, the bands are found to consist of normal-appearing amnionic epithelium with its connective tissue. There are few signs of degeneration, and inflammation is absent; there is also no evidence that bands may derive by a mechanism of "adhesions," as suggested by Lockwood et al. (1989). Because the amnion does not completely attach itself to the chorion until the 12th week (Boyd & Hamilton, 1970), we assume that in the typical amnionic band syndrome cases the rupture of the amnion occurred before the 3rd month. It would then allow the fetus to escape into the chorionic sac and to become entangled in the amnionic remains when moving. The amnion, whose growth it appears is mediated by stretching of an enlarging sac, shrivels when

ruptured; its remains then produce the amnionic adhesions. The fetus may not always entangle, but one finds only rarely spontaneously denuded placentas without fetal amputations. They then usually relate to the disruptions occurring in the process of labor, and the entire amnion is present and not, as in the band syndrome, only small portions thereof. Torpin (1968, 1969) made the point that it is at times difficult to identify band formation on the placental surface. He advocated that the placenta be studied under water, which enhances the detection of placental structural abnormalities. He also described the case of a fetus from whose mouth a 94-cm-long piece of amnionic band was extracted (Torpin et al., 1964).

The etiology of these bands has stimulated the interest of obstetricians and dysmorphologists. We and others have questioned patients extensively as to possible traumatic or other significant events of early pregnancy, always with negative results. We have seen a set of twins who may shed some light on this question. A woman with previous salpingectomy had in vitro fertilization with transfer of five ova. Three of the ova "took," and the pregnancy was followed closely by sonography. At 6 weeks an abdominal catastrophe was diagnosed as uterine rupture from placenta percreta of one triplet that had nested near the tubal stump. It was resected, and the pregnancy went to term. One placenta was normal; the other had an opaque surface and the remnants of a shriveled amnion around the cord with a small extension of band. The newborn had a single finger constriction. It was speculated that the amnion disruption occurred at the time of uterine rupture or during its repair. Many of these aspects were well discussed in Torpin's book (1968) and by Street and Cunningham (1964). Rarely have toxins such as lysergic acid diethylamide (LSD) been implicated (Blanc et al., 1971). As a rule, the mothers do not recall anything unusual in their pregnancy. The few exceptions of antenatal trauma have been well documented in Torpin's classic book (1968). It must be emphasized that the event typically occurs spontaneously. It is an open question whether excessive fetal activity or defective amnion development are causes of such rupture. Garza and colleagues (1988) concluded that amnionic bands are not hereditary. Only one study suggested that it may rarely occur in families repetitively (Lubinsky et al., 1983). These authors described two families with possible band-related amputations and reviewed the sparse literature. Torpin (1968) also suggested from his large experience that recurrence would be an exceptional event. Hereditary collagen defects (Ehlers-Danlos syndrome and osteogenesis imperfecta) were implicated by Young et al. (1985), but we have seen several cases of both conditions with entirely normal membranes; moreover, in one reported case of Ehlers-Danlos type III no untoward membrane complication was reported (Atalla & Page, 1988).

It must be cautioned, however, that it is the **fetus** who must be affected with this collagen defect to exhibit possible ill effects from this condition. There is thus the report by Barabas (1966) that reviewed the gestational history of 18 patients with this syndrome. In his series, 14 of 18 patients (78%) were born prematurely secondary to premature rupture of the membranes. This large number suggests strongly, as did the author, that membrane integrity in this genotype may be adversely affected. Likewise, Levick (1989) found an increased number of miscarriages and intrauterine fetal deaths in families, even in those where the father had the disease. She studied three families with this defect and attributed miscarriage to "cervical laxity or premature rupture of fetal membranes." In neither report were bands described. Most authors consider that amnionic bands represent a sporadic event without recurrence risk; the usual discordance in monozygotic twins is further support. Some authors have described occasional families with possible band-related recurrent amputations, but it is exceptional (see also Lockwood et al., 1989). The notion that once the amnion has ruptured in early life the chorion allows fluid transfer and oligohydramnios, as suggested by Lockwood et al. (1989), has no merit. Nor has their suggestion that possible ensuing oligohydramnios leads to fetal skin abrasions. Amnionic bands have been described in monkeys at least twice (Tarantal & Hendrickx, 1987), and we have been shown a chimpanzee with typical finger amputations.

The nomenclature of modern dysmorphologists refers to these anomalies as the ADAM complex (amnionic deformities, adhesions, mutilation). The **incidence** of amnionic bands is difficult to assess. An epidemiologic study was undertaken in Atlanta to identify the prevalence of TEARS (the early amnion rupture sequence). It was found to be 1.16 per 10,000 births among 388,325 live births assessed (Garza et al., 1988). These authors identified 45 cases of these severe, disruptive injuries. The incidence was higher in blacks and correlated with low maternal age. There was a 30% mortality rate. On occasion, amnionic bands have been recognized by sonography; more commonly, however, the amnionic sheets are seen sonographically. It has also been suggested that amniocentesis might be the cause of early amnion disruption and of bands (Rehder & Weitzel, 1978; Moessinger et al., 1981), but this must be uncommon. Amniocentesis is also generally done too late in gestation to detach the amnion from the chorion. Christiaens and colleagues (1989) provided evidence that CVS may occasionally be held responsible for such injury. Although this point has been debated in the literature, it is the sense that only very early CVS may be related to this anomaly (see Chapter 21). Seeds et al. (1982) also described such occurrence. Moessinger et al. (1981) found an arm constriction in an aborted fetus after complicated CVS with chorioamnionitis ensuing. Lage et al. (1988) have also been skeptical of the role of amniocentesis in the causation of amnionic bands. Moreover, the experimental studies just cited suggest that the sequelae of early fluid withdrawal differ from what is observed clinically in this syndrome, which is frequently referred to as "Streeter's bands," after his early (1930) description. There are also bands that completely encircle the abdomen or an extremity (see Fig. 11.41), and that have caused deep furrows and produced sloughing of skin. Finally, there are cases in which the circulation of the umbilical cord has been interrupted by bands composed of amnion (see Figs. 11.37 and 11.39) (Kohler & Collins, 1972; Ashkenazy et al., 1982; Yang, 1990). Furthermore, in some cases bands have caused fusion of fingertips, with a space remaining at their base. All these varieties cannot be rationally explained by "germ plasm defects"; the primacy of the simple bands from sac disruption makes much more sense. We admit that the limb–body wall complexes do not have similar amputations and, as a rule, they lack amputations. Their pathogenesis is different, and the broad amnionic sheet adhesions are surely the reason for their short umbilical cords. Some authors have suggested that short cords are not a related feature, but that has not been our experience and it is certainly not the case in the review by Moerman et al. (1992). The complete review of pathogenesis and associated features provided in the report of two cases by Seidman et al. (1989) should be consulted. Lockwood and his colleagues (1988, 1989) provided suggestions on how to make the diagnosis of amnionic bands in twins, and they also considered their pathogenesis. They reviewed 15 cases of amnionic bands in twin gestations, all of them in monochorionic ("identical") twins. The absence of this syndrome in dizygotic (dichorionic twins), and other considerations led these authors to reject an "exogenous" etiology. The spectrum of anomalies in these twins, however, makes it clear that no single entity is being discussed.

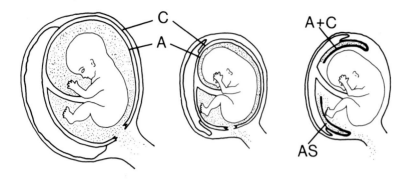

FIGURE 11.44. Extramembranous pregnancy. A, amnion; C, chorion; AS, amnionic sac. (*Source*: Perlman et al., 1980, with permission from the American College of Obstetricians and Gynecologists.)

Extramembranous Pregnancy

Not only may the amnion rupture, with the fetus developing outside the amnion although still contained within the chorion, but also the entire chorion (laeve) may rupture. The fetus then lies in the endometrial cavity, and the pregnancy is referred to as "extramembranous" (Fig. 11.44). Although several previous cases were well described, the first observation made in situ was by Hofbauer (1929), who provided an excellent picture. The patient had hysterectomy for mistaken diagnosis and gave a history of repeated prenatal hemorrhage to have been a major problem. Torpin (1968) collected 100 such cases and illustrated them well. These cases are rare circumstances, usually associated with prolonged "amniorrhea" (actually representing periodic fetal urination). Commonly there are severe positional deformities of the fetus associated with extramembranous gestation, and pulmonary hypoplasia is a characteristic sequela (Benirschke, 1977). Occasionally, such fetuses have survived, as in the cases reported by Perlman et al. (1980) (Fig. 11.44). These authors collected the few cases reported since Torpin's (1968) review; we witnessed three cases during the 1980s and have seen others since then. We are impressed with the uniformity of the placental findings. The placenta is typically circumvallate (Fig. 11.45); the cords are short, and in the membranes one finds substantial quantities of posthemorrhagic hemosiderin. There may be sparse amnion nodosum over the placental tissue, but it is not striking. The remaining edge of the membranes is relatively normal, as was depicted by Perlman and his colleagues (1980). Most of these pregnancies abort or terminate prematurely. They are occasionally associated with infection. Evidence that the fetus must have escaped out of the membranes much earlier is manifested by the diminutive hole that usually remains in the membranes. The hole may barely admit the umbilical cord, let alone fetal parts (Fig. 11.46). As in the other cases of bands and membrane rupture, the etiology

remains obscure. It is nevertheless interesting to reflect on fetal life within the endometrium and to ponder the pathogenesis of circumvallate placentation. The placental membranes that have folded over appear essentially normal (Fig. 11.47), with the exception of some minor degree of amnion nodosum and hemosiderin. Panayiotis and Grunstein (1979) have reported that one of dichorionic twins suffered prolonged amniorrhea and was born with severe growth retardation (1600 g) and typical Potter syndrome–like features. The placenta was characteristically circumvallate, and the co-twin (2150 g) survived. Extramembranous development was reported by Vago and Chavkin (1980) as having occurred after amniocentesis that led to amniorrhea. Despite deformities and some pulmonary hypoplasia, the 1520-g neonate survived. The placenta was typical. Occasionally, extramembranous pregnancy occurs with multiple gestations. Baergen et al. (1995) have described such a case in dichorionic twins. The unusual feature of that case was that the extramem-

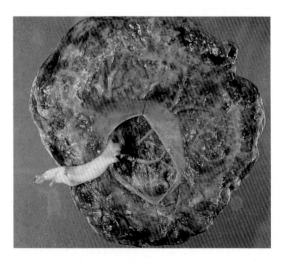

FIGURE 11.45. Extramembranous pregnancy. Note the circumvallate nature of the surface and the diminutive opening through which the cord emerges. Infant died of pulmonary hypoplasia.

FIGURE 11.46. Extramembranous pregnancy with fetus. Note the size of fetus and the membrane opening. There is a circumvallate placenta and marked pulmonary hypoplasia.

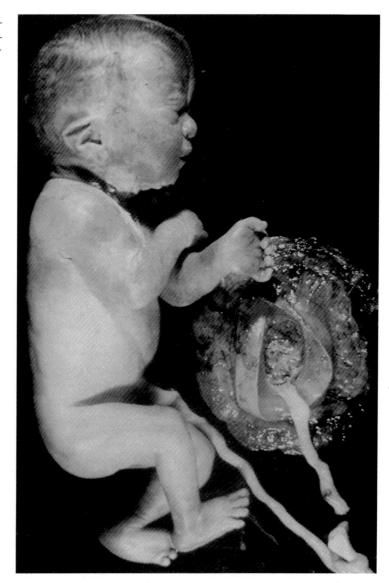

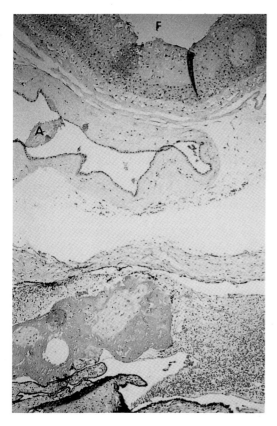

FIGURE 11.47. Membrane insertion in the extramembranous pregnancy shown in Figure 11.46. Below is villous tissue; membranes are folded at the right, and the fetus lay in space F. Much necrotic debris and inflammatory exudate are present at the margin. A, focal amnion nodosum. H&E ×64.

branous twin had significantly less evidence of prenatal compression, presumably because of "cushioning" by the second, fluid-filled amnionic sac.

References

Abramovich, D.R. and Gray, E.S.: Physiologic fetal defecation in midpregnancy. Obstet. Gynecol. **60**:294–296, 1982.

Abu-Yousef, M.M., Bleicher, J.J., Williamson, R.A. and Weiner, C.P.: Subchorionic hemorrhage: sonographic diagnosis and clinical significance. AJR **149**:737–740, 1987.

Acosta, R., Oyachi, N., Lee, J.L., Lakshmanan, J., Atkinson, J.B. and Ross, M.G.: Mechanisms of meconium passage: Cholinergic stimulation of electromechanical coordination in the fetal colon. J. Soc. Gynecol. Inv. **12**:169–173, 2005.

Ahmed, M.N., Killam, A., Thompson, K.H. and Qumsiyeh, M.B.: Unconjugated estriol as an indication for prenatal diagnosis of steroid sulfatase deficiency by in situ hybridization. Obstet. Gynecol. **92**:687–689, 1998.

Akgur, F.M. and Olguner, M.: Amniotic fluid beta-endorphin: a prognostic marker for gastroschisis. J. Pediatr. Surg. **39**:506–507, 2004.

Akle, C.A., Adinolfi, M., Welsh, K.I., Leibowitz, S. and McColl, I.: Immunogenicity of human amniotic epithelial cells after transplantation into volunteers. Lancet **2**:1003–1005, 1981.

Alger, L.S., Kisner, H.J. and Nagey, D.A.: The presence of a meconium-like substance in second-trimester amniotic fluid. Amer. J. Obstet. Gynecol. **150**:380–385, 1984.

Allen, R.: The significance of meconium in midtrimester genetic amniocentesis. Am. J. Obstet. Gynecol. **152**:413–417, 1985.

Al-Nuaim, L., Chowdhury, N. and Adelusi, B.: Subchorionic hematoma in threatened abortion: sonographic evaluation and significance. Ann. Saudi Med. **16**:650–653, 1996.

Altshuler, G. and Hyde, S.: Meconium induced vasoconstriction: a potential cause of cerebral and other fetal hypoperfusion and of poor pregnancy outcome. J. Child Neurol. **4**:137–142, 1989.

Altshuler, G. and McAdams, A.J.: The role of the placenta in fetal and perinatal pathology. Amer. J. Obstet. Gynecol. **113**:616–626, 1972.

Altshuler, G., Arizawa, M. and Molnar-Nadasdy, G.: Meconium-induced umbilical cord vascular necrosis and ulceration: a potential link between the placenta and poor pregnancy outcome. Obstet. Gynecol. **79**:760–766, 1992.

Al-Zaid, N.S., Bou-Resli, M.N. and Goldspink, G.: Bursting pressure and collagen content of fetal membranes. Br. J. Obstet. Gynaecol. **87**:227–229, 1980.

Anderson, H.C., Merker, P.C. and Fogh, J.: Formation of tumors containing bone after intramuscular injection of transformed human amnion cells (FL) into cortisone treated mice. Amer. J. Pathol. **44**:507–519, 1964.

Antonowicz, I. and Schwachman, H.: Meconium in health and in disease. Yearbook of Pediatrics, pp. 275–310, 1979. Yearbook Publishers, Chicago.

Aplin, J.D. and Allen, T.D.: The extracellular matrix of human amniotic epithelium: ultrastructure, composition and deposition. J. Cell Sci. **79**:119–136, 1985.

Aplin, J.D. and Campbell, S.: An immunofluorescence study of extracellular matrix associated with cytotrophoblast of the chorion laeve. Placenta **6**:469–479, 1985.

Aplin, J.D., Campbell, S. and Allen, T.: Human amnion epithelial extracellular matrix: ultrastructure, composition, and deposition. J. Cell Sci. **79**:119–136, 1985.

Aplin, J.D., Campbell, S., Donnai, P., Bard, J.B.L. and Allen, T.D.: Importance of vitamin C in maintenance of the normal amnion: an experimental study. Placenta **7**:377–389, 1986.

Appelman, Z., Zalel, Y., Fried, S. and Caspi, B.: Delayed fusion of amnion and chorion: a possible association with trisomy 21. Ultrasound Obstet. Gynecol. **11**:303–304, 1998.

Ariel, I.B. and Landing, B.H.: A possible distinctive vacuolar change of the amniotic epithelium associated with gastroschisis. Pediatr. Pathol. **2**:283–289, 1985.

Armstrong, W.D., Wilt, J.C. and Pritchard, E.T.: Vacuolation in the human amnion cell studied by time-lapse photography and electron microscopy. Amer. J. Obstet. Gynecol. **102**:932–948, 1968.

Artal, R., Sokol, R.J., Neuman, M., Burstein, A.H. and Stojkov, J.: The mechanical properties of prematurely and non-prematurely ruptured membranes: methods and preliminary results. Amer. J. Obstet. Gynecol. **125**:655–659, 1976.

Artal, R., Burgeson, R.E., Hobel, C.J. and Hollister, D.: An in vitro model for the study of enzymatically mediated biomechanical changes in the chorioamniotic membranes. Amer. J. Obstet. Gynecol. **133**:656–659, 1979.

Arts, N.F.T.: Investigations on the vascular system of the placenta. Part II. The maternal vascular system. Amer. J. Obstet. Gynecol. **82**:159–166, 1961.

Ashkenazy, M., Borenstein, R., Katz, Z. and Segal, M.: Constriction of the umbilical cord by an amniotic band after midtrimester amniocentesis. Acta Obstet. Gynecol. Scand. **61**:89–91, 1982.

Atalla, A. and Page, I.: Ehlers-Danlos syndrome type III in pregnancy. Obstet. Gynecol. **71**:508–509, 1988.

Azegami, M. and Mori, N.: Amniotic fluid embolism and leukotrienes. Amer. J. Obstet. Gynecol. **155**:1119–1124, 1986.

Baergen, R.N., Boue, D.R. and Mannino, F.: Placental pathology case book. J. Perinatol. **15**:510–513, 1995.

Bain, A.D., Smith, I.I. and Gauld, I.K.: Newborn after prolonged leakage of liquor amnii. Br. Med. J. **2**:598–599, 1964.

Baker, C.J. and Rudolph, A.J.: Congenital ring constriction and intrauterine amputations. Amer. J. Dis. Child. **121**:393–400, 1971.

Ballantyne, J.W.: Manual of Antenatal Pathology and Hygiene. The Embryo. Wm. Greene & Sons, Edinburgh, 1904.

Barabas, A.P.: Ehlers-Danlos syndrome: associated with prematurity and premature rupture of foetal membranes; possible increase in incidence. Br. Med. J. **2**:682–684, 1966.

Barnes, A.C. and Seeds, A.E.: The Water Metabolism of the Fetus. Thomas, Springfield, 1972.

Barss, V.A., Benacerraf, B.R. and Frigoletto, F.D.: Second trimester oligohydramnios, a predictor of poor fetal outcome. Obstet. Gynecol. **64**:608–610, 1984.

Bartels, H. and Wang, T.: Intercellular junctions in the human fetal membranes. Anat. Embryol. (Berl.) **166**:103–120, 1983.

Bartman, J. and Blanc, W.A.: Ultrastructure of human fetal placental membranes in chorio-amnionitis and meconium exposure. Obstet. Gynecol. **35**:554–561, 1970.

Bartman, J. and Driscoll, S.G.: Amnion nodosum and hypoplastic cystic kidneys: an electron microscopic and microdissection study. Obstet. Gynecol. **32**:700–705, 1968.

Battaglia, F.C., Hellegers, A.E., Meschia, G. and Barron, D.H.: In vitro investigations of the human chorion as a membrane system. Nature (Lond.) **196**:1061–1063, 1962.

Battaglia, F.C., Behrman, R.E., Meschia, G., Seeds, A.E. and Bruns, P.D.: Clearance of inert molecules, Na, and Cl ions across the primate placenta. Amer. J. Obstet. Gynecol. **102**:1135–1143, 1968.

Bautzmann, H.: Fruchthüllenmotorik und Embryokinese: Ihre Natur und ihre Bedeutung für eine physiologische Embryonalentwicklung bei Tier und Mensch. Arch. Gynäkol. **187**:519–545, 1956.

Bautzmann, H. and Hertenstein, C.: Zur Histogenese und Histologie des menschlichen fetalen und Neugeborenen-Amnion. Z. Zellforsch. **45**:589–611, 1957.

Bautzmann, H. and Schröder, R.: Studien zur funktionellen Histologie und Histogenese des Amnions beim Hühnchen und beim Menschen. Z. Anat. Entwicklungsgesch. **117**:166–214, 1953.

Bautzmann, H. and Schröder, R.: Vergleichende Studien über Bau und Funktion des Amnions. Neue Befunde am menschlichen Amnion mit Einschluß seiner freien Bindegewebs- oder sog. Hofbauerzellen. Z. Anat. **119**:7–22, 1955.

Bautzmann, H., Schmidt, W. and Lemburg, P.: Experimental electron- and light-microscopic studies on the function of the amnion-apparatus of the chick, the cat and man. Anat. Anz. **108**:305–310, 1960.

Baxi, L.V. and Pearlstone, M.M.: Subchorionic hematomas and the presence of autoantibodies. Am. J. Obstet. Gynecol. **165**:1423–1424, 1991.

Beaufort, A.J. de, Pelikan, D.M.V., Elferink, J.G.R. and Berger, H.M.: Effect of interleukin 8 in meconium on in vitro neutrophil chemotaxis. Lancet **352**:102–105, 1998.

Bedin, M., Weil, D., Fournier, T., Cedard, L. and Frezal, J.: Biochemical evidence for non-inactivation of the steroid sulfatase locus in human placenta and fibroblasts. Hum. Genet. **59**:256–258, 1981.

Beham, A., Denk, H. and Desoye, G.: The distribution of intermediate filament proteins, actin and desmoplakins in human placental tissue as revealed by polyclonal and monoclonal antibodies. Placenta **9**:479–492, 1988.

Behzad, F., Dickinson, M.R., Charlton, A. and Aplin, J.D.: Brief communication: Sliding displacement of amnion and chorion following controlled laser wounding suggests a mechanism for short-term sealing of ruptured membranes. Placenta **15**:775–778, 1994.

Beller, F.K., Douglas, G.W., Debrovner, C.H. and Robinson, R.: The fibrinolytic system in amniotic fluid embolism. Amer. J. Obstet. Gynecol. **87**:48–55, 1963.

Bendon, R.W. and Ray, M.B.: The pathologic findings of the fetal membranes in very prolonged amniotic fluid leakage. Arch. Pathol. Lab. Med. **110**:47–50, 1986.

Benedetti, W.L., Sala, M.A. and Alvarez, H.: Histochemical demonstration of enzymes in the umbilical cord and membranes of human term pregnancy. Eur. J. Obstet. Gynecol. Reprod. Biol. **3**:185–189, 1973.

Benedetto, M.T., de Cicco, F., Rossielli, F., Nicosia, A.L., Lupi, G. and Dell'Acqua, S. Oxytocin receptor in human fetal membranes at term and during labor. J. Steroid Biochem. **35**:205–208, 1990.

Benirschke, K.: Effects of placental pathology on the embryo and the fetus. In, Handbook of Teratology, Vol. 3. J.G. Wilson and F.C. Fraser, eds., pp. 79–115. Plenum Press, New York, 1977.

Benirschke, K.: Placenta pathology: questions to the perinatologist. J. Perinatol. **14**:371–375, 1994.

Benirschke, K.: Fetal consequences of amniotic fluid meconium. Contemp. Obstet. Gynec. **46**:76–83, 2001.

Benson, M.D. and Lindberg, R.E.: Amniotic fluid embolism, anaphylaxis, and tryptase. Amer. J. Obstet. Gynecol. **175**:737, 1996.

Bernstein, I.M., Barth, R.A., Miller, R. and Capeless, E.L.: Elevated maternal serum alpha-fetoprotein: association with placental sonolucencies, fetomaternal hemorrhage, vaginal bleeding, and pregnancy outcome in the absence of fetal anomalies. Obstet. Gynecol. **79**:71–74, 1992.

Bieber, F.R., Mostoufi-Zadeh, M., Birnholz, J.C. and Driscoll S.G.: Amniotic band sequence associated with ectopia cordis in one twin. J. Pediatr. **105**:817–819, 1084.

Bilic, G., Ochsenbein-Kölble, N., Hall, H., Huch, R. and Zimmermann, R.: In vitro lesion repair by human amnion epithelial and mesenchymal cells. Amer. J. Obstet. Gynecol. **190**:87–92, 2004.

Blackwell, S.C., Hallak, M., Hotra, J.W., Refuerzo, J., Sokol, R.J. and Sorokin, Y.: Prolonged in utero meconium exposure impairs spatial learning in the adult rat. Amer. J. Obstet. Gynecol. **190**:1551–1556, 2004.

Blanc, W.A.: Vernix granulomatosis of amnion ("amnion nodosum") in oligohydramnios: lesion associated with urinary anomalies, retention of dead fetuses, and prolonged leakage of amniotic fluid. N.Y. State J. Med. **61**:1492–1496, 1961.

Blanc, W.A., Apperson, J.W. and McNally, J.: Pathology of the newborn and of the placenta in oligohydramnios. Bull. Sloane Hosp. Women **7**:51–64, 1962.

Blanc, W.A., Mattison, D.R., Kane, R. and Chauhan, P.: L.S.D., intrauterine amputations, and amniotic-band syndrome. Lancet **2**:158–159, 1971.

Bohle, A. and Hienz, H.A.: Zellkernmorphologische Geschlechtsbestimmung an der Placenta. Klin. Wochenschr. **34**:981–985, 1956.

Boll, H.U., Forssmann, W.G. and Taugner, R.: Studies on the juxtaglomerular apparatus. IV. Freeze-fracturing of membrane surfaces. Cell Tissue Res. **161**:459–469, 1975.

Borlum, K.-G.: Second-trimester chorioamniotic separation and amniocentesis. Eur. J. Obstet. Gynecol. Reprod. Biol. **30**:35–38, 1989.

Bou-Resli, M.N., Al-Zaid, N.S. and Ibrahim, M.E.A.: Full-term and prematurely ruptured fetal membranes. Cell Tissue Res. **220**:263–278, 1981.

Boué, A., Muller, F., Briard, M.L. and Boué, J.: Interest of biology in the management of pregnancies where a fetal malformation has been detected by ultrasonography. Fetal Ther. **3**:14–23, 1988.

Bourne, G.L.: The microscopic anatomy of the human amnion and chorion. Am. J. Obstet. Gynecol. **79**:1070–1073, 1960.

Bourne, G.L.: The Human Amnion and Chorion. Lloyd-Luke, London, 1962.

Bourne, G.L. and Lacy, D.: Ultrastructure of human amnion and its possible relation to the circulation of amniotic fluid. Nature (Lond.) **168**:952–954, 1960.

Boyd, J.D. and Hamilton, W.J.: The Human Placenta. Heffer, Cambridge, 1970.

Breed, A., Mantingh, A., Govaerts, L., Booger, A., Anders, G. and Laurini, R.: Abnormal karyotype in the chorion, not confirmed in a subsequently aborted fetus. Prenat. Diagn. **6**:375–377, 1986.

Brown, D.R., Doshi, N. and Taylor, P.M.: Oligohydramnios and fatal pulmonary hypoplasia without amnion nodosum. J. Reprod. Med. **20**:293–296, 1978.

Brusis, E., Nitsch, B. and Wengeler, H.: Fruchtwasser und Amnion. In, Klinik der Frauenheikunde und Geburtshilfe, Vol. 4. G. Döderlein and K.H. Wulf, eds., pp. 667–750. Urban & Schwarzenberg, Munich, 1975.

Bryant-Greenwood, G.D.: The extracellular matrix of the human fetal membranes. Structure and function. Placenta **19**:1–11, 1998.

Bryant-Greenwood, G.D., Rees, M.C.P. and Turnbull, A.C.: Immunohistochemical localization of relaxin, prolactin and prostaglandin synthase in human amnion, chorion and decidua. J. Endocrinol. **114**:491–496, 1987.

Bühler, F.R.: Randbildungen der menschlichen Placenta. Acta Anat. (Basel) **59**:47–76, 1964.

Bullen, B., Bloxam, D., Ryder, T.A., Mobberley, M.A. and Bax, C.M.: Two-sided culture of human placental tropho-blast. Morphology, immunohistochemistry and permeability properties. Placenta **11**:431–450, 1990.

Burgess, A.M. and Hutchins, G.M.: Inflammation of the lungs, umbilical cord, and placenta associated with meconium passage in utero: review of 123 autopsied cases (abstract 4). Modern Pathol. **7**(1):1P, 1994.

Butler, W.J., Schwartz, C.E., Sauer, S.M., Wilson, J.T. and McDonough, P.G.: Discordance in deoxyribonucleic acid analysis of fetus and trophoblast. Am. J. Obstet. Gynecol. **158**:642–645, 1988.

Byrne, D.L. and Gau, G.: In utero meconium aspiration: an unpreventable cause of neonatal death. Br. J. Obstet. Gynaecol. **94**:813–814, 1987.

Cajal, C.L.R.y and Martinez, R.O.: Defecation in utero: A physiologic fetal function. Amer. J. Obstet. Gynecol. **188**:153–156, 2003.

Campbell, S., Allen, T.D., Moser, B.B. and Aplin, J.D.: The translaminal fibrils of the human amnion basement membrane. J. Cell Sci. **94**:307–318, 1989.

Campos, G.A., Guerra, F.A. and Israel, E.J.: Effects of cholic acid infusion in fetal lambs. Acta Obstet. Gynecol. Scand. **65**:23–26, 1986.

Cane, F.E.: The functions of the amnion. Lancet **2**:1274, 1888.

Casey, M.L., Delgadillo, M., Cox, K.A., Niesert, S. and MacDonald, P.C.: Inactivation of prostaglandins in human decidua vera (parietalis) tissue: substrate specificity of prostaglandin dehydrogenase. Amer. J. Obstet. Gynecol. **160**:3–7, 1989.

Casey, M.L., Word, R.A. and MacDonald, P.C.: Endothelin-1 gene expression and regulation of endothelin mRNA and protein biosynthesis in avascular human amnion. J. Biol. Chem. **266**:5762–5768, 1991.

Charpin, C., Kopp, F., Pourreau-Schneider, N., Lissitzky, J.C., Lavaut, M.N., Martin, P.M. and Toga, M.: Laminin distribution in human decidua and immature placenta: an immunoelectronmicroscopic study (avidin-biotin-peroxidase complex method). Amer. J. Obstet. Gynecol. **151**:822–826, 1985.

Chaurasia, B.D.: Amniochorionic bands and adhesions with fetal deformities. Anat. Anz. **144**:158–162, 1978.

Cheung, P.Y., Walton, J.C., Tai, H.H., Riley, S.C. and Challis, J.R.: Immunocytochemical distribution and localization of 15-hydroxyprostaglandin dehydrogenase in human fetal membranes, decidua, and placenta. Amer. J. Obstet. Gynecol. **163**:1445–1449, 1990.

Chez, R.A., Josimovich, J.B. and Schultz, S.G.: The transfer of human placental lactogen across isolated amnion-chorion. Gynecol. Invest. **1**:312–318, 1970.

Christiaens, G.C.M.L., van Baarlen, J., Huber, J. and Leschot, N.J.: Fetal limb constriction: a possible complication of CVS. Prenat. Diagn. **9**:67–71, 1989.

Clark, P. and Duff, P.: Inhibition of neutrophil oxidative burst and phagocytosis by meconium. Amer. J. Obstet. Gynecol. **173**:1301–1305, 1995.

Clark, S.L.: Arachidic acid metabolites and the pathophysiology of amniotic fluid embolism. Semin. Reprod. Endocrinol. **3**:253–257, 1985.

Clark, S.L.: Amniotic fluid embolism and leukotrienes. Amer. J. Obstet. Gynecol. **158**:681, 1988.

Clark, S.L., Pavlova, Z., Greenspoon, J., Horenstein, J. and Phelan, J.P.: Squamous cells in the maternal pulmonary circulation. Amer. J. Obstet. Gynecol. **154**:104–106, 1986.

Clark, S.L., Cotton, D.B., Gonik, B., Greenspoon, J. and Phelan, J.P.: Central hemodynamic alterations in amniotic fluid embolism. Amer. J. Obstet. Gynecol. **158**:1124–1126, 1988.

Clark, S.L., Hankins, G.D.V., Dudley, D.A., Dildy, G.A. and Porter, T.F.: Amniotic fluid embolism: analysis of the national registry. Amer. J. Obstet. Gynecol. **172**:1158–1169, 1995.

Clayton, E.M., Waller, D.H. and Foster, E.B.: The significance of heme pigments in amniotic fluid. Obstet. Gynecol. **34**:641–647, 1969.

Clement, D., Schifrin, B.S. and Kates, R.B.: Acute oligohydramnios in postdate pregnancy. Amer. J. Obstet. Gynecol. **157**:884–886, 1987.

Cooperberg, P.L., Wright, V.J. and Carpenter, C.W.: Ultrasonographic demonstration of a placental maternal lake. J. Clin. Ultrasound **7**:62–64, 1979.

Corridan, M., Kendall, E.D. and Begg, J.D.: Cord entanglement causing premature placental separation and amniotic fluid embolism: case report. Br. J. Obstet. Gynaecol. **87**:935–940, 1980.

Coston, H.R.: Report of a case of ichthyosis fetalis; placenta and membranes involved. Amer. J. Obstet. Dis. Women Child. **58**:650–654, 1908.

Crane, J.P. and Cheung, S.W.: An embryonic model to explain cytogenetic inconsistencies observed in chorionic villus versus fetal tissue. Prenatal. Diagn. **8**:119–129, 1988.

Craven, C.M. and Ward, K.: Premature rupture of the amniotic membranes diagnosed by placental bed biopsy. Arch. Pathol. Lab. Med. **121**:167–168, 1997.

Crescimanno, C., Mühlhauser, J., Castellucci, M., Rajaniemi, H., Parkkila, S. and Kaufmann, P.: Immunocytochemical expression patterns of carbonic anhydrase isoenzymes in human placenta, cord and membranes. Placenta **14**:A11, 1993.

Danforth, D.N. and Hull, R.W.: The microscopic anatomy of the fetal membranes with particular reference to the detailed structure of the amnion. Amer. J. Obstet. Gynecol. **75**:536–550, 1958.

Danforth, D.N., Elin, T.W. and Stanes, M.N.: Studies on fetal membranes. I. Bursting tension. Amer. J. Obstet. Gynecol. **65**:480–490, 1953.

Davis, G.E., Blaker, S.N., Engvall, E., Varon, S., Manthorpe, M. and Gage, F.H.: Human amnion membrane serves as a substratum for growing axons in vitro and in vivo. Science **236**:1106–1109, 1987.

Davis, J.R. and Penny, R.J.: Improved fluorescence method for identifying sex chromatin in formalin-fixed tissue. Amer. J. Clin. Pathol. **75**:731–733, 1981.

Davis, R.O., Philips J.B., III, Harris, B.A., Wilson, E.R. and Huddleston, J.F.: Fatal meconium aspiration syndrome occurring despite airway management considered appropriate. Amer. J. Obstet. Gynecol. **151**:731–736, 1985.

Déglon, P.: Lésions placentaires et foetales dans 100 cas d'oligohydramnios. Thesis, University of Lausanne, 1978.

de Ikonicoff, L.K. and Cedard, L.: Localization of human chorionic gonadotropic and somatomammotropic hormones by the peroxidase immuno-enzymologic method in villi and amniotic epithelium of human placenta (from six weeks to term). Amer. J. Obstet. Gynecol. **116**:1124–1132, 1973.

De Myer, W. and Baird, I.: Mortality and skeletal malformations from amniocentesis and oligohydramnios in rats: cleft palate, clubfoot, microstomia, and adactyly. Teratology **2**:33–38, 1969.

DeSa, D.J.: Rupture of fetal vessels on placental surface. Arch. Dis. Child. **46**:495–501, 1971.

Desmond, M.M., Lindley, J.E., Moore, J. and Brown, C.A.: Meconium staining of newborn infants. J. Pediatr. **49**:540–549, 1956.

Dickey, R.P., Olar, T.T., Curole, D.N., Taylor, S.N. and Matulich, E.M.: Relationship of first-trimester subchorionic bleeding detected by color Doppler ultrasound to subchorionic fluid, clinical bleeding, and pregnancy outcome. Obstet. Gynecol. **80**:415–420, 1992.

Dominguez, R., Segal, A.J. and O'Sullivan, J.A.: Leukocytic infiltration of the umbilical cord: manifestation of fetal hypoxia due to reduction of blood flow in the cord. JAMA **173**:346–349, 1960.

Donskikh, N.V.: New views on vascularity of the human amnion. Akusn. Ginekol. (Mosc.) **33**:93–94, 1957 (in Russian).

Dooley, S.L., Pesavento, D.J., Depp, R., Socol, M.L., Tamura, R.K. and Wiringa, K.S.: Meconium below the vocal cords at delivery: correlation with intrapartum events. Amer. J. Obstet. Gynecol. **153**:767–770, 1985.

Dye, T., Aubry, R., Gross, S. and Artal, R.: Amnioinfusion and the intrauterine prevention of meconium aspiration. Amer. J. Obstet. Gynecol. **171**:1601–1605, 1994.

Editorial: Anyone for amnion? Lancet **1**:719, 1984.

Enders, A.C. and King, B.F.: Formation and differentiation of extraembryonic mesoderm in the rhesus monkey. Amer. J. Anat. **181**:327–340, 1988.

Evaldson, G.R., Larsson, B. and Jiborn, H.: Is collagen content reduced when the fetal membranes rupture? A clinical study of term and prematurely ruptured membranes. Gynecol. Obstet. Invest. **24**:92–94, 1987.

Falciglia, H.S.: Failure to prevent meconium aspiration syndrome. Obstet. Gynecol. **71**:349–353, 1988.

Falciglia, H.S., Kosmetatos, N., Brady, K. and Wesseler, T.A.: Intrauterine meconium aspiration in an extremely premature infant. Amer. J. Dis. Child. **147**:1035–1037, 1993.

Faulk, W.P., Hsi, B.-L., Yeh, C.-J.G., McIntyre, J.A. and Stevens, P.J.: Epidermolysis bullosa letalis: an immunogenetic disease of extraembryonic extoderm? Amer. J. Obstet. Gynecol. **158**:150–157, 1988.

Fitch, N. and Lachance, R.C.: The pathogenesis of Potter's syndrome of renal agenesis. Can. Med. Assoc. J. **107**:653–656, 1972.

Fleischer, A.C., Kurtz, A.B., Wapner, R.J., Ruch, D., Sacks, G.A., Jeanty, P., Shah, D.M. and Boehm, F.H.: Elevated alpha-fetoprotein and a normal fetal sonogram: association with placental abnormalities. AJR **150**:881–883, 1988.

Florio, P., Michetti, F., Bruschettini, M., Lituania, M., Bruschettini, P., Severi, F.M., Petraglia, F. and Gazzolo, D.: Amniotic fluid S100B protein in mid-gestation and intrauterine fetal death. Lancet **364**:270–272, 2004.

Foltz, C.M., Russo, R.G., Terranova, V.P. and Liotta, L.A.: Interactions of tumour cells with whole basement membrane in the presence or absence of endothelium. In, Interaction of Platelets and Tumour Cells. G.A. Jamieson and A.R. Scipio, eds., pp. 353–371. Liss, New York, 1982.

Forssmann, W.G. and Taugner, R.: Studies on the juxtaglomerular apparatus. V. The juxtaglomerular apparatus in Tupaia with special reference to intercellular contacts. Cell Tissue Res. **177**:291–305, 1977.

Fort, A.T.: Prenatal intrusion into the amnion. Amer. J. Obstet. Gynecol. **110**:432–455, 1971.

Fortunato, S.J., Menon, R. and Lombardi, S.J.: Collagenolytic enzymes (gelatinases) and their inhibitors in human amnio-chorionic membrane. Amer. J. Obstet. Gynecol. **177**:731–741, 1997.

Foster, H.W. and Das, S.K.: Study of lipids in human amnion and chorion. Am. J. Obstet. Gynecol. **149**:670–673, 1984.

Fox, H. and Butler-Manuel, R.: A teratoma of the placenta. J. Pathol. Bacteriol. **88**:137–140, 1964.

Frank, H.G., Malekzadeh, F., Kertschanska, S., Crescimanno, C., Castellucci, M., Lang, I., Desoye, G. and Kaufmann, P.: Immunohistochemistry of two different types of placental fibrinoid. Acta Anat. Basel. **150**:55–68, 1994.

Franqoual, J., Lindenbaum, A., Benattar, C., Dehan, M., Cohen, H. and Leluc, R.: Importance of simultaneous determination of coproporphyrin and hemoglobin in contaminated amniotic fluid. Clin. Chem. **32**:877–878, 1986.

Franqué, O. v.: Zur Kenntnis der Amnionanomalien. Monatsschr. Geburtsh. Gynäkol. **6**:36–41, 1897.

Frels, W.I., Rossant, J. and Chapman, V.M.: Maternal X chromosome expression in mouse chorionic ectoderm. Dev. Genet. **1**:123–132, 1979.

Fuchs, A.R., Periysamy, S., Alexandrova, M. and Soloff, M.: Correlation between oxytocin receptor concentration and responsiveness to oxytocin in pregnant myometrium: effects of ovarian steroids. Endocrinology **113**:742–749, 1983.

Fujikura, T. and Klionsky, B.: The significance of meconium staining. Am. J. Obstet. Gynecol. **121**:45–50, 1975.

Garcia, A.G.P., Consorte, S.M., Lana, A.M.A. and Friede, R.: Amnion nodosum and congenital ichthyosis. Amer. J. Clin. Pathol. **67**:567–572, 1977.

Garza, A., Cordero, J.F. and Mulinare, J.: Epidemiology of the early amnion rupture spectrum of defects. Amer. J. Dis. Child. **142**:541–544, 1988.

Gaus, G., Funayama, H., Huppertz, B., Kaufmann, P. and Frank, H.G.: Parent cells for trophoblast hybridization I: Isolation of extravillous trophoblast cells from human term chorion laeve. Trophoblast Res. **10**:181–190, 1997.

Gautray, J.P., Jolivet, A., Vielh, J.P. and Guillemin, R.: Presence of immunoassayable β-endorphin in human amniotic fluid: Elevation in cases of fetal distress. Amer. J. Obstet. Gynecol. **129**:211–212, 1977.

Ghidini, A. and Spong, C.Y.: Severe meconium aspiration syndrome is not caused by aspiration of meconium. Amer. J. Obstet. Gynecol. **185**:931–938, 2001.

Gibb, W. and Lavoie, J.C.: Effects of glucocorticoids on prostaglandin formation by human amnion. Can. J. Physiol. Pharmacol. **68**:671–676, 1990.

Gilbert, W.M., Eby-Wilkens, E. and Tarantal, A.F.: The missing link in rhesus monkey amniotic fluid volume regulation: Intramembranous absorption. Obstet. Gynecol. **89**:462–465, 1997.

Goetzman, B.W.: Meconium aspiration. Amer. J. Dis. Child. **146**:1282–1283, 1992.

Golbus, M.S. and Stephens, J.D.: Prenatal diagnosis, chromosomal abnormalities and neural tube defects. Clin. Perinatol. **6**:245–254, 1979.

Goodlin, R.C.: Meconium aspiration. Obstet. Gynecol. **32**:94–95, 1968.

Gossrau, R., Graf, R., Ruhnke, M. and Hanski, C.: Proteases in the human full-term placenta. Histochemistry. **86**:405–413, 1987.

Grafe, M.J. and Benirschke, K.: Ultrastructural study of the amniotic epithelium in a case of gastroschisis. Pediatr. Pathol. **10**:95–101, 1990.

Griffiths, D.M. and Burge, D.M.: When is meconium stained liquor actually bile stained vomitus? Arch. Dis. Child. **63**: 201–202, 1988.

Grimes, L.D. and Cassady, G.: Fetal gastrointestinal obstruction. Amer. J. Obstet. Gynecol. **106**:1196–1200, 1970.

Grosser, O.: Frühentwicklung, Eihautbildung und Placentation des Menschen und der Säugetiere. Bergmann, Munich, 1927.

Guidotti, R.J., Grimes, D.A. and Cates, W.: Fatal amniotic fluid embolism during legally induced abortion, United States, 1972 to 1978. Amer. J. Obstet. Gynecol. **141**:257–261, 1981.

Haddad, F.S.: Amniotic fluid embolism: a review of the literature and a case report with recovery. J. Indian Med. Assoc. **17**:76–79, 1985.

Hamilton, W.J. and Boyd, J.D.: Development of the human placenta in the first three months of gestation. J. Anat. **94**: 297–328, 1960.

Hankins, G.D.V., Rowe, J., Quirk, J.G., Trubey, R. and Strickland, D.M.: Significance of brown and/or green amniotic fluid at the time of second trimester genetic amniocentesis. Obstet. Gynecol. **64**:353–358, 1984.

Harrison, K.B. and Warburton, D.: Preferential X-chromosome activity in human female placental tissue. Cytogenet. Cell Genet. **41**:163–168, 1986.

Hartwig, N.G., Vermej-Keers, C.H.R., de Vries, H.E., Kagie, M. and Kragt, H.: Limb body wall malformation complex: an embryologic etiology? Hum. Pathol. **20**:1071–1077, 1989.

Hebertson, R.M., Hammond, M.E. and Bryson, M.J.: Amniotic epithelial ultrastructure in normal, polyhydramnic, and oligohydramnic pregnancies. Obstet. Gynecol. **68**:74–79, 1986.

Hempel, E.: Die ultrastrukturelle Differenzierung des menschlichen Amnionepithels unter besonderer Berücksichtigung des Nabelstranges. Anat. Anz. **132**:356–370, 1972.

Herendael, B.J. v., Oberti, C. and Brosens, I.: Microanatomy of the human amniotic membranes: a light microscopic, transmission, and scanning electron microscopic study. Amer. J. Obstet. Gynecol. **131**:872–880, 1978.

Hertig, A.T.: On the development of the amnion and exocoelomic membrane in the previllous human ovum. Yale J. Biol. Med. **18**:107–115, 1945.

Hertig, A.T.: Human Trophoblast. Thomas, Springfield, 1968.

Hertig, A.T. and Rock, J.: Two human ova of the previllous stage having an ovulation age of about eleven and twelve days respectively. Contrib. Embryol. Carnegie Inst. **29**:127–156, 1941.

Hessle, H. and Engvall, E.: Type VI collagen. J. Biol. Chem. **259**:3955–3961, 1984.

Hessle, H., Sakai, L.Y., Hollister, D.W., Burgeson, R.E. and Engvall, E.: Basement membrane diversity detected by monoclonal antibodies. Differentiation **26**:49–54, 1984.

Hieber, A.D., Corcino, D., Motosue, J., Sandberg, L.B., Roos, P.J., Yeh Yu, S., Csiszar, K., Kagan, H.M., Boyd, C.D. and Bryant-Greenwood, G.D.: Detection of elastin in the human fetal membranes. Proposed molecular basis for elasticity. Placenta **18**:301–312, 1997.

Higginbottom, M.C., Jones, K.L., Hall, B.D. and Smith, D.W.: The amniotic band disruption complex: timing of amnion rupture and variable spectra of consequent defects. J. Pediatr. **95**:544–549, 1979.

Hills, B.A.: Further studies of the role of surfactant in premature rupture of the membranes. Amer. J. Obstet. Gynecol. **170**: 195–201, 1994.

Hinrichsen, K.: Embryogenese, Äußere Körperform und Nabelbildung. In, Humanembryologie, K. Hinrichsen, ed. Springer-Verlag, Heidelberg, 1990.

Hofbauer, J.: Extrachoriale Fruchtentwicklung, in situ beobachtet. Arch. Gynäkol. **135**:332–333, 1929.

Hogge, W.A., Schonberg, S.A. and Golbus, M.S.: Prenatal diagnosis by chorionic villus sampling: lessons of the first 600 cases. Prenat. Diagn. **5**:393–400, 1985.

Holcberg, G., Huleihel, M., Katz, M., Segal, D., Sapir, O., Mazor, M., Malek, A. and Schneider, H.: Vasoconstrictive activity of meconium stained amniotic fluid in the human placental vasculature. Europ. J. Obstet. Gynecol. Reprod. Biol. **87**:147–150, 1999.

Hong, C.Y. and Simon, M.A.: Amniotic bands knotted about umbilical cord: a rare cause of fetal death. Obstet. Gynecol. **22**:667–670, 1963.

Houben, J.J. and Huygens, R.: Subcellular effects of experimental oligohydramnios on the developing rat limb. Teratology **36**:107–116, 1987.

Hoyes, A.D.: Fine structure of human amniotic epithelium in early pregnancy. J. Obstet. Gynaecol. Br. Commonw. **75**: 949–962, 1968a.

Hoyes, A.D.: Ultrastructure of the epithelium of human umbilical cord. J. Anat. **103**:388–389, 1968b.

Hoyes, A.D.: Ultrastructure of the human mesenchymal layers of the human chorion in early pregnancy. Amer. J. Obstet. Gynecol. **106**:557–566, 1970.

Hoyes, A.D.: Ultrastructure of the mesenchymal layers of the human chorion laeve. J. Anat. **109**:17–30, 1971.

Hoyes, A.D.: Fine structure of human amnionic epithelium following short term preservations in vitro. J. Anat. **111**:43–54, 1972.

Hsieh, T.T., Hsieh, C.C., Hung, T.H., Chiang, C.H., Yang, F.P. and Pao, C.C.: Differential expression of interleukin-1β and interleukin-6 in human fetal serum and meconium-stained amniotic fluid. J. Reprod. Immunol. **37**:155–161, 1998.

Huppertz, B., Kertschanska, S., Frank, H.G., Gaus, G., Funayama, H. and Kaufmann P.: Extracellular matrix components of the placental extravillous trophoblast: immunohistochemistry and ultrastructural distribution. Histochem. Cell Biol. **106**: 291–301, 1996.

Ibrahim, M.E.A., Bou-Resli, M.N., AI-Zaid, N.S. and Bishay, L.F.: Intact fetal membranes: morphological predisposal to rupture. Acta Obstet. Gynecol. Scand. **62**:481–485, 1983.

Itskovitz, J., Abramovici, H. and Brandes, J.M.: Oligohydramnion, meconium and perinatal death concurrent with indomethacin treatment in human pregnancy. J. Reprod. Med. **24**:137–140, 1980.

Jacques, S.M. and Qureshi, F.: Subamnionic vernix caseosa. Pediatr. Pathol. **14**:585–593, 1994.

Jazayeri, A., Politz, L., Tsibris, J.C.M., Queen, T. and Spellacy, W.N.: Fetal erythropoietin levels in pregnancies complicated by meconium passage: Does meconium suggest fetal hypoxia? Amer. J. Obstet. Gynecol. **183**:188–190, 2000.

Jenkins, D.M., O'Neill, M., Matter, M., France, V.W., Hsi, B.L. and Faulk, W.P.: Degenerative changes and detection of plasminogen in fetal membranes that rupture prematurely. Br. J. Obstet. Gynaecol. **90**:841–846, 1983.

Jonas, E.G. and Caunt, A.E.: Clinical evaluation of human amnion tissue culture. Br. Med. J. **1**:898–901, 1965.

Jones, S.A. and Challis, J.R.: Local stimulation of prostaglandin production by corticotropin-releasing hormone in human fetal membranes and placenta. Biochem. Biophys. Res. Commun. **159**:192–199, 1989.

Jones, S.A., Brooks, A.N. and Challis, J.R.: Steroids modulate corticotropin-releasing hormone production in human fetal membranes and placenta. J. Clin. Endocrinol. Metab. **68**: 825–830, 1989.

Joseph, T.J. and Vogt, P.J.: Placental teratomas. Obstet. Gynecol. **41**:574–578, 1973.

Kakinuma, R., Shimizu, H. and Ogawa, Y.: Effect of meconium on the rate of in vitro subtype conversion of swine pulmonary surfactant. Europ. J. Pediatr. **161**:31–36, 2002.

Kallakury, B., Kelty, R., Ross, J.S. and Amyot, K.: Prevalence, histological characteristics and clinical significance of meconium in placentas (abstract 26). Modern Pathol. (Pediatr. Pathol.) **6**:5P, 1993.

Kalousek, D.: Amniotic band syndrome in previable fetuses. Pediatr. Pathol. **7**:488, 1987.

Kalousek, D.K. and Bamforth, S.: Amnion rupture sequence in previable fetuses. Amer. J. Med. Genet. **31**:63–73, 1988.

Kalousek, D.K. and Dill, F.J.: Chromosomal mosaicism confined to the placenta in human conceptions. Science **221**:665–667, 1983.

Kaltenbach, F.J. and Sachs, W.: The uptake of tritiated thymidine in human fetal membranes during the last third of pregnancy. Z. Geburtshilfe Perinatol. **183**:285–295, 1979.

Kanayama, N., Terao, T., Kawashima, Y., Horiuchi, K. and Fujimoto, D.: Collagen types in normal and prematurely ruptured amniotic membranes. Amer. J. Obstet. Gynecol. **153**:899–903, 1985.

Kaplan, C.: Placental pathology in perinatal disease. In, Gynecology and Obstetrics, Vol. 3. J.J. Sciarra, ed., pp. 1–21. Harper & Row, Hagerstown, 1980.

Kaplan, M.: Fetal breathing movements: an update for the pediatrician. Amer. J. Dis. Child. **137**:177–181, 1983.

Karimi-Nejad, M.H., Khajavi, H., Gharavi, M.J. and Karimi-Nejad, R.: Neu-Laxova syndrome: report of a case and comments. Amer. J. Med. Genet. **28**:17–23, 1987.

Karp, L.E. and Schiller, H.S.: Meconium staining of amniotic fluid at midtrimester amniocentesis. Obstet. Gynecol. **50**: 47s–49s, 1977.

Kaspar, H.G., Abu-Musa, A., Hannoun, A., Seoud, M., Shammas, M., Usta, I. and Khalil, A.: The placenta in meconium staining: lesions and early neonatal outcome. Clin. Exp. Obstet. Gynecol. **27**:63–66, 2000.

Katz, V.L. and Bowes, W.A.: Meconium aspiration syndrome: reflections on a murky subject. Amer. J. Obstet. Gynecol. **166**:171–183, 1992.

Kaufmann, P.: Entwicklung der Plazenta. In, Die Plazenta des Menschen. V. Becker, T.H. Schiebler and F. Kubli, eds. Thieme, Stuttgart, 1981.

Kearney, M.S.: Chronic intrauterine meconium aspiration causes fetal lung infarcts, lung rupture, and meconium embolism. Ped. Devel. Pathol. **2**:544–551, 1999.

Kearney, M.S. and Mortensen, E.: Intrauterine meconium aspiration in the second trimester fetus. Ped. Devel. Pathol. **3**: 394–403, 2000 (abstract).

Keene, D.R., Sakai, L.Y., Lunstrum, G.P., Morris, N.P. and Burgeson, R.E.: Type VII collagen forms an extended network of anchoring fibrils. J. Cell Biol. **104**:611–621, 1987.

Kilbride, H.W., Thibeault, D.W., Yeast, J., Maulik, D. and Grundy, H.O.: Fetal breathing is not a predictor of pulmonary hypoplasia in pregnancies complicated by oligohydramnios. Lancet **1**:305–306, 1988.

Kim, C.K., Naftolin, F. and Benirschke, K.: Immunohistochemical studies of the "X cell" in the human placenta with anti-human chorionic gonadotropin and anti-human placental lactogen. Am. J. Obstet. Gynecol. **111**:672–676, 1971.

King, B.F.: Developmental changes in the fine structure of rhesus monkey amnion. Amer. J. Anat. **157**:285–307, 1980.

King, B.F.: Developmental changes in the fine structure of the chorion laeve (smooth chorion) of the rhesus monkey placenta. Anat. Rec. **200**:163–175, 1981.

King, B.F.: Cell surface specializations and intercellular junctions in human amnionic epithelium: an electron microscopic and freeze-fracture study. Anat. Rec. **203**:73–82, 1982.

King, B.F.: Distribution and characterization of anionic sites in the basal lamina of developing human amniotic epithelium. Anat. Rec. **212**:57–62, 1985.

King, L.A., MacDonald, P.C. and Casey, M.L.: Regulation of metallothionein expression in human amnion epithelial and mesenchymal cells. Amer. J. Obstet. Gynecol. **177**:1496–1501, 1997.

Kino, Y.: Reductive malformations of the limbs in the rat fetus following amniocentesis. Congenital Anom. (Japan) **12**:35–44, 1972.

Kinoshita, K., Satoh, K. and Sakamoto, S.: Human amniotic membrane and prostaglandin biosynthesis. Biol. Res. Pregnancy Perinatol. **5**:61–67, 1984.

Kisalus, L.L. and Herr, J.C.: Immunocytochemical localization of heparan sulfate proteoglycan in human decidual cell secretory bodies and placental fibrinoid. Biol. Reprod. **39**:419–430, 1988.

Kisalus, L.L., Herr, J.C. and Little, C.D.: Immunolocalization of extracellular matrix proteins and collagen synthesis in first-trimester human decidua. Anat. Rec. **218**:402–415, 1987.

Kjaeldgaard, A., Pschera, H., Larsson, B., Gaffney, P. and Astedt, B.: Plasminogen activators and inhibitors in amniotic fluid. Fibrinolysis **3**:203–206, 1989.

Klima, G., Zerlauth, B., Richter, J. and Schmidt, W.: Die Mikrotextur von Amnion- und Chorionbindegewebe. Anat. Anz. (Jena) **168**:395–400, 1989.

Klima, G., Zerlauth, B., Wolf, H.J. and Schellnast, R.: A study of lectin bindings to the fetal membranes. Anat. Anz. (Jena) **173**:87–91, 1991.

Klinger, H.P. and Schwarzacher, H.G.: XY/XXY and sex chromatin positive cell distribution in a 60mm human fetus. Cytogenetics **1**:266–290, 1962.

Kohler, H.G.: An unusual case of sirenomelia. Teratology **6**: 295–302, 1972.

Kohler, H.G. and Collins, M.L.: Ligation of the umbilical cord by torn amniotic membrane. J. Obstet. Gynaecol. Br. Commonw. **79**:183–184, 1972.

Kowalewska-Kantecka, B.: Motilin in umbilical blood. Rocz. Akad. Med. Bialymstoku **40**:662–666, 1995.

Kratzsch, E. and Grygiel, I.-H.: †ber das Vorkommen eines spezifischen Enzyms der Glucuronsäurebildung im menschlichen Amnion. Z. Zellforsch. **123**:566–571, 1972.

Küster, J.: Adultes Teratom ("Dermoid") der Placenta. Arch. Gynäkol. **133**:93–99, 1928.

Lage, J.M., van Marter, L.J. and Bieber, F.R.: Questionable role of amniocentesis in the formation of amniotic bands. J. Reprod. Med. **33**:71–73, 1988.

Landing, B.H.: Amnion nodosum: a lesion of the placenta apparently associated with deficient secretion of fetal urine. Amer. J. Obstet. Gynecol. **60**:1339–1342, 1950a.

Landing, B.H.: The pathogenesis of amniotic-fluid embolism. N. Engl. J. Med. **243**:590–596, 1950b.

Laufer, A., Polishuk, W.Z., Boxer, J. and Ganzfried, R.: Studies of amniotic membranes. J. Reprod. Fertil. **12**:99–105, 1966.

Lauweryns, J., Bernat, R., Lerut, A. and Detournay, G.: Intrauterine pneumonia. An experimental study. Biol. Neonate. **22**:215–231, 1973.

Lavery, J.P. and Miller, C.E.: The viscoelastic nature of chorioamniotic membranes. Obstet. Gynecol. **50**:467–472, 1977.

Lavery, J.P., Miller, C.E. and Johns, P.: Effect of meconium on the strength of chorioamniotic membranes. Obstet. Gynecol. **56**:711–715, 1980.

Lavery, J.P., Miller, E. and Knight, R.D.: The effect of labor on the rheologic response of chorioamniotic membranes. Obstet. Gynecol. **60**:87–92, 1982.

Leary, O.C. and Hertig, A.T.: Pathogenesis of amniotic fluid embolism. I. Possible placental factors-aberrant squamous cells in placenta. NEJM **243**:588–590, 1950.

Legge, M.: Dark brown amniotic fluid-identification of contributing pigments. Br. J. Obstet. Gynaecol. **88**:632–634, 1981.

Lei, H., Furth, E.E., Kalluri, R., Chiou, T., Tilly, K.I., Elkon, K.B., Jeffrey, J.J. and Strauss, J.F.: A program of cell death and extracellular matrix degradation is activated in the amnion before onset of labor. J. Clin. Invest. **96**:1971–1978, 1996.

Leivo, I. and Engvall, E.: C3d fragment of complement interacts with laminin and binds to basement membranes of glomerulus and trophoblast. J. Cell Biol. **103**:1091–1100, 1986.

Lembel, A., Gaddipati, R., Gordon, R., Selam, B., Berkowitz, R.I. and Salafia, C.: Meconium induced vascular smooth muscle necrosis: timing and ultrastructure. Amer. J. Obstet. Gynecol. **182**:abstract 442, 2000.

Levick, K.: Pregnancy loss and fathers with Ehlers-Danlos syndrome. Lancet **II**:1151, 1989.

Lewis, M.P., Clements, M., Takeda, S., Kirby, P.L., Seki, H., Lonsdale, L.B., Sullivan, M.H.F., Elder, M.G. and White, J.O.: Partial characterization of an immortalized human trophoblast cell-line, TCL-1, which possesses a CSF-1 autocrine loop. Placenta **17**:137–146, 1996.

Linnala, A., Balza, E., Zardi, L. and Virtanen, I.: Human amnion epithelial cells assemble tenascins and three fibronectin isoforms in the extracellular matrix. FEBS Lett. **317**:74–78, 1993.

Linton, G. and Lilford, R.J.: False-negative finding on chorionic villus sampling. Lancet **2**:630, 1986.

Liotta, L.A., Lee, C.W. and Morakis, D.J.: New method for preparing large surfaces of intact human basement membrane for tumor invasion studies. Cancer Lett. **11**:141–152, 1980.

Lister, U.M.: Ultrastructure of the human amnion, chorion and fetal skin. J. Obstet. Gynaecol. Br. Commonw. **75**:327–341, 1968.

Lloyd, S.J., Garlid, K.D., Reba, R.C. and Seeds, A.E.: Permeability of different layers of the human placenta to isotopic water. J. Appl. Physiol. **26**:274–276, 1969.

Lockwood, C., Ghidini, A. and Romero, R.: Amniotic band syndrome in monozygotic twins: prenatal diagnosis and pathogenesis. Obstet. Gynecol. **71**:1012–1016, 1988.

Lockwood, C., Ghidini, A., Romero, R. and Hobbins, J.C.: Amniotic band syndrome: reevaluation of its pathogenesis. Amer. J. Obstet. Gynecol. **160**:1030–1033, 1989.

Lockwood, C.J., Bach, R., Guha, A., Zhou, X., Miller, W.A. and Nemerson, Y.: Amniotic fluid contains tissue factor, a potent initiator of coagulation. Am. J. Obstet. Gynecol. **165**: 1335–1341, 1991.

Longo, S., Towers, C., Strauss, A., Asrat, T. and Freeman, R.: Meconium has no L or S but affects the L/S ratio. Amer. J. Obstet. Gynecol. **174**:383 (abstract), 1996.

Lopez Bernal, A., Hansell, D.J., Khong, T.Y., Keeling, J.W. and Turnbull, A.C.: Prostaglandin E production by the fetal membranes in unexplained preterm labour and preterm labour associated with chorioamnionitis. Br. J. Obstet. Gynaecol. **96**:1133–1139, 1989.

Lubinsky, M., Sujansky, E., Sanger, W., Salyards, P. and Severn, C.: Familial amniotic bands. Amer. J. Med. Genet. **14**:81–87, 1983.

Lucas, A., Christofides, N.D., Adrian, T.E., Bloom, S.R. and Aynsley-Green, A.: Fetal distress, meconium, and motilin. Lancet **1**:718, 1979a.

Lucas, A., Adrian, T.E., Aynsley-Green, A. and Bloom, S.R.: Gut hormones in fetal distress. Lancet 2:968, 1979b.

Luckett, P.: The origin of extraembryonic mesoderm in the early human and rhesus monkey embryos. Anat. Rec. 169:369–370, 1971.

Luckett, W.P.: Amniogenesis in the early human and rhesus monkey embryos. Anat. Rec. 175:375, 1973.

Ludwig, H., Metzger, H., Korte, M. and Wolf, H.: Die freie Oberfläche des Amnionepithels. Rasterelektronenmikroskopische Studie. Arch. Gynäkol. 217:141–154, 1974.

Luna, L.G., ed.: Luna-Ishak stain. In, Manual of Histologic Staining Methods of the Armed Forces Institute of Pathology, 3rd Ed., pp. 74–75. McGraw-Hill Book New York, 1968.

MacLachlan, T.B.: A method for the investigation of the strength of the fetal membranes. Amer. J. Obstet. Gynecol. 91:309–313, 1965.

Macri, C.J., Schrimmer, D.B., Leung, A., Greenspoon, J.S. and Paul, R.H.: Prophylactic amnioinfusion improves outcome of pregnancy complicated by thick meconium and oligohydramnios. Am. J. Obstet. Gynecol. 167:117–121, 1992.

Madri, J.A, Williams, S.K., Wyatt, T. and Mezzio, C.: Capillary endothelial cell cultures: phenotypic modulation by matrix components. J. Cell Biol. 97:153–165, 1983.

Maher, J.E., Wenstrom, K.D., Hauth, J.C. and Meis, P.J.: Amniotic fluid embolism after saline amnioinfusion: two cases and review of the literature. Obstet. Gynecol. 83:851–854, 1994.

Mahieu-Caputo, D., Muller, F., Jouvet, P., Thalabard, J.C., Jouannic, J.M., Nihoul-Fekete, C., Dumez, Y. and Dommergues, M.: Amniotic fluid beta-endorphin: a prognostic marker for gastroschisis? J. Pediatr. Surg. 37:1602–1606, 2004.

Mahmoud, E.L., Benirschke, K., Vaucher, Y.E. and Poitras, P.: Motilin levels in term neonates who have passed meconium prior to birth. J. Pediatr. Gastroenterol. Nutr. 7:95–99, 1988.

Mahony, B.S., Filly, R.A., Callen, P.W. and Golbus, M.S.: The amniotic band syndrome: antenatal sonographic diagnosis and potential pitfalls. Amer. J. Obstet. Gynecol. 152:63–68, 1985.

Malak, T.M. and Bell, S.C.: Distribution of fibrillin-containing microfibrils and elastin in human fetal membranes: a novel molecular basis for membrane elasticity. Amer. J. Obstet. Gynecol. 171:195–205, 1994a.

Malak, T.M. and Bell, S.C.: Structural characteristics of term human fetal membranes: a novel zone of extreme morphological alterations within the rupture site. Br. J. Obstet. Gynaecol. 101:375–386, 1994b.

Malak, T.M. and Bell, S.C.: Fetal membranes structure and prelabour rupture. Fetal Matern. Med. Rev. 8:143–164, 1996.

Malak, T.M., Ockleford, C.D., Bell, S.C., Dalgleish, R., Bright, N. and MacVicar, J.: Confocal immunofluorescence localization of collagen type-I, type-III, type-IV, type-V and type-VI and their ultrastructural organization in term human fetal membranes. Placenta 14:385–406, 1993.

Manabe, Y., Himeno, N. and Fukumoto, M.: Tensile strength and collagen content of amniotic membrane do not change after the second trimester or during delivery. Obstet. Gynecol. 78:24–27, 1991.

Manchanda, R., Vora, M. and Gruslin, A.: Influence of postdatism and meconium on fetal erythropoietin. J. Perinatol. 19:479–482, 1999.

Mann, S.E., Nijland, M.J.M. and Ross, M.G.: Mathematic modeling of human amniotic fluid dynamics. Amer. J. Obstet. Gynecol. 175:937–944, 1996.

Mann, S.E., Ricke, E.A., Yang, B.A., Verkman, A.S. and Taylor, R.N.: Expression and localization of aquaporin 1 and 3 in human fetal membranes. Amer. J. Obstet. Gynecol. 187:902–907, 2002.

Maradny, E.E.: Urinary trypsin inhibitor has a protective effect on the amnion. Gynecol. Obstet. Invest. 38:169–172, 1994.

Martinez-Frias, M.L.: Clinical and epidemiological characteristics of infants with body wall complex with and without limb deficiency. Amer. J. Med. Genet. 73:170–175, 1997a.

Martinez-Frias, M.L.: Epidemiological characteristics of amnionic band sequence (ABS) and body wall complex (BWC): are they two different entities? Amer. J. Med. Genet. 73:176–179, 1997b.

Masson, J.C., Philippe, E., Korn, R., Irrmann, M., Dehalleux, J.M. and Gandar, R.: Amnion nodosum. Rev. Fr. Gynécol. Obstét. 61:701–707, 1966.

Matsubara, S. and Tamada, T.: Ultracytochemical study of the permeability of the human amniotic epithelium. Acta Obstet. Gynaecol. Jpn. 43:641–646, 1991.

Mazor, M., Furman, B., Wiznitzer, A., Shoham-Vardi, I., Cohen, J. and Ghezzi, F.: Maternal and perinatal outcome of patients with preterm labor and meconium-stained amniotic fluid. Obstet. Gynecol. 86:830–833, 1995.

McCoshen, J.A., Tulloch, H.V., Johnson, K. and Odowichuk, C.: Evidence of a differential chorionic influence on prostaglandin E2 release by human amnion before and after term labour. Placenta 7:479, 1986.

McGregor, J.A., French, J.I., Lawellin, D., Franco-Buff, A., Smith, C. and Todd, J.K.: Bacterial protease-induced reduction of chorioamniotic membrane strength and elasticity. Obstet. Gynecol. 69:167–174, 1987.

McParland, P.C., Taylor, D.J. and Bell, S.C.: Mapping of zones of altered morphology and chorionic connective tissue cellular phenotype in human fetal membranes (amniochorion and decidua) overlying the lower uterine pole and cervix before labor at term. Amer. J. Obstet. Gynecol. 189:1481–1488, 2003.

Mercer, L.J. and Brown, L.G.: Fetal outcome with oligohydramnios in the second trimester. Obstet. Gynecol. 67:840–842, 1986.

Meirowitz, N.B., Smulian, J.C., Hahn, R.A., Zhou, P., Shen-Schwarz, S., Lambert, G.H., Gerecke, D. and Gordon, M.K.: Collagen messenger RNA expression in the human amniochorion in premature rupture of membranes. Amer. J. Obstet. Gynecol. 187:1679–1685, 2002.

Metz, J., Weihe, E. and Heinrich, D.: Intercellular junctions in the full term human placenta. I. Syncytiotrophoblastic layer. Anat. Embryol. (Basel) 158:41–50, 1979.

Meudt, R.: Beitrag zur Festigkeit der menschlichen Eihaut. Gynaecologia 162:430–434, 1966.

Michael, H., Ulbright, T.M. and Brodhecker, C.: Magma reticulare-like differentiation in yolk sac tumor and its pluripotential nature. Mod. Pathol. 1:63A, 1988.

Millar, L.K., Stollberg, J., DeBuque, L. and Bryant-Greenwood, G.: Fetal membrane distention: Determination of the intrauterine surface area and distention of the fetal membranes preterm and at term. Amer. J. Obstet. Gynecol. 182:128–134, 2000.

Miller, P.W., Coen, R.W. and Benirschke, K.: Dating the time interval from meconium passage to birth. Obstet. Gynecol. **66**:459–462, 1985.

Mitchell, M.D.: Sources of eicosanoids within the uterus during pregnancy. In, The Onset of Labor: Cellular and Integrative Mechanisms. D. McNellis, ed., pp. 165–181. Perinatology Press, Ithaca, 1988.

Mitchell, J., Schulman, H., Fleischer, A., Farmakides, G. and Nadeau, D.: Meconium aspiration and fetal acidosis. Obstet. Gynecol. **65**:352–355, 1985.

Modesti, A., Kalebic, T., Scarpa, S., Togo, S., Grotendorst, G., Liotta, L.A. and Triche, T.J.: Type V collagen in human amnion is a 12-nm fibrillar component of the pericellular interstitium. Eur. J. Cell Biol. **35**:246–255, 1984.

Moerman, P., Fryns, J.-P., Vandenberghe, K. and Lauweryns, J.M.: Constrictive amniotic bands, amniotic adhesions, and limb-body wall complex: discrete disruption sequences with pathogenetic overlap. Am. J. Med. Genet. **42**:470–479, 1992.

Moessinger, A.C., Blanc, W.A., Byrne, J., Andrews, D., Warburton, D. and Bloom, A.: Amniotic bank syndrome associated with amniocentesis. Amer. J. Obstet. Gynecol. **141**:588–591, 1981.

Moirot, H., Thomine, E., Martin, M., Labadie, C., Fessard, C., Ensel, P., Pellerin, A., Ducastelle, T., Hemet, J., Bourreille, M.C. and Boullie, M.C.: Amniotic anomalies and lamellar ichthyosis. A case report (abstract). In, Placental Communication: Biochemical, Morphological and Cellular Aspects. L. Cedard, E. Alsat, J.C. Challier, G. Chaouat and A. Malassine, eds. INSERM, Libbey Eurotext **199**:281, 1990.

Morhaime, J.L., Park, K., Benirschke, K. and Baergen, R.N.: Disappearance of meconium pigment in placental specimens on exposure to light. Arch. Pathol. Lab. Med. **127**:711–714, 2003.

Mühlhauser, J., Crescimanno, C., Rajaniemi, H., Parkkila, S., Castellucci, M., Milovanov, A.S. and Kaufmann, P.: Immuno-histochemistry of carbonic anhydrase in the human placenta and fetal membranes. Histochemistry **101**:91–98, 1994.

Muir, R. and Niven, J.S.F.: The local formation of blood pigments. J. Pathol. **41**:183–197, 1935.

Mukaida, T., Yoshida, K., Kikyokawa, T. and Soma, H.: Surface structure of the placental membranes. J. Clin. Electron Microsc. **10**:447–448, 1977.

Naeye, R.L.: Factors that predispose to premature rupture of the fetal membranes. Obstet. Gynecol. **60**:93–98, 1982.

Nanbu, Y., Fujii, S., Konishi, I., Nonogaki, H. and Mori, T.: CA 125 in the epithelium closely related to the embryonic ecto-derm: the periderm and the amnion. Amer. J. Obstet. Gynecol. **161**:462–467, 1989.

Nathan, L., Leveno, K.J., Carmody, T.J., Kelly, M.A. and Sherman, M.L.: Meconium: a 1990s perspective on an old obstetric hazard. Obstet. Gynecol. **83**:329–332, 1994.

Nemeth, E., Tashima, L.S., Yu, Z. and Bryant-Greenwood, G.D.: Fetal membrane distention. I. Differentially expressed genes regulated by acute distention in amniotic epithelial (WISH) cells. Amer. J. Obstet. Gynecol. **182**:50–59, 2000a.

Nemeth, E., Tashima, L.S., Yu, Z. and Bryant-Greenwood, G.D.: Fetal membrane distention. II. Differentially expressed genes regulated by acute distention in vitro. Amer. J. Obstet. Gynecol. **182**:60–67, 2000b.

Nickell, K.A. and Stocker, J.T.: Placental teratoma: a case report. Pediatr. Pathol. **7**:645–650, 1987.

Nieland, M.L., Parmley, T.H. and Woodruff, J.D.: Ultrastructural observations on amniotic fluid cells. Amer. J. Obstet. Gynecol. **108**:1030–1042, 1970.

Nolan, D.G., Martin, L.S., Natarajan, S. and Hume, R.F.: Fetal compromise associated with extreme fetal bile acidemia and maternal primary sclerosing cholangitis. Obstet. Gynecol. **84**:695–695, 1994.

Novak, R. and Kokomoor, F.: Placental pathology of meconium-stained premature infants (abstract 35). Mod. Pathol. **1**:7p, 1988.

Nyberg, D.A., Mahony, B.S. and Pretorius, D.H.: Diagnostic Ultrasound of Fetal Anomalies: Text and Atlas. Year Book, Chicago, 1990.

Ockleford, C.D., Malak, T., Hubbard, A., Bracken, K., Burton, S.A., Bright, N., Blakey, G., Goodliffe, J., Garrod, D. and d'Lacey, C.: Human amniochorion cytoskeletons at term. Placenta **14**:A56, 1993.

Ockleford, C., Bright, N., Hubbard, A., d'Lacey, C., Smith, J., Gardiner, L., Sheikh, T., Albentosa, M. and Turtle, K.: Micro-trabeculae, macro-plaques or mini-basement membranes in human term fetal membranes. Philos. Trans. R. Soc. Lond. B **342**:121–136, 1994.

Ohyama, M., Ogasawara, M., Itani, Y., Ijiri, R., Tanaka, Y. and Hori, K.: Letter to the editors. [On neonatal death with ulcer-ated cord]. Europ. J. Obstet. Gynecol. Reprod. Biol. **87**:101, 1999.

Ohyama, M., Itani, Y., Yamanaka, M., Imaizumi, K., Nishi, T., Ijiri, R. and Tanaka, Y.: Umbilical cord ulcer: a serious in utero complication of intestinal atresia. Placenta **21**:432–435, 2000.

Okamoto, E., Takagi, T., Azuma, C., Kimura, T., Tokugawa, Y., Mitsuda, N., Saji, F. and Tanizawa, O.: Expression of the cor-ticotropin-releasing hormone (CRH) gene in human placenta and amniotic membrane. Horm. Metab. Res. **22**:394–397, 1990.

Okazaki, T., Casey, M.L., Okita, J.R., MacDonald, P.C. and Johnston, J.M.: Initiation of human parturition. XII. Biosynthesis and metabolism of prostaglandins in human fetal membranes and uterine decidua. Am. J. Obstet. Gynecol. **139**:373–381, 1981a.

Okazaki, T., Sagawa, N., Bleasdale, J.E., Okita, J.R., MacDonald, P.C. and Johnston, J.M.: Initiation of human parturition: XIII. Phospholipase C, phospholipase A2, and diacylglycerol lipase activities in fetal membranes and decidua vera tissues from early and late gestation. Biol. Reprod. **25**:103–109, 1981b.

Oláh, K.S., Gee, H., Rushton, I. and Fowlie, A.: Massive subcho-rionic thrombohaematoma presenting as a placental tumor. A case report. Br. J. Obstet. Gynaecol. **94**:995–997, 1987.

Olson, D.M. and Smieja, Z.: Arachidonic acid incorporation into lipids of term human amnion. Am. J. Obstet. Gynecol. **159**:995–1001, 1988.

Olson, D.M., Skinner, K. and Challis, J.R.: Prostaglandin output in relation to parturition by cells dispersed from human intrauterine tissues. J. Clin. Endocrinol. Metab. **57**:694–699, 1983.

Opitz, H. and Bernoth, E.: Strukturuntersuchungen der mensch-lichen Eihaut nach vor- und rechtzeitigem Blasensprung. Arch. Gynäkol. **196**:435–446, 1962.

Ostrea, E.M. and Naqvi, M.: The influence of gestational age on the ability of the fetus to pass meconium in utero: clinical implications. Acta Obstet. Gynecol. Scand. **61**:275–277, 1982.

Panayiotis, G. and Grunstein, S.: Extramembranous pregnancy in twin gestation. Obstet. Gynecol. **53**:34S–35S, 1979.

Paterson, W.G., Grant, K.A., Grant, J.M. and McLean, N.: The pathogenesis of amniotic fluid embolism with particular reference to transabdominal amniocentesis. Eur. J. Obstet. Gynecol. Reprod. Biol. **7**:319–324, 1977.

Patten, R.M., Allen, M.V., Mack, L.A., Wilson, D., Nyberg, D., Hirsch, J. and Viamont, T.: Limb-body wall complex: in utero sonographic diagnosis of a complicated fetal malformation. Amer. J. Radiol. **146**:1019–1024, 1986.

Patterson, T.J.S.: Amniotic bands. In, The Human Amnion and Chorion. Bourne, G.L., ed. Lloyd-Luke, London, 1962, pp. 250–264.

Pearlstone, M. and Baxi, L.: Subchorionic hematoma: a review. Obstet. Gynecol. Surv. **48**:65–68, 1993.

Pedersen, J.F. and Mantoni, M.: Prevalence and significance of subchorionic hemorrhage in threatened abortion: a sonographic study. AJR **154**:535–537, 1990.

Perlman, M., Tennenbaum, A., Menash, M. and Ornoy, A.: Extramembranous pregnancy: maternal, placental, and perinatal implications. Obstet. Gynecol. **55**:34S–37S, 1980.

Petry, G.: Die Bedeutung der Embryonalhüllen bei der Frage nach der Herkunft alkalischer Phosphatase im menschlichen Fruchtwasser. Z. Geburtshilfe Gynäkol. **158**:171–180, 1962.

Phelan, J.P. and Ahn, M.O.: Perinatal observations in forty-eight neurologically impaired term infants. Amer. J. Obstet. Gynecol. **171**:424–431, 1994.

Phelan, J.P., Ahn, M.O., Kirkendall, C. and Lee, F.: Meconium is not a sign of fetal distress. Obstet. Gynecol. **93**:23S, 1999.

Philippe, E., Dourov, N., Muller, P. and Fruhling, L.: Le substratum morphologique de l'embolie amniotique. A propos de deux observations d'incoagulabilité sanguine par embolie amniotique. Ann. Anat. Pathol. **6**:479–496, 1961.

Pilgram, H.: Die Zotten und Karunkeln des menschlichen Amnion. Marburg, **1889**. [Cited by Blanc et al. (1962).]

Platt, L.D., DeVore, G.R. and Gimovsky, M.L.: Failed amniocentesis: the role of membrane tenting. Amer. J. Obstet. Gynecol. **144**:479–480, 1982.

Poggi, S., Leak, N., Ghidini, A., Hodor, J., Meck, J. and Salafia, C.: Meconium staining of placenta may be later than conventionally thought. Amer. J. Obstet. Gynecol. **189**: abstract 483, 2003.

Poisner, A.M., Wood, G.W., Poisner, R. and Inagami, T.: Localization of renin in trophoblasts in human chorion laeve at term pregnancy. Endocrinology **109**:1150–1155, 1981.

Polano, O.: Beiträge zur Anatomie und Physiologie des menschlichen Amnions. Z. Anat. Entwicklungsgesch. **63**:539–553, 1922.

Polet, H.: The effect of hydrocortisone on the membranes of primary human amnion cells in vitro. Exp. Cell Res. **41**: 316–323, 1966.

Polishuk, W.Z., Konhane, S. and Peranio, A.: The physical properties of fetal membranes. Obstet. Gynecol. **20**:204–210, 1962.

Polishuk, W.Z., Kohane, S. and Hader, A.: Fetal weight and membrane tensile strength. Amer. J. Obstet. Gynecol. **20**: 204–250, 1964.

Polishuk, W.Z., Boxer, J. and Granzfried, R.: Lipid in amniotic membranes. Amer. J. Obstet. Gynecol. **91**:61–64, 1965.

Pomerance, W., Biezenski, J.J., Moltz, A. and Goodman, J.: Origin of amniotic fluid lipids. II. Abnormal pregnancy. Obstet. Gynecol. **38**:379–382, 1971.

Porreco, R.P., Young, P.E., Resnik, R., Cousins, L., Jones, O.W., Richards, T., Kernahan, C. and Matson, M.: Reproductive outcome following amniocentesis for genetic indications. Amer. J. Obstet. Gynecol. **143**:653–660, 1982.

Pritchard, E.T., Armstrong, W.D. and Wilt, J.C.: Examination of lipids from amnion, chorion, and vernix. Amer. J. Obstet. Gynecol. **100**:289–298, 1968.

Prusa, A.-R., Marton, E., Rosner, M., Bettelheim, D., Lubec, G., Pollack, A., Bernaschek, G. and Hengstschläger, M.: Neurogenic cells in human amniotic fluid. Amer. J. Obstet. Gynecol. **191**:309–314, 2004.

Pysher, T.J.: Discordant congenital malformations in monozygous twins. The amniotic bank disruption complex. Diagn. Gynecol. Obstet. **2**:221–225, 1980.

Queenan, J.T., Thompson, W., Whitfield, C.R. and Shah, S.I.: Amniotic fluid volumes in normal pregnancies. Amer. J. Obstet. Gynecol. **114**:34–38, 1972.

Rajabi, M.R., Dean, D.D. and Woessner, J.F.: Changes in active and latent collagenase in human placenta around time of parturition. Amer. J. Obstet. Gynecol. **163**:499–505, 1990.

Randel, S.B., Filly, R.A., Callen, P.W., Anderson, R.L. and Golbus, M.S.: Amniotic sheets. Radiology **166**:633–636, 1988.

Rao, C.V. and Lei, Z.M.: The presence of gonadotropin receptors in human placenta, amnion, chorion and decidua. Placenta **10**:458, 1989.

Rao, C.V., Carman, F.R., Chegini, N. and Schultz, G.S.: Binding sites for epidermal growth factor in human fetal membranes. J. Clin. Endocrinol. Metab. **58**:1034–1042, 1984.

Rao, S., Pavlova, Z., Incerpi, M.H. and Ramanathan, R.: Meconium-stained amniotic fluid and neonatal morbidity in near-term and term deliveries with acute histologic chorioamnionitis and/or funisitis. J. Perinatol. **21**:537–540, 2001.

Rapoport, S. and Buchanan, D.J.: The composition of meconium: isolation of blood group specific polysaccharides, abnormal composition of meconium in meconium ileus. Science **112**:150–153, 1950.

Rastan, S., Kaufman, M.H., Handyside, A.H. and Lyon, M.F.: X-chromosome inactivation in extraembryonic membranes of diploid parthenogenetic mouse embryos demonstrated by differential staining. Nature (Lond.) **288**:172–173, 1980.

Reale, E., Wang, T., Zaccheo, D., Maganza, C. and Pescetto, G.: Junctions on the maternal blood surface of the human placental syncytium. Placenta **1**:245–258, 1980.

Redline, R.W. and O'Riordan, M.A.: Placental lesions associated with cerebral palsy and neurologic impairment following term birth. Arch. Pathol. Lab. Med. **124**:1785–1791, 2000.

Redmond, A.D.: Amnion dressing. Lancet **1**:902, 1984.

Rees, M.C.P., di Marzo, V., Lopez Bernal, A., Tippins, J.R., Morris, H.R. and Turnbull, A.C.: Leukotriene release by human fetal membranes, placenta and decidua in relation to parturition. J. Endocrinol. **118**:497–500, 1988.

Rehder, H. and Weitzel, H.: Intrauterine amputations after amniocentesis. Lancet **1**:382, 1978.

Reisfield, D.R.: Congenital defect in the fetal membranes: a condition simulating spontaneous rupture. Bull. Sloane Hosp. Women **4**:16–18, 1958.

Reshef, E., Lei, Z.M., Rao, C.V., Pridham, D.D., Chegini, N. and Luborsky, J.L.: The presence of gonadotropin receptors in nonpregnant human uterus, human placenta, fetal membranes, and decidua. J. Clin. Endocrinol. Metab. **70**:421–430, 1990.

Resnik, R., Swartz, W.H., Plumer, M.H., Benirschke, K. and Stratthaus, M.E.: Amniotic fluid embolism with survival. Obstet. Gynecol. **47**:295–298, 1976.

Richey, S.D., Ramin, S.M., Bawdon, R.E., Roberts, S.W., Dax, J., Roberts, J. and Gilstrap, L.C.: Markers of acute and chronic asphyxia in infants with meconium-stained amniotic fluid. Amer. J. Obstet. Gynecol. **172**:1212–1215, 1995.

Robb, S.A. and Hytten, F.E.: Placental glycogen. Br. J. Obstet. Gynaecol. **83**:43–53, 1976.

Roberts, J.S., McCraken, J.A., Gavagan, J.E. and Soloff, M.S.: Oxytocin-stimulated release of prostaglandin $F_{2\alpha}$ from ovine endometrium in vitro: correlation with estrous cycle and oxytocin-receptor binding. Endocrinology **99**:1107–1114, 1976.

Rogers, B.B., Widness, J.A., Coustan, D.R. and Singer, D.B.: Fetal acidosis and placental pathology (abstract 498). Mod. Pathol. **3**(1):85A, 1990.

Romero, R., Hanaoka, S., Mazor, M., Athanassiadis, A.P., Callahan, R., Hsu, Y.C., Avila, C., Nores, J. and Jimenez, C.: Meconium-stained amniotic fluid: a risk factor for microbial invasion of the amniotic cavity. Amer. J. Obstet. Gynecol. **164**:859–862, 1991.

Ropers, H.H., Wolff, G. and Hitzeroth, H.W.: Preferential X inactivation in human placenta membranes: is the paternal X inactive in early embryonic development of female mammals? Hum. Genet. **43**:265–273, 1978.

Rossant, J. and Croy, B.A.: Genetic identification of tissue of origin of cellular populations within the mouse placenta. J. Embryol. Exp. Morphol. **86**:177–189, 1985.

Rote, N.S., Menon, R., Swan, K.F., Lyden, T.W. and Fortunato, S.J.: Expression of IL-1b and IL-6 protein and mRNA in amniochorionic membrane. Placenta **14**:A63, 1993.

Rubovits, W.H., Taft, E. and Neuwelt, F.: The pathologic properties of meconium. Amer. J. Obstet. Gynecol. **36**:501–505, 1938.

Sakbun, V., Ali, S.M., Greenwood, F.C. and Bryant-Greenwood, G.D.: Human relaxin in the amnion, chorion, decidua parietalis, basal plate, and placental trophoblast by immunocytochemistry and northern analysis. J. Clin. Endocrinol. Metab. **70**:508–514, 1990a.

Sakbun, V., Ali, S.M., Lee, Y.A., Jara, C.S. and Bryant-Greenwood, G.D.: Immunocytochemical localization and messenger ribonucleic acid concentrations for human placental lactogen in amnion, chorion, decidua, and placenta. Am. J. Obstet. Gynecol. **162**:1310–1317, 1990b.

Sala, M.A. and Matheus, M.: Histochemical study of the fetal membranes in the human term pregnancy. Gegenbaurs Morphol. Jahrb. **130**:699–705, 1984.

Salazar, H., Kanbour, A.I. and Pardo. M.: Amnion nodosum. Ultrastructure and histopathogenesis. Arch. Pathol. **98**:39–46, 1974.

Santiago-Schwarz, F. and Fleit, H.B.: Identification of nonadherent mononuclear cells in human cord blood that differentiate into macrophages. J. Leukocyte Biol. **43**:51–59, 1988.

Schindler, A.E.: Hormones in human amniotic fluid. Monogr. Endocrinol. **21**:1–158, 1982.

Schindler, P.D.: Nuclear deoxyribonucleic acid (DNA) content, nuclear size and cell size in the human amnion epithelium. Acta Anat. (Basel) **44**:273–285, 1961.

Schmidt, W.: Der Feinbau der reifen menschlichen Eihäute. Z. Anat. Entwicklungsgesch. **119**:203–222, 1956.

Schmidt, W.: Struktur und Funktion des Amnionepithels von Menschen und Huhn. Z. Zellforsch. **61**:642–660, 1963.

Schmidt, W.: Untersuchungen zur Frage des paraplazentaren Stofftransportes beim Menschen. Anat. Anz. **115**:161–163, 1965a.

Schmidt, W.: Über den paraplacentaren, fruchtwassergebundenen Stofftransport beim Menschen. I. Histochemische Untersuchung der in den Eihäuten angereicherten Stoffe. Z. Anat. Entwicklungsgesch. **124**:321–334, 1965b.

Schmidt, W.: Über den paraplacentaren, fruchtwassergebundenen Stofftransport beim Menschen. II. Nachweis der vom Amnion abgegebenen Lipide im Fruchtwasser und im Dünndarm des Keimes. Z. Anat. Entwicklungsgesch. **126**: 276–288, 1967.

Schmidt, W.: The amniotic fluid compartment: the fetal habitat. Adv. Anat. Embryol. Cell Biol. **127**:1–100, 1992.

Schmidt, W., Eberhagen, D. and Svejcar, J.: Über den paraplazentaren, fruchtwassergebundenen Stofftransport beim Menschen. III. Quantitative und qualitative Analyse der im Fruchtwasser enthaltenen Stoffe. Z. Anat. Entwicklungsgesch. **135**:210–221, 1971.

Schulze, B., Schlesinger, C.H. and Miller, K.: Chromosomal mosaicism confined to chorionic tissue. Prenatal Diagn. **7**:451–453, 1987.

Schwarzacher, H.G.: Beitrag zur Histogenese des menschlichen Amnion. Acta Anat. (Basel) **43**:303–311, 1960.

Schwarzacher, H.G. and Klinger, H.P.: Die Entstehung mehrkerniger Zellen durch Amitose in Amnionepithel des Menschen und die Aufteilung des chromosomalen Materials auf deren einzelne Kerne. Z. Zellforsch. **60**: 741–754, 1963.

Scott, H., Walker, M. and Gruslin, A.: Significance of meconium-stained amniotic fluid in the preterm population. J. Perinatol. **21**:174–177, 2001.

Seeds, A.E., Eichhorst, B.C. and Stolee, A.: Factors determining human chorion laeve permeability in vitro. Am. J. Obstet. Gynecol. **128**:13–21, 1977.

Seeds, J.W., Cefalo, R.C. and Herbert, W.N.P.: Amniotic band syndrome. Amer. J. Obstet. Gynecol. **144**:243–248, 1982.

Seidman, J.D., Abbondanzo, S.L., Watkin, W.G., Ragsdale, B. and Manz, H.J.: Amniotic band syndrome: report of two cases and review of the literature. Arch. Pathol. Lab. Med. **113**:891–897, 1989.

Sepkowitz, S.: Influence of the legal imperative and medical guidelines on the incidence and management of the meconium-stained newborn. Amer. J. Dis. Child. **141**:1124–1127, 1987.

Sepúlveda, W.H., Gonzalez, C., Cruz, M.A. and Rudolph, M.I.: Vasoconstrictive effect of bile acids on isolated human placental chorionic veins. Eur. J. Obstet. Gynecol. Reprod. Biol. **42**:211–215, 1991.

Shanklin, D.R. and Scott, J.S.: Massive subchorial thrombohaematoma (Breus' mole). Br. J. Obstet. Gynaecol. **82**:476–487, 1975.

Shareef, M.J., Lawlor-Klean, P., Kelly, K.A., LaMear, N.A. and Schied, M.J.: Collodion baby: a case report. J. Perinatol. **4**: 267–269, 2000.

Shephard, T.H., Fantel, A.G., Fujinaga, M. and Fitzsimmons, J.: Amniotic band disruption syndrome: why do their faces look alike? (abstract). Congenital Anom. (Japan) **37**:491–492, 1988.

Shimizu, T., Dudley, D.K.L., Borodchack, P., Belcher, J., Perkins, S.L. and Gibb, W.: Effect of smoking on fibronectin production by human amnion and placenta. Gynecol. Obstet. Invest. **34**:142–145, 1992.

Shipp, T.D., Genest, D. and Benacerraf, B.R.: A case of fetal decapitation. J. Ultrasound Med. **15**:535–537, 1996.

Sieber-Blum, M. and Grim, M.: The adult hair follicle: Cradle for pluripotent neural crest stem dells. Birth Defects Res. (Part C) **72**:162–172, 2004.

Sienko, A. and Altshuler, G.: Meconium-induced umbilical vascular necrosis in abortuses and fetuses: a histopathologic study for cytokines. Obstet. Gynecol. **94**:415–420, 1999.

Silver, M.M., Thurston, W.A. and Patrick, J.E.: Perinatal pulmonary hyperplasia due to laryngeal atresia. Hum. Pathol. **19**:110–113, 1988.

Singh, G. and Singh, S.: Hemorrhage induced by amniocentesis and vascular clamping in the limbs of rat fetuses. Congenital Anom. (Japan) **18**:89–93, 1978.

Singhas, C.A.: Lectin histochemistry of the human amniochorionic membrane complex. Placenta **13**:523–534, 1992.

Sinha, A.A.: Ultrastructure of human amnion and amniotic plaques of normal pregnancy. Z. Zellforsch. **122**:1–14, 1971.

Skinner, K.A. and Challis, J.R.: Changes in the synthesis and metabolism of prostaglandins by human fetal membranes and decidua at labor. Amer. J. Obstet. Gynecol. **151**:519–523, 1985.

Skinner, S.J., Campos, G.A. and Liggins, G.C.: Collagen content of human amniotic membranes: effect of gestation length and premature rupture. Obstet. Gynecol. **57**:487–489, 1981.

Smadja, A., Hoang Ngoc Minh and Nguyen, T.L.: Conception nouvelle sur la physiologie de la circulation amniotique. Rev. Fr. Gynécol. **69**:111–114, 1974.

Smieja, Z., Zakar, T., Walton, J.C. and Olson, D.M.: Prostaglandin endoperoxide synthase kinetics in human amnion before and after labor at term and following preterm labor. Placenta **14**:163–175, 1993.

Smith, G.C.S., Wood, A.M., Pell, J.P., White, I.R., Crossley, J.A. and Dobbie, R.: Second-trimester maternal serum levels of alpha-fetoprotein and subsequent risk of sudden infant death syndrome. NEJM **351**:978–986, 2004.

Smith, L.A. and Pounder, D.J.: A teratoma-like lesion of the placenta: a case report. Pathology **14**:85–87, 1982.

Sonek, J., Gabbe, S.G., Iams, J.D. and Kniss, D.A.: Morphologic changes in the human amnion epithelium that accompany labor as seen with scanning and transmission electron microscopy. Amer. J. Obstet. Gynecol. **164**:1174–1180, 1991.

Spinillo, A., Fazzi, E., Capuzzo, E., Stronati, M., Piazzi, G. and Ferrari, A.: Meconium-stained amniotic fluid and risk for cerebral palsy in preterm infants. Obstet. Gynecol. **90**:519–523, 1997.

Spinillo, A., Capuzzo, E., Stronati, M., Ometto, A., de Santolo, A. and Acciano, S.: Obstetric risk factors for periventricular leukomalacia among preterm infants. Br. J. Obstet. Gynaecol. **105**:865–871, 1998.

Spirt, B.A., Gordon, L.P. and Silverman, R.K.: Letter to the editor. J. Ultrasound Med. **3**:167–168, 1993.

Starck, D.: Embryologie. Thieme, Stuttgart, 1975.

Steer, P.J., Eigbe, F., Lissauer, T.J. and Beard, R.W.: Interrelationships among abnormal cardiotocograms in labor, meconium staining of the amniotic fluid, arterial cord blood pH, and Apgar scores. Obstet. Gynecol. **74**:715–720, 1989.

Steiner, P.E. and Lushbaugh, C.C.: Maternal pulmonary embolism by amniotic fluid as cause of obstetric shock and unexpected deaths in obstetrics. J.A.M.A. **117**:1245–1254, 1340–1345, 1941.

Stempel, L.E. and Nelson, D.M.: Retained chorionic membrane following repeated amniocenteses. Amer. J. Obstet. Gynecol. **142**:242–243, 1982.

Street, D.M. and Cunningham, F.: Congenital anomalies caused by intra-uterine bands. Clin. Orthop. **37**:82–97, 1964.

Streeter, G.L.: Focal deficiencies in fetal tissues and their relation to intrauterine amputations. Contrib. Embryol. Carnegie Inst. **22**:1–15, 1930.

Streuli, C.H. and Aplin, J.D.: Editorial: Life and death at labor. J. Clin. Invest. **98**:1947–1948, 1996.

Sutcliffe, R.G.: The nature and origin of the soluble protein in human amniotic fluid. Biol. Rev. **50**:1–33, 1975.

Symchych, P.S. and Winchester, P.: Animal model: amniotic fluid deficiency and fetal lung growth in the rat. Amer. J. Pathol. **90**:779–782, 1978.

Symonds, E.M., Skinner, S.L., Stanley, M.A., Kirkland, J.A. and Ellis, R.C.: An investigation of the cellular source of renin in human chorion. J. Obstet. Gynaecol. Br. Commonw. **77**: 885–890, 1970.

Szendi, B.: Experimentelle Untersuchungen beim Menschen Über den Austausch und die intrauterine Rolle des Fruchtwassers. Arch. Gynäkol. **170**:205–227, 1940.

Talmi, Y.P., Sigler, L., Inge, E., Finkelstein, Y. and Zohar, Y.: Antibacterial properties of human amniotic membranes. Placenta **12**:285–288, 1991.

Tarantal, A.F. and Hendrickx, A.G.: Amniotic band syndrome in a rhesus monkey: a case report. J. Med. Primatol. **16**: 291–299, 1987.

Teodoro, W.R., Andreucci, D. and Palma, J.A.: Short communication: placental collagen and premature rupture of fetal membranes. Placenta **11**:549–551, 1990.

Thiede, H.A. and Choate, J.W.: Chorionic localization in the human placenta by immunofluorescent staining. II. Demonstration of hCG in the trophoblast and amnion epithelium of immature and mature placentas. Obstet. Gynecol. **22**:433–443, 1963.

Thomas, C.E.: The ultrastructure of human amnion epithelium. J. Ultrastruct. Res. **13**:65–84, 1965.

Thompson, V.M.: Amnion nodosum. J. Obstet. Gynaecol. Br. Emp. **67**:611–614, 1960.

Thorburn, M.J.: Sex-chromatin in a 13-day embryo. Lancet **1**:277–278, 1964.

Thureen, P.J., Hall, D.M., Hoffenberg, A. and Tyson, R.W.: Fatal meconium aspiration in spite of appropriate perinatal airway management: pulmonary and placental evidence of prenatal disease. Amer. J. Obstet. Gynecol. **176**:967–975, 1997.

Tibboel, D., Vermey-Keers, C., Klück, P., Gaillard, J.L.J., Kloppenberg, J. and Molenaar, J.C.: The natural history of gastroschisis during fetal life: development of the fibrous coating on the bowel loops. Teratology **33**:267–272, 1986.

Torpin, R.: Fetal Malformations Caused by Amnion Rupture During Gestation. Thomas, Springfield, 1968.

Torpin, R.: The Human Placenta. Its Shape, Form, Origin and Development. Thomas, Springfield, 1969.

Torpin, R. and Faulkner, A.: Intrauterine amputation with the missing member found in the fetal membranes. JAMA **198**:185–187, 1966.

Torpin, R., Goodman, L. and Gramling, Z.W.: Amnion string swallowed by fetus. Amer. J. Obstet. Gynecol. **90**:829–830, 1964.

Toth, P. and Rao, C.V.: Direct novel regulation of cyclooxygenase (COX) and prostacyclin synthase (PGI$_2$-S) by hCG in human amnion. Placenta **13**:A63, 1992.

Toth, P., Li, X. and Rao, C.V.: Expression of hCG/LH receptor gene and its functional coupling to the regulation of cyclooxygenase-1 and -2 enzymes in human fetal membranes. Placenta **14**:A78, 1993.

Trasler, D.G., Walker, B.E. and Fraser, F.C.: Congenital malformations produced by amniotic-sac puncture. Science **124**:439, 1956.

Trimmer, K.J. and Gilstrap, L.C.: "Meconiumcrit" and birth asphyxia. Amer. J. Obstet. Gynecol. **165**:1010–1013, 1991.

Tuller, M.A.: Amniotic fluid embolism, afibrinogenemia, and disseminated fibrin thrombosis. Case report and review of the literature. Amer. J. Obstet. Gynecol. **73**:273–287, 1957.

Uhing, M.R., Bhat, R., Philobos, M. and Raju, T.N.K.: Value of amnioinfusion in reducing meconium aspiration syndrome. Amer. J. Perinatol. **10**:43–45, 1993.

Unger, J.: Placental teratoma. Amer. J. Clin. Pathol. **92**:371–373, 1989.

Uotila, P.J. and Kääpä, P.O.: Cyclooxygenase-2 expression in human monocytes stimulated by meconium. Lancet **351**:878, 1988.

Usher, R.H., Boyd, M.E., McLean, F.H. and Kramer, M.S.: Assessment of fetal risk in postdate pregnancies. Amer. J. Obstet. Gynecol. **158**:259–264, 1988.

Usta, I.M., Mercer, B.M., Aswad, N.K. and Sibai, B.M.: The impact of a policy of amnioinfusion for meconium-stained amniotic fluid. Obstet. Gynecol. **85**:237–241, 1995.

Uyehara, C.F.T. and Claybaugh, J.R.: Vasopressin metabolism in the amniotic sac of the fetal guinea pig. Endocrinology **123**:2040–2047, 1988.

Vadillo-Ortega, F., Gonzales-Avila, G., Furth, E.E., Leih, H.Q., Muschel, R.J., Stetler-Stevenson, W.G. and Strauss, J.F.: 92-kd type IV collagenase (matrix metalloproteinase-9) activity in human amniochorion increases with labor. Amer. J. Pathol. **146**:148–156, 1995.

Vadillo-Ortega, F., Hernandez, A., Gonzales-Avila, G., Bermejo, L., Iwata, K. and Strauss, J.F.: Increased matrix metalloproteinase activity and reduced tissue inhibitor of metalloproteinases-1 levels in amniotic fluids from pregnancies complicated by premature rupture of membranes. Amer. J. Obstet. Gynecol. **174**:1371–1376, 1996.

Vago, T. and Chavkin, J.: Extramembranous pregnancy: an unusual complication of amniocentesis. Amer. J. Obstet. Gynecol. **137**:511–512, 1980.

van Bogaert, L.-J., Maldague, P. and Staquet, J.-P.: Morphologic changes in the amniotic epithelium in relation to

placental weight and fetal maturity. Arch. Gynecol. **226**: 241–245, 1978.

Vantrappen, G., Janssens, J., Peeters, T.L., Bloom, S.R., Christofides, N.D. and Hellemans, J.: Motilin and the interdigestive migrating motor complex in man. Amer. J. Digest. Dis. **24**:497–500, 1979.

Verbeek, J.H., Robertson, E.M. and Haust, M.D.: Basement membranes (amniotic, trophoblastic, capillary) and adjacent tissue in term placenta. Amer. J. Obstet. Gynecol. **99**: 1136–1146, 1967.

Verjaal, M., Leschot, N.J., Wolf, N.J. and Treffers, P.E.: Karyotypic differences between cells from placenta and other fetal tissues. Prenatal Diagn. **7**:343–348, 1987.

Verma, I.C. and Ghai, O.P.: Study of sex chromatin in amniotic membranes of newborns. Indian J. Med. Res. **59**:1660–1665, 1971.

Vijayakumar, P. and Koh, T. When is meconium-stained cord actually bile-stained cord? Case report and literature review. J. Perinatol. **21**:467–468, 2001.

Wagner, G. and Tygstrup, I.: Oligohydramnios and urinary malformations in early human pregnancy. Acta Pathol. Microbiol. Scand. **59**:273–278, 1963.

Wang, T.: Fetalmembranen des Menschen. Fortschr. Med. **46**:1185–1188, 1984.

Wang, T. and Schneider, J.: Myofibroblasten im Bindegewebe des menschlichen Amnions. Z. Geburtshilfe Perinatol. **186**: 164–168, 1982.

Wang, T. and Schneider, J.: Cellular junctions on the free surface of human placental syncytium. Arch. Gynecol. **240**:211–216, 1987.

Wehbeh, H., Fleisher, J., Karimi, A., Mathony, A. and Minkoff, H.: The relationship between the ultrasonographic diagnosis of innocent amniotic band development and pregnancy outcomes. Obstet. Gynecol. **81**:565–568, 1993.

Weitzner, J.S., Strassner, H.T., Rawlins, R.G., Mack, S.R. and Anderson, R.A.: Objective assessment of meconium content of amniotic fluid. Obstet. Gynecol. **76**:1143–1144, 1990.

Welsh, J.B., Yi, E.S., Pretorius, D.H., Scioscia, A., Mannino, F.L. and Masliah, E.: Amnion rupture sequence and severe congenital high airway obstruction. J. Perinatol. **20**:387–389, 2000.

Wentworth, P. and Turnbull, I.: Bilateral renal agenesis (Potter's syndrome) J. Reprod. Med. **3**:87–91, 1969.

Weser, H. and Kaufmann, P.: Lichtmikroskopische und histochemische Untersuchungen an der Chorionplatte der reifen menschlichen Placenta. Arch. Gynaekol. **225**:15–30, 1978.

Wewer, U.M., Faber, M., Liotta, L.A. and Albrechtsen, R.: Immunochemical and ultrastructural assessment of the nature of pericellular basement membrane of human decidual cells. Lab. Invest. **53**:624–633, 1985.

Wigglesworth, J.S. and Desai, R.: Is fetal respiratory function a major determinant of perinatal survival? Lancet **1**:264–267, 1982.

Wiswell, T.E., Foster, N.H., Slayter, M.V. and Hachey, W.E.: Management of a piglet model of the meconium aspiration syndrome with high-frequency or conventional ventilation. Amer. J. Dis. Child. **146**:1287–1293, 1992.

Wolf, H.J. and Desoye, G.: Immunohistochemical localization of glucose transporters and insulin receptors in human fetal membranes at term. Histochemistry **100**:379–385, 1993.

Wolf, H.J. and Schmidt, W.: Histochemical study of carbohydrate metabolism in fetal membranes. Acta Histochem. **91**: 3–11, 1991.

Wolf, H.J., Schmidt, W. and Drenckhahn, D.: Immunocytochemical analysis of the cytoskeleton of the human amniotic epithelium. Cell Tissue Res. **266**:385–389, 1991.

Wong, F.W.S., Loong, E.P.L. and Chang, A.M.Z.: Ultrasound diagnosis of meconium-stained amniotic fluid. Amer. J. Obstet. Gynecol. **150**:359, 1985.

Woolnough, H.C.: Amniotic band syndrome (abstract). Teratology **36**:150, 1987.

Woyton, J.: Encephalocele attached to the placenta. Am. J. Obstet. Gynecol. **81**:1028–1032, 1961.

Wyatt-Ashmead, J. and Ashmead, A.: Placental membrane bursting pressures. Modern Pathol. **17**:275 (abstract 41), 2004.

Wynn, R.M.: Morphology of the placenta. In, Biology of Gestation. N.S. Assali, ed. Academic Press, New York, 1968.

Wynn, R.: Ultrastructural development of the human decidua. Amer. J. Obstet. Gynecol. **118**:652–670, 1974.

Wynn, R.M. and French, G.L.: Comparative ultrastructure of the mammalian amnion. Obstet. Gynecol. **31**:759–774, 1968.

Wynn, R.M., Sever, P.S. and Hellman, L.M.: Morphologic studies of the ruptured amnion. Amer. J. Obstet. Gynecol. **99**: 359–367, 1967.

Yamaguchi, Y., Isemura, M., Yosizawa, Z., Kurosawa, K., Yoshinaga, K., Sato, A. and Suzuki, M.: Changes in the distribution of fibronectin in the placenta during normal human pregnancy. Amer. J. Obstet. Gynecol. **152**:715–718, 1985.

Yang, S.S.: ADAM sequence and innocent amniotic band: manifestations of early amnion rupture. Amer. J. Med. Genet. **37**:562–568, 1990.

Yeomans, E.R., Gilstrap, L.C., Leveno, K.J. and Burris, J.S.: Meconium in the amniotic fluid and fetal acid-base status. Obstet. Gynecol. **73**:175–178, 1989.

Yoder, B.A.: Meconium-stained amniotic fluid and respiratory complications: Impact of selective tracheal suction. Obstet. Gynecol. **83**:77–84, 1994.

Yoshimura, S., Nishimura, T. and Yoshida, Y.: The morphometry of the Sudan-III-positive granules in the cytoplasm of the human amniotic epithelium. Acta Cytol. (Baltimore) **224**: 44–48, 1980.

Young, I.D., Lindenbaum, R.H., Thompson, E.M. and Pembrey, M.E.: Amniotic bands in connective tissue disorders. Arch. Dis. Child. **60**:1061–1063, 1985.

Yurchenco, P.D. and Ruben, G.C.: Basement membrane structure in situ: evidence for lateral associations in the type IV collagen network. J. Cell Biol. **105**:2559–2568, 1994.

Zorn, E.M., Hanson, F.W., Greve, L.C., Phelps-Sandall, B. and Tennant, F.R.: Analysis of the significance and origin of the discolored amniotic fluid detected at midtrimester amniocentesis. Amer. J. Obstet. Gynecol. **154**:1234–1240, 1986.

12
Anatomy and Pathology of the Umbilical Cord

DEVELOPMENT

The development of the umbilical cord is closely related to that of the amnion (see Chapter 11). Throughout the last days of the second week postcoitus (p.c.), the blastocystic cavity is filled by a loose meshwork of mesoderm cells, the extraembryonic mesoblast, which surrounds the embryoblast (Fig. 12.1, day 13). The embryoblast at that time is composed of two vesicles: the amnionic vesicle and the primary yolk sac. When these two vesicles are in contact with each other, they form the double-layered embryonic disk. During the following days the extraembryonic mesoderm cells are rearranged in such a way that they line the inner surface of the trophoblastic shell as chorionic mesoderm. They also cover the surface of the two embryonic vesicles (Fig. 12.1, day 18). Between the two mesoderm layers the exocoelom cavity forms. It largely separates the embryo and its mesodermal cover from the chorionic mesoderm. The exocoelom is bridged by the mesoderm in only one place, which lies basal to the amnionic vesicle. This mesenchymal connection is referred to as the connecting stalk (Fig. 12.1, day 18). It fixes the early embryo to the membranes and is the forerunner of the umbilical cord. During the same period (around day 18 p.c.), a duct-like extension of the yolk sac, originating from the future caudal region of the embryo, develops into the connecting stalk. This structure is the transitory allantois, the primitive extraembryonic urinary bladder. Heifetz (1996) estimated that some 20% of umbilical cords at term contain remnants of allantoic or omphalomesenteric duct, primarily near the fetal end.

The three subsequent weeks are characterized by three developmental processes:

1. The embryo rotates in such a way that the yolk sac vesicle, originally facing the region opposite the implantation site, is turned toward the implantation pole.
2. The amnionic vesicle enlarges considerably, extending around the embryo.
3. The originally flat embryonic disk is bent in the anteroposterior direction and rolled up in the lateral direction. It thus "herniates" into the amnionic vesicle. As the embryo bends, it subdivides the yolk sac into an intraembryonic duct (the intestines) and an extraembryonic part (the omphaloenteric or omphalomesenteric duct), which is dilated peripherally to form the extraembryonic yolk sac vesicle.

Both the allantois and the extraembryonic yolk sac extend into the mesenchyme of the connecting stalk (Fig. 12.1, day 22). Between days 28 and 40 p.c., the expanding amnionic cavity has surrounded the embryo so far that the connecting stalk, the allantois, and the yolk sac are compressed to a slender cord, which is then covered by amnionic epithelium (Fig. 12.1, day 28). They thus form the umbilical cord. The cord lengthens as the embryo "prolapses" backward into the amnionic sac (Hertig, 1962). During the same process of expansion, the amnionic mesenchyme locally touches and finally fuses with the chorionic mesoderm, thus occluding the exocoelomic cavity. This process persists until the end of the first trimester when, at approximately 12 weeks, the amnionic cavity completely occupies the exocoelom so that amnionic and chorionic mesenchyme have fused everywhere.

During the 3rd week p.c. the extraembryonic yolk sac, the omphalomesenteric duct that connects with the embryonic intestines, and the allantois become supplied with fetal vessels. All mammals use either allantoic or yolk sac vessels for the vascularization of the placenta. The human allantoic vessels, two allantoic arteries originating from the internal iliac arteries, and one allantoic vein that enters the hepatic vein, invade the placenta and become connected to the villous vessels. The allantoic participation in placental vascularization is the reason for the term **chorioallantoic** placenta. In contrast, in the choriovitelline or vitelline placentation (e.g., that of rodents and bats), the yolk sac vessels establish fetoplacental vascular connections.

The development of the cord has been treated in detail in the classical text by Cullen (1916). Unfortunately, this book is so inaccessible that it is rarely cited, let alone read. Another major review with special reference to comparative anatomy is that by Arvy and Pilleri (1976a). This volume brings together an enormous amount of material and is of particular interest because so many features considered to be abnormal in human placentas are normal features in some other species. Thus, many animals have pronounced squamous metaplasia on the cord's surface and nodules, not only near its abdominal end, that make the surface feel somewhat sandy. Blackburn and Cooley (1993) have also contributed a major review of all aspects of umbilical cord anatomy and pathology that should be consulted for additional considerations. It is richly illustrated and has major relevance to the relationship of cord anomalies to congenital malformations of the fetus.

Amnionic Epithelium

The cord is covered by amnionic epithelium. Near the umbilicus, a largely unkeratinized, stratified squamous epithelium provides the transition from the abdominal wall to the cord's surface. Farther away from the umbilicus, the epithelium transforms into a stratified columnar epithelium (two to eight layers) and finally into a simple columnar epithelium (Hoyes, 1969; Sinha, 1971; Hempel, 1972). The latter continues developing into the simple columnar to cuboidal epithelium of the placental amnionic surface. The basal cells of the stratified parts of the amnion resemble the amnionic epithelium of the membranes, whereas the superficial cells sometimes are squamous, poor in organelles, and pyknotic (Bourne, 1962). Parry and Abramovich (1970) found two principal cell types, with intermediates. In contrast to earlier theories, they suggested that these cells do not have any water-regulatory function. Thus, if there is larger water content in the proximal portion of the cord it must have other underlying causes. In this context it is interesting to note that Gebrane-Younes and coworkers (1986), based on the ultrastructure of the umbilical endothelium and other wall components, have suggested a considerable fluid transudation out of the umbilical vessels into the amnionic fluid.

In general, the amnion of the cord is structurally similar to that described in the membranes; and there are no indications that this is different for its basic functions (see Chapter 11). In contrast to the amnion that covers the chorionic surface of the placenta, however, and that of the membranes where it is easily detached, the amnion of the cord grows firmly into the central connective tissue core. It cannot be dislodged.

Wharton's Jelly

The connective tissue of the cord, or Wharton's jelly, is derived from the extraembryonic mesoblast. McKay et al. (1955) referred to this jelly-like material of the exocoelom as a "thixotropic gel" because it liquefies when touched (see also Bacsich & Riddell, 1945). The incorporation of this mesenchyme into the cord substance and the subamnionic layers probably accounts for their mucoid and compressible structures. The importance of this faculty was stressed by Reynolds (1952). He likened the compressed (by distended fetal vessels) Wharton's jelly to erectile tissue. It is clearly true that a filled umbilical cord is a relatively firm, rigid structure and that, with expansion and contraction of the vasculature, its thickness and turgidity vary. Strong (1997a) reviewed this protective function of Wharton's jelly. This jelly is composed of a ground substance of open-chain polysaccharides (hyaluronic acid: Graumann, 1964; carbohydrates with glycosyl and mannosyl groups: Yamada & Shimizu, 1976), distributed in a fine network of microfibrils. Immunohistochemically, the interstitial collagens types I, III, and VI, as well as the basal lamina molecules collagen type IV, laminin, and heparan sulfate were found (Nanaev et al., 1992, 1997). Immunoreactivities for these extracellular matrix molecules were accumulated around cleft-like territories ("stromal clefts") in Wharton's jelly; the stromal clefts themselves were occupied by homogeneous ground substance, which was devoid of collagens and basal lamina

molecules but probably contained ample proteoglycans. These fiber-free stromal clefts must not be misunderstood as lymphatic vessels that exist neither in the cord nor in the placenta.

Wharton's jelly contains evenly distributed spindle-shaped fibroblasts with long extensions (Parry, 1970) and numerous mast cells. These cells can be stained selectively, surround the vessels densely, and are also found underneath the cord surface (Moore, 1956). Electron microscopic and immunohistochemical studies by Takechi and coworkers (1993) revealed that the stromal cells embedded into the collagen meshwork were myofibroblasts rather than typical fibroblasts. Myofibroblasts are fiber-producing cells that have contractile properties similar to those of smooth muscle cells. These data were supported and further extended by Nanaev and coworkers (1997). According to these authors, the stromal cells of Wharton's jelly depending on their location within the cord, show different degrees of differentiation from mesenchymal cells to myofibroblasts:

- The most immature, still proliferating cells are located close to the amnionic surface. These undifferentiated cells very likely correspond to cells isolated from Wharton's jelly, which proliferate well in vitro and contain stem cells that differentiate into neurons and glia (Mitchell et al., 2003).
- With increasing distance of the amnionic surface, the stromal cells acquire cytoskeletal features of contractile cells, including desmin, α-smooth muscle actin and partly also γ-smooth muscle actin.
- In close proximity to the umbilical vessels highly differentiated myofibroblasts expressing additionally smooth muscle myosin were found.

The myofibroblasts and their less differentiated precursors line the jelly-filled, stromal clefts of Wharton's jelly (Nanaev et al., 1997). The authors speculated that jelly-filled stromal spaces together with the surrounding meshwork of contractile cells serve as a mechanism for turgor regulation of the cord, avoiding compression of umbilical veins and counteracting bending of the cord.

There are surprisingly few macrophages in the umbilical cord. Even when the cord is deep green due to meconium staining and when meconium-filled macrophages are readily seen in the membranes, only relatively few activated and pigmented macrophages are seen in the cord substance. Similarly, after intrafunicular bleeding, hemosiderin is not formed in situ.

The tensile properties of the cord have been reported by Ghosh et al. (1984). No significant differences in the tensile parameters with respect to the sex of the baby were found, but there was a significant positive correlation between the tensile breaking load and the birth weight of the baby. The average tensile breaking load is

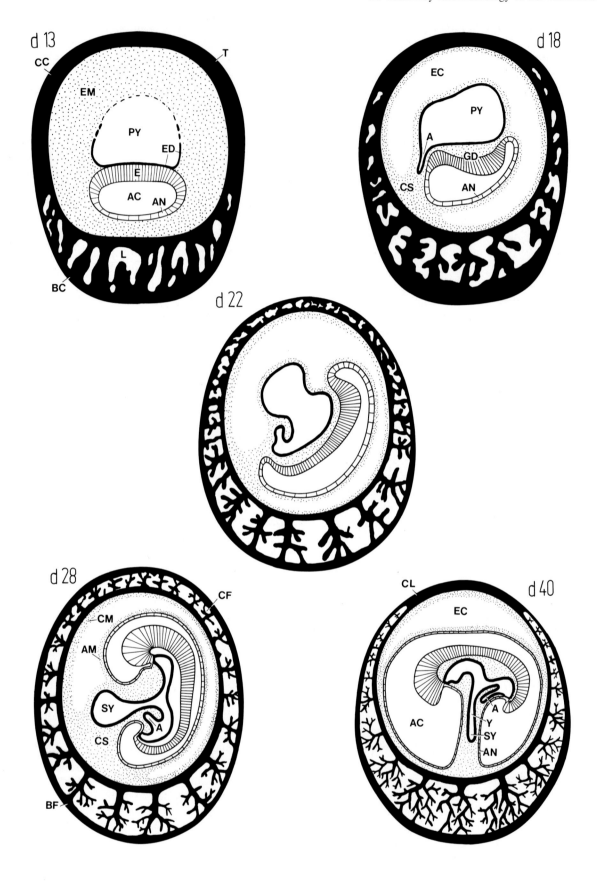

2.49 times the weight of the baby at birth. Additional biomechanical data on the mechanical strength of cord vessels and Wharton's jelly may be found in the paper by Pennati (2001).

Recent studies by sonographers have concerned the variable thickness (diameter) of the umbilical cord as it varies considerably and, at times, can be shown to have prognostic value. Needless to say, the diameter increases with gestational age to about 32 weeks (Ghezzi et al., 2001a) and has led these investigators to create nomograms (Ghezzi et al., 2001b). The same group of obstetricians has also found that chromosomally abnormal fetuses and those with other placental abnormalities had larger volumes of cords (Ghezzi et al., 2002; Raio et al., 2004). Cysts, for instance may cause much enlargement (vide infra) and make the cord heavier, and in many placentas of pregnancies in diabetics the cord appears thicker and more water-logged. Cysts are relatively frequent (2.1% according to Ghezzi et al., 2003) and may be single (good prognosis) or multiple (aneuploidy, miscarriage).

Structure of Umbilical Vessels

There are normally two arteries and one vein in the human umbilical cord (Fig. 12.2). An originally developed second umbilical vein atrophies during the second month of pregnancy. In rare cases—1% according to Boyd and Hamilton (1970)—there is only one umbilical artery (vide infra), an anomaly that may be associated with multiple fetal malformations (Lemtis, 1966, 1968). Local fusion of the two arteries has also been reported (Kelber, 1976). The arrangement is different in many other species. For example, two arteries and two veins are found in the nine-banded armadillo, with many subtle variations (Benirschke et al., 1964) and, as indicated earlier, other animals may have an admixture of yolk sac (vitelline) vessels. Cats may have four vessels of each type. The notion of a

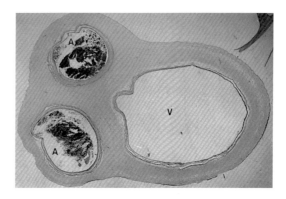

FIGURE 12.2. Cross section of mature umbilical cord, near its placental insertion. Wharton's jelly is compressed by the expanded umbilical vein (V) and two arteries (A). (*Source:* Schiebler & Kaufmann, 1981, with permission.) H&E ×10.

"double umbilicus" (Reeves, 1916) is based on a single observation of a somewhat displaced, doubled umbilical vein found in an adult, with puckering of the skin. In another case, described by Murdoch (1966), there were two umbilical veins, and a portion of the cord was separated, giving it a partially split appearance. Hill and associates (1994b) also described the persistence of a second (right) umbilical vein within frequently (18%) malformed fetuses. They did not report upon the possible persistence of a second vein in the umbilical cord itself, however. Thus, the findings are limited to sonographic intrafetal findings. The topic was reviewed by Bell et al. (1986), who found a second vein in a severely anomalous fetus but it was not present in the umbilical cord. The mean intravital diameter of the arteries is around 3 mm, with a slight tendency to increase toward the placenta. The venous diameter is around twice this size (Fig. 12.2).

Human umbilical vessels differ in many ways from the major vessels of the body. The endothelial cells of both the arteries and the veins are unusually rich in organelles

---

FIGURE 12.1. Simplified representation of the development of the umbilical cord and amnion. Day (d) 13 postcoitus (p.c.): The embryonic disk consists of two epithelial layers: the ectoderm (E), which is contiguous with the amnionic epithelium (AN), and the endoderm (ED), which partially surrounds the primary yolk sac cavity (PY). Both vesicles are surrounded by the extraembryonic mesoderm (EM). Day 18 p.c.: At this stage, the endoderm has become closely applied to the periphery of the yolk sac; and at the presumptive caudal end of the germinal disk, the allantoic invagination (A) has occurred. In the extraembryonic mesoderm, the exocoelom (EC) has cavitated. A mesenchymal bridge, the "connecting stalk" (CS), has developed that will ultimately form the umbilical cord. Day 28 p.c.: The embryo has begun to rotate and fold. The primary yolk sac is being subdivided into the intraembryonic intestinal tract and the secondary

(extraembryonic) yolk sac (SY). Secondary yolk sac and allantois extrude from the future embryonic intestinal tract into the connecting stalk. The amnionic sac largely surrounds the embryo because of its folding and rotation. Villous formation has occurred at the entire periphery of the chorionic vesicle, forming the chorion frondosum (CF). Day 40 p.c.: The embryo has now fully rotated and folded. It is completely surrounded by the amnionic cavity and is attached to the umbilical cord. The latter has developed from the connecting stalk as it has become covered by amnionic membrane. The exocoelom has become largely compressed by the expansion of the amnionic cavity. At the abembryonic pole of the chorionic vesicle, the recently formed placental villi gradually atrophy, thus forming the chorion laeve (CL). Only that portion that retains villous tissue, that which has the insertion of the umbilical cord develops into the placental disk.

(Parry & Abramovich, 1972; Las Heras & Haust, 1981) and thus structurally different from the endothelium of the villous vessels. Gebrane-Younes et al. (1986) have given a careful account of the ultrastructure of the endothelium. They described ultrastructural evidence that transudation of fluid through the umbilical vessel walls contributes to the formation of amnionic fluid.

Despite all differences among umbilical and villous endothelium, human umbilical vein-derived endothelial cells (HUVECs) are often used for cell culture as models for "placental endothelium." The findings by Lang et al. (1993) suggested to us that we should be careful with the interpretation of such experiments. The latter authors described considerable differences among umbilical and villous endothelium with respect to cell surface markers and receptors for transferrin and immunoglobulin G (IgG).

Slender endothelial extensions, penetrating the basal lamina, may interdigitate with the neighboring muscle cells and form an endotheliomuscular system (Nikolov & Schiebler, 1973). The arteries possess no internal elastic membrane and have much less elastica in general than other arteries (Boyd & Hamilton, 1970; Nikolov & Schiebler, 1973). The vein, on the other hand, has an elastic subintimal layer (Fig. 12.3). The muscular coat of the arteries consists of a system of crossing spiraled fibers (von Hayek, 1936; Goerttler, 1951; Scheuner, 1964). Desmin-positive smooth muscle cells are largely concentrated on the outer layer of the media (Nanaev et al., 1991). In contrast, the inner media smooth muscle cells are poorly differentiated with few myofilaments (Meyer et al., 1978; Sexton et al., 1996). They hardly can contribute actively to postpartal closure of the cord arteries. The venous muscular coats are thinner than those of the arteries and composed of more separate layers of longitudinal or circular fibers. Media smooth muscle cells of the cord and adjacent chorionic vessels are major placental storage sites for glycogen; only minor quantities were found in the surrounding stromal myofibroblasts. Glycogen levels showed a strong direct correlation with fetal birth weight (Mvumbi et al., 1996).

Cardoso and colleagues (1992) have analyzed the extracellular matrix of isolated umbilical arteries. In general, hyaluronic acid was increased, whereas heparan sulfate and chondroitin 4- and 6-sulfate were reduced in normal umbilical arteries as compared to normal adult systemic arteries. Following hypertension in pregnancy, the total glycosaminoglycan and collagen content of the umbilical arteries were reduced; these changes were unlikely to impair the hemodynamic properties of the cord vessels. Each umbilical vessel is surrounded by crossing bundles of spiraled collagen fibers that form a kind of adventitia. The umbilical vessels of human umbilical cords lack vasa vasorum. Fetuses beyond 20 weeks of gestation, however, have vasa vasorum in the intraabdominal portions of their umbilical arteries (Clarke, 1965).

INNERVATION

There is general agreement about the findings by Spivack (1943) that no nerves traverse the umbilical cord from fetus to placenta, and that the placenta has no neural supply. A number of investigators, however, have since investigated this apparent lack of nerves, and some have come to different conclusions. Thus, Kernbach (1963) studied the amnion with Cajal stains and considered the powdery Nissl substance of extravillous trophoblast cells to represent sympathicoblasts with nerve fibers. He also believed that he had identified nerves in the amnion (Kernbach, 1969). Ten Berge (1963) reviewed the older literature on this topic and found only three authors who claimed to have demonstrated nerves by "persevering techniques." Ten Berge was unable to obtain convincing preparations with a variety of stains. He believed, however, that the responsiveness to oxygen perfusion and a variety of pharmacologic agents argues in favor of innervation. Fox and Jacobson (1969) stained various segments of umbilical cords from abortuses and term placentas with methylene blue and observed fibers in all segments of all cords. The fibers were most easily seen in Wharton's jelly but surrounded and entered the vascular walls. Fox and Jacobson interpreted the fibers to be neural elements. It is possible that these structures relate to the vagal fibers described in embryos by Pearson and Sauter

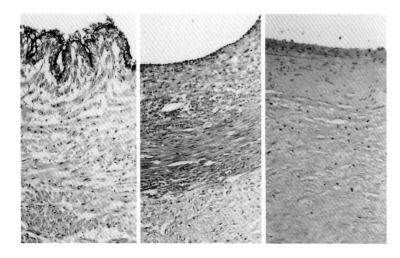

FIGURE 12.3. Umbilical cord sections of a stillborn with necrosis (from thrombosis) of one umbilical artery (right) and a normal artery (middle) and vein (left). In these sections, one may observe the presence of a delicate subendothelial elastica only in the vein at left. von Gieson ×160.

(1969), which are thought to be instrumental in closing the ductus venosus after birth. The same authors subsequently investigated the sacral portions of embryos and found convincing evidence of neural supply of umbilical arteries (Pearson & Sauter, 1970). Some neural elements terminate before entering the cord, whereas others penetrate it. This report was contrary to the older literature, which was reviewed.

Ellison (1971) then took up the topic and studied the cords with a thiocholine technique. He demonstrated acetylcholinesterase-positive nerve endings in the proximal 20 cm of umbilical cord, but the placental side invariably gave negative results. The illustrations of tiny nerves present around the umbilical vessels appear convincing. Because they frequently showed degenerative changes, they were interpreted as having a primarily prenatal function. Ellison (1971) was unable to confirm the assertion by Fox and Jacobson (1969) of a subamnionic neural plexus and interpreted it as an artifact. Electron-microscopic search for innervation of the human umbilical cord has generally been negative (Nadkarni, 1970). Fox (1978), who cited other studies, believed that the topic may be controversial because of the paucity of fibers. Lachenmayer (1971) examined guinea pig and human cords, as well as the intrafetal portions of vessels for formaldehyde-induced fluorescence, considered to be specific for catecholamines. He found no evidence of nerve fibers in the cord vessels, but they were present within the fetus and the immediate vicinity of the umbilicus. He considered the cord to be a model of a nerve-free effector organ. Later studies, for example those by Nikolov and Schiebler (1973), Papaloucas et al. (1975), and Reilly and Russel (1977), have corroborated this view. Immunohistochemical examination of cords obtained from the first, second, and third trimester and using a panel of antibodies directed against neural and glial structures, also failed to identify any nerve tissues in the middle and placental segment of the human umbilical cord (Fox & Khong, 1990).

Contractility of Umbilical Vessels

There has been much interest in the mechanisms of closure of umbilical vessels after birth (Editorial, 1966). Yao et al. (1977) observed umbilical cords after delivery and witnessed that irregular constrictions of arteries occurred at irregular intervals. Davignon et al. (1965) showed that increased transmural pressures exerted on the umbilical arteries led to vasoconstriction. This finding is usual in the guinea pig also. Throughout the last 2 weeks of pregnancy, the cord vessels show increasing responsiveness to mechanical irritation, which is not present during the preceding periods of pregnancy. This response and other mechanisms indirectly confirm the absence of a neural mechanism operating in cord vessels (Shepherd, 1968).

Electron-microscopic observations led Röckelein and Scharl (1988) to the assumption that an endotheliomuscular interaction, mediated by the endotheliomuscular interdigitations (Nikolov & Schiebler, 1973), may play an important role. As a consequence of muscular contraction, the authors described a cytoplasmic prolapse of smooth muscle cells into the endothelial cells, thus causing a kind of "hydrops" of the latter. Seemingly hydropic endothelial cells of umbilical arteries deeply protruding into the arterial lumens and partly occluding those have been seen by many authors. Sometimes they have been interpreted as a pathologic finding, for example, in the allantoic vessels obtained from HIV-positive mothers (Jimenez et al., 1988). According to Röckelein and Hey (1985; Hey & Röckelein, 1989) this phenomenon is more likely to be a result of either postpartal muscle contraction or even an artifact due to delayed fixation. And this is our experience as well.

The vessels are exquisitely sensitive to various endocrine mediators, such as serotonin, angiotensin, and oxytocin (LeDonne & McGowan, 1967; Dyer, 1970; Winters, 1970). Moreover, smooth muscle contractility of the vessel walls is influenced in paracrine loops by substances produced within the neighboring endothelial cells. Among these mediators, prostaglandins have been shown to be produced within the umbilical vascular endothelium. Despite earlier observations to the contrary, it is now known that the endothelium of the umbilical vein produces far more prostaglandins than does that of the arteries (Harold et al., 1988). There is, however, little production of prostaglandins in placental surface vessels. Karbowski and coworkers (1991) have cultured umbilical vein endothelial cells from smoking and from diabetic mothers, and they found that the synthetic rate of prostaglandins PGI_2 and PGE_2 was significantly reduced as compared to those from normal control mothers. Because both prostaglandins are potent vasodilators and platelet aggregation inhibitors, the authors concluded that impaired placental perfusion in smoking and diabetic mothers may be mediated by the altered umbilical endothelium. Ulm et al. (1995) observed similar defective prostacyclin production of umbilical arterial response in cords delivered to cigarette smoking mothers. McCoshen et al. (1989) found by incubation experiments that the cord (presumably its amnionic surface) is the major source of PGE_2 in the gestational sac during labor.

Another vasodilator that has attracted much attention is nitric oxide—identical with the endothelium-derived relaxing factor from the older literature (Pinto et al., 1991; Mildenberger et al., 2003)—which is produced from the conversion of L-arginine to citrulline by nitric oxide synthase (NOS). This enzyme has been detected immunohistochemically not only in villous syncytiotrophoblast but also in fetal villous and umbilical endothelium (Myatt et al., 1993). A reduction in this enzyme's activity has been correlated with abnormal umbilical artery waveforms (Giles et al., 1997). Atrial natriuretic peptide (ANP) is another potent vasodilator that additionally seems to be involved in fetal fluid hemostasis. Its binding sites have been detected in umbilical smooth muscle cells (Salas et al., 1991). Immunoreactivity for the peptide itself and its messenger RNA have been found in the umbilical endothelium (Cai et al., 1993a,b) even though Inglis and colleagues (1993) questioned the local umbilical synthesis. They suggested an endocrine action of the peptide that would be released from the fetal heart into the circulation (for review see Macara et al., 1993); messenger RNA for ANP is present in cardiomyocytes of fetuses as early as 19 weeks (Gardner et al., 1989).

Vasoconstrictor substances found in umbilical endothelium comprise angiotensin II, 5-hydroxytryptamine (5-HT) and thromboxane (see Macara et al., 1993), neuropeptide Y (NPY) (Cai et al., 1993a), as well as endothelin-1 (Hemsen et al., 1991). Gu and coworkers (1991), however, detected endothelins-1 and -2 only in fibroblasts and amnionic epithelium of human cords rather than in endothelium. Bindings sites for endothelin-1 have been described in the media of umbilical vessels, the activity of the arteries exceeding that of the vein (Rath et al., 1993). The functions of these vasoconstrictors are still under discussion. NPY and angiotensin II, which are found most abundantly in the endothelial cells, cause relatively weak or no responses on the term umbilical artery in vitro (White, 1989). When White compared the effects of various vasoactive agents on the arteries in premature and term placentas, significant differences were found. Immature vessels were more sensitive to angiotensin II, arachidonic acid, and oxytocin; term vessels reacted more to vasopressin, norepinephrine, PGD_2, and PGE_2. In vitro, 5-HT and endothelin-1 were found to be powerful vasoconstrictors on all levels of fetoplacental circulation (Maclean et al., 1992). The latter substances are also under discussion as mediators of closure of placental circulation at birth (Hemsen et al., 1991).

These findings shed new light on the highly complex mechanisms of autoregulation, not only of the umbilical circulation, but also of the villous circulation, as most of these mediators have been described also in the walls of the larger chorionic and villous vessels (for reviews see Macara et al., 1993; Okatani et al., 1995). Further studies will have to elucidate the complicated interactions of these substances, as they are very likely to be involved in abnormal conditions, such as intrauterine growth restriction (IUGR) and a high Doppler resistance index.

The vessels of patients with preeclampsia, growth-retarded fetuses, and diabetes, as well as those of smoking mothers, show reduced prostacyclin production (Busacca et al., 1982; Dadak et al., 1982; Jogee et al., 1983; Mäkilä et al., 1983). Similar effects have been found in vitro by Karbowski et al. (1991). Degeneration of endothelium from umbilical vessels had earlier been shown to occur in smoking mothers (Asmussen & Kjeldsen, 1975). Other effects of smoking on the placenta have been discovered as well; most are discussed in Chapter 19. One example is that the steroid production is altered (Mochizuki et al., 1984); others are trophoblastic degeneration, microvascular changes, and several other effects have been observed (Wigger et al., 1984). Although it is attractive to consider that prostaglandins are the principal mediators of umbilical vascular responses, some evidence has been adduced

that there may be considerable differences among species (Dyer, 1970). Alcohol leads to a dose-dependent contractile response in umbilical arteries in vitro (Yang et al., 1986). Estrogens dilate the vessels (de Sa & Meirelles, 1977).

Hyrtl's Anastomosis, False Knots, and Hoboken Nodes

An important macroscopic feature of umbilical arteries is the presence of an anastomosis between the two arteries near the surface of the placenta. The older literature (Hyrtl, 1870; Fig. 12.4) and more recent studies have shown that 96% of cords have some sort of arterial anastomosis (Priman, 1959; Arts, 1961). Most were seen 1.5 cm from the placental insertion and were either truly anastomotic vessels, or the two arteries fused. On rare occasions, two such communicating vessels exist. Fujikura (2003) measured the distance of the anastomosis from the placental surface—0.5 to 6 cm. Like Hyrtl (1870), who attached much importance to this communication, we believe it to be meaningful for an equalization of flow and pressures between the two arteries and for the uniform distribution of blood to the different lobes of the placenta. A better understanding of the functional importance of Hyrtl's anastomosis has come from numerous sonographic studies that employed Doppler flow evaluation. These have taken on a significant importance in prenatal evaluations now and have, for instance, detected a difference in the size of the two arteries (Dolkart et al., 1992) and are commonly used to anticipate fetal growth and its impairment (e.g., Raio et al., 2003). In a study to evaluate Hyrtl's anastomosis, Raio et al. (2001) showed that it was present in 36 of 41 cases they studied, and a fusion existed in the remaining five. Greater impedance occurred when the anastomosis was oblique rather than straight across the arteries, and they also came to conclude that it served as a means to equalize pressures and circulation. Ullberg et al. (2001) studied 67 placentas and found an anastomosis in 60, two connections in one, and absence of four cords. Its relevance to an understanding of single umbilical artery, the commonest macroscopic anomaly of the placenta, is discussed below. Young (1972), who provided an admirable review of the literature, studied this anastomosis in many primate species and prepared an elaborate classification scheme for the different types observed. He found that "lower" primates (e.g., lemurs) lacked it; New World monkeys had it in some 30% of cords, and Old World monkeys showed an 80% incidence. It is apparently a recent evolutionary development. Ullberg et al. (1994) studied 83 placentas with barium sulfate injection and found 76 to have an anastomosis. Of the seven others, three had a single umbilical artery and four had true absence. They found

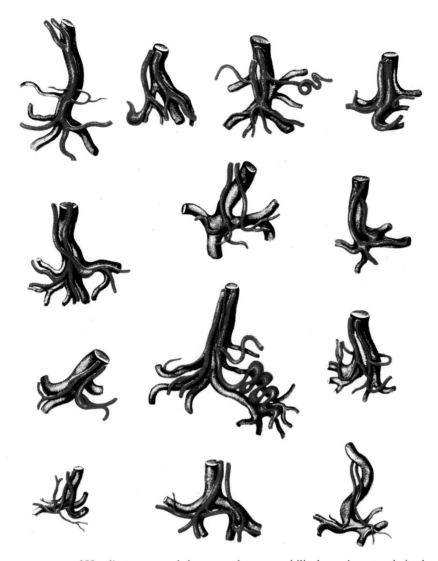

FIGURE 12.4 Various arrangements of Hyrtl's anastomosis between the two umbilical arteries near their placental insertion. [Injection studies of Hyrtl (1870); reproduced with permission.© Wilhelm Braumüller, Wien 1870.]

no correlation with fetal growth. When Predanic et al. (1998) sonographically studied blood flow velocities in parallel umbilical arteries, they found a substantial number with markedly different flow and arterial resistance. This was more pronounced at earlier gestational ages and tended to diminish toward term. They speculated that the aberrant cases may have lacked Hyrtl's anastomosis, but did not examine for its presence.

Often the looping of umbilical vessels is the cause for "false knots" of the cord. In most cases, local loops of the arteries, or sometimes even the vein, cause knot-like dilation of the cord. Sometimes focal varicosities of the veins or perivascular accumulations of connective tissue result in a similar external appearance. Finally, there are the "valves (nodes) of Hoboken" (Hoboken, 1669; Spivack, 1936), named after a 17th-century Dutch anatomist.

Malpas and Symonds (1966) concluded that these crescentic folds in the inner wall of umbilical arteries are present after delivery, but that they do not exist in vivo. Reynolds (1952) was not so sure and depicted some of these vascular indentations. He speculated that they resulted from muscular constriction, a view that has been corroborated by electron-microscopic studies. Thus, Röckelein and Scharl (1988) and Röckelein et al. (1990) speculated on the occurrence of some interference with postnatal closure of the cord vessels. On the other hand, most other observers believe that the folds have no physiologic significance, as was inferred by Spivack (1936). They cautioned that incisive observations have to be made immediately after cesarean section because the folds form quickly. Ideally, their presence in vivo should be studied with sonography before birth.

Allantois

The allantoic duct, a minute connection to the fetal bladder is frequently found in the proximal portions of the umbilical cord. Remnants may exist discontinuously throughout the cord. Complete obliteration of the duct is normally achieved by 15 weeks' gestation (Janosco et al., 1977). In the fetus, the rudiment is referred to as the median umbilical ligament. The remains of this connection in the umbilical cord are always located centrally between the two umbilical arteries, and they usually consist of a collection of epithelial cells without lumens (Fig. 12.5). The epithelium, when present, is generally of the transitional, bladder type. Mucin-producing epithelium is also found occasionally, perhaps because of the proximity to the yolk sac during development. Rarely is the allantoic tissue accompanied by muscle and even more uncommonly is the duct patent. Nevertheless, urination from the clamped umbilical stump has been reported, and cysts may even persist into adult life (Kreibich, 1947). A patent duct ("urachus") on the abdominal wall may complicate pregnancy. Nielsen et al. (1982) reviewed 12 such cases from the literature and reported on an additional patient. Their patient had a discharge from the umbilicus during pregnancy. Her bladder became infected, and pyelonephritis ensued. Infection is a common complication of this rare condition. An abscess of the allantoic duct remnant was described by Baill et al. (1989). It was found in the placenta of a 22 weeks' gestation placenta that was involved with chorioamnionitis and funisitis.

The allantoic remnant may be symptomatic at birth, presenting as a "giant umbilical cord" (Ente et al., 1970). In one of the two patients of these authors, the cord was tense and swollen to a 5-cm diameter. Urine discharged from it. The second patient also had an enlarged cord but only after the cord had separated during the neonatal period did urine pass through the duct. The authors

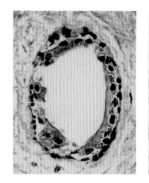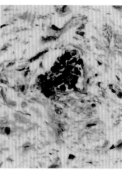

FIGURE 12.5. Two remnants of allantoic duct: left patent, right obliterated. Note the absence of the muscular coat. H&E ×525. (Courtesy of G.L. Bourne.)

stressed the association with a tense, "giant" cord swelling and contrasted it to that found with omphalomesenteric remnants. That was also the finding in a case reported by Chantler and his colleagues (1969), where a single umbilical artery ("fusion") was an associated anomaly. Browne (1925) described a cyst in the umbilical cord originating from the allantois that is very similar to the one depicted here. It measured 14 cm in diameter and weighed 300 g. The neonate did well after initial depression. De Sa (1984) described a small cyst and likened its appearance to the cell nests of von Brunn, which are characteristic for bladder epithelium. Such a case is shown in Figure 12.5. This stillborn had a prenatally diagnosed swelling at the abdomen. At delivery, the "giant", edematous cord (Fig. 12.6) weighed 180 g (the average normal weight of the cord is 40 to 45 g). Sections showed that the urachus extended deep into the umbilical cord; it was accompanied by normal bladder musculature and was located in its usual place between the two arteries (Fig. 12.7). The remarkable feature of this umbilical cord was that it had numerous vasa aberrantia. These vessels cannot be classified as vasa vasorum because they were similarly distributed around vessels and the urachus. Normally, vasa

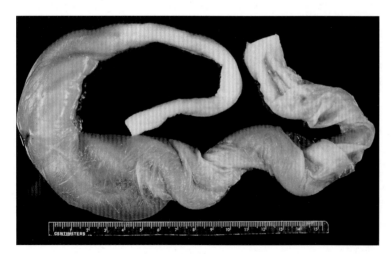

FIGURE 12.6. Edematous umbilical cord of a 32-week fetus with a large urachal extension into the cord. It was correctly diagnosed by sonography before birth. This cord weighed 180 g (compared with a normal weight of about 40 g). (Courtesy of Dr. S. Kassel, Fresno, California.)

FIGURE 12.7. A: Histologic appearance of the umbilical cord shown in Figure 12.6. The urachus is at the arrow. Note the presence of small vessels and vasa aberrantia around the vein and one artery. H&E ×6. B: Vasa aberrantia around the umbilical vein in the same case. H&E ×64.

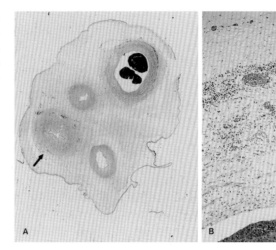

vasorum are confined to the intraabdominal portions of these structures. Furthermore, around all these small vessels were numerous islands of extramedullary hematopoiesis. The fetus presumably died because venous return was compressed by this large cyst in the cord.

Even if there are no macroscopic or clinical suggestions for the presence of allantoic vestiges, careful histologic examination may reveal their presence. When studying the placental extremities of 1000 cords, Jauniaux and coworkers (1989a) found such remnants in 14.6% of the cases. The overall incidence of a truly patent urachus, however, is estimated as uncommonly as once in 200,000 births, and it is more frequent in males (Costakos et al., 1992). Remnants have also been described as presenting with a cord cyst. Such a case was recognized sonographically in a case of trisomy 18 by Ramirez et al. (1995), although the true nature of the cystic cavity was not described.

OMPHALOMESENTERIC DUCT

The omphalomesenteric (vitelline) duct arises through the lengthening of the umbilical stalk when the embryo retracts ("herniates" or "prolapses") into the amnionic cavity. While the embryo is folding and the cord becomes established, the connection between the gut and the yolk sac lengthens. From the primary yolk sac develops the secondary structure that is connected to the fetal intestines. Gonzales-Crussi and Roth (1976) and Ukeshima et al. (1986) have provided detailed morphologic descriptions of the intact, nonregressive yolk sac during the early stages

of pregnancy. The yolk sac has a three-layered wall, consisting of an inner resorptive endodermal epithelium and an outer mesothelium that are joined by some mesenchyme. Erythropoiesis was found in the mesenchyme from 6 to 8 weeks of gestation (Jones et al., 1993).

When the gut rotates and withdraws to its original cavity, this duct atrophies. Atrophy is usually complete by the 7th to 16th weeks (Janosco et al., 1977). Jones et al. (1993) described generalized degenerative changes for the 10th week. Meckel's diverticulum, a small outgrowth of the ileum, is a frequent remnant of this connection in the fetus. Only in exceptional cases can a larger duct be found. It then connects the ileum with the proximal part of the cord. Having thus an endodermal origin, it is not surprising that in remnants of this duct one may find liver, pancreas, stomach, and intestinal structures.

Minute vitelline ducts are frequently found on histologic study in the umbilical cord. At the placental extremities, the incidence seems to be lower; of 1000 mature cords studied, only 1.5% showed remnants of the omphalomesenteric duct, whereas vitelline vessels were present in about 7% (Jauniaux et al., 1989b). Clinically, these vestiges are unimportant unless the occasional direct communication with fetal bowel is explored by curious investigators (Hinson et al., 1997). The blood vessels that may accompany the vitelline duct are always tiny and may even contain red blood cells. It is noteworthy, however, that these vessels always lack a muscular coat; this, we believe, develops only under the influence of blood pressure. Thus, when in sirenomelia the omphalomesenteric artery is probably converted to the sole umbilical artery (because the allantoic vessels failed to develop), this vessel acquires a "normal" muscular investment. Usually, vitelline vessels are composed only of endothelium. There are other points of view with respect to the single artery in sirens, and they are discussed at the end of this chapter.

Cysts of vitelline origin have been described many times. In contrast to the allantoic duct remnants, they often have muscular coats (Fig. 12.8) and may occur in duplicate (Fig. 12.9). True intestinal walls,

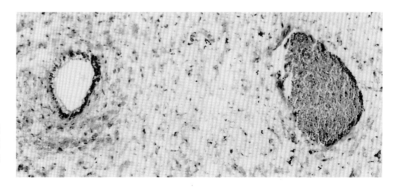

FIGURE 12.8. Omphalomesenteric duct remnant at left with mucus-producing epithelium and a small amount of musculature in the wall. At right are the remains of the vitelline vein. H&E ×100.

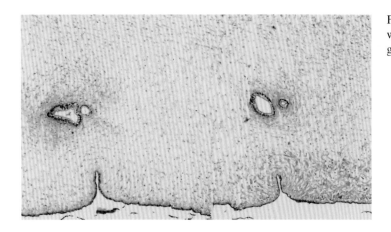

FIGURE 12.9. Microscopic section of term pregnancy cord with four remnants of omphalomesenteric duct. The marginal position of such vestiges is typical. H&E ×50.

including ganglion cells, may be present. Browne (1925) referred to a report of one such cyst as having caused fetal death, presumably due to compression of the allantoic vessels. Three cases were reported by Heifetz and Rueda-Pedraza (1983a), one of which had many other anomalies. These authors reviewed six previously described cases and extensively discussed the embryology. Heifetz and Rueda-Pedraza made the point that the cysts (0.4 to 6.0 cm) are frequently surrounded by a plexus of small vessels (Fig. 12.10) and that they usually lie in the proximal portion of the cord. Males outnumber females 4:1. Although these vitelline remnants are not particularly common and usually have no clinical significance, this is not always the case, and the question of what to do when such an anomaly is found is not always easy to answer. Heifetz and Rueda-Pedraza (1983a) thought that exploration of the neonate's abdomen is not indicated. Schellong and Pfeiffer (1967), however, described a child with intestinal obstruction that developed after the umbilical stump had fallen off. A "wart-like" swelling had developed at the navel. Because it was later identified as the severed intestine that had entered the cord for some distance, they favored exploration when such structures are found.

Remnants of distended omphalomesenteric ducts can be associated with atresia of the small intestine and can be a rare cause of abdominal distension (Petrikovsky et al., 1988). One experienced obstetrician stated to me that he had severed the normal-appearing cord of a neonate who was later found to have nearly the entire length of small bowel within that cord. King (1968) described similar cases and

referred to them as ileal "prolapse," a normal feature in early embryos (Fig. 12.11). Such remnants of intestine may be seen on the surface of the umbilical cord. Lee and Aterman (1968) reported an intestinal polyp arising 5 cm from the end of the cord. Dombrowski et al. (1987) described intestinal epithelium on the surface of the umbilical cord that was associated with a hemangioma of the cord. Harris and Wenzl (1963) reported the only other similar case, in which they found pancreatic tissue within the anomaly. No islets of Langerhans, however, were present in that pancreatic remnant. In neither case was abdominal exploration necessary. Fetal death occurred as a rather unusual complication of such an embryologic remnant in the interesting case described by Blanc and Allan (1961). Ectopic adrenal tissue, liver, and nevus cells were identified in umbilical cords by Sotelo et al. (2001). Ulceration of the cord with fetal hemorrhage has been observed by Ohyama et al. (2000) in several cases, some associated with intestinal atresia. Bile acids were found in amnionic fluid and the authors suggested that bile vomiting may have been responsible. Prenatal exsanguinating hemorrhage had taken place into the amnionic sac from a "tear" in the umbilical cord, near the fetal surface. Because of the proximity of vitelline structures, including gastric mucosa, it was inferred that the umbilical vein had ulcerated owing to erosive activity within this location. Calcific masses accompanied this lesion. On other occasions, a fibrous band has emanated from the end of Meckel's diverticulum and neonatal demise with obstruction of intestines. Two such cases were described in detail by Pfalzgraf et al. (1988). When there is per-

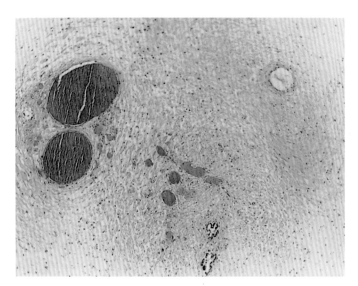

FIGURE 12.10. A plexus of small vitelline vessels accompanies the duct remnants (bottom center) in term cord. At top right is the dilated allantoic duct. H&E ×64.

FIGURE 12.11. Cross section of an umbilical cord of a 4-cm crown-to-rump embryo from a tubal pregnancy. The large space (extraembryonic coelom) contains a loop of intestine; below it are the two umbilical arteries (right) with tiny allantoic remnants below and between. At left bottom is the umbilical (allantoic) vein. H&E ×25.

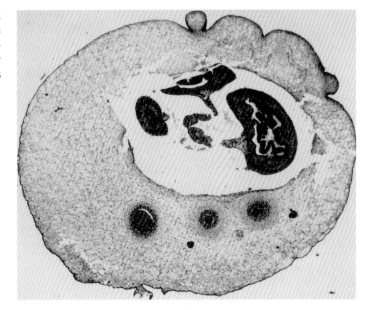

sistence of the vitelline duct and it opens upon the abdomen, a fistula with bowel discharge may develop and can be demonstrated radiographically (Ankola & Pradham, 2000).

The finding of liver tissue at the umbilicus (Shaw & Pierog, 1969) is rare and probably relates more to exomphalos (omphalocele) than to the vestiges herein described. Patel et al. (1989) reported a newborn with a markedly swollen umbilical cord (70-mm circumference) at its abdominal attachment that contained herniated bowel. Because of having seen this case, they determined the normal circumference of the umbilical cord in 191 neonates at different fetal ages and of various weights. The normal circumference was found to be 37.7 ± 7.3 mm. They cautioned that clamping large cords may cause bowel obstruction.

After regression of the omphalomesenteric duct, remainders of the detached yolk sac persist in many cases and can be found as 3- to 5-mm white-yellow disks in the chorionic plate (see Chapter 11). Meyer (1904) found them to measure up to 15 mm and wondered how such atrophic structures could become so large while degenerating. The yolk sac remnant is almost invariably located near the margin of the term placenta. It lies underneath the amnion and has a somewhat pasty consistency. This vestige must not be interpreted as being abnormal or

perhaps as representing the site of former inflammation. Histologically, it stains deeply purple with hematoxylin. It appears to be calcified but is probably mostly a deposit of pasty calcium phosphates (Fig. 12.12). The calcareous nature of this material was discussed at length by Meyer (1904). Our own x-ray microanalysis studies (courtesy Dr. Lee Hagey) revealed the predominance of calcium phosphates in the remainders of the yolk sac. The yolk sac can be visualized as a small sac during early pregnancy (Reece et al., 1987). Ferrazzi et al. (1988) reported an overall success of 97% with this visualization, at 7 weeks' gestation. Minute omphalomesenteric vessels may also accompany these yolk sac remnants. They can be seen coursing toward the umbilical cord (Fig. 12.13). The yolk sac can be visualized as a small sac during early pregnancy (Reece et al., 1987). Ferrazzi et al. (1988) reported an overall success of 97% with this visualization, at 7 weeks' gestation.

It is now well recognized that the vessels are exquisitely sensitive to various mediators, for example, serotonin, angiotensin, and oxytocin (LeDonne & McGowan, 1967; Dyer, 1970; Winters, 1970). The cord and certainly the placenta are here considered as having no functional neural investment, a conclusion that is shared by most authors (e.g., Lauweryns et al., 1969).

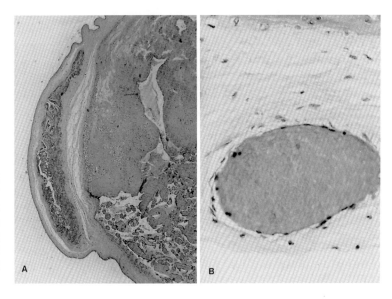

FIGURE 12.12. A: Microscopic appearance of a yolk sac remnant in a term placenta. It consists of irregular fragments of calcium phosphate deposits, underneath which are remains of omphalomesenteric vessels. The amnion is above, the chorion below. H&E ×50. B: Remains of a vitelline vessel in the proximal part of the cord. Note the squamous metaplasia on the cord surface. H&E ×400.

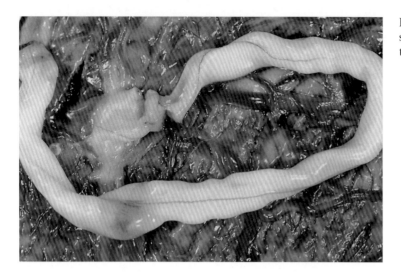

FIGURE 12.13. Vitelline vessels coursing from a yolk sac remnant (not seen) on the cord surface of a normal term placenta.

Spiral Turns of the Cord

The umbilical cord is usually spiraled, a quality referred to as "chirality" (Fletcher, 1993). A counterclockwise spiral (left) exceeds that of the opposite direction by a ratio of 7:1. The helices may be seen by ultrasonographic examination as early as during the first trimester of pregnancy (Figs. 12.14 and 12.15; Dudiak et al., 1995). Lacro et al. (1987) have studied this phenomenon in greater detail, efforts that evidently are not appreciated by everyone. For instance, Eastman (1967) stated, "As far as I am aware, knowledge about these helices is of no practical value whatsoever." Helices are readily seen by the 9th week of gestation. They usually number up to 40, but as many as 380 turns have been described. The number is already well established early in pregnancy, and it increases only insignificantly during the third trimester.

It therefore follows that the cord length grows not by increased spiraling but by increasing the pitch between each turn of the spiral. It is uncommon to find an absence of spirals in the cord but when this occurs, it has an ominous prognosis (Strong et al., 1993). These authors found that 4.3% of newborns lacked cord twists and that these had a significantly higher increase in perinatal mortality and other problems. Later, the same authors suggested that the umbilical coiling index (number of coils divided by length of cord; average 0.21/cm) may identify the fetus at risk (Strong et al., 1994). When the index fell below the 10th percentile, more chromosomal errors, fetal distress, and meconium staining were identified. A subsequent study by Rana et al. (1995) examined this proposition. They found that excessive coiling was associated with cocaine usage and increased frequency of premature labor. Reduced coiling was a predictor of problems

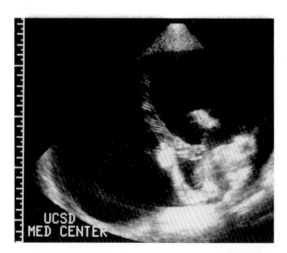

FIGURE 12.14. Sonographic appearance of a left umbilical helix in one of monochorionic twins with the transfusion syndrome at 22 weeks' gestation. (Courtesy of Dr. G.R. Leopold.)

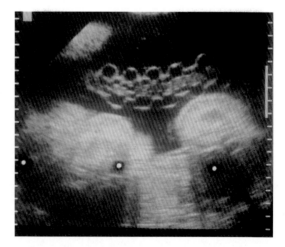

FIGURE 12.15. The helical nature of the distended blood vessels in the umbilical cord is shown in this sonograph of a pregnancy at 38 weeks' gestation. (Courtesy of Dr. G.R. Leopold.)

with labor and delivery. Uncoiled cords were present in 4.9%; their mean coiling index was 0.19/cm, and the cords of the uncoiled specimens were not unusually short. Del Valle et al. (1995) had similar results and suggested prenatal sonographic detection of chirality as an important desirability (see Degani et al., 1995; Lewinsky et al., 1996). In the study undertaken by Weeks et al. (1995), it was found that black patients had significantly less coiling than white patients. Infants with fixation of their bodies to the placental surface (due to amnionic bands) have not only relatively short cords but also few or no umbilical helices (Spatz, 1968). Likewise, Drut and Drut (2003) described a complex fetal anomaly with undercoiled, short umbilical cord and suggested decreased fetal motion to have occurred. The same is true for species with elongated embryos in elongated uterine horns (e.g., whales), a situation that hinders embryonic rotation (Slijper, 1960; Arvy & Pilleri, 1976b). This point causes us to infer that the turns must be induced by fetal rotations. Furthermore, because the left spirals outweigh the right spirals by approximately the same frequency as the distribution of handedness, Lacro et al. (1987) reasoned that the cerebral organization is the cause of the direction of spirals. The authors subsequently found that this hypothesis is incorrect, and that there was no correlation between the handedness of the fetus (and that of the mother) and the direction of spirals (Table 12.1). Furthermore, twins were found to have spirals in the same or opposite directions, although in general they had fewer twists than singletons and a different ratio. Monozygotic twins may have helices in different directions, an observation often made before. Only infants with single umbilical arteries had a significant reduction of spirals. No other anomalous development correlated, and one or the other twist was not more commonly associated with perinatal morbidity or mortality. It is interesting that an occasional cord may have helices in opposite directions (Fig. 12.16). Shen-Schwarz et al. (1997a) found that cords were more often not coiled

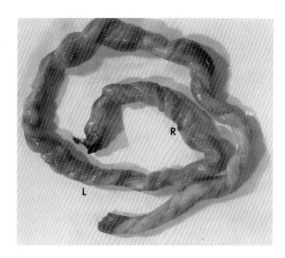

FIGURE 12.16. Umbilical cord with helices pointing to the right and left directions. Normal infant, 52-cm cord, circumvallation.

in twin gestations, irrespective of their chorionicity. The spirals of the cord have been studied in 5000 cords by morphometry and histology (Blackburn et al., 1988). A left twist was found in 79% with a left/right ratio of 3.7:1.0; in twins, the left direction was found in 61%, and mixed spiraling occurred in 26%. In contrast to the findings of Lacro et al. (1987), Blackburn et al. (1988) always found identical twins to spiral in the same directions. Fetuses with single umbilical arteries had a 1.5:1.0 left/right ratio. These authors also gave figures for cord dry mass and weight/length ratios. Fletcher (1993) found a 76.5% left-handed spiral in patients at Abu Dhabi, a right-handed twist in 15.5%, mixed in 6.5%. They found no sex difference. When Atalla et al. (1998) correlated neonatal acid–base findings with cord status, they found that there was a linear relation between venous and arterial pH, PCO_2, and length of cord, spiraling index, and other macroscopic characteristics of the cord structure.

Most authors have concluded that spiraling of the cord is the result of some fetal activity, and that the lack of spiraling may reflect fetal inactivity and possibly central nervous system (CNS) disturbances. Thus, reduced coiling has a poor prognosis (Strong et al., 1993). We have seen absent twists not only in many stillborns but also in various chromosomal errors and congenital syndromes such as the Pena Shokeir syndrome, and others. Another suggestion for the occurrence of spirals is that they are governed by the earth's rotational forces and that, like the familiar bathtub vortex (Sibulkin, 1983), there are differences in the chirality of cords between the hemispheres. This postulate has been disproved by our study of chirality in the Northern and Southern hemispheres. Edmonds (1954) and Lacro et al. (1987) considered in detail the various theories that are the basis for umbilical cord spiraling. The causes remain unknown. In our experience, Schordania's (1929a) notion that long cords are

TABLE 12.1. Distribution of the direction of the umbilical cord helix

| Source of cord | Direction of the cord helix | | | |
	Left (%)	Right (%)	None (%)	Left/right ratio
Live-born singletons	7.8	83	12	5
All twins (combined data for 290 sets)	3.7	66	18	11
Monochorionic twins	7.8	82	11	7
Dichorionic twins	4.8	77	16	8
Intrauterine deaths	8.7	73	8	18
Single umbilical artery (SUA)	2.8	63	22	15
SUA with problems	1.1	44	39	17
SUA without problems	5.2	72	14	5.2
Placental singletons ($n = 14,070$)	7.5	75	10	15

more spiraled is correct, although it contradicts the findings of Chaurasia and Agarwal (1979), who studied only a small number of specimens. The higher fetal mortality seen with intense spiraling (Fig. 12.17) has been discussed.

The fact that frequently, but not always, the spirals represent distended umbilical arteries is well seen in Figure 12.18. This helical arrangement of vessels has been helpful in the diagnosis of fetal death, as in some such pregnancies gas can then be visualized in an helical arrangement (Gruber, 1967). Several investigators have suggested that differential pressures of different-size umbilical arteries are the forces that produce the helices. The findings on single umbilical arteries (Lacro et al., 1987) tend to negate this notion. It may be that we are failing to differentiate true umbilical cord twists from changes in which the umbilical arteries are merely wound around a less spiraled vein. Whether arteries are wound around the vein (Smart, 1962) or the vein winds around arteries (Potter, 1961) is irrelevant. Both arrangements can be seen in the same cord (Fig. 12.18). The many arrangements that exist have been depicted by Hyrtl (1870) and Arvy and Pilleri (1976a), among others. These authors made numerous corrosion preparations of cords to investigate these features. Dado et al. (1997) deduced from their perfusion studies of cords that coiling had little effect on resistance when external pressure was applied or the cords were stretched. They felt that "differences in morbidity associated with umbilical cord coiling should not be attributed simply to mechanical factors, and other mechanisms should be sought."

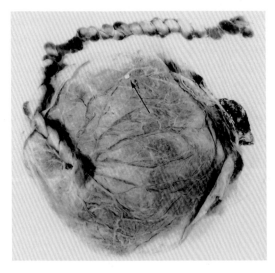

FIGURE 12.17. Term placenta of a stillborn infant with an intensely twisted umbilical cord. The cause of death was inferred to be the twisted cord as there were no other findings. Note also the remains of the yolk sac (arrow).

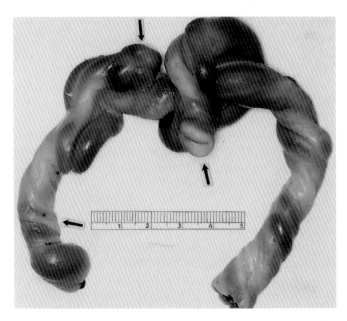

FIGURE 12.18. Umbilical cord with true and false knots in a live infant. The arteries wind around the vein (left arrow); in the knot, the vein winds about the artery. False knots with vessels (top arrow) and with only Wharton's jelly (central arrow) are apparent as well.

Length of the Cord

The length of the umbilical cord has been the topic of numerous studies. Most authors agree that excessively short and long cords correlate well with a variety of fetal problems and have been adequately summarized by Gilbert-Barness et al. (1993). The normal length at term has been cited by Grosser (1927), who utilized data from various older studies, but standards for measuring the length were supplied later (e.g., Mills et al., 1983). These authors and Naeye (1985) used the very large number of cord measurements from the Collaborative Perinatal Study and provided smoothed curves from 34 to 43 weeks' gestation. These data are not significantly different from ours (provided at the end of this book in tabular form). The mean length of 59.44 cm was determined by one of us (8000 measurements, ranging from 24 to 146 cm); another author found it to be 66.54 cm (12,000 measured). When circled once about the neck the cord was 76.5 cm long, and when circled twice about the neck it was 93.5 cm. Thus, wide variations were detected. As was suggested by Leonardo da Vinci, the umbilical cord has usually the same length as the baby. Figure 12.19 gives values for cord lengths as determined by a variety of authors. Manci et al. (1993), however, found that the length of the cord shrinks up to 7 cm in the first few hours following delivery. Thus, accurate recording at birth is preferable.

There have been numerous other studies. Malpas (1964), stimulated by the birth of a baby with a 129-cm-

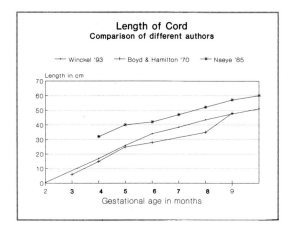

FIGURE 12.19. Length of umbilical cord as determined by different authors. When exact numbers were not given, the approximate number was entered.

long cord, measured 538 normal cords at term. He found a normal distribution, with an average length of 61 cm (30 to 129 cm). There was slight correlation with fetal and placental weights. Gardiner (1922) obtained an average length of 55 cm for normal cords. He considered less than 32 cm as "absolutely" short, and more than 32 cm as "relatively" short. He also suggested what the length of the cord *should* be if it were to allow a normal delivery with cephalic or breech presentations with looping (he also gave quantitative accounts of the frequency of coiling). He assumed that the length of the cord was determined by the amount of amnionic fluid and depended also on fetal movements. The complete findings of Malpas just cited supported the notion of Walker and Pye (1960) (average 54.1 cm, maximum values ranging from 17.8 to 121.9 cm) that most of the cord's length is achieved by the 28th week of pregnancy. During the 41st day p.c., the developing cord, the amnionic covering of which is still incomplete, has a mean length of about 0.5 cm. By the 4th lunar month it has grown to between 16 and 18 cm and, by the 6th month, to between 33 and 35 cm. It was also suggested that there may be a relation to umbilical arterial pressures, but this point was not well supported. In a series of 37 pairs of monozygotic twins studied, little difference was found when they were compared to singletons. Naeye (1985) based his findings on the measurements of cords at birth from the Collaborative Perinatal Study (35,779 cases) and found that the cord grows progressively from 32 cm at 20 weeks to 60 cm at term. Although growth slowed progressively, it never ceased. Ultrasonographic measurements have also been published that describe the length of the umbilical cord in early gestation. Thus, Hill et al. (1994a) studied 53 normal fetuses and 15 with fetal death between 6 and 11 weeks' gestation. The cord lengths of 60% of the dead fetuses was significantly shorter. These finding suggested to the

authors that demise is preceded by reduced fetal activity. The normal fetuses' cords grew linearly. The measurements are depicted in tabular form in Chapter 28. Weissman et al. (1994) studied the diameters of cord and its vessels of 368 normal gestations of between 8 and 40 weeks and ascertained smooth curves of growth for all data. More recently, the recognition of a relationship between fetal movements and fetal well-being have resulted in "kick-counts"; the results are summarized in an early contribution by Grant et al. (1989) and in many publications since. They have also been charted extensively and followed with advancing gestational age (ten Hof et al., 1999). These studies are difficult and analysis is complex because of the irregularities in the occurrence of movements, the minor and major bursts that occur, the length of observation, etc. Increased length between bursts was observed with advancing age.

Abnormal Length, Nuchal Cord

Although it in known that short cords (less than 40 cm) are correlated with neonatal problems and depressed intelligence quotient (IQ) values, the essential question, however, remains whether the length of the cord is determined by prenatal CNS problems or whether the CNS problems that are so well correlated, result from perinatal problems attending the delivery with a short cord. This question is of interest because it has been shown not only that short cords are more common with a variety of congenital anomalies but also that the length of the cord is usually determined by fetal movements in early fetal life. When the fetus is constrained, as occurs for instance with amnionic adhesions and in ectopic pregnancies, the cord is short (Miller et al., 1981). The possible relation between long cords and excessive fetal movements is more difficult to assess because of the deficiency of quantitative data on prenatal movements. It would also be of great interest to obtain more information as to whether children associated with long umbilical cords remain to be "hyperactive" in later life; the contribution by Naeye and Tafari (1983) suggests that this may be so.

Moessinger and his colleagues (1982) have investigated the question of the cord's length experimentally in rats. They injected curare (short cords), placed the rat fetuses in an extrauterine position (long cords), and produced oligohydramnios (short cords). It has also been learned that infants with Down syndrome (trisomy 21) have significantly shorter cords (45.1 cm versus 57.3 cm for controls), speculated to be due to the reduced fetal activity in utero (Moessinger et al., 1986). Likewise, with breech presentations, the cord is shorter by some 4.5 cm than with births from a vertex presentation, and 7.9 cm shorter in twins (Soernes & Bakke, 1986). These authors also confirmed other investigators' findings that males have slightly longer cords than females (58.46 cm versus 56.90 cm in vertex; 53.78 versus 52.51 cm in breech). Snider (1997) examined the length of umbilical cords associated with lethal bony malformations such as osteogenesis imperfecta. All had significantly reduced cord lengths. Four additional cases with similar findings came from Dr. M. Grafe (personal communication, 1997) and many more cases have since come to our attention. It was inferred that because the presumed pain felt with movements the fetuses did not move normally. This is also one explanation for the pulmonary hypoplasia (lack of chest movements) and reduced motion is also the finding during sonography of such fetuses. In Chapter 11 we discussed the possible relationship of pain to endorphin levels in amnionic fluid, and suggested that such studies should be encouraged to be pursued in the future. Correlations such as these have led to experiments in animals, where it was found that prenatal alcohol administration to rats shortens the cords (Barron et al., 1985), as does atenolol (a beta-blocker) given to rabbits (Katz et al., 1987). Shorter cords have since been found in offspring who suffer the fetal alcohol syndrome (Calvano et al., 2000). Contrary to these views, Fujinaga et al. (1990) have opined that the "stretch hypothesis" is faulty. Their findings verified that umbilical cords of humans and rats steadily increase with gestational age, but in some of their cases with oligohydramnios long cords were found. Moreover, their tenet was that the amount of amnionic fluid decreases with advancing gestational age and that, therefore, "fetuses should be less active." This is not the place to argue extensively over the merits of one or the other theory; suffice it to say that oligohydramneic fetuses may be just as active as those in normal environments and thus may be able to stretch their cords. It is also important to know how long

the oligohydramnios had existed and how severe it was. Moreover, because cords grow substantially early in fetal life (before for instance endorphin secretion in cases of osteogenesis imperfecta (OI) and urinary deficiency may have influenced the growth of cords, the finding of longer cords in some cases of oligohydramnios is not surprising. Further data are definitely needed. Naeye and Tafari (1983) found that neonates with long cords were relatively hyperkinetic when compared with those that had shorter cords. Malicki et al. (1997) analyzed retrospectively data from 38,224 placental studies and concluded that excessively long cords (3.95%) were significantly more common with right spirals, with excessive spiraling, true knots, thromboses in fetal vessels, congestion, and meconium staining. Male fetuses were also overrepresented. Kalish et al. (2003) also found a deleterious effect of right twisting (placenta previa and hemorrhage).

An interesting study of equine abortions comes from Hong et al. (1993). They found that torsion of an excessively long umbilical cord is an important cause of fetal wastage in horses, making up some 4.5% of 1211 cases. The normal cord length in horses was found to be 52 cm whereas that of abortuses with torsion was 72 cm. Excellent photographs accompany this description and are further considered below.

There are rare cases of "achordia", which have mostly been associated with abdominal wall defects (Giacoia, 1992), as in Figure 12.20, or with acardiac fetuses (see Chapter 25). Most of these infants actually have a diminutive cord rather than no cord at all. Rupture of short cords and of cords with entanglement have been reported by Szécsi (1955). Several authors have delineated a "short cord syndrome" that includes a variety of associated anomalies (Gilbert, 1986; Grange et al., 1987). In the

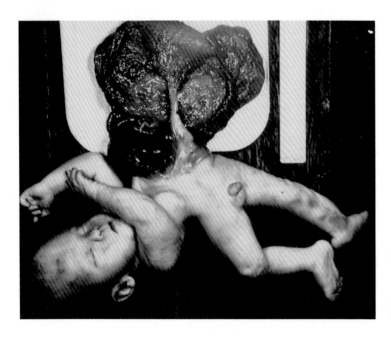

FIGURE 12.20. Excessively short umbilical cord at term with an abdominal wall defect (gastroschisis).

latter study, cords less than 15 cm were often associated with abdominal wall defects and evisceration, spinal and limb deformities, and other lesions. The authors thought of it as a "primary malformation."

An excessively long cord poses problems because the fetus may become entangled in it or the cord may prolapse, especially after the membranes rupture. The successful clinical management of gestations with long cords has been detailed by Katz et al. (1988). In general, long cords have more pronounced spiraling and it may be inferred from this fact also that the excessive length results from increased fetal movements. Umbilical cords measuring up to 300 cm have been reported (Arvy & Pilleri, 1976a). The greatest length we have measured was 165 cm. One would think that such excessively long and spiraled cords would also require greater perfusion pressure, but this has not been confirmed, and some studies suggest that it is not true.

Looping about the neck and extremities was found in 23% of overall obstetrical cases by Earn (1951) and it was more common with excessively long cords. He once found the cord to be wound eight times around the neck. The fetus in Figure 12.21 had died because its cord was entwined around the neck three times; there was obstruction of venous return from the placenta. The constriction of the cord shown in Figure 12.22 led to its reduced size. It had been wound around the arm and the depression of the arm was clearly discernible and bore testimony to this entwinement having caused the fetal death. We have subsequently seen similar compression of an extremity due

to cord pressure, but the fetus survived. Although it simulated grossly the constriction of amnionic bands, it was much wider. Nelson and Grether (1998) found that a statistically significant correlation exists between the presence of tight nuchal cords at delivery and the occurrence of otherwise unexplained spastic cerebral palsy (quadriplegia, not diplegia), to be discussed next.

To find an entanglement of cords with extremities and bodies of young fetuses establishes that these abnormalities are not just features of labor and term pregnancy. Javert and Barton (1952) also made such observations. They studied 1000 spontaneous abortions, of which 297 cases had sufficiently well-preserved cords for study. Of these, 104 (35%) were abnormal, compared with a rate of 4.8% in a control group of "therapeutic" abortions; 13.4% were of excessive length and had looping. In those cases, excessive fetal activity had often been observed before fetal death occurred. A case reported by Williams and colleagues (1981) is of considerable interest here. They had a patient with fetal growth retardation at 38 weeks' gestation in whom an emergency cesarean section was performed because of flat fetal heart rate tracings. The normally long umbilical cord was wound five times about the severely compressed and bruised neck. Various clinical findings, including oligohydramnios and a lack of fetal movements led them to suspect that this cord entanglement had been present for at least 2 months. Lin et al. (1999) showed an impressive indenture of the abdomen of a monoamnionic twin neonate due to encircling by the umbilical cord. It disappeared spontaneously.

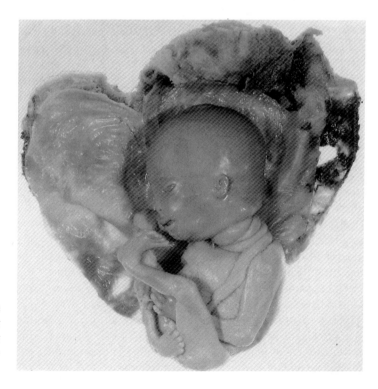

FIGURE 12.21. Stillborn fetus with cord wrapped three times about its neck. Death presumably came about by obstruction to venous return from the placenta, not by obstruction to vessels of the fetal head. Note the congestion of the head.

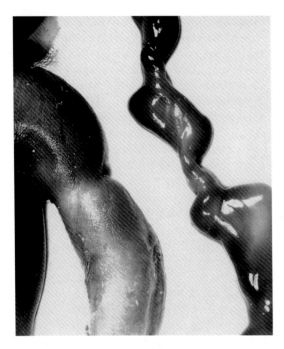

FIGURE 12.22. Umbilical cord and arm of a stillborn fetus. There is marked constriction of the arm and cord where the latter had wound firmly about the arm. The specimen was received with the amnion unruptured, so fetal motion alone must have caused the entanglement.

There have been numerous investigations to ascertain whether nuchal cords may cause fetal death or asphyxia during labor. Crawford (1962) found its incidence to be as high as 34% in vaginal vertex deliveries. He surmised that the significantly increased morbidity was related to deprivation of placental perfusion after expulsion of the fetus. In later analysis of his data, Crawford concluded that the incidence of nuchal cords rises steeply after 38 weeks of gestation, perhaps secondary to greater fetal activity or because of decreasing amnionic fluid volume (1964). A somewhat similar incidence of nuchal cords and its complications was found by Kan and Eastman (1957) (one coil 20.6%, two coils 2.5%, three coils 0.5%), Reiss (1964), Horwitz et al. (1964), and others. McCurdy et al. (1994) were able to identify the presence of nuchal cords sonographically, confirming other radiologists' impressions. In their study, the presence of nuchal cords led to more admissions to the neonatal intensive care unit (NICU) and to cesarean section. Schaefer et al. (1998) saw nuchal cords in 26 of 316 (8.23%) sonographically examined fetuses at 10 to 14 weeks' gestation, but most had disappeared at term. Collins et al. (1991) and Collins (1997) separated two types of nuchal cords, to be distinguished at delivery, much as Giacomello had done (1988): "Type A encircles the neck in an unlocked pattern; Type B encircles the neck in a locked pattern." Type B is found to be associated with breech delivery and is considered to be as having more severe consequences for fetal

outcome (see also Collins, 2002). In 850 deliveries, type B was found three times, two of whom had fetal distress and one was stillborn. In another study of nuchal cords of 231 prenatally studied patients, Collins et al. (1995) found that nuchal cords can be present as early as at 20 weeks' gestation. Of 36 cases, 11 resolved before delivery, one with triple encirclement resolved to a single loop around the neck. A nuchal cord may form, they found, when the umbilical cord is four fifths as long as the fetus. That nuchal cords may be associated with or cause fetal growth restriction was demonstrated by Soernes (1995) in 11,201 deliveries. In 19% of deliveries one encirclement was found, 5.3% had two loops, 1.2% had three, and 0.2% had four cord encirclements. In statistical analysis, Soernes found a detrimental effect of nuchal cord encirclement upon fetal weight and a similar relation to increasing length of the umbilical cord. From this he inferred that encirclement must have existed for long periods in utero and cautions that inferences of poor fetal outcome with nuchal cords may reflect long-standing prenatal events (see also Nelson & Grether, 1998).

Some authors, however, deny any relation to fetal distress and poor fetal outcome from problems of cord length. Sinnathuray (1966) and Kan and Eastman (1957) found no increase in perinatal mortality. Dippel (1964) wrote that nuchal cords are much "maligned" and observed only a significant increase in the frequency of irregular fetal heart rates and the need for resuscitation when they were present. He opined that a hasty delivery is rarely required. Spellacy and coauthors (1966) studied this phenomenon in 17,190 deliveries from the Collaborative Perinatal Study. They concluded that nuchal coils occurred in 20.4% of deliveries and that there was entwinement about the body in 2%, and knots occurred in 1%. There were more complications with long cords, and with "tight" cords, that is, cords that were functionally short. Entanglement was the cause of depressed 1-minute Apgar scores but did not cause low 5-minute scores. Length of cord was also not correlated with the 1-year neurologic status; stillbirths, though, were increased with true knots. McLennan et al. (1988) undertook a prospective study of 1115 vaginal deliveries to ascertain the frequencies of knots and encirclement. Six knots (0.5%) and 158 cases with encirclement (14.2%) were found, with cords ranging from 27 to 122 cm in length. No warning of such knots or entanglements was identified in the gravidas, and the offspring had no problems, although the authors admitted that they are the cause of 10% of fetal deaths above 2500 g. In their experience, the average cord length was 52 cm, the 10th percentile was 40 cm, and the 90th percentile 69 cm. Giacomello (1988) reported the detection of nuchal cord in a large proportion of breech presentations by ultrasonography. He cautioned that an assessment of the postdelivery incidence of nuchal cords is unreliable and minimally requires description of the nature of the nuchal cord. He depicted two types, locked and not locked, much as Collins (1997) did subsequently. The following photographs impressively demonstrate the consequences of severe spiraling that led to thrombosis of surface vessels with fetal demise (Figs. 12.23 and 12.24).

In recent years, obstetrical care has frequently involved extensive monitoring of fetal heart rates. Cord entanglement, the now uncommon cord prolapse (Panter & Hannah, 1996), and other abnormalities during labor have thus become better correlated with compromised cord perfusion. Rayburn et al. (1981), for instance, reviewed some of these findings. They studied 536 term deliveries in an effort to correlate the findings of fetal heart rate monitoring with cord length. They defined a short cord as all cords measuring less than 35 cm in length and a long cord as measuring more than 80 cm. Of the 32 cases with "cord accidents," 20 (62.5%) were found with long cords. The monitor tracings had cord compression patterns. These authors advocated measuring cord length routinely after delivery, a recommendation since strongly repeated (Benirschke, 1991). Fribourg (1981) objected to this measurement as an idle enterprise because there are "no current means of performing measurements before the fact." But this situation is changing with improved sonographic techniques and with the development of velocimetry (Feinstein et al., 1985; Guidetti et al., 1987). A better understanding of the correlations just described is deemed especially important for infants whose poor outcome is otherwise unexplained. This consideration particularly concerns medical litigation.

It was mentioned earlier that infants born with nuchal cords are more often deprived of placental blood transfusion because their cords are severed by the obstetrician before extraction. Shepherd et al. (1985) identified that newborns with nuchal cords are significantly more anemic than controls, presumably because of reduced venous return from the placenta secondary to compression of the umbilical vein. Vanhaesebrouck et al. (1987) suggested that tight nuchal cords may be the cause of hypovolemic shock of the newborn. They observed two newborns with anemia and cord entanglement and suggested that entanglement occurs as often as in some 20% of births. That nuchal cord entanglement may have serious sequelae for the fetus was shown in the retrospective study of Nelson and Grether (1998). They found cerebral palsy as a probable consequence of this prenatal problem. Fetomaternal hemorrhage was ruled out by Kleihauer stains on maternal blood to have caused the anemia. These authors also suggested that problems of venous return from the placenta allowed pooling of blood in the placenta. Thus, "fetoplacental" hemorrhage is the mode they used to explain the neonatal anemia in their cases. Anagnostakis and coauthors (1974) conjectured that the two neonatal deaths with pulmonary hemorrhages they saw may have resulted from increased pulmonary perfusion because of tight nuchal cords. This argument is difficult to accept, as nuchal cords are so common and lethal pulmonary hemorrhages rare.

Premature separation of the cord with fetal bleeding may occur with short cords and when a "relative" short cord is induced by entangling. An interesting suggestion has been made by Akiyama et al. (1981), who were concerned with ascertaining clinically when the placenta had detached from the uterus so as to allow its delivery. When they clamped the cord immediately after delivery of the infant, pinched the placental end of the cord, and then squeezed the blood toward the placenta for 10 to 15 cm, they could assess the backflow of blood in their fingers when slowly releasing the pressure. When backflow was sensed, the placenta had not yet separated.

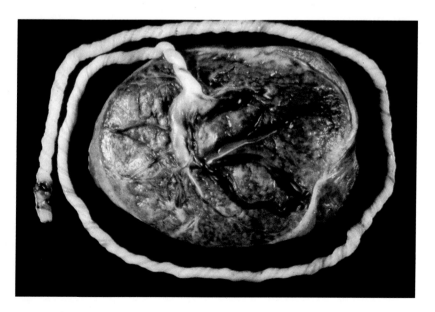

FIGURE 12.23. Marked spiraling of umbilical cord with surface vessel thrombosis (see next figure). Intrauterine fetal demise.

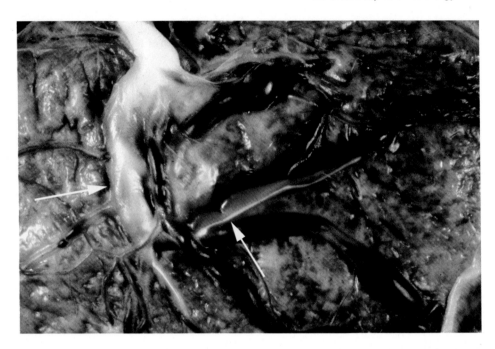

FIGURE 12.24. Marked spiraling of umbilical cord with surface vessel thrombosis (see previous figure). Intrauterine fetal demise. The partially calcified thrombosis of surface veins is indicated by arrows.

Eastman and Hellman (1961) emphasized that the absolute and relative lengths of cords are the important factors, not the actual measurement of the cord length. It is obvious that a long cord, wound about the neck five times, may in fact be a relatively short cord during fetal descent with delivery. Dislodgment of the placenta may then occur, which may cause bleeding. In the case described by Corridan and coauthors (1980), this complication was associated with fatal amnionic fluid embolism. The reader is also referred to Fox's (1978, 1997) book on the placenta for additional references. Fox as well as de Sa (1984) were not impressed with the opinion that mechanical factors such as traction play an important role in fetal compromise when short cords are present. Perhaps vascular spasm (Camilleri, 1964) is the important event. This hypothesis is supported by our finding a nuchal cord with fetal death in an otherwise well developed extrauterine (tubal) fetus. The umbilical cord of this fetus was occluded, yet it was clearly stationary.

Prolapse of the cord is associated more often with multiparity, premature labor, multiple gestation, and with cords that are longer than those of normal length. At times, this situation has grave prognostic significance for the fetus and Uchide et al. (1997), who diagnosed it sonographically, suggested that its recognition by Doppler sonography is mandatory for a good outcome. Widholm and Nieminen (1963) recorded cord prolapse in 0.41% of 7500 deliveries with a 13.4% perinatal mortality. This figure is similar to the results published by Brant and Lewis (1966), who urged that a prolapsed cord be kept

warm so as to avoid spasm of vessels. Another review of the topic was provided by Levy et al. (1984), who also found this complication more often in multiparous women. One half of their study group had fetal malpresentations, one third had premature onset of labor, and a variety of other abnormal factors was present. Good obstetrical management usually gave a good fetal outcome so long as the fetus was alive on admission. Dildy and Clark (1993) found that cord prolapse occurred in 1 of 275 deliveries and that the risk was greatest with artificial rupture of membranes with high presenting fetal parts. It has been cautioned that many cases of fatal cord prolapse result from amniotomy, and that some occur after external fetal version (Lehman, 1983). It is now possible to make the diagnosis antenatally with ultrasonography, particularly when malposition and hydramnios suggest this possibility (Lange et al., 1985). A large study on causes of, or associations with cord prolapse was undertaken by Critchlow et al. (1994). Their findings indicated a high cesarean section rate, a 10% mortality, and high prematurity and breech rates, but data on length of cord were not available. The hemodynamic response with fetal heart rate monitoring has been detailed by Lee and Hon (1963) and is of particular importance for the cases with occult prolapse. These authors found prompt, marked bradycardia when the umbilical arteries were occluded and believed that this probably resulted from increased fetal blood pressure. This finding has come to be looked at as being pathognomonic for the detection of cord compression during monitored labor. The compressed umbilical cord may show profound pathologic changes, such as hemorrhage, and even rupture at the site of compression. It leads occasionally to thrombosis, found when multiple sections are taken, but thrombi ensue more commonly in the surface chorionic vessels. That cord compression may have serious fetal neurologic consequences is one of the reasons for taking the cord compression pattern of fetal heart monitoring so seriously. Its effects on CNS damage have been amply studied in fetal sheep (Mallard et al., 1992; Kaneko et al., 2003). They detected that even short arterial occlusion may cause damage, predominantly in the hippocampal area. We have seen a stillbirth at 19 weeks' gestation from an excessively long prolapsed cord with an extremely pale placenta. The villous tissue had the appearance of being exsanguinated and was similar to the hydropic placenta of erythroblastosis. Instead, the umbilical arteries had constricted from presumed cold exposure, with labor leading to the return of placental blood to the polycythemic fetus.

A few other findings may be mentioned briefly. Thus, when all factors contributing possibly to intrauterine fetal death, Karin et al. (2002) found that cord problems accounted for 9% (infection 24%, growth restriction 22%, abruption 19%, maternal conditions 12%, anomalies 10%). Williams and O'Brien (2000a) found that cord entanglement was associated more frequently with a larger placental mass and decreased fetal/placental ration in a cohort of 37,014 infants they reviewed. In a second contribution (Williams & O'Brien, 2000b) they concluded that nuchal cords and tight loops did not cause significant peripartum morbidity but appeared to be related to chronic rather than acute stress. Clapp et al. (2003) determined the occurrence of nuchal cords prospectively from 24 weeks on and found it to increase from 12% to 37%. They thought of it as a chance phenomenon that bears little relation to perinatal morbidity. An interesting sonographic study by Habek et al. (2003) recorded the grasping of the umbilical cord by the fetus. They observed seven cases and all had normal outcome ultimately but had flow-related abnormalities during the event. Camann and Marquardt (2003) produced a fine picture of a compound knot of the umbilical cord with normal outcome but variable decelerations before birth. Hershkovitz et al. (2001) emphasized the need for careful study of the cord in pregnancies with fetal distress; they described a 1.2% incidence of knots (in 69,139 gestations) and higher perinatal morbidity. Hydramnios and male fetuses had a greater propensity. Finally, a statistical study of 926 cases with excessively long cords (70+cm) was performed by Baergen et al. (2001). They found a "significantly increased risk of brain imaging abnormalities and/or abnormal neurological follow-up." In addition, mothers with a history of an excessively long umbilical cord are at increased risk of a second long cord. Our experience with excessively long and short cords and their presumed causes are provided in Figures 12.28 and 12.29.

Site of Cord Insertion

The umbilical cord normally inserts on the placental tissue itself, more often near or at the center than elsewhere, as shown in Figure 12.25. In nearly 7% of term placentas, it has a marginal insertion, which, in the English-language literature, is often referred to as a "Battledore" placenta. In about 1% of placentas the umbilical cord inserts on the membranes, referred to as velamentous or membranous insertion. Here, the umbilical vessels course over the free membranes and, having lost their protection by Wharton's jelly, are more vulnerable to trauma and disruption.

Not only are the sites of insertion variable, the insertion itself may take an abnormal shape. Thus, the branching of vessels can occur before the cord comes to the surface of the placenta in the "furcate cord" insertion (Ottow, 1923; see Fig. 12.27). At times, the cord runs parallel to the placental surface or in the membranes before its vessels branch, the "interposition" (Ottow, 1922). The fetal end of the umbilical cord may also be anomalous, as is found primarily in infants with gastroschisis (short cords) (see Fig. 12.20) or with omphaloceles. These conditions can now be diagnosed prenatally and assume a greater importance in management than they did in the past (Didolkar et al., 1981). Some of these anomalies are associated with significant disturbances in fetal growth or during delivery and are thus of importance. Moreover, the formal genesis has interested students of the placenta so that they may obtain a better insight into the factors that regulate placental growth. We have seen typical interposition in a case of trisomy 13, associated with a severely malformed fetus and extensive thrombosis of fetal vessels. The umbilical vein of the interposed segment had mural thrombosis and old calcifications in the wall; the fetus had intestinal arterial thrombi.

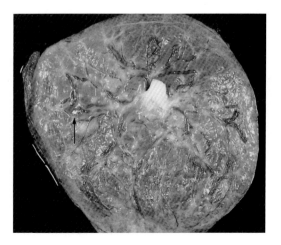

FIGURE 12.25. Normal term placenta with near-central insertion of the umbilical cord. Note the disperse distribution of vessels, marginal membranes, and calcified yolk sac remnant (arrow).

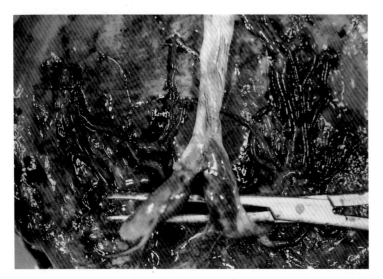

FIGURE 12.26. Furcate cord insertion with thrombosis. (Courtesy of Dr. S. Lewis, Miami, Florida.)

Furcate Cord Insertion

Furcate cord insertion is a rare abnormality in which the umbilical vessels separate from the cord substance prior to reaching the surface of the placenta. They lose the protection afforded by Wharton's jelly and are prone to thrombosis and injury. The condition was first described in three patients by Hyrtl (1870) and has received more attention from Herberz (1938) (six cases) and Swanberg and Wiqvist (1951) (stillborn, hemorrhage). Four of

Herberz's cases were associated with normal infants, and much discussion was devoted to its differentiation from velamentous insertion. Kessler (1960) also described fatal hemorrhage associated with this condition and supplied an extensive literature of intrapartum hemorrhage on request. The manner of insertion and the dissociation of vessels from the cord substance and membranes are well seen in Figures 12.25 and 12.26. This placenta was associated with normal outcome. The infant whose placenta is shown in Figure 12.30, however, was growth-restricted and had low Apgar scores. The furcate and velamentous cord had varices and numerous mural thrombi; many of the placental vessels had degenerations and calcifications in their walls. This case illustrates why the conditions furcate and velamentous have often posed semantic problems of classification.

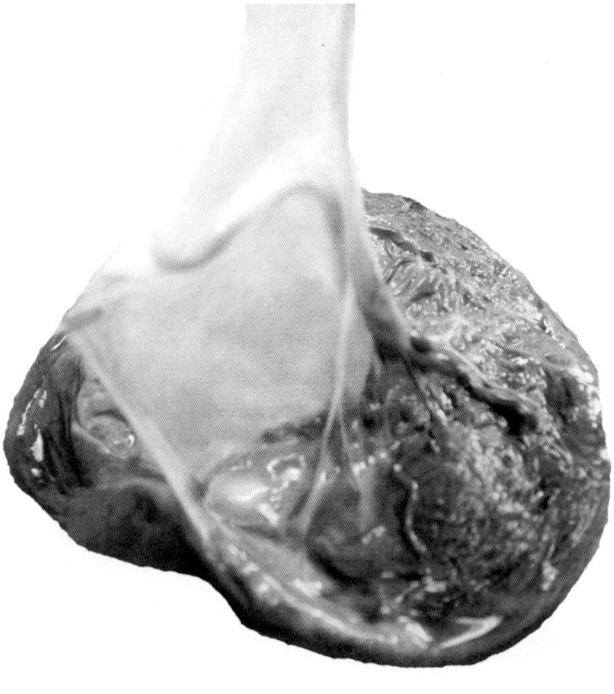

FIGURE 12.27. Furcate insertion and interposition of umbilical cord. The vessels divide and spread prior to their insertion on the placental surface and course in amnion.

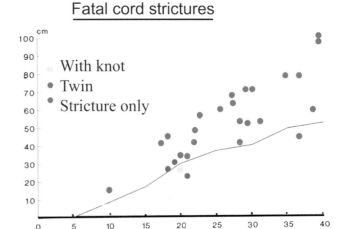

FIGURE 12.28. Diagram to show the relation of knots, twin cords, and excessively long cords in prenatal deaths. Knots and fatal strictures are nearly always found with cords of excessive length. (Line depicts expected normal length.)

Length of umbilical cord

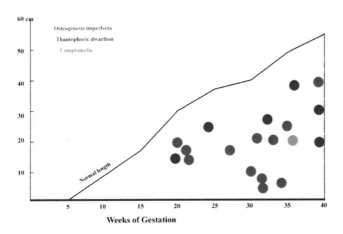

FIGURE 12.29. The length of umbilical cord in our cases of osteogenesis imperfecta, thanatophoric dwarfism and camptomelia. All have shorter umbilical cords, presumably because of "fear to move" in utero because of pain or inability to move.

Velamentous Cord Insertion

Because of its relative frequency and importance to the course of pregnancy and delivery, velamentous or membranous insertion of the umbilical cord has been studied by many investigators. Complications include rupture of membranous vessels and vasa previa. Moreover, vasa previa may be compressed during labor and cause fetal distress (Cordero et al., 1993). Velamentously inserted

TABLE 12.2. Large series' frequencies of cord insertions in singletons

Authors	No.	Marginal (%)	Velamentous (%)	Normal (%)
Benirschke 1972–1975	4,601	8.5	1.5	90
Nöldeke (1934)	10,000	ng	1.1	
Grieco (1936)	23,469	?	0.41	
Earn (1951)	5,412	15	1.0	84
Di Terlizzi and Rossi (1955)	15,416	?	1.0	
Scott (1960)	3,161	2	1.5	96.5
Corkill (1961)	12,695	ng	0.024	
Eastman and Hellman (1961)	2,000	7	1.25	91
Thomas (1963)	18,316	5.2	1.3	93.5
Krone et al. (1965)	2,868	7.9	1.8	90.3
Scheffel and Langanke (1970)	37,963	ng	0.22	
Uyanwah-Akpom and Fox (1977)	1,000	5.6	1.6	92.8
Robinson et al. (1983)	44,677	8.5	1.5	90
This series (1984–1987)	12,787	9.17	1.27	89.6
Total	194,365	6.89	1.11	90.9

ng, not given.

cords are associated with twinning and single umbilical artery (SUA). The incidence of various types of cord insertion varies throughout numerous reported series because the interpretation of what is truly a marginal or already a velamentous insertion, or merely an excessively eccentric one, differs in the eyes of the beholder. Nevertheless, Table 12.2 shows that most observers agree that

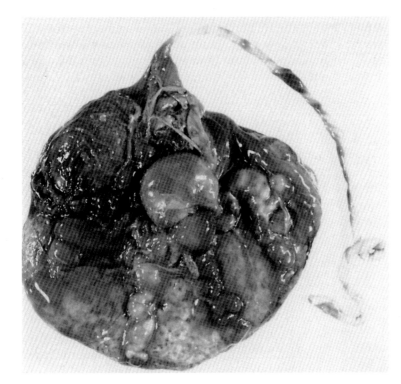

FIGURE 12.30. Velamentous and furcate insertion of the cord in a growth-restricted infant with low Apgar scores. There are numerous aneurysms, extensive mural thrombosis, and vessel wall calcifications. (Courtesy of Dr. M. Rockwell.)

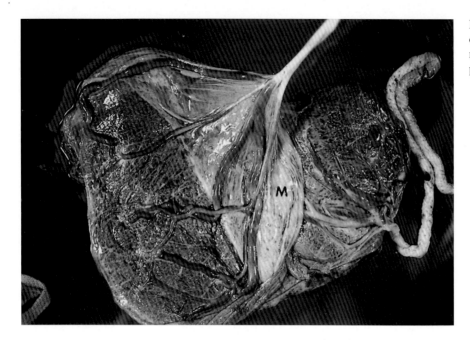

FIGURE 12.31. Velamentous insertion of umbilical cord on the dividing membranes (M) of dichorionic twin placenta.

its frequency is around 1% of singleton term deliveries. The cord may insert reasonably close to the edge of the placenta or far away from it. The close insertion is much more common than the extreme situation, where the cord inserts at the apex of the membranous sac. In the latter configuration, the long membranous course of the vessels makes them even more vulnerable to injury. It should be pointed out though that a membranous course of fetal blood vessels is not reserved to a velamentous insertion of the cord. Quite often there are such membranous vessels issuing from marginally inserted cords, and they have the same serious prognosis. Also, membranous fetal vessels are not synonymous with vasa previa. The latter condition exists only when the membranous vessels course over the internal os uteri, previous to (ahead of)

the fetal head during delivery. In multiple gestations, the velamentous cord insertion often arises on the dividing membranes (Fig. 12.31) and the membranous vessels are then similarly prone to disruption. Fries et al. (1993) found that velamentous cord insertion is more common in placentas of the twin-to-twin transfusion syndrome and suggested that this may impact the severity of the growth restriction to the donor twin.

Thrombosis of arteries (Fig. 12.32) and veins (Fig. 12.33) has both been seen in this insertional anomaly, and thrombi may be associated with neonatal purpura and fetal death. Hemorrhages arise most commonly from the veins, and they are the most frequent complications of membranous vessels. Hemorrhages may even commence in utero, before labor has begun (Bilek et al., 1962). In

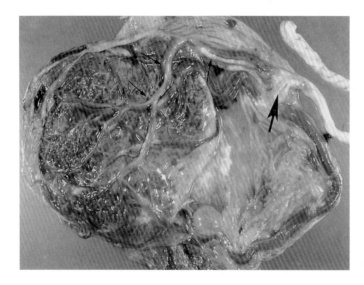

FIGURE 12.32. Velamentous (membranous) insertion of the umbilical cord (large arrow) with several calcified arterial thrombi (small arrows). Apgar scores were 1/9.

FIGURE 12.33. Velamentous insertion of the umbilical cord with sudden fetal death at 37 weeks. Note the large venous thrombi (arrows). The different ages of thrombi are seen in darker and lighter colors, indicating different degrees of hemolysis.

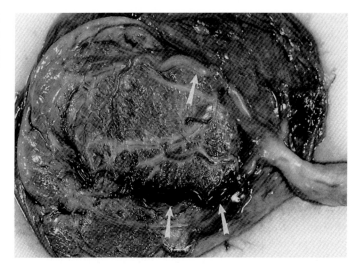

several cases that we have seen there were numerous hemosiderin-laden macrophages around the necrotic, thrombosed artery, presumably derived from the hemolysis of extravasated blood. In addition, it has been our observation that there is older medial necrosis of the muscular wall than of its periphery. We have sought to explain this by better oxygen supply from the periphery (through the cord substance). Thrombosis and arterial necrosis occasionally follow arterial spasm after cordocentesis, perhaps in response to the release of vasoactive substances measured by Rizzo et al. (1996). Depending on whether a Hyrtl anastomosis is present, large areas of placental tissue may also infarct. We have seen such isolated thrombosis also in two cases with excessively spiraled umbilical cords. Cook et al. (1995) discovered thrombosis by sonography at 31 weeks' gestation when the fetus had decreased movements. The thrombus originated from the aorta and embolization to umbilical vessels was suggested. It resolved spontaneously after birth, without an etiology having been ascertained. The more distal consequences of fetal artery thromboses were studied by McDermott and Gillan (1995a). They found that, macroscopically, isolated areas of the placenta assumed pallor and, microscopically, granular iron-containing incrustations located at the trophoblastic basement membrane. Similar incrustations are frequent in spontaneous abortion. In subsequent studies of infarcts (McDermott and Gillan, 1995b), these authors affirmed such deposits in placental infarcts and inferred disturbed maternofetal transfer as their cause.

Thromboses and disruptions are more often found when the membranous vessels course over the internal os and are, as vasa previa, broken by the exiting fetal head or by the obstetrical attendant who ruptures the membranes (Quek & Tan, 1972). Obolensky (1967) provided a description of the differential diagnosis of fetal (versus maternal) blood, in such unsuspected vaginal bleeding.

The manner by which fetal blood can be distinguished from maternal blood is discussed in greater detail in the discussion on hemorrhage due to placenta previa and in Chapter 17. Exsanguination from ruptured vasa previa can proceed within minutes. We have seen fatalities occur within 3 minutes of disruption through unrecognized velamentous vessels. Experience of successful immediate blood transfusion has also been reported (Mitchell et al., 1957). The frequency of hemorrhages is difficult to assess but has been estimated by Quek and Tan (1972) to be 1 in 50 cases of velamentous insertions. The mortality rate from intrapartum rupture and hemorrhage was given as 58% by Rucker and Tureman (1945) in their report of three cases and in their comprehensive literature review. Remarkably, the mortality has been 73% when the hemorrhage occurred before delivery (Torrey, 1952). Pent (1979) went so far as to state that "an active obstetric service can expect to have one perinatal death each year due to vasa previa."

Hemorrhages have on occasion been recognized by palpation of vasa previa, by amnioscopy, and even by sonography (Gianopoulos et al., 1987). Vasa previa were diagnosed by ultrasonography (color Doppler) prior to hemorrhage and thus leading to elective section (Meyer et al., 1993). The aberrant vessels coursed toward a succenturiate lobe. When the velamentous vessels are compressed during labor, this may be recognized by a sinusoidal fetal heart rate pattern much as in cord prolapse. An example is the twin pregnancy described by Antoine et al. (1982). These authors reviewed the dismal experience with vasa previa in twin pregnancies. Obstetricians have also occasionally made the diagnosis of bleeding from vasa previa by examining vaginal blood during labor or color Doppler sonographic study (Harding et al., 1990). Diagnostic methods have included Kleihauer stains and other techniques to detect fetal blood (Bergström, 1963; Carp et al., 1979; Vandriede & Kammeraad, 1981;

Silva et al., 1985; Jones et al., 1987). Because of the ability to ascertain fetal blood in vaginal bleeding from vasa previa, it has become a topic for litigation, but Messer et al. (1987) surveyed 100 community hospitals and concluded that such testing is currently not a standard of care in the United States.

As already stated, vasa previa are not confined to velamentous insertions. At times, a marginally inserted cord may have aberrant branches that course over the membranes; even cords with a more central position can have such vessels. Vasa previa may also occur with succenturiate lobes (Radcliffe et al., 1961) and in bilobed placentas (Waidl, 1960; Kouyoumdjian, 1980). Scheuner (1965) studied the histologic characteristics of nine term velamentous cord insertions and discussed the rich literature of this condition in detail. He found that membranous vessels are firmly anchored to the chorion by collagenous fibers, which explains why it is that the vessels rupture so readily when the chorion breaks.

It has been of great interest to understand the pathogenesis of velamentous and marginal insertions of the umbilical cord. There are two mutually contradictory theories: abnormal primary implantation (polarity theory), and trophotropism. Arguments have been brought to bear for both of these points of view. We favor the second and believe that it derives stronger support from the various placental constellations one finds associated with this condition.

The primarily abnormal implantation theory postulates that, at the nidation of the blastocyst, the embryo does not face the endometrium; rather, that it is located at the opposite side, or that it is obliquely oriented. Thus, when the vascular stalk develops, this trunk has to seek its connection with the future area of placentation by extending its vessels from the embryo to the base of implantation. Eventually, the vessels must thereby become membranous in location. This view was championed, among others, by Hertig (1968), despite the fact that in virtually all of the normal early embryos that he discovered and described in meticulous detail, the embryo had a normal (endometrial) position. Carnegie specimen 8671 (his Figure 65), however, had a somewhat oblique orientation, which might have caused a marginal insertion of the cord. Beer (1954) suggested that the cord arises "from the most vascular portion of the decidua," an opinion that is difficult to comprehend. If that were the case, one would perhaps expect to find as high a frequency (or a higher one) of velamentous and marginal cords during the first trimester as that which occurs later in gestation—which is not the case.

Monie (1965) found 15.3% of velamentous and 14.7% of marginal cords among 183 specimens of 9- to 13-week abortuses. He confirmed that velamentous insertion was highly correlated with congenital anomalies (marginal cords were in between) and provided a particularly good discussion and diagrams of the various notions published by earlier investigators. Monie acknowledged the frequency of velamentous cords in South American monkeys that have a superficial implantation. This finding negated earlier suggestions by Torpin (1953) that too deep an implantation may be the cause of velamentous cord insertion. Monie also reviewed the two types of velamentous insertion: normal and interpositional. Parenthetically, it may be mentioned that the umbilical cords of gorillas have nearly always been found to be marginal and also to be relatively long, about 100 cm (Ludwig, 1961). Hathout (1964) searched for cord insertion sites in 131 abortions, to 28 weeks' gestation. He found velamentous cords in 8.1% (three twins); 21.5% had marginal cords (one twin). It was central/eccentric in 70%. Because the abnormal cords were from midtrimester abortions, one might consider that the factors involved in trophotropism were also the cause of abortion. This contention is not supported by the extensive mathematical analysis of McLennan (1968), who sided with the theory of primarily disturbed placentation.

The case for trophotropism was first presented in detail by Strassmann (1902) in his large study of placenta previa and associated placental anomalies. The etiologic role of trophotropism is supported by cogent considerations: Velamentous and marginal cords are much more common in twins and are almost invariably present in higher multiple births. They are common when intrauterine devices (IUDs) are found in the placental membranes. Some of these pregnancies have led to prenatal hemorrhages and abortion (Golden, 1973). Moreover, one can sonographically observe eccentric expansion of the placenta during the course of advancing pregnancy, which would leave the cord insertion site behind. The distribution of cord insertions of some consecutive twin placentas are recorded in Table 12.3. It can be seen that, with the exception of diamnionic/dichorionic separate twin placentas, all others have an excessively high rate of abnormal cord insertions.

Finally, a series of successively undertaken ultrasonographs has shown that the placenta may "wander," called dynamic placentation (King, 1973). That is, when during early pregnancy a placenta previa was unmistakenly diagnosed (in 5.3% of patients), it often converted to a marginal or higher-lying placenta with progressing pregnancy; a placenta previa was found at term in only 0.58% (Rizos et al., 1979). In the series published by Meyenburg (1976), which supports these observations, the point is made that an opposite migration never takes place. Regrettably, in none of these studies is the location of the umbilical cord mentioned—neither at the time when the placenta was first localized nor after delivery. It would be desirable to collect this information in the future. The placental movement is not accomplished by the placenta unseating and

TABLE 12.3. Distribution of cord insertion in twin placentas past 20 weeks

Type of placenta	Pairs No.	Infants No.	Marginal twin A	Marginal twin B	Velamentous twin A	Velamentous twin B	Eccentric or central	Marginal (%)	Velamentous (%)	Dead (No.)	Dead (%)
MoMo	15	30	5	5	2	3	15	33	16	9	30
DiMo	247	494	69	77	36	29	283	30	13	110	22
DiDi fused	188	376	48	43	15	21	249	24	10	28	7.4
DiDi sep.	241	482	30	27	8	7	410	2	3	1	8.5
Total	691	1,382	152	152	61	60	957	21.9	8.7		

MoMo, monoamnionic/monochorionic; DiMo, diamnionic/monochorionic; DiDi, diamnionic/dichorionic.

relocating itself, but rather through marginal atrophy on one side and expansion on the other, as well as through the development and thinning of the lower uterine segment. This mechanism is also the best one to explain the sickle-shaped, marginal placental atrophy that has been observed (Winter, 1978). Young (1978), who studied a large number of such early placentas previa, referred to the process as an "amoeba-like growth."

The most extensive writings on this topic come from Krone. In 1962 this author began studies showing that marginal and velamentous cords tend to correlate with fetal anomalies. In his early contributions, Krone (1960) presented data to show that 9% of normal infants had a markedly eccentric cord, as did 28% of malformed babies. Marginal and velamentous cord insertion was present in 6% and 26%, respectively. In a later study of 2868 placental examinations, Krone et al. (1965) found that such cord insertional anomalies correlated with advanced maternal age and multiparity, and that they often followed abortions and curettage. He believed that the abnormal placentas could not be the cause of fetal anomalies because final placental shape occurs only *after* the "teratogenetic termination period" of Schwalbe (1906).

These placentas, however, direct our attention to the existence of an abnormal nidation/placentation process (Krone, 1967). Our own studies of fetal anomalies and cord insertion clearly showed such a relation and it has been noted by others as well (Robinson et al., 1983). The suggestion by Shanklin (1970) that abnormal cord insertion correlates with low birth weight was not supported by the study of Woods and Malan (1978), who evaluated 940 placentas with marginal or central cords. Shen-Schwarz et al. (1997b), however, found a significant reduction of birth weights with velamentous cord insertion in diamnionic/monochorionic (DiMo) twins, but not in diamnionic/dichorionic (DiDi) twins. Although we have not done a statistical study of the topic, our findings also suggest reduced birth weight to be associated with velamentous cord insertion. Similar findings come from a large retrospective study by Heinonen et al. (1996). They detected significantly more low birth weight fetuses, growth retardation, low Apgar scores, and abnormal fetal heart rate patterns with velamentous insertions. Rarely were they able to identify the cause sonographically, and they called for new diagnostic modalities, such as Doppler study, in order to detect the correct cord insertion site. Nöldeke (1934) found that abnormally inserted cords occur more often in prematurely delivered infants. He noted increased difficulty of placental separation, as did Earn (1951). Their findings were not confirmed, however, by the study of Uyanwah-Akpom and Fox (1977). In all these considerations one must remember that twins have to be excluded from any study so as to make the data truly comparable. This is often not done; thus, from many of the original papers it is impossible to discern the extent to which twins were present within the data sets and thereby increased the numbers of velamentous cords. Therefore, the numbers in Table 12.2 and in the reports must be interpreted with some caution.

Eddleman and colleagues (1992) reviewed the sonograms of the 82 cases of velamentous cord insertions seen in their 4-year experience (77 singletons). In none of them had the diagnosis been made before birth, including the three cases of vasa previa later identified. The infants born to these women had lower birth weights than controls and more intrapartum complications, but the mothers did not have higher parity or more frequently prior cesarean sections as is often assumed. Importantly, the study showed that, sonographically, this diagnosis cannot be expected to be made routinely.

Placental Surface Vessels

It is convenient to consider the placental vascular tree at this point, as future discussion of the thrombotic events of the cord often interrelate to those of the vasculature on the surface of the placenta. The distribution of the blood vessels across the placenta is not random, although we do not understand the mechanisms that govern their growth. Two principal patterns of vessel distribution have been described in the literature, and admixtures exist occasionally. The disperse pattern has a fine network of vessels that course from the cord insertion to the various

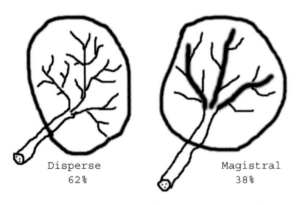

FIGURE 12.34. Disperse and magistral distributions of placental arterial vessels.

placental cotyledons. The magistral pattern has arteries that course across the placental surface nearly to the edge without diminishing their diameters. The arteries have a fairly uniform diameter, and they have many branches. These two types are shown in Figure 12.34. They have been delineated by injection and corrosion techniques that employ a variety of materials, including lead salts and plastics (Hyrtl, 1870; Schordania, 1929b; Bacsich & Smout, 1938; Smart, 1962; Kishore & Sarkar, 1967; and others cited by these authors). Schordania (1929b), who is responsible for the aforementioned terminology, advanced the theory that the magistral type of vascularity leads to better-developed fetuses. This theory was not affirmed by the studies of Crawford (1959), however; and Bacsich and Smout (1938) failed to identify the arterial anastomoses in the periphery of the placenta that were delineated by Hyrtl (1870) and others. The same observation was made by Priman (1959). The superficial arteries are end-arteries to which feature Bacsich and Smout (1938), incorrectly we believe, attributed the occurrence of white infarcts near term. The disperse type of vessel distribution is more commonly present (61.8%), with the magistral type occurring in 38.2% (Kishore & Sarkar, 1967). The latter authors found no association with placental size or anomalies but noted that the disperse type was more frequent in placentas with centrally inserted cords. There is no racial influence on these features (Andrade, 1968).

At the periphery, the arteries individually supply a single cotyledon ("placentone"), turning abruptly toward the maternal surface, then branching repeatedly and finally becoming capillaries; the blood is then returned from the capillary loops of the cotyledon to the umbilical cord by veins that merge. It is crucial to recognize that, in the overwhelming majority of cotyledons, there is a 1:1 relation between artery and vein at the periphery. Otherwise, the transfusion syndrome of monochorial twins could not be understood. It is further remarkable that at least the larger arteries always cross over the veins, par-

ticularly nearer the cord insertion (Smart, 1962). Wentworth (1965) reported that only about 3% show the opposite condition. Also, Bhargava and colleagues, in a series of studies (Bhargava & Raja, 1969), suggested that veins may occasionally cross over arteries. They undertook a quantitative analysis of these features. In their material, this reversal of the normal pattern correlated significantly with abnormal fetal development and with hydramnios. However, according to Boyd and Hamilton (1970) the superficial position of one or few veins at points of arteriovenous crossing is not unusual even in normal placentas. They can thus be readily identified by macroscopic examination. Histologically, it is nearly impossible to make this distinction (Fig. 12.35). What makes these vessels assume this pattern so uniformly? Because we understand genetic influences on the placenta very poorly at this point, it is our belief that when the earliest embryonic vessels grow into the placental surface, the subsequent perfusion, at first sluggish, determines the vascular pattern that ultimately results. It may well be subject to trophic or mechanical (pressure) forces. For a better comprehension of the complexities of the vascularity in twin placentation, it would be helpful to have a better understanding of these vascular phenomena.

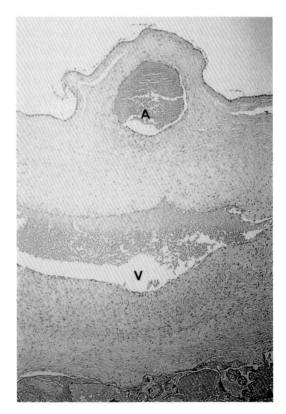

FIGURE 12.35. Microscopic appearance of the surface of the placenta with the artery (A) above the vein (V). Note that the fetal side of both vessels has a much thinner muscular wall and that the artery lies on top of the vein. H&E ×60.

It is further remarkable that the circumferential architecture of the placental surface vessels is asymmetrical (Fig. 12.36). This area has been studied by Fujikura and Carleton (1968), who found that the thinning of the muscular wall of arteries (80%) commences after 12 weeks of gestation. Of the two theories they advanced (trophic growth of muscle and hemodynamic thinning), we favor the latter and believe that the pressure buckles and thins the superficial portions of the vessels, whereas the fixed portions resist this pressure. This phenomenon of thinning of the superficial aspect of chorionic vessels (also shared with cord vessels) may actually be a sequel of amnionic rupture and a change in intraamnionic pressure relation **after** that event of membrane rupture. Contrary to the observations of Fujikura and Carleton (1968), we believe this property to be shared by veins (Fig. 12.35), a feature Fujikura and Hosoda (1990) have now acknowledged. Unilateral thickening of the muscular walls of large chorionic veins (>1.0mm diameter) on the chorionic side is a usual finding in all normal placentas after 17 weeks of gestation. The ratio of amnionic to chorionic wall thickness may be 1:3 to 1:4. It is caused by muscular hyperplasia rather than by arteriosclerotic changes. Fujikura and Hosoda (1990) concluded that differences in wall movement were the etiologic factors.

Surface arteries and veins are subject to spontaneous rhythmic contractions and to the influences of various

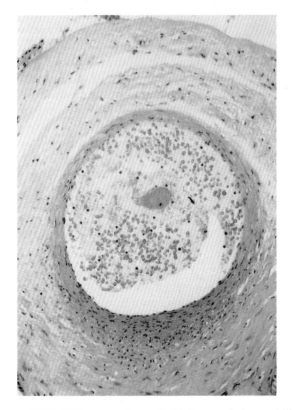

FIGURE 12.36. Differences in wall thickness of the umbilical vein branch at term. H&E ×240.

mediators, such as serotonin, prostaglandins, atrial natriuretic peptide, nitric oxide and endothelin-1 (Panigel, 1962; Panizza et al., 1981; Robaut et al., 1991; Salas et al., 1991; Omar et al., 1992; Myatt et al., 1993; Rath et al., 1993). Methyldopa, for instance, was found to decrease the placental vascular resistance in maternal hypertensive disease when Doppler velocimetry was done (Rey, 1992). Isolated fetal placental arteries dilated experimentally when exposed to nitric oxide (Learmont & Poston, 1996). In general, the larger chorionic and stem vessels seem to behave like the umbilical vessels (see above) (Macara et al., 1993). Endothelin, on the other hand, is said to increase resistance in the arterial bed (Bodelsson et al., 1992).

Studies have also endeavored to correlate umbilical artery flow waveforms with abnormalities in the vascular beds of tertiary villi (McCowan et al., 1987). When the cord arterial pulsatility index is high, indicating peripheral vascular resistance, the peripheral arterial vessel count is low, a finding that is strongly correlated with growth-restricted fetuses (Hitschold et al., 1993). Similar studies by Doppler waveform analysis of umbilical cord flow showed that, during preterm labor, ritodrine (but not magnesium sulfate) affected umbilical vascular resistance (Brar et al., 1988). When, with serial determinations, different patterns of flow were thus determined, the placenta was subsequently found to have one large infarcted lobe, supplied by one artery; and the authors believed that the infarction may have been the reason for the difference (Trudinger & Cook, 1988). The pattern of umbilical blood velocity waveforms changes abruptly at about 12 weeks' gestation. Prior to that time, there are no end-diastolic frequencies (EDFs), which, in later life, would be held to be an abnormal feature of fetal circulation. Fisk et al. (1988) and Loquet et al. (1988) simultaneously reported that no EDFs were observed before 12 weeks (as is normal in peripheral arteries), and that their appearance at the second trimester perhaps signals the development of vessels in the tertiary villi and the disappearance of the membranous circulation. It signals the sudden decrease of placental villous flow resistance. Interesting observations of fetuses grasping and constricting the umbilical cords in utero are referred to in letters by Petrikovsky and Kaplan (1993), Collins (1995a), and Habek et al. (2003).

A variety of disease processes affect placental surface vessels. The easiest to understand is hemorrhage after traumatic laceration. Disruption of chorionic vessels is commonest after amniocentesis and may lead to rapid fetal exsanguination (Goodlin & Clewell, 1974) and intraamnionic bleeding. It has been recognized by sonography during amniocentesis as a spurt. We have seen three such lacerations of surface vessels due to amniocentesis in a patient with diabetes, done to assess fetal maturity (Fig. 12.37). The infant survived. In another case,

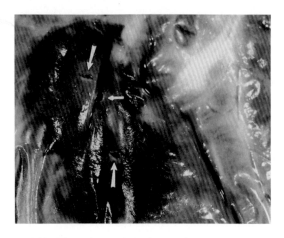

FIGURE 12.37. Three lacerations (arrows) from amniocentesis at 38 weeks' gestation in a patient with diabetes, performed to assess fetal maturity. Cesarean section, live birth.

where amniocentesis was performed at 12 weeks to obtain genetic information, the anterior placenta had one surface vessel ruptured, and blood dissected underneath the amnion. When a stillborn fetus was eventually delivered, hemosiderin and nucleated red blood cells were found along the well-defined needle track. Intraamnionic bleeding has been studied with sonographic surveillance and correlation with Kleihauer tests, so as to adjudicate the amount of RhoGAM needed for Rh-negative patients (Lenke et al., 1985). It was found that bleeding occurred most commonly when, in anterior placentas, the placenta needed to be traversed by the needle. No correlation with fetal-to-maternal hemorrhage has been found. A case was referred to us with a posterior placenta that exsanguinated through a transverse laceration of a surface artery. The amniocentesis needle had caused this lesion after much amnionic fluid had been withdrawn, perhaps because the posterior placenta had then come closer. Considerable search may be required to identify such defects, but the pallor of the placental tissue is the first sign of blood loss, the suspicion of which then leads to a detailed inspection for an explanation. Needle puncture of the fetus at amniocentesis has also been reported. When it occurs during early diagnostic procedures fetal scars may result (Broome et al., 1975, 1976); in later gestations, hemorrhage may ensue (Galle & Meis, 1982). The practice of cordocentesis may also cause hematoma and other injury to the umbilical cord. Jauniaux et al. (1989b) found, among 50 cases studied, one giant hematoma of the cord and four small hematomas that encircled the walls of the arteries. The needle puncture sites were readily visible in 37 cases. Thrombosis was not found, and these authors suspected that the injured vessel was repaired within 1 week. In a fortuitous section, de Sa (1984) depicted (his Figures 5 to 8) the disruption of an umbilical vein within a cord hematoma. We have seen several such hematomas after cordocentesis, occasionally

so massive that they required delivery. In others, repeated (×6) cordocentesis left only small defects in the amnion.

In recent years, the practice of prenatal transfusion of blood at the site of cord insertion has become more commonly practiced. It has also led to some disastrous results. Weiner et al. (1991) analyzed the results of 594 cordocenteses and 156 transfusions and found that the results differed with the type of procedure. Ney et al. (1989) deduced from in vitro studies that amnionic fluid had coagulative properties that prevent massive hemorrhage, whereas Chénard et al. (1990) depicted the circumstances of a rapidly developing fatal hematoma in a 29-week fetus. It must be cautioned, however, that subamnionic fresh blood is commonly found in placentas. It may then be the result of traction (with disruption) of the cord for delivery of the placenta or, more commonly perhaps, because neonatologists have drawn blood from placental surface vessels for pH determination, and the site continued to ooze blood thereafter. It is of historic interest to review the practice of traction on the cord for placental delivery (Rehstein, 1969), as it was a feared practice in the past because of the possibility of uterine inversion. Now, with oxytocics that better contract the uterus, this is rarely observed. Khoury et al. (1991) compared cord pH and gases from blood obtained before delivery (in cesarean sections) and after delivery and found significant differences.

More frequent perhaps are hemorrhages that occur after laceration of velamentous vessels and vasa previa. This subject is discussed later in this chapter. A remarkable case was described by Tuggle and Cook (1978): An infant had experienced massive bleeding from a surface vein that led to cesarean section; no therapeutic intervention could be blamed for this spontaneous rupture. Because of the unusually long fingernails of the newborn, it was conjectured that the nails of the fetus may have caused the tear.

Nucleated Red Blood Cells (NRBCs)

A really important observation needs to be made when examining the fetal blood within chorionic vessels, easiest done in the blood of the larger vessels on the fetal surface, or in the umbilical cord. That observation is to gain an appreciation of the presence of nucleated red blood cells (NRBCs) in the fetal circulation. In normal term pregnancies, very few red blood cells with nuclei are visible in the fetal blood during placental examination. There is, however, considerable controversy about how many NRBCs may be found in truly normal neonates. When many NRBCs are seen in the absence of anemia or erythroblastosis, it is a distinctly abnormal finding and the pathologist should endeavor to ascertain the reason for their presence. There exists an extensive literature on this topic and its findings are not always in agreement. One reason for discrepant results may be that, especially in older citations, the authors have not always excluded infants who suffered hypoxia or other causes for the presence of NRBCs. This aspect is fully discussed in Chapter 8, and by Korst et al., 1996.

Cysts and Edema

Aside from the aforementioned cysts, we have seen a small amnionic epithelial inclusion cyst in a fetus with 47, XXX chromosome constitution. It was filled with clear fluid. And then, on rare occasion cysts arise within Wharton's jelly. They are most obvious in the edematous umbilical cords that have been associated with some cases of the respiratory distress syndrome of newborns (Coulter et al., 1975). Coulter and colleagues found 10% of babies to have edematous cords; the occurrence is more common in premature infants. These authors related the edema to reduced oncotic pressure. Edema is apparent in the markedly swollen, glistening umbilical cord shown in Figure 12.38. It resembles the condition of "mucoid degeneration," described by Bergman et al. (1961). These investigators believed that one of their patients died as a result of this degeneration. Whether this is truly a degenerative event, however, remains to be ascertained. Rolschau (1978), on the other hand, found that edema of the cord had no influence on fetal development and well-being. This pathologic change may be diffusely distributed, as happens for instance in some cases of severe funisitis, or it occur focally as cysts. Usually, the cysts in Wharton's jelly are not accompanied by fetal disease, and there is a normal fetal outcome. Severe distention, up to 5 cm diameter, occurs for unknown reason

occasionally and may then be accompanied by hydramnios and an excessive number of mast cells (Howorka & Kapczynski, 1971). Walz (1947) has studied this phenomenon in more detail when he observed a growth-retarded infant with a normal placenta but "arm-thick" umbilical cord that was difficult to ligate. It also had calcifications that will be discussed shortly. The cord was 46 cm long and 7 cm thick. Histologically, it was edematous and had acute inflammatory cell infiltration, mural thrombi, and many areas of degeneration. Walz reviewed the older literature on this finding. Occasionally, the cord has a complete lack of Wharton's jelly, which is usually a sign of fetal growth retardation (Scott & Jordan, 1972). The association is not a strict one, however, and many infants with IUGR (e.g., renal agenesis) have normal cords. Nevertheless, experienced obstetricians regard lean cords as a sign of dysmaturity (Goodlin, 1987). A large cyst of the umbilical cord is depicted in Figure 12.6. Degeneration of cord substance, with an absence of Wharton's jelly, has also been reported by Labarrere et al. (1985). They found three cases of meconium-stained term neonates who died shortly after birth in whom the umbilical arteries were detached from the cord substance. Much of the amnionic epithelium of the cord was defective, as was Wharton's jelly. They speculated that there may have been incomplete fusion of amnion with cord and likened the condition's etiology to that of furcate insertion. The pathologic change may be diffusely distributed or occur focally as cysts (Figures 12.5 and 12.39). The relationship to meconium was disputed by Thomson and Hoo (1996), who described such a case of "linear disruption of the umbilical cord" in a severely retarded child, but in whose delivery notes meconium was not described as having been present. We have seen such degenerated cords, most often associated with prolonged meconium staining, but not always associated with bad fetal outcome, and a relevant

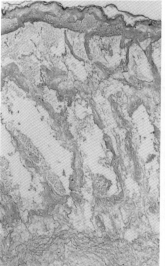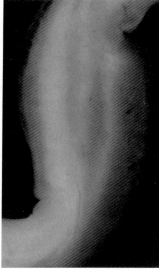

Figure 12.38. Marked edema in the umbilical cord of a normal newborn infant. Note the dissociation of fibrous tissue underneath the surface of the cord. H&E ×160.

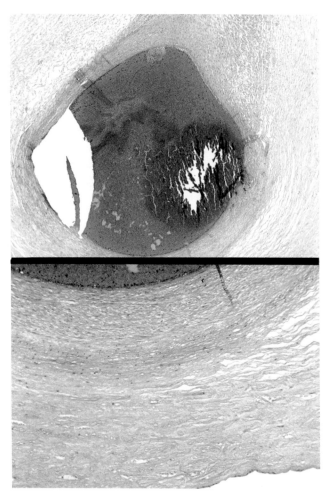

FIGURE 12.39. Umbilical artery after meconium damage. Note the apparent acellularity of the cord, due to toxicity, and the thinned portion of umbilical cord. This is the result of meconium damage penetrating from the outside.

case with normal outcome is depicted in Chapter 11. A typical example of meconium-induced necrosis of portions of the umbilical arterial wall is shown in Figure 12.39. It will be noted that the necrosis is confined toward the cord's surface whence the toxic meconium originated. The dissociated vessels in many of such damaged arteries, however, have often been severely inflamed; our opinion is that this is most often the result of meconium toxicity and does not represent a congenital anomaly. More discussion of meconium-induced arterial toxicity follows later in this chapter and is also to be found in Chapter 11.

The water content of the umbilical cord has been studied in great detail by Scott and Wilkinson (1978). Edematous cords had a water content of 93.5%, and wrinkled cords had 89.2% water. The correlation with cystic spaces such as those of Figure 12.38 is then excel-lent. There is a tendency for the amount of Wharton's jelly or its water content to decrease with advancing gestation. Bender et al. (1978) provided a particularly useful review of the older literature on this topic and studied the relation of the amount of jelly to outcome. They found that infants with much jelly and more spiraling of vessels have better outcomes than those who do not. In the still-born with a markedly spiraled, jelly-poor cord, it can be argued that the jelly has disappeared because of vascular compression. It is not proved that Wharton's jelly was primarily absent; in general, we are ignorant of the mechanisms that provide cord jelly and its water content. Realizing that the amnionic fluid decreases with advancing gestational age and that there may be a correlation with cord thickness, R.K. Silver et al. (1987) sonographically studied the cord thickness and circumference after birth. The cord diameter varied from 1.25 to 2.00cm and its circumference from 2.4 to 4.4cm. Fetal monitoring inferred to be compression patterns increased in frequency with decreasing fluid content of the cord. It may also be mentioned that experimental evidence has indicated that, in fetal lambs, intermittent partial cord occlusion leads to cerebral necrosis (Clapp et al., 1988; Mallard et al., 1992). Gill and Jarjoura (1993) measured the quantity of jelly in umbilical cords; they found a positive relation to male fetuses, increased prepartum maternal weight and heavier birth weight.

Excessively thin umbilical cords are abnormal and potential causes of fetal problems. This has been referred to as the "thin cord syndrome" by Hall (1961). It may involve the entire cord and also only portions of the umbilical cord. The latter examples are most often those cases in which the cord has become extremely thinned near the abdominal surface of the fetus due to torsion, the so-called coarctation. It frequently leads to fetal death and abortion (see Fig. 12.47). In the prototype of an abnormally thin cord, there is a deficiency of Wharton's jelly and compression of vessels is a greater possibility than when they are protected. Thin cords occur more often with growth-restricted fetuses and in preeclampsia, but unknown causes exist as well. Labarrere et al. (1985) presented three cases in which Wharton's jelly was deficient with arteries free next to the umbilical cords and causing fetal demise. As mentioned earlier, meconium is often present and it may be able to cause the degenerative changes. It is of parenthetic interest again to recall that similar fetal deaths due to excessively long umbilical cords with marked coiling occur in race horses (Whitwell, 1975; Giles et al., 1993; Hong et al., 1993). Microscopic calcification was often present in the vessels of these abnormal cords. Because the longitudinal orientation of equine fetuses prevents turning in later stages of pregnancy, here too, early motion of the fetus must be held responsible for the excessive lengths and twisting.

Single Umbilical Artery

Single umbilical artery (SUA) is the commonest true congenital anomaly of humans. An enormous literature has been created in efforts to explain its nature and significance. Our file contains more than 80 articles dealing with SUA, and many more are reviewed and critically analyzed in the review articles by Heifetz (1984) and Leung and Robson (1989). These reports can be consulted for all of the relevant literature.

Single umbilical artery was apparently first described by Vesalius. It did not attract further notice until the 40 cases listed by Otto (1830) and the later attention by Hyrtl (1870), who summarized 70 cases in his interesting monograph. Considering its incidence of about 1% in newborns (Heifetz compiled all data and reported there being a 0.63% frequency), it is surprising that its relation to anomalous fetal development was overlooked for so long, until we drew attention to it again (Benirschke & Brown, 1953; Benirschke & Bourne, 1960). Since then, there has been a veritable flood of information on SUA (Table 12.4). Single umbilical artery can now be detected prenatally by ultrasonography (Tortora et al., 1984; Herrmann & Sidiropoulos, 1988), and Jones et al. (1993) make the point that it is unforgivable if it is not ascertained at birth. Raio et al. (1999) found that SUA is more commonly associated with reduced amounts of Wharton's jelly, irrespective of its association with chromosomal disorders. Among the seven patients of Tortora et al. (1984), four had hydramnios, two were growth-retarded, two died, two survived with anomalies, and three were normal infants. Herrmann and Sidiropoulos (1988) found SUA in four cases and drew attention to the growth restriction of the neonates. The relation of SUA to growth restriction has also been studied by Rolschau (1978). He found that SUA correlated with circumvallation of the placenta, and that marginal cord insertion was moderately well correlated with small placentas and fetuses. Velamentous insertion of the cord, however, had a strong negative effect on fetal and placental weights. Leung and Robson (1989) found SUA in 159 of 56,919 infants. Twins had an incidence of 8.8%, and it was usually the smaller twin who had the anomaly. Single umbilical artery was associated with diabetes, epilepsy, preeclampsia, antepartum hemorrhage, hydramnios, and oligohydramnios. Anomalies were detected in 44.7% of the associated infants, and other placental abnormalities were found in 16.4%. Because of the frequency of renal anomalies (18.5%), these authors recommended that neonatal renal sonography be performed when SUA is found. Abuhamad et al. (1995) found sonographically that in 73% of 77 cases of SUA the defect locates to the left artery and that cytogenetic and complex anomalies were associated nearly exclusively with the left-sided absence. Theirs is the largest prospective series, and they found a 30% associated anomaly incidence. Growth retardation was found in 8% of cases. Parilla et al. (1995) deduced from their 50 cases that an isolated SUA (without other sonographic anomalies) did not affect outcome and should not alter obstetric management. Conversely, when Pavlopoulos et al. (1998) studied infants with SUA they found a significantly higher frequency of hollow organ pathology, especially intestinal atresia, and cautioned sonographers to pay special attention to the intestines before birth when SUA is identified. A meta-analysis of cases with SUA was conducted by Thummala et al. (1998) that showed that in otherwise apparently normal neonates, SUA is associated with only a slight increase in renal anomalies and does "not justify extensive urologic radiographic investigation." Benoit et al. (2002) came to similar conclusions more recently.

Absence of one umbilical artery may occur as aplasia or as the consequence of atrophy of one artery. The latter mechanism is probably more frequent and can be seen to have occurred in many specimens when histologic examination is undertaken (Fig. 12.40). Degeneration of one artery occasionally occurs late in pregnancy but when it

TABLE 12.4. Frequency of single umbilical artery (SUA) in various populations

Series of prospective deliveries	SUA		
	No.	No.	%
Review	332,067	2,099	0.63
Autopsies	18,614	357	1.92
Twin deliveries	1,323	51	3.9
Twin Infants	2,399	56	2.3

Source: Data from Heifetz (1984).

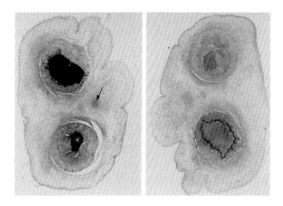

FIGURE 12.40. Umbilical cord from a placenta with marginal cord insertion. A degenerating second artery is seen (arrow). Elastic tissue stain (right) shows the internal elastica of the umbilical vein and absence in both arteries. H&E (left), von Gieson (right). ×10.

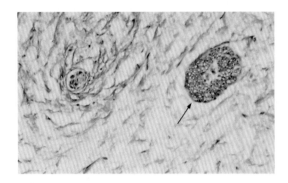

FIGURE 12.41. Muscular remnant of a vanished second umbilical artery (arrow); the other is a remnant of an allantoic duct. H&E ×60.

took place some longer time before birth, the arterial lumen gradually vanishes, and only a tiny muscular remnant then remains (Fig. 12.41). We have seen a relevant case that bears on this question: A patient had decreased fetal movements and was studied repeatedly sonographically; eventually she delivered at 35 weeks an infant who did well after having had initial problems. One umbilical artery was completely thrombosed and the wall was autolyzing with hemoglobin staining of the jelly. Remarkably, there was an inflammatory response from artery and vein toward the degenerating vessel and not, as is usual, toward the cord's surface; also there was no chorioamnionitis. Hyrtl's anastomosis was absent. The Gravida 5 Para 1 patient had anticardiolipin titers, but it is not certain that these relate to the thrombosis. The newer Doppler techniques have now allowed prenatal diagnosis of discordant umbilical arterial size (Raio et al., 1998). The smaller vessel was found to have an increased resistance index and, remarkably, five of the 14 cases analyzed lacked Hyrtl's anastomosis.

The question of whether SUA from aplasia has a prognosis different from that from atrophy was examined in a large study by Altshuler et al. (1975). These authors found 19 placentas with SUA among 4138 consecutive deliveries (0.46%). Altogether, they analyzed 48 children with this anomaly and found no significant difference "in congenital malformations or neonatal mortality." The more frequent detection of SUA in term placentas than in placentas of early gestation further supports the view that the etiology involves arterial atrophy. On the other hand, early embryos with SUA have also been seen, and SUA has been observed associated with many chromosomal anomalies and exposure to such teratogens as thalidomide. It has even occurred in baboons so treated experimentally. Single umbilical artery is also found almost regularly in association with sirenomelia and is present in the cords of most acardiac fetuses (malformed monozygotic twins; see Chapter 25), which also supports

the notion of occasional aplasia as its origin. Perez-Aytes et al. (1997) described a relevant case in which the single artery of a sirenomelic fetus was directly continuous with the aorta.

It must be cautioned that SUA may be found at one end of the cord and not the other. We have therefore suggested that, to verify its existence, one must sample three areas of the umbilical cord. At times, the arteries fuse far above the cord insertion on the placenta (Kelber, 1976) in a manner that is similar to their normal communication near the placenta. An interesting question is what happens when there is no communicating artery during early development, as is the case in some 4% of term umbilical cords (Priman, 1959). Because each artery supplies a portion of placental tissue, the area supplied by an atrophying artery would then presumably undergo atrophy. Such atrophic changes may explain the much higher frequency of SUA in multiple births. Trophotropic expansion and pressures from one twin placenta may then affect the placental expansion of the other placenta (Thomas, 1961). Such considerations may also relate to the finding that SUA is associated with lower birth weight, as the amount of some placental area would be reduced by the placental atrophy. This concept has been supported by the experimental ligation of one artery in sheep fetuses (Hobel et al., 1970). Bhargava et al. (1971) found a higher frequency of the magistral pattern of chorial blood vessels with SUA, and the vascular pattern of SUA differs from that of cords with fused arteries.

Much has been made of the significance of SUA with respect to other congenital anomalies in the fetus and how seriously one should look for such anomalies. It can now be said that there is no predilection for any specific type of fetal anomaly. Moreover, SUA is often found in perfectly healthy infants who eventually attain normal size and development. Therefore, an extraordinary or invasive study of infants born with SUA is not warranted. To be sure, the pediatrician should be notified of its existence and then should make certain by doing a more detailed physical examination that the infant has no hidden anomalies. We do not perform radiographic or invasive studies.

The SUA is commoner in European whites than in Orientals, in multiple births, in autopsy series (because of associated anomalies), in spontaneous abortions, with other placental anomalies [velamentous cord and choriangioma: 2.70% and 0.65%, respectively (Froehlich & Fujikura, 1966); perhaps circumvallates], and chromosomal errors; it has no familial or genetic tendency. The suggested relation to the development of inguinal hernias has been disputed. Infants with SUA have lower birth weights and are more often prematurely born. When one considers all the details of the enormous study produced by Heifetz (1984), it is apparent that the diagnosis of SUA is usually made at birth and, when found, one proceeds with cautious further studies in an attempt to find its possible cause and relevance. There is no reason, however, to change our view from that expressed earlier (Benirschke & Driscoll, 1967) that the "indiscriminate association of the absence of one umbilical artery with various and quite diverse chromosomal disorders indicates how limited the placenta is in expressing a variety of constitutional defects." Most likely, SUA is either part of a constellation of multiple anomalies, not its cause, or it develops during pregnancy by atrophy and then it may be the reason for restricted fetal growth (small for gestational age, SGA). The importance of abnormal cord insertion in SUA is borne out, for instance, in the study of Matheus and Sala (1980), who reported an incidence of 0.95%. Of their 42 cases, 11.9% had velamentous insertion, and 33.3% were associated with abnormal fetuses. Kaplan et al. (1990) have suggested that SUA may be associated with cord accidents during labor. They reported on four infants with SUA who died suddenly in utero, presumably because of cord accidents, but these were not growth-restricted because of SUA.

Sireniform fetuses (sympodia) form perhaps a special case of SUA; it is nearly invariably found in this condition. The question posed by this finding is whether the single umbilical artery, arising usually directly from the aorta and immediately distal to the celiac artery, is of enteric (omphalomesenteric, vitelline) nature or whether it is an allantoic vessel, as would be normal for the cord. This anomaly (sympus) has occasionally been referred to as caudal regression syndrome, but this term is inappropriately used; frequently there is no evidence for regression, particularly in the cases that are so descriptive of diabetic embryopathy (Benirschke, 1987). In any event, we have suggested that this vessel "steals" blood from the lower aortic blood flow and is thus responsible for the caudal maldevelopment (Stevenson et al., 1986). The older literature on this topic has been considered in this study of 11 sireniform fetuses. This review and the papers cited by Heifetz (1984) can be consulted when further insight into this phenomenon is desired. The dispute is not totally resolved, however, as studies in mice with this anomaly suggest the vessel to be allantoic in nature; it is thought only to take an abnormal course, with fusion of the two arteries (Schreiner & Hoornbeek, 1973). How complex these embryologic considerations are can be seen in the study by Monie and Khemmani (1973). They induced SUA in rat fetuses with retinoic acid and described the vitello-umbilical anastomosis in the embryos. After due consideration, they could not rule out the occasional existence of such anastomoses in human embryos; it is their opinion, however, that the SUA of symmelia represents a remaining allantoic vessel. These considerations are of interest only in that the view of persisting vitelline vessels would support the notion that, when these vessels become dominant, they can acquire

muscular coats. This is not the case in the usual persistence of omphalomesenteric vessels; they are composed essentially of only endothelium.

More than three umbilical vessels are normal for many species (Benirschke et al., 1964), but this is rare in human umbilical cords. Painter and Russell (1977) described a stillborn with ectopia cordis and other anomalies; there were two umbilical veins, the right umbilical vein having persisted. Hathout (1964) mentioned that one of his cases had five vessels due to "division of both arteries" and one had four and a nodular embryo. One must take care, when assessing an increased number of vessels, not to be misled by the frequent looping that occurs in many cord vessels.

Placental Transfusion

When the fetus is delivered, the umbilical cord may break by the mechanisms discussed above, and bleeding ceases shortly thereafter. More commonly now, the attending obstetrician clamps the cord. With vaginal deliveries the amount of fetal blood remaining in the placenta is 2.5% of fetal body weight, even with prompt cord ligation. With cesarean section, that figure is 4.5% (Gruenwald, 1969). It has become customary to clamp both sides of the cord, even though the loss of placental fetal blood might be thought irrelevant. One reason for clamping has been the realization that, on occasion, an unrecognized twin may be present; that twin may exsanguinate quickly through inter-twin arterial anastomoses of monochorial placentas. Moreover, the continuous blood issuing from the cut end of the cord is messy. On the other hand, a less turgid, deflated placenta may separate more readily when the uterus contracts.

Walsh (1968) found that postpartum hemorrhage and retained secundines are significantly more common when early clamping is practiced. The amount of fetal blood contained within the placenta varies. It is generally between 50 and 100 mL but is significantly greater in pregnancies of diabetic mothers (Kjeldsen & Pedersen, 1967; Klebe & Ingomar, 1974a,b). Newton and Moody (1961) estimated that 9.4 mL of fetal blood per 100 g of placenta remained after delivery when the cord was ligated immediately, and there were 9.6 mL maternal blood. The latter quantity did not change with delivery and clamping practices. When the cord was ligated after pulsations ceased, only 5 mL fetal blood remained. They estimated that the term neonate may receive as much as 10% of his blood volume (26.6 mL) when cord ligation is delayed and the placental vessels allowed to empty. The presence of fetal blood is what imparts the red color to the villous tissue, not the maternal intervillous blood content. That has largely been squeezed out by uterine contractions.

Numerous studies have been conducted to ascertain whether it is best to allow as much blood to drain from the placenta into the fetus as possible (under the influence of maternal uterine contractions) before the cord is ligated and severed. Vardi (1965) reviewed the older literature and advocated that the delivered placenta be held above the infant but advised against stripping the cord. His studies showed that it is beneficial for the hematologic and iron requirements of the infant to let as much blood drain into the fetus as possible. Yao et al. (1968) found marked hematologic changes with different clamping times, studied up to 3 minutes. They thought that the maximum transfer had taken place by that time. Later, these investigators studied the fetal/placental blood volume changes (Yao et al., 1969). When the cord was clamped within 5 seconds of birth, the infant/placental volume distribution was 67%/33%; by 3 minutes it was 87%/13%. In later studies, which included a complete summary of their findings, Yao and Lind (1974, 1982) evaluated the consequences of cord clamping at various times after birth with respect to the development and behavior of the newborn infant. Special attention was paid to the occasional hypervolemia resulting from late clamping. Their recommendation was that, for vaginal deliveries clamping be done within 30 seconds, provided that the baby is not elevated. With cesarean section, elevation of the infant is to be avoided; and when there is no distress, the cord be handled as for vaginal births.

Fetal-to-maternal red blood cell transfer during labor is not influenced by the timing of cord ligation (Dunn et al., 1966; Moncrieff et al., 1986). An interesting study of residual placental fetal blood content and neonatal outcome was done by Philip et al. (1969). They found that, compared with normal newborns, asphyxiated neonates had already received more blood prenatally, irrespective of postnatal transfusions. There are other complex questions of cord clamping time, for example, the increased frequency of neonatal hyperbilirubinemia with draining of the placental blood into the fetus; but they are beyond the scope of this chapter (see Philip, 1973).

The spontaneous detachment of the umbilicus from the infant is variable, with a mean of 7.4 days according to Oudesluys-Murphy et al. (1987), and 13.9 days as per Novack et al. (1988). Numerous studies have endeavored to ascertain its causes, which remain unresolved, but drying and bacterial colonization have been held responsible. Cesarean section delays it by several days, immature cords separate later than mature ones, and infection may delay separation but does not always do so. Cesarean sectioned infants separated their cord stumps slightly later (Anhalt et al., 1992). It was found by Ronchera-Oms et al. (1994) that bacterial colonization enhances separation, antiseptic therapy prolongs the interval.

Knots

Excessively long umbilical cords are apt to become knotted. We have seen three true knots in a 76-cm-long cord with which the fetus suffered severe cerebral palsy. He was born without fibrinogen and had widespread petechiae. Much venous distention was evident behind the first knot. Collins (1993; Collins et al., 1993) also described triple knots associated with fetal demise and other cord abnormalities, such as torsion. Knots in the umbilical cord may not only cause fetal death (see Fig. 12.43), but they may lead to significant prepartum hypoxia with lasting damage. A study by Maher and Conti (1996), however, suggested that true knots were not significantly associated with fetal acidemia. These authors also reviewed the controversial aspect of the time when knots are first formed in the umbilical cord.

There are thus some important questions: Does every knot cause some damage (Fig. 12.42)? If not, when are umbilical cord knots clinically significant? Although knots are important clinical findings, with an associated fetal mortality of around 10% (Scheffel & Langanke, 1970), it is surprising how little has been written about them. Perhaps the topic is too obvious to demand the attention of many investigators. Browne (1925) reported that true knots occur with a frequency of 0.4% to 0.5%. He performed perfusion experiments to ascertain the resultant perfusion pressure that presumably follows the presence of knots. The normal pressure in the umbilical vein (10mm Hg) was raised to 20mm by one slack knot; two knots raised it to 60mm. If a weight of 100g was used to cause increased tension on the one knot, the perfusion pressure was raised to 100mm. These findings were partially contradicted by the investigations of Chasnoff and Fletcher (1977), who did not find that elevated pressure for perfusion was required when a loose knot was laid; only when more than a 20g weight was applied did the pressure requirements for perfusion rise markedly. They saw a 0.35% incidence of true knots among 2000 consecutive deliveries: one was stillborn, one had low Apgar scores, five were normal.

The venous stasis that occurs with true knots of the umbilical cord often results in thrombosis of placental surface veins. Mural thrombosis or complete occlusion may be found, some even being calcified. In addition, the veins are frequently thickened and may exhibit "cushions." These frequent lesions have long been recognized and were beautifully depicted by Becker (1962). He inferred that their frequency was related to the unusual construction of the placental vessels, especially their deficiency of an elastic membrane. Therefore, he writes, such lesions develop; but their precise etiology was not demonstrated. De Sa (1973) clearly identified these lesions in surface veins of abnormal placentas in which an "elevation of umbilical venous pressure" must be inferred. These

FIGURE 12.42. Knot in the umbilical cord (actually two loops) that had no untoward sequelae.

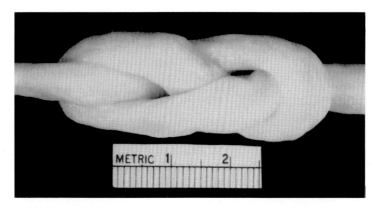

are myxoid-appearing, irregular areas of thickening of blood vessels (Fig. 12.44), similar to those that pathologists find in the pulmonary vessels of patients with pulmonary hypertension. Because they are associated with (inferred) venous hypertension and often have mural thrombi overlying them, we believe them to result from blood stasis. They are commonest in placental surface veins, but cushions may also be found in major villous stem vessels. Some of these cushions are undoubtedly organized thrombi; others may merely reflect the reaction of blood vessels to hypertension. We think it likely that cushions form first and then, after much distention and further exposure to elevated pressure, their endothelial surface degenerates and mural thrombosis forms locally (Fig. 12.44). We have also encountered these cushions in vessels of the twin-to-twin transfusion syndrome and

found no fibrin within them; antibodies to actin, myosin heavy chain antigens and collagen IV, as well as vimentin stained them readily, while they lacked endothelial markers (S.C. Emery, personal observations).

Knots cause compression of Wharton's jelly at the site of knotting. When examined microscopically, one often finds mural thrombosis in the vein. Venous distention distal to the knot is a characteristic finding in knots with clinical significance, as is the tendency of the unknotted cord to curl if the knot had been present for some time. Parenthetically, it may be mentioned that stillbirth due to a cord knot has also been recorded in an African green monkey (Brady, 1983). Its cord was unusually long, and there was congestion behind the knot. Chimpanzees and orangutans have also been reported to have true knots in some cords (Naaktgeboren & Wagtendonk, 1966).

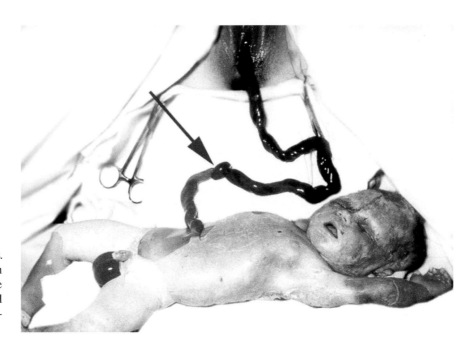

FIGURE 12.43. Macerated stillborn fetus. Death was due to a true knot with obstruction of venous return from the placenta 10 cm from the abdomen. Total length was 65 cm. Note the marked congestion of the cord distal to the knot.

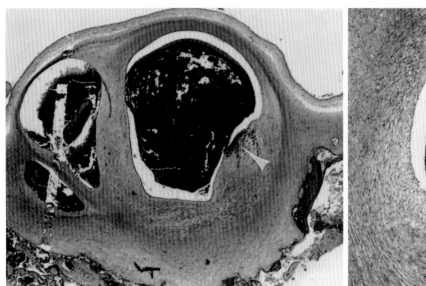
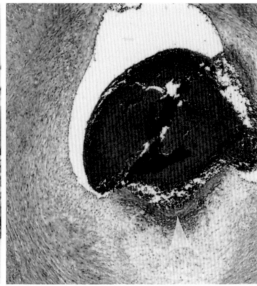

FIGURE 12.44. Mural thrombi in surface veins of case shown in Figure 12.43. Mural thrombi are shown at sites of marked wall thickening, the cushions. Note pallor of thickened vein wall on right. H&E ×16, left; Masson trichrome ×64, right.

False Knots

False knots should not be listed as knots at all. This term has become so customary, however, that it merits brief discussion. One such structure is shown in Figure 12.45. These anomalies are local redundancies of umbilical vessels (mostly the vein), rather than knots, and they are often large. Their vasculature has been depicted by Hyrtl (1870), Arvy and Pilleri (1976a), and others. A rarely used term for these changes is **nodus spurious vasculosus**. When an excessive amount of Wharton's jelly is present, the term **nodus spurious gelatinosus** has been used. So far as can be determined, these structures have absolutely no clinical importance. Of course, there may be the occa-

sional clot formed in this area, and it is conceivable that they might bleed. Despite their clinical irrelevancy, questions persist just why these redundancies appear at all. What are the forces that regulate the growth of fetal vessels in the first place and do the false knots merely signify a temporal discrepancy of vascular growth with inadequate cord lengthening? Answers to these questions elude us at present.

A completely forgotten notion, the angle of insertion (*Insertionswinkel*) to which Hyrtl (1870) tried to draw attention, suggests that one may infer the position held in utero, and reflecting trophotropic departure of the placenta from its original site of implantation. This angle was between 0 and 90 degrees in the original observations

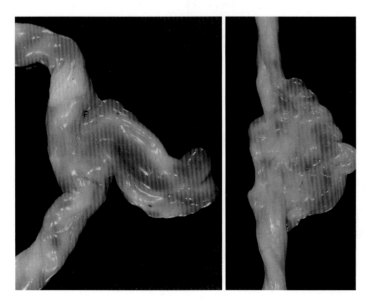

FIGURE 12.45. False knots, representing vascular redundancies.

and is clearly variable when one examines placentas. Strassmann (1902) regretted that in his studies on placenta previa he failed to take note of this feature, which might have enhanced his conviction of trophotropism.

Strictures

Significant reductions in the size of the umbilical cord are referred to as stricture, torsion, and coarctation (Figs. 12.46 and 12.47). These abnormalities are not uncommon and are especially frequently found on the abdominal surfaces of macerated fetuses with long, heavily spiraled cords (Benirschke, 1994). Javert and Barton (1952) have also depicted this problem in several of their illustrations. One must assume that the fetus has been so active as to have sheared off the blood supply at the site of torsion. In the first edition of this book we were skeptical about the significance of this lesion and some of the case reports. Since then we have seen many additional cases that have convinced us it is a real phenomenon. One may even see much congestion on one side of the torsion and find thrombi in placental surface veins. Because they are often macerated fetuses, the demonstration of thrombi is hampered. Moreover, coagulation is inadequately developed in embryos. Nevertheless, the constriction near the fetal abdominal surface often shows the vein to be severely compressed. Heifetz (1996) had a different opinion. He argued that strictures at the fetal abdomen were secondary to gradually diminishing Wharton's jelly at that end of the cord, and that they were not the cause of fetal (embryonic) demise. The fact that this lesion is associated with excessively long cords, with heavy spiraling, with frequent placental surface venous thrombi and cushions, makes us believe in the primacy of the constriction as cause of fetal demise. Heifetz points out that the association with many small vessels at the abdominal portion of the cord is a normal feature. These vessels ultimately aid in the healing ("organization") of the cord stump after birth.

A typical case of cord constriction is shown in Figure 12.46, and several authors have provided single and multiple case reports (King, 1926; Weber, 1963; Quinlan, 1965; Virgilio & Spangler, 1978; Robertson et al., 1981; Glanfield & Watson, 1986; Herman et al., 1991; Sun et al., 1995; Masliah & Wahl, 2004). These authors have shown that the phenomenon is not confined to abortions or to the fetal end of the cord. Glanfield and Watson (1986) reported a case with a fresh thrombus at the site of torsion at the twisted placental end of the cord that led to fetal death at 35 weeks of gestation. They also reviewed the sparse literature of this anomaly whose etiology is not known. Nevertheless, Weber (1963) stated that the constriction is rarely reported although it is not uncommon, and described five cases. Dargent et al. (2002) described an interesting arrangement of markedly twisted blood vessels ("cork-

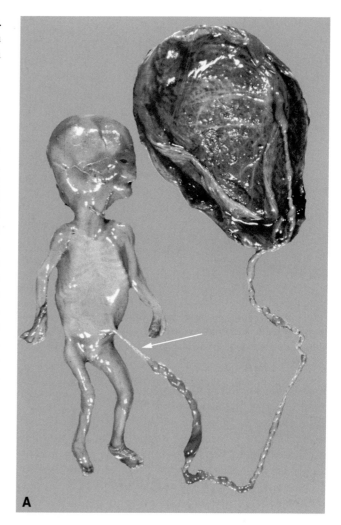

A

FIGURE 12.46. 12 weeks' gestation fetus with velamentous cord insertion, excessive length and excessive spiraling of the umbilical cord. The fetus died because of the constriction near the fetal end (arrow). This is not due to a deficiency of Wharton's jelly but it is the result of spiraling and consequent dissipation of jelly; it is often inappropriately referred to as "coarctation". This cause of death in abortion specimens is usually overlooked by pathologists.

screw-like twist") in a set of monoamnionic twins. Of course, cord entanglement and often knotting are commonly observed in monoamnionic/monochorionic (MoMo) twins and a cause for their excessive mortality.

Robertson et al. (1981) surmised that the cause of constriction is a primary deficiency of Wharton's jelly, a true coarctation. These investigators lost two fetuses with this lesion soon after amniocentesis. Hersh and Buchino (1988), who observed two successive deaths in one family from torsion of the cord, also believed that primary absence of Wharton's jelly is the cause of this lesion. They had previously seen two similar cases in one family and hinted at the possibility that the recurrence risk is greater than what had been thought. There is normally a gradually

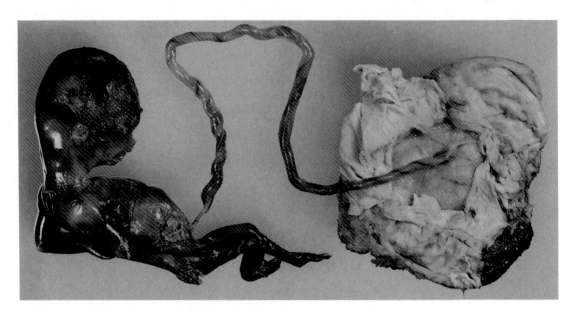

FIGURE 12.47. Both of these two spontaneous abortuses, at 12 and 14 weeks gestation respectively, had markedly spiraled umbilical cords and severe constrictions of the cords ("coarctation", torsion) near the fetal surfaces that led to their deaths. This is not a deficiency of Wharton's jelly and it is commonly overlooked by pathologists.

diminishing amount of Wharton's jelly near the abdominal surface. It may be for this reason that the stricture is most commonly seen at that site. We have had such a case, with a 64-cm umbilical cord in a stillborn; the two umbilical arteries exhibited significant, long-standing degenerative changes at this site. It was the cause of the fetal death. Collins (1995b) proposed severe torsion as a cause of nonimmune hydrops (see also Poeschmann et al., 1991). Colgan and Luk (1982), who reported the death of one MoMo twin from such a torsion, found thrombi in all three vessels at that site. Very frequently, the stricture is associated with an excessively long umbilical cord that is markedly spiraled throughout as well. Again, it is our opinion that the absence of Wharton's jelly is secondary to being squeezed out by the twisting. Although future studies will have to confirm this assumption, we believe that undue movements of the early fetus lead to the lengthening of the cord and its twisting. Remarkably, the excessive twisting with fetal demise can occur repetitively. Thus, Bakotic et al. (2000) found it in three successive gestations and depict it well. Wiedersberg et al. (2001) found strictures ("thin cord syndrome" they called it) often as cause of fetal demise and abortion. Singh et al. (2003) confirmed this for early abortion specimens. The entire topic has been thoroughly reviewed by Benirschke (1994).

Rupture

It is not surprising that short cords may avulse from the placenta during descensus, particularly during a precipitous delivery. The cord may rupture completely or partially, and it may bleed or form hematomas. Bahary et al.

(1965) reported a severely anemic newborn whose marginally inserted short cord (24 cm) had ruptured during descensus. They believed that velamentous cord insertion was the most frequent antecedent of this complication. Rhen and Kinnunen (1962) lost a fetus with a 50-cm cord before labor due to a ruptured umbilical vein. It occurred spontaneously after tumultuous movements by the fetus. Foldes (1957) reported a stillbirth after rupture in which the normally long cord was wound tightly around the neck. These authors reviewed older literature of this rare event. Bleeding from the injured cord after amniocentesis has been recorded by ultrasonography (Romero et al., 1982); and the development of a cord hematoma following in utero transfusion, with bradycardia secondary to arterial spasm, was observed by Moise et al. (1987).

Such experiences and the question as to how much traction may be applied to the cord during delivery have stimulated systematic studies on the tensile strength of the umbilical cord (e.g., Crichton, 1973). Crichton tested 200 normal term umbilical cords without having their blood drained. He thus obtained a nearly normal distribution of breaking weights. Most cords ruptured when 12 pounds were applied, the extremes being 4 and 24 pounds. There was no correlation with fetal weight, length of cord, or placental weight. Although the cord ruptured most often (22.5%) at the site of its placental attachment, rupture could occur anywhere (Siddall, 1925). It must be said, however, that spontaneous complete rupture is an uncommon event; most ruptures are partial and cause local hematomas or hemorrhage. Leinzinger (1972) reported such a case in association with hydramnios and reviewed the relevant literature, but the case reported by Golden (1973) must not be cited as one of umbilical cord rupture. In his patient the cord separated when traction was applied to it after the child was delivered; the hematoma was at the site of detachment, and there was an adjacent IUD (Lippe's loop). The photograph he supplied suggests that the cord was either marginal or in a velamentous insertion, a finding that is frequently made when IUDs remain during pregnancy. The IUD was certainly not within the amnionic sac and had nothing directly to do with the traumatic postnatal cord separation. More likely, the cord ruptured through velamentous vessels.

Hematoma

Hemorrhages into the cord substance are more common than complete rupture, and they may be similarly life-threatening. Figure 12.48 shows such an example, associated with a slightly shorter than average cord (42 cm). It has been conjectured in the past that such hemorrhages occur because of fatty degeneration of the cord (Browne, 1925), but we have not seen such changes. In our experience, spontaneous cord hematomas are associated with short cords, trauma, and with entangling. At times there are associated thrombi. Whichever event is the primary one is then unknown. Vu et al. (1984) reported on five cases; they stated that inflammation eventually occurs when the hemorrhage is not lethal. This finding is also contrary to our experience. Hemorrhage may be recognized sonographically (Sutro et al., 1984) and fetal heart rate problems have been reported with hematomas (Ballas et al., 1985).

It is a common practice for the obstetrician to use a clamp to apply gentle traction to the cord after delivery. This may induce local hematoma formation, and such a history must be ascertained before the diagnosis of spontaneous hematoma is entertained. Hematomas due to cord clamping is often obvious because the serrations of

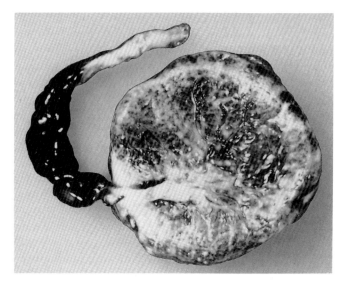

FIGURE 12.48. Stillbirth because of rupture (hematoma) of a 46-cm-long umbilical cord.

a clamp remain visible. Traumatic injury to cord vessels during amniocentesis has often been reported (James & Nickerson, 1976; Gassner & Paul, 1976; Bobitt, 1979). This potential hazard, when it occurs, demands emergency attention.

Ruvinsky et al. (1981), reviewing the entire literature (57 cases), found that hematomas of the cord are associated with a 50% fetal mortality. They described a case that was diagnosed by at 32 weeks by ultrasonography. The hematoma measured $6 \times 9 \times 3$ cm and was estimated to contain 100 mL of blood. The cord was 52 cm long and had a ruptured vein from which the sac-like extension of the hematoma took place. The fetus exsanguinated; it did not die from compression of vessels. In the cord shown in Figure 12.49, the aneurysmally distended vein was so huge that the arteries were compressed and the fetus stillborn. Remarkably, the external appearance was not one of

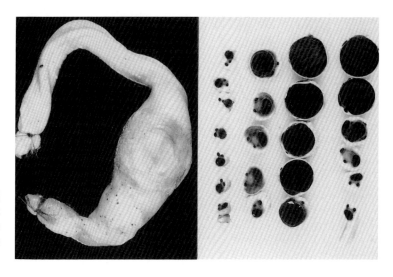

FIGURE 12.49. Aneurysmal dilatation of the umbilical vein with fatal compression of arteries. Stillborn at term after a normal pregnancy and delivery. No cause was identified for this lesion. There were also no thrombi.

hemorrhage. A similar case, but involving the umbilical artery, has been described by Fortune and Östör (1978). It was a 36-week spontaneous intrauterine death. The two umbilical arteries were looped and one had an 8×3 cm aneurysmal dilatation that had obstructed the blood flow through the other vessels. There was no thrombosis and no underlying pathology existed. Gerlach (1968) had previously described a cherry-sized aneurysm of the umbilical artery, in its abdominal portion of a child with anomalies. He concluded that it was part of a dysmorphic condition. The wall of that vessel was partially calcified. Two similar cases were described by Rissmann (1931); one was a stillborn, and the other lived. The classical report of cord hematoma is that of Dippel (1940), who found 36 cases. He believed that congenital thinning, fatty and mucoid degeneration of the vein wall, varices, and looping of a long cord are instrumental in the cause. Schreier and Brown (1962) depicted such a defect in the vein of a child who survived a large hematoma. When elastic stains are done on such cords it has been repeatedly found that the elastic fibers of the vein are focally deficient. Remarkably, the infant of the cord shown in Figure 12.50 survived, even though much clotted blood was found in the distorted Wharton's jelly. Although the disruptive lesion is usually located in the vein (Dippel cited a 9:1 ratio), one of the cases described by Gardner and Trussell (1964) involved an artery in a patient who had a prolapsed cord. Other case reports have stressed that the overall mortality rate is around 50%, that hematomas may occur with long and short cords, with and without inflammation, and that their primary cause remains generally unknown (Irani, 1964; Ratten, 1969; Clare et al., 1979; Dillon & O'Leary, 1981; Feldberg et al., 1986). Although funisitis renders the cords generally slightly more friable (Summerville et al., 1987), it was an infrequent finding. Syphilis, once thought to be a major cause, was specifically ruled out by Dippel (1940), and Fox (1978) also agreed with the unimportant contribution of infection to hematomas. He lamented that the main etiology is usually obscure but considered deficient Wharton's jelly as possibly important, particularly as hematomas are relatively more frequent in prolonged pregnancy. We have seen one case of cord hematoma with fatal prenatal myocardial infarct of the fetus. Aneurysms of cord and placental surface vessels are considered below. Cordocentesis may lead to hemorrhage into the umbilical cord as well (see above). In a case we saw, the umbilical artery had been aspirated at cordocentesis for presumed thrombocytopenia with thrombosis ensuing. The artery had become completely obliterated and its wall was necrotic. Hemosiderin-laden macrophages were adjacent to the hemolyzing blood in this artery. The neonate suffered cerebral palsy. In another case, spontaneous thrombosis of one umbilical artery, with necrosis of its wall, was accompanied by a longitudinal hematoma-like streak of hemolysis in Wharton's jelly. The fetus had exhibited decreased reactivity and reduced movements, but survived. The villous tissue showed chorangiosis, and many nucleated red blood cells were present in fetal vessels.

Several investigators have attempted ultrastructural delineation of the vessels' unusual structure. We once saw an apparently normal umbilical artery that had two well-defined lumens. Spiteri et al. (1966) were anxious to state that there was no sign of senescence in term arteries when they were compared with those of 7-week-old fetuses. This finding is in contrast to the expected degenerative changes seen in the aging intraabdominal portions of the umbilical arteries (Takagi et al., 1984).

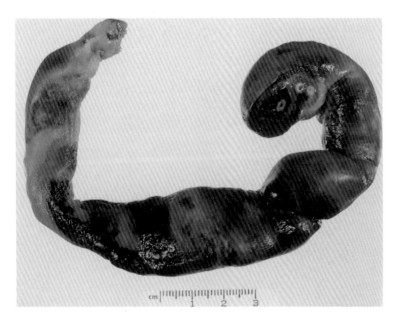

Figure 12.50. Large, 90-cm-long umbilical cord with hematoma and surviving 5300-g infant. Despite the large hematoma, the vascular lumens were patent and had no thrombus, as also described by Bret and Bardiaux (1956).

Vascular structure and changes induced in the umbilical vein by maternal smoking were investigated by Asmussen (1978). These studies showed damage to the intima, elastic subintimal membrane, and media. There are also edema, deficiency of collagen, and myocyte proliferation. A peculiar feature of these large and thick umbilical vessels is that they allow penetration of many polymorphonuclear leukocytes in the usual inflammatory reaction of the amnionic sac infection syndrome. This trait is so striking and so different from other vessels that it is discussed in more detail in the consideration of chorioamnionitis. It may be related to the absence of a true adventitia, as it is seen in systemic blood vessels. Moreover, in the umbilical cord, the extensions of Wharton's jelly penetrate in the muscular walls of the arteries and vein, which may enhance transport of signals, such as leukotaxins.

Varices and Aneurysms

As happens with umbilical cords, surface vessels may have aneurysms that can bleed, thrombose, and rupture (Fig. 12.51). Six such placentas with subamnionic hemorrhages from partially thrombosed chorionic vessels were described by de Sa (1971). He made the point that such thrombi are often associated with fetal growth retardation, diabetes, diffuse thromboses, and organized cushions. These lesions must be differentiated from tears induced during delivery. It must also be cautioned that the obstetrician and neonatologist often draw blood from the chorionic vessels after birth, and the vessels may subsequently leak blood. Thus, when a pathologist observes these surface hematomas, he or she must make sure that they are not artifacts of handling. Varices must not be confused with hemorrhagic subchorial cysts originating from degenerating trophoblastic cell islands. Note,

however, that a number of cases have been described that are difficult to trace. They are instances where blood was found in the amnionic space and in which subamnionic hemorrhages had occurred before birth. They originated from small lesions in vessels that could be demonstrated only by an injection study (Gad, 1968). Their etiology was often obscure. Such a case was reported by Leff (1931). The most detailed study of placental aneurysms derived from the examination of 1000 consecutive placentas reported by Lemtis (1968), whose article was accompanied by exemplary photographs. Lemtis found these lesions in 24 cases, one of which was a partial hydatidiform mole that had numerous aneurysms. Lemtis classified the anomalies into several types. The aneurysms were usually associated with atypical insertion of the cord, SUA, fetal growth retardation, or other placental anomalies; therefore, Lemtis considered them to be true developmental errors. In a set of dizygotic twins we saw, one twin's placenta had two chorionic venous aneurysms. This twin expired from completely spontaneous rupture during labor. Because rupture and exsanguination have been reported only during labor, it is our conviction that the aforementioned distention of the surface half of chorionic vessels after membrane rupture leads to this thinning and the vulnerability of potential aneurysms. Other large aneurysms we have seen have been described as "cirsoid." They were huge dilatations of surface vessels, often partially thrombosed and associated with thrombocytopenia of the neonate. A relevant case of cirsoid or serpentine aneurysm has been described by us (Zhang & Benirschke, 2000). Characteristically, there were many thrombi and some infarction with this anomaly. In one such case, the subjacent main stem vessels had a mole-like myxoid distention. Similarly, Lee et al. (1991) described a huge placenta (1490 g) with a typical cirsoid angiomatous configuration that arose from the umbilical vein of an otherwise normal cord. The umbilical cord of

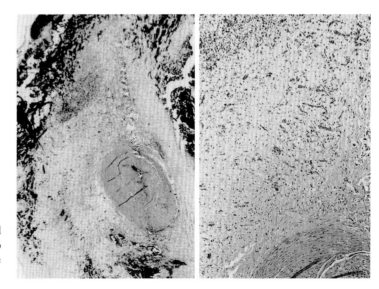

FIGURE 12.51. Umbilical cord of a patient with a palsied infant and hematoma. Numerous capillaries testify to probable earlier, intrauterine traumatic hemorrhage with "organization." H&E ×40, left; ×160, right.

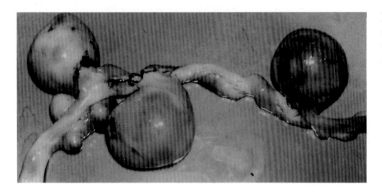

FIGURE 12.52. Multiple aneurysms of the umbilical cord associated with a single umbilical artery. The child was well at 3 years. (Courtesy of R.E. Wybel, Bakersfield, California.)

this growth-restricted neonate had a membranous insertion. The infant was anemic and did well after transfusion. Some of the veins had massive aneurysmal dilatation but lacked thrombotic deposits. The so-called mesenchymal dysplasia that is frequently associated with cirsoid aneurysms and chorangiomas is discussed in greater detail in Chapter 24. Siddiqi and colleagues (1992) described a classic umbilical arterial aneurysm in a two-vessel cord. It was noted to grow in repeated sonographic studies and had a partially calcified wall. It measured 13×5 cm and was 15 cm from the fetus; although it had no thrombus, the cardiac hypertrophy found in the stillborn infant suggested that it had circulatory consequences. Reinhardt et al. (1999) described sonographic findings with mural thrombosis of subchorionic aneurysms that could be confused with chorangiomas. Vandevijver et al. (2000) lost an infant during labor at 41 weeks due to a large aneurysm of the umbilical vein and deduced that excessive thinning (absence of muscle) was the cause of the aneurysm.

Varicosities in the umbilical cord are much more common than aneurysms. An example is illustrated in Figure 12.45. Real varix formations, such as are seen in Figures 12.52 and 12.53 are rare. A case was described by Leinzinger (1969), who also reviewed the sparse literature. Leinzinger observed during a normal delivery a 70-cm-long umbilical cord that had a peach-sized varix of the umbilical vein that was largely thrombosed. He drew attention to the focally marked thinning of the wall of the umbilical vein. This has also been reported to be associated with necrosis of muscle wall and has attracted greater interest recently (Qureshi & Jacques, 1994). Altshuler and Hyde (1989) first depicted necrosis of umbilical vessel walls and suggested that it is the occasional result of chronic and severe meconium exposure. These authors also demonstrated, in vitro, that meconium may induce a significant contraction when strips of umbilical vein are exposed to solutions of meconium. The vasoconstrictive effect of cholic acids was later confirmed when Sepúlveda et al. (1991) experimentally exposed chorionic surface vein samples to these agents. Their interest derived from the poor fetal outcomes in the condition known as cholestasis of pregnancy (Laatikainen et al., 1978). Bile aci-

demia for other reasons than cholestasis of pregnancy is thought to have similar consequences (Nolan et al., 1994). Figure 12.54 shows a somewhat similar thinning of the vein wall as described by Altshuler and Hyde in a child with cerebral palsy. Note that this thinning did not take place in a varix; there is no thrombus, nor is the thinned wall toward the cord surface, which might be expected if mechanical pressure had been the cause of this marked diminution in vessel wall thickness. Such areas of degeneration not only occur in the vein but also may affect arteries for still unknown reasons. To be sure, on occasion they are the sequelae of thrombosis, but they may occur without it. It may also be that constriction is mediated by interleukin-1, as demonstrated to occur in meconium staining (Baergen et al., 1994). Within the stillborn whose umbilical artery is shown in Figure 12.55, a thin segment of artery had numerous rounded, degenerating myocytes. This process was confined to only one artery, it lay under the cord surface, and there was mild phlebitis. The short cord was loosely wound around the neck, but no reason-

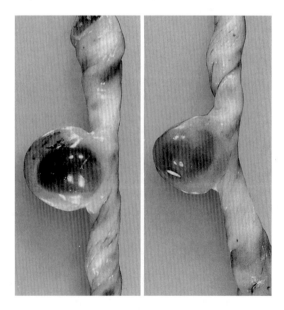

FIGURE 12.53. Partially thrombosed varix near the fetal end of the cord. Normal infant, 65-cm-long cord.

FIGURE 12.54. Segmental thinning toward the middle of the cord in an umbilical vein (arrows). The child suffered cerebral palsy. A cause for this anomaly was not detected. H&E ×60, left; ×160, right.

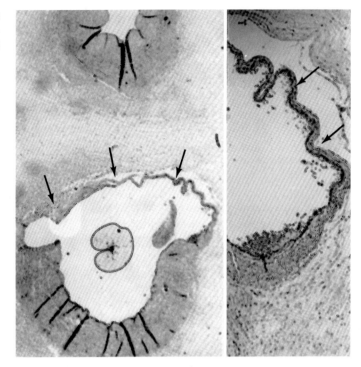

able cause of the lesion was identified. Similar hypoplasia of segments of umbilical vessels, usually veins, has been reported a few times in the literature. It is usually associated with rupture of the cord or hematomas (Bender et al., 1978). Severe venous distention of the umbilical vein, detected sonographically, has been used as an indicator of severe hemolytic disease in the fetus (DeVore et al., 1981). In recent years, there have been many reports of umbilical arterial necrosis associated with meconium staining in which the meconium toxicity is held responsible, even though the exact toxic moiety of this material is unknown (see Chapter 11). Bendon et al. (1991) described such necrosis with ulceration in association with intestinal atresia and suggested this to be a new syndrome. Similarly, Khurana (1995) found duodenal atresia in a fetus with ulcerated umbilical arteries. The amnionic fluid was bloody at the time of delivery, at 35 weeks' gestation. The neonate died with numerous infarctive lesions. Because the duodenum had two areas of obliteration, the only explanation for meconium-induced arterial wall degeneration would be prenatal bilious vomiting had occurred.

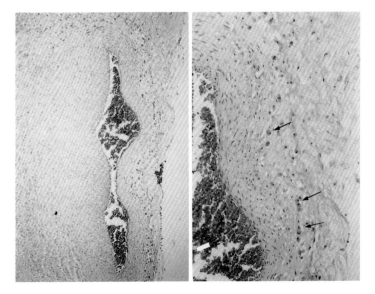

FIGURE 12.55. Segmental thinning of one umbilical arterial wall with degenerating rounded myocytes (arrows) under the surface. Stillborn infant, short nuchal cord. H&E ×60, left; ×160, right.

Thrombosis of the Umbilical Vessels

Thrombi of vessels in the umbilical cord are common, and they occur most often in surface veins. They may take place already during early pregnancy and then lead to SUA; but this is not very likely because of the difficulty in fetal clotting during early pregnancy. More frequently, thrombi occur near term. The formation of thrombi with velamentous insertion of the cord is readily understandable. Here the membranous vessels course in the chorion, unprotected by Wharton's jelly; they are thus prone to injury from compression and are also subject to tears. Neonatal thrombocytopenia and bruising has been witnessed on several such occasions.

Severe inflammatory reactions of the cord often cause mural thrombi as well. Such a case with a surviving, bruised infant has been described by Wolfman et al. (1983). The umbilical vein of this premature infant of an otherwise uncomplicated pregnancy was inflamed and nearly completely thrombosed. In addition, there was one peculiar lesion of the cord with old inflammatory exudate surrounding the vessels. These lesions are often calcified, and macroscopically resemble the precipitation ring in Ouchterlony plates. This unusual entity is further discussed in Chapter 20. Thrombi are frequent in this condition.

It is also easy to understand that thrombosis of cord vessels may occur in varices (Figs. 12.53 and 12.56), and from looping and knotting of the umbilical cord. Likewise, the entangling of cords in monoamnionic twins, with vascular obstruction ensuing, and that from amnionic bands are mechanical reasons for thrombosis. Thrombosis has also followed intravascular exchange transfusion and was there associated with an intrafunicular hematoma (Seeds et al., 1989). These situations can all compromise the circulation and lead to fetal death, and experimentally, cord occlusion in fetal lambs has been shown to cause neuropathologic changes (Ikeda et al.,

1998). The thrombi may break off and potentially embolize to the fetus or to the placenta, where they may cause infarction. Thrombosis can become so extensive that they so compromise the circulation and lead to fetal death. Myocardial infarction with prenatal tamponade has been reported from embolism (Wolf et al., 1985).

Thrombi have been held responsible for amputations (Hoyme et al., 1982) and for a generalized bleeding tendency due to disseminated intravascular coagulation (DIC) or consumption coagulopathy (Williams & Benirschke, 1978). More remarkable are the thrombi that occur in the absence of all of these more readily understood complications, and they are perhaps the most common. We have seen many such cases that resulted in fetal death, and others in children who developed cerebral palsy. In retrospect, there is often no good explanation for their genesis (Fig. 12.57). There are numerous case reports on the subject; often the pathologist is unable to explain the origin of thrombi. Very frequently thromboses of vessels in the cord are associated with similar events in the villous ramifications. From finding occasionally deposits of calcium salts in such vessel walls, and because of the apparent organization of these thrombosed vessels, it must be inferred that the clots have been present for days, if not weeks. Doshi and Klionsky (1979) also found it to be a frequent problem in severely ill newborns. They described 40 cases of DIC with thromboses in placental vessels, at least six of which had a prenatal onset. Coagulation problems caused by activated protein C resistance (factor V Leiden mutation) or S deficiency are sometimes suspected (Kraus, 1996), but they have only recently been proved to exist. The cases of Seligsohn et al. (1984) and Marcianiak et al. (1985) of familial protein C deficiency supported this notion. The neonatal purpura fulminans of protein C deficiency was reviewed by Dreyfus et al. (1991) and depicted by Hartman et al. (1990). In these pedigrees, prenatal thrombosis was not reported, although the condition at birth is summarized

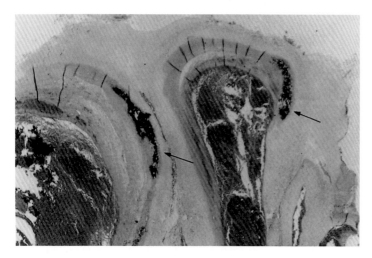

FIGURE 12.56. Partially calcified vessel walls (arrows) in the cord of a stillborn. Cord also had varices but no inflammation. H&E ×60.

FIGURE 12.57. Nearly occlusive venous thrombus with fetal death. Long cord. H&E ×40.

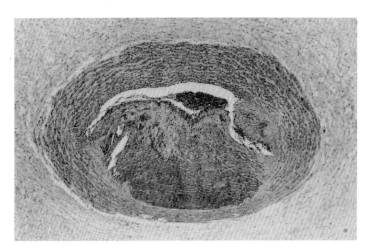

by the latter authors. In three cases of neonatal CNS disorders, Thorarensen et al. (1997) found thrombosis because of inherited Leiden heterozygosity. One of these infants had placental multiple thromboses, was born with seizures and had extensive CNS lesions. DNA analysis on the infant showed it to possess the mutation. Because factor V Leiden mutation is now recognized as perhaps the most important cause of familial thrombophilia, future placental vascular disease needs to be studied with this in mind (see Chapter 21). The possibility of making the genetic diagnosis of a factor V Leiden mutation was demonstrated by Newman et al. (1998). They purified DNA from paraffin blocks of a neonate dying with aortic thrombosis and unequivocally diagnosed the mutation. Maternal thrombotic events have also often been ascribed to activated protein-C resistance, as by Rotmensch et al. (1997), who found extremely poor obstetric outcomes. It must be appreciated, however, that normally pregnancy is associated with an increase in activated protein-C resistance (Walker et al., 1997). One case of protein-S deficiency in pregnancy has been reported (Tharakan et al., 1993). The pregnancy of this patient ended in a stillbirth with placental vascular thrombosis and the patient had a pulmonary embolus. After anticoagulation, she had a successful pregnancy. Unfortunately, the state of the placenta in each of these four newborns with massive venous thrombosis and fulminant purpura developing shortly after birth was not reported. Heifetz (1988) has reviewed three patient populations, in addition to 68 cases gathered from the literature. The incidence of thrombosis was 1 in 1300 deliveries, 1 in 1000 perinatal autopsies, and 1 in 250 high-risk gestations. Venous thromboses were more common than thromboses in one or both arteries, but the latter was more often lethal.

Protein C deficiency was found to be associated with the 11 neonatal cases reported by Marco-Johnson et al. (1988). They established that the protein C levels are very low in newborns, and that an inherited deficiency to explain neonatal thrombosis must be carefully docu-

mented. The relatives of their patients were not heterozygotes and, after successful therapy with heparin in four patients, their protein C levels gradually rose to normal. Five of their patients were one of twins; one of these twins was the recipient of the transfusion syndrome and the co-twin had died at birth; one patient had a diabetic mother. Four infants had aortic thromboses (one also had renal thrombosis), and one had CNS thrombosis. The mechanism of this presumably acquired absence of protein C in these neonates remained unknown, and the placentas were not described.

In two other cases of arterial thrombosis we have witnessed, one umbilical artery had a completely necrotic wall, and many thrombi were found in the fetal chorionic vascular ramifications. One child died during the neonatal period with prenatal thrombosis of one pulmonary artery and an infarcted lung; the other survived but developed severe cerebral palsy. Maternal diabetes, which is occasionally associated with thromboses, was not present, and no other morphologic or clinical features helped to explain the cause of this fetal vascular coagulation.

It is often desirable to estimate the age of the thrombi. When calcification accompanies them, they are clearly old; for younger clots, the table derived from the detailed investigations on aging of thrombi by Leu and Leu (1989) is helpful.

There was such massive calcification in the walls of some umbilical cord blood vessels in a few cases (Rust, 1937; Walz, 1947; Perrin & Bel, 1965; Pekarske, 1995) that it occasionally became difficult to ligate the cord (Fig. 12.56). Two of these infants survived. In others, the calcification affected fetal arteries with lethal consequences (Ivemark et al., 1962). Schiff et al. (1976) were the first to recognize a calcified cord antenatally. The three vessels were calcified virtually over the entire length of the cord and attended by much inflammation; the neonate died with pulmonary hypoplasia. There are some reports of venous thrombosis associated with severe fetal distress (Eggens & Bruins, 1984), cerebral palsy, massive fetomaternal hemorrhage (Hoag, 1986), and other complications. Occasionally, maternal smoking and diabetes have been implicated. Abrams et al. (1985) were able to make the diagnosis by sonography, and there are many other case reports, too numerous to list, that attest to thromboses as being an important problem in perinatology. It stands to reason that such occlusions, particularly when associated with villous vascular disease, raise fetal blood pressure and, like the experimental obliteration of placental vessels by microembolization (Trudinger et al., 1987), they may have abnormal sonographic consequences. Thrombi may also lead to fetal growth restriction. In an occasional case, one may observe strange phenomena that clearly betray long-standing prenatal problems, as shown later in Figure 12.63. Here, the cord of an infant with renal agenesis can be seen to be unusually long (77 cm) for an oligohydramneic pregnancy (Fig. 12.58). The placenta had many thrombi in its surface vessels, and the partially calcified umbilical vein had ruptured. Squamous debris (vernix caseosa) had dissected underneath the cord surface, all of which suggested that the process had been ongoing for weeks prior to delivery. Parenthetically, it may be mentioned that fatal air embolization has been reported when, during cesarean section, the placenta had to be incised (Allen et al., 1969). In addition, the frequent amnion nodosum of the placental surface seen in renal agenesis or in other causes of severe oligohydramnios is rarely present on the cord's surface.

Khong and Dilly (1989) reviewed the topic of the rare calcifications in umbilical arteries and presented five new cases. These authors were of the opinion that the calcifications fall into two classes: those with calcific thrombi, and those with evidence of funisitis, inflammation of the amnionic sac, or both. They described two complete thromboses of one artery with calcification. In one, the mother had a lupus-like disease and there was 20% infarction of the placenta, with a liveborn at 35 weeks. In the other, a mother with a skin rash at 28 weeks' gestation gave birth to a severely growth-retarded (940 g) macerated fetus at 34 weeks with apparent amnionic bands, with amputations and cord constriction. The other three cases (one living) had associated inflammation without recognized microorganisms.

Thrombosis of the Placental Vascular Tree

Mural and occlusive thrombi occur frequently in the superficial placental vessels and their villous ramifications. They are variably located across the fetal surface and within the placenta, and only occasionally are they accompanied by thrombi in the umbilical cord. Often these vascular occlusions have grave consequences. Surface thrombi are usually recognized during careful gross examination. When the vessel is hugely distended, as that shown in Figure 12.59A, the identification of thrombosis is easy. Much more frequently overlooked are such thrombi as seen in Figures 12.60 and 12.61. When thrombi are fresh, their gross appearance is that of a slightly enlarged vessel that may have an unusual color. It is not so shiny and blue as normal vessels. One is also unable to move the blood mechanically in thrombosed vessels and of course histologically they are easily diagnosed (Fig. 12.62). Older thrombi become white or yellow.

Mural thrombosis is much more frequent than complete obliteration of the vessel. Such thromboses often

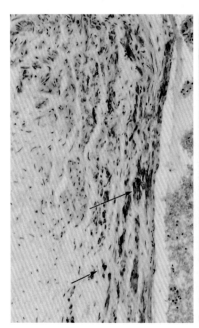
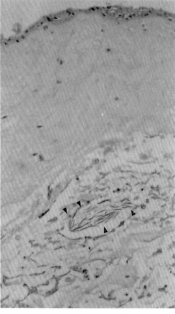

FIGURE 12.58. Umbilical cord (77 cm) in renal agenesis with partial calcification of the vein wall (left, arrows) and vernix dissection (right, arrows). H&E ×160.

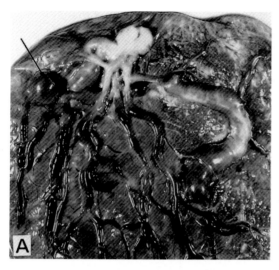

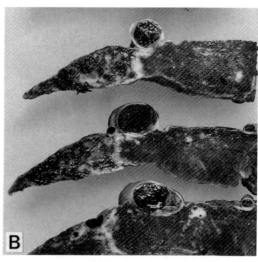

FIGURE 12.59. A: Varix in a surface chorionic vein branch (arrow) and hugely distended, thrombosed umbilical vein tributary (at right). Neonatal death with umbilical vein thrombosis, renal necrosis, and possible maternal diabetes. B: The layered thrombi are apparent in the cross sections.

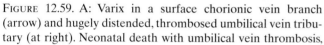

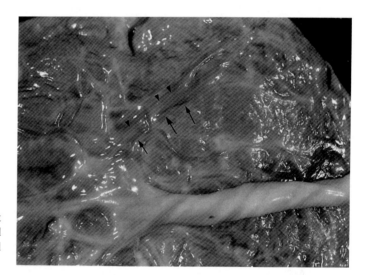

FIGURE 12.60. Thrombosis of an umbilical vein tributary at arrows. Note the discoloration (hemolysis). The infant had disseminated intravascular coagulation (DIC), exhibited schistocytes, and developed cerebral palsy.

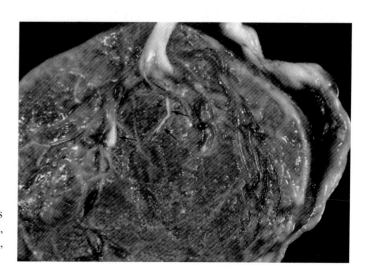

FIGURE 12.61. Partially calcified thrombi in artery branches (arrows) of a child with renal agenesis, a long cord (77 cm), calcification of the umbilical vein wall, and amnion nodosum, a rare feature of cord surfaces.

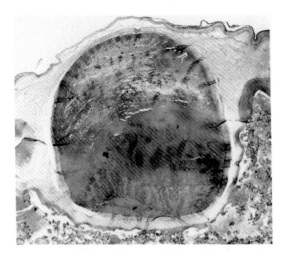

FIGURE 12.62. Layered thrombus in a dilated chorionic vein tributary. Stillbirth, long cord, sacrococcygeal teratoma. H&E ×16.

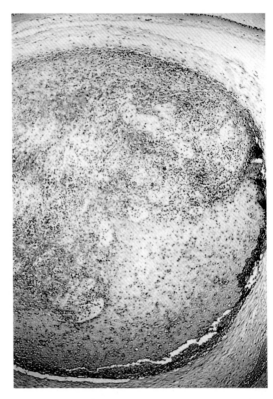

FIGURE 12.63. Unexplained thrombus with partial calcification (right margin) of surface vein in a stillborn infant. H&E ×26.

calcify (Fig. 12.63) but variations are frequent; and when thrombosis has occurred a long time before examination, the vessel may obliterate completely. It then appears as a fibrous strand that may be difficult to recognize as once having been a vessel. We have seen such thrombi in placentas of trisomy 18 and associated with cytomegalovirus infection, excessively long cords with and without excessive spiraling, cord knots, velamentous cord insertion, amputation necrosis in the fetus, severe chorioamnionitis, neonatal purpura, generalized fetal thrombosis, and many other conditions. They are not rare events and clearly bespeak a pathologic prenatal environment. They may occur in arteries as well as (more commonly) in veins, and the vascular wall may show various stages of degeneration or calcification. Thrombi are generally not a cause of local inflammation. The topic has been discussed extensively in a study of umbilical cord lesions (Benirschke, 1994).

Similar thrombosis of the further ramifications of the vascular tree exist (Fig. 12.64). If the thrombi have been occlusive for a prolonged time, the entire villous tree may

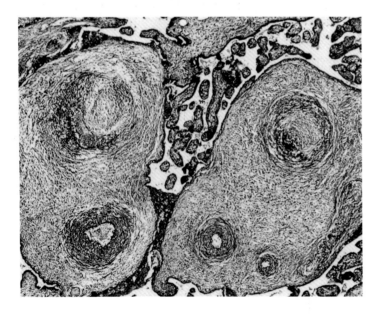

FIGURE 12.64. Muscular hypertrophy and old occlusions in several of many stem vessels of a child with unexplained mid-forearm amputation. H&E ×260.

become avascular and atrophy, undergo fibrosis (Fig. 12.65). It does not infarct; true infarction of villous tissue occurs only when the maternal blood supply is interrupted. The villous tissue merely atrophies over time. Localized thrombosis with early blanching of the affected villous district has been well illustrated by Fox (1966).

In the blood of neonates whose placental vessels had thrombi, one may detect schistocytes and find hematologic derangements such as fibrinogen and platelet deficiencies. Kristiansen and Nielsen (1985) described three cases with fatal thromboses; they concluded that, most often, mechanical factors are the cause. The relation of thrombi to fetal deaths was evaluated by Cook et al. (1987). They found thrombi in 98% of fetal deaths, which is much in excess of our observations; moreover, we disagree with their interpretation of organization of the thrombotic material. In fact, true organization of dead tissues, as the pathologist knows it from renal or splenic infarcts, is rare in all placental degenerative lesions. That is, removal of debris by phagocytes and the ingrowth of granulation tissue with fibrous tissue substitution are phenomena not seen in true placental infarcts, nor do they occur in thrombosed placental vessels. Rather, these lesions shrink, and some phagocytes may appear; but eventually they either become calcified (Pekarske, 1995), or the vessel atrophies. It may eventually disappear completely, becoming unrecognizable as having been a vessel.

As indicated, thromboses extend occasionally into the major ramifications of villous vessels. They may be occlusive; their walls and the extensions of Wharton's jelly may calcify also. When many placentas are examined histologically, one finds these lesions more often than they are suspected macroscopically. They are not always associated with recognizable surface thrombi (Fig. 12.66), and often the etiology of the lesions remains unknown. They are frequently associated with fetal growth restriction,

intrauterine demise, and occasionally with neonatal coagulation disorders. When associated with excessively long cords, Boué et al. (1995) found occasional cerebral degenerative changes, and Kraus (1997) has drawn attention to its frequent relevance in medicolegal cases. We have speculated that they may be the result of prenatal insults, such as virus infections or perhaps even trauma due to fetal motions, but the etiology remains often obscure. Cytomegalovirus infection is definitely an occasional cause of these vascular calcifications. It is common to find occlusions of placental vessels with stillborns but to differentiate thrombi from autolytic degeneration may be difficult. Caution must be exercised when these large stem villi are evaluated. Collagenous trabeculae therein have much the same appearance as old occlusive thrombi.

Obliterative vascular changes were probably first described by Merttens (1894). They have since been discussed at length by Becker and Dolling (1965), who believed them to be the sequelae of infections in earlier fetal life. These authors found neovascularization and other phenomena that they thought to be indications of organization. The former notion of a syphilitic endovasculitis as the etiology was negated. Other authors cited by these investigators and by Fox (1966) found such vascular obliterations unduly commonly in diabetic pregnancies, 3.6% single arterial stem thrombi in liveborn infants. Fox (1966) also observed them much more commonly in the placentas of stillborns.

Apparently dissatisfied with the varied literature of this topic, Fox (1967) studied fetal stem arteries from 682 placentas, 36 of which were from stillbirths. He observed three lesions: obliterative endarteritis, fibromuscular sclerosis, and thrombosis. These lesions were common in patients with diabetes (23%) and hypertension (about 30%). From a comparison of material from live and dead infants he asserted that the "sclerosis" of vessel walls was a postmortem change. Similar vascular changes were held

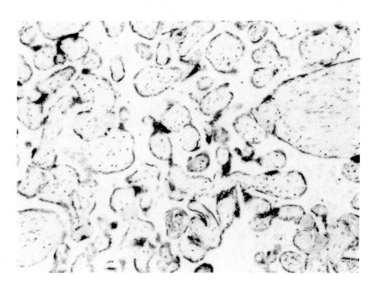

FIGURE 12.65. Diffuse atrophy (degeneration and disappearance) of villous vessels in a placenta with extensive surface thromboses. Fetal growth retardation was evident, and the infant had low Apgar scores. H&E ×60.

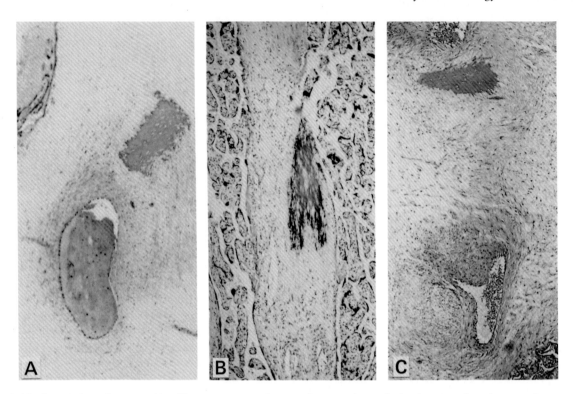

FIGURE 12.66. Composite of cases with villous stem vascular lesions. A: Growth retardation, wavy ribs, 29 weeks' gestation. B: Neonate with phocomelia. C: Growth retardation, purpura, pulmonary hypoplasia, degenerations in several organs, neonatal death. All have calcified deposits in stem vessel walls, and some have thrombi or muscular lesions. H&E ×60.

to be of postmortem nature by Theuring (1968) in his study of placentas from stillborns. He considered that the placenta continues to live after fetal death and that the vessels live in a tissue-culture-like environment to attain such occlusions. The longer the fetal death, the more extensive the occlusions. A similar position was taken by Altemani (1987) who concluded that, because the placental perfusion after fetal death keeps the tissue alive, many of the vascular occlusions seen in stillborns were of postmortem origin. He believed that true organization occurs in these vessels and alluded to the relation of vascular occlusions to hemorrhagic endovasculitis (HEV). The vascular changes found in diabetics were discussed by Fox (1967) and thought to be true in vivo lesions, as had been suggested by Fujikura and Benson (1964) earlier, an observation that was supported by others. Dolff (1978) studied the phenomenon in serial sections, mostly in placentas of stillborn infants. Having duly considered the two principal theories (postnatal change versus prenatal endarteritis obliterans), Dolff came to the conclusion that (1) this lesion is an in vivo phenomenon of importance, and (2) the dynamics that lead to recanalization of the affected vessels is the function of the paracapillary network of the placental stem vessels. Altemani and Lopes de Faria (1987) made a thorough study of the muscular and endothelial changes of main stem blood vessels in 50 stillborns and 50 controls. In their opinion,

the occlusive changes seen were mostly a postmortem phenomenon that was not the cause of fetal demise. Becker and Röckelein (1989) saw in the endarteritis obliterans a common end stage of infections (syphilis, rubella) but also believed that diabetes and preeclampsia have pathogenic importance. In our view this vascular lesion of main stem villous vessels is not a true inflammation, but results most often from thrombosis of more proximal vessels or occasionally represents a postmortem phenomenon. Fok et al. (1990) and other authors (reviewed by Divon, 1996) correlated abnormal Doppler velocimetry studies with occlusive or constrictive placental stem villous arterial lesions. Growth restriction was commonly found. Hitschold (1998) now found that Doppler flow velocity of umbilical arteries accurately correlates with intravillous blood volume in term gestations. In his study of postmortem changes of the placenta, Genest (1992) was able to time the vascular events and confirmed that most endothelial abnormalities occurred after fetal death. Karyorrhexis of villous capillaries occurred in 6 hours, stem villus vascular septation and complete obliteration took 2 days or longer, and fibrosis of terminal villi took weeks to occur.

Such studies have recently become more interesting as prenatal Doppler studies identify frequently abnormal fetal blood flow and correlations are sought to endothelial damage of placental vessels. Thus, Wang et al. (2002,

2003) have obtained plasma from such abnormal fetuses and exposed a culture of fetal endothelial cells to this medium. They found that there was a significant increase in endothelial cell apoptosis due to fetal cytokines apparently released with the abnormal Doppler findings. Importantly, this was independent of maternal preeclampsia that did not have this effect. This is relevant because Trollmann et al. (2003) have demonstrated upregulation of the fetal vascular endothelial growth factor in preeclampsia, speculating that it may be a "potential early indicator of severe birth asphyxia." It is further relevant because fetal villous obliteration and capillary thromboses are by some considered to be indicators of sequelae of "poor maternal intervillous perfusion."

These considerations are important because the entity "hemorrhagic endovasculitis" (Sander, 1980) has aroused so much controversy. Briefly stated, this concept evolved from the study of many formalin-fixed placentas seen in a registry of placentas collected from perinatal deaths and infants with perinatal problems. It was hypothesized that HEV may play an important role in the etiology of these tragedies and that it may be caused by a specific viral or other infectious agent. Hemosiderin was found in some cases to indicate the presumed antiquity of the lesion. HEV is not one lesion; it is a microangiopathy that etiologically and pathologically resembles the glomerulopathy of the hemolytic uremic syndrome. A proliferative, inflammatory vasculitis is not present. The pathologic changes consist in endothelial degeneration, thrombosis, and diapedesis of red blood cells (Fig. 12.67). Stevens and Sander (1984) found HEV to be present in 52% of stillborns and in 22% of liveborn infants. They found associations with preeclampsia, prolonged pregnancy, meconium staining, and with growth retardation. In a later study,

Sander et al. (1997) described recurrence in 28% of subsequent pregnancies. Other investigators (Shen-Schwarz et al., 1986, 1988) found a much lower incidence of this lesion (0.67% after 20 weeks), and associated it with nuchal cords, meconium staining, and postmaturity. Many of these associations did not involve infection, and many infants survived. Also, ultrastructural investigations have not shown organisms. Therefore, the etiology must be considered to include hypoxia, acidosis, and perhaps the DIC associated with the Shwartzman phenomenon.

M.M. Silver et al. (1987, 1988) have done a complete analysis of HEV and confirmed the findings of Ornoy et al. (1976) that the fetal vascular occlusions are most frequently seen in the placentas of macerated stillborns. They presumed it to be a postmortem development. For that reason, they cultured villous tissue in vitro and sampled it at regular intervals for light and electron-microscopic study. They saw a similar lesion develop, in time, when organ explants were allowed to degenerate, thus confirming their original assumption. They believed that it is the sequela of focal or uniform postmortem autolysis of vessel walls. Our own assessment is that HEV is not a specific entity. Clearly, thrombotic lesions of villous stem vessels occur, and often they are associated with cord lesions and surface thrombi. They can be seen in a variety of clinical circumstances, as we have indicated. The occlusion of vessels after death, however, so much mimic degenerative lesions that they may be over-interpreted. Moreover, we now believe the vascular anomaly (proliferation of vessels in an abortus) shown in their Figure 276 (Benirschke & Driscoll, 1967), to be a typical, albeit unusual postmortem phenomenon. In short, although HEV does exist, it does not represent a specific disease entity.

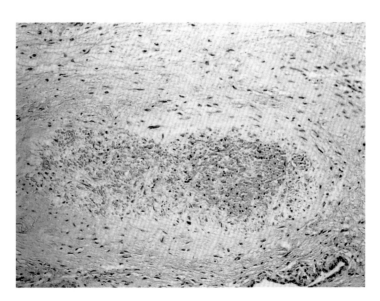

Figure 12.67. Hemorrhagic endovasculitis (HEV) in a main stem villous vessel of a stillborn monozygotic twin. The other twin was well. H&E ×160.

Tumors of the Umbilical Cord

Aside from the tumor-like swellings of aneurysms discussed above, only two true tumors occur in the umbilical cord: angiomas of great variety and significance and, much more rarely, teratomas.

As early as 1939 Marchetti was able to summarize 209 cases of placental angioma (chorangioma) and added eight cases of his own, and Fortune and Östör (1980) summarized 58 cases. A cord angioma was not among this large group. Frequently, the fetus dies when large tumors exist in the cord; hemangiomas or other anomalies may coexist in the fetus (Barry et al., 1951; Corkill, 1961). Some authors have found myxoma-like Wharton's jelly in such tumors (Benirschke & Dodds, 1967; Fortune & Östör, 1980), or have interpreted them to be hamartomas. These neoplasms are never malignant and have a uniform appearance (Figs. 12.68 and 12.69). Death often occurs because of obstruction of blood flow. Occasionally, an associated atrophic artery signifies their long existence before birth. Heifetz and Rueda-Pedreza (1983b) have summarized much of the literature; they noted that angiomas tend to occur at the placental end of the cord and arise from one or more umbilical vessels. Unlike chorangiomas, angiomas of the cord are also usually not associated with hydramnios. Thus, the large angioma described by Barents (1953) was not associated with hydramnios and resulted in a normal infant. Mishriki et al. (1987) described an exception.

Resta et al. (1988) have described an angioma of the cord in association with extremely high (887 to 1030 IU/mL) α-fetoprotein (AFP) levels in the maternal serum at 16 weeks' gestation. The lesion was unsuccessfully biopsied, and the fetus died 1 week later. A 3.2 × 1.8 × 2.0 cm angioma was found, in addition to severe narrowing of the cord at the fetal end. Resta et al. found 22 cases of funicular angioma in the literature. Transplacental bleeding was excluded as possibly accounting for this 30-fold elevation. The neoplasms may attain rather large size, such as the 9 × 7 × 6 cm lesion found by Nieder and Link (1970) or that reported by Yavner and Redline (1989). The angiomyxoma of theirs was associated with a slightly elevated AFP level and was diagnosed sonographically at 19 weeks' gestation. The infant was delivered at 38 weeks and was normal. The large tumor (5.0 × 9.5 cm, 900 g) included a large cystic mass. Its location was typically near the fetal end of the cord. Other large tumors have been diagnosed prenatally. A cord angioma measuring 18 cm in length and associated with a cord that measured 9 cm in width was responsible for nonimmune hydrops of one of dichorionic twins successfully treated during the neonatal period and reported by Seifert et al. (1985). These authors postulated that the cause of the nonimmune hydrops was high-output cardiac failure. Dombrowski et al. (1987) reported a case of severe fetal hemorrhage from the angiomatous cord. Interestingly, this specimen also had intestinal epithelium on the cord's surface. Another case of cystic angiomyxoma reported by Wilson et al. (1994) was followed sonographically during pregnancy and decompressed prior to delivery. At 36 weeks, 350 mL fluid were aspirated from the cyst, decreasing its volume by one half. When the mass increased in size again, delivery was accomplished with good outcome. The angioma was 14 cm in greatest diameter with a 5-cm solid component and was located near the fetal end of the 39-cm-long umbilical cord. An unusual arteriovenous malformation of the umbilical cord was diagnosed sonographically in the distal end (5 cm) of a fetus by Richards et al. (1995). Funipuncture allowed the diagnosis of fetal DIC with low hematocrit due to hemolytic anemia. The neonate was appropriately treated and did well; there was, however, an echogenic hepatic focus associated with

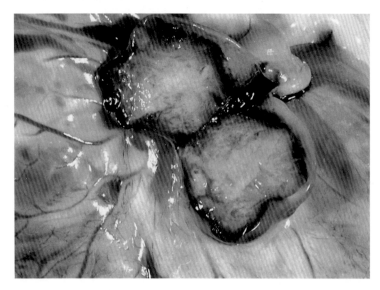

FIGURE 12.68. Angioma at the insertion of the cord in one of twins.

FIGURE 12.69. Histologic appearance of a hemangioma of the umbilical cord. H&E ×20. (*Source:* Benirschke & Dodds, 1967, with permission.)

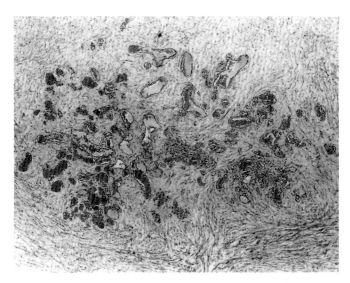

umbilical vein thrombosis. The angiomatous mass had areas of thrombosis and calcification.

Teratomas are much less common than angiomas. Browne (1925) discussed the semantics of teratoma and dermoid. He reported one teratoma and one dermoid, with an anencephalic fetus. Smith and Majmudar (1985) presented a case of a term fetus with bladder exstrophy who also had a pendulous 1.8 × 0.6 cm tumor that was 30 cm from the placental surface. It was focally calcified and contained skin with appendages, colonic epithelium, smooth muscle, and connective tissue. The authors found four previously reported cases in the literature, and six cases in which the lesions were located on the placental surface, the largest measuring 7.5 cm. All were benign. Kreczy and colleagues (1994) reported another case and reviewed the sparse literature of cord teratomas. Their 210-g skin-covered tumor was attached to the cord 2 cm from the neonate's abdominal surface, which also had an omphalocele. The authors discussed the difficult differential diagnosis, especially the distinction from acardiac twins. They came to the conclusion that, lacking a skeletal axis, their lesion represented a true tumor.

One still wonders if these teratomas represent variations of acardiac twins. The latter, however, usually have some longitudinal differentiation and should have their own, separate umbilical cords. Nevertheless, the possibility that teratomas of the cord may represent a form of acardiac fetus has been considered by several authors. Thus, Kreyberg (1958) observed a stillborn premature infant with a 36-cm cord that had, 16 cm from its insertion, a bulky tumor with cystic cavities and a variety of tissues (platysma?, sebaceous glands, hair, myelinated nerves, glia). He cited other similar tumors, one the size of a child's head. Heckmann et al. (1972) illustrated their finding of a 9 × 7 cm tumor that was situated 25 cm from

the fetal end of the cord and 45 cm from the placenta. It had an epidermoid surface and several chambers lined by skin and intestinal epithelium, as well as cartilage and lymphatic remnants. The child did well. The authors considered displaced germ cells as its origin.

References

Abrams, S.L., Callen, P.W. and Filly, R.A.: Umbilical vein thrombosis: sonographic detection in utero. J. Ultrasound Med. **4**:283–285, 1985.

Abuhamad, A., Shaffer, W., Mari, G., Copel, J., Hobbins, J. and Evans, A.: Single umbilical artery: does it matter which artery is missing? Amer. J. Obstet. Gynecol. **173**:728–732, 1995.

Akiyama, H., Kohzu, H. and Matsuoka, M.: An approach to detection and expulsion with new clinical sign: a study based on hemodynamic method and ultrasonography. Amer. J. Obstet. Gynecol. **140**:505–511, 1981.

Allen, J.R., Carrera, G.M. and Weed, J.C.: Neonatal death due to embolism. JAMA **207**:756–757, 1969.

Altemani, A.M.: Thrombosis of fetal placental vessels: a quantitative study in placentas of stillbirths. Pathol. Res. Pract. **182**:685–689, 1987.

Altemani, A.M. and Lopes de Faria, J.: Non-thrombotic changes of fetal placental vessels. A qualitative and quantitative study. Pathol. Res. Pract. **182**:676–683, 1987.

Altshuler, G.: Some placental considerations related to neurodevelopmental and other disorders. J. Child Neurol. **8**:78–94, 1993.

Altshuler, G. and Hyde, S.: Meconium induced vasoconstriction: a potential cause of cerebral and other fetal hypoperfusion and of poor pregnancy outcome. Child Neurol. **4**:137–142, 1989.

Altshuler, G., Tsang, R. and Ermocilla, R.: Single umbilical artery: correlation of clinical status and umbilical cord histology. Amer. J. Dis. Child. **129**:697–700, 1975.

Anagnostakis, D., Kazlaris, E., Xanthou, M. and Maounis, F.: Umbilical cord entanglement: A cause of neonatal pulmonary hemorrhage? Helv. Paediatr. Acta 29:167–171, 1974.

Andrade, A.: Anatomical and radiographic study on the anastomosis and branching of the umbilical arteries in white and non-white Brazilians. Acta Anat. (Basel) 70:66–75, 1968.

Anhalt, H., Marino, R.V. and Rosenfeld, W.: Retained umbilical stump: clinical approaches and separation anxiety. Amer. J. Dis. Childr. 146:1413–1414, 1992.

Ankola, P.A. and Pradham, G.: Radiology casebook. J. Perinatol. 3:196–197, 2000.

Antoine, C., Young, B.K., Silverman, F., Greco, M.A. and Alvarez, S.P.: Sinusoidal fetal heart rate pattern with vasa previa in twin pregnancy. J. Reprod. Med. 27:295–300, 1982.

Arts, N.F.T.: Investigations on the vascular system of the placenta. I. General introduction and the fetal vascular system. Amer. J. Obstet. Gynecol. 82:147–158, 1961.

Arvy, L. and Pilleri, G.: Le Cordon Ombilical. Funis Umbilicalis. Verlag Hirnanatomisches Institut, Ostermundigen (Bern), Switzerland, 1976a.

Arvy, L. and Pilleri, G.: The cetacean umbilical cord; studies of the umbilical cord of two Platanistoidea: Platanista gangetica and Pontoporia blainvillei. In, Volume VII: Investigations on Cetacea, G. Pilleri, ed. Brain Anatomy Institute, Berne, Switzerland, pp. 91–103, 1976b.

Asmussen, I.: Ultrastructure of human umbilical veins. Acta Obstet. Gynecol. Scand. 57:253–255, 1978.

Asmussen, I. and Kjeldsen, K.: Intimal ultrastructure of human umbilical arteries: observations on arteries from newborn children of smoking and nonsmoking mothers. Circ. Res. 36:579–589, 1975.

Atalla, R.K., Abrams, K., Bell, S.C. and Taylor, D.J.: Newborn acid-base status and umbilical cord morphology. Obstet. Gynecol. 92:865–868, 1998.

Bacsich, P. and Riddell, W.J.B.: Structure and nutrition of the cornea, cartilage and Wharton's jelly. Nature 155:271, 1945.

Bacsich, P. and Smout, C.F.V.: Some observations on the foetal vessels of the human placenta with an account of the corrosion technique. J. Anat. 72:358–364, 1938.

Baergen, R., Benirschke, K. and Ulich, T.R.: Cytokine expression in the placenta. The role of interleukin 1 and interleukin 1 receptor antagonist expression in chorioamnionitis and parturition. Arch. Pathol. Lab. Med. 118:52–55, 1994.

Baergen, R.N., Malicki, D., Behling, C. and Benirschke, K.: Morbidity, mortality, and placental pathology in excessively long umbilical cords: retrospective study. Pediatr. Developm. Pathol. 4:144–153, 2001.

Bahary, C.M., Gabbai, M. and Eckerling, B.: Rupture of the umbilical cord: report of a case. Obstet. Gynecol. 26:130–132, 1965.

Baill, I.C., Moore, G.W. and Hedrick, L.A.: Abscess of allantoic duct remnant. Amer. J. Obstet. Gynecol. 161:334–336, 1989.

Bakotic, B.W., Boyd, T., Poppiti, R. and Pflueger, S.: Recurrent umbilical cord torsion leading to fetal death in 3 subsequent

pregnancies. A case report and review of the literature. Arch. Pathol. Lab. Med. 124:1351–1355, 2000.

Balls, S., Gitstein, S. and Kharash, J.: Fetal heart rate variation with umbilical haematoma. Postgrad. Med. J. 61:753–755, 1985.

Barents, J.W.: Over tumoren van de navelstreng en de placenta. Nederl. Tijdschr. Verlosk. Gynaecol. 52:243–251, 1953.

Barron, S., Riley, E.P., Smotherman, W.P. and Kotch, L.E.: Umbilical cord length in rats is altered by prenatal alcohol exposure. Teratology 31:49A–50A, 1985.

Barry, F.E., McCoy, C.P. and Callahan, W. P.: Hemangioma of the umbilical cord. Amer. J. Obstet. Gynecol. 62:675–680, 1951.

Becker, V.: Funktionelle Morphologie der Placenta. Arch. Gynäkol. 198:1–28, 1962.

Becker, V.: Plazenta bei Totgeburt. In, Die Plazenta des Menschen. V. Becker, Th.H. Schiebler and F. Kubli, eds., Thieme, Stuttgart, pp. 305–308, 1981.

Becker, V. and Dolling, D.: Gefäßverschlüsse in der Placenta von Totgeborenen. Virchows Arch. [Pathol. Anat.] 338:305–314, 1965.

Becker, V. und Röckelein, G.: Pathologie der weiblichen Genitalorgane I. Pathologie der Plazenta und des Abortes. Springer-Verlag, Heidelberg, New York, 1989.

Beer, D.C.: Vasa previa: review of current concepts of management and report of a case. Obstet. Gynecol. 3:595–597, 1954.

Bell, A.D., Gerlis, L.M. and Variend, S.: Persistent right umbilical vein—case report and review of literature. Intern. J. Cardiol. 10:167–176, 1986.

Bender, H.G., Werner, C. and Karsten, C.: Zum Einfluß der Nabelschnurstruktur auf Schwangerschafts- und Geburtsverlauf. Arch. Gynäkol. 225:347–362, 1978.

Bendon, R.W., Tyson, R.W., Baldwin, V.J., Cashner, K.A., Momouni, F. and Miodovnik, M.: Umbilical cord ulceration and intestinal atresia: a new association? Amer. J. Obstet. Gynecol. 164:582–586, 1991.

Benirschke, K.: You need a sympathetic pathologist! The borderline of embryology and pathology revisited. Teratology 36:389–393, 1987.

Benirschke, K.: College of American Pathologists conference XIX on examination of the placenta: Summary. Arch. Path. Lab. Med. 115:720–721, 1991.

Benirschke, K.: Obstetrically important lesions of the umbilical cord. J. Reprod. Med. 39:262–272, 1994.

Benirschke, K. and Bourne, G.L.: The incidence and prognostic implication of congenital absence of one umbilical artery. Amer. J. Obstet. Gynecol. 79:251–254, 1960.

Benirschke, K. and Brown, W.H.: A vascular anomaly of the umbilical cord: the absence of one umbilical artery in the umbilical cords of normal and abnormal fetuses. Obstet. Gynecol. 6:399–404, 1953.

Benirschke, K. and Dodds, J.P.: Angiomyxoma of the umbilical cord with atrophy of an umbilical artery. Obstet. Gynecol. 30:99–102, 1967.

Benirschke, K. and Driscoll, S.G.: The Pathology of the Human Placenta. Springer-Verlag, New York, 1967.

Benirschke, K., Sullivan, M.M. and Marin-Padilla, M.: Size and number of umbilical vessels: a study of multiple pregnancy in man and the armadillo. Obstet. Gynecol. **24**:819–834, 1964.

Benoit, R., Copel, J. and Williams, K.: Does single umbilical artery (SUA) predict IUGR? Amer. J. Obstet. Gynecol. **187**:208 (abstract 546), 2002.

Bergman, P., Lundin, P. and Malmström, T.: Mucoid degeneration of Wharton's jelly: an umbilical cord anomaly threatening foetal life. Acta Obstet. Gynecol. Scand. **40**:372–378, 1961.

Bergström, H.: Intrauterin fosterdöd genom förblödning. Nord. Med. **4**:592–593, 1963.

Bhargava, I. and Raja, P.T.K.: Arteriovenous crossings on the chorial surface of the human placenta in abnormal pregnancy and development. Experientia **25**:831–832, 1969.

Bhargava, I., Chakravarty, A. and Raja, P.T.K.: Anatomy of foetal blood vessels on the chorial surface of the human placenta. IV. With absence of one umbilical artery. Acta Anat. (Basel) **80**:620–635, 1971.

Bilek, K., Roth, K. and Piskazeck, K.: Insertio-velamentosa-Blutung vor dem Blasensprung. Zentralbl. Gynäkol. **84**:1536–1541, 1962.

Blackburn, W. and Cooley, N.R.: The umbilical cord. In, Human Malformations and Related Anomalies, Volume II R.E. Stevenson, J.G. Hall and Goodman, R.M., eds. Oxford Monographs on Medical Genetics, Oxford University Press, New York and Oxford, pp. 1081–1141, 1993.

Blackburn, W., Cooley, N.R. and Manci, E.A.: Correlations between umbilical cord structure-composition and normal and abnormal fetal development. In, Proceedings of the Greenwood Genetics Conference Vol. 7. R.A. Saul, ed., pp. 180–181. Jacobs Press, Clinton, SC, 1988.

Blanc, W.A. and Allan, G.W.: Intrafunicular ulceration of persistent omphalomesenteric duct with intra-amniotic hemorrhage and fetal death. Amer. J. Obstet. Gynecol. **82**:1392–1396, 1961.

Bobitt, J.R.: Abnormal antepartum fetal heart rate tracings, failure to intervene, and fetal death: review of five cases reveals potential pitfalls of antepartum monitoring programs. Amer. J. Obstet. Gynecol. **133**:415–421, 1979.

Bodelsson, G., Sjöberg, N.-O. and Stjernquist, M.: Contractile effect of endothelin in the human uterine artery and autoradiographic localization of its binding sites. Amer. J. Obstetr. Gynecol. **167**:745–750, 1992.

Boué, D.R., Stanley, C. and Baergen, R.N.: Placental pathology casebook. J. Perinatol. **15**:429–431, 1995.

Bourne, G.L.: The Human Amnion and Chorion. Lloyd-Luke, London, 1962.

Boyd, J.D. and Hamilton, W.J.: The Human Placenta. W. Heffer & Sons, Cambridge, 1970.

Brady, A.G.: Knotted umbilical cord as a cause of death in a Cercopithecus aethiops fetus. Lab. Anim. Sci. **33**:375–376, 1983.

Brant, H.A. and Lewis, B.V.: Prolapse of the umbilical cord. Lancet **2**:1443–1445, 1966.

Brar, H.S., Medearis, A.L., DeVore, G.R. and Platt, L.D.: Maternal and fetal blood flow velocity waveforms in patients with preterm labor: effect of tocolytics. Obstet. Gynecol. **72**:209–214, 1988.

Bret, A.J. and Bardiaux, M.: Hématome du cordon. Rev. Fr. Gynécol. Obstét. **55**:240–249, 1956.

Broome, D.L., Kellogg, B., Weiss, B.A. and Wilson, M.G.: Needle puncture of the fetus during amniocentesis. Lancet **2**:604, 1975.

Broome, D.L., Wilson, M.G., Weiss, B. and Kellogg, B.: Needle puncture of the fetus: a complication of second-trimester amniocentesis. Amer. J. Obstet. Gynecol. **126**: 247–252, 1976.

Browne, F.J.: On the abnormalities of the umbilical cord which may cause antenatal death. J. Obstet. Gynaecol. Brit. Emp. **32**:17–48, 1925.C

Busacca, M., Dejana, E., Balconi, G., Olivieri, S., Pietra, A., Vergara-Dauden, M. and de Gaetano, G.: Reduced prostacyclin production by cultured endothelial cells from umbilical arteries of babies born to women who smoke. Lancet **2**:609–610, 1982.

Cai, W.Q., Bodin, P., Sexton, A., Loesch, A. and Burnstock, G.: Localization of neuropeptide Y and atrial natriuretic peptide in the endothelial cells of human umbilical blood vessels. Cell Tissue Res. **272**:175–181, 1993a.

Cai, W.Q., Terenghi, G., Bodin, P., Burnstock, G. and Polak, J.M.: In situ hybridization of atrial natriuretic peptide mRNA in the endothelial cells of human umbilical vessels. Histochemistry **100**:277–283, 1993b.

Calvano, C.J., Hoar, R.M., Mankes, R.F., Lefevre, R., Reddy, P.P., Moran, M.E. and Mandell, J.: Experimental study of umbilical cord length as a marker of fetal alcohol syndrome. Teratology **61**:184–188, 2000.

Camilleri, A.P.: Umbilical cord. Brit. Med. J. **2**:757, 1964.

Camman, W. and Marquardt, J.: Complex umbilical-cord knot. NEJM **349**:159, 2003.

Cardoso, L.E.M., Erlich, R.B., Rudge, M.C., Peracoli, J.C. and Mourao, P.A.S.: A comparative analysis of glycosaminoglycans from human umbilical arteries in normal subjects and in pathological conditions affecting pregnancy. Lab. Invest. **67**:588–595, 1992.

Carp, H.J.A., Mashiach, S. and Serr, D.M.: Vasa previa: a major complication and its management. Obstet. Gynecol. **53**:273–275, 1979.

Chantler, C., Baum, J.D. and Scopes, J.W.: Giant umbilical cord associated with a patent urachus and fused umbilical arteries. J. Obstet. Gynaecol. Brit. Commonw. **76**:273–274, 1969.

Chasnoff, I.J. and Fletcher, M.A.: True knot of the umbilical cord. Amer. J. Obstet. Gynecol. **127**:425–427, 1977.

Chaurasia, B.D. and Agarwal, B.M.: Helical structure of the umbilical cord. Acta Anat. (Basel) **103**:226–230, 1979.

Chénard, E., Bastide, A. and Fraser, W.D.: Umbilical cord hematoma following diagnostic funipuncture. Obstet. Gynecol. **76**:994–996, 1990.

Clapp, J.F., Peress, N.S., Wesley, M. and Mann, L.I.: Brain damage after intermittent partial cord occlusion in the chronically instrumented fetal lamb. Amer. J. Obstet. Gynecol. **159**:504–509, 1988.

Clapp, J.F., III, Stepanchak, W., Hashimoto, K., Ehrenberg, H. and Lopez, B.: The natural history of antenatal nuchal cords. Amer. J. Obstet. Gynecol. **189**:488–493, 2003.

Clare, N.M., Hayashi, R. and Khodr, G.: Intrauterine death from umbilical cord hematoma. Arch. Pathol. Lab. Med. **103**:46–47, 1979.

Clarke, J.A.: An x-ray microscopic study of the vasa vasorum of the human umbilical arteries. Z. Zellforsch. **66**:293–299, 1965.

Colgan, T.J. and Luk, S.C.: Umbilical-cord torsion, thrombosis, and intrauterine death of a twin. Arch. Pathol. Lab. Med. **106**:101, 1982.

Collins, J.C.: Umbilical cord accidents: human studies. Seminars Perinatol. **26**:79–82, 2002.

Collins, J.C., Muller, R.J. and Collins, C.L.: Prenatal observation of umbilical cord abnormalities: a triple knot and torsion of the umbilical cord. Amer. J. Obstetr. Gynecol. **169**:102–104, 1993.

Collins, J.H.: Two cases of multiple umbilical cord abnormalities resulting in stillbirth: prenatal observation with ultrasonography and fetal heart rates. Amer. J. Obstetr. Gynecol. **168**:125–128, 1993.

Collins, J.H.: Fetal grasping of the umbilical cord. Reply. Amer. J. Obstet. Gynecol. **172**:1071, 1995a.

Collins, J.H.: Prenatal observation of umbilical cord torsion with subsequent premature labor and delivery of a 31-week infant with mild nonimmune hydrops. Amer. J. Obstet. Gynecol. **172**:1048–1049, 1995b.

Collins, J.H.: Nuchal cord type A and type B. Amer. J. Obstet. Gynecol. **177**:94, 1997.

Collins, J.H., Geddes, D., Collins, C.L. and De Angelis, L.: Nuchal cord: a definition and a study associating placental location and nuchal cord incidence. J. Louisiana State Med. Soc. **143**:18–23, 1991.

Collins, J.H., Collins, C.L., Weckwerth, S.R. and De Angelis, L.: Nuchal cords: timing of prenatal diagnosis and duration. Amer. J. Obstet. Gynecol. **173**:768, 1995.

Cook, F.G., Taylor, R. and Gillan, J.E.: Placental venous thrombosis—a clinically significant finding in intrauterine death. Lab. Invest. **56**:1P, 1987.

Cook, V., Weeks, J., Brown, J. and Bendon, R.: Umbilical artery occlusion and fetoplacental thromboembolism. Obstet. Gynecol. **85**:870–872, 1995.

Cordero, D.R., Helfgott, A.W., Landy, H.J., Reik, R.F., Medina, C. and O'Sullivan, M.J.: A non-hemorrhagic manifestation of vasa previa: a clinicopathologic case report. Obstet. Gynecol. **82**:698–700, 1993.

Corkill, T.F.: The infant's vulnerable life-line. Aust. N.Z. J. Obstet. Gynaecol. **1**:154–160, 1961.

Corridan, M., Kendall, E.D. and Begg, J.D.: Cord entanglement causing premature separation and amniotic fluid embolism: case report. Brit. J. Obstet. Gynaecol. **87**:935–940, 1980.

Costakos, D.T., Williams, A.C., Love, L.A. and Wood, B.P.: Patent urachal duct. Amer. J. Dis. Childr. **146**:951–952, 1992.

Coulter, J.B.S., Scott, J.M. and Jordan, M.M.: Oedema of the umbilical cord and respiratory distress in the newborn. Brit. J. Obstet. Gynaecol. **82**:453–459, 1975.

Crawford, J.M.: A study of human placental growth with observations on the placenta in erythroblastosis foetalis. J. Obstet. Gynaecol. Brit. Emp. **66**:885–896, 1959.

Crawford, J.S.: Cord round the neck: incidence and sequelae. Acta Paediatr. (Stockh.) **51**:594–603, 1962.

Crawford, J.S.: Cord around the neck: Further analysis of incidence. Acta Paediatr. (Stockh.) **53**:553–557, 1964.

Crichton, J.L.: Tensile strength of the umbilical cord. Amer. J. Obstet. Gynecol. **115**:77–80, 1973.

Critchlow, C.W., Leet, T.L., Benedetti, T.J. and Daling, J.R.: Risk factors and infant outcomes associated with umbilical cord prolapse: a population-based case-control study among births in Washington State. Amer. J. Obstet. Gynecol. **170**:613–618, 1994.

Cullen, T.S.: Embryology, Anatomy, and Disease of the Umbilicus Together with Diseases of the Urachus. Saunders, Philadelphia, 1916.

Dadak, C., Kefalides, A., Sinzinger, H. and Weber, G.: Reduced umbilical artery prostacyclin formation in complicated pregnancies. Amer. J. Obstet. Gynecol. **144**:792–795, 1982.

Dado, G.M., Dobrin, P.B. and Mrkvicka, R.S.: Venous flow through coiled and noncoiled umbilical cords. Effects of external compression, twisting and longitudinal stretching. J. Reprod. Med. **42**:576–580, 1997.

Dargent, J.-L., Makke, M., Valaeys, V., Verdebout, J.-M., Thomas, D. and Barlow, P.: Corkscrew-like umbilical cord twist. Pediatr. Develop. Pathol. **5**:103–104, 2002.

Davignon, J., Lorenz, R.R. and Shepherd, J.T.: Response of human umbilical artery to changes in transmural pressure. Amer. J. Physiol. **209**:51–59, 1965.

Degani, S., Lewinsky, R.M., Berger, H. and Spiegel, D.: Sonographic estimation of umbilical coiling index and correlation with Doppler flow characteristics. Obstet. Gynecol. **86**:990–993, 1995.

Del Valle, G.O., Santerini, K., Sanchez-Ramos, L., Gaudier, F.L. and Delke, I.: The straight umbilical cord: Significance and perinatal implications. Amer. J. Obstet. Gynecol. **172**:286 (abstract 83), 1995.

De Sa, D.J.: Rupture of fetal vessels on placental surface. Arch. Dis. Child. **46**:495–501, 1971.

De Sa, D.J.: Intimal cushions in foetal placental veins. J. Pathol. **110**:347–352, 1973.

De Sa, D.J.: Diseases of the umbilical cord. In, Pathology of the Placenta. E.V.D.K. Perrin, ed. Churchill Livingstone, New York, 1984.

De Sa, M.F. and Meirelles, R.S.: Vasodilating effect of estrogen on the human umbilical artery. Gynecol. Invest. **8**:307–313, 1977.

DeVore, G.R., Mayden, K., Tortora, M., Berkowitz, R.L. and Hobbins, J.C.: Dilation of the umbilical vein in rhesus hemolytic anemia: a predictor of s severe disease. Amer. J. Obstet. Gynecol. **141**:464–466, 1981.

Didolkar, S.M., Hal, J., Phelan, J., Gutberlett, R. and Hill, J.L.: The prenatal diagnosis and management of a hepatoomphalocele. Amer. J. Obstet. Gynecol. **141**:221–222, 1981.

Dildy, G.A. and Clark, S.L.: Umbilical cord prolapse. Contemp. Ob/Gyn. **38**:23–31, 1993.

Dillon, W.P. and O'Leary, L.A.: Detection of fetal cord compromise secondary to umbilical cord hematoma with the nonstress test. Amer. J. Obstet. Gynecol. **141**:102–1103, 1981.

Dippel, A.L.: Hematomas of the umbilical cord. Surg. Gynecol. Obstet. **70**:51–57, 1940.

Dippel, A.L.: Maligned umbilical cord entanglements. Amer. J. Obstet. Gynecol. **88**:1012–1018, 1964.

Divon, M.Y.: Umbilical artery Doppler velocimetry: clinical utility in high-risk pregnancies. Amer. J. Obstet. Gynecol. **174**:10–14, 1996.

Di Terlizzi, G. and Rossi, G.F.: Studio clinico-statistico sulle anomalie del funiculo. Ann. Obstet. Ginecol.**77**:459–474, 1955. [see Fox, 1978.]

Dolff, M.: Die sogenannten Rekanalisationen der Stammzottengefäße bei Endarteritis obliterans der Plazentagefäße. Arch. Gynecol. **226**:325–332, 1978.

Dolkart, L.A., Reimers, F.T. and Kuonen, C.A.: Discordant umbilical arteries: ultrasonographic and Doppler analysis. Obstet. Gynecol. **79**:59–63, 1992.

Dombrowski, M.P., Budev, H., Wolfe, H.M., Sokol, R.J. and Perrin, E.: Fetal hemorrhage from umbilical cord hemangioma. Obstet. Gynecol. **70**:439–442, 1987.

Doshi, N. and Klionsky, B.: Pathology of disseminated intravascular coagulation in the newborn. Lab. Invest. **40**:303, 1979.

Dreyfus, M., Magny, J.F., Bridey F., Schwarz, H.P., Planché, C., Dehan, M. and Tchernia, G.: Treatment of homozygous protein C deficiency and neonatal purpura fulminans with a purified protein C concentrate. NEJM **325**:1565–1568, 1991.

Drut, R. and Drut, R.M.: Pathology of the umbilical cord in adrenal fusion syndrome. Pediatr. Pathol. Molec. Med. **22**:243–246, 2003.

Dudiak, C.M., Salomon, C.G., Posniak, H.V., Olson, M.C. and Flisak, M.E.: Sonography of the umbilical cord. RadioGraphics **15**:1035–1050, 1995.

Dunn, P.M., Fraser, I.D. and Raper, A.B.: Influence of early cord ligation on the transplacental passage of foetal cells. J. Obstet. Gynaecol. Brit. Commonw. **73**:757–760, 1966.

Dyer, D.C.: Comparison of the constricting actions produced by serotonin and prostaglandins on isolated sheep umbilical arteries and veins. Gynecol. Invest. **1**:204–209, 1970.

Earn, A.A.: The effect of congenital abnormalities of the umbilical cord and placenta on the newborn and mother: a survey of 5676 consecutive deliveries. J. Obstet. Gynaecol. Brit. Emp. **58**:456–459, 1951.

Eastman, N.J.: Editorial comments. Surg. Gynecol. Obstetr. **22**:16, 1967.

Eastman, N.J. and Hellman, L.M., eds.: Williams Obstetrics 12th ed. Appleton, New York, 1961.

Eddleman, K.A., Lockwood, C.J., Berkowitz, G.S., Lapinski, R.H. and Berkowitz, R.L.: Clinical significance and sonographic diagnosis of velamentous umbilical cord insertion. Amer. J. Perinatol. **9**:123–126, 1992.

Editorial: Closure of umbilical blood-vessels. Lancet **2**:381, 1966.

Edmonds, H.W.: The spiral twist of the normal umbilical cord in twins and in singletons. Amer. J. Obstet. Gynecol. **67**:102–120, 1954.

Eggens, J.H. and Bruins, H.W.: An unusual case of fetal distress. Amer. J. Obstet. Gynecol. **148**:219–220, 1984.

Ellison, J.P.: The nerves of the umbilical cord in man and the rat. Amer. J. Anat. **132**:53–60, 1971.

Ente, G., Penzer, P.H. and Kenigsberg, K.: Giant umbilical cord associated with patent urachus. Amer. J. Dis. Child. **120**:82–83, 1970.

Feinstein, S.J., Lodeiro, J.G., Vintzileos, A.M., Weinbaum, P.J., Campbell, W.A. and Nochimson, D.J.: Intrapartum ultrasound diagnosis of nuchal cord as a decisive factor in management. Amer. J. Obstet. Gynecol. **153**:308–309, 1985.

Feldberg, D., Ben-David, M., Dicker, D., Samuel, N. and Goldman, J.: Hematoma of the umbilical cord with acute antepartum fetal distress. A case report. J. Reprod. Med. **31**:65–66, 1986.

Ferrazzi, E., Brambati, B., Lanzani, A., Oldrini, A., Stripparo, L., Guerneri, A. and Makowski, E.L.: The yolk sac in early pregnancy failure. Amer. J. Obstet. Gynecol. **158**:137–142, 1988.

Fisk, N.M., Maclachlan, N., Ellis, C., Tannirandorn, Y., Tonge, H.M. and Rodeck, C.H.: Absent end-diastolic flow in first trimester umbilical artery. Lancet **2**:1256–1257, 1988.

Fletcher, S.: Chirality in the umbilical cord. Brit. J. Obstetr. Gynaecol. **100**:234–236, 1993.

Fok, R.Y., Pavlova, Z., Benirschke, K., Paul, R.H. and Platt, L.D.: The correlation of arterial lesions with umbilical artery Doppler velocimetry in placentas of small-for-dates pregnancies. Obstet. Gynecol. **75**:578–583, 1990.

Foldes, J.J.: Spontaneous intrauterine rupture of the umbilical cord: report of a case. Obstet. Gynecol. **9**:608–609, 1957.

Fortune, D.W. and Östör, A.G.: Umbilical artery aneurysm. Amer. J. Obstet. Gynecol. **131**:339–340, 1978.

Fortune, D.W. and Östör, A. G.: Angiomyxomas of the umbilical cord. Obstet. Gynecol. **55**:375–378, 1980.

Fox, H.: Thrombosis of foetal arteries in the human placenta. J. Obstet. Gynaecol. Brit. Commonw. **73**:961–965, 1966.

Fox, H.: Abnormalities of the foetal stem arteries in the human placenta. J. Obstet. Gynaecol. Brit. Commonw. **74**:734–738, 1967.

Fox, H.: Pathology of the Placenta. Saunders, London, 1978.

Fox, H.: Pathology of the Placenta. 2nd edition. Saunders, London, 1997.

Fox, H. and Jacobson, H.N.: Innervation of the human umbilical cord and umbilical vessels. Amer. J. Obstet. Gynecol. **103**:384–389, 1969.

Fox, H. and Khong, T.Y.: Lack of innervation of human umbilical cord. An immunohistochemical and histochemical study. Placenta **11**:59–62, 1990.

Fribourg, S.: Cord length and complications. Obstet. Gynecol. **58**:533, 1981.

Fries, M.H., Goldstein, R.B., Kilpatrick, S.J., Golbus, M.S., Callen, P.W. and Filly, R.A.: The role of velamentous cord insertion in the etiology of twin-twin transfusion syndrome. Obstet. Gynecol. **81**:569–574, 1993.

Froehlich, L.A. and Fujikura, T.: Significance of a single umbilical artery: report from the collaborative study of cerebral palsy. Amer. J. Obstet. Gynecol. **94**:274–279, 1966.

Fujikura, T.: Fused umbilical arteries near placental cord insertion. Amer. J. Obstet. Gynecol. **188**:765–767, 2003.

Fujikura, T. and Benson, R.C.: Placentitis and fibrous occlusion of fetal vessels in the placenta of stillborn infants. Amer. J. Obstet. Gynecol. **89**:225–229, 1964.

Fujikura, T. and Carleton, J. H.: Unilateral thickening of fetal arteries on the placenta resembling arteriosclerosis. Amer. J. Obstet. Gynecol. **100**:843–845, 1968.

Fujikura, T. and Hosoda, Y.: Unilateral thickening of placental fetal veins. Placenta **11**:241–245, 1990.

Fujinaga, M., Chinn, A. and Shepard, T.H.: Umbilical cord growth in human and rat fetuses: evidence against the "stretch hypothesis." Teratology. 41:333–339, 1990.

Gad, C.: A case of haemorrhage in labour from a placental vessel causing foetal death. Acta Obstet. Gynecol. Scand. 47:342–344, 1968.

Galle, P.C. and Meis, P.J.: Complications of amniocentesis: a review. J. Reprod. Med. 27:149–155, 1982.

Gardiner, J.P.: The umbilical cord: normal length; Length in cord complications; etiology and frequency of coiling. Surg. Gynecol. Obstet. 34:252–256, 1922.

Gardner, D.G., Hedges, B.K., Lapointe, M.C. and Deschapper, C.F.: Expression of the atrial natriuretic peptide gene in human fetal heart. J. Clin. Endocrinol. Metab. 69:729–737, 1989.

Gardner, R.F.R. and Trussell, R.R.: Ruptured hematoma of the umbilical cord. Obstet. Gynecol. 24:791–793, 1964.

Gassner, C.B. and Paul, R.H.: Laceration of umbilical cord vessels secondary to amniocentesis. Obstet. Gynecol. 48:627–630, 1976.

Gebrane-Younes, J., Minh, H.N. and Orcel, L.: Ultrastructure of human umbilical vessels: a possible role in amniotic fluid formation? Placenta 7:173–185, 1986.

Genest, D.R.: Estimating the time of death in stillborn fetuses: II. Histologic evaluation of the placenta; a study of 71 stillborns. Obstet. Gynecol. 80:585–592, 1992.

Gerlach, H.: Kongenitales Nabelarterienaneurysma. Z. Allg. Pathol. 111:420–423, 1968.

Ghezzi, F., Raio, L. Di Naro, E., Franchi, M., Balestreri, D. and D'Addario, V.: Nomogram of Wharton's jelly as depicted in the sonographic cross section of the umbilical cord. Ultrasound Obstet. Gynecol. 18:121–125, 2001a.

Ghezzi, F., Raio, L., Di Naro, E., Franchi, M., Bruhwiler, H., D'Addario, V. and Schneider, H.: First-trimester sonographic umbilical cord diameter and the growth of the human embryo. Ultrasound Obstet. Gynecol. 18:348–351, 2001b.

Ghezzi, F., Raio, L., Di Naro, E., Franchi, M., Buttarelli, M. and Schneider, H.: First-trimester umbilical diameter: a novel marker of fetal aneuploidy. Ultrasound Obstet. Gynecol. 19:235–239, 2002.

Ghezzi, F., Raio, L., Di Naro, E., Franchi, M., Cromi, A. and Durig, P.: Single and multiple umbilical cord cysts in early gestation: two different entities. Ultrasound Obstet. Gynecol. 21:215–219, 2003.

Ghosh, K.G., Ghosh, S.N. and Gupta, A.B.: Tensile properties of human umbilical cord. Indian J. Med. Res. 79:538–541, 1984.

Giacoia, G.P.: Body stalk anomaly: Congenital absence of the umbilical cord. Obstet. Gynecol. 80:527–529, 1992.

Giacomello, F.: Ultrasound determination of nuchal cord in breech presentation. Amer. J. Obstet. Gynecol. 159:531–532, 1988.

Gianopoulos, J., Carver, T., Tomich, P.G., Karlman, R. and Gadwood, K.: Diagnosis of vasa previa with ultrasonography. Obstet. Gynecol. 69:488–491, 1987.

Gilbert, E.: The short cord syndrome. Pediatr. Pathol. 5:96, 1986.

Gilbert-Barness, E., Drut, M.R., Grange, D.K. and Opitz, J.M.: Developmental abnormalities resulting in short umbilical cord. Birth Defects: Original Article Series 29(1):113–140, 1993.

Giles, R.C., Donahue, J.M., Hong, C.B., Tuttle, P.A., Petrites-Murphy, M.B., Poonacha, K.B., Roberts, M.S., Tramontin, R.R., Smith, B. and Swerczek, T.W.: Causes of abortion, stillbirth, and perinatal death in horses: 3,527 cases (1986–1991). J. Amer. Vet. Med. Assoc. 203:1170–1175, 1993.

Giles, W., O'Callaghan, S., Read, M., Gude, N., King, R. and Brennecke, S.: Placental nitric oxide synthase activity and abnormal umbilical artery flow velocity waveforms. Obstet. Gynecol. 89:49–52, 1997.

Gill, P. and Jarjoura, D.: Wharton's jelly in the umbilical cord: a study of its quantitative variations and clinical correlates. J. Reprod. Med. 38:611–614, 1993.

Glanfield, P.A. and Watson, R.: Intrauterine death due to umbilical cord torsion. Arch. Pathol. Lab. Med. 110:357–358, 1986.

Goerttler, K.: Die Bedeutung der funktionellen Struktur der Gefäßwand. I. Untersuchungen an der Nabelschnurarterie des Menschen. Gegenbaurs Morphol. Jahrb. 91:368–393, 1951.

Golden, A.S.: Umbilical cord-Placental separation: a complication of IUD failure. J. Reprod. Med. 11:79–80, 1973.

Gonzalez-Crussi, F. and Roth, L.M.: The human yolk sac and yolk sac carcinoma. Hum. Pathol. 7:675–691, 1976.

Goodlin, R.C.: Fetal dysmaturity, "lean cord", and fetal distress. Amer. J. Obstet. Gynecol. 156:1357, 1987.

Goodlin, R.C. and Clewell, W.H.: Sudden fetal death following amniocentesis. Amer. J. Obstet. Gynecol. 118:285–288, 1974.

Grange, D.K., Arya, S., Opitz, J.M., Laxova, R., Herrmann, J. and Gilbert, E.F.: The short umbilical cord. Birth Defects 23:191–214, 1987.

Grant, A., Elbourne, D., Valentin, L. and Alexander, S.: Routine formal fetal movement counting and risk of antepartum late death in normally formed singletons. Lancet. ii:345–349, 1989.

Graumann, W.: Polysaccharide. Ergebnisse der Polysaccharidhistochemie: Mensch und Säugetier. In, Handbuch der Histochemie, Vol. II/2. W. Graumann and K. Neumann, eds. Fischer, Stuttgart, 1964.

Grieco, A.: Rilievi clinico-statistici sulla inserzione velamentosa ed a racchetta del cordone ombellicale. Monit. Ostet.-Ginecol. Endocrin. Metabol. 8:89–102, 1936.

Grosser, O.: Frühentwicklung, Eihautbildung und Placentation des Menschen und der Säugetiere. J.F. Bergmann, München, 1927.

Gruber, F.H.: Gas in the umbilical vessels as a sign of fetal death. Radiology 89:881–882, 1967.

Gruenwald, P.: The amount of fetal blood remaining in the placenta at birth. Proc. Soc. Exp. Biol. Med. 130:326–329, 1969.

Gu, J., Pinheiro, J.M.B., Yu, C.Z., D'Andrea, M., Muralidharan, S. and Malik, A.: Detection of endothelin-like immunoreactivity in epithelium and fibroblasts of the human umbilical cord. Tissue and Cell 23:437–444, 1991.

Guidetti, A.A., Divon, M.Y., Cavaleri, R.L., Langer, O. and Merkatz, I.R.: Fetal umbilical artery flow velocimetry in postdate pregnancies. Amer. J. Obstet. Gynecol. **157**:1521–1523, 1987.

Habek, D., Habek, J.C., Barbir, A., Barbir, M. and Granic, P.: Fetal grasping of the umbilical cord and perinatal outcome. Arch. Gynecol. Obstet. **268**:274–277, 2003.

Hall, S.P.: The thin cord syndrome. A review with a report of two cases. Obstet. Gynecol. **18**:507–509, 1961.

Harding, J.A., Lewis, D.F., Major, C.A., Crade, M., Patel, J. and Nageotte, M.P.: Color glow Doppler—a useful instrument in the diagnosis of vasa previa. Amer. J. Obstet. Gynecol. **163**:1566–1568, 1990.

Hartman, K.R., Rawlings, J.S. and Feingold, M.: Protein C deficiency. Amer. J. Dis. Child. **144**:1353–1354, 1990.

Harold, J.G., Siegel, R.J., Fitzgerald, G.A., Satoh, P. and Fishbein, M.C.: Differential prostaglandin production by human umbilical vasculature. Arch. Pathol. Lab. Med. **112**:43–46, 1988.

Harris, L.E. and Wenzl, J.E.: Heterotopic pancreatic tissue and intestinal mucosa in the umbilical cord. NEJM **268**:721–722, 1963.

Hathout, H.: The vascular pattern and mode of insertion of the umbilical cord in abortion material. J. Obstet. Gynaecol. Brit. Commonw. **71**:963–964, 1964.

Heckmann, U., Cornelius, H.V. and Freudenberg, V.: Das Teratom der Nabelschnur. Ein kasuistischer Beitrag zu den echten Tumoren der Nabelschnur. Geburtsh. Frauenheilk. **32**:605–607, 1972.

Heifetz, S.A.: Single umbilical artery: a statistical analysis of 237 autopsy cases and review of the literature. Perspect. Pediatr. Pathol. **8**:345–378, 1984.

Heifetz, S.A.: Thrombosis of the umbilical cord: analysis of 52 cases and literature review. Pediatr. Pathol. **8**:37–54, 1988.

Heifetz, S.A.: The umbilical cord: obstetrically important lesions. Clin. Obstet. Gynecol. **39**:571–587, 1996.

Heifetz, S.A. and Rueda-Pedraza, M.E.: Omphalomesenteric duct cysts of the umbilical cord. Pediatr. Pathol. **1**:325–335, 1983a.

Heifetz, S.A. and Rueda-Pedraza, M.E.: Hemangiomas of the umbilical cord. Pediatr. Pathol. **1**:385–398, 1983b.

Heinonen, S., Ryynänen, M., Kirkinen, P. and Saarikoski, S.: Perinatal diagnostic evaluation of velamentous umbilical cord insertion: clinical, Doppler, and ultrasonic findings. Obstet. Gynecol. **87**:112–117, 1996.

Hempel, E.: Die ultrastrukturelle Differenzierung des menschlichen Amnionepithels unter besonderer Berücksichtigung des Nabelstrangs. Anat. Anz. **132**:356–370, 1972.

Hemsen, A., Gillis, C., Larsson, O., Haegerstrand, A. and Lundberg J.M.: Characterization, localization and actions of endothelins in umbilical vessels and placenta. Acta Physiol. Scand. **143**:395–404, 1991.

Herberz, O.: Über die Insertio furcata funiculi umbilicalis. Acta Obstet. Gynecol. Scand. **18**:336–351, 1938.

Herman, A., Zabow, P., Segal, M., Ron-el, R., Bukovsky, Y. and Caspi, E.: Extremely large number of twists of the umbilical cord causing torsion and intrauterine fetal death. Intern. J. Gynaecol. Obstet. **35**:165–167, 1991.

Herrmann, U.J. and Sidiropoulos, D.: Single umbilical artery: prenatal findings. Prenat. Diagn. **8**:275–280, 1988.

Hersh, J. and Buchino, J.J.: Umbilical cord torsion/constriction sequence. In, Proceedings of the Greenwood Genetics Conference Vol. **7**. R.A. Saul, ed., pp. 181–182, Jacobs Press, Clinton, SC, 1988.

Hershkovitz, R., Silberstein, T., Sheiner, E., Shoham-Vardi, I., Holcberg, G., Katz, M. and Mazor, M.: Risk factors associated with true knots of the umbilical cord. Europ. J. Obstet. Gynecol. Reprod. Biol. **98**:36–39, 2001.

Hertig, A.T.: The placenta: Some new knowledge about an old organ. Obstet. Gynecol. **20**:859–866, 1962.

Hertig, A.T.: Human Trophoblast. Charles C Thomas, Springfield, IL, 1968.

Hey, A. und Röckelein, G.: Die sogenannten Endothelvakuolen der Plazentagefäße—Physiologie oder Krankheit. Pathologe **10**:66–67, 1989.

Hill, L.M., DiNofrio, D.M. and Guzick, D.: Sonographic determination of first trimester umbilical cord length. J. Clin. Ultrasound **22**:435–438, 1994a.

Hill, L.M., Mills, A., Peterson, C. and Boyles, D.: Persistent right umbilical vein: sonographic detection and subsequent neonatal outome. Obstet. Gynecol. **84**:923–925, 1994b.

Hinson, R.M., Biswas, A., Mizelle, K.M. and Tunnessen, W.W.: Persistent omphalomesenteric duct. Arch. Pediatr. Adolesc. Med. **151**:1161–1162, 1997.

Hitschold, T.P.: Doppler flow velocity waveforms of the umbilical arteries correlate with intravillous blood volume. Amer. J. Obstet. Gynecol. **179**:540–543, 1998.

Hitschold, T., Weiss, E., Beck, T., Hüntefering, H. and Berle, P.: Low target birth weight or growth retardation? Umbilical Doppler flow velocity waveforms and histometric analysis of fetoplacental vascular tree. Amer. J. Obstetr. Gynecol. **168**:1260–1264, 1993.

Hoag, R.W.: Fetomaternal hemorrhage associated with umbilical vein thrombosis. Amer. J. Obstet. Gynecol. **154**:1271–1274, 1986.

Hobel, C.J., Emmanouilides, G.C., Townsend, D.E. and Yashiro, K.: Ligation of one umbilical artery in the fetal lamb: experimental production of fetal malnutrition. Obstet. Gynecol. **36**:582–588, 1970.

Hoboken, W.: Anatomia secundinae. Ribbium, Ultrajecti, 1669.

Hof, J. ten, Nijhuis, I.J.M., Nijhuis, J.G., Narayan, H., Taylor, D.J., Visser, G.H.A. and Mulder, E.J.H.: Quantitative analysis of fetal general movements: methodological considerations. Early Human Devel. **56**:57–73, 1999.

Hong, C.B., Donahue, J.M., Giles, R.C., Petrites-Murphy, M.B., Poonacha, K.B., Roberts, A.W., Smith, B.J., Tramontin, R.R., Tuttle, P.A. and Swerczek, T.W.: Equine abortion and stillbirth in central Kentucky during 1988 and 1989 foaling seasons. J. Vet. Diagn. Invest. **5**:560–566, 1993.

Horwitz, S.T., Finn, W.F. and Mastrota, V.F.: A study of umbilical cord encirclement. Amer. J. Obstet. Gynecol. **89**:970–974, 1964.

Howorka, E. and Kapczynski, W.: Unusual thickness of the fetal end of the umbilical cord. J. Obstet. Gynaecol. Brit. Commonw. **78**:283, 1971.

Hoyes, A.D.: Ultrastructure of the epithelium of the human umbilical cord. J. Anat. **105**:149–162, 1969.

Hoyme, H.E., Jones, K.L., Allen, M.I.V., Saunders, B.S. and Benirschke, K.: Vascular pathogenesis of transverse limb reduction defects. J. Pediatr. **101**:839–843, 1982.

Hyrtl, J.: Die Blutgefäße der menschlichen Nachgeburt in normalen und abnormen Verhältnissen. Braumüller, Wien, 1870.

Ikeda, T., Murata, Y., Quilligan, E.J., Choi, B.H., Parer, J.T., Dol, S. and Park, S.D.: Physiologic and histologic changes in near-term fetal lambs exposed to asphyxia by partial umbilical cord occlusion. Amer. J. Obstet. Gynecol. **178**:24–32, 1998.

Inglis, C.G., Kingdom, J.C.P. and Nelson D.M.: Atrial natriuretic hormone: a paracrine or endocrine role within the human placenta? JCEM **76**:1014–1018, 1993.

Irani, P.K.: Haematoma of the umbilical cord. Brit. Med. J. **ii**:1436–1437, 1964.

Ivemark, B.I., Lagergren, C. and Ljungqvist, A.: Generalized arterial calcification associated with hydramnios in two stillborn infants. Acta Paediatr. [Suppl.] (Stockh.) **135**:103–110, 1962.

James, J.D. and Nickerson, C.W.: Laceration of umbilical artery and abruptio placentae secondary to amniocentesis. Obstet. Gynecol. **48s**:44s–45s, 1976.

Janosco, E.O., Lona, J.Z. and Belin, R.P.: Congenital anomalies of the umbilicus. Amer. Surg. **43**:177–185, 1977.

Jauniaux, E., Donner, C., Simon, P., Vanesse, M., Hustin, J. and Rodesch, F.: Pathological aspects of the umbilical cord after percutaneous umbilical blood sampling. Obstet. Gynecol. **73**:215–218, 1989a.

Jauniaux, E., De Munter, C., Vanesse, M., Wilkin, P. and Hustin, J.: Embryonic remnants of the umbilical cord: morphologic and clinical aspects. Hum. Pathol. **20**:458–462, 1989b.

Javert, C.T. and Barton, B.: Congenital and acquired lesions of the umbilical cord and spontaneous abortion. Amer. J. Obstet. Gynecol. **63**:1065–1077, 1952.

Jimenez, E., Unger, M., Vogel, M., Lobeck, H., Wagner, G., Schwiermann, J., Schäfer, A. und Grosch-Wörner, I.: Morphologische Untersuchungen an Plazenten HIV-positiver Mütter. Pathologe **9**:228–234, 1988.

Jogee, M., Myatt, L. and Elder, M.G.: Decreased prostacyclin production by placental cells in culture from pregnancies complicated by fetal growth retardation. Brit. J. Obstet. Gynaecol. **90**:247–250, 1983.

Jones, C.J.P., Jauniaux, E. and Campbell, S.: Development and degeneration of the secondary human yolk sac. Placenta **14**:A32, 1993.

Jones, K.P., Wheater, A.W. and Musgrave, W.: Simple test for bleeding from vasa previa. Lancet **2**:1430–1431, 1987.

Jones, T.B., Sorokin, Y., Bhatia, R., Zador, I.E. and Bottoms, S.F.: Single umbilical artery: Accurate diagnosis? Amer. J. Obstet. Gynecol. **169**:538–540, 1993.

Kalish, R.B., Hunter, T., Sharma, G. and Baergen, R.N.: Clinical significance of the umbilical cord twist. Amer. J. Obstet. Gynecol. **189**:736–739, 2003.

Kan, P.S. and Eastman, N.J.: Coiling of the umbilical cord around the foetal neck. J. Obstet. Gynaecol. Brit. Emp. **64**:227–228, 1957.

Kaneko, M., White, S., Homan, J. and Richardson, B.: Cerebral blood flow and metabolism in relation to electrocortical activity with severe umbilical cord occlusion in the near-term ovine fetus. Amer. J. Obstet. Gynecol. **188**:961–972, 2003.

Kaplan, C., August, D. and Mizrachi, H.: Single umbilical artery and cord accidents. Modern Pathol. **3**(1):4P (Abstract No. 17), 1990.

Karbowski, B., Bauch, H.J. and Schneider, H.P.G.: Functional differentiation of umbilical vein endothelial cells following pregnancy complicated by smoking or diabetes mellitus. Placenta **12**:405, 1991.

Katz, V., Blanchard, G., Dingman, C., Bowes, W.A. and Cefalo, R.C.: Atenolol and short umbilical cords. Amer. J. Obstet. Gynecol. **156**:1271–1272, 1987.

Katz, Z., Shosham, Z., Lancet, M., Blickstein, I., Mogilner, B.M. and Zalel, Y.: Management of labor with umbilical cord prolapse: a 5-year study. Obstet. Gynecol. **72**:278–280, 1988.

Kelber, R.: Gespaltene "solitäre" Nabelschnurarterie. Arch. Gynäkol. **220**:319–323, 1976.

Kernbach, M.: Das neuroektoblastische System der Plazenta des Menschen. Anat. Anz. **113**:259–269, 1963.

Kernbach, M.: Existe-t-il du tissu nerveux dans le placenta? Rev. Fr. Gynécol. **64**:357–361, 1969.

Kessler, A.: Blutungen aus den Nabelschnurgefässen in der Schwangerschaft. Gynaecologia **150**:353–365, 1960.

Khong, T.Y. and Dilly, S.A.: Calcification of umbilical artery: two distinct lesions. J. Clin. Pathol. **42**:931–934, 1989.

Khoury, A.D., Moretti, M.L., Barton, J.R., Shaver, D.C. and Sibai, B.M.: Fetal blood sampling in patients undergoing elective cesarean section: a correlation with cord blood gas values obtained at delivery. Amer. J. Obstet. Gynecol. **165**:1026–1029, 1991.

Khurana, A., Huettner, P.C. and Cole, F.S.: Umbilical cord ulceration as a cause of hypoxic-ischemic encephalopathy: report of a case and review of the literature. J. Perinatol. **15**:423–425, 1995.

King, D.L.: Placental migration demonstrated by ultrasonography: a hypothesis of dynamic placentation. Radiology **109**:167–170, 1973.

King, E.L.: Intrauterine death of the fetus due to abnormalities of the umbilical cord: report of three cases. Amer. J. Obstet. Gynecol. **12**:812–816, 1926.

King, S.: Patent omphalomesenteric duct. Arch. Surg. **96**:545–548, 1968.

Kishore, N. and Sarkar, S.C.: The arterial patterns of placenta. A postpartum radiological study. J. Obstet. Gynaecol. India **17**:9–13, 1967.

Kjeldsen, J. and Pedersen, J.: Relation of residual placental blood-volume to onset of respiration and the respiratory-distress syndrome in infants of diabetic and non-diabetic mothers. Lancet **1**:180–184, 1967.

Klebe, J.G. and Ingomar, C.J.: Placental transfusion in infants of diabetic mothers elucidated by placental residual blood volume. Acta Paediatr. (Stockh.) **63**:59–64, 1974a.

Klebe, J.G. and Ingomar, C.J.: The influence of the method of delivery and the clamping technique on the red cell volume in infants of diabetic and non-diabetic mothers. Acta Paediatr. (Stockh.) **63**:65–69, 1974b.

Korst, L.M., Phelan, J.P., Ahn, M.O. and Martin, G.I.: Nucleated red blood cells: An update on the marker for fetal asphyxia. Amer. J. Obstet. Gynecol. **175**:843–846, 1996.

Kouyoumdjian, A.: Velamentous insertion of the umbilical cord. Obstet. Gynecol. **56**:737–742, 1980.

Kraus, F.T.: Placenta: thrombosis of fetal stem vessels with fetal thrombotic vasculopathy and chronic villitis. Pediatr. Pathol. **16**:143–148, 1996.

Kraus, F.T.: Cerebral palsy and thrombi in placental vessels of the fetus: insights from litigation. Human Pathol. **28**:246–248, 1997.

Kreczy, A., Alge, A., Menardi, G., Gassner, I., Gschwendtner, A. and Mikuz, G.: Teratoma of the umbilical cord. Case report with review of the literature. Arch. Pathol. Lab. Med. **118**:934–937, 1994.

Kreibich, Dr.: Über eine grosse Urachuscyste bei einer 80 jährigen Frau. Zentralbl. Gynäkol. **69**:523–528, 1947.

Kreyberg, L.: A teratoma-like swelling in the umbilical cord possibly of acardiac nature. J. Pathol. Bacteriol. **75**:109–112, 1958.

Kristiansen, F.V. and Nielsen, V.T.: Intra-uterine fetal death and thrombosis of the umbilical vessels. Acta Obstet. Gynecol. Scand. **64**:331–334, 1985.

Krone, H.-A.: Die Bedeutung der Nidationsstörungen für die Pathologie der Embryonalentwicklung. Bibl. Microbiol. Fasc. **1**:111–116, 1960 (Wiener Colloqium: Pränatale Infektionen, 1959).

Krone, H.-A.: Die Bedeutung der Plazenta für die Entstehung von Mißbildungen. Wien. Med. Wochenschr. **117**:393–397, 1967.

Krone, H.A., Jopp, H. and Schellerer, W.: Die Bedeutung anamnestischer Befunde für die verschiedenen Formen des Nabelschnuransatzes. Z. Geburtsh. Gynäkol. **163**:205–213, 1965.

Laatikainen, T.J., Lehtonen, P.J. and Hesso, A.E.: Fetal sulfated and nonsulfated bile acids in intrahepatic cholestasis of pregnancy. J. Lab. Clin. Med. **92**:185–193, 1978.

Labarrere, C., Sebastiani, M., Siminovich, M., Torassa, E. and Althabe, O.: Absence of Wharton's jelly around the umbilical arteries: an unusual cause of perinatal mortality. Placenta **6**:555–559, 1985.

Lachenmayer, L.: Adrenergic innervation of the umbilical vessels: light- and fluorescence microscopic studies. Z. Zellforsch. **120**:120–136, 1971.

Lacro, R.V., Jones, K.L. and Benirschke, K.: The umbilical cord twist: origin, direction, and relevance. Amer. J. Obstet. Gynecol. **157**:833–838, 1987.

Lang, I., Hartmann, M., Blaschitz, A., Dohr, G., Skofitsch, G. and Desoye, G.: Immunohistochemical evidence for the heterogeneity of maternal and fetal vascular endothelial cells in human full-term placenta. Cell Tissue Res. **274**:211–218, 1993.

Lange, I.R., Manning, F.A., Morrison, I., Chamberlain, P.F. and Harman, C.R.: Cord prolapse: is antenatal diagnosis possible. Amer. J. Obstet. Gynecol. **151**:1083–1085, 1985.

Las Heras, J. and Haust, D.: Ultrastructure of fetal stem arteries of human placenta in normal pregnancy. Virchows Arch. **393**:133–144, 1981.

Lauweryns, J.M., deBruyn, M., Peuskens, J. and Bourgeois, N.: Absence of intrinsic innervation of the human placenta. Experientia **25**:432, 1969.

Learmont, J.G. and Poston, L.: Nitric oxide is involved in flow-induced dilation of isolated human small fetoplacental arteries. Amer. J. Obstet. Gynecol. **174**:583–588, 1996.

LeDonne, A.T. and McGowan, L.: Effect of an oxytocic on umbilical cord venous pressure. Obstet. Gynecol. **30**:103–107, 1967.

Lee, G.K., Chi, J.G. and Cha, K.S.: An unusual venous anomaly of the placenta. Amer. J. Clin. Pathol. **95**:48–51, 1991.

Lee, M.C.L. and Aterman, K.: An intestinal polyp of the umbilical cord. Amer. J. Dis. Child. **116**:320–323, 1968.

Lee, S.T. and Hon, E.H.: Fetal hemodynamic response to umbilical cord compression. Obstet. Gynecol. **22**:553–562, 1963.

Leff, M.: Hemorrhage from a ruptured varicosity in the placenta causing the death of the fetus. Amer. J. Obstet. Gynecol. **22**:117–118, 1931.

Lehman, R.E.: Umbilical cord prolapse following external cephalic version with tocolysis. Amer. J. Obstet. Gynecol. **146**:963–964, 1983.

Leinzinger, E.: Varixthrombose der Nabelschnur. Z. Geburtsh. Gynäkol. **171**:82–87, 1969.

Leinzinger, E.: Totaler Nabelschnurabriss intra partum bei Hydramnion. Zentralbl. Gynäkol. **94**:1233–1238, 1972.

Lemtis, H.: Über eine seltene Nabelschnurmißbildung. Geburtsh. Frauenh. **26**:986–993, 1966.

Lemtis, H.: Über Aneurysmen im fetalen Gefäßapparat der menschlichen Plazenta. Arch. Gynäkol. **206**:330–347, 1968.

Lenke, R.R., Ashwood, E.R., Cyr, D.R., Gravett, M., Smith, J.R. and Stenchever, M.A.: Genetic amniocentesis: significance of intraamniotic bleeding and placental location. Obstet. Gynecol. **65**:798–801, 1985.

Leu, A.J. and Leu, H.J.: Spezielle Probleme bei der histologischen Altersbestimmung von Thromben und Emboli. Pathologe **10**:87–92, 1989.

Leung, A.K.C. and Robson, W.L.M.: Single umbilical artery: a report of 159 cases Amer. J. Dis. Child. **143**:108–111, 1989.

Levy, H., Meier, P.R. and Makowski, E.L.: Umbilical cord prolapse. Obstet. Gynecol. **64**:499–502, 1984.

Lewinsky, R.M., Degani, S., Berger, H. and Spiegel, D.: Umbilical venous flow may be dependent on umbilical coiling. Amer. J. Obstet. Gynecol. **174**:456 (abstract 539), 1996.

Lin, A.E., Genest, D.R. and Brown, D.L.: Circumferential abdominal skin defect possibly due to umbilical cord encirclement. Teratology **60**:258–259, 1999.

Loquet, P., Broughton-Pipkin, F., Symonds, E.M. and Rubin, P.C.: Blood velocity waveforms and placental vascular formation. Lancet **2**:1252–1253, 1988.

Ludwig, K.: Ein weiterer Beitrag zum Bau der Gorilla-Placenta. Acta Anat. (Basel) **46**:304–310, 1961.

Macara, L.M., Kingdom, J.C.P. and Kaufmann, P.: Control of the fetoplacental circulation. Fetal Maternal Med. Rev. **5**:167–179, 1993.

Maclean, M.R., Templeton, A.G.B. and McGrath, J.C.: The influence of endothelin-1 on human foeto-placental blood vessels: a comparison with 5-hydroxytryptamine. Brit. J. Pharmacol. **106**:937–941, 1992.

Mäkilä, U.M., Jouppila, P., Kirkinen, P., Viinikka, L. and Ylikorkala, O.: Relation between umbilical prostacyclin production and blood-flow in the fetus. Lancet **1**:728–729, 1983.

Malicki, D., Behling, C.A., Benirschke, K. and Baergen, R.N.: The excessively long umbilical cord: a clinicopathologic study of 924 cases. Modern Pathol. **10**:156A (abstract 923), 1997.

Maher, J.T. and Conti, J.A.: A comparison of umbilical cord blood gas values between newborns with and without true knots. Obstet. Gynecol. **88**:863–866, 1996.

Mallard, E.C., Gunn, A.J., Williams, C.E., Johnston, B.M. and Gluckman, P.D.: Transient umbilical cord occlusion causes hippocampal damage in fetal sheep. Amer. J. Obstet. Gynecol. **167**:1423–1430, 1992.

Malpas, P.: Length of the umbilical cord at term. Brit. Med. J. **1**:673–674, 1964.

Malpas, P. and Symonds, E.M.: Observations on the structure of the human umbilical cord. Surg. Obstet. Gynecol. **123**:746–750, 1966.

Manci, E.A., Ulmer, D.R., Nye, D.M., Shah, A. and Mvumbi, L.: Variations in normal umbilical cord length following birth. Modern Pathol. **6**:p6p, abstract 33, Pediatric Pathol., 1993.

Marchetti, A.A.: A consideration of certain types of benign tumors of the placenta. Surg. Gynecol. Obstet. **68**:733–743, 1939.

Marcianiak, E., Wilson, H.D. and Marlar, R.A.: Neonatal purpura fulminans: a genetic disorder related to the absence of protein C in blood. Blood **65**:15–20, 1985.

Marco-Johnson, M.J., Marlar, R.A., Jacobson, L.J., Hays, T. and Warady, B.A.: Severe protein C deficiency in newborn infants. J. Pediatr. **113**:359–363, 1988.

Masliah, E. and Wahl, C.: Umbilical cord stricture in a 21-week fetus. J. Perinatol. **24**:48–49, 2004.

Matheus, M. and Sala, M.A.: The importance of placental examination in newborns with single umbilical artery. Z. Geburtsh. Perinatol. **184**:231–232, 1980.

McCoshen, J.A., Tulloch, H.V. and Johnson, K.A.: Umbilical cord is the major source of prostaglandin E_2 in the gestational sac during term labor. Amer. J. Obstet. Gynecol. **160**:973–978, 1989.

McCowan, L.M., Mullen, B.M. and Ritchie, K.: Umbilical artery flow velocity waveforms and the placental vascular bed. Amer. J. Obstet. Gynecol. **157**:900–902, 1987.

McCurdy, C., Anderson, C., Borjon, N., Brzechffa, P., Miller, H., McNamara, M., Newman, A. and Seeds, J.: Antenatal sonographic diagnosis of nuchal cord. Amer. J. Obstet. Gynecol. **170**:(abstract 329), 366, 1994.

McDermott, M. and Gillan, J.E.: Trophoblast basement membrane haemosiderosis in the placental lesion of fetal artery thrombosis: A marker for disturbance of maternofetal transfer? Placenta **16**:171–178, 1995a.

McDermott, M. and Gillan, J.E.: Chronic reduction in fetal blood flow is associated with placental infarction. Placenta **16**:165–170, 1995b.

McKay, D.G., Roby, C.C., Hertig, A.T. and Richardson, M.V.: Studies of the function of early human trophoblast. II. Preliminary observations on certain chemical constituents of chorionic and early amniotic fluid. Amer. J. Obstet. Gynecol. **69**:735–741, 1955.

McLennan, J.E.: Implications of the eccentricity of the human umbilical cord. Amer. J. Obstet. Gynecol. **101**:1124–1130, 1968.

McLennan, H., Price, E., Urbanska, M., Craig, N. and Fraser, M.: Umbilical cord knots and encirclements. Aust. N.Z. J. Obstet. Gynaecol. **28**:116–119, 1988.

Merttens, J.: Beiträge zur normalen und pathologischen Anatomie der menschlichen Placenta. Z. Geburtsh. Gynäkol. **30**:1–97, 1894.

Messer, R.H., Gomez, A.R. and Yambao, T.J.: Antepartum testing for vasa previa: current standard of care. Amer. J. Obstet. Gynecol. **156**:1459–1462, 1987.

Meyenburg, M.: Gibt es Veränderungen des Plazentasitzes im Bereich kaudaler Uterusabschnitte während der Schwangerschaft? Eine echographische Verlaufsstudie. Geburtsh. Frauenheilk. **36**:715–721, 1976.

Meyer, A.W.: On the structure of the human umbilical vesicle. Amer. J. Anat. **3**:155–166, 1904.

Meyer, W.J., Blumenthal, L., Cadkin, A., Gauthier, D.W. and Rotmensch, S.: Vasa previa: Prenatal diagnosis with transvaginal color Doppler flow imaging. Amer. J. Obstet. Gynecol. **169**:1627–1629, 1993.

Meyer, W.W., Rumpelt, H.J., Yao, A.C. and Lind, J.: Structure and closure mechanisms of the human umbilical artery. Eur. J. Pediatr. **128**:247–259, 1978.

Mildenberger, E., Biesel, B., Siegel, G. and Versmold, H.T.: Nitric oxide and endothelin in oxygen-dependent regulation of vascular tone of human umbilical vein. Amer. J. Physiol. Heart Circ. Physiol. **285**:H1730–H1737, 2003.

Miller, M.E., Higginbottom, M. and Smith, D.A.: Short umbilical cord: its origin and relevance. Pediatrics **67**:618–621, 1981.

Mills, J.L., Harley, E.E. and Moessinger, A.C.: Standards for measuring umbilical cord length. Placenta **4**:423–426, 1983.

Mishriki, Y.Y., Vanyshelbaum, Y., Epstein, H. and Blanc, W.: Hemangioma of the umbilical cord. Pediatr. Pathol. **7**:43–49, 1987.

Mitchell, A.P.B., Anderson, G.S. and Russell, J.K.: Perinatal death from foetal exsanguination. Brit. Med. J. **1**:611–614, 1957.

Mitchell, K.E., Weiss, M.L., Mitchell, B.M., Martin, P., Davis, D., Morales, L., Helwig, B., Beerenstrauch, M., Abou-Easa, K., Hildreth, T., Troyer, D. and Medicetty, S.: Matrix cells from Wharton's jelly form neurons and glia. Stem Cells **21**:50–60, 2003.

Mochizuki, M., Maruo, T., Masuko, K. and Ohtsu, T.: Effects of smoking on fetoplacental-maternal system during pregnancy. Amer. J. Obstet. Gynecol. **149**:413–420, 1984.

Moessinger, A.C., Blanc, W.A., Marone, P.A. and Polsen, D.C.: Umbilical cord length as an index of fetal activity: experimental study and clinical implications. Pediatr. Res. **16**:109–112, 1982.

Moessinger, A.C., Mills, J.L., Harley, E.E., Ramakrishnan, R., Berendes, H.W. and Blanc, W.A.: Umbilical cord length in Down's syndrome. Amer. J. Dis. Child. **140**:1276–1277, 1986.

Moise, K.J., Carpenter, R.J., Huhta, J.C. and Deter, R.L.: Umbilical cord hematoma secondary to in utero intravascular transfusion for Rh isoimmunization. Fetal Ther. **2**:65–70, 1987.

Moncrieff, D., Parker-Williams, J. and Chamberlain, G.: Placental drainage and fetomaternal transfusion. Lancet **2**:453, 1986.

Monie, I.W.: Velamentous insertion of cord in early pregnancy. Amer. J. Obstet. Gynecol. **93**:276–281, 1965.

Monie, I.W. and Khemmani, M.: Absent and abnormal umbilical arteries. Teratology **7**:135–142, 1973.

Moore, R.D.: Mast cells of the human umbilical cord. Amer. J. Pathol. **32**:1179–1183, 1956.

Murdoch, D.E.: Umbilical-cord doubling. Obstet. Gynecol. **27**:555–557, 1966.

Mvumbi, L., Manci, E.A., Ulmer, D. and Shah, A.K.: Glycogen levels in human term placental disks, umbilical cords, and membranes. Pediatr. Path. Lab. Med. **16**:597–605, 1996.

Myatt, L., Brockman, D.E., Eis, A.L.W. and Pollock, J.S.: Immunohistochemical localization of nitric oxide synthase in the human placenta. Placenta **14**:487–495, 1993.

Naaktgeboren, C. and van Wagtendonk, A.M.: Wahre Knoten in der Nabelschnur nebst Bemerkungen über Plazentophagie bei Menschenaffen. Z. Säugetierk. **31**:376–382, 1966.

Nadkarni, B.B.: Innervation of the human umbilical artery: an electron-microscope study. Amer. J. Obstet. Gynecol. **107**:303–312, 1970.

Naeye, R.L.: Umbilical cord length: clinical significance. J. Pediatr. **107**:278–281, 1985.

Naeye, R.L. and Tafari, N.: Noninfectious disorders of the placenta, fetal membranes and umbilical cord. In, Risk Factors in Pregnancy and Disease of the Fetus and Newborn. Williams and Wilkins, Baltimore, pp. 145–172, 1983.

Nanaev, A.K., Shirinsky, V.P. and Birukov, K.G.: Immunofluorescent study of heterogeneity in smooth muscle cells of human fetal vessels using antibodies to myosin, desmin and vimentin. Cell Tissue Res. **266**:535–540, 1991.

Nanaev, A.K., Domogatsky, S.P. and Milovanov, A.P.: Immunohistochemical study of the extracellular matrix and intermediate filaments in the human umbilical cord. Placenta **13**:A48, 1992.

Nanaev, A.K., Kohnen, G., Milovanov, A.P., Domogatsky, S.P. and Kaufmann, P.: Stromal differentiation and architecture of the human umbilical cord. Placenta **18**:53–64, 1997.

Nelson, K.B. and Grether, J.K.: Potentially asphyxiating conditions and spastic cerebral palsy in infants of normal birth weight. Amer. J. Obstet. Gynecol. **179**:507–513, 1998.

Newman, R.S., Spear, G.S. and Kirschbaum, N.: Postmortem DNA diagnosis of factor V Leiden in a neonate with systemic thrombosis and probable antithrombin deficiency. Obstet. Gynecol. **92**:702–705, 1998.

Newton, M. and Moody, A.R.: Fetal and maternal blood in the human placenta. Obstet. Gynecol. **18**:305–308, 1961.

Ney, J.A., Fee, S.C., Dooley, S.L., Socol, M.L. and Minogue, J.: Factors influencing hemostasis after umbilical vein puncture in vitro. Amer. J. Obstet. Gynecol. **160**:424–426, 1989.

Nieder, J. and Link, M.: Ein Beitrag zur Pathologie der Nabelschnurgeschwülste. Z. Gynäkol. **92**:420–428, 1970.

Nielsen, T.P., Nelson, R.M., Lee-Green, B., Lowe, P.N. and Reese, L.A.: Patent urachus complicating pregnancy: a review and report of a case. Amer. J. Obstet. Gynecol. **143**:61–68, 1982.

Nikolov, S.D. and Schiebler, T.H.: Über das fetale Gefäßsystem der reifen menschlichen Placenta. Z. Zellforsch. **139**:333–350, 1973.

Nolan, D.G., Martin, L.S., Natarajan, S. and Hume, R.F.: Fetal compromise associated with extreme fetal bile acidemia and maternal primary sclerosing cholangitis. Obstet. Gynecol. **84**:695–696, 1994.

Nöldeke, H.: Geburtskomplikationen bei Insertio velamentosa. Zentralbl. Gynäkol. **58**:351–356, 1934.

Novack, A.H., Mueller, B. and Ochs, H.: Umbilical cord separation in the newborn. Amer. J. Dis. Child. **142**:220–223, 1988.

Obolensky, W.: Durch Blasensprung bedingte Blutung aus dem Fötalkreislauf, ihre Erkennung und Verhütung. Gynaecologia **164**:279–282, 1967.

Ohyama, M., Itani, Y., Yamanaka, M., Imaizumi, K., Nishi, T., Ijiri, R. and Tanaka, Y.: Umbilical cord ulcer: a serious in utero complication of intestinal atresia. Placenta **21**:432–435, 2000.

Okatani, Y., Taniguchi, K. and Sagara, Y.: Amplifying effect of endothelin-1 on serotonin-induced vasoconstriction of human umbilical artery. Amer. J. Obstet. Gynecol. **172**:1240–1245, 1995.

Omar, H.A., Figueroa, R., Omar, R.A. and Wolin, M.S.: Properties of an endogenous arachidonic acid-elicited relaxing mechanism in human placental vessels. Amer. J. Obstetr. Gynecol. **167**:1064–1070, 1992.

Ornoy, A., Crone, K. and Altshuler, G.: Pathological features of the placenta in fetal death. Arch. Pathol. Lab. Med. **100**:367–371, 1976.

Otto, A.W.: Lehrbuch der pathologischen Anatomie des Menschen und der Thiere. Ruecker, Berlin, 1830.

Ottow, B.: Interpositio velamentosa funiculi umbilicalis, eine bisher übersehene Nabelstranganomalie, ihre Entstehung und klinische Bedeutung. Arch. Gynäkol. **116**:176–199, 1922.

Ottow, B.: Über die Insertio furcata der Nabelschnur. Arch. Gynäkol. **118**:378–382, 1923.

Oudesluys-Murphy, A.M., Eilers, G.A.M. and deGroot, C.J.: The time of separation of the umbilical cord. Eur. J. Pediatr. **146**:387–389, 1987.

Painter, D. and Russell, P.: Four-vessel umbilical cord associated with multiple congenital anomalies. Obstet. Gynecol. **50**:505–507, 1977.

Panigel, M.: Réactions vaso-motrices de l'arbre vasculaire foetal au cours de la perfusion de cotylédons placentaires isolés maintenus en survie. C. R. Acad. Sci. (Paris) **255**:3238–3240, 1962.

Panizza, V.H., Alvarez, H. and Benedetti, W.L.: The in vitro contractility of the human placental chorial vessels. J. Reprod. Med. **26**:478–482, 1981.

Panter, K.R. and Hannah, M.E.: Umbilical cord prolapse: so far so good? Lancet **347**:74, 1996.

Papaloucas, A., Avgoustiniatos, J. and Paisios, P.: Innervation of the umbilical cord in full term foetuses. IRCS Med. Sci. Anat. Hum. Biol. **3**:117–118, 1975.

Parilla, B.V., Tamura, R.K., MacGregor, S.N., Geibel, L.J. and Sabbagha, R.E.: The clinical significance of a single umbilical artery as an isolated finding on prenatal ultrasound. Obstet. Gynecol. **85**:570–572, 1995.

Parry, E.W.: Some electron microscope observation on the mesenchymal structures of full-term umbilical cord. J. Anat. **107**:505–518, 1970.

Parry, E.W. and Abramovich, D.R.: Some observations on the surface layer of full-term human umbilical cord epithelium. J. Obstet. Gynaecol. Brit. Commonw. **77**:878–884, 1970.

Parry, E.W. and Abramovich, D.R.: The ultrastructure of human umbilical vessel endothelium from early pregnancy to full term. J. Anat. **111**:29–42, 1972.

Patel, D., Dawson, M., Kalyanam, P., Lungus, E., Weiss, H., Flaherty, E. and Nora, E.G.: Umbilical cord circumference at birth. Amer. J. Dis. Child. **143**:638–639, 1989.

Pavlopoulos, P.M., Konstantinidou, A.E., Agapitos, E., Christodoulou, C.N. and Davaris, P.: Association of single umbilical artery with congenital malformations of vascular etiology. Pediat. Development. Pathol. **1**:487–493, 1998.

Pearson, A.A. and Sauter, R.W.: The innervation of the umbilical vein in human embryos and fetuses. Amer. J. Anat. **125**:345–352, 1969.

Pearson, A.A. and Sauter, R.W.: Nerve contributions to the pelvic plexus and the umbilical cord. Amer. J. Anat. **128**:485–498, 1970.

Pekarske, S.L.: Placental pathology casebook. J. Perinatol. **15**:81–83, 1995.

Pennati, G.: Biomechanical properties of the human umbilical cord. Biorheology **38**:355–366, 2001.

Pent, D.: Vasa previa. Amer. J. Obstet. Gynecol. **134**:151–155, 1979.

Perez-Aytes, A., Montero, L., Gomez, J. and Paya, A.: Single aberrant umbilical artery in a fetus with severe caudal defects: Sirenomelia or caudal dysgenesis. Amer. J. Med. Genet. **69**:409–412, 1997.

Perrin, E.V.D. and Bel, J.K-V.: Degeneration and calcification of the umbilical cord. Obstet. Gynecol. **26**:371–376, 1965.

Petersson, K., Bremme, K., Bottinga, R., Hofsjö, A., Hulthén-V., I., Kublickas, M., Norman, M., Papadogiannakis, N., Wàonggren, K. and Wolff, K.: Diagnostic evaluation of intrauterine fetal deaths in Stockholm 1998–1999. Acta Obstet. Gynecol. Scand. **81**:284–292, 2002.

Petrikovsky, B. and Kaplan, G.: Fetal grasping of the umbilical cord causing variable fetal heart rate decelerations. J. Clin. Ultrasound **21**:642–644, 1993 (and Amer. J. Obstet. Gynecol. **172**:1071, 1995).

Petrikovsky, B.M., Nochimson, D.J., Campbell, W.A. and Vintzileos, A.M.: Fetal jejunoileal atresia with persistent omphalomesenteric duct. Amer. J. Obstet. Gynecol. **158**:173–175, 1988.

Pfalzgraf, R.R., Zumwalt, R.E. and Kenny, M.R.: Mesodiverticular band and sudden death in children. Arch. Pathol. Lab. Med. **112**:182–184, 1988.

Philip, A.G.S.: Further observations on placental transfusion. Obstet. Gynecol. **42**:334–343, 1973.

Philip, A.G., Yee, A.B., Rosy, M., Surti, N., Tsamtsouris, A. and Ingall, D.: Placental transfusion as an intrauterine phenomenon in deliveries complicated by foetal distress. Brit. Med. J. **1**:11–13, 1969.

Pinto, A., Sorrentino, R., Sorrentino, P., Guerritore, T., Miranda, L., Biondi, A. and Martinelli, P.: Endothelial-derived relaxing factor released by endothelial cells of human umbilical vessels and its impairment in pregnancy-induced hypertension. Amer. J. Obstet. Gynecol. **164**:507–513, 1991.

Poeschmann, R.P., Verheijen, R.H.M. and Dongen, P.W.J.: Differential diagnosis and causes of non-immunological hydrops fetalis: a review. Obstet. Gynecol. Surv. **46**:223–231, 1991.

Potter, E.L.: Pathology of the Fetus and Infant. Yearbook Medical Publishers, Chicago, 1961.

Predanic, M., Kolli, J., Yousefzadeh, P. and Pennisi, J.: Disparate blood flow patterns in parallel umbilical arteries. Obstet. Gynecol. **91**:757–760, 1998.

Priman, J.: A note on the anastomosis of the umbilical arteries. Anat. Rec. **134**:1–5, 1959.

Quek, S.P. and Tan, K.L.: Vasa previa. Aust. N.Z. J. Obstet. Gynaecol. **12**:206–209, 1972.

Quinlan, D.K.: Coarctation in cord of twenty-one-week-old fetus, with atresia, fibrosis, secondary torsion. S. Afr. J. Obstet. Gynaecol. **3**:1–2, 1965.

Qureshi, F. and Jacques, S.M.: Marked segmental thinning of the umbilical cord vessels. Arch. Pathol. Lab. Med. **118**:826–830, 1994.

Radcliffe, P.A., Sindelair, P.J. and Zeit, P.R.: Vasa previa with marginal placenta previa of an accessory lobe: report of a case. Obstet. Gynecol. **16**:472–475, 1961.

Raio, L., Ghezzi, F., Di Naro, E., Gomez, R., Saile, G. and Brühwiler, H.: The clinical significance of antenatal detection of discordant umbilical arteries. Obstet. Gynecol. **91**:86–91, 1998.

Raio, L., Ghezzi, F., Di Naro, E., Franchi, M., Bruhwiler, H. and Luscher, K.P.: Prenatal assessment of Wharton's jelly in umbilical cords with single artery. Ultrasound Obstet. Gynecol. **14**:42–46, 1999.

Raio, L., Ghezzi, F., Di Naro, E., Franchi, M., Balestreri, D., Dürig, P. and Schneider, H.: In-utero characterization of the blood flow in the Hyrtl anastomosis. Placenta **22**:597–601, 2001.

Raio, L., Ghezzi, F., Di Naro, E., Duwe, D.G., Cromi, A. and Schneider, H.: Umbilical cord morphologic characteristics and umbilical artery Doppler parameters in intrauterine growth-restricted fetuses. J. Ultrasound Med. **22**:1341–1347, 2003.

Raio, L., Ghezzi, F., Cromi, A., Nelle, M., Durig, P. and Schneider, H.: The thick heterogeneous (jellylike) placenta: a strong predictor of adverse pregnancy outcome. Prenat. Diagn. **24**:182–188, 2004.

Ramirez, P., Haberman, S. and Baxi, L.: Significance of prenatal diagnosis of umbilical cord cyst in a fetus with trisomy 18. Amer. J. Obstet. Gynecol. **173**:955–957, 1995.

Rana, J., Ebert, G.A. and Kappy, K.A.: Adverse perinatal outcome in patients with an abnormal umbilical coiling index. Obstet. Gynecol. **85**:573–577, 1995.

Rath, W., Osterhage, G., Kuhn, W., Gröne, H.J. and Fuchs, E.: Visualization of ^{125}I-endothelin-1 binding sites in human placenta and umbilical vessels. Gynecol. Obstet. Invest. **395**:209–213, 1993.

Ratten, G.J.: Spontaneous haematoma of the umbilical cord. Aust. N.Z. J. Obstet. Gynaecol. **9**:125–126, 1969.

Rayburn, W.F., Beynen, A. and Brinkman, D.L.: Umbilical cord length and intrapartum complications. Obstet. Gynecol. **57**:450–452, 1981.

Reece, E.A., Pinter, E., Green, J., Mahoney, M.J., Naftolin, F. and Hobbins, J.C.: Significance of isolated yolk sac visualised by ultrasonography. Lancet **1**:269, 1987.

Reeves, T.B.: A double umbilicus. Anat. Rec. **10**:15–18, 1916.

Rehsteiner, H.P.: Die Leitung der Placentarperiode—Der Zug an der Nabelschnur. Gynaecologia **167**:185–196, 1969.

Reilly, F.D. and Russell, P.T.: Neurohistochemical evidence supporting an absence of adrenergic and cholinergic innervation in the human placenta and umbilical cord. Anat. Record **188**:277–286, 1977.

Reinhart, R.D., Wells, W.A. and Harris, R.D.: Focal aneurysmal dilatation of subchorionic vessels simulating chorioangioma. Ultrasound Obstet. Gynecol. **13**:147–149, 1999.

Reiss, H.E.: Umbilical cord. Brit. Med. J. **2**:511, 1964.

Resta, R.G., Luthy, D.A. and Mahony, B.S.: Umbilical cord hemangioma associated with extremely high alpha-fetoprotein levels. Obstet. Gynecol. **72**:488–491, 1988.

Rey, E.: Effects of methyldopa on umbilical and placental artery flow velocity waveforms. Obstetr. Gynecol. **80**:783–787, 1992.

Reynolds, S.R.M.: The proportion of Wharton's jelly in the umbilical cord in relation to distention of the umbilical arteries and vein, with observations on the folds of Hoboken. Anat. Rec. **113**:365–377, 1952.

Rhen, K. and Kinnunen, O.: Ante-partum rupture of the umbilical cord. Acta Obstet. Gynecol. Scand. **41** 86–89, 1962.

Richards, D.S., Lutfi, E., Mullins, D., Sandler, D.L. and Raynor, B.D.: Prenatal diagnosis of fetal disseminated intravascular coagulation associated with umbilical cord arteriovenous malformation. Obstet. Gynecol. **85**:860–862, 1995.

Rissmann, Dr.: Aneurysma der Nabelschnurarterie. Zentralbl. Gynäkol. **55**:550–551, 1931.

Rizos, N., Doran, T.A., Miskin, M., Benzie, R.J. and Ford, J.A.: Natural history of placenta previa ascertained by diagnostic ultrasound. Amer. J. Obstet. Gynecol. **133**:287–291, 1979.

Robaut, C., Mondon, F., Bandet, J., Ferre, F. and Cavero. I.: Regional distribution and pharmacological characterization of [^{125}I]endothelin-1 binding sites in human fetal placental vessels. Placenta **12**:55–67, 1991.

Robertson, R.D., Rubinstein, L.M., Wolfson, W.L., Lebherz, T.B., Blanchard, J.B. and Crandall, B.F.: Constriction of the umbilical cord as a cause of fetal demise following midtrimester amniocentesis. J. Reprod. Med. **26**:325–327, 1981.

Robinson, L.K., Jones, K.L. and Benirschke, K.: The nature of structural defects associated with velamentous and marginal insertion of the umbilical cord. Amer. J. Obstet. Gynecol. **146**:191–193, 1983.

Röckelein, G. and Hey, A.: Ultrastrukturelle Untersuchungen der Vakuolenbildung in arteriellen Choriongefäßen der reifen menschlichen Plazenta. Z. Geburtsh. Perinat. **189**:65–68, 1985.

Röckelein, G. and Scharl, A.: Scanning electron microscopic investigations of the human umbilical artery intima: a new conception on postnatal arterial closure mechanism. Virchows Arch. [A] **413**:555–561, 1988.

Röckelein, G., Kobras, G. and Becker, V.: Physiological and pathological morphology of the umbilical and placental circulation. Path. Res. Pract. **186**:187–196, 1990.

Rolschau, J.: The relationship between some disorders of the umbilical cord and intrauterine growth retardation. Acta Obstet. Gynecol. Scand. [Suppl.] **72**:15–21, 1978.

Romero, R., Chervenak, F.A., Coustan, D., Berkowitz, R.L. and Hobbins, J.C.: Antenatal sonographic diagnosis of umbilical cord laceration. Amer. J. Obstet. Gynecol. **143**:719–720, 1982.

Ronchera-Oms, C., Hernandez, C. and Jimenez, N.V.: Antiseptic cord care reduces bacterial colonisation but delays cord detachment. Arch. Dis. Childh. **70**:F70, 1994.

Rotmensch, S., Liberati, M., Mittelmann, M. and Ben-Rafael, Z.: Activated protein C resistance and adverse pregnancy outcome. Amer. J. Obstet. Gynecol. **177**:170–173, 1997.

Rucker, M.P. and Tureman, G.R.: Vasa previa. Va. Med. Monthly **72**:202–207, 1945.

Rust, W.: Seltsame Veränderungen an den Nabelschnurgefässen. Arch. Gynäkol. **165**:58–62, 1937.

Ruvinsky, E.D., Wiley, T.L., Morrison, J.C. and Blake, P.G.: In utero diagnosis of umbilical cord hematoma by ultrasonography. Amer. J. Obstet. Gynecol. **140**:833–834, 1981.

Salas, S.P., Power, R.F., Singleton, A., Wharton, J., Polak, J.M. and Brown, J.: Heterogeneous binding sites for α-atrial natriuretic peptide in human umbilical cord and placenta. Amer. J. Physiol. **261**:R633–R638, 1991.

Sander, C.H.: Hemorrhagic endovasculitis and hemorrhagic villitis of the placenta. Arch. Pathol. Lab. Med. **104**:371–373, 1980.

Sander, C.M., Gilliland, D., Flynn, M.A. and Swart-Hills, L.A.: Risk factors for recurrence of hemorrhagic endovasculitis of the placenta. Obstet. Gynecol. **89**:569–576, 1997.

Schaefer, M., Laurichesse-Delmas, H. and Ville, Y.: The effect of nuchal cord on nuchal translucency measurement at 10–14 weeks. Ultrasound Obstetr. Gynecol. **11**:271–273, 1998.

Scheffel, T. and Langanke, D.: Die Nabelschnurkomplikationen an der Universitäts-Frauenklinik von 1955 bis 1967. Zentralbl. Gynäkol. **92**:429–434, 1970.

Schellong, G. and Pfeiffer, R.A.: Persistierender Ductus omphalo-mesentericus als Ursache ungewöhnlicher Komplikationen bei der Austauschtransfusion. Arch. Kinderheilk. **175**:204–209, 1967.

Scheuner, G.: Über die Verankerung der Nabelschnur an der Plazenta. Morphol. Jahrb. **106**:73–89, 1964.

Scheuner, G.: Über die mikroskopische Struktur der Insertio velamentosa. Zentralbl. Gynäkol. **87**:38–49, 1965.

Schiebler, T.H. and Kaufmann, P.: Reife Plazenta. In, Die Plazenta des Menschen. V. Becker, T.H. Schiebler and F. Kubli, eds. Thieme, Stuttgart, 1981.

Schiff, I., Driscoll, S.G. and Naftolin, F.: Calcification of the umbilical cord. Amer. J. Obstetr. Gynecol. **126**:1046–1048, 1976.

Schordania, J.: Über das Gefäßsystem der Nabelschnur. Z. Ges. Anat. **89**:696–726, 1929a.

Schordania, J.: Der architektonische Aufbau der Gefässe der menschlichen Nachgeburt und ihre Beziehungen zur Entwicklung der Frucht. Arch. Gynäkol. **135**:568–598, 1929b.

Schreier, R. and Brown, S.: Hematoma of the umbilical cord: report of a case. Obstet. Gynecol. **20**:798–800, 1962.

Schreiner, C.A. and Hoornbeek, F.K.: Developmental aspects of sirenomelia in the mouse. J. Morphol. **141**:345–358, 1973.

Schwalbe, E.: Allgemeine Mißbildungslehre (Teratologie). Gustav Fischer, Jena, 1906.

Scott, J.M. and Jordan, J.M.: Placental insufficiency and the small-for-dates baby. Amer. J. Obstet. Gynecol. **113**:823–832, 1972.

Scott, J.M. and Wilkinson, R.: Further studies on the umbilical cord and its water content. J. Clin. Pathol. **31**:944–948, 1978.

Scott, J.S.: Placenta extrachorialis (placenta marginata and placenta circumvallata). J. Obstet. Gynaecol. Brit. Emp. **67**:907–918, 1960.

Seeds, J.W., Chescheir, N.C., Bowes, W.A. and Owl-Smith, F.A.: Fetal death as a complication of intrauterine intravascular transfusion. Obstet. Gynecol. **74**:461–463, 1989.

Seifert, D.B., Ferguson, J.E., Behrens, C.M., Zemel, S., Stevenson, D.K. and Ross, J.C.: Nonimmune hydrops fetalis in association with hemangioma of the umbilical cord. Obstet. Gynecol. **66**:283–286, 1985.

Seligsohn, U., Berger, A., Abend, M., Rubin, L., Attias, D., Zivelin, A. and Rapaport, S.I.: Homozygous protein C deficiency manifested by massive venous thrombosis in the newborn. NEJM **310**:559–562, 1984.

Sepúlveda, W.H., González, C., Cruz, M.A. and Rudolph, M.I.: Vasoconstrictive effect of bile acids on isolated human placental chorionic veins. Eur. J. Obstetr. Gynecol. Reprod. Biol. **42**:211–215, 1991.

Sexton, A.J., Turmaine, M., Cai, W.Q. and Burnstock, G.: A study of the ultrastructure of developing human umbilical vessels. J. Anat. **188**:75–85.

Shanklin, D.R.: The influence of placental lesions on the newborn infant. Pediatr. Clin. North America **17**:25–42, 1970.

Shaw, A. and Pierog, S.: "Ectopic" liver in the umbilicus: an unusual focus of infection in a newborn infant. Pediatrics **44**:448–450, 1969.

Shen-Schwarz, S., Macpherson, T. and Mueller-Heubach, E.: Hemorrhagic endovasculitis of the placenta: incidence and clinical features in an unselected population. Pediatr. Pathol. **5**:112, 1986.

Shen-Schwarz, S., Macpherson, T.A. and Mueller-Heubach, E.: The clinical significance of hemorrhagic endovasculitis of the placenta. Amer. J. Obstet. Gynecol. **159**:48–51, 1988.

Shen-Schwarz, S., Ananth, C.V., Smulian, J.C. and Vintzleos, A.M.: Umbilical cord twist patterns in twin gestations. Amer. J. Obstet. Gynecol. **176**:S154 (abstract 538), 1997a.

Shen-Schwarz, S., Smulian, J.C., Ananth, C.V., Lai-Ling, Y. and Vintzileos, A.M.: Placental cord insertion in relation to birth weight and placental weight discordancy in twin gestations. Amer. J. Obstet. Gynecol. **176**:S134, abstract 457, 1997b.

Shepherd, A.J., Richardson, C.J. and Brown, J.P.: Nuchal cords as a cause of neonatal anemia. Amer. J. Dis. Child. **139**:71–73, 1985.

Shepherd, J.T.: Bayliss response in the umbilical artery. Fed. Proc. **27**:1408–1409, 1968.

Sibulkin, M.: A note on the bathtub vortex and the earth's rotation. Amer. Sci. **71**:352–353, 1983.

Siddall, R.S.: Spontaneous rupture of the umbilical cord. Amer. J. Obstet. Gynecol. **10**:836–840, 1925.

Siddiqi, T.A., Bendon, R., Schultz, D.M. and Miodovnik, M.: Umbilical artery aneurysm: Prenatal diagnosis and management. Obstet. Gynecol. **80**:530–533, 1992.

Silva, P. de, Stoskopf, C.G., Keegan, K.A. and Murata, Y.: Use of fetal scalp hematocrit in the diagnosis of severe hemorrhage from vasa previa. Amer. J. Obstet. Gynecol. **153**:307–308, 1985.

Silver, M.M., Yeger, H. and Lines, L.D.: Hemorrhagic endovasculitis-like lesion in placental organ culture. Lab. Invest. **56**:6P, 1987.

Silver, M.M., Yeger, H. and Lines, L.D.: Hemorrhagic endovasculitis-like lesion induced in placental organ culture. Hum. Pathol. **19**:251–256, 1988.

Silver, R.K., Dooley, S.L., Tamura, R.K. and Depp, R.: Umbilical cord size and amniotic fluid volume in prolonged pregnancy. Amer. J. Obstet. Gynecol. **157**:716–720, 1987.

Singh, V., Khanum, S. and Singh, M.: Umbilical cord lesions in early intrauterine fetal demise. Arch. Pathol. Lab. Med. **127**:850–853, 2003.

Sinha, A.A.: Ultrastructure of human amnion and amniotic plaques of normal pregnancy. Z. Zellforsch. **122**:1–14, 1971.

Sinnathuray, T.A.: The nuchal cord incidence and significance. J. Obstet. Gynaecol. Brit. Commonw. **73**:226–231, 1966.

Slijper, E.J.: Die Geburt der Säugetiere. In, Handbuch der Zoologie, Vol. 8. W. Kükenthal, ed., pp. 1–108. de Gruyter, Berlin, 1960.

Smart, P.J.G.: Some observations on the vascular morphology of the foetal side of the human placenta. J. Obstet. Gynaecol. Brit. Commonw. **69**:929–933, 1962.

Smith, D. and Majmudar, B.: Teratoma of the umbilical cord. Hum. Pathol. **16**:190–193, 1985.

Snider, W.: Placental pathology casebook. J. Perinatol. **17**:327–329, 1997.

Soernes, T.: Umbilical cord encirclements and fetal growth restriction. Obstet. Gynecol. **86**:725–728, 1995.

Soernes, T. and Bakke, T.: The length of the human umbilical cord in vertex and breech presentations. Amer. J. Obstet. Gynecol. **154**:1086–1087, 1986.

Sotelo, A.K., Sotelo, C., Hathaway, C.S. and Vogler, C.A.: Incidental ectopic tissues in the placenta. Placenta **22**(7):A29, 2001.

Spatz, W.B.: Nabelschnur-Längen bei Insektivoren und Primaten. Z. Säugetierk. **33**:226–239, 1968.

Spellacy, W.N., Gravem, H. and Fisch, R.O.: The umbilical cord complications of true knots, nuchal coils, and cords around the body. Amer. J. Obstet. Gynecol. **94**:1136–1142, 1966.

Spiteri, M., Anh, N.H. and Panigel, M.: Ultrastructure du muscle lisse des artères du cordon ombilical humain. Pathol. Biol. **14**:348–357, 1966.

Spivack, M.: On the anatomy of the so-called 'valves' of umbilical vessels, with especial reference to the valvulae Hobokenii. Anat. Rec. **66**:127–148, 1936.

Spivack, M.: On the presence or absence of nerves in the umbilical blood vessels of man and guinea pig. Anat. Rec. **85**:85–109, 1943.

Stevens, N.G. and Sander, C.H.: Placental hemorrhagic endovasculitis: risk factors and impact on pregnancy outcome. Lab. Invest. **50**:57A, 1984.

Stevenson, R.E., Jones, K.L., Phelan, M.C., Jones, M.C., Barr, M., Clericuzio, C., Harley, R.A. and Benirschke, K.: Vascular steal: the pathogenetic mechanism producing sirenomelia and associated defects of the viscera and soft tissues. Pediatrics **78**:451–457, 1986.

Strassmann, P.: Placenta praevia. Arch. Gynäkol. **67**:112–275, 1902.

Strong, T.H.: Factors that provide optimal umbilical protection during gestation. Contemporary Obstet. Gynecol. **42**:82–105, 1997.

Strong, T.H., Elliott, J.P. and Radin, T.R.: Non-coiled umbilical blood vessels: A new marker for the fetus at risk. Obstet. Gynecol. **81**:409–411, 1993.

Strong, T.H., Jarles, D.L., Vega, J.S. and Feldman, D.B.: The umbilical coiling index. Amer. J. Obstet. Gynecol. **170**:29–32, 1994.

Summerville, J.W., Powar, J.S. and Ueland, K.: Umbilical cord hematoma resulting in intrauterine fetal demise. A case report. J. Reprod. Med. **32**:213–216, 1987.

Sun, Y., Arbuckle, S., Hocking, G. and Billson, V.: Umbilical cord stricture and intrauterine fetal death. Pediatr. Pathol. Lab. Med. **15**:723–732, 1995.

Sutro, W.H., Tuck, S.M., Loesewitz, A., Novotny, P.L., Archbald, F. and Irwin, G.A.L.: Prenatal observation of umbilical cord hematoma. AJR **142**:801–802, 1084.

Swanberg, H. and Wiqvist, N.: Rupture of the umbilical cord during pregnancy. Acta Obstet. Gynecol. Scand. **30**:323–337, 1951.

Szécsi, K.: Beiträge zur spontanen Zerreißung der zu kurzen Nabelschnur. Zentralbl. Gynäkol. **77**:1024–1028, 1955.

Takagi, T., Toda, T., Leszczynski, D. and Kummerow, F.: Ultrastructure of aging human umbilical artery and vein. Acta Anat. (Basel) **119**:73–79, 1984.

Takechi, K., Kuwabara, Y. and Mizuno, M.: Ultrastructural and immunohistochemical studies of Wharton's jelly umbilical cord cells. Placenta **14**:235–245, 1993.

Ten Berge, B.S.: Nervenelemente in Plazenta und Nabelschnur. Gynaecologia **156**:49–53, 1963.

Tharakan, T., Baxi, L.V. and Diuguid, D.: Protein S deficiency in pregnancy: A case report. Amer. J. Obstet. Gynecol. **168**:141–142, 1993.

Theuring, F.: Fibröse Obliterationen an Deckplatten- und Stammzottengefäßen der Placenta nach intrauterinem Fruchttod. Arch. Gynäkol. **206**:237–251, 1968.

Thomas, J.: Untersuchungsergebnisse über die Aplasie einer Nabelarterie unter besonderer Berücksichtigung der Zwillingsschwangerschaft. Geburtsh. Frauenh. **21**:984–992, 1961.

Thomas, J.: Die Entwicklung von Fetus und Placenta bei Nabelgefäßanomalien. Arch. Gynäkol. **198**:216–223, 1963.

Thomson, L.L. and Hoo, J.J.: Linear disruption of umbilical cord: A rare anomaly of the cord associated with acute fetal distress and perinatal death/pronounced psychomotor retardation. Amer. J. Med. Genet. **62**:348–349, 1996.

Thorarensen, O., Ryan, S., Hunter, J. and Younkin, D.P.: Factor V Leiden mutation: An unrecognized cause of hemiplegic cerebral palsy, neonatal stroke, and placental thrombosis. Ann. Neurol. **42**:372–375, 1997.

Thummala, M.R., Raju, T.N. and Langenberg, P.: Isolated single umbilical artery anomaly and the risk for congenital malformations: a meta-analysis. J. Pediatr. Surg. **33**:580–585, 1998.

Torpin, R.: Classification of human pregnancy based on depth of intrauterine implantation of ovum. Amer. J. Obstet. Gynecol. **66**:791–800, 1953.

Torrey, W.E.: Vasa previa. Amer. J. Obstet. Gynecol. **63**:146–152, 1952.

Tortora, M., Chervenak, F.A., Mayden, K. and Hobbins, J.C.: Antenatal sonographic diagnosis of single umbilical artery. Obstet. Gynecol. **63**:693–696, 1984.

Trollmann, R., Amann, K., Schoof, E., Beinder, E., Wenzel, D., Rascher, W. and Dötsch, J.: Hypoxia activates the human placental vascular endothelial growth factor system in vitro and in vivo: Up-regulation of vascular endothelial growth factor in clinically relevant hypoxic ischemia in birth asphyxia. Amer. J. Obstet. Gynecol. **188**:517–523, 2003.

Trudinger, B.J. and Cook, C.M.: Different umbilical artery flow velocity waveforms in one patient. Obstet. Gynecol. **71**:1019–1021, 1988.

Trudinger, B.J., Stevens, D., Connelly, A., Hales, J.R.S., Alexander, G., Bradley, L., Fawcett, A. and Thompson, R.S.: Umbilical artery flow velocity waveforms and placental resistance: the effects of embolization of the umbilical circulation. Amer. J. Obstet. Gynecol. **157**:1443–1448, 1987.

Tuggle, A.Q. and Cook, W.A.: Laceration of a placental vein: an injury possibly inflicted by the fetus. Amer. J. Obstet. Gynecol. **131**:220–221, 1978.

Uchide, K., Ueno, H., Inuyama, R., Murakami, K. and Terada, S.: Cord presentation with posterior placenta previa. Lancet **350**:1448, 1997.

Ukeshima, A., Hayashi, Y. and Fujimoto, T.: Surface morphology of the human yolk sac: endoderm and mesothelium. Arch. Histol. Jpn. **49**:483–494, 1986.

Ullberg, U., Sandstedt, B. and Lingman, G.: Hyrtl's anastomosis occurrence, morphology and relation to umbilical artery blood flow waveforms and fetal growth. Placenta **15**:Abstract A.71, 1994.

Ullberg, U., Sandstedt, B. and Lingman, G.: Hyrtl's anastomosis, the only connection between the two umbilical arteries. A study in full term placentas from AGA infants with normal umbilical artery blood flow. Acta Obstet. Gynecol. Scand. **80**:1–6, 2001.

Ulm, M.R., Plöckinger, B., Pirich, C., Gryglewski, R.J. and Sinzinger, H.F.: Umbilical arteries of babies born to cigarette smokers generate less prostacyclin and contain less arginine and citrulline compared with those of babies born to control subjects. Amer. J. Obstet. Gynecol. **172**:1485–1487, 1995.

Uyanwah-Akpom, P.O. and Fox, H.: The clinical significance of marginal or velamentous insertion of the cord. Brit. J. Obstet. Gynaecol. **84**:941–943, 1977.

Vandevijver, N., Hermans, R.H., Schrander-Stumpel, C.C., Arends, J.W., Peeters, L.L. and Moerman, P.L.: Aneurysm of the umbilical vein: case report and review of literature. Eur. J. Obstet. Gynecol. Reprod. Biol. **89**:85–87, 2000.

Vandriede, D.M. and Kammeraad, L.A.: Vasa previa: case report, review and presentation of a new diagnostic method. J. Reprod. Med. **26**:577–580, 1981.

Vanhaesebrouck, P., Vanneste, K., de Praeter, C. and van Trappen, Y: Tight nuchal cord and neonatal hypovolemic shock. Arch. Dis. Child. **62**:1276–1277, 1987.

Vardi, P.: Placental transfusion: an attempt at physiological delivery. Lancet **2**:12–13, 1965.

Virgilio, L.A. and Spangler, D.B.: Fetal death secondary to constriction and torsion of the umbilical cord. Arch. Pathol. Lab. Med. **102**:32–33, 1978.

von Hayek, H.: Der funktionelle Bau der Nabelarterien und des Ductus Botalli. Z. Anat. Entwicklungsgesch. **105**:15–24, 1936.

Vu, T., Baldwin, V.J., Perrin, E.V.D.K. and Shanklin, D.R.: Major umbilical vessel rupture in utero. Pediatr. Pathol. **2**:494, 1984.

Waidl, E.: Zur Genese und Klinik der Insertio velamentosa. Zentralbl. Gynäkol. **82**:1902–1906, 1960.

Walker, C.W. and Pye, B.G.: The length of the umbilical cord; a statistical report. Brt. Med. J. **1**:546–548, 1960.

Walker, M.C., Garner, P.R., Keely, E.J., Rock, G.A. and Reis, M.D.: Changes in activated protein C resistance during normal pregnancy. Amer. J. Obstet. Gynecol. **177**:162–169, 1997.

Walsh, S.Z.: Maternal effects of early and late clamping of the umbilical cord. Lancet **1**:996–997, 1968.

Walz, W.: Über das Ödem der Nabelschnur. Zentralbl. Gynäkol. **69**:144–148, 1947.

Wang, X., Yi, S., Athayde, N. and Trudinger, B.: Endothelial cell apoptosis is induced by fetal plasma from pregnancy with umbilical placental vascular disease. Amer. J. Obstet. Gynecol. **186**:557–563, 2002.

Wang, X., Athayde, N. and Trudinger, B.: Fetal plasma stimulates endothelial cell production of cytokines and the family of suppressor of cytokine signaling in placental vascular disease. Amer. J. Obstet. Gynecol. **188**:510–516, 2003.

Weber, J.: Constriction of the umbilical cord as a cause of foetal death. Acta Obstet. Gynecol. Scand. **42**:259–268, 1963.

Weeks, J.W., Smith, A., Hogue, T., Spinnato, J.A. and Gall, S.A.: The umbilical coiling index and feto-placental characteristics. Amer. J. Obstet. Gynecol. **172**:32v (abstract 211), 1995.

Weiner, C.P., Wenstrom, K.D., Sipes, S.L. and Wiliamson, R.A.: Risk factors for cordocentesis and fetal intravascular transfusion. Amer. J. Obstet. Gynecol. **165**:1020–1025, 1991.

Weissman, A., Jakobi, P., Bronshtein, M. and Goldstein, I.: Sonographic measurements of the umbilical cord and vessels during normal pregnancies. J. Ultrasound Med. **13**:11–14, 1994.

Wentworth, P.: Some anomalies of the foetal vessels of the human placenta. J. Anat. **99**:273–282, 1965.

White, R.P.: Pharmacodynamic study of maturation and closure of human umbilical arteries. Amer. J. Obstet. Gynecol. **160**:229–237, 1989.

Whitwell, K.E.: Morphology and pathology of the equine umbilical cord. J. Reprod. Fertil., Suppl. **23**:599–603, 1975.

Widholm, O. and Nieminen, U.: Prolapse of umbilical cord. Acta Obstet. Gynecol. **42**:21–29, 1963.

Wiedersberg, E., Wittstock, G. and Wiedersberg, H.: Pathologie der Nabelschnur in Abhängigkeit vom Gestationsalter. Befunde bei 4267 fetalen und neonatalen Autopsien. Verh. Dtsch. Ges. Pathol. **85**:175–192, 2001.

Wigger, H.J., Kiu, T.W., Moessinger, A.C., Marboe, C.C. and Blanc, W.A.: Effect of cigarette smoking on the ultrastructure of the placenta. Lab. Invest. **50**:14P, 1984.

Williams, J.H. and Benirschke, K.: Chorionic vessel thrombosis: a possible etiology of neonatal purpura. J. Reprod. Med. **20**:285–288, 1978.

Williams, J., Katzman, G.H. and Kripke, S.S.: Neck compression by nuchal cord. Amer. J. Obstet. Gynecol. **140**:345–346, 1981.

Williams, M. and O'Brien, W.: Umbilical cord entanglements are associated with increased placental mass and decreased fetal placental ration. Amer. J. Obstet. Gynecol. **187**:p.S93 (abstract 114), 2000a.

Williams, M. and O'Brien, W.: Multiple or tight nuchal cord loops are not associated with significant perinatal morbidity. Amer. J. Obstet. Gynecol. **187**:p.S93 (abstract 113), 2000b.

Wilson, R.D., Magee, J.F., Sorensen, P.H.B. and Johnson, A.: In utero decompression of umbilical cord angiomyxoma followed by vaginal delivery. Amer. J. Obstet. Gynecol. **171**:1383–1385, 1994.

Winter, R.: Die Rolle regressiver Veränderungen der Plazenta bei der sogenannten Plazentamigration. Geburtsh. Frauenheilk. **38**:1093–1098, 1978.

Winters, R.H.: Unique vascular relationship in human umbilical cord. Nature **226**:656, 1970.

Wolf, P.L., Jones, K.L., Longway, S.R., Benirschke, K. and Bloor, C.: Prenatal death from acute myocardial infarction and cardiac tamponade due to embolus from the placenta. Amer. Heart J. **109**:603–605, 1985.

Wolfman, W.L., Purohit, D.M. and Self, S.E.: Umbilical vein thrombosis at 32 weeks' gestation with delivery of a living infant. Amer. J. Obstet. Gynecol. **146**:468–470, 1983.

Woods, D.L. and Malan, A.F.: The site of umbilical cord insertion and birth weight. Brit. J. Obstet. Gynaecol. **85**:332–333, 1978.

Yamada, K. and Shimizu, S.: Concanavalin a-peroxidase-diaminobenzidine (Con A-PO-DAB)-alcian blue (AB): a reliable method for dual staining of complex carbohydrates. Histochemistry **47**:159–169, 1976.

Yang, H.Y., Shum, A.Y.C., Ng, H.T. and Chen, C.F.: Effect of ethanol on human umbilical artery and vein in vitro. Gynecol. Obstet. Invest. **21**:131–135, 1986.

Yao, A.C. and Lind, J.: Placental transfusion: review. Amer. J. Dis. Child. **127**:128–141, 1974.

Yao, A.C. and Lind, J.: Placental transfusion. A Clinical and Physiological Study. Charles C. Thomas, Springfield, 1982.

Yao, A.C., Hirvensalo, M. and Lind, J.: Placental transfusion-rate and uterine clamping. Lancet **1**:380–383, 1968.

Yao, A.C., Moinian, M. and Lind, J.: Distribution of blood between infant and placenta after birth. Lancet **2**:871–873, 1969.

Yao, A.C., Lind, J. and Lu, T.: Closure of the human umbilical artery: a physiological demonstration of Burton's theory. Eur. J. Obstet. Gynecol. Reprod. Biol. **7**:365–368, 1977.

Yavner, D.L. and Redline, R.W.: Angiomyxoma of the umbilical cord with massive cystic degeneration of Wharton's jelly. Arch. Pathol. Lab. Med. **113**:935–937, 1989.

Young, A.: The primate umbilical cord with special reference to the transverse communicating artery. J. Hum. Evol. **1**:345–359, 1972.

Young, G.B.: The peripatetic placenta. Radiology **128**:183–188, 1978.

Zhang, P. and Benirschke, K.: Placental pathology casebook. J. Perinatol. **1**:163–65, 2000.

13
Placental Shape Aberrations

In recent years, it has become practical to record and follow the location of the placenta during the course of gestation by sonography. This methodology has shown that a "dynamic placentation" occurs. That is to say, the original location of the implanting blastocyst may be modified during the course of its development to becoming a term placenta. This chapter discusses these concepts, the various types of abnormal placental development, and the morphology of placenta accreta, percreta, and ectopic implantation.

The factors that determine the site of nidation of the human blastocyst are not fully understood. The human blastocyst implants normally in the upper portion of the uterus; nevertheless, abnormal implantation is frequent and may lead to pregnancy complications, such as placenta previa. It has been suggested, for instance, that the site of placental implantation influences the frequency of fetal malpresentation. Wingate and Pauls (1968) studied this using chromium 51 as tracer in placental localization in 85 patients. They found no correlation between either fundal or lower uterine implantation and fetal malpresentations. Previous authors, on the other hand, had suggested that an abnormal location of the blastocyst in the endometrium may lead to abnormal forms of the mature placenta. An early proponent of such thoughts was Schatz (1886), who envisaged normal, broad, and superficial implantations. Later, these ideas were particularly strongly championed by Torpin (1969a), who related the depth of implantation and its location in the uterus to the development of circumvallate placentation. The location of the implantation may be important and can be better correlated now with sonography. Thus, we have seen two circumvallate placentas in cornual implantations. Others have suggested that the placental location is instrumental in triggering the normal impulse for the initiation of labor and that it is correlated with the length of gestation.

SITE OF PLACENTAL ATTACHMENT

There are several means by which investigators have approached localization of the implantation and the ultimate placental site. Hertig and Rock (1973) summarized their findings from the successful search of 34 early human ova; they obtained the following results:

Tubal location	1
Free in uterus	7
Implanted, normal	17
Implanted, abnormal	9

The normal embryos were more often on the posterior wall than were the implantations of abnormal blastocysts.

When the placental site is determined by postpartum palpation, as was done by Booth et al. (1962) in 200 patients, the following distribution emerged:

Anterior	53%
Posterior	39%
Lateral	8%

When these data are expressed with respect to the height of placental location, the following distributions were found:

Fundal position	2%
Fundal and upper segment	42%
Upper segment	47%
Upper and lower segments	9%

A fundal attachment was found in 44% of primigravidae and 20% of multigravidae; preeclampsia was twice as common in fundal placentas, which may merely reflect the fact that this condition is commoner in a first pregnancy. There was no relation to the length of pregnancy and labor. Scipiades and Burg (1930), in an extensive study on placentation, cited Orsini (1928), who found an anterior placenta in 26.6%, a posterior implantation in 41.6%, a fundal site in 2.2%, a lower uterus site in 23%, and at other sites in 3.5%. Later methods have used the distance of the membrane rupture site to the edge of the placenta as an indicator of placental localization (Little, 1962; Little & Friedman, 1964). This method needs to take into consideration that the placenta must be carefully extracted and not disturbed after delivery. Among the 10,101 placentas correlated during the evaluation by Little and Friedman (1964), the mean rupture site was between 5 and 9 cm in 39.3%. In 11% it was 0 cm (possible marginal placenta previa), and in only 0.3% was it more than 19 cm. These authors were unable to confirm the relation of high uterine position and preeclampsia but did not make a distinction with the parity of their patients. They found a twofold higher frequency of vaginal bleeding with low-lying placentas, but otherwise no influence on the length of labor, type of delivery, or neonatal outcome was identified. Torpin (1958) used his method of distending the membranous sac in a bucket of water after birth and determined, in 147 cases, that when the placenta had implanted in the "crease made by the reflection of the anterior and posterior uterine walls, the resulting placenta is almost invariably bilobate."

Indium isotope scanning and sonography were employed by Harris (1975) in 401 patients for placental localization in an effort to ascertain whether localization over the putative uterine "pacemaker" (Larks et al., 1959) influences the length of pregnancy. It was found in the right upper quadrant in about the same frequency as in the left (85%/79%), although the former had statistically slightly significantly shorter pregnancies. This finding disagrees with the theory that the location in the right upper quadrant lengthens pregnancy.

More incisive results come from studies using sonographic localization of the placenta (Gottesfeld et al., 1966), which is now almost routinely ascertained during the course of pregnancy. Taipale et al. (1997) found that when transvaginal sonographic screening was done at between 12 and 16 weeks of gestation, and the placenta then extended 15 mm over the internal os, the probability of a placenta previa at delivery was 5.1%. Studies such as these have stimulated interest in the past on the mechanism of the outcome of low placentation. King (1973) was the first to show that a placenta previa of early pregnancy changes to one that does not require surgery for placenta previa at term, and that this change takes place in most cases. He termed this phenomenon "dynamic placentation." In none of his 14 cases of marginal placenta previa, observed near mid-gestation, was there a true placenta previa at term, although several had a near cervical implantation. He reasoned that this change in position comes about largely by uterine growth and its changing shape as gestation advances. Nearly the same conclusions were arrived at independently by Meyenburg (1976) and have since been confirmed by many other investigators (e.g., Winters, 1978). Young (1978), who studied the same features with arteriography, located the placenta twice as often in the upper uterine segment than as a placenta previa. He also noted the disappearance of most placentas previa with term approaching. He suggested that those placentas that do not move may represent accretas, but there was no histologic support for this concept. In a large study of ultrasonographic findings prior to amniocentesis between 16 and 18 weeks, Rizos et al. (1979) found the following locations:

Site	Previas (%)	All placentas (%)
Anterior	69	37
Posterior	10	24
Anterior and posterior	21	5
Fundal	0	34

Their incidence of placenta previa at midterm was 5.3%, and it converted to a nonprevia in 90.4% by term. Their overall term previa incidence was 0.58%, similar to that of other studies.

A similar, large study of placental localization by sonography was reported by Fried (1978). When he followed the location over the three trimesters, he observed the following:

Site	10–20 weeks (%)	21–31 weeks (%)	32–40 weeks (%)
Anterior	25	41	44
Posterior	37	28	26
Anterior-fundal	9	6	8
Posterior-fundal	17	18	15
Fundal	12	7	7

In other words, little change occurred in the overall location of placentas. Parenthetically, he found many more cephalic presentations with anterior than posterior placentas. Castro et al. (1995) found that 77% of initially low-lying placentas moved upward, whereas 68% of fundal implantations extended downward as pregnancy progressed; laterally located placentas tended to move the least.

Gallagher et al. (1987) performed sonography during the second trimester of pregnancy in 1239 women and found a central placenta previa in three patients and marginal or partial previa in 48 (5%). At term, only four (0.3%) of the following patients had a placenta previa: the three patients with the central previa previously identified and one with marginal previa found during the second trimester. The authors chose, therefore, to name this condition "potential previa" when it is so identified during mid-gestation in order to clearly distinguish this sonographic condition from the true placenta previa at term. Studies have shown that transvaginal ultrasonography is informative with respect to the presence of placenta previa when third trimester hemorrhage necessitates diagnosis (Lim et al., 1989). Of considerable interest is the study by Guy et al. (1990) on patients with antepartum bleeding. They showed by transvaginal sonography of many patients with persistent previas that the intervillous blood flow is predominantly "lacunar." These patients also had a greater requirement for blood replacement subsequent to delivery. Oppenheimer et al. (1994) documented the "migration" by transvaginal sonography during the third trimester. When more migration occurred, then cesarean section was much less often needed. Magann et al. (1998) studied the "migration" of singleton placentas (n = 2526) at 18 weeks. They found that posterior implantation is more common than anterior (45.1% vs. 42.1%) and that these are more likely to migrate fundally than anterior-located implantations; they related it to a putative greater growth of the posterior uterus with advancing gestation. In contrast, Ghourab and Al-Jabari (2000) found that when a posterior placenta previa lay within 1 cm of the internal os or when it was a complete previa, it did not migrate in the third trimester. We have studied the rates of placental "migration" in low-lying placentas and placental previa (unpublished). Those patients who had placenta previa at delivery had slower rates of placental migration and more often had a deceleration pattern of placental migration. This suggests that abnormalities in the rates of placental migration may have more effect on the presence of placental previa than the original site of implantation. Higher rates of placenta accreta and manual removal of the placenta were also seen.

An incisive study of localization by indium scintigraphy and cobalt cervical marker comes from Nordlander et al. (1977; see also Nelp & Larson, 1967; Gustafson et al., 1974). Their rather clear-cut data are redrawn in Figure 13.1; they showed an anterior placenta in 98 instances and a posterior placenta in 80. An anterior placenta had a significantly greater chance of being low-lying, and the distance of the placental edge from the uterine internal cervical os increased with the age of the gestation. Attempts at making the exact diagnosis of placenta

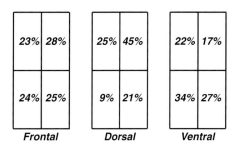

FIGURE 13.1. Distribution of placental location in quadrants when viewed from side (frontal) and with respect to anterior and posterior portions of the uterus. (*Source:* After Nordlander et al., 1977.)

previa during early gestation have ramifications for therapy. Thus, Arias (1988) reported that the use of cervical cerclage in the treatment of vaginal bleeding from placenta previa has merits as a temporary measure.

Volumetric Growth

Sonography has also remedied the absence of data about growth of the human placenta. In 1967 Boyd and Hamilton lamented that few studies on the in situ placenta were published. They presented their findings of 151 such specimens beyond the third month of gestation and found striking variations in the thickness of the placentas; they also reviewed the published data from many countries on placental growth. Their findings refuted the then prevalent thought of Grosser (1927) that placental expansion ceases after the 4th month of gestation. In their study, it was evident that continuous growth of the placental diameter could be measured up to 17.2 cm, with a surface area of 23,245 mm^2 at term. Conversely, Bleker et al. (1977), who measured the placental volume from 23 weeks on and expressed it from sonographic determinations of cross sections, found that growth in volume ceased well before term, peaking at 250 days and then even decreasing. Hoogland et al. (1980) suggested from their sonographic study of placental size at 150 days' menstrual age that this methodology is reliable only when the placenta occupies an anterior position. It is interesting to note that small size of the placenta foreshadowed low birth weight even at that early age. Reliable data on placental volume were also obtained sonographically by Wolf et al. (1979), who compared their measured volume with that of the delivered placenta in a water bath. Habib (2002) estimated volumetric growth sonographically and deduced that a placental diameter of less than 18 cm and

thickness of 2 cm at 36 weeks are prognostic indicators of growth restriction.

Abnormal Shapes ("Errors in Outline")

The term **error in outline** (Shanklin, 1958) is a rather descriptive and appropriate designation for a variety of placental forms. The placenta is rarely truly circular. More often it is oval, and not infrequently it has an irregular, often triangular shape that is presumably determined by its site of location, areas of atrophy, and perhaps the manner of its original implantation. The most striking abnormality is the placenta bilobata, two lobes being separated by a segment of membranes (Fig. 13.2). It stands to reason that these membranous vessels occasionally thrombose, or that they present clinically as vasa previa with bleeding. The second lobe is not always as large as the main lobe; it varies, becoming occasionally a much smaller lobe, which is then called a succenturiate (accessory) lobe. When the placental halves are connected by a broad or even a narrow band, one may classify the misshapen organ differently, according to the whim of the observer. Firm rules do not exist. It must also be acknowledged that vasa previa may bleed and still cause fetal problems because of compression of the vessels (Cordero et al., 1993).

Succenturiate lobes may occur singly or multiply, have a tendency to infarct, may present as placenta previa (Roth, 1957; Fig. 13.3), and they may be retained in utero after delivery. A wide spectrum of abnormalities exists here, and the incidence differs with the series published. Thus, Fujikura et al. (1970) found a "bipartite" (duplex) placenta in 4.2% of 8505 specimens collected in the Collaborative Perinatal Study. They found both multiparity

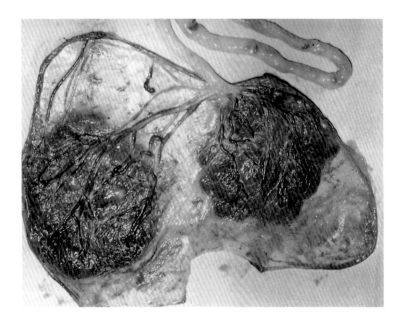

FIGURE 13.2. Bilobed placenta (duplex; bipartite). One disk was attached anteriorly, and the other was on the posterior wall of the uterus. Membranous vessels course from the characteristically velamentous insertion of the umbilical cord.

FIGURE 13.3. Succenturiate lobes in an immature placenta. Some of these lobes are infarcted (pallor) and would atrophy in time.

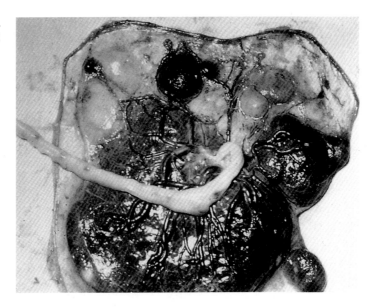

and relative sterility overrepresented in these women, as well as prenatal bleeding, placenta previa (Fig. 13.4), and retained placentas. They also commented on the fact that the cord usually inserts between the two lobes, as in Figure 13.4. Torpin and Barfield (1968), who clearly had the greatest interest in this condition, found that in one third of bilobed placentas the cord inserts on the larger lobe, and in two thirds it has a velamentous insertion. Occasionally, though, it takes its position on the smaller lobe (Fig. 13.5). Torpin and Hart (1941) had twice the incidence (8.6%) in their extensive historical review and reported on 355 cases. Usually, the placental lobes of bilobed organs had an anterior and a posterior location, and the larger lobe was usually marginate. The collar-shaped placenta reported by Keeler and Cope (1963) is but a variation of the theme. Likewise, the "pendulous

placental polyp" described by Thomas (1962), although unusual, probably merely represents an exceptional succenturiate lobe.

In our experience, succenturiate lobes occur in 5% to 6% of routinely examined placentas. One third of them are associated with some type of infarction of placental tissue, and occasional atrophy occurs between the extra lobe and the main placenta. This situation contrasts with the 13% overall incidence of infarcts without succenturiate lobes. Succenturiate lobes have been recognized by ultrasonography (Hata et al., 1988).

Other unusual shapes occur. Thus, Bergman (1961) reported on a placenta whose surface looked as though it was a loosely tied sac (a circumvallate placenta) and found that it was caused by a bicornuate uterus. Figure 13.6 shows a placenta fenestrata, one in which a central

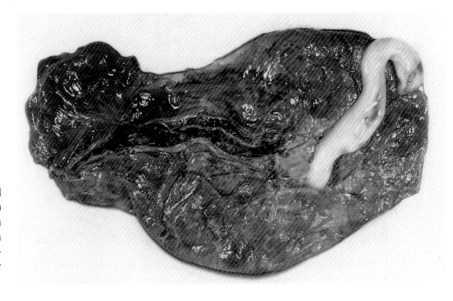

FIGURE 13.4. Succenturiate lobe (attached to the main placenta by a broad bridge) having necessitated cesarean section because it was positioned as a placenta previa. It is one of a number of such specimens. The accessory lobe is remarkably hemorrhagic.

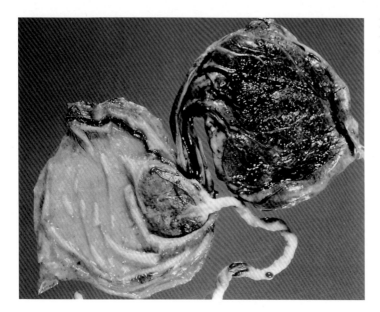

FIGURE 13.5. Large succenturiate (accessory) lobe from which the cord arises. No complications are evident. (Courtesy of Drs. Farsad and Gore, Birmingham, Alabama.)

portion is atrophied sufficiently to appear like the membranes. There was no cotyledon missing, and the cause (myoma?, possible site of cornual tubal orifice?) could not be ascertained. A similar condition must have prevailed in Greig's (1950) case of a central placenta previa with bulging membranes and hemorrhage. Another case of "placenta fenestrata" has since come to my attention. In this 29 weeks' gestation the fenestrated area was underlain by clot and located over the internal os, obviously having been a placenta previa at one time (courtesy of Dr. L. Matsumoto, 2004).

The mechanism by which succenturiate lobes and duplex placentas develop is unclear. It is relevant, however, that this placentation occurs nearly regularly in many catarrhine monkeys and has best been studied in the rhesus monkey. Torpin (1969b) found 75% of rhesus monkey placentas to be bidiscoid, whereas the other 25% had a single lobe, and he observed that the connecting vessels always course laterally, never otherwise. He made the important notation that atrophic villi are found in the membranes, implying that the blastocyst must have originally implanted interstitially and not, as had been

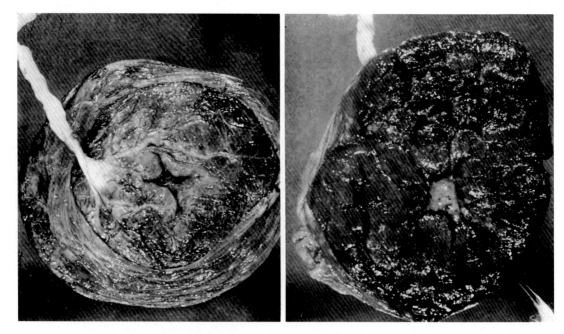

FIGURE 13.6. Placenta fenestrata. The central area of the placenta has a distinct defect, only chorionic membranes being present. No explanation was evident. (Courtesy of Dr. L.F. Moreno, Caracas, Venezuela.)

assumed, only superficially so as to reach both uterine surfaces. Because baboons are close relatives—indeed may mate and hybridize with rhesus monkeys—but have a single-disked placenta, their placental evolution was of interest to Chez et al. (1972). These authors found single disks in 22% of the 121 rhesus monkey placentas studied. They suggested that implantation is partially under genetic influence because some males were much more prone to father the single placentas. A clear-cut mode of genetic transmission was absent, but they searched for membranous villi, as did we (Benirschke & Miller, 1982), and found none. They concluded that these monkeys (but also baboons) have a more superficial implantation, supporting Heuser and Streeter's (1941) finding that the primary disk implants on day 9, and the secondary disk on day 14, but on the opposite side of the uterus. This differs clearly from human placentation and to date, then, a decisive answer of the origin of placentas with accessory lobes is outstanding. It is interesting, however, that at least half of the placentas with succenturiate lobes have areas of atrophy or frank infarction. This finding much supports the notion of a secondary conversion from more normal placentation. As with other anomalies, we await studies of the births of offspring from such abnormal placentas in order to ascertain possible genetic causes.

The condition "capped placenta" has been described by Defoort and Thiery (1988). This abnormal shape is characterized by having a cup or bell shape, and curvatures in two axes. These investigators studied the uncommon (0.8%) feature of bleeding during the second trimester. Previously, bleeding at that time had been considered to be most frequently a feature of a placenta previa-like implantation. Defoort and Thiery did not find it to be so. Circumvallate placentation, succenturiate lobes, low-lying placentas, and retroamnionic bleeding were found instead. In addition, 17 of their 63 cases (27%) were due to "capped placentas"—placentas with implantation on lateral, anterior, and posterior walls of the uterus. The lower portion of the placenta did not reach the uterine isthmus. Round or oval placentas are clearly the predominant forms of human placentas, abnormalities are rare. This is particularly the case for zonary (annular) placentas, which are the regular shapes of many carnivores. Steemers et al. (1995) described an annular placenta, sonographically diagnosed and with a velamentous cord insertion. It is likely that it derived from focal atrophy of low-lying villous tissue.

Placenta Previa

The term **placenta previa** refers to the location of the placenta over the internal os. The placenta is thus being "previous" to the delivering part of the baby. Low implantation is the cause, and the condition is of great medical concern. Placenta previa is the principal cause of third trimester bleeding, and it often necessitates an emergency cesarean section. Both mother and fetus may bleed in a life-threatening manner. The incidence is variably given as between 0.3% and 1.0% (even 3.0%) since the first publication of a large database by Strassmann (1902). Abnormal cord insertion and circumvallation are frequently present as well. Nielsen and colleagues (1989) found an incidence of 0.33% among 26,644 patients of placenta previa that necessitated abdominal delivery. The risk was 0.25% in "unscarred" uteri, compared to 1.22% in patients with previous cesarean section(s). These authors concluded that previous cesarean section predisposes to placenta previa and antenatal hemorrhage, a notion that was confirmed in the large review by Hemminki and Meriläinen (1996). Nevertheless, when Taylor et al. (1994) reexamined this relation and eliminated confounding factors, they found only a small influence of prior section as a cause. A large National statistical review by Iyasu et al. (1993) describes the overall incidence of placenta previa to be 4.8 per 1000 deliveries with a fatality of 0.03% of the cases; it was higher in black women than in white women. In addition, these authors ascertained a higher risk for abruptio, fetal malpresentation, postpartum hemorrhage, and cesarean section. For some as yet to be explained reason, placenta previa is reported as being more frequent in Asian women living in the United States (Taylor et al., 1995). When Miller et al. (1997a) examined the risk for placenta previa and accreta in 155,670 deliveries, they found that placenta accreta occurred in 29% when the placenta implanted over a previous section scar (6.5% when it was not there located). Their overall incidence of placenta accreta was 1:2500 deliveries, as compared with 10% in placenta previa.

Placenta previa has been the topic of a large body of literature. Many authors are concerned with optimal clinical management (Kellogg, 1943; Schmitz et al., 1954; Scott, 1964; Brenner et al., 1978; Khashoggi, 1995, and many others). Some investigators concern themselves mostly with the origin of the blood in the vaginal hemorrhage (Bartholomew et al., 1953; Hartemann et al., 1962; McShane et al., 1985). Yet others address fetal prematurity, early diagnosis, and its causes and relation to cervical pregnancy and placenta accreta. Ananth et al. (2003) found a 2.8% frequency in live births with a 10.7 rate of neonatal mortality compared to 2.5 in normal implantation when the pregnancy was >37 weeks, but not so in younger gestations. Salihu et al. (2003) studied the outcome of 3,773,369 live births in the U.S. and found a tripling of neonatal mortality with placenta previa.

It has become customary to subdivide placenta previa into several categories, such as "central" (total) and "partial" (lateral or marginal) placenta previa. Strassmann (1902) criticized rigid subdivisions and questioned their terminology. Despite this criticism, everyone understands the terms **central previa** and **marginal previa.** The former generally poses the greater threat and requires early diagnosis. Schmitz et al. (1954) separated their 112 cases (0.6%) into 31% total, 27% partial, and 42% low-lying previas. (The latter are somewhat dubiously included in this group.)

Tatum and Mulé (1965) evolved a complex "overlay" method of grading the previas (depending on cervical canal coverage if the cervix were allowed to completely efface). They found that their classification did not correlate well with effective clinical management. The term **low-lying previa** therefore is not a well-defined entity.

Brenner et al. (1978) surveyed 31,070 pregnancies (185 previas) and found an 0.6% overall frequency, with 0.12% of total previas. They confirmed the long-suspected correlation with multiparity (also older women), previous abortion, multiple births, and male infant. Surprisingly, prolapsed cord was also three times more common. Fetal and placental weights were not affected when corrected for fetal age. There was a significant association with fetal mortality, fetal anomalies, and low Apgar scores. Francois et al. (2003) found no increase of placenta previa with multiple gestations. Gabert (1971) also found normal fetal weights. Jopp and Krone (1966), on the other hand, reported significant fetal weight depression and increases in placental weight, which they attributed to compensatory placental hyperplasia. Higginbottom et al. (1975) also found lower than expected fetal weights and associated dysmaturity.

It is easy to understand that the maternal hemorrhage may originate from the placental margin or the disrupted intervillous space. There is, however, also significant neonatal anemia associated with the birth from a placenta previa, and it is the case more so when the maternal bleeding has been excessive (Wickster, 1952; McShane et al., 1985). This anemia is clearly due to the well recognized, but rarely recorded, fetal bleeding that occurs from disrupted placental villous vessels during labor (Bromberg et al., 1957; Hartemann et al., 1962; Bar-David et al., 1984). However, it may be difficult to detect the defects by placental examination (Wiener, 1948). Some authors found that fetomaternal bleeding also occurs (Zilliacus, 1964; Huntington, 1968). The neonatal anemia can result from the disruption that occurs when the placenta is cut during cesarean section, aspects that are well discussed by Schellong (1969).

The early diagnosis of placenta previa was once accomplished by arteriography (Borell et al., 1963) but is now readily made sonographically. Evidence for the frequent finding of previa placentation during early pregnancy and the subsequent "conversion" of such placentas previa to low-lying, nonprevias is reviewed in the section above. Wexler and Gottesfeld (1977, 1979) went so far as to consider this previa position as a "normal" variant of placentation, and Ballas et al. (1979) stated that it fre-

quently causes midtrimester vaginal bleeding. From their evaluation of the location of the placenta, these authors prognosticated the ultimate outcome by the extent of previa placental tissue. Many other investigators (e.g., Comeau et al., 1983) subsequently addressed this topic with an aim to improve fetal outcome in this common condition. Bartholomew et al. (1953) suggested a novel mechanism of bleeding in central placenta previa. They observed that in the central villous portion of the tissue that overlies the internal os there were numerous old clots, apparently from former bleeding episodes. They held these clots to be evidence of placental villous disruption and assumed that it is not the detachment of placenta from the decidua that causes the bleeding. Moreover, at the edge of the placenta, disruption of the "marginal sinus" may take place in marginal placenta previa, and thus lead to bleeding when the endocervix dilates during late gestation. These findings are currently supported by sonographic appearances (vide infra).

Marginal bleeding occurs frequently in ascending infection and chorioamnionitis (see Chapter 20); it then also often separates the edges of the placenta in the low-lying portion and is occasionally referred to as "abruptio." Harris (1988) reviewed this topic and considered it to be a distinct entity that is associated with minimal bleeding and prematurity. He distinguished it from placenta previa; in our opinion this is principally decidual bleeding that is secondary to deciduitis.

The pathology of placenta previa is easy to understand. The membranes have no free margin in the vaginally delivered placenta, and the edge of the placenta is frequently disrupted and hemorrhagic. Because there are often old clots at this site, these may vary from being laminated and brown, friable loose blood to partly decomposed material that is sometimes green from hemosiderin (Figs. 13.7 and 13.8; also see Fig. 13.16). The fetal vessels of the chorionic surface, when at the edge, may be disrupted.

According to Strassmann (1902), one often encounters some degree of circumvallation or margination. It is rarely reported in other series and is also not our experience. Strassmann also correlated the insertion of the umbilical cord with previas and found that the cord may insert anywhere but is more often near the site of the cervical os. That problem is certainly not the case in the placenta shown in Figure 13.7, and examples of the eccentric placental growth that made Strassmann such an ardent champion of the trophotropic expansion theory of placental tissue (expanding toward the better endometrial grounds above) are not often clearly seen.

Low-lying portions of placenta are occasionally either atrophied or infarcted. It is most often the case when the initially marginal previa has failed to develop, has undergone atrophy, and has thus become a "marginal" previa or better, a low-lying placenta. An intact uterus with an immature fetus from a placenta previa complication is

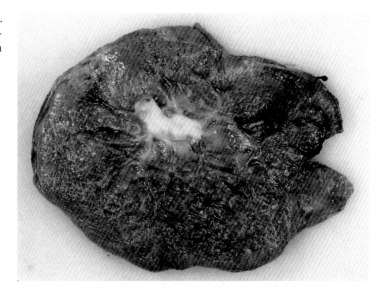

FIGURE 13.7. Placenta previa from cesarean section. Note the disruption and discoloration of the right, previa-pole of the placenta. The cord is centrally inserted in a "disperse vasculature" arrangement.

seen in Figure 13.9. The cervical canal and the forelying placental tissue betray the bleeding that had occurred. That the bleeding can be due to a succenturiate placental lobe has been described several times (Radcliffe et al., 1961; Van Huysen, 1961), and the condition has been observed in a variety of animals as well. These reports even included cases where placenta previa caused fetal exsanguination (Kingsley & Martin, 1979).

The cause of placenta previa is perhaps the most widely debated aspect of this anomaly. Obstetricians of the last century suggested much the same pathophysiology that we know today. It is aptly summarized in the long article by Strassmann (1902). Multiparity, advanced maternal age, previous abortions, and rapid succession of pregnancies are the principal factors. Studies have been contradictory as to whether induced abortions were (Barrett et al., 1981) or were not (Grimes & Techman, 1984) precursors of placenta previa. Grimes and Techman reviewed

the early literature that reported no such correlation; they also found no risk from preceding curettage. Thus, there is still dispute as to the main reasons for this condition. Strassmann believed that the placenta implanted low because of unsuitability of the fundal endometrium. He reasoned that in rapidly successive pregnancies the endometrium had not reconstituted sufficiently to become a site of implantation. His discussion included the putative *Haftfleck* (point of attachment) of Schatz that was disturbed by a previous pregnancy or abortion. Similar notions were reiterated by Nieminen and Klinge (1963), who discussed Iffy's (1962) theory of abnormal endocrine support. Although occasionally disputed, the dependence of placenta previa on maternal age and parity has been solidly supported by the findings of Penrose (1939) and Kalmus (1947). It has often been stated that placenta previa is significantly more common after a prior cesarean section, and the more sections, the greater the prob-

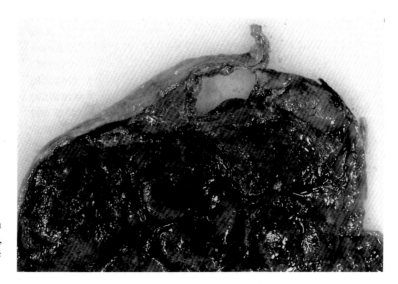

FIGURE 13.8. Maternal surface of the placenta in Figure 13.7. The old marginal clot is brown and friable, and the edge of the placenta is disrupted; the membranes are torn.

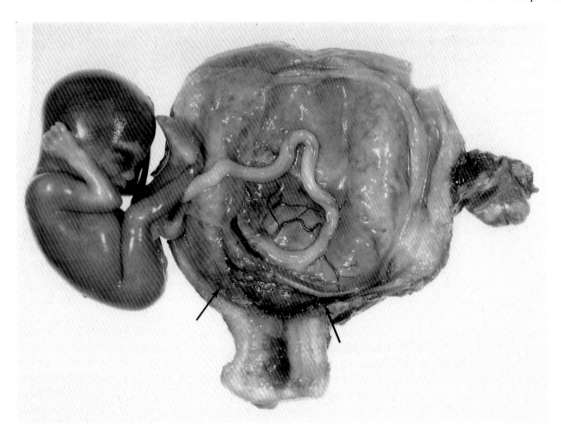

FIGURE 13.9. Placenta previa accreta. Hysterectomy was done at approximately 14 weeks (fetus is 10 cm crown–rump length). Note the endocervical blood and congested sickle-shaped previa (arrows).

ability of a previa (To & Leung, 1995; Ananth et al., 1997). Strangely, placenta previa is also said to be more common in users of cocaine (Macones et al., 1997). Rarely is a placenta previa found in association with incompetent cervix, but such may be difficult to diagnose as an independent condition when the previa has already led to hemorrhage (Ringrose, 1976). An extensive analysis of correlative factors has emerged from the oft-mentioned Collaborative Perinatal Study and was published by Naeye (1978). This author found no increase in fetal anomalies, and there was no association with maternal age in placenta previa. There was a relatively high perinatal mortality (11%) and increased fetal hematopoiesis (anemia?, stress?) as well as growth restriction were found. Moreover, contrary to many earlier reports, the placentas and fetal organs were lighter. The placental villi were interpreted to show hyperplasia. Nielsen et al. (1989) found a greater incidence after cesarean section in a large cohort.

There can be no doubt, however, that placenta previa is often associated with placenta accreta. In placenta accreta, the placenta fails to dislodge from the uterus after delivery of the newborn. When such a uterus is studied histologically, it is found that the villous tissue had not been attached to decidua, but that it had grown

onto the myometrium without intervening decidua. There is good evidence that placenta accreta is due to the failure of normal decidua to form, usually because the endometrium is deficient and cannot transform. Kistner et al. (1952) stated that the absence of the "spongious layer" of the decidua is the important feature. Thus, the trophoblast does not stop invading when it should, and it penetrates more broadly into muscle than is normal. Placenta accreta is also a regular finding in abdominal and tubal pregnancies, where there is also no normal endometrium to transform into decidua. A similar situation arises in the lower uterine segment and endocervix. Despite the thick nature of the endocervical mucosa, it does not follow the normal hormonal signals for decidualization, and when implantation occurs here, a placenta accreta forms. Although placenta previa accreta and cervical pregnancy are relatively rare, many reports (reviews by Kistner et al., 1952; Friesen, 1961) attest to the importance of this condition, which may endanger the mother's life because of afibrinogenemia, aside from the hemorrhage that takes place (Rosa et al., 1956; Koren et al., 1961; Khashoggi, 1995). Some authors note the frequency of prior cesarean section and curettage as being important (Rubenstone & Lash, 1963; Clark et al., 1985). Clark et al. believed that placenta previa and its variants are not rare, and cited a steady rise in case reports, whereas Comstock et al. (2004) stated that the condition of placenta accreta can be detected as early as at 15 to 20 weeks' gestation because of the sonographic "visualization of irregular vascular spaces within the placenta (placental lacunae)." More discussion is to be found in Chapter 9.

It is then surprising to find the study from Khong and Robertson (1987), which purported to negate the previous theories on the pathogenesis of placenta accreta and placenta previa accreta. Their novel view, which requires more discussion, is based on study of the placental bed in placenta accreta (inappropriately referred to as "creta"). Here they found a deficiency of the usual placental bed giant cells, a preponderance of uninuclear trophoblast, and a difference in the maternal vasculature in the areas of adherence. Moreover, they (as did other investigators) found that accretas may be focal and that, next to areas of adherence, there may be normal decidua, and that the decidua parietalis of such cases is also normal. From these findings they deduced that "there is a defective interaction between maternal tissues, particularly decidua, and migratory trophoblast in early stages of placentation, resulting in undue adherence of the placenta or penetration into the uterus coupled with the development of an abnormal uteroplacental circulation." In other words, they believed that absent decidua is not the primary event, as is our opinion and that held by most previous students of the matter. This concept is contrary to all other findings made in studies of this disease. Similar findings of accreta placentation are regularly made with ectopic pregnancy, in both the tubal and abdominal varieties. Although occasional decidualization of tubal mucosa does occur, it is uncommon, and true decidua in ectopic pregnancy is rare. One must be able to differentiate decidual cells from X

cells (extravillous trophoblast), which is not always easy for pathologists. A recent study by Kim et al. (2004) suggests that an excess of intermediate trophoblast is found in accretas, and the authors suggested a relationship of this excess to the development of accretas. They examined 56 hysterectomy specimens, 34 with and 22 without accreta, using immunohistochemistry with the cell adhesion molecule marker CD146 that is expressed by these X cells. They found a significant increase in confluent masses of extravillous trophoblast with the myometrium in accretas, as in ectopic tubal gestations and related this to the development of accretas. There was no significant increase in multinuclear trophoblastic cells. In addition, they reviewed older theories of deficient or increased enzymes as being the principal cause of the formation of placenta accreta. Our belief is that the really primary aspect is the deficient decidua basalis, and that in that deficiency, the infiltrating trophoblast assumes different behaviors. It is not unusual, however, to find a few myometrial fibers in the basal plate of delivered placenta near spiral arteries and especially in prematurely delivered organs (9.5% by Sherer et al., 1996), without this representing true accretas. Minimal accretas, not necessitating hysterectomy, were found occasionally by Jacques et al. (1996) in careful placental studies, especially following previous cesarean sections (see also Sarantopoulos & Natarajan, 2002) (Fig. 13.10). Placenta accreta is also an occasional finding during evacuation in the second trimester (Rashbaum et al., 1995), and Ophir et al. (1999) found an increase in creatine kinase with these conditions. Mussalli et al. (2000) suggested conservative therapy for accretes with methotrexate.

Placenta accreta is also typical for endocervical implantation and in uteri that were altered focally by curettage or by the scars of cesarean section. Khong and Robertson

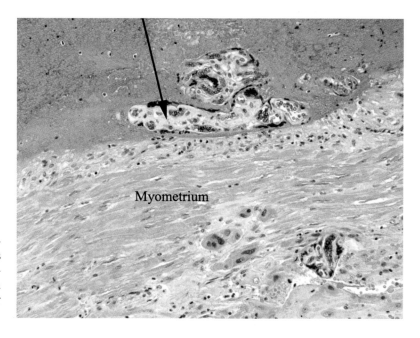

FIGURE 13.10. Microscopic region of focal placenta accreta showing absence of decidua basalis and extravillous trophoblast infiltrating myometrium. Otherwise this is a normal term placenta and there was no history of former curettage or cesarean section.

(1987) dismissed the analogy of deficient decidua in tubal pregnancy by saying that these pregnancies rarely go to term. [Augensen (1983) described an exception and reviewed the literature; *vide infra*. Similarly, Steyn and Gebhardt (1999) had a stillbirth at 35 weeks—2250 g—from a ruptured tubal gestation and stated that this is not so infrequent in South Africa because of the frequency of salpingitis.] True enough, but the reason for the usual failure of ectopic pregnancies to reach term is that the accretas of tubal pregnancy usually become placentas percretas with bleeding. This point has also been emphasized by Pauerstein et al. (1986), who recommended local resection on that basis. Moreover, many term tubal pregnancies have indeed been observed (e.g., Frachtman, 1953; Miller, 1987).

In our opinion, the adherent placental bed morphology betrays the ill-understood interactions between trophoblast and normal decidua. After all, why is it that not every pregnancy results in placenta accreta? The trophoblast stops destroying the endometrium or decidua at a given point in placentation and leaves (in humans) a portion of decidua basalis untouched. It is not so in all species, as in the *Dasypodidae*, where the superficial myometrium is also differently constructed. This failure to destroy all of the decidua basalis in human gestations may be related to temporal changes in the trophoblast's behavior, carefully timed genetically; or it may be that the decidua plays a specific role in this delimitation of the advancing invasion by trophoblastic cells (see Chapter 5). This is not to say that some of the advancing trophoblast does not reach deeper into the mouths of vessels and into the myometrium; it certainly does. A primary deficiency of decidual transformation or of the depth of endometrium/decidua, however, still best explains the placenta accreta. The findings described by Khong and Robertson (1987) may be explained as sequelae of absent decidua rather than as its cause. Parenthetically, we agree with their statement that the presence of adenomyosis as a basis of placenta accreta has been vastly overrated in the past.

Cramer (1987) described a placenta increta that had invaded and partially destroyed the leiomyoma on which it rested. From this finding he deduced that accretas/incretas are due to overly aggressive trophoblast, rather than decidual deficiency. He believed it to be the cause, not only in this case but also of other accretas. He reasoned that the ability of decidua to produce laminin, fibronectin, collagen type IV, and proteoglycans (Wewer et al., 1986) may be defective, and suggested that the normal balance of the placental invasiveness and the decidua to resist invasion may be disturbed in accretas. Rice et al. (1989), who studied pregnancies complicated by leiomyomas, found that retroplacental tumors were significantly frequently complicated by abruptio placentae. It might be mentioned here parenthetically that Arcangeli and Pasquarette (1997) observed the rupture of a uterus at 26

weeks' gestation after laparoscopic myolysis of a leiomyoma had been done months before pregnancy. Spontaneous rupture of an unscarred uterus seldom occurs (review by Miller et al., 1997b). In this connection, **placenta percreta** needs to be discussed separately and in more detail because of the apparent increase reported in the recent literature and because of our increasing concern with this formerly rare condition. It is frequently associated with uterine rupture, major maternal problems, stillbirths, and placenta accreta/increta. There is little doubt that structural abnormalities of the uterus can lead to uterine rupture during pregnancy without it having been "scarred" earlier; but that is uncommon. Much the most frequent antecedent condition is prior cesarean section with dehiscence of the scar and thus mimicking a "percreta." Because this relates to the overall conditions subsumed under trophoblastic invasion, the topic is covered extensively in Chapter 9; it is of great current relevance.

Placenta Membranacea

Placenta membranacea is an unusual abnormality of placental form. Although some authors have estimated its occurrence to be 1 in 3300 pregnancies, this approximation is a gross overestimate. Although the entity was described as early as 1807, only a handful of references can be found on placenta membranacea. Many cases are hidden in the literature on placenta accreta. Thus, of the 622 cases of placenta accreta gathered by Fox (1972) for his report, seven were placentas membranacea. Although it is true that some membranaceae are also accretas, it is not the case for all. The placenta membranacea (diffusa) is an organ in which all, or nearly all, of the circumference of the fetal sac is covered by villous tissue. The placental mass is generally thin (1 to 2 cm), and it is often disrupted (Figs. 13.11 and 13.12). Although one may suggest that placenta membranacea is a variant of extensive succenturiate lobe formation, we do not believe it to be the case. There is never a separation or even a hint of segregation of tissue from a main placental disk; the tissue is uniformly thin. This type of placental anomaly has been likened to the placenta found in Suidae, Equidae, and Cetacea. It is not an appropriate comparison, however, because these orders of mammals do not have an invasive placenta. Only a superficial macroscopic similarity to the animals' placentas exists, and it is thus not appropriate to speak of "atavism."

Placenta membranacea manifests frequently clinically as early bleeding and placenta previa. Affected pregnancies often also terminate in premature delivery, but not invariably. They also may incur difficulties with placental separation after delivery. The literature on placenta membranacea has been reviewed by Finn (1954) and Janovski and Granowitz (1961); later cases were reported by

FIGURE 13.11. Placenta membranacea at 35 weeks' gestation. Virtually no free membranes are seen: the placenta is very thin. Patient had recurrent bleeding necessitating hysterotomy.

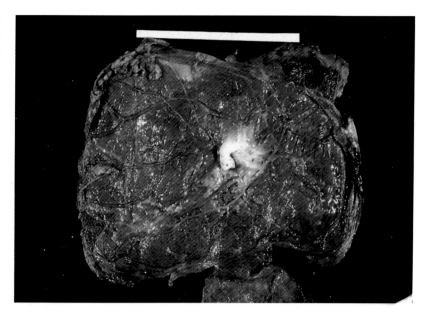

Mathews (1974), Las Heras et al. (1982), and Hurley and Beischer (1987). A complete review of this unusual anomaly comes from Ekoukou et al. (1995), who found only 36 cases to be reported. More recently, Ahmed and Gilbert-Barness (2003) described three cases without finding an etiologic factor. In fact, the etiology of placenta membranacea is not understood. It is easy to state that those villi that are destined to become the chorion laeve do not atrophy normally and that there is endometrial hypoplasia on "constitutional" or other grounds; but, in general, no author has presented support for these hypotheses. The fact that the anomaly often presents with middle trimester bleeding and is thus often diagnosed with placenta accreta may merely reflect that placenta membranacea also overlies the internal os and thereby has a chance of becoming a placenta previa accreta. Occasional cases, such as the one depicted in the previous edition of this book, may have other areas of accretion. Most reported patients delivered their placentas without evidence of accreta. There has not been any associated fetal growth restriction.

One of the cases, described by Finn (1954), is of particular interest. He was the obstetrician for this "infant" 27 years after her birth. She delivered a macerated, stillborn fetus at 5 months, after several weeks of bleeding. This placenta, just like that associated with her own birth, was a typical placenta membranacea (Finn, personal communication, 1976). Thus, either genetic influences determined

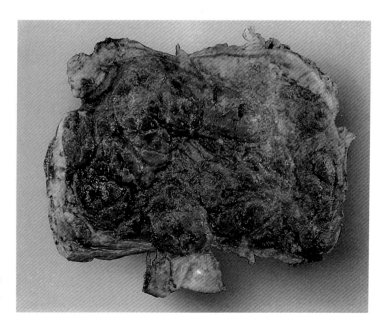

FIGURE 13.12. Maternal surface of Figure 13.11, showing old clot but the absence of accreta in this placenta membranacea.

this abnormal placenta, or it was the result of an abnormal uterine environment that was under genetic control. It seems highly improbable that such a rare anomaly would occur twice within this one pedigree by accident.

Circumvallate Placenta (Extrachorial, Circummarginate Placentas)

Some writers have regarded the circumvallate placenta to be clinically important; others have stated that it is a clinically meaningless deviation from normal. In circumvallate placentas, the membranes of the chorion laeve insert not at the edge of the placenta but at some inward distance from the margin, toward the umbilical cord. At the margin, one usually finds variable amounts of fibrin, with recent and old blood. At times, a striking number of such deposits are present. In typical circumvallates, there is a truly complete circumferential ring that severely restricts the total surface of the chorion frondosum. At the periphery, "naked" placental tissue protrudes, which is the reason for the designation **placenta extrachorialis.** This condition should not be confused with the placenta accompanying an extramembranous fetus, a placental anomaly that occurs after early rupture of the membranes with the fetus lying in the endometrial cavity and outside the membranous sac. This situation is not the case with ordinary circumvallate placentas, although, as is seen in the considerations of the extramembranous pregnancy, in that condition there is also a striking circumvallation present (see Chapter 11). When no typical plication of the membranes occurs at the margin, and when the edge of the protruding placenta is covered only by some fibrin, we speak of a circummarginate placenta.

These two forms blend into each other, and partial circumvallation is common. The incidence of these

TABLE 13.1. Reported frequency of circumvallate and circummarginate placentas

Authors	No. of studies	Circumvallate (%)	Circummarginate (%)
Scott (1960)	3,161	18.3% extrachorial	
Ziel (1963)	40,143	0.62	
Wilson and Paalman (1967)	10,927	1.0	
Wentworth (1968)	895	6.5	25.5
Benson and Fujikura (1969)	39,514	3.6 (whites) 2.0 (blacks)	3.3 (whites) 3.4 (blacks)
Fox and Sen (1972)	3,000	2.4	22
Benirschke (this series)	13,537	5.25	

common conditions is listed in Table 13.1, which was compiled from several large prospectively and retrospectively collected series. Circumvallates are rarely found during the first trimester, although Meyer (1909) and Torpin (1966) depicted uteri at 3.5 months with intact circumvallate placentas. Most authors agree that circumvallation is often complicated by prenatal bleeding and premature delivery.

Two characteristic circumvallate placentas with different amounts of extrachorial tissue are illustrated in Figures 13.13 and 13.14, and Figure 13.15 shows a typical circummarginate placenta. Variations between these degrees are frequent. Gross examination of such placentas often shows yellow-brown discolored marginal fibrin, testifying to its origin from hematomas. In cases where this anomaly is the cause of midtrimester hemorrhage and premature delivery, one may find a substantial amount of blood at the margin. It may undermine the margin of the placenta and may thus initiate a clinical picture of abruptio placentae. Although much of this

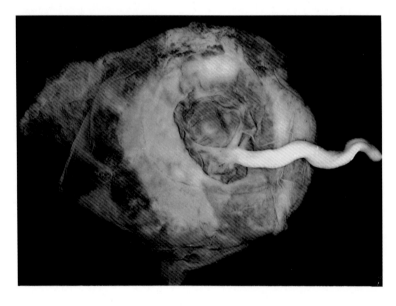

FIGURE 13.13. Typical circumvallate placenta at approximately 35 weeks' gestation. Note the small surface area of the remaining chorion frondosum and large white fibrin ring at the periphery.

FIGURE 13.14. There is a lesser degree of circumvallation than in Figure 13.13.

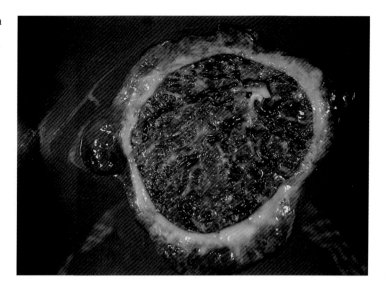

blood comes from the maternal vessels, the bleeding may be so significant that it elevates the chorion laeve from the site of its insertion and then disrupts the fetal vessels (Fig. 13.16). Thus, the hematoma and vaginal bleeding are frequently of mixed maternal and fetal origin. In some cases, it is the mechanism of neonatal anemia (Mitchell et al., 1957). Scott (1960) superbly investigated the structure of the margins of extrachorial pregnancies and found evidence that the chorion, once upon a time, must have been more marginally inserted. When he injected placental vessels with radiopaque dye and placed a wire around the insertion sites of the membranes, he found pictures such as that shown in Figure 13.17. Here one can see that the fetal surface vessels pursue a horizontal course way past the wire circumference before they dip vertically

into the placental tissue. It indicates that the vessels must have been running in chorion initially, before this membrane was dislodged by the hematoma; this is dramatically shown in Figure 13.16. The bleeding was so acute in this case that many fetal vessels were severed. This old blood accumulated at the margin, hemolyzed, and changed into fibrin-like deposits that cover up the old horizontal vessels. It is also the cause of the discoloration. Hemosiderin is often found in the more extensive cases. This fibrin causes the plica to form that is so characteristic of circumvallates (Figs. 13.18 and 13.19). The amnion may follow the chorion into this plica, or most commonly, it flatly covers the plica without infolding.

Because circumvallation is so frequent, this anomaly has been investigated many times to explain its formal

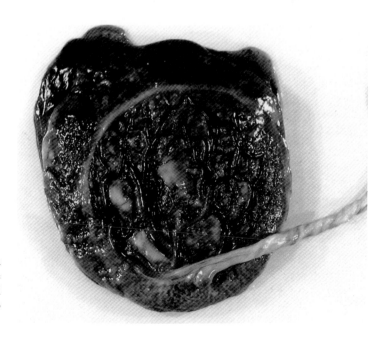

FIGURE 13.15. Sickle-shaped circummarginate placenta with free villous tissue protruding beyond the membrane insertion. This point, combined with the near-marginal insertion of the cord at the opposite end, is considered to reflect trophotropism.

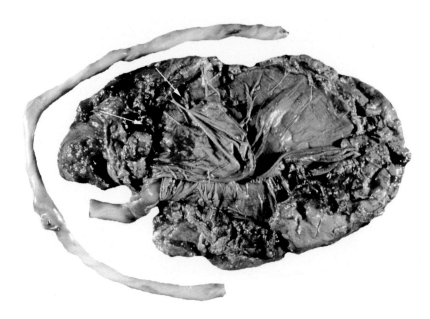

FIGURE 13.16. Immature placenta from an exsanguinated premature infant. Massive old and recent blood clot was circumferentially present; it has been partially removed to show the stretched and occasionally interrupted fetal vessels (arrows) through which the fetus bled. The membranes were brown from deposits of hematoidin and hemosiderin, and from hemolyzed blood.

genesis. As a result, numerous theories have been proposed. Several opposing ideas have been presented without, it is fair to say, firm resolution that would be acceptable to all. Schatz (1886) reviewed older writings with which he strongly disagreed. He contended that circumvallates arise because the embryonic mass implants too superficially. That concept was supported by Hertig and Gore (1969). The opposite view has been defended by Torpin (1953, 1955, 1965, 1966). He confessed a life-long preoccupation with understanding the etiology of these abnormal placental forms. Torpin believed that the evidence points to excessively deep implantation of the blastocyst into a "fungating," hyperplastic decidua. He concurred with Gottschalk's (1891) opinion. That view-

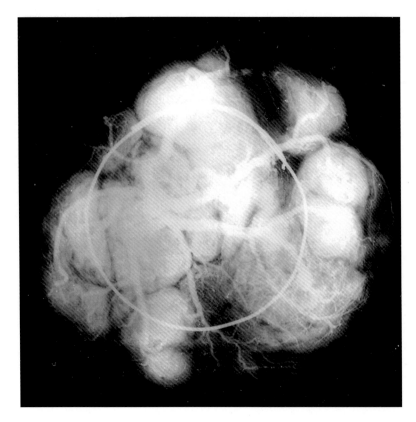

FIGURE 13.17. Radiograph of placenta "extrachorialis" (circumvallate) whose fetal vessels were injected with barium sulfate. The circular wire marks the edge of the chorionic plate. Note the many chorionic vessels pursuing a straight course past the edge of the membranes' insertion. (*Source:* Scott, 1960, with permission.)

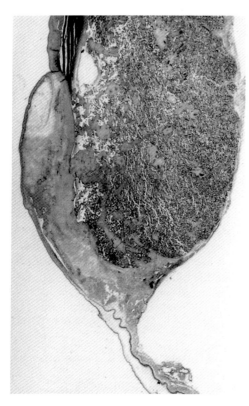

FIGURE 13.18. Margin of circumvallate placenta. The gray, homogeneous material under the plica represents fibrin and degenerating clot. Note that the amnion is not infolding with the chorion in this example, as is otherwise so often the case. H&E. ×4.

point, expressed many years earlier, was a dissenting voice against Schatz's superficial ("polypoid") placentation theory. Nevertheless, this superficial implantation theory has become the predominant thought in our texts, perhaps because of the eminence of Schatz (1886) and Meyer (1909). Likewise, the pronouncements of Williams (1927) carried much weight in the United States. Williams

had done a study of circumvallate placentas and opined that "all had been said" about the theories of its genesis. He further suggested that we discard the term **marginata** (circummarginate). His opinions included claims that true circumvallation occurs in less than 2% of deliveries, and he supported the notion of superficial implantation.

A challenging consideration of pathogenesis is that which was originally enunciated by Liepmann (1906). He saw several early circumvallates, one of which clearly related to premature loss of amnionic fluid. Exactly the same mechanism takes place in all extramembranous pregnancies, which are some of the most classical examples of circumvallate placentation (see Chapter 12). Liepmann proposed that the marginal infolding derives from *Stauchung* (impaction, collision, jamming), the failure of the sac to be held open. Later students have either confirmed Torpin's view (Wentworth, 1968) or were noncommittal (Scott, 1960).

All theories seem to suggest that there is only one way for circumvallates to originate, whereas in fact there may be different types and origins. Reduced amnionic fluid pressure distending the sac in extramembranous pregnancy clearly speaks as an etiologic moment in those cases. When significant hemorrhage occurs circumferentially, as can happen with middle trimester abortion, it may be the primary cause of circumvallation. When a middle trimester placenta previa changes to a marginal insertion at the lower segment and the fundal portion expands, it may be the origin of the sickle-shaped, so-called marginatas. The terms **placenta marginata** and **circummarginate placenta** are poor ones, and most authors consider these placentas to be part of the spectrum of circumvallation. These terms should be abandoned. When the apposing membranous sacs of twins exert differential pressures on one another, the meeting point is often discordant with the placental bed. That is, the membranes often do not meet exactly over the place where the respective placental areas terminate. They are frequently

FIGURE 13.19. Plica of the circumvallate margin with a wire holding up the overhanging margin of the membrane insertion, showing the simultaneous infolding of the amnion.

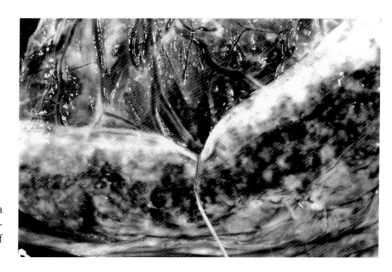

pushed away from this "equator," and "bare" placental tissue exists; at least it is covered by the membranes of the other twin. It, too, is a form of extrachorial placenta. If, as has been suggested, a polypoid, superficial implantation were the cause of circumvallation, one might find fewer atrophied villi in the chorion laeve. This possibility had already been entertained by Torpin (1969a), and we have looked for such a possible deficiency in rolled membranes of normal and circumvallate placentas as well. We found that there was a high degree of variation in the number of villi so discovered, but circumvallates often did have such atrophic villi. Harbert et al. (1970) described three circumvallates in rhesus monkeys that had only a single disk (instead of their normal two-disked placenta). Harbert et al. evaluated the respective interrelations of these anomalies and concluded that if they were indeed related it would mean that the cause must have been aberrant trophoblastic behavior before the 17th day of pregnancy. Johnson et al. (1978) had two similar cases in stumptailed macaques. Suzuki (1971), however, found two circumvallates in two-disked rhesus placentas. This finding negates the hypothesis of Harbert and colleagues (1970). Because of the relative frequency of single-disked placentas in macaques (25%), the concurrences of the two conditions may be merely happenstance.

As stated earlier, "true" circumvallates are correlated with prenatal bleeding, premature termination of pregnancy, multiparity, abruptio, and early fluid loss (Ziel, 1963; Naftolin et al., 1973), and occasionally it is familial (Deacon et al., 1974). For a consideration of clinical significance, it must be cautioned that the term **circumvallate** is not used uniformly by all pathologists and obstetricians, which is perhaps one reason for the marked differences in the reported incidence (1% to 7%) and for the confusion with the so-called marginatas. Moreover, many circumvallates masquerade clinically as abruptios. Elliott et al. (1998) have written about chronic abruption with oligohydramnios, representing perhaps one end of the spectrum of this entity. Our data include only cases such as are shown in Figures 13.13, 13.14, and 13.16, but not Figure 13.15. Lademacher et al. (1981), who favored a genetic etiology of this anomaly, identified significantly higher frequencies of perinatal death (11% versus 3%), premature deliveries (37% versus 13%), congenital anomalies (15% versus 4%), and single umbilical artery (SUA) with circumvallate placentation. It was true also for circummarginates, where the figures were 3%, 25%, and 4%, respectively. In a study of 3000 consecutive deliveries, Fox and Sen (1972) again suggested that circummarginates have no clinical importance but that circumvallates associate significantly frequently with threatened abortion, premature labor, and fetal growth restriction. To this list some authors (Morgan, 1955) have added that circumvallation is associated with a higher maternal morbidity rate due to postpartum hemorrhage

and the more frequent need for manual removal of the placenta. Repeated occurrence of circumvallate placentas in successive pregnancies has been reported occasionally (Wilson & Paalman, 1967).

Benson and Fujikura (1969) concluded, after an exhaustive analysis of the 39,514 pregnancies in the Collaborative Perinatal Study, that "despite some well-documented obstetric-pediatric complications, extrachorial placenta is an uncommon, rarely serious clinical problem." They further believed that "our finding of minimal correlation between these morphologic variations and clinical abnormalities is due to the prospective nature of the study." We doubt that everyone would agree with this statement. Rolschau (1978), for instance, found this placentation to be correlated with single umbilical artery, growth restriction, and an increased incidence of prematurity. Other authors found similar results from large studies of prospectively collected placentas.

References

Ahmed, A. and Gilbert-Barness, E.: Placenta membranacea: a developmental anomaly with diverse clinical presentation. Pediat. Developm. Pathol. **6**:201–202, 2003.

Ananth, C.V., Smulian, J.C. and Vintzileos, A.M.: The association of placenta previa with history of cesarean delivery and abortion: A metaanalysis. Amer. J. Obstet. Gynecol. **177**:1071–1078, 1997.

Ananth, C.V., Smulian, J.C. and Vintzileos, A.M.: The effect of placenta previa on neonatal mortality: A population-based study in the United States, 1989 through 1997. Amer. J. Obstet. Gynecol. **188**:1299–1304, 2003.

Arcangeli, S. and Pasquarette, M.M.: Gravid uterine rupture after myolysis. Obstet. Gynecol. **89**:857, 1997.

Arias, F.: Cervical cerclage for temporary treatment of patients with placenta previa. Obstet. Gynecol. **71**:545–548, 1988.

Augensen, K.: Unruptured tubal pregnancy at term with survival of mother and child. Obstet. Gynecol. **61**:259–261, 1983.

Ballas, S., Gitstein, S., Jaffa, A.J. and Peyser, M.R.: Midtrimester placenta previa: normal or pathologic finding. Obstet. Gynecol. **54**:12–14, 1979.

Bar-David, J., Piura, B., Leiberman, J.R. and Kaplan, H.: Discrimination between fetal and maternal blood. Amer. J. Obstet. Gynecol. **148**:352, 1984.

Barrett, J.H., Boehm, F.H. and Killam, A.P.: Induced abortion: a risk factor for placenta previa. Amer. J. Obstet. Gynecol. **141**:769–772, 1981.

Bartholomew, R.A., Colvin, E.D., Grimes, W.H., Fish, S.S. and Lester, W.M.: Hemorrhage in placenta previa: a new concept of its mechanism. Obstet. Gynecol. **1**:41–45, 1953.

Benirschke, K. and Miller, C.J.: Anatomical and functional differences in the placenta of primates. Biol. Reprod. **26**:29–53, 1982.

Benson, R.C. and Fujikura, T.: Circumvallate and circummarginate placenta. Unimportant clinical entities. Obstet. Gynecol. **34**:799–804, 1969.

Bergman, P.: Accidental discovery of uterus bicornis on examination of placenta. Obstet. Gynecol. **17**:649, 1961.

Bleker, O.P., Kloosterman, G.J., Breur, W. and Mieras, D.J.: The volumetric growth of the human placenta: a longitudinal ultrasonic study. Amer. J. Obstet. Gynecol. **127**:657–661, 1977.

Booth, R.T., Wood, C., Beard, R.W., Gibson, J.R.M. and Pinkerton, J.H.M.: Significance of site of placental attachment in uterus. Brit. Med. J. **1**:1732–1734, 1962.

Borell, U., Fernström, I. and Ohlson, L.: Diagnostic value of arteriography in cases of placenta previa. Amer. J. Obstet. Gynecol. **86**:535–547, 1963.

Boyd, J.D. and Hamilton, W.J.: Development and structure of the human placenta from the end of the 3rd month of gestation. J. Obstet. Gynaecol. **74**:161–226, 1967.

Brenner, W. E., Edelman, D.A. and Hendricks, C.H.: Characteristics of patients with placenta previa and results of "expectant management." Amer. J. Obstet. Gynecol. **132**:180–191, 1978.

Bromberg, Y.M., Salzberger, M. and Abrahamov, A.: Foetal blood in genital haemorrhage due to placenta praevia and abruptio placentae. Lancet **1**:767, 1957.

Castro, L.C., Hobel, C.J., Walla, C., Ortiz, L. and Platt, L.D.: Placental migratory patterns and birthweight. Amer. J. Obstet. Gynecol. **172**:346 (abstract 309), 1995.

Chez, R.A., Schlesselman, J.J., Salazar, H. and Fox, R.: Single placentas in the rhesus monkey. J. Med. Primatol. **1**:230–240, 1972.

Clark, S.L., Koonings, P.P. and Phelan, J.P.: Placenta previa/accreta and prior cesarean section. Obstet. Gynecol. **66**:89–92, 1985.

Comeau, J., Shaw, L., Marcell, C.C. and Lavery, J.P.: Early placenta previa and delivery outcome. Obstet. Gynecol. **61**:577–580, 1983.

Comstock, C.H., Love, J.J., Bronsteen, R.A., Lee, W., Vettraino, I.M., Huang, R.R. and Lorenz, R.P.: Sonographic detection of placenta accreta in the second and third trimesters of pregnancy. Amer. J. Obstet. Gynecol. **190**:1135–1140, 2004.

Cordero, D.R., Helfgott, A.W., Landy, H.J., Reik, R.F., Medina, C. and O'Sullivan, M.J.: A non-hemorrhagic manifestation of vasa previa: A clinicopathologic case report. Obstet. Gynecol. **82**:698–700, 1993.

Cramer, S.F.: Letter to the editor: case report. Pediatr. Pathol. **7**:473–475, 1987.

Deacon, J.S.R., Gilbert, E.F., Visekul, C., Herrmann, J. and Opitz, J.M.: Polyhydramnios and neonatal hemorrhage in three sisters: a circumvallate placenta syndrome. Birth Defects **10**:41–49, 1974.

Defoort, S.S. and Thiery, W.M.: Capping placenta: A new etiologic factor in midtrimester bleeding. Z. Geburtshilfe Perinatol. **192**:33–35, 1988.

Ekoukou, D., Tin, L.N.W., Nere, M.B., Bourdet, O., Elaloui, Y. and Bazin, C.: Placenta membranacea. Revue de la literature, a propos d'un cas. J. Gynecol. Obstet. Biol. Reprod. **78**:189–193, 1995.

Elliott, J.P., Gilpin, B., Strong, T.H.Jr. and Finberg, H.J.: Chronic abruption—oligohydramnios sequence. J. Reprod. Med. **43**: 418–422, 1998.

Finn, J.L.: Placenta membranacea. Obstet. Gynecol. **3**:438–440, 1954.

Fox, H.: Placenta accreta, 1945–1969. Obstet. Gynecol. Surv. **27**: 475–490, 1972.

Fox, H. and Sen, D.K.: Placenta extrachorialis. A clinico-pathologic study. J. Obstet. Gynaecol. Brit. Commonw. **79**:32–35, 1972.

Frachtman, K.G.: Unruptured tubal term pregnancy. Amer. J. Surg. **86**:161–168, 1953.

Francois, K., Johnson, J.M. and Harris, C.: Is placenta previa more common in multiple gestations? Amer. J. Obstet. Gynecol. **188**:1226–1227, 2003.

Fried, A.M.: Distribution of the bulk of the normal placenta: review and classification of 800 cases by ultrasonography. Amer. J. Obstet. Gynecol. **132**:675–680, 1978.

Friesen, R.F.: Placenta previa accreta. Can. Med. Assoc. J. **84**:1247–1253, 1961.

Fujikura, T., Benson, R.C. and Driscoll, S.G.: The bipartite placenta and its clinical features. Amer. J. Obstet. Gynecol. **107**: 1013–1017, 1970.

Gabert, H.A.: Placenta previa and fetal growth. Obstet. Gynecol. **38**:403–406, 1971.

Gallagher, P., Fagan, C.J., Bedi, D.G., Winsett, M.Z. and Reyes, R.N.: Potential placenta previa: definition, frequency, and significance. A.J.R. **149**:1013–1015, 1987.

Ghourab, S. and Al-Jabari, A.: Placental migration and mode of delivery in placenta previa: Transvaginal sonographic assessment during the third trimester. Ann. Saudi Med. **20**:382–385, 2000.

Gottesfeld, K.R., Thompson, H.E., Holmes, J.H. and Taylor, E. D.: Ultrasonic placentography—a new method for placental localization. Amer. J. Obstet. Gynecol. **96**:538–547, 1966.

Gottschalk, S.: Weitere Studien über die Entwicklung der menschlichen Placenta. Arch. Gynäkol. **40**:169–244, 1891.

Greig, C.: Central placenta previa with bulging bag of membranes. J. Obstet. Gynaecol. Brit. Emp. **57**:251–252, 1950.

Grimes, A.A. and Techman, T.: Legal abortion and placenta previa. Amer. J. Obstet. Gynecol. **149**:501–504, 1984.

Grosser, O.: Frühentwicklung, Eihautbildung und Placentation des Menschen und der Säugetiere. Bergmann, München, 1927.

Gustafson, H., Nordlander, S., Westin, B. and Asard, P.-E.: Placenta praevia and abruptio placentae. Acta Obstet. Gynecol. Scand. **53**:235–241, 1974.

Guy, G.P., Peisner, D.P. and Timor-Tritsch, I.E.: Ultrasonographic evaluation of uteroplacental blood flow patterns of abnormally located and adherent placentas. Amer. J. Obstet. Gynecol. **163**:723–727, 1990.

Habib, F.A.: Prediction of low birth weight infants from ultrasound measurement of placental diameter and placental thickness. Ann. Saudi Med. **22**:312–314, 2002.

Harbert, G.M., Martin, C.B. and Ramsey, E.M.: Extrachorial (circumvallate) placentas in rhesus monkeys. Amer. J. Obstet. Gynecol. **108**:98–104, 1970.

Harris, B.A. Jr.: Peripheral placental separation: a review. Obstet. Gynecol. Surv. **43**:577–581, 1988.

Harris, V.G.: Relation between placental site and length of gestation. Brit. J. Obstet. Gynaecol. **82**:581–584, 1975.

Hartemann, J., Dellestable, P. and Pierce, A.: L'anémie des enfants de placenta praevia. Bull. Féd. Soc. Gynécol. Fr. **14**:422–424, 1962.

Hata, K., Hata, T., Aoki, S., Takamori, H., Takamiya, O. and Kitao, M.: Succenturiate placenta diagnosed by ultrasound. Gynecol. Obstet. Invest. **25**:273–276, 1988.

Hemminki, E. and Meriläinen, J.: Long-term effects of cesarean sections: ectopic pregnancies and placental problems. Amer. J. Obstet. Gynecol. **174**:1569–1574, 1996.

Hertig, A.T. and Gore, H.: Die Implantation, die Frühentwicklung des befruchteten Eies und ihre Störungen. In, Gynäkologie und Geburtshilfe. Vol. I. O. Käser, V. Friedberg, K.G. Ober, K. Thomsen and J. Zander, eds. pp. 565–584. Georg Thieme, Stuttgart, 1969.

Hertig, A.T. and Rock, J.: Searching for early fertilized human ova. Gynecol. Invest. **4**:121–139, 1973.

Heuser, C.H. and Streeter, G.L.: Development of the macaque embryo. Contrib. Embryol. Carnegie Inst. **29**:15–55, 1941.

Higginbottom, J., Slater, J. and Porter, G.: The low-lying placenta and dysmaturity. Lancet **1**:859, 1975.

Hoogland, H.J., deHaan, J. and Martin, C.B.: Placental size during early pregnancy and fetal outcome: a preliminary report of a sequential ultrasonographic study. Amer. J. Obstet. Gynecol. **138**:441–443, 1980.

Huntington, K.M.: Foetal cells in antepartum haemorrhage. Lancet **2**:682, 1968.

Hurley, V.A. and Beischer, N.A.: Placenta membranacea: case reports. Brit. J. Obstet. Gynaecol. **94**:798–802, 1987.

Iffy, L.: Contribution to the etiology of placenta previa. Amer. J. Obstet. Gynecol. **83**:969–975, 1962.

Iyasu, S., Saftlas, A.K., Rowley, D.L., Koonin, L.M., Lawson, H.W. and Atrash, H.K.: The epidemiology of placenta previa in the United States, 1979 through 1987. Amer. J. Obstet. Gynecol. **168**:1424–1429, 1993.

Jacques, S.M., Qureshi, F., Trent, V.S. and Ramirez, N.C.: Placenta accreta: mild cases diagnosed by placental examination. Internat. J. Gynecol. Pathol. **15**:28–33, 1996.

Janovski, N.A. and Granowitz, E.T.: Placenta membranacea: report of a case. Obstet. Gynecol. **18**:206–212, 1961.

Johnson, W.D., Hughes, H.C. and Stenger, V.G.: Placenta extrachorialis in the stumptailed macaque (*Macaca arctoides*). Lab. Anim. Sci. **28**:81–84, 1978.

Jopp, H. and Krone, H.: Das Verhältnis zwischen Kindesgewicht und Plazentagewicht bei Placenta praevia. Geburtshilfe Frauenheilk. **26**:403–408, 1966.

Kalmus, H.: The incidence of placenta praevia and antepartum haemorrhage according to maternal age and parity. Ann. Eugen. **13**:283–290, 1947.

Keeler, F.J. and Cope, P.H.: Placenta of unusual shape. Obstet. Gynecol. **22**:679, 1963.

Kellogg, F.S.: Eight years of placenta previa at the Boston Lying-in Hospital. Med. Rec. Ann. Houston **37**:502–507, 1943.

Khashoggi, T.: Maternal and neonatal outcome in major placenta previa. Ann. Saudi Med. **15**:313–316, 1995.

Khong, T.Y. and Robertson, W.B.: Placenta creta and placenta praevia creta. Placenta **8**:399–409, 1987.

Kim, K.-R., Jun, S.-Y., Kim, J.-Y. and Ro, J.Y.: Implantation site intermediate trophoblasts in placenta cretas. Modern Pathol. **17**:1483–1490, 2004.

King, D.L.: Placental migration demonstrated by ultrasonography. Radiology **109**:167–170, 1973.

Kingsley, S.R. and Martin, R.D.: A case of placenta praevia in an orangutan. Vet. Rec. **104**:56–57, 1979.

Kistner, R.W., Hertig, A.T. and Reid, D.E.: Simultaneously occurring placenta previa and placenta accreta. Surg. Gynecol. Obstet. **94**:141–151, 1952.

Koren, Z., Zuckerman, H. and Brzezinski, A.: Placenta previa accreta with afibrinogenemia: report of 3 cases. Obstet. Gynecol. **18**:138–145, 1961.

Lademacher, D.S., Vermeulen, R.C.W., Harten, J.J.v.d. and Arts, N.F.: Circumvallate placenta and congenital anomalies. Lancet **1**:732, 1981.

Larks, S.D., Dasgupta, K., Assali, N.S. and Morton, D.G.: The human electrohysterogram: electrical evidence for the existence of pacemaker function in the parturient uterus. J. Obstet. Gynaecol. Brit. Emp. **66**:229–238, 1959.

Las Heras, J.L., Harding, P.G. and Haust, M.D.: Recurrent bleeding associated with placenta membranacea partialis: report of a case. Amer. J. Obstet. Gynecol. **144**:480–482, 1982.

Liepmann, W.: Beitrag der Placenta circumvallata. Arch. Gynäkol. **80**:439–454, 1906.

Lim, B.H., Tan, C.E., Smith, A.P.M. and Smith, N.C.: Transvaginal ultrasonography for diagnosis of placenta praevia. Lancet **1**:444, 1989.

Little, W.A.: Toxaemia and placental attachment. Brit. Med. J. **2**:387, 1962.

Little, W.A. and Friedman, E.A.: Significance of the placental position: a report from the collaborative study of cerebral palsy. Obstet. Gynecol. **23**:804–809, 1964.

Macones, G.A., Sehdev, H.M., Parry, S., Morgan, M.A. and Berlin, J.A.: The association between maternal cocaine use and placenta previa. Amer. J. Obstet. Gynecol. **177**:1097–1100, 1997.

Magann, E.F., Evans, S.F. and Newnham, J.P.: Placental implantation at 18 weeks and migration throughout pregnancy. South. Med. J. **91**:1025–1027, 1998.

Mathews, J.: Placenta membranacea. Aust. N.Z. J. Obstet. Gynaecol. **14**:45–47, 1974.

McShane, P.M., Heyl, P.S. and Epstein, M.F.: Maternal and perinatal morbidity resulting from placenta previa. Obstet. Gynecol. **65**:176–182, 1985.

Meyenburg, M.: Gibt es Veränderungen des Plazentasitzes im Bereich kaudaler Uterusabschnitte während der Schwangerschaft? Eine echographische Verlaufsstudie. Geburtsh. Frauenheilk. **36**:715–721, 1976.

Meyer, R.: Zur Anatomie und Entstehung der Placenta marginata s. partim extrachorialis. Arch. Gynäkol. **89**:542–573, 1909.

Miller, D.A., Chollet, J.A. and Goodwin, T.M.: Clinical risk factors for placenta previa–placenta accreta. Amer. J. Obstet. Gynecol. **177**:210–214, 1997a.

Miller, D.A., Goodwin, T.M., Gherman, R.B. and Paul, R.H.: Intrapartum rupture of the unscarred uterus. Obstet. Gynecol. **89**:671–673, 1997b.

Miller, E.D.: A 2000 gm tubal pregnancy. Amer. J. Obstet. Gynecol. **156**:1152–1153, 1987.

Mitchell, A.P.B., Anderson, G.S. and Russell, J.K.: Perinatal death from foetal exsanguination. Brit. Med. J. **1**:611–614, 1957.

Morgan, J.: Circumvallate placenta. J. Obstet. Gynaecol. Brit. Emp. **62**:899–900, 1955.

Mussalli, G.M., Shah, J., Berck, D.J., Elimian, A., Tejani, N. and Manning, F.A.: Placenta accrete and methotrexate therapy: Three case reports. J. Perinatol. **5**:331–334, 2000.

Naeye, R.L.: Placenta previa: predisposing factors and effects on the fetus and surviving infants. Obstet. Gynecol. **52**:521–525, 1978.

Naftolin, F., Khudr, G., Benirschke, K. and Hutchinson, D.L.: The syndrome of chronic abruptio placentae, hydrorrhea, and circumvallate placenta. Amer. J. Obstet. Gynecol. **116**:347–350, 1973.

Nelp, W.B. and Larson, S.M.: Diagnosis of placenta praevia by photoscanning with albumin labeled with technetium Tc 99m. JAMA **200**:158–162, 1967.

Nielsen, T.F., Hagberg, H. and Ljungblad, U.: Placenta previa and antepartum hemorrhage after previous cesarean section. Gynecol. Obstet. Invest. **27**:88–90, 1989.

Nieminen, U. and Klinge, E.: Placenta praevia and low implantation of the placenta. Acta Obstet. Gynecol. Scand. **42**:339–357, 1963

Nordlander, S., Sundberg, B., Westin, B. and Asard, P.-E.: Scintigraphic studies of uterine and placental growth and placental migration during pregnancy. Acta Obstet. Gynecol. Scand. **56**:483–486, 1977.

Ophir, E., Tendler, R., Odeh, M., Khouri, S. and Oettinger, M.: Creatine kinase as a biochemical marker in diagnosis of placenta increta and percreta. Amer. J. Obstet. Gynecol. **180**:1039–1040, 1999.

Oppenheimer, L.W., Mackenzie, F., Girard, J., Dabrowski, A. and Yossef, E: Migration rate of low lying placenta in the third trimester—can it predict outcome? Amer. J. Obstet. Gynecol. **170**:361, abstract 309, 1994.

Orsini, A.: La sede della placenta nella specie umana. Riv. Ital. Ginecol. **8**:19–63, 1928.

Pauerstein, C.J., Croxatto, H.B., Eddy, C.A., Ramzy, I. and Walters, M.D.: Anatomy and pathology of tubal pregnancy. Obstet. Gynecol. **67**:301–308, 1986.

Penrose, L.S.: Maternal age, order of birth and developmental abnormalities. J. Ment. Sci. **85**:1141–1150, 1939.

Radcliffe, P.A., Sindelair, P.J. and Zeit, P.R.: Vasa previa with marginal placenta previa of an accessory lobe: report of a case. Obstet. Gynecol. **16**:472–475, 1961.

Rashbaum, W.K., Gates, E.J., Jones, J., Goldman, B., Morris, A. and Lyman, W.D.: Placenta accreta encountered during dilation and evacuation in the second trimester. Obstet. Gynecol. **85**:701–703, 1995.

Rice, J.P., Kay, H.H. and Mahony, B.S.: The clinical significance of uterine leiomyomas in pregnancy. Amer. J. Obstet. Gynecol. **160**:1212–1216, 1989.

Ringrose, C.A.: Placenta previa in association with an incompetent cervix. Amer. J. Obstet. Gynecol. **124**:659, 1976.

Rizos, N., Doran, T.A., Miskin, M., Benzie, R.J. and Ford, J.A.: Natural history of placenta previa ascertained by diagnostic ultrasound. Amer. J. Obstet. Gynecol. **133**:287–291, 1979.

Rolschau, J.: Circumvallate placenta and intrauterine growth retardation. Acta Obstet. Gynecol. Scand. [Suppl.] **72**:11–14, 1978.

Rosa, P., Ghilain, A. and Dumont, A.: Placenta praevia accreta et afibrinogénémie secondaire. Bull. Soc. R. Belge Gynecol. Obstet. **26**:588–594, 1956.

Roth, L.G.: Central placenta previa due to a succenturiate lobe. Amer. J. Obstet. Gynecol. **74**:447–449, 1957.

Rubenstone, A.I. and Lash, S.R.: Placenta previa accreta. Amer. J. Obstet. Gynecol. **87**:198–202, 1963.

Salihu, H.M., Li, Q., Rouse, D.J. and Alexander, G.R.: Placenta previa: neonatal death after live births in the United States. Amer. J. Obstet. Gynecol. **188**:1305–1309, 2003.

Sarantopoulos, G.P. and Natarajan, S.: Placenta accreta. Arch Pathol. Lab. Med. **126**:1557–1558, 2002.

Schatz, F.: Die Gefässverbindungen der Placentarkreisläufe eineiiger Zwillinge, ihre Entwicklung und ihre Folgen. Arch. Gynäkol. **27**:1–72, 1886.

Schellong, G.: Anämie und Schock beim Neugeborenen durch fetalen Blutverlust. Monatsschr. Kinderheilk. **117**:578–579, 1969.

Schmitz, H.E., O'Dea, N.J. and Isaacs, J.H.: Placenta previa: a survey at the Lewis Memorial Maternity Hospital. Obstet. Gynecol. **3**:3–10, 1954.

Scipiades, E. and Burg, E.: Über die Morphologie der menschlichen Placenta mit besonderer Rücksicht auf unsere eigenen Studien. Arch. Gynäkol. **141**:577–619, 1930.

Scott, J.S.: Placenta extra-chorialis (placenta marginata and circumvallata): a factor in antepartum haemorrhage. J. Obstet. Gynaecol. Brit. Emp. **67**:904–918, 1960.

Scott, J.: Antepartum haemorrhage-2. Brit. Med. J. **1**:1231–1234, 1964.

Shanklin, D.R.: The human placenta: a clinicopathologic study. Obstet. Gynecol. **11**:129–138, 1958.

Sherer, D.M., Salafia, C.M., Minior, V.K., Sanders, M., Ernst, L. and Vintzileos, A.M.: Placental basal plate myometrial fibers: Clinical correlations of abnormally deep trophoblast invasion. Obstet. Gynecol. **87**:444–449, 1996.

Steemers, N.Y., Rop, C. de, Assche, A. van: Zonary placenta. Intern. J. Gynecol. Obstet. **51**:251–253, 1995.

Steyn, P.S. and Gebhardt, G.S.: Advanced extra-uterine pregnancy—a case of fimbrial expulsion of the fetus with complete placental development in the fallopian tube. Europ. J. Obstet. Gynecol. Reprod. Biol. **87**:167–168, 1999.

Strassmann, P.: Placenta praevia. Arch. Gynäkol. **67**:112–275, 1902.

Suzuki, K.: Concomitant occurrence of circumvallate placenta with single disc and bidiscoid placentas. Amer. J. Obstet. Gynecol. **110**:1147–1148, 1971.

Taipale, P., Hilesmaa, V. and Ylöstalo, P.: Diagnosis of placenta previa by transvaginal sonographic screening at 12–16 weeks in a nonselected population. Obstet. Gynecol. **89**:364–367, 1997.

Tatum, H.J. and Mulé, J.G.: Placenta previa: a functional classification and a report on 408 cases. Amer. J. Obstet. Gynecol. **93**:767–774, 1965.

Taylor, V.M., Kramer, M.D., Vaughan, T.L. and Peacock, S.: Placenta previa and prior Cesarean delivery: How strong is the association? Obstet. Gynecol. **84**:55–57, 1994.

Taylor, V.M., Peacock, S., Kramer, M.D. and Vaughan, T.L.: Increased risk of placenta previa among women of Asian origin. Obstet. Gynecol. **86**:805–808, 1995.

Thomas, J.: Der gestielte Plazentarkotyledo-eine Bauanomalie der Nachgeburt. Zentralbl. Gynäkol. **84**:684–690, 1962.

Torpin, R.: Classification of human pregnancy based on depth of intrauterine implantation of the ovum. Amer. J. Obstet. Gynecol. **66**:791–800, 1953.

Torpin, R.: Placenta circumvallata and placenta marginata. Obstet. Gynecol. **6**:277–284, 1955.

Torpin, R.: Human placental anomalies: etiology, evolution and historical background. Mo. Med. **55**:353–357, 1958.

Torpin, R.: An explanation of placental marginal infarct rings: a significant summary of a life-long evaluation of a concept of placental formation. J. Med. Assoc. Ga. **54**:274–276, 1965.

Torpin, R.: Evolution of a placenta circumvallata. Obstet. Gynecol. **27**:98–101, 1966.

Torpin, R.: The Human Placenta. Its Shape, Form, Origin and Development. Charles C Thomas, Springfield, IL, 1969a.

Torpin, R.: Placentation in the rhesus monkey (Macaca mulatta). Obstet. Gynecol. **34**:410–413, 1969b.

Torpin, R. and Barfield, W.E.: Placenta duplex. J. Med. Assoc. Ga. **57**:78–80, 1968.

Torpin, R. and Hart, B.F.: Placenta bilobata. Amer. J. Obstet. Gynecol. **42**:38–49, 1941.

Van Huysen, W.T.: Placenta previa of a succenturiate lobe. NEJM **265**:284–286, 1961.

Wentworth, P.: Circumvallate and circummarginate placentas. Amer. J. Obstet. Gynecol. **102**:44–47, 1968.

Wewer, U.W., Faber, M., Liotta, L.A. and Albrechtsen, R.: Immunochemical and ultrastructural assessment of the nature of the pericellular basement membrane of human decidual cells. Lab. Invest. **53**:624–633, 1986.

Wexler, P. and Gottesfeld, K.R.: Second trimester placenta previa: an apparently normal placentation. Obstet. Gynecol. **50**:706–709, 1977.

Wexler, P. and Gottesfeld, K.R.: Early diagnosis of placenta previa. Obstet. Gynecol. **54**:231–234, 1979.

Wickster, G.Z.: Posthemorrhagic shock in the newborn. Amer. J. Obstet. Gynecol. **63**:524–537, 1952.

Wiener, A.S.: Diagnosis and treatment of anemia of the newborn caused by occult placental hemorrhage. Amer. J. Obstet. Gynecol. **56**:717–722, 1948.

Williams, J.W.: Placenta circumvallata. Amer. J. Obstet. Gynecol. **13**:1–16, 1927.

Wilson, D. and Paalman, R.J.: Clinical significance of circumvallate placenta. Obstet. Gynecol. **29**:774–778, 1967.

Wingate, M.B. and Pauls, F.: Effect of the placental site on fetal presentation at term. Can. Med. Assoc. J. **99**:531–532, 1968.

Winters, R.: Die Rolle regressiver Veränderungen der Plazenta bei der sogenannten Plazentamigration. Geburtsh. Frauenheilk. **38**:1093–1098, 1978.

Wolf, H., Oosting, H. and Treffers, P.E.: Placental volume measurements by ultrasonography: evaluation of the method. Amer. J. Obstet. Gynecol. **156**:1191–1194, 1979.

Young, G.B.: The peripatetic placenta. Radiology **128**:183–188, 1978.

Ziel, H.A.: Circumvallate placenta, a cause of antepartum bleeding, premature delivery, and perinatal mortality. Obstet. Gynecol. **22**:798–802, 1963.

Zilliacus, H.: The detection of foetal blood in haemorrhage of late pregnancy. Gynaecologia **157**:103–109, 1964.

14
Histopathologic Approach to Villous Alterations

How to Assess Villous Histopathology

Evaluation of the placental villous tissue during the routine evaluation of the placenta is important to gain an overall understanding of the normalcy of the placenta and to ascertain possible disorders. If the villous structure is abnormal, this helps to direct one's attention to certain pregnancy disturbances that may require further study.

In addition, one needs to consider the influences on the villous structure between delivery and preparation of tissue sections, such as the time and mode of cord clamping (Bouw et al., 1976) and the method of fixation (see Chapter 28, Tables 28.8 to 28.10). Different fixatives produce different histologic appearances with which one needs to be familiar. Moreover, the rapidity of fixation is important if such features as edema are to be evaluated properly (Voigt et al., 1978; Kaufmann, 1985). All these findings are crucial for a proper microscopic evaluation of villous tissue, which is peculiarly subject to artifacts.

The placental examination can then lead to significant insight as to the pathogenesis of many disorders. Salafia et al. (1992), Macara et al. (1996), and Todros et al. (1998) found, for instance, an excellent correlation of various features with intrauterine growth restriction (IUGR). Importantly, the associated or causative villous pathology was chronic villitis, infarcts, so-called hemorrhagic endovasculitis, thromboses, and fetoplacental vascular maldevelopment. In their quantitative study of placentas from undefined growth-retarded newborns and appropriate controls, Wong and Latour (1966) found only minor changes that would not allow characterization by ordinary microscopy. It was, however, possible only to show that the placentas of growth-retarded neonates had a reduced villous surface area when quantitative measurement of villi and trophoblast were made. Since then, however, a much better understanding of IUGR has been gained and one cannot help but believe that the cases studied by these authors had a very mixed etiology. Like-

wise, one must then presume that the placental changes might differ markedly.

Such scrutiny presupposes a considerable familiarity with the normal structure of the placenta and also that sufficient tissue samples have been collected for this study. For instance, it must be appreciated that the center of placental lobules differs in its villous appearance from that of the lobular periphery. In the central areas and under the chorion the villi are more widely separated, and they may have quite a different appearance from the villi at the periphery of a lobule (see Chapter 7, Fig. 7.18). This organization of the "placentone," as the German histologists have named this area (Schuhmann, 1981), is particularly well shown in Figure 24 of Becker and Röckelein (1989). Misinterpretation of that feature alone may lead to an assessment of the so-called dysmaturity of villi. Altshuler and Herman (1989) characterized villous dysmaturity thus: "Third trimester placentas that have large villi with numerous stromal cells, a lack of syncytiotrophoblast, and syncytiotrophoblastic knots . . . examples are chorangiosis, diabetes, and immunohemolytic anemia." It must be said, however, that there is no unifying hypothesis to define, let alone explain, "dysmaturity." We prefer not to use this term at all because it is not sufficiently specific. Rather, we employ the term **villous maldevelopment** to mean similar abnormalities in structure when no specific cause is apparent. What is meant is that the villous architecture is admixed; there are perhaps mature villi mixed with edematous or hypercellular immature villi, scarred avascular villi with chorangiosis (Figs. 14.1 to 14.3), and so on. Dysmaturity is not a precise diagnosis and it would be better to describe the abnormality specifically rather than to use the poorly defined term **dysmaturity**.

Assessment of Villous Maturation

Other considerations concerning errors in villous development have been summarized by Vogel (1996). He suggested that these maturational disturbances occur as

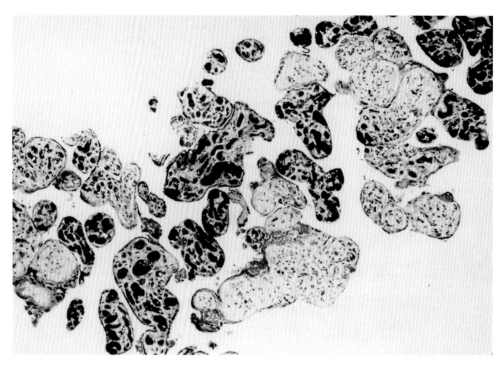

FIGURE 14.1. Chorangiosis (grade 2 according to Altshuler, 1984), associated with villitis of unknown origin. H&E ×90. (Courtesy of Dr. G. Altshuler, Oklahoma City, Oklahoma.)

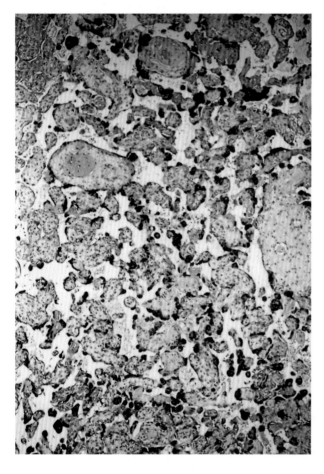

FIGURE 14.2. Tenney-Parker changes at 25 weeks' gestation. This placenta is from a preeclamptic pregnancy and shows features of accelerated maturation. Large numbers of syncytial knots (Tenney-Parker) are everywhere present. H&E ×64.

FIGURE 14.3. Marked congestion of villous capillaries and veins in a 30-week placenta of preeclampsia. Note association with increased knotting. Similar congestion of capillaries and veins is usually found after preterm rupture of membranes; it is probably caused by cord compression due to loss of amnionic fluid. H&E ×100.

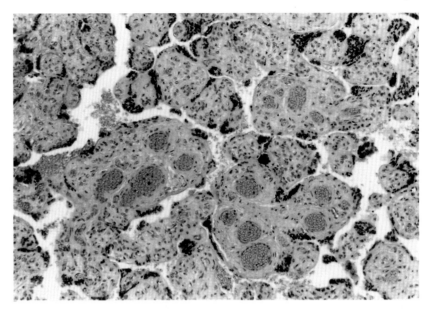

often as in 25% of otherwise normal placentas, albeit only in confined, small areas of the placentone. Most did not have a known fetal impact, although their frequency was much increased in problem pregnancies. As there exists no uniform, agreed-upon terminology, Vogel (1996) produced the following table:

Becker (1981a)	Schweikhart (1985)	Kloos and Vogel (1974)	Vogel (1984)
Normal maturation	Synchronous maturation	Mature, age-corresponding	Mature gestation, age-appropriate
Delayed maturation		Discontinuous vascularization	Dissociated villous maturation, mostly mature
Retarded maturation	Terminal villi deficiency	Concordant retarded villi	Dissociated villous maturation, mostly immature
Arrested maturation	Persisting immaturity	Persisting embryonal structure	Arrest of villous maturation
Premature maturation	Asynchronous postterm maturity	Premature maturation	Villous premature maturation
Chorangiosis		Chorangiomatosis	Chorangiosis, type I
Pseudochorangiosis		Angiomatosis	Chorangiosis, type II
Chorangiomatosis		Chorangiosis	

The term placental dysfunction was perhaps first used by Clifford (1954), when he described the features of **postmature** gestations. He suggested that postmature delivery occurred then as often as in 5% of gestations, and he indicated that perinatal mortality increased significantly after term. He was emphatic that much of this mortality reflected intrauterine fetal demise and suggested that it resulted from the supposed decrease of placental function. Clifford addressed fetal function but had little to say about placental findings. Meconium discharge, deficient water transfer, and meconium aspiration seem to have been the principal aspects of postmaturity he considered, although oxygen deficiency was inferred. From the pathologist's point of view there are no truly characteristic histologic findings that allow one to make the diagnosis of postmaturity in placental examination. Rather, two different features can be found:

1. In the first group of cases, one finds persisting immaturity with scarcity of terminal villi and prevalence of immature intermediate villi, resembling placentas from the early third trimester (Fox, 1968d; Kemnitz & Theuring, 1974; Mikolajczak et al., 1987) (cf. Chapter 8). Other pathologic findings are generally absent. The delay of villous maturation in these cases suggests that postterm delivery was due to absence of placental signals inducing labor. According to Becker (1981a) there was no indication that, from a placental point of view, there was no urgency of delivery.

2. Another quite different entity of postterm placentas shows full villous maturity or even "hypermaturity" with prevalence of mature intermediate and terminal villi and complete absence of immature villous types. The picture may also include increased syncytial knotting (Tenney-Parker changes). Statistically speaking, this type of post-

mature placenta is more calcified, but because not all postmature placentas have an excess of calcification, this is a difficult parameter to judge. These placentas are also more frequently meconium stained, and they have more often chorioamnionitis (Naeye, 1992), but not all are so altered (see Chapter 1).

The same heterogeneity of findings is typical for **premature** deliveries:

1. The inexperienced pathologist, when studying the histology of a prematurely delivered placenta, expects prevalence of large-caliber, lightly stained immature villous types and scarcity of terminal villi. Surprisingly, this is the case in only 33% of the respective placentas; the immature villous maturational state corresponds to the premature stage of pregnancy (synchronous villous immaturity) (Schweikhart et al., 1986).
2. The majority of spontaneous preterm deliveries show more advanced villous maturation. Fully mature villous trees or even abnormal-appearing villi showing increased degrees of capillarization occur frequently in prematurely delivered placentas of preeclamptic women. They are primarily manifest as an increase of syncytial knots (Tenney-Parker changes), smaller villi, and perhaps an increase in the cross sections of capillary lumens (Fig. 14.2). Schweikhart et al. (1986) were impressed with the proliferation of terminal villi in premature placentas, likening their architecture to "bonsai" trees; they found "hypermature" placentas as often as in 42% of placentas delivered between 29 and 32 weeks. In the case of preeclampsia, the incidence was raised to 60%. This frequent combination of premature delivery with villous maturity has been called accelerated maturation or maturitas praecox placentae (Becker, 1960), to indicate that some villous features indicated greater development than expected for the gestational age. Naeye (1992), however, made the point that this concept of accelerated maturation has often led to confusion and that it is difficult to define precisely. Becker (1981a) proposed that full maturity of the placenta is needed to be responsible for a spontaneous induction of labor ("placental need for delivery").

In summary, these data suggest that spontaneous induction of labor requires the coincidence of placental maturation with extraplacental signals. Various mixtures of these two factors allow for five different combinations, all of which have been described:

1. Normal villous maturation and extraplacental signals at term: **term** delivery with normal **maturity** of villi.
2. Normal villous maturation, but delayed or missing extraplacental signals for delivery: **postterm** delivery with **hypermaturity** of the placenta.
3. Normal villous maturation, but premature induction of labor: **preterm** delivery with **immaturity** of villi (synchronous immaturity).
4. Delayed maturation of villi, delayed or missing spontaneous induction of labor: **postterm** delivery with **immaturity** of villi (persisting immaturity).
5. Premature maturation of villi, with preterm induction of labor: **preterm** delivery with full maturity or even **hypermaturity** of villi.

Placental Insufficiency

The term **placental insufficiency** is a most difficult one to define precisely. One might expect that placental weight bears on this question, and placental weight has often been used to suggest that the placental function is "adequate" or "insufficient." Ratios to fetal weight have then been used to correlate placental function. Sinclair (1948) found the placental weight to increase linearly as gestation progresses; he was unable to account for the great microscopic variability among placentas. He indicated also that birth weights were lower when a marginal insertion of the umbilical cord was present, a feature that is often neglected in published studies because the cord insertion is usually not recorded. This feature is easiest to observe in dizygotic twin pregnancies, where marked discrepancies in size and development can occur.

Garrow and Hawes (1971) examined the proposition of placental weight increases in some detail. They showed that after 42 weeks there was no accumulation of structural proteins in the placenta but that the increasing weight resulted from pooling of fetal blood, a variable that also needs to be carefully controlled for meaningful analysis. After much effort at quantitative analysis they concluded that studies such as the ones reported are "a laborious task, and the yield of additional information is relatively small." Mayhew and colleagues (1994) assessed placental growth from 12 weeks to term and showed linear growth by "hyperplasia" rather than by ultimate hypertrophy. Generally, the weight ratio given for such comparisons is that of fetus/placenta. Normally, this ratio is between 7 and 7.5, but alterations of the ratio are so frequent that one cannot deduce placental dysfunction from an altered ratio. It is now possible to ascertain sonographically the placental volume (thickness and circumference) and to relate it to fetal growth. Perhaps more appropriate correlations will be made in the future with this modality. That these parameters are more useful was impressively shown by early results of studies by Jauniaux et al. (1994).

A consideration of the entity placental insufficiency fits well into the context of this discussion. As can be imagined, we prefer not to use this term. It implies a specific placental disease when in fact the malady is usually caused by one of a variety of factors. These include an abnormal fetal genome, chronic infection, and a large number of maternal diseases; they may also relate to the localization of the placenta in the uterus. A good case in point to illuminate the semantic complexity is the discussion by Fejgin et al. (1993). These authors suggested that the low gonadotropin secretion of triploid placentas was caused by placental insufficiency. A much more cogent and persuasive argument was supplied by Goshen and Hochberg (1994). They explained the secretory levels as being caused by the genetic contribution in the two different types of partial hydatidiform moles (PHMs), and in complete hydatidiform moles (CHMs). Thus, two **maternal** genomes (in triploidy) leads to low human chorionic gonadotropin (hCG) values, and two **paternal** genomes (in some cases of PHM, and usually in CHM) leads to excessive secretion of this hormone because of the genetic expression of specific genes.

For somewhat different reasons, others have also spoken against the use of this all-inclusive term (Gille, 1985; Kuss, 1987), as was quoted in some detail by Vogel (1996). Conversely, Becker and Röckelein (1989) made cogent pleas to retain the term **placental insufficiency**. They then produced a complex tabular account of the possible causes of placental insufficiency and stated that an insufficient placenta is one of critical reduction of placental exchange membrane. This entity then encompasses all those features discussed under their special headings, such as preeclamptic changes, chorangiosis, tumors, avascular villi, and excessive fibrin deposits. We prefer to specify and name the lesions rather than to embrace them all in the imprecise terminology of placental insufficiency.

For routine examination of the histologic picture it is important to study various areas in the placenta as they do not all have the same appearance. For example, the peripheral edge of the placenta often has some increased fibrinoid deposition as a normal feature, and some degree of infarction may be present that is not representative of the remainder of the organ. The villi beneath the chorionic plate are also more widely spaced than those of the floor, and this anatomic difference often leads to focal coagulation that is not necessarily pathologic. At the margin of the placenta, infarction and excessive fibrin deposits are common and should be considered to be normal events, if that is the only location of these changes.

Examination of Fetal Stem Vessels

In assessing the adequacy of villous tissue for fetal growth, it is our practice to proceed in an orderly fashion with the examination so that all aspects are inspected and evaluated. We begin with the assessment of the **umbilical cord and its vessels**. It is of interest to know whether the vasculature is congested, whether there is a sufficient amount of blood within the vessels, and, importantly, whether there are nucleated red blood cells (NRBCs) within the fetal blood. The presence of NRBCs is abnormal and connotes anemia, previous hypoxia of some duration, or fetal growth disturbances (Bernstein et al., 1997). When NRBCs are found, we make it a practice to check the newborn blood smear to enumerate these cells (see Chapter 8). At this time we also examine the vessels of the umbilical cord for thrombi, inflammation, and possible meconium damage.

The vascular system is next studied in the **surface of the placenta**. Here, the presence or absence of thrombi is carefully assessed. These frequent, important aspects of prenatal pathology are most commonly found in the veins. These surface veins are difficult to differentiate from arteries by histologic study alone. Veins lie usually below the arteries, but it is best to identify them macroscopically. When thrombi are very old, they transform ultimately into "cushions" (see Chapter 12) (de Sa, 1973), organized thickenings of the venous vascular wall. It must be emphasized that some of these cushions are readily misinterpreted as they may represent bifurcations of vessels. The thrombi may be occlusive, and they may also calcify; this change is prominently found in cytomegalovirus (CMV) infections and also when the thrombi are very old. Calcification also occurs in the walls of vessels when thrombi have been long-standing.

Similar cushions have been described in walls of umbilical arteries, chorionic arteries, and occasionally also in those of larger villous arteries (Emmrich, 1991). Altshuler (1993) stated that he found cushions "associated with clinically diagnosed neonatal asphyxia." Becker (1981a) introduced the term asphyxial infiltrates. This view has been contradicted by Emmrich et al. (1998a,b), who did not find any correlation between incidence of arterial cushions and signs of hypoxia or acidosis in the neonate.

More often than obliterative thrombosis, one finds only mural fibrin deposits. These usually betray long-standing diseases and correlate primarily with stasis from cord problems such as knots, entangling, or prolapse. Occasionally, mural thrombosis of surface veins results solely from marked twisting of the umbilical cord.

The **main stem villous vessels** are next inspected. It is in these vessels that hemorrhagic endovasculitis (HEV) is most commonly seen (Sander, 1980), which is primarily a feature associated with stillbirths. It represents in our opinion a postmortem or postthrombotic phenomenon; the lesion is discussed in greater detail in Chapter 12 (see Thrombosis of the Placental Vascular Tree).

Examination of the Fetal Capillary Bed

The number of capillaries in the terminal villi is next evaluated. They may be markedly congested when the cord has been clamped soon after delivery of the neonate and also when maternal diabetes has complicated the pregnancy. **Congestion** as shown in Figure 14.3, however, must not be confused with the more ominous condition known as **chorangiosis** (Altshuler, 1984). The designation chorangiosis makes reference to a numerical increase of capillaries within the peripheral placental villi. Although chorangiosis can be a very impressive feature, it does not relate to neoplastic changes such as angiomas, as has been suggested. This condition is presently underrated as an indicator of chronic prenatal hypoxia. In studying the placentas of infants that were admitted to the neonatal intensive care unit of his hospital, Altshuler found that 5.5% had chorangiosis in their placentas. He provided criteria for the evaluation that have not yet been challenged.

What is important about chorangiosis is its relative rarity and that it is strongly correlated with perinatal mortality and a wide variety of pregnancy and placental disorders. It is definitely a pathologic feature. The appearance is characteristic, and it is obvious that weeks must be required for the degree of capillary proliferation to take place that produces chorangiosis. It is perhaps for these reasons that the lesion had been termed chorangiomatosis in the past (see Chapter 24).

Chorangiosis occurs also in women who have pregnancies at very high altitude (Reshetnikova et al., 1994) and in severely anemic mothers (Kadyrov et al., 1998). That the proliferation of villous capillaries is an adaptation to chronic oxygen deficiency is further supported by the experimental results in guinea pigs described by Scheffen et al. (1990). They demonstrated such increase of capillaries when guinea pigs were chronically (45 days) deprived of normal oxygen tension in their environment. This point is relevant also to the long history of placental studies at high altitude, where the smaller size of infants and placentas found has much interested investigators. Jackson and her coworkers (1987) have studied the placenta of women at high altitude in Bolivia and compared them with those at sea level. The total villous length was smaller at high altitude, and capillary cross sections were increased. Thus, an altered capillary/villus ratio emerged as being characteristic.

The terminal villi may lack all capillaries, markedly reducing the available exchange area, and its quantity needs to be estimated. Such **avascular villi** are most common following chronic villitis, as in CMV infection. Next most commonly, avascular villi result from main stem and surface vessel thrombosis (Fig. 14.4) (Altshuler & Herman, 1989). In similar degenerative events, McDermott and Gillan (1995) have shown that a chronic reduction of fetal blood flow precedes villous infarction. They suggested that siderosis of villous basement membranes, seen so prominently in cases with arterial thrombosis, was a good marker for this reduced flow. Calcifications of villous basement membranes, having a similar appearance, are discussed next.

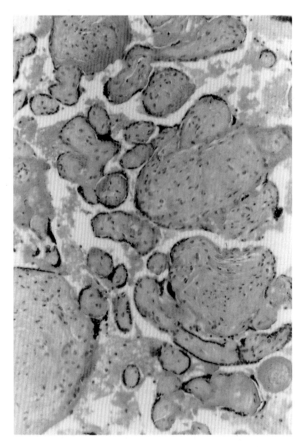

FIGURE 14.4. Marked fibrosis and "avascularity" of villous district caused by obliteration of a large surface vessel. Note the extremely thin trophoblastic cover of villi and pyknotic nuclei. H&E ×160.

Villous Architecture and Fibrinoid

Having studied the vasculature, we prefer next to evaluate the low-power appearance of the villous architecture. It is at this time that structural abnormalities are identified that have an only focal distribution. Focal edema (Naeye et al., 1983; Shen-Schwarz et al., 1989; Naeye, 1992; Altshuler, 1993) is easiest to identify at this time and its abundance can then be estimated. Naeye et al. (1983) had described **villous edema** to occur especially in placentas affected by chorioamnionitis but believed it to correlate best with fetal hypoxia. The extent of edema also correlated with low Apgar scores and other features leading to perinatal mortality. Naeye (1992) specifically suggested that severe villous edema may interfere with oxygen delivery to the fetus by compression of capillaries within villi. Edema would also allow one to recognize possibly increased numbers of Hofbauer cells, especially in Rh incompatibility, chronic infections, and maternal diabetes. It is important to note that not all lightly stained villi represent truly edematous villi. Rather normal immature intermediate villi may be misinterpreted as such, as their reticular stromal core has only a low affinity for conventional histologic stains (see following, and Immature Intermediate Villi in Chapter 7).

During this survey with low-power inspection of the villous tissue, the **maturity of villi** is adjudicated, perhaps representing the most difficult task in placental examination for the novice. It must be admitted that it is often impossible to accomplish this task accurately, mostly because of preparative problems. Thus, the diagnosis of postmature villi cannot easily be made correctly from villous examination alone. Maternal factors, fixation, and storage all strongly affect the histologic villous appearance and must be weighed. The influence of maternal conditions is perhaps best seen in preeclampsia when the reduced intervillous blood flow leads to the "Tenney-Parker changes" (Tenney & Parker, 1940). These changes are exemplified by a diffuse increase in syncytial knotting and a decreased size of terminal villi caused by lack of interstitial fluid.

An examination of the villous tissue under low power also allows one to identify irregular maturation of villi, foci of fibrosis, and the quantity of **fibrin** or **fibrinoid** deposited. A diffuse increase of perivillous fibrin is sometimes interpreted as reflecting chronic intervillous perfusional problems (Altshuler, 1993). Alternatively, excessive fibrinoid deposition is a striking feature of the so-called maternal floor infarction syndrome (see Chapter 9). In this condition, not only is the decidual floor heavily infiltrated by "fibrinoid," but also this material often disseminates throughout the villous tissue and is associated with proliferation of extravillous trophoblast. The villous tissue in such cases is stiff during macroscopic study, is diffusely penetrated with gray fibrin masses (*Gitterinfarkt*), and may show many microcysts in the increased extravillous trophoblast deposits. Microscopically, the fibrin encases villi that are being strangled, consequently lack vessels, and ultimately die. It strongly correlates with fetal growth retardation and intrauterine fetal demise. Naturally, true infarcts are also noted during this survey and their age is estimated as well (see Infarcts in Chapter 19).

Intervillous Space, Infarcts

Finally, the intervillous space is evaluated. Does it contain **thrombi**, especially beneath the chorionic plate? Are they fresh or old, and are they the possible sites of fetal bleeding? Are there tumor metastases or other abnormal features that need study with higher magnification? And are the maternal red blood cells perhaps sickled? Subchorionic thrombi are common, as was discussed extensively in Chapter 12. Sonographers have often referred to the subchorionic space as being "lucent" and have speculated that sonographic lucencies are meaningful abnormalities of placentation. There is some indication also that lucencies are a possible warning sign of placenta accreta or

placenta percreta. In most, the sonographically identified subchorionic lucencies disappear with delivery. Nevertheless, large laminated thromboses may occur in this location that can interfere with fetal development. Growth retardation, vascular compromise, and lateral expansion of these thrombi with abruptio have all been described and were discussed in some detail earlier (see Chapter 9). What is not clear from the current literature is the etiology of large "thrombohematomas," as the larger of these abnormalities have been referred to. Some authors consider them to be related to abruptio placentae, whereas others have likened them to Breus' mole. We consider it possible that they are accidental expansions of the normal subchorionic thrombi that make up the fibrinous plaques of term placental surface and which arise most likely by eddying and rheologic aberrations in the intervillous circulation. None of these lesions are related to angiomas, even though sonographically they may have similar appearances.

Also evaluation of the **width of the intervillous space** may give important hints: An unusually wide intervillous space combined with abnormally small villous calibers (see Figs. 14.8 and 15.7) is a usual finding in postplacental hypoxia (Kingdom & Kaufmann, 1997) (see Types of Hypoxia and Its Effects on Villous Development in Chapter 7). Clinically, this condition is characterized by intrauterine growth restriction combined with absent or reverse end-diastolic umbilical flow (Macara et al., 1996; Kingdom et al., 1997). In contrast, an extremely narrow, cleft-like intervillous space combined with irregularly shaped, highly branched terminal villi and impressive Tenney-Parker changes (see Fig. 15.5) is characteristic for villi with increased numbers of highly branched capillaries (excessive branching angiogenesis, chorangiosis). It is often found in severe preplacental hypoxia (maternal anemia; Kadyrov et al., 1998) and in uteroplacental hypoxia (IUGR with preserved end-diastolic flow in the umbilical arteries, with or without preeclampsia, Todros et al., 1999).

True placental infarcts result from occlusion of maternal vascular supply. They have different qualities sonographically and are also clearly different from thromboses. They involve actual placental tissue, whereas the thromboses push the villous structures aside. There may be some infarction of villi adjacent to the thromboses, but that is not a major feature. Infarcts are generally the result of disturbances of intervillous circulation, usually secondary to obstruction of maternal arteries in the placental floor. They also accompany most abruptios. In a true infarct, the trophoblast dies first and subsequently the stroma, vessels, and all other components of the villi undergo necrosis. Initially, there is still some nuclear dusting from karyorrhexis, but eventually that disappears too. Early infarcts still possess some fetal red blood cells with hemoglobin and they are therefore red; later the hemoglobin lyses and the infarcts turn white or yellowish. Eventually, infarcts atrophy remarkably and may focally calcify. In the adjacent villous tissue there is frequently some degree of Tenney-Parker change because of the circulatory disturbance and the ensuing local hypoxia. Virtually all infarcts have the same appearance, and it is uncommon that their microscopic evaluation makes a useful contribution to the understanding of the placental pathology. Although we have recommended that few of them be examined microscopically and, rather, that more noninfarcted tissue be sampled in placentas affected by infarcts, this is not always prudent. Numerous cases of unsuspected choriocarcinoma in situ have now been described in term placentas that have the macroscopic appearance of ordinary infarcts (see Chapter 23). One usually can reliably identify infarcts macroscopically, and then make a judgment as to their volumetric contribution to the whole organ.

Abruptio Placentae

More problematic is the evaluation of abruptio placentae. When it is very fresh, no histopathology may be visible. The retroplacental hematoma may have the same appearance as that blood which normally follows placental detachment. Older abruptios tend to compress the villous tissue and are then more easily identified microscopically. The blood cells are degenerating, there is laminated fibrin, pigmented macrophages may be present after a few days, and the decidua basalis is degenerated and often replaced by the hematoma. Indeed, this destruction of the decidua basalis usually makes it impossible to identify the maternal blood vessels and the atherosis or thrombosis within them that were responsible for the abruptio.

It is noteworthy that small areas of abruptio placentae are much more common than is usually stated (Benirschke & Gille, 1977). The reason for this is that most retroplacental hemorrhages do not produce the usually cited clinical symptomatology of sudden abdominal pain and bleeding. Their contribution to fetal well-being may also be much less significant than is that of the large retroplacental hemorrhage with detachment of a major portion of placental tissue. Because most abruptios are considered to be the result of trauma or maternal vascular disease, an assessment of the decidual spiral arterioles is desirable. In the locale of the abruption, however, this is usually impossible. The vessels here are often destroyed by the process or have remained behind during the delivery of the placenta. Therefore, one must look in adjacent portions of decidua, and especially in the decidua capsularis. Atherosis and thrombosis are often well displayed in these vessels, but it must be cautioned that their absence is not meaningful. These lesions are often very irregularly distributed, and to ascertain their status with certainty requires blunt curettage after delivery of the placenta.

That procedure is not a favorite part of obstetrical care and thus it is not often undertaken. It is therefore frequently impossible to rule out vascular changes as a cause of abruptions, and therefore their etiology remains obscure.

Major Histopathologic Findings

This brief survey lists the major histopathologic observations that should be made in placental microscopy.

Syncytiotrophoblast

The syncytiotrophoblastic cover of the villous trees usually shows considerable variations in thickness, distribution of nuclei, and structure of nuclei. Extremely thin anuclear areas (epithelial plates) and accumulations of nuclei (syncytial knots) are arranged in a mosaic-like pattern. **Homogeneous trophoblastic thickness**, combined with numerous Langhans' cells (villous cytotrophoblast), are found in immature placentas (see Fig. 6.13), in persisting villous immaturity, erythroblastosis (see Fig. 15.10), and in most placentas from diabetic mothers (see Fig. 19.6).

Homogeneous trophoblastic thickness, combined with loss of villous cytotrophoblast, is a typical feature of post-placental hypoxia that is discussed in detail in Chapter 15 (see Fig. 15.17) (Fig. 14.5). Extremely thin syncytiotrophoblast with evenly distributed pyknotic nuclei locally forming large knots (Figs. 14.4 and 14.6; also see Fig. 12.60) are additional important features. Most of the latter are indications of accumulation and shedding of apoptotic nuclei (cf. Chapter 6). When they are combined with the absence of villous cytotrophoblast, this usually points to deficient fetal perfusion of the villi (e.g., fetal death, thrombosis of stem vessels). This malperfusion leads to an increased intravillous oxygen partial pressure and failure of villous cytotrophoblast to proliferate and to regenerate the syncytium (see Oxygen and Oxygen-Controlled Growth Factors as Regulators of Villous Development in Chapter 7).

Knotting of the Syncytiotrophoblast

Increased numbers of syncytial knots, sprouts, and bridges are called syncytial knotting, or Tenney-Parker changes. As discussed in Chapter 15 (see Syncytial Knotting), these features have to be interpreted with care because they are influenced by the thickness of the section. Küstermann (1981), Burton (1986a,b), and Cantle et al. (1987) have shown that most of these nuclear accumulations are flat sections of irregularly shaped villous surfaces. An **increased incidence of syncytial knotting** thus points to abnormal villous shapes (increased branching and bulging

FIGURE 14.5. Persisting immaturity near term. Note the slender, straight sections of mature intermediate villi are arranged in parallel and the absence of terminal villi with sinusoidally dilated capillaries. In normal pregnancy, this feature would correspond to the 32nd to 34th week of gestation. It is also a common feature of postmature placentas, combined with IUGR. H&E ×30.

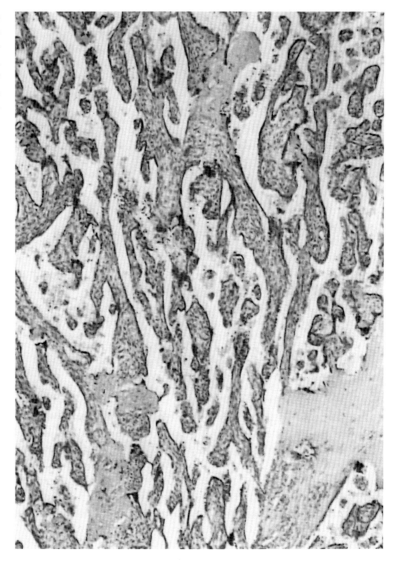

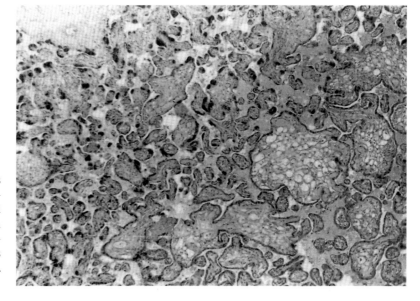

FIGURE 14.6. Immature placenta at 30 weeks from a patient with preeclampsia. Note the accelerated maturity (at left) with numerous syncytial knots (Tenney-Parker change) associated with small terminal villi and large immature intermediate villi at right. The latter are not edematous in nature but, rather, display a reticular stroma. H&E ×64.

of villi) (see Chapter 15), and they can usually be found under hypoxic conditions. Typical clinical examples include hypertensive disorders (Alvarez et al., 1969) (Fig. 14.6), maternal anemia (Piotrowicz et al., 1969), and pregnancy at high altitude (Jackson et al., 1987). Also, some cases of prolonged pregnancy (see Fig. 15.14) (Essbach & Röse, 1966; Emmrich & Mälzer, 1968) and many cases of preterm delivery (maturitas precox placentae) (Becker, 1981a; Schweikhart et al., 1986) show similar features. When groups of small terminal villi with increased knotting alternate with groups of severely immature villi (Fig. 14.6), preeclampsia is a prominent possibility (see Chapter 19).

The syncytial knots caused by trophoblastic flat sectioning just discussed are usually concentrated in groups of terminal villi. Similar trophoblastic features around the surfaces of immature villous types represent, in most cases, **villous sprouting**. Abnormal degrees of this phenomenon can be seen in moles and in several of the chromosomal aberrations (see Chapter 21, Fig. 21.27, and Chapter 22).

Langhans' Cells

The villous cytotrophoblast is difficult to identify in routine paraffin sections. Despite the fact that Langhans' cells are present at about 20% of the villous surfaces at term, one usually finds only one clearly identifiable Langhans' cell per cross section of any peripheral villus. **Lower frequencies of Langhans' cells** (in routine paraffin histology: fewer than a mean of one visible in two peripheral villous cross sections) are found in postplacental hypoxia (e.g., IUGR with absent end-diastolic flow in the umbilical arteries) (Macara et al., 1996) (see Chapter 15), and in fetally malperfused villi (fetal death, thrombosis of stem vessels) (see Placental Surface Vessels in Chapter 12).

In contrast, **increased numbers of Langhans' cells** (in routine paraffin histology: more than two visible per peripheral villous cross section) are usual findings in immature placentas; they also exist in "persisting immaturity" (Becker & Röckelein, 1989) (see Chapter 15), erythroblastosis (Wentworth, 1967; Pilz et al., 1980) (see Chapter 16), maternal anemia (Kosanke et al., 1998) (see Chapter 19), and maternal diabetes mellitus (Werner & Schneiderhan, 1972) (see Chapter 19). It is said that their number increases with the severity and duration of preeclampsia (Fox, 1997).

Vasculosyncytial Membranes

Vasculosyncytial membranes are the result of sinusoidal dilatation of the terminal villous capillaries, which bulge against the trophoblastic surfaces and attenuate them to thin lamellae (see Figs. 6.4A and 6.7A). The incidence is closely related to fetal villous vascularization. Imma-

ture placentas and cases of "persisting immaturity" (Fig. 14.5; also see Chapter 15) show reduced villous capillarization and, consequently, a **paucity of vasculosyncytial membranes**.

On the other hand, an increased capillarization of terminal villi is found at high altitude (Jackson et al., 1987; Reshetnikova et al., 1994) and in some other hypoxic disorders (preeclampsia, maternal heart failure, maternal anemia) (Beischer et al., 1970; Alvarez et al., 1970, 1972; Kadyrov et al., 1998) (see Control of Villous Development in Chapter 7). It results in an **increase of the vasculosyncytial membranes**; it can come about only when these conditions have existed for some time. In IUGR with absent end-diastolic umbilical blood flow, similar features are observed. Here, abnormally long, unbranched capillaries are combined with reduced diameters of terminal villi (Krebs et al., 1996; Macara et al., 1996). Finally, fetal villous congestion (see Fig. 14.1) can increase vasculosyncytial membranes.

Trophoblastic Basement Membrane

In routine paraffin sections of normal villi, the trophoblastic basement membrane is usually only seen when special stains are applied, such as aldehyde-fuchsin, periodic acid-Schiff (PAS), and immunohistochemistry for collagen IV or laminin. **Marked thickening** of the basement membrane that becomes clearly visible has been described under various pathologic conditions, such as preeclampsia and essential hypertension (Fox, 1968c), maternal diabetes (Liebhart, 1971, 1974), and IUGR with absent end-diastolic umbilical blood flow (Macara et al., 1996). The reason for these basement membrane changes presumably is that constituents of the basal lamina are secretory products of the villous trophoblast; the increased thickness indicates an altered trophoblastic activity, for example, increased secretion or decreased turnover of basal lamina molecules.

Perivillous Fibrinoid

Most perivillous fibrinoid is a blood clotting product. It is found in defects of the villous trophoblastic cover (see Perivillous Fibrinoid in Chapter 6) and here may act as a substitute for damaged trophoblast. The deposition of perivillous fibrinoid is a regular phenomenon, occurring in every placenta, and the amount increases with advancing pregnancy. This increase is particularly true for the stem villi, whose trophoblastic surface is largely replaced by fibrinoid at term (see Figs. 8.11 and 8.12). One normally finds some increase of fibrin encasing larger groups of villi below the chorionic plate (subchorionic laminated fibrin, bosselation), and also in the marginal zone.

Macroscopically visible deposits that embed larger parts of villous trees are abnormal. These are referred to as *Gitterinfarkts* (Becker & Röckelein, 1989), whereas increased amounts of fibrinoid at the base of the placenta belong to the entity known as **maternal floor infarction**, an important placental disease (see Maternal Floor Infarction in Chapter 9). In obstructing large parts of the maternofetal exchange surface, these deposits may endanger fetal growth and survival. Otherwise, **disseminated perivillous fibrinoid deposition** has no pathologic significance (Fox, 1967, 1997).

Intravillous Fibrinoid

This different type of fibrinoid has also been referred to as villous fibrinoid necrosis. It must not be confused with the perivillous fibrinoid just discussed. It is a fibrinoid patch that replaces villous stroma and vasculature underneath a more or less intact trophoblastic cover (see Fig. 3.2F). It occurs occasionally in normal mature placentas, but its incidence is increased in placentas from diabetic mothers and in cases of erythroblastosis fetalis (Fox, 1968a). Its genesis has been discussed in context with immune attacks (Burstein et al., 1973).

Villous Calcification

Villous calcifications are relatively uncommon and quite different from the minute calcium deposits in fibrinoid that occur with advancing gestation. The latter is found mostly in the floor and septa and was discussed in Chapter 9. **Villous calcification** may occur when villi have been destroyed by processes of the past such as thrombosis, CMV infection, and infarction (Fig. 14.7). Calcifications of villous tissues are also observed in some retained placental fragments or when the placenta of a fetus papyraceus is retained to term. Quantitatively they play no important role in placental pathology.

An entirely different type of calcification is the finely granular deposition of purple-staining **calcium precipitate in basement membranes** of abortuses. It is currently not certain that this represents calcium salts, as other salts have similar staining characteristics. This fine stippling is perhaps the result of deficient transport of materials through the trophoblast but not consumed after fetal death with its cessation of capillary flow. It has no known etiologic role.

Stem Vessels

It was suggested that the number of arteries in peripheral stem villi is decreased in association with umbilical Doppler high resistance (Giles et al., 1985). Since then, the topic of fetal villous arteries has attracted much attention. Studies by other investigators have not corroborated this finding (Jackson et al., 1995; Macara et al., 1995).

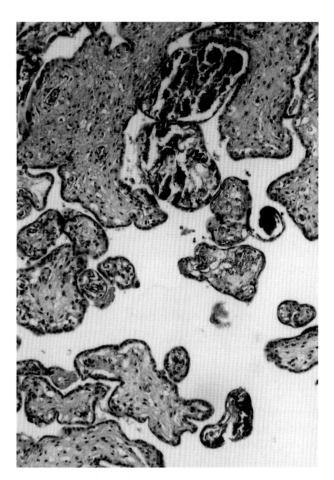

FIGURE 14.7. Immature placenta with degenerated villi that contain conspicuous areas of calcification (black, irregular, and fragmented intravillous foci). H&E ×160.

The most conspicuous pathologic changes of fetal stem vessels comprise **thromboses**. These are common features and affect mostly superficial veins. Laminated mural thrombi are our most common finding. They result primarily from obstruction of venous return to the fetus (cord knots, spirals, and prolapse) and velamentous insertion, and accompany long-standing chorioamnionitis and CMV infection. The main stem vessels and further distal vascular structures may atrophy or disappear completely. Thrombosis may thus lead to complete atrophy of portions of the villous tissue (see Fig. 12.60). Thrombosis of large arteries is less common, and usually it remains unclear what the etiology might have been. Protein C and S deficiencies have been entertained as possible causes but have never been proved. They are extremely serious for fetal development and survival.

Obliterative endarteritis (see Fig. 13.14) and especially **hemorrhagic endovasculitis (HEV)** (see Fig. 12.62) are prominent aspects of this area. HEV is found nearly exclusively in stillborn infants and most often results from postmortem dissolution of the large blood vessels and those of stem villi. Identical changes accompany local obliterations (velamentous vessels); there is no convincing evidence that they represent an infection (see Chapter 12).

Other vascular phenomena, such as **fibromuscular sclerosis**, also occur in stem vessels, primarily arteries. They are extensively discussed by Fox (1997) and other placentologists. We see them as secondary features of vascular phenomena and usually find them in the "localized" form. It is very uncommon to identify such lesions in widespread distribution. They are then related to Doppler flow anomalies and growth restriction (Fok et al., 1990), but a precise etiology has not been identified. Occlusions of this type are found after infarcts and primarily in long-standing thrombosis. Indeed, when they occur in infarcts we find it unlikely that they are "proliferative" in nature; rather, it is more probable that they come about by the condensation of dying tissues. These obliterations are usual findings in placentas associated with fetal demise. We believe them to be secondary features because other diseases nearly always explain the fetal death. In the presence of absent or reversed end-diastolic velocity in Doppler flow studies, and fetal growth retardation, NRBCs are elevated, and Bernstein et al. (1997) presumed the stem vessel lesions to have derived from thromboses. These were held to be responsible for increased impedance and, thus, growth restriction. By contrast, Krebs et al. (1996) and Macara et al. (1996) studied the vascularization of peripheral villi of growth-restricted neonates and absent end-diastolic flow velocity by scanning and transmission electron microscopy. They found significant villous abnormalities caused by abnormal capillarization, which they declared to be the reason for growth restriction of the fetus. Concentric thickening of media and intima of the tertiary villous vessels were found by Harvey-Wilkes and her colleagues (1996). Associated with this, they observed elevated endothelin levels and used these findings to explain an increased placental resistance and the fetal growth restriction. But what the original etiology for most of these changes is remains speculative, although thrombosis remains the most attractive hypothesis. For that reason, microembolism studies were undertaken in sheep (Gagnon et al., 1996); the results are similar to the spontaneous occurrence in human placentas.

The extensive discussion of endarteritis obliterans by Fox (1997) includes a photograph (see Fig. 6.23) of a vessel depicting "endothelial swelling." Others have called similar features **endothelial edema**. It very likely represents an artifact and has no relationship to endarteritis. Similar discussions occurred in considerations of HIV-related vascular alterations (see Contractility of Umbilical Vessels in Chapter 12). Indeed, the entity has been widely discussed as occurring in diabetes, pre-eclampsia, erythroblastosis, and other conditions. Rapid fixation and the use of Bouin's solution usually prevents "endarteritis" from being recognizable. It must also be said that the peripheral districts of so-called endarteritis are usually not disturbed, negating its importance as a primary disease of the placenta.

Nucleated Red Blood Cells

The fetal blood vessels may contain NRBCs. This is a normal finding in gestations of less than 3 months' duration (see Fig. 3.1C). These elements are abnormal in the last trimester, however, especially when they are identified in routine histology. They then betray the fetal response to erythropoietin (EPO), a hormone that is now frequently measured in neonates. When NRBCs are present one must enumerate them in neonatal blood smears as they rapidly decline after birth. They signify fetal anemia, infection, erythroblastosis, transplacental hemorrhage, or, importantly, prenatal hypoxia. Because it takes time for the secretion of these cells from precursor stores (liver, marrow) through the intervention of EPO and perhaps other signals, the presence of NRBCs suggests that fetal tissue hypoxia of whatever type has occurred many hours, perhaps days, before birth. The topic is covered more extensively in Chapter 8 (see Nucleated Red Blood Cells).

Villous Capillarization

The vasculature of villi is difficult to adjudicate because the capillaries tend to collapse after delivery. The degree of collapse depends on the mode of delivery, the mode of cord clamping, the time elapsed between cessation of umbilical circulation and fixation, and the composition of the fixative (see Tables 28.8 to 28.10). Moreover, when the tissue is fixed in inadequate volumes of fixative the tissue becomes compressed. Thus, asymmetrical compression or distortion of the placenta during fixation may cause considerable shifts of intravascular volume with complete collapse in one part of the fetal vascular bed and apparent overdistention in another. Conclusions concerning villous capillarization, therefore, must always take these potential errors into consideration.

Reduced capillarization of the terminal villous tree is found in slightly immature placentas (see Figs. 14.5 and 15.9). This feature is combined with a uniform trophoblastic cover of the mature intermediate villi that show unusually straight and parallel sections because terminal side branches are largely missing (Fig. 14.5; see Chapter 15).

Complete atrophy of capillaries can be found peripheral to obstructive lesions in the stem vessels (see Placental Surface Vessels in Chapter 12). Small groups of avascular villi are seen in every placenta (Fig. 14.4), but a higher incidence is often combined with IUGR or intrauterine fetal death.

Hypercapillarization may show different features, some of these have already been considered. Cases of **hypoxic hypercapillarization** are usually characterized by numerous but small capillary cross sections in clusters of aggregated terminal villi. The latter are often connected to each other by trophoblastic flat sections. This feature is often referred to as chorangiosis (see Figs. 14.1, 15.6, and 15.16, and Chapter 24) (Bacon et al., 1984; Jackson et al., 1985, 1988). Three-dimensional reconstruction revealed richly branched capillary nets (Scheffen et al., 1990) resulting from branching angiogenesis. Branching angiogenesis is driven by vascular endothelial growth factor (VEGF), the expression of which is upregulated by low oxygen partial pressures (see Chapter 7). Typical examples of hypoxic hypercapillarization are found in maternal anemia (Kadyrov et al., 1998), and in IUGR with preserved end-diastolic umbilical flow with or without preeclampsia (Todros et al., 1999).

One sometimes finds cases in which very few (usually only two) but locally dilated capillary cross sections occupy extremely small terminal villi (see Fig. 15.13). These villi have long, unbranched capillary loops (see Figs. 7.17 and 15.6) resulting from **excessive nonbranching angiogenesis**. The respective terminal villi rarely aggregate, forming clusters of villi connected by syncytial knotting. Rather, they represent a mixture of single villous cross sections measuring only 40 to 60 μm in diameter, together with few filiform longitudinal sections (Fig. 14.8). These features often exist among premature deliveries (Schweikhart et al., 1986). We observed the most impressive cases of this kind associated with severe IUGR with absent umbilical end-diastolic blood flow (Krebs et al., 1996; Macara et al., 1996; Kingdom et al., 1997) (Fig. 14.8). This condition is thought to be caused by abnormally high intervillous oxygen partial pressures (postplacental hypoxia) (Kingdom & Kaufmann, 1997).

These features are not always easy to differentiate from **villous congestion** (see Fig. 14.3), also resulting in overdistended peripheral vessels. The presence of overdistended veins in stem villi, the normalcy of villous caliber distribution, the loss of plasma between the erythrocytes, extravasations, and signs of hemolysis may be helpful for the diagnosis. Congestion may be the result of cord complications (see the sections Knots and Thrombosis of the Placental Vascular Tree in Chapter 12) and also of thrombosis of major villous stem veins. Finally, we have often observed congestion in cases of premature rupture of the membranes, perhaps because of loss of amnionic fluid thus altering venous umbilical blood flow.

Stromal Architecture and Stromal Fibrosis

Fibrosis of stem villi is a good indicator of placental maturity (see Chapter 8, Figs. 8.2 to 8.12). Fibrosis starts on about the 15th week postmenstruation (p.m.), begins

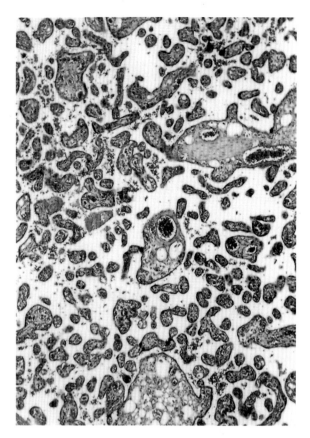

FIGURE 14.8. Placenta at 29 weeks' gestation associated with severe fetal growth retardation (neonatal death), showing marked accelerated maturation of the terminal villous branches. The small diameter of terminal villi and the absence of syncytial knotting suggest this is a case of nonbranching angiogenesis in terminal villi caused by postplacental hypoxia (cf. Chapter 15). As is typical for many cases of accelerated maturation, stem villi remain in their normal immature condition. Their appearance must not be confused with edema. H&E ×64.

around the stem vessels, and should be complete a few weeks before term. When reticular, unfibrosed connective tissue persists under the trophoblastic membrane, as in Figures 8.5 and 8.6, it signifies immaturity.

Extensive stromal fibrosis is abnormal, especially when it is not restricted to the stem villi (i.e., those with media-endowed vessels). It can be found in "intrauterine growth retardation combined with absent umbilical end-diastolic blood flow" (Macara et al., 1996), in avascular villi following stem vessel obstruction or fetal death (see Fig. 14.4) (Becker, 1981b; Veen et al., 1982), in CMV infection, and in a few other conditions. It has been speculated that increased intravillous oxygen partial pressure stimulates collagen synthesis when it occurs in the maternally well oxygenated but fetally malperfused placenta (for review, see Kaufmann et al., 1993; Kingdom & Kaufmann, 1997). In contrast, intraplacental hypoxia has been inferred to be responsible for reduced villous fibrosis (Fox, 1968b,

1997), for example, unfibrosed, immature villi in preeclampsia (see Fig. 14.6).

Hofbauer Cells (Macrophages)

These cells can easily be seen within the stromal channels of the immature intermediate villi (see Figs. 7.4 and 7.9). When one uses immunohistochemical markers for macrophages (CD68 antibodies), it becomes evident that they are present in all villous types throughout all stages of pregnancy, although they may be difficult to see. Therefore, the impression of increased numbers of Hofbauer cells is usually the result of increased numbers of immature intermediate villi. It thus points to an immature placenta or persisting immaturity in a term organ. Other associations are unknown.

An apparent deficiency of macrophages is observed in moles and some chromosomal aberrations, especially in their large, pale villi that otherwise have the appearance of immature intermediate villi. In these cases, the pale stroma is very loose and hydropic and does not belong to the reticular type, that which has stromal channels and contains macrophages (see Chapters 21 and 22, Figs. 21.5, 22.9, and 22.21).

Inflammatory Changes

Villi may participate in infectious diseases by infiltration of mononuclear and polymorphonuclear leukocytes (polys). Polys are rarely within villi; they are most common in the amnionic sac infection syndrome, chorioamnionitis. When polys are present within villi, this signifies an acute infectious bacterial disease. **Acute villitis** is a prominent feature of listeriosis, a disease that is disseminated by maternal septicemia. Other maternal bacterial infections, such as staphylococcal sepsis and other bacterial septicemias, are extremely uncommon. They all produce abscesses in the placenta with dissolution of villous tissue.

Much the commonest placental infection recognized is that with **cytomegalovirus** (CMV). The picture this virus produces is extremely variable. When one finds plasma cells concentrated in a few villi, especially when they are accompanied by hemosiderin-laden macrophages and villous sclerosis, then CMV infection is likely. One may then have to search for the typical inclusion bodies, a sometimes difficult task, or stain with immunoprobes or identify the virus with the polymerase chain reaction (PCR) technique. Typical "owl-eye" cells may be found in endothelium, trophoblast, and unidentified stromal cells (see Fig. 20.48). Other chronic villitides are caused by toxoplasma and syphilis; they are rarely due to rubella and other recognized viruses (see Chapter 20).

Much the most problematic is the entity known as **villitis of unknown etiology** (VUE), which is also discussed at length in Chapter 20. In this villitis chronic inflamma-

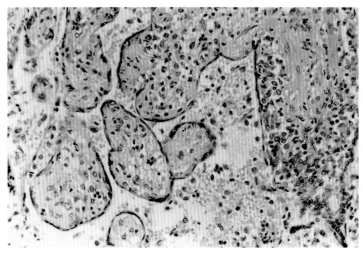

FIGURE 14.9. Placenta from a patient with villitis of unknown etiology (VUE) at 36 weeks' gestation. The infant was stillborn. Note marked infiltration of chronic inflammatory cells and simultaneous destruction of villous integrity (right). H&E ×250.

tory cells predominate but plasma cells and polys are generally absent. The villi, however, may disintegrate as Figure 14.9 shows. Villitis of unknown etiology is frequent and has no known etiology. It may recur in subsequent gestations and, when extensive, it may cause fetal death. No microorganisms have been discovered as its cause and recent suggestions of the possible infiltration with maternal immunocytes are too inconclusive still. They may signal immune recognition of the fetal antigen, but that is far from certain.

Villous Edema or Immaturity

Many authors call every large, pale-staining villus an edematous villus following the description by Naeye et al. (1983). It is our experience that most of these villi are in fact normal immature intermediate villi (Fig. 14.10) (Pilz et al., 1980; Kaufmann et al., 1987). They may cause diagnostic problems, as their reticular stromal core has only a weak affinity for conventional stains because it lacks collagen. The resulting histologic picture is that of a seemingly edematous villus that had accumulated much interstitial fluid.

True **edematous villi** indeed exist, however, as well. They are particularly impressive in hydatidiform moles and hydatid degeneration of abortion specimens (Fig. 14.11), but some are found occasionally in infections such as syphilis, toxoplasmosis, CMV infection, and a variety of cases of hydrops (Fig. 14.12). Placentas from erythroblastosis and other causes of hydrops may show a combination of the two features, as most villi display a retarded maturation and many are additionally edematous (Fig. 14.13).

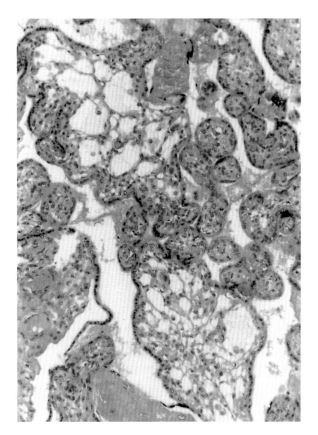

FIGURE 14.10. Placenta at 26 weeks' gestation of a case of congenital epidermolysis bullosa. The villous architecture, appropriate for this gestational age, is composed of immature intermediate villi with reticular stroma. They are surrounded by small mesenchymal villi. H&E ×160.

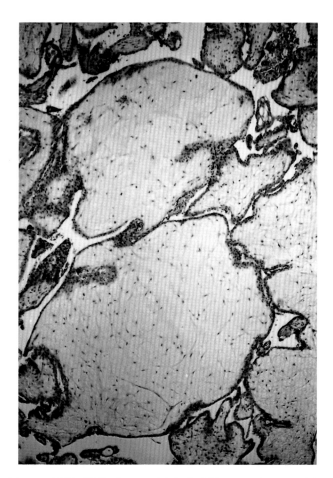

FIGURE 14.11. Villi of a partial hydatidiform mole caused by triploidy. There is marked villous distention with edema fluid. On first glance, this appearance is similar to that of immature intermediate villi (Figs. 14.10 and 14.13), but the macrophages of normal intermediate villi are lacking. H&E ×64.

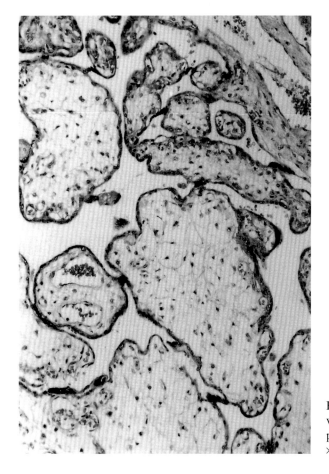

FIGURE 14.12. Villi of hydropic fetus with Finnish nephrosis. Most villi are severely hydropic, but they are not different from villi in placentas of other hydrops cases. Compare with Figure 14.11. H&E ×160.

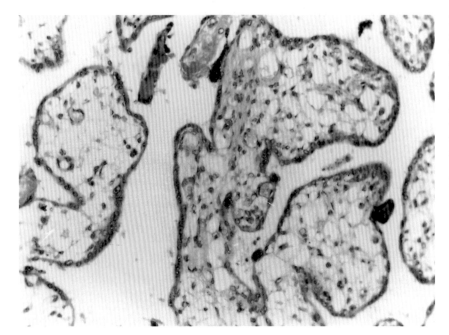

FIGURE 14.13. Immature placenta of a pregnancy with hydrops fetalis caused by fetal endocardial fibroelastosis. The placenta shows a combination of normal immaturity with edema. The villi exhibit partly normal immature reticular stroma with an abundance of macrophages (Hofbauer cells, dark cells in reticular spaces), which is normal for immature intermediate villi. In other villi the reticular pattern is partially destroyed by various degrees of edema. H&E ×256.

Small numbers of **immature intermediate villi** are found in the centers of the villous trees in nearly every mature placenta (see Fig. 7.18). These are the still proliferating villi and may represent a kind of growth reserve. When they occur in disseminated fashion, or even when there is only a prevalence of this villous type, this indicates immaturity, synchronous or asynchronous. It may be found in many cases of preterm delivery (Schweikhart et al., 1986) and of prolonged pregnancy (Fox, 1968d; Kemnitz & Theuring, 1974; Mikolajczak et al., 1987).

References

Altshuler, G.: Chorangiosis: an important placental sign of neonatal morbidity and mortality. Arch. Pathol. Lab. Med. **108**:71–74, 1984.

Altshuler, G.: Some placental considerations related to neuro-developmental and other disorders. J. Child Neurol. **8**:78–94, 1993.

Altshuler, G. and Herman, A.A.: The medicolegal imperative: placental pathology and epidemiology. In, Fetal and Neonatal Brain Injury: Mechanisms, Management and the Risk of Malpractice. D.K. Stevenson and P. Sunshine, eds., pp. 250–263. Decker, Toronto, 1989.

Alvarez, H., Morel, R.L., Benedetti, W.L. and Scavarelli, M.: Trophoblast hyperplasia and maternal arterial pressure at term. Amer. J. Obstet. Gynecol. **105**:1015–1021, 1969.

Alvarez, H., Benedetti, W.L., Morel, R.L. and Scavarelli, M.: Trophoblast development gradient and its relationship to placental hemodynamics. Amer. J. Obstet. Gynecol. **106**:416–420, 1970.

Alvarez, H., Medrano, C.V., Sala, M.A. and Benedetti, W.L.: Trophoblast development gradient and its relationship to placental hemodynamics. II. Study of fetal cotyledons from the toxemic placenta. Amer. J. Obstet. Gynecol. **114**:873–878, 1972.

Bacon, B.J., Gilbert, R.D., Kaufmann, P., Smith, A.D., Trevino, F.T. and Longo, L.D.: Placental anatomy and diffusing capacity in guinea pigs following long-term maternal hypoxia. Placenta **5**:475–487, 1984.

Becker, V.: Über maturitas praecox placentae. Verh. Deutsche Gesellsch. Pathol. **44**:256–260, 1960.

Becker, V.: Pathologie der Ausreifung der Plazenta. In, Die Plazenta des Menschen. V. Becker, T.H. Schiebler and F. Kubli, eds., pp. 266–281. Thieme, Stuttgart, 1981a.

Becker, V.: Plazenta bei Totgeburt. In, Die Plazenta des Menschen. V. Becker, T.H. Schiebler and F. Kubli, eds., pp. 305–308. Thieme, Stuttgart, 1981b.

Becker, V. and Röckelein, G.: Pathologie der weiblichen Genitalorgane I. Pathologie der Plazenta und des Abortes. Springer-Verlag, Heidelberg, 1989.

Beischer, N.A., Sivasamboo, R., Vohra, S., Silpisornkosal, S. and Reid, S.: Placental hypertrophy in severe pregnancy anaemia. J. Obstet. Gynaecol. Br. Commonw. **77**:398–409, 1970.

Benirschke, K. and Gille, J.: Placental pathology and asphyxia. In, Intrauterine Asphyxia and the Developing Fetal Brain. L. Gluck, ed. Year Book, Chicago, 1977.

Bernstein, P.S., Minior, V.K. and Divon, M.Y.: Neonatal nucleated red blood cell counts in small-for-gestational age fetuses with abnormal umbilical artery Doppler studies. Amer. J. Obstet. Gynecol. **177**:1079–1084, 1997.

Bouw, G.M., Stolte, L.A.M., Baak, J.P.A. and Oort, J.: Quantitative morphology of the placenta. 1. Standardization of sampling. Europ. J. Obstet. Gynecol. Reprod. Biol. **6**:325–331, 1976.

Burstein, R., Frankel, S., Soule, S.D. and Blumenthal, H.T.: Aging of the placenta: autoimmune theory of senescence. Am. J. Obstet. Gynecol. **116**:271–276, 1973.

Burton, G.J.: Intervillous connections in the mature human placenta: Instances of syncytial fusion or section artifacts? J. Anat. **145**:13–23, 1986a.

Burton, G.J.: Scanning electron microscopy of intervillous connections in the mature human placenta. J. Anat. **147**:245–254, 1986b.

Cantle, S.J., Kaufmann, P., Luckhardt, M. and Schweikhart, G.: Interpretation of syncytial sprouts and bridges in the human placenta. Placenta **8**:221–234, 1987.

Clifford, S.H.: Postmaturity-with placental dysfunction. Amer. J. Obstet. Gynecol. **44**:1–13, 1954.

de Sa, D.J.: Intimal cushions in foetal placental veins. J. Pathol. **110**:347–352, 1973.

Emmrich, P.: Pathologie der Plazenta. VII. Asphyxieinfiltrate der Plazenta. Zentralbl. Pathol. **137**:479–485, 1991.

Emmrich, P. and Mälzer, G.: Zur Morphologie der Plazenta bei Übertragung. Pathol. Microbiol. **32**:285–302, 1968.

Emmrich, P., Dalitz, H. and Rother, P.: Genesis and significance of so-called asphyxial infiltrates of the placenta. I. Histological findings. Ann. Anat. **180**:123–130, 1998a.

Emmrich, P., Friedrich, T. and Dalitz, H.: Genesis and significance of so-called asphyxial infiltrates of the placenta. I. Immunohistochemical findings. Ann. Anat. **180**:203–209, 1998b.

Essbach, H. and Röse, I.: Plazenta und Eihäute. Fischer, Jena, 1966.

Fejgin, M.D., Amiel, A., Goldberger, S., Barnes, I., Zer, T. and Kohn, G.: Placental insufficiency as a possible cause of low maternal serum human gonadotropin and low maternal serum unconjugated estriol levels in triploidy. Amer. J. Obstet. Gynecol. **167**:766–767, 1993.

Fok, R.Y., Pavlova, Z., Benirschke, K., Paul, R.H. and Platt, L.D.: The correlation of arterial lesions with umbilical artery Doppler velocimetry in the placentas of small-for-dates pregnancies. Obstet. Gynecol. **75**:578–583, 1990.

Fox, H.: Perivillous fibrin deposition in the human placenta. Am. J. Obstet. Gynecol. **98**:245–251, 1967.

Fox, H.: Fibrinoid necrosis of placental villi. J. Obstet. Gynaecol. Br. Commonw. **75**:448–452, 1968a.

Fox, H.: Fibrosis of placental villi. J. Pathol. Bacteriol. **95**:573–579, 1968b.

Fox, H.: Basement membrane changes in the villi of the human placenta. J. Obstet. Gynaecol. Br. Commonw. **75**:302–306, 1968c.

Fox, H.: Villous immaturity in the term placenta. Obstet. Gynecol. **31**:9–12, 1968d.

Fox, H.: Pathology of the Placenta. 2nd Ed. Saunders, London, 1997.

Gagnon, R., Johnston, L. and Murotsuki, J.: Fetal placental embolization in the late-gestation ovine fetus: alterations in umbilical blood flow and fetal heart rate patterns. Amer. J. Obstet. Gynecol. **175**:63–72, 1996.

Garrow, J.S. and Hawes, S.F.: The relationship of the size and composition of the human placenta to its functional capacity. J. Obstet. Gynaecol. Br. Commonw. **78**:22–28, 1971.

Giles, W.B., Trudinger, B.J. and Baird, P.J.: Fetal umbilical artery flow velocity waveforms and placental resistance: pathological correlation. Br. J. Obstet. Gynaecol. **92**:31–38, 1985.

Gille, J.: Kritische Gedanken zur "Plazentainsuffizienz". Med. Klin. **80**:148–152, 1985.

Goshen, R. and Hochberg, A.A.: The genomic basis of the §-subunit of human chorionic gonadotropin diversity in triploidy. Amer. J. Obstet. Gynecol. **170**:700–701, 1994.

Harvey-Wilkes, K., Nielsen, H.C. and D'Alton, M.E.: Elevated endothelin levels are associated with increased placental resistance. Amer. J. Obstet. Gynecol. **174**:1599–1604, 1996.

Jackson, M.R., Joy, C.F., Mayhew, T.M. and Haas, J.D.: Stereological studies on the true thickness of the villous membrane in human term placentae: a study of placentae from high altitude pregnancies. Placenta **6**:249–258, 1985.

Jackson, M.R., Mayhew, T.M. and Haas, J.D.: Morphometric studies on villi in human term placentae and the effects of altitude, ethnic grouping and sex of newborn. Placenta **8**:487–495, 1987.

Jackson, M.R., Mayhew, T.M. and Haas, J.D.: On the factors which contribute to thinning of the villous membrane in human placentae at high altitude. II. An increase in the degree of peripheralization of fetal capillaries. Placenta **9**:9–18, 1988.

Jackson, M.R., Walsh, A.J., Morrow, R.J., Mullen, J.B.M., Lye, S.J. and Ritchie, J.W.K.: Reduced placental villous tree elaboration in small-for-gestational-age pregnancies: relationship with umbilical artery Doppler waveforms. Amer. J. Obstet. Gynecol. **172**:518–525, 1995.

Jauniaux, E., Ramsay, B. and Campbell, S.: Ultrasonographic investigation of placental morphologic characteristics and size during the second trimester of pregnancy. Amer. J. Obstet. Gynecol. **170**:130–137, 1994.

Kadyrov, M., Kosanke, G., Kingdom, J. and Kaufmann, P.: Increased fetoplacental angiogenesis during first trimester in anaemic women. Lancet **352**(9142):1747–1749, 1998.

Kaufmann, P.: Influence of ischemia and artificial perfusion on placental ultrastructure and morphometry. Contrib. Gynecol. Obstet. **13**:18–26, 1985.

Kaufmann, P., Luckhardt, M., Schweikhart, G. and Cantle, S.J.: Cross-sectional features and three-dimensional structure of human placental villi. Placenta **8**:235–247, 1987.

Kaufmann, P., Kohnen, G. and Kosanke, G.: Wechselwirkungen zwischen Plazentamorphologie und fetaler Sauerstoffversorgung. Versuch einer zellbiologischen Interpretation pathohistologischer und experimenteller Befunde. Gynäkologe **26**:16–23, 1993.

Kemnitz, P. and Theuring, F.: Makroskopische, licht- und elektronenmikroskopische Plazentabefunde bei Uebertragung. Zentralbl. Allg. Pathol. **118**:43–54, 1974.

Kingdom, J.C.P. and Kaufmann, P.: Oxygen and placental villous development: origins of fetal hypoxia. Placenta **18**:613–621, 1997.

Kingdom, J.C.P., Macara, L.M., Krebs, C., Leiser, R. and Kaufmann, P.: Pathological basis for abnormal umbilical artery Doppler waveforms in pregnancies complicated by intrauterine growth restriction. Trophoblast Res. **10**:291–309, 1997.

Kloos, K. and Vogel, M.: Pathologie der Perinatalperiode. Thieme, Stuttgart, 1974.

Kosanke, G., Kadyrov, M., Korr, H. and Kaufmann, P.: Maternal anemia results in increased proliferation in human placental villi. Trophoblast Res. **11**:339–357, 1998.

Krebs, C., Macara, L.M., Leiser, R., Bowman, A.W., Greer, I.A. and Kingdom, J.C.P.: Intrauterine growth restriction with absent end-diastolic flow velocity in the umbilical artery is associated with maldevelopment of the placental terminal villous tree. Amer. J. Obstet. Gynecol. **175**:1534–1542, 1996.

Küstermann, W.: Über "Proliferationsknoten" und "Syncy-tialknoten" der menschlichen Placenta. Anat. Anz. **150**:144–157, 1981.

Kuss, E.: Was ist "Das Plazentainsuffizienzsyndrom"? Geburtsh. Frauenheilkd. **47**:664–670, 1987.

Liebhart, M.: The electron microscopic pattern of placental villi in diabetes of the mother. Acta Med. Pol. **12**:133–137, 1971.

Liebhart, M.: Ultrastructure of the stromal connective tissue of normal placenta and of placenta in diabetes mellitus of mother. Pathol. Eur. **9**:177–184, 1974.

Macara, L.M., Kingdom, J.C.P., Kohnen, G., Bowman, A.W., Greer, I.A. and Kaufmann, P.: Elaboration of stem villous vessels in growth restricted pregnancies with abnormal artery Doppler waveforms. Br. J. Obstet. Gynaecol. **102**:807–812, 1995.

Macara, L.M., Kingdom, J.C.P., Kaufmann, P., Kohnen, G., Hair, J., More, I.A.R., Lyall, F. and Greer, I.A.: Structural analysis of placental terminal villi from growth-restricted pregnancies with abnormal umbilical artery Doppler waveforms. Placenta **17**:37–48, 1996.

Mayhew, T.M., Wadrop, E. and Simpson, R.A.: The proliferative versus hypertrophic growth in tissue subcompartments of human placental villi during gestation. J. Anat. **184**:535–543, 1994.

McDermott, M. and Gillan, J.E.: Chronic reduction of fetal blood flow is associated with placental infarction. Placenta **16**:165–170, 1995.

Mikolajczak, J., Ruhrberg, A., Fetzer, M., Kaufmann, P. and Goecke, C.: Irreguläre Zottenreifung bei Frühgeburtichkeit und Übertragung, und ihre Darstellbarkeit im Ultraschall. Gynaekol. Rundsch. **27**:145–146, 1987.

Naeye, R.L.: Disorders of the Placenta, Fetus, and Neonate. Diagnosis and Clinical Significance. Mosby Year Book, St. Louis, 1992.

Naeye, R.L., Maisels, J., Lorenz, R.P. and Botti, J.J.: The clinical significance of placental villous edema. Pediatrics **71**:588–594, 1983.

Pilz, I., Schweikhart, G. and Kaufmann, P.: Zur Abgrenzung normaler, artefizieller und pathologischer Strukturen in reifen menschlichen Plazentazotten. III. Morphometrische Untersuchungen bei Rh-Inkompatibilität. Arch. Gynecol. Obstet. **229**:137–154, 1980.

Piotrowicz, B., Niebroj, T.K. and Sieron, G.: The morphology and histochemistry of the full term placenta in anaemic patients. Folia Histochem. Cytochem. **7**:436–444, 1969.

Reshetnikova, O.S., Burton, G.J. and Milovanov, A.P.: Effects of hypobaric hypoxia on the fetoplacental unit: the morphometric diffusing capacity of the villous membrane at high altitude. Amer. J. Obstet. Gynecol. **171**:1560–1565, 1994.

Salafia, C.M., Vintzileos, A.M., Silberman, L., Bantham, K.F. and Vogel, C.A.: Placental pathology of idiopathic intrauterine growth retardation at term. Amer. J. Perinatol. **9**:179–184, 1992.

Sander, C.H.: Hemorrhagic endovasculitis and hemorrhagic villitis of the placenta. Arch. Pathol. Lab. Med. **104**:371–373, 1980.

Scheffen, I., Kaufmann, P., Philippens, L., Leiser, R., Geisen, C. and Mottaghy, K.: Alterations of the fetal capillary bed in the guinea pig placenta following long-term hypoxia. Adv. Exp. Med. Biol. **277**:779–790, 1990.

Schuhmann, R.: Plazenton: Begriff, Entstehung, funktionelle Anatomie. In, Die Plazenta des Menschen. V. Becker, T.H. Schiebler and F. Kubli, eds., pp. 192–207. Thieme, Stuttgart, 1981.

Schweikhart, G.: Morphologie des Zottenbaumes der menschlichen Plazenta. Orthologische und pathologische Entwicklung und ihre klinische Relevanz. Thesis, Medical Faculty of University Mainz, 1985.

Schweikhart, G., Kaufmann, P. and Beck, T.: Morphology of placental villi after premature delivery and its clinical relevance. Arch. Gynecol. **239**:101–114, 1986.

Shen-Schwarz, S., Ruchelli, E. and Brown, D.: Villous oedema of the placenta: a clinicopathological study. Placenta **10**:297–307, 1989.

Sinclair, J.G.: Significance of placental and birthweight ratios. Anat. Rec. **102**:245–258, 1948.

Tenney, B. and Parker, F.: The placenta in toxemia of pregnancy. Amer. J. Obstet. Gynecol. **39**:1000–1005, 1940.

Todros, T., Sciarrone, A., Piccoli, E., Guiot, C., Kaufmann, P. and Kingdom, J.: Umbilical Doppler waveforms and placental villous angiogenesis in pregnancies complicated by fetal growth restriction. Obstet. Gynecol. **93**:499–503, 1999.

Veen, F., Walker, S. and Fox, H.: Endarteritis obliterans of the fetal stem arteries of the human placenta: an electron microscopic study. Placenta **3**:181–190, 1982.

Vogel, M.: Pathologie der Schwangerschaft, der Plazenta und des Neugeborenen. In, Pathologie, Vol. 3. Remmele, W. ed. Springer-Verlag, Heidelberg, 1984.

Vogel, M.: Atlas der Morphologischen Plazentadiagnostik. 2nd Ed. Springer-Verlag, Heidelberg, 1996.

Voigt, S., Kaufmann, P. and Schweikhart, G.: Zur Abgrenzung normaler, artefizieller und pathologischer Strukturen in reifen menschlichen Plazentazotten. II. Morphometrische Untersuchungen zum Einfluß des Fixationsmodus. Arch. Gynäkol. **226**:347–362, 1978.

Wentworth, P.: The placenta in cases of hemolytic disease of the newborn. Amer. J. Obstet. Gynecol. **98**:283–289, 1967.

Werner, C. and Schneiderhan, W.: Plazentamorphologie und Plazentafunktion in Abhaengigkeit von der diabetischen Stoffwechselfuehrung. Geburtsh. Frauenheilkd. **32**:959–966, 1972.

Wong, T.-C. and Latour, J.P.A.: Microscopic measurement of the placental components in an attempt to assess the malnourished newborn infant. Amer. J. Obstet. Gynecol. **94**:942–950, 1966.

15
Classification of Villous Maldevelopment

Three-Dimensional Interpretation of Two-Dimensional Sections

The histopathology of villous maldevelopment is based on the light microscopy of paraffin sections. Thus, the normal and pathologic features of the placenta are usually described in terms of the two dimensions apparent by light microscopy. These two-dimensional findings very often do not reflect the underlying three-dimensional malformation of villi, as becomes particularly obvious when considering the pathologically meaningful finding of "syncytial knotting" (Tenney-Parker changes).

Syncytial Knotting: Artifact or Meaningful Pathologic Finding

In past decades several studies have revealed that the two-dimensional impression does not always reflect the three-dimensional structure. Küstermann (1981) used reconstructions of serial paraffin sections to show that most sprouts and bridges are in fact flat sections of irregularly shaped villous surfaces. Burton (1986a,b, 1987), who worked with plastic serial sections, and Cantle et al. (1987) and Kaufmann et al. (1987), who compared light microscopic findings of villous sections with scanning electron microscopy of the identical material (Fig. 15.1), arrived at similar conclusions. All three groups concluded that most of the syncytial knots, syncytial sprouts, and syncytial bridges, summarized as syncytial knotting or Tenney-Parker changes (for definition, see Chapter 6) proved to be only tangential sections of the villous surface. The true interpretation is of considerable importance for aspects of placental pathology, as the histologic appearance of syncytial knotting is widely accepted as a diagnostic indicator of placental ischemia, for example, in preeclampsia (Tenney & Parker, 1940; Alvarez et al., 1964, 1969, 1970; Schuhmann & Geier, 1972).

Küstermann's (1981) statement that all sprouts, knots, and bridges of the mature placenta must be interpreted as sectional artifacts brought about the question whether the histopathologic experience should be abandoned. Küstermann's results were largely corroborated by the studies of Burton (1986a) and Cantle et al. (1987). At the same time, it became apparent (Kaufmann et al., 1987) that despite this new interpretation, the diagnostic value of syncytial knotting, even in most cases representing artifacts, was still useful. As is described next, they are significant artifacts that point to a characteristic deformation of the terminal villi. This deformation is usually caused by abnormal villous angiogenesis resulting from abnormal placental oxygenation (see Fig. 15.6). Therefore, the final conclusions drawn by Alvarez et al. (1969, 1970) are generally correct: the diagnostic value of the two-dimensional findings of syncytial knotting remains.

Interpretation of Syncytial Knotting

Küstermann (1981) and Burton (1986a) used three-dimensional reconstructions of serial sections to verify that most knots, sprouts, and bridges are only flat sections (see Fig. 15.4), a point that can be demonstrated even more impressively in two other ways. Cantle et al. (1987) prepared 10-μm epoxy resin sections stained with toluidine blue. This dye does not infiltrate the resin and stains it only superficially. The resulting light microscopic picture corresponds to that of a semithin section of 0.5 to 1.0 μm (Fig. 15.2A). When studying the same section with phase contrast microscopy, one obtains a view of the complete 10-μm section of the identical material. When comparing the two pictures of the same section shown in Figure 15.2B, one easily realizes that the thin section does not show any sprouts, whereas the thick section reveals three apparent sprouts that were obviously tangential sections of the trophoblastic surface.

This finding is in agreement with the experience of all electron microscopists who have studied the placenta:

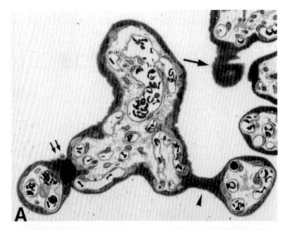

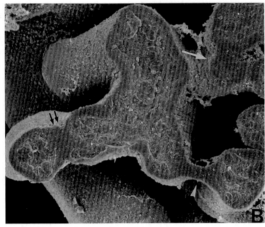

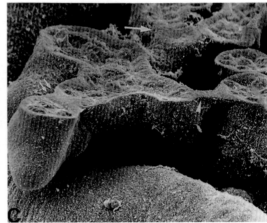

FIGURE 15.1. Term placenta. After preparing a semithin section (A), the epoxy resin has been removed from the remaining tissue block. The latter was prepared for scanning electron microscopy. Identical villi are shown in a semithin section (A) and scanning electron micrographs in vertical (B) and nearly horizontal orientations (C). The arrowhead points to a true syncytial bridge, histologically characterized by its smooth surface, whereas the other "bridge" (double arrow), characterized by its irregular histologic appearance, proves to be a tangential section of a curved villous portion. The large arrow marks an artificial "sprout" that can easily be identified as a tangential section. ×265. (*Source:* Cantle et al., 1987, with permission.)

knots, sprouts, and bridges are common in paraffin sections (5–10 μm), rare in semithin sections (0.5–1.0 μm), and mostly absent in the ultrathin sections (0.05–0.1 μm) prepared for electron microscopy. The situation is schematically depicted in Figure 15.3.

Similar conclusions were deduced when we prepared semithin sections for light microscopy and subsequently removed the epoxy resin from the remaining tissue block. The remaining villi were studied with the scanning electron microscope and compared to the semithin section (Fig. 15.1) (Cantle et al., 1987). Using this method, real sprouts and bridges as well as flat-sectioned villous surfaces can easily be identified and compared to the sectional picture of this tissue. It became evident from such material that branching, twisting, and coiling of villi (e.g., as a result of hypoxia) enhances the chance of tangential sectioning of trophoblastic surfaces and thus increases

the number of artificial knots, sprouts, and ridges (see Fig. 15.6).

On the other hand, scanning electron microscopic proof was presented by Schiebler and Kaufmann (1981), Burton (1986b, 1987), and Cantle et al. (1987) that not all sprouts, knots, and bridges are sectional artifacts; rather, few real such trophoblastic specializations do exist. They may serve (1) as first steps of villous sprouting, that is, formation of new villi (trophoblastic or syncytial sprouts) (Boyd & Hamilton, 1970; Cantle et al., 1987; Castellucci et al., 1990); (2) as a mechanism of extrusion of old syncytial nuclei (Martin & Spicer, 1973; Jones & Fox, 1977), most of the latter meanwhile identified as being apoptotic in nature (Huppertz et al., 1998); or (3) as simple mechanical aids to establish junctions between neighboring villi (syncytial bridges) (Cantle et al., 1987). Based on the findings by Cantle et al. (1987) and Huppertz et al.

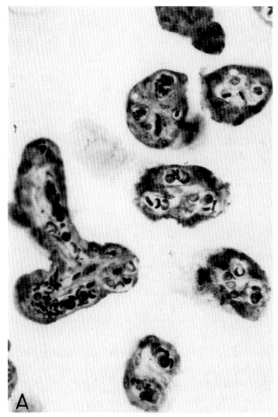
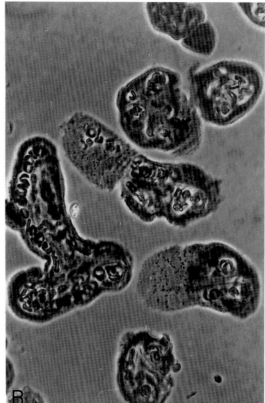

FIGURE 15.2. Term placenta from a patient with preeclampsia. A: A 10–μm epoxy resin section is stained only superficially with toluidine blue, comparable to a semithin section of about 1–μm thickness. B: The same section as in A is observed with phase contrast microscopy and now represents the full section thickness of 10μm. It shows three sprout-like structures, obviously tangential sections of the trophoblastic surface and not visible in the "thinner" section. It demonstrates the influence of the thickness of the section on the appearance of so-called sprouts and knots, caused by trophoblastic tangential sectioning. ×380. (*Source:* Cantle et al., 1987, with permission.)

(1998) we suggest the following criteria for discriminating between true trophoblastic specializations and tangential sections (Fig. 15.5):

- **True syncytial sprouting** resulting from trophoblastic proliferation is usually characterized by smooth surfaces with well-developed microvilli and loosely scattered, ovoid nuclei (see Fig. 6.11A,B). Only incidentally do they fuse with neighboring villi to form syncytial bridges (see Figs. 6.12A,B and 15.1A).

- Degenerative, **apoptotic knotting** results in knot- or sprout-like structures showing smooth surfaces, mostly devoid of microvilli; the densely packed nuclei show highly condensed chromatin, the most peripheral nuclei usually displaying annular chromatin condensation (see Figs. 6.10A, 6.18, and 6.22).
- Flat sections (**syncytial knotting, Tenney-Parker changes**) result in knots, sprouts, and bridges that are irregularly shaped and notched (see Figs. 6.10C and 15.1A); they are characterized by heterogeneous nuclear shapes as these are typical for syncytiotropho-

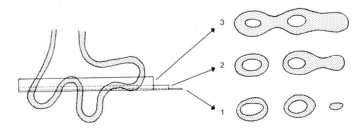

FIGURE 15.3. Influence of section thickness on the structural appearance of villi in the microscope. 1, electron microscopic ultrathin section that normally shows only few sprout- and knot-like structures; 2, light microscopic semithin section; 3, light microscopic paraffin section in which, because of its thickness, "syncytial knotting" is a frequent feature.

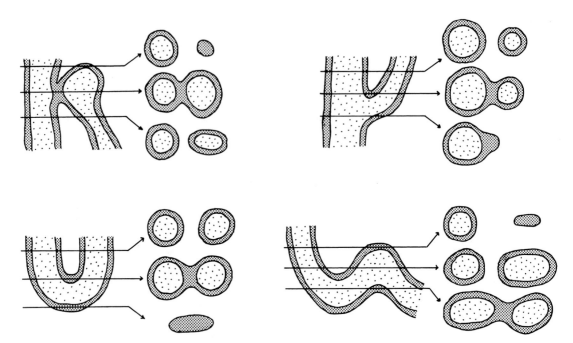

FIGURE 15.4. Ways by which the appearance of apparent syncytial fusion between villi may arise. Only in the first case (top left) is there true syncytial fusion, whereas in the other three cases the histologic appearance of sprouting and bridging is of artifactual nature. (*Source:* Adapted from Burton, 1986a, with permission.)

blast. The apparent numerical density of nuclei increases with section thickness.

Not only the structural features but also the stage of pregnancy and the type of villi involved, may be helpful for discrimination between the true sprouting, apoptotic shedding, and trophoblastic flat sectioning (Fig. 15.5).

Generally, in paraffin sections of the **young placenta** most sprouts attached to immature intermediate and mesenchymal villi are signs of villous sprouting; less often are they sites of extrusion of apoptotic nuclei. Only a minority is artificially produced by trophoblastic flat sectioning. In contrast, in paraffin sections of the **mature placenta**, most knots, sprouts, and bridges are caused by flat sectioning; this is particularly true for those found in conglomerates of terminal villi. Far fewer are sites of accumulation of apoptotic nuclei. Only a very small minority, mostly arising from immature intermediate villi located in the centers of the villous trees, represents real villous sprouting.

Artificial Knotting as Related to Villous Shapes in Paraffin Sections

The question of how to interpret knots, sprouts, and bridges relates to the more relevant question of how to interpret villous shapes and branching patterns three-dimensionally. Figure 15.4 based on a drawing by Burton (1986a) and the diagrammatic reconstruction in Figure 15.6, show that three factors increase the chance of tangential sectioning of villi: branching, curving, and superficial notching:

1. Long, slender, stretched villi, such as those derived from a slightly immature placenta of about 32 to 36 weeks menstrual age (see Figs. 8.9, 8.10, and 15.9) or from intrauterine growth restriction (IUGR) with absent or reversed end-diastolic umbilical flow (postplacental hypoxia) (see Figs. 15.6C to 15.17) have a low incidence of tangential sectioning.

2. Thicker, bulbous, and partly notched villi, as during the early stages of pregnancy (see Fig. 15.8), gestational diabetes mellitus (see Fig. 15.18), persisting immaturity at term, and rhesus incompatibility (see Fig. 15.10), show a few more tangential sections.

3. The normal mature placenta, which has numerous short terminal villi branching from the curved surfaces of the mature intermediate villi (see Figs. 15.6B and 15.11), has a higher incidence of tangential sectioning.

4. The hypoxic, hypercapillarized placenta (preplacental or uteroplacental hypoxia; e.g., maternal anemia as well as most cases of preeclampsia) is characterized by multiply branched, short, fist-like terminal villi (see Figs. 15.6A, 15.15, and 15.16). It shows such a degree of flat sectioning (syncytial knotting, Tenney-Parker changes)

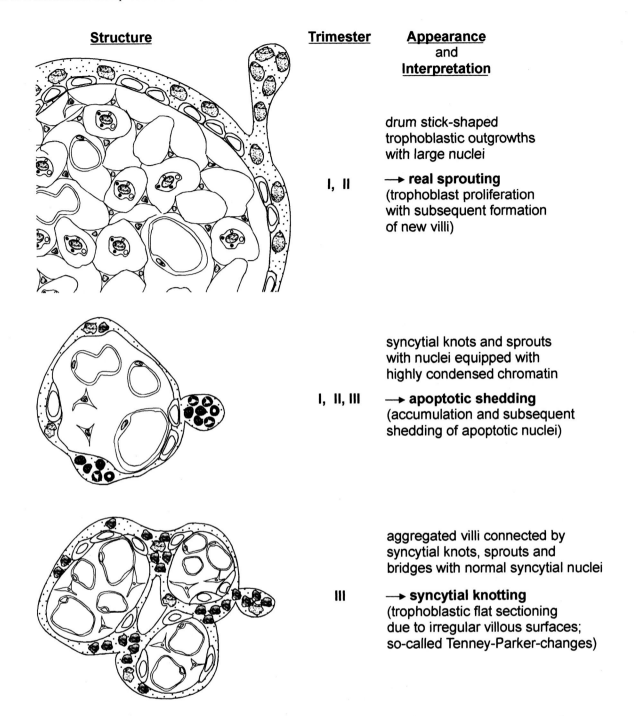

Structure   **Trimester**   **Appearance**
                                                     and
                                              Interpretation

drum stick-shaped
trophoblastic outgrowths
with large nuclei

I, II   → **real sprouting**
(trophoblast proliferation
with subsequent formation
of new villi)

syncytial knots and sprouts
with nuclei equipped with
highly condensed chromatin

I, II, III   → **apoptotic shedding**
(accumulation and subsequent
shedding of apoptotic nuclei)

aggregated villi connected by
syncytial knots, sprouts and
bridges with normal syncytial nuclei

III   → **syncytial knotting**
(trophoblastic flat sectioning
due to irregular villous surfaces;
so-called Tenney-Parker-changes)

FIGURE 15.5. Diagrammatic aid for the interpretation of tro-phoblastic knotting, sprouting, and bridging. Upper panel: Sprouts characterized by loosely arranged, large nuclei with homogeneously distributed chromatin are attached to the surfaces of immature intermediate and mesenchymal villi and are results of real trophoblastic sprouting. These true syncytial sprouts prevail throughout the first two trimesters of pregnancy. Middle panel: Knot- and sprout-like structures equipped with densely packed small nuclei with highly condensed, partly annular chromatin represent stages of extrusion of apoptotic nuclei; they can be found along the surfaces of all villous types in all stages of pregnancy. Lower panel: Aggregates of nuclei forming knots, sprouts, and bridges between densely packed third trimester terminal villi are likely to be the result of tro-phoblastic flat sectioning. Their nuclei display the same variability of chromatin condensation as is found along all villous surfaces of third trimester placentas.

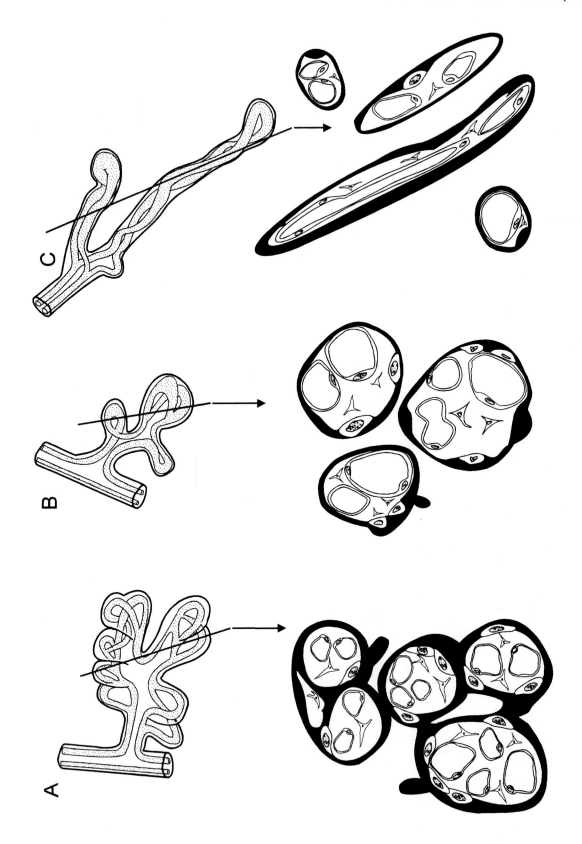

that the two-dimensional picture may achieve a net-like appearance in which most terminal villi are seemingly connected to each other by syncytial "bridges" (see Fig. 15.15B).

Conclusions Concerning Knotting

Three different phenotypes of syncytial knotting have been described: syncytial knots are local accumulations of syncytial nuclei in a moderately thickened syncytial layer, syncytial sprouts are multinucleated, fungiform protrusions of the syncytiotrophoblast into the intervillous space, and syncytial bridges are multinucleated syncytiotrophoblast connections between neighboring villous cross sections.

Unfortunately, all three definitions are sometimes used for mere structural description. In other cases, their use implies a functional meaning, such as trophoblastic sprouting, nuclear extrusion, or flat sectioning. In our experience, there is no histopathologic need to identify every multinucleated structure. Rather, it is important to decide for every placenta how to interpret the majority of its respective structures. For this purpose we suggest the following practical nomenclature (see Fig. 15.5):

- Use of the term **syncytial sprouting** is recommended only when describing true syncytial sprouts protruding from immature villous types, the former representing early stages of villous growth and branching.
- The term **apoptotic knotting** is justified when referring to local knot- or sprout-like intrasyncytial accumulations of aged or apoptotic nuclei characterized by high degrees of chromatin condensation.
- Local accumulations of syncytial knots, sprouts, and bridges in groups of irregularly shaped terminal villi are very likely to represent **trophoblastic flat sectioning** and should be referred to as **syncytial knotting** or **Tenney-Parker changes**. They are usually restricted to third trimester placentas.

Classification of Villous Maldevelopment

Based on these considerations, the following sections briefly consider typical cases of villous maldevelopment and their three-dimensional branching patterns and the diagnostic problems they cause in histologic sections. This chapter is not the place for a detailed discussion of their pathogenetic and clinical background.

The primary finding in placentas with villous maldevelopment is an abnormal numerical composition of otherwise largely normal villous types (Kaufmann et al., 1987):

- This is true for **immature intermediate villi** and the **mesenchymal villi** branching off, and for the **mature intermediate villi** and the **terminal villi** branching off. The villous trees in the case of villous maldevelopment differ from the mature villous trees at term by predominance of only one of these villous types at the expense of others. Furthermore, they differ concerning the type of capillarization of terminal villi.
- In contrast, the structure and the number of **stem villi** seem to be largely independent of the pathologic conditions. Rather, they are influenced by the stage of maturation (Macara et al., 1995; Todros et al., 1999). Therefore, even in cases of severe villous maldevelopment, they can be easily used for determination of gestational age (Kaufmann & Castellucci, 1995) (Table 15.1).

Summarizing Diagram of Villous Maldevelopment

Systematic analysis of the various cases of villous maldevelopment has shown that the balance among the various villous types is affected mainly by two different factors: the degree of placental maturation (Castellucci et al.,

---

FIGURE 15.6. Capillary branching patterns and their effects on terminal villous shapes in histologic cross sections. A: Predominance of branching angiogenesis results in highly branching capillary nets and in short, knob-like, multiply indented terminal villi. In paraffin sections these irregularly shaped terminal villi cause increased trophoblastic flat sectioning. The resulting villous profiles are connected to each other by syncytial "bridges" and show increased numbers of syncytial knots and sprouts (so-called syncytial knotting or Tenney-Parker changes). B: Groups of grape-like terminal villi with smooth surfaces are the result of a balanced mixture of branching and nonbranching

angiogenesis. The resulting histologic sections reveal less trophoblastic flat sectioning than shown in A. The terminal villi are rather large and equipped with sinusoidally dilated capillaries. C: Prevalence of nonbranching angiogenesis causes long poorly branched, slightly coiled capillaries in long, filiform terminal villi. Because of the absence of parallel capillary loops within one villus, the villi have unusually small diameters, ranging between 30 and 40 μm. Histologically, these features result in isolated villous cross sections intermingled with a few longitudinal villous profiles, both showing unusually small calibers.

TABLE 15.1. Villous maturation scores in normoxic villous development

Score	Distribution of villous types	Maturation of stem villi	Usually found in pregnancy at weeks
Normal maturation			
00	Predominance of immature intermediate villi	Stem villi are only partly fibrosed	Weeks 8 to 23[a]
01	Predominance of immature intermediate villi, but few newly formed mature intermediate villi; terminal villi still absent	Only stem villi measuring <300 mm in caliber are completely fibrosed	Weeks 24 to 28[a]
10	Predominance of mature intermediate villi, immature intermediate villi less common, few terminal villi	Only small stem villi (caliber <200 mm) are completely fibrosed	Weeks 29 to 32[a]
11	Predominance of mature intermediate villi, few terminal villi, immature intermediate villi restricted to isolated foci	Only small stem villi (caliber <200 mm) are completely fibrosed; larger stems superficially still have reticular stroma	Weeks 32 to 34[a]
12	Predominance of mature intermediate villi, increasing numbers of normally capillarized terminal villi; very few immature intermediate villi, locally restricted	Most stem villi are fully fibrosed; those partly fibrosed lack reticular stroma	Weeks 34 to 36[a]
21	Balance between mature intermediate villi and terminal villi; very few immature intermediate villi, locally restricted	Large-caliber stem villi show an unfibrosed, highly cellular subtrophoblastic rim; little perivillous fibrinoid replacing the trophoblast	Weeks 36 to 37[a]
22	Fully mature, normally capillarized villous trees with predominance of terminal villi; many mature intermediate villi; only accidental foci with immature intermediate villi	All stem villi fully fibrosed; trophoblast focally replaced by perivillous fibrinoid	Weeks 38 to 41[a]
34	Hypermature villous trees in postmature pregnancies, showing a mixture of enhanced branching (33) and nonbranching angiogenesis (44) (see Table 15.2)	Stem villi are usually fully fibrosed	>42 weeks[b]
Delayed maturation			
02	Mixture of immature intermediate villi with largely mature villous types (specific feature of placentas following asynchronous maturation)	Mostly poorly fibrosed, largely immature stem villi	Usually term placentas[c]
20	Largely mature villous trees with locally increased numbers of immature intermediate villi	Locally poorly fibrosed, partly immature stem villi	Usually term placentas[d]
00, 01, 10, 11, 12	Structurally similar to earlier stages of normal maturation, but now persisting in later stages	As described for the respective scores	Term or preterm pregnancies
Accelerated maturation			
22, rarely 12, 02	Fully or nearly mature features	Larger stem villi usually show[a] subtrophoblastic layer with reticular stroma	<36 weeks
34	Hypermature villous trees showing a mixture of enhanced branching (33) and nonbranching angiogenesis (44)	Stem villi are usually fully fibrosed	Term or near-term pregnancies

Normal maturation (scores **00** through **22**) is compared to delayed maturation (persisting immaturity) and accelerated maturation.

[a] Data are valid only for normal pregnancies.
[b] "Hypermaturity" in prolonged pregnancy.
[c] Unusual mixture of villi in normal pregnancies; more common in cases of persisting villous immaturity.
[d] Usual feature in persisting villous immaturity and sometimes even in normal term pregnancies.

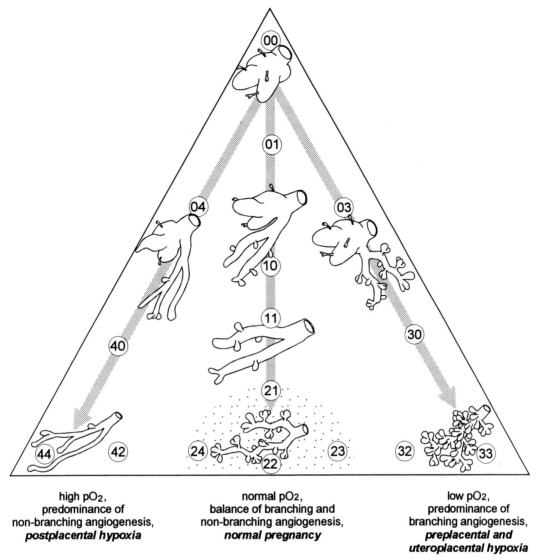

high pO₂,
predominance of
non-branching angiogenesis,
postplacental hypoxia

normal pO₂,
balance of branching and
non-branching angiogenesis,
normal pregnancy

low pO₂,
predominance of
branching angiogenesis,
*preplacental and
uteroplacental hypoxia*

FIGURE 15.7. Classification of normal and abnormal villous ramification patterns at term. Because villous maldevelopment affects mainly immature and mature intermediate as well as terminal villi, the stem villi are neglected in this diagram. The left arrow represents villous development from the first trimester (**00**, upper corner) until term (**44**, lower-left corner) with prevailing nonbranching angiogenesis, as is found in cases of postplacental hypoxia. This type of maldevelopment results in scarce, poorly branched, filiform terminal villi. The right arrow illustrates villous development in placental hypoxia, resulting in branching angiogenesis with multiply branched, fist-like terminal villi (**33**, lower-right corner). The central arrow represents normal villous development from prevalence of immature intermediate villi (**00**) via prevalence of mature intermediate villi (**11**) to the normal term situation with prevalence of terminal villi with some admixture of mature intermediate villi (**22**). The two-digit scores define the composition of the villous trees: **0,** prevalence of immature intermediate villi; **1,** prevalence of mature intermediate villi; **2,** prevalence of terminal villi with balanced angiogenesis; **3,** prevalence of terminal villi with branching angiogenesis; **4,** prevalence of terminal villi with non-branching angiogenesis. The point-shaded area indicates those features that usually are found in combination with normal pregnancy outcome at term. (*Source:* Modified from Kaufmann et al., 1987, with permission.)

1990), and the degree of oxygenation (Macara et al., 1996; Kingdom & Kaufmann, 1997; Todros et al., 1999). Figure 15.7 summarizes the resulting types of maldevelopment as a diagnostic aid:

1. The vertical axis of the diagram represents the **degree of maturation**, resulting in changes in numerical composition of the villous trees. From the first trimester (top) until term (bottom), a developmental shift occurs

from immature intermediate villi toward mature intermediate and finally terminal villi.

2. The horizontal axis of the diagram represents the **degree and type of fetoplacental angiogenesis**, controlled by intraplacental oxygen levels. The fetoplacental angiogenesis influences the numbers and shapes of terminal villi.

3. The left route of maturation represents villous features resulting from **placental oxygenation that is better than normal** ("postplacental hypoxia"; cf. Fig. 7.19). It is characterized by the predominance of nonbranching angiogenesis resulting in poorly developed, long, filiform terminal villi with long, largely unbranched capillary loops (see Fig. 15.6C).

4. The right route of maturation is the result of **intraplacental hypoxia** ("preplacental hypoxia" and "uteroplacental hypoxia"; cf. Fig. 7.19). The low oxygen levels induce branching angiogenesis (cf. Chapter 7), resulting in clusters of richly developed, short, highly branched and notched terminal villi, showing intense Tenney-Parker changes (see Fig. 15.6A).

5. The intermediate route of villous maturation is the result of **normal oxygenation of the placenta**. It is characterized by a balance between branching and nonbranching angiogenesis in terminal villi. The latter are grape-like in shape and poorly branched. Large numbers of such fungus-shaped terminal villi branch off from long, multiply bending mature intermediate villi (see Fig. 15.6B).

VILLOUS MATURATION SCORE

In our experience, villous cross-sectional patterns are difficult to define. Moreover, descriptions provided by different histopathologists are rarely comparable. In our hands, a simple two-digit code (villous maturation score) proved to be useful. It summarizes the developmental status of the villous trees including its numerical composition of the various villous types as well as the kind of terminal villous capillarization. As discussed earlier, number and differentiation of stem villi remain unconsidered.

00 signifies uniform predominance of immature intermediate villi
11 codes for general predominance of mature intermediate villi
22 characterizes normally matured villous trees composed of normally capillarized mature intermediate and terminal villi
33 denotes predominance of clustered terminal villi connected to each other by intense syncytial knotting, pointing to branching angiogenesis caused by preplacental or uteroplacental hypoxia
44 codes for predominance of loosely arranged, extremely small, filiform terminal villi, resulting from nonbranching angiogenesis

Scores with mixed digits such as **23**, **32**, **01**, or **40** describe features intermediate between the above extremes, the dominating feature represented by the first digit and the secondary feature by the second digit. For example, the score **23** codes for a more or less normally matured villous tree with a slight touch of Tenney-Parker changes, pointing to the existence of very mild hypoxia; in contrast, the score **32** denotes a similar situation with more pronounced Tenney-Parker changes.

Using this score, the different pathways of villous development and maldevelopment can be described as follows (see Table 15.1):

- The **normal maturation** of villous trees described by this score starts with **00** [pregnancy weeks 8–23 postmenstruation (p.m.)] and proceeds via **01** (weeks 24–28), **10** (weeks 29–32), **11** (weeks 32–34), **12** (weeks 34–36), **21** (weeks 36–37) to **22** (weeks 38–41). The scores **21** and **22** represent the normal range of villous maturational patterns at term. If delivery is delayed (prolonged pregnancies), the villi may even reach excessive degrees of branching and nonbranching angiogenesis with respective terminal villus formation, summarized by the score **34** or **43**, depending on the prevailing type of angiogenesis.
- **Persisting villous immaturity** can be described by the actual villous maturational stage as compared to the age-appropriate maturational score, given in parentheses: the score **00 (21)** codes for a slightly preterm delivered placenta (weeks 36–37; expected age-appropriate score, **21**) composed of immature intermediate villi, resembling a placenta from week 23 or earlier; the score **11 (22)** codes for a placenta delivered at term, composed of stem and mature intermediate villi, but largely lacking terminal villi, thus resembling a placenta about weeks 32 to 34.
- **Accelerated villous maturation** can be coded accordingly by characterizing the actual developmental status as compared to the score expected for that particular stage of pregnancy (in parentheses): the score **22 (12)** describes a structurally fully mature placenta delivered between weeks 34 and 36 (preterm maturation, maturitas praecox placentae); the score **34 (22)** codes for a placenta delivered at term, but displaying "hypermature" features composed of a mixture of enhanced branching and nonbranching angiogenesis.

The developmental pathways resulting from abnormal degrees of placental oxygenation can also be characterized by the villous maturation score (Table 15.2):

- Villous trees in **severely hypoxic placentas** (preplacental and uteroplacental hypoxia), such as maternal anemia, high altitude, or preeclampsia, are characterized by scores proceeding from **00** via **03** and **30** to **33**: The respective histologic features show syncytial knotting (Tenney-Parker changes) clearly exceeding normal degrees. Typically, in this developmental pathway mature intermediate villi (coded by the digit **1**) do not dominate the sections in any stage.
- **Less severe cases of placental hypoxia** result in villous features with less expressive knotting and are coded by **32** or **23**, the latter entity still belonging to the normal range of full-term placentas.
- Cases of **severe postplacental hypoxia** (e.g., IUGR with absent end-diastolic flow in the umbilical arteries) are coded by scores proceeding from **00** via **04** and **40** to **44**. The typical histologic features comprise increased numbers of filiform terminal villi of minimum diameters with absence of capillary branching. Also in these cases, the paucity of mature intermediate villi is highly characteristic; at the transition from the second to the third trimester, immature intermediate villi mix with terminal villi (stages **04** or **40**).
- **Less severe cases of postplacental hypoxia** lead to a mixture of normally matured terminal villi with filiform terminal villi resulting from nonbranching angiogenesis, coded by **42** to **24**, the latter feature still belonging to the normal full-term range of villous development.

Clearly, not all cases of villous maldevelopment can be coded accordingly. This condition is particularly valid for those abnormalities in which the quality of villous differentiation is affected rather than the numerical composition of the villous trees, including the types of angiogenesis. Typical examples comprise placentas from diabetic mothers, from heavy smokers, and cases with chromosomal aberrations.

TABLE 15.2. Villous maturation scores in cases of abnormal oxygenation

Score	Distribution of villous types	Maturation of stem villi	Usually found in pregnancy at weeks
Prevailing branching angiogenesis			
03	Predominance of immature intermediate villi; small groups of clustered terminal villi with Tenney-Parker changes	Only stem villi with calibers <300mm are completely fibrosed	Weeks 24 to 28[a]
30	Prevalence of clustered, knotted terminal villi (moderate Tenney-Parker changes); numerous small capillary cross sections; many immature intermediate villi	Only small stem villi (caliber <200mm) are completely fibrosed; larger stems superficially still have reticular stroma	Weeks 28 to 34[a]
33	Predominance of clustered, highly knotted terminal villi (severe Tenney-Parker changes); numerous small capillary cross sections; immature intermediate villi absent	All stem villi fully fibrosed; trophoblast focally replaced by perivillous fibrinoid	Weeks 34 to 40[a]
32	Less severe form: mixture of **33** with **22**, predominance of **33**	Most stem villi fully fibrosed; trophoblast focally replaced by fibrinoid	Weeks 34 to 40[b]
23	Mild form: mixture of **33** with **22**, predominance of **22**		Weeks 34 to 40[c]
Prevailing nonbranching angiogenesis			
04	Predominance of immature intermediate villi; small groups of extremely small, filiform terminal villi with long, wide capillary loops; locally intense superficial capillarization of immature intermediate villi	Only stem villi with calibers <300mm are completely fibrosed	Weeks 20 to 40[d]
40	Large groups of extremely small, filiform terminal villi with long, wide capillary loops; still some evenly distributed, highly capillarized immature intermediate villi	Only small stem villi (caliber <200mm) are completely fibrosed; the larger ones still have subtrophoblastic reticular stroma	Weeks 24 to 28[d]
44	Predominance of extremely small, filiform terminal villi with long, wide capillary loops; obvious gap in calibers between the unusually small terminal villi and the larger stem villi	Most stem villi are fully fibrosed; trophoblast is focally replaced by perivillous fibrinoid	Weeks 28 to 34[d]
42	Less severe form: mixture of **44** with **22**, predominance of **44**	Most stem villi are fully fibrosed; the trophoblast is focally replaced by perivillous fibrinoid	Weeks 32 to 38[e]
24	Mild form: mixture of **44** with **22**, predominance of **22**		Weeks 36 to 40[f]

Maturation during preplacental and uteroplacental hypoxia with prevailing branching angiogenesis (scores **03** through **33**) is compared with the maturation during postplacental hypoxia with prevailing nonbranching angiogenesis (scores **04** through **44**).

[a] Characteristic feature for cases of severe maternal anemia, pregnancies in high altitude or IUGR/preeclampsia with preserved end-diastolic flow in the umbilical arteries.
[b] Milder cases of maternal anemia, high altitude, or IUGR/preeclampsia with preserved end-diastolic flow in the umbilical arteries.
[c] Usual feature also in normal term pregnancies.
[d] Characteristic feature for IUGR with absent or reverse end-diastolic flow in the umbilical arteries.
[e] Less severe cases of IUGR with absent or reverse end-diastolic flow in the umbilical arteries.
[f] Usual feature also in normal term pregnancies.

TABLE 15.3. Comparison of different terminologies concerning villous maldevelopment

Villous maturation score (as compared to age-appropriate score)	Author's nomenclature	Becker and Röckelein, 1989	Becker, 1981; Vogel, 1984, 1996	Schweikhart, 1985
Normal maturation				
Ideally 22, but also 20, 21, 23, 24	Synchronous villous maturity	Maturitas iusta (normal maturation)	Mature gestation, age-appropriate	Synchronous maturity
00, 01, 10, 11, 12	Synchronous villous immaturity	—	—	Synchronous immaturity
Delayed maturation				
12 (22)	Persisting immaturity, very mild form	Maturitas tarda (delayed maturation)	Dissociated villous maturation, mostly mature	Mild form of terminal villus deficiency
11 (22) 10 (22)	Persisting villous immaturity, Moderate form	Maturitas retardata (retarded maturation)	Dissociated villous maturation, mostly immature	Terminal villus deficiency
00 (22) 01 (22)	Persisting villous immaturity, Severe form	Arrested maturation	Arrest of villous maturation	Persisting immaturity
Accelerated maturation				
22 (12) 22 (11)	Preterm villous maturation	Maturitas praecox (premature maturation)	Premature maturation	Asynchronous maturation
34 (22)	Hypermaturity	—	—	Hypermaturity
Abnormal angiogenesis				
33 (22)	Terminal villi with prevalence of branching angiogenesis	—	—	Hypercapillarization
44 (22) 40 (10 or 01)	Terminal villi with prevalence of nonbranching angiogenesis	—	Intermediate villus deficiency	Terminal villus deficiency?

Note that for the pathologic villous maturation scores listed in the left column the age-appropriate normal scores are given in parentheses.

Our villous maturation score is not the first attempt to classify villous maldevelopment. In Table 15.3 we have tried to compare our classification with the terminologies introduced by other authors (Becker, 1981; Vogel, 1984, 1996; Schweikhart, 1985; Becker & Röckelein, 1989).

Cases of Villous Maldevelopment

Synchronous Villous Immaturity

The term **synchronous** is used for histologic features of immature villous trees that correspond to what we expect to be normal for the respective stage of pregnancy (Schweikhart et al., 1986). For a normal baseline, we refer to the pictures and data provided by Boyd and Hamilton (1970), Kaufmann (1981), Vogel (1986), Stoz et al. (1988), and Vogel (1996), and to the data presented in Chapter 8.

From the 8th to 24th week p.m., the immature villous trees are composed of uniformly thick, bulbous, immature intermediate villi (villous maturation score **00**). Until week 28 these are completed by some newly formed mature intermediate villi (score **01**). The trophoblastic surface of the immature intermediate villi is unevenly curved and distended (Fig. 15.8A). Terminal villi are virtually absent. The numerous side branches of small caliber are composed of real sprouts and newly produced mesenchymal villi. For geometrical reasons, the chance of obtaining flat sections depends on the villous diameter and decreases with increasing villous caliber. Therefore,

the rare event of tangential sectioning of such immature cases with prevailing large villi does not give an incorrect impression of sprouting (Fig. 15.8B).

In later stages of villous development (weeks 29–36; villous maturation scores **10–12**), increasing amounts of mature intermediate villi are formed. In particular, in weeks 32 to 34, when these villi clearly dominate the histologic section, they are characterized by rather large, homogeneous calibers (150–250 μm) and a highly cellular stroma (Fig. 15.9; also see Fig. 8.9). The number of terminal villi slowly increases throughout this period. By definition, placentas showing synchronous villous immaturity can be found only in cases of premature deliveries. On the other hand, as discussed in Chapter 14, in only 33% of premature deliveries are the placentas in fact structurally immature (Schweikhart et al., 1986); rather, most prematurely delivered cases are characterized by fully mature or even "hypermature" features. Becker and Röckelein (1989) suggested this to be responsible for preterm onset of labor. This, however, still remains speculative.

Persisting Villous Immaturity and Rhesus Incompatibility

Persisting immaturity of unknown etiology is a usual feature in postterm pregnancies (Fox, 1968; Kemnitz &

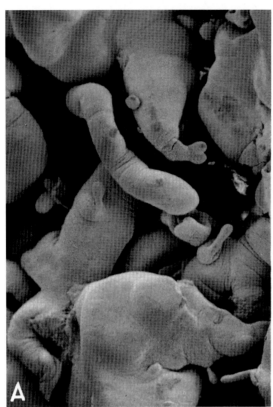

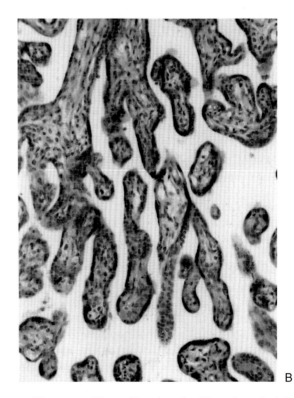

FIGURE 15.8. Immature placenta, 20th week of gestation. The immature intermediate villi are devoid of terminal villi. Large-caliber villi prevail. The numerous true sprouts, clearly visible in the scanning electron micrograph (A), are rarely seen (arrows) in the corresponding cross-sectional picture (B). ×66. (*Source:* Part A from Kaufmann et al., 1987, with permission.)

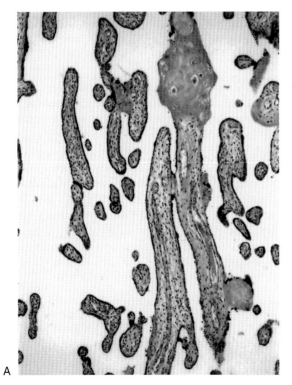

A

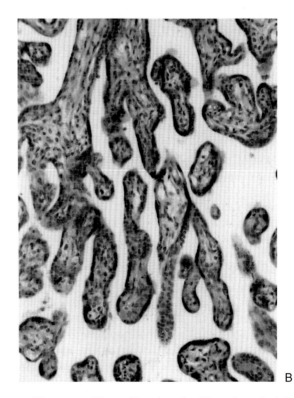

B

FIGURE 15.9. Immature placenta, 34th week of pregnancy. Long, straight, mature intermediate villi with calibers ranging from 150 to 250μm prevail. Due to the paucity of terminal villi branching off, the mature intermediate villi are arranged in parallel and do not show the zigzag course of mature intermediate villi at term. The uniformity of calibers is typical for this stage of pregnancy. Similar features can be found in postterm pregnancies combined with slight persisting immaturity; in this condition this feature has been called "terminal villus deficiency." A: ×60; B: ×125.

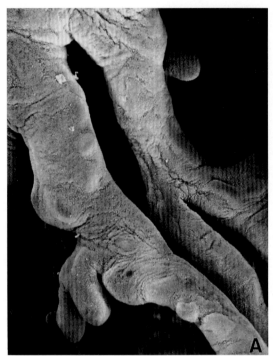 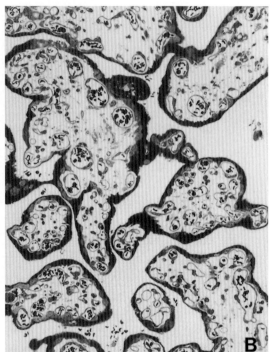

FIGURE 15.10. Placenta from a case of severe rhesus incompatibility, near term. Immature intermediate villi with a large caliber prevail. Only a few smaller side branches (terminal or mesenchymal villi) arise from the surfaces (A). True syncytial sprouting comparable to that seen in normal immature intermediate villi is rare. The occasional "sprouts" and "bridges" visible in semithin sections (B) are mostly artifacts caused by tangential sectioning of the irregular, notched outer surface of the immature intermediate villi. These villi are much better vascularized in rhesus incompatibility than are those of normal early pregnancy. In well-stained, thin histologic sections, one can easily identify that the large caliber of the villi is the result of villous immaturity rather than of villous edema. ×195. (*Source:* From Kaufmann et al., 1987, with permission.)

Theuring, 1974) (for details, see Chapter 14). Villous maturation features in most cases resemble synchronous developmental stages from the 26th to 32nd week of pregnancy (villous maturation scores **01** or **10**); the villous trees are composed mainly of immature intermediate villi with various degrees of admixture of mature intermediate villi.

Severe cases of persisting immaturity are regular features following rhesus immunization (scores **00**, **01**, or **10**). It is generally considered that villous maturation is retarded in this condition (Wentworth, 1967; Werner et al., 1973; Fox, 1997; Pilz et al., 1980), but it is still disputed whether the villous features are further complicated by edema. In our experience, the villous features are influenced by a delay in villous maturation at an unduly early stage of development; thus, immature intermediate villi of large caliber persist (Fig. 15.10A). As is characteristic for this villous type, terminal branches are uncommon and depend on the degree of isoimmunization. There are, however, some differences when compared to cases of synchronous villous immaturity. True syncytial sprouts are less common (compare Figs. 15.8 and 15.10). This finding is in agreement with the pathogenetic concept that villous maturation, and thus the formation of new villi, is decelerated in this condition. Moreover, cases of persisting immaturity at term or of severe maturational arrest in patients with erythroblastosis exhibit better fetal vascularization (Fig. 15.10B) than cases of synchronous immaturity. In accordance with the straight course of the large villi and their intensively notched surfaces seen in scanning electron micrographs (Fig. 15.10A), the histologic sections (Fig. 15.10B) usually reveal large-caliber villi of varying sizes, with occasional signs of syncytial knotting. Most of the latter structures are caused by tangential sectioning.

Normal Mature Placenta

In the normal, term placenta, the dominant structures are long, slender, mature intermediate villi from which short, grape-like terminal villi branch (Fig. 15.11A; also see Fig. 7.7). As long as the terminal villi are short and only poorly branched, as in the cases depicted, the incidence of tangential sectioning is low. Most of the peripheral villous cross sections have calibers ranging from 60 to 150 mm (Figs. 15.11B,C), except for some occasional stem and

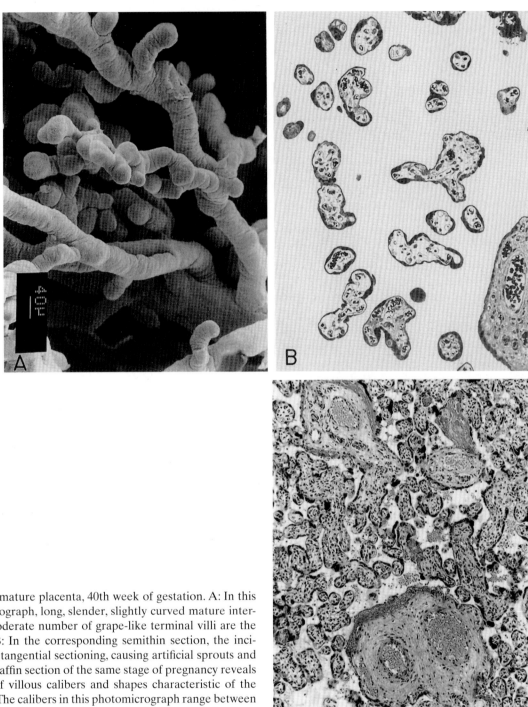

FIGURE 15.11. Normal mature placenta, 40th week of gestation. A: In this scanning electron micrograph, long, slender, slightly curved mature intermediate villi with a moderate number of grape-like terminal villi are the dominating features. B: In the corresponding semithin section, the incidence of trophoblastic tangential sectioning, causing artificial sprouts and bridges, is low. C: A paraffin section of the same stage of pregnancy reveals the colorful mixture of villous calibers and shapes characteristic of the normal term placenta. The calibers in this photomicrograph range between 40 and 250 μm without obvious predominance of a single group of calibers (compare with Figs. 15.9 and 15.17B). A,B: ×120; C ×85. (*Source:* A,B from Kaufmann et al., 1987, with permission.)

immature intermediate villi. Usually, the latter villi accumulate in the centers of the villous trees and should not be misunderstood as signs of persisting immaturity (Fig. 15.12; compare parts A and B).

Trophoblastic tangential sectioning resulting in the incorrect impression of sprouting is a rare event in thin plastic sections (Fig. 15.11B); this picture is seen some-

what more frequently in the thicker paraffin sections (see Figs. 8.11 and 8.12) (Becker, 1981; Fox, 1997). Only some of these "typical signs of villous maturation" (*Reifezeichen* of Becker, 1981) have a real structural basis. We estimate that less than 5% of sprout-like structures seen in paraffin sections are true trophoblastic outgrowths, that is, signs of trophoblastic sprouting or extrusion of apoptotic

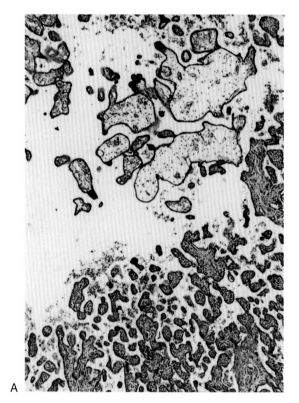
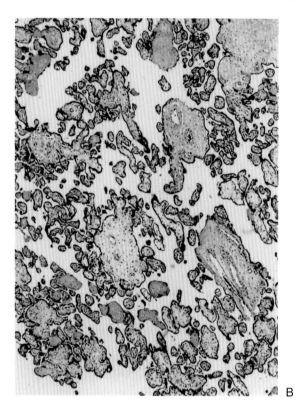

FIGURE 15.12. Comparison of immature intermediate villi in two different types of term placentas. A: In the center of the villous tree of a normal, term placenta, the immature intermediate villi together with sprouts and mesenchymal side branches form an isolated group surrounded by ample intervillous space belonging to the central cavity. This normal feature should not be confused with the more homogeneously distributed immature intermediate villi as shown in part B, which represents a case of persisting immaturity at term. ×15.

nuclei; the remaining 95% are artifacts from sectioning. Despite this fact, they can be regarded as reliable signs of full maturation in paraffin sections (see Fig. 8.12). Their artificial genesis points to the existence of mature villous shapes. When studying the thinner semithin sections (1 mm) (see Fig. 15.11B), one must exercise care because to the inexperienced observer the reduced incidence of artificial "sprouting" may wrongly suggest an organ that is not yet fully mature.

In the ideal case of full, normal villous maturation, the villous trees are composed as outlined here, corresponding to a villous maturation score of **22**. It is, however, the general histopathologic experience that uncomplicated term pregnancies with normal fetal outcome very often are combined with less ideally structured placentas. These may include (1) slightly increased numbers of immature intermediate villi (score **20**), (2) a certain prevalence of large-caliber mature intermediate villi (score **21**), (3) locally restricted admixtures of clusters of villi with intense knotting (score **23**), and (4) a certain number of long, filiform, unbranched terminal villi with minimum diameters as typical results of nonbranching angiogenesis (score **24**).

Preterm Villous Maturation and Villous Hypermaturity

In 50% of placentas of preterm deliveries from the 29th to 32nd week of pregnancy and in 33% of those of preterm deliveries from the 33rd to 37th week, Schweikhart et al. (1986) found a villous maturational state that corresponded to the normal mature placenta. Becker (1981) used the term **maturitas praecox placentae** when the villous maturation is accelerated and reaches structurally normal term features (score **22**) considerably before the 40th week. In other cases, the villi even displayed degrees of formation of terminal villi exceeding those in normal maturity, resulting in "hypermaturity" (score **34**) (Salvatore, 1968). According to the results of Schweikhart et al. (1986), hypermaturity is an even more common finding in cases of preterm delivery than is maturitas praecox. Becker (1981) concluded that the prematurely matured placenta may induce labor (cf. Chapter 14).

Preterm villous maturation is characterized by normal villous features that under normal conditions would have been reached only in later stages of pregnancy. In contrast, the more severe form of this entity, hypermaturity, is struc-

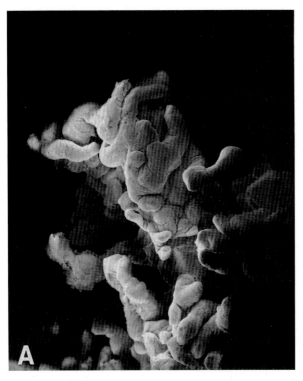

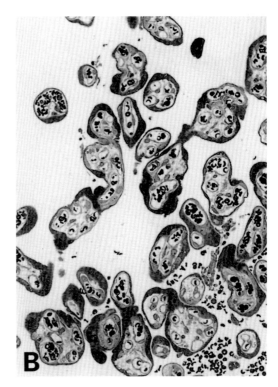

FIGURE 15.13. Prematurely delivered placenta (37th week of pregnancy) from a pregnancy complicated by preeclampsia and IUGR. A: Scanning electron micrograph shows the typical feature of preterm maturation (or hypermaturity), with long, twisted, partly branched terminal villi that are aggregated around the hidden mature intermediate villus. The underlying pathogenesis is likely to be a severe alteration of terminal villous capillarization, showing local variations from nonbranching to prevailing branching angiogenesis (villous maturation score, **34**). B: In a plastic section, this feature results in the appearance of numerous small cross sections of highly capillarized terminal villi, locally intermingled with increased trophoblastic flat sectioning. A: ×125; B: ×200. (*Source:* Part A from Kaufmann et al., 1987, with permission.)

turally characterized by a mixture of two different types of abnormal terminal villi: (1) long, unbranched, and twisted small-diameter terminal villi, corresponding to those found in cases of postplacental hypoxia (scores **42** and rarely even **44**); these terminal villi largely hide the central mature intermediate villus from which they branch (Fig. 15.13A); and (2) short, highly branched, fist-like terminal villi with increased branching angiogenesis showing increased incidence of knotting (Tenney-Parker changes) in paraffin sections. These villi resemble those displayed in preplacental hypoxia and uteroplacental hypoxia (villous maturation scores **32** or even **33**). Accordingly, the features typical for hypermaturity may overlap with those found following preplacental hypoxia (e.g., maternal anemia), or they are displayed by postplacental hypoxia (IUGR with absent end-diastolic umbilical flow). Usually a mixture of both types of terminal villi, caused by mixtures of branching and nonbranching angiogenesis, is found (score **34**). In histologic sections, complicated networks of narrow capillaries are accompanied in parallel by long, winding dilated capillaries. The corresponding branching patterns of the terminal villi, as seen by scanning electron microscopy (Fig.

15.13A), showed partly long winding, partly short, and multiply indented villi. Histologically, this situation results in complex pictures with partly isolated villous sections having dilated capillaries and partly net-like villous conglomerates (Fig. 15.13B).

The coexistence of these features suggests that overstimulated angiogenesis (branching or nonbranching type) is one of the underlying pathogenetic mechanisms for hypermature villous maturation. This concept agrees with the experience that these pregnancies often are complicated by hypertensive disorders as well as intrauterine growth retardation. At present it is still difficult to differentiate between cause and effect. The molecular basis of the obvious alteration of villous angiogenesis is not yet understood.

Prolonged Pregnancy

For decades, most "prolonged pregnancies" have actually been miscalculated term pregnancies (Fox, 1997); however, careful ultrasound examination throughout pregnancy now has allowed more precise dating. Placen-

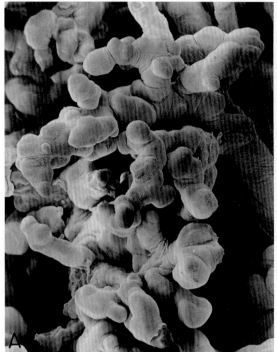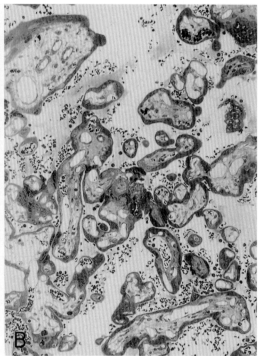

FIGURE 15.14. Placenta in prolonged pregnancy, 43rd week of gestation. This case shows a mixture of hypermature and hypoxic changes of the terminal villi, both resulting in hypercapillarization and overproduction of terminal branches. A: Scanning electron micrograph shows complicated convolutions of long, branched, and multiply notched and indented terminal villi, completely hiding the central mature intermediate axis. B: The semithin section is a mixture of small terminal villus cross sections (as in the case of postplacental hypoxia; see Fig. 15.17) with tangentially sectioned, web-like arrangement of terminal villi (as in pre- and uteroplacental hypoxia; see Figs. 15.15 and 15.16). ×115. (*Source:* Kaufmann et al., 1987, with permission.)

tas from true 42 and 43 weeks' gestations (postmaturity) usually are characterized by one of two contrasting histological features:

1. The usual finding is slight immaturity: dominance of mature intermediate villi with deficiency of terminal villi (Kaufmann et al., 1987) (scores **11** and **12**) (see Fig. 14.5) or even more severe cases of persisting immaturity (Fox, 1968; Kemnitz & Theuring, 1974; Mikolajczak et al., 1987) (scores **10**, **01**, and **00**). In the latter cases, the villous maturation features resemble synchronous developmental stages from the 26th to 32nd week of pregnancy, the villous trees being composed mainly of immature intermediate villi with various degrees of admixture of mature intermediate villi. Many placenta pathologists had already pointed to this correlation with abnormal villous maturation before ultrasound confirmation of pregnancy length (Becker, 1963; Emmrich & Mälzer, 1968; Kemnitz & Theuring, 1974; Kloos & Vogel, 1974).

2. By contrast, a certain percentage of prolonged pregnancies is characterized by normal mature villous patterns (score **22**) or even "hypermature" features characterized by increased branching angiogenesis (scores **32**, **33**, **34**) (Fig. 15.14). According to Schweikhart (1985),

hypermaturity amounts to about 12% of postterm pregnancies (see Preterm Villous Maturation and Villous Hypermaturity, above): these data are generally in agreement with those of Essbach and Röse (1966), Emmrich and Mälzer (1968), and Mikolajczak et al. (1987).

Placentas at High Altitude and Maternal Anemia (Preplacental Hypoxia)

There is general agreement that hypoxia is responsible for the placental changes in women with anemia (Piotrowicz et al., 1969; Beischer et al., 1970; Kadyrov et al., 1998; Kosanke et al., 1998) and those women living at high altitude (Jackson et al., 1987, 1988a,b; Reshetnikova et al., 1993). Corresponding features have also been observed in placentas from mothers with cyanotic heart disease. All three conditions have been characterized as preplacental hypoxia (Kingdom & Kaufmann, 1997). Experimental studies have supported the view that deficiency of oxygen is the decisive pathogenetic mechanism in this group of disorders. Studies of the in vitro influence of hypoxia on villous explants (Tominaga & Page, 1966; Fox, 1970; Amaladoss & Burton, 1985; Burton et al., 1989;

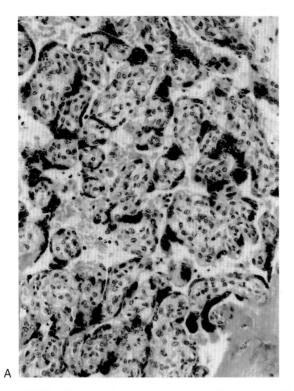

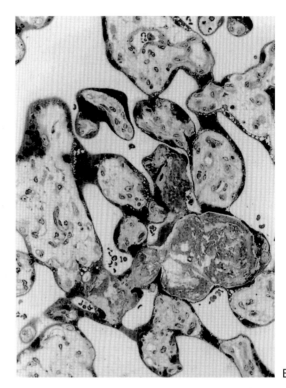

FIGURE 15.15. Placenta from maternal anemia at term. The chronic preplacental hypoxia causes prevalence of branching angiogenesis, resulting in multiply branched and indented terminal villi, as shown in Fig. 15.16A. The corresponding paraffin section (A) reveals intense trophoblastic knotting (Tenney-Parker changes) as a result of increased flat sectioning across irregular villous surfaces. A higher magnified plastic section (B) demonstrates even better artifactually caused syncytial knotting and bridging. A: ×120; B: ×300.

Ong & Burton, 1991) and experimental studies on long-term effects of hypoxia on pregnant guinea pigs (Bacon et al., 1984; Geisen et al., 1990; Scheffen et al., 1990) and pregnant ewes (Krebs et al., 1997) have reported comparable structural features.

All these studies indicate that increased trophoblastic proliferation and increased villous capillary branching are the typical placental responses to long-term hypoxia (see Fig. 7.17). Branching angiogenesis is probably caused by stimulated expression of vascular endothelial growth factor (VEGF) and its two receptors, flt-1 and KDR (see Chapter 7). Hypoxia results in richly branched, net-like capillary beds that are easy to perfuse, as their structure provides less flow resistance than comparably large capillary beds composed of longer, less branched capillaries. This situation is compatible with the decrease in capillary diameter that was found in related animal experiments (Bacon et al., 1984; Scheffen et al., 1990) and which seemed to be highly characteristic for hypoxic villi in the studies on human placentas from high altitude performed by Jackson et al. (1987, 1988a,b). It must be pointed out, however, that Reshetnikova et al. (1993) in this particular respect arrived at opposite conclusions; in their group of placentas from women who lived and delivered in high

altitude, they observed a general increase in capillary diameters as compared to lowland pregnancies.

The richly branched capillaries from hypoxic placentas (see Figs. 7.17 and 15.6A) are responsible for a characteristic deformation of the outer shape of the terminal villi (Fig. 15.15; also see Fig. 15.6A). These are usually short, knob-like, and have multiply indented surfaces that resemble fists (compare Fig. 15.16A). Histologic sections of such villi show increased areas of flat sectioning of trophoblast, histologically appearing as increased syncytial knotting (Tenney-Parker changes). Groups of villi are connected to each other by syncytial bridges (Figs. 15.6 and 15.15). Often a net-like appearance is achieved, the extent of which depends on the thickness of the section. The respective villous maturation scores are **03**, **30**, or **33**, depending on the stage of pregnancy.

Intrauterine Growth Restriction with Preserved End-Diastolic Umbilical Flow in the Third Trimester, with or Without Late-Onset Preeclampsia (Uteroplacental Hypoxia)

A great variety of pathologic correlates has been found in cases of IUGR, such as small placenta, persisting

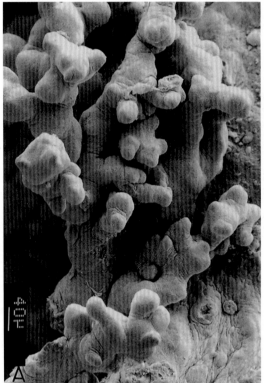
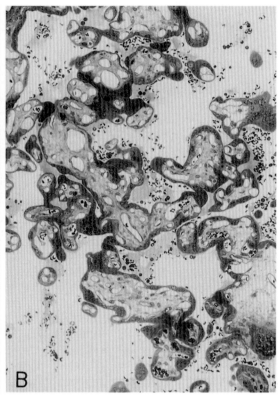

Figure 15.16. Placenta from a patient with severe preeclampsia, near term. Because of long-lasting uteroplacental hypoxia, the branching pattern of the villi in this case is similar to that in maternal anemia (see Fig. 15.15). A: The multiply branched, short capillary loops (cf. Fig. 15.6A) cause short, knob-like, indented villous surfaces. B: The corresponding semithin section shows a conglomeration of terminal villi with apparent syncytial "bridging" and "sprouting" artifactually, caused by tangential sectioning. Sometimes it results in a net-like appearance. ×125. (*Source:* Part B from Kaufmann et al., 1987, with permission.)

placental immaturity, high degree of placental infarction, fetoplacental vasculopathy, villous hypermaturity, deficiency of terminal villus, etc. (for reviews, see Chapter 19; also Vogel, 1996; Fox, 1997; Kingdom et al., 1997). The pathogenesis is thought to be a consequence of failing trophoblast invasion and consequently falling dilatation of the uteroplacental arteries (Brosens et al., 1967; Brosens, 1988). This loss results in maternal malperfusion of the placenta. Different from the preplacental hypoxia that is found in maternal anemia, for example, in IUGR, the mother is generally normoxic and due to the underlying maladaptation of the uteroplacental arteries only the intrauterine compartment, that is, placenta and fetus, may become hypoxic ("uteroplacental hypoxia").

In a certain percentage of cases, IUGR becomes complicated by preeclampsia. Originally, this disease was thought to be a direct consequence of failing trophoblast invasion of uteroplacental arteries (Brosens et al., 1970). Meanwhile there is general agreement that the direct consequence of the latter is malperfusion of the placenta resulting in IUGR; whether the latter becomes additionally complicated by preeclampsia or not seems to be a question of whether villous trophoblast turnover is impaired by placental malperfusion or not (Black et al., 2002; Huppertz et al., 2002; 2003; Sibley et al., 2002; Kaufmann et al., 2003).

Histologic evaluation of placentas in IUGR resulted in extremely heterogeneous features. These features become more homogeneous, classifying the cases according to the presence or absence of end-diastolic flow in the umbilical arteries (Macara et al., 1995, 1996; Todros et al., 1998). The placentas derived from pregnancies with IUGR with abnormal but still preserved end-diastolic (PED) flow in the umbilical arteries, irrespective of whether complicated by preeclampsia or not, show the same, very homogeneous histologic structure as has been described for preplacental hypoxia (maternal anemia, high altitude) (Todros et al., 1998): Richly branched, net-like capillary beds with mostly narrow capillaries are responsible for the characteristic fist-like deformation of the terminal villi (Fig. 15.16). They are short, knob-like, and multiply indented. Histology displays increased knotting, and Tenney-Parker changes (flat sectioning) (Alvarez et al., 1964, 1970). The respective villous maturation scores are **03**, **30**, **32**, or **33**, depending on severity and stage of pregnancy. As a consequence of increased terminal villus branching, the intervillous space is abnormally narrow and sometimes difficult to identify.

An alternative view for the Tenney-Parker change is that the increased knotting relates to deficient water transfer from mother to baby. Neonates of such pregnancies are generally dehydrated and have elevated hematocrits; the placentas are thin, appear dark on sectioning, and the villi are small and composed primarily of capillaries. It is also possible that the syncytium "buckles" because of this deficient water transfer, thus causing increased knotting in histologic preparations.

Intrauterine Growth Restriction Combined with Absent or Reverse End-Diastolic Umbilical Blood Flow in the Second Trimester, with or without Early-Onset Preeclampsia (Postplacental Hypoxia)

When fetal IUGR in the second trimester of pregnancy is combined with absent or reverse end-diastolic (ARED) umbilical blood flow, as judged by Doppler examination, the histopathologic findings are very homogeneous, but surprisingly quite different from those obtained in IUGR with PED (Macara et al., 1995, 1996; Krebs et al., 1996; Kingdom & Kaufmann, 1997; Kingdom et al., 1997; Todros et al., 1999). Also in this entity, as in IUGR with PED, whether or not the case is complicated by preeclampsia does neither influence villous maturation patterns or fetoplacental vascularization, or other gross pathohistologic features.

In general, the histopathologic features resemble those described earlier as "terminal villi deficiency," a type of villous maldevelopment that is clinically characterized by imminent fetal asphyxia (Schweikhart & Kaufmann, 1983, 1987; Schweikhart et al., 1986; Kaufmann et al., 1987). It is likely that the two entities are basically identical, even though we have to admit that the cases of "terminal villus deficiency" were not defined by Doppler ultrasound and probably were mixed up with cases of mild persisting immaturity (cf. Prolonged Pregnancy, above).

Scanning electron microscopy (Kaufmann et al., 1987; Krebs et al., 1996) revealed that the mature intermediate villi together with their terminal villous continuations are extremely long, largely unbranched, filiform structures (Fig. 15.17A; also see Fig. 15.6C). Terminal villous side branches of the mature intermediate villi are largely missing. The terminal capillary loops, resulting from nonbranching angiogenesis (see Figs. 7.17 and 15.6C), are

long, slender, and usually unbranched, thus explaining the high Doppler resistance index (Kingdom et al., 1997).

Further findings, according to Macara et al. (1996), include (1) thinning of villous trophoblast; (2) numerical reduction of cytotrophoblast and reduction of cytotrophoblastic proliferation; (3) increased incidence of apoptotic trophoblastic nuclei and syncytial knotting with extrusion of nuclei; (4) increased amounts of stromal collagen I, collagen IV, and laminin; and (5) wide intervillous space as a consequence of reduced peripheral villous branching.

The straight course of the largely unbranched, filiform terminal villi results in predominance of villous cross sections of minimum diameters (30–60 μm) with admixture of some longitudinal sections (Figs. 15.6C and 15.17B). The prevalence of smallest villous diameters, in combination with occasional unbranched, filiform, small-caliber villous sections, absence of syncytial knotting (Tenney-Parker changes), an obvious caliber gap between small-caliber terminal villi and stem villi, and an unusually wide intervillous space, make this condition easily identifiable. The villous maturation scores are **04**, **40**, and **44**, and in less severe cases **42**, depending on the stage of pregnancy. In agreement with the experimental findings of Panigel and Myers (1972), these features were interpreted as signs of intraplacental oxygen levels higher than normal, possibly caused by decreased oxygen extraction by the fetally malperfused villi (Kingdom & Kaufmann, 1997; Kingdom et al., 1997).

Casts of the fetoplacental villous vessels, prepared from such specimens and studied in the scanning electron microscope, revealed long, poorly branched capillaries (Krebs et al., 1996) (compare Figs. 7.17 and 15.6C). Focal sinusoidal dilatation is only sometimes present; it can be interpreted as an attempt at compensation for the increase in blood flow impedance in these long capillary loops. The Doppler measurement cited provided evidence that the resulting blood flow impedance was considerably increased, despite sinusoidal dilatation. In some parts of the fetoplacental vascular bed the flow of blood obviously came to a standstill; histologically, one may find aggregation of fetal erythrocytes caused by stasis (Macara et al., 1996). Ultrastructurally, the erythrocytes showed damage to their membranes and partial lysis, which can be interpreted as signs of fetal circulatory decompensation. Clinically the Doppler findings were considered in all these cases as evidence of fetal compromise with need for immediate termination of pregnancy (Macara et al., 1996; Kingdom et al., 1997).

The relative or absolute scarcity of mature intermediate villi in this condition has led Vogel (1996) to call this entity "deficiency of intermediate villi"; in fact, seen histologically, well-fibrosed stem villi and perfectly capillarized terminal villi are the prevailing structures.

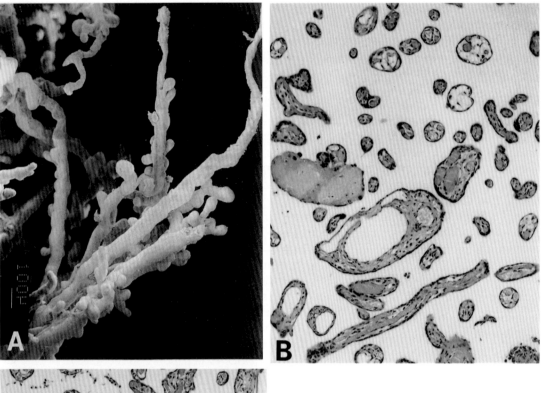

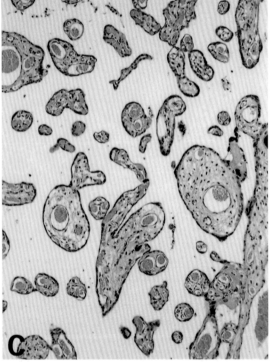

FIGURE 15.17. Placenta from a patient with IUGR with absent or reverse end-diastolic (ARED) flow in the umbilical arteries (postplacental hypoxia), 40th week of gestation. A: Scanning electron micrograph shows long, poorly branched bundles of mostly filiform terminal villi. Before definition of the entity IUGR with ARED, these villi were misunderstood as mature intermediate villi and the entity was called "terminal villi deficiency." B: On first glance, the corresponding histologic section resembles that of a normal term placenta; the diagnosis "postplacental hypoxia," however, can be deduced from the striking predominance of smallest villous calibers, appearing as a mixture of tiny cross sections and filiform longitudinal profiles, together with the scarcity of intermediate villous calibers (80–120 μm) and the unusually wide intervillous space (villous maturation score, **44**). C: Similar case from 30 weeks of gestation: the villous calibers are slightly larger. Few lightly stained immature intermediate villi (center) in combination with terminal villi of smallest diameter (villous maturation score, **40**) led to the correct diagnosis. A,B,C: ×55. (*Source:* Part A from Kaufmann et al., 1987, with permission.)

Preeclampsia

As already described above, the presence or absence of preeclampsia does not influence either villous maturational patterns or fetoplacental capillarization. Rather, these features are defined by the type of IUGR, which is normally combined with preeclampsia:

• IUGR with PED accompanying late-onset preeclampsia in the third trimester is characterized by the features of uteroplacental hypoxia: richly branched, net-like villous capillary beds with mostly narrow capillaries resulting in short, knob-like, and multiply indented villi, which in scanning electron microscopy have a fist-like appearance (see Fig. 15.16). Histology displays increased knotting and Tenney-Parker changes (flat sectioning) (Alvarez et al., 1964, 1970). The respective villous maturation scores are **03**, **30**, **32**, or **33**, depending on severity and stage of pregnancy. Due to increased villous branching, the intervillous space is abnormally narrow. The amount of villous cytotrophoblast is increased as the thickness of syncytiotrophoblast is.

- IUGR with ARED accompanying early-onset preeclampsia at the transition of the second to the third trimester shows extremely long, largely unbranched, filiform villi (Figs. 15.6C and 15.17A). Terminal villous side branches are largely missing. The terminal capillary loops, resulting from nonbranching angiogenesis (see Figs. 7.17 and 15.6C), are long, slender, and usually unbranched, thus explaining the high Doppler resistance index (Kingdom et al., 1997). Villous cytotrophoblast is scarce; the thickness of villous syncytiotrophoblast is dramatically decreased. As a consequence of reduced peripheral villous branching, the intervillous space is abnormally wide.

- Preeclampsia without obvious IUGR and with normal umbilical Doppler patterns usually also shows normal villous branching patterns.

Despite the fact that gross villous maturational patterns are only influenced by the type of IUGR accompanying preeclampsia, there seems to be one parameter that is directly correlated with the presence or absence of this hypertensive disorder: the amount and extent of necrotic foci in villous syncytiotrophoblast (Black et al., 2002; Huppertz et al., 2002, 2003). Due to the absence of immunohistochemical markers for trophoblast necrosis, it is still impossible to quantify trophoblast necrosis. The visual impression of increased necrosis, however, is underlined by the facts (a) that cell-free fetal DNA is increased in the blood of mothers with preeclampsia (Hahn & Holzgreve, 2002) and (b) that experimental data suggest that this cell-free DNA is derived from increased trophoblast necrosis (Black et al., 2002; Huppertz et al., 2002). Under normal pregnancy conditions daily up to 3g of aged, apoptotic syncytiotrophoblast are shed into the maternal circulation. These trophoblast fragments are sealed by membranes, are trapped by maternal macrophages in the maternal lung, and do not induce any adverse maternal reactions. If, by contrast, apoptotic discharge of trophoblast due to adverse local energy supply becomes impossible, the aging trophoblast is discharged into the maternal circulation by necrosis: in this case trophoblastic compounds such as fetal DNA, free globular actin, and other fetal proteins are directly set free into the maternal circulation and cause an inflammatory response including maternal macrophage activation and maternal endothelial damage (Stepan et al., 2004; Zhong et al., 2004) (for details see Chapter 6).

HELLP Syndrome (Postplacental Hypoxia)

To our best knowledge, data on the placental histology in the case of HELLP (hemolysis, elevated liver enzymes, low platelets) syndrome have never been published. We, too, have analyzed only very few cases of acute HELLP syndrome, resulting in C-section between 28 and 32 weeks of pregnancy. These cases showed a surprising structural homogeneity. All of them were characterized by features of postplacental hypoxia, similar to those described above for IUGR with ARED, combined with early-onset preeclampsia: Mature intermediate villi and terminal villi were extremely long, thin, filiform, and largely unbranched. Terminal villous side branches are largely missing. Consequently, intervillous space is abnormally wide (Fig. 15.18A,B). The terminal capillary loops, resulting from nonbranching angiogenesis are long, slender, and usually unbranched (Fig. 15.18D). Their geometry explains the abnormally high umbilical Doppler resistance indices. As in postplacental hypoxia, villous cytotrophoblast is barely undetectable. Accordingly, in spite of ample immunoreactivities for proliferation marker MIB-1 in the villous stroma, proliferating cytotrophoblast is missing. The thickness of villous syncytiotrophoblast is dramatically decreased. Signs of apoptotic knotting and respective TUNEL reactivity are largely missing, whereas disintegration of the apical plasmalemma, accumulation of trophoblastic debris in the intervillous space, as wells as fresh intervillous blood clot and perivillous fibrinoid are universally visible.

Because most placentas in HELLP syndrome are delivered at the beginning of the third trimester, local areas with obvious synchronous villous immaturity are found (Fig. 15.18C). These are in striking contrast to the otherwise prematurely differentiated villi.

These preliminary findings support the view that HELLP syndrome is a hypertensive disorder of the late second trimester and therefore shows features similar to those of early-onset preeclampsia combined with IUGR with ARED (see above). As already indicated above, our findings are based on only a few cases. Two findings from the literature suggest, however, that the general structural features described above may be representative:

- Our findings of numerical reduction of villous cytotrophoblast and increased syncytiotrophoblast necrosis suggest a decreased rate of syncytial fusion. This is in agreement with the data by Knerr et al. (2002), who showed that syncytin expression in these placentas is reduced (cf. Chapter 6).

- Prevalence of nonbranching angiogenesis in the placental villi, as described above, is supported by the findings by Zhou et al. (2002), who found reduced VEGF but normal placental growth factor (PlGF) expression, by cytotrophoblast from HELPP placentas, both in situ and in vivo. This is a combination of angiogenetic

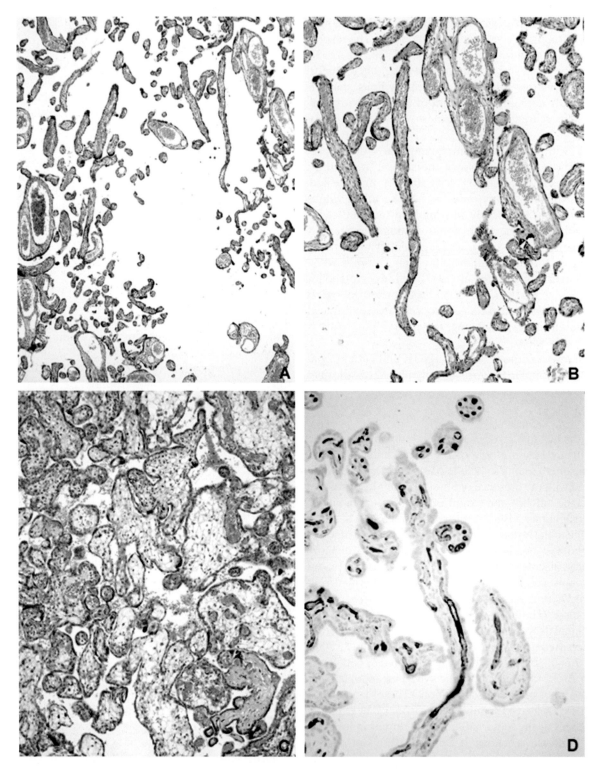

FIGURE 15.18. Placenta from a patient with severe HELLP syndrome showing typical features of postplacental hypoxia, 30th week of gestation. A: Paraffin survey picture. Note the long, poorly branched bundles of mostly filiform terminal villi with an extremely wide intervillous space. ×25. B: In higher magnification the unusually small diameter of the majority of terminal villi becomes evident. ×50 C: The center of a villous tree of the same case still shows synchronous immaturity, which reflects the stage of pregnancy. ×50. D: QBend10 staining of the same case reveals few, mostly undilated, poorly branched capillaries (brown). This feature is highly characteristic for postplacental hypoxia. ×140.

growth factors that are thought to be responsible for the development of excessive nonbranching angiogenesis in placental villi (for review see Charnock-Jones et al., 2004 and Kaufmann et al., 2004).

Maternal Diabetes Mellitus

The villi associated with maternal diabetes mellitus have usually been described as being immature (Greco et al., 1989; Vogel, 1996; Fox, 1997). A more detailed evaluation reveals several differences when compared to synchronous immature villi or to those of persisting immaturity and rhesus incompatibility. Werner and Schneiderhan (1972), Emmrich et al. (1975), Gödel and Emmrich (1976), and Fox (1997) have all described characteristic features in diabetes, including increased villous diameters, stromal fibroblastic proliferation (Fig. 15.19A,B), increased basal lamina thickness, an excess of Langhans' cells, and

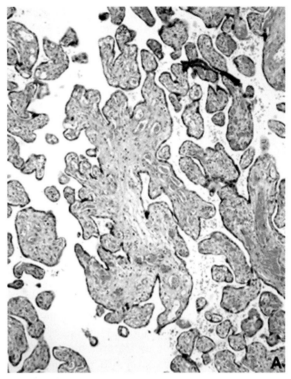

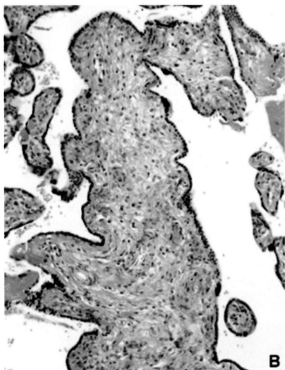

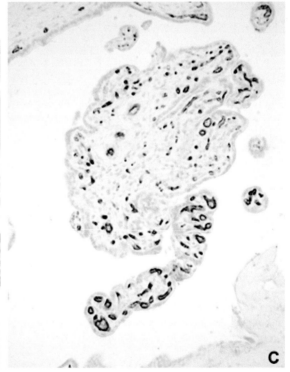

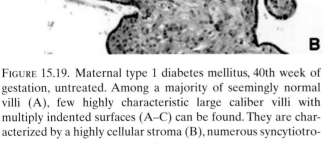

FIGURE 15.19. Maternal type 1 diabetes mellitus, 40th week of gestation, untreated. Among a majority of seemingly normal villi (A), few highly characteristic large caliber villi with multiply indented surfaces (A–C) can be found. They are characterized by a highly cellular stroma (B), numerous syncytiotro- phoblastic nuclei (B), and large numbers of small capillaries, which are evenly distributed throughout the stroma. A: ×25; B: ×50; C: QBend10 staining, ×50. (Courtesy of Dr. Berthold Huppertz, Aachen, Germany.)

decreased fetal vascularization with increased maternofetal diffusion distances. On the other hand, we also observed large, hypercellular villi from diabetic pregnancies that showed unusually dense capillarization (Fig. 15.19C). We agree with Vogel (1996), who pointed to the local and interindividual variability of the villous patterns, which can be only partly explained by various degrees of illness or success of treatment.

The scanning electron microscopic appearance is similar to that of cases of synchronous immaturity but different from that of persisting immaturity and rhesus incompatibility. The number of drumstick-shaped true trophoblastic sprouts increases with increasing diameter of the immature villi, suggesting considerable proliferative activity. Because of their small size, the incidence of true sprouts is moderate in histologic sections. The diagnosis can be based on the large caliber of the villi, which often show fist-like indented surface (Fig. 15.19). Moreover, unusual amounts of villous cytotrophoblast and voluminous stromal cells are significant findings. The villous maturation score is not applicable to these villous features because qualitative alterations of villous structure prevail, rather than alterations of the numerical composition of villous trees.

References

Alvarez, H., De Bejar, R. and Aladjem, S.: La placenta human. Aspectos morfologicos y fisio-patologicos. In, 4th Uruguayan Congress for Obstetrics and Gynecology, Vol. 1, pp. 190–261, 1964.

Alvarez, H., Morel, R.L., Benedetti, W.L. and Scavarelli, M.: Trophoblast hyperplasia and maternal arterial pressure at term. Amer. J. Obstet. Gynecol. **105**:1015–1021, 1969.

Alvarez, H., Benedetti, W.L., Morel, R.L. and Scavarelli, M.: Trophoblast development gradient and its relationship to placental hemodynamics. Amer. J. Obstet. Gynecol. **106**:416–420, 1970.

Amaladoss, A.S.P. and Burton, G.J.: Organ culture of human placental villi in hypoxic and hyperoxic conditions: a morphometric study. J. Dev. Physiol. (Oxf.) **7**:113–118, 1985.

Bacon, B.J., Gilbert, R.D., Kaufmann, P., Smith A.D., Trevino, F.T. and Longo, L.D.: Placental anatomy and diffusing capacity in guinea pigs following long-term maternal hypoxia. Placenta **5**:475–488, 1984.

Becker, V.: Funktionelle Morphologie der Plazenta. Arch. Gynäkol. **198**:3–28, 1963.

Becker, V.: Pathologie der Ausreifung der Plazenta. In, Die Plazenta des Menschen. V. Becker, T.H. Schiebler and F. Kubli, eds., pp. 266–281. Thieme, Stuttgart, 1981.

Becker, V. and Röckelein, G.: Pathologie der Plazenta und des Abortes. Springer, Heidelberg, 1989.

Beischer, N.A., Sivasamboo, R., Vohra, S., Silpisornkosal, S. and Reid, S.: Placental hypertrophy in severe pregnancy anaemia. J. Obstet. Gynaecol. Br. Commonw. **77**:398–409, 1970.

Black, S., Huppertz, B., Pötgens, A.J.G., Adzic, J., Kadyrov, M. and Kaufmann, P.: Trophoblast shedding causes endothelial apoptosis: implications for preeclampsia. Placenta **23** (Suppl. A): A.37, 2002.

Boyd, J.D. and Hamilton, W.J.: The Human Placenta. Heffer, Cambridge, 1970.

Brosens, I.: The utero-placental vessels at term-the distribution and extent of physiological changes. Trophoblast Res. **3**:61–68, 1988.

Brosens, I., Robertson, W.B. and Dixon, H.G.: The physiological response of the vessels of the placental bed to normal pregnancy. J. Pathol. Bacteriol. **93**:569–579, 1967.

Brosens, I.A., Robertson, W.B. and Dixon, H.G.: The role of the spiral arteries in the pathogenesis of pre- eclampsia. J. Pathol. **101**:177–191, 1970.

Burton, G.J.: Intervillous connections in the mature human placenta: Instances of syncytial fusion or section artifacts? J. Anat. **145**:13–23, 1986a.

Burton, G.J.: Scanning electron microscopy of intervillous connections in the mature human placenta. J. Anat. **147**:245–254, 1986b.

Burton, G.J.: The fine structure of the human placental villus as revealed by scanning electron microscopy. Scanning Microsc. **1**:1811–1828, 1987.

Burton, G.J., Mayhew, T.M. and Robertson, L.A.: Stereological re-examination of the effects of varying oxygen tensions on human placental villi maintained in organ culture for up to 12 h. Placenta **10**:263–273, 1989.

Cantle, S.J., Kaufmann, P., Luckhardt, M. and Schweikhart, G.: Interpretation of syncytial sprouts and bridges in the human placenta. Placenta **8**:221–234, 1987.

Castellucci, M., Scheper, M., Scheffen, I., Celona, A. and Kaufmann, P.: The development of the human placental villous tree. Anat. Embryol. (Berl.) **181**:117–128, 1990.

Charnock-Jones, D.S., Kaufmann, P. and Mayhew, T.M.: Aspects of Human fetoplacental vasculogenesis and angiogenesis. I. Molecular regulation. Placenta **25**:103–113, 2004.

Emmrich, P. and Mälzer, G.: Zur Morphologie der Plazenta bei Übertragung. Pathol. Microbiol. **32**:285–302, 1968.

Emmrich, P., Gödel, E., Amendt, P. and Müller, G.: Schwangerschaft bei Diabetikerinnen mit diabetischer Angiolopathie. Klinische Ergebnisse in Korrelation zu morphologischen Befunden an der Plazenta. Zentralbl. Gynäkol. **97**:875–883, 1975.

Essbach, H. and Röse, I.: Plazenta und Eihäute. Fischer, Jena, 1966.

Fox, H.: Villous immaturity in the term placenta. Obstet. Gynecol. **31**:9–12, 1968.

Fox, H.: Effect of hypoxia on trophoblast in organ culture. Amer. J. Obstet. Gynecol. **107**:1058–1064, 1970.

Fox, H.: Pathology of the Placenta. 2nd Ed. Saunders, London, 1997.

Geisen, C., Mottaghy, K., Scheffen, I. and Kaufmann, P.: Effect of long-term hypoxia on oxygen transport properties of blood in pregnant guinea pigs. In, Oxygen Transport to Tissue, Vol. XII. J. Piiper, T.K. Goldstick and D. Meyer, eds., pp. 767–777. Plenum Press, New York, 1990.

Gödel, E. and Emmrich, P.: Morphologie der Plazenta und Qualität der metabolischen Kontrolle während der Schwangerschaft bei Diabetes mellitus. Zentralbl. Gynäkol. **98**: 1307–1311, 1976.

Greco, M.A., Kamat, B.R. and Demopolulos, R.I.: Placental protein distribution in maternal diabetes mellitus: an immunocytochemical study. Pediatr. Pathol. **9**:679–690, 1989.

Hahn, S. and Holzgreve, W.: Fetal cells and cell-free DNA in maternal blood: new insights into pre-eclampsia. Hum. Reprod. Update **8**:501–508, 2002.

Huppertz, B., Frank, H.G., Kingdom, J.C.P., Reister, F. and Kaufmann, P.: Villous cytotrophoblast regulation of the syncytial apoptotic cascade in the human placenta. Histochem. Cell Biol. **110**:495–508, 1998.

Huppertz, B., Black, S., Kadyrov, M., Kaufmann, P. and Groten, T. In late-onset preeclampsia the amount of shed trophoblast and maternal immune cells is increased in the intervillous space. Placenta **23**(Suppl. A):A.37, 2002.

Huppertz, B., Kingdom, J., Caniggia, I., Desoye, G., Korr, H. and Kaufmann, P.: Hypoxia favors necrotic versus apoptotic shedding of placental syncytiotrophoblast into the maternal circulation. Implications for the pathogenesis of preeclampsia. Placenta **24**:181–190, 2003.

Jackson, M.R., Mayhew, T.M. and Haas, J.D.: Morphometric studies on villi in human term placentae and the effects of altitude, ethnic grouping and sex of newborn. Placenta **8**:487–495, 1987.

Jackson, M.R., Mayhew, T.M. and Haas, J.D.: On the factors which contribute to thinning of the villous membrane in human placentae at high altitude. I. Thinning and regional variation in thickness of trophoblast. Placenta **9**:1–8, 1988a.

Jackson, M.R., Mayhew, T.M. and Haas, J.D.: On the factors which contribute to thinning of the villous membrane in human placentae at high altitude. II. An increase in the degree of peripheralization of fetal capillaries. Placenta **9**:9–18, 1988b.

Jones, C.J.P. and Fox, H.: Syncytial knots and intervillous bridges in the human placenta: an ultrastructural study. J. Anat. **124**:275–286, 1977.

Kadyrov, M., Kosanke, G., Kingdom, J. and Kaufmann, P.: Increased fetoplacental angiogenesis during first trimester in anaemic women. Lancet **352**:1747–1749, 1998.

Kaufmann, P.: Entwicklung der Plazenta. In, Die Plazenta des Menschen. V. Becker, T.H. Schiebler and F. Kubli, eds., pp. 13–50. Thieme, Stuttgart, 1981.

Kaufmann, P. and Castellucci, M.: Development and anatomy of the placenta. Fox, H. and Wells, M. Haines and Taylor: Obstetrical and Gynaecological Pathology. IVth edition, 1437–1476. 1995.

Kaufmann, P., Luckhardt, M., Schweikhart, G. and Cantle, S.J.: Cross-sectional features and three-dimensional structure of human placental villi. Placenta **8**:235–247, 1987.

Kaufmann, P., Black, S. and Huppertz, B.: Endovascular trophoblast invasion: implications fort the pathogenesis of intrauterine growth retardation and preeclampsia. Biol. Reprod. **69**:1–7, 2003.

Kaufmann, P., Mayhew, T.M. and Charnock-Jones, D.S.: Aspects of human fetoplacental vasculogenesis and angiogenesis. II. Changes during normal pregnancy. Placenta **25**:114–126, 2004.

Kemnitz, P. and Theuring, F.: Makroskopische, licht- und elektronenmikroskopische Plazentabefunde bei Übertragung. Zentralbl. Allg. Pathol. **118**:43–54, 1974.

Kingdom, J.C.P. and Kaufmann, P.: Oxygen and placental villous development: origins of fetal hypoxia. Placenta **18**:613–621, 1997.

Kingdom, J.C.P., Macara, L.M., Krebs, C., Leiser, R. and Kaufmann, P.: Pathological basis for abnormal umbilical artery Doppler waveforms in pregnancies complicated by intrauterine growth restriction. Trophoblast Res. **10**:291–309, 1997.

Kloos, K. and Vogel, M.: Pathologie der Perinatalperiode. Grundlage, Methodik und erste Ergebnisse einer Kyematopathologie. Thieme, Stuttgart, 1974.

Knerr, I., Beinder, E. and Rascher, W.: Syncytin, a novel human endogenous retroviral gene in human placenta: Evidence for its dysregulation in preeclampsia and HELLP syndrome. Amer. J. Obstet. Gynecol. **186**:210–213, 2002.

Kosanke, G., Kadyrov, M., Korr, H. and Kaufmann, P.: Maternal anemia results in increased proliferation in human placental villi. Trophoblast Res. **11**:339–357, 1998.

Krebs, C., Macara, L.M., Leiser, R., Bowman, A.W., Greer, I.A. and Kingdom, J.C.P.: Intrauterine growth restriction with absent end-diastolic flow velocity in the umbilical artery is associated with maldevelopment of the placental terminal villous tree. Amer. J. Obstet. Gynecol. **175**:1534–1542, 1996.

Krebs, C., Longo, L.D. and Leiser, R.: Term ovine placental vasculature: comparison of sea level and high altitude conditions by corrosion cast and histomorphometry. Placenta **18**:43–51, 1997.

Küstermann, W.: Über "Proliferationsknoten" und "Syncytialknoten" der menschlichen Placenta. Anat. Anz. **150**:144–157, 1981.

Macara, L., Kingdom, J.C.P., Kaufmann, P., Kohnen, G., Hair, J., More, I.A.R., Lyall, F. and Greer, I.A.: Structural analysis of placental terminal villi from growth-restricted pregnancies with abnormal umbilical artery Doppler waveforms. Placenta **17**:37–48, 1996.

Martin, B.J. and Spicer, S.S.: Ultrastructural features of cellular maturation and aging in human trophoblast. J. Ultrastruct. Res. **43**:133–149, 1973.

Mikolajczak, J., Ruhrberg, A., Fetzer, M., Kaufmann, P. and Goecke, C.: Irreguläre Zottenreifung bei Frühgeburtlichkeit und Übertragung, und ihre Darstellbarkeit im Ultraschall. Gynäkol. Rundsch. **27**:145–146, 1987.

Mohr, H.: Zur Histologie der übertragenen Plazenta. Zentralbl. Gynäkol. **72**:1530, 1950.

Ong, P.J. and Burton, G.J.: Thinning of the placental villous membrane during maintenance in hypoxic organ culture: structural adaptation or syncytial degeneration? Eur. J. Obstet. Gynecol. Reprod. Biol. **39**:103–110, 1991.

Panigel, M. and Myers, R.E.: Histological and ultrastructural changes in rhesus monkey placenta following interruption of fetal placental circulation by fetectomy or interplacental umbilical vessel ligation. Acta Anat. (Basel) **81**:481–506, 1972.

Pilz, I., Schweikhart, G. and Kaufmann, P.: Zur Abgrenzung normaler, artefizieller und pathologischer Strukturen in reifen menschlichen Plazentazotten. III. Morphometrische Untersuchungen bei Rh-Inkompatibilität. Arch. Gynecol. Obstet. **229**:137–154, 1980.

Piotrowicz, B., Niebroj, T.K. and Sieron, G.: The morphology and histochemistry of the full term placenta in anaemic patients. Folia Histochem. Cytochem. (Krakow) **7**:435–444, 1969.

Reshetnikova, O.S., Burton, G.J. and Milovanov, A.P.: The effects of hypobaric hypoxia on the terminal villi of the human placenta. J. Physiol. (Lond.) **459**:308P, 1993.

Salvatore, C.A.: The placenta in acute toxemia. A comparative study. Amer. J. Obstet. Gynecol. **102**:347–353, 1968.

Scheffen, I., Kaufmann, P., Philippens, L., Leiser, R., Geisen, C. and Mottaghy, K.: Alterations of the fetal capillary bed in the guinea pig placenta following long-term hypoxia. In, Oxygen Transfer to Tissue, Vol. XII. J. Piiper, T.K. Goldstick and D. Meyer, eds., pp. 779–790. Plenum Press, New York, 1990.

Schiebler, T.H. and Kaufmann, P.: Reife Plazenta. In, Die Plazenta des Menschen. V. Becker, T.H. Schiebler and F. Kubli, eds., pp. 51–111. Thieme, Stuttgart, 1981.

Schuhmann, R. and Geier, G.: Histomorphologische Placentabefunde bei EPG-Gestose. Arch. Gynäkol. **213**:31–47, 1972.

Schweikhart, G.: Morphologie des Zottenbaumes der menschlichen Plazenta-Orthologische und pathologische Entwicklung und ihre klinische Relevanz. Thesis, Medical Faculty, University of Mainz, 1985.

Schweikhart, G. and Kaufmann, P.: Histologie und Morphometrie der Plazenta bei intrauteriner Mangelentwicklung des Feten. Arch. Gynäkol. **235**:566–567, 1983.

Schweikhart, G. and Kaufmann, P.: Endzottenmangel und klinische Relevanz. Gynäkol. Rundsch. **27**(Suppl. 2):147–148, 1987.

Schweikhart, G., Kaufmann, P. and Beck, T.: Morphology of placental villi after premature delivery and its clinical relevance. Arch. Gynecol. Obstet. **239**:101–114, 1986.

Sibley, C.P., Pardi, G., Cetin, I., Todros, T., Piccoli, E., Kaufmann, P., Huppertz, B., Bulfamante, G., Cribiu, F.M., Ayuk, P., Glazier, J. and Radaelli, T.: Pathogenesis of intrauterine growth restriction (IUGR)—conclusions derived from a European Union Biomed 2 Concerted Action Project: importance of oxygen supply in intrauterine growth restricted pregnancies—a workshop report. Placenta **23**(Suppl. A):S75–S79, 2002.

Stepan, H., Faber, R., Froster, U.G., Heinritz, W., Wallaschofski, H., Dechend, R., Walther, T. and Huppertz, B.: Pre-eclampsia as a "three stage problem"—a workshop report. Placenta **25**:585–587, 2004.

Stoz, F., Schuhmann, R.A. and Schebesta, B.: The development of the placental villus during normal pregnancy: morphometric data base. Arch. Gynecol. Obstet. **244**:23–32, 1988.

Tenney, B. and Parker, F.: The placenta in toxemia of pregnancy. Amer. J. Obstet. Gynecol. **39**:1000–1005, 1940.

Todros, T., Sciarrone, A., Piccoli, E., Guiot, C., Kaufmann, P. and Kingdom, J.: Umbilical Doppler waveforms and placental villous angiogenesis in pregnancies complicated by fetal growth restriction. Obstet. Gynecol. **93**:499–503, 1999.

Tominaga, T. and Page, E.W.: Accommodation of the human placenta to hypoxia. Amer. J. Obstet. Gynecol. **94**:679–691, 1966.

Vogel, M.: Pathologie der Schwangerschaft, der Plazenta und des Neugeborenen. In, Pathologie, Vol. 3. Remmele, W., ed. Springer-Verlag, Heidelberg, 1984.

Vogel, M.: Histologische Entwicklungsstadien der Chorionzotten in der Embryonal- und der frühen Fetalperiode (5. bis 20. SSW). Pathologe **7**:59–61, 1986.

Vogel, M.: Atlas der morphologischen Plazentadiagnostik. 2nd Ed. Springer, Berlin, 1996.

Wentworth, D.: The placenta in cases of hemolytic disease of the newborn. Amer. J. Obstet. Gynecol. **98**:283–289, 1967.

Werner, C. and Schneiderhan, W.: Plazentamorphologie und Plazentafunktion in Abhängigkeit von der diabetischen Stoffwechselführung. Geburtsh. Frauenheilkd. **32**:959–966, 1972.

Werner, C., Göbel, U., Kramartz, N., Werners, P. and Haering, M.: Plazentareifungsstörungen und Schweregrad des Morbus haemolyticus neonatorum. Geburtsh. Frauenheilkd. **33**:776–785, 1973.

Zhong, X.Y., Wang, Y., Chen, S., Labu, Pubuzhuoma, Gesangzhuogab, Ouzhuwangmu, Pan, X., Zhu, N., Hahn, C., Huppertz, B., Holzgreve, W. and Hahn, S.: Circulating fetal DNA in maternal plasma is increased in pregnancies at high altitude and is further enhanced by preeclampsia. Clin. Chem. **50**:2403–2405, 2004.

Zhou, Y., Mcmaster, M., Woo, K., Janatpour, M., Perry, J., Karpanen, T., Alitalo, K., Damsky, C., Fisher, S.J.: Vascular endothelial growth factor ligands and receptors that regulate human cytotrophoblast survival are dysregulated in severe preeclampsia and hemolysis, elevated liver enzymes, and low platelets syndrome. Amer. J. Pathol. **160**:1405–1423, 2002.

16
Erythroblastosis Fetalis and Hydrops Fetalis

ERYTHROBLASTOSIS FETALIS

Erythroblastosis fetalis, or hemolytic disease of the newborn, is a condition caused by specific antibodies of the mother, directed against red cell antigens of the fetus. These are largely Rh–(D) antigens, but rare cases of sensitization against other antigens (e.g., Kell), and of ABO incompatibility with fetal hemolytic disease have been described. Leventhal and Wolf (1956) have presented Kell-isoimmunization as a cause of fatal erythroblastosis fetalis (EF). This was also found in the well-illustrated case of Ivemark et al. (1959). Anti-K antibodies usually arise as a result of transfusion and the fetal disease is usually mild. Of 194 pregnancies complicated by this antibody constellation, only 16 affected babies were identified, of which three were severely affected by hemolytic disease (Leggat et al., 1991). The difficulty in this situation is the identification of the pregnancies at risk, an aspect discussed in some detail in an editorial in *Lancet* (1991). Anti-K hemolytic disease does not differ histopathologically from anti-D–caused erythroblastosis. However, there may be a difference in the response to this antibody. Vaughan et al. (1998) showed that they specifically inhibit growth of K-positive erythroid precursors and may thus lead to severe fetal anemia. Relatively few cases of typical, severe EF have been described as being due to ABO incompatibility. These were summarized by Freda and Carter (1962), and a fatal case is delineated by Miller and Petrie (1963), but usually, the hemolytic disease of ABO-incompatibility is mild. The pathologic findings of infant and placenta are the same as those in EF due to Rh incompatibility; in their case, the placenta weighed 900 g and had typical features of erythroblastosis. Other types of hemolysis occur which also produce similar pathologic features of infant and placenta. Thus, hemolysis in fetal blood may rarely result because of glucose-6-phosphate dehydrogenase (G-6-PD) deficiency, virus infection, and for other uncommon reasons. These causes of fetal hemolysis must be differentiated from the classic erythroblastosis.

As RhoGAM prophylaxis (Mittendorf & Williams, 1991) has become more widespread, the typical disease has become relatively uncommon in this country. Pathologists and clinicians are now more challenged to unravel the causes and therapy of "nonimmunologic hydrops fetalis" (vide infra) and of other causes of prenatal anemia, such as transplacental bleeding (vide infra and Chapter 17). From a pathologist's point of view, these conditions are often indistinguishable, and additional tests need to be employed to identify the many specific disease entities that comprise this complex fetal condition. It is worth mentioning that the fetal genotype (RhD+) is now commonly made in Europe from free DNA in maternal serum (Gautier et al. 2005).

The cause of typical erythroblastosis is the transplacental transfer of maternal antibodies that cause hemolysis in the fetus. As a consequence, the fetus attempts to repair this loss of red blood cells by overproduction and premature dissemination of immature red cell precursors (nucleated red blood cells, NRBCs). The hematopoietic tissue becomes increasingly activated in the fetus and the peripheral blood thus contains an increased number of NRBCs and erythroblasts, elegantly demonstrated by Nicolaides et al. (1988a,b). They performed reticulocyte counts in 127 pregnancies with isoimmunization, from 17 to 36 weeks, and also suggested that it may be the extensive hepatic red cell production that may cause the hydrops, by obstruction of sinusoidal blood flow. In our opinion, this is not the most likely mechanism for hydrops to develop. We believe that fetal cardiac failure is the main cause of hydrops and of the placental changes. The high-output congestive heart failure results from anemia and is the presumed cause of cardiomegaly and heart failure in EF (Naeye, 1967). The issue is not completely resolved, however, as there is no strict correlation between the severity of anemia and cardiac hypertrophy (Carter et al., 1990). From the frequently extensive hemolysis, large iron stores may occur in the liver and spleen, whereas the fetus becomes progressively anemic. When the hematocrit falls much below 15%, edema, ascites, and eventually anasarca develop—the condition known as hydrops fetalis (Saltzman et al., 1989). Normative values for hemoglobin and NRBC and reticulocyte counts, ascertained by cordocentesis, are to be found in the contribution by Nicolaides et al. (1989). They discovered that hemoglobin and red blood cell counts increased linearly from 17 to 40 weeks' gestation. Importantly, the "erythroblast count decreased exponentially from a mean of 83/100 leukocytes at 17 weeks to 4/100 leukocytes at 40 weeks." Similar values obtained by other investigators were reviewed by Weiner et al. (1992), who also measured protein levels, enzymes, pH, and gases, as well as venous pressure. Thilaganathan and collaborators (1992) found that erythropoietin (EPO) levels were significantly increased only in severe fetal anemia. Moya and his colleagues (1993) found that EPO levels were elevated in erythroblastosis also, but before 24 weeks' gestation this response was much smaller.

Fetal hydrops is now readily diagnosed sonographically (Saltzman et al., 1989); if it is due to hemolysis, the hydrops may be quickly and completely reversed when the anemic fetus is transfused intravascularly before birth (abdominally or by cordocentesis), thus restoring oxygenation (Socol et al., 1987; Grannum et al., 1988). The latter authors documented the impressive changes in protein and hemoglobin levels that occur. Nicolaides et al. (1988) who provided the normative values for fetal hemoglobin levels from 17 to 40 weeks' gestation (11–15 g/dL), found that hydropic fetuses had hemoglobin values of 7 to 10 g/dL. A study investigating the possible mechanism of fetal death occurring in such pregnancies during transfusion showed that acute increases in hematocrit were associated with substantial mortality (Radunovic et al., 1992), whereas Nicolini et al. (1989) implicated increases in venous pressure during transfusion. The bilirubin, liberated by hemolysis, is effectively exchanged transplacentally and the neonate rarely has much jaundice. This is a later, usually neonatal development in erythroblastosis.

Other fetal changes are worth mentioning. Hepatosplenomegaly is prominent; usually the infants have some hypoproteinemia. They also often suffer severe thrombocytopenia (Harman et al., 1988) and display increased beta-cell activity of their islets of Langerhans. The islet cell hyperplasia, which is combined with a greater islet insulin content (Driscoll & Steinke, 1967), was explained to result from insulin binding by the circulating hemoglobin (Steinke et al., 1967). The occasional presence of large maternal ovarian lutein cysts with hydrops fetalis is more difficult to explain. These cysts are clearly associated with an usually enlarged placenta, as was shown by Burger (1947), Christie (1961), Rabinowitz et al. (1961), and Hatjis (1985). Ovarian lutein cysts are also found in nonimmune hydrops, and they occasionally accompany fetal triploidy as well. These varied observations have led to the suggestion that, similar to the ovaries of women with hydatidiform moles, the fetal ovarian cysts result from elevated titers of human chorionic gonadotropin (hCG), produced because of the enlargement of the placentas with increased trophoblastic mass. Christie (1961) and Hatjis (1985) have determined that the maternal serum levels of hCG are significantly above normal with fetal hydrops. Initially, this elevation of hCG titers was thought to result from the persistent presence of the Langhans layer of trophoblast, or from its exaggerated appearance. Now that the origin of hCG has clearly been determined to be the syncytium, the abundance of hCG with fetal hydrops must be assumed to result from placental enlargement alone. In this connection, it is relevant to point out that human placental lactogen (hPL) and placental protein 5 (PP5) are also elevated in fetal hydrops (Lee et al., 1984). Although the elevation of hPL and hCG levels may relate to a larger placental mass, as suggested by Lee et al. (1984), the increase of PP5 levels is not so readily understood.

Placental Pathology in Erythroblastosis

The striking features of the placenta in erythroblastosis fetalis are its pallor, uniform enlargement, presence of bone marrow elements in the fetal circulation, and the villous "immaturity" (Fig. 16.1). Because of the edema and enlargement, placentas of erythroblastosis are also very friable. The changes were delineated early by Hellman and Hertig (1937), prior to a knowledge of the nature of the disease. They enumerated syncytial degeneration, persistence of Langhans' layer, prominence of Hofbauer cells, presence of erythropoietic cells in the vascular spaces, and stromal edema of villi. Since then, many studies have been conducted, all with essentially the same findings. Of comparative interest is that the hematopoiesis proceeds within the villous blood vessels (Alenghat & Esterly, 1983), in contrast to the villous arrangement in marmoset monkeys where it also proceeds in the villous stroma. It is now apparent that the placental alterations are largely secondary to the fetal anemia and to cardiac failure. Wentworth (1967) studied the placentas with the Gough large-section technique and affirmed that "the more severely the baby was affected, the larger the placenta was in relation to the baby." In the severe cases, the placentas were extremely pale and more friable than normal. Additional diagnostic histologic features in the placenta were a marked decrease in the number of fetal vessels and an increase in the number of NRBC in these vessels. Langhans' layer persisted in all cases but in itself it was not considered to be a specific change. Wentworth believed that the pathologic changes resulted from a direct effect of antibodies on the placenta. Montemagno et al. (1966) suggested from immunofluorescent antibody studies, that the syncytium possesses the Rh antigen and that antibodies localize to these antigens. Thus, the antibodies were believed to damage the syncytium and thereby produce the pathologic changes seen in the placenta of EF. More detailed examination of this question by Benachi et al. (1998), however, revealed decisively that the RhD antigen is not expressed by syncytiotrophoblast.

On occasion, one may find small amounts of hemosiderin deposited in chorionic macrophages betraying the long-standing hemolysis. It is not a prominent finding,

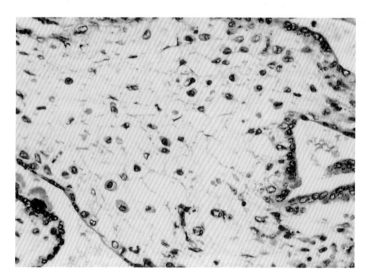

FIGURE 16.1. Villus in stillborn with typical erythroblastosis fetalis showing edema, abundance of Hofbauer cells, and persistent cytotrophoblast. Because of fetal demise, the fetal vessels are obliterated. H&E ×250.

however. We presume that the affinity for iron of fetuses is too great for substantial hemosiderin accumulation to take place in the placenta. Rarely, one observes some icteric staining of placental surface vessels and umbilical cord. We now know that these are nonspecific changes that are essentially similar in placentas of unrelated types of hydrops fetalis (e.g., α-thalassemia). We believe that it is impossible, without history or specific immunologic tests, to make the specific diagnosis of EF from a placental examination alone, an opinion similar to that expressed by Bouissou et al. (1969), who suggested, however, that the crowding of hematopoietic elements in the hepatic parenchyma may cause the fetal edema, which is contrary to our views. It is noteworthy that with the polymerase chain reaction (PCR) to ascertain fetal Rh genotype, the diagnosis is now readily achieved from blood and by the usage of amnionic fluid (Veyer & Moise, 1996; Veyer et al., 1996). The possible importance of vascular endothelial growth factor (VEGF) distribution in the placenta was investigated by Shiraishi et al. (1997). Because Rh disease is uncommon in Japan, they studied primarily the placentas of nonimmune hydrops by immunohistochemistry of this placentally active cytokine (Jackson et al., 1994). VEGF was found in syncytiotrophoblast of all placentas and in stromal cells (fibroblasts) during the first trimester of normal placentas, but not later. In the hydropic organs, however, stromal cells remained positive in 12 of 18 cases, those whose outcome was poor. They confirmed also that hydropic placentas are composed of hypovascular villi and made reference to the persistence of β-hCG, lactogen, and phosphatase expression throughout pregnancy in hydrops fetalis (Kamat et al., 1989). Their suggestion is that, functionally as well as structurally, hydropic placentas remain immature and that VEGF may have a regulatory function in the vasculogenesis of these abnormal placentas.

Wentworth (1967) provided an excellent photograph of the anemic and normal placental portions of a set of dizygotic (DZ) twins in which only one twin was affected. Becker and Bleyl (1961) performed fluorescence microscopy on such placentas and believed that these demonstrated the increased permeability of the erythroblastotic placentas. The authors showed a "condensation of . . . the interfibrillary substance of the connective tissue" of villi and believed it to be due to an increase in interfibrillary substance. This, we believe is largely the result of edema and of the accumulation of Hofbauer cells. It has occasionally been suggested that extramedullary hematopoiesis also takes place within the villous stroma. We believe that this is not the case. To be sure, the abundance of erythroblasts in some cases so much crowds the fetal capillaries that a villous production site is simulated. There is normally a large number of bone marrow–like elements in the fetal capillaries in EF; Alenghat and Esterly (1983) even found some of these cells to contain

mitoses in abortions specimens. Burstein and Blumenthal (1962) found that the abundance of syncytial knots was about the same as that found in normal controls but that the villi were much expanded; by their method, this resulted in a decreased villus count. They also emphasized the occurrence of fetal capillary proliferative lesions. There was no mention as to whether any of the placentas came from stillborn infants. Apparently similar pathologic findings were presented in a Russian article that was not accessible to us (Iakovtsova, 1964). Busch and Vogel (1972) provided a complete review of the historical aspects "of the placental changes theretofore described" and added their own observations of 58 cases. They found that these related to the severity of the hemolytic disease, that is, the degree of anemia, and emphasized the occurrence of "maturational changes of villi." Finally, they found that about one third of their cases had intervillous thrombi. This is indeed a common lesion in the placentas of erythroblastosis fetalis, and it is not easily or satisfactorily explained. One may postulate that intervillous thrombi are the sequel of an increased hydrostatic pressure within the fetal capillaries, and resultant bleeding. This would be supported by finding many nucleated red blood cells within the thrombi (Fig. 16.2). Intervillous thrombi, however, are also extremely frequent in hydatidiform moles that have no fetal vasculature. We believe that the mechanism of the formation of intervillous thromboses in both conditions may be similar. The villous edema so alters the intervillous blood flow as to cause local eddying and stasis, with thrombosis being the end result. Nevertheless, because NRBC are often found in the thrombi, fetal bleeding must occur at times. It may result from local villous hypoxic injury, as it has been repeatedly demonstrated that distention of fetal vessels and necrosis at the surface of the villi take place. This is further discussed in Chapter 17 in considerations of fetal hemorrhage. Busch and Vogel (1972) contended that the placental enlargement was the result of real growth. The investigations by Vidyasagar and Haworth (1973), however, negated this explanation. They found no differences when they compared the weights of non-EF placentas with those from nonhydropic cases of EF. Their decidual surfaces, and DNA, water, and protein contents all were similar.

An electron microscopic study of the placentas from erythroblastotic infants was undertaken by Jones and Fox (1978). These investigators found characteristic syncytial necrosis, cytotrophoblastic hyperplasia, thickening of basement membranes of villi and vessels, and immature endothelial cells. They did not identify a distinct pathogenesis of these alterations, but ruled out immunologically mediated changes. Rather, they felt that the syncytial degeneration was the result of villous enlargement with consequent decrease of the intervillous space. The most detailed study of villous alterations in EF comes from the

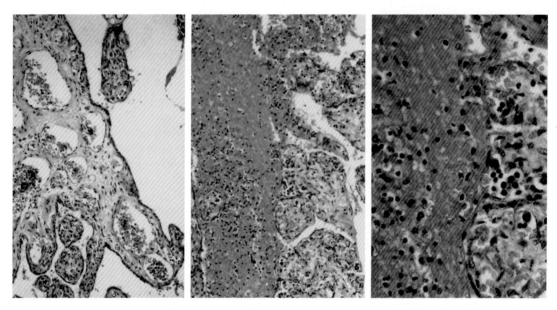

FIGURE 16.2. Immature placenta of live infant with edema. Marked villous vascular distention, numerous erythroblasts in the fetal circulation (left). Intervillous thrombi with nucleated red blood cells in same placenta (middle, right). H&E ×60; ×40; ×160.

investigations by Pilz et al. (1980). They insisted that, in order to obtain reproducible results, it is necessary for protocols to provide specific fixation and other data. They obtained their material from in situ aspiration biopsies of eight cases of EF, and compared them with 20 normal organs. Their morphometry showed an enlargement of intermediate villi that depended upon the severity of the disease. They also observed an increase in cytotrophoblast; the terminal villi were not altered, and there was an increase in Hofbauer cells. These investigators believed that the increased number and size of Hofbauer cells probably related to the increased antigen-antibody reaction that must take place in the stroma of villi. They were unable to find the alterations in capillary lumens that were suggested to exist by other authors. There was no chorangiosis. They further emphasized that the changes that they observed may represent a true maturational disturbance of the villi. In this regard, it is noteworthy that calcifications of the placenta are very uncommon in EF.

Modern management of the isoimmunized gravida requires supervision of fetal progress. This includes sonography for the detection of edema, evaluation of amnionic bilirubin concentration, and the ascertainment of umbilical vein diameter. When these parameters were correlated, Reece et al. (1988) showed that umbilical venous dimension does not parallel the other time-honored methods of prenatal evaluation. Prenatal intraabdominal transfusion for the therapy of affected fetuses (e.g., Queenan & Douglas, 1965) is gradually being displaced by intravascular transfusion with cordocentesis. This is usually done near the site of cord insertion on the placental surface (Rodeck et al., 1984;

Schumacher & Moise, 1996), a technique that allows sampling of fetal blood and estimation of total blood volume (Macgregor et al., 1988). The survival of transfused blood in the fetus is approximately similar with the two techniques (Pattison & Roberts, 1989; Van Kamp et al., 2005). With the introduction of transfusion by cordocentesis, newly observed pathologic features have been witnessed in the placenta. Berkowitz et al. (1986) presented their results of 18 such transfusions, weighed the advantages and disadvantages of cordocentesis, and drew attention to the problems that ensue from the need for repeated puncture. The complications mainly involved injury to the umbilical cord; they witnessed stillbirth as a result. Pielet et al. (1988) also drew attention to the possible dangers accruing from cordocentesis. They found two stillbirths without recognizable cord injury; in another neonate with postnatal developmental delay, however, one umbilical artery was clotted after transfusion had been performed into the umbilical vein. A similar case is shown in Figure 16.3. This patient had unsuccessful cord blood sampling at 28 weeks' gestation. At 29½ weeks successful transfusion of 45 mL of blood was accomplished into the vein. At 32 weeks, another transfusion was attempted; it ended with infusion of blood into the cord, and emergency cesarean section was necessary. The child survived. The cord had a superficial hematoma that extended onto the placental surface. The entire cord was stained with hemolyzed blood; hemosiderin was found in the chorionic macrophages. One umbilical artery was necrotic and had old obliterative thrombosis. Interestingly, there was a line of polymorphonuclear leukocytic exudation extending between the vein and the occluded artery, in the absence of chorioamnionitis. We concluded that the degenerating

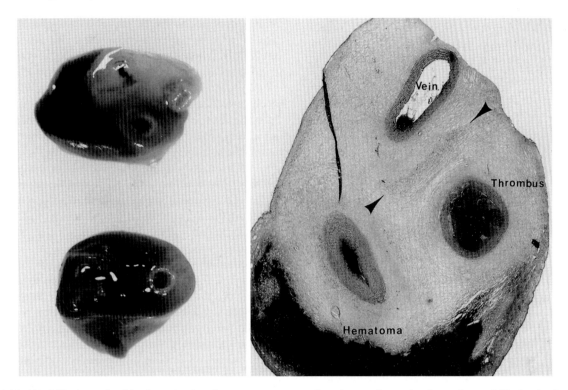

FIGURE 16.3. Umbilical cord with thrombosis of one artery, following cordocentesis 3 weeks earlier. A new attempt caused infusion of blood into the cord substance. A line of leukocytic exudate (arrows), coming from the umbilical vein, has formed between vein and the occluded artery, whose wall is dead. H&E ×3.

vessel caused the (sterile) inflammation. This occlusion had presumably occurred 3 weeks earlier.

Figure 16.4 shows the result of needle puncture of the fetal surface in a relevant case. During amniocentesis, the posterior-located placenta was accidentally injured, and an "upwelling" of blood was seen sonographically. Two weeks later, a stillborn fetus was delivered. The placental surface showed the site of needle injury to a surface vessel. We have also seen a stillborn fetus whose third transfusion was given into the cord. During that procedure, bradycardia developed after the needle was inserted. The procedure was stopped and abdominal blood was given instead, but the fetus succumbed. There was a tense, placental portion of the cord with hematoma, and fresh occlusive thrombi were found within superficial arterial ramifications. Moreover, within this thrombotic material, typical squames were identified (Fig. 16.5), presumably introduced by the needle from the amnionic cavity. Our interpretation was that, after needle insertion, a cord hematoma and vascular spasm ensued, which were followed by arterial thrombosis. Seeds and his colleagues (1989) asserted that the demonstration of "echogenic venous turbulence" was an important feature of successful intravascular transfusion. When they found it absent in a case that developed bradycardia, a hematoma of the cord was found to have developed. In another case one artery thrombosed but the fetus survived. Other hemorrhagic and thrombotic complications of cordocentesis are

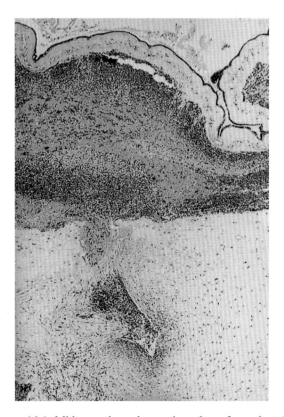

FIGURE 16.4. Mid-gestation placental surface, 2 weeks after amniocentesis. The needle injured the chorionic vessel below. Fresh hematoma, with hemosiderin, and attempted repair of vascular wall. H&E ×16.

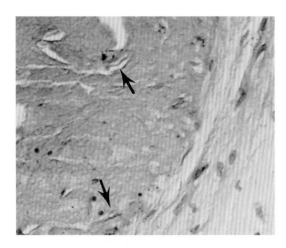

FIGURE 16.5. Arterial thrombus of placental surface in hydropic stillborn, days after cordocentesis for transfusion. Typical squames are seen (arrows), presumably introduced by the needle during transfusion. H&E ×256.

discussed in Chapter 12. James (1970) measured villous size in EF placentas after intrauterine (abdominal) transfusions had been given, and correlated the findings with hemoglobin levels. Normal values were found when the hemoglobin was above 11 g/dL, but the mean villous volume was increased in more severely affected infants. Houston and Brown (1966) reported a case of fetal gasbacillus infection after fetal transfusion; the edematous placenta was colonized by large numbers of grampositive bacterial rods and there was chorioamnionitis.

When it is necessary to traverse the placenta to gain access to the fetus, it may be injured and may bleed from the villous tissue. This may then enhance maternal immunization. These aspects were described by Friesen et al. (1967), who identified puncture marks in the placenta in such cases. These investigators found significant bleeding into the mother in 7.5% of cases when transgression of an anterior placenta was necessary to gain access to the amnionic sac.

As Figure 16.8 shows, the placenta of severe erythroblastosis has a remarkable macroscopic appearance but the correct diagnosis cannot be made solely on account of the severe anemia, and the other causes of fetal anemia to be discussed subsequently need to be included in the differential diagnosis.

Twins may also be discordant (Figs. 16.6 to 16.8) or concordant for EF. When discordant, the severity of the disease often differs markedly (Beischer et al., 1969). In one such case with marked discrepancy, a difference in ABO compatibility was held to be responsible. The authors postulated that undetermined factors may be operative in producing discordance. A similarly discordant set of DZ twins with EF was detailed by Wiener et al. (1962). Manning et al. (1985) reported on the prenatal transfusions in a number of such twins. It is further remarkable that maternal Rh isoimmunization may occur after fetal demise. Stedman et al. (1988) described three cases. They assumed that transplacental bleeding had occurred early during this unsuccessful pregnancy, and was thus causally related to the fetal demise by the pro-

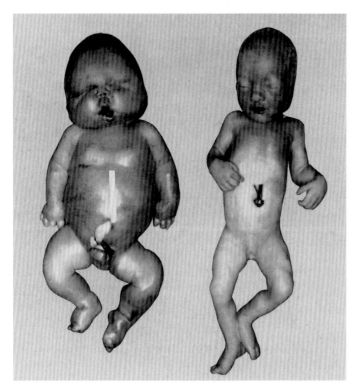

FIGURE 16.6. Immature, fraternal twins, one with erythroblastosis, the other normal. The placenta of the erythroblastotic twin (Fig. 16.6) is markedly enlarged and is unusually pale.

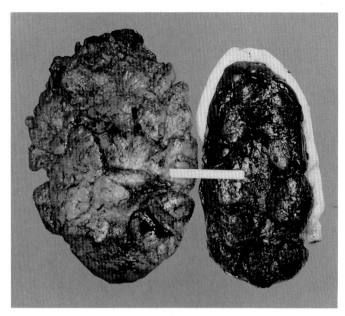

FIGURE 16.7. Normal term placenta (right) and placenta of erythroblastosis (left). Note the marked pallor and disruption of the erythroblastotic placenta.

duction of antibodies. This is most likely to have been true in their first patient who had torsion of the umbilical cord; the others had negative placental findings. This observation brings into question the mechanism of primary immunization against Rh antigens, usually held to occur most frequently at the time of delivery, or imme-

diately thereafter. It is the rationale for postpartum RhoGAM prophylaxis that has been extremely effective in preventing isoimmunization. Injury to the placenta, such as occurs during manual removal of the placenta and during Cesarean section, enhances fetal blood transfer. Queenan and Nakamoto (1964) found that spontaneous placental delivery and previous drainage of cord blood minimize the probability of isoimmunization. Although it is possible that occasional fetal bleeding in early pregnancy may lead to immunization of primigravidae, the commonest time of sensitization is at delivery (Scott et al., 1977).

Maternal bleeding into a female fetus presumably accounts only for very few immunizations in their future gestations, when an Rh-negative infant is delivered to an Rh-positive mother (Taylor, 1967). Such mother-to-fetus transfer of blood, however, is said to occur as often as in 43% of samples analyzed by Luca et al. (1978). This feature of maternal–fetal blood exchange is further discussed in Chapter 17.

The amount of immunogen needed for isoimmunization has been debated. Attempts to elucidate this with experimental findings have been made in Rh-negative volunteers. Zipursky and Israels (1967) suggested that repeated injections of as little as 0.1 mL ABO compatible Rh-positive blood will suffice to immunize Rh-negative individuals. That is an amount that is presumably frequently attained in normal pregnancies. Mollison (1968) opined that the minimum amount needed for immunization is 0.25 mL of fetal blood.

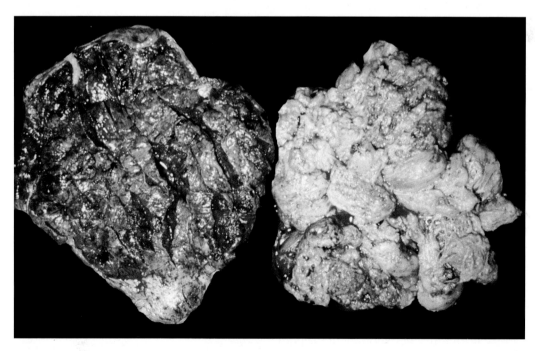

FIGURE 16.8. Placentas of twins as in Figure 17.7. The enlarged, edematous placenta of the diamnionic/dichorionic (DiDi) twins, one with erythroblastosis (left), shows the pallor and bulky cotyledons.

These deliberations are particularly important when one considers whether a hydatidiform mole, spontaneous abortion, or ectopic pregnancy can immunize an Rh-negative woman. Price (1968) reported a case of hydatidiform mole, followed by a normal pregnancy, in which antibodies were detected at about 6 months; the neonate succumbed from EF. The assumption was made that the mole had immunized the primigravida. It seems unlikely to us that a bloodless structure is capable of Rh immunization, unless the original tissue was a partial mole with triploidy and the possibility of fetal blood content. Alternatively, it is now proven that early hydatidiform moles may possess some fetal red blood cells, to disappear later (Baergen et al., 1996; Fisher et al., 1997; Paradinas et al., 1997); perhaps their detection by such a mother led to antibody formation. It has also been debated why, in patients having an abortion, it sometimes becomes necessary to provide RhoGAM to patients. Freda et al. (1970) came to the conclusion that this was indicated only after the second month of pregnancy. Regrettably, their data do not specify whether the abortions they studied were terminations of pregnancy, or whether they were true spontaneous abortions. The vast majority of the latter cases have no circulating fetal blood as they are due to chromosomal errors that led to embryonic death earlier. They would not be expected to deliver sufficient antigen for sensitization; there is no doubt, however, that embryonic erythrocytes are capable of immunization. Examples of this are the cases of therapeutic terminations of early pregnancy studied by Matthews et al. (1969), Jorgensen (1969), Murray and Barron (1971), and Eklund (1981). To be sure, the risk of sensitization is small and it depends also on the type of instrumentation used in the termination of pregnancy, such as suction vs. dilatation and curettage. And it also depends on fetal age. Ectopic pregnancies present a significantly higher risk for isoimmunization than that which occurs with spontaneous abortion (Grimes et al., 1981), presumably because of their less frequent cytogenetic abnormality and fewer embryonic deaths. Whether chorionic villus sampling (CVS) presents a risk, is yet to be determined. When Warren et al. (1985) studied α-fetoprotein (AFP) levels and Kleihauer-Betke stains following CVS, they found AFP levels to rise. They felt that the Kleihauer technique was not sufficiently sensitive to detect possible fetal bleeding. But to our knowledge, the risk incurred for isoimmunization from CVS has not been sufficiently investigated. It is generally thought that Rh-positive fetal red blood cells represent the only immunogen to Rh-negative women; trophoblastic cells were once thought to contain Rh antigen and also produce sensitization, but the later studies detailed above show this not to be the case. Besides, then every Rh-positive gestation should lead to isoimmunization because of the massive transportation of syncytium to the maternal lung and its subsequent destruction. Direct immunofluorescent studies with fluorescent anti-Rh D-antibodies have shown that fluorescence may localize to the syncytium (Jarkowski et al., 1964). Goto et al. (1980) extended these studies. They impressively demonstrated, with appropriate controls, that the amount of trophoblastic Rh-antigen decreases with advancing gestation, in contrast to the increasing prevalence on fetal red blood cells. They also showed that it localizes on trophoblastic surfaces, and that it is present in hydatidiform mole. Whether it can be the cause of sensitization remains elusive for reasons alluded to. The newest observations negate such a possibility. The studies by Benachi et al. (1998) have now revealed decisively that the RhD antigen is not expressed by syncytiotrophoblast. There is no answer to the obvious question as to why it is that not all Rh-negative women with Rh-positive conceptuses become immunized. Although the trophoblastic embolization to the maternal lung in all pregnancies was formerly thought to have relevance in this respect, this is no longer held to be so. With the definitive exclusion of the Rh antigen from syncytium, this speculation fails. Complete absence of AB antigens from trophoblast was also demonstrated by the early studies of Szulman (1972), who did, however, readily identify the antigen in fetal epithelium and in placental capillaries, including in a chorangioma.

NONIMMUNE HYDROPS

In the majority of cases of hydrops fetalis, the etiology is different from that EF, discussed above. Santolaya et al. (1992) found that of the 76 fetuses with hydrops (among 12,572 ultrasound examinations), only 10 were due to immunologic causes and 66 had nonimmune hydrops fetalis. They were unable to assign a cause in 17 cases. Some of the other hydropic fetuses resulted from fetal anemia and heart failure, trisomies, and other abnormalities. But many other hydropic fetuses are "idiopathic," a euphemism for our lack of knowledge of their precise etiology. It must also be cautioned that ascites alone is insufficient for the diagnosis of hydrops, in which case there is generalized edema, and fluid exists in all cavities. This fluid accumulation in the pleural spaces often leads to pulmonary hypoplasia, a condition that is not the cause of the hydrops, however (Green et al., 1990). The placental pathology is similar to that of EF, but substantial differences are also identified in individual cases. Novak et al. (1991) described cases of what they considered to be "hemorrhagic endovasculitis" of the placental vessels with fetal hydrops, although they did not claim causality. This entity is more fully discussed elsewhere (Chapter 12). They depicted obliterated main stem vessels amidst rather nonhydropic villi; usually this is regarded as a postmortem phenomenon. Eight of their 14 cases were stillborn, and most were complicated by hydramnios. In some unexplained cases of fetal hydrops, pathologists may be able to exclude specific causes. Often, they are confronted with a stillborn, frequently a macerated, hydropic fetus, and are asked to provide an idea as to the mechanism that led to the fetal hydrops. In the following pages we review many of the currently known entities of nonimmunologic hydrops, and then discuss idiopathic hydrops fetalis. Larger series dealing with causes of hydrops fetalis are the following reports: Macafee et al. (1970), Moerman et al. (1982), Hutchison et al. (1982), Nakamura et al. (1987), Machin (1989), Villaespesa et al. (1990), and Lallemand et al. (1999). Watson and Campbell (1986) provided a detailed management protocol for such pregnancies. A large review of 600 cases is provided by Jauniaux et al. (1990), who ascertained that more than 35% of cases could be ascribed to a genetically transmitted disease, similar to that of Lallemand et al. (1999) who thought that 38% of their 94 cases had a chromosomal origin. Chromosomal disorders also ranked first in Jauniaux's series, with 15.7%, α-thalassemia was second (10.3%), and a wide variety of anomalies followed. They suggested that chromosomal analysis was needed in such cases. Mallmann and colleagues (1991) suggested that perhaps 49 of their 324 cases of nonimmune hydrops represent an expression of immunologic rejection. Quite uncommonly prenatal trauma (e.g., a motor vehicle accident) has been held responsible for fetal hydrops, and even transitory events have been reported (see Chapter 17).

α-Thalassemia

Normal adult hemoglobin molecules contain two unlike pairs of polypeptide (globin) chains, the α-chains and the β-chains. In embryonic and fetal life, special forms of hemoglobin are prevalent at different and carefully scheduled times. Abnormal construction of the globin chains that make up fetal hemoglobin results in altered hemoglobins that may be deficient in oxygen-carrying capacity. This, in turn, can lead to abnormal red blood cell shapes, such as occurs in sickle cell disease. In the thalassemias (α- and β-thalassemias), anemic disorders result from a decreased production of normal hemoglobin. These disorders are classified according to the chain, which is depressed. Examples include α-, β-, δ-, and γ-thalassemia (Nathan, 1973).

α-Thalassemia is an inherited abnormality of hemoglobin structure that often causes hydrops fetalis and that was lethal until the event of intrauterine blood replacement. Carr et al. (1995) have now shown in an afflicted Filipina that repeated transfusions before birth can yield a surviving, transfusion-dependent child. α-Thalassemia was also the first type of nonimmunologic hydrops for which an innovative explanation was identified. This complication of pregnancy has occupied much greater attention in this country in recent years because of the immigration of Indochinese with this genetic background. It is also a model for which prenatal marrow transplantation and gene therapy are being considered. Thus, diagnosis is important, as the homozygous condition is lethal and recurrence rate is at least 1 in 4. Detailed screening methods (cresyl blue staining, erythrocyte indices, and iron study) have been described for the couples at risk for this disease (Skogerboe et al., 1992). The pathology seen in the newborn is essentially identical to that of Rh disease. Lie-Injo and her colleagues (1959, 1962, 1968) reported the association of hydrops fetalis and Bart's (Bartholomew) hemoglobin, in Indonesian families. Since then, this disease has been recognized in Filipinos (Pearson et al., 1965; Nakayama et al., 1986), Thais (Pootrakul et al., 1967; Thumasathit et al., 1968), Chinese (Kan et al., 1967), Germans (Rönisch & Kleihauer, 1967), and Canadian Orientals (with hemoglobin-H disease: Ing et al., 1968; Gray et al., 1972). It probably occurs in other races. The α-thal₁ gene has been identified in Kurdish Jews (Horowitz et al., 1966) and in Ashkenazi Jews, but it has there not been associated with hydrops (Goldschmidt et al., 1968). The same is true of American blacks. The frequency of this deletion of α-chain genes is greatest in Indonesians and Chinese (Zeng & Huang, 1985). Hydrops is caused by the homozygous presence of the gene for Bart's hemoglobin. The four α-chains are herein replaced by four τ-chains. The γ-chains are often heterogeneous (Vedvick et al., 1979), and different chain composition causes different severities of the disease. In hemoglobin-Bart's disease, the α-thalassemia, the defective hemoglobin is unable to release its oxygen effectively, which causes tissue hypoxia, fetal cardiac failure, and hydrops (Orkin & Nathan, 1976). It is essentially lethal at birth or very shortly thereafter. The fetal red blood cells in this disorder are frequently misshapen; for example, they may be sickled. Cardiac hypertrophy is often striking, as is the extensive and widespread extramedullary hematopoiesis. The substitution of various types of hemoglobin chains during development, and the location of their production in the fetus are complex and have been lucidly portrayed by Nalbandian et al. (1971). Orkin and Michelson (1980) showed, by DNA sequence analysis, that the 5'-portion of the α-globin structural gene was deleted in a case of α-thalassemia.

The switching of hemoglobins in embryonic development is regulated in a complex manner; it has been studied by Peschle et al. (1985), and by Wood and his colleagues (1985). Different states of DNA-methylation have been identified, but the mechanism that initiates this switch remains unknown. Many other types of neonatal hemoglobinopathies are known, as for instance hemoglobin-H disease, in which four β-chains constitute the molecule. This particular hemoglobinopathy is prevalent in Orientals and has a wide spectrum of severity, including occasional hydrops. It causes neonatal anemia, and hydrops was described later (Milner et al., 1971; Chen et al., 2000). A comprehensive analysis of the various genetic deletions and substitutions of the α-globin gene in hemoglobin-H disease is found in Chen et al. (2000), who studied Chinese patients from different regions in Asia. Hydrops fetalis is uncommon of unheard of in sickle cell anemia and sickle cell β-thalassemia. Both are associated with poor reproductive outcome, however, but generally do not feature hydrops as a complication (Laros & Kalstone, 1971). A detailed review of many of these considerations was provided by Jonxis (1965). He described details on the switching from embryonic to fetal, and from fetal to adult hemoglobins, and also listed the then known abnormal hemoglobins.

Louderback and Shanbrom (1967) indicated that hemoglobin electrophoresis is perhaps the simplest and most widely available tool for the differential diagnosis of the various types of cord blood hemoglobin. Sexauer et al. (1975) described a simple and rapid electrophoretic method for the analysis of cord bloods. They found that 11% of their 7500 cord blood samples from black newborns contained an abnormal hemoglobin. The methods for genetic diagnosis have now been considerably simplified (Lebo et al., 1990), and they have been successfully applied to prenatal diagnosis as well. Kan et al. (1976) accomplished this by molecular hybridization. Rubin and Kan (1985) presented a rapid and decisive method, based on slot-blot analysis. Williamson et al. (1981) and Chang and Kan (1981) showed that, with CVS biopsy, it is easily possible to make the accurate diagnosis of sickle cell disease in the fetus, and of many cases of thalassemia by direct globin gene analysis. It is important to state that appropriate samples of blood must be saved for such studies at autopsy when the etiology of hydrops is uncertain. The aforementioned methods also much facilitate the diagnosis of heterozygotes that was previously so difficult to accomplish (Terheggen & Kleihauer, 1968). Unusual causes of hemolytic disease of the newborn, such as the γ-β-thalassemia reported by Kan et al. (1972), are also thus delineated.

The placenta in thalassemia does not differ very much from that of children with classical erythroblastosis, and histology alone cannot make the correct differential diagnosis. The placenta, however, is usually even more enlarged than in erythroblastosis; it is pale, friable, and edematous. The cytotrophoblast is prominent and, in the much enlarged fetal circulation, large numbers of red-cell precursors are found (Figs. 16.9 and 16.10). Hemosiderin is occasionally seen within chorionic macrophages, but it may also be bilirubin pigment from bilirubinuria and liver damage. Hemosiderosis of the placenta has also been a feature of β-thalassemia (Birkenfeld et al., 1989), although Knisely (1990a) cautions that iron occurs in many placentas. On the whole, Birkenfeld and colleagues were probably correct in their interpretation, because

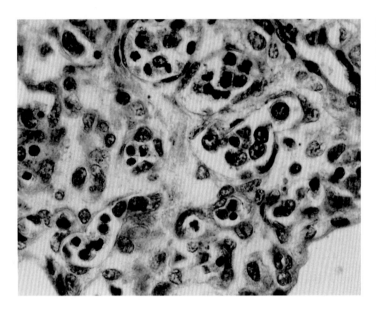

FIGURE 16.9. Placenta in α-thalassemia with fetal hydrops. This placenta weighed 1900 g and had macroscopic features such as the organ in Figure 16.8. Note the large number of marrow-like elements in the fetal capillaries. H&E ×640.

total iron content was compared with the normal and was elevated. The placental enlargement in thalassemia has often been massive. Thus, the placenta shown in Figure 16.9 weighed 1900 g. Lie-Injo et al. (1968) described weights up to 3500 g (!), most of which is water. They observed a set of fraternal twins, wherein one of the placentas was normal and the other was abnormal. This conclusively established that the pathologic changes in the placenta have a fetal cause. Pregnancy-induced hypertension (preeclampsia) is a frequent corollary of this condition, presumably because of the massive placental enlargement (Suh, 1994). This author also showed hematopoiesis in the fetal dermis and, by electrophoresis, that 91.2% of the fetal hemoglobin was abnormal.

It is of related interest to be aware of the complex relationships that exist between placental weight (and edema) to fetal and to maternal anemia. These aspects have been studied by Beischer and his colleagues (1968). These investigators found that the placental weight of mothers with various types of anemia was in an approximately normal range whereas the placental weight in cases of EF was much more increased, even when compared with the enhanced placental weight found usually in the pregnancies of diabetic mothers. Other aspects of clinical management are important. Thus, Guy and colleagues (1985) studied five pregnant Oriental women sonographically and found that sonographic surveillance for hydrops was an invaluable tool in clinical management (see also Saltzman et al., 1989 for criteria). These investigators emphasized that the pregnancies were frequently complicated by preeclampsia, and by retained placentas that necessitated manual removal. Miller et al.

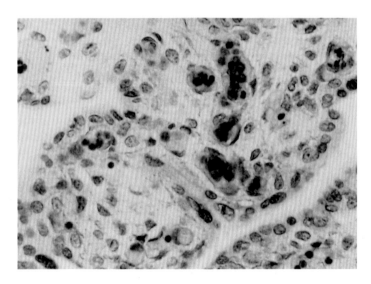

FIGURE 16.10. Villi of macerated, hydropic fetus showing edema and numerous hyperchromatic cells intravascularly. Neuroblastoma was suspected but could not be proved. H&E ×350.

(1987) reported theca-lutein cysts in a Vietnamese mother who had hydramnios and an hydropic 1290-g infant who died immediately after birth. The placenta weighed 1600 g. The ovarian cysts are attributed to elevated hCG levels from the enlarged placenta. The mother's β-chain hCG levels were 1,120,000 mIU/mL. The gonadotropin levels fell rapidly to 83.8 mIU/ml within 15 days, and her ovarian masses disappeared. This is not unlike the cases of ovarian cysts that may accompany EF. Mouse models of this disorder have been described. Their potential usefulness for the elucidation of yet unknown aspects of this disease was discussed by Whitney and Popp (1984). With the increasing population of Vietnamese and other Orientals in this country, α-thalassemia is seen more frequently and must be routinely considered in the differential diagnosis of hydrops (Suh, 1994). As more prenatal sonography is now being practiced, new methods are being sought in early diagnosis of these diseases. Thus, Lam et al. (1999) found that the cardiothoracic ratio may be significantly elevated in α-thalassemia as early as at 12 to 13 weeks' gestation.

New hematologic disorders have come onto the horizon as the genome is being explored in greater detail. Thus, Gallagher et al. (1995) described the occurrence of fatal anemia in two children (due to red cell membrane instability) with hydrops. The instability was the result of a homozygous mutation of the β-spectrin gene, producing the spectrin "Providence." The Diamond-Blackfan anemia was found to be the cause of hydrops in two children described by Rogers et al. (1997). One child survived after prenatal transfusions and needs lifelong transfusion. The other, born with a hematocrit of 10% and a hydropic placenta, died neonatally. Interestingly, the islets of Langerhans were much enlarged, a condition here assumed to be secondary to anemia. Methemoglobinemia was the cause of hydrops in a case described by Özmen et al. (1995). The pregnancy was terminated and the placenta was not described.

Fetal Hemorrhage

Hydrops fetalis has repeatedly been the result of massive and usually chronic fetomaternal hemorrhage, and it is for that reason that it has been our practice to examine maternal blood for fetal cells (Kleihauer-Betke technique, see Chapter 17) in all cases of unexplained stillbirths. As in EF, when the hemoglobin levels fall below a certain point (about 7 g/dL, or a hematocrit of approximately 15% or less), cardiac failure may cause hydrops. When the fetal exsanguination is rapid, it does not produce hydrops so quickly and may result more likely in fetal death. It requires ensuing heart failure and transudation for hydrops to occur. This complex aspect of adjustments was discussed in the case presented by

Herman et al. (1987), with a fetal hematocrit of 15% and hemoglobin of 3 g/dL at term. In that case, the mother had a 2.8% Kleihauer test result (which equals approximately 150 mL fetal blood) and no placental abnormalities were found. Bowman et al. (1984) considered transplacental hemorrhage to be an exceptional cause of fetal hydrops. They reviewed the few cases from the literature and described a neonate in whom large and chronic, bidirectional blood exchange must have occurred. The placenta showed major fetal vessels to have ruptured that were believed to explain this phenomenon, and there were also many placental infarcts. The placenta was not markedly enlarged (560 g). No untoward accidents had occurred until 31 weeks, when the mother experienced a rapidly increasing abdominal girth. The authors suggested that the hydrops resulted from fetal hypervolemic heart failure. Cardwell (1988) described an hydropic 2750-g liveborn infant who had been treated by prenatal transfusion at 21 weeks' gestation. The Kleihauer test had been 0.4%, which corresponded to a 50% loss of fetal blood. The finding of NRBCs in the fetal circulation is herein also an important pathologic finding (Fox, 1967). Villaespesa and colleagues (1990), who investigated 59 cases of nonimmune hydrops, felt that right-sided cardiovascular failure should be investigated, as 50% of their cases were due to this mechanism. This is borne out by direct measurements of venous pressures in hydropic fetuses (Johnson et al., 1992).

We have now seen many hydropic neonates with verified fetomaternal hemorrhage. One had the hemorrhage after an amniocentesis, which was done to ascertain fetal maturity (0.3% Kleihauer; hematocrit 19% 3 days later). Another fetus exsanguinated for no known reason (shown in Chapter 17). A third newborn had an 18% hematocrit at birth, and could not be revived. Many NRBCs were found in villous vessels. All three placentas were extremely pale and edematous, but were not so overtly hydropic as in thalassemia. Other cases have since surfaced and I believe that this is not so uncommon a cause of hydrops (certain fetal demise) as had once been believed. It is important, however, to note that ABO incompatibility between mother and fetus may rapidly remove the fetal red blood cells on which (by Kleihauer test) we rely to make the diagnosis of transplacental hemorrhage. This is an important consideration that will be further elaborated upon in Chapter 17. Zwi and Becroft (1986) reported a patient with ulcerative colitis who was on prednisone and sulfasalazine therapy; the fetus developed hydrops fetalis at 24 weeks' gestation, after 4 weeks of vaginal bleeding. No fetal red cells were identified in this blood, but a marginal separation of a 460-g edematous placenta had occurred. The macerated fetus weighed 1070 g. It had a dilated and enlarged heart, and there was complete absence of hematopoiesis in the liver and bone marrow. The latter finding led the authors to suggest that aplastic anemia was the cause of the fetal hydrops and placentomegaly. The cause of the anemia was not determined, but it is noteworthy that the mother's sulfasalazine therapy had been discontinued in early pregnancy.

Fetal Tumors

Congenital neuroblastoma has repeatedly been shown to cause fetal death. Birner (1961) described such a fetus and found an unusually enlarged placenta (1240 g). The 3925-g fetus was slightly edematous and macerated, but the placenta did not contain neuroblastoma cells. The villi were enlarged, edematous, and had an increased number of Hofbauer cells. Additionally, Langhans' cells had persisted to term. Strauss and Driscoll (1964) were the first authors to draw attention to the involvement of the placenta with neuroblastoma metastases. Their first fetus was edematous and resembled an erythroblastotic infant. The placenta was markedly enlarged and friable, and it also resembled that of EF. Cords of neuroblastoma cells were found in fetal capillaries. Their second infant was born at term, and it was accompanied by a 1030-g placenta. Typical neuroblastoma cells and erythroblasts crowded the fetal capillaries (Figs. 16.10 and 16.11). The fetal heart was enlarged. The first mother had theca lutein cysts, similar to those mentioned earlier in this chapter. Other cases of fetal hydrops with congenital neuroblastoma and placentomegaly have since been described (Anders et al., 1973; Moss & Kaplan, 1978; Slikke & Balk, 1980; Perkins et al., 1980; Smith et al., 1981; Newton et al., 1985). A possible immune hypothesis for the development of the hydrops was entertained by Strauss and Driscoll (1964), but most authors have now discounted this possibility. Hydrops and placentomegaly were present in Birner's case (1961), but there was no placental neoplasm. This finding suggested that it was not the plugging of fetal capillaries with tumor cells that causes the placentomegaly and this could thus not be the etiology of hydrops. The case of Newton et al. (1985) may have relevance to the considerations of pathogenesis. Their case was associated with maternal hypertension, which was presumed to be caused by the production of catecholamines from the fetal neuroblastoma. Perhaps, similar changes of blood pressure occur in the fetus and contribute to fetal heart failure. Perkins et al. (1980) found, in a case of congenital neuroblastoma, that the villous tissue, too, was infiltrated by neuroblastoma cells and that these contained cytoplasmic granules, which, electron microscopically, were typical of neuroblastoma cells.

We have seen placental hydrops with a severely hydropic and macerated fetus in whose placental vessels there were many malignant small cells. A positive diagnosis of the neoplasm was impossible (Fig. 16.12). No tumor mass existed in the fetus. The most recent review of the 11 cases of placental neuroblastoma with fetal hydrops reported comes from Lynn et al. (1997). They concluded that, after careful review of all factors, the pathogenesis of hydrops remains to be identified. They ruled out secretory products from the neuroblasts as mechanism and provided guidelines for a differential diagnosis, as they showed the tumor cells to be positive for neuron-specific enolase, negative for cytokeratin, desmin, synaptophysin, and bcl-2. Determinations of atrial natriuretic factor and aldosterone concentrations showed them to be elevated in hydrops fetalis due to anemia (Ville et al., 1994a,b). Perhaps future studies need to concentrate on such determinations for an explanation of the development of hydrops fetalis in general. It should be pointed out also that not all cases of congenital neuroblastoma are associated with hydrops. This was shown, for instance, in the two patients described by Ohyama et al. (1999) whose tumors were diagnosed by placental examination. These authors also referred to additional congenital cases and described additional differential diagnostic tests.

Very similar in its placental manifestation was the hydropic pregnancy described by Doss et al. (1998) that was the result of a fetal hepatoblastoma. The villous capillaries of this enlarged placenta (1190 g at 33 weeks) were filled with immature cells, metastatic from the hepatic lesion. The tumor cells stained positively for α-fetoprotein. Oetama et al. (2001) described fetal hydrops due to an epithelioid hemangioendothelioma of the fetal bone marrow space. Uniform monocyte-like cells dominated the blood smear, and there was a large number of NRBCs as well. This is a difficult diagnosis to make and it would be even harder in macerated fetuses.

Sacrococcygeal teratomas also produce placentomegaly and fetal edema. They are frequently accompanied by hydramnios and elevated hCG levels (Barentsen, 1975). In the first two such cases described, the placental edema and large number of NRBCs in the villous capillaries were identical to that seen in placental erythroblastosis (Kohga et al., 1980). When we wrote this paper, we suggested that high-output cardiac failure produced the hydrops. This was confirmed by the study of Langer et al.

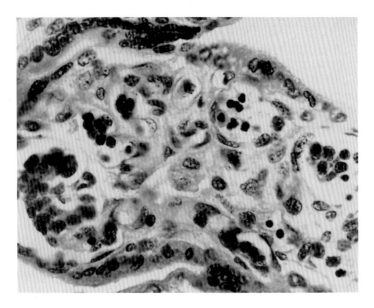

FIGURE 16.11. Villus of case with congenital neuroblastoma. The enlarged villus has numerous neuroblastoma cells in fetal vessels, some of which show some rosetting. H&E ×400.

FIGURE 16.12. Placenta from macerated stillborn with presumed leukemia. The villous capillaries are packed with leukemic cells, and some stromal infiltration is also seen. (Courtesy of Dr. E.V. Perrin.) H&E ×60; ×160.

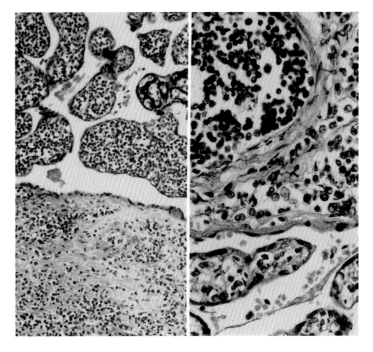

(1989). These authors observed such a tumor at 21 weeks' gestation with hydrops and placental edema. After they attempted to remove the tumor they observed a diminution of hydrops and a reduction in placental thickness. Other cases of sacrococcygeal teratoma, hydramnios, hydrops and placentomegaly (occasionally associated with preeclampsia) are reviewed in this publication and those of Perlin et al. (1981), Feige et al. (1982), Holzgreve et al. (1987), Kuhlmann et al. (1987), Pringle et al. (1987), Bock et al. (1990), and in an intrapericardial teratoma by Sklansky et al. (1997). These reports present additional cases that may be consulted for completeness. The usual prenatal recognition of this tumor has now also led to successful therapy. Adzick et al. (1997) found in a fetus with such a tumor that the hydrops and placentomegaly markedly increased between 20 and 25 weeks. The tumor was then resected in utero, whereupon the hydrops disappeared and the 29-week-gestation child was electively delivered by cesarean section and did well.

Fetal placental leukemia is rare. Macroscopically, it resembles erythroblastosis fetalis and causes placentomegaly. Figure 16.12 shows a 1000-g placenta in presumed fetal leukemia that came with a severely macerated fetus that was not autopsied. We have seen only one other similar case, which involved a fetus with trisomy 21.

Various angiomas have repeatedly caused hydrops fetalis and placentomegaly (see Chapter 24). For instance, Imakita et al. (1988) described a patient with severe hydramnios at 31 weeks' gestation; there were sonographic features of hydrops fetalis and a large chorangioma. After an amniocentesis, the patient delivered 2 days later but the infant died at 2 days of age. The neonate's

hemoglobin content was 15 g/dL; there was hypoproteinemia but no evidence of iso-immunization. The fetal heart was markedly hypertrophied and dilated, and the 840 g placenta had a 5.5 × 4.5 × 3 cm chorangioma. The authors conjectured that the location of the angioma may have been such as to have obstructed the venous return from the placenta. They also reviewed many previously reported cases of the association of chorangioma with hydrops. No doubt, in this case also, high-output cardiac failure of the fetus was responsible for the hydramnios and the placentomegaly. An interesting case of fetal hydrops, resulting from a complex hemangioma of the umbilical cord, was presented by Seifer et al. (1985). This occurred in one of dichorionic female twins who weighed 2100 g at birth but who lost her edema over the course of the first month of life. The birth weight of the co-twin was 1670 g. High-output failure was thought to have been caused by an angioma in the umbilical cord that measured 9 cm in diameter and 18 cm (!) in length. This enlargement was mainly due to edema, however. The placenta was otherwise normal. Hepatic angiomas of the fetus are occasionally so large as to cause fetal heart failure (Gonen et al., 1989; Skopec & Lakatua, 1989) and may be associated with significant neonatal thrombocytopenia. We have seen such a case in which the left lobe of the liver was replaced by a cavernous angioma. The remainder of liver had extensive centrolobular ischemic necrosis, and the kidneys were acutely infarcted. The neonate had cardiomegaly, a markedly hydropic placenta (1050 g), and an increase in NRBCs (Fig. 16.13). The neonate expired in 2 days. In cases of prenatally recognized nonimmune hydrops fetalis, sonographic study may

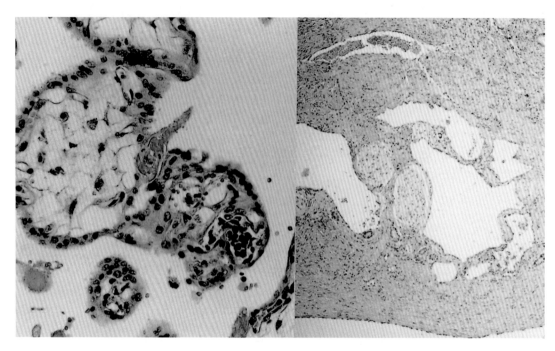

FIGURE 16.13. Edematous villi with capillaries stuffed with red cells precursors (left) in hydropic patient with cavernous hepatic angioma (right). H&E ×250; ×60.

identify such tumors as a cause of hydrops. In the past, Dr. A. James McAdams had shown us a 7-month-old child with a presumed hepatic "hamartoma" in whom the hydropic placenta had weighed 1320g. Of course, acardiac twins may present so much of a hemodynamic burden to the normal "donor" that hydrops can occur in that donor twin. It is an indication for prenatal ablation of the acardiac. Such a circumstance was recorded by Harkavy and Scanlon (1978) and is further discussed in Chapter 25.

Maternal disease, other than hydramnios, has occasionally occurred with large chorangiomas. Thus, Dorman and Cardwell (1995) observed a patient with a large placental angioma who suffered Ballantyne syndrome, a combination of severe edema, hypertension, and eclamptic fits that resolved promptly after elective delivery. Interestingly, the pregnancy was not accompanied by hydramnios. Three additional patients were described by Selm et al. (1991), who discussed the possible etiology of this complex but rare syndrome.

Cystic-adenomatoid malformation (CAM) of the lung, while not a true neoplasm, is another well-recognized cause of fetal hydrops and placental edema. Figure 16.15 shows the markedly hydropic placenta of the case published by Gottschalk and Abramson (1957). In this case, autopsy findings indicated that the mediastinum had shifted and had thus caused a chronic impediment to venous return from the placenta. The fetal heart was one-half the expected size; the placenta was edematous and weighed 1105g, at 27 weeks' gestation. The authors cited

additional similar cases. We saw such a case sonographically in one twin, with shift of the mediastinum, and Bromley et al. (1992) reported a similar set of twins. An infant with anasarca, whose placenta was not described, had a successful removal of such a large "tumor" (Aslam et al., 1970). Clark et al. (1987) even operated successfully on a hydropic child with cystic adenomatoid malformation after having placed an intrathoracic shunt prenatally. Ascites and subcutaneous edema disappeared, and the child delivered normally 17 weeks later. The tumor was removed on the first day of life. These authors and Kohler and Rymer (1973) cited additional cases of hydrops with adenomatoid malformations of the fetal lung. Occasional other tumors may also be associated with hydrops or cause fetal hydrops; some only produce polyhydramnios. Thus, Gray (1989) reported the latter condition with a mesoblastic nephroma. Fung et al. (1995) also found polyhydramnios associated with a fetal mesoblastic nephroma and believed the calciuria to have been responsible for the polyhydramnios. In neither case was the placenta described.

Congenital Anomalies and Hydrops Fetalis

Aside from the adenomatoid malformation of the lung, numerous other congenital anomalies have been causally or otherwise related to the development of fetal hydrops.

Benacerraf and Frigoletto (1986) diagnosed the presence of a diaphragmatic hernia and then drained a large right hydrothorax; the fetus survived and was born without further complications. The placenta was not described. The Klippel-Trenaunay syndrome (angio-osteohypertrophy) has occurred with hydrops fetalis (Mor et al., 1988). The placenta weighed 760 g and was bulky and friable. The newborn had giant port-wine nevi and high-output cardiac failure. Seward and Zusman (1978) reported the case of a hydropic newborn that had fetal anemia, perhaps due to a small bowel volvulus. Brinson and Goldsmith (1988) reported a child with intrauterine intussusception and intestinal perforation; hypoproteinemia was therein presumed to have caused the hydrops. Pulmonary sequestration has often caused nonimmune hydrops (Weiner et al., 1986), presumably also because of an obstructed venous return to the heart. The placenta in this case was normal. Several cases of hydrops in Noonan's syndrome have been described (Bawle & Black, 1986; Oudesluys-Murphy, 1987); the associated placentas were not mentioned. Koffler et al. (1978) described two cases of chylothorax that were associated with hydramnios, in the absence of hydrops; the placenta was not mentioned. Both infants survived. A similar case comes from Sacks et al. (1983), who stated that the placenta was not enlarged. Chylothorax and lymphangiectasis are occasionally the causes of hydrops. Abnormal development of lymphatics may be responsible for generalized edema (Windebank et al., 1987). These authors identified abnormal connections of lymphatics and vessels in an hydropic infant. They were also associated with cystic hygroma, a feature that may be at the basis of the edema in 45,X fetuses (Turner syndrome). Alternatively, coarctation of the aorta may be causative (Lacro et al., 1988). But the placenta in Turner's syndrome is not truly hydropic. If anything, it is smaller in size, and occasionally has the features of a Breus' mole (subchorionic tuberous hematoma). We have observed a set of monozygotic twins with abnormal chromosomes; one was 46,XX and normal, the other was 45,X and had massive edema, ascites, and cervical hygroma. A similar set of discordant monozygotic (MZ) twins (46,XY and 45,X) with hydrops in the latter twin was reported by Gonsoulin et al. (1990). Many reports on chromosomal trisomies suggest that these anomalies are an occasional cause of hydrops. Landrum et al. (1986) found that 17 cases of hydrops with trisomy 21, six with trisomy 18, and two with trisomy 13 had been reported. They added three cases with trisomy 21, and one with trisomy 13 of their own. Hendricks et al. (1993) also found two cases of hydrops with trisomy 21 and an associated but transitory myeloproliferative disorder, and anemia. It is of interest to note here that, in a case of chromosome 18p- syndrome, the fetal hydrops was probably due to complete heart block, resulting from calcifications in the atrioventricular node (Bridge et al., 1989). Schwanitz and colleagues (1988) have reported hydrops fetalis in a child with duplications of the long arms of chromosomes 15 and 17, offspring of a parent with balanced 15/17 translocation. They suggested that a chromosomal analysis should be undertaken in every case of nonimmune hydrops in which the cause has remained obscure. The cause of hydrops in these infants is unknown (see also Watson & Campbell, 1986), and the placenta is rarely discussed. Greenberg et al. (1983) described hygromas and hydrops in a fetus with trisomy 13 and cautioned that hygromas are not necessarily due to monosomy X; the macerated fetus had many other anomalies, but the placenta was not described. Gropp (1984) found similar conditions of edema in the experimentally induced mouse trisomy. He evaluated the various reported suggestions that seek to explain the fetal hydrops. The Neu-Laxova syndrome is another cause of hydrops; it is accompanied by multiple anomalies, hydramnios, and occasional placental edema (Broderick et al., 1988). It has also been reported that congenital myotonic dystrophy may lead to hydrops and pleural effusions but the status of the placenta was not described (Curry et al., 1988). Tuberous sclerosis has also been implicated in the genesis of hydrops fetalis. Östör and Fortune (1978) described such a case, but did not mention the placenta. The hydrops was presumably secondary to the cardiac rhabdomyoma present.

Congenital Heart Disease

Numerous cases of congenital heart disease have been described as being accompanied by hydrops fetalis. Best known among these perhaps are Ebstein's anomaly of the tricuspid valve (Moller et al., 1966), endocardial fibroelastosis (Ben Ami et al., 1986), premature closure of the foramen ovale (Rodin & Nichols, 1975; Olson et al., 1987), and some forms of hypoplastic left heart (Leake et al., 1973). Many other types of anomalies have been listed, too numerous for this discussion. Some are listed by Kleinman et al. (1982), who did not have any cases of idiopathic hydrops. They reported 10 cases of cardiovascular anomalies, and three with supraventricular tachycardia. These authors emphasized the importance of fetal echocardiography. McFadden and Taylor (1989), in their review of a large series of congenital heart disease and nonimmune hydrops, expressed the view that the coincidence of the two conditions was not causally related. They were especially emphatic in pointing out that premature closure of the foramen ovale was not a cause of hydrops fetalis. Graves and Baskett (1984) reviewed 26 cases of nonimmune hydrops fetalis. They found 11 cases with anomalies and five with primary heart malformation. There were also four cases of the twin transfusion syndrome. In a set of twins whose placenta did not show anastomoses, Mogilner et al. (1982) attributed the hydrops to prolonged maternal indomethacin therapy and ductal closure. There is even a report of a massively edematous rhesus monkey fetus with hydrops fetalis due to a complex anomaly of the heart (Cukierski et al., 1986). The placenta was circumvallate, monodiscoid, and had numerous infarcts and features of placenta previa. The fetus was no longer edematous at autopsy, long after fetal death, but its thickened, edematous features had been identified sonographically. Rare cases of hydrops with generalized arterial calcification (Williams syndrome) have occurred (Jones et al., 1972; Carles et al., 1992). Pulmonary hemorrhage (blood clot) was believed to be the cause in the last case. In one such fetus, prenatal blood sampling allowed the diagnosis of fetal hypercalcemia (Westgren et al., 1988). Its placenta was markedly edematous. In other cases, calcifications extended along the cord and placental vessels. In a case with massive calcifications of the placental villous cores that we saw, fetal fructokinase deficiency was diagnosed. It is unknown as to whether this was the cause of hydrops.

Cardiac Arrhythmias

A variety of arrhythmias have been documented to cause anasarca and placentomegaly, as just mentioned. Some of these, when recognized by sonography or other means, have been treated successfully before birth. Fetal heart block and other rhythm disturbances have occasionally been attributed to specific antibodies, such as occur in lupus, Sjögren's syndrome, and other autoimmune diseases. Vetter and Rashkind (1938) have summarized this. Specific morphologic alterations in the atrioventricular (AV) node, localized deposits of antibodies and other globulins, have occasionally been thus identified. Veille et al. (1985) described such a child in a mother with Sjögren's syndrome, wherein antinuclear antibodies against the Ro (SSA) and La (SSB) antigens were detected during pregnancy. Despite fetal heart block, a normal child was born; the placenta was apparently normal. Taylor et al. (1986) showed that these antibodies cross the placental barrier. In fatal cases, the authors found the antibodies localized in all portions of the fetal hearts. Scheib and Waxman (1989) described recurrent congenital heart block without hydrops. Supraventricular tachycardia has often caused hydrops and placental enlargement. This is particularly important for pathologists to appreciate because, in such stillborns, no specific pathologic findings will explain the placentomegaly and hydrops. Clinical observations are necessary for the diagnosis. One of the first cases described with severe hydrops, hydramnios, and placentomegaly (1025 g) is that by Silber and Durnim (1969). The reduced cardiac output was believed to result in the fetal edema.

Lingman et al. (1986) reviewed 113 cases of fetal cardiac arrhythmia. Ninety-four cases had supraventricular arrhythmias, consisting mostly of extrasystoles. None had heart failure. Five cases had heart block; of these fetuses, three died from congestive heart failure. Fourteen cases had ventricular arrhythmias. In 2%, there were associated congenital anomalies; 13.5% had fetal distress, and there was an 0.7% mortality. Four fetuses required in utero therapy for congestive heart failure. In 72% of cases, the arrhythmias disappeared spontaneously in the perinatal period. Additional cases with successful prenatal therapy were detailed by Copel et al. (1995) and Anandakumar et al. (1996). Vintzileos et al. (1985) found that atrial flutter complicated a case of familial vitamin D–resistant rickets, in which edema and placentomegaly were observed prenatally. The fetus was resistant to therapy. The authors reviewed the previously described cases of prenatally recognized atrial flutter. Fetal hydrops was rare among them, whereas cardiomegaly and hepatomegaly were common.

Since the initial report by Klein et al. (1979) of attempted cardioversion with propranolol, numerous hydropic fetuses with atrioventricular tachycardia have been successfully treated before birth. The treatment was primarily with digitalis (Hallak et al., 1991), but also with quinidine (Guntheroth et al., 1985), verapamil, and other agents (review by Wiggins et al., 1986; DeLia & Emery, 1986). An important consideration is that with severely hydropic fetuses, placental drug transport may be insufficient for effective digitalization (Younis & Granat, 1987). Direct fetal injections have also been given (Weiner & Thompson, 1988). In some of the many reported case, disappearance of hydrops and placental enlargement have been seen sonographically. This indicates that the placental edema results from fetal heart failure. Hydrops and its subsequent resolution have also been induced experimentally in fetal sheep by atrial pacing (Stevens et al., 1982; Nimrod et al., 1987).

Placental edema and enlargement have also been reported following periods of acute fetal tachypnea (Manning et al., 1981). Such rapid respirations are probably the result of the edema rather than its cause.

Nephrotic Syndrome

Congenital nephrosis is another well-recognized cause of fetal hydrops with placentomegaly. It is an autosomal-recessive condition characterized by anasarca, hypoproteinemia, and albuminuria. Despite the commonly used designation as "Finnish type" of nephrosis, the first case was probably described from Switzerland in 1942 (Giles et al., 1957). The familial nature, a frequent Finnish background of families, and electron-microscopic findings

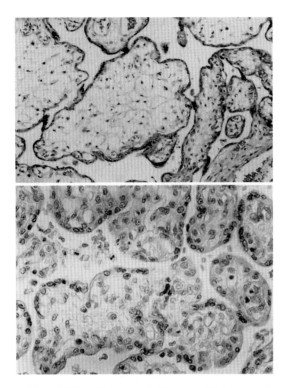

FIGURE 16.14. Villi with hydropic fetus in "Finnish nephrosis." All villi are severely hydropic, but not different from hydropic placentas in other types of hydrops. The cytotrophoblast (Langhans' layer) is unusually prominent. H&E ×160; ×400.

have been summarized by Hoyer et al. (1967, 1973) and Seppälä et al. (1976). The latter authors found that over one half of the more than 200 cases reported came from Finnish ancestry, where the incidence is said to be as high as 1:8000 (Hogge et al., 1992). They also reported that amnionic fluid AFP levels are elevated in this condition, whereas Hogge et al. (1992) found their index cases

through high maternal AFP levels combined with normal acetylcholinesterase levels; fetal death may occur. Although the placenta in their case was described to be grossly and microscopically normal, that of a Chinese patient reported by Hung et al. (1977) was enlarged (700 g) and edematous. Milunsky et al. (1977) also saw a normal placenta with an aborted specimen at 14 weeks' gestation. Kaplan et al. (1985), who reported several cases and did electron microscopy of the glomeruli (see also Hogge et al., 1992), found only mild placental edema. Presumably, the placentomegaly that has been observed occasionally is dependent on the degree of hypoproteinemia in the fetus. There are no characteristic features in the placental pathology (Fig. 16.14). Dr. G. Altshuler kindly provided me with an electron micrograph of the placental barrier in a case with recurrent congenital nephrosis. The patient had a therapeutic abortion at 19 weeks (see Fig. 16.17). No abnormalities were present in the fetus or placenta, grossly or microscopically. The kidneys showed the typical abnormality of the glomeruli.

Parvovirus Anemia

Pattison et al. (1981) recognized that human parvovirus B19 infection may cause severe anemia and a hypoplastic crisis in patients with sickle cell anemia. Using modern techniques, Essary et al. (1998) reported that 16% of nonimmune hydrops cases are estimated to be due to this infection, whereas maternal infection in pregnancy is estimated to be 1 in 400. A succinct review of the diseases caused by this virus may be found in the editorial by Anderson and Török (1989) and a book edited by Anderson and Young (1997), and Rodis et al. (1998) described the management of the infection during pregnancy. Infec-

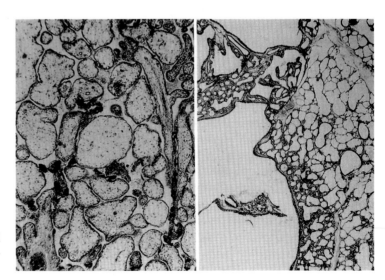

FIGURE 16.15. Edematous villi (left) in 27-week-old fetus with hydrops due to cystic adenomatoid malformation of lung (right). H&E ×150; ×100.

tion with this highly contagious virus is now known to be one of the more important causes of second trimester abortion and hydrops fetalis. Prospective studies have shown that viral transmission from mother to fetus occurs in approximately 25% to 33% of women with acute infection during pregnancy and that serious fetal disease results in 9% of these cases (Public Health, 1990). The probability of infection is highest from the gravida's own child (Harger et al., 1998) and the risk of fetal hydrops is low. Infections by many different types of parvoviruses have been reviewed by Anderson and Pattison (1984). In children, infection with parvovirus B19 causes the so-called fifth disease, or erythema infectiosum (Pillay et al., 1992). The affliction is commonly referred to as "slapped cheeks (or face)" syndrome because of the facial appearance of infected children, a disease that is usually self-limited, and 40% to 60% of adults have antibodies (immunoglobulin G, IgG) from previous infection. Asymptomatic women (often schoolteachers) may transmit the virus to their fetuses, and anemia and hydrops may thus result (Brown et al., 1984). These authors cited other infectious causes of hydrops as well, including Chagas' disease and cytomegalovirus infection, which will be discussed in Chapter 20. Similarly, listeriosis has been an occasional cause of nonimmune hydrops (Gembruch et al., 1987).

Parvovirus infection does not always cause maternal symptoms, nor does maternal infection always lead to fetal hydrops (Public Health, 1990; Harger et al., 1998). In the fetus, however, the infection can cause hydrops and profound anemia (Figs. 16.16 and 16.18). It can also usually be diagnosed by the typical ground-glass inclusion bodies of NRBCs it produces. These are composed of crystals of the small, 20-nm virus particles. The inclusion bodies may also be seen in stillborn hydropic fetuses, as they are resistant to autolysis and often, but not always, they can be identified in their placentas, as was pointed out in the review by Rogers (1992) (Fig. 16.19). It has been pointed out, however, that care must be exercised when interpreting inclusions. De Krijger et al. (1998) impressively showed many artifactual "inclusions" that were similar to parvovirus crystals, but for which there was no DNA support. They emphasized that PCR studies need to be done to verify the true nature of inclusion bodies. Additionally, one often observes hemosiderin in chorionic macrophages. Among other cases, we have seen a macerated fetus with this condition, with typical placental pathology and whose intestines had ruptured before birth. Bond et al. (1986) reported on a woman with this infection at 15 weeks' gestation. She had a skin rash, and 12 weeks later she delivered an hydropic fetus. DNA hybridization studies and electron microscopy showed many parvovirus particles in the placenta. Some were coated with antibody. Knisely et al. (1988) have also shown that the virions are readily identified in erythroid precursor cells by electron microscopy, even when only formalin-fixed tissues were available. The virus has a preferential attraction to hemopoietic (erythroid) precursor cells (Srivastara & Lu, 1988), but inclusion bodies have been observed in other tissues (e.g., hepatocytes, myocardium, endothelium; see Knisely, 1990b). But not all infections lead to hydrops, even when they may prove lethal to the fetus (Tolfvenstam et al., 2001). Moreover, in some infections it may be primarily diagnosed by increased nuchal translucency (Markenson et al., 2000).

The characteristic feature of this infection, then, is the presence of lightly staining, eosinophilic intranuclear inclusion bodies in circulating normoblasts (identification from fetal cord samples by Nerlich et al., 1991), and in their precursors in fetal organs (Anand et al., 1987). Cordocentesis has also been employed by Peters and Nicolaides (1990) for the identification of the virus by DNA hybridization. Immunoglobulins were negative, and the hydrops from fetal parvovirus infection resolved following prenatal transfusions. Other cases of successful intrauterine transfusion have been presented. It may then be impossible to identify the virus in circulating blood, and only by DNA hybridization of marrow cells may it be recovered (Brown et al., 1994). Kovacs et al. (1992), working with fetal blood samples and amnionic fluid, developed a sensitive and rapid PCR test for the detection of the antigen. An even more sensitive method for detection (by nested PCR) was advocated by Yamakawa et al. (1995). The inclusion bodies contain the B19 antigen, whose serologic detection is now widely available (Gray, 1987). Rogers and colleagues (1996) provided a protocol with which to identify viral DNA from archival material. In general, elevated IgG titers in maternal blood denote former infection, whereas an elevated IgM titer diagnoses recent or active disease. Diagnostic criteria on histologic material from marrow are well described and beautifully depicted by Krause et al. (1992). The diagnosis is feasible even in autolyzed specimens because of the resistance of the virus particles. Generally, the fetal tissues show little or no inflammatory reaction. Elsacker-Niele and collaborators reported an exception. They found two aborted fetuses; in one fetus, tissues other than the erythroid cells were involved, and in a terminated pregnancy they discovered extensive ocular malformations and inflammation of all fetal and placental tissues. One wonders if this could have been another infection superimposed on parvovirus disease. Although this virus was believed to lack teratogenicity, Weiland et al. (1987) also found an infected fetus with myocarditis and ocular anomalies. Other case descriptions with the identification of the virus are by Briner et al. (1987), and Franciosi and Tattersall (1987), who used paraffin-embedded tissue for DNA hybridization. Carrington et al. (1987) and Bernstein and Capeless (1989) found elevated maternal serum AFP-levels in this condition. Rogers et al. (1993) and Mark et al. (1993)

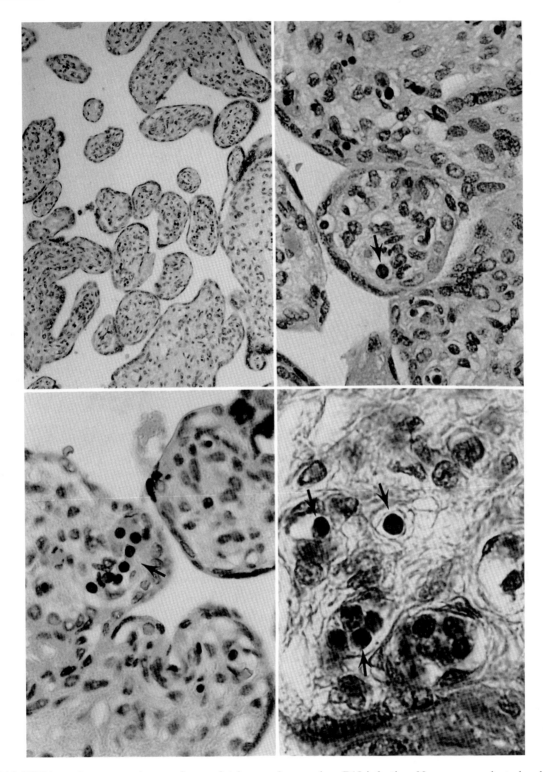

FIGURE 16.16. Villi in an immature placenta from a fatal case of parvovirus B19 infection. Numerous nucleated red-blood cells with inclusion bodies are seen at the arrows. H&E ×160, 200, 200, 400.

reviewed their 32 past cases of hydrops fetalis and found 16% to have been due to this infection. Sections of liver were most productive, whereas only two of five placentas had diagnostic inclusions. In their analysis, the inclusion bodies were so characteristic that PCR with DNA hybridization was unnecessary. Jordan (1996) conducted a retrospective study of previously unresolved cases of hydrops fetalis and found that 18% had positive signals of parvo-

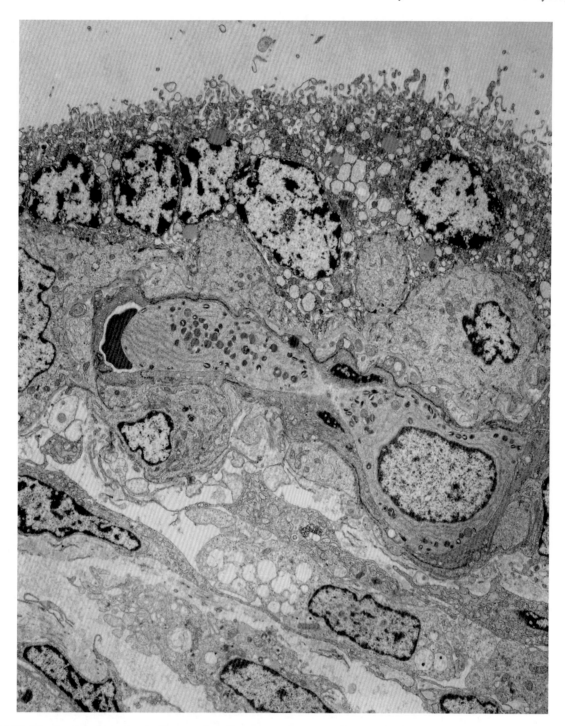

FIGURE 16.17. Electronmicrograph of villous surface in a case with fetal hydrops due to the nephrotic syndrome. Villous surface (above), microvilli, basement membranes, fetal capil-lary, are all normal. (Courtesy of Dr. G. Altshuler, Oklahoma City, Oklahoma.) ×4800.

virus B19. Similarly high-incidence figures for prenatal infection were discussed by Swain and Cameron (1997), who suggested that a parvovirus epidemic in 1993 may be partly responsible for these findings.

The reason for the severe anemia of fetuses was explored by Gray et al. (1987) and by Kinney et al. (1988)

in prospective studies of cord bloods during an outbreak of the infection. The investigation of the frequency of stillbirths, occurring during an outbreak, showed that the risk of stillbirth or abortion is not great. Similar prospective studies come from Hall et al. (1990) in England, and Rodis et al. (1990) in the United States.

FIGURE 16.18. Cross section of a normal placenta above; below is the cross section of a placenta of a fetus with parvovirus B19 infection and hydrops.

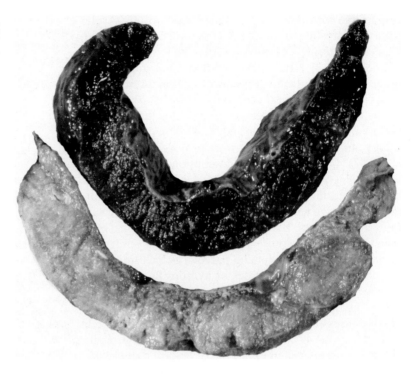

These studies indicated a rather low risk of fetal hydrops development. Although intrauterine transfusion therapy has been shown to be beneficial (Soothill, 1990; Sahakian et al., 1991), recovery from this infection has also been witnessed without therapy. Humphrey et al. (1991) observed one such case with recovery from hydrops after a 26-week infection, whereas Pryde et al. (1992) observed two cases that resolved spontaneously. A similar case with ascites and spontaneous resolution was described early by Morey and colleagues (1991), and two others observed by Sheikh et al. (1992) had normal postnatal development. Maeda et al. (1988) depicted the intense hepatic iron deposits in these hydropic infants, perhaps only related to the hemolysis. Schwarz et al. (1988), who observed 42 pregnancies with parvovirus infection, found that the infection was inapparent in one third of the gravidas. In about one quarter, there were fetal complications; the authors felt that the ascites, rather than the anemia, leads to fetal death. In a later contribution (1991) these investigators found parvovirus infection to be

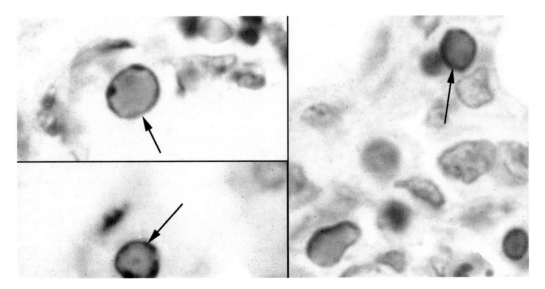

FIGURE 16.19. Hydrops caused by fetal human parvovirus B19 infection. The villi were edematous and the fetal capillaries filled with normoblasts. Many normoblast nuclei have smudged amphophilic, intranuclear inclusion bodies (arrows). H&E ×400; ×640.

responsible for numerous spontaneous abortions. Aside from the so-called lantern cells (the inclusions resemble Chinese lanterns), the authors identified the DNA by hybridization in NRBCs. Myocardium and most other tissue were negative; hydrops was found in 14 of the 15 spontaneous abortuses occurring between 20 and 30 weeks. Further, these investigators suggested that mothers are asymptomatic in 75% of fetal infections. Other case reports and literature review were provided by Vogel et al. (1997). Of interest is the description of dichorionic twins by Pustilnik and Cohen (1994). One twin developed hydrops and died, and the other remained negative for the infection. A fetus papyraceus accompanied a normal fetus and placenta. Burton and Caul (1988) emphasized that the placenta represents "a most fruitful source of nucleated red cells containing parvovirus inclusions and is worthy of study in all cases of hydrops fetalis caused by infection with human parvovirus B19."

Macroscopically, the placenta is not different from that in other cases of hydrops fetalis. It is pale, friable, enlarged, and edematous. A complete review of the topic is available elsewhere (Anand et al., 1987). Rodis et al. (1988), in their study of pregnant women during an outbreak in Connecticut, drew attention to the potential dangers of this disease for pregnant teachers because of their contact with infected children. Further annotations are provided by Stocker and Singer (1988). Anderson et al. (1988) reported a hydrops due to this infection, and Porter et al. (1988) showed by immunohistochemistry that fetal myocardial nuclei are also infected, whereas Metzman and colleagues (1989) showed that this infection may cause severe liver disease. They reported a neonatal death with growth retardation and severe hepatic destruction in an infected infant whose mother suffered a rash during the 21st week of pregnancy. It has now also been reported that villous destruction may be the result of parvovirus infection. Samra et al. (1989), who reviewed the world literature of this fetal infection, observed that there is "a high risk to the fetus once the virus crosses the placenta." Their 20 weeks' gestation hydropic stillborn was accompanied by a placenta that showed villous necrosis and calcification.

Hydrops of Unknown Etiology

As the previous discussion has indicated, more and more causes of fetal edema and hydrops have become known. Therefore, this baffling entity is shrinking rapidly and the indications are that, with careful prenatal sonographic surveillance and with the help of more sophisticated genetic and autopsy techniques, this entity may vanish in the future. The recognition of syphilis as one such occasional cause (Barton et al., 1992) is representative of the many unusual etiologies one must consider. We believe that the term **idiopathic hydrops fetalis** should be used with restraint. It merely betrays that we have not as yet discovered its etiology and must probe further to assign a specific cause. Drogendijk (1963), who considered this topic in some detail, was of the opinion that hydrops of unknown etiology probably results from some placental malfunction.

He illustrated trophoblastic mitoses and other microscopic alterations of villi, but it is our conviction that these are all secondary to the fetal condition and that placental edema follows fetal decompensation. Mostoufi-Zadeh et al. (1985) have compiled a thoughtful review of the topic and brought together much of the literature of this "challenge to the perinatal pathologist." Other reviews and a presentation of 11 cases (Evron et al., 1985; Rodriguez et al., 2002) consider many different types of defects, including diabetes, hygroma, congenital heart disease (CHD), twin-to-twin transfusion syndrome (TTTS), arteriovenous anomalies, etc. Congenital herpes virus 6 was later added as a possible cause of fetal hydrops (Ashshi et al., 2000). Both cases also had chromosomal anomalies and it remains speculative which caused the edema. Some of the rarer entities identified to cause fetal hydrops are discussed by Gloster et al. (1984). These include the Beckwith-Wiedemann syndrome with omphalocele and unusual tumors. Hydrops and placentomegaly in Beckwith-Wiedemann syndrome were also described by Lage (1991) and Drut and Drut (1996). Lage found it in one definite and two suspected cases of Beckwith-Wiedemann syndrome; remarkably, the villi had lacunar, hydropic expansion and focal chorangiomatosis. Flow cytometry showed all of them to be diploid. Similarly, McCowan and Becroft (1994) found placentomegaly and focal hydatid changes in stem villi (once) that were sonographically visible in three cases of this syndrome they studied. In one of their cases the grape-like villous tissue was detached from the main placental mass. The authors thought of it as a specific placental feature of Beckwith-Wiedemann syndrome and also drew attention to an association with proteinuric hypertension. The Druts identified the frequent and characteristic trisomy 11p15 in placental slides with the fluorescent in situ hybridization (FISH) methodology, a useful adjunct in differential diagnosis. We have seen four placentas of definite Beckwith-Wiedemann syndrome (Fig. 16.20). In one singleton and two twins there were venous thrombi (one calcified) in surface vessels; three discordant monozygotic twins were among this group, with one normal twin and one with the syndrome. None had gross or microscopic villous vesicles. Drut and colleagues (1998) found two nodules of a yolk sac tumor in the enlarged placenta of a 4200-g neonate with Beckwith-Wiedemann syndrome.

Ginsburg and Groll (1973) and Rice et al. (1984) found fetal Gaucher's disease as a cause. Godra et al. (2003) incriminated sialidosis III as a cause, and Davis (1982) presented a long list for the differential diagnosis. It included fetal G-6-PD deficiency (in male fetuses) with hemolysis resulting from maternal ingestion of fava beans and ascorbic acid (Mentzer & Collier, 1975) or sulfonamides (Perkins, 1971), myocarditis, renal vein thrombosis, achondroplasia, and other conditions. Glycogenosis IV was the cause in three familial cases of hydrops and arthrogryposis described by Cox et al. (1999). We have seen a case of myocarditis causing hydrops in an 18 weeks' gestation pregnancy. The mother had a "bad cold" in early pregnancy. In the fetus, myocarditis and thyroiditis were present with many plasma cells. The placenta was edematous but otherwise normal. Coxsackie B_5 virus infection was believed to be responsible (Benirschke et al., 1986). Ravindranath et al. (1987) identified glucose-phosphate-isomerase deficiency as a cause of hydrops fetalis. Appelman et al. (1988) found I-cell disease (mucolipidosis type II; see Chapter 18), pterygium syndrome, and α-thalassemia as causes of hydrops and suggested that elevated optical density levels (ΔOD_{450}) may be associated with hydrops fetalis of nonimmune etiology. Other essays on hydrops of nonimmune etiology have been provided by Verger et al. (1963), Giacoia (1980), and Maidman et al. (1980). The latter authors encountered five cases in 12,830 deliveries (1:2566) and suggested management principles, as did McCoy et al. (1995). A case of hydrops with unknown etiology was successfully managed by abdominal albumen injection (Shimokawa et al., 1988). Several perplexing instances of recurrent hydrops of unknown etiology have been reported by Silverstein and Kanbour (1981). We have seen such a case in which there were large thrombi in the umbilical cord vessels whose ultimate etiology remained elusive. Cumming (1979) had two recurrent cases. We autopsied three imma-

FIGURE 16.20. Villous alteration in the Beckwith-Wiedemann syndrome. Massive cistern, chorangiosis, congestion, placentomegaly (600 g at 36 weeks). There was a 69-cm-long cord with true knot, thrombosis of veins with calcification, and the neonate had adrenal cytomegaly and pancreatic nesidioblastosis. Masson trichrome ×160.

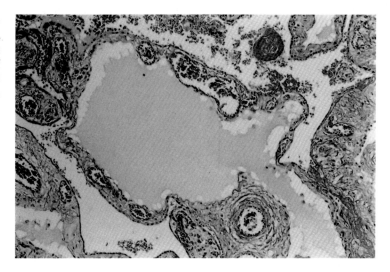

ture infants with hydrops in whose livers (only) there was massive and unexplained iron deposition. The anemic fetuses had numerous prenatally acquired encephaloclastic lesions, although in one the hematocrit was 23%. This condition may be similar to the perinatal hemochromatosis described by Silver et al. (1989) and Hardy et al. (1990) in several sibships. Although some of their cases had neonatal edema and ascites, hydrops was not described. The placentas of four of their cases was described as being hydropic, with numerous NRBCs in vessels. The iron and copper contents were not increased in them. Schwartz et al. (1981) had two of their four cases in a sibship; they suggested that hypoproteinemia is an important aspect and that this is perhaps the reason for successful therapy with albumen. Turski et al. (1978) also found marked decrease in serum albumen in a case of unexplained hydrops with hepatosplenomegaly and a 1900-g edematous placenta. Although it may have been speculated that fetal deficiency of AFP could be a cause of fetal hydrops, this has not been found to be so in two cases with such deficiency described by Greenberg et al. (1992). Seeds et al. (1984) attempted, unsuccessfully, to prevent pulmonary hypoplasia in an hydropic fetus with single umbilical artery. They placed a shunt from the peritoneum to the amnionic sac, at 29 weeks' gestation. The measured amniotic fluid pressure ranged from 17 to 26 cm H_2O. The investigators determined various constituents in the ascitic fluid as well. Other genetic metabolic diseases have been associated with hydrops, but it is not always certain that the disorder was also the true cause of the hydrops. Thus, Meizner et al. (1990) found it in Niemann-Pick disease, Uno et al. (1973) reported hydrops in Wolman's disease, Gillan et al. (1984) found it in another lysosomal storage disorder, and glucuronidase deficiency has been the apparent cause in cases described by Nelson et al. (1982) and Irani and colleagues (1983). Apparently thyrotoxicosis can be a cause of fetal hydrops as well. Thus, Watson and Fiegen (1995) detail the development of fetal thyrotoxicosis and hydrops development in a euthyroid mother who had radioactive ablation of the thyroid for Graves' disease, presumably because of the transplacental transfer of maternal IgG antibodies that ultimately lead to fetal tachycardia. Treadwell et al. (1996) described another such patient whose previous three fetuses died in utero with hydrops, secondary to her Graves' disease. In the next pregnancy, propylthiouracil therapy led to resolution of fetal tachycardia and the resulting hydrops. We were shown the placenta of a 29 weeks' gestation with Graves' disease, necessitating thyroidectomy. The fetus suffered fetal tachycardia and thyrotoxicosis; the neonate died. There was thrombosis of one umbilical artery, massive necrosis of arteries in the cord from meconium damage (see Chapter 11), and an excessive number of NRBCs. Because meconium discharge does not otherwise occur that early in gestation, one wonders if it was the result of thyrotoxicosis.

References

Adzick, N.S., Crombleholme, T.M., Morgan, M.A. and Quinn, T. M.: A rapidly growing fetal teratoma. Lancet **349**:538, 1997.

Alenghat, E. and Esterly, J.R.: Intravascular hematopoiesis in chorionic villi. Amer. J. Clin. Pathol. **79**:225–227, 1983.

Anand, A., Gray, E.S., Brown, T., Clewley, J.P. and Cohen, B.J.: Human parvovirus infection in pregnancy and hydrops fetalis. NEJM **316**:183–186, 1987.

Anandakumar, C., Biswas, A., Chew, S.S.L., Chia, D., Wong, Y. C. and Ratnam, S.S.: Direct fetal therapy for hydrops secondary to congenital atrioventricular heart block. Obstet. Gynecol. **87**:835–837, 1996.

Anders, D., Kindermann, G. and Pfeifer, U.: Metastasizing fetal neuroblastoma with involvement of the placenta simulating fetal erythroblastosis. J Pediatr. **82**:50–53, 1973.

Anderson, L.J. and Török, T.J.: Human parvovirus B 19. NEJM **321**:536–538, 1989.

Anderson, L.J. and Young, N.S.: Human Parvovirus B19. Monographs in Virology, Karger, Basel, 1997.

Anderson, M.J. and Pattison, J.R.: The human parvoviruses: Brief review. Arch. Virol. **82**:137–148, 1984.

Anderson, M.J., Khousam, M.N., Maxwell, D.J., Gould, S.J., Happerfield, L.C. and Smith, W.J.: Human parvovirus B19 and hydrops fetalis. Lancet **i**:535, 1988.

Appelman, Z., Blumberg, B.D., Golabi, M. and Golbus, M.S.: Nonimmune hydrops fetalis may be associated with an elevated delta OD_{450} in the amniotic fluid. Obstet. Gynecol. **71**:1005–1008, 1988.

Aslam, P.A., Korones, S.B., Richardson, R.L. and Pate, J.W.: Congenital cystic adenomatoid malformation with anasarca. JAMA **212**:622–624, 1970.

Baergen, R.N., Kelly, T., McGinnis, M.J., Jones, O.W. and Benirschke, K.: Complete hydatidiform mole with coexisting embryo. Human Pathol. **27**:731–734, 1996.

Barentsen, R.: Sacrococcygeal teratoom en hydramnion. Nederl. Tidschr. Geneesk. **119**:1168–1169, 1975.

Barton, J.R., Thorpe, E.M., Shaver, D.C., Hager, W.D. and Sibai, B.M.: Nonimmune hydrops fetalis associated with maternal infection with syphilis. Amer. J. Obstet. Gynecol. **167**:56–58, 1992.

Bawle, E.V. and Black, V.: Nonimmune hydrops fetalis in Noonan's syndrome. Amer. J. Dis. Childr. **140**:758–760, 1986.

Becker, V. und Bleyl, U.: Placentarzotte bei Schwangerschafts-toxikose und fetaler Erythroblastose im fluorescenzmikros-kopischen Bilde. Virchows Arch. Pathol. Anat. **334**:516–527, 1961.

Beischer, N.A., Holsman, M. and Kitchen, W.H.: Relation of various forms of anemia to placental weight. Amer. J. Obstet. Gynecol. **101**:801–809, 1968.

Beischer, N.A., Pepperell, R.J. and Barrie, J.U.: Twin pregnancy and erythroblastosis. Obstetr. Gynecol. **34**:22–29, 1969.

Benacerraf, B.R. and Frigoletto, F.D.: In utero treatment of a fetus with diaphragmatic hernia complicated by hydrops. Amer. J. Obstet. Gynecol. **155**:817–818, 1986.

Benachi, A., Garritsen, H.S.P., Howard, C.M., Bennett, P. and Fisk, N.M.: Absence of expression of RhD by human trophoblast cells. Amer. J. Obstet. Gynecol. **178**:294–299, 1998.

Ben-Ami, M., Shalev, E., Romano, S. and Zuckerman, H.: Midtrimester diagnosis of endocardial fibroelastosis and atrial septal defect: A case report. Amer. J. Obstet. Gynecol. **155**:662–663, 1986.

Benirschke, K., Swartz, W.H., Leopold, G. and Sahn, D.: Hydrops due to myocarditis in a fetus. Amer. J. Cardiovasc. Pathol. **1**:131–133, 1986.

Berkowitz, R.L., Chitkara, U., Goldberg, J.D., Wilkins, I., Chervenak, F.A. and Lynch, L.: Intrauterine intravascular transfusions for severe red blood cell isoimmunization: Ultrasound-guided percutaneous approach. Amer. J. Obstetr. Gynecol. **155**:574–581, 1986.

Bernstein, I.M. and Capeless, E.L.: Elevated maternal serum alpha-fetoprotein and hydrops fetalis in association with fetal parvovirus B-19 infection. Obstet. Gynecol. **74**:456–457, 1989.

Birkenfeld, A., Mordel, N. and Okon, E.: Direct demonstration of iron in a term placenta in a case of β-thalassemia. Amer. J. Obstet. Gynecol. **160**:562–563, 1989.

Birner, W.F.: Neuroblastoma as a cause of antenatal death. Amer. J. Obstet. Gynecol. **82**:1388–1391, 1961.

Bock, B., Riess, R., Wünsch, P.H. und Feige, A.: Pränatale Diagnostik eines Steißbeinteratoms mit Hydrops fetalis und Plazentahypertrophie—Konsequenzen für den weiteren Schwangerschaftsverlauf. Geburtsh. Frauenheilk. **50**:647–649, 1990.

Bond, P.R., Caul, E.O., Usher, J., Cohen, B.J., Clewley, J.P. and Field, A.M.: Intrauterine infection with human parvovirus. Lancet **i**:448–449, 1986.

Bouissou, H., Kanoun, T., Bierme, S. et Bierme, R.: Foie et placenta au cours de la maladie hémolytique par iso-immunisation Rh. (Étude histologique et déductions). Pathol. Biol. **17**:109–120, 1969.

Bowman, J.M., Lewis, M. and de Sa, D.J.: Hydrops fetalis caused by massive maternofetal transplacental hemorrhage. J. Pediatr. **104**:769–772, 1984.

Bridge, J.A., McManus, B.M., Remmenga, J. and Cuppage, F.P.: Complete heart block in the 18p- syndrome. Congenital cal-cification of the atrioventricular node. Arch. Pathol. Lab. Med. **113**:539–541, 1989.

Briner, J., Hassam, S., Girsberger, M. and Tratschin, J.D.: Dem-onstration of parvovirus infection in human fetuses and infants by in situ hybridization. Pediatr. Pathol. **7**:479–480, 1987.

Brinson, R.A. and Goldsmith, J.P.: Nonimmune hydrops fetalis associated with intrauterine intussusception. J. Perinatol. **8**:225–227, 1988.

Broderick, K., Oyer, R. and Chatwani, A.: Neu-Laxova syn-drome: A case report. Amer. J. Obstet. Gynecol. **158**:574–575, 1988.

Bromley, B., Frigoletto, F.D., Estroff, J.A. and Benacerraf, B.R.: The natural history of oligohydramnios/polyhydramnios sequence in monochorionic diamniotic twins. Ultrasound Obstet. Gynecol. **2**:317–320, 1992.

Brown, K.E., Green, S.W., de Mayolo, J.A., Bellanti, J.A., Smith, S.D., Smith, T.J. and Young, N.S.: Congenital anaemia after transplacental B19 parvovirus infection. Lancet **343**:895–896, 1994.

Brown, T., Anand, A., Ritschie, L.D., Clewley, J.P. and Reid, T. M.S.: Intrauterine parvovirus infection associated with hydrops fetalis. Lancet **ii**:1033–1034, 1984.

Burger, K.: Mit Hydrops foetus et placentae einhergehende Luteinzysten. Zbl. Gynäkol. **69**:533–536, 1947.

Burstein, R.H. and Blumenthal, H.T.: Vascular lesions of the placenta of possible immunogenic origin in erythroblastosis fetalis. Amer. J. Obstetr. Gynecol. **83**:1062–1068, 1962.

Burton, P.A. and Caul, E.O.: Fetal cell tropism of human parvo-virus B 19. Lancet **i**:767, 1988.

Busch, W. und Vogel, M.: Die Plazenta beim "Morbus haemo-lyticus neonatorum". Z. Geburtsh. Perinatol. **176**:17–28, 1972.

Cardwell, M.S.: Successful treatment of hydrops fetalis caused by fetomaternal hemorrhage: A case report. Amer. J. Obstet. Gynecol. **158**:131–132, 1988.

Carles, D., Serville, F., Dubecq, J.-P., Alberti, E.M., Horowitz, J. and Weichwold, W.: Idiopathic arterial calcification in a still-born complicated by pleural hemorrhage and hydrops fetalis. Arch. Pathol. Lab. Med. **116**:293–295, 1992.

Carr, S., Rubin, L., Dixon, D., Star, J. and Dailey, J.: Intrauterine therapy for homozygous α-thalassemia. Obstet. Gynecol. **85**:876–879, 1995.

Carrington, D., Gilmore, D.H., Whittle, M.J., Aitken, D., Gibson, A.A.M., Patrick, W.J.A., Brown, T., Caul, E.O., Field, A.M., Clewley, J.P. and Cohen, B.J.: Maternal serum α-fetoprotein—a marker of fetal aplastic crisis during intrauterine human parvovirus infection. Lancet **i**:433–435, 1987.

Carter, B.S., DiGiacomo, J.E., Balderston, S.M., Wiggins, J.W. and Merenstein, G.B.: Disproportionate septal hypertrophy associated with erythroblastosis. Amer. J. Dis. Child. **144**: 1225–1228, 1990.

Chang, J.C. and Kan, Y.W.: Antenatal diagnosis of sickle cell anaemia by direct analysis of the sickle mutation. Lancet **ii**:1127–1129, 1981.

Chen, F.E., Ooi, C., Ha, S.Y., Cheung, B.M.Y., Todd, D., Liang, R., Chan, T.K. and Chan, V.: Genetic and clinical features of hemoglobin H disease in Chinese patients. NEJM **343**:544–550, 2000.

Christie, R.W.: Lutein cysts of ovaries associated with erythroblastotic hydrops fetalis. Assay of gonadotropin in serum of Rh-sensitized women in later stages of pregnancy. Amer. J. Clin. Pathol. **36**:518–523, 1961.

Clark, S.L., Vitale, D.J., Minton, S.D., Stoddard, R.A. and Sabey, P.L.: Successful fetal therapy for cystic adenomatoid malformation associated with second-trimester hydrops. Amer. J. Obstet. Gynecol. **157**:294–295, 1987.

Copel, J.A., Buyon, J.P. and Kleinman, C.S.: Successful in utero therapy of fetal heart block. Amer. J. Obstet. Gynecol. **173**:1384–1390, 1995.

Cox, P.M., Brueton, L.A., Murphy, K.W., Worthington, V.C., Bjelorglic, P., Lazda, E.J., Sabire, N.J. and Sewry, C.A.: Early-onset fetal hydrops and muscle degeneration in siblings due to a novel variant of type IV glycogenosis. Amer. J. Med. Genet. **86**:187–193, 1999.

Cukierski, M.A., Tarantal, A.F. and Hendrickx, A.G.: A case of nonimmune hydrops fetalis with a rare cardiac anomaly in a rhesus monkey. J. Med. Primatol. **15**:227–234, 1986.

Cumming, D.C.: Recurrent nonimmune hydrops fetalis. Obstet. Gynecol. **54**:124–126, 1979.

Curry, C.J.R., Chopra, D. and Finer, N.N.: Hydrops and pleural effusions in congenital myotonic dystrophy. J. Pediatr. **113**:555–557, 1988.

Davis, C.L.: Diagnosis and management of nonimmune hydrops fetalis. J. Reprod. Med. **27**:594–600, 1982.

De Krijger, R.R., van Elsacker-Niele, A.M.W., Mulder-Stapel, A., Salimans, M.M.M., Dreef, E., Weiland, H.T., van Krieken, J.H.J.M. and Vermeij-Keers, C.: Detection of parvovirus B 19 infection in first and second trimester fetal loss. Pediatr. Pathol. Lab. Med. **18**:23–34, 1998.

DeLia, J.E. and Emery, M.G.: Digoxin therapy in the fetus. Amer. J. Dis. Childr. **140**:974–975, 1986.

Dorman, S.L. and Cardwell, M.S.: Ballantyne syndrome caused by a large placental chorioangioma. Amer. J. Obstet. Gynecol. **173**:1632–1633, 1995.

Doss, B.J., Vicari, J., Jacques, S.M. and Qureshi, F.: Placental involvement in congenital hepatoblastoma. Pediat. Development. Pathol. **1**:538–542, 1998.

Driscoll, S.G. and Steinke, J.: Pancreatic insulin content in severe erythroblastosis fetalis. Pediatrics **39**:449–450, 1967.

Drogendijk, A.C.: The pathogenesis of foetal hydrops. Gynaecologia **156**:129–139, 1963.

Drut, R.M. and Drut, R.: Nonimmune fetal hydrops and placenomegaly: Diagnosis of familial Wiedemann-Beckwith syndrome with trisomy 11p15 using FISH. Amer. J. Med. Genet. **62**:145–149, 1996.

Drut, R., Mortera, M. and Drut, R.M.: Yolk sac tumor of the placenta in Wiedemann-Beckwith syndrome. Pediat. Development. Pathol. **1**:534–537, 1998.

Editorial: Dangers of anti-Kell in pregnancy. Lancet **337**:1319–1320, 1991.

Eklund, J.: Embryonic rhesus-positive red cells stimulating a secondary response after early abortion. Lancet ii:748, 1981.

Elsacker-Niele, A.M.W., Salimans, M.M.M., Weiland, H.T., Vermey-Keers, C., Anderson, M.J. and Versteeg, J.: Fetal pathology in human parvovirus B19 infection. Brit. J. Obstet. Gynaecol. **96**:768–775, 1989.

Essary, L.R., Vnencak-Jones, C.L., Manning, S.S., Olson, S.J. and Johnson, J.E.: Frequency of parvovirus B19 infection in nonimmune hydrops fetalis and utility of three diagnostic methods. Hum. Pathol. **29**:696–701, 1998.

Evron, S., Yagel, S., Samueloff, A., Margaliot, E., Burstein, P. and Sadovsky, E.: Nonimmunologic hydrops fetalis: a review of 11 cases. J. Perinat. Med. **13**:147–151, 1985.

Feige, A., Gille, J., Maillot, K.v. und Mulz, D.: Pränatale Diagnostik eines Steißbeinteratoms mit Hypertrophie der Plazenta. Geburtsh. Frauenheilk. **42**:20–24, 1982.

Fisher, R.A., Paradinas, F.J., Soteriou, B.A., Foskett, M. and Newlands, E.S.: Diploid hydatidiform moles with fetal red blood cells in molar villi. 2—genetics. J. Pathol. 181189–195, 1997.

Fox, H.: The incidence and significance of nucleated erythrocytes in the foetal vessels of the mature human placenta. J. Obstet. Gynaecol. Brit. Cwlth. **74**:40–43, 1967.

Franciosi, R. and Tattersall, P.: Human parvovirus (B19) causing hydrops fetalis. Pediatr. Pathol. **7**:485–486, 1987.

Freda, V.J. and Carter, B.-A.: Placental permeability in the human for anti-A and anti-B isoantibodies. Amer. J. Obstetr. Gynecol. **84**:1351–1367, 1962.

Freda, V.J., Gorman, J.G., Galen, R.S. and Treacy, N.: The threat of Rh immunisation from abortion. Lancet i:147–148, 1970.

Friesen, R.F., Bowman, J.M., Barnes, P.H., Grewar, D., Mcinnis, C. and Bowman, W.D.: Intrauterine transfusions for erythroblastosis. Amer. J. Obstetr. Gynecol. **97**:343–339, 1967.

Fung, T.Y., Fung, Y.M.H., Ng, P.C., Yeung, C.K. and Chang, M. Z.A.: Polyhydramnios and hypercalcemia associated with congenital mesoblastic nephroma: case report and a new appraisal. Obstet. Gynecol. **85**:815–817, 1995.

Gallagher, P.G., Weed, S.A., Tse, W.T., Benoit, L., Morrow, J.S., Marchesi, S.L., Mohandas, N. and Forget, B.G.: Recurrent fatal hydrops fetalis associated with a nucleotide substitution in the erythrocyte β-spectrin gene. J. Clin. Invest. **95**:1174–1182, 1995.

Gautier, E., Benachi, A., Giovangrandi, Y., Ernault, P., Olivi, M., Gaillon, T. and Costa, J.-M.: Fetal RhD genotyping by maternal serum analysis: a two-year experience. Amer. J. Obstet. Gynecol. **192**:666–669, 2005.

Gembruch, U., Niesen, M., Hansmann, M. and Knöpple, G.: Listeriosis: A cause of non-immune hydrops fetalis. Prenat. Diagn. **7**:277–282, 1987.

Giacoia, G.P.: Hydrops fetalis (Fetal edema). A survey. Clin. Pediatr. **19**:334–339, 1980.

Giles, H.M., Ough, R.C.B., Darmady, E.M., Stranack, F. and Woolf, L.I.: The nephrotic syndrome in early infancy: A report of three cases. Arch. Dis. Childh. **32**:167–180, 1957.

Gillan, J.E., Lowden, J.A., Gaskin, K. and Cutz, E.: Congenital ascites as a presenting sign of lysosomal storage disease. J. Pediatr. **104**:225–231, 1984.

Ginsburg, S.J. and Groll, M.: Hydrops fetalis due to infantile Gaucher's disease. J. Pediatr. **82**:1046–1048, 1973.

Gloster, E.S., Jimenez, J.F., Godoy, G., Burrows, P., Hill, D., Mollitt, D.L. and Grunow, W.A.: Nonimmune hydrops fetalis: the Arkansas Children's Hospital experience for 1982–1983. Lab. Invest. **50**:3P, 1984.

Godra, A., Kim, D.U. and D'Cruz, C.: A 5-day-old boy with hydrops fetalis. Arch. Pathol. Lab. Med. 1271051–1052, 2003.

Goldschmidt, E., Cohen, T., Isacsohn, M. and Freier, S.: Incidence of hemoglobin Bart's in a sample of newborn from Israel. Acta Genet. (Basel) 18:361–368, 1968.

Gonen, R., Fong, K. and Chiasson, D.A.: Prenatal sonographic diagnosis of hepatic hemangioendothelioma with secondary nonimmune hydrops fetalis. Obstet. Gynecol. 73:485–487, 1989.

Gonsoulin, W., Copeland, K.L., Carpenter, R.J., Hughes, M.R. and Elder, F.B.: Fetal blood sampling demonstrating chimerism in monozygotic twins discordant for sex and tissue karyotype (46,XY and 45,X). Prenat. Diagn. 10:25–28, 1990.

Goto, S., Nishi, H. and Tomoda, Y.: Blood group Rh-D factor in human trophoblast determined by immunofluorescent method. Amer. J. Obstetr. Gynecol. 137:707–712, 1980.

Gottschalk, W. and Abramson, D.: Placental edema and fetal hydrops. A case of congenital cystic and adenomatoid malformation of the lung. Obstet. Gynecol. 10:626–631, 1957.

Grannum, P.A.T., Copel, J.A., Moya, F.R., Scioscia, A.L., Robert, J.A., Winn, H.N., Coster, B.C., Burdine, C.B. and Hobbins, J. C.: The reversal of hydrops fetalis by intravascular intrauterine transfusion in severe isoimmune fetal anemia. Amer. J. Obstetr. Gynecol. 158:914–919, 1988.

Greenberg, F., Carpenter, R.J. and Ledbetter, D.H.: Cystic hygroma and hydrops fetalis in a fetus with trisomy 13. Clin. Genet. 24:389–391, 1983.

Grimes, D.A., Geary, F.H. and Hatcher, R.A.: Rh immunoglobulin utilization after ectopic pregnancy. Amer. J. Obstetr. Gynecol. 140:246–249, 1981.

Groves, G.R. and Baskett, T.F.: Nonimmune hydrops fetalis: Antenatal diagnosis and management. Amer. J. Obstet. Gynecol. 148:563–569, 1984.

Gray, E.S.: Human parvovirus infection. J. Pathol. 153:310–311, 1987.

Gray, E.S.: Mesoblastic nephroma and non-immunological hydrops fetalis. Letter to the editor. Pediatr. Pathol. 9:607–609, 1989.

Gray, E.S., Davidson, R.J.L. and Anand, A.: Human parvovirus and fetal anaemia. Lancet i:1144, 1987.

Gray, G.R., Towell, M.E., Wright, V.J. and Hardwick, D.F.: Thalassemic hydrops fetalis in two Chinese-Canadian families. Canad. Med. Assoc. J. 107:1186–1190, 1972.

Green, D.W., Donovan, E.F. and Wood, B.P.: Radiological cases of the month. Amer. J. Dis. Child. 144:93–94, 1990.

Greenberg, F., Faucett, A., Rose, E., Bancalari, L., Kardon, N.B., Mizejewski, G., Haddon, J.E. and Alpert, E.: Congenital deficiency of α-fetoprotein. Amer. J. Obstet. Gynecol. 167:509–511, 1992.

Gropp, A.: Fetal hydrops in chromosome disorders as principle of damage in developmental pathology. Clinical observations in man and experimental studies in the mouse. Chapter 8 in, One Medicine, O.A. Ryder and M.L. Byrd, eds. pp 84–95. Springer-Verlag, New York, 1984.

Guntheroth, W.G., Cyr, D.R., Mack, L.A., Benedetti, T., Lenke, R.R. and Petty, C.N.: Hydrops from reciprocating atrioventricular tachycardia in a 27-week fetus requiring quinidine for conversion. Obstet. Gynecol. 66:29S–33S, 1985.

Guy, G., Coady, D.J., Jansen, V., Snyder, J. and Zinberg, S.: α-Thalassemia hydrops fetalis: Clinical and ultrasonographic considerations. Amer. J. Obstet. Gynecol. 153:500–504, 1985.

Hall, S.M., Cohen, B.J., Mortimer, P.P., Caul, E.O., Cradock-Watson, J., Anderson, M.J., Pattison, J.R., Shirley, J.A. and Peto, T.E.A.: Prospective study of human parvovirus (B 19) infection in pregnancy. Brit. Med. J. 300:1166–1170, 1990.

Hallak, M., Neerhof, M.G., Perry, R., Nazir, M. and Hulka, J.C.: Fetal supraventricular tachycardia and hydrops fetalis: Combined intensive, direct, and transplacental therapy. Obstet. Gynecol. 78:523–525, 1991.

Hardy, L., Hansen, J.L., Kushner, J.P. and Knisely, A.S.: Neonatal hemochromatosis. Genetic analysis of transferrin-receptor, H-apoferritin, and L-apoferritin loci and of the human leukocyte antigen class I region. Amer. J. Pathol. 137:149–153, 1991.

Harger, J.H., Adler, S.P., Koch, W.C. and Harger, G.F.: Prospective evaluation of 618 pregnant women exposed to parvovirus B19: Risks and symptoms. Obstet. Gynecol. 91:413–420, 1998.

Harkavy, K.L. and Scanlon, J.W.: Hydrops fetalis in a parabiotic, acardiac twin. Amer. J. Dis. Child. 132:638–639, 1978.

Harman, C.R., Bowman, J.M., Menticoglou, S.M., Pollock, J.M. and Manning, F.A.: Profound fetal thrombocytopenia in rhesus disease: Serious hazard at intravascular transfusion. Lancet ii:741–742, 1988.

Hatjis, C.G.: Nonimmunologic fetal hydrops associated with hyperreactio luteinalis. Obstetr. Gynecol. 65:11S–13S, 1985.

Hellman, L.M. and Hertig, A.T.: Pathological changes in the placenta associated with erythroblastosis of the fetus. Amer. J. Pathol. 14:111–120, 1937.

Hendricks, S.K., Sorensen, T.K. and Baker, E.R.: Trisomy 21, fetal hydrops, and anemia: Prenatal diagnosis of transient myeloproliferative disorder? Obstet. Gynecol. 82:703–705, 1993.

Herman, A., Bukovsky, Y., Benson, L., Weinraub, Z. and Caspi, E.: Intrapartum use of fetal scalp hematocrit in the diagnosis of profound fetal anemia caused by fetomaternal hemorrhage. Amer. J. Obstet. Gynecol. 157:1182–1183, 1987.

Hogge, W.A., Hogge, J.S., Schnatterly, P.T., Sun, C.J. and Blitzer, M.G.: Congenital nephrosis: Detection of index cases through maternal serum α-fetoprotein screening. Amer. J. Obstet. Gynecol. 167:1330–1333, 1992.

Holzgreve, W., Miny, P., Anderson, R. and Golbus, M.S.: Experience with 8 cases of prenatally diagnosed sacrococcygeal teratomas. Fetal Therapy 2:88–94, 1987.

Horowitz, A., Cohen, T., Goldschmidt, E. and Levene, C.: Thalassemia among Kurdish Jews in Israel. Brit. J. Haematol. 12:555–568, 1966.

Houston, C.S. and Brown, A.B.: An unusual complication of intrauterine transfusion. Canad. Med. Ass. J. 94:1274–1277, 1966.

Hoyer, J.R., Michael, A.F., Good, R.A. and Vernier, R.L.: The nephrotic syndrome of infancy: Clinical, morphologic, and immunologic studies of four infants. Pediatrics 40:233–246, 1967.

Hoyer, J.R., Mauer, S.M., Kjellstrand, C.M., Buselmeier, T.J., Simmons, R.L., Michael, A.F., Najarian, J.S. and Vernier, R.L.: Successful renal transplantation in 3 children with congenital nephrotic syndrome. Lancet i:1410–1413, 1973.

Humphrey, W., Magoon, M. and O'Shaughnessy, R.: Severe non-immune hydrops secondary to parvovirus B-19 infection: Spontaneous reversal in utero and survival of a term infant. Obstet. Gynecol. **78**:900–902, 1991.

Hung, P.-L., Huang, C.-C. and Huang, T.-S.: Nephrotic syndrome in a Chinese infant. Amer. J. Dis. Childr. **131**:557–559, 1977.

Hutchison, A.A., Drew, J.H., Yu, V.Y.H., Williams, M.L., Fortune, D.W. and Beischer, N.A.: Nonimmunologic hydrops fetalis: A review of 61 cases. Obstet. Gynecol. **59**:347–352, 1982.

Iakovtsova, A.G.: Morphologic changes in the placenta in iso-antigenic incompatibility of maternal and fetal blood. Pediatr. Akhush. Ginekol. **1**:53–55, 1964.

Imakita, M., Yutani, C., Ishibashi-Ueda, H., Murakami, M. and Chiba, Y.: A case of hydrops fetalis due to placental chorangioma. Acta Pathol. Japan **38**:941–945, 1988.

Ing, R.Y.K., Crookston, J.H., Dworatzek, J.A. and Burnie, K.L.: Alpha thalassemia: Five cases of hemoglobin H disease in Oriental-Canadian families. Canad. Med. Ass. J. **99**:49–56, 1968.

Irani, D., Kim, H.S., El-Hibri, H., Dutton, R.V., Beaudet, A. and Armstrong, D.: Postmortem observations on β-glucuronidase deficiency presenting as hydrops fetalis. Ann. Neurol. **14**: 486–490, 1983.

Ivemark, B.I., Högman, C., Rudert, P.O. and Andersen, B.: Kell-iso-immunization as the cause of fatal erythroblastosis fetalis. Acta Pathol. Microbiol. Scand. **45**:193–202, 1959.

Jackson, M.R., Carney, E.W., Lye, S.J. and Knox Ritchie, J.W.: Localization of two angiogenic growth factors (PDECGF and VEGF) in human placentae throughout gestation. Placenta **15**:341–353, 1994.

James, G.B.: Histology of the placenta after repeated intrauterine transfusions. Proc. Roy. Soc. Med. **63**:54, 1970.

Jarkowski, T.L., Rosenblatt, M., Wolf, P. and Pearson, B.: Tissue-fixed antigens of the Rh blood group system in placentae and fetuses; with particular reference to hemolytic disease of the newborn. Lab. Invest. **13**:937, 1964.

Jauniaux, E., Maldergem L.v., Munter, C.de, Moscoso, G. and Gillerot, Y.: Nonimmune hydrops fetalis associated with genetic abnormalities. Obstet. Gynecol. **75**:568–572, 1990.

Johnson, P., Sharland, G., Allan, L.D., Tynan, M.J. and Maxwell, D.J.: Umbilical venous pressure in nonimmune hydrops fetalis: Correlation with cardiac size. Amer. J. Obstet. Gynecol. **167**:1309–1313, 1992.

Jones, C.J.P. and Fox, H.: An ultrastructural study of the placenta in materno-fetal rhesus incompatibility. Virchows Arch. Pathol. Anat. Histol. **379**:229–241, 1978.

Jones, D.E.D., Pritchard, K.I., Gioannini, C.A., Moore, D.T. and Bradford, W.D.: Hydrops fetalis associated with idiopathic arterial calcification. Obstet. Gynecol. **39**:435–440, 1972.

Jonxis, J.H.P.: The development of hemoglobin. Pediatr. Clinics North Amer. **12**:535–550, 1965.

Jordan, J.A.: Identification of human parvovirus B19 infection in idiopathic nonimmune hydrops fetalis. Amer. J. Obstet. Gynecol. **174**:37–42, 1996.

Jorgensen, J.: Rhesus-antibody development after abortion. Lancet **ii**:1253–1254, 1969.

Kamat, B.R., Greco, M.A. and Demopoulos, R.I.: Immunocyto-chemichal staining patterns of placentas associated with hydrops fetalis. Int. J. Gynecol. Pathol. **8**:246–254, 1989.

Kan, Y.W., Allen, A. and Lowenstein, L.: Hydrops fetalis with alpha thalassemia. NEJM **276**:18–23, 1967.

Kan, Y.W., Forget, B.G. and Nathan, D.G.: Gamma-beta thalassemia: A cause of hemolytic disease of the newborn. NEJM **286**:129–134, 1972.

Kan, Y.W., Golbus, M.S. and Dozy, A.M.: Prenatal diagnosis of α-thalassemia: Clinical application of molecular hybridization. NEJM **295**:1165–1167, 1976.

Kaplan, C., Lane, B., Miller, F., Baker, D. and Trunca, C.: Renal pathology of prenatally diagnosed nephrosis. Pediatr. Pathol. **3**:271–281, 1985.

Kinney, J.S., Anderson, L.J., Farrar, J., Strikas, R.A., Kumar, M.L., Kliegman, R.M., Sever, J.L., Hurwitz, E.S. and Sikes, R.K.: Risk of adverse outcomes of pregnancy after human parvovirus B19 infection. J. Infect. Dis. **157**:663–667, 1988.

Klein, A.M., Holzman, I.R. and Austin, E.M.: Fetal tachycardia before the development of hydrops-attempted cardioversion: a case report. Amer. J. Obstet. Gynecol. **134**:347–348, 1979.

Kleinman, C.S., Donnerstein, R.L., Devore, G.R., Jaffe, C.C., Lynch, D.C., Berkowitz, R.L., Talner, N.S. and Hobbins, J.C.: Fetal echocardiography for evaluation of in utero congestive heart failure. A technique for study of nonimmune hydrops. NEJM **306**:568–575, 1982.

Knisely, A.S.: Placental siderosis in maternal β-thalassemia. Amer. J. Obstet. Gynecol. **162**:1638–1639, 1990a.

Knisely, A.S.: Parvovirus B19 infection in the fetus. Lancet **336**:443, 1990b.

Knisely, A.S., O'Shea, P., McMillan, P., Singer, D.B. and Magid, M.S.: Electron microscopic identification of parvovirus virions in erythroid-line cells in fatal hydrops fetalis. Pediatr. Pathol. **8**:163–170, 1988.

Koffler, H., Papile, L.-A. and Burstein, R.: Congenital chylothorax: two cases associated with maternal polyhydramnios. Amer. J. Dis. Childr. **132**:638, 1978.

Kohga, S., Nambu, T., Tanaka, K., Benirschke, K., Feldman, B.H. and Kishikawa, T.: Hypertrophy of the placenta and sacrococcygeal teratoma. Report of two cases. Virchows Arch. A Pathol. Anat. Histol. **386**:223–229, 1980.

Kohler, H.G. and Rymer, B.: Congenital cystic malformation of the lung and its relation to hydramnios. J. Obstet. Gynaecol. Brit. Cwlth. **80**:130–134, 1973.

Kovacs, B.W., Carlson, D.E., Shahbahrami, M.S. and Platt, L.D.: Prenatal diagnosis of human parvovirus B 19 in nonimmune hydrops fetalis by polymerase chain reaction. Amer. J. Obstet. Gynecol. **167**:461–466, 1992.

Krause, J.R., Penchansky, L. and Knisely, A.S.: Morphological diagnosis of parvovirus B19 infection. Arch. Pathol. Lab. Med. **116**:178–180, 1992.

Kuhlmann, R.S., Warsof, S.L., Levy, D.L., Flake, A.J. and Harrison, M.R.: Fetal therapy **2**:95–100, 1987.

Lacro, R.V., Jones, K.L. and Benirschke, K.: Coarctation of the aorta in Turner syndrome: a pathologic study of fetuses with nuchal hygromas, hydrops fetalis, and female genitalia. Pediatrics **81**:445–451, 1988.

Lage, J.M.: Placentomegaly with massive hydrops of placental stem villi, diploid DNA content, and omphaloceles: possible association with Beckwith-Wiedemann syndrome. Human Pathol. **22**:591–597, 1991.

Landrum, B.G., Johnson, D.E., Ferrara, B., Boros, S.J. and Thompson, T.R.: Hydrops fetalis and chromosomal trisomies. Amer. J. Obstet. Gynecol. **154**:1114–1115, 1986.

Langer, J.C., Harrison, M.R., Schmidt, K.G., Silverman, N.H., Anderson, R.L., Goldberg, J.D., Filly, R.A., Crombleholme, T.M., Longaker, M.T. and Golbus, M.S.: Fetal hydrops and death from sacrococcygeal teratoma: rationale for fetal surgery. Amer. J. Obstet. Gynecol. **160**:1145–1150, 1989.

Lallemand, A.V., Doco-Fenzy, M. and Gaillard, D.A.: Investigation of nonimmune hydrops fetalis: multidisciplinary studies are necessary for diagnosis—review of 94 cases. Ped. Developm. Pathol. **2**:432–439, 1999.

Lam, Y.-H., Tang, M.H.-Y., Lee, C.-P. and Tse, H.-Y.: Prenatal ultrasonographic prediction of homozygous type 1 α-thalassemia at 12 to 13 weeks of gestation. Amer. J. Obstetr. Gynecol. **180**:148–150, 1999.

Laros, R.K. and Kalstone, C.E.: Sickle cell β-thalassemia and pregnancy. Obstet. Gynecol. **37**:67–71, 1971.

Leake, R.D., Strimling, B. and Emmanouilidis, G.C.: Intrauterine cardiac failure with hydrops fetalis. Case report in a twin with the hypoplastic left heart syndrome and review of the literature. Clin. Pediatr. **12**:649–651, 1973.

Lebo, R.V., Saiki, R.K., Swanson, K., Montano, M.A., Erlich, H.A. and Golbus, M.S.: Prenatal diagnosis of α-thalassemia by polymerase chain reaction and dual restriction enzyme analysis. Hum. Genet. **85**:293–299, 1990.

Lee, J.-N., Huang, S.-C., Ouyang, P.-C. and Chard, T,: Circulating placental proteins in pregnancies complicated by Rh isoimmunization. Obstetr. Gynecol. **64**:131–132, 1984.

Leggat, H.M., Gibson, J.M., Barron, S.L. and Reid, M.M.: Anti-Kell in pregnancy. Brit. J. Obstetr. Gynaecol. **98**:162–165, 1991.

Leventhal, M.L. and Wolf, A.M.: Erythroblastosis (hydrops) fetalis from Kell sensitization. Amer. J. Obstetr. Gynecol. **71**:452–454, 1956.

Lie-Injo, L.E.: Haemoglobin of new-born infants in Indonesia. Nature **183**:1125–1126, 1959.

Lie-Injo, L.E.: Alpha-chain thalassemia and hydrops fetalis in Malaysia; report of 5 cases. Blood **20**:581–590, 1962.

Lie-Injo, L.E., Lopez, C.G. and Dutt, A.K.: Pathological findings in hydrops foetalis due to alpha-thalassemia: a review of 32 cases. Trans. Roy. Soc. Tropical Med. Hyg. **62**:874–879, 1968.

Lingman, G., Lundström, N.R., Marsal, K. and Ohrlander, S.: Fetal cardiac arrhythmia-clinical outcome in 113 cases. Acta Obstet. Gynecol. Scand. **65**:263–267, 1986.

Louderback, A.L. and Shanbrom, E.: Hemoglobin electrophoresis. JAMA **202**:718–719, 1967.

Luca, E.C. de, Casadei, A.M., Pascone, R., Tardi, C. and Pacioni, C.: Maternofetal transfusion during delivery and sensitization of newborn against the rhesus D-antigen. Vox Sanguinis **34**:241–243, 1978.

Lynn, A.A.A., Parry, S.I., Morgan, M.A. and Mennuti, M.T.: Disseminated congenital neuroblastoma involving the placenta. Arch. Pathol. Lab. Med. **121**:741–744, 1997.

Macafee, C.A.J., Fortune, D.W. and Beischer, N.A.: Non-immunological hydrops fetalis. J. Obstet. Gynaecol. Brit. Cwlth. **77**:226–237, 1970.

Machin, G.A.: Hydrops revisited: Literature review of 1,414 cases published in the 1980s. Amer. J. Med. Genet. **34**:366–390, 1989.

Macgregor, S.N., Socol, M.L., Pielet, B.W., Sholl, J.T. and Minogue, J.P.: Prediction of fetoplacental blood volume in isoimmunized pregnancy. Amer. J. Obstetr. Gynecol. **159**: 1493–1497, 1988.

Maeda, H., Shimokawa, H., Saton, S., Nakano, H. and Nunoue, T.: Nonimmunologic hydrops fetalis resulting from intrauterine human parvovirus B-19 infection: report of two cases. Obstet. Gynecol. **72**:482–485, 1988.

Maidman, J.E., Yeager, C., Anderson, V., Makabali, G., O'Grady, J.P., Arce, J. and Tishler, D.M.: Prenatal diagnosis and management of nonimmunologic hydrops fetalis. Obstet. Gynecol. **56**:571–576, 1980.

Mallmann, P., Gembruch, U., Mallmann, R. and Hansmann, M.: Investigations into a possible immunological origin of idio-pathic non-immune hydrops fetalis and initial results of pro-phylactic immune treatment of subsequent pregnancies. Acta Obstet. Gynecol. Scand. **70**:35–40, 1991.

Manning, F.A., Heaman, M., Boyce, D. and Carter, L.J.: Intrauterine fetal tachypnea. Obstet. Gynecol. **58**:398–400, 1981.

Manning, F.A., Bowman, J.M., Lange, I.R. and Chamberlain, P. F.: Intrauterine transfusion in an Rh-immunized twin pregnancy: a case report of successful outcome and a review of the literature. Obstetr. Gynecol. **65**:2S–6S, 1985.

Mark, Y., Rogers, B.B. and Oyer, C.E.: Diagnosis and incidence of fetal parvovirus infection in an autopsy series: II. DNA amplification. Pediatr. Pathol. **13**:381–386, 1993.

Markenson, G., Correia, L.A., Cohn, G., Bayer, L. and Kanaan, C.: Parvoviral infection associated with increased nuchal translucency: a case report. J. Perinatol. **2**:129–131, 2000.

Matthews, C.D., Matthews, A.E.B. and Gilbey, B.E.: Antibody development in rhesus-negative patients following abortion. Lancet **ii**:318–319, 1969.

McCowan, L.M.E. and Becroft, D.M.O.: Beckwith-Wiedemann syndrome, placental abnormalities, and gestational protein-uric hypertension. Obstet. Gynecol. **83**:813–817, 1994.

McCoy, M.C., Katz, V.L., Gould, N. and Kuller, J.A.: Non-immune hydrops after 20 weeks' gestation: review of 10 years' experience with suggestions for management. Obstet. Gynecol. **85**:578–582, 1995.

McFadden, D.E. and Taylor, G.P.: Cardiac abnormalities and nonimmune hydrops fetalis: a coincidental, not causal, relationship. Pediatr. Pathol. **9**:11–17, 1989.

Meizner, I., Levy, A., Carmi, R. and Robinsin, C.: Niemann-Pick disease associated with nonimmune hydrops fetalis. Amer. J. Obstet. Gynecol. **163**:128–129, 1990.

Mentzer, W.C. and Collier, E.: Hydrops fetalis associated with erythrocyte G-6-PD deficiency and maternal ingestion of fava beans and ascorbic acid. J. Pediatr. **86**:565–567, 1975.

Metzman, R., Anand, A., DeGiulio, P.A. and Knisely, A.S.: Hepatic disease associated with intrauterine parvovirus B19 infection in a newborn premature infant. J. Pediat. Gastroen-terol. Nutr. **9**:119–114, 1989.

Miller, D.F. and Petrie, S.J.: Fatal erythroblastosis fetalis secondary to ABO incompatibility. Obstetr. Gynecol. **22**:773–777, 1963.

Miller, P.D., Smith, B.C. and Marinoff, D.N.: Theca-lutein ovarian cysts associated with homozygous α-thalassemia. Amer. J. Obstet. Gynecol. **157**:912–914, 1987.

Milner, P.F., Clegg, J.B. and Weatherall, D.J.: Haemoglobin-H disease due to a unique haemoglobin variant with an elongated α-chain. Lancet **i**:729–732, 1971.

Milunsky, A., Alpert, E., Frigoletto, F.D., Driscoll, S.G., McCluskey, R.T. and Colvin, R.B.: Prenatal diagnosis of the congenital nephrotic syndrome. Pediatrics **59**:770–773, 1977.

Mittendorf, R. and Williams, M.A.: RH₀(D) immunoglobulin (RhoGAM): How it came into being. Obstetr. Gynecol. **77**:301–303, 1991.

Moerman, P., Fryns, J.P., Goddeeris, P. and Lauweryns, J.M.: Nonimmunologic hydrops fetalis. A study of ten cases. Arch. Pathol. Lab. Med. **106**:635–640, 1982.

Mogilner, B.M., Ashkenazy, M., Borenstein, R. and Lancet, M.: Hydrops fetalis caused by maternal indomethacin treatment. Acta Obstet. Gynecol. Scand. **61**:183–185, 1982.

Moller, J.H., Lynch, R.P. and Edwards, J.E.: Fetal cardiac failure resulting from congenital anomalies of the heart. J. Pediatr. **68**:699–703, 1966.

Mollison, P.L.: Suppression of Rh-immunization by passively administered anti-Rh. Br. J. Haematol. **14**:1–4, 1968.

Montemagno, U., Stefano, M.di e Cardone, A.: Aspetti istoimmunologici della placenta nella incompatibilita Rh. In, Simpos. sui Problemi Ostetrico-Pediatrici della Sofferenza Fetale. Offic. Grafiche Stianti-Sanscasciano, Siena, Italy, 1966. pp. 649–655.

Mor, Z., Schreyer, P., Wainraub, Z., Hayman, E. and Caspi, E.: Nonimmune hydrops fetalis associated with angioosteohypertrophy (Klippel-Trenaunay) syndrome. Amcr. J. Obstet. Gynecol. **159**:1185–1186, 1988.

Morey, A.L., Nicolini, U., Welch, C.R., Economides, D., Chamberlain, P.F. and Cohen, B.J.: Parvovirus B 19 infection and transient fetal hydrops. Lancet **337**:496, 1991.

Moss, T.J. and Kaplan, L.: Association of hydrops fetalis with congenital neuroblastoma. Amer. J. Obstet. Gynecol. **132**:905–906, 1978.

Mostoufi-Zadeh, M., Weiss, L.M. and Driscoll, S.G.: Nonimmune hydrops fetalis: a challenge in perinatal pathology. Human Pathol. **16**:785–789, 1985.

Moya, F.R., Grannum, P.A.T., Widness, J.A., Clemons, G.K., Copel, J.A. and Hobbins, J.C.: Erythropoietin in human fetuses with immune hemolytic anemia and hydrops fetalis. Obstet. Gynecol. **82**:353–358, 1993.

Murray, S. and Barron, S.L.: Rhesus isoimmunization after abortion. Brit. Med. J. **iii**:87–89, 1971.

Naeye, R.L.: New observations in erythroblastosis fetalis. JAMA **200**:105–110, 1967.

Nakamura, Y., Komatsu, Y., Yano, H., Kitazono, S., Hosokawa, Y., Fukuda, S., Kawano, S., Nagasue, N., Matsunaga, T., Aiko, Y., Hashimoto, T. and Morimatsu, M.: Nonimmunologic hydrops fetalis: a clinicopathological study of 50 autopsy cases. Pediatr. Pathol. **7**:19–30, 1987.

Nakayama, R., Yamada, D., Steinmiller, V., Hsia, E. and Hale, R.W.: Hydrops fetalis secondary to Bart hemoglobinopathy. Obstet. Gynecol. **67**:176–180, 1986.

Nalbandian, R.M., Henry, R.L., Camp, F.R., Wolf, P.L. and Evans, T.N.: Embryonic, fetal, and neonatal hemoglobin synthesis: relationship to abortion and thalassemia. Obstet. Gynecol. Survey **26**:185–191, 1971.

Nathan, D.G.: Thalassemia: a progress report on applied molecular biology. NEJM **288**:1122–1123, 1973.

Nelson, A., Peterson, L.A., Frampton, B. and Sly, W.S.: Mucopolysaccharidosis VII (β-glucuronidase deficiency) presenting as nonimmune hydrops fetalis. J. Pediatr. **101**:574–576, 1982.

Nerlich, A., Schwarz, T.F., Roggendorf, M., Roggendorf, H., Ostermeyer, E., Schramm, T. and Gloning, K.-P.: Parvovirus B19–infected erythroblasts in fetal cord blood. Lancet **337**:310, 1991.

Newton, E.R., Louis, F., Dalton, M.E. and Feingold, M.: Fetal neuroblastoma and catecholamine-induced maternal hypertension. Obstet. Gynecol. **65**:49S–52S, 1985.

Nicolaides, K.H., Soothill, P.W., Clewell, W.H., Rodeck, C.H., Mibashan, R.S. and Campbell, S.: Fetal haemoglobin measurement of red cell isoimmunization. Lancet **i**:1073–1075, 1988a.

Nicolaides, K.H., Thilaganathan, B., Rodeck, C.H. and Mibashan, R.S.: Erythroblastosis and reticulocytosis in anemic fetuses. Amer. J. Obstet. Gynecol. **159**:1063–1065, 1988b.

Nicolaides, K.H., Thilaganathan, B. and Mibashan, R.S.: Cordocentesis in the investigation of fetal erythropoiesis. Amer. J. Obstetr. Gynecol. **161**:1197–1200, 1989.

Nicolini, U., Talbert, D.G., Fisk, N.M. and Rodeck, C.H.: Pathophysiology of pressure changes during intrauterine transfusion. Amer. J. Obstetr. Gynecol. **160**:1139–1145, 1989.

Nimrod, C., Davies, D., Harder, J., Iwanicki, S., Kondo, C., Takahashi, Y., Maloney, J., Persaud, D. and Nicholson, S.: Ultrasound evaluation of tachycardia-induced hydrops in the fetal lamb. Amer. J. Obstet. Gynecol. **157**:655–659, 1987.

Novak, P.M., Sander, M., Yang, S.S. and Oeyen, P.T.v.: Report of fourteen cases of nonimmune hydrops fetalis in association with hemorrhagic endovasculitis of the placenta. Amer. J. Obstet. Gynecol. **165**:945–950, 1991.

Oetama, B.K., Tucay, R.F. and Morgan, D.L.: Nonimmune hydrops in a newborn. Arch. Pathol. Lab. Med. **125**:1609–1610, 2001.

Ohyama, M., Kobayashi, S., Aida, N., Toyoda, Y., Ijiri, R. and Tanaka, Y.: Congenital neuroblastoma diagnosed by placental examination. Med. Ped. Oncol. **33**:430–431, 1999.

Olson, R.W., Nishibatake, M., Arya, S. and Gilbert, E.F.: Nonimmunologic hydrops fetalis due to intrauterine closure of fetal foramen ovale. In, Genetic Aspects of Developmental Pathology. E.F. Gilbert, ed. Birth Defects: Original Article Series. 23(1):433–442, 1987. Alan R. Liss, New York.

Orkin, S.H. and Michelson, A.: Partial deletion of the α-globin structural gene in human α-thalassemia. Nature **286**:538–540, 1980.

Orkin, S.H. and Nathan, D.G.: Current concepts in genetics. NEJM **295**:710–714, 1976.

Östör, A.G. and Fortune, D.W.: Tuberous sclerosis initially seen as hydrops fetalis. Report of a case and review of the literature. Arch. Pathol. Lab. Med. **102**:34–39, 1978.

Oudesluys-Murphy, A.M.: Nonimmune hydrops fetalis in Noonan's syndrome. Amer. J. Dis. Childr. **141**:478–479, 1987.

Özmen, S., Seçkin, N., Turhan, N.Ö., Dilmen, G. and Dilmen. U.: Fetal methemoglobinemia: a cause of nonimmune hydrops. Amer. J. Obstet. Gynecol. **173**:232–233, 1995.

Paradinas, F.J., Fisher, R.A., Browne, P. and Newlands, E.S.: Diploid hydatidiform moles with fetal red blood cells in molar villi. 1—pathology, incidence, and prognosis. J. Pathol. **181**:183–188, 1997.

Pattison, J.R., Jones, S.E., Hodgson, J., Davis, L.R., White, J.M., Stroud, C.E. and Murtoza, L.: Parvovirus infections and hypoplastic crisis in sickle-cell anaemia. Lancet i:664–665, 1981.

Pattison, N. and Roberts, A.: The management of severe erythroblastosis fetalis by fetal transfusion: survival of transfused adult erythrocytes in the fetus. Obstetr. Gynecol. 74:901–904, 1989.

Pearson, H.A., Shanklin, D.R. and Brodine, C.R.: Alphathalassemia as cause of nonimmunological hydrops. Amer. J. Dis. Childr. 109:168–172, 1965.

Perkins, D.G., Kopp, C.M. and Haust, M.D.: Placental infiltration in congenital neuroblastoma: a case study with ultrastructure. Histopathol. 4:383–389, 1980.

Perlin, B.M., Pomerance, J.J. and Schifrin, B.S.: Nonimmunologic hydrops fetalis. Obstet. Gynecol. 57:584–588, 1981.

Perkins, R.P.: Hydrops fetalis and stillbirth in a male glucose-6-phosphate dehydrogenase-deficient fetus possibly due to maternal ingestion of sulfisoxazole. Amer. J. Obstet. Gynecol. 111:379–381, 1971.

Peschle, C., Mavilio, F., Care, A., Migliaccio, G., Migliaccio, A. R., Salvo, G., Samoggia, P., Petti, S., Guerriero, R., Marinucci, M., Lazzaro, D., Russo, G. and Mastroberardino, G.: Haemoglobin switching in human embryos: asynchrony of ʃ → α and epsilon → gamma-globin switches in primitive and definitive erythropoietic lineage. Nature 313:235–238, 1985.

Peters, M.T. and Nicolaides, K.H.: Cordocentesis for the diagnosis and treatment of human fetal parvovirus infection. Obstet. Gynecol. 75:501–504, 1990.

Pielet, B.W., Socol, M.L., Macgregor, S.N., Ney, J.A. and Dooley, S.L.: Cordocentesis: an appraisal of risks. Amer. J. Obstet. Gynecol. 159:1497–1500, 1988.

Pillay, D., Patou, G., Hurt, S., Kibbler, C.C. and Griffiths, P.D.: Parvovirus B19 outbreak in a children's ward. Lancet 339:107–109, 1992.

Pilz, I., Schweikhart, G. und Kaufmann, P.: Zur Abgrenzung normaler, artefizieller und pathologischer Strukturen in reifen menschlichen Plazentarzotten. III. Morphometrische Untersuchungen bei Rhesus-Inkompabilität. Arch. Gynecol. 229:137–154, 1980.

Pootrakul, S., Wasi, P. and Na-Nakorn, S.: Haemoglobin Bart's hydrops foetalis in Thailand. Ann. Hum. Genet. 30:293–311, 1967.

Porter, H.J., Quantrill, A.M. and Flehming K.A.: B19 parvovirus infection of myocardial cells. Lancet i:535–536, 1988.

Price, J.R.: Rh sensitization by hydatidiform mole. NEJM 278:1021, 1968.

Pringle, K.C., Weiner, C.P., Soper, R.T. and Kealey, P.: Sacrococcygeal teratoma. Fetal Therapy 2:80–87, 1987.

Pryde, P.G., Nugent, C.E., Pridjian, G., Barr, M. and Faix, R.G.: Spontaneous resolution of nonimmune hydrops fetalis secondary to human parvovirus B19 infection. Obstet. Gynecol. 79:859–861, 1992.

Public Health Laboratory Service Working Party on Fifth Disease: prospective study of human parvovirus (B-19) infection in pregnancy. Brit. Med. J. 300:1166–1170, 1990.

Pustilnik, T.B. and Cohen, A.W.: Parvovirus B19 infection in a twin pregnancy. Obstet. Gynecol. 83:834–836, 1994.

Queenan, J.T. and Douglas, G.R.: Intrauterine transfusion: a preliminary report. Obstetr. Gynecol. 25:308–321, 1965.

Queenan, J.T. and Nakamoto, M.: Postpartum immunization: the hypothetical hazard of manual removal of the placenta. Report of a study. Obstetr. Gynecol. 23:392–395, 1964.

Rabinowitz, P., Harris, e.J. and Friedman, I.S.: Theca-lutein cysts of the ovaries. A case of erythroblastosis with abruptio placentae and acute renal failure. JAMA 177: 509–510, 1961.

Radunovic, N., Lockwood, C.J., Alvarez, M., Plecas, D., Chitkara, U. and Berkovitz, R.L.: The severely anemic and hydropic isoimmune fetus: changes in fetal hematocrit associated with intrauterine death. Obstetr. Gynecol. 79:390–393, 1992.

Ravindranath, Y., Paglia, D.E., Warrier, I., Valentine, W., Nakatani, M. and Brockway, R.A.: Glucose phosphate isomerase deficiency as a cause of hydrops fetalis. NEJM 316:258–261, 1987.

Reece, E.A., Gabrielli, S., Abdalla, M., O'Connor, T.Z. and Hobbins, J.C.: Reassessment of the utility of fetal umbilical vein diameter in the management of isoimmunization. Amer. J. Obstetr. Gynecol. 159:937–938, 1988.

Rice, G.E., Mostoufi-Zadeh, M., Kolodny, E.H. and Driscoll, S.G.: Hydrops fetalis in Gaucher's disease. Teratology 29:53A–54A, 1984.

Rodeck, C.H., Nicolaides, K.H., Warsof, S.L., Fysh, W.J., Gamsu, H.R. and Kemp, J.R.: The management of severe rhesus isoimmunization by fetoscopic intravascular transfusions. Amer. J. Obstetr. Gynecol. 150:769–774, 1984.

Rodin, A.E. and Nichols, M.M.: Congestive heart failure in the fetus and during the first day of life. Texas Med. 72:44–48, 1975.

Rodis, J.F., Hovick, T.J., Quinn, D.L., Rosengren, S.S. and Tattersall, P.: Human parvovirus infection in pregnancy. Obstet. Gynecol. 72:733–738, 1988.

Rodis, J.F., Quinn, D.L., Gary, G.W., Anderson, L.J., Rosengren, S., Cartter, M.L., Campbell, W.A. and Vintzileos, A.M.: Management and outcomes of pregnancies complicated by human B19 parvovirus infection: a prospective study. Amer. J. Obstet. Gynecol. 163:1168–1171, 1990.

Rodis, J.F., Borgida, A.F., Wilson, M., Egan, J.F.X., Leo, M.V., Odibo, A.O. and Campbell, W.A.: Management of parvovirus infection in pregnancy and outcomes of hydrops: a survey of members of perinatal obstetricians. Amer. J. Obstet. Gynecol. 179:985–988, 1998.

Rodriguez, M.M., Chaves, F., Romaguera, R.L., Ferrer, P.L., Guardia, C. de la and Bruce, J.H.: Value of autopsy in nonimmune hydrops fetalis: series of 51 stillborn fetuses. Pediatr. Devel. Pathol. 5:365–374, 2002.

Rönisch, P. und Kleihauer, E.: Alpha-Thalassämie mit HbH und Bart's in einer deutschen Familie. Klin. Wchschr. 45:1193–1200, 1967.

Rogers, B.B.: Histopathologic variability of finding erythroid inclusions with intranuclear parvovirus B19 infection. Pediatr. Pathol. 12:883–889, 1992.

Rogers, B.B., Mark, Y. and Oyer, C.E.: Diagnosis and incidence of fetal parvovirus infection in an autopsy series: I. Histology. Pediatr. Pathol. 13:371–379, 1993.

Rogers, B.B., Rogers, Z.R. and Timmons, C.F.: Polymerase chain reaction amplification of archival material for parvovirus B19 in children with transient erythroblastopenia of childhood. Pediatr. Pathol. Lab. Med. 16471–478, 1996.

Rogers, B.B., Bloom, S.L. and Buchanan, G.R.: Autosomal dominantly inherited Diamond-Blackfan anemia resulting in nonimmune hydrops. Obstet. Gynecol. **89**:805–807, 1997.

Rubin, E.M. and Kan, Y.W.: A simple sensitive prenatal test for hydrops fetalis caused by α-thalassemia. Lancet **i**:75–77, 1985.

Sacks, L.M., Polin, J.I. and Breckenridge, J.: Congenital chylothorax presenting as hydrops fetalis. A case report. J. Reprod. Med. **28**:341–344, 1983.

Sahakian, V., Weiner, C.P., Naides, S.J., Williamson, R.A. and Scharosch, L.L.: Intrauterine transfusion treatment of nonimmune hydrops fetalis secondary to human parvovirus B19 infection. Amer. J. Obstet. Gynecol. **164**:1090–1091, 1991.

Saltzman, D.H., Frigoletto, F.D., Harlow, B.L., Barss, V.A. and Benacerraf, B.R.: Sonographic evaluation of hydrops fetalis. Obstet. Gynecol. **74**:106–111, 1989.

Samra, J.S., Obhrai, M.S. and Constantine, G.: Parvovirus infection in pregnancy. Obstet. Gynecol. **73**:832–834, 1989.

Santolaya, J., Alley, D., Jaffe, R. and Warsof, S.L.: Antenatal classification of hydrops fetalis. Obstet. Gynecol. **79**:256–259, 1992.

Scheib, J.S. and Waxman, J.: Congenital heart block in successive pregnancies: a case report and evaluation of risk with therapeutic consideration. Obstet. Gynecol. **73**:481–484, 1989.

Schumacher, B. and Moise, K.J.: Fetal transfusion for red blood cell alloimmunization. In pregnancy. Obstet. Gynecol. **88**:137–150, 1996.

Schwanitz, G., Zerris, K., Niesen, M., Haverkamp, F. and Schmid, G.: Hydrops fetalis as an indication for prenatal chromosome analysis with the example of the diagnosis of a duplication 15q11 and 17q25 due to familial translocation 15/17. Ann. Genet. **31**:186–189, 1988.

Schwartz, S.M., Visekul, C., Laxova, R., McPherson, E. and Gilbert, E.F.: Idiopathic hydrops fetalis report of 4 patients including 2 affected sibs. Amer. J. Med. Genet. **8**:59–66, 1981.

Schwarz, T.F., Roggendorf, M., Hottenträger, Deinhardt, B., Enders, G., Gloning, K.P., Schramm, T. and Hansmann, M.: Human parvovirus B19 infection in pregnancy. Lancet **ii**:566–567, 1988.

Schwarz, T.F., Nerlich, A., Hottenträger, B., Jäger, G., Wiest, I., Kantimm, S., Roggendorf, H., Schultz, M., Gloning, K.P., Schramm, T., Holzgreve, W. and Roggendorf, M.: Parvovirus B19 infection of the fetus. Histology and in situ hybridization. Amer. J. Clin. Pathol. **95**:121–126, 1991.

Scott, J.R., Beer, A.E., Guy, L.R., Liesch, M. and Elbert, G.: Pathogenesis of Rh immunization in primigravidas. Fetomaternal versus maternofetal bleeding. Obstetr. Gynecol. **49**:9–14, 1977.

Seeds, J.W., Herbert, W.N.P., Bowles, W.A. and Cefalo, R.C.: Recurrent idiopathic fetal hydrops: results of prenatal therapy. Obstet. Gynecol. **64**:30S–33S, 1984.

Seeds, J.W., Bowes, W.A. and Chescheir, N.C.: Echogenic venous turbulence is a critical feature of successful intravascular transfusion. Obstetr. Gynecol. **73**:488–490, 1989.

Seifer, D.B., Ferguson, J.E., Behrens, C.M., Zemel, S., Stevenson, D.K. and Ross, J.: Nonimmune hydrops fetalis in association with hemangioma of the umbilical cord. Obstet. Gynecol. **66**:283–286, 1985.

Selm, M.V., Kanhai, H.H.H. and Gravenhorst, J.B.: Maternal hydrops syndrome: a review. Obstetr. Gynecol. Surv. **46**:785–788, 1991.

Seppälä, M., Aula, P., Rapola, J., Karjalainen, O., Huttunen, N.-P. and Ruoslahti, E.: Congenital nephrotic syndrome: prenatal diagnosis and genetic counselling by estimation of amniotic-fluid and maternal serum alpha-fetoprotein. Lancet **i**:123–125, 1976.

Seward, J.F. and Zusman, J.: Hydrops fetalis associated with small-bowel volvulus. Lancet **ii**:52–53, 1978.

Sexauer, C.L., Graham, H.L., Starling, K.A. and Fernbach, D.J.: A test for abnormal hemoglobins in umbilical cord blood. Amer. J. Dis. Childr. **130**:805–806, 1976.

Sheikh, A.U., Ernest, J.M. and O'Shea, M.: Long-term outcome in fetal hydrops from parvovirus B 19 infection. Amer. J. Obstet. Gynecol. **167**:337–341, 1992.

Shimokawa, H., Hara, K., Fukuda, A. and Nakano, H.: Idiopathic hydrops fetalis successfully treated in utero. Obstet. Gynecol. **71**:984–986, 1988.

Shiraishi, S., Kinukawa, N., Nakano, H. and Sueishi, K.: Immunohistochemical distribution of vascular endothelial growth factor in the human placenta associated with hydrops fetalis. Pediatr. Pathol. Lab. Med. **17**:65–81, 1997.

Silber, D.L. and Durnim, R.E.: Intrauterine atrial tachycardia. Associated with massive edema in a newborn. Amer. J. Dis. Childr. **117**:722–726, 1969.

Silver, M.M., Beverley, D.W., Valberg, L.S., Cutz, E., Phillips, M.J. and Shaheed, W.A.: Perinatal hemochromatosis. Clinical, morphologic, and quantitative iron studies. Amer. J. Pathol. **128**:538–554, 1989.

Silverstein, A.J. and Kanbour, A.I.: Repetitive idiopathic fetal hydrops. Obstet. Gynecol. **57**:18S–21S, 1981.

Sklansky, M., Greenberg, M., Lucas, V. and Gruslin-Giroux, A.: Intrapericardial teratoma in a twin fetus: diagnosis and management. Obstet. Gynecol. **89**:807–809, 1997.

Skogerboe, K.J., West, S.F., Smith, C., Terashita, S.T., LeCrone, C.N., Detter, J.C. and Tait, J.F.: Screening for α-thalassemia. Correlation of hemoglobin H inclusion bodies with DNA-determined genotype. Arch. Pathol. Lab. Med. **116**:1012–1018, 1992.

Skopec, L.L. and Lakatua, D.J.: Non-immune fetal hydrops with hepatic hemangioendothelioma and Kasabach-Merritt syndrome: a case report. Pediatr. Pathol. **9**:87–93, 1989.

Slikke, J.W. v.d. and Balk, A.G.: Hydramnios with hydrops fetalis and disseminated fetal neuroblastoma. Obstet. Gynecol. **55**:250–253, 1980.

Smith, C.R., Chan, H.S.L. and DeSa, D.J.: Placental involvement in congenital neuroblastoma. J. Clin. Pathol. **34**:785–789, 1981.

Socol, M.L., Macgregor, S.N., Pielet, B.W., Tamura, R.K. and Sabbagha, R.E.: Percutaneous umbilical transfusion in severe rhesus isoimmunization: resolution of fetal hydrops. Amer. J. Obstetr. Gynecol. **157**:1369–1375, 1987.

Soothill, P.: Intrauterine blood transfusion for non-immune hydrops fetalis due to parvovirus B19 infection. Lancet **336**:121–122, 1990.

Srivastara, A. and Lu, L.: Replication of B19 parvovirus in highly enriched haematopoietic progenitor cells from normal human bone marrow. J. Virol. **62**:3059–3063, 1988.

Stedman, C.M., Quinlan, R.W., Huddleston, J.F., Cruz, A.C. and Kellner, K.R.: Rh sensitization after third-trimester fetal death. Obstetr. Gynecol. **71**:461–463, 1988.

Steinke, J., Gries, F.A. and Driscoll, S.G.: In vitro studies of insulin inactivation with reference to erythroblastosis fetalis. Blood **30**:359–363, 1967.

Stevens, D.C., Hilliard, J.K., Schreiner, R.L., Hurwitz, R.A., Murrell, R., Mirkin, L.D., Bonderman, P.W. and Nolen, P.A.: Supraventricular tachycardia with edema, ascites, and hydrops in fetal sheep. Amer. J. Obstet. Gynecol. **142**:316–322, 1982.

Stocker, J.T. and Singer, D.B.: Human parvovirus B19 infection, hydrops fetalis, and possibly myocarditis. Annotated bibliography. Pediatr. Pathol. **8**:356–358, 1988.

Strauss, L. and Driscoll, S.G.: Congenital neuroblastoma involving the placenta. Reports of two cases. Pediatrics **34**:23–31, 1964.

Suh, Y.K.: α-Thalassemia—differential diagnosis. J. Perinatol. **14**:319–321, 1994.

Swain, S. and Cameron, A.D.: Establishing the cause of nonimmune hydrops. Amer. J. Obstet. Gynecol. **176**:951, 1997.

Szulman, A.E.: The A, B and H blood-group antigens in human placenta. NEJM **286**:1028–1031, 1972.

Taylor, J.F.: Sensitization of Rh-negative daughters by their Rh-positive mothers. NEJM **276**:547–551, 1967.

Taylor, P.V., Scott, J.S., Gerbis, L.M., Esscher, E. and Scott, O.: Maternal antibodies against fetal cardiac antigens in congenital complete heart block. NEJM **315**:667–672, 1986.

Terheggen, H.G. und Kleihauer, E.: Die α-Thalassämie. Eine kasuistische Mitteilung. Z. Kinderh. **103**:182–191, 1968.

Thilaganathan, B., Salvesen, D.R., Abbas, A., Ireland, R.M. and Nicolaides, K.H.: Fetal plasma erythropoietin concentration in red blood cell-isoimmunized pregnancies. Amer. J. Obstetr. Gynecol. **167**:1292–1297, 1992.

Thumasathit, B., Nondasuta, A., Silpisornkosol, S., Lousuebsakul, B., Unchalipongse, P. and Mangkornkanok, M.: Hydrops fetalis associated with Bart's hemoglobin in northern Thailand. J. Pediatr. **73**:132–138, 1968.

Tolfvenstam, T., Papadogiannakis, N., Norbeck, O., Petersson, K. and Broliden, K.: Frequency of human parvovirus B19 infection in intrauterine death. Lancet **357**:1494–1497, 2001. (see also Correspondence. Lancet **358**:1180–1181, 2001).

Treadwell, M.C., Sherer, D.M., Sacks, A.j., Ghezzi, F. and Romero, R.: Successful treatment of recurrent non-immune hydrops secondary to fetal hyperthyroidism. Obstet. Gynecol. **87**:838–840, 1996.

Turski, D.M., Shahidi, N., Visekul, C. and Gilbert, E.: Nonimmunologic hydrops fetalis. Amer. J. Obstet. Gynecol. **131**:586–587, 1978.

Uno, Y., Taniguchi, A. and Tanaka, E.: Histochemical studies in Wolman's disease—report of an autopsy case accompanied with a large amount of milky ascites. Acta Pathol. Jpn. **23**:779–790, 1973.

Van Kamp, I.L., Klumper, F.J.C.M., Oepkes, D., Meerman, R.H., Scherjon, S.A., Vandenbussche, F.P.H.A. and Kanhai, H.H.H.: Complications of intrauterine intravascular transfusion for fetal anemia due to re-cell alloimmunization. Amer. J. Obstet. Gynecol. **192**:171–177, 2005.

Vaughan, J.I., Manning, M., Warwick, R.M., Letsky, E.A., Murray, N.A. and Roberts, I.A.G.: Inhibition of erythroid progenitor cells by anti-Kell antibodies in fetal alloimmune anemia. NEJM **338**:798–803, 1998.

Vedvick, T.S., Wheeler, S.A. and Koenig, H.M.: Heterogeneity of fetal hemoglobin in severe α-thalassemia. Biol. Neonate **36**:181–184, 1979.

Veille, J.C., Sunderland, C. and Bennett, R.M.: Complete heart block in a fetus associated with maternal Sjögren's syndrome. Amer. J. Obstet. Gynecol. **151**:660–661, 1985.

Verger, P., Martin, C., Dubecq, J.-P., Kermarec, Y. et Lomazzi, R.: Étude pathologique et therapeutique de l'anasarque foeto-placentaire. Arch. Franc. Pediatr. **20**:417–436, 1963.

Vetter, V.L. and Rashkind, W.J.: Congenital complete heart block and connective-tissue disease. NEJM **309**:236–238, 1983.

Veyer, I.B.v.d. and Moise, K.J.: Fetal RhD typing by polymerase chain reaction in pregnancies complicated by rhesus alloimmunization. Obstet. Gynecol. **88**:1061–1067, 1996.

Veyer, I.B.v.d., Subramanian, S.B., Hudson, K.M., Werch, J., Moise, K.J. and Hughes, M.R.: Prenatal diagnosis of the RhD fetal blood type on amniotic fluid by polymerase chain reaction. Obstet. Gynecol. **87**:419–422, 1996.

Vidyasagar, D. and Haworth, J.C.: Placental dimensions, cell size, and cell number in erythroblastosis fetalis. Amer. J. Obstetr. Gynecol. **115**:267–270, 1973.

Villaespesa, A.R., Mier, M.P.S., Ferrer, P.L., Baleriola, I.A. and Gonzalez, J.I.R.: Nonimmunologic hydrops fetalis: An etiopathogenetic approach through the postmortem study of 59 patients. Amer. J. Med. Genet. **35**:274–279, 1990.

Ville, Y., Proudler, A., Abbas, A. and Nicolaides, K.: Atrial natriuretic factor concentration in normal, growth-retarded, anemic, and hydropic fetuses. Amer. J. Obstet. Gynecol. **171**:777–783, 1994a.

Ville, Y., Proudler, A., Kuhn, P. and Nicolaides, K.: Aldosterone concentration in normal, growth-retarded, anemic, and hydropic fetuses. Obstet. Gynecol. **84**:511–514, 1994b.

Vintzileos, A.M., Campbell, W.A., Soberman, S.M. and Nochimson, D.J.: Fetal atrial flutter and X-linked dominant vitamin D-resistant rickets. Obstet. Gynecol. **65**:39S–44S, 1985.

Vogel, H., Kornman, M., Ledet, S.C., Rajagopalan, L., Taber, L. and McClain, K.: Congenital parvovirus infection. Pediatr. Pathol. Lab. Med. **17**:903–912, 1997.

Warren, R.C., Butler, J., Morsman, J.M., Mckenzie, C. and Rodeck, C.H.: Does chorionic villus sampling cause fetomaternal hemorrhage? Lancet **i**:691, 1985.

Watson, J. and Campbell, S.: Antenatal evaluation and management in nonimmune hydrops fetalis. Obstet. Gynecol. **67**:589–593, 1986.

Watson, W.J. and Fiegen, M.M.: Fetal thyrotoxicosis associated with nonimmune hydrops. Amer. J. Obstet. Gynecol. **172**:1039–1040, 1995.

Weiland, H.T., Vermey-Keers, C., Salimans, M.M.M., Fleuren, G.J., Verwey, R.A. and Anderson, M.J.: Parvovirus B19 associated with fetal abnormality. Lancet **i**:682–683, 1987.

Weiner, C.P and Thompson, I.B.: Direct treatment of fetal supraventricular tachycardia after failed transplacental therapy. Amer. J. Obstet. Gynecol. **158**:570–573, 1988.

Weiner, C., Varner, M., Pringle, K., Hein, H., Williamson, R. and Smith, W.L.: Antenatal diagnosis and palliative treatment of nonimmune hydrops fetalis secondary to extralobar sequestration. Obstet. Gynecol. **68**:275–280, 1986.

Weiner, C.P., Sipes, S.L. and Wenstrom, K.: The effect of fetal age upon normal fetal laboratory values and venous pressure. Obstetr. Gynecol. **79**:713–718, 1992.

Wentworth, P.: The placenta in cases of hemolytic disease. Amer. J. Obstetr. Gynecol. **98**:283–289, 1967.

Westgren, M., Eastman, W.N., Ghandourah, S. and Woodhouse, N.: Intrauterine hypercalcaemia and non-immune hydrops fetalis—relationship to the Williams syndrome. Prenatal Diagnosis **8**:333–337, 1988.

Whitney, J.B. and Popp, R.A.: Thalassemia. Alpha-thalassemia in laboratory mice. Amer. J. Pathol. **116**:523–525, 1984.

Wiener, A.S., Wexler, I.B. and Schutta, E.J.: A pair of male fraternal twins with contrasting manifestations of Rh hemolytic disease. Acta Genet. Med. Gemell. **11**:17–28, 1962.

Wiggins, J.W., Bowes, W., Clewell, W., Manco-Johnson, M., Manchester, D., Johnson, R., Appareti, K. and Wolfe, R.R.: Echocardiographic diagnosis and intravenous digoxin management of fetal tachyarrhythmias and congestive heart failure. Amer. J. Dis. Childr. **140**:202–204, 1986.

Williamson, R., Eskdale, J., Coleman, D.V., Niazi, M., Loeffler, F.E. and Modell, B.M.: Direct gene analysis of chorionic villi: a possible technique for first-trimester antenatal diagnosis of haemoglobinopathies. Lancet **ii**:1125–1127, 1981.

Windebank, K.P., Bridges, N.A., Ostman-Smith, I. and Stevens, J.E.: Hydrops fetalis due to abnormal lymphatics. Arch. Dis. Childh. **62**:198–200, 1987.

Wood, W.G., Bunch, C., Kelley, S., Gunn, Y. and Breckon, G.: Control of haemoglobin switching by a developmental clock? Nature **313**:320–323, 1985.

Yamakawa, Y., Oka, H., Hori, S., Arai, T. and Izumi, R.: Detection of human parvovirus B19 DNA by nested polymerase chain reaction. Obstet. Gynecol. **86**:126–129, 1995.

Younis, J.S. and Granat, M.: Insufficient transplacental digoxin transfer in severe hydrops fetalis. Amer. J. Obstet. Gynecol. **157**:1268–1269, 1987.

Zeng, Y.-T. and Hunag, S.-Z.: α-Globin gene organisation and prenatal diagnosis of α-thalassemia in Chinese. Lancet **i**:304–307, 1985.

Zipursky, A. and Israels, L.G.: The pathogenesis and prevention of Rh immunization. Canad. Med. Assoc. J. **97**:1245–1257, 1967.

Zwi, L.J. and Becroft, D.M.O.: Intrauterine aplastic anemia and fetal hydrops: a case report. Pediatr. Pathol. **5**:199–205, 1986.

17
Transplacental Hemorrhage, Cell Transfer, Trauma

Transplacental Blood and Cell Transfer

In the 19th century ago, considerable controversy raged as to whether the fetal and maternal circulations were united or separate. In an interesting essay, von Baer (1828) discussed this dispute in great detail and, in order to settle the issue "once and for all," he performed experiments on dogs. These showed conclusively that the two vascular beds are separate one from another and illustrated his findings well. The history of this topic is covered in excellent detail in the historical review of de Witt (1959).

Although transfer of maternal cells to the fetus is an exceptional event, the fetus often bleeds into the maternal circulation, despite the anatomic separation of the two circulations. The reason for this fetal bleeding is often obscure. It is an important aspect of placentation, however, whose pathogenesis must be further explored. Pathologists who examine placentas must make the appropriate observations at placental examination, as will soon be explained. They must also be familiar with the methodology that enables them to make a positive diagnosis of fetal blood loss, and they may then be in the position to add new knowledge about the mechanism of transplacental fetal bleeding from the detailed study of relevant cases.

Trauma

A very large retrospective study of trauma in pregnancy has been published by Kady et al. (2004). It enumerates the frequency of fractures to mother and fetus, suicides, fetal death, etc. in a California population from 1991 to 1999 and emphasizes the need to carefully evaluate falls in pregnancy. Fetal bleeding across the placenta occurs for many different known reasons, one of which that has been well substantiated is trauma to the placenta. In fact, **transplacental fetal bleeding** and **abruptio placentae** are the two major complications of severe trauma during pregnancy. It has been alleged that "blunt abdominal trauma during pregnancy occurs in 0.62 per 1000 deliveries, with 26% of such cases involving assault" (Rodgers et al., 1992). These authors presented such a case in which a conviction for negligent homicide was obtained. A 60-mL (46%) fetomaternal hemorrhage had occurred after the patient had been kicked in the abdomen. A complete overview of blunt trauma during pregnancy can be found in the review by Pearlman et al. (1990a). The same group of authors also undertook a prospective study of 85 women with trauma during pregnancy (Pearlman et al., 1990b). They found significantly more fetomaternal hemorrhages than in controls, especially when the placenta was located anterior in the uterus. Abruptio occurred also frequently and could not be predicted by the severity of the trauma. Dahmus and Sibai (1993), on the other hand, found in 233 hospitalizations for blunt trauma to the pregnant abdomen preterm delivery in 1%, fetal distress in 1.7%, and 2.6% of abruptio. In their experience, Kleihauer tests were not predictive of outcome, and Dhanraj and Lambers (2004) found positive Kleihauer tests to be as frequent in a control population. They suggested that "a positive KB [Kleihauer-Betke] test alone does not necessarily indicate pathologic fetal–maternal hemorrhage in patients with trauma." Williams et al. (1990) found that preterm labor was the principal sequela of trauma during pregnancy. They studied 84 relevant cases and observed abruptio and rupture of uterus but found no cases of delayed abruptio. Premature labor occurred in 28% of their cases, but there were no fetal injuries. Schultze et al. (1998) described fetal death from abruptio occurring despite deployment of an airbag in an automobile accident.

On the other hand, it has been substantiated that the fetus may sustain injuries, such as skull fracture, or that it may have significant brain damage, even after seemingly minor accidents (Anquist et al., 1994). The placenta itself may also actually rupture from various insults.

Buchsbaum (1968, 1979) and Crosby (1974) have competently reviewed the numerous descriptions from the literature. Buchsbaum pointed out that abruptio is only rarely caused by trauma (0.49% to 1.30%). Much more commonly it is the result of maternal vascular disease, appearing as a complication of preeclampsia. These studies must be consulted for a comprehensive overview of the topic; they are not restricted to physical trauma but include topics such as hypovolemia and sports injuries. Crosby emphatically stated that if abruptio from accidents leads to fetal demise, it usually occurs within 48 hours. Moreover, it was his opinion that a causal relation between trauma and fetal injury is often difficult to establish. Extreme care must be exercised, however, in being categorical in such judgments. Thus, a serious central nervous system (CNS) injury occurred to a 29-week fetus following a minor car accident that had even deployed an airbag (Karimi et al., 2004). Goodwin and Breen (1990) studied 205 patients with noncatastrophic trauma during pregnancy and found complications in 18 (8.8%). Premature labor was seen in 10, abruptio in five, fetal injury in one, and fetal death in two. Although fetal hemorrhage occurred significantly more commonly than in a control population, the authors opined that when no obstetric complications are evident, the quantitation of transplacental bleeding is unnecessary.

Amniocentesis is a frequently discussed topic when considering placental trauma, as transplacental hemorrhage not infrequently occurs after amniocentesis. It happens not only when amniocentesis is done for genetic diagnosis during the second trimester (Blajchman et al., 1974; Goodlin & Clewell, 1974; Young et al., 1977; Lele et al., 1982) but also near term, when it is done to determine fetal maturity or to evaluate the status of Rh disease (Zipursky et al., 1963a,b). With improved localization of the placenta by sonography, this hazard has diminished. Nevertheless, it remains an important complication that may lead to fetal exsanguination, stillbirth, and maternal immunization against fetal Rh antigens (Bowman & Pollock, 1985). Herrmann and Sidiropoulos (1986) found a 1.5% incidence of transplacental bleeding when amniocentesis was done in the second trimester (vide infra), whereas Bombard et al. (1995) reported that risk to the fetus is not greater when the placenta is transgressed during a tap. They found a 1.3% overall loss rate in 1000 procedures.

Examination of the placenta in such cases may be rewarding, as is shown in Chapter 12, Figure 12.37. In that patient, repeated amniocentesis for the assessment of fetal maturity in a diabetic patient had led to several disruptions of the fetal surface vessels; it eventually necessitated cesarean section because of fetal bleeding. Bleeding of the fetus may take place into the amnionic cavity or transplacentally into the mother. For its avoidance, the value of placental localization prior to amnio-

centesis has been well established. Pauls and Boutros (1970) localized the placenta with chromium-51–tagged red blood cells. They found that bleeding of the fetus occurred much more frequently when the placenta had not been localized (11% versus 0%). Ultrasonographic localization has achieved the same results but is more easily accomplished (Gottesfeld et al., 1966; Mennuti et al., 1983). Herrmann and Sidiropoulos (1986) evaluated their results in 209 Rh-negative women who came to amniocentesis during the second trimester. Significant hemorrhages occurred in three patients, that is, Kleihauer-positive findings of more than 2 per 100 cells in the maternal circulation. There was no correlation with anterior placentas and bloody amnionic fluid. It was the authors' opinion that the rarity of this occurrence, the ability to predict sensitization accurately with Kleihauer stains, and the use of prophylactic RhoGAM therapy have made amniocentesis a safe procedure.

A positive Kleihauer-Betke test (Kleihauer et al., 1957) quickly establishes the presence of fetal blood in the maternal circulation. Assessment of maternal serum α-fetoprotein (MSAFP) levels also reflecting fetal blood transfer, as done by Mennuti et al. (1983), is perhaps preferable. Lele et al. (1982) found this test to be more sensitive than the Kleihauer technique. For example, when maternal/fetal major blood group incompatibilities exist, the fetal red blood cells may quickly lyse in the mother's circulation, which causes misleading results in Kleihauer tests. Other studies also indicated that raised MSAFP levels often result from fetomaternal hemorrhage (Los et al., 1979; Christmas et al., 1994). Placental injury following amniocentesis has also been described by Goodlin and Clewell (1974). They found two defects in a large placental surface vein from which the fetus had exsanguinated into the amnionic cavity. Figure 17.1 shows the placenta of a stillborn fetus at 30 weeks. This fetus was transfused 4 days before delivery as therapy for Rh

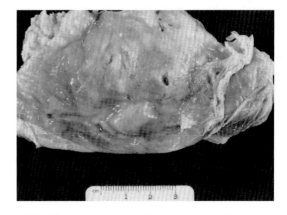

FIGURE 17.1. Fetal surface of a placenta from a 30–week gestation with three holes through which exsanguination occurred. The fetus had been transfused 4 days earlier. There were many hemosiderin-laden macrophages in the chorion and amnion that obscure the vascular architecture.

disease. Three large defects (holes) were found on the fetal surface. Exsanguination had thus occurred. The placenta had a posterior (!) uterine location; hemosiderin macrophages were located near the sites of injury. Retromembranous hematomas have also been identified following amniocentesis, a complication that is discussed in Chapter 11.

Fetal bleeding into the mother often occurs during **therapeutic abortion**, even in early pregnancy (Voigt & Britt, 1969; Walsh & Lewis, 1970; Lakoff et al., 1971; Leong et al., 1979). Because there is complete disruption of the placenta, the bleeding is not surprising. Curettage for abortion of Rh-negative women is thus now routinely followed by prophylactic RhoGAM therapy. Warren et al. (1985), in a study of 161 chorionic villus sampling (CVS) procedures, found that fetomaternal hemorrhage occurred as often as in 49%. They found all Kleihauer-test evaluations to be negative and therefore judged this procedure to be too insensitive. Positive results were obtained by measuring α-fetoprotein levels in maternal blood before and after the curettage. Los et al. (1993) observed the first case of fetal demise following transabdominal CVS, occurring 1 week after the procedure, while Pozniak et al. (1988) observed rapid retromembranous bleeding during CVS from "venous lakes." However, it was apparently composed of maternal blood. Litwak et al. (1970) reported that 32% of patients with spontaneous abortion had fetal bleeding. More surprising is that 11% of women with threatened abortion before 20 weeks' gestation had a positive Kleihauer test, as opposed to 4% of the controls (Stein et al., 1992). Fernandez-Rocha and Oullette (1976) depicted the placenta in a fetal hemorrhage, produced by insertion of a pressure catheter. In an effort to secure fetal monitoring, the catheter was introduced with a stiff guide. The amnionic cavity contained much blood and the fetal surface had disrupted vessels and contained a hematoma.

That the placenta bleeds into the mother during labor and delivery has long been recognized (Lloyd et al., 1980), and it is the reason for prophylactic, passive immunization with RhoGAM. In 14.5% of the patients reported by Lloyd et al., fetal cells were recognized in postpartum maternal blood; in 1% of deliveries a larger hemorrhage was diagnosed. Manual removal of the placenta was even more disruptive.

Doolittle (1963) studied placentas after delivery to identify the nature of the fetal vascular disruptions. He first cannulated the umbilical veins during labor and then measured pressures of 30 to 60 mm Hg, which increased to 90 to 115 mm Hg just prior to extrusion of the placenta. The cannulated placentas were then insufflated with air under water while the pressures exerted were recorded. In 23% of these placentas, air leaks were identified, usually near the chorionic surface. Pressures of up to 300 mm Hg did not burst the villous circulation within intact vessels. Doolittle opined that traction on the cord was a probable mechanism of the frequent placental disruption that leads to fetal bleeding. He suggested that most such bleeding would be prevented by opening the cord clamp before extrusion of the placenta. This measure, in his experience, allowed an average of 70 mL of fetal blood to escape.

Cesarean section may also allow fetal bleeding to occur from the placenta. This fact was recognized as early as 1888 according to Smith and Benjamin (1968). Feldman and her collaborators (1990) found that in 18% of patients undergoing cesarean section some fetal hemorrhage occurred, with 2.5% losing more than 30 mL of blood. They discussed at some length the possible mechanism of this bleeding and could exclude that blood loss occurred during manual separation of the placenta. Alternatively, since Pilkington et al. (1966) had identified fetal bleeding **before** cesarean section, the possibility remains that the clinical reasons for the section are in part responsible for the hemorrhage. The important aspect of this study is to recognize that a single dose of RhoGAM may not suffice for immunoprophylaxis after cesarean section.

Pollack (1968) first found that external fetal version, done for breech presentation, may injure the placenta with fetal bleeding into the mother. This report described a pregnancy at 35 weeks' gestation in which the patient experienced hemoglobinuria 4 hours after version. The placenta showed "a small area of separation." This cause of fetal bleeding is an infrequent but serious event. To prevent the risk of exsanguination, external fetal rotation is now commonly followed by fetal monitoring and Kleihauer studies. Gjode et al. (1980) found that, in the first attempt of version, which they investigated in 50 women, 28% had fetal hemorrhage of between 0.1 and 1.5 mL. In Rh-negative women, therefore, prophylaxis is needed. A fatal case of transplacental bleeding after fetal version was described by Luyet et al. (1976). In a case of "spontaneous" massive fetomaternal hemorrhage with a meconium-stained but otherwise normal placenta, the fetus developed extensive infarctions of various organs (Naeye et al., 1964).

Buchsbaum and Staples (1985) reported two patients with self-inflicted **gunshot injuries** that caused fetal death, and they reviewed many other similar cases. The placenta was not described in this report but, in Buchsbaum's extensive summary of 1968, several placental injuries from gunshot wounds were cited. Awwad et al. (1994) reviewed 14 cases of penetrating wounds of the pregnant uterus. Two women died and one half of the fetuses were stillborn. Fetal fractures were witnessed; abruptio placentae and placental tears were also seen. Overstreet et al. (2002) described a gunshot wound in a 27-week pregnancy that led to surgery within 2 hours. The 1000-g fetus suffered wounds with humerus fracture that proved nonfatal; the placenta was not injured. Interestingly, there were two old hematomas with hemosiderin deposits in the membranes from former spouse abuse.

Automobile accidents are now the commonest cause of traumatic transplacental hemorrhages. Skull fractures, fetal death, and vaginal bleeding were reviewed with a case reported by Theurer and Kaiser (1963), but the placenta of that case was not discussed. In a case of apparently minor trauma sustained in an automobile accident reported by Anquist et al. (1994) that resulted in severe cerebral damage, the placenta was reported only as being small and diffusely calcified. Brill (1995) took exception to this interpretation, saying it was unproven. Abruptio placentae and uterine disruption led to fetal death in a case reported by Eaton and Danzinger (1967). Exsanguination into the amnionic sac from a complete radial tear of the placenta occurred in the case of Peyser and Toaff (1969). We have documented another case of blunt trauma received in an automobile accident during the 34th week of a normal pregnancy (Benirschke & Gille, 1977). Fetal heart tones were absent 3 hours after the accident. The uterus and spleen were lacerated, and the placenta had a 50% retroplacental hematoma with early infarction 2 days after the accident. Figure 17.2 shows a relevant case. This term pregnancy eventuated in the precipitous birth of a stillborn infant with cardiac arrest and intraventricular hemorrhage. A 7-cm fresh retroplacental hematoma was found that had compressed a large portion of placenta, causing it to be acutely infarcted. The mother had worn a seat belt.

Crosby and Costiloe (1971) found that pregnant women who are involved in car accidents have a high fetal loss. Separation of the placenta was found to be the most common cause of fetal death when the mother lived. Fetal death was commonest in car accidents as a result of maternal demise. The question of the efficacy of wearing seat belts to avoid possible uterine injury was also answered in this study of Crosby and Costiloe. They concluded that, despite occasional fetal loss from abruptio,

seat belts should be worn by pregnant mothers. Crosby (1968) had earlier found that abortion occurred in 20% of patients pregnant 20 weeks or less when they were in automobile accidents. Pearlman and Phillips (1996) found that only one third of women use seat belts or wear them incorrectly during pregnancy. In unselected cases of car accidents, fetal loss was 25%, but 50% of these were due to maternal death. In an apparently trivial car accident near term, suffered by a patient described by Cumming and Wren (1978), multiple fetal surface placental hemorrhages were identified, and fetal skull fracture led to fetal death. Larroche (1986) has provided evidence of a relation between car accidents and prenatal encephaloclastic lesions. A 75% placental abruptio, with a surviving immature infant, occurred in a pregnancy in which a delayed retroplacental hemorrhage had developed. The patient had not worn a seat belt and suffered a steering wheel injury to the abdomen (Lavin & Miodovnik, 1981). Delayed abruptio was also reported by Higgins and Garite (1984). It occurred 5 days after an automobile accident, and there was old, clotted blood behind the placenta. Kettel et al. (1988) reported varying amounts of abruption in three patients who were in car accidents. Crosby (1974) had opined that abruptio following trauma usually leads to fetal demise within 48 hours or not at all. Parida et al. (1999) reported bowel injury in two fetuses following car accidents. Regrettably, as in most case reports, the placentas were not described, but many additional cases were cited by these authors.

Murray (1964) described a patient with fetal death, who delivered 6 hours after a car accident and where the mother suffered severe fibrinogenopenia, presumably from consumption coagulopathy. Because defibrination with disseminated intravascular coagulation is often a sequela of eclampsia, and hypotheses relating the two have been formed, it is relevant to emphasize that this patient had no evidence of preeclampsia. She was a gravida 14 without hypertension. Chibber et al. (1984) have docu-

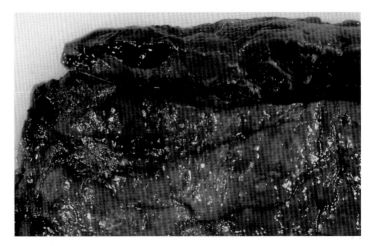

FIGURE 17.2. Retroplacental hematoma after an automobile accident at term. The infant was stillborn with intraventricular hemorrhage. The placental area of abruptio is depressed and there is early infarction. See text.

mented that inapparent placental injury during a car accident may lead to transplacental bleeding with rhesus immunization. The placenta of their case was not described. In a woman who delivered a 2100-g infant, a transplacental hemorrhage of 42% estimated blood volume occurred after a car accident; despite this bleeding, Bickers and Wennberg (1983) judged the placenta to be normal, grossly and microscopically. Stafford et al. (1988) described eight cases of fetal death following automobile accidents; they found four abruptios, three placentas with severe infarction, and miscellaneous lacerations. Umbilical thrombosis was present in one fetus. Cardwell and Snyder (1989), in reply, drew attention to the perhaps more important aspect of transplacental hemorrhage in such cases. A patient with whom we are familiar had a car accident with immediate cessation of fetal movements. The patient received a blow to the right abdomen, whereupon she noted the fetus to have shifted to the left. She was admitted to the hospital 12 hours later, where fetal monitoring recorded a sudden drop of heart rate. An emergency cesarean section was performed 6 hours after the accident. The 7 months' gestation fetus was stillborn, and a small laceration of uterus and placental contusions were noted. No abruptio was found, and there was no blood in the amnionic sac. Portions of the placenta were dark (Fig. 17.3). The mother had been wearing a lap belt and cross-chest seat belt. This fetus clearly exsanguinated into the mother, as the Kleihauer stain yielded 2.05% of fetal red blood cells in the maternal circulation, representing 60 to 75 mL of fetal blood; his hematocrit was 36%.

The nature of placental injury that may lead to transplacental bleeding in car accidents is depicted in Figure 17.4. This patient had an automobile accident at 33 weeks'

gestation; she was admitted and was found to have normal fetal heart tones. She was then discharged, but precipitous labor ensued and she delivered 14 hours after the accident. The infant's depressed Apgar scores (5/5), subsequent stormy course, and intraventricular hemorrhage presumably stemmed from the acute anemia (hemoglobin 8 g/dL, hematocrit 24%). Some nucleated red blood cells in the fetal circulation indicated the fetal response to anemia. There was a large bruise of villous tissue with focal massive intravillous hemorrhage. In addition, an intervillous hematoma and small laceration of the placenta were found. If Kleihauer studies had been done shortly after the accident, they would have forewarned the treating physician of the fetal blood loss. Low and his colleagues (1996) also saw a patient with blunt trauma from a car accident and delivered the child 2 hours later. Her hematocrit was 30%, Kleihauer-Betke 12%, retroplacental hematoma. The neonate died at 28 hours with extensive CNS damage.

Fetal hemorrhage occurred in 28% of patients who experienced **other types of abdominal trauma**, such as falling. Rose et al. (1985) reviewed this subject in one of the few reports with case controls. The extent of bleeding (average volume 16 mL) was not related to the nature of the trauma or to the gestational age. Fort and Harlin (1970) produced similar figures and discussed the poor fetal prognosis of such trauma. When reading these various reports, one is impressed by the frequency with which relatively minor trauma can cause fetal transplacental hemorrhage. "Spontaneous" hemorrhage also occurs. We have always believed that such spontaneous hemorrhages may result from trauma to the placenta inflicted by the fetus, such as by kicking. This assumption

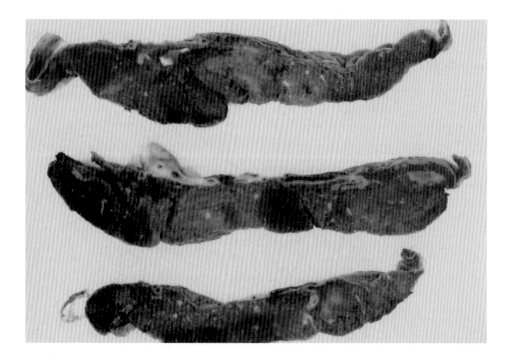

FIGURE 17.3. Placenta at 37 weeks after an automobile accident 6 hours earlier, with fetal death from exsanguination. Note the dark, hemorrhagic areas of the villous tissue that had intravillous hemorrhages. Bleeding into the decidua basalis had also occurred, although there was no abruptio. Fetal hematocrit was 36%. (Courtesy of Dr. D.J. Carlson, Exeter, New Hampshire.)

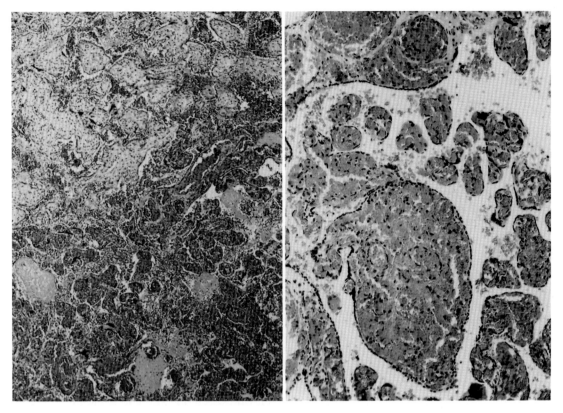

FIGURE 17.4. Massive, focal villous hemorrhage ("bruise") in an immature placenta 14 hours after an automobile accident. The mother had been discharged, but fetal hemorrhage into the mother led to severe, disabling anemia. H&E ×40 (left); ×160 (right).

was strengthened when Eden (1987) reported two cases of maternal vaginal bleeding during pregnancy, associated with severe pain that was caused by fetal movements. Upon sonographic study, it became apparent that the fetus was "punching" the area of the placenta from which (marginal) bleeding occurred. Rare cases of umbilical cord hemorrhage and laceration, following trauma, have been summarized by Buchsbaum (1968). The management of trauma during pregnancy has been detailed by Higgins (1988).

Quintero et al. (1993) have searched for fetal trauma by embryoscopy. They found hemorrhagic lesions of the fetus, especially of the skull, in 30% of cases during CVS. Thrombi were not seen. Shulman and colleagues (1990) felt that it was the amount of villous tissue sampled, rather than the method employed, that correlated with the extent of fetal—maternal bleeding during CVS. Unfortunately, in most cases the cause of spontaneous transplacental hemorrhage remains obscure. Punching or turning by the fetus may injure the placenta, much as the placenta is occasionally injured with external version of a fetus in breech presentation. We have seen a stillbirth in a near-term pregnancy that was complicated by sudden maternal hemoglobinuria. A Kleihauer-Betke stain was done and 15 mL of fetal blood were detected in the maternal circulation. The baby died shortly thereafter. It was blood group A+, and the mother was O Rh-negative. The placenta was very pale and had several intervillous thromboses but no other lesions to account for the transplacental hemorrhage.

Other causes of transplacental hemorrhage include placental disease, such as chorangioma, choriocarcinoma in situ (placental choriocarcinoma), placenta previa, and abruptio placentae. Perhaps other conditions exist that need yet to be identified. Huff (1988) found that "fetal" (placental) bleeding occurred more often after cesarean section when the placenta had not been "drained" of fetal blood from the cord. Parenthetically it should be mentioned that occasionally fetal brain may be deported to the placental vasculature (Baergen et al., 1997). In this, and rare other cases described, head trauma was presumably incurred during forceps delivery and embolic brain tissue was also found in the fetal lung. More often such deportation has been seen in fetal lung sections, but Silver and Newman (1998) reported cerebellar embolism to placental vessels with a surviving normal infant. There had been a skull fracture. Other causes are discussed with four cases, especially relative to alloimmunization by Zizka et al. (2001), but the publication is difficult to access.

Placenta in Hemorrhage

One should suspect transplacental bleeding when the villous tissue of the placenta is unusually pale. This observation presupposes that the examiner is familiar with the "normal" color of the placental tissue at the different stages of gestation. Immature placentas are paler than are those at term. The presence of intervillous thrombi may be another clue signaling that bleeding through the placenta has occurred; the thrombi may even signify the point of origin of hemorrhage and should be noted for that reason. The temporal aspects of the development of fetal anemia from transplacental hemorrhage are usually not known. One might think that a given hematocrit and hemoglobin value of the newborn should give detailed information as to the precise time when the hemorrhage took place. This is, unfortunately, not true, as specific studies to ascertain the decrease of hematocrit have not been made. It would be desirable to collect information in cases where the timing is well known (from trauma) and the amount estimated (from Kleihauer stains), in order to estimate just how long it takes to reduce the hematocrit to a given level. This would aid in assessing doubtful cases, some of which end in litigation. When placental or neonatal anemia are apparent, the maternal blood must be studied promptly for the possible presence of fetal red blood cells, and perhaps also for α-fetoprotein levels.

Another concern is how rapid the response of red cell replacement is when blood is lost. It is known that **nucleated red blood cells** (NRBCs) appear in the circulation of anemic fetuses, best exemplified by erythroblastosis fetalis. The same happens when acute blood loss occurs and when fetuses are hypoxic. This feature plays an important role in current medicolegal decisions. What we need to know is how rapid the response of the appearance of NRBCs is to the loss of red cells and hypoxia, and whether this response is quantitatively reflected in the number of the NRBCs in the circulation. Considerable confusion exists as to the number of NRBCs in the neonatal circulation. It is our opinion that in the histologic evaluation of placentas NRBCs should not be observed in the term placenta. When NRBCs are present in the fetal blood, and it is obviously important that they be diagnosed correctly, it is a distinctly abnormal finding. The pathologist should then try to find the reason for their presence. Geissler and Japha (1901) stated emphatically that, "contrary to the dogma," NRBCs are not found in young children. Ryerson and Sanes (1934) undertook incisive studies of NRBCs in placentas. They attempted to ascertain the parameters that allowed one to decide the age of gestation histologically. All NRBCs had disappeared at the end of the third month of pregnancy, and if more than 1% NRBC are found, this indicated to them immaturity. Fox (1967) also published on this phenome-non and related NRBCs to hypoxia or asphyxia. We concur with the interpretation of a relationship to fetal tissue hypoxia; indeed, it is our practice to take note of the presence of NRBCs when examining placentas. Green and Mimouni provided criteria and suggested that "a value $> 1 \times 10^9$/L. should be considered as a potential index of intrauterine hypoxia." Normally, there were no NRBCs in term neonates, and the 95th percentile had 1.7 in absolute counts. Diabetic mothers' babies had increased numbers, as did infants with hypoxia and growth-retarded neonates. Shurin (1987) concluded that there are about 200 to 600 NRBCs/mm^3 and 10,000 to 30,000 WBCs; she also stated that the normal infant has 4% to 5% of NRBCs in cord blood samples, which is higher than is our experience. Shurin reflected that this number indicates the erythroid hyperplasia due to high levels of erythropoietin (EPO) production. In general, it is our belief that because of the complex sequence of signals to initiate erythropoiesis and release of NRBCs, many hours have to pass from a hypoxic (anemic) stimulus to the appearance of NRBCs in the circulation. Thus, the identification of NRBCs suggests a significant fetal problem many hours prior to birth. Quantitative and temporal sequences must be obtained in future studies, and two relevant cases that provide some guide are discussed in Chapter 26. Shields et al. (1993), in the laboratory of R.A. Brace, have reviewed what is known of this aspect of red cells restoration after hemorrhage in sheep. Despite an initial rise in EPO level, a significant hemorrhage (40%) is not followed by a significant increase in reticulocyte count, nor are the former blood volume and hematocrit restored before birth. In a later study, Shields et al. (1996) further showed the recovery from hemorrhage with an expanding red cells mass, elevation of reticulocytes and EPO, correlated with iron availability, but nucleated red cells were not addressed. Similar temporal findings as recorded here urgently need to be collected for human fetuses, as the ovine model may not be entirely adequate to understand the physiology of this important topic (see Chapter 8 for further information on nucleated red blood cells).

Jauniaux et al. (1990) have made an important clinicopathologic correlation in a case of significant fetal–maternal hemorrhage. They observed sonographically a 3×3 cm heterogeneic, hypoechoic placental lesion when, at 18 weeks' gestation, a pregnant patient was found to have elevated MSAFP levels. The Kleihauer test was positive. At 22 weeks there was only peripheral turbulent flow around the lesion, which, at about 30 weeks' gestation, was found to represent a laminated white lesion of fibrin. It was the presumed area of intervillous thrombosis whence the fetal hemorrhage occurred.

It should also be mentioned that intervillous thromboses are not necessarily due to fetal–maternal hemorrhages. When the bloods are compatible, agglutination may not take place. Conversely, intervillous hematomas may occur for entirely different reasons also. They can result when the intervillous perfusion is significantly altered, as for instance because of the presence of placental edema (erythroblastosis, Chapter 15; hydatidiform moles, Chapter 22), and also for local, structural reasons. This type of intervillous thrombosis is considered in greater detail in Chapter 9.

TECHNIQUE FOR IDENTIFICATION OF FETAL RED BLOOD CELLS

Fetal red blood cells in the maternal blood are best identified with a technique named after the inventors, Kleihauer and Betke (Kleihauer et al., 1957). Since that seminal contribution, the original method has undergone many refinements. Moreover, there are several commercial kits available for the detection of fetal cells in the maternal circulation (e.g., Boehringer Mannheim; Simmler, St. Louis, MO; Fetaldex of Ortho Diagnostics, Raritan, NJ; Sure-tech Diagnostics Associates, Inc. St. Louis [ST 101-C], and others). Some of these were mentioned by Virgilio and Simon (1977), who evaluated several different methods. Simon et al. (1978) used two techniques to evaluate the risk of fetal bleeding in 200 Rh-negative women. Six women experienced significant fetal hemorrhages that necessitated RhoGAM administration. The Fetaldex and Kleihauer techniques compared favorably in the assessment. For the purposes of rapidly identifying mothers in need of RhoGAM immunoprophylaxis, Nance and her colleagues (1989) have presented a flow cytometry methodology that is effective in identifying quickly and accurately the contamination with D+ cells in maternal blood. The use of flow cytometry has now frequently been preferred to the more cumbersome enumeration of red cells in blood smears. It compares favorably with the older method as a detailed contribution by Pelikan et al. (2004) has shown.

The Kleihauer-Betke technique depends on the fact that fetal hemoglobin, in an acid milieu of a pH 3, is less soluble than maternal (adult) hemoglobin. For its execution, air-dried maternal blood films are first fixed in 80% alcohol for 5 minutes and then eluted in one of several possible buffers for 7 to 10 minutes. Usually, the buffer is freshly made from 0.2M Na_2PO_4 and 0.1M citric acid. The slides are rinsed twice with water, stained for 10 minutes in hematoxylin solution, rinsed, and covered with a 1% eosin solution (or a similar dye) for 10 minutes. They are then rinsed in water and air dried. Palliez et al. (1970) suc-

cessfully used 1% safranin and a 1:20 dilution of Ziehl fuchsin. Fetal red blood cells maintain their color but, because the maternal hemoglobin is largely eluted, the maternal cells appear as mere shadows (Fig. 17.5). From counts at 250× magnification of 10 fields of these respective cell populations, the quantity of fetal blood loss can be estimated as follows: If the total number of fetal red cells counted is 25 among 4000 maternal red blood cells, the ratio would be 0.006. Total maternal blood volume (RBC + plasma) at term is approximately 5000 mL. One can thus calculate:

$$\frac{\text{Fetal red blood cells [25]}}{\text{Maternal red blood cells [4000]}} = \frac{X \text{ (mL fetal blood in maternal circulation) [in this case 30m]}}{\text{Maternal blood volume [about 5000 mL at term]}}$$

Mollison (1972) also suggested a formula that simplified for him the estimation of fetal blood loss. In this careful survey of stains, executed under standard conditions by various laboratories, Mollison emphasized that any enumeration of the fetal (stained) cells alone underestimates the fetal blood loss, since only 90% of fetal cells stain positively; the remainder already possesses hemoglobin A. He recommended a standardized approach to the estimation of fetal blood loss, as otherwise large errors would invalidate the results. The method of enumeration used by Kleihauer, for instance, would underestimate the amount of fetal blood lost. Mollison suggested that five fields be counted under low power and compared with an appropriate reference slide. If more than 10 darkly stained cells are found in a field, then a quantitative analysis was recommended. Grobbelaar (1968) also quantitated the red cell contamination of maternal blood and recommended that 50 mm^2 of blood film be scanned, and that reports give the precise methodology of enumeration; it is recommended lest the results not be interpretable. In a thoughtful review of the results of 523 Kleihauer-Betke procedures done in their institution, Emery et al. (1995) evaluated its usefulness. They suggested that a prevailing opinion exists that this test may have little value for clinical management but concluded that the test should be performed when a positive screening test exists in Rh-negative women with Rh-positive fetuses and in trauma cases. Unexplained increased maternal α-fetoprotein levels, fetal distress with abnormal heart tracings, fetal demise, and unexplained fetal anemia constituted other recommended applications of the technique, whereas abruptio placentae was not a condition for which the Kleihauer reaction

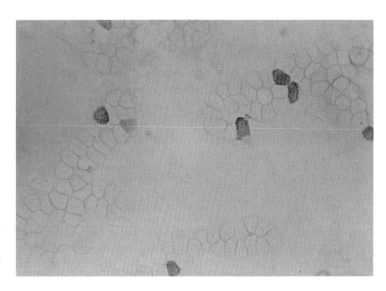

FIGURE 17.5. Kleihauer stain of maternal blood. The darkly stained cells are fetal erythrocytes. The percentage of fetal cells in this blood film is approximately 5%. Eosin stain; Kleihauer preparation ×1000.

was found to be of benefit. In another study, Veyver et al. (1993) also ascertained that Kleihauer tests were useful for ascertainment of fetal hemorrhage in trauma cases but that the clinical therapeutic decision had usually been made by the time the test result was known. In England, Kleihauer tests were done after delivery of every RhD-negative woman gives birth to an RhD-positive infant. To evaluate the efficacy of various techniques, Bromilow and Duguid (1997) compared three types of Kleihauer tests and two flow cytometry techniques. Although considerable differences were found, a simple stain was judged to be helpful; flow cytometry, however, was most efficient for quantitative assessment of the hemorrhage.

Zipursky et al. (1959) found that 21% of postpartum patients had fetal cells in the circulation, but other authors have found that a much greater percentage of postpartum women has fetal red cell contamination (McLarey & Fish, 1966; Sullivan & Jennings, 1966). Fraser and Raper (1962) made the important observation that ABO-incompatible cells disappear much more rapidly than do compatible cells. Their finding was affirmed later by the results of a study by Palliez et al. (1970). Indeed, Zilliacus (1963) found occasional agglutinated and partially disintegrated packets of fetal cells in maternal blood in women who had experienced transplacental hemorrhage from the fetus. An important study of fetal blood transfer to the mother comes from Owen et al. (1989). These investigators undertook a prospective analysis of Kleihauer stains before and after normal delivery in 66 patients. They found that "three patients (4.6%) had a massive fetomaternal hemorrhage. None of the postdelivery stains showed evidence of a significant fetomaternal hemorrhage unless results of the antepartum stain had also been positive. We conclude that the delivery process itself does not stimulate a massive fetomaternal hemorrhage in cases of fetal death." Massive fetal hemorrhage occurring in three women presented as decreased fetal movements, nonreactive fetal heart rates, and positive Kleihauer tests (Kosasa et al., 1993). This led the authors to recommend immediate delivery for such pregnancies. The cause of the hemorrhage remained unknown.

Some authors have doubted that the Kleihauer test truly evaluates fetal cells in the maternal circulation. This aspect was studied, and the techniques verified, by the large investigation undertaken by Freese and Titel (1963). They made some modification of the Kleihauer technique and reviewed improvements of methods from other authors that they collected from the literature. As with other investigators, these authors found a high incidence of fetal blood contamination in postpartum maternal circulating blood, and they established a quantitative relationship of this contamination to the ABO status of mother and infant. When the mother was blood group O and the fetus A, B, or AB, then the fetal cells disappeared more rapidly from the maternal blood. Other authors have demonstrated frequent but small "leaks" of fetal blood; they have also made modifications of the technique (Lewi et al., 1961; Browne & Cowles, 1963; Keenan & Pearse, 1963; Fielding, 1968). Virgilio and Simon (1977) provided a quantitative assessment of the number of red cells and compared commercial kits with the original method. Two reports specifically evaluated the methods that enumerate very small numbers of contaminating fetal red cells. Thus, Schneider and Ludwig (1963) showed that they were able to quantitate fetal blood volumes of between $50\,mm^3$ and 50 mL in the maternal circulation with the Kleihauer technique. Jones (1969) described a simple "machine" that obtains comparably thin blood films for the better quantitation of fetal blood loss. Stonehill and LaFerla (1986) emphasized that in 25% of pregnancies, from 10 to 28 weeks' gestation, the maternal blood contains increasing amounts of fetal hemoglobin, a finding originally emphasized as a possible cause of erroneous Kleihauer tests by Pembrey et al. (1973). During that gestational period, maternal cells with fetal hemoglobin should not be confused with fetal cells. Woodrow and Finn (1966) also studied the staining reaction of red cells in pregnant and nonpregnant women. They concluded that, because of occasional staining of cells in nonpregnant women, only findings of more than two cells per 50 low-power fields are of significance. They found

no increased transplacental bleeding in the third trimester, and suggested that most cases of Rh-isoimmunization take place during labor. Finally, Leiberman et al. (1989) also noted that 25% of pregnant women produce hemoglobin F. Other interfering factors are the prevalence of -thalassemia minor, which occurs in 1.4% of African Americans, and the fact that 1.7% of white Americans may have increased numbers of hemoglobin F containing red blood cells. These findings make it mandatory that elevated Kleihauer results be carefully evaluated. They have also suggested the use of the more sensitive measurement of α-fetoprotein for an evaluation of cases with presumed transplacental bleeding. The possible confusion here, in cases of fetal anomalies that may be another cause of elevated α-fetoprotein levels, is obvious.

That errors in assessment of transplacental bleeding occur was shown in a case described by LaFerla et al. (1981) and these errors are the reason why the authors recommended that the Kleihauer test be supported with findings from other tests. These other techniques, however, have fully validated the concept of transplacental bleeding. This is true for the test developed by Ness (1982), an enzyme-linked antiglobulin reaction, which can also be useful for evaluation of the potential recipients of Rh-immune globulin. Tomoda (1964) demonstrated that fluorescent antibodies against fetal hemoglobin can be employed to enumerate the fetal cells in the maternal circulation. Streiff et al. (1964) used a variety of techniques to demonstrate fetal cells in the maternal system; Zilliacus et al. (1975) found that fluorescent-Y chromosome stains often showed fetal (male) lymphocytes in pregnant mothers' blood; and Lee and Vazquez (1962) showed that fluorescent antibodies against the A and B blood groups stained appropriately marked fetal cells in maternal blood with blood group O. Thus, the warning issued by Stonehill and La Ferla (1986) may have been too cautious. It is imperative that the quantity of fetal cells be assessed accurately for the judgment of quantities of antiglobulin administration in rhesus-negative mothers (Eich & Tripoldi, 1974).

The transfer of fetal cells into the maternal circulation has taken on greater importance with the recognition that the fetal karyotype may be ascertained from the study of DNA of fetal NRBCs lifted from the maternal circulation. A symposium publication reviewed the principal mechanisms and results (Simpson & Elias, 1994). Aside from NRBCs, maternal blood has long been known to contain syncytial cells, swept from the placenta to the maternal lung. The process is described in detail in Chapter 19. Studies suggest that some of these cells may escape pulmonary entrapment and serve as possible precursors for DNA amplification (Hawes et al., 1994). Gänshirt-Ahlert et al. (1992b) showed that umbilical vein blood contained the same ratio of fetal/maternal DNA as did peripheral maternal blood, paving the way for further fetal DNA study. Elegant techniques have since been devised for the enrichment and study of this fetal DNA from maternal blood, relying principally on NRBCs, as they will not be perpetuated into future pregnancies, as lymphocytes might be (Adkinson et al., 1994; Bianchi et al., 1994, and many others). The survival of fetal cells into adult life is now being considered as possible basis of systemic sclerosis (scleroderma) (see Chapter 19). The rate of disappearance of fetal NRBCs from the maternal circulation was documented by Hamada et al. (1995). Three months after delivery, NRBCs would have disappeared, even after fetomaternal hemorrhage.

The life span of fetal cells in the maternal circulation has been studied by Kleihauer and Brandt (1964). It is often stated that fetal red blood cells have a decreased longevity, but these authors determined that fetal cells can be maintained for a long time in the maternal circulation. Although the life span of fetal cells in the maternal circulation is somewhat shorter than that of normal cells, the cause of neonatal anemia from transplacental bleeding may be ascertained for as long as 4 to 6 weeks after delivery, by Kleihauer tests alone, so long as no ABO incompatibility exists. Fetal red blood cells can also be identified in amnionic fluid and vaginal blood with the aforementioned techniques (e.g., in cases of presumed placenta previa).

Occasional failure to identify fetal red blood cells by the Kleihauer technique, in cases that strongly suggest their presence, has led to the development of alternate methods. Thus, failing to identify fetal cells in blood-stained amnionic fluid in a patient with elevated α-fetoprotein levels, led Ahmed and Brown (1986) to perform hemoglobin electrophoresis; they thereby identified predominantly fetal hemoglobin. Chamberlain et al. (1982) compared the results from Kleihauer stains with α-fetoprotein levels. They found that the latter method gave more accurate results. In this connection, the **Apt test** is occasionally mentioned, without there generally being a clear understanding of the usefulness of this test. The Apt-Downey test was primarily designed to differentiate between fetal and maternal blood in the stomachs of newborns; it has also been used for the examination of vaginal blood. Apt and Downey (1955) first described the method to allow a rapid determination of the origin of blood in stool of neonates (melena). The method is generally less satisfactory than the others mentioned for distinguishing fetal red blood cells from maternal cells. The procedure depends on alkali-denaturation of hemoglobin. Crissinger et al. (1987) described it as follows: "Specimen is mixed with tap water (1 part of hemorrhagic fluid to 5 parts water), centrifuged, and 1 mL of 0.25 M sodium hydroxide is added to 5 mL of the supernatant. Brown-yellow color indicates adult hemoglobin, and pink indicates fetal hemoglobin."

Another method for the identification of fetal red blood cells was employed by Kaplan et al. (1982). These investigators were interested in ascertaining whether placental intervillous thrombi (IVT) are composed of fetal or maternal erythrocytes. Potter (1948) had earlier assumed them to be made up of mainly maternal cells. She based her deduction on macroagglutination findings with differing ABO blood groups of mother and fetus. Cells that were presumably NRBCs were interpreted as lymphocytes. Javert and Reiss (1952) had shown that the so-called red infarcts of earlier nomenclature were intervillous coagulation events. Because they found in 48.7% of these thrombi NRBCs, they discouraged the use of the term *intervillous thrombus*. Kaplan et al. (1982) used Sternberger's technique of peroxidase labeling to study histologic sections with intervillous coagulation. They found that over 85% of intervillous thrombi contained irregularly distributed fetal erythrocytes (Fig. 17.6). Often, they were present in large numbers, and the authors deduced from these findings that intervillous thrombi may be one entry point for fetal cells into the maternal circulation. Devi et al. (1968) had previously established that a good correlation exists between the presence of fetal red blood cells in the maternal circulation and the number of intervillous thrombi.

Significant Transplacental Hemorrhage

The diagnosis of anemia in the newborn, due to occult hemorrhage, was first seriously considered by Wiener (1948). He had observed three newborns with low hemoglobin values, two of them being 6.5 and 8.7 g. One patient had been delivered by cesarean section for a placenta previa, one was born normally, and the third patient was an unusual case of erythroblastosis, a disease that was under intensive study at that time, and whose cause was then being defined. There was much interest in this new phenomenon of a putative transplacental passage of fetal blood to the mother. Wiener stated, "The main objection to this concept is the difficulty of demonstrating such postulated placental defects in pathologic specimens." He referred to the known hemorrhages from vasa previa, but found no good explanation for his observations of neonatal anemia. This "interesting and recent hypothesis" was discussed by Wickster (1952). He reviewed some cases of abruptio and placenta previa. He also presented the case of an unexplained fetal blood loss, enough to cause shock in the neonate, but recent enough not to have caused isoimmunization of the mother. Only after Chown's papers were published in 1954 and 1955 did wider interest develop in the topic of prenatal bleeding. Chown (1954) reported two cases of neonatal anemia. I (K.B.) examined the placentas and found intervillous thrombi, and noted also many NRBCs in the fetal circulation. A transfusion reaction had occurred in one mother; the other suffered "pain at 8 months gestation."

It is now widely recognized that significant fetomaternal hemorrhages may cause fetal anemia, even exsanguination, hydrops fetalis, maternal isoimmunization, and fetal cardiac rhythm irregularities, and that fetal death may result from it (Saber, 1977; Shahar et al., 1981; Laube

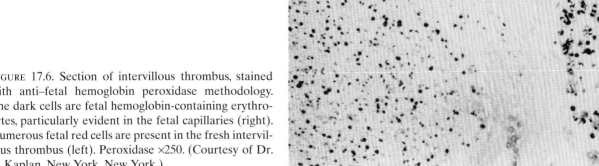

FIGURE 17.6. Section of intervillous thrombus, stained with anti–fetal hemoglobin peroxidase methodology. The dark cells are fetal hemoglobin-containing erythrocytes, particularly evident in the fetal capillaries (right). Numerous fetal red cells are present in the fresh intervillous thrombus (left). Peroxidase ×250. (Courtesy of Dr. C. Kaplan, New York, New York.)

& Schauberger, 1982; Fay, 1983; Almeida & Bowman, 1994). Indeed, there is a report of a patient who had at least three consecutive pregnancies complicated by this event, without explanation for the recurrence of their significant transplacental hemorrhage (Catalano & Capeless, 1990). It is also not an uncommon cause of fetal demise. Biankin et al. (2003) estimated that such significant fetomaternal hemorrhage occurs once in 2800 pregnancies. Samadi et al. (1996) surveyed their 319 cases of fetal demise (above 500 g weight) in which Kleihauer-Betke tests had been done. They found massive hemorrhage (more than 1% Kleihauer positive cells) in 4.7% of these stillborns. The neonate often displays significant morbidity; severe anemia and shock are common in the neonatal period (Moya et al., 1987; Li & Bromham, 1988; vide infra). It has also been reported that cerebral palsy has resulted from prenatal hemorrhage (Fay, 1983; Kirkendall et al., 2001) presumably due to acute hypotension, and neonatal death is frequent (Griffin, 1969; others). The documentation of fetal microcephaly following such an event is especially important. Del Valle and colleagues (1992) documented a fascinating event of this nature. The patient sustained a motor vehicle accident at 27 weeks with fetal distress ensuing. Kleihauer tests were negative but amniocentesis yielded bloody fluid, and cordocentesis disclosed a hematocrit of 17%. The fetus was transfused and a mature fetus delivered at 37 weeks. Its Apgar scores were 8/9 and the hematocrit 50%. There was a 25% infarction of the placenta that the authors believed to have been caused by a rupture of a fetal vessel at the time of the accident. It may well also have been the cause of hemorrhage and the CNS insult. Direct trauma to the fetus from stabbing at 29 weeks' gestation with CNS injury and bleeding was described by Avenarius et al. (1999). The frequency and magnitude of transplacental hemorrhage were well evaluated in a large study by Almeida and Bowman (1994). They stated in their comprehensive study that "there appear to be two important factors in clinical outcome: the amount of and rate of bleeding." Montgomery et al. (1995) identified 6% Kleihauer positive cells in the maternal circulation and a hydropic fetus with hematocrit of 16.4%. They transfused the fetus five times intraperitoneally and intravascularly over 24 days, and also supplied platelets. They delivered a healthy premature infant who needed no blood replacement. The cause of transplacental hemorrhage was not established and, except for hydropic changes, the placenta appeared normal. Interestingly, after the last transfusion, fever developed and gram-positive rods were observed at amniocentesis, leading to cesarean section delivery. Rijhsingani and Smith (1997) described a patient at 31 weeks' gestation following a severe rear-end collision. The fetus developed transient hydrops 2 days after the accident and the maternal blood contained 1.6% Kleihauer-positive cells (96 mL fetal blood). Also, clots

were found in the amnionic cavity. And abruptio was suspected, the fetus was delivered (hematocrit 27%) and did well. The placenta was not described. Pourbabak et al. (2004) emphasized that major transplacental hemorrhage may occur with the absence of clinical suspicion. While they described the identification of fetal red cells (Kleihauer, flow cytometry) of their three cases in some detail, they did not mention placental findings.

To make the precise diagnosis of fetal hemorrhage prenatally may be difficult in the clinical arena. Cardwell (1987) has reviewed this aspect and also provided management suggestions (see Leiberman et al., 1989). Similarly, Mor-Yosef and his colleagues (1984) considered the sinusoidal rhythm of fetal heart tracings as being the result of massive transplacental hemorrhage near term. The anemic neonate had a marked reticulocytosis and elevated globin synthesis; the cause may have been an exceedingly tightly entangled cord. Ellis and Kohler (1976) found marked thymic atrophy in these neonates at autopsy. The thymic atrophy certainly is not specific for hemorrhage, but is found in a wide variety of infants who have experienced prenatal "stress." It should be considered a result of adrenocorticotropic hormone (ACTH)-cortisol stimulation, as is also the maturation found in the fetal adrenal cortex. Following an initial review of the topic by Fynaut (1960), Renaer et al. (1976) gathered many of the reported cases of significant prenatal hemorrhage into a large review article. There were 11 cases of massive transplacental transfusion. The reviewers concluded that the incidence of transfer of blood increases with gestational age, and that it is as common as in 1 of 300 pregnancies. The phenomenon accounts for the fetal death in approximately 1:2,000 deliveries. Renaer et al. (1976) also observed one maternal transfusion reaction, and described a wide range of hematocrits and hemoglobin values of the newborns. Etiologic factors included cesarean section, external fetal version, amniocentesis, placement of a Drew-Smythe catheter, trauma, and tumultuous labor (see also Zipursky et al., 1963a,b; Finn et al., 1963). A catalogue of other associated or causative conditions, including the large number of European references, may be found in Rosta's review (1978).

Separate from the aforementioned literature, many other cases have been described in individual case reports. Gunson (1957) provided six such observations. Borum et al. (1957) reported two cases, one of which had a normal placenta, and in the other a cord that was wrapped twice around the neck. Perhaps the venous congestion from this obstruction caused the transplacental bleeding. Mannherz (1960) observed a neonatal RBC count of 2.05 million and 7.3% Kleihauer-positive cells in the maternal circulation. He estimated that, over time, the fetus must have lost 250 mL of blood. The placental surface was brownish and the villous tissue pale. Grimes and Wright (1961) reported an anemic, distressed newborn from an uncomplicated pregnancy. They drew attention to a case in which the mother suffered hemolysis, fibrinogenopenia, and acute renal tubular necrosis. In that case, there was an ABO incompatibility between mother and fetus. Donaldson (1962) found a recently stillborn, postmature baby who had died from transplacental hemorrhage and whose placenta had a large retroplacental hematoma. In this case, the retroplacental bleeding occurred in the absence of toxemia. Rudolph et al. (1962) had a fetal death in whose placenta an intervillous thrombus was locally accompanied by hemosiderin deposits. Paros (1962) described an anemic term infant in whom he estimated that 400 mL of fetal blood had been lost into the maternal circulation over a period of time. Willis and Foreman (1988) observed massive, chronic fetal bleeding with fetal cardiac irregularities and later, persistent late decelerations. The Kleihauer-Betke stains showed 14.5% fetal cells in the maternal circulation, an estimated 700 mL of fetal blood; the fetus had a hematocrit of 17%, hemoglobin of 5.1 g/dL, and was meconium-stained, but had a normal neonatal course. It must have bled over a prolonged time period. These authors reviewed several other cases not listed here, and found an essentially normal placenta in their case. No untoward events had been noted during the 38-week pregnancy. Rouse and Weiner (1990) saw the development of fetal hydrops and attempted treatment with serial transfusions. The placenta they found was large, but it had no characteristic lesions to explain the fetal hemorrhage. Other cases of significant fetal—maternal hemorrhage treated with repeated transfusion were reported by Fischer et al. (1990) and Lipitz et al. (1997). In the first case, a sinusoidal pattern of heart tracings was observed; the fetus's movements improved immediately after transfusions. The placenta had a subchorionic hematoma 2 cm from the cord insertion, perhaps from needle insertion. Thrombi were found in stem vessels of the placenta. The second case took place following blunt trauma from falling; bleeding had not occurred. The Kleihauer test yielded 3% to 5% of fetal cells in the maternal circulation (at 27 weeks!) and treatment with 30 mL packed red blood cells was performed. The fetus did well. Van Kamp et al. (2005) reviewed intrauterine transfusion results of 254 fetuses and found it to be a safe procedure. They had 89% survival.

Cohen et al. (1964) stated that the placenta rarely accomplishes a perfect separation of maternal from fetal blood streams, and estimated that 1% of pregnancies are complicated by significant fetal bleeding. Despite these repetitious reports in the literature, Keller et al. (1980) still considered this entity to be a frequently overlooked cause of perinatal morbidity and mortality. They reported on five cases with two deaths, and one of the infants had cerebral infarcts at birth. Schellong (1969), who discussed the causes and therapy of neonatal anemia, felt that

transfusion of the neonate is indicated only when the observed neonatal hemoglobin value falls below 8% to 10% of normal. Shiller (1957) observed shock in an anemic neonate whose placenta had a retroplacental blood clot. He drew attention to the presence of many NRBCs in the fetal circulation, in a maternal vein, and in the intervillous space. Because of the known risk factors for transplacental bleeding (cesarean section, trauma, etc.), Ness et al. (1987) prospectively studied a cohort of D-negative women for fetal hemorrhage and isoimmunization. The investigators were unable to predict reliably the occurrence of such hemorrhage, nor were they able to use historical events from the patient to form a basis for the administration of prophylactic antibodies (RhoGAM). Fliegner et al. (1987) also felt that occult fetomaternal hemorrhage was an important cause of fetal mortality and morbidity that should be investigated in otherwise unexplained stillbirths.

Fetal Consequences of Massive Hemorrhage Across the Placenta

Severe fetal anemia is a prominent sequela of transplacental hemorrhage. A cross section of the placenta from such a case is shown in Figure 17.7. The villous tissue is unusually thick and pale, and one large, fresh intervillous hematoma is seen within the middle section depicted. The villous capillary bed of this placenta was markedly distended and had the appearance of chorangiosis. This was the first pregnancy of a patient whose 2040-g infant had Apgar scores of 8/8, a neonatal hemoglobin level of 4.5 g, and a hematocrit of 14%. An excessive number of NRBCs was present in the fetal blood. The maternal and fetal blood groups were compatible. The child was edematous and had cardiomegaly but improved markedly after prompt transfusions were given. By Kleihauer stains, there were 3% to 5% of fetal cells in the maternal circulation. No history of trauma or other untoward event had occurred during the pregnancy that could have been held responsible for the massive fetal bleeding. Many cases like this have been reported in the literature (e.g., Debelle et al., 1977; Pourbabak et al., 2004), and every perinatal pathologist has seen cases of this entity (review by Freese, 1965; McGowan, 1968; Smith & Benjamin, 1968; Pai et al., 1975). For example, Carper and O'Donnell (1967) described a neonate with shock attributable to protracted fetal anemia; there were 4.5% positive cells in Kleihauer stains of maternal blood. The mother and fetus were blood group compatible, and the infant survived after transfusion. The placenta was not overtly unusual, but the mother had sustained two falls in pregnancy that may have been the cause of trauma to the placenta. Naeye et al. (1964) observed a neonate with prenatal exsanguination, manifested by a hematocrit of 15%, hemoglobin of

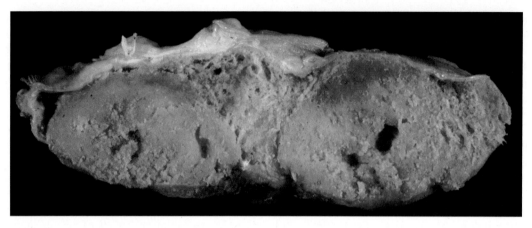

FIGURE 17.7. One slice of formalin-fixed placenta of neonate with edema and severe anemia (hemoglobin 4.5 g; hematocrit 14%) from transplacental hemorrhage. Note the thickness of the placenta, the severe pallor and the large intervillous hematoma.

7.4 g%, and 48 NRBCs per 100 WBCs. Despite therapy, the infant died. Autopsy findings included widespread infarctive necroses in many organs. The placenta was meconium stained, but was not otherwise described. It is important to emphasize in this connection that it may be very difficult for the pathologist to identify fetal anemia in a stillborn at autopsy. Thus, in every stillborn coming to autopsy, the possibility of fetal transplacental hemorrhage should be considered, and it must be properly excluded if such cases are not to be missed. This is the point of the contribution by Laube and Schauberger (1982). They found that 3.4% of all fetal deaths and 0.04% of all births among 9223 deliveries were due to this cause. Walter et al. (1965) found a severely anemic 3100-g newborn, rapidly and successfully treated with transfusion, whose placenta weighed 1920 g. It had no specific lesions, other than distention of all villous vessels. Because transplacental bleeding may result in necrosis of a variety of fetal organs, including the brain, its documentation is of particular importance at a time when medicolegal claims abound. Reference to such cases has been made in an earlier portion of this chapter. It must be remembered also that fetal blood is often transferred across the placenta at the time of delivery. This is the basis for the RhoGAM prophylaxis after delivery. Owen et al. (1989), conscious of the possible misinterpretation of fetal hemorrhage (as evidenced by Kleihauer stains) in being the cause of prenatal death, compared predelivery vs. postdelivery Kleihauer stain results. Their findings indicated that puerperal collection of blood for Kleihauer stains is satisfactory. Their contribution and others suggested that 10% to 15% of otherwise unexplained fetal deaths and perhaps 4% of all fetal deaths were the result of massive transplacental hemorrhage. Only Biankin et al. (2003) produced a series of five autopsy findings in massive hemorrhage (between 443 and 104 mL). There were few findings other than a marked increase in NRBCs in all organs and placental tissue. Intervillous hematomas with NRBCs

and collapse of veins were seen, as well as thrombosis of placental vessels.

Prenatal blood loss has been associated with the clinical identification of some very specific prenatal disturbances. Thus, Clark and Miller (1984) observed a sinusoidal fetal heart rate patterns during labor that they associated with the occurrence of a fetal to maternal hemorrhage. The mother had spontaneous rupture of membranes and, because of the fetal heart rate patterns, a cesarean section was performed. The neonate had a hematocrit of 16%, and Kleihauer stains showed 7.6% fetal cells in the maternal circulation. Because of the large quantity of fetal blood in the mother (265 mL), a chronic hemorrhage was suspected. In a pregnancy where fetal tachycardia, atrial dilatation, and atrial fibrillation were present, Bacevice et al. (1985) observed 45 to 60 mL of fetal red cells in the maternal circulation, before birth. This led to digitalization, cesarean section, and the delivery of an infant with a 37% hematocrit. Unfortunately, the placenta was not described. There had been no risk factors associated with the fetal hemorrhage.

In the cases of fetal bleeding that complicates **cordocentesis** (Feinkind et al., 1990; Ghidini et al., 1993), local hemorrhage or abruptio can sometimes be identified. It is the risk of this procedure that can lead to exsanguination and also to tachycardia (Seligman & Young, 1996). Usually it is a benign procedure with little bleeding, but depending on whether the procedure is done for transfusion or blood sampling, fetal sequelae differ substantially (Pielet et al., 1988). It also carries an increased risk of transplacental hemorrhage and, thus, the possibility of maternal alloimmunization (Bowman et al., 1994). These authors recommended that cord puncture for genotyping be done only when vessels are of sufficient size to allow immediate transfusion, if needed. It is often impossible to clearly identify, by detailed pathologic examination, the site of fetal hemorrhage. Most of the pathologic changes found in their placenta **result** from the fetal anemia, rather than being their **cause**. The pallor, the edema, the chorangiosis, and the placentomegaly all result from prolonged fetal cardiac failure. Many of the placentas cannot be shown to have overt abnormalities that could be the cause of the fetal bleeding. This was, for instance, the case in the well-studied infant described by Láwi et al. (1965). This infant had a neonatal hematocrit of only 17% and a hemoglobin concentration of 4.8 g%. Likewise, Desbuquois et al. (1962) observed a normal placenta associated with fetal anemia in a 3400-g neonate; they cited similar cases from the literature. We have observed an exsanguinated, term stillborn infant in whose subamnionic space a large amount of fresh blood separated the amnion (4 cm) from the chorion. At cesarean section, 500 mL of blood could be removed, and the placenta was 50% abrupted. No risk factors were identified. To be sure, many of the placentas of cases with fetal exsanguinations also possess intervillous thrombi. These have often been thought of as the possible sites of the fetal bleeding; as suspected in the earliest cases described by Chown (1955), the case of Debelle et al. (1977), and in the case illustrated in Figure 17.7. Devi et al. (1968) studied the placentas of 120 normal deliveries, 264 complicated deliveries, and 98 pregnancies of Rh-negative women without and 35 Rh-negative patients with antibodies. Their findings indicated that the so-called Kline's hemorrhages (vide infra) positively correlated with the presence of fetal cells in the maternal circulation. The more frequently such lesions were present, the greater was the size of the transplacental hemorrhage. The authors presented their findings in several tables. Those results impressively support the notion that Kline's lesions, intervillous thrombi, operative delivery, infarcts and abruptio placentae statistically correlate with fetal bleeding.

Kline had described in 1948 that specific microscopic lesions in the placenta correlate with bleeding of the fetus. In the placentas of 15 erythroblastotic fetuses, he found "numerous breaks," with NRBCs in the adjacent intervillous space. He deduced that these breaks occurred in the peripheral capillaries, or even in larger blood vessels. After agglutination of red cells and deposition of fibrin, the overlying trophoblastic epithelium appeared to degenerate, serving as a nidus for clots to form. We believe that this alleged causality of the capillary occlusion is incorrect. In many fetal vascular occlusions, there is no trophoblastic degeneration, nor can breaks in blood vessels and villous surfaces be identified. It is also noteworthy that, despite the presence of a 2.7-cm spherical "cyst" with NRBCs in one of Chown's cases (1955), no trophoblastic damage was found on the villous surfaces. The integrity of the villous surface trophoblast is dependent solely on the intervillous circulation (e.g., hydatidiform moles). It is not dependent on the fetal circulation. Occlusions of fetal capillaries do not cause trophoblastic necrosis; they cause the villus to atrophy, occasionally to

become edematous, and eventually they make it fibrotic. Nevertheless, the term **Kline hemorrhage** has become associated with the putative lesions that are believed to initiate transplacental hemorrhage. When defects in the trophoblast occur, fibrinoid deposits across the defects; the trophoblast disruptions increase in frequency with advancing gestation normally, as does the fibrin (see Chapter 9). The fibrin so deposited may calcify and eventually become part of the diffuse microcalcification of term placentas. Breaks of villi also occur frequently throughout gestation. Presumably, they are "healed" by this maternal fibrin deposition.

We believe that, in vivo, the fetal blood flow and its pressure maintain the placental villi in an "erected" position (accounting for the thicker placenta seen sonographically as compared to when dissected). They are thus more susceptible to injury from fetal kicking than if they are empty, or "deflated." We can readily envisage that small breaks can then occur spontaneously and when the villi are injured by the fetus. To us, this more readily explains the frequency of fetal bleeding in otherwise normal placentas. Wentworth (1964) has advocated the use of flat and large ("Gough") sections of the delivered, and formalin-fixed, placenta for the observation of Kline hemorrhages. The cases he studied were correlated with Kleihauer stains of maternal blood, and the Kline hemorrhages could be evaluated by gross inspection. A positive correlation between the number of Kline lesions and the finding of positive Kleihauer stains was observed by Wentworth. Some of the illustrated "lesions" indicate that the author considered the normal villous lakes to be Kline lesions. These are the sites of primary injection of the maternal jets, the "holes" one observes in most delivered placentas. Wentworth (1964) found no correlation with infarcts, calcification, or other placental lesions.

Large intervillous thrombi may occur during labor (Fig. 17.8). They are then fresh clots, and without structure. There may be older, laminated clots with a similar appearance (Figs. 17.9 to 17.11). When these contain fetal cells, their older age may be revealed by the presence of macrophages that have engulfed fetal red blood cells (Fig. 17.12). We are here referring to intervillous thrombi that occur in the centers of the villous mass, and that do not relate to lesions in the floor of the placenta, such as those shown in Figs. 17.9 and 17.10. The latter intervillous thrombi are associated with maternal vascular lesions, often occur in preeclampsia, and are frequently laminated and pale. They differ from infarcts, which are granular in macroscopic appearance and invariably involve villi. Typical intervillous thrombi merely displace adjacent villi. If intervillous thrombi become large, or if they are of longer duration, the compressed adjacent villous tissue will also become infarcted. Other intervillous thrombi occur beneath the fetal surface. Those subchorionic fibrin masses increase with gestation and result from

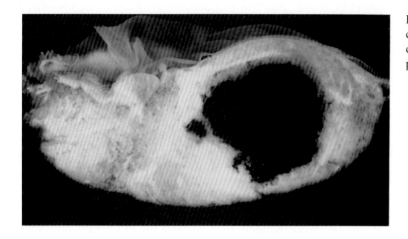

FIGURE 17.8. Fresh intervillous thrombus in the center of villous tissue and presumed to have occurred during the delivery. Note the extreme pallor of this placenta from an erythroblastotic infant.

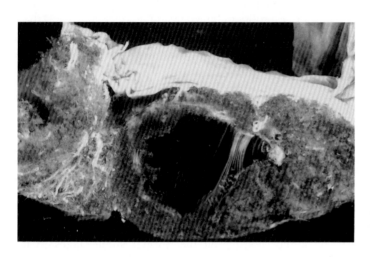

FIGURE 17.9. Somewhat older intervillous thrombus in center of term placenta. Note the laminated fibrin at right.

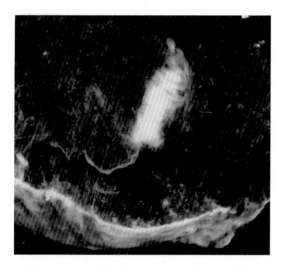

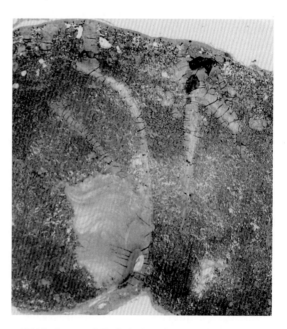

FIGURE 17.10. Layered fibrin residue of old intervillous thrombus originating from cotyledonary septum.

FIGURE 17.11. Layered fibrin in basal type of intervillous thrombus, associated with decidual necrosis and thrombosis of decidual vein. There is no adjacent infarction yet. H&E ×6.

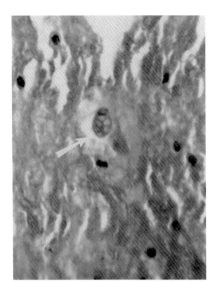

FIGURE 17.12. Old intervillous thrombus. At arrow is a maternal erythrocytophagocytic macrophage. H&E ×400.

never manifests the fibrous tissue ingrowth, and the neovascularization that occurs in other organs, whose infarcts organize and become scars. Even the larger thrombi of surface vessels and in the umbilical cord do not "organize" frequently.

In occasional cases of fatal fetomaternal bleeding, the placenta has exhibited specific lesions that may explain the hemorrhage. Thus, Santamaria et al. (1987) found a choriocarcinoma in situ in the pale placenta of an otherwise normal stillborn. The trophoblast was clearly invasive and had presumably caused some fetal vascular discontinuity. More importantly perhaps, the lesion was not identifiable by macroscopic examination as a tumor. Small "infarcts" were seen and sampled, but they were not deemed grossly to be exceptional. The discovery of this (and other) placental choriocarcinomas in situ was fortuitous (see Chapter 23). Perhaps other "unexplained" transplacental hemorrhages would have yielded similar lesions, had the placenta been examined in more detail. A small chorangioma of the placenta was found in another fetus with transplacental hemorrhage (Fig. 17.13). There was no tumorous destruction of villi in this case, but the adjacent vessels were severely distended. These may have bled. Stiller and Skajish (1986) also reported on transplacental hemorrhage in association with a chorangioma of the placenta, fetal distress, and maternal hemolysis. Brown (1963) found that very large placentas, and excessively calcified organs, have an increased association with transplacental hemorrhage. Pollack and Montague (1968), on the other hand, stated that postmature placentas did not allow fetal hemorrhage to occur more frequently. The occurrence of fetal hemoglobin (>5%) in retroplacental hematomas was demonstrated in 29 of 93 cases by Oehlert et al. (1960).

eddying of the intervillous blood as it is reflected beneath the chorion. In some placentas, they protrude into the amnionic cavity and may become so-called Breus' moles. These features are discussed in Chapter 9. Finally, more remarkable subchorionic fibrin deposits occur in some maternal cardiac diseases. These are shown in the Chapter 19. In addition, subchorionic fibrin deposits are regularly present in the immature placentas delivered after intra-amnionic saline and urea instillation for therapeutic abortion. It is of parenthetic interest here to note that intervillous thrombi and placental infarcts never undergo the repair process known to pathologists as "organization." That is to say, unlike other organs, the placenta

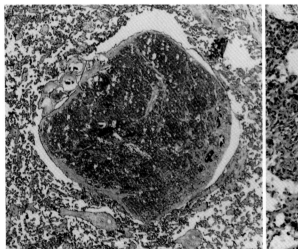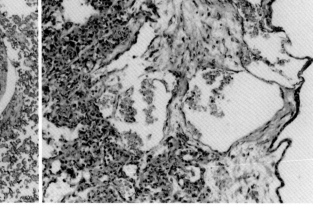

FIGURE 17.13. Small chorangioma in mature placenta (maternal sickle cell disease) having caused transplacental hemorrhage (hematocrit 22%; 120-mL blood loss). Markedly distended fetal vessels seen at right with extreme thinning of their walls, possibly the sites of hemorrhage. H&E ×12.5 (left); ×50 (right).

Other Fetal Blood Elements Passing Through the Placenta

Although transplacental red blood cell passage may have the most serious consequences (anemia, immunization), transplacental white blood cell transfer is also of interest and has now become important because of the sequelae of the developing maternal microchimerism. For instance, do tumor cells readily pass the placental villi? As is reviewed in Chapter 19, maternal leukemia cells do not usually pass the placental "barrier" but on occasion have led to neonatal demise (Maruko et al., 2004). Of the solid neoplasms, only occasional melanoma cells are known to have traversed the placenta to the fetus with certainty. It is thus surprising to learn that some studies have suggested that lymphocyte traffic may occur across the placenta, and that it is alleged to take place in both directions. The topic has been reviewed in some detail by Schröder (1975), who concluded that the question of fetal leukocytes in the maternal circulation was still controversial, at least it was at that time. In part, the results of such studies are difficult to interpret because the mitotic inhibition of maternal leukocytes, when admixed with fetal lymphocytes, prevents ready identification of fetal cells (Olding et al., 1974). The conclusion, however, of Schröder was that fetal lymphocytes frequently pass to the mother, and that they probably do so in most normal pregnancies. They may be found up to years postpartum in the maternal blood or bone marrow, but they do not respond to the usual mitogens (Schröder et al., 1977). Selypes and Lorencz (1988) have developed a new methodology with which to identify fetal lymphocytes in the maternal circulation. They used this technique for the identification of fetal sex and diagnosis of possibly aberrant fetal karyotypes. Even newer techniques are now being pursued for the identification of fetal cells in the maternal blood.

Adinolfi et al. (1989), and Lo et al. (1989) used polymerase chain reaction (PCR) for DNA amplification and the identification of Y-chromosome–bearing cells in maternal venous blood. No contamination with fetal cells was found in six samples of pregnancies between 24 and 36 weeks' gestation by the first investigators, although deported syncytiotrophoblast was trapped in the maternal lung. Their deportation had long been known (Schmorl, 1893, 1905; Raafat et al., 1975). When we studied lungs from a patient dying shortly after pregnancy, numerous apparent syncytiotrophoblastic cells were present in pulmonary capillaries, but staining with anti–human chorionic gonadotropin (hCG) antibodies failed because the cells had already lost their cytoplasm. There was neither a reaction nor thrombosis associated with these deported placental cells (Fig. 17.14). In the investigation by Lo et al. (1989), Y-sequences were found in the cells of all 12 women with male conceptuses, but in none of those seven cases with female fetuses. The possibility of contamination in this study was criticized by Holzgreve et al. (1990). Isolation of fetal DNA from maternal blood, contaminated by fetal NRBCs has been amply documented also by Bianchi et al. (1990). In later studies she suggested that these cells traverse the placenta at different times (Bianchi et al., 1991). The reliability of Lo's technique was further questioned by the study of Suzumori et al. (1992). On the other hand, a carefully designed and cautiously executed study of peripheral blood for Y-specific ZFY sequences showed conclusively that nucleated fetal cells nearly regularly contaminate maternal blood (Kao et al., 1992). In a prospective study, Hamada et al. (1993) found by fluorescent in situ hybridization (FISH) in 50 male conceptuses that NRBCs were regularly found in the maternal circulation after 15 weeks. In the first trimester there were 1:100,000 nucleated cells, whereas 1:10,000 were seen at term. Elias and colleagues (1992) have even made

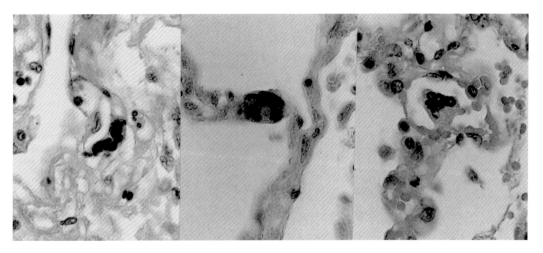

FIGURE 17.14. Syncytiotrophoblastic cells trapped in pulmonary capillaries of patient, dead from pulmonary hypertension shortly after delivery. The syncytial cells have lost their cytoplasm. H&E ×400.

the diagnosis of trisomy 21 and trisomy 18 by the FISH method, the demonstration of three fluorescent markers in nucleated cells from maternal blood. Cell sorting of nucleated cells and other techniques are now in use to enrich the fetal cells contaminating the maternal blood (Gänshirt-Ahlert et al., 1992a,b). Very surprisingly, Bertero et al. (1988) have found some maternal (definitely **not** fetal) antigens on the surface of these circulating cells. They deduced from this that the prenatal diagnosis of β-thalassemia they attempted was not feasible. When the fetal DNA, however, was amplified from only a few NRBCs in the maternal circulation, sickle cell disease and β-thalassemia were successfully diagnosed prenatally by Cheung et al. (1996). Other single gene disorders are similarly susceptible. The topic of prenatal diagnosis from maternal blood contaminated by fetal cells continues to be under intense study. As indicated above, many different types of approaches were evaluated at the conference edited by Simpson and Elias (1994). It seems likely that the nearly regular, if small contamination of NRBCs in the maternal circulation even in early pregnancy will be most suitable for this purpose. Concentration methods steadily improve, clinical trials are ongoing, and verification of the cells under study as being cells from the current fetus are assured. Less optimal, because somewhat invasive, are the methods to obtain cells from washings of the endocervical canal.

MOTHER-TO-FETUS TRANSFER OF CELLS

Although occasional cases of such cellular exchange have been well documented, much less good evidence has been adduced that maternal cells frequently pass to the fetus in significant numbers. Schröder (1975), in the same review mentioned above, recited the observation of Kadowaki et al. (1965) of the prenatally incurred lymphocytic chimerism, in a neonate with presumed immunologic incompetence. This child later developed graft-versus-host disease as a result of his lymphocyte chimerism. Similar chimerism, induced by prenatal maternal lymphocyte transfer in a child with thymic alymphoplasia, reported by Githens et al. (1969), had no ill effect. More deleterious consequences were described from transfer of malignant maternal cells into immunocompromised fetuses by Barth et al. (1972) and Pollack et al. (1982). Oehme et al. (1966) were able to show maternal leukocyte transfer to the rabbit fetus, with striking accumulation of these cells in the fetal lung. A few other reports of 46,XX cells in the circulation of male fetuses have been forthcoming (El-Alfi & Hathout, 1969; Moszkowski et al., 1971). Such passage is clearly exceptional, and graft-versus-host rejection of the immunologically compromised fetus, as in Kadowaki's case, must be exceedingly uncommon. Moreover, when lymphocyte cocultivation of maternal and fetal cells is experimentally studied, the maternal cell response is markedly reduced (Kawagoe et al., 1971; Olding et al., 1974). This may also have been the cause of Olding's failure to identify 46,XX cells in the cord blood of male infants (1972).

Interestingly, there have been occasional reports of fetal plethora that were apparently due to mother-to-fetus blood transfer. Wong and Cann (1972) described a fatal transfusion reaction with fetal renal tubular necrosis in such a putative case of maternal–fetal transfusion. The child was born at 43 weeks' gestation, after a normal pregnancy, and the placenta was not infarcted or abrupted. The neonatal hemoglobin concentration was 16.8 g%, there was hemoglobinuria, and the fetal blood did not clot. Immunologic studies of the fetal red blood cells suggested that maternal cells were circulating at birth. Chronic maternofetal transfusion was found in a case of hydrops fetalis described by Bowman et al. (1984). The mother had received fetal cells transplacentally (5.4% Kleihauer positive cells). The hydropic infant was plethoric, with a hemoglobin of 20.5 g and a hematocrit of 63%. The placenta accompanying this fetus had extensive areas of infarction and intervillous thrombi, and microscopically there were torn fetal vessels. The authors concluded that such cases must be exceedingly rare, and they were able to refer to only one previously described report with fetal plethora, that of Michael and Mauer (1961). They suggested that this bidirectional exchange was possible only because of the disrupted large fetal placental vessels, an otherwise uncommon phenomenon. Michael and Mauer found three newborns of normal pregnancies with hematocrits of 73%, 79%, and 80% respectively, and hemoglobin values of 21.2, 21.8, and 24.6 g%. In two of these, the fetal and maternal blood groups differed, and differential agglutination allowed proof of maternal red cell transfer to the fetus. The placentas were not described, and the mechanism of transplacental transfer was only speculated upon. There are, however, numerous studies that affirm the nearly regular transfer of **some** maternal red blood cells to the fetus, albeit in smaller numbers than those needed to induce fetal plethora. They are not accompanied by abnormal placentas, have also been found to occur in mice (Holliday & Barnes, 1973), and they obviously embody the importance of possible fetal Rh-isoimmunization, when the fetus is Rh-negative and the mother is Rh-positive (Jennings & Clauss, 1978). Messer et al. (1966) found that parenteral administration of carbazochrome to the mother decreased the transfer. Red cell transfer from mother to fetus was affirmed by Smith et al. (1961) and Zarou et al. (1964) using chromium-labeled red blood cells. Macris et al. (1958) and Fujikura and Klionsky (1975) identified such transfer with the marker being sickled erythrocytes. Many other studies are summarized by additional investigators (Megapanos et al., 1966; Eimer & Weiland, 1969). These leave no doubt that this is a relatively frequent and perhaps an occasionally important phenomenon. Mayer et al. (1956) demonstrated in an impressive electron micrograph the apparent passage of a red blood cell through a fetal villous capillary.

References

Adinolfi, M., Camporeses, C. and Carr, T.: Gene amplification to detect fetal nucleated cells in pregnant women. Lancet **ii**:328–329, 1989.

Adkinson, L.R., Andrews, R.H., Vowell, N.L. and Koontz, W.L.: Improved detection of fetal cells from maternal blood with polymerase chain reaction. Amer. J. Obstet. Gynecol. **170**:952–955, 1994.

Ahmed, J. and Brown, C.: Failure of the Kleihauer test to detect red blood cells in amniotic fluid. Lancet **i**:1393, 1986.

Almeida, V.de and Bowman, J.M.: Massive fetomaternal hemorrhage: Manitoba experience. Obstet. Gynecol. **83**:323–328, 1994.

Anquist, K.W., Parnes, S., Cargill, Y. and Tawagi, G.: An unexpected fetal outcome following a severe maternal motor vehicle accident. Obstet. Gynecol. **84**:656–659, 1994.

Apt, L. and Downey, W.S.: "Melena" neonatorum: The swallowed blood syndrome. A simple test for the differentiation of adult and fetal hemoglobin in bloody stools. J. Pediatr. **47**:6–12, 1955.

Avenarius, S., Föhe, K., Schultz, H., Canzler, E. and Wood, B.P.: Radiological case of the month. Arch. Ped. Adolesc. Med. **153**:1103–1104, 1999.

Awwad, J.T., Azar, G.B., Seoud, M.A., Mroueh, A.M. and Karam, K.S.: High-velocity penetrating wounds of the gravid uterus: review of 16 years of civil war. Obstet. Gynecol. **83**:259–264, 1994.

Bacevice, A.E., Dierker, L.J. and Wolfson, R.N.: Intrauterine atrial fibrillation associated with fetomaternal hemorrhage. Amer. J. Obstet. Gynecol. **153**:81–82, 1985.

Baer, K.E.V.: Untersuchungen ueber die Gefaessverbindungen zwischen Mutter und Frucht in den Saeugethieren. L. Voss, Leipzig, 1828.

Baergen, R.N., Castillo, M.M., Mario-Singh, B., Stehly, A.J. and Benirschke, K.: Embolism of fetal brain tissue to the lungs and the placenta. Pediatr. Pathol. Lab. Med. **17**:159–167, 1997.

Barth, F.B., Khurana, S.K., Vergara, G.G. and Lowman, J.T.: Rapidly fatal familial histiocytosis associated with eosinophilia and primary immunological deficiency. Lancet **2**:503–506, 1972.

Benirschke, K. and Gille, J.: Placental pathology and asphyxia. In, Intrauterine Asphyxia and the Developing Fetal Brain. L. Gluck, ed. pp. 117–136. Year Book Medical Publishers, Chicago, 1977.

Bertero, M.T., Camaschella, C., Serra, A., Bergui, L. and Caligaris-Cappio, F.: Circulating trophoblast cells in pregnancy have maternal genetic markers. Prenat. Diagn. **8**:585–590, 1988.

Bianchi, D.W., Flint, A.F., Pizzimenti, M.F., Knoll, J.H.M. and Latt, S.A.: Isolation of fetal DNA from nucleated erythrocytes in maternal blood. Proc. Natl. Acad. Sci. USA **87**:3279–3283, 1990.

Bianchi, D.W., Stewart, J.E., Garber, M.F., Lucotte, G. and Flint, A.F.: Possible effect of gestational age on the detection of fetal nucleated erythrocytes in maternal blood. Prenat. Diagn. **11**:523–528, 1991.

Bianchi, D.W., Shuber, A.P., DeMaria, A., Fougner, A.C. and Klinger, K.W.: Fetal cells in maternal blood: Determination of purity and yield by quantitative polymerase chain reaction. Amer. J. Obstet. Gynecol. **171**:922–926, 1994.

Biankin, S.A., Arbuckle, S.M. and Graf, N.S.: Autopsy findings in a series of five cases of fetomaternal haemorrhages. Pathology **35**:319–324, 2003.

Bickers, R.G. and Wennberg, R.P.: Fetomaternal transfusion following trauma. Obstet. Gynecol. **61**:258–259, 1983.

Blajchman, M.A., Maudsley, R.F., Uchida, I. and Zipursky, A.: Diagnostic amniocentesis and fetal-maternal bleeding. Lancet **1**:993, 1974.

Bombard, A.T., Powers, J.F., Carter, S., Schwartz, A. and Nitowsky, H.M.: Procedure-related fetal losses in transplacental genetic amniocentesis. Amer. J. Obstet. Gynecol. **172**:868–872, 1995.

Borum, A., Loyd, H.O. and Talbot, T.R.: Possible fetal hemorrhage into maternal circulation. Report of two cases. JAMA **164**:1087–1088, 1957.

Bowman, J.M. and Pollock, J.M.: Transplacental fetal hemorrhage after amniocentesis. Obstet. Gynecol. **66**:749–754, 1985.

Bowman, J.M., Lewis, M. and de Sa, D.J.: Hydrops fetalis caused by massive maternofetal transplacental hemorrhage. J. Pediatr. **104**:769–772, 1984.

Bowman, J.M., Pollock, J.M., Peterson, L.E., Harman, C.R., Manning, F.A. and Menticoglou, S.M.: Fetomaternal hemorrhage following funipuncture: Increase in severity of maternal red-cell alloimmunization. Obstet. Gynecol. **84**:839–843, 1994.

Brill, C.B.: An unexpected fetal outcome following a severe maternal motor vehicle accident. Obstet. Gynecol. **85**:319, 1995.

Bromilow, I.M. and Duguid, J.K.M.: Measurement of fetomaternal haemorrhage: a comparative study of three Kleihauer techniques and two flow cytometry methods. Clin. Lab. Haematol. **19**:137–142, 1997.

Brown, E.S.: Foetal erythrocytes in the maternal circulation. Brit. Med. J. **i**:1000–1001, 1963.

Brown, W.E. and Cowles, G.T.: Fetal cells in maternal blood. South. Med. J. **56**:782–783, 1963.

Buchsbaum, H.J.: Accidental injury complicating pregnancy. Amer. J. Obstet. Gynecol. **102**:752–769, 1968.

Buchsbaum, H.J.: Trauma in Pregnancy. Saunders, Philadelphia, 1979.

Buchsbaum, H.J. and Staples, P.P.: Self-inflicted gunshot wound to the pregnant uterus: report of two cases. Obstet. Gynecol. **65**:32S-65S, 1985.

Cardwell, M.S.: Fetomaternal hemorrhage. When to suspect, how to manage. Postgrad. Med. **82**:127–130, 1987.

Cardwell, M.S. and Snyder, S.W.: Feto-maternal hemorrhage—possible cause of fetal distress. Amer. J. Obstet. Gynecol. **161**:1744, 1989.

Carper, J.M. and O'Donnell, W.M.: Severe neonatal anemia due to massive transplacental hemorrhage. Amer. J. Clin. Pathol. **47**:444–447, 1967.

Catalano, P.M. and Capeless, E.L.: Fetomaternal bleeding as a cause of recurrent fetal morbidity and mortality. Obstet. Gynecol. **76**:972–73, 1990.

Chamberlain, E.M., Scott, J.R., Wu, J.T., Rote, N.S. and Egger, M.J.: A comparison of acid-elution techniques and alpha-fetoprotein levels for the detection of fetomaternal bleeding. Amer. J. Obstet. Gynecol. **143**:912–917, 1982.

Cheung, M.C., Goldberg, J.D. and Kan, Y.W.: Prenatal diagnosis of sickle cell anaemia and thalassaemia by analysis of fetal cells in maternal blood. Nature Genet. **14**:264–268, 1996.

Chibber, G., Zacher, M., Cohen, A.W. and Kline, A.J.: Rh immunization following abdominal trauma: a case report. Amer. J. Obstet. Gynecol. **149**:692, 1984.

Chown, B.: Anaemia from fetal bleeding of the fetus into the mother's circulation. Lancet **i**:1213–1215, 1954.

Chown, B.: The fetus can bleed. Three clinicopathological pictures. Amer. J. Obstet. Gynecol. **70**:1298–1308, 1955.

Christmas, J.T., Vanner, L.V., Daniels, R.M., Bodurtha, J.N., Hays, P.M. and Redwine, F.O.: The effect of fetomaternal bleeding on the risk of adverse pregnancy outcome in patients with elevated second-trimester maternal serum α-fetoprotein levels. Amer. J. Obstet. Gynecol. **171**:315–320, 1994.

Clark, S.L. and Miller, F.C.: Sinusoidal fetal heart rate pattern associated with massive fetomaternal transfusion. Amer. J. Obstet. Gynecol. **149**:97–99, 1984.

Cohen, F., Zuelzer, W.W., Gustafson, D.C. and Evans, M.M.: Transplacental bleeding from the fetus. Blood **23**:621–646, 1964.

Crissinger, K.D., Ryckman, F.C. and Balisteri, W.F.: Necrotizing enterocolitis and gastrointestinal hemorrhage. In,

Neonatal-Perinatal Medicine. Diseases of the Fetus and Infant. A.A. Fanaroff and R.J. Martin eds., C.V. Mosby Company, St. Louis. pp. 928–932, 1987.

Crosby, W.M.: Pathology of obstetric injuries in pregnant automobile-accident victims. In, Accident Pathology. Proceedings of an International Conference. K.M. Brinkhous, ed. pp. 204–207. US Government Printing Office, Washington, D.C. 1968.

Crosby, W.M.: Trauma during pregnancy: maternal and fetal injury. Obstet. Gynecol. Surv. 29:683–699, 1974.

Crosby, W.M. and Costiloe, J.P.: Safety of lap-belt restraint for pregnant victims of automobile collisions. NEJM 284:632–636, 1971.

Cumming, D.C. and Wren, F.D.: Fetal skull fracture from an apparently trivial motor vehicle accident. Amer. J. Obstet. Gynecol. 132:342–343, 1978.

Dahmus, M.A. and Sibai, B.M.: Blunt abdominal trauma: Are there any predictive factors for abruptio placentae or maternal-fetal distress? Amer. J. Obstet. Gynecol. 169:1054–1059, 1993.

Debelle, G.D., Gillam, G.L. and Tauro, G.P.: A case of hydrops foetalis due to foeto-maternal haemorrhage. Austral. Paediatr. J. 13:131–133, 1977.

Desbuquois, G., Boulard, P. et Grenier, B.: Hemorrhage foetale dans la circulation maternelle. Arch. Franç. Pédiatr. 19:1341–1346, 1962.

Devi, B., Jennison, R.F. and Langley, F.A.: Significance of placental pathology in transplacental hemorrhage. J. Clin. Pathol. 21:322–331, 1968.

De Witt, F.: An historical study on theories of the placenta to 1900. J. Hist. Med. & Allied Sci. 14:360–374, 1959.

Dhanraj, D. and Lambers, D.: The incidences of positive Kleihauer-Betke test in low-risk pregnancies and maternal trauma patients. Amer. J. Obstet. Gynecol. 190:1461–1463, 2004.

Donaldson, I.: Intrauterine haemorrhage as a cause of foetal death. Lancet i:1351, 1962.

Doolittle, J.E.: Placental vascular integrity related to third-stage management. Obstet. Gynecol. 22:468–472, 1963.

Eaton, C.J. and Danzinger, R.F.: Traumatic disruption of pregnancy: report of a case and its legal implications. Obstet. Gynecol. 30:16–22, 1967.

Eden, J.A.: Fetal-induced trauma as a cause of antepartum hemorrhage. Amer. J. Obstet. Gynecol. 157:830–831, 1987.

Eich, F.G. and Tripoldi, D.: Screening and quantitating fetal-maternal hemorrhages. Amer. J. Clin. Pathol. 61:192–198, 1974.

Eimer, H. und Weiland, A.: Untersuchungen über die Placentapassage mütterlicher Erythrocyten. Arch. Gynäkol. 208:113–122, 1969.

El-Alfi, O. and Hathout, H.: Maternofetal transfusion: Immunologic and cytogenetic evidence. Amer. J. Obstet. Gynecol. 103:599–600, 1969.

Elias, S., Price, J., Dockter, M., Wachtel, S., Tharapel, A., Simpson, J.L. and Klinger, K.W.: First trimester prenatal diagnosis of trisomy 21 in fetal cells from maternal blood. Lancet 340:1033, 1992.

Ellis, J. and Kohler, H.G.: Small infant thymus in cases of fatal feto-maternal transfusion. Brit. Med. J. i:694, 1976.

Emery, C.L., Morway, L.F., Chung-Park, M., Wyatt-Ashmed, J., Sawady, J. and Beddow, T.D.: The Kleihauer-Betke Test.

Clinical utility, indication, and correlation in patients with placental abruption and cocaine use. Arch. Pathol. Lab. Med. 119:1032–1037, 1995.

Fay, R.A.: Feto-maternal haemorrhage as a cause of fetal morbidity and mortality. Brit. J. Obstet. Gynaecol. 90:443–446, 1983.

Feinkind, L., Nanda, D., Delke, I. and Minkoff, H.: Abruptio placentae after percutaneous umbilical cord sampling: a case report. Amer. J. Obstet. Gynecol. 162:1203–1204, 1990.

Feldman, N., Skoll, A. and Sibai, B.: The incidence of significant fetomaternal hemorrhage in patients undergoing cesarean section. Obstet. Gynecol. 163:855–858, 1990.

Fernandez-Rocha, L. and Oullette, R.: Fetal bleeding: An unusual complication of fetal monitoring. Amer. J. Obstet. Gynecol. 125:1153–1154, 1976.

Fielding, J.: Detecting foetal cells. Lancet i:202, 1968.

Finn, R., Harper, D.T., Stallings, S.A. and Krevans, J.R.: Transplacental hemorrhage. Transfusion 3:114–124, 1963.

Fischer R.L., Kuhlman, K., Grover, J., Montgomery, O. and Wapner, R.J.: Chronic, massive fetomaternal hemorrhage treated with repeated fetal intravascular transfusions. Amer. J. Obstet. Gynecol. 162:203–204, 1990.

Fliegner, J.R.H., Fortune, D.W. and Barrie, J.U.: Occult fetomaternal hemorrhage as a cause of fetal mortality and morbidity. Austral. New Zeal. J. Obstet. Gynecol. 27:158–161, 1987.

Fort, A.T. and Harlin, R.S.: Pregnancy outcome after non-catastrophic maternal trauma during pregnancy. Obstet. Gynecol. 35:912–915, 1970.

Fox, H.: The incidence and significance of nucleated erythrocytes in the foetal vessels of the mature human placenta. J. Obstet. Gynaecol. Brit. Commonw. 74:40–43, 1967.

Fraser, I.D. and Raper, A.B.: Observation of compatible and incompatible foetal red cells in the maternal circulation. Brit. Med. J. ii:303–304, 1962.

Freese, U.E.: Massive fetal hemorrhage into the maternal circulation. Obstet. Gynecol. 26:848–851, 1965.

Freese, U.E. and Titel, J.H.: Demonstration of fetal erythrocytes in maternal circulation. Obstet. Gynecol. 22:527–532, 1963.

Fujikura, T. and Klionsky, B.: Transplacental passage of maternal erythrocytes with sickling. J. Pediatr. 87:781–783, 1975.

Fynaut, J.: Anémie par hémorragie transplacentaire. Bull. Soc. Roy. Belge Gynécol. d'Obstet. 30:198–206, 1960.

Gänshirt-Ahlert, D., Burschyk, M., Garritsen, H.S.P., Helmer, L., Miny, P., Horst, J., Schneider, H.P.G. and Holzgreve, W.: Magnetic cell sorting and the transferrin receptor as potential means of prenatal diagnosis from maternal blood. Amer. J. Obstet. Gynecol. 166:1350–1355, 1992a.

Gänshirt-Ahlert, D., Basak, N., Aidynli, K. and Holzgreve, W.: Fetal DNA in uterine vein blood. Obstet. Gynecol. 80:601–603, 1992b.

Geissler, Dr. and Japha, A.: Beitrag zu den Anämieen junger Kinder. Jahrb. Kinderh. 56:627–647, 1901.

Ghidini, A., Sepulveda, W., Lockwood, C.J. and Romero, R.: Complications of fetal blood sampling. Amer. J. Obstet. Gynecol. 168:1339–1344, 1993.

Githens, J.H., Muschenheim, F., Fulginiti, V.A., Robinson, A. and Kay, H.E.M.: Thymic alymphoplasia with XX/XY lymphoid chimerism secondary to probable maternal-fetal transfusion. J. Pediatr. 75:87–94, 1969.

Gjode, P., Rasmussen, T.B. and Jorgensen, J.: Fetomaternal bleeding during attempts at external version. Brit. J. Obstet. Gynaecol. **87**:571–573, 1980.

Goodlin, R.C. and Clewell, W.H.: Sudden fetal death following diagnostic amniocentesis. Amer. J. Obstet. Gynecol. **118**:285–288, 1974.

Goodwin, T.M. and Breen, M.T.: Pregnancy outcome and fetomaternal hemorrhage after noncatastrophic trauma. Amer. J. Obstet. Gynecol. **162**:665–671, 1990.

Gottesfeld, K.R., Thompson, H.E., Holmes, J.H. and Taylor, E. D.: Ultrasonic placentography—a new method for placental localization. Amer. J. Obstet. Gynecol. **96**:538–547, 1966.

Green, D.W. and Mimouni, F.: Nucleated erythrocytes in healthy infants and in infants of diabetic mothers. J. Pediatr. **116**:129–131, 1990.

Griffin, W.T.: Occult fetal-maternal transfusion. Amer. J. Obstet. Gynecol. **105**:993, 1969.

Grimes, H.G. and Wright, F.S.: Fetomaternal transfusion. A case report. Amer. J. Obstet. Gynecol. **82**:1371–1374, 1961.

Grobbelaar, B.G.: Transplacental haemorrhage in Rh-haemolytic disease. Brit. Med. J. **i**:300, 1968.

Gunson, H.H.: Neonatal anemia due to fetal hemorrhage into the maternal circulation. Pediatrics **20**:3–6, 1957.

Hamada, H., Arinami, T., Kubo, T., Hamaguchi, H. and Iwasaki, H.: Fetal nucleated cells in maternal peripheral blood: frequency and relationship to gestational age. Hum. Genet. **91**:427–432, 1993.

Hamada, H., Arinami, T., Hamaguchi, H. and Kubo, T.: Fetal nucleated cells in maternal peripheral blood after delivery in cases of fetomaternal hemorrhage. Obstet. Gynecol. **85**:449–451, 1995.

Hawes, C.S., Suskin, H.A., Petropoulos, A., Latham, S.E. and Mueller, U.W.: A morphologic study of trophoblast isolated from peripheral blood of pregnant women. Amer. J. Obstet. Gynecol. **170**:1297–121300, 1994.

Herrmann, U. und Sidiropoulos, D.: Amniocentese bei rhesus-negativen Frauen: Häufigkeit und Konsequenzen fetomaternaler Transfusionen. Arch. Gynecol. **239**:241–243, 1986.

Higgins, S.D.: Trauma in pregnancy. J. Perinatol. **8**:288–292, 1988.

Higgins, S.D. and Garite, T.J.: Late abruptio placenta in trauma patients: implications for monitoring. Obstet. Gynecol. **63**:10S–12S, 1984.

Holliday, J. and Barnes, R.D.: The normal transplacental passage of maternal red cells in mice. Cell Tissue Kinet. **6**:455–459, 1973.

Holzgreve, W., Gänshirt-Ahlert, D., Burschyk, M., Horst, J., Miny, P., Gal, A. and Pohlschmidt, M.: Detection of fetal DNA in maternal blood by PCR. Lancet **335**:1220–1221, 1990.

Huff, D.L.: Fetal-maternal hemorrhage and management of the third stage of labor at Cesarean section—A prospective study. Oklahoma Obstet. Gynecol. J. Club. **4**:92, 1988.

Jauniaux, E., Gibb, D., Moscoso, G. and Campbell, S.: Ultrasonographic diagnosis of a large placental intervillous thrombosis associated with elevated maternal serum α-fetoprotein level. Amer. J. Obstet. Gynecol. **163**:1558–1560, 1990.

Javert, C.T. and Reiss, C.: The origin and significance of macroscopic intervillous coagulation hematomas (red infarcts) of the human placenta. Surg. Gynecol. Obstet. **94**:257–269, 1952.

Jennings, E.R. and Clauss, B.: Maternal-fetal hemorrhage: Its incidence and sensitizing effects. Amer. J. Obstet. Gynecol. **131**:725–727, 1978.

Jones, P.: Assessment of size of small volume foeto-maternal bleeds. A new method of quantification of the Kleihauer technique. Brit. Med. J. **i**:85–88, 1969.

Kadowaki, J., Thompson, R.I., Zuelzer, W.W., Wooley, P.V., Brough, A.J. and Gruber, D.: XX/XY lymphoid chimaerism in congenital immunological deficiency syndrome with thymic aplasia. Lancet **ii**:1152–1156, 1965.

Kady, D.E., Gilbert, W.M., Anderson, J., Danielsen, B., Towner, D. and Smith, L.H.: Trauma during pregnancy: An analysis of maternal and fetal outcomes in a large population. Amer. J. Obstet. Gynecol. **190**:1661–1668, 2004.

Kao, S.-M., Tang, G.-C., Hsieh, T.-T., Young, K.-C., Wang, H.-C. and Pao, C.C.: Analysis of peripheral blood of pregnant women for the presence of fetal Y chromosome-specific ZFY gene deoxyribonucleic acid sequences. Amer. J. Obstet. Gynecol. **166**:1013–1019, 1992.

Kaplan, C., Blanc, W.A. and Elias, J.: Identification of erythrocytes in intervillous thrombi: A study using immunoperoxidase identification of hemoglobins. Human Pathol. **13**:554–556, 1982.

Karimi, P., Ramus, R., Urban, J. and Perlman, J.M.: Extensive brain injury in a premature infant following a relatively minor maternal motor vehicle accident with airbag deployment. J. Perinatol. **24**:454–457, 2004.

Kawagoe, K., Koresawa, M., Ohama, K. and Kadotani, T.: A preliminary study of immunological tolerance in human newborn baby based on mixed leucocyte cultures. Japan J. Genet. **46**:191–194, 1971.

Keenan, H. and Pearse, W.H.: Transplacental transmission of fetal erythrocytes. Amer. J. Obstet. Gynecol. **86**:1096–1098, 1963.

Keller, J.L., Baker, D.A. and Clemmons, J.J.: Massive fetal-maternal hemorrhage: An overlooked cause of perinatal morbidity and mortality. Lab. Invest. **42**:32, 1980.

Kettel, L.M., Branch, D.W. and Scott, J.R.: Occult placental abruption after maternal trauma. Obstet. Gynecol. **71**:449–453, 1988.

Kirkendall, C., Romo, M. and Phelan, J.: Fetomaternal hemorrhage in fetal brain injury. Amer. J. Obstet. Gynecol. **185**:S153 (abstract 268), 2001.

Kleihauer, E. und Brandt, G.: Zur Lebensdauer fetaler Erythrocyten im mütterlichen Kreislauf nach fetomaternaler Transfusion. Klin. Wschr. **42**:458–459, 1964.

Kleihauer, E., Braun, H. und Betke, K.: Demonstration von fetalem Hämoglobin in den Erythrocyten eines Blutausstriches. Klin. Wschr. **35**:637–638, 1957.

Kline, B.S.: Microscopic observations of the placental barrier in transplacental erythrocytotoxic anemia (erythroblastosis fetalis) and in normal pregnancy. Amer. J. Obstet. Gynecol. **56**:226–237, 1948.

Kosasa, T.S., Ebesugawa, I., Nakayama, R.T. and Hale, R.W.: Massive fetomaternal hemorrhage preceded by decreased fetal movement and a nonreactive fetal heart rate pattern. Obstet. Gynecol. **82**:711–714, 1993.

LaFerla, J.J., Butch, S.H. and Cooley, J.R.: Utilization of specific mixed agglutination in a case of apparent fetomaternal hemorrhage. Amer. J. Obstet. Gynecol. **141**:581–582, 1981.

Lakoff, K.M., Klein, J., Bolognese, R.J. and Corson, S.L.: Transplacental hemorrhage during voluntary interruption of pregnancy. J. Reprod. Med. **6**:260–261, 1971.

Larroche, J.-C.: Fetal encephalopathies of circulatory origin. Biol. Neonate **50**:61–74, 1986.

Laube, D.W. and Schauberger, C.W.: Fetomaternal bleeding as a cause for "unexplained" fetal death. Obstet. Gynecol. **60**:649–651, 1982.

Lavin, J.P. and Miodovnik, M.: Delayed abruption after maternal trauma as a result of an automobile accident. J. Reprod. Med. **26**:621–624, 1981.

Lee, R.E. and Vazquez, J.J.: Immunocytochemical evidence for transplacental passage of erythrocytes. Lab. Invest. **11**:580–584, 1962.

Leiberman, J.R., Mazor, M. and Cohen, A.: Detection of fetal blood. Amer. J. Obstet. Gynecol. **161**:257–258, 1989.

Lele, A.S., Carmody, P.J., Hurd, M.E. and O'Leary, J.A.: Fetomaternal bleeding following diagnostic amniocentesis. Obstet. Gynecol. **60**:60–64, 1982.

Leong, M., Duby, S. and Kinch, R.A.H.: Fetal-maternal transfusion following early abortion. Obstet. Gynecol. **54**:424–426, 1979.

Léwi, S., Barrier, J., Ducas, P. et Clarke, T.K.: Nouvelle observation de transfusion foeto-maternelle. Bull. Féd. Soc. Gynécol. Obstétr. **17**:130–136, 1965.

Léwi, S., Clarke, T.K., Guéritat, Walker, P. et Mayer, M.: Less érythrocytes foetaux dans la circulation maternelle. Bull. Gynécol. d'Obstet. **13**:535–545, 1961.

Li, T.C. and Bromham, D.R.: Fetomaternal macrotransfusion in the Yorkshire region. 2. Perinatal outcome. Brit. J. Obstet. Gynaecol. **95**:1152–1158, 1988.

Lipitz, S., Achiron, R., Horoshovski, D., Rotstein, Z., Sherman, D. and Schiff, E.: Fetomaternal haemorrhage discovered after trauma and treated by fetal intravascular transfusion. Europ. J. Obstetr. Gynaecol. Repro. Biol. **71**:21–22, 1997.

Litwak, O., Taswell, H.F., Banner, E.A. and Keith, L.: Fetal erythrocytes in maternal circulation after spontaneous abortion. JAMA **214**:531–534, 1970.

Lloyd, L.K., Miya, F., Hebertson, R.M., Kochenour, N.K. and Scott, J.R.: Intrapartum fetomaternal bleeding in Rh-negative women. Obstet. Gynecol. **56**:285–288, 1980.

Lo, Y.-M.D., Patel, P., Wainscoat, J.S., Sampietro, M., Gillmer, M.D.G. and Fleming, K.A.: Prenatal sex determination by DNA amplification from maternal peripheral blood. Lancet **ii**:1363–1365, 1989.

Los, F.J., de Wolf, B.T.H.M. and Huisjes, H.J.: Raised maternal serum-alpha-fetoprotein levels and spontaneous fetomaternal transfusion. Lancet **ii**:1210–1212, 1979.

Los, F.J., Jahoda, M.G.J., Wladimiroff, J.W. and Brezinka, C.: Fetal exsanguination by chorionic villus sampling. Lancet **342**:1559, 1993.

Low, J.A., Ludwin, S.K. and Fisher, S.: Severe fetal asphyxia associated with neuropathology. Amer. J. Obstet. Gynecol. **175**:1385–1385, 1996.

Luyet, F., Schmid, J., Maroni, E. and Duc, G.: Massive feto-maternal transfusion during external version with fatal outcome. Arch. Gynäkol. **221**:273–275, 1976.

Macris, N.T., Hellman, L.M. and Watson, R.J.: Transmission of transfused sickle-trait cells from mother to fetus. Amer. J. Obstet. Gynecol. **76**:1214–1218, 1958.

Mannherz, K.H.: Feto-maternale Blutung als Ursache von Neugeborenenanämie. Zbl. Gynäkol. **82**:1252–1257, 1960.

Maruko, K., Maeda, T., Kamitomo, M., Hatae, M. and Sueyoshi, K.: Transplacental transmission of maternal B-cell lymphoma. Amer. J. Obstet. Gynecol. **191**:380–381, 2004.

Mayer, M.M., Anh, J.N.H. et Panigel, M.M.: Observation au microscope électronique du passage d'hématies a travers la paroi des capillaires foetaux dans le placenta humain. Compt. Rend. Acad. Sc. Paris. **260**:4605–4606, 1965.

McGowan, G.W.: Massive transplacental hemorrhage with neonatal death. JAMA **203**:599–601, 1968.

McLarey, D.C. and Fish, S.A.: Fetal erythrocytes in the maternal circulation. Amer. J. Obstet. Gynecol. **95**:824–830, 1966.

Megapanos, E.N., Rettos, A.S., Sfontouris, I.G. et Statholoulos, A.I.: La perméabilité du placenta aux érythrocytes maternels au terme grossesse. Gynécol. Obstet. (Paris) **65**:233–240, 1966.

Mennuti, M.T., DiGaetano, A., McDonnell, A., Cohen, A.W. and Liston, R.M.: Fetal-maternal bleeding associated with genetic amniocentesis: real-time versus static ultrasound. Obstet. Gynecol. **62**:26–30, 1983.

Messer, R.H., Pearse, W.H. and Keenan, H.: Effect of carbazochrome salicylate on transplacental transmission of fetal erythrocytes. Obstet. Gynecol. **27**:83–88, 1966.

Michael, A.F. and Mauer, A.M.: Maternal-fetal transfusion as a cause of plethora in the neonatal period. Pediatrics **28**:458–461, 1961.

Mollison, P.L.: Quantitation of transplacental haemorrhage. Brit. Med. J. **iii**:31–34, 1972. (Correction p. 115).

Montgomery, L.D., Belfort, M.A. and Adam, K.: Massive fetomaternal hemorrhage treated with serial combined intravascular and intraperitoneal fetal transfusions. Amer. J. Obstet. Gynecol. **173**:234–235, 1995.

Mor-Yosef, S., Granat, M., Cividalli, G. and Peleg, O.: Acute feto-maternal transfusion—Diagnostic considerations. Austr. N.Z.J. Obstetr. Gynaecol. **24**:219–222, 1984.

Moszkowski, E.F., Eby, B., Shocket, C. and Givila, V.: Cytogenetic evidence for materno-fetal transfusion of polymorphonuclears. J. Reprod. Med. **6**:49–51, 1971.

Moya, F.R., Perez, A. and Reece, E.A.: Severe fetomaternal hemorrhage. A report of four cases. J. Reprod. Med. **32**:243–246, 1987.

Murray, D.J.: Severe abruptio placentae initiated by trauma and associated with hypofibrinogenemia. Can. Med. Assoc. J. **91**:1316–1317, 1964.

Naeye, R.L., Lambert, K.C. and Durfee, H.A.: Widespread infarcts following fetomaternal hemorrhage. Report of case. Obstet. Gynecol. **23**:115–117, 1964.

Nance, S.J., Nelson, J.M., Arndt, P.A., Lam, H.-T. C. and Garratty, G.: Quantitation of fetal-maternal hemorrhage by flow cytometry. A simple and accurate method. Amer. J. Clin. Pathol. **91**:288–292, 1989.

Ness, P.M.: The assessment of fetal-maternal hemorrhage by an enzyme-linked antiglobulin test for Rh-immune globulin recipients. Amer. J. Obstet. Gynecol. **143**:788–792, 1982.

Ness, P.M., Baldwin, M.L. and Niebyl, J.R.: Clinical high-risk designation does not predict excess fetal-maternal hemorrhage. Amer. J. Obstet. Gynecol. **156**:154–158, 1987.

Oehlert, G., Mohrmann, J.E. und Michel, C.F.: Untersuchungen zur Plazentapassage fetaler Blutelemente. Zbl. Gynäkol. **82**:1544–1551, 1960.

Oehme, J., Hundeshagen, H. und Eschenbach, C.: Über die Passage markierter Leukocyten vom Muttertiere zum Feten —zugleich ein Beitrag zur Runt-Disease. Klin. Wchschr. **44**:430–433, 1966.

Olding, L.: The possibility of materno-foetal transfer of lymphocytes in man. Acta Paediatr. Scand. **61**:73–75, 1972.

Olding, L., Benirschke, K. and Oldstone, M.B.A.: Inhibition of mitosis of lymphocytes from human adults by lymphocytes from human newborns. Clin. Immunol. Immunopathol. **3**:79–89, 1974.

Overstreet, K., Mannino, F.L. and Benirschke, K.: The role of placental pathology in the evaluation of interpersonal violence: a case of abdominal gunshot wound in a 27-week gravid uterus. J. Perinatol. **22**:675–678, 2002.

Owen, J., Stedman, C.M. and Tucker, T.L.: Comparison of predelivery versus postdelivery Kleihauer-Betke stains in cases of fetal death. Amer. J. Obstet. Gynecol. **161**:663–666, 1989.

Pai, M.K.R., Bedritis, I. and Zipursky, A.: Massive transplacental hemorrhage: clinical manifestations in the newborn. Canad. Med. Assoc. J. **112**:585–589, 1975.

Palliez, R., Delecour, M., Monnier, K.-C., Hutin, A. et Abdelatif, M.: Passage transplacentaire des hématies foetales durant la grossesse et dans le post-partum. Rev. Franç. Gynécol. **65**:579–584, 1970.

Parida, S.K., Kriss, V.M. and Pulito, A.R.: Fetal morbidity and mortality following motor vehicle accident: Two case reports. J. Perinatol. 19:144–146, 1999.

Paros, N.L.: Case of foetal anaemia due to transplacental bleeding seen in general practice. Brit. M. J. **i**:839–840, 1962.

Pauls, F. and Boutros, P.: The value of placental localization prior to amniocentesis. Obstet. Gynecol. **35**:175–177, 1970.

Pearlman, M.D. and Phillips, M.E.: Safety belt use during pregnancy. Obstet. Gynecol. **88**:1026–1029, 1996.

Pearlman, M.D., Tintinalli, J.E. and Lorenz, R.P.: Blunt trauma during pregnancy. NEJM **323**:1609–1613, 1990a.

Pearlman, M.D., Tintinalli, J.E. and Lorenz, R.P.: A prospective controlled study of outcome after trauma during pregnancy. Amer. J. Obstet. Gynecol. **162**:1502–1510, 1990b.

Pelikan, D.M., Scherjon, S.A., Mesker, W.E., de Groot-Swings, G.M., Brouwer-Mandema, G.G., Tanke, H.J. and Kanhai, H. H.; Quantification of fetomaternal hemorrhage: a comparative study of the manual and automated microscopic Kleihauer-Betke tests and flow cytometry in clinical samples. Amer. J. Obstet. Gynecol. **191**:551–557, 2004.

Pembrey, M.E., Weatherhall, D.J. and Clegg, J.B.: Maternal synthesis of haemoglobin F in pregnancy. Lancet **i**:1350–1355, 1973.

Peyser, M.R. and Toaff, R.: Traumatic rupture of the placenta: a rare cause of fetal death. Obstet. Gynecol. **34**:561–563, 1969.

Pielet, B.W., Socol, M.L., MacGregor, S.N., Ney, J.A. and Dooley, S.L.: Cordocentesis: an appraisal of risks. Amer. J. Obstet. Gynecol. **159**:1497–1500, 1988.

Pilkington, R., Knoz, E.G., Russell, J.K. and Walker, W.: Foetal-maternal transfusion and rhesus sensitisation. J. Obstet. Gynaecol. Brit. Cwlth. **73**:909–916, 1966.

Pollack, M. and Montague, A.C.W.: Transplacental hemorrhage in postterm pregnancies. Amer. J. Obstet. Gynecol. **102**:383–387, 1968.

Pollack, M.S., Kirkpatrick, D., Kapoor, N., Dupont, B. and O'Reilly, R.J.: The identification by HLA typing of intrauterine-derived maternal T cells in four patients with severe immunodeficiency. NEJM **307**:662–666, 1982.

Pollock, A.: Transplacental haemorrhage after external cephalic version. Lancet **1**:612, 1968.

Potter, E.L.: Intervillous thrombi in the placenta and their possible relation to erythroblastosis fetalis. Amer. J. Obstet. Gynecol. **56**:959–961, 1948.

Pourbabak, S., Rund, C.R. and Crookston, K.P.: Three cases of massive fetomaternal hemorrhage presenting without clinical suspicion. Arch. Pathol. Lab. Med. **128**:463–465, 2004.

Pozniak, M.A., Cullenward, M.J., Zickuhr, D. and Curet, L.B.: Venous lake bleeding: a complication of chorionic villus sampling. J. Ultrasound Med. **7**:297–299, 1988.

Quintero, R.A., Romero, R., Mahoney, M.J., Abuhamad, A., Vecchio, M., Holden, J. and Hobbins, J.C.: Embryoscopic demonstration of hemorrhagic lesions on the human embryo after placental trauma. Amer. J. Obstet. Gynecol. **168**: 756–759, 1993.

Raafat, M., Brayton, J.B., Apgar, V. and Borgaonkar, D.S.: A new approach to prenatal diagnosis using trophoblastic cells in maternal blood. Birth Defects Original Article Series **11**:295–302, 1975.

Renaer, M., Putte, I.V. de and Vermylen, C.: Massive fetomaternal hemorrhage as cause of perinatal mortality and morbidity. Europ. J. Obstet. Gynecol. Reprod. Biol. **6**:125–140, 1976.

Rijhsinghani, A. and Smith, D.: Self-limiting nonimmune hydrops and acute fetal small bowel distention following maternal trauma. Obstetr. Gynecol. **90**:700–701, 1997.

Rodgers, B.D., Marusak, J.J. and Rodgers, D.E.: Criminal prosecution for prenatal injury. Obstet. Gynecol. **80**:522–523, 1992.

Rosc, P.G., Strohm, P.L. and Zuspan, F.P.: Fetomaternal hemorrhage following trauma. Amer. J. Obstet. Gynecol. **153**:844–847, 1985.

Rosta, J.: Feto-maternal hemorrhage during pregnancy and delivery. In, Perinatal Medicine, Part II. E. Kerpel-Fronius, P.V. Véghelyi and J. Rosta, eds. Akademiai Kiado, Budapest, 1978.

Rouse, D. and Weiner, C.: Ongoing fetomaternal hemorrhage treated by serial fetal intravascular transfusions. Obstet. Gynecol. **76**:974–975, 1990.

Rudolph, A.J., Abrahamov, A.A. and deVenecia, J.F.: Another case of fetomaternal transfusion. J. Philipp. Med. Assoc. **38**:134–137, 1962.

Ryerson, C.S. and Sanes, S.: The age of pregnancy. Histologic diagnosis from percentage of erythroblasts in chorionic capillaries. Arch. Pathol. **17**:548–651, 1934.

Saber, R.S.: Stillbirth due to extensive feto-maternal transfusion. N.Y. State J. Med. **77**:2249–2250, 1977.

Samadi, R., Miller, D., Settlage, R., Gvazda, I, Paul, R. and Goodwin, T.M.: Massive fetomaternal hemorrhage and fetal death: Is it predictable? Amer. J. Obstet. Gynecol. **174**:391 (abstr. 294), 1996.

Santamaria, M., Benirschke, K., Carpenter, P.M., Baldwin, V.J. and Pritchard, J.A.: Transplacental hemorrhage associated with placental neoplasms. Pediatr. Pathol. **7**:601–615, 1987.

Schellong, G.: Anämie und Schock beim Neugeborenen durch fetalen Blutverlust. Monatsschr. Kinderh. **117**:578–579, 1969.

Schmorl, G.: Pathologisch-Anatomische Untersuchungen über Puerperale Eklampsie. F.C.W. Vogel, Leipzig, 1893.

Schmorl, G.: Über das Schicksal embolisch verschleppter Plazentarzellen. Verhandl. Deutsch. Pathol. Gesellsch. **8**:39–46, 1905.

Schneider, J. und Ludwig, G.A.: Eine neue Zählmethode zur quantitativen Erfassung kleinster Mengen fetaler, in den mütterlichen Kreislauf eingeschwemmter Erythrocyten. Klin. Wschr. **41**:563–565, 1963.

Schröder, J.: Review article: Transplacental passage of blood cells. J. Med. Genet. **12**:230–242, 1975.

Schröder, J., Schröder, E. and Cann, H.M.: Fetal cells in the maternal blood. Lack of response of fetal cells in maternal blood to mitogens and mixed leukocyte culture. Hum. Genet. **38**:91–97, 1977.

Schultze, P.M., Stamm, C.A. and Roger, J.: Placental abruption and fetal death with airbag deployment in a motor vehicle accident. Obstet. Gynecol. **92**:719, 1998.

Seligman, S.P. and Young, B.K.: Tachycardia as the sole fetal heart rate abnormality after funipuncture. Obstet. Gynecol. **87**:833–834, 1996.

Selypes, A. and Lorencz, R.: A noninvasive method for determination of the sex and karyotype of the fetus from the maternal blood. Hum. Genet. **79**:357–359, 1988.

Shahar, E., Birenbaum, E., Inbar, D. and Brish, M.: Hypovolemic shock at birth due to extensive fetomaternal hemorrhage. Israel J. Med. Sci. **17**:441–444, 1981.

Shields, L.E., Widness, J.A. and Brace, R.A.: Restoration of fetal red blood cells and plasma proteins after a moderately severe hemorrhage in the ovine fetus. Amer. J. Obstet. Gynecol. **169**:1472–1478, 1993.

Shields, L.E., Widness, J.A. and Brace, R.A.: The hematologic and plasma iron responses to severe fetal hemorrhage in the ovine fetus. Amer. J. Obstet. Gynecol. **174**:55–61, 1996.

Shiller, J.G.: Shock in the newborn caused by transplacental hemorrhage from fetus to mother. Pediatrics **20**:7–11, 1957.

Shulman, L.P., Meyers, C.M., Simpson, J.L., Andersen, R.N., Tolley, E.A. and Elias, S.: Fetomaternal transfusion depends on amount of chorionic villi aspirated but not on method of chorionic villus sampling. Amer. J. Obstet. Gynecol. **162**:1185–1188, 1990.

Shurin, S.B.: The blood and the hematopoietic system. In, A.A. Fanaroff & R.J. Martin, eds. Neonatal-Perinatal Medicine. Chapter 32 I. C.V. Mosby Co., St. Louis, 1987. pp. 826–827.

Silver, M.M. and Newman, C.: Letter to the editor. Pediatr. Developm. Pathol. **1**:172–173, 1998.

Simon, N.V., Virgilio, L.A., Beaverson, M.L. and Deveney, L.B.: Detection of large fetal-maternal transfusions. Obstet. Gynecol. **52**:249–252, 1978.

Simpson, J.L. and Elias, S.: Fetal Cells in Maternal Blood. Prospects for noninvasive prenatal diagnosis. Ann. N.Y. Acad. Sci. **731**:1–270, 1994.

Smith, J.J. and Benjamin, F.: Post-hemorrhagic anemia and shock in the newborn at birth. Obstet. Gynecol. Surv. **23**:511–521, 1968.

Smith, K., Duhring, J.L., Greene, J.W., Rochlin, D.B. and Blakemore, W.S.: Transfer of maternal erythrocytes across the human placenta. Obstet. Gynecol. **18**:673–676, 1961.

Stafford, P.A., Biddinger, P.W. and Zumwalt, R.E.: Lethal intrauterine fetal trauma. Amer. J. Obstet. Gynecol. **159**:485–489, 1988.

Stein, G.A.V., Munsick, R.A., Stiver, K. and Ryder, K.: Fetomaternal hemorrhage in threatened abortion. Obstet. Gynecol. **79**:383–386, 1992.

Stiller, A.G. and Skafish, P.R.: Placental chorangioma: a rare cause of fetomaternal transfusion with maternal hemolysis and fetal distress. Obstet. Gynecol. **67**:296–298, 1986.

Stonehill, L.L. and LaFerla, J.J.: Assessment of fetomaternal hemorrhage with Kleihauer-Betke test. Amer. J. Obstet. Gynecol. **155**:1146, 1986.

Streiff, F., Peters, A. et Vincent, D.: La perméabilité placentaire aux hématies. Pathologie-Biologie **12**:963–972, 1964.

Sullivan, J.F. and Jennings, E.R.: Transplacental fetal-maternal hemorrhage. Amer. J. Pathol. **46**:36–42, 1966.

Suzumori, K., Adachi, R., Okada, S., Narukawa, T., Yagami, Y. and Sonta, S.: Fetal cells in the maternal circulation: Detection of Y-sequence by gene amplification. Obstet. Gynecol. **80**:150–154, 1992.

Theurer, D.E. and Kaiser, I.H.: Traumatic fetal death without uterine injury. Report of a case. Obstet. Gynecol. **21**:477–480, 1963.

Tomoda, Y.: Demonstration of foetal erythrocyte by immunofluorescent staining. Nature **202**:910–911, 1964.

Valle, Del G.O., Joffe, G.M., Izquierdo, L.A., Smith, J.F., Kasnic, T., Gilson, G.J., Chatterjee, M.S. and Curet, L.B.: Acute posttraumatic fetal anemia treated with fetal intravascular transfusion. Amer. J. Obstet. Gynecol. **166**:127–129, 1992.

Van Kamp, I.L., Klumper, F.J.C.M., Oepkes, D., Meerman, R.H., Scherjon, S.A., Vandenbussche, F.P.H.A. and Kanhai, H.H.H.: Complications of intrauterine intravascular transfusion for fetal anemia due to re-cell alloimmunization. Amer. J. Obstet. Gynecol. **192**:171–177, 2005.

Veyver, I.V.D., Saade, G., Lockett, L., Hudson, K. and Moise, K.: The use of Kleihauer-Betke stain in pregnant patients with abdominal trauma. Amer. J. Obstet. Gynecol. **168**:432 (abstr. 492), 1993.

Virgilio, L.A. and Simon, N.V.: Measurement of fetal cells in the maternal circulation. Obstet. Gynecol. **50**:364–366, 1977.

Voigt, J.C. and Britt, R.P.: Feto-maternal haemorrhage in therapeutic abortion. Br. Med. J. **2**:395–396, 1969.

Walsh, J.J. and Lewis, B.V.: Transplacental haemorrhage due to termination of pregnancy. J. Obstet. Gynaecol. Br. Commonw. **77**:133–136, 1970.

Walter, P., Lewi, S., Loewe-Lyon, S. et Clarke, T.K.: Transfusion foeto-maternelle avec hypertrophie du placenta. Gynecol. Obstet. (Paris) **64**:103–110, 1965.

Warren, R.C., Butler, J., Morsman, J.M., McKenzie, C. and Rodeck, C.H.: Does chorionic villus sampling cause fetomaternal haemorrhage? Lancet **1**:691, 1985.

Wentworth, P.: A placental lesion to account for foetal haemorrhage into the maternal circulation. J. Obstet. Gynaecol. Brit. Cwlth. **71**:379–387, 1964.

Wickster, G.Z.: Posthemorrhagic shock in the newborn. Amer. J. Obstet. Gynecol. **63**:524–537, 1952.

Wiener, A.S.: Diagnosis and treatment of anemia of the newborn caused by occult placental hemorrhage. Amer. J. Obstet. Gynecol. **56**:717–722, 1948.

Williams, J.K., McCalin, L., Rosemurgy, A.S. and Colorado, N. M.: Evaluation of blunt abdominal trauma in the third trimester of pregnancy: maternal and fetal considerations. Obstet. Gynecol. **75**:33–37, 1990.

Willis, C. and Foreman, C.S.: Chronic massive fetomaternal hemorrhage: a case report. Obstet. Gynecol. **71**:459–461, 1988.

Wong, T.T.T. and Cann, M.C.K.: Transfusion reaction following ABO-incompatible maternofetal transfusion. J. Pediatr. **80**:479–483, 1972.

Woodrow, J.C. and Finn, R.: Transplacental haemorrhage. Brit. J. Haematol. **12**:297–309, 1966.

Young, P.E., Matson, M.R. and Jones, O.W.: Fetal exsanguination and other vascular injuries from midtrimester amniocentesis. Amer. J. Obstet. Gynecol. **129**:21–24, 1977.

Zarou, D.M., Lichtman, H.C. and Hellman, L.M.: The transmission of chromium-51 tagged maternal erythrocytes from mother to fetus. Amer. J. Obstet. Gynecol. **88**:565–571, 1964.

Zilliacus, H.: Agglutinated incompatible fetal erythrocytes in the maternal circulation. Amer. J. Obstet. Gynecol. **86**:1093–1095, 1963.

Zilliacus, R., Chapelle, A. de la, Schröder, J., Tilikainen, A., Kohne, E. and Kleihauer, E.: Transplacental passage of foetal blood cells. Scand. J. Haematol. **15**:333–338, 1975.

Zipursky, A., Hull, A., White, F.D. and Israel, L.G.: Foetal erythrocytes in the maternal circulation. Lancet **i**:451–452, 1959.

Zipursky, A., Pollock, J., Chown, B. and Israels, L.G.: Transplacental foetal haemorrhage after placental injury during delivery or amniocentesis. Lancet **ii**:493–494, 1963a.

Zipursky, A., Pollock, J., Neelands, P., Chown, B. and Israels, L. G.: The transplacental passage of foetal red blood-cells and the pathogenesis of Rh immunisation during pregnancy. Lancet **ii**:489–493, 1963b.

Zizka, Z., Calda, P., Zlatohlavkova, B., Haakova, L., Cerna, M., Jirasek, J.E., Fait, T., Hajek, Z. and Kvasnicka, J.: Massive fetomaternal transplacental hemorrhage as a perinatology problem, role of ABO fetomaternal compatibility—case studies. Med. Sci. Monit. **7**:308–311, 2001.

18
Fetal Storage Disorders

Many of the so-called errors in metabolism, the storage diseases, produce inclusions or vacuoles in the tissues of affected individuals. The placenta is often similarly involved, and chorionic villus sampling (CVS) biopsy is now more often employed to make the diagnosis prenatally, as for instance in diagnosing lipofuscinosis (Rapola et al., 1990). Electron microscopy and special enzyme studies are usually helpful for the precise diagnosis of the defect involved. Thus, appropriate fixation is needed when such disease is suspected and it must also be anticipated at the time of CVS, as many of the inclusions are highly water and lipid-solvent soluble. Because many of these diseases are the cause of fetal hydrops, the cases of nonimmune hydrops fetalis warrant special attention. An excellent ultrastructural study of 11 cases has been published by Jones et al. (1990) that details procedures and findings, and Fox (1997) has shown other material. These publications depict the findings in admirable detail and provide additional literature. Table 18.1 summarizes the current status of placental studies in various storage disorders.

Gaucher's disease, as mentioned in Chapter 16, may cause fetal hydrops. It is a heterogeneous disease whose genetics and clinical manifestations were well described by Sidransky and Ginns (1993). In the case described by Ginsburg and Groll (1973), polyhydramnios complicated the second pregnancy of a patient in the second trimester. At 34 weeks, she delivered a macerated, hydropic fetus. The large and edematous placenta had the macroscopic features of erythroblastosis fetalis. The mother's third pregnancy also resulted in neonatal demise due to Gaucher's disease. The fetal findings were characteristic of type II Gaucher's disease in the hydropic 21-week fetus described by Rice et al. (1984). The placenta was not described. Gillan et al. (1984) and Bouvier and Maire (1997) provided additional insight with numerous diverse cases. Soma et al. (2000) illustrated a characteristic case with recurrent hydrops fetalis in a Japanese pedigree.

Mucolipidosis type II, or **I-cell disease,** is a rare and fatal disorder whose genetic transmission is autosomal recessive. Gellis and Feingold (1977) delineated the principal features of affected children. Hanai et al. (1971) emphasized the abundance of periodic acid-Schiff (PAS)-positive lysosomal inclusions in the cells of affected children. In 1974, Granström et al. and Rapola et al. separately reported that affected newborns may have coarse features similar to those of patients with Hurler's syndrome, and demonstrated inclusions in leukocytes. Aula et al. (1975) made the first prenatal diagnosis of this disease from an increase of amnionic fluid hydrolases. Later, they used fibroblasts of the aborted fetus to confirm the diagnosis. The investigators emphasized that paraffin sections do not allow the visualization of the inclusions; they are obvious, however, in epoxy-embedded material. The inclusions of this disorder are preferentially located in kidney and mesenchymal cells. Terashima et al. (1975) presented an extensive differential diagnosis of these inclusions in their description of three cases. Placental involvement with inclusion-bearing cells was first demonstrated in a case report of Powell et al. (1976). The syncytium and Hofbauer cells were primarily affected; the vacuoles of formerly mucolipid-containing lysosomes were readily apparent in paraffin sections of the placenta (Figs. 18.1 and 18.2), but the features were much enhanced by processing the tissues in epoxy resin. The authors of this paper emphasized that only **fetal** cells contained the vacuoles. Affected tissue included the X cells of cell columns and the placental floor. There were no inclusions in decidual cells, and they used this to further identify X cells as being of fetal origin. The placenta was grossly pale and somewhat enlarged; the fetus was not hydropic. The same report contained three additional and similar storage diseases that affected the placenta but the precise nature of their storage disorders could not be identified. Abe et al. (1976) and Nagashima et al. (1977) described other morphologic studies. Several investigators further elaborated on placental aspects of mucolipidosis type II.

TABLE 18.1. Summary of placental findings in various storage diseases

Disease	Findings	Reference
Glycogen storage type II Pompe's disease	Vacuoles full of glycogen in EM in stroma, endothelium, cytotrophoblast, lysosomes	Bendon and Hug, 1985 Jones et al., 1990 Roberts et al., 1991
Mucopolysaccharidosis Hurler's disease	Vacuolization of fibroblasts and syncytium	Jones et al., 1990
Sanfilippo's disease	Vacuolated syncytium, absent heparin-N-sulfatase in CVS	Jones et al., 1990 Kleijer et al., 1986
Morquio's disease, type IV	Edema of villi	Applegarth et al., 1987
β-glucuronidase deficiency	Hofbauer cell vacuolization, hydrops	Nelson et al., 1993
Sialic acid storage Salla's disease	Vacuolated syncytium and Hofbauer cells with amorphous and fibrillar material, vacuolated extravillous trophoblast and amnionic epithelium	Gillan et al., 1984 Jauniaux et al., 1987 Jones et al., 1990 Roberts et al., 1991
Gaucher's disease	Hydrops	Ginsburg and Groll, 1973 Gillan et al., 1984 Rice et al., 1984 Sidransky and Ginns, 1993
Sphingomyelin storage Niemann-Pick's disease types A and C; Type B may have inclusions	Vacuolization and laminated inclusions (myelin bodies) in syncytium, stroma, Hofbauer cells, umbilical cord fibrocytes, hydrops	Sarrut and Belamich, 1983 Vanier et al., 1989 Meizner et al., 1990 Schoenfeld et al., 1985
Gangliosidoses GM 2, gangliosidosis type I, Tay-Sachs' disease	Vacuolated trophoblast and Hofbauer cells, amnion Absent hexosaminidase in CVS	Lowden et al., 1973 Grebner et al., 1983 Roberts, 1991 Benirschke and Kaufmann, 1995
Type II Sandhoff's disease	Multiple parallel arrays in lysosomes of stroma, vacuolated syncytium, myelin bodies	Fox, 1997
Fabry's disease Glycosphingolipidosis	Lamellar lysosomal inclusions in decidual cells, chorionic cells normal, in heterozygous carrier	Popli et al., 1990
Mucolipidoses Type I Sialidosis	Vacuolated trophoblast and stroma, normal amnion	Riches and Smuckler, 1983 Laver et al., 1983 Stevenson et al., 1983 Gillan et al., 1984 Baldwin et al., 1985 Mahmood and Haleem, 1989 Bouvier and Maire, 1997
Type II I-cell disease	Vacuolated syncytium, vacuolated Hofbauer and X cells Occasional myelin figures in EM	Powell et al., 1976 Rapola and Aula, 1977 Sarrut and Belamich, 1983
Type IV	Vacuolated stroma with lamellar inclusions of endothelium	Sekeles et al., 1978
Galactosialidosis	Vacuolated trophoblast and stroma, hydrops	Scully, 1997
Neuronal ceroid lipofuscinosis	Vacuoles in syncytium, amnion, endothelium with "fingerprint" inclusions	Rapola et al., 1988 Conradi et al., 1989

CVS, chorionic villus sampling; EM, electron microscopy.

Thus, Rapola and Aula (1977) beautifully demonstrated the ultrastructural changes of the syncytium and suggested that the diagnosis could easily be made from this material alone (Fig. 18.3). With CVS biopsy, this would now be possible without having to resort to enzymatic study. Gehler et al. (1976) reported biochemical studies of I-cell disease. The differential diagnosis of mucolipidosis types I and III was discussed in a study by Herd et al. (1978). Hug et al. (1984) have shown that maternal serum hexosaminidase levels are increased in pregnancies affected by I-cell disease, which allows diagnosis without uterine invasion. We strongly disagree with the interpretation of Cozzutto (1983), however, who reported on a macerated stillborn whose placenta also had extensive vacuolar changes. The placenta was structurally typical of I-cell disease. Cozzutto found vacuolated "stromal decidual cells," but he did not depict these. He interpreted the changes as "convincingly demonstrating" that the foam cells are a transformation secondary to edema or fetal death. In our experience, such vacuolation never results

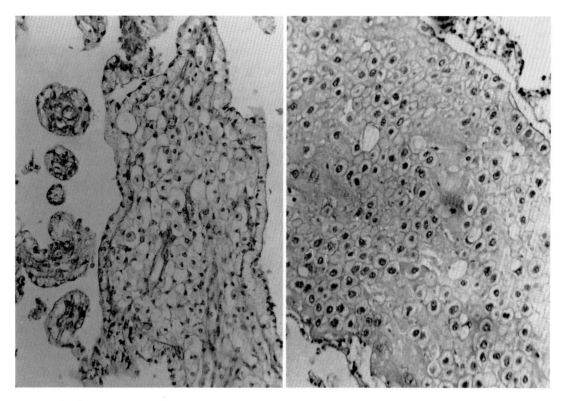

FIGURE 18.1. Villus (left) and X-cell column of placenta, affected by mucolipidosis II (I-cell disease). Note the abundance of vacuoles in the syncytium and Hofbauer cells; similar inclusions are present in the cytoplasm of X cells. H&E ×240.

from fetal death or edema. The abundance of foam cells, the disposition of trophoblastic vacuoles, and irregular calcifications observed by him (and us as well) all are indicative of an unidentified fetal storage disorder. Because the cellular glycolipids are highly water-soluble, the empty appearance of the vacuoles is the usual finding in many fetal storage disorders. We saw another case with

extensive and typical syncytial vacuolization (courtesy of S. Romansky, Los Angeles). The neonate was well and had no signs of disease when 4 months old. The enlarged placenta had also numerous vascular lesions, mostly in the villous stem arteries, varying from fibrinoid necrosis to complete obliteration, with occasional histologic findings of the nonspecific "hemorrhagic endovasculitis". In

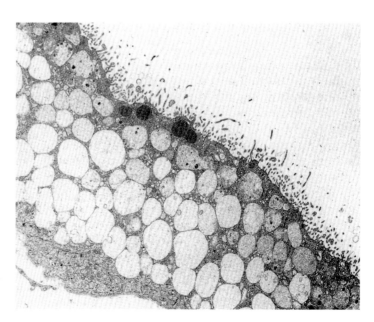

FIGURE 18.2. Syncytium in case of I-cell disease. Note the extensive, fine vacuolation, the storage site of washed-out glycolipids in the syncytial cytoplasm. EM ×6700. (Courtesy of Dr. J. Rapola, Helsinki, Finland.)

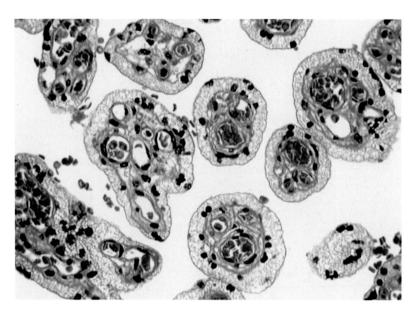

FIGURE 18.3. Appearance of villi in I-cell disease (mucolipidosis II). The syncytium is characteristically uniformly finely vacuolated. (Courtesy of Dr. Scott Hyde, 1999.)

addition, there were numerous foci of villous calcifications. Because of the simultaneous presence of numerous myelin figures in electron micrographs, the diagnosis of I-cell disease was thought unlikely; moreover, neonatal screening tests were negative. Follow-up with skin biopsies at herniorrhaphy at age 8 months showed vacuolar changes in fibroblasts and coarse facial features became evident. Very high levels of lysosomal enzymes were then found and I-cell disease was diagnosed. The infant became severely retarded.

Hurler's syndrome (mucopolysaccharidosis I) showed "striking vacuolation of stromal cells," including Hofbauer cells (Jones et al., 1990).

Other storage diseases affect fetal and placental tissue. By amniocentesis at 14 weeks, Lowden et al. (1973) identified, the absence of β-galactosidase. That absence is diagnostic of type 1 G_{M1} **gangliosidosis**. The pregnancy was terminated; typical inclusions (zebra bodies) were ultrastructurally identified in the fetal ganglion cells. Although other fetal cells were unremarkable in paraffin sections, vacuoles were seen in epon-embedded material. The placenta showed numerous "empty vacuoles" in the syncytial cytoplasm, extravillous trophoblast, and Hofbauer cells (Roberts et al., 1991). They were visible even in paraffin sections. Presumably, these contain the water-soluble storage product, and galactose-rich mucopolysaccharide. Other case descriptions of the disease do not include descriptions of the placenta (Giugliani et al., 1985).

Absence of α-galactosidase A results in **Fabry's disease**, a disorder of glycosphingolipid metabolism. The tissues accumulate ceramide trihexose. A pregnancy in a patient with this disease was described by Popli et al. (1990) after she had received a renal allograft. The placenta of the

term fetus was normal but the decidual cells contained argyrophilic granules that electron micrographically had the appearance similar to zebra bodies. The fetal portions of the placenta were normal. O'Brien (1982) reviewed many lysosomal disorders and their enzymatic deficiencies and provided details of the enzymatic defect.

In the studies by Jones et al. (1990), **Tay Sachs'** disease (G_{M2}-gangliosidosis type I) was found to produce vacuolation of syncytiotrophoblast, with occasional myelin bodies in villous stromal cells. In **Sandhoff's disease** (type II), "the most striking feature ... was the occurrence of parallel membranous arrays in occasional lysosomes within stromal cells." Myelin bodies were found in trophoblast and endothelium.

Mucolipidosis IV (Morquio syndrome type B) is due to the deficiency of β-galactosidase and also referred to as G_{M1}-gangliosidosis. This disease has been diagnosed from cultured amnionic fluid cells by Kohn et al. (1977). The amnion cells contained multiple single-membrane bounded inclusions. Mesodermal elements, however, were negative. Although it may appear superficially that this disease is similar to I-cell disease, in this condition the amnion, not syncytium and Hofbauer cell, has the vacuolation. The placenta of a case we saw was much enlarged (950 g) and much paler and softer than normal. Its amnionic epithelium, trophoblast, Hofbauer cells, and circulating lymphocytes showed striking vacuolation, similar to those of I-cell disease. Calcified thrombi were found in large surface vessels. The 4050-g neonate had massive ascites but no organomegaly. Another case of mucolipidosis IV, supplied by Dr. P. J. Cera, also had surface vessel calcified thrombi, ascites, and massive trophoblastic vacuolization. We have seen endothelial damage, perhaps secondary to lipid accumulation, in other cases of storage disease. In a case of G_{M1} gangliosidosis (mucolipidosis IV) fetal endothelial vacuolization was demonstrable in villous stem vessels (K. Winn, personal communication, 1974).

Morquio's disease (mucopolysaccharidosis type IV A) has also been diagnosed from enzyme analysis of chorionic villus biopsy (Applegarth et al., 1987). Within the family reported by these authors, nonimmune hydrops fetalis had occurred in previous pregnancies. The authors drew attention to previous reports of hydrops with Gaucher's, Wolman's, and Salla's diseases, with sialidosis and mucopolysaccharidosis type VII. In their family, they had a hydropic fetus with a bulky placenta. Vacuolar villous edema and prominent Hofbauer cells were found, but there was no histologic evidence of storage products in the trophoblast.

Maroteaux et al. (1978) and See et al. (1978) have described the general features of **sialidosis** ("nephrosialidosis"; mucolipidosis type I). They depicted the inclusions in the neuraminidase-deficient cells, but did not describe the placenta. In other case reports (Aylsworth et al., 1980; Stevenson et al., 1983), the inclusions of tissues and cultured cells are all well depicted, but these authors did not describe the associated placentas either. Laver et al. (1983) found typical storage vacuoles in Hofbauer cells and the villous syncytium. Amniocyte morphology in this disease has been reported to be normal by electron microscopic study (Stevenson et al., 1983). In a similar disorder, hydrops fetalis resulted in two pregnancies from a combined deficiency of neuraminidase and β-galactosidase (Kleijer et al., 1979). The placenta of these fetuses was not described. Gillan et al. (1984), who discussed congenital ascites in various storage disorders (sialidosis, Salla's disease, gangliosidosis, Gaucher's disease), depicted a placental villus with vacuolated syncytial cytoplasm of a fetus with Salla's disease.

Niemann-Pick disease (type C) does not result in visible storage products of the placenta. When tissue is obtained from CVS and cultured under special conditions, however, the tissue-cultured cells of affected fetuses have been shown to accumulate laminated inclusions of nonesterified cholesterol (myelin bodies), which can then be stained with filipin for unesterified cholesterol, and the diagnosis may thus be secured (Vanier et al., 1989; Jones et al., 1990). Nonimmune hydrops with hydramnios, commencing at 19 weeks' gestation, has been described by Meizner et al. (1990) in Niemann-Pick disease. Fetal death occurred at 36 weeks and the inclusions were identified electron microscopically in the enlarged spleen. The placenta was not described. Niemann-Pick disease type A, due to sphingomyelin diphosphodiesterase deficiency, can be diagnosed from absent enzyme in amnionic fluid. Unusual echogenic densities in the placentas of several cases that also had thick chorionic plates

were sonographically demonstrated by Schoenfeld et al. (1985). Vacuolated syncytium, Hofbauer cells, and fibrocytes of the umbilical cords contained accumulations of sphingomyelin, as did the chorion laeve.

Desai et al. (1985) found lysosomal lipid deposits in **cholesterol ester storage disease** in which the fetal adrenal glands had foci of necrosis and many other tissues possessed a vacuolated cytoplasm. In a detailed Cabot Case description in the *New England Journal of Medicine,* Scully (1997) described a child with hydrops of unknown etiology whose placenta had extensive vacuolation of the syncytium and stromal cells. Because of deficient levels of β-galactosidase and α-neuramidase from cultured cells obtained at amniocentesis the diagnosis of galactosialidosis was established. This discussion included a consideration of the pathogenesis of the fetal hydrops that is still not clarified for most storage diseases.

Bendon and Hug (1985) reported placental abnormalities in five cases of **Pompe's disease** (glycogen storage disease type II; α-1,4-glucosidase deficiency). In routine examination of the placenta, the only unusual finding was the cytoplasmic vacuolation of amnionic connective tissue cells and the villous capillary endothelial cells (Roberts et al., 1991). Electron microscopy, however, showed typical membrane-bounded, glycogen-filled inclusions in capillary endothelial cells and in the villous stroma. They were present even in middle trimester abortuses. Hug et al. (1991) described the diagnosis from CVS at 10 weeks. The previous pregnancy had resulted in an affected child. Electron-microscopic examination 5 days after biopsy identified the typical glycogen-packed membrane-enclosed inclusions in many fetal cells, including fibrocytes that appear as vacuoles in histologic study. These authors insisted that the demonstration of vacuoles alone is insufficient for the diagnosis. Jones and her collaborators (1990) made similar findings of lysosomal glycogen accumulation. These were seen in cytotrophoblast, endothelium, fibrocytes, and pericytes. We have seen the placenta of a neonate with **glycogen storage disease, type IV** (amylopectinase deficiency). It had vacuoles in amnionic epithelium, but no specific lesions were identified. There were none of those cells that had been identified in Pompe's disease. The pregnancy was complicated by hydramnios. The newborn had Lafora bodies in heart, liver, and muscle, had pleural transudate, was dysmorphic, and suffered fatal pulmonary hypoplasia. The placenta was enlarged. A second pregnancy was similarly involved.

Similarly, in **sialic acid storage disease**, Jones et al. (1990) identified the Hofbauer cells, endothelium, and syncytium to be packed with clear, membrane-bound vacuoles (Jauniaux et al., 1987). Roberts et al. (1991) also found vacuolization in extravillous trophoblast and amnionic epithelium. And from chorionic villus biopsy material, more sophisticated culture methods we can anticipate more complex storage diseases to be identified in the future, just as had been anticipated by Nadler and Gerbie many years earlier (1970). Thus, Menkes' disease was diagnosed by the absence of copper from CVS samples (Tønnesen et al., 1985).

It is apparent from these descriptions that many congenital enzyme deficiencies can be diagnosed from amnionic fluid cultures, and chorionic villus samples, and that they may be accompanied by placental manifestations. The location and type of inclusion cannot always be anticipated. Thus, the inclusions of lipofuscinosis were mainly in the fetal capillary endothelium, although they had earlier been suggested to be in syncytiotrophoblast (Rapola et al., 1990). The villus specimens, therefore, should be processed for optimal ultrastructural studies. Chorionic villus biopsy has become of great value in selected cases, especially for prenatal counseling. In this area of research, some published animal models closely parallel the human disease. Most known animal models of storage disease and spontaneous occurrences of inborn errors of metabolism were reviewed by Jolly and Walkley (1997). Their use may be of value, particularly in attempts at therapy, but also for the study of their placentas (Baker et al., 1976).

References

Abe, K., Matsuda, I., Arashima, S., Mitsuyama, T., Oka, Y. and Ishikawa, M.: Ultrastructural studies in fetal I-cell disease. Pediatr. Res. **10**:669–676, 1976.

Applegarth, D.A., Toone, J.R., Wilson, R.D., Long, S.L. and Baldwin, V.J.: Morquio disease presenting as hydrops fetalis and enzyme analysis of chorionic villus tissue in a subsequent pregnancy. Pediatr. Pathol. **7**:593–599, 1987.

Aula, P., Rapola, J., Autio. S., Raivio, K. and Karjalainen, O.: Prenatal diagnosis and fetal pathology of I-cell disease (Mucolipidosis Type II). J. Pediatr. **87**:221–226, 1975.

Aylsworth, A.S., Thomas, G.H., Hood, J.L., Malouf, N. and Libert, J.: A severe infantile sialidosis: clinical, biochemical, and microscopic features. J. Pediatr. **96**:662–668, 1980.

Baker, H.J., Mole, J.A., Lindsey, J.R. and Creel, R.M.: Animal models of human ganglioside storage diseases. Fed. Proceed. **35**:1193–1201, 1976.

Baldwin, V.J., Applegarth, D.A., Pantzar, T.R., Smyth, J. and McGillivray, B.C.: Congenital sialidosis. Lab. Invest. **52**:1P (abstract), 1985.

Bendon, R.W. and Hug, G.: Morphologic characteristics of the placenta in glycogen storage disease type II (β-1,4-glucosidase deficiency). Amer. J. Obstet. Gynecol. **152**:1021–1026, 1985.

Benirschke, K. and Kaufmann, P.: Pathology of the Human Placenta. Third edition. Springer-Verlag, New York, 1995.

Bouvier, R. and Maire, I.: Fetal presentation of 23 cases of lysosomal storage disease. A collaborative study of the French Society of Fetal Pathology. Pediatr. Pathol. Lab. Med. **17**:675, 1997.

Conradi, N.G., Uverbrandt, P. Hökegård, K.-H., Wahlströmm T. and Mellqvist, L.: First-trimester diagnosis of juvenile neuro-

nal ceroid lipofuscinosis by demonstration of fingerprint inclusions in chorionic villi. Prenat. Diagn. **9**:283–287, 1989.

Cozzutto, C.: Case report. Foamy degeneration of placenta. Virchows Arch. Pathol. Anat. **401**:363–368, 1983.

Desai, P.K., Astrin, K.H., Gordon, R.E., Thung, S., Strauss, L. and Desnick, R.J.: Cholesterol ester storage disease: prenatal diagnosis and fetal pathology. Lab. Invest. **52**:4P, 1985.

Fox, H.: Pathology of the Placenta. 2nd edition. W.B. Saunders, London, 1997.

Gehler, J., Cantz, M., Stoeckenius, M. and Spranger, J.: Prenatal diagnosis of mucolipidosis II (I-cell disease). Europ. J. Pediatr. **122**:201–206, 1976.

Gellis, S.S. and Feingold, M.: Picture of the month. I-cell disease (mucolipidosis II). Amer. J. Dis. Childr. **131**:1137–1138, 1977.

Gillan, J.E., Lowden, J.A., Gaskin, K. and Cutz, E.: Congenital ascites as a presenting sign of lysosomal storage disease. J. Pediatr. **104**:225–231, 1984.

Ginsburg, S.J. and Groll, M.: Hydrops fetalis due to infantile Gaucher's disease. J. Pediatr. **82**:1046–1048, 1973.

Giugliani, R., Dutra, J.C., Pereira, M.L.S., Rotta, N., Drachler, M.d.L., Ohlweiler, L., Neto, J.M.d.P., Pinheiro, C.E. and Breda, D.J.: GM$_1$ gangliosidosis: Clinical and laboratory findings in eight families. Hum. Genet. **70**:347–354, 1985.

Granström, M.-L., Aula, P. ja Rapola, J.: Kliinis-patologinen kokousselostus XY. Kudosviljelyn avulla selvitetty aineenvaihduntasairaus. Duodecim **90**:421–430, 1974.

Grebner, E.E., Wapner, R.J., Barr, M.A. and Jackson, L.G.: Prenatal Tay-Sachs diagnosis by chorionic villi sampling. Lancet **ii**:286–287, 1983.

Hanai, J., Leroy, J. and O'Brien, J.S.: Ultrastructure of cultured fibroblasts in I-cell disease. Amer. J. Dis. Childr. **122**:34–38, 1971.

Herd, J.K., Dvorak, A.D., Wiltse, H.E., Eisen, J.D., Kress, B.C. and Miller, A.L.: Mucolipidosis type II. Multiple elevated serum and urine enzyme activities. Amer. J. Dis. Childr. **132**:1181–1186, 1978.

Hug, G., Bove, K.E., Soukup, S., Ryan, M., Bendon, R., Babcock, D., Warren, N.S. and Dignan, P.S.J.: Increased serum hexosaminidase in a woman pregnant with a fetus affected by mucolipidosis II (I-cell disease). NEJM **311**:988–989, 1984.

Hug, G., Chuck, G., Chen, Y.-T., Kay, H.H. and Bossen, E.H.: Chorionic villus ultrastructure in type II glycogen storage disease (Pompe's disease). NEJM **324**:342–343, 1991.

Jauniaux, E., Vamos, E., Libert, J., Elkhazen, N., Wilkin, P. and Hustin, J.: Placental electron microscopy and histochemistry in a case of sialic acid storage disorder. Placenta **8**:433–442, 1987.

Jolly, R.D. and Walkley, S.U.: Lysosomal storage diseases of animals: an essay in comparative pathology. Vet. Pathol. **34**:527–548, 1997.

Jones, C.J.P., Lendon, M., Chawner, L.E. and Jauniaux, E.: Ultrastructure of the human placenta in metabolic storage disease. Placenta **11**:395–411, 1990.

Kleijer, W.J., Hoogeveen, A., Verheijen, F.W., Niermeijer, M.F., Galjaard, H., O'Brien, J.S. and Warner, T.G.: Prenatal diagnosis of sialidosis with combined neuraminidase and β-galactosidase deficiency. Clin. Genet. **16**:60–61, 1979.

Kleijer, W.J., Janse, H.C., Vosters, R.P.L., Niermeijer, M.F. and v.d. Kamp, J.J.P.: First-trimester diagnosis of mucopolysaccharidosis IIIA (Sanfilippo A disease). NEJM **314**:185–186, 1986.

Kohn, G., Livni, N., Ornoy, A., Sekeles, E., Beyth, Y., Legum, C., Bach, G. and Cohen, M.M.: Prenatal diagnosis of mucolipidosis IV by electron microscopy. J. Pediatr. **90**:62–66, 1977.

Laver, J., Fried, K., Beer, S.I., Iancu, T.C., Heyman, E., Bach, G. and Zeiger, M.: Infantile lethal neuraminidase deficiency (sialidosis). Clin. Genet. **23**:97–101, 1983.

Lowden, J.A., Cutz, E., Conen, P.E., Rudd, N. and Doran, T.A.: Prenatal diagnosis of G_{M1}-gangliosidosis. NEJM **288**:225–228, 1973.

Mahmood, K. and Haleem, A.: Placental morphology in sialidosis: report of a case. Ann. Saudi Med. **9**:302–304, 1989.

Maroteaux, P., Humbel, R., Strecker, G., Michalski, J.-C. and Mande, R.: Un nouveau type de sialidose avec atteinte rénale: La nephrosialidose. Arch. Franç. Pédiatr. **35**:819–829, 1978.

Meizner, I., Levy, A., Carmi, R. and Robinsin, C.: Niemann-Pick disease associated with nonimmune hydrops fetalis. Amer. J. Obstet. Gynecol. **163**:128–129, 1990.

Nadler, H.L. and Gerbie, A.B.: Role of amniocentesis in the intrauterine detection of genetic disorders. NEJM **282**:596–599, 1970.

Nagashima, K., Sakakibara, K., Endo, H., Konishi, Y., Nakamura, N., Suzuki, Y. and Abe, T.: I-cell disease (mucolipidosis II). Pathological and biochemical studies of an autopsy case. Acta Pathol. Jap. **27**:251–264, 1977.

Nelson, J., Kenny, B., O'Hara, D., Harper, A. and Broadhead, D.: Foamy changes of placental cells in probable beta glucuronidase deficiency associated with hydrops fetalis. J. Clin. Pathol. **46**:370–371, 1993.

O'Brien, J.F.: The lysosomal storage diseases. Mayo Clin. Proceed. **57**:192–197, 1982.

Popli, S., Leehey, D.J., Molnar, Z.V., Nawab, Z.M. and Ing, T.S.: Demonstration of Fabry's disease deposits in placenta. Amer. J. Obstet. Gynecol. **162**:464–465, 1990.

Powell, H.C., Benirschke, K., Favara, B.E. and Pflueger, O.H.: Foamy changes of placental cells in fetal storage disorders. Virchows Arch. A Pathol. Anat. Histol. **369**:191–196, 1976.

Rapola, J. and Aula, P.: Morphology of the placenta in fetal I-cell disease. Clin. Genet. **11**:107–113, 1977.

Rapola, J., Autio, S., Aula, P. and Nanto, V.: Lymphocytic inclusions in I-cell disease. J. Pediatr. **85**:88–90, 1974.

Rapola, J., Santavuori, P. and Heiskala, H.: Placental pathology and prenatal diagnosis of infantile type of neuronal ceroid-lipofuscinosis. Amer. J. Med. Genet. Suppl. **5**:99–103, 1988.

Rapola, J., Salonen, R., Ämmälä, P. and Santavuori, P.: Prenatal diagnosis of the infantile type of neuronal ceroid lipofuscino-

sis by electron microscopic investigation of human chorionic villi. Prenat. Diagn. **10**:553–559, 1990.

Rice, G.E., Mostoufi-Zadeh, M. and Driscoll, S.G.: Hydrops fetalis in Gaucher's disease. Teratology **29**:53A–54A, 1984.

Riches, W.G. and Smuckler, E.A.: A severe infantile mucolipidosis. Clinical, biochemical, and pathologic features. Arch. Pathol. Lab. Med. **107**:147–152, 1983.

Roberts, D.J., Ampola, M.G. and Lage, J.M.: Diagnosis of unsuspected fetal metabolic storage disease by routine placental examination. Pediatr. Pathol. **11**:647–656, 1991.

Sarrut, S. and Belamich, P.: Étude du placenta dans trois observations de dyslipide à révélation neonatale. Arch. D'Anat. Cytol. Pathol. **31**:187–189, 1983.

Schoenfeld, A., Abramovici, A., Klibanski, C. and Ovadia, J.: Placental ultrasonographic biochemical and histochemical studies in human fetuses affected with Niemann-Pick disease Type A. Placenta **6**:33–44, 1985.

Scully, R.E. (Ed.): Cabot case No. 23-1997. NEJM **337**:260–267, 1997.

See, G.L., Stanescu, R. and Lyon, G.: Un nouveau type de sialidose avec atteinte rénale: la nephrosialidose. Arch. Franç. Pédiatr. **35**:830–844, 1978.

Sekeles, E., Ornoy, A., Cohen, R. and Kohn, G.: Mucolipidosis IV: fetal and placental pathology. A report on two subsequent interruptions of pregnancy. Monogr. Human Genet. **10**:47–50, 1978.

Sidransky, E. and Ginns, E.I.: Clinical heterogeneity among patients with Gaucher's disease. JAMA **269**:1154–1157, 1993.

Stevenson, R.E., Lubinsky, M., Taylor, H.A., Wenger, D.A., Schroer, R.J. and Olmstead, P.M.: Sialic acid storage disease with sialuria: clinical and biochemical features in the severe infantile type. Pediatrics **72**:441–449, 1983.

Soma, H., Yamada, K., Osawa, H., Hata, T., Oguro, T. and Kudo, M.: Identification of Gaucher cells in the chorionic villi associated with recurrent hydrops fetalis. Placenta **21**:412–416, 2000.

Terashima, Y., Tsuda, K., Isomura, S., Sugiura, Y. and Nogami, H.: I-cell disease. Report of three cases. Amer. J. Dis. Childr. **129**:1083–1090, 1975.

Tønnesen, T., Horn, N., Søndergaard, F., Boué, J., Damsgaard, E. and Heydorn, K.: Measurement of copper in chorionic villi for first-trimester diagnosis of Menkes' disease. Lancet **i**:1038–1039, 1985.

Vanier, M.T., Rousson, R.M., Mandon, G., Choiset, A., Lake, B.D. and Pentchev, P.G.: Diagnosis of Niemann-Pick disease type C on chorionic villus biopsy. Lancet **i**:1014–1015, 1989.

19
Maternal Diseases Complicating Pregnancy: Diabetes, Tumors, Preeclampsia, Lupus Anticoagulant

Numerous diseases may complicate pregnancy. The most important of those that affect placental development and function are herein reviewed. Our own experience with some of these entities is cited. With some of these complications of pregnancy, the placental findings may simply be confirmatory of the disease. With others, placental pathology may be the first indication of an abnormality. Despite many reports of diseases that complicate pregnancy, associated placentas are often not examined, or they are not reported in the descriptions. That is unfortunate because those placentas could aid in diagnosis and knowledge of the pathogenesis of these conditions. Moreover, a better understanding of the placenta could allow us better insight into the mechanisms of the effects that certain conditions have on the fetus. Burrow and Ferris (1988) have written a comprehensive text on medical complications of pregnancy but have also almost totally excluded placental considerations; the general texts on obstetrics and perinatology should also be consulted. Because of their particular importance, some entities (e.g., Rh-isoimmunization disease and hydrops, pyelonephritis, and infections in general), are presented in separate chapters.

Maternal Diseases

Scleroderma, also called systemic sclerosis, is characterized by the deposition of fibrous tissue in many organs and the production of autoimmune antibodies. Its etiology is currently under very active study. This disease has been reported on many occasions to occur in pregnancy, although the usually late onset of scleroderma makes it an uncommon association. Slate and Graham (1968) observed six patients with generalized scleroderma and followed their nine pregnancies. When reviewing all pregnancies of their scleroderma patients, irrespective of the time of onset of the disease before or during pregnancy, stillbirths, abortions, and premature births were found to

be common. Pregnancies occurring after the onset of scleroderma ended in two premature births, two stillborns, and 12 abortions. When they reviewed the literature, these authors also found five maternal deaths among 72 women. These investigators thought that preeclampsia was not an unduly common complication of scleroderma. In the discussion following their paper, additional cases were presented. None, however, was accompanied by a placental description.

Spellacy (1964), who reported a case with premature labor, found that the placenta had small infarcts, and he gathered 11 additional cases from the literature. Abruptio placentae was described in a case by Hayes et al. (1962). Maternal (decidual) vascular changes have not been described with scleroderma, which is remarkable because scleroderma is occasionally complicated by lupus erythematosus, and abruptios have been reported to occur with scleroderma. The two patients in whom we saw extensive fibrinoid deposits gave the appearance of "maternal floor infarction." One such placenta is shown in Figure 19.1. This 34-year-old gravida IV, para I, aborta II, had a precipitous labor at 38 weeks' gestation. Her obstetricians suspected abruptio placentae. The pregnancy terminated with a growth-restricted stillbirth. The placenta was also unusually small (310 g) and had numerous infarcts and X-cell proliferations. Many nucleated red blood cells (NRBCs) were present in the fetal circulation, and marked X-cell proliferation was accompanied by many cysts. A similarly cystic placenta had been seen by us previously in scleroderma, but that pregnancy was associated with a normal child. Neither placenta had decidual vascular lesions. Gunther and Harer (1964) observed three pregnancies in a patient with scleroderma. Each was complicated by placenta previa. Doss et al. (1998) observed 13 placentas from eight women with scleroderma. They found decidual vasculopathy commonly, lesions that simulated those found in maternal hypertensive disorders. In addition, abruptio, infarcts, and decidual fibrin deposits were more frequently observed than in normal placentas.

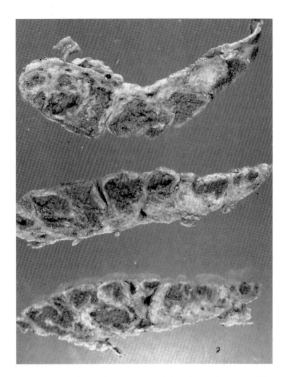

FIGURE 19.1. Placenta of a patient with scleroderma at 38 weeks' gestation. Numerous infarcts, "gitterinfarkts," maternal floor infarction, and X-cell proliferation were seen. The placenta and stillborn fetus were growth-restricted. (Courtesy of Dr. Bonnie Bobzien.)

Studies to further elucidate the etiology of scleroderma have taken an unexpected turn with the finding by Artlett et al. (1998) that the disease may be the result of fetal graft-versus-host disease (GVHD) rejection. They identified fetal DNA (by demonstration of Y-specific sequences) in women who had previous male births and suggested that competent fetal lymphocytes (CD3 cells) had traveled transplacentally to set up colonization of the mother. This is an attractive hypothesis for a condition with some features having a resemblance to cases with known GVHD, and it further delineates "microchimerism" (Mullinax, 1998; Nelson, 1998, 2004; Nelson et al., 1998). Murata et al. (1999), in contrast, found no Y-chromosomal signals in Japanese patients with systemic sclerosis. Perhaps other autoimmune diseases fall into the same category, as transplacental transfer of fetal cells to the mother is common (see Chapter 17) and there is also an excess of autoimmune diseases in women. This has been proven for postpartum thyroiditis and, remarkably, in one patient even the thyroid epithelium was "repaired" by fetal cells, most likely deriving from stem cells (Srivatsa et al., 2001; Ando & Davies, 2003). This is an exciting new field and several diseases are under suspicion of being caused by the transplacentally developing microchimerism.

Dermatomyositis, another autoimmune disease with primarily cutaneous expression, was reported during pregnancy by Barnes and Link (1983). The patient became ill at age 15, had a therapeutic abortion at age 22, and developed significant subcutaneous calcinosis while being treated. The successful pregnancy occurred at age 24, 3 months after cessation of methotrexate medication. Vaginal spotting took place at 3 months, but she remained normotensive and had no proteinuria. A cesarean section was performed at 42 weeks with a healthy infant delivered. The placenta had "subamnionic necrosis and hemorrhage involving 30% of the fetal surface." There also was an infarct, but no decidual arteriolopathy was present. The authors referred to a few other case reports, with similar findings of infarcts in the placenta the only pathologic lesions. We saw the placenta of such a patient who had spontaneous demise of a growth-restricted fetus at 38 weeks. The placenta had the typical appearance of massive Gitterinfarkts (see Chapter 9).

Ehlers-Danlos syndrome is not a homogeneous disease entity. Many types have been differentiated, and a foundation concerned with this disease collects data, including those of pregnancy. One or another form occurs occasionally during pregnancy. Atalla and Page (1988) estimated Ehlers-Danlos disease to occur once in 150,000 pregnancies, of which 35% were of type II. Barabas (1966) found that 14 of his 18 patients delivered prematurely because of premature rupture of the membranes. He suggested that the membranes were exceptionally fragile, but there are no actual measurements of the strength of membranes, nor are there pathologic data. Normal members of the families did not suffer from this putative lack of membrane strength. In the pedigrees reported by Barabas, the premature membrane ruptures were nearly always restricted to affected fetuses. Atalla and Page (1988) reported a case of Ehlers-Danlos syndrome type III with pregnancy and reviewed the sparse literature. Their patient never developed abdominal striae, but because of increasing pains during pregnancy, she had a cesarean section at 35 weeks' gestation. Her membranes were then ruptured artificially. Thus, with the possible exception of a true increased fragility of the fetal membranes in affected offspring, the placenta has not been reported to be abnormal.

Rheumatoid arthritis has rarely been observed during pregnancy, according to the report of Duhring (1970). He described the successful outcome of pregnancy in a para III patient who had suffered the disease for 17 years. The fetus was markedly growth-restricted, and the placenta was small, infarcted, and calcified. The umbilical cord was grossly virtually devoid of Wharton's jelly, but a histologic study was not reported.

Nine cases of **periarteritis nodosa** had been reported before Nagey et al. (1983) described another case. Their patient was a 28-year-old woman who had experienced many complications of the disease for 5 years. This mother had one previous abortion, and her pregnancy was therapeutically terminated at 16 weeks. The placenta appeared to be normal by light and electron microscopic examination. Decidual vessels, however, were not present in the specimen. Previous reports had commented on the high risk for maternal survival but did not include descriptions of the placenta. Owen and Hauth (1989) reported another case, but they did not include a description of the placenta.

A report of maternal **Takayasu's arteritis** complicating pregnancy indicates that normal gestation may yield a normal infant. Winn et el. (1988) observed a woman who had this disease diagnosed 3 years earlier and who had significant arterial disease as a consequence. She was delivered of a healthy infant at 33 weeks. The placenta was not described.

A patient with progressive, severe **myositis ossificans** posed serious problems in pregnancy management but the mother delivered a healthy neonate. The pregnancy was complicated by premature rupture of membranes and infection with group B β-hemolytic streptococci. The placenta was not described (Thornton et al., 1987).

Patients in **acute renal failure** from whatever cause not only may now survive pregnancy and have normal infants when appropriately managed, but their placentas are found to be normal (Soyannwo et al., 1966; Jones & Hayslett, 1996). This is the case only when the renal failure is independent of pregnancy-induced hypertension and its frequently accompanying decidual vascular disease. Renal injury may occur after spider (Martinez, 1967) and snake bites (James, 1985). The latter author suggested that the venom may cross the placenta and kill the fetus. Renal failure and abruptio placentae have also been produced by the bite of *Bothrops jararaca*, a species of snake (Zugaib et al., 1985). This accident occurred during the 32nd week of gestation and, despite antiserum administration within 6 hours, the fetus died in utero from a 75% abruption. Mushroom poisons (amatoxins) have been described to cause maternal intoxication, but they do not cross the placenta. A fetus appeared to progress normally after such intoxication, and there was no detectable amnionic fluid toxin; the placenta was not described (Belliardo et al., 1983).

Pregnant women with **chronic renal failure** have a high perinatal mortality rate (Hou, 1985). Many placental lesions are found. Most notable among them is retarded growth of the placenta, presumably secondary to maternal decidual vascular disease and hypertension.

Patients with successful **renal transplantation** have a 30% incidence of preeclampsia during pregnancy and suffer occasional rejection of the transplant (Penn et al., 1980; Davison, 1987). It is interesting that toxemia of pregnancy develops so frequently in these patients who usually are medicated with steroids and immunosuppres-sive agents. Intercurrent infection is a serious hazard, but cyclosporine immunosuppression apparently does not interfere with placentation. The placenta, however, is rarely described (Burrows et al., 1988). Beller et al. (1976) made efforts to differentiate the clinical identification of **malignant nephrosclerosis** from preeclampsia but did not provide information on the placentas in the two patients they described.

Although **acute fatty liver of pregnancy** has a dismal outcome (the survival rate has improved to between 18% to 23%), placental abnormalities remain undescribed (Kaplan, 1985). Hemolysis, coagulation, and other disturbances occur clinically, and toxemia may result with its complications, but the primary disease does not apparently affect the placenta. When maternal bilirubin is high, gross examination of the placenta can identify the pigmentation, particularly in the perivascular connective tissue of the fetal surface. Microscopically, however, no abnormalities are detected, and visible pigment-laden macrophages are rare.

Cholestasis of pregnancy has been associated with a high rate of stillbirth and other perinatal complications. Fisk and Storey (1988) reviewed 83 such cases and found meconium staining in 45%, preterm labor in 44%, and fetal distress in 22%. In their opinion, the low mortality achieved (three of 83) was due to intensive monitoring of the end stages of pregnancy and the result of judicious intervention. Other than the frequent meconium staining of the placenta, there were no abnormal placental findings. One wonders whether some of the "meconium-staining" may not have been bilirubin-staining. Matos et al. (1997), who lost a fetus at 37 weeks, found that it had extensive cerebral hemorrhage, presumably related to the cholestasis. The placenta was entirely normal and not abrupted.

Patients with **hyperemesis gravidarum** who were treated with total parenteral alimentation were studied by Levine and Esser (1988). Their fetuses all matured to at least 38 weeks' gestation and were not growth-restricted. Examination of the placentas showed no lipid deposits or other abnormalities.

A direct effect of **alcohol** on the placenta is disputed, although fetal growth restriction and other consequences of the fetal alcohol syndrome are well delineated in the offspring of patients with alcohol abuse during pregnancy (Jones et al., 1973). Several studies have shown that the placenta is smaller than that of controls. Kaminski et al. (1978) found the placentas to weigh 591 g when 45 to 67 mL of alcohol were consumed daily, and 581 g when more than 67 mL were consumed daily. Control placental weights were 611 g for less than 44 mL daily alcohol consumption. That the placenta transports alcohol readily has been shown on numerous occasions (Ditts, 1970), with fatal fetal intoxication having been reported (Jung et al., 1980). The influence of alcoholism on the length of umbilical cords (shortening in experimental systems) was mentioned in Chapter 12. Baldwin et al. (1982) reviewed placentas of pregnancies with alcohol abuse and found an increased incidence of chorioamnionitis, chronic villitis, meconium staining, chorangiomas, and, especially, with persistence of embryologic remnants in the umbilical cords. The significance of these lesions is unknown. The inflammatory complications indicate that the social circumstances of the population differed from those of the controls. Other investigators (Sokol et al., 1980) observed no abnormalities in placentas of alcoholics. Marbury et al. (1983), on the other hand, found a significant increase in the incidence of abruptio placentae and a correlation with the amount of alcohol consumed. Blakley (1983), who reviewed the topic extensively, referred to evidence that alcohol consumption leads to fetal hypoxia and compensatory placental enlargement.

The use of **cocaine** (benzoylmethylecgonine) and crack (the free-base smokable form of cocaine) during pregnancy has continues. A survey conducted in Florida indicated that some 15% of pregnant women tested positive for urinary metabolites of controlled substances (Chasnoff et al., 1990), but in a community study of South Carolina it was only 1% (Weathers et al., 1993). Consuming cocaine in pregnancy has been linked to abruptio placentae (Acker et al., 1983; Chasnoff et al., 1985; Dombrowski et al., 1991; Hoskins et al., 1991). In vitro enzymatic studies by Roe et al. (1990) showed that placental microsomal fractions biotransform cocaine to inactive compounds. Fetal growth restriction, transient hypertension, severe placental vasoconstriction (Lederman et al., 1978), and other deleterious outcomes of pregnancy are reported (Cregler & Mark, 1986). Mercado et al. (1989) observed a patient with repeated abruptios, abortions, and continued cocaine use who ultimately had a postpartum cerebral hemorrhage, presumably from hypertension. Page et al. (1989) found in the placentas of 20 crack users that 12 of them had abruptio placentae (10 with large clots, one with retroplacental depression, six with recent and old clots). Eight had normal placentas, and 10 of the abrupted placentas had liveborn babies; two had placenta previa and five had chorioamnionitis. Much of the effect of cocaine, at least during pregnancy, seems to be mediated through its known hypertensive and vasoconstrictive activity (Woods et al., 1987). A large retrospective study by Sprauve et al. (1997) showed that only decreased birth weight resulted when confounders were removed; abruptio was not increased. Specific effects on placental structure have not been reported, nor have they been present in our experience; moreover, the frequency of abruptio placentae is, in our experience, not as excessive as given in the many reports (Gilbert et al., 1990). The reported series of abruptio placentae that are a complication of cocaine exposure (occasionally remote exposure!) do not provide data on the pathologic examination of the pla-

centas. Thus, it cannot be ascertained whether the alleged abruptios are recent or old, and whether they are related to chorioamnionitis, as this is more frequent in these patients. A study by Miller et al. (1995) found a significant excess of abruptio, vaginal bleeding, marked growth restriction and premature rupture of membranes (PROMs). Moreover, there was a strong association with maternal smoking, which may have additive effects on lowering fetal weight. Chorioamnionitis, as discussed in Chapter 20, often causes marked deciduitis with bleeding and clots from that site that mimics abruptio, but it is a different mechanism. Therefore, we are still skeptical that cocaine exposure produces abruptio placentae often (Gilbert et al., 1990). Moreover, the vasculature that might be affected by the putative constriction of cocaine, the spiral arterioles, should be inviolate because of the structural change from trophoblast infiltration. However, there is no question of the increased frequency of fetal growth restriction. Little et al. (1989), who studied outcome in 53 cocaine abusers, found a significant increase only of prematurity and preeclampsia. There was also a slight increase of congenital heart disease, but in contrast to other studies they reviewed and that showed more abruptios, this was not found in their population. The authors suggested that it may be due to the fact that placentas are not routinely examined or are examined only when stillbirths occur. It must be admitted also, and was commented on by these investigators, that cocaine abuse is often combined with alcohol and other drug abuse and with maternal cigarette smoking; this has also been pointed out by Donvito (1988), Frank et al. (1988), Miller et al. (1995), and Ness et al. (1999). Moreover, the social makeup of the population may predispose to intrauterine infection. The vasoconstriction caused by these agents may be transmitted to the fetus, in whom cerebral infarction has occasionally been observed (Chasnoff et al., 1986). In a study of 75 pregnant women with cocaine use, the patterns of preterm delivery, growth restriction, and abruptio were affirmed, but the cause of abruptio was questioned (Chasnoff et al., 1989). When women stopped using cocaine after the first trimester, there was no reduction in the incidence of abruptio placentae. Fulroth et al. (1989) reported a significantly higher incidence (34%) of meconium staining when compared with that (10%) of a control population. The cardiovascular effect of cocaine injection has been studied in pregnant sheep by Moore et al. (1986). They found a rise of maternal arterial pressure (32% to 37%), combined with a 36% to 42% reduction of uterine blood flow, lasting 15 minutes after injection, at levels comparable to those seen with human usage. Fetal arterial pressure also rose to 12.6%. Chávez et al. (1989) reported that offspring of cocaine abusers suffer an increased risk of urinary tract anomalies, but that has not been our experience. Bailey (1997) found that cocaine is strongly bound to placental homogenates and suggested that the placenta might serve as a reservoir for cocaine. Shiono et al. (1995) found few adverse effects from cocaine and **marijuana** usage during pregnancy and attributed most reduction of birth weight to cigarette smoking.

Effects on pregnancy somewhat similar to those seen with cocaine usage have been seen with maternal **heroin** abuse. Naeye et al. (1973) studied this complication of pregnancy in detail and found that 60% of these mothers had intrauterine infection (chorioamnionitis) as the principal finding. Also, there was frequent meconium staining of the fetus and placenta, and growth restriction.

LSD (lysergic acid diethylamide) administration during pregnancy is associated with an increased abortion rate (McGlothlin et al., 1970), but the placenta has not been described to be abnormal. The abortions and fetal damage have been inferred to be secondary to chromosome breakage (Warren et al., 1970). Later studies have negated this effect. An extensive investigation of drug-related injury on the placenta was undertaken by Freese (1978). He found that no consistent changes take place, and that any effect is one of direct action on the fetus, rather than on the placenta. Blanc et al. (1971) described a case of amnionic bands with amputations of digits in an LSD user. This finding prompted their review of six malformed infants born to LSD users and led them to caution that a causal relation may exist between LSD and amnionic bands.

Smoking during pregnancy has been the topic of numerous studies and many have yielded contradictory results. Two comprehensive, useful reviews were written by Werler (1997) and Page et al. (1997). Smoking is often considered to be the cause of an increased frequency of abortions (Kline et al., 1977), low birth weight, and some minor morphologic placental changes. A study of 7651 patients from California indicated that smokers' placentas had more calcifications and more subchorionic fibrin deposits (Christianson, 1979). This investigator found the placental weight not to be decreased, as did so many other authors. He likened the result to placentas of higher altitude and made reference to the self-selection of smokers and the difficulties inherent in ascertaining true alterations that might be due only to smoking. An early review of the topic (Editorial, 1968) suggested that the adverse effects may be mediated through reduced blood flow to placenta and fetus. When umbilical and uterine blood flow velocities were studied, the effect on fetal growth appeared to result from a highly significant rise in fetal placental vascular resistance (Morrow et al., 1988). Studies on isolated stem villous arteries shows them to be more responsive by constriction when exposed to endothelin-1 and other vasoactive peptides (Clausen et al., 1999). Other causes (hypoxia and cation changes) have also been held responsible. The data relating to reduction of birth weight, often considered as being

controversial, were reviewed by Murphy et al. (1977) and Alberman et al. (1977). Asmussen (1979) found fetal weight to be reduced by 325 g and the placenta by 123 g, similar to the later findings of Wen et al. (1990). The relative hypoxia was incriminated as a cause of significantly elevated fetal erythropoietin levels with maternal smoking (Jazayeri et al., 1998). In addition to growth restriction, Raymond and Mills (1993) found abruptio placentae significantly increased, as well as congenital heart disease. Studies of the endothelium obtained from umbilical arteries and vein showed widening of the basement membrane; in heavy smokers this change is said to have been visible even by light microscopy. Additionally, there were deposition of other materials, edema, reduction of the smooth endoplasmic reticulum of muscle cells, and loss of intercellular junctions between endothelial cells. Heavy smokers had marked dilatation of the rough endoplasmic reticulum. The microvillous surface of the syncytial cells was reduced, and there was a reduction in cytotrophoblastic elements. The villi had decreased vascularization and increased collagen content. The authors inferred that similar changes may take place in the vessels of the fetus. Wingerd et al. (1976) reported that the placental/fetal ratio was increased in smokers, presumably due to the reduced fetal weight. On the other hand, Teasdale and Ghislaine (1989), who undertook a careful quantitative morphometric study with appropriate controls, found only minor changes in the placenta. There was a "tendency for the placentas ... to contain proportionally more nonparenchymal and less parenchymal tissue." The authors concluded that the effect of smoking was more related to ischemic or toxic effects of several compounds in tobacco smoke than to significant alterations in the functional structure of the placenta. This opinion was also voiced in an editorial (Anonymous, 1989b), whose author pleaded that "it is dishonest to say there is serious evidence that her fetus is at risk if she does not give up smoking." Jauniaux and Burton (1992), on the other hand, found that smokers developed increased mean thicknesses of the villous membrane and trophoblast. They believed that these changes may account for the biologic disturbances in gestation. Isaksen et al. (2004) reported a relation to trophoblast apoptosis. Horn et al. (1994) are the only authors to suggest that chorangiosis is a sequel of smoking (and of the fetal demise they reported). Unexpectedly, a huge study from the Swedish Medical Birth Register (Cnattingius et al., 1997) indicated that smoking reduces the incidence of toxemia of pregnancy. When it was found in smokers, however, then the perinatal mortality, abruptio placentae, and number of small-for-gestational-age (SGA) neonates were increased.

Naeye (1978) has reported an increased frequency of single umbilical artery (SUA) and abnormal cord insertions in the anomalous fetuses of smokers. Kuhnert et al. (1987a) showed that placental cadmium and zinc levels were increased in smokers, with a 9% reduction in zinc levels of fetal red blood cells (and a decrease in fetal weight) (Kuhnert et al., 1987b). A significant reduction of umbilical arterial prostacyclin production was reported by Dadak et al. (1981) in the umbilical cords of smoking mothers. They likened this effect to a similar finding in women with preeclampsia and speculated that this potent vasodilator may be involved in growth restriction of the fetus. The immunohistologic study of Sanyal et al. (1993) indicated that smokers' placentas have an increased activity of hydrocarbon hydroxylase within the trophoblast, presumably stimulated by the toxins within the smoke. Rubin et al. (1986), as well as some other authors, have reported that significant passive smoking has a similar deleterious effect on fetal development. The difficulties of such correlation were examined by Chen et al. (1989), who conducted a study in Chinese women. They did not find that passive smoking posed a risk to the fetus.

A variety of ultrastructural observations were made on the umbilical blood vessels in smoking women's pregnancies. Thus Asmussen (1978) found the intima and media of the vein to be edematous, and the elastic membranes were partially destroyed. Fewer changes were identified in the umbilical arteries (Asmussen, 1982a); but in heavy smokers, scanning electron microscopy delineated more general changes (Bylock et al., 1979). Intercellular "holes" were seen in the intima that were interpreted to result from cellular injury, and Asmussen (1982b) found glycogen and lipid accumulation in the muscular wall cells. He also reported an increase of mitochondria in the endothelial cells of arteries of smoking mothers (Asmussen, 1984). In the villous basement membranes of such pregnancies, this author observed thickening and an increase in villous stromal collagen (Asmussen, 1980). Pinette et al. (1989) reported that the placentas of smoking mothers had increased maturation, as graded by sonographic scanning methodology. Pfarrer et al. (1999) also used scanning electron microscopy of freshly injected capillary beds of placentas from women who smoked more than 20 cigarettes daily. They found an increased capillary bed and increased branching of capillaries, presumably in response to smoking.

Additionally, there have been numerous investigations concerning the putative relation of abruptio placentae to smoking; most of these have suggested that a relation exists. It is troublesome, however, that very few of these studies have actually examined the placentas, that an increased frequency of premature rupture of membranes was also found, and that it is thus possible that chorioamnionitis may be the mechanism of possible so-called abruptio. Voigt et al. (1990) did a population-based case-control study of smoking and abruptio, using data from birth certificates, that endeavored to ascertain if smoking, abruptio, and SGA status were correlated. Importantly,

the placentas were not examined. An increased frequency of abruptio was found with smoking and an increase of SGA infants, but the latter was not correlated with smoking. These authors suggested that 38% of abruptios were "attributable to maternal smoking." Perhaps the first authors to suggest an increase of "accidental hemorrhage" (abruptio) with smoking were Andrews and McGarry (1972), whose paper is replete with a variety of tabular information. Goujard et al. (1975) opined that abruptios were perhaps due to "serious spasm, the release of which, by surge of blood, would cause arterial rupture." Their point is difficult to follow as the rate of stillbirth in smokers was much increased (250%) in their study population but the rate of abruptios was lower than in controls. In a later study (Goujard et al., 1978) the authors provided additional evidence for a relation to stillbirths and made further correlation with alcohol intake. But, as is true for most studies, the placentas were not studied for inflammation and the cause of true abruptio is thus difficult to evaluate. Meyer and Tonascia (1977) found a dose-related increase in abruptio, placenta previa, and premature rupture of membranes. Most of the abruptios occurred before 32 weeks' gestation, which leads us to consider that inflammation, rather than true retroplacental bleeding, may be the significant problem. The increase in placental ratio in smokers, studied by Wingerd et al. (1976), was found to be the result of lower fetal weights, rather than larger placentas. Naeye et al. (1977) reviewed the data from the Collaborative Study for the influence of smoking on placental/fetal development. They found an increase of abruptios, infarcts, and lighter placentas in smokers. All in all, there appears to be a large body of evidence to suggest that smoking has some deleterious effect upon placenta and fetal development, but that it is not a large one. Bernstein et al. (2000) opined from their study of growth-restricted infants of smoking mothers that the effect was most pronounced on abdominal circumference.

Few other **drugs** have shown well-recorded effects on placental structure, the notable exception being **methotrexate** (Li et al., 1956; Goldstein & Berkowitz, 1987) with its severe trophoblast toxicity. Severe fetal growth restriction occurred with a patient who attempted to cause abortion by taking much **aminopterin**; the placenta was not described (Shaw & Rees, 1980). Alkylating agents have been used successfully for the therapy of malignancies during pregnancy, and usually they have been attended without ill-effect. Lacher and Geller (1966) reported a successful gestation in a pregnant patient with Hodgkin's disease who was given therapeutic doses of cyclophosphamide and vinblastine. The placenta was not specifically mentioned. The size of the infant (3060 g) and its development, however, suggested that the placenta must have been normal. Hennessey and Rottino (1963) concluded from personal observations on 35 patients with **Hodgkin's disease** complicating pregnancy that there was no need to interrupt the pregnancy. They did not describe the associated placentas. Knörr et al. (1969) found no abnormalities of placental structure after therapy with alkylating agents during pregnancy, and Nordlund et al. (1968) also found that pregnancy progresses without fetal toxicity. Nicholson (1968) reviewed the cytotoxic agents used during pregnancy. In the villi of a therapeutic abortion of an **epileptic** patient medicated with **diphenylhydantoin**, large clusters of lymphocytes were found in the fetal capillaries; it is unknown if this finding resulted from the lymphoproliferative effect of the drug (Greco et al., 1973), as the specimen did not contain an embryo.

Irradiation during pregnancy is usually avoided because of the deleterious effects it has on the fetus. In two gestations complicated by squamous cell carcinoma of the cervix, Driscoll et al. (1963) reported the effects of therapeutic irradiation on two fetuses, 16 and 22 weeks' gestational age. In the first, hydronephrosis was present, and the decidua showed foci of necrosis and inflammation, as well as necrosis of the amnion and chorion laeve. In the older fetus, scattered degenerative changes were observed, but the placenta was normal. Likewise, when rat placentas were irradiated with the fetus shielded, the exposure had no effect on fetal growth. Relative "radioresistance" of the gestationally older placenta was inferred from these experiments (see also Brent, 1960).

Whether treatment with the β-adrenergic blocking agent **propranolol** has an effect on placental development is uncertain. Fiddler (1974) described the pregnancy of a patient who had been taking 30 mg of propranolol three times daily for 3 years for treatment of obstructive hypertrophic cardiomyopathy. The patient delivered a severely growth-restricted infant accompanied by a 200-g placenta. He quoted other authors who found no ill-effect from this medication and yet others who witnessed spontaneous abortions. Reduction of maternal cardiac output was speculated to have caused this fetal growth restriction, but the disease itself may also have been causative.

The consequences that maternal **heart disease** has on pregnancy have been the topic of many studies. Because of their complexity, the outcome of fetal growth and placental development is variable. Only one of five patients with aortic stenosis was reported to have fetal growth restriction (Easterling et al., 1988). McFaul et al. (1988) found no increased fetal mortality, growth restriction, or congenital anomalies among 519 pregnancies of 405 women treated for heart disease during pregnancy. Feraboli (1951) described placental infarcts and intervillous thromboses in six patients with "cardiopathy" and opined that the lesions are not specific but resulted from "slowing of the general circulation." He suggested that the fetal vessels were sclerosed, and that placental villous

fibrosis occurred. We have seen several placentas of patients with severe rheumatic cardiac disease, especially with mitral stenosis, in whose placentas there were large subchorionic intervillous thromboses. In some of them adjacent infarcts were present. Nuñez (1963) studied 15 placentas of women with cardiac disease properly classified according to New York Heart Association standards. He performed a quantitative assessment of villous structures and found the villous surface to be reduced, with simultaneous reduction of the fetal/maternal placental weight ratio. Because the villous capillary bed was expanded, Nuñez inferred that there was an expanded fetal blood volume. Kerber et al. (1968) found a normal placenta and normal-sized fetus with choanal atresia in a patient who was being treated with warfarin and heparin for a prosthetic mitral valve.

Pregnancy complicated by **hypercholesterolemia** resulted in an entirely normal placenta, despite fetal growth restriction (Barss et al., 1985). Cholesterol deposits were sought but not found. In **hypobetalipoproteinemia** also, a normal placenta was found (Parker et al., 1986). Numerous lipid-laden macrophages were present in the intervillous space of a patient with extreme **hyperlipemia** that complicated pregnancy (Nielsen et al., 1973). The foam cells measured up to 35 μm in diameter and were concentrated at the maternal floor of the placenta. No foam cells were found within the placental villi. The infant delivered normally, had a birth weight of 3650 g, and was normal. The placenta also had a normal gross appearance. The placenta of a patient with "well-controlled" **phenylketonuria**, provided by Dr. B.H. Landing, was entirely normal. In a case of **Gordon's syndrome** (short stature, defective dentition, hyperkalemic hyperchloremic acidosis, and chronic hypertension), Kirshon et al. (1987) reported normal fetal development and, it is assumed, a normal placenta. We have seen a patient with **Smith-Lemli-Opitz syndrome** whose pregnancy ended prematurely (courtesy of Dr. S. Sadowinski, Los Angeles). The placenta showed slight edema but had no other findings of note. As is regrettably so often the case, the placental findings were not documented in a case of **cystic fibrosis**, reported by Rosenow and Lee (1968). The infant developed normally. So did two term infants in a patient with **Wilson's disease**, but the placenta was not reported (Dreifuss & McKinney, 1966). Oga et al. (1993) reported on the birth of a child who had hepatomegaly from this maternal disease and continued to suffer abnormal liver function tests. The "maternal side of the placenta" had an increased copper content. Their illustration suggests that the copper is contained in the cytoplasm of the decidua basalis cells.

With **pruritus gravidarum**, the associated cholestasis is frequently accompanied by premature birth and fetal death; the placenta is commonly meconium-stained (Sasseville et al., 1981). The same authors discussed many other dermatoses in pregnancy and reported that **impetigo herpetiformis** is associated with frequent stillbirths and "placental insufficiency." With **papular dermatitis of pregnancy**, it has been suggested that the lesions are due to a "hypersensitivity reaction to an abnormal placenta." High human chorionic gonadotropin (hCG) levels are believed to reflect this abnormality, but the evidence does not appear to be firm. Moreover, in subsequent pregnancies, this dermatologic disorder does not recur. **Pruritus** during pregnancy (of undefined etiology) was thought to be the cause of hyperplacentosis (placentas of more than 600 g) with increased hCG levels (Goodlin et al., 1985). This association, however, also seems ill-defined, and specific placental lesions were not reported. We have observed the placenta from a patient whose hCG levels were 260,000 IU in the last half of pregnancy; she had developed huge cystic follicles and elevated testosterone levels. Placenta and offspring were normal and the patient's hCG titer fell rapidly. The reason for this elevated titers remained unexplained.

Several contributions have elucidated the pathology of **sarcoidosis** during pregnancy. This is a chronic granulomatous inflammation of systemic nature but life-limiting primarily because of pulmonary granulomatosis. The individual granulomas have a superficial similarity to tuberculosis but organisms have not been identified. Altchek et al. (1955) found uterine involvement by sarcoidosis granulomas and established that, despite active, widespread sarcoidosis, normal pregnancy may ensue. Dines and Banner (1967) and other authors they quoted found that the pulmonary complication of sarcoidosis may improve during pregnancy. From his review of 54 pregnancies, O'Leary (1968) was unable to agree. Kelemen and Mándi (1969) were the first authors to report typical sarcoid granulomas in the term placenta of a normal infant. Small, grossly visible granulomas were seen in the floor of that placenta. Boggess et al. (1995) found little ill-effect on pregnancies from restrictive maternal lung disease but did not observe placentas.

In maternal **cystinosis** that had much earlier been complicated by nephropathy and renal allografts at age 8, normal fetal development occurred. The maternal cells in the decidua capsularis had numerous vacuolated, cystine-containing cells. The placenta was normal (Reiss et al., 1988). **Cystinuria**, on the other hand, has occasionally been associated with mild fetal growth restriction. **Fetal cystinosis** may be diagnosed from placental specimens. Smith et al. (1989) found that homozygous cystinosis patients' placentas had significantly elevated cystine content, as did fetal leukocytes; heterozygotes could not be clearly distinguished from normals. Maternal **hyperhomocysteinemia** is associated with intrauterine growth restriction (IUGR), thromboembolism, pregnancy-induced hypertension (PIH), and abortion. The placenta of seven such pregnancies showed nonspecific changes, such as atherosis, small placenta, thromboses, and accelerated maturation (Khong & Hague, 1997).

Maternal **Gaucher's disease** (a storage disease due to enzyme deficiency; see Chapter 18) complicating pregnancy has been associated with hemorrhagic complications that resulted from thrombocytopenia. Houlton and Jackson (1978) described it to be due to extensive infiltration with foamy macrophages throughout the marrow spaces. In another case (Addleman & Gold, 1963) with good outcome, the placenta appeared grossly normal (Addleman, personal communication, 1963). Watov and de Sandre (1964) reported another four pregnancies, two of which resulted in placenta previa. The authors did not report the placental histology. These reports referred to other cases in the literature, but a definitive study of the placenta with maternal Gaucher's disease has only recently come to our attention. It describes 43 patients (17 treated; 26 untreated) with 66 pregnancies and, additionally, it presents a complete overview of reported cases (Elstein et al., 2004). In general, treated patients had fewer abortions but more postpartum hemorrhage and infection; overall live birth rates were 78.3% in the treated and 86% in the untreated group.

Maternal **Niemann-Pick disease** (another genetic storage disorder) has been reported perhaps only once (Porter et al., 1997) and was not associated with placental or fetal disease. When the fetus suffers this disease, extensive placental lesions have been reported and are reviewed in Chapter 18.

Pheochromocytoma complicating pregnancy has serious implications for the fetus and mother. A review made in our department (Russo, personal communication, 1986) encountered 120 case reports with 45% fetal deaths, 12% abortions, and 25% maternal mortality. Thrombosis of the umbilical cord was found in one case (Fox et al., 1969) and abruptio placentae in four cases (Pestelek & Kapor, 1963). Most of the deaths could not be adequately explained. The disease is often mistaken for toxemia of pregnancy because of the hypertension and frequent albuminuria (Cannon, 1958). Cannon described several abortions that occurred in a patient with pheochromocytoma. Combs et al. (1989) found that there was a marked fall (40%) in cardiac output during paroxysmal attacks due to pheochromocytoma and suggested that it may compromise the fetus. Others have seen few complications with pregnancy, even with a recurrent pheochromocytoma (after adrenalectomy) (Sweeney & Katz, 1994). This tumor occurs as part of Sipple's (multiple endocrinopathy) syndrome, which, absent this tumor, has no placental or pregnancy-related complications (Wax et al., 1997).

In a case of **fetal Letterer-Siwe's disease** described by Ahnquist and Holyoke (1960), the placenta was entirely normal. The stillborn fetus had widespread involvement of reticuloendothelial cell proliferation with numerous giant cells. The mother had been vaccinated against poliomyelitis and influenza during pregnancy, but the authors considered a causal relation unlikely.

Hematologic Disorders

Sickle cell anemia occurs, with few exceptions, in Blacks. It is characterized by the presence of sickle-shaped red blood cells, which result from crystallization into "tactoids" of the abnormal hemoglobin S, particularly under conditions of reduced oxygen tension. Formalin fixation usually allows the microscopic identification of sickle cells in histologic sections (Fig. 19.2), and often NRBCs can be found in the intervillous space. Fujikura and Froehlich (1968) suggested that the hypoxia of postpartum placental separation induces sickling in the intervillous space. They examined 2117 placentas of black women and found sickling in 9.4%. They remarked that formalin fixation was superior for preservation; Bouin's solution causes too much red blood cell lysis, and Zenker's solution causes a reversal of the sickling phenomenon. No associated pathologic findings were reported in their large study. It has been our experience that placental infarcts are more common in maternal sickle cell disease; Pantanowitz et al. (2000) found a chorangioma with a normally grown infant and impressively showed the sickled red cells in the intervillous space.

The heterozygous condition ("trait") of S hemoglobinopathy occurs with a frequency of 9% in the United States African-American population and is as high as 45% in central Africa. In infants with sickle cell thalassemia (hemoglobin SC disease), infarcts of the placenta have been reported (Bentsi-Enchill & Konotey-Ahulu, 1969).

Patients with the homozygous sickle cell disease have many serious problems. Urinary tract infection (45%), preeclampsia (25%), and puerperal sepsis (20%) are the main complications. In heterozygotes, these complications are significantly less frequent and less severe (Winston & Mastroianni, 1953). Whalley et al. (1963) found no difference in the outcome of pregnancy in heterozygotes when compared to controls. Platt (1971) found increased perinatal mortality, and Brown et al. (1972) observed lower birth weights. Fetal growth restriction was also a finding (21%) in the large study summarized by Smith et al. (1996). Mortality was not increased. They did not report on placentas. "Blister cells" (erythrocytes with vacuoles) were found in a patient with sickle cell disease who died after giving birth to a growth-restricted child (Krayalcin et al., 1972). Prophylactic transfusion reduces the frequency of painful crises but does not secure a beneficial pregnancy outcome (Koshy et al., 1988), presumably because the significant placental lesions have already been produced prior to this therapy.

The placentas of patients with hemoglobin SS disease may have "Tenney-Parker" changes, infarcts, increased fibrin, abruptios, and villous edema (Anderson et al., 1960; Shanklin, 1976; Koshy et al., 1988; Dunn et al., 1989). These placentas are relatively small, and the associated fetuses have growth restriction. Fox (1978) did not encounter those lesions; he reported that most of the changes are the histologic alterations of the intervillous red blood cells. A single pregnancy with hemoglobin SE disease has been reported, but the placenta was not described (Ramahi et al., 1988). The 2310-g neonate had hydrocephalus. Fujikura (personal communication, 1976) found that maternal sickle cells occasionally traverse the placenta to the fetal side. He indicated that in about half

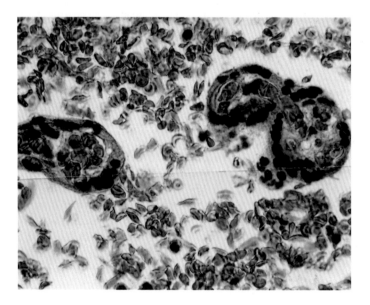

FIGURE 19.2. Sickle-shaped red blood cells in the intervillous space of a patient with hemoglobin SS disease at term. The **fetal** capillaries contain normal red blood cells, with mostly fetal hemoglobin. H&E ×640.

of the placentas examined sickle cells were found in aspirated cord blood; in addition, he identified occasional deported villi (Fig. 19.3) in this blood. Doubtless, it is a traumatic feature of delivery of the placenta and has no bearing on normal fetal life.

Mordel et al. (1989) reviewed the literature of pregnancy complicated by maternal β-**thalassemia**. Their patient was transfusion-dependent but delivered a normal term infant. They referred to other patients who suffered fetal growth restriction and abortion. A larger study by Aessopos et al. (1999) of well-treated patients with this disease showed little ill-effect from this hemoglobin defect. The placentas of both studies, however, were not described.

Idiopathic thrombocytopenia (ITP) is a rare complication of pregnancy. It carries with it the risk of postpartum hemorrhage and, less commonly, it has neonatal hemorrhagic complications (Jones et al., 1961; Payne et al., 1997). The latter may be a hazard when obtaining fetal scalp samples for the purpose of fetal pH determination. Cordocentesis has been practiced successfully in maternal thrombocytopenic states so as to assess the fetal platelet counts (Kaplan et al., 1990). That cordocentesis is not without risk, however, was detailed by Paidas et al. (1995) in their study of **fetal alloimmune thrombocytopenia** (Bussel et al., 1997). Fetal platelet counts were significantly depressed and exsanguination was observed after cordocentesis. We saw a similar event and one with complete obstruction and death of one artery. On rare occa-

sion the placenta has had intervillous thrombi in maternal thrombocytopenia, but most commonly the disease is not associated with placental lesions (Kaibara et al., 1985). In a few other cases, infarcts and decidual vascular lesions have been reported in the placenta (Scott, 1966; Mercer et al., 1988). It is not clear, however, whether they were caused by the ITP or were perhaps the result of preeclampsia and steroid therapy (Schenker & Polishuk, 1968).

Thrombotic thrombocytopenic purpura (TTP) during pregnancy has been described by Wurzel (1979). The pregnancy ended with a macerated fetus. The placenta showed many "hyaline thrombi" in the decidual arterioles that presumably caused the fetal death. Thrombotic thrombocytopenic purpura is a serious disease and carries a high mortality rate. Fewer than 70 cases have been described, according to Ambrose et al. (1985). Often the disease is mistaken for severe preeclampsia; perhaps some aspects of their clinical presentations are shared because of the similarity of their occlusive vascular lesions. In a case of maternal TTP we have seen fibrin deposits in decidual vessels, resembling atherosis. An apparently normal placenta with an infant having no thrombocytopenia was described in the first report of **Evans syndrome** during pregnancy (Silverstein et al., 1966).

Neonatal thrombocytopenia has many causes, including the transfer of maternal **human leukocyte antigen (HLA) antibodies** (Sharon & Amar, 1981; Sørensen et al.,

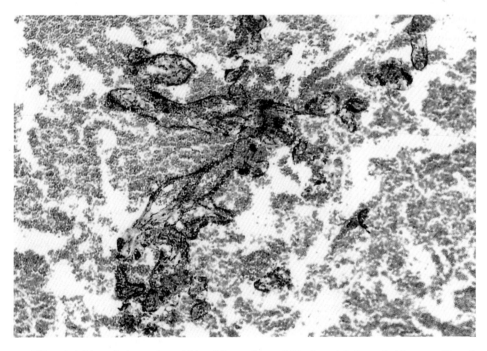

FIGURE 19.3. Mature villi and sickle cells in aspirated blood from the umbilical cord. It is probably an artifact that occurred during the delivery of the placenta. H&E ×150. (Courtesy of Dr. T. Fujikura.)

1982; Morales & Stroup, 1985), maternal **thiazide** administration (Rodriguez et al., 1964), and **alloimmunization** (Deaver et al., 1986). The latter condition has special dangers of fetal intracranial hemorrhage and is now being treated with prenatal platelet transfusions (Daffos et al., 1988; Mueller-Eckhardt et al., 1988). Despite these advances, the placenta remains usually unstudied or it was found to be normal.

Messer (1987) and Handin (1981) have reviewed **bleeding disorders** during pregnancy. **Leukoagglutinins** cause neonatal neutropenia but have no known effect on the placenta (Payne, 1964). Pregnancies complicated by **von Willebrand's disease** were reported by Leone et al. (1975) and Watanabe et al. (1997), but the placentas were not reported; the infants were normal and, with adequate therapy, the patients did well. A patient with **factor VII deficiency** was successfully treated by Fadel and Krauss (1989), whose main concern was possible abruptio. A retrospective study of pregnancy outcome of 32 patients with **hemorrhagic hereditary telangiectasia** showed a slightly higher frequency of abortions. The placentas were not reported (Goodman et al., 1967). **Protein C deficiency** during pregnancy was studied by Vogel et al. (1989). They reported no complications to have occurred. In a pedigree that contained 15 pregnancies no excess fetal loss but an increased incidence of thrombosis were observed (Trauscht-Van Horn et al., 1992). The effect of various **thrombophilic defects** (factor V Leiden, deficiency of antithrombin, protein C, protein S) upon fetal losses was studied by Preston et al. (1996). They found no increased losses when the father had the condition, and from the **factor V Leiden mutation**. Younis et al. (2000a,b, 2003; Sarig et al., 2002), however, found increased fetal losses in patients with "activated protein C resistance" (APCR), whereas Göpel et al. (2001) determined that successful in vitro fertilization (IVF) is increased when the factor V Leiden mutation is present. Lakasing et al. (1999) found no increase in poor pregnancy outcomes when the antiphospholipid syndrome exists in their immunocytochemical study of villi with antibodies to thrombomodulin and annexin V, similar to the retrospective review undertaken by Mooney et al. (2003), which correlated "cushions" and mural thromboses in the placentas of 72 cases of neonatal encephalopathy. Subsequently, these authors (McDonald et al., 2004) found neonatal encephalopathy to be related to fetal thromboses and, especially, to infection and meconium staining. To complicate matters, Infante-Rivard et al. (2002) found no relation to IUGR and thrombophilia and, in a large study of gene polymorphism and intrauterine fetal death (IUFD), Hefler et al. (2004) were adamant that "our data represent the largest study and . . . we challenge the importance of thrombophilia and vascular gene polymorphism in the pathogenesis of this condition." The problems of understanding these relations are also borne out by the

meta-analysis of 31 studies undertaken by Rey et al. (2003). They found that "exclusion of women with other pathologies that could explain fetal loss strengthened the association between factor V Leiden and recurrent fetal loss." Another meta-analysis was undertaken by Howley et al. (2005) from which they concluded that "factor V Leiden and prothrombin gene variant both confer an increased risk of giving birth to an intrauterine growth restricted infant, although this may be driven by small, poor-quality studies that demonstrated extreme associations. Large well-controlled prospective studies are required to determine definitively whether an association between thrombophilia and intrauterine growth restriction is present." Martinelli et al. (2000) saw tripling of late fetal losses when factor V Leiden and the prothrombin gene mutations were present and found 24% of placentas to be normal, and in the remainder were thrombi, decidual vascular lesions, necrosis, and infarcts. We have also found thrombi, decidual vascular lesions, chronic deciduitis, infarcts, and increased perivillous fibrin in placentas of mothers with various thrombophilias (Baergen et al., 2001). An interesting report of three pregnancy losses with thrombophilia comes from Heller et al. (2003). They found large subchorionic hematomas as the cause of fetal demises and suggested that this was the result of increased maternal coagulability. It is especially relevant because these subchorionic hematomas are otherwise relatively uncommon but are observed now sonographically. The lesion is occasionally described as a Breus' mole and has been associated primarily with chromosomal errors, but that may need to be reconsidered, as the accumulated blood has now been shown to be definitely of maternal origin (Wright et al., 1999). Thus, there are still outstanding issues to be understood for a conclusive interpretation of various types of thrombophilia and their effect on gestational success. When the **fetus** has evidence of thrombophilic mutations, no placental lesions or thromboses were found (Ariel et al., 2004).

Other conditions, especially when combining as thrombophilia, elevated the fetal loss rate in the study by Preston et al. (1996). Regrettably, there is no report on the placentas of the study population. Greer (1999) indicated that thrombosis in pregnancy has much increased in England and reviewed the fetal and maternal consequences. The single commonest cause of deep vein thrombosis is activated protein C resistance (APCR), due to a point mutation in the factor V gene and referred to as "factor V Leiden" (Ridker et al., 1995). There has been much interest in this mutation, and the worldwide distribution has been assessed by Rees et al. (1995). The allele frequency is highest in Europeans (especially Greeks), while it is absent from many non-European populations. Several groups (Gratton et al., 1997; Walker et al., 1997) have warned that activated protein C resistance (factor V Leiden) rises in pregnancy and that falsely high levels may be misinterpreted. Because of reduced intervillous flow and increased fibrin deposition, so hypothesize Dizon-Townson et al. (1996), there is a significant increase in the predisposition to preeclampsia in women with factor V Leiden. Dizon-Townson et al. (1997) reported a significantly higher Leiden carriage with occurrence of repeat abortion, and even more increase in the fetal side of the placenta when numerous infarcts were present (see also Wiener-Megnagi et al., 1998; Kupferminc et al., 1999). Pauer et al. (1998), however, found no such correlation in their material. From the fetal vantage point, Goodwin et al. (1995) found that even heterozygous protein C deficiency can lead to serious peripartum thrombosis in the fetus. Thus, a somewhat different outcome may occur in fetal protein C deficiency (and protein S deficiency); they are discussed in Chapter 12 (see Thromboses of the Fetal Circulation). The histologic features of placental specimens with thrombophilias were recently presented by Horn et al. (2004) and Baergen et al. (2001). These reports provide an overview of the lesions identified (infarcts, decidual necrosis, inflammation, thrombosis) and suggest that the features are nonspecific and "may not differentiate between women with antiphospholipid syndrome and antiphospholipid-like syndromes." Alonso et al. (2002) considered thrombophilias to be important causes of fetal losses in a Spanish population and drew special attention to the frequency of placental infarcts, whereas McCowan et al. (2003) did not consider these conditions as being responsible for IUGR gestations. An excellent review of all aspects of the pathophysiology of the antiphospholipid syndrome may be found in Levine et al. (2002). It includes features to be found with therapeutic measures. We conclude from this array of conflicting reports that much additional information is needed before firm conclusions can be drawn as to the direct effects of the various types of thrombophilia on placental structure and fetal outcome.

Milo et al. (1989) reported on a patient with acute intermittent **porphyria** during pregnancy believed to be secondary to the antiemetic drug metoclopramide. When the drug was discontinued, the symptoms disappeared and a normal infant was delivered. We saw a case of alleged porphyria developing during pregnancy that, after examination of the placenta, was shown to be due to acute cytomegalovirus infection.

Folate deficiency has been incriminated in many complications of pregnancy, including abortion, abruptio placentae, and other diseases (Streiff & Little, 1967; Hibbard & Hibbard, 1968). In two large studies of women with folic acid deficiency severe enough to cause megaloblastic anemia in the mother, no measurable effect on fetal well-being or placentation was observed (Kitay, 1968; Pritchard et al., 1970).

Beischer et al. (1970) evaluated the effect of **anemia** on pregnancy and the placenta. They prospectively studied a large number of placentas that were obtained from different localities. The investigators found that severe maternal anemia caused highly significant placental enlargement. In their interpretation, the "anemia causes inadequate oxygenation of the fetoplacental unit, which in turn, in a proportion of patients, evokes a physiological response which results in compensatory placental hypertrophy." Some placentas weighed in excess of 700 g. We have seen, however, placentas of severely anemic patients, with hemoglobin values of 4 g/dL, that were small and had pronounced "Tenney-Parker changes," that is, increased knotting of the syncytium. An enlargement of placentas and an increased placental ratio were confirmed in mild maternal iron-deficiency anemia and thalassemia trait by Lao and Wong (1997). Enlargement was largely dependent on maternal hemoglobin concentration and it correlated with gestational age. In an histomorphometric study of placentas in women with iron-deficiency anemia, Reshetnikova et al. (1995) found no placentomegaly. In fact, they found a reduction in size of the villous tree, with thinning of the diffusion membrane. To explain the difference of their finding from that reported in the literature (enlargement), the authors suggested that simultaneously existing malnutrition may be the answer, as it is nearly always associated with severe anemia.

The finding of placental hypertrophy with anemia has raised the question as to what changes may be observed in placentas of chronic oxygen deficiency at **high altitude**. Metcalfe et al. (1966) have summarized the adaptation of the pregnant organism to the rarified atmosphere; placental changes were not then identified with certainty. Alzamora (1958), on the other hand, has reported that the placenta at high altitude is considerably larger than normal. This point is of particular interest, in relation to the important studies carried out by Tominaga and Page (1966). These investigators experimentally studied placental effects of oxygen deprivation. They exposed explanted human placental tissue to low and high oxygen tension in vitro, and found that low oxygen exposure led to increased syncytial "knotting" (the Tenney-Parker change of preeclampsia). Contrary to the findings of later investigators (Ong & Burton, 1991), they found a reversibility of this phenomenon. This trophoblastic change was believed to cause thinning of the exchange membrane and was thus considered to enhance oxygen transfer to the fetus. Quantitative studies on the effect of high altitude on the placenta were carried out by Jackson et al. (1987, 1988) and their results are quite different. They also reviewed the relevant literature and found that infants at high altitude were smaller, but that the placental weight was not enlarged (at 3600 m in Bolivia). There was, however, a histologic (measured and quantitated) alteration in the disposition of villous capillaries. Mean villous length was reduced at high altitude, whereas villous capillaries were thinner and cross sections of capillaries more numerous. This effect (presumably due to chronic hypoxia) led to an altered capillary/villous ratio at high altitude in these Bolivian samples. The capillaries were also more closely applied to the trophoblastic surface than is the case at sea level. This finding was particularly evident in the histometric study of Reshetnikova et al. (1996). These investigators found a significantly larger capillary volume in placentas of high altitude; the findings were at times similar to chorangioma, presumably representing chorangiosis (see Chapter 24). Kaufmann et al. (1993) reviewed this topic in some detail and suggested that a first effect of hypoxia is an effect on cytotrophoblast with its proliferation, to be followed by syncytiogenesis ("knots"). They suggested that various cytokines of yet undetermined nature and sequence affect the connective tissue of the villi (perhaps Hofbauer cells) to mediate these effects.

Endocrine Disorders

Thyroid diseases have no direct known impact on placental structure and function but many thyroid disorders enhance the probability of preeclampsia. Placental infarcts and abruptio are thus found more commonly than normal. Scott (1966) stated that hyperthyroidism is not infrequent during pregnancy and mentioned that hydramnios occasionally complicates such pregnancies. Davis et al. (1989) found an incidence of hyperthyroidism of one per 2000 deliveries. Vulsma et al. (1989) suggested that substantial amounts of maternal thyroxine may be transferred to the fetus; however, Bachrach and Burrows (1989) provided evidence that the amounts transferred in fact may be much smaller than was suggested. Infants of hyperthyroid patients may be growth-restricted or hyperthyroid (Elsas et al., 1967; Cove & Johnson, 1985). They also more frequently have prenatal distress, meconium staining, and fetal demise (Page et al., 1988). These authors encountered chronic villitis in one of their perinatal deaths, but it probably bears no relation to the maternal hyperthyroidism. Diabetes is also more frequent in hyperthyroid patients during pregnancy (Bruner et al., 1988). All aspects of the physiology of thyroid metabolism and thyroid diseases are well reviewed elsewhere (American College of Obstetricians and Gynecologists, 1993). Hydrops fetalis has been reported in a number of patients with treated Graves' disease (Watson & Fiegen, 1995). Apparently maternal immunoglobin G (IgG) thyroid antibodies are transmitted transplacentally, induce fetal hyperthyroidism and tachycardia (see Chapter 16). The placental physiology of iodine and thyroxine handling is discussed by Burrow et al. (1994).

Untreated hypothyroidism renders most patients anovulatory. It is therefore not often encountered as a complication of pregnancy. Davis et al. (1988) reviewed 14 pregnancies in overtly hypothyroid patients. Anemia (31%), toxemia (44%), abruptio (19%), and postpartum hemorrhage (19%) were found. Fetal death occurred in 12% and growth restriction in 31%. The frequent abortions, congenital anomalies, and maternal infertility associated with hypothyroid states were discussed in some detail by Hoet et al. (1960). When pregnancy is complicated by **Sipple's syndrome**, the outcome is good, so long as pheochromocytoma has not occurred (Wax et al., 1997).

Cushing's disease rarely complicates pregnancy. Grimes et al. (1973) adequately reviewed the literature of 26 reported pregnancies that resulted in only 11 term births. There were four abortions and four stillbirths; premature deliveries made up the remainder. The placentas of these pregnancies were not reported. Likewise, Aron et al. (1990), in an extensive review of complications of this disease, failed to indicate if placental pathologic features are seen. These authors, as well as Buescher et al. (1992) suggested that the adrenocorticotropic hormone (ACTH)-like material from the placenta and its corticotropin-releasing hormone–like compound may exacerbate the clinical state of Cushing's disease during pregnancy. Occasionally, Cushing's disease has its onset during pregnancy and disappears after its termination. Wieland et al. (1971) reported such a case and referred to others in the literature. Upon termination of pregnancy during the 14th week, their patient improved remarkably. Normal placental tissue was obtained.

Diabetes insipidus is also a most uncommon disease during pregnancy. Hanson and colleagues (1997) have reported such a patient who presented with the classic symptoms of the disease and severe oligohydramnios. Treatment with desmopressin acetate promptly relieved symptoms and oligohydramnios; the disease was assumed to be a congenital hypoplasia of the posterior pituitary. The placenta was not described.

Zollinger-Ellison syndrome is compatible with normal fetal development and represents a rare complication of pregnancy (Harper et al., 1995). Apparently no adverse influence on the placenta takes place.

Diabetes Mellitus During Pregnancy

Abnormalities of glucose metabolism, such as gestational and overt insulin-dependent diabetes, are among the commonest medical complications of pregnancy. These conditions cause increased fetal wastage such as abortion, prematurity, macrosomia, and some types of congenital anomalies (Cheung et al., 1990; White & Beischer, 1990). A comprehensive review of these complications with a classification of the disease is to be found in Viscarello et al. (1993). The consequences of maternal diabetes for the placenta are reviewed in detail by Desoye and Shafrir

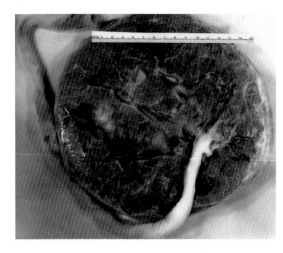

FIGURE 19.4. Plethoric, thick, and somewhat edematous placenta of a patient with treated class A diabetes.

(1964, 1996). Susa et al. (1984) were able to mimic most of the fetal consequences of maternal diabetes in rhesus monkeys fetuses infused with excess amounts of insulin.

The placenta of women with diabetes is often severely abnormal (Singer, 1984). The results of placental investigations, however, must be considered with caution as they are subject to many variations, mostly the degree of diabetic control during gestation. There have been dramatic changes in the management of maternal diabetes and in surveillance for gestational diabetes over the years. Thus, the results of older placental studies are not necessarily expected to be found currently. Also, because of the high fetal mortality during the last 2 weeks of pregnancy, most pregnant diabetic patients are now delivered before term, which perhaps helps explain why most diabetic mothers' placentas are not so calcified in current observations; older publications state that diabetic mothers' placentas showed increasing amounts of calcium deposits. We have the impression, however, that the usual

calcifications in the floor of the placenta and in the septa are decreased in diabetics' placentas. Perhaps for the same reasons we see these placentas to be less frequently meconium stained. Haust (1981) provided a comprehensive review of diabetic pregnancies, fetal outcome, anomalies, and placental changes. It is thoroughly referenced and illustrated, and contains a large section on placental changes in maternal diabetes. In particular, there is a detailed consideration of the ultrastructural pathology of the associated placenta.

The placenta of most poorly controlled diabetics is enlarged, thick, and plethoric (Fig. 19.4), which are generally thought to be manifestations of fetal hypervolemia and maternal hyperglycemia. The hypervolemia is also reflected in the considerably higher residual blood volume of the delivered placenta (Kjeldsen & Pedersen, 1967; Klebe & Ingomar, 1974a,b). An altered fetal cardiac activity and blood flow were observed sonographically by Rizzo et al. (1995) and may result from fetal cardiac hypertrophy. When diabetes is well controlled during pregnancy, the placental weight does not deviate from that of normal organs (Clarson et al., 1989) and the villous structure is normal (Fox, 1978). By contrast, in other cases the villous structure of the placenta in maternal diabetes may be focally "dysmature" or relatively immature-appearing; increased numbers of villous trophoblast cells, pointing to increased incidence of trophoblast proliferation, may be observed (Fox, 1997). An increased frequency of cytotrophoblastic mitoses may be observed. These placentas are also sometimes edematous, and their appearance has occasionally been likened to that of placentas from erythroblastotic pregnancies (Maqueo et al., 1965), although the fetuses lack the anemia. Maqueo et al. also observed a high frequency of preeclampsia in this population, which is not our observation. There is frequently some degree of chorangiosis in the placentas of diabetic patients (Figs. 19.5 and 19.6). In the offspring,

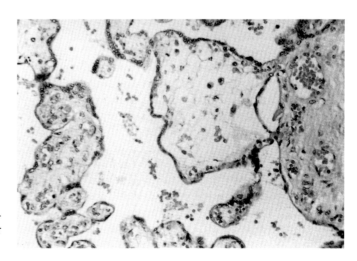

FIGURE 19.5. Focal immaturity and villous edema of the placenta in class A diabetic mother. Note the large Hofbauer cells in the edematous villus. H&E ×160.

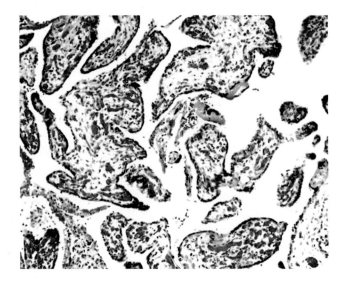

FIGURE 19.6. Placenta of a diabetic mother with marked plethora and chorangiosis. H&E ×160.

there is a slight increase in the frequency of single umbilical artery (3% to 5% in diabetic progeny compared to a ~1% average incidence; Driscoll, 1965). This is particularly so in gestations that were complicated by acidosis (Emmrich et al., 1974). When the pregnancy is complicated by nephropathy (class F diabetes), fetal growth restriction and placental infarcts may be found with increased frequency. Infarcts are otherwise uncommon in diabetic mothers' placentas. It is our opinion that none of these changes is specific for maternal diabetes and that they reflect primarily the altered glucose availability and fetal adjustments to the intermittent excessive glucose load. Perhaps most characteristic of diabetes is the greater probability of fetal and placental vascular thrombosis. This problem is occasionally reflected in fetal renal and adrenal vein thrombosis, and it may also be the cause of thromboses in the fetal placental surface and mainstem vessels. The umbilical cord is usually more "edematous" or, more accurately, it contains more Wharton's jelly. Since Mvumbi et al. (1996) observed that the midportion of umbilical cords contains normally the highest glycogen content (in the fibrocytes), one may speculate that the thicker cords are related to that storage, but it has not been studied. No specific placental anomalies are associated with the one highly characteristic fetal anomaly of maternal diabetes, sacral agenesis (the so-called caudal regression syndrome). Not all cases of this anomaly, however, are the result of maternal diabetes; some may have an environmental toxic heritage (Rojansky et al., 2002). Salafia and Silberman (1989) made the point that funisitis is common in diabetic pregnancies and that it is correlated with irregular fetal heart rate patterns. The placentas they studied were also heavier.

There is no longer doubt that the placenta possesses specific insulin-binding receptors (Haour & Bertrand, 1974), and that these receptors are reduced in number in placentas of SGA babies (Potau et al., 1981). By contrast, in insulin-treated diabetes, but not when treated with diet alone, more insulin receptors were found on the maternal surface of the placental villi, that is, the trophoblast plasma membrane; this was verified also in isolated trophoblast preparations (Desoye et al., 1992). It is unclear whether the increased number of receptors is elicited by insulin-treatment of the mothers, or whether they are a response to other factors in the circulation that are altered on diabetes. The consequences of the greater receptor density on the trophoblast are also unknown, because no clear-cut effect of insulin on the placenta has been identified yet. At present it remains an open question whether or not the expression of insulin receptors located at the surface facing the fetal circulation, that is, the endothelium (Desoye et al., 1994), shows respective changes in maternal diabetes mellitus. Despite earlier assertions that transplacental insulin traffic occurs (Gitlin et al., 1965), it is now clear that insulin does not normally pass the placenta in quantities sufficient to have a metabolic effect (Adam et al., 1969; Wolf et al., 1969; Kalhan et al., 1975). There is, however, antibody-bound insulin transferred in significant quantities and this correlates with fetal macrosomia (Menon et al., 1990). This suggested to the authors that immunogenic insulin should not be used in pregnancy, a recommendation that meanwhile is followed in nearly all civilized countries. Another interpretation of the data was provided by Kimmerle and Chantelau (1991). Glucose passes the placenta readily, and the fetus responds to hyperglycemia with hyperplasia of the islets of Langerhans (Driscoll, 1965) and increased insulin secretion (Jørgensen et al., 1966; Thomas et al., 1967), the primary reason for fetal overweight in maternal diabetes. The hyperplastic islets contain an increased amount of insulin (Steinke & Driscoll, 1965). Periodic hyperglycemia was thought to be the cause of fetal polyuria and hydramnios. That this assertion is probably an oversimplification has been demonstrated by the ultrasonographic study of fetal urination in the presence of diabetes-induced hydramnios (Wladimiroff et al., 1975).

A paradoxical finding is the increased deposition of glycogen in the placenta of diabetics (Desoye et al., 1992), whereas in all other organs diabetes results in a decreased glycogen content. Robb and Hytten (1976) have rigorously studied placental glycogen content throughout gestation and in maternal diabetes. They found that glycogen concentrations normally decrease toward term, when it was around 1.5 mg/g of blood-free placental tissue. There were no significant changes when diabetic mothers' placentas were compared with those of normal pregnancies (for review see Shafrir & Barash, 1991) or those from toxemic gestations (see also Fischer & Horky, 1966). Thus, the larger size of the placenta is not attributable to glycogen storage, but the results of Mvumbi et al. (1996) should be considered before definitive conclusions are drawn. Most of the large fetal size is due to obesity. A valuable test to ascertain maternal hyperglycemia during pregnancy is the concentration of glycohemoglobin in maternal blood. It adequately reflects the degree of maternal control, and higher concentrations significantly correlate with abortions in diabetics (Miodovnik et al., 1985). When strict control is exercised, pregnant diabetics are no more liable to lose a pregnancy than normal women, and they have normal amounts of glycosylated hemoglobin in their circulation (Mills et al., 1988). In pregnancies complicated by maternal diabetes, there is also much enhanced secretion of hCG by the placenta, as reflected in blood and amnionic fluid levels. Elkind-Hirsch and colleagues (1989) have found that the placenta of diabetics contains more gonadotropin-releasing hormone than do normal placentas. The hCG concentration, on the other hand, was not elevated. Greco et al. (1989) asserted from their immunocytochemical studies of proteins in diabetic placentas that β-hCG staining was increased, while other proteins (PLAP, SP1, and hPL) were decreased. It must be cautioned that the evaluation of these staining reactions is subjective and visual only. Moreover, the endocrine data are very likely to depend on the control of the diabetes, as does the villous structure.

Thomsen and Lieschke (1958) were among the earliest investigators to study the placental structure in maternal diabetes. They found increased weight, plethora, calcifications, and "villous regenerations." The latter manifests as "immaturity" of the villi, more abundant and obvious cytotrophoblastic investment of villi, and villous edema. These nonspecific changes were found randomly distributed throughout the placenta. Burstein et al. (1963) claimed that major fetal vessels of the placenta have insulin bound to their walls. They studied diabetic placentas using insulin antibodies and fluorescence microscopy. They observed that placentas from diabetics had increased knotting of the syncytium. Aladjem (1967a,b) examined villi with phase contrast microscopy and found no specific changes in diabetes, although many minor placental alterations were described. Vogel (1967), on the other hand, believed that he found changes that he considered to be so characteristic that he coined the term **plakopathia diabetica**. This condition consists of persistent embryonic villi, discordant maturation of villous structure, disorders of villous ramification, and chorangiosis. Decreases in collagen content and mucopolysaccharides in diabetic mothers' placentas were found by Liebhardt (1968). We also believe that collagen content is much decreased, as these placentas are remarkably friable. The basement membrane may be thicker in diabetes as compared to normal pregnancies, probably because of a higher degree of nonenzymatic glycosylation (Iioka et al., 1987) or due to an increased amount of the most prominent type of basal lamina collagen, that is, type IV (Laureti et al., 1982; Leushner et al., 1986). Greater contents of DNA, triglycerides, phospholipids, and cholesterol are also characteristic features of the placenta in diabetes (for review see Desoye & Shafrir, 1996).

Winick and Noble (1967) observed that an increase in the number of normal-sized cells caused increased placental size. In the study of 48 placentas from diabetic mothers, Fox (1969) observed some abnor-

malities of villous maturation, as well as "obliterative endarteritis of fetal stem arteries," thickening of trophoblast membrane, and an increase in villous fibrinoid necrosis. He speculated that these changes may result from "an immunologic reaction." Thickening of stem arterial walls was shown by Samaan et al. (1974); they correlated it with the degree of the diabetic metabolic disturbance. Jácomo et al. (1976) described similar vascular changes and attempted to quantitate them. In our experience quantitation is a difficult endeavor, and to evaluate villous vessels without establishing some rigid criteria for measurement produces problematic results. Thus we do not believe that they are "real" changes, and most certainly none is specific for maternal diabetes. If they were real, they could be related only to fetal hypervolemia, perhaps to a higher fetal blood pressure.

Differences of opinion and interpretation, reflected in a voluminous literature on the placenta of diabetic pregnancies, have been reviewed by Teasdale (1981, 1983, 1984), who studied, with carefully controlled quantitative tools, the histomorphometry of placentas of diabetics from classes A, B, and C, classified according to White (1978). Teasdale's principal findings were that the placental exchange membrane (fetal vascular and villous surfaces) increases with maternal diabetes, but that few other significant changes (other than enlargement) could be detected.

Somewhat similar findings of an increased surface membrane for exchange were observed with planimetry by Björk and Persson (1984). These investigators paid particular attention to the taking of samples from similar areas of the placenta, as the villous structure differs so much in the center of a cotyledon from that at its periphery. This normally orderly organization of the cotyledonary structure was found to be somewhat disrupted in diabetic mothers' placentas. Driscoll (1965) found that the weight increase of placentas from class F diabetics was smaller than that from nondiabetics. This difference of class A to C from class F placentas is mostly subject to the influence of maternal renal disease. Driscoll also observed that the decidua is often unusually thick, and with preeclampsia and hypertension the decidual vessels show characteristic arteriolar angiopathy (see also Horký, 1968). Parenthetically, it may be mentioned that the placentas of experimentally induced diabetes in rats share the enlarged size with the human counterpart (Pitkin et al., 1971). In addition, Padmanabhan et al. (1988) found cystic degeneration in the labyrinthine area. They interpreted it to result from glycogen depletion and coalescence of cellular degenerations. Both investigators observed preservation of normal architecture when insulin therapy was instituted. The cystic degenerations occurred even in the placentas of spontaneously diabetic BB-Wistar rats (Brownscheidele & Davis, 1981).

A number of electron-microscopic studies have been undertaken to gain a better understanding of the morphologic alterations of diabetic mothers' placentas. Okudaira et al. (1966) found no specific changes in these placentas. Minor, irregular degenerative changes were recorded, such as mitochondrial and endoplasmic reticulum degeneration in the syncytial cells. Some thickening of the basement membranes was observed, but it was not uniform. Widmaier (1970) added the finding of persistence of a nearly complete Langhans' cytotrophoblastic layer. Jones and Fox (1976) were more emphatic about ultrastructural changes in placentas of diabetics. Although they investigated mainly gestational diabetes, these investigators described patchy syncytial necrosis, dilated rough endoplasmic reticulum, cytotrophoblastic hyperplasia, focal thickening of basement membranes, and narrowing of small vessels. Others had reported dilatation of capillaries to be a prominent finding. Jones and Fox (1976) suggested that the changes they observed may occur only patchily, and that they were similar to those of overt diabetes. Interestingly, at the ultrastructural level in diabetes, glycogen deposits greater than normal were found in the endothelium of placental capillaries in diabetes (Jones & Desoye, 1993). Laurini et al. (1984) reported that, despite strict control of diabetes during pregnancy, ultrastructural changes in the placenta—"blebs," thickened basement membranes, endothelial proliferation, and increased collagen content—continue to persist. Their deduction was that the commonest pathologic feature is "dysmaturity," defined as relative immaturity of the placenta. Kaufmann and Stark (1977) also reported that characteristic placental alterations occur in maternal diabetes. During cesarean section, they obtained biopsies of the placenta for electron microscopy. In these tissues they observed the following characteristic features: 75-Å-thick intratrophoblastic filaments, an abundance of smooth endoplasmic reticulum, and collapsed mitochondria in relatively edematous cells. Thus, there is good evidence that the placenta, in a somewhat variable fashion, undergoes some minor morphologic alterations in response to maternal diabetes. The significance of these findings remains uncertain, especially vis-à-vis their relation to the altered physiologic states experienced by mothers and infants affected by this condition.

Congenital, hereditary **fructose intolerance** during pregnancy was studied by Marks et al. (1989), who also discussed the difficult management of such patients. Two children succumbed neonatally, and the most recent pregnancy was associated with a livebirth and a "calcified placenta."

Maternal Neoplasms

Many maternal neoplasms have complicated pregnancy and some have caused placental disease. Pulitzer et al. (1985) have even reported that, on rare occasion, implantation takes place upon endometrial adenocarcinoma; there was no associated placental development, however. Implantation over leiomyomas caused abruptio placentae in 57% of cases observed by Rice et al. (1989). We have seen placenta accreta in such locations. Carcinoma of the breast and cervix, gastrointestinal neoplasms, and melanoma has occurred during pregnancy, in that order of frequency (Donegan, 1963). Delerive et al. (1989) reported the metastasis of a pulmonary oat cell carcinoma to the placenta. In their review they found that 39% of the 38 cases of placental metastases reported were of melanoma. The tumor of their case lay free in the intervillous space and had not invaded the villi; the neonate was free of disease. Macroscopically, the placenta was entirely normal. In our experience, metastasis to the fetus is rare. Although metastases of several cancers and lymphomas have been found in the placenta, and in leukemias the intervillous space may be filled with leukemic cells, few neoplasms have traversed the placental "barrier" and seeded to the fetus. This is well described in the report by Lentz et al. (1998). In their maternal lymphoma case, the intervillous space was crowded with malignant cells, but the villi were devoid of these cells. Conversely, the fetal circulation was crowded with malignant cells in a fetal proliferative disorder, not the intervillous space. Only Barth et al. (1972) and Pollack et al. (1982) have reported rapidly fatal fetal disease, transferred from maternal lymphoproliferative disorders, assuming that the fetal immune incompetence allowed

proliferation of the cells. Since then a few other reports have shown that maternal tumor cells can travel to the fetus through the placenta. Catlin et al. (1999) reported the transplacental transmission of a natural killer (NK) cell lymphoma. It caused neonatal demise in 2 months and was not "rejected" by the neonate presumably because of similarity of HLA markers. There were tumor cells in the decidua of the placental specimen, and, by special techniques (only), some tumor cells were later shown to exist in villous capillaries. No obvious neoplastic cells were evident in the placental examination. In addition, a metastatic B-cell lymphoma arising in the mother and filling the intervillous space has been described by Maruko et al. (2004). In this case, the neoplasm infiltrated the villi in a major fashion, disseminated into the fetus and eventually caused its neonatal demise.

The most important of these neoplasms is **malignant melanoma**. A melanoma metastasis was described and well illustrated by Holland (1949); Reynolds (1955) also found a placental metastasis of another malignant melanoma. The placenta appeared grossly normal but contained many microscopic amelanotic nodules. The infant remained normal for at least 10 months. George et al. (1960) reviewed 115 cases of melanoma that complicated pregnancy. They found two cases with placental metastases; all of the infants remained normal. The difficulty cells have in traversing the placenta was studied experimentally. Working with experimental melanoma cell lines, Retik et al. (1962) were able to induce widespread maternal metastases, but the placenta and fetuses remained free of tumor. Cavell (1963) identified melanoma metastases in an infant of 2 months. Apparently, the infant had acquired the metastases transplacentally from the mother, but they disappeared spontaneously. The placenta was described as having been scarred and infarcted, but it did not undergo microscopic study. Aronson (1963) observed a muscular swelling that contained melanin pigment in an infant whose mother died from melanoma 4 days after parturition. Those lesions also disappeared spontaneously. Another case of transplacental metastatic melanoma was described by Brodsky et al. (1965). In umbilical cord blood, cells were identified that were consistent with melanoma, and many placental intervillous spaces were filled with melanoma cells. The maternal surface of the placenta appeared brown, with "rare foci of black pigmentation." Both mother and infant died with widespread metastases.

Heite and Kaden (1972) collected 27 cases of metastatic placental cancer, three of which were placental melanoma metastases, of which two metastasized to the fetus. A case of metastatic amelanotic melanoma in the placenta, the ninth reported melanoma of the placenta, was published by Sokol et al. (1976). These authors found that 28 cases of metastatic cancer in the placenta had been reported, five of which had involved the fetus. Their patient had undergone a cesarean section at 31 weeks. She died with widespread tumor 8 days postpartum. The neonate, who died from respiratory disease, had no tumor. Multiple firm nodules, 0.5 cm in diameter, were found in the villous tissue. They were composed of cells that contained melanin and were similar to the maternal tumor cells. The placental villi were focally invaded by the neoplasm.

The placental melanoma metastasis shown in Figure 19.7 was as described in a patient by Freedman and McMahon (1960). Despite villous infiltration with melanophages and some tumor cells, no fetal metastases were found, nor did the infant have melanuria. Widespread placental metastases from a maternal melanoma were found by Stephenson et al. (1971). The infant developed hepatomegaly, but metastatic tumor was never found. Melanoma metastases in the placenta were identified immunohistochemically with the S-100 protein probe by Machin (1987). The infant was growth-restricted but had no evidence of tumor. A maternal melanoma was first diagnosed by placental metastases in the case described by Anderson et al. (1989). The tumor was metastatic to the intervillous space and present in villi; the infant remained normal, but the mother died 6 months after delivery. The authors suggested in their review of 16 cases that a more unfavorable prognosis exists when the maternal age is under 30, when the tumor is present in the lower extremity, and when the neoplastic disease commenced during the 3 years before the affected pregnancy. They asserted that the extent of villous involvement had no influence on prognosis.

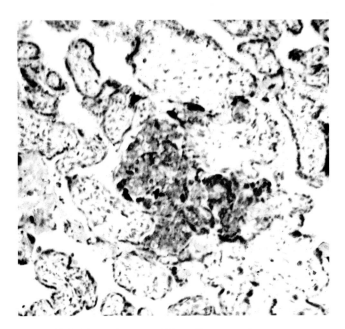

FIGURE 19.7. Term placenta with malignant melanoma metastasis. Pigmented tumor cell invade the villous tissue, and many pigmented Hofbauer cells are present. H&E ×160.

Placental metastases from an ocular choroidal melanoma were described by Marsh and Chu (1996). The only microscopically discovered pigmented tumor cells were found in the intervillous space and had not invaded villi; the neonate was free of tumor. A comprehensive review of melanoma metastatic to the placenta comes from Baergen et al. (1997). Our patient with extensive metastases died soon after delivery, but the fetus remained normal. We summarized the world literature of 19 cases in this report, with five neonatal deaths due to transplacentally acquired melanoma.

Fetal giant pigmented nevi were described by Holaday and Castrow (1968) and later by Demian et al. (1974), and then by Campbell et al. (1987). In the placenta of the first case, multiple foci of pigmented nevus cells were present in the villi. The neoplasm was considered to be benign despite these deposits. In the second case of extensive **fetal** giant nevus, the placenta was grossly unremarkable but was extensively involved microscopically (Fig. 19.8). Because of this large amount of placental tumor, the authors suggested that the cells had arrived there by early neural crest cell migration. The last case may actually have been a malignant melanoma. At autopsy, metastases were found in the fetus. Its skin lesion, a large "nevus," was detected sonographically. By light microscopy, the enlarged but grossly normal placenta was densely infiltrated with neoplastic cells. In contrast to the finding of maternal melanoma, these cells were confined to the villi. They did not invade the intervillous space, nor were they metastatic to the mother.

An example of metastatic **breast carcinoma** is depicted in Figure 19.9. It was confined to the intervillous space. Similar cases have been described by Cross et al. (1951) and Rewell and Whitehouse (1966). Many adenocarcinomas of the breast have metastasized to the placenta, according to the reviews of Freedman and McMahon (1960), McGowan (1964), Lemtis and Hörmann (1969), Potter and Schoeneman (1970), Salamon et al. (1994), and Ackerman and Gilbert-Barness (1997a). The latter authors reviewed all metastatic lesions to the placenta, and Lemtis and Hörmann (1969) drew attention to the absence of vascularization of these intervillous tumor colonies. For that reason, they suggested that these deposits be called "pseudometastases." Many authors have commented on the finding of a grossly normal placenta riddled with metastatic lesions. Therefore, it is recommended that patients suffering from tumors in the past have placental examination when they become pregnant. It appears that those patients with advanced disease and thus a large tumor load are most likely to develop placental metastases. This explains the frequency of metastatic melanoma in placental metastases in spite of the rarity of melanoma in pregnancy women. The following other **solid tumors** have been found in the placenta:

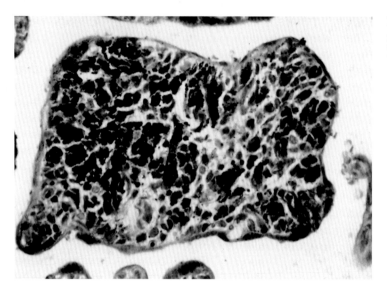

FIGURE 19.8. Widely disseminated **fetal** giant cell nevus cells in placental villi. H&E ×250. (Courtesy of Dr. G. Monif.)

1. Pancreas (Smythe et al., 1976)
2. Lung (Jones, 1969; Read & Platzer, 1981)
3. Ovary (Horner, 1960)
4. Rectum (Rothman et al., 1973)
5. Skin: squamous cell carcinoma (Orr et al., 1982)
6. Medulloblastoma (Pollack et al., 1993)
7. Rhabdomyosarcoma from the orbit (O'Day et al., 1994)

Several of these reviewers referred to single additional cases of rare other tumors that were present in the placenta but that did not metastasize to the fetus. With the exception of melanoma, no documented case of transplacental seeding by a malignant maternal neoplasm has been identified. Hörmann and Lemtis (1965a,b) gathered a number of cases of metastatic tumors. They opined that the placenta has "remarkable defense mechanisms" against passing neoplasms from the mother to the fetus. A report by Sironi et al. (1994) on a placental teratoma represents in our opinion an acardiac amorphous twin and will be discussed in Chapter 25.

In the rare cases where **multiple myeloma** has complicated pregnancy, the placentas were not described. The associated fetuses and infants developed normally, despite maternal chemotherapy with urethane (Kosova & Schwartz, 1966; Rosner et al., 1968). When **Hodgkin's disease** was treated during pregnancy, the infants also developed normally. Of the 35 cases reviewed by

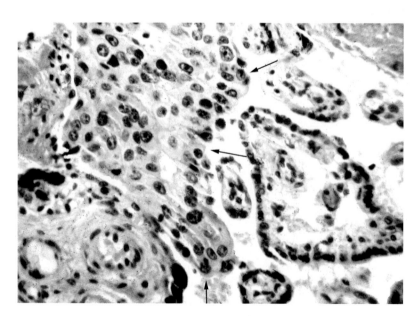

FIGURE 19.9. Adenocarcinoma of the breast, metastatic to the intervillous space (arrow). Note the absence of vascularization of the tumor cells nests. H&E ×160.

Hennessy and Rottino (1963), the placenta was not studied, except in the case of non-Hodgkin's lymphoma described by Tsujimura et al. (1993). The placenta showed numerous yellow, partially necrotic lesions and the tumor had massively invaded the intervillous space; the premature infant succumbed. It is unknown whether the placental substance was invaded and whether the fetus became affected by the tumor. On occasion, though, it has been described that the fetus has acquired the disease transplacentally (Priesel & Winkelbauer, 1926). A pregnancy complicated by a diffuse cavernous **hemangioma of the uterus** was described by Lotgering et al. (1989). They delivered the patient at 35 weeks and found the placenta to separate only with difficulty and with much loss of blood. Possible hemorrhage from placental invasion of the angioma is a possibility in this condition, although placenta accreta is more likely.

Many reports have dealt with the question of transplacental transfer of cells in maternal **leukemia**. At times the intervillous space is filled with leukemic cells (Fig. 19.10), and yet no malignant cells can be identified in the fetal vessels of the placenta. Usually, these cells are not present in blood aspirated from the umbilical cord. Extreme idiopathic maternal leukocytosis occasionally occurs during pregnancy only to disappear after parturition. The intervillous spaces may then be crowded with maternal leukocytes, giving the appearance of leukemia. Care must thus be taken to differentiate this phenomenon from maternal leukemia. Bierman et al. (1956) found 50 reported cases

of maternal leukemia during pregnancy. Not a single infant had been affected with the disease. In their case of acute lymphocytic leukemia, the maternal white blood cell count at birth was 154,000 mm³, but that of the neonate was only 3300 mm³. The placenta had extensive leukemic cell infiltration that was confined to the intervillous space. Similarly, Chrisomalis et al. (1996), who described the unusual event of chronic lymphocytic leukemia in a pregnant young woman, found the intervillous space to be crowded with tumor cells, but a normal infant. Ask-Upmark (1964) followed six children born to leukemic mothers for 9 to 41 years. Leukemia developed in none. Rigby and his colleagues (1964) quinacrine-labeled the buffy coat cells of a mother with acute myelogenous leukemia and reinjected them before birth. They then examined the fetal blood 7 hours after injection, when the infant had delivered. Occasional fluorescing forms were seen. Such findings, however, are not convincing evidence of transplacental transfer of leukemic cells. Diamandopoulos and Hertig (1963) studied the placenta of a leukemic patient and the offspring of 48 pregnancies. They did not find any transfer of cells. These authors estimated that about 400 patients with leukemia complicating pregnancy had been reported. Only a few cases of transplacental transmission seemed possible, but they were not well supported. One such case is that of a mother who was diagnosed as having lymphocytic leukemia postpartum. Her child developed leukemia at age 9 months (Cramblett et al., 1958). The placenta and neonatal studies

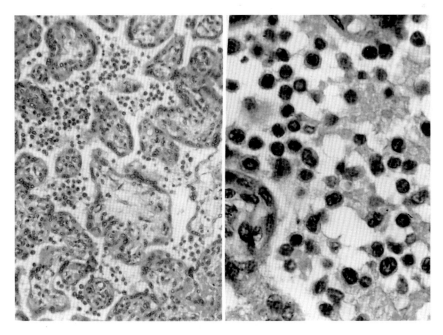

FIGURE 19.10. Placenta at 36 weeks' gestation of patient who died from acute myelogenous leukemia the day after cesarean section. The white blood cell count at delivery was 147.200/mm³.

The child was well at 10 years. Note the large number of leukemic cells in the intervillous space but not within the villi. H&E ×160 (left); ×640 (right).

were not described. Thus, there can be only speculation as to transplacental transfer of leukemic cells in that particular case. Other larger reviews of the literature also have shown no fetal acquisition of the disease, despite the presence of large numbers of leukemia cells in the intervillous space and despite the fact that a variety of maternal leukemia types were studied (Ask-Upmark, 1961; Lee et al., 1962; Johnson, 1972; Nummi et al., 1973). In another case, despite massive intervillous invasion by myeloid leukemia cells, the villi of a partial hydatidiform mole were not invaded (Honoré & Brown, 1990). That some maternal cells do pass the placenta occasionally is discussed in Chapter 17, and by Nelson et al. (1998).

Primary fetal leukemia has been reported only rarely, the Cabot case No. 37-1976 of myelogenous leukemia in a neonate being a good example (Scully et al., 1976). Finally, intrauterine growth restriction and a meconium-stained placenta were found by Ohba et al. (1988) in a patient with adult T-cell leukemia/lymphoma. On the other hand, transient fetal leukemia associated often with fetal hydrops occurs characteristically in some cases of trisomy 21. In one of our cases, the neonate had 940 NRBCs/100 WBCs. The cause of hydrops is so far obscure (see also Zipursky et al., 1997).

Hypertensive Disorders

Preeclampsia

This common disease of pregnancy is now most frequently referred to as pregnancy-induced hypertension (PIH). The terms are interchangeable and it must be stated that not all PIH cases are equivalent to preeclampsia, as is usually assumed. One other reason to be as specific as possible about the terminology is that the disease process may produce symptoms similar to those of circulating lupus anticoagulant, discussed below. Moreover, our veterinary colleagues denote "toxemia" as a different disorder, usually a condition of ruminants. In fact, classic PIH is uncommon in animals. It has there been diagnosed primarily in some catarrhine primates, especially in Patas monkeys (Gille et al., 1977; Palmer et al., 1979), but its effects are seen in other primate species, such as gorilla, chimpanzee, and langurs. Chesley (1985), a master of this disease, is adamant that strict criteria should be used in the definition of this condition. He asserted that many patients with mild preeclampsia later suffer eclampsia. He also emphasized that all of the abnormal clinical findings in the pregnancy-induced disease disappear after gestation and that there are no sequelae to be expected in renal or vascular involvement in the future lives of the patient. This contrasts with the report of Epstein (1964), who found that women with a history of PIH had a significantly higher risk of developing "late hypertension."

An extensive review of prevalent theories to explain the pathogenesis has been published by Beek and Peeters (1998). More recently, Sibai et al. (2005) inclusively reviewed in great detail the theories that have been advanced and are especially helpful in the immunologic considerations.

Two classifications of preeclampsia and hypertensive disorders of pregnancy have been devised. These include a relatively simple definition, primarily based on blood pressure changes and put forth by Redman and Jefferies (1988), and the more complex systematics published by Davey and MacGillivray (1988). Both proposals are aimed at providing a better delineation of the various hypertensive diseases, so that the effect of treatment can be more meaningfully assessed. These classifications may simplify diverse designations of the past and make some order of chaos, but that they are unlikely to be generally useful has been the topic of an editorial (Anonymous, 1989a), and correspondence by Davey and MacGillivray, Roberts, and Lilford (1989). Whether hypertension is primary or due to an impaired removal of placental serotonin production was explored by Gujrati et al. (1996). These investigators found that in preeclampsia and eclampsia monoamine oxidase was reduced in syncytial cytoplasm and translocated into nuclei, thus perhaps inducing a hyperserotonomic state.

Pregnancy-induced hypertension presents clinically as hypertension, edema, and proteinuria. Typically, after the uterus has been emptied of fetus and placenta, the disease ceases. Indeed, Hunter et al. (1961) found that an immediate postpartum curettage of the placental bed causes maternal blood pressures to return to normal much more quickly than when curettage was not done. Inasmuch as PIH occurs in the absence of a fetus (as in hydatidiform moles), it is clearly dependent on the presence of placental tissue. The ultimate pathogenesis of PIH, however, has not yet been fully defined. Easterling and Benedetti (1989) have suggested that the disease is the result of a "hyperdynamic condition in which the characteristic hypertension and proteinuria are mediated by renal hyperperfusion." Numerous other possible etiologic factors exist, and these were analyzed by these authors. Zhou et al. (1997) proposed that the basic defect lies in an inadequate "epithelial-to-endothelial conversion" of the invading trophoblast, which is also emphasized in the review by Burton and Jauniaux (2004). The implanting cellular trophoblast, normally replacing the endothelium of the spiral arterioles was shown to change a number of epithelial markers [platelet endothelial cellular adhesion molecule (PECAM), vascular endothelial (VE)-cadherin, vascular cell adhesion molecule-1 (VCAM-1), several integrins] and assume endothelial characters. Absence of this conversion is thought to be the basis for the disease. Indeed, currently this endothelial disease is in the foreground of considerations that attempt to explain the etiology of PIH. Chaiworapongsa et al. (2004) found a significant increase in vascular endothelial growth factor receptor-1 (VEGFR-1) in the plasma of PIH patients and found that the quantity corresponded to the severity of the disease. Other studies of the intricate relationships between endothelium, vascular growth and circulating cytokines in PIH have come from Levine et al. (2004), who found a decrease in VEGF and increased levels of a tyrosine kinase in PIH; they relate these and suggest a possible causal mechanism for PIH. The role of complement activation in the pathophysiology of preeclampsia is currently under investigation. There are so many factors now isolated that a clear understanding of the ultimate mechanism for PIH still eludes us. We found of interest the demonstration by Taylor et al. (2003) that placental serum growth factors were reduced in PIH, relating it to villous angiogenesis and, secondarily to IUGR of the fetuses, whereas Leach et al. (2002) had postulated that their finding of a fivefold reduction of the epidermal growth factor–like growth factor (heparin-binding (HB)-EGF) expression in placentas of PIH might be the cause of cytotrophoblastic underperformance (deficient arterial remodeling and invasion). Similarly, Graham and McCrae (1996) showed that an altered expression of gelatinase and surface-associated plasminogen activator activity of trophoblastic cells characterizes preeclamptic pregnancies, perhaps being instrumental in altered invasiveness of the cells. The most recent entrant in this confusing array of factor that could have a causal or mediating effect on the development of PIH is "syncytin." This gene derives from a retroviral entry after the separation of platyrrhine primates from the catarrhine primates. It has the postulated ability to fuse cells and lead to the trophoblastic syncytium whose nuclei, as a consequence, have then become unable to divide. Knerr et al. (2002) promptly found markedly reduced gene expression in PIH (see letters by Keith et al., 2002). One may cautiously state that this enthusiasm for involvement of new proteins, genes, or their expression is understandable mostly because a clear-cut understanding of what causes PIH is yet elusive.

ANIMAL MODELS

Because of the frequency of toxemia, and to better understand its pathogenesis, several animal models have been used with the intent to simulate the human disease. This has been a difficult undertaking, and many of these models have primarily addressed the mechanism of abruptio placentae. Haynes (1963) induced abruptio placentae in the rabbit by temporary occlusion of the inferior vena cava. Fibrinoid degeneration and aneurysmal dilatation were produced in the decidual vessels; this simulated human toxemic pathology. An interesting discussion of the paper further elucidated this relationship. Abitbol et al. (1976a) have used the rabbit in a more extensive model study. They constricted the lower aorta; this caused hypertension, proteinuria, and fetal growth restriction. They also demonstrated changes in liver and kidney, similar to those of human PIH. The placenta contained infarcts and other changes resembling PIH, but these were also seen in some animals that did not exhibit toxemic symptoms (Abitbol et al., 1976b).

Two decades before, Howard and Goodson (1953) produced abruptio placentae in dogs when they ligated their lower vena cava in pregnancy. Combs et al. (1993) constricted the aorta in rhesus monkeys and also produced a "syndrome resembling preeclampsia," presumably because of the reduced lower aortic blood pressure. Interestingly, this group of investigators found that in these animals the depth of cytotrophoblastic infiltration into the endomyometrium was markedly enhanced (Zhou et al., 1993). When Hodari (1967) constricted uterine arteries of dogs before their pregnancy occurred, progressive hypertension and proteinuria were produced, which ceased after delivery. Abitbol et al. (1976c) also used strictures (of aortas) before dogs became pregnant; they observed proteinuria, hypertension, and some fluid retention. The placentas of these animals showed diffuse hemorrhagic infarction; in addition, typical renal lesions were induced. Many investigators have attempted to produce PIH and placental abruption in nonhuman primates. Thus, Myers and Fujikura (1968), in the course of studies on the effect of ligation of intercotyledonary vessels in rhesus monkeys, found that ablation of the "accessory lobe" invariably led to fetal death. They found that ligation of intercotyledonary vessels caused placental villi to continue their growth, and to develop increased syncytial knotting, a common feature of PIH. Wallenburg et al. (1973b) identified and ligated from one to four uteroplacental arteries in the floor of rhesus monkey placentas. This was invariably followed by necrosis and typical infarction. The earliest identifiable lesions occurred 23 hours after ligation. The infarction closely resembled that seen in human placentas with PIH. Cavanagh et al. (1974) have long worked to develop a suitable model in baboons, and placed clips about uterine arteries before pregnancy. Primarily renal lesions were thus produced. In later experiments, the investigators obtained hypertension and proteinuria that simulated human PIH (Cavanagh et al., 1977). When they subsequently constricted aortic blood flow in baboons, fetal and placental growth restriction and a reduction of amnionic fluid were induced; the placental morphology was not described (Cavanagh et al., 1985). Abitbol et al. (1977) also induced PIH in rhesus monkeys. They restricted aortic flow only in the last month of gestation. Resultant lesions included diffuse hemorrhagic infarction of the placenta, aside from renal and hepatic lesions. In general, the primate models more closely simulated the disease of PIH of women; certainly the placental infarcts and glomerular lesion were identical. Spiral arterioles in the placental bed, characteristically altered in human PIH, however, have usually not been investigated in these experiments. In the sporadic cases of primate toxemia that we have seen, the atherosis lesions were not fully expressed.

Placental Pathology of Preeclampsia

The principal pathologic changes of the placenta in PIH include (1) decidual arteriolopathy, (2) infarcts and ischemic change in central portions of the placenta, (3) abruptio placentae, (4) "Tenney-Parker changes," and (5) restricted fetal growth. These pathologic features are not all invariably present but they are significantly overrepresented in PIH, whereas chorioamnionitis is decreased in frequency (Moldenhauer et al., 2003). Also, one observes occasional cases with severe placental changes, in which no maternal symptoms relative to PIH have been elicited. Fetal and placental growth restriction, Couvelaire uterus, defibrination, and the nephropathy of "glomerular capillary endotheliosis" are frequently encountered manifestations of PIH and some are perhaps secondary features. Pampus et al. (1999) found that "hemostatic abnormalities" with the risk of thrombosis are much overrepresented in patients with severe PIH, and PIH is much commoner with multiple pregnancy (Sibai et al., 2000). Wynn (1977) concluded correctly that "conventional gross and histologic examinations of the fetal portion of the placenta have not uncovered a pathognomonic lesion of preeclampsia." This statement is particularly pertinent now that the lesions of "lupus anticoagulant" have been found to be identical to those previously ascribed solely to toxemia. Sletnes et al. (1992) studied preeclamptic women and found that 19% had antiphospholipid antibodies, with growth restriction of the offspring a prominent feature. A central question in the understanding of pathologic changes in PIH is whether these placental features allow a clean differentiation of PIH from other states of hypertensive disease. Wynn's review is one of the most critical essays that examines this question. Other reviews may be consulted. For example, that by Muller et al. (1971) is based on their study of 168 cases of PIH. They attempted to make a correlation of the villous changes with the severity of PIH. The studies by Schuhmann and Geier (1972) and Hölzl et al. (1974) also examined the severity of the clinical disease in relation to perfusional and villous alterations. Another review of the placenta in toxemia came from Soma and his colleagues (1982). It gives the following tabular presentation of placental lesions in 53 cases of severe toxemia:

Lesions	%	Controls (%)
Infarcts	54.7	32.8
Intervillous thrombi	20.7	10
Circumvallation	26.4	10
Abruptio	11.3	0
Decidual necrosis	16.9	9.6
Abnormal cord insertion	12.1	4.1
Meconium staining	18.9	12.8

Decidual Arteriopathy

Hertig (1945) was the first investigator to describe the pathologic changes of PIH in the spiral arterioles at the implantation site. Since then, "atherosis" has become one of the hallmarks of the disease, and it is generally believed that the other major placental changes are the result of specifically altered placental bed arterial vessels (Figs. 19.11 and 19.12). Zeek and Assali (1950) found "acute atherosis" in the placental bed of 34 toxemic patients; none was present in 37 other cases, and only three of 143 nontoxemic patients had early atherosis. Eighteen nontoxemic hypertensive patients did not have atherosis. They considered the lesion to be an early change of the spiral arterioles; fibrinoid necrosis and lumen obstruction by thrombosis were considered to be later events. Zeek and Assali believed this lesion to be the primary cause of placental infarcts. They also emphasized that the fetal circulation does not maintain the integrity of the placental villous tissue; rather, this integrity is contingent upon the intervillous blood flow. This is the maternal blood supply, bringing oxygen and nutrients. When the fetal circulation is obliterated, the villi merely shrink. Only much later do they atrophy and degenerate, with typical hyalinization of the stroma. The typical infarcts, however, have a maternal vascular disruption as their cause. Many other investigators have made the same observations, and they have summarized the vast literature of this topic. Here, the systematic studies of Marais (1962, 1963) must be mentioned. He was the first investigator to describe the appearance of spiral arteries in some detail, using the colposcope. Marais determined, by simultaneous injections of maternal and fetal circulations of an intact uterus, the nature of intervillous flow; he reaffirmed the independence of the two circulations. He delineated atherosis, fibrin deposition, and

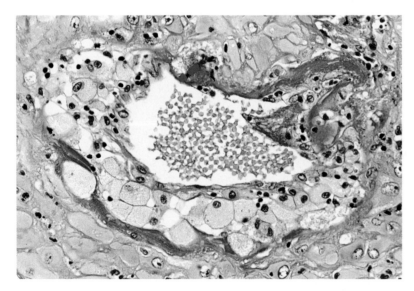

FIGURE 19.11. Atherosis in decidual arteriole of patient with preeclampsia. Note that the vessel wall has been replaced by fibrin, the intima is replaced by cholesterol-laden macrophages, and there is mural thrombosis. H&E ×250.

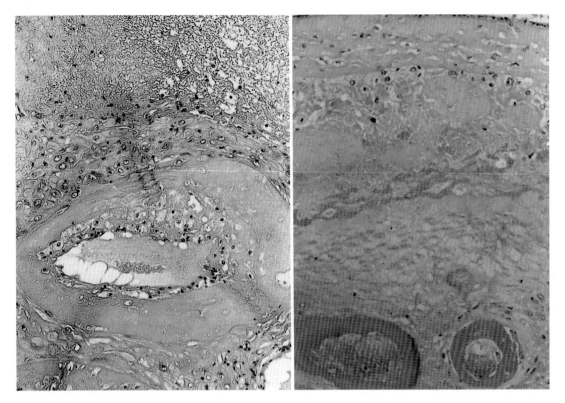

FIGURE 19.12. Hyalinized vessels with thrombosis and old atherosis in decidua capsularis; adjacent decidual necrosis. Pregnancy at 33 weeks (920 g small for age infant), severe pregnancy-induced hypertension (PIH), abruptio. H&E ×60.

arteriosclerosis, and contended that acute thrombosis of placental bed vessels is the principal lesion that ultimately leads to placental ablation. Because he observed obliterative lesions in the absence of hypertension, Marais also concluded that the obliterative changes of these vessels were not caused by the maternal hypertension. Nadji and Sommers (1973) found decidual vascular changes in 14% of induced first-trimester abortuses and suggested that they represent precursors of future PIH lesions. Likewise, Lichtig et al. (1984) described atherosis in the first trimester of pregnancy, whose significance also remains uncertain. Shanklin and Sibai (1989) undertook a systematic electron-microscopic study of maternal vessels in PIH with controls. They found extensive endothelial injury especially in placental site venules, with some fibrin deposition. No relationship to degree of hypertension could be established, and they found no atherosis. They emphasized that the lesions they found were venous endothelial, and not confined to the placental site, let alone the arterioles. Most recently, Schmidt et al. (2005) studied placentas of PIH in 350 patients. Lesions were seen in 21.4% and they were most readily identified in the decidua capsularis of the membrane roll, not the decidua basalis. Nevertheless, 130 of 350 had villous infarcts. When Salafia and her colleagues (1995) examined a variety of histologic factors associated with preterm preeclampsia, they were impressed by the frequency of

inflammatory changes they found, such as vasculitis, chronic villitis, and "hemorrhagic endovasculitis." From this they argued for an immunopathologic, vasculo-occlusive process to occur in PIH. Indeed, inflammation and activation complement may also play a role in the vascular damage and sequelae seen in PIH and antiphospholipid antibody syndrome (Salmon et al., 2001).

The decidual vascular changes are not always easily found, especially in the delivered placenta, or in the decidua capsularis of the rolled membranes. For that reason, Khong and Chambers (1992) proposed an improved method for sampling. They suggested the preparation of en face sections of the maternal floor in order to obtain more cross sections of maternal arterioles. While this makes intuitive sense, we have practiced this methodology for some time and found it not to enhance our ability to diagnose atherosis or other lesions.

Brosens et al. (1967, 1972) and Robertson et al. (1967) have led a major group of investigators who studied the pathogenesis of the decidual vascular lesions in PIH. They documented the normal response to implantation of placental bed vessels, and the alterations that occur in hypertensive pregnancies. The principal tenet of these investigators is that, under physiologic conditions, trophoblast of the placental shell infiltrates the arterial beds of decidua and myometrium, and destroys the walls with fibrinoid changes. This infiltration of the 100 or so arterial mouths of the implantation site ultimately renders these vessels incapable of reacting to mediators by constriction, as they normally would have. In preeclampsia, on the other hand, the invasion of the proximal, myometrial branches is impeded, a feature that was supported with in vitro experiments by Pijnenborg et al. (1996). They found that trophoblast of preeclamptic women's placentas had a reduced in vitro capacity for attachment to fibronectin and vitronectin. De Groot et al. (1996) studied CA 125 and insulin-like growth factor binding protein-1 concentrations in plasma from preeclamptic patients and found them to be reduced when compared to those of normal controls. Whether this failure of the "second wave" of invading cells is an intrinsic trophoblastic failure or is mediated by maternal (decidual) influences, is still unknown. In PIH, trophoblast merely penetrates the decidual vessels, but it fails to alter the myometrial vasculature's constrictive reactivity to mediators. Under "physiologic" conditions, the arteries are changed into "large, tortuous channels by replacement of the normal musculoelastic wall with a mixture of fibrinoid material and fibrous tissue" (Brosens et al., 1967). This is illustrated by Kim et al. (2001), who found abnormal transformation frequently in patients with preterm labor and intact membranes. The interactions of toxemia with or without preexisting hypertension were also detailed and well illustrated by Brosens and his investigators (1967). The changes and interpretations are complex and hypothetical. They must be read in the original text or in the summary review (Brosens et al., 1972). Similar findings were made in subsequent investigations by Gerretsen et al. (1981). De Wolf et al. (1975) made electron-microscopic studies of the decidual vasculature in PIH. Their findings are important as they illustrated the imbibition of plasma constituents, proliferative activity of intimal and muscle cells, and the damage to the vascular endothelium. Labarrere and Faulk (1994) made the important observation that the vascular invasion of trophoblast expresses completely different staining characteristics in preeclamptic vessels when compared to normal vessels and provided thus a means of clearly differentiating these populations of cells. Fatty infiltration was first observed in the endothelial cells; later, macrophages phagocytose fat from degenerating lipid-laden myogenic foam cells; eventually, medial necrosis occurs. Haust et al. (1977) also found that muscle cells accumulate lipid in PIH. Their description, however, is not quite clear. Although they refer to myometrial cells as having accumulated lipid droplets, the electron micrograph suggests this to occur in the muscular wall of the arterioles at the decidual–myometrial interface of the placental bed. The difficulties of differentiating smooth muscle cells from lipid-laden macrophages in atherosclerotic lesions have been further investigated by Schaffner et al. (1980). At present it is not absolutely certain, we believe, that the altered elements in atherosis represent typical muscle cells, rather than macrophages. The conclusion that the lipid-laden cells are mostly, if not totally, composed of macrophages was also reached in the immunologic studies conducted by Klurfeld (1985) on atheromatous plaques. In further studies of the vascular damage of PIH, Khong et al. (1992) observed that the normal endothelial coat of uteroplacental vessels is disrupted in eight of 10 patients with PIH. Pijnenborg et al. (1991) observed vascular changes in 47 hypertensive and 17 normal pregnancies. Various states of hypertensive disease, not only PIH, were a cause of atherosis. It had been suggested that the transformation is mediated by expression of PECAM-1, but a detailed study by Lyall et al. (2001) failed to confirm this. Zhou et al. (1993) showed in rhesus monkeys with aortic ligatures that the depth of cytotrophoblastic invasion was enhanced, perhaps being mediated by blood pressures.

Because there is so much apparent "fibrinoid" deposition at this site (Fig. 19.13), Kitzmiller and Benirschke (1973) undertook fluorescent labeling studies of placental beds from normal patients and from those with PIH. They found a heavy deposition of gamma globulin and complement C3 in the vascular lesions of PIH (Fig. 19.14). Some fibrin could also be demonstrated, but neither Hageman factor nor albumin was found here. Two hypertensive patients without preeclampsia, and a diabetic primigravida also showed negative staining. In subsequent studies of PIH, Kitzmiller et al. (1981) invalidated the possibility that these deposits were the result of an immunologic "rejection" phenomenon. Only 53% of patients with PIH had such lesions, and some non-PIH patients with hypertension or diabetes had indistinguishable vascular changes. Similar investigations published by Weir (1981) also showed very variable deposits and a predominance of fibrin and C3, but no immunoglobulins. Parenthetically, it may be mentioned here that skin biopsies in patients with PIH have shown deposits of immune complexes (Houwert de Jong et al., 1982). The review by Wells and Bulmer (1984) should be consulted for additional considerations of the possible immunologic delineation of atherosis. Also, Branch et al. (1989) have shown that patients with severe, early-onset toxemia have circulating antibodies to phospholipids. They drew analogies to the lupus anticoagulant syndrome (vide infra), further enhancing the notion that this common disorder has an immune-mediated background. Parenthetically it might be pointed out that the term **lupus anticoagulant** is a misnomer, as the majority of patients with systemic lupus erythematosus (SLE) lack this antibody (Ackerman et al., 1999) and coagulation is more commonly an issue.

Although the decidual blood vessels in PIH are often accompanied by a sparse number of lymphoid cells, plasma cells are conspicuously absent (Fig. 19.15). Bradeguez et al. (1991) studied the T-lymphocyte population in 62 primigravidae. They found a significant decrease

FIGURE 19.13. Acute atherosis, fibrinoid degeneration, early mural thrombosis of decidual vessel in PIH. H&E ×160.

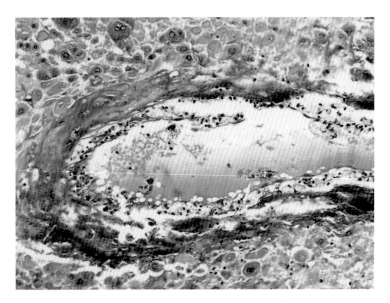

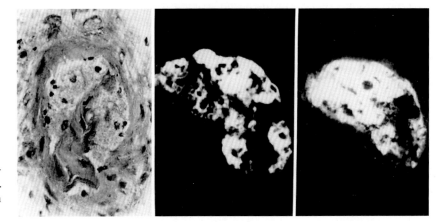

FIGURE 19.14. Atherosis and mural thrombosis in decidual vessel of patient with PIH. (*Source:* Kitzmiller & Benirschke, 1973, with permission.) H&E ×800.

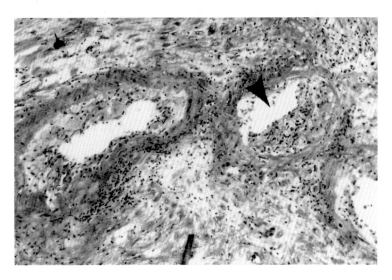

FIGURE 19.15. Decidual vessels in PIH with lymphocyte and macrophage infiltration, atherosis, and old mural thrombosis (arrowhead). Globulin and complement were localized in these vessels. H&E ×250.

in T-helper cells in the second trimester of those women who later developed PIH. This decrease occurred long before clinical symptoms became evident and disappeared 6 to 10 weeks postpartum. Other immune response studies are cited by these authors. Absence of a significant lymphocyte population from the decidua of PIH patients was the finding in the ultrastructural study of Shanklin and Sibai (1989). On occasion, we have observed a granulomatous reaction at this site (Fig. 19.16). This is exceptional and may be explained on the basis of a possible immune vasculitis, and not related to PIH. The occasional presence of lymphoid cells at the implantation site and many other features of PIH, have repeatedly suggested an immunologic basis for this disease. Gusdon et al. (1977), therefore, studied the percentage distribution of T and B cells in normal and toxemic patients. They found no significant differences between the two populations. With the recent greater interest in genetic factors of disease, many studies of antigen expression and reactions thereto have been undertaken and were reviewed by Roberts and Cooper (2001) without resolution. Esplin et al. (2001) found that "both men and women who were the product of a pregnancy complicated by preeclampsia were significantly more likely than control men and women to have a child who was the product of a pregnancy complicated by preeclampsia." O'Shaughnessy and colleagues (2000) found concordance of PIH expression among monozygotic twins. One can also argue that the

known much greater risk of first pregnancy to develop PIH has an immunologic reason and it is thus of interest that women who had never been exposed to the sperm antigens and conceived with IVF had a much increased risk for PIH (Wang et al., 2002). Chaiworapongsa et al. (2002) suggested from the increase of CD45RO+ lymphocytes and decrease of CD45RA+ cells that patients with PIH had an earlier antigenic exposure of unknown nature. Ariel et al. (2001) used microarrays to survey 588 genes in pregnant women and found that 79 were expressed in toxemic women but not in normal patients. Moses et al. (2002) find a locus on chromosome 2 that perhaps exposes to PIH susceptibility. Recurrence of PIH in second gestations was lower with the same paternity and smoking, but higher with longer intervals, diabetes, and other variables (Mostello et al., 2002).

Many studies of the vascular lesions in the placenta of patients with PIH have been made of the decidua capsularis that accompanies the membranes (Fig. 19.12), rather than on the decidua basalis. The latter is often markedly altered and, at times, it is necrotic and thus less useful for investigation. These findings of often-significant atherosis in the decidua capsularis brings into question whence their perfusion derives. In our view this is not the decidua vera of the opposite site from implantation, and therefore the great variability of positive findings may find an explanation. Placental bed biopsies have been examined to great advantage. The results from a three-center study,

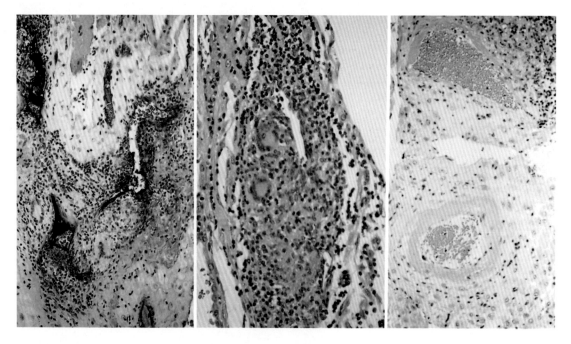

FIGURE 19.16. Granulomatous reaction around decidual vessels in 21-year-old patient with eclampsia following severe preeclampsia at 31 weeks' gestation. Anti–factor VIII stains (left) show the association with vessels. In the center several multi-nucleated giant cells are present; at right are typical toxemia changes. (Anti-VIII, and H&E ×160, ×240. (Courtesy of Dr. R. V. O'Toole, Columbus, Ohio.)

and extending over 30 years, have been published by Robertson et al. (1986). They emphasized that such biopsies, usually taken at cesarean section, should include the myometrium. They gave precise details as to how the biopsy should be obtained and processed in order for it to be useful. Even in their experienced hands, decidual bed biopsies were acceptable for interpretation in only 70%. These investigators found the decidua vera to be the most useful tissue for the observation of atherosis and, remarkably, they consider the membrane-associated decidua to be decidua vera. This group of investigators pays special attention to the lack of physiologic vascular changes in the myometrial vessels, and to the occurrence of vascular thickening ("spasm") in PIH (Fig. 19.17). Similar changes have been reported in otherwise unexplained fetal growth restriction. When considering all these reports, it must be remembered that the findings made in patients with lupus anticoagulant (vide infra) may explain some of the still inexplicable results of the past. In these studies, they have not yet been considered as possibly confounding the results. Robson et al. (2002) took placental bed biopsies successfully transcervically before terminations and from cesarean section placental beds without ill effects. They also summarized the previous results of such efforts, illustrated in color with the normal vessels, but they did not address the altered arterioles.

Khong et al. (1987) attempted a statistical analysis from the study of decidual vessels in 39 patients with PIH. They were unable to relate the lesions to parity, degree of proteinuria, severity and duration of hypertension, or its therapy, and found an incidence of 46% atherosis in PIH. This is similar to that of other workers cited. Stillbirths, SGA infants, and fetal distress occurred slightly more often in pregnancies whose placentas had atherosis.

These results differ from the findings of some other studies, wherein there was a more appreciable increase of pregnancy complications (McFayden et al., 1986). Khong et al. (1987) reaffirmed their conviction that hypertension was not the cause of atherosis and suggested that inappropriate immune reactions may be causative. They also found that the presence of atherosis did not affect fetal outcome. The final pathogenesis of this lesion, however, remains unresolved.

Labarrere (1987) also found macrophage and T-cell infiltration, as well as deposits of immunoglobulins and complement around the spiral arterioles of PIH decidual beds. His observations challenge some of the assertions made by Robertson et al. (1986). They mainly indicate that the pathogenesis of atherosis, as well as that of PIH, is still unresolved. Gerretsen et al. (1983) observed, in placental bed biopsies, that the physiologic change of spiral arteries was present in 95% of normal pregnancies, but occurred in only 19% of those that were complicated by PIH or fetal growth restriction. They observed, nevertheless, that the trophoblastic syncytial giant cell infiltration of the uterine wall in PIH, occurring adjacent to the uterine vessels, was of normal magnitude. The findings of Gerretsen et al. (1983) reaffirmed that pregnancy alterations of the uterine vascular walls are not due to ingrowth of trophoblast from the outside. Rather, this physiologic change of vessels is accomplished by upstream growth of cells that originate at the mouths of these vessels. The histochemical studies performed by these investigators confirmed that the cells in the vascular walls are not of the syncytial type but that they represent extravillous trophoblast or X cells. We have seen a patient who died from eclampsia and who had typical lesions of atherosis and thrombosis in the central portion of the myometrium under the placental bed. This indicated to us that, on

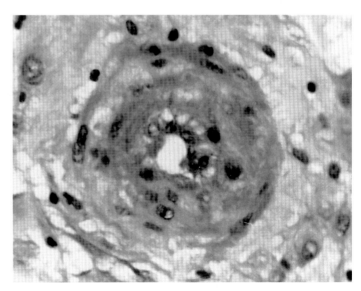

FIGURE 19.17. Myometrial vessel of case in Figure 19.12 showing the thickened artery, presumably exhibiting "spasm,", as suggested by Robertson et al. (1986). H&E ×220.

occasion, the second wave infiltration of X cells takes place in patients who develop preeclampsia. As mentioned earlier, atherosis, infarcts, and IUGR all can take place long before clinical manifestations allow the diagnosis of preeclampsia.

Infarcts

Placental infarcts are the commonest and most conspicuous lesions observed by the pathologist. They represent necrotic villous tissue. There is no longer any doubt that the tissue has died because of deficient intervillous (maternal) circulation. Infarcts are firm, condensed dead areas of villous tissue that often encompass the entire thickness of the placenta (Fig. 19.18). More frequently, however, they involve mainly the base of the placenta and are particularly common at the placental edge. Here, they signify that the placental edge is "plastic." That is to say, placental edges often atrophy in later gestation, with the histologic picture of infarction ensuing (Fig. 19.19). Thus the underlying etiology of these peripheral lesions is fundamentally different from that of central lesions, which represent true infarction. When infarcts are found in the central portions of the placenta, and particularly when they are randomly thus distributed, PIH or the condition of circulating lupus anticoagulant with anticardiolipins are almost invariably present. This is particularly true when infarcts are found in the first and second trimesters, at which time they are otherwise extremely uncommon. The earlier in pregnancy they appear, the more likely the lupus anticoagulant syndrome is to be expected. Placental infarcts differ grossly from intervillous thrombi. They have a granular surface and are much firmer. Intervillous thrombi, in contrast, are either fresh red clots and shiny, or they are laminated and light tan-gray. Their periphery

commonly has some infarction of villous tissue. These disturbances of placental perfusion can now be evaluated by echoplanar imaging (Francis et al., 1998).

Placental infarcts are initially dark red. They can be distinguished from living tissue by their firmness and by their lack of a spongy texture (Fig. 19.20). As they age, infarcts lose their fetal hemoglobin and become yellow, and then tan-gray. Unlike infarcts of other organs (kidney, spleen), they are never invaded by "organizing" fibrous tissue; in their subsequent evolution, they only become atrophic. Hemosiderin is sometimes found in early infarcts. The color changes ("red and white infarcts") have been especially studied by Bartholomew and his colleagues (1961), who advocated a special method of examining the placenta for the presence of infarcts. They suggested that the entire organ be fixed in formalin and later serially sliced. The value of this method is supported by the studies of Steigrad (1952), in his evaluation of 716 unselected placentas. He suggested a complex division of infarcts, grading them from types A to H, and attempted a correlation with PIH, especially with its nephropathy. Shanklin (1959), who studied 767 unselected placentas, found no relationship of "white or red" infarcts to toxemia. This is very inconsistent with the experience of other authors. He was correct, however, when he emphasized the occurrence of increased trophoblastic knotting ("senescence," as he called it) in PIH, the "Tenney-Parker change." Javert and Reiss (1952) studied "red infarcts" (intervillous thrombi); they found them most frequently in erythroblastosis, but in toxemia, their 49% incidence was substantially increased over the average of 17.6%. These investigators pleaded that the designation "intervillous thrombus" is a misnomer. Because of the frequent (48.7%) contamination with NRBCs, they wished to draw attention to the admixture of maternal and fetal cellular

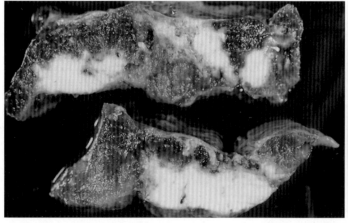
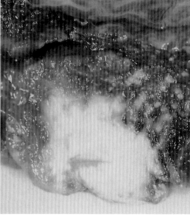

FIGURE 19.18. Macroscopic aspects of "white" infarcts, scattered throughout the placental tissue and amounting to 40% in this patient with PIH. Note that most infarcts involve primarily the placental floor.

FIGURE 19.19. Macroscopic and histologic aspects of old marginal infarct that is not related to preeclampsia. H&E ×10.

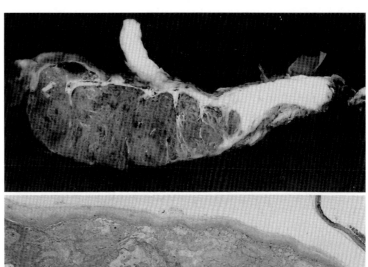

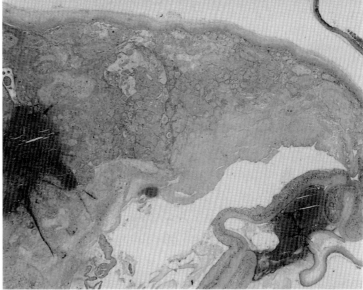

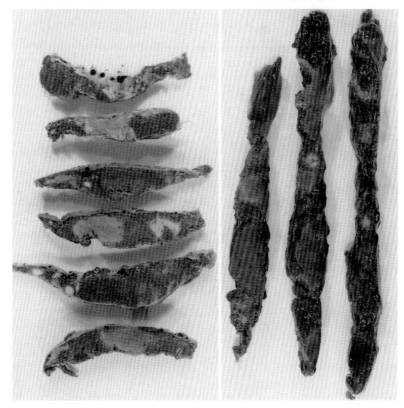

FIGURE 19.20. Macroscopic aspect of multiple infarcts in placenta of patient with severe PIH and stillborn fetus. Varying ages of infarcts are shown as dark red (fresh), dark gray (intermediate), and white (old). Patient eventually had abruptio placentae.

components (further discussed in Chapter 17). Fox (1963) asserted that the term "white infarct" should be abolished because it is often confused with laminated fibrin/clot accumulation. He found a percentage of subchorionic fibrin plaques (15%), perivillous fibrin (28%), true infarcts (22%), central intervillous thrombus (12%), and basal intervillous thrombus (6%) in a series of 200 normal pregnancies. Huber et al. (1961) also found that intervillous thrombi result from a disturbance of decidual vein perfusion, but suggested that they represent different lesions from true infarcts. Bartholomew differed with this view in the discussion of this paper. Marais (1962c) illustrated the lesions in excellent color photographs and succinctly described their pathogenesis. Carter et al. (1963a) presented excellent photomicrographs and affirmed the villous dependence on maternal oxygen supply via the intervillous circulation. In a subsequent contribution (1963b), the same authors presented a complex classification of infarcts and described a novel entity, the "divergent villous lesion." We believe that there is no need to make such complex distinctions, as they do not aid in prediction or understanding of infarcts, nor do they aid in diagnosis of maternal disease. The "divergent" lesion described is simply an expanding intervillous thrombus with adjacent villous infarction. Torpin and Swain (1966) interpreted laminated subchorial intervillous thrombi as "infarcts" and thereby confused the nomenclature even more. Stark and Kaufmann (1974) have studied the early changes of placental infarction and examined them with fine structural methods and enzymatic analysis. They found that an early process in the genesis of infarcts is the development of "plasma polyp" formation from the syncytium and beautifully demonstrated this by scanning electron microscopy.

Several investigators have attempted to relate the presence of infarcts to preeclampsia. Thus, Budliger (1964)

reviewed the older literature and made a planimetric and histologic study of 95 formalin-fixed placentas. Hemorrhagic and white infarcts were significantly more common and they were larger in PIH than in controls. Intervillous thrombi were not more common but, when present, they were also larger. This author deduced from his findings that a minimum of 190 g of placental tissue is needed for fetal survival. Wentworth (1967) examined 679 consecutive placentas with a large section technique, after prolonged formalin fixation. Of these, 77 came from patients with mild PIH and 12 from those with severe PIH. He found the following: red infarcts, 1.3%; old, true infarcts, 6.2%. There was a significant increase of infarcts (67%) in the severely toxemic patients, whereas the mildly toxemic patients had only a 11.7% incidence of infarction. Some of the villi adjacent to infarcts showed also impressive chorangiosis (Figs. 19.21 and 19.22; see Chapter 24). In fact, the massive congestion seen in these early lesions is a necrobiotic change and it often results in villous hemorrhage before complete infarction takes place. Wallenburg (1969) also found a significant increase of infarcts with toxemia and noted that the infarcts are commonly found centrally in the placenta. He also noted a significant correlation with low Apgar scores and low birth weight. In a later contribution, this group of investigators concluded that an infarct represents the death of a fetal cotyledon due to the occlusion of a single decidual blood vessel (Wallenburg et al., 1973a) (Fig. 19.23). Brosens and Renaer (1972) found in their placental bed biopsy study of the spiral arterioles underlying infarcts that the lesions lacked normal trophoblastic invasion (and thus the physiologic reaction of myometrial vessels), and had occlusive thrombosis.

The most ambitious study of the relationship of infarcts to perinatal outcome comes from Richard Naeye (1977). He evaluated 31,494 placentas from the prospective Col-

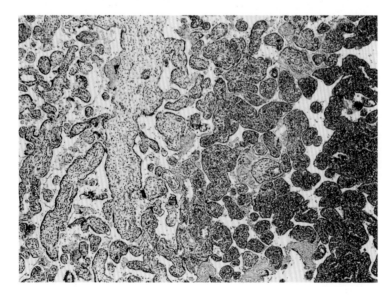

FIGURE 19.21. Very fresh infarct (right) with marked congestion and villous hemorrhages at 27 weeks' gestation in patient with PIH and abruptio two days earlier. H&E ×60.

FIGURE 19.22. A patient with PIH and fetal growth restriction. Intermediate aged infarct (left) and older infarct (right) are shown. H&E ×260.

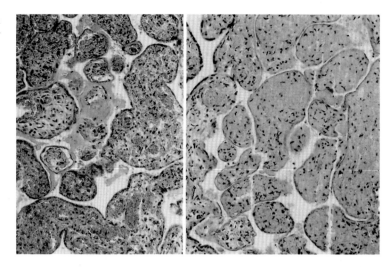

laborative Study and endeavored to separate infarction from abruptio placentae, and then to determine their influence on fetal outcome. He deduced that placental infarction caused 2.26/1000 perinatal deaths. "Fatal infarcts were strongly associated with diastolic pressures over 90 mm Hg in the gravida," and this was augmented when accompanied by proteinuria. Moreover, fatal infarcts were five times commoner in abruptio placentae, and they were also more common in older and overweight gravidas. He believed that infarcts often serve as a nidus for the inception of abruptio. It may also be mentioned here that infarcts and abruptios are not infrequent in patients with sicklemia.

Abruptio Placentae

Abruptio placentae, the detachment of the placenta from its decidual seat, has had many different names. Holmes (1908) called it ablatio placentae; it has also been referred to as accidental hemorrhage, premature separation of the normally situated placenta, and perhaps other names. Gruenwald et al. (1968) suggested that the terms **abruptio** and **premature separation** should not be used interchangeably. He proposed that the former be used only for the cases recognized before birth, and the latter be reserved for the pathologically diagnosed cases. Overlaps occur, which Gruenwald and colleagues acknowledged, and we consider the terms to be identical. It is commonly assumed that this complication of pregnancy represents a sudden and very painful event. In total abruptio, or when a very large retroplacental hematoma suddenly forms, there may indeed be pain due to sudden stretching of the uterine peritoneal covering. More often, abruptio is partial and painless. These cases would be classified as "premature separation," according to Gruenwald et al. (1968). Notelvitz et al. (1979) described three cases of "painless abruptio placentae," characterized by vaginal bleeding and accompanied by backache and a nontender uterus. Because ultrasonographic recognition of this placental separation prevented fetal mortality in their cases, the authors advocated this for diagnostic evaluation.

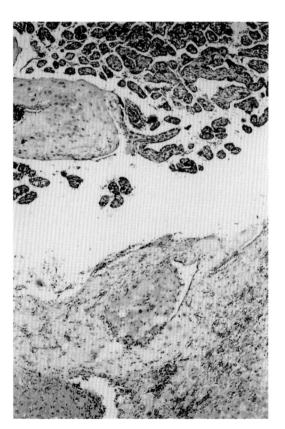

FIGURE 19.23. Same patient as in Figure 19.22. The decidual vessel is nearly completely occluded by an old thrombus. H&E ×60.

There are many causes of abruptio, such as trauma from accidents or amniocentesis, abnormal uterine structure, separation at the edge in partial placenta previa and, prominently, preeclampsia. In an occasional placenta, one may also recognize the abnormal shape of a bicornuate or otherwise irregular uterus by the configuration of the abrupted placenta (Fig. 19.24). Kramer et al. (1997) enumerated the many factors that are correlated with or can cause abruptio placentae. They suggested that about 1% of pregnancies are complicated by detachment of the placenta. An unusual cause, congenital hypofibrinogenemia, with recurrent abruptio placentae was described by Ness et al. (1983). In our experience, when one half or more of the placenta detaches suddenly, the fetus dies. Lemtis (1967) has referred to similar estimates. He made reference to the very rare case of fetal survival with as much as five-sixths abruption. Lemtis places much reliance on the irregular nature of placental perfusion for survival of the fetus. Delivery should be accomplished rapidly in cases of recognized abruptio. If placental detachment takes place over a long period of time, in stages and with infarcts ensuing, then the fetus may survive but will suffer from deficient transplacental oxygen and nutrient supply. It has been shown that trophoblast releases a factor that inhibits platelet aggregation (O'Brien et al., 1987) and it has been postulated that this factor is needed for normal placental blood flow. When it is decreased, abruptio may take place. Toivonen et al. (2004) found that the low-activity haplotype C-A (His113-His139) of the microsomal epoxide hydrolase gene was less frequent in women with abruptio.

The frequency of abruptio placentae in unselected series of pregnancies is estimated to be between 0.17% and 0.96% (Waddington, 1957; Halberstadt et al., 1969). Such figures reflect the obstetrician's ability to make the clinical diagnosis; they are not based on recognition by placental examination. It must be admitted at the outset, however, that the pathologist cannot recognize reliably the presence of a very acute abruptio placentae; thus, the overall incidence is underestimated by anatomic review. The diagnosis of a very recent abruption can only be made clinically. The pathologist relies on alterations in placental structure, and on color changes of the retroplacental blood clot. These take time to develop. When we studied 7038 consecutive placentas past the 20th week of pregnancy, 3.75% of them were found to have features of some degree of abruptio placentae (Benirschke & Gille, 1977). Niswander and Gordon (1972) found evidence of abruption in 2.12% among the prospectively collected cases of the Collaborative Study. They were usually described as "retroplacental hematomas." Because not all abruptios bleed externally (the "concealed hemorrhage") or produce the classical signs of a painful, rigid abdomen, the clinical diagnosis is bound to be made less frequently. Our series encountered trauma of various kinds only rarely, whereas preeclampsia and eclampsia were present in 13%; nevertheless, clinically uncomplicated pregnancies predominated (Fig. 19.25). Trauma and, recently, allegedly cocaine abuse are thought to be frequent causes of abruptio. They are covered in other chapters of this book. With regard to trauma, we here relate findings of an important case. The patient had been in a car accident. Her newborn delivered at 37 weeks, had an Apgar score

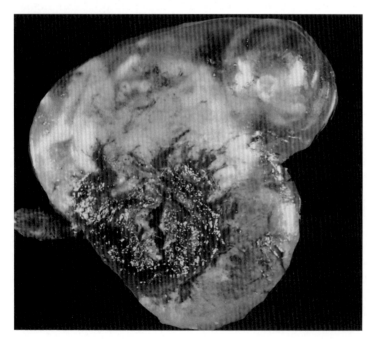

FIGURE 19.24. Delivery of baby "en caul," with abruptio of a growth-restricted placenta. The bicornuate nature of the uterus is reflected in the abnormally shaped membranes.

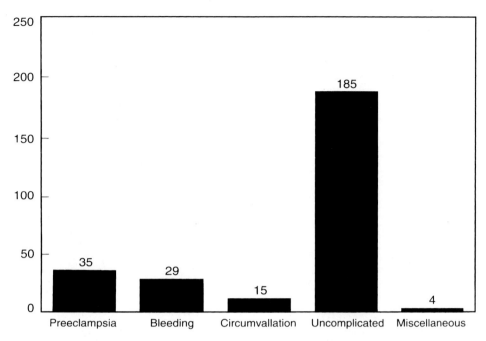

FIGURE 19.25. Causes of abruptio placentae, pathologically identified.

of 0/1 and a hematocrit of 17%, and required transfusion. The maternal Kleihauer test was negative. A fresh, large retroplacental hematoma contained 60% fetal cells. Higgins and Garite (1984) impressively demonstrated that late abruptio is an important sequel of trauma in pregnancy. It may even occur after deployment of airbags (Schultze et al., 1998). Abdella et al. (1984) found that abruptio was most common with eclampsia (23%), chronic hypertension (10%), and preeclampsia (2.3%). Clinical "abruptio" is also mimicked by active peripheral bleeding that ultimately leads to circumvallation, by marginal hemorrhage associated with severe ascending infection, and by the unusual entity of "marginal sinus thrombosis" (Fig. 19.26). The mechanism of marginal sinus thrombosis was explored and well depicted by Bartholomew (1961). He believed this to be the outstanding cause of first trimester bleeding, but it was also frequent in later pregnancy. In marginal abruptions, Harris et al. (1985) felt that the site of bleeding was venous in nature. In other cases, though, it is undoubtedly related to decidual necrosis and inflammation (Fig. 19.27). Elliott et al. (1998) went so far as to create a new syndrome: chronic abruption–oligohydramnios sequence (CAOS). They found a high frequency of prematurity and premature rupture of membranes, but were unable to explain the etiology of the new entity.

That abruptio is not diagnostic of preeclampsia, as was earlier contended, has been emphasized by many investigators (Tatum, 1953; Dyer & McCaughey, 1959; Hibbard

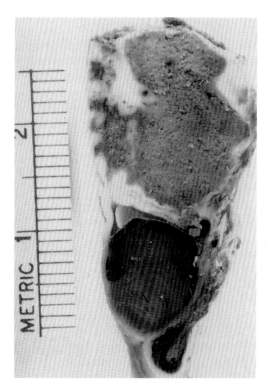

FIGURE 19.26. "Marginal sinus thrombosis," actually a marginal abruption with layered blood clot in an immature placenta.

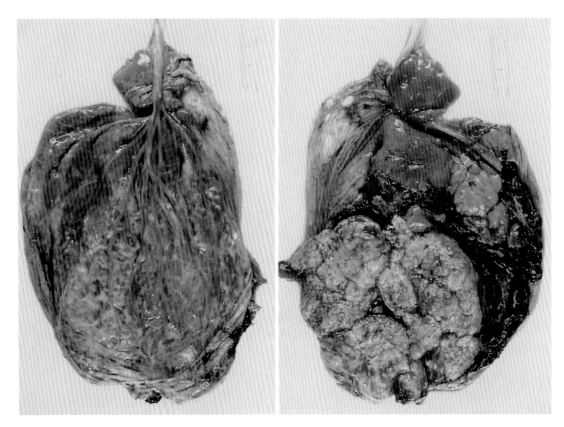

FIGURE 19.27. Immature placenta with velamentous insertion of the cord and long-standing abruption beneath the cord insertion. Clot is of different ages and has brown, yellow, and red color; there is associated chorioamnionitis.

& Hibbard, 1963). Tatum (1953) discussed the wide spectrum of associated pain and symptoms, whereas Dyer and McCaughey (1959) were more concerned with the appropriate therapy. Hibbard and Hibbard (1963) also denied the overwhelming frequency of toxemia as the etiology of abruptio placentae; they considered folic acid deficiency and grand multiparity to be important etiologic factors. Morgan and his colleagues (1994) found that neonatal outcome of infants with abruptio due to toxemia is not better than that from other causes, a long disputed point.

The placenta in classic abruptio placentae has fresh clot attached at the maternal surface. The villous tissue may be compressed and, because of the frequent association with toxemia, infarcts are often additionally found. Placental abruptios are most prominent beneath a gradually developing infarct and frequently they are associated with well-formed infarcts in other portions of the placenta (Fig. 19.28). The clot may be firm, if the ablation is older. It may be dry, and become brown after many hours. Eventually, the clot retracts and has the appearance of fibrinous strands. Initially, there is a depression with the clot, but this disappears as the overlying placenta infarcts and then atrophies. In very old and small abruptions, only minor color changes and infarcts will be

seen at the maternal aspect of the placenta. When toxemia is the cause of abruptio, the hemorrhage presumably begins with the decidual vascular lesions described above. Thrombosis of the decidual arterioles may lead to decidual necrosis and to subsequent venous hemorrhage (see also Harris et al., 1985). Although rough estimates can be made about how long the retroplacental clot has existed, exact figures cannot be given, despite frequent legal questions. Boe (1959) illustrated the rupture of a spiral arteriole with thrombosis, as the cause of a case of abruptio. The patient was not described as being preeclamptic, and several smaller decidual hemorrhages were found. When Hill and Brunton (1968) performed arteriography in pregnant patients, their results suggested that future abruptios could be anticipated because of poor vascular perfusion. It is now agreed that abruptio placentae occurs with increasing frequency in patients with chronic hypertension. Whether the ablation is due to hypertension or from a putative release of vasoactive agents after abruption has been discussed by several investigators. Abdella et al. (1984) favor the hypertension as causing the hemorrhage, a point that we also espouse. It is further supported by the relatively common findings of abruptios attending pregnancies that are complicated by pheochromocytomas.

FIGURE 19.28. Abruptio placentae with layered retroplacental clots and several infarcts (yellow to white) in preeclampsia. With this much acute abruption, the fetus dies.

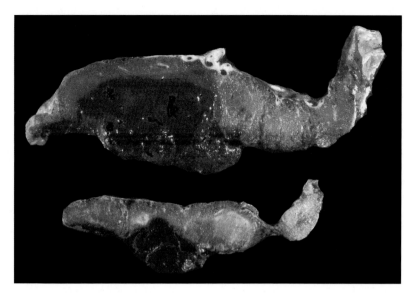

Because abruptio poses a major threat to fetal and maternal survival, therapeutic regimens have been carefully considered. Sholl (1987) suggested that treatment should be given according to the gestational age at which the abruptio occurs. Preterm abruptions, which often are associated with poor obstetric history and with maternal smoking, may respond to tocolysis; but this is a complex clinical problem, not easily discussed fully in this context. Sholl found that his overall fetal mortality was 17%. He advised the use of ultrasonography. Cardwell (1987) also made the diagnosis by ultrasound examination in eight patients, and found significant fetal–maternal hemorrhage with the abruptio. One fetus lost 72 mL into the maternal circulation. Coen et al. (1974) described the remarkable survival of a 1630-g premature infant delivered after 75 minutes of complete abruption. They believed that the attending hypothermia may have aided this infant. Equally remarkable is the patient described by Lopez-Zeno et al. (1990). In their case, the fatal injury to the mother occurred 47 minutes before cesarean delivery, and the infant was born 22 minutes after maternal cardiac arrest had occurred. Follow-up at 18 months revealed no neurologic deficit, although focal central nervous system (CNS) infarction was seen by computed tomography (CT) scan at 5 weeks. Neonatal shock, from anemia or hypoxia, is often the life-threatening problem for the fetus (Haupt, 1963). Waddington (1957) found 254 abruptios of normally implanted placentas among 26,358 deliveries (1:104). There was a maternal death and an 83.5% fetal survival when aggressive management was used, but only a 72.7% fetal survival with passive management. Waddington observed three cases of Couvelaire uterus (enlarged uterus with massive interstitial hemorrhage) and one coagulation defect, in this group of patients. In a prospective study, Naeye et al. (1977) found an incidence of 3.96 per 1000 perinatal deaths due to abruptio. They identified a high usage of cigarettes in the mothers and poor maternal weight gains during pregnancy. Fetuses often suffered growth restriction. Important maternal complications are defibrination (Wisot, 1969) and renal necrosis from disseminated intravascular coagulation (DIC) (Sanerkin & Evans, 1965; Carter, 1967). Impressive deposits of fibrin may be found in the renal vessels as well as in other organs of such patients (Schmorl, 1893; Schneider, 1951). Endotoxin shock is often observed. This has led to considerations that toxemia of pregnancy results from a generalized Shwartzman reaction (McKay et al., 1959). Vassalli et al. (1963) observed deposits of fibrin and some gamma globulin in the glomeruli of patients with preeclampsia. The clinical relevance of this was discussed by Dunlop et al. (1978), who found no coagulation problems in patients with essential hypertension.

Kåregård and Gennser (1986) reported an 0.44% incidence of abruptio in a large Swedish cohort, with a 20.2% fetal mortality. Of interest in this study is that a history of abruptio increased the risk for a subsequent abruptio 10.2-fold. Male conceptuses and twins were overrepresented in abruptios. In discussion of this paper, Grossman and Goldberg (1987) suggested that recurrence rate may relate to high anti-H-Y antibodies, which they found in a patient with three abruptios. On a rare occasion, abruptio with defibrination may occur long after fetal death has occurred (Schneider, 1953). One type of abruptio that has been referred to in the obstetric literature is that associated with marked prematurity and chorioamnionitis (Vintzileos et al., 1987). We believe that this is misdiagnosed as "abruptio" because of the presence of a clot accompanying the placenta. When the placenta is carefully examined one finds that the hemorrhage and clot came from the inflamed decidua capsularis, rather than from a retroplacental location. Thus, the appellation abruptio is inappropriate.

Fetal Effects of Abruptio Placentae

Older studies have suggested that maternal eclampsia may result in vascular damage of their fetuses (König, 1956). This author demonstrated hyalinization and coagulation of small cerebral vessels in such an infant. In a study of 34 cases of placenta previa and 64 cases of abruptio placentae, Robbins et al. (1967) found a high incidence of late cerebral abnormalities of the infants at 1 year of age. Haile (1940) described an infant with "eclamptic liver necrosis" and referred to the few other reports in the literature of similar injuries. The kidneys were normal, and it is doubtful to us that a similar coagulation disorder existed in the fetus as that observed in maternal DIC. It is not uncommon for neonates, dying from many different disorders, to suffer DIC, as was shown by Bleyl and Büsing (1969) and other authors. There are many sporadic reports, however, of thrombocytopenia and other hematologic disorders in neonates of mothers with preeclampsia (Mirro & Brown, 1982; Schmidt et al., 1986). Severe defibrination (unmeasurable levels) following abruptio was reported by Edson et al. (1968). The relationship of fetal coagulation events in preeclampsia was studied more systematically by Weiner and Keller (1986). They found lowered antithrombin III activity and higher fibrinopeptide A concentrations in preeclamptic women; paired samples from fetuses showed normal values. Lau et al. (1964) found abruptio primarily with toxemia, and reported a 68% fetal mortality and 35 maternal mortality in their 100 cases studied.

Other Placental Changes in Preeclampsia

Aside from the liability of infarcts, abruptio, and the frequent decidual vascular alterations, the placenta of toxemia of pregnancy undergoes some additional and mostly minor structural changes. More often than not, the placenta is smaller and "drier" than expected for that gestational age. When sectioned, the toxemic patient's placenta is much darker than normal organs, reflecting the hemoconcentration of the fetus. Siegel (1962), who unsuccessfully attempted to correlate preeclamptic retinal changes with the degree of toxemia, depicted most of the classic degenerative changes in the placenta. Teasdale (1985) performed histomorphometric studies of the placentas in patients with severe preeclampsia and with moderate fetal growth restriction. He measured a variety of structural features and found only minor quantitative differences from normal controls. Schumann and Lehmann (1973) correlated maternal urinary estriol excretion, DHA-conversion and placental morphology,

with fetal outcome. They found a lack of any such predictability for fetal outcome and suggested that the outcome is primarily dependent on clinical management. Considerably lighter placentas and fetuses were found in hypertensive patients in a study of Cibils (1974). He made teased villous preparations and observed them with a stereomicroscope. There was considerably increased budding of the syncytium in these placentas, representative of the Tenney-Parker change discussed.

Prominence of syncytial buds has been observed ever since Schmorl (1893) first drew attention to these cells in the pulmonary vessels of patients who died from eclampsia. Earlier, these cells had been interpreted as necrotic, embolized liver cells, but this was not borne out by Schmorl's detailed studies. Syncytial embolism to the lung is now accepted to be a normal feature of all pregnancies (Bardawil & Toy, 1959; Attwood & Park, 1961). Because these cells have no reproductive potential, they die in situ, after first losing their cytoplasm. Remarkably, there is neither fibrin deposition nor an inflammatory reaction. Perhaps all this happens because of the normal apoptosis that is proceeding in these cells. Trophoblastic apoptosis in PIH has now been the topic of several incisive studies. Thus, Huppertz and Kingdom (2004) accepted it as a normal feature of trophoblast turnover and suggested that "during preeclampsia there seems to be an altered balance between proliferation and apoptosis of villous trophoblast leading to a dysregulation of the release from the syncytiotrophoblast." They called it "aponecrotic shedding." Other studies by Crocker et al. (2003) and Ishihara et al. (2002) made similar incisive observations in toxemia and growth restriction, whereas the results by Battistelli et al. (2004) are less convincing that apoptosis is a significant ingredient of IUGR. Many et al. (2000) related this phenomenon to oxidative stress (see also DiFederico et al., 1999). Jauniaux et al. (2003) examined Doppler flow in abnormal placentation and found restricted flow with oxidative damage in "shallow" implantations and placental damage as a result.

In toxemia, and particularly in eclampsia, there is enhanced embolization of syncytial cells and it is likely that the much increased level of fetal DNA in the maternal circulation (Cotter et al., 2004) is its result although these authors, cautiously, interpreted the finding to increased fetal transplacental cell traffic. Occasional authors have even suggested that excessive pulmonary embolization with syncytial buds may be a cause of maternal death (Marcuse, 1954; Roffman & Simons, 1969). The association of these giant cells in these cases with fibrin thrombi is impressive but does not prove that they have been the cause of DIC in the patients. Jäämeri et al. (1965) found a markedly increased number of circulating syncytial cells in the blood of toxemic patients when compared to that in normal pregnant women. Iklé (1961, 1964) provided a methodology for the isolation of these cells from the blood and estimated that approximately 100,000 such cells are liberated daily in pregnancy. More recent quantitative studies are discussed elsewhere. Wagner (1967) and Wagner et al. (1964) felt that release of these cells was uncommon, unless the uterus was "manipulated," and showed an impressive degree of embolization during curettage for hydatidiform mole. Tedeschi and Tedeschi (1963) showed experimentally that these cells were swiftly disposed of in the lung. These cells have been studied with flow cytometry, and their DNA content displayed, and the suggestion has been made that they might serve as means for prenatal cytogenetic diagnosis (Covone et al., 1984). Rushton (1984) rightly pointed out, however, that the syncytium has no reproductive potential and is, at present at least, incapable of serving this cytogenetic purpose. It could serve for polymerase chain reaction (PCR) and fluorescent in situ hybridization (FISH), but the cells rarely traverse the lung to become accessible in peripheral blood. Cameron and Park (1965) showed embolized decidua in the lung at necropsy of two pregnant women. Cockell et al. (1997) showed that in preeclamptic patients deported trophoblastic microvilli impair the maternal vascular relaxation response to acetylcholine, which suggests an altered endothelial response in the omental vessels obtained during cesarean section.

Tenney and Parker (1940) had emphasized that the increased budding of placental syncytium is very characteristic of preeclampsia. It is so significant and common in PIH that we now call this finding the "Tenney-Parker change." It features bunching of syncytial cytoplasm and agglomeration of nuclei. This produces characteristic "knots" at the villous surface (Fig. 19.29). Although some

such knots are normally found in preterm and term placentas, their number is much increased in toxemia. In addition, these knots are often larger and contain more nuclei than those found in the term placenta. Often, this change has been referred to as "premature aging" of the villous tissue, incorrectly we believe, as there is only the microscopic appearance, not real aging. Stallmach et al. (2001) examined "defective placental maturation" with respect to late fetal mortality in archival material and suggested it to be the cause of hypoxia. The knots may result initially from the loss of villous fluid, and secondary buckling of the covering trophoblast follows; apoptosis has also been demonstrated. There are also changes of the amount of cytotrophoblast proliferation with subsequent proliferation of syncytium, as discussed earlier. The mechanism of this villous change was studied in vitro by Tominaga and Page (1966). They perfused human placental tissue and observed the response to varying oxygen concentrations of the perfusate. Hypoxia led to vasodilatation of fetal capillaries, and high O_2-saturation produced fetal capillary vasoconstriction. In long-term organ culture, the reduction of oxygen saturation from 26% to 6% led to the bunching of syncytial nuclei and thinning of the villous trophoblastic covering. This change was found to be reversible when oxygen was increased again. Others have not been able to repeat the reversibility aspect of these experiments (Ong & Burton, 1991). There are light-microscopic similarities between the maternal vascular disease of preeclampsia and that of circulating lupus anticoagulant. It must be emphasized that these changes of toxemia are also present in very immature placentas in which, ordinarily, little syncytial budding would be seen. In our experience, when more than 30%

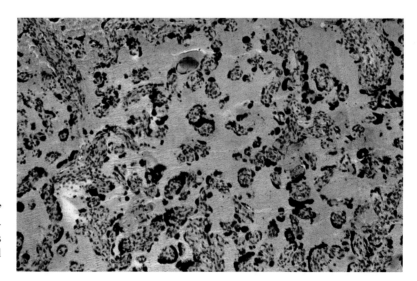

FIGURE 19.29. Excessive syncytial "knotting" (budding, sprouting) in 30-week-gestation preeclamptic patient. Almost every tertiary villus has a densely clumped agglomeration of syncytial nuclei, possessing little cytoplasm. H&E ×160.

of tertiary villi possess syncytial buds, especially in the premature placenta, this is diagnostic of a perfusional compromise. Such features may be associated with abruptio placentae (Fig. 19.30), and can also be seen in the vicinity of fresh infarcts (Fig. 19.31). Alvarez and his colleagues (1967, 1969, 1970) related knotting to an altered maternal arterial pressure and further supported the notion that this is a diagnostic feature of toxemia; they also quantitated the budding by use of phase contrast microscopy. Aladjem (1967b) made similar observations, but they suggested that this syncytial change is not caused by cell degeneration. There is also no occlusion of fetal vessels. The sprouting is considered to be an adaptive change to altered maternal blood flow or oxygen content of intervillous blood. Aladjem differentiated between "buds" and "sprouts," and called this phenomenon "sprouting." Fox (1970) kept villi in organ culture for 10 days; he found markedly increased tritiated thymidine incorporation into cytotrophoblast when the organ culture was hypoxic. This suggested to him that the response represents repair of damaged syncytium. A later study by Howard et al. (1987) showed that cotyledons, perfused in vitro, responded to hypoxia with acute vasoconstriction, rather than the earlier suggested dilatation. This accords well with findings by Doppler velocimetry, in which maternal and umbilical arterial blood flows were found to be reduced in hypertensive patients who ultimately delivered growth-restricted infants (Giles et al., 1985; Ducey et al., 1987; Hanretti et al., 1988; and critique by Pearce & McParland, 1988). Indeed, evidence has been obtained now that an abnormal umbilical artery waveform strongly predicts bad neonatal outcome in preeclamptic patients (Yoon et al., 1994). Such clinical studies have led to new insight and a more reliable categorization of risk in hypertensive pregnancies. Rauramo and Forss (1988) have used Doppler velocimetry to show that exercise in toxemia and in pregnancy diabetes may have significant deleterious effect on uterine blood flow. Lin et al. (1995), likewise, have shown by Doppler velocimetry abnormal uterine artery flow velocity in toxemia, and related this to abnormal trophoblast invasion into the spiral arterioles. When Matijevic et al. (1995) studied flow in spiral arterioles in early pregnancy, they found that remodeling is finished at 17 weeks of pregnancy. And, because nitric oxide (NO) regulates placental blood flow, Myatt et al. (1997) studied the expression of endothelial NO in placentas of growth-restricted pregnancies and preeclampsia. They found "significantly more basal distribution of endothelial nitric oxide synthase (eNOS) in syncytiotrophoblast . . . [while] it was intense in the endothelium of. . . . IUGR and preeclampsia." They interpreted this as an adaptive response to increased resistance and poor perfusion. Ghabour et al. (1995) had made similar observations in their earlier studies, and Pascoal et al. (1998) investigated the pharma-

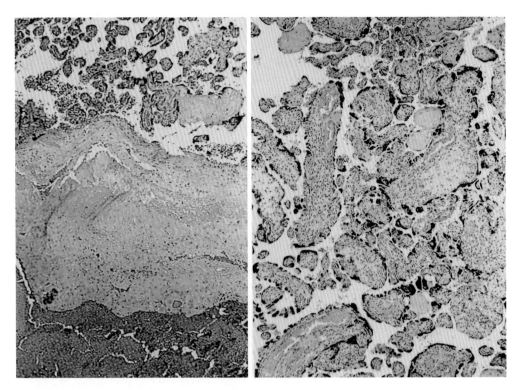

FIGURE 19.30. Placenta of 30 weeks' gestation with preeclampsia and abruptio placentae (left). Typical "Tenney-Parker" change is present in the prematurely "aged" villi. H&E ×16 (left); ×100 (right).

FIGURE 19.31. Very fresh placental infarct, perhaps 1 day old. Intervillous space is obliterated, many villi lack circulation, and a preexisting syncytial knotting (Tenney-Parker change) is present. Patient had toxemia of pregnancy. H&E ×16.

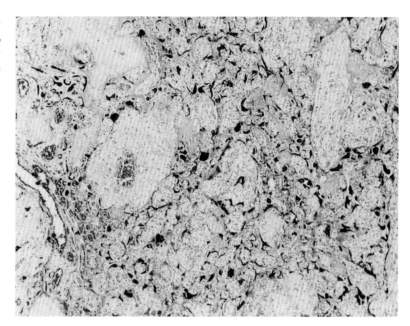

cologic response of omental vessels in this condition. A large review by Granger et al. (2002) links the placental ischemia to microvascular dysfunction and incriminates various cytokines and endothelial factors to PIH.

Maternal fibronectin levels are elevated in preeclampsia, but Anunciado et al. (1987) showed, with fluorescent antibodies, that the villous vascular fibronectin content is decreased. By the use of histochemical techniques, Wielenga and Willighagen (1966) demonstrated that toxemic placentas have characteristic losses of enzymes; this was apparent in areas that required histochemical methods for detection of tissue ischemia. In severe toxemia, the disease process was manifested by increased placental lactate production (Ginsburg & Jeacock, 1967). Further, there are profound microangiopathic alterations of maternal erythrocytes (Cunningham et al., 1985).

Several electron-microscopic studies have compared villi of normal placentas with those from preeclamptic patients. No characteristic findings were made in the PIH study reported by Zacks and Blazar (1963). Anderson and McKay (1966) found an increase in cytotrophoblast, thickening of villous basement membranes, and an increase in "bulbous syncytial microvilli." They suggested that only quantitative changes occur, but none that characterize the diseased organ. When MacLennan et al. (1972) kept villous tissue in culture for prolonged periods, degenerative changes occurred in the syncytium. The appearance resembled hypoxic alterations seen in preeclampsia. To avoid secondary artifacts, Pavelka et al. (1979) took biopsies of preeclampsia patients' placentas at cesarean section. They observed a loss of architecture, fibrin deposition, reduction in microvilli, and dilatation of endoplasmic reticulum and of the Golgi apparatus of the syncytium. Their photographs provided superior detail.

Similar results were obtained by Jones and Fox (1980); like most authors, they came to the conclusion that the lesions are all explicable on the basis of reduced perfusion by maternal blood.

ETIOLOGY OF TOXEMIA, PREGNANCY-INDUCED HYPERTENSION, OR PREECLAMPSIA

Preeclampsia is a common complication of pregnancy (7% to 10% of primigravidae) that is characterized by elevated blood pressure, edema, and proteinuria. Although characteristically all three components are present, they are variably expressed. The clinical manifestations may come about slowly or, occasionally, explosively. If untreated, preeclampsia (also known as pregnancy-induced hypertension, PIH) may result in eclampsia, that is, convulsions. The disease is infinitely more common in first pregnancy, in very young gravidas, and in multiple pregnancy as indicated earlier. The fetus is commonly growth-restricted because of fairly characteristic placental alterations that result from a disturbed interaction of trophoblast with maternal uterine blood vessels. Placental delivery nearly always terminates the illness abruptly. Preeclampsia has many serious complications, such as placental infarction, abruptio placentae, and fetal demise. Because of cerebral hemorrhage or DIC, preeclampsia can lead to maternal demise. PIH can also become associated with the HELLP syndrome (Fagan, 1994) and it has also become a compartment of the so-called syndrome X, hypertension with hyperinsulinemia (Roberts, 1994; Duda, 1996; Martinez et al., 1996; Himmelmann et al., 1997). An important and inclusive review comes from Sibai et al. (2005).

The principal cause of preeclampsia is still unknown, although inroads are being made by the employment of modern molecular tools (Duda, 1996). Heterogeneous causes as the etiology of PIH (such as preexisting maternal conditions, reduced placental perfusion) have been suggested by Ness and Roberts (1996) and were subsequently discussed in letters to the editor. Although it is certain that the disease relates to the presence of placental tissue, the proximate cause is still obscure. The fact, however, that the delivery of the placenta (or hydatidiform mole) ends the disease process speaks for this causal relationship, and many theories have been advanced to explain the mechanism that leads to the symptomatology and pathologic features of toxemia. We will briefly describe only the most recent hypotheses and give references to the general literature. General reviews of etiology and pathogenesis are those by Cunningham and Lindheimer (1992) and Duda (1996).

Lueck et al. (1983) proposed that preeclampsia was the result of an infection by a worm-like "agent." They identified these structures from the peripheral blood of toxemic patients. In a later paper (Aladjem et al., 1983), the authors believed they have shown that they induced a toxemia-like syndrome in dogs, by injecting these animals with blood from toxemic patients. These observations caused much subsequent work and provoked intense discussion. Several investigators then found that males have similar structures in the serum (Gau et al., 1983). The structures are now considered to be artifacts of the preparative procedures (Long et al., 1984; Ayala et al., 1986). They do not represent the cause of preeclampsia.

The possibility that toxemia of pregnancy represents an immune-mediated disorder has long been an attractive consideration. As was previously discussed in this chapter, immune complexes have been localized in the spiral arterioles of the placental bed and in the renal glomeruli of patients with preeclampsia. Moreover, the lesions of lupus anticoagulant, a condition with identifiable "irregular" antibodies, are often indistinguishable from those of toxemia of pregnancy. Hulka and Brinton (1963) suggested that circulating fluorescein-conjugated antibodies localize on trophoblast and signify an immunologic conflict. That subsequent pregnancies of patients with toxemia in their first gestation are usually not affected, was overlooked. Sophian (1964) appropriately criticized this simplistic explanation. Much conflicting evidence of the alleged immunopathologic etiology has since been gathered in efforts to clarify this situation. Kitzmiller et al. (1973), Balasch et al. (1981), and Rote and Caudle (1983) all found no elevation of complement titers in toxemic pregnancies. This was countered by studies of Vasquez-Escobosa et al. (1982) and Massobrio et al. (1985), who found significant levels of various immunoglobulins and also of immune complexes in patients with severe toxemia. Alanen et al. (1984), on the other hand, found only a slight increase in circulating immune complexes in patients with severe preeclampsia. Perhaps the tests are not sensitive enough, or they are too dissimilar for the consistent demonstration of an immune reaction. At present, they do not offer much support for the idea that toxemia has an immunologic origin.

Two large reviews in 1976 weighed the evidence for and against an immunologic disorder. Although Scott and Beer found some relationship to a disturbance in the blocking antibodies that, normally, are believed to protect against placental rejection, their conclusion was that there is no major immunologic etiology to explain toxemia. Reid (1998) provided some additional considerations for a better understanding of the nonrejection of the placenta. Simultaneously, he seeks an explanation for how the maternal–fetal balance is disturbed that enhances the occurrence of some unusual infections to occur in pregnancy. Scott and Jenkins (1976) elicited evidence for a genetic predisposition; they concluded that the disease probably has a "multifactorial" etiology. Some support for a genetic predisposition also came from the findings of Redman et al. (1978), who found that toxemia occurred more often in women who had only one HLA-B antigen locus. Perhaps homozygosity at the HLA locus enhances the possibility of developing the disease. Against a simple genetic etiology is the finding of occasional discordance in monozygotic twins and other observations recorded by Thornton and Sampson (1990). Thornton and Onwude (1991) suggested from their retrospective survey of putatively monozygotic twins that the frequent discordance of PIH speaks against a simple genetic disorder. Totally unexplored was the HLA status of the respective husbands and other aspects one would want to know if an immunologic model as the basis for PIH were to be scrutinized. It has been shown, however, that the level of HLA-G expression in placental tissue is reduced in patients with preeclampsia, apparently related to the quantity of trophoblast (Colbern et al., 1994). Now some evidence has been generated that there is an alteration of the messenger RNA (mRNA) splice forms in PIH (Emmer et al., 2004) that affects the remodeling of spiral arterioles.

Blaschitz et al. (2001) and Le Bouteiller et al. (2003) have also investigated the variable expression of HLA-G by extravillous trophoblast. This topic is now under very active investigation and it is too early to say whether this altered HLA antigen mechanism is the principal reason for placental nonrejection. Future findings from more detailed studies of paternal and fetal HLA antigens and maternal response should provide more definitive answers as to this possible mechanism that may be altered in PIH. Scott and Jenkins (1976) and Willems (1977) postulated a relationship to an inadequate production of blocking antibodies in PIH and suggested a possible immunization procedure for the prevention of preeclampsia. Circulating antigen-antibody complexes were sought in toxemic patients by Knox et al. (1978), but none was found. McLaughlin et al. (1979), on the other hand, did find circulating complexes in toxemic women and offered suggestions for a resolution of the discrepancies that exist in the literature. We have been interested to find that in dichorionic twin placentas or those of higher multiples, the severity of the alterations (infarcts, Tenney Parker change) often differs in their placental portions. Perhaps this relates to some differences in antigen presentation by dizygotic twins; others have been less impressed with such differences. There is no doubt, however, that twin- and higher multiple pregnancies are much more frequently complicated by (a somewhat abnormal) form of preeclampsia. Hardardottir et al. (1996) reviewed this topic and summarized the experience published earlier of incidences from 6% to 46%. Also discussed was the probably erroneous notion that the explanation for this increase simply lies in the presentation of more placental mass. An altered immunologic maternal response is also suggested by the studies of Robillard et al. (1994). An increased exposure to multiple sperm before first pregnancy, they suggested, so alters the immunologic response to trophoblastic invasion into spiral arterioles (that usually exists) that PIH is avoided. The topic is further explored in an editorial by Clark (1994) and is an attractive way of interpreting the complex disease process that was earlier mentioned from the study by Wang et al. (2002).

Much attention was then directed toward the study of the great variety of cellular components at the placental/uterine interface. Scott et al. (1978) reviewed that evidence. They found many articles to support the notion that a disturbed lymphocyte function exists in toxemia. Specifically, it was suggested that patients who exhibit the disease have a high degree of immunologic compatibility with their fetus. Thus, Hoff and Bixler (1984), from ABO-antigen studies of a large cohort, deduced that "the greater the potential for an immune response of the mother to the ABO and HY antigens, the lower is the likelihood of preeclampsia developing in the first pregnancy. . . ." The extensive reviews by Daunter (1992) and MacLean et al. (1992) should be read for greater details to explain the unusual immunologic phenomenon of placentation. Slukvin et al. (1998) discussed in some detail the confusing elements of the various classes of major histocompatibility complex (MHC) antigens, especially HLA-G and their recognition by the mother. Birkeland and Kristofferson (1979) observed that, in toxemia, there is a marked hyporesponsiveness of maternal lymphocytes to phytohemagglutinin (PHA) stimulation. Subsequently, similar findings by Griffin and Wilson (1979) favored the interpretation that this alteration in lymphocyte behavior "may be a consequence rather than the cause of their clinical disease." It should be noted, however, that Musci et al. (1988) found in the serum of preeclamptic patients an increased amount of mitogen. They postulated that this is the result of release from damaged endothelium occurring in this disease. Although Sridama et al. (1983) found a significant decrease in circulating T cells with preeclampsia, there was no good correlation of the severity of the disease with the number of T cells. Moreover, the ratio of helper to suppressor cells was undisturbed. Toder et al. (1983) found the NK cell activity to be increased with toxemia, and that these cells had been preactivated. The question of a change in lymphocyte populations was addressed by Gusdon et al. (1984), with monoclonal antibodies against specific subpopulations of cells. They found that the OKM1 population was normally significantly reduced in the third trimester, but not in preeclamptic patients.

These cells mediate NK cell activity and antibody-dependent cellular cytotoxicity. Khong (1987) investigated the in situ population of cells that infiltrates the placental attachment site. He was unable to identify any quantitative or qualitative difference between the populations in normal vs. preeclamptic patients and suggested that the large population of macrophages may downregulate a maternal immunologic response. Many other contradictory investigations could be cited that only serve to emphasize that the simple notion of toxemia as an immunologic disorder may be erroneous. Kilpatrick (1987) effectively summarized some of these arguments. It should also be noted that evidence shows that the "labor-related stress significantly decreases the total number of neonatal T-lymphocytes and the CD4 (helper) T-cell subpopulation in cord blood" (Pittard et al., 1989). Finally, it has been suggested that placental isoferritin, known to be located in the syncytiotrophoblast, acts as an immune mediator in pregnancy. Maymon et al. (1989) found that, in preeclampsia, placental isoferritin concentration in serum was low (7.5 U/mL), as compared to 81.6 U/mL in normal pregnancy, and 54.8 U/mL in term delivery. They suggested this as a useful marker for toxemia.

More attention is now being paid to the possibility that preeclampsia may be the result of reduced prostacyclin production or at least that an imbalance of prostaglandin secretion exists. Moreover, as Brosens et al. (1974) pointed out, the response of uterine vessels to vasoactive agents may be significantly different in toxemia, because the "second wave" of trophoblast invasion fails to alter myometrial vessels and thereby leaves them responsive to constrictive agents. Specifically, lowered prostacyclin production by the placenta and enhanced thromboxane A_2 production, have been delineated in numerous detailed studies. Prostacyclin binding and its half-life are reduced in pregnancy. O'Brien et al. (1988) have shown that this decrease is variable, perhaps accounting for some of the conflicting results obtained in the past. There is a significant decrease of prostacyclin in hypertensive pregnancy, which may explain some of the clinical findings in this disease. These aspects have been reviewed, and Ylikorkala and Mäkilä (1985) and Mäkilä et al. (1986) discussed their clinical implications. In a more recent review of the remodeling of spiral arterioles, especially in the endometrial/myometrial junction zone, Brosens et al. (2002) suggested that the normal decidual alteration of the spiral arterioles (endothelial edema, separation of the musculoelastic layer–complex cytokine-regulated changes) is disrupted and leads to "a cascade of events resulting in failed deep implantation."

Demers and Gabbe (1976) found that placentas from preeclamptic women have significantly less prostaglandin E (PGE), and vasoconstrictive PGF is much increased. A marked reduction of prostacyclin production was found in growth-restricted neonates whose mothers had suffered hypertension and preeclampsia (Stuart et al., 1981). Importantly, this reduction was not confined to patients with toxemia. A review of prostaglandins in pregnancy (Anonymous, 1982) brought all findings together and suggested that experimental prostacyclin infusion in preeclampsia may have a beneficial effect. In this review it was suggested that "if normal pregnancy, like normal processes in general, is under the fine control of enzyme systems, abnormal pregnancy, like many other disease states, may reflect the relatively uncontrolled activity of free radicals." Hollister et al. (1988), on the other hand, found that prostacyclin infusion into pregnant sheep did not increase placental vasodilation. Mäkilä et al. (1984) showed that the deficiency of prostacyclin (PGI_2) in preeclampsia is specific for the disease and that it is not the result of the mode of delivery or anesthesia. Erskine et al. (1985) found evidence to suggest that altered ratios of certain plasma phospholipids may be a useful predictor for the likely development of preeclampsia. In a detailed study of prostacyclin production by placenta, amnion, and chorion, Walsh et al. (1985) showed a marked reduction of the toxemic placenta to produce this enzyme; amnion and chorion did not show this alteration. Jeremy et al. (1986) confirmed this study and offered comments. The deficiency of prostacyclin in toxemia correlates well with its known platelet aggregation effect and hypertension.

Prostacyclin has the effect of preventing both of these. Walsh (1985) had suggested that preeclampsia represents an imbalance of prostacyclin ($\downarrow$) and thromboxane A_2 ($\uparrow$) production. He supported this with experimental findings. The recognition of these complex interactions has led to successful preventive therapy by Beaufils et al. (1985). Early in pregnancy, they gave antiplatelet medication (150 mg aspirin and 300 mg dipyridamole daily) to mothers who were at high risk for toxemia. They suggested that this treatment prevented toxemia and fetal growth restriction. More extensive studies have borne this out, selectively suppressing maternal platelet thromboxane B_2 (or A_2) production (Benigni et al., 1989; Schiff et al., 1989; Uzan et al., 1991). It has also been found that low-dose aspirin inhibits the production of thromboxane from placental surface arteries, whereas the production of prostacyclin is not disturbed (Thorp et al., 1988). Friedman (1988) provided a comprehensive review of all these aspects concerning mediators and their relationship to PIH. Rosenfeld (1988) added to this review; he pointed out that, during pregnancy, angiotension is vasoconstrictive rather than vasodilatory. The primary derangement of these enzymatic changes remains unknown. The interactions of endothelial cell prostanoid release with leukotrienes and complement are probably important (Lundberg et al., 1986; Pober, 1988; Fitzgerald et al., 1990). These topics are most actively being investigated in an attempt to unravel the mysteries of this common disease.

Other theories concerning the etiology of PIH are too numerous to mention. The idea of excessive salt intake as a cause of toxemia was reviewed by Robinson (1958), and Chalmers (1988) has commented about this. The conclusion is that, although salt regulation in pregnancy has not been accorded needed attention, its causal role for PIH is not secure. Bartholomew et al. (1957) opined that the toxemic aspects of the disease were due to necrosis of placental tissue. This is most unlikely, because many patients with severe toxemia may have few or even no placental infarcts at the time of their first symptoms, and the death of one twins' placenta does not induce the disease. Redman and his colleagues (1999) believe that the endothelial damage and pathologic changes result from a more generalized inflammatory reaction that involves the clotting system and they summarize studies that support this notion. Importantly, they opined that the abnormal placentation is secondary to these disturbances.

Lupus Erythematosus and Lupus Anticoagulant

Lupus Erythematosus

Systemic lupus erythematosus (SLE) occurs primarily in young women and it occasionally complicates pregnancy. It has been speculated that this autoimmune disorder is so much more common in women than in men (10:1) because of their sensitization to nuclear antigens to which they are exposed during menstruation (Dameshek, 1958; Grimes et al., 1985; Hulka, 1985). Estrogens exacerbate the disease, because they have a "potent influence on the immune system and therefore an effect on disease processes" (Hayslett & Reece, 1985). These authors reviewed reports of the influence of pregnancy on the course of SLE and found that, in 25% to 50% of patients with SLE, the disease exacerbates or relapses with pregnancy. In addition, their review indicates that fetal survival is reduced because of an increased number of abortions, maternal renal insufficiency, and placental pregnancy complications. They suggested treatment regimens for women with SLE and pregnancy. It is now believed that pregnancy itself does not constitute a risk to patients with SLE. Low-dose aspirin therapy is being used but is not very effective (Editorial, 1991). Mund et al. (1963) found a 30% abortion rate when SLE began after conception, as opposed to a 14% rate when the disease was already established. A 66% fetal loss in SLE was reported by Schenker et al. (1972), who asserted that toxemia and renal disease were the most common complications.

Systemic lupus erythematosus (LE) is accompanied by a variety of circulating antibodies, the best known of which is the antinuclear antibody (ANA) that also elicits the LE phenomenon. That the destruction of nuclei and DNA is due to this antibody has been shown by Bennett et al. (1986). These authors identified a "functionally defective receptor for DNA" in the majority of patients with SLE and were able to induce this defect by incubating healthy mononuclear cells with the circulating antibodies of patients with SLE. The defect was manifest by an impaired binding of exogenous DNA to the surfaces of peripheral mononuclear cells. It must be remembered, however, that up to 50% clinically normal, pregnant women have ANAs at least once during the course of their pregnancy (Rosenberg et al., 1986). Lymphocytotoxic antibodies have been found in about 80% of patients with SLE (Pritchard et al., 1978). Other investigators have reported that these antibodies possess antitrophoblastic activity. This may possibly explain the poor pregnancy outcome that attends the disease (Bresnihan et al., 1977). This idea was particularly attractive because other inflammatory diseases such as rheumatoid arthritis and scleroderma do not have a high rate of abortion. When Ornoy et al. (2003) used the IgG purified sera of patients with lupus erythematosus and the antiphospholipid syndrome for the culture of rat embryos and placentas, they observed damage to the yolk sac and reduced trophoblastic growth with increased apoptosis.

The placentas of five patients with SLE were studied by Grennan et al. (1978). They identified fluorescent antibodies against complexes to nuclear antigens on placental villous basement membranes. Grimmer et al. (1988) have undertaken further studies to define this antitrophoblastic activity. They found IgM antitrophoblast antibodies in a patient with thrombocytopenia and a rash, who also experienced circulating lupus anticoagulant activity, twins, and an intrauterine fetal demise. By immunofluorescent antibody techniques, they localized the factor to the placental syncytium and found C3 to be deposited on the basement membranes of villi. The studies were done with the patient's placenta as well as with normal placentas; small vessel deposition of the antibodies was also observed. IgG, IgA, and C3 deposits were not localized to these areas. The twin placenta of this pregnancy was 10% infarcted and had decidual necrosis, but it lacked vascular disease. Perhaps the absence of vascular disease was due to sampling technique, but the authors were cautious in interpreting the findings as having an etiologic relationship to the fetal demise. This is particularly pertinent because deposits of C3 on the villous basement membranes have been observed in normal placentas (Johnson et al., 1977). The recognition of other circulating antibodies in SLE as possible causes of pregnancy mishaps will be discussed below. It must be said, however, that despite all the findings of abnormal placentas in SLE, one encounters occasional patients who have neither decidual vascular lesions nor infarcts or fetal growth restriction with this condition. Presumably, these patients are in remission, despite the presence of specific antibodies. The SLE patients who have no anticoagulant antibodies have fewer abortions (24.7%) than do those with such antibodies (58.7%), according to the retrospective study of Loizoll et al. (1988). In an immunologic study of placentas from a variety of patients with immunologic disorders, Ackerman and Gilbert-Barness (1997b) found fluorescent antibody localization (fibrinogen, IgG, IgM, IgA, and C3) to the trophoblastic basement membranes. Electron microscopically the basement membrane was thickened. In a subsequent contribution on placentas in maternal connective tissue diseases (Ackerman et al., 1999), five SLE, one rheumatoid arthritis, and two with mixed connective tissue disorders were described. Decidual vasculopathy or thrombosis was not seen, but three SLE patients' placenta showed thickening of the trophoblastic basement lamina electron miscroscopically. Magid et al. (1998) prospectively studied 40 placentas from 33 women with SLE. The decidual vasculopathy (17%), VUE (28%), and infarcts (18%) were principally associated with the simultaneous presence of antiphospholipid antibodies. Ischemic/hypoxic changes (diminutive and sparse villi) were prominent and depicted by these authors.

Some antibodies of patients with SLE are transferred to the fetus, which is often growth-restricted. These antibodies may cause thrombocytopenia, discoid lupus, and a variety of other conditions, including the LE phenomenon. We have seen a full-term infant weighing 2000 g of a mother with discoid lupus whose placenta possessed many infarcts and weighed only 320 g. There was intensive chronic deciduitis in the decidua basalis and decidua vera, with foci of old abruptio placentae. Atherosis was absent, but most decidual vascular walls were infiltrated by chronic inflammatory cells, among which plasma cells predominated. There also was diffuse, moderate chronic villitis. Beck et al. (1966) observed ANA titers in neonates of women with SLE, at approximately the same titers as in the mother. Despite this, the three neonates they observed remained healthy. The LE cells were repeatedly observed in the neonates of mothers with SLE, as reported by Mijer and Olsen (1958) and Gött (1969). These cells disappeared within 7 weeks after delivery, and the infants subsequently developed normally. Jackson (1964) described a third case of a newborn with discoid lupus, delivered by a mother with SLE. The neonatal lesions disappeared within 5 months but left small scars. Congenital heart block in such offspring has caused concern and is estimated to occur in 1 of 60 SLE pregnancies (Editorial, 1991). Hull et al. (1966) reported a neonatal death; the mother had suffered SLE for 13 years and had been treated with chloroquine throughout pregnancy. The 2500-g neonate was hydropic at birth, had a complete heart block (45/168 ventricular to atrial contractions), and had skin lesions. At autopsy, there was patchy fibrosis of the myocardium. The placenta was bilobed, edematous, and "fibrous-friable." This constellation is now considered to be the neonatal lupus syndrome. Provost et al. (1987) described two cases and reviewed the literature. In almost all cases, neonatal complications are associated with anti-U_1RNP antibodies, and the mother has anti-La(SS-B) or anti-Ro(SS-A) IgG antibodies. For this and other reasons, fetal surveillance has been recommended (Druzin et al., 1987). Another case of heart block was documented by Richards et al. (1990). Their primigravida was not known to have SLE when her fetus developed a complete heart block at 23 weeks' gestation and ascites at 26 weeks. Her ANA titers were then found to be 1:1024. Incipient hydrops led to treatment with betamethasone and was followed by reduction of signs of fluid accumulation, which the authors attributed to transplacental steroid antiinflammatory action. The neonate delivered at 37 weeks with retained heart block but did well. Another case of fetal heart block was detailed by Silver et al. (1992a). It caused fetal death, presumably secondary to the very extensive placental infarction (>80%) found. Thrombosed vessels with and without atherosis were present in the decidua basalis. In the atrial septum near Koch's triangle, dense fibrosis and calcification were identified and believed to have been responsible for the heart block. The mother possessed anti-Ro and anti-La antibodies. Seip (1960) and Cruveiller et al. (1970), among other investigators, have observed hemolytic anemia, rashes, thrombocytopenia, and leukopenia in neonates of mothers with SLE. Klippel et al. (1974) found inexplicable tubuloreticular cytoplasmic inclusions in the lymphocytes of neonates whose mothers had SLE.

The placenta of patients with SLE may be normal. More often it shows changes that are frequently impossible to differentiate from the lesions of preeclampsia (Magid et al., 1998). It must be appreciated, however, that preeclampsia is also more frequently seen in patients with SLE. It is thus difficult, at times, to know whether the placental pathology is due to preeclampsia or to SLE. The infarctions and retarded placental growth are the result of decidual vascular lesions that, in turn, are the cause of the fetal growth restriction of SLE. Abramowsky and his colleagues (1980) studied 10 placentas from patients with SLE, and one placenta of a patient with discoid lupus. They found vascular lesions in five placentas. Two placentas had over 25% infarction; others showed only discolorations. The outstanding lesion was decidual arteriopathy, with fibrinoid necrosis and infiltration by inflammatory cells. Some vessels appeared aneurysmally dilated and had atherosis. No abruptions were seen grossly, but microscopic study indicated this in two cases. Infarction and "premature aging of villi" were the only other pathologic findings. In two patients, immunofluorescent study showed massive deposition of IgM, and a lesser amount of C3 in the decidual vascular walls. We have had similar experiences with SLE (Benirschke & Driscoll, 1967) and have suggested that the decidual lesions are best observed in retroplacental curettings. Alternatively, the place to find most decidual arterioles with these pathologic changes is in the decidua capsularis of the membrane roll. These vessels have lesions that are similar to those in the maternal floor of the placenta. They are usually less readily found in the decidua basalis that comes with the delivered placenta because not enough of that decidua separates with delivery of the placenta. Moreover, in the floor of the placenta, fibrin and old clot from partial abruptions usually preclude adequate study. One would need to do postpartum curettage or placental bed biopsy in order to obtain sufficient material for proper evaluation. But that is not often practical and should probably be avoided because of the potential for creating future accretas. Vascular lesions, including atherosis and thrombosis, are clearly the cause of the placental infarcts, the associated abruptions, and the reduced weights of placenta and fetus. Between the infarcts of affected placentas, the villous tissue displays Tenney-Parker changes, the increased syncytial knotting, best known in preeclampsia and due to reduced maternal perfusion of the intervillous space. This histologic state is often referred to as "enhanced aging," but it is simply a reflection of reduced oxygen availability from the decreased intervillous blood flow. Thus, there is no need to postulate that specific antitrophoblastic antibodies exert an additional or specific destructive effect. Figure 19.32 shows the macroscopic appearance of the placenta in a patient with SLE. It has numerous infarcts (55%), which caused fetal death. The placenta was multilobulated because numerous infarcts had caused atrophy of many areas. The placenta of the case described by Hull et al. (1966) was bilobate, perhaps for the same reasons. Our patient had a previous spontaneous abortion, and a placenta with many decidual vascular lesions. Figures

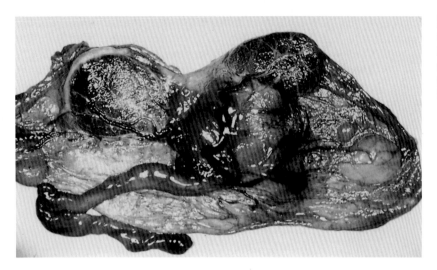

FIGURE 19.32. Placenta in systemic lupus erythematosus (SLE) near term. The placenta has many infarcts (55%) of varying ages, separated lobules (succenturiate lobes), and, microscopically, many arteriolar lesions. The fetus was stillborn and growth restricted.

19.33 to 19.36 illustrate vascular lesions of two other patients with SLE. In both cases, fetal death occurred at about 19 weeks' gestation. The macerated fetuses showed no lesions. The placentas were extensively infarcted and had several areas of abruptio and Tenney-Parker changes. Although this change is most common in preeclampsia, it is usually not seen until the third trimester when pure preeclampsia complicates pregnancy most commonly. There was no clinical evidence of preeclampsia in these patients. Interestingly, with one of these cases, mural thrombi were present in vessels of the umbilical cord and of the placental surface. Branch and Rodgers (1993) found that thrombosis occurred most likely as the result of antibodies to endothelial tissue factor expression.

Because many of these patients have had prednisolone therapy, it may be conjectured that some of the pathologic changes might be attributed to this therapy. This was investigated by Warrell and Taylor (1968). They studied

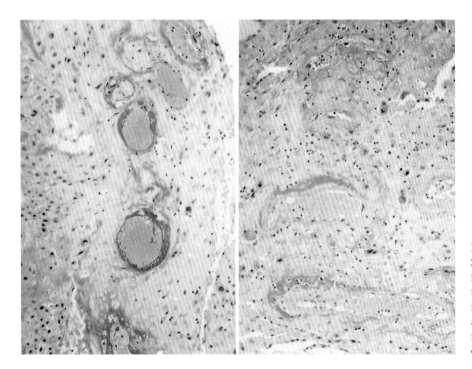

FIGURE 19.33. Decidual arteriopathy of SLE in decidua capsularis. There are fibrin infiltration of the wall, mural thrombosis, and minimal leukocytic infiltration. The pregnancy terminated at 21 weeks with stillbirth of a 215-g (!) macerated fetus. The placenta weighed only 60 g. H&E ×16 (left); ×160 (right).

FIGURE 19.34. Another case of decidual arteriopathy in SLE at 19 weeks' gestation with stillborn, macerated fetus. Several types of vascular lesions are seen in these vessels of the decidua basalis and capsularis: mural thrombosis, hyalinization, inflammation, thickening of spiral arterioles, organized old thromboses, and fresh thrombi with decidual necrosis. The fetal vessels also had mural thrombi. H&E ×160 (left); ×250 (right).

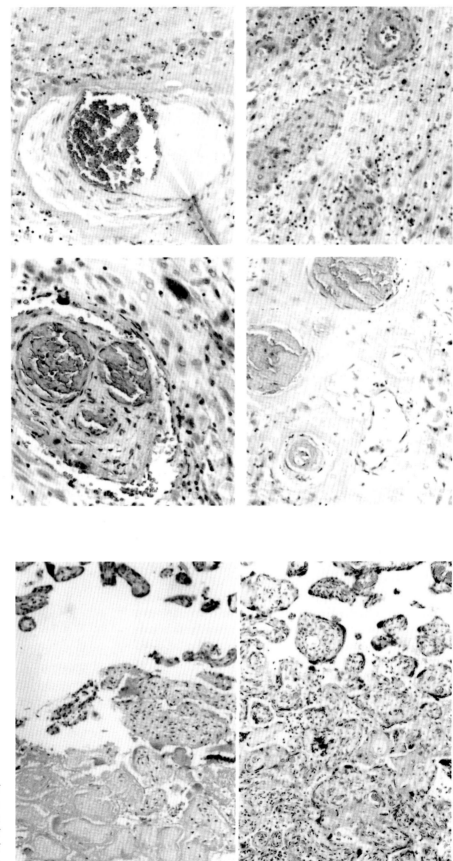

FIGURE 19.35. Microscopic aspect of villous tissue in SLE of previous case (Fig. 19.34) showing old and recent infarcts and Tenney-Parker change of viable villi. They have the appearance of term villi because of the loss of water and shrinkage. H&E ×160.

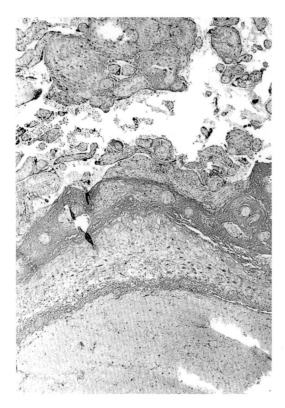

FIGURE 19.36. Fresh abruptio placentae in SLE with minimal infarction of villous tissue (same case as Fig. 19.33). The retro-placental clot below is elevating the decidua basalis. These changes usually preclude one from observing the vascular lesions in the decidua basalis. H&E ×60.

34 pregnancies of 30 women receiving prednisolone for asthma (18), ulcerative colitis (2), SLE (4), eczema/urti-caria (7), and arthritis/sarcoidosis (3). There were eight fetal deaths, and nine fetuses that were at risk of "placental insufficiency." The authors concluded that the enhanced risk to the fetus may be explained by the experimental findings of Blackburn et al. (1965). These investigators had given large doses of prednisolone to pregnant rats and observed smaller placentas, fetal deaths, and "increased aging of the placenta." No decidual vascular lesions were seen, but the decidua was significantly under-developed. It is likely that the findings of Warrell and Taylor (1968) represent changes that are not related to SLE or its therapy. Why not all patients with full-blown SLE exhibit identical vascular lesions and destructive placental infarcts may relate to the severity of the disease or perhaps to the therapeutic regimen and its efficacy.

Lupus Anticoagulant

This is the most commonly observed of several antiphos-pholipid antibodies; there are also anticardiolipin and antiphosphatidylserine. Aside from the ANAs mentioned above, in SLE there exists a variety of less well defined immunoglobulins whose origin and determinants have been superbly reviewed by experts in this complex field (Asherson et al., 1989). The best known of these antibod-ies are the "lupus anticoagulant" and "anticardiolipin," a type of antiphospholipid antibody. The topic is difficult and has many contradictions. It is perhaps best to begin with a quote from Gleicher (1997): "Antiphospholipid antibodies are present in virtually every individual . . . at higher levels in females." Thus, care is needed in interpre-tation of tests used for their determination, levels, types of antibody, and controls employed in critical studies. Moreover, when Kutteh and Franklin (2004) studied the results of assay findings from 10 different laboratories, only mild to moderate reliability was demonstrated. Averbuch et al. (1987) have found elevated levels of lupus anticoagulant in about 20% of SLE cases. Feinstein (1985) has incisively pointed out in his review that the term **anticoagulant** is clearly a misnomer. He writes, "It has become clear that the lupus anticoagulant is more fre-quently encountered in patients without lupus, and it is not associated with abnormal bleeding in most patients except when hypoproteinemia, thrombocytopenia, or a qualitative platelet defect is present." This antibody pro-longs phospholipid-dependent coagulation tests by binding to epitopes on the phospholipid portion of pro-thrombinase (factors Xa and Va, calcium, and phospho-lipid). It was first described by Bowie et al. (1963) in four patients with SLE who had thrombotic complications. Since then it has been recognized that women with his-tories of repeated abortion and premature births often possess "circulating lupus anticoagulants" that may indi-rectly be held responsible for this excessive fetal wastage. For instance, Kowal-Vern et al. (1996) suggested, from reviewing the literature, that anticardiolipin antibodies are present (cause?) in 3% to 10% of women with recur-rent pregnancy losses. Because of the variety of antibod-ies found, it has become customary to speak of the circulating lupus anticoagulant syndrome (CLAS). The heterogeneity of the antibodies and the difficulty in defin-ing them have been presented in some detail by Triplett et al. (1985). They found that 2% of patients screened for activated partial thromboplastin times had this antibody, and they provided a detailed discussion of the tests avail-able for the definition of the antibodies. In a later con-tribution, Triplett (1993) summarized the thrombotic sequelae of these antiphospholipid antibodies, especially those in the arterial circulation, and other reviews have been summarized above. Triplett went on to describe the placental anticoagulant protein-1 (PAP-1) with the poten-tial of inducing thrombosis. Lazarchick and Kizer (1989) have given specific details of laboratory procedures nec-essary for the establishment of this diagnosis, an impor-tant issue. They found that dilute Russell viper venom time and the tissue thromboplastin inhibition test are sensitive assays. Nevertheless, in several patients, the discordance of test results necessitated measurements of specific coagulation factors in order to establish the diagnosis. Apparently wide differences exist in laboratories reporting test results (Peaceman et al., 1992), which must be taken into consideration when prevalence figures and treatment results are evaluated. The antibodies are usually IgG molecules, but may be also be IgM and IgA, or combinations. They interfere with the phospholipid-dependent coagulation assays (see also Brandt et al., 1987). Usually considered to be in vitro phenomena (Woodhouse, 1984), their presence may be indicative of diverse clinical states, such as thromboses, pregnancy wastage, polyneuritis, and sundry others. As indicated, a comprehensive review of this complex topic has been provided by Triplett (1989, 1993), and another comes from Rote et al. (1998). The former papers not only summarize the basis for the action of various antibodies (see also Reece et al., 1990) but also provide a list of reports on pregnancies with and without therapy.

Numerous complications have attended pregnancies with CLAS antibodies, but then there are other cases in which no pathology is observed. At present there is no conclusive resolution of this complex topic; especially lacking are concrete results that link recurrent abortion to the existence of the antibodies. Indeed, the case-control study by Infante-Rivard (1991) indicated that "there is no apparent justification for considering lupus anticoagulants or IgG anticardiolipins to be risk factors for fetal loss among women who present with spontaneous abortion or fetal death and have had no previous spontaneous fetal loss." Balasch et al. (1997) came to similar conclusions. El-Roeiy and colleagues (1990) ascertained that in normal pregnancies, elevated levels of antiphospholipid antibodies are not observed. Their study also suggested that when these exist in low titers, they have little or no effect on pregnancy wastage; growth restriction of the fetus may be a sequel, however (Gleicher, 1997). Aside from fetal wastage, now recognized in some of these gestations, a maternal death (following fetal death) has also occurred. This happened in a patient who, one day following the diagnosis of fetal death, suffered disseminated small-vessel thrombosis. Myocarditis and pericarditis were present in the mother, who also had sickle trait and presumably "occult" SLE (Bendon et al., 1987). Farquharson et al. (1985) had reported life-threatening thrombosis that necessitated therapeutic abortion in a pregnant patient. The authors suggested that immunosuppressive therapy may have to be initiated before pregnancy occurs in order to avoid such complications. Other cases of severe maternal thrombotic events in this antibody syndrome are by Hochfeld et al. (1994) and Kupferminc et al. (1994). But not all such patients have clinical symptoms. When abnormal immunologic findings with irregular antibodies are present in pregnant patients,

such as an unexpectedly positive Venereal Disease Research Laboratory (VDRL) test, further investigation is required. This necessitates especially a search for the presence of lupus anticoagulant and anticardiolipins. In the patient just described, many myometrial vessels had lesions at the placental floor; one third of the placenta had infarcts (30%), and an abruptio placentae was found. The mother also had myocardial and renal lesions. Lockshin et al. (1989) evaluated therapy in 21 patients with high antiphospholipid antibodies and one prior fetal death. They concluded that prednisone does not improve outcome but in fact may worsen it. Branch et al. (1989) showed that an association of antiphospholipid antibodies exists also with severe toxemia of pregnancy and suggested that this is one more reason to consider an immune hypothesis for both diseases.

Although there is this well-known relationship of such "irregular" antibodies to recurrent fetal wastage, the prevalence of the various types has been disputed and, most importantly, it had not been known whether the existence of one or the other types of antibody spells a more sinister prognosis. The study conducted by Lockwood et al. (1989) corrected this deficiency. They ascertained the presence of lupus anticoagulant and anticardiolipin antibodies in a low-risk population and found two of 737 patients to have lupus anticoagulants and recurrent abortions. Conversely, 16 of 737 patients had anticardiolipins, and four of these had uncomplicated pregnancies. Twelve had various complications. They concluded that the presence of antiphospholipid antibodies was correlated with unfavorable pregnancy outcome, and that their prevalence is in the range of 0.3%. Two cases of fetal stroke, recognized only later in the neonatal period, were attributed by Silver et al. (1992b) to result from anticardiolipin antibodies. Many subsequent studies have tried to clarify the situation. Regrettably, few have availed themselves of a systematic examination of the placenta from the study population. For instance, Oshiro et al. (1996), who found that antiphospholipid antibodies correlated with fetal demise rather than early trimester abortion, did not evaluate the pathology, even though they referred to the proverbial "placental insufficiency." Branch et al. (1997) concluded that women with recurrent losses are no more likely to possess antiphospholipid antibodies once anticoagulant and anticardiolipins are excluded. They did not evaluate placentas. When such study was undertaken in patients with anticardiolipin antibodies (Kowal-Vern et al., 1996), no abnormal changes were detected. Thus, one needs to exercise caution in attributing many or all recurrent pregnancy losses to placental lesions in this syndrome. To better understand the effect of these antibodies on placental function, Silver et al. (1997a,b) have passively immunized mice with some of these human antibodies. Some fetal demises and resorptions were observed, but no clear relation was found to explain the result; nevertheless, they provided a first insight into possible effects on intervillous circulation. More light comes from the investigation by Rand and coworkers (1997), who provided a basis for understanding that anticoagulants have a coagulative ability in the placenta. They found an interaction of the antibodies from three affected women with the annexin V (placental anticoagulant protein I) residing on the surface of cells of a trophoblast cell line. Their results suggest that the annexin levels are reduced after antibody exposure and that this may be the mechanism that leads to the thrombosis in the intervillous space in recurrent fetal losses. To understand these issues is especially important for potential preventive therapy in such patients, as Cowchock (1997) discussed in an editorial. Prednisone is thus less likely to be beneficial than heparin or anticoagulation of other types.

Investigations regarding the nature of the CLAS began with the identification of a patient by Nilsson et al. (1975). That mother experienced pregnancies with three intrauterine deaths and she had circulating lupus anticoagulants. The authors indicated that a relation may exist between this antibody and placental infarction. McVerry et al. (1980) then reported two patients with deficient prostacyclin (PGI_2) production and SLE. Soon after, this was followed by a report of a patient with history of arterial thromboses, fetal death at 23 weeks, and CLAS (Carreras et al., 1981a). Decreased prostacyclin release could be elicited from that mother's IgG fraction, when aortic strips were incubated. The same authors found that two of 24 women with repeated abortions, intrauterine fetal growth restriction, and fetal death had lupus anticoagulants (Carreras et al., 1981b). Many reports of essentially similar findings have since followed, as for instance the demonstration by Xu et al. (1990) of the prevalence of low-titer ANA-positive serum in patients with pregnancy losses. There was also a controlled multicenter study by Out et al. (1992), which demonstrated conclusively that possession of antiphospholipid antibodies was "a risk factor for adverse pregnancy outcome." In their analysis of 47 placentas with intrauterine death, 16 had antiphospholipid antibodies (Out et al., 1991). Fibrosis in infarcts, areas of thrombosis, and Tenney-Parker changes were prominent findings. Buchanan et al. (1992), who investigated 100 lupus pregnancies with concurrent antiphospholipid antibodies, found an 81% pregnancy loss.

Once the causative relationship of CLAS to repetitive pregnancy failure had been suggested, various forms of therapy were tried. Lubbe et al. (1983), who treated six CLAS patients, successfully achieved suppression of the anticoagulant by prednisone therapy. On the other hand, Prentice et al. (1984) managed 15 patients who had three successful pregnancies without immunosuppressive therapy, whereas the results published by Carp et al.

(1989) were much less optimistic. This emphasizes the erratic nature of CLAS antibodies in predicting outcome and possibly differences in laboratory evaluation of these tests. In a later publication, Lubbe and Liggins (1985) reviewed their experience with 49 patients who had 160 unsuccessful pregnancies. They recommended prednisone (40–60 mg/day) and aspirin (75 mg/day) therapy for the management of such pregnancies. Prednisone and aspirin medication, beginning 4 weeks prior to ovulation, was shown to be effective in preventing recurrent early pregnancy failure in the study conducted by Geva et al. (1998). Rouget et al. (1982) observed a familial case of anticoagulant in mother and daughter. Branch et al. (1985) reported the frequency of preeclampsia in these patients, and recommended steroid and aspirin therapy to improve fetal outcome. The addition of immunoglobulin infusion in the therapy of such patients has been advocated by Wapner et al. (1989). Unander et al. (1987) studied the sera of 99 patients with habitual abortion and found elevated anticardiolipin antibodies in 42 patients. There was concomitant low C4 activity. Because it is well known that protein C deficiency may lead to thromboses, Cariou et al. (1986) studied the interaction of anticoagulants and protein C. They found inhibition of protein C activation by the antibodies and suggested that this acts against thrombomodulin or its phospholipid moiety. Considerations of the mechanisms of action of the different antibodies in CLAS have been reviewed by Reece et al. (1984) and Lockwood et al. (1986). Two reports have suggested that treatment with high doses of gamma globulin (IgG) not only lowers the levels of antiphospholipid antibodies but also results in improved fetal salvage in severely compromised patients (Carreras et al., 1988; Scott et al., 1988). A most interesting "natural experiment" was reported by Stormorken et al. (1988). A patient who had four consecutive miscarriages with the anticoagulant syndrome had a normal, term pregnancy because the mother had spontaneously developed antifactor II antibody. This had led to hypoprothrombinemia with marked anticoagulation. The authors suggested that one should infer from this case the need for anticoagulation in the usual cases of lupus anticoagulant that complicates pregnancy. Randomized trials and prospective studies of the efficacy of various modes of treatment have shown that low-dose aspirin is a preferable method over prednisone (Cowchock et al., 1992) and that fewer placental infarcts occurred with heparin therapy (Rosove et al., 1990). It has also been suggested that the frequently premature rupture of membranes is related to prednisone medication. Recent studies using a mouse model have also demonstrated a critical role of complement activation in pathophysiology of the antiphospholipid antibody syndrome (Salmon et al., 2003). In this model, significant fetal loss was associated with experimentally induced antiphospholipid antibody syndrome. Treatment with heparin and other anticoagulants caused reversal of this fetal loss and growth restriction. The authors postulated that activation of complement leads to placental tissue injury and subsequent fetal loss and growth restriction. Likewise, Bose et al. (2004) found heparin to be helpful in preventing placental apoptosis in patients with lupus anticoagulant sera.

In most studies it has been shown that the placenta in patients with CLAS is morphologically indistinguishable from that of patients with severe preeclampsia. In CLAS, the extensive placental infarctions and decidual vascular lesions are often found at much younger gestational ages than is the case for preeclampsia. Frequently, the lesions occur before the 20th week of pregnancy. De Wolf et al. (1982) first drew attention to the decidual vascular lesions in this condition. They found multiple microthrombi and typical atherosis in a placenta that had 50% infarction. The authors suggested that, because prostacyclin ordinarily is the most important inhibitor of platelet aggregation, antibodies to this agent may be held responsible for the thrombosis. Gleicher and Friberg (1985) and Silver (1988) also reported CLAS associated with atherosis and massive placental infarction. The reviews by Triplett (1989, 1993) provide a good chronology of these discoveries. As was mentioned earlier, there is probably no need to incriminate the antitrophoblastic antibodies detected by Grimmer et al. (1988) in the causality of fetal demise. The degree of infarction and compromise of the intervillous circulation adequately explain resultant stillbirth and growth restriction (Polzin, 1991). It now needs to be learned whether this intervillous coagulation relates to the reduction of annexin V, as suggested by the study of Rand et al. (1997). Thus, sophisticated concomitant placental examinations should be undertaken. An example of such an abnormal placenta is shown in Figure 19.37.

This is the placenta of a severely growth-restricted fetus (30 weeks, 700 g) with placental abruptio and 50% infarction, in addition to a velamentous insertion of the umbilical cord. There were many decidual vessels with atherosis, thrombosis and hyalinization of the thickened walls. The mother had anticardiolipin antibodies but no symptoms of SLE, and the fetus survived. We have also seen atherosis in the decidual vessels of a patient with CLAS, whose pregnancy was considered to have been successfully treated; thus the degree of recognizable vascular lesions in the decidua often does not correspond precisely to the degree of growth restriction of fetus and placenta. Although the finding of vascular lesions confirms the diagnosis of CLAS when preeclampsia is absent, it is probably the extent of decidual compromise that determines the fetal and placental growth and pregnancy outcome. But, the degree of vasculopathy is highly variable. It is often difficult to assess quantitatively, unless one has adequate placental site curettings available for interpretation. Figure 19.38 shows mild arteriopathy in the floor of an extensively infarcted placenta. The fetus was stillborn at 25 weeks, but the extent of atherosis poorly correlated with the 25% infarction found in the placenta. Several reviews of the vascular control of placental blood flow are available, especially those by Ylikorkala and Mäkilä (1985) and Mäkilä et al. (1986). These authors suggested that, because decidual spiral arterioles are already optimally dilated in pregnancy, two agents, prostacyclin and thromboxane A_2, are used in regulating the intervillous blood flow. A disturbance of their finely tuned balance, as accomplished by the anti-prostacyclin activity of lupus anticoagulant, may be the principal cause of hypoperfusion of placenta and the subsequent infarction of placental tissue. This is also the best explanation for the efficacy of treatment with

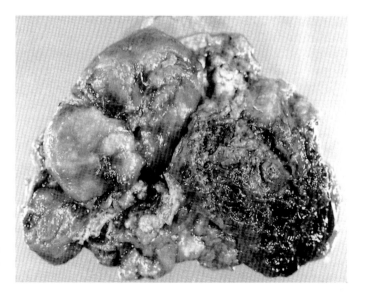

FIGURE 19.37. Retroplacental hemorrhage with 50% infarction of 30 weeks' gestation placenta with maternal anticardiolipin antibodies. The 700-g infant survived.

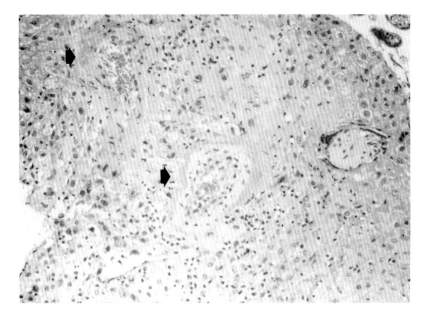

FIGURE 19.38. Decidua basalis of patient with lupus anticoagulant at 25 weeks' gestation. Decidual arterioles (arrows) show mild mural thrombosis and fibrin deposits, although the placenta was 25% infarcted. H&E ×160.

aspirin (150 mg/day) and dipyridamole (300 mg/day) in preeclampsia and in CLAS. Peaceman and Rehnberg (1993) showed that with incubation of the immunoglobulin G fraction of patients having lupus anticoagulant, with placental extracts from normal gestations, thromboxane was significantly increased.

As recently as 2004, Kujovich reviewed the literature and found that although thrombophilia has a negative influence on pregnancy outcome, "definition of the magnitude of risk will require prospective longitudinal studies." In addition to decidual vessels with thromboses, vascular occlusions have also been observed in the fetus, when maternal CLAS was present. Sheridan-Pereira et al. (1988) reported a neonate with aortic thrombosis. We know of a similar case where the fetus had carotid artery obliteration and consequent brain necrosis. As mentioned earlier, Silver et al. (1992b) attributed the cerebral infarction in two infants to transplacentally transmitted antibodies. In line with what has been reported by Darnige et al. (2004), this is unusual. These investigators showed the occurrence of thrombocytopenia in the offspring of a mother with antiphospholipid syndrome. Trudinger et al. (1988) suggested that the abnormal umbilical artery flow velocity waveforms that they identified were the result of "vascular sclerosis evident in the small arteries of the tertiary villi." We have not been able to observe such lesions in the many cases of CLAS we have seen. In our opinion, the degree of infarction and shrinkage of surviving villi that are associated with the decidual arteriopathy are sufficient to explain the abnormal blood flow. Clearly, much more needs to be known of the numerous antibodies now identified and their effect on fetus and newborn before the issue is completely resolved.

References

Abdella, T.N., Sibai, B.M., Hays, J.M. and Anderson, G.D.: Relationship of hypertensive disease to abruptio placentae. Obstet. Gynecol. **63**:365–370, 1984.

Abitbol, M.M., Gallo, G.R., Pirani, C.L. and Ober, W.B.: Production of experimental toxemia in the pregnant rabbit. Amer. J. Obstetr. Gynecol. **124**:460–470, 1976a.

Abitbol, M.M., Driscoll, S.G. and Ober, W.B.: Placental lesions in experimental toxemia in the rabbit. Amer. J. Obstetr. Gynecol. **125**:942–948, 1976b.

Abitbol, M.M., Pirani, C.L., Ober, W.B., Driscoll, S.G. and Cohen, M.W.: Production of experimental toxemia in the pregnant dog. Obstetr. Gynecol. **48**:537–548, 1976c.

Abitbol, M.M., Ober, W.B., Gallo, G.R., Driscoll, S.G. and Pirani, C.L.: Experimental toxemia of pregnancy in the monkey, with a preliminary report on renin and aldosterone. Amer. J. Pathol. **86**:573–590, 1977.

Abramowsky, C.R., Vegas, M.E., Swinehart, G. and Gyves, M.T.: Decidual vasculopathy of the placenta in lupus erythematosus. NEJM **303**:668–672, 1980.

Acker, D., Sachs, B.P., Tracey, K.J. and Wise, W.E.: Abruptio placentae associated with cocaine use. Amer. J. Obstet. Gynecol. **146**:220–221, 1983.

Ackerman, J. and Gilbert-Barness, E.F.: Malignancy metastatic to the products of conception: a case report with review of the literature. Pediatr. Pathol. Lab. Med. **17**:577–586, 1997a.

Ackerman, J. and Gilbert-Barness, E.F.: An immunological study of the placenta in maternal connective tissue disease. Pediatr. Pathol. Lab. Med. **17**:513–514, 1997b.

Ackerman, J., Gonzalez, E.F. and Gilbert-Barness, E.: Immunological studies of the placenta in maternal connective tissue disease. Pediat. Development. Pathol. **2**:19–24, 1999.

Adam, P.A.J., Teramo, K., Raiha, N., Gitlin, D. and Schwartz, R.: Human fetal insulin metabolism early in gestation: response to acute elevation of the fetal glucose concentration and placental transfer of human insulin-I-131. Diabetes **18**: 409–416, 1969.

Addleman, W. and Gold, S.: Gaucher's disease and pregnancy. Can. Med. Assoc. J. **89**:821–823, 1963.

Aessopos, A., Karabatsos, F., Farmakis, D., Katsantoni, A., Hatziliami, A., Youssef, J. and Karagiorga, M.: Pregnancy in patients with well-treated thalassemia: outcome for mothers and newborn infants. Amer. J. Obstet. Gynecol. **180**:360–365, 1999.

Ahnquist, G. and Holyoke, J.B.: Congenital Letterer-Siwe disease (reticuloendotheliosis) in a term stillborn infant. J. Pediatr. **57**:897–904, 1960.

Aladjem, S.: Morphologic aspects of the placenta in gestational diabetes seen by phase-contrast microscopy. Amer. J. Obstet. Gynecol. **99**:341–349, 1967a.

Aladjem, S.: The syncytial knot: a sign of active syncytial proliferation. Amer. J. Obstet. Gynecol. **99**:350–358, 1967b.

Aladjem, S., Lueck, J. and Brewer, J.I.: Experimental induction of a toxemia-like syndrome in the pregnant beagle. Amer. J. Obstetr. Gynecol. **145**:27–38, 1983.

Alanen, A., Kekomäki, R., Kero, P., Lindström, P. and Wager, O.: Circulating immune complexes in hypertensive disorders of pregnancy. J. Reprod. Immunol. **6**:133–140, 1984.

Alberman, E., Pharoah, P. and Chamberlain, G.: Smoking and the fetus. Lancet **2**:36–37, 1977.

Alonso, A., Soto, I., Urgellés, M.F., Corte, J.R., Rodriguez, M.J. and Pinto, C.R.: Acquired and inherited thrombophilia in women with unexplained fetal loss. Amer. J. Obstet. Gynecol. **187**:1337–1342, 2002.

Altchek, A., Gaines, J.A. and Siltzbach, L.E.: Sarcoidosis of the uterus. Amer. J. Obstet. Gynecol. **70**:540–547, 1955.

Alvarez, H.: Prolifération du trophoblaste et sa relation avec l'hypertension artérielle de la toxémie gravidique. Gynecol. Obstet. (Paris) **69**:581–588, 1970.

Alvarez, H., Benedetti, W.L. and DeLeons, V.K.: Syncytial proliferation in normal and toxemic pregnancies. Obstetr. Gynecol. **29**:637–643, 1967.

Alvarez, H., Morel, R.L., Benedetti, W.L. and Scavarelli, M.: Trophoblast hyperplasia and maternal arterial pressure at term. Amer. J. Obstet. Gynecol. **105**:1015–1021, 1969.

Alzamora, O.: Algunas observaciones sobre las alteraciones de la placenta human en la altura. Rev. Asoc. Med. Prov. Yauli. **3**:75, 1958.

Ambrose, A., Welham, R.T. and Cefalo, R.C.: Thrombotic thrombocytic purpura in early pregnancy. Obstet. Gynecol. **66**:267–272, 1985.

American College of Obstetricians and Gynecologists: Thyroid disease in pregnancy. ACOG Technical Bulletin No. **181**:1–6, 1993.

Anderson, W.R. and McKay, D.G.: Electron microscope study of the trophoblast in normal and toxemic placentas. Amer. J. Obstetr. Gynecol. **95**:1134–1148, 1966.

Anderson, M., Went, L.N., MacIver, J.E. and Dixon, H.G.: Sickle cell disease in pregnancy. Lancet **2**:516–521, 1960.

Anderson, J.F., Kent, S. and Machin, G.A.: Maternal malignant melanoma with placental metastasis: a case report with literature review. Pediatr. Pathol. **9**:35–42, 1989.

Ando, T. and Davies, T.F.: Clinical review 160: postpartum autoimmune thyroid disease: the potential role of fetal microchimerism. J. Clin. Endocrinol. Metab. **88**:2965–2971, 2003.

Andrews, J. and McGarry, J.: A community study of smoking in pregnancy. J. Obstetr. Gynaecol. Brit. Cwlth. **79**:1057–1073, 1972.

Anonymous: Pregnancy and the arachidonic-acid cascade. Lancet **i**:997–998, 1982.

Anonymous: Classification of hypertensive disorders of pregnancy. Lancet **i**:935–936, 1989a.

Anonymous: Smoke screen round the fetus. Lancet **2**:1310–1311, 1989b.

Anunciado, A.N., Stubbs, T.M., Pepkowitz, S.H., Lazarchick, J., Miller III, C.M. and Pilia, P.: Altered villus vessel fibronectin in preeclampsia. Amer. J. Obstetr. Gynecol. **156**:898–900, 1987.

Ariel, I., Anteby, E., Schneider, T., Pinar, H., Ayesh, S., Hansen, K., Singer, D.B., deGroot, N. and Hochberg, A.: The placental gene expression profile in pre-eclampsia. Pediatr. Devel. Pathol. **4**:313, 2001.

Ariel, I., Anteby, E., Hamani, Y. and Redline, R.W.: Placental pathology in fetal thrombophilia. Hum. Pathol. **35**:729–733, 2004.

Aron, D.C., Schnall, A.M. and Sheeler, L.R.: Cushing's syndrome and pregnancy. Amer. J. Obstet. Gynecol. **162**:244–252, 1990.

Aronson, S.: A case of transplacental tumor metastasis. Acta Paediatr. (Stockh.) **52**:123–124, 1963.

Artlett, C.M., Smith, J.B. and Jimenez, S.A.: Identification of fetal DNA and cells in skin lesions from women with systemic sclerosis. NEJM **338**:1186–1191, 1998.

Asherson, R.A., Khamashta, M.A., Ordi-Ros, J., Derksen, R.H.D.M., Machin, S.J., Barquinero, J., Outt, H.H., Harris, E.N., Vilardell-Torres, M. and Hughes, G.R.V.: The "primary" antiphospholipid syndrome: Major clinical and serological features. Medicine **68**:366–374, 1989.

Ask-Upmark, E.: Leukemia and pregnancy. Acta Med. Scand. **170**:635–658, 1961.

Ask-Upmark, E.: Another follow-up study of children born of mothers with leukemia. Acta Med. Scand. **175**:391–394, 1964.

Asmussen, I.: Ultrastructure of human umbilical veins: observations on veins from newborn children of smoking and nonsmoking mothers. Acta Obstet. Gynecol. Scand. **57**: 253–255, 1978.

Asmussen, I.: Effects of maternal smoking on the cardiovascular system. Cardiovasc. Med. **4**:777–790, 1979.

Asmussen, I.: Ultrastructure of the villi and fetal capillaries in placentas from smoking and nonsmoking mothers. Brit. J. Obstet. Gynaecol. **87**:239–245, 1980.

Asmussen, I.: Ultrastructure of the umbilical artery from a newborn delivered at term by a mother who smoked 80 cigarettes per day. Acta Pathol. Microbiol. Immunol. Scand. [A] **90**:397–404, 1982a.

Asmussen, I.: Ultrastructure of human umbilical arteries from newborn children of smoking and non-smoking mothers. Acta Pathol. Microbiol. Immunol. Scand. [A] **90**:375–383, 1982b.

Asmussen, I.: Mitochondrial proliferation in endothelium: observations on umbilical arteries from newborn children of smoking mothers. Atherosclerosis **50**:203–208, 1984.

Atalla, A. and Page, I.: Ehlers-Danlos syndrome type III in pregnancy. Obstet. Gynecol. **71**:508–509, 1988.

Attwood, H.D. and Park, W.W.: Embolism to the lungs by trophoblast. J. Obstetr. Gynaecol. Brit. Cwlth. **68**:611–617, 1961.

Averbuch, M., Koifman, B. and Levo, Y.: Lupus anticoagulant, thrombosis and thrombocytopenia in systemic lupus erythematosus. Amer. J. Med. **293**:2–5, 1987.

Ayala, A.R., De La Fuente, F.R., Loyola, F.D., Gonzalez, E. and Kunhardt, J.: Evidence that a toxemia-related organism (*Hydatoxi lualba*) is an artifact. Obstetr. Gynecol. **67**:47–50, 1086.

Bachrach, L.K. and Burrows, G.N.: Maternal-fetal transfer of thyroxine. NEJM **321**:1549, 1989.

Baergen, R.N., Johnson, D., Moore, T. and Benirschke, K.: Maternal melanoma metastatic to the placenta. A case report and review of the literature. Arch. Pathol. Lab. Med. **121**:508–511, 1997.

Baergen, R.N., Chacko, S.A., Edersheim, T., Etingin, O, Hutson, J.M. and Pirog, E.: The placenta in thrombophilias: a clinicopathologic study. Modern Pathol. **14**: 213A, 2001.

Bailey, D.N.: Cocaine and cocaethylene binding to human placenta in vitro. Amer. J. Obstet. Gynecol. **177**:527–531, 1997.

Balasch, J., Mirapeix, E., Borche, L., Vives, J. and Gonzalez-Merlo, J.: Further evidence against preeclampsia as an immune complex disease. Obstetr. Gynecol. **58**:435–437, 1981.

Balasch, J., Reverter, J.C., Fábregues, F., Tàssies, D., Rafel, M., Creus, M. and Vanrell, J.A.: First-trimester repeated abortion is not associated with activated protein resistance. Human Reprod. **12**:1094–1097, 1997.

Baldwin, V.J., MacLeod, P.M. and Benirschke, K.: Placental findings in alcohol abuse in pregnancy. Birth Defects **18**:89–94, 1982.

Barabas, A.P.: Ehlers-Danlos syndrome: associated with prematurity and premature rupture of foetal membranes; possible increase in incidence. Brit. Med. J. **2**:682–684, 1966.

Bardawil, W.A. and Toy, B.L.: The natural history of choriocarcinoma: problems of immunity and spontaneous regression. Ann. N.Y. Acad. Sci. **80**:197–261, 1959.

Bardeguez, A.D., McNerney, R., Frieri, M., Verma, U.L. and Tejani, N.: Cellular immunity in preeclampsia: Alterations in T-lymphocyte subpopulations during early pregnancy. Obstet. Gynecol. **77**:859–862, 1991.

Barnes, A.B. and Link, D.A.: Childhood dermatomyositis and pregnancy. Amer. J. Obstet. Gynecol. **146**:335–336, 1983.

Barss, V., Phillippe, M., Greene, M.F. and Covell, L.: Pregnancy complicated by homozygous hypercholesterolemia. Obstet. Gynecol. **65**:756–757, 1985.

Barth, F.B., Khurana, S.K., Vergara, G.G. and Lowman, J.T.: Rapidly fatal familial histiocytosis associated with eosinophilia and primary immunological deficiency. Lancet **2**:503–506, 1972.

Bartholomew, R.A.: Hemorrhages of late pregnancy. With emphasis on placental circulation and the mechanism of bleeding. Postgraduate Med. **30**:397–406, 1961.

Bartholomew, R.A., Colvin, E.D., Grimes, W.H., Fish, J.S., Lester, W.M. and Galloway, W.H.: Facts pertinent to the etiology of eclamptogenic toxemia. Amer. J. Obstet. Gynecol. **74**:64–84, 1957.

Bartholomew, R.A., Colvin, E.D., Grimes, W.H., Fish, J.S., Lester, W.M. and Galloway, W.H.: Criteria by which toxemia of pregnancy may be diagnosed from unlabeled formalin-fixed placentas. Amer. J. Obstet. Gynecol. **82**:277–290, 1961.

Battistelli, M., Burattini, S., Pomini, F., Scavo, M., Caruso, A. and Falcieri, E.: Ultrastructural study on human placenta from intrauterine growth retardation cases. Microscopy Res. Techn. **65**:150–158, 2004.

Beaufils, M., Uzan, S., Donsimoni, R. and Colau, J.C.: Prevention of pre-eclampsia by early antiplatelet therapy. Lancet **i**:840–842, 1985.

Beck, J.S., Oakley, C.L. and Rowell, N.R.: Transplacental passage of antinuclear antibody. Arch. Dermatol. **93**:656–663, 1966.

Beek, E.v. and Peeters, L.L.H.: Pathogenesis of preeclampsia: a comprehensive model. Obstet. Gynecol. Survey **53**:233–239, 1998.

Beischer, N.A., Sivasamboo, R., Vohra, S., Silpisornkosal, S. and Reid, S.: Placental hypertrophy in severe pregnancy anaemia. J. Obstet. Gynaecol. Brit. Commonw. **77**:398–409, 1970.

Beller, F.K., Intorp, H.W., Losse, H., Loew, H., Moenninghoff, W., Schmidt, E.H. and Grundmann, E.: Malignant nephrosclerosis during pregnancy and in the postpartum period (the uremic hemolytic syndrome). Amer. J. Obstet. Gynecol. **125**:633–639, 1976.

Belliardo, F., Massano, G. and Accomo, S.: Amatoxins do not cross the placental barrier. Lancet **1**:1381, 1983.

Bendon, R.W., Wilson, J., Getahun, B. and Bel-Kahn, J.v.d.: A maternal death due to thrombotic disease associated with anticardiolipin antibody. Arch. Pathol. Lab. Med. **111**:370–373, 1987.

Benigni, A., Gregorini, G., Frusca, T., Chiabrando, C., Ballerini, S., Valcamonico, A., Orisio, S., Piccinelli, A., Pinciroli, V., Fanelli, R., Gastaldi, A. and Remuzzi, G.: Effect of low-dose aspirin on fetal and maternal generation of thromboxane by platelets in women at risk for pregnancy-induced hypertension. NEJM **321**:357–362, 1989.

Benirschke, K. and Gille, J.: Placental pathology and asphyxia. In, Intrauterine Asphyxia and the Developing Fetal Brain, L. Gluck, ed.. Year Book Medical Publishers, Chicago, 1977.

Bennett, R.M., Peller, J.S. and Merritt, M.M.: Defective DNA-receptor function in systemic lupus erythematosus and related diseases: evidence for an autoantibody influencing cell physiology. Lancet **i**:186–188, 1986.

Bentsi-Enchill, K.K. and Konotey-Ahulu, F.I.D.: Thirteen children from twelve pregnancies in sickle-cell thalassemia. Brit. Med. J. **2**:762, 1969.

Bernstein, I.M., Plociennik, K., Stahle, S., Badger, G.J. and Secker-Walker, R.: Impact of maternal cigarette smoking on fetal growth and body composition. Amer. J. Obstet. Gynecol. **183**:883–886, 2000.

Bierman, H. R., Aggeler, P.M., Thelander, H., Kelly, K.H. and Cordes, F.L.: Leukemia and pregnancy. JAMA **161**:220–223, 1956.

Birkeland, S.A. and Kristofferson, K.: Pre-eclampsia—a state of mother-fetus immune imbalance. Lancet **ii**:720–723, 1979.

Björk, O. and Persson, B.: Villous structure in different parts of the cotyledon in placentas of insulin-dependent diabetic women. Acta Obstet. Gynecol. Scand. **63**:37–43, 1984.

Blackburn, W.R., Kaplan, H.S. and McKay, D.G.: Morphologic changes in the developing rat placenta following prednisolone administration. Amer. J. Obstet. Gynecol. **92**:234–246, 1965.

Blakley, P.M.: Experimental teratology of ethanol. In, Issues and Reviews in Teratology. H. Kalter, ed., pp. 237–282. Plenum Press, New York, 1983.

Blaschitz, A., Hutter, H. and Dohr, G.: HLA class I protein expression in the human placenta. Early Pregnancy **5**:67–69, 2001.

Blanc, W.A., Mattison, D.R., Kane, R. and Chauhan, P.: L.S.D., intrauterine amputations, and amniotic-band syndrome. Lancet **2**:158–159, 1971.

Bleyl, U. und Büsing, C.M.: Disseminierte intravasale Gerinnung und perinataler Schock. Verhandl. Deutsche Gesellsch. Pathol. **53**:495–501, 1969.

Boe, F.: Vascular changes in premature separation of the normally implanted placenta. Acta Obstetr. Gynecol. Scand. **38**:441–443, 1951.

Boggess, K.A., Easterling, T.R. and Raghu, G.: Management and outcome of pregnant women with interstitial and restrictive lung disease. Amer. J. Obstet. Gynecol. **173**:1007–1014, 1995.

Bose, P., Black, S., Kadyrov, M., Bartz, C., Shlebak, A., Regan, L. and Huppertz, B.: Adverse effects of lupus anticoagulant positive blood sera on placental viability can be prevented by heparin in vitro. Amer. J. Obstet. Gynecol. **191**:2125–2131, 2004.

Bouteiller, P. Le, Pizzato, N., Barakonyi, A. and Solier, C.: HLA-G, pre-eclampsia, immunity and vascular events. J. Reprod. Immunol. **59**:219–234, 2003.

Bowie, E.J., Thompson, J.H., Pascuzzi, C.A. and Owen, C.A.: Thrombosis in systemic lupus erythematosus despite circulating anticoagulants. J. Lab. Clin. Med. **62**:416–430, 1963.

Branch, D.W. and Rodgers, G.M.: Induction of endothelial cell tissue factor activity by sera from patients with antiphospholipid syndrome: a possible mechanism of thrombosis. Amer. J. Obstet. Gynecol. **168**:206–210, 1993.

Branch, D.W., Scott, J.R., Kochenour, N.K. and Hershgold, E.: Obstetric complications associated with the lupus anticoagulant. NEJM **313**:1322–1326, 1985.

Branch, D.W., Andres, R., Digre, K.B., Rote, N.S. and Scott, J.R.: The association of antiphospholipid antibodies with severe preeclampsia. Obstet. Gynecol. **73**:541–545, 1989.

Branch, D.W., Silver, R., Pierangeli, S., Leeuwen, I. van and Harris, E.N.: Antiphospholipid antibodies other than lupus anticoagulant and anticardiolipin antibodies in women with recurrent pregnancy loss, fertile controls, and antiphospholipid syndrome. Obstet. Gynecol. **89**:549–555, 1997.

Brandt, J.T., Triplett, D.A., Musgrave, K. and Orr, C.: The sensitivity of different coagulation reagents to the presence of lupus anticoagulants. Arch. Pathol. Lab. Med. **111**:120–124, 1987.

Brent, R.L.: The indirect effect of radiation on embryonic development. II. Irradiation of the placenta. Amer. J. Dis. Child. **100**:103–108, 1960.

Bresnihan, B., Grigor, R.R., Oliver, M., Lewkonia, R.M., Hughes, G.R.V., Lovins, R.E. and Faulk, W.P.: Immunological mechanism for spontaneous abortion in systemic lupus erythematosus. Lancet **ii**:1205–1207, 1977.

Brodsky, I., Baren, M., Kahn, S.B., Lewis, G. and Tellem, M.: Metastatic malignant melanoma from mother to fetus. Cancer **18**:1048–1054, 1965.

Brosens, I. and Renaer, M.: On the pathogenesis of placental infarcts in pre-eclampsia. J. Obstetr. Gynaecol. Brit. Cwlth. **79**:794–799, 1972.

Brosens, I., Robertson, W.B. and Dixon, H.G.: The physiological response of the vessels of the placental bed to normal pregnancy. J. Pathol. Bacteriol. **93**:569–579, 1967.

Brosens, I.A., Robertson, W.B. and Dixon, H.G.: The role of the spiral arteries in the pathogenesis of preeclampsia. In, Obstetrics and Gynecology Annual: 1972, R.M. Wynn, ed. Vol. I. 177–191, 1972. Appleton-Century-Crofts, New York.

Brosens, I., Dixon, H.G. and Robertson, W.B.: Prostaglandins and pre-eclampsia. Lancet **ii**:412–413, 1974.

Brosens, J.J., Pijnenborg, R. and Brosens, I.A.: The myometrial junctional zone spiral arteries in normal and abnormal pregnancies. Amer. J. Obstet. Gynecol. **187**:1416–1423, 2002.

Brown, S., Merkow, A., Wiener, M. and Khajezadeh, J.: Low birth weight in babies born to mothers with sickle cell trait. JAMA **221**:1404–1405, 1972.

Brownscheidele, C.M. and Davis, D.L.: Diabetes in pregnancy: a preliminary study of the pancreas, placenta and malformations in the BB Wistar rat. Placenta [Suppl.] **3**:203–216, 1981.

Bruner, J.P., Landon, M.B. and Gabbe, S.: Diabetes and Graves' disease in pregnancy complicated by maternal allergies to antithyroid medication. Obstet. Gynecol. **72**:443–445, 1988.

Buchanan, N.M.M., Khamashta, M.A., Morton, K.E., Kerslake, S., Baguley, E. and Hughes, G.R.V.: A study of 100 high risk lupus pregnancies. Amer. J. Reprod. Immunol. **28**:192–194, 1992.

Budliger, H.: Plazentarveränderungen und ihre Beziehung zur Spättoxikose und perinatalen kindlichen Sterblichkeit. Fortschr. Geburtsh. Gynäkol. **17**:86–110, 1964.

Buescher, M.A., McClamrock, H.D. and Adashi, E.Y.: Cushing syndrome in pregnancy. Review. Obstet. Gynecol. **79**:130–137, 1992.

Burrow, G.N. and Ferris, T.F.: Medical Complications during Pregnancy. Saunders & Harcourt Brace Jovanovich, Philadelphia, 1988.

Burrow, G.N., Fisher, D.A. and Larsen, P.R.: Maternal and fetal thyroid function. NEJM **331**:1072–1078, 1994.

Burrows, D.A., O'Neil, T.J. and Sorrells, T.L.: Successful twin pregnancy after renal transplant maintained on cyclosporin A immunosuppression. Obstet. Gynecol. **72**:459–461, 1988.

Burstein, R., Berns, A.W., Hirata, Y. and Blumenthal, H.T.: A comparative histo- and immunopathological study of the placenta in diabetes mellitus and in erythroblastosis fetalis. Amer. J. Obstet. Gynecol. **86**:66–76, 1963.

Burton, G.J. and Jauniaux, E.: Placental oxidative stress: from miscarriage to preeclampsia. J. Soc. Gynecol. Investig. **11**:342–352, 2004.

Bussel, J.B., Zabusky, M.R., Berkowitz, R.L. and McFarland, J.G.: Fetal alloimmune thrombocytopenia. NEJM **337**:22–26, 1997.

Bylock, A., Bondjers, G., Jansson, I. and Hansson, H.-A.: Surface ultrastructure of human arteries with special reference to the effects of smoking. Acta Pathol. Microbiol. Scand. [A]. **87**:201–209, 1979.

Cameron, H.M. and Park, W.W.: Decidual tissue within the lung. J. Obstetr. Gynaecol. Brit. Cwlth. **72**:748–754, 1965.

Campbell, W.A.: Fetal malignant melanoma: ultrasound presentation and review of the literature. Obstet. Gynecol. **70**:434–439, 1987.

Cannon, J.F.: Pregnancy and pheochromocytoma. Obstet. Gynecol. **11**:43–48, 1958.

Cardwell, M.S.: Ultrasound diagnosis of abruptio placentae with fetomaternal hemorrhage. Amer. J. Obstetr. Gynecol. **157**:358–359, 1987.

Cariou, R., Tobelem, G., Soria, C. and Caen, J.: Inhibition of protein C activation by endothelial cells in the presence of lupus anticoagulant. NEJM **314**:1193–1194, 1986.

Carp, H.J.A., FrenkeL, Y., Many, A., Menashe, Y., Mashiach, S., Nebel, L., Toder, V. and Serr, D.M.: Fetal demise associated with lupus anticoagulant: clinical features and results of treatment. Gynecol. Obstet. Invest. **28**:178–184, 1989.

Carreras, L.O., Defreyn, G., Machin, S.J., Vermylen, J., Deman, R., Spitz, B. and Assche, A.v.: Arterial thrombosis, intrauterine death and "lupus" anticoagulant: detection of immunoglobulin interfering with prostacyclin formation. Lancet **i**:244–246, 1981a.

Carreras, L.O., Vermylen, J., Spitz, B. and Assche, A.v.: "Lupus" anticoagulant and inhibition of prostacyclin formation in patients with repeated abortion, intrauterine growth retardation and intrauterine death. Brit. J. Obstet. Gynaecol. **88**:890–894, 1981b.

Carreras, L.O., Perez, G.N., Vega, H.R. and Casavilla, F.: Lupus anticoagulant and recurrent fetal loss: Successful treatment with gammaglobulin. Lancet **ii**:393–394, 1988.

Carter, B.: Premature separation of the normally implanted placenta. Six deaths due to gross bilateral cortical necrosis of the kidneys. Obstetr. Gynecol. **29**:30–33, 1967.

Carter, J.E., Vellios, F. and Huber, C.P.: Histologic classification and incidence of circulatory lesions of the human placenta, with a review of the literature. Amer. J. Clin. Pathol. **40**:374–378, 1963a.

Carter, J.E., Vellios, F. and Huber, C.P.: Circulatory factors governing the viability of the human placenta, based on a morphologic study. Amer. J. Clin. Pathol. **40**:363–373, 1963b.

Catlin, E.A., Roberts, J.D., Erana, R., Preffer, F.I., Ferry, J.A., Kelliher, A.S., Atkins, L. and Weinstein, H.J.: Transplacental transmission of natural-killer-cell lymphoma. NEJM **341**:85–91, 1999.

Cavanagh, D., Rao, P.S., Tung, K.S.K. and Gastoni, L.: Eclamptogenic toxemia: the development of an experimental model in the subhuman primate. Amer. J. Obstetr. Gynecol. **120**:183–196, 1974.

Cavanagh, D., Rao, P.S., Tsai, C.C. and O'Connor, T.C.: Experimental toxemia in the pregnant primate. Amer. J. Obstetr. Gynecol. **128**:75–85, 1977.

Cavanagh, D., Rao, P.S., Knuppel, R.A., Desai, U. and Balis, J.U.: Pregnancy-induced hypertension: Development of a model in the pregnant primate (*Papio anubis*). Amer. J. Obstet. Gynecol. **151**:987–999, 1985.

Cavell, B.: Transplacental metastasis of malignant melanoma: report of a case. Acta Paediatr. [Suppl.] **146**:37–40, 1963.

Chaiworapongsa, T., Gervasi, M.-T., Refuerzo, J., Espinoza, J., Yoshimatsu, J., Berman, S. and Romero, R.: Maternal lymphocyte subpopulations (CD45RA+ and CD45RO+) in preeclampsia. Amer. J. Obstet. Gynecol. **187**:889–893, 2002.

Chaiworapongsa, T., T., Romero, R., Espinoza, J., Bujold, E., Kim, Y.M., Gonçalves, L.F., Gomez, R. and Edwin, S.: Evidence supporting a role for blockade of the vascular endothelial growth factor system in the pathophysiology of preeclampsia. Amer. J. Obstet. Gynecol. **190**:1541–1550, 2004.

Chalmers, I.: Salt, pregnancy, hypertension—and literature searches. Lancet **ii**:1146, 1988.

Chasnoff, I.J., Burns, W.J., Schnoll, S.H. and Burns, K.A.: Cocaine use in pregnancy. NEJM **313**:666–669, 1985.

Chasnoff, I.J., Bussey, M.E., Savich, R. and Stack, C.M.: Perinatal cerebral infarction and maternal cocaine use. J. Pediatr. **108**:210–213, 1986.

Chasnoff, I.J., Griffith, D.R., MacGregor, S., Dirkes, K. and Burns, K.A.: Temporal patterns of cocaine use in pregnancy: perinatal outcome. JAMA **261**:1741–1744, 1989.

Chasnoff, I.J., Landress, H.J. and Barrett, M.E.: The prevalence of illicit-drug or alcohol use during pregnancy and discrepancies in mandatory reporting in Pinellas County, Florida. NEJM **322**:1202–1206, 1990.

Chávez, G.F., Mulinare, J. and Cordero, J.F.: Maternal cocaine use during early pregnancy as a risk factor for congenital urogenital anomalies. JAMA **262**:795–798, 1989.

Chen, Y., Pederson, L.L. and Lefcoe, N.M.: Passive smoking and low birthweight. Lancet **2**:54–55, 1989.

Chesley, L.C.: Diagnosis of preeclampsia. Obstetr. Gynecol. **65**:423–425, 1985.

Cheung, T.H., Leung, A. and Chang, A.: Macrosomic babies. Austr. N. Z. J. Obstetr. Gynaecol. **30**:319–322, 1990.

Chrisomalis, L., Baxi, L.V. and Heller, D.: Chronic lymphocytic leukemia in pregnancy. Amer. J. Obstet. Gynecol. **175**:1381–1382, 1996.

Christianson, R.E.: Gross differences observed in the placentas of smokers and nonsmokers. Amer. J. Epidemiol. **110**:178–187, 1979.

Cibils, L.A.: The placenta and newborn infant in hypertensive conditions. Amer. J. Obstetr. Gynecol. **118**:256–268, 1974.

Clark, D.A.: Does immunological intercourse prevent preeclampsia? Lancet **344**:969–970, 1994.

Clarson, C., Tevaarwerk, G.J.M., Harding, P.G.R., Chance, G.W. and Haust, M.D.: Placental weight in diabetic pregnancies. Placenta **10**:275–281, 1989.

Clausen, H.V., Jorgensen, J.C. and Ottesen, B.: Stem villous arteries from the placentas of heavy smokers: Functional and mechanical properties. Amer. J. Obstet. Gynecol. **180**:476–482, 1999.

Cnattingius, S., Mills, J.L., Yuen, J., Eriksson, O. and Ros, H.S.: The paradoxical effect of smoking in preeclamptic pregnancies: Smoking reduces the incidence but increases the rates of perinatal mortality, abruptio placentae, and intrauterine growth retardation. Amer. J. Obstet. Gynecol. **177**:156–161, 1997.

Cockell, A.P., Learmont, J.G., Smárason, A.K., Redman, C.W.G., Sargent, I.L. and Poston, L.: Human placental syncytiotrophoblast microvillous membranes impair maternal vascular endothelial function. Brit. J. Obstet. Gynaecol. **104**:235–240, 1997.

Coen, R.W., Papile, L.-A., Figueroa, R. and Henderson, V.M.: Infant survival following protracted fetoplacental separation. Pediatrics 53:760–761, 1974.

Colbern, G.T., Chiang, M.H. and Main, E.K.: Expression of the nonclassic histocompatibility antigen HLA-G by preeclamptic placenta. Amer. J. Obstet. Gynecol. 170:1244–1250, 1994.

Combs, C.A., Easterling, T.R., Schmucker, B.C. and Benedetti, T.J.: Hemodynamic observations during paroxysmal hypertension in a pregnancy with a pheochromocytoma. Obstet. Gynecol. 74:439–441, 1989.

Combs, C.A., Katz, M.A., Kitzmiller, J.L. and Brescia, R.J.: Experimental preeclampsia of the lower aorta: Validation with longitudinal blood pressure measurements in conscious rhesus monkeys. Amer. J. Obstet. Gynecol. 169:215–223, 1993.

Cotter, A.M., Martin, C.M., O'Leary, J.J. and Daly, S.F.: Increased fetal DNA in the maternal circulation in early pregnancy is associated with an increased risk of preeclampsia. Amer. J. Obstet. Gynecol. 191:515–520, 2004.

Cove, D.H. and Johnson, P.: Fetal hyperthyroidism: experience of treatment in four siblings. Lancet 1:430–432, 1985.

Covone, A.E., Mutton, D., Johnson, P.M. and Adinolfi, M.: Trophoblast cells in peripheral blood from pregnant women. Lancet ii:841–843, 1984.

Cowchock, F.S., Reece, E.A., Balaban, D., Branch, D.W. and Plouffe, L.: Repeated fetal losses associated with antiphospholipid antibodies: a collaborative randomized trial comparing prednisone with low-dose heparin treatment. Amer. J. Obstet. Gynecol. 166:1318–1323, 1992.

Cowchock, S.: Autoantibodies and pregnancy loss. Editorial. NEJM 337:197–198, 1997.

Cramblett, H.G., Friedman, J.L. and Najjar, S.: Leukemia in an infant born of a mother with leukemia. NEJM 259:727–729, 1958.

Cregler, L.L. and Mark, H.: Medical complications of cocaine abuse. NEJM 315:1495–1500, 1986.

Crocker, I.P., Cooper, S., Ong, S.C. and Baker, P.N.: Differences in apoptotic susceptibility of cytotrophoblasts and syncytiotrophoblasts in normal pregnancy to those complicated with preeclampsia and intrauterine growth restriction. Amer. J. Pathol. 162:637–643, 2003.

Cross, R.G., O'Connor, M.H. and Holland, P.J.: Placental metastasis of a breast carcinoma. J. Obstet. Gynaecol. Brit. Emp. 58:810–811, 1951.

Cruveiller, J., Harpey, J.-P., Vernon, P., Cannat, A., Delattre, A., Hervet, E., Lafourcade, J. et Turpin, R.: Lupus érythémateux systémique. Transmission de manifestations cliniques et de facteurs biologiques de la mère au nouveu-né. Arch. Franc. Pediatr. 27:195–209, 1970.

Cunningham, F.G. and Lindheimer, M.D.: Hypertension in pregnancy. NEJM 326:927–932, 1992.

Cunningham, F.G., Lowe, T., Guss, S. and Mason, R.: Erythrocyte morphology in women with severe preeclampsia. Preliminary observations with scanning electron microscopy. Amer. J. Obstetr. Gynecol. 153:358–363, 1985.

Dadak, C., Leithner, C., Sinzinger, H. and Silberbauer, K.: Diminished prostacyclin formation in umbilical arteries of babies born to women who smoke. Lancet 1:94, 1981.

Daffos, F., Forester, F. and Kaplan, C.: Prenatal treatment of fetal alloimmune thrombocytopenia. Lancet 2:910, 1988.

Dameshek, W.: Systemic lupus erythematosus: a complex autoimmune disorder? Ann. Intern. Med. 48:707–730, 1958.

Darnige, L., Boutignon, H., Arvieux, J., Benhamou, E. and Kaplan, C.: Immune thrombocytopenia in a newborn from a mother with primary antiphospholipid syndrome. Amer. J. Hematol. 75:119–120, 2004.

Daunter, B.: Immunology of pregnancy: towards a unifying hypothesis. Eur. J. Obstet. Gynecol. Reprod. Med. 43:81–95, 1992.

Davey, D.A. and MacGillivray, I.: The classification and definition of the hypertensive disorders of pregnancy. Amer. J. Obstetr. Gynecol. 158:892–898, 1988.

Davey, D.A. and MacGillivray, I.: Classification of hypertensive disorders of pregnancy. Lancet ii:112, 1989.

Davis, L.E., Leveno, K.J. and Cunningham, F.G.: Hypothyroidism complicating pregnancy. Obstet. Gynecol. 72:108–112, 1988.

Davis, L.E., Lucas, M.J., Hankins, G.D.V., Roark, M.L. and Cunningham, F.G.: Thyrotoxicosis complicating pregnancy. Amer. J. Obstet. Gynecol. 160:63–70, 1989.

Davison, J.M.: Renal transplantation and pregnancy. Amer. J. Kidney Dis. 9:374–380, 1987.

Deaver, J.E., Leppert, P.C. and Zaroulis, C.G.: Neonatal alloimmune thrombocytopenic purpura: a case report. Amer. J. Obstet. Gynecol. 154:153–155, 1986.

Delerive, C., Locquet, F., Mallart, A., Janin, A. and Gosselin, B.: Placental metastasis from maternal bronchial oat cell carcinoma. Arch. Pathol. Lab. Med. 113:556–558, 1989.

Demers, L.M. and Gabbe, S.G.: Placental prostaglandin levels in pre-eclampsia. Amer. J. Obstetr. Gynecol. 126:137–139, 1976.

Demian, S.D.E., Donnelly, W.H., Frias, J.L. and Monif, G.R.G.: Placental lesions in congenital giant pigmented nevi. Amer. J. Clin. Pathol. 61:438–442, 1974.

Desoye, G. and Shafrir, E.: Placental metabolism and its regulation in health and diabetes. Molecular Aspects of Medicine 15:505–682, 1994.

Desoye, G. and Shafrir, E.: The human placenta in diabetic pregnancy. Diabetes Reviews 4:70–89, 1996.

Desoye, G., Hoffmann, H.H. and Weiss, P.A.M.: Insulin binding to trophoblast plasma membranes and placental glycogen content in well-controlled gestational diabetic women treated with diet or insulin, in well-controlled overt diabetic patients and in healthy control subjects. Diabetologia 35:45–55, 1992.

Diamandopoulos, G.Th. and Hertig, A.T.: Transmission of leukemia and allied diseases from mother to fetus. Obstet. Gynecol. 21:150–154, 1963.

DiFederico, E., Genbacev, O. and Fisher, S.J.: Preeclampsia is associated with widespread apoptosis of placental cytotrophoblasts within the uterine wall. Amer. J. Pathol. 155:293–301, 1999.

Dines, D.E. and Banner, E.A.: Sarcoidosis during pregnancy. Improvement in pulmonary function. JAMA 200:726–727, 1967.

Ditts, P.V.: Placental transfer of ethanol. Amer. J. Obstet. Gynecol. 112:1195–1198, 1970.

Dizon-Townson, D.S., Nelson, L.M., Easton, K. and Ward, K.: The factor V Leiden mutation may predispose women to severe preeclampsia. Amer. J. Obstet. Gynecol. 175:902–905, 1996.

Dizon-Townson, D.S., Meline, L., Nelson, L.M., Varner, M. and Ward, K.: Fetal carriers of the factor V Leiden mutation are prone to miscarriage and placental infarction. Amer. J. Obstet. Gynecol. **177**:402–405, 1997.

Dombrowski, M.P., Wolfe, H.M., Welch, R.A. and Evans, M.I.: Cocaine abuse is associated with abruptio placentae and decreased birth weight, but not shorter labor. Obstet. Gynecol. **77**:139–141, 1991.

Donegan, W.L.: Cancer and pregnancy. CA **33**:194–214, 1983.

Donvito, M.T.: Cocaine use during pregnancy: Adverse perinatal outcome. Amer. J. Obstet. Gynecol. **159**:786–787, 1988.

Doss, B.J., Jacques, S.M., Atty, S., Mayes, M.D. and Qureshi, F.: Maternal scleroderma: Placental findings and perinatal outcome. Modern Pathol. **11**:103A (abstract 593), 1998.

Dreifuss, F.E. and McKinney, W.M.: Wilson's disease (hepatolenticular degeneration) and pregnancy. JAMA **195**:960–962, 1966.

Driscoll, S.G.: The pathology of pregnancy complicated by diabetes mellitus. Med. Clin. North Amer. **49**:1053–1067, 1965.

Driscoll, S.G., Hicks, S.P., Copenhaver, E.H. and Easterday, C.L.: Acute radiation injury in two human fetuses. Arch. Pathol. **76**:113–119, 1963.

Druzin, M.L., Lockshin, M., Edersheim, T.G., Hutson, J.M., Krauss, A.L. and Kogut, E.: Second-trimester fetal monitoring and preterm delivery in pregnancies with systemic lupus erythematosus and/or circulating anticoagulant. Amer. J. Obstet. Gynecol. **157**:1503–1510, 1987.

Ducey, J., Schulman, H., Farmakides, G., Rochelson, B., Bracero, L., Fleischer, A., Guzman, E., Winter, D. and Penny, B.: A classification of hypertension in pregnancy based on Doppler velocimetry. Amer. J. Obstetr. Gynecol. **157**:680–685, 1987.

Duda, J.: Preeclampsia. Still an enigma. West. J. Med. **164**:315–320, 1996.

Duhring, J.L.: Pregnancy, rheumatoid arthritis, and intrauterine growth retardation. Amer. J. Obstet. Gynecol. **108**:325–326, 1970.

Dunlop, W., Hill, L.M., Landon, M.J., Oxley, A. and Jones, P.: Clinical relevance of coagulation and renal changes in preeclampsia. Lancet **ii**:346–349, 1978.

Dunn, D.T., Poddar, D., Serjeant, B.E. and Serjeant, G.R.: Fetal haemoglobin and pregnancy in homozygous sickle cell disease. Brit. J. Haematol. **72**:434–438, 1989.

Dyer, I. and McCaughey, E.V.: Abruptio placentae: a ten-year survey. Amer. J. Obstetr. Gynecol. **77**:1176–1184, 1959.

Easterling, T.R. and Benedetti, T.J.: Preeclampsia: a hyperdynamic disease model. Amer. J. Obstetr. Gynecol. **160**:1447–1453, 1989.

Easterling, T.R., Chadwick, H.S., Otto, C.M. and Benedetti, T.J.: Aortic stenosis in pregnancy. Obstet. Gynecol. **72**:113–118, 1988.

Editorial: Smoking during pregnancy. Brit. Med. J. **2**:339–340, 1968.

Editorial: Systemic lupus erythematosus in pregnancy. Lancet **338**:87–88, 1991.

Edson, J.R., Blaese, R.M., White, J.G. and Krivit, W.: Defibrination syndrome in an infant born after abruptio placentae. Amer. J. Obstet. Gynecol. **72**:342–346, 1968.

Elkind-Hirsch, K.E., Raynolds, M.V. and Goldzieher, J.W.: Comparison of immunoreactive gonadotropin-releasing hormone and human chorionic gonadotropin in term placentas from normal women and those with insulin-dependent and gestational diabetes. Amer. J. Obstet. Gynecol. **160**:71–78, 1989.

Elliott, J.P., Gilpin, B., Strong, T.H.Jr. and Finberg: Chronic abruption—oligohydramnios sequence. J. Reprod. Med. **43**:418–422, 1998.

El-Roeiy, A., Myers, S.A. and Gleicher, N.: The prevalence of autoantibodies and lupus anticoagulant in healthy pregnant women. Obstet. Gynecol. **75**:390–396, 1990.

Elsas, L.J., Whittemore, R. and Burrow, G.N.: Maternal and neonatal Graves' disease. JAMA **200**:250–252, 1967.

Elstein, Y., Eisenberg, V., Granovsky-Grisaru, S., Rabinovitz, R., Samueloff, A., Zimran, A. and Elstein, D.: Pregnancies in Gaucher disease: a 5-year study. Amer. J. Obstet. Gynecol. **190**:435–441, 2004.

Emmer, P.M., Joosten, I., Schut, M.H., Zusterzeel, P.L.M., Hendriks, J.C.M. and Steegers, E.A.P.: Shift in expression of HLA-G mRNA spliceforms in pregnancies complicated by preeclampsia. J. Soc. Gynecol. Investig. **11**:220–226, 2004.

Emmrich, P., Amendt, P. and Gödel, E.: Morphologie der Plazenta und neonatale Acidose bei mütterlichem Diabetes mellitus. Pathol. Microbiol. **40**:100–114, 1974.

Epstein, F.H.: Late vascular effects of toxemia of pregnancy. NEJM **271**:391–395, 1964.

Erskine, K.J, Iversen, S.A. and Davies, R.: An altered ratio of 18:2(9,11) to 18:2(9,12) linoleic acid in plasma phospholipids as a possible predictor of pre-eclampsia. Lancet **i**:554–555, 1985.

Esplin, M.S., Fausett, M.B., Fraser, A., Kerber, R., Mineau, G., Carrillo, J. and Varner, M.W.: Paternal and maternal components of the predisposition to preeclampsia. NEJM **344**:867–872, 2001.

Fadel, H.E. and Krauss, J.S.: Factor VII deficiency and pregnancy. Obstet. Gynecol. **73**:453–454, 1989.

Fagan, E.A.: Diseases of liver, biliary system, and pancreas. In, Maternal-Fetal Medicine. Principles and Practice. R.K. Creasy and R. Resnik, eds. W.B. Saunders, Philadelphia, 1994.

Farquharson, R.G., Compston, A. and Bloom, A.L.: Lupus anticoagulant: a place for pre-pregnancy treatment? Lancet **ii**:842–843, 1985.

Feinstein, D.I.: Lupus anticoagulant, thrombosis, and fetal loss. NEJM **313**:1348–1350, 1985.

Feraboli, M.: La placenta nelle cardiopatie. Quad. Clin. Ostet. Ginecol. (Genoa) **6**:219–230, 1951.

Fiddler, G.I.: Propranolol and pregnancy. Lancet **2**:722–723, 1974.

Fischer, U. and Horký, Z.: Vorläufige Untersuchungen zum Glykogengehalt sowie Sauerstoff- und Glukoseverbrauch der Plazenta in vitro bei Diabetes mellitus. In, Schwangerschaft und Neugeborenes der zuckerkranken Frau. (IV. Intern. Symp. Diabetesfragen). G. Mohnike, ed., Berlin, pp. 82–88, VEB Verlag Volk u. Gesundheit 1966.

Fisk, N.M. and Storey, G.N.B.: Fetal outcome in obstetric cholestasis. Brit. J. Obstet. Gynaecol. **95**:1137–1143, 1988.

Fitzgerald, D.J., Rocki, W., Murray, R., Mayo, G. and Fitzgerald G.A.: Thromboxane A_2 synthesis in pregnancy-induced hypertension. Lancet **335**:751–754, 1990.

Fox, H.: White infarcts of the placenta. J. Obstetr. Gynaecol. Brit. Cwlth. **70**:980–991, 1963.

Fox, H.: Pathology of the placenta in maternal diabetes mellitus. Obstet. Gynecol. **34**:792–798, 1969.

Fox, H.: Effect of hypoxia on trophoblast in organ culture. Amer. J. Obstetr. Gynecol. **107**:1058–1064, 1970.

Fox, H.: Pathology of the Placenta. Saunders, London, 1978.

Fox, L.P., Grandi, J., Johnson, A.H., Watrous, W.G. and Johnson, M.J.: Pheochromocytoma associated with pregnancy. Amer. J. Obstet. Gynecol. **104**:288–294, 1969.

Francis, S.T., Duncan, K.R., Moore, R.J., Baker, P.N., Johnson, I.R. and Gowland, P.A.: Non-invasive mapping of placental perfusion. Lancet **351**:1397–1399, 1998.

Frank, D.A., Zuckerman, B.S., Amaro, H., Aboagye, K., Bauchner, H., Cabral, H., Fried, L., Hingson, R., Kayne, H., Levenson, S.M., Parker, S., Reece, H. and Vinci, R.: Cocaine use during pregnancy: prevalence and correlates. Pediatrics **82**:888–895, 1988.

Freedman, W.L. and McMahon, F.J.: Placental metastasis: review of the literature and report of a case of metastatic melanoma. Obstet. Gynecol. **16**:550–560, 1960.

Freese, U.E.: A placental evaluation of drug addiction in pregnancy. J. Reprod. Med. **20**:307–315, 1978.

Friedman, S.A.: Preeclampsia: a review of the role of prostaglandins. Obstetr. Gynecol. **71**:122–137, 1988.

Fujikura, T. and Froehlich, L.: Diagnosis of sickling by placental examination. Amer. J. Obstet. Gynecol. **100**:1122–1124, 1968.

Fulroth, R., Phillips, B. and Durand, D.J.: Perinatal outcome of infants exposed to cocaine and/or heroin in utero. Amer. J. Dis. Child. **143**:905–910, 1989.

Gau, G.S., Bhundia, J., Napier, K. and Ryder, T.A.: The worm that wasn't. Lancet **i**:1160–1161, 1983.

George, P.A., Fortner, J.G. and Pack, G.T.: Melanoma with pregnancy: a report of 115 cases. Cancer **13**:854–859, 1960.

Gerretsen, G., Huisjes, H.J. and Elema, J.D.: Morphological changes of the spiral arteries in the placental bed in relation to pre-eclampsia and fetal growth retardation. Brit. J. Obstetr. Gynaecol. **88**:876–881, 1981.

Gerretsen, G., Huisjes, H.J., Hardonk, M.J. and Elema, J.D.: Trophoblastic alterations in the placental bed in relation to physiological changes in spiral arteries. Brit. J. Obstetr. Gynaecol. **90**:34–39, 1983.

Geva, E., Amit, A., Lerner-Geva, L. and Lessing, J.B.: Prevention of early pregnancy loss in autoantibody seropositive women. Lancet **351**:34–35, 1998.

Ghabour, M.S., Eis, A.L.W., Brockman, D.E., Pollock, J.S. and Myatt, L.: Immunohistochemical characterization of placental nitric oxide synthase expression in preeclampsia. Amer. J. Obstet. Gynecol. **173**:687–694, 1995.

Gilbert, W.M., Lafferty, C.M., Benirschke, K. and Resnik, R.: Lack of specific placental abnormality associated with cocaine use. Amer. J. Obstetr. Gynecol. **163**:998–999, 1990.

Giles, W.B., Trudinger, B.J. and Baird, P.J.: Fetal umbilical artery blood flow velocity waveforms and placental resistance: pathological correlation. Brit. J. Obstetr. Gynaecol. **92**:31–35, 1985.

Gille, J.H., Moore, D.G. and Sedgwick, C.J.: Placental infarction: a sign of preeclampsia in a Patas monkey (*Erythrocebus patas*). Lab. Animal Sci. **27**:120–121, 1977.

Ginsburg, J. and Jeacock, M.K.: Placental lactate production in toxemia of pregnancy. Amer. J. Obstetr. Gynecol. **98**:239–244, 1967.

Gitlin, D., Kumate, J. and Morales, C.: Placental insulin transport. Pediatrics **33**:65–69, 1965.

Gleicher, N.: Antiphospholipid antibodies and reproductive failure: what they do and what they do not do; how to, and how not to treat! Human Reprod. **12**:13–16, 1997.

Gleicher, N. and Friberg, J.: IgM gammopathy and the lupus anticoagulant syndrome in habitual aborters. JAMA **253**: 3278–3281, 1985.

Goldstein, D.P. and Berkowitz, R.S.: Single-agent chemotherapy. In, Gestational Trophoblastic Disease. A.E. Szulman and H.J. Buchsbaum, eds., pp. 135–145. Springer-Verlag, New York, 1987.

Goodlin, R.C., Anderson, J.C. and Skiles, T.L.: Pruritus and hyperplacentosis. Obstet. Gynecol. **66**:36S–38S, 1985.

Goodman, R.M., Gresham, G.E. and Roberts, P.L.: Outcome of pregnancy in patients with hereditary hemorrhagic telangiectasia: a retrospective study of 40 patients and 80 matched controls. Fertil. Steril. **18**:272–277, 1967.

Goodwin, T.M., Gazit, G. and Gordon, E.M.: Heterozygous protein C deficiency presenting as severe protein C deficiency and peripartum thrombosis: successful treatment with protein C concentrate. Obstet. Gynecol. **86**:662–664, 1995.

Göpel, W., Ludwig, M., Junge, A.K., Kohlmann, T., Diedrich, K. and Möller, J.: Selection pressure for the factor-V-Leiden mutation and embryo implantation. Lancet **358**:1238–1239, 2001.

Gött, E.: Lupus erythematodes disseminatus: Schwangerschaft und Geburt. Deutsch. Med. Wschr. **94**:274–279, 1969.

Goujard, J., Rumeau, E. and Schwartz, D.: Smoking during pregnancy, stillbirth and abruptio placentae. Biomedicine **23**:20–22, 1975.

Goujard, J., Kaminski, M., Rumeau-Rouquette, C. and Schwartz, D.: Maternal smoking, alcohol consumption, and abruptio placenta. (Letter to the editor). Amer. J. Obstet. Gynecol. **130**:738–739, 1978.

Graham, C.H. and McCrae, K.R.: Altered expression of gelatinase and surface-associated plasminogen activator activity by trophoblast cells isolated from placentas of preeclamptic patients. Amer. J. Obstet. Gynecol. **175**:555–562, 1996.

Granger, J.P., Alexander, B.T., Llinas, M.T., Bennett, W.A. and Khalil, R.A.: Pathophysiology of preeclampsia: linking placental ischemia/hypoxia with microvascular dysfunction. Microcirculation **9**:147–160, 2002.

Gratton, R.J., Knight, S., Heine, R.P., Laifer, S.A., Harger, J.H., Bontempo, F.A. and Hassett, A.C.: Activated protein C resistance (APCr) in normal pregnancy. Amer. J. Obstet. Gynecol. **176**:SPO abstract S172; #603; 1997.

Greco, M.A., Klein, S. and Bigelow, B.: Lymphocytosis in the first-trimester placenta of a mother taking diphenylhydantoin. NEJM **289**:867–868, 1973.

Greco, M.A., Kamat, B.R. and Demopoulos, R.I.: Placental protein distribution in maternal diabetes mellitus: an immunocytochemical study. Pediatr. Pathol. **9**:679–690, 1989.

Greer, I.A.: Thrombosis in pregnancy: maternal and fetal issues. Lancet **353**:1258–1265, 1999.

Grennan, D.M., McCormick, J.N., Wojtacha, D., Carty, M. and Behan, W.: Immunological studies of the placenta in systemic lupus erythematosus. Ann. Rheum. Dis. **37**:129–134, 1978.

Griffin, J.F.T. and Wilson, E.W.: Pre-eclampsia: a state of mother-fetus immune imbalance. Lancet **ii**:1366–1367, 1979.

Grimes, E.M., Fayez, J.A. and Miller, G.L.: Cushing's syndrome and pregnancy. Obstet. Gynecol. **42**:550–559, 1973.

Grimes, D.A., LeBolt, S.A., Grimes, K.R. and Wingo, P.A.: Systemic lupus erythematosus and reproductive function: a case-control study. Amer. J. Obstet. Gynecol. **153**:179–186, 1985.

Grimmer, D., Landas, S. and Kemp, J.D.: IgM antitrophoblast antibodies in a patient with a pregnancy-associated lupuslike disorder, vasculitis, and recurrent intrauterine fetal demise. Arch. Pathol. Lab. Med. **112**:191–193, 1988.

Groot, C.J.M. de, O'Brien, T.J. and Taylor, R.N.: Biochemical evidence of impaired trophoblastic invasion of decidual stroma in women destined to have preeclampsia. Amer. J. Obstet. Gynecol. **175**:24–29, 1996.

Grossman, R.A. and Goldberg, E.H.: Incidence and recurrence rate of abruptio placentae in Sweden. Obstetr. Gynecol. **69**:280–281, 1987.

Gruenwald, P., Levin, H. and Yousem, H.: Abruption and premature separation of the placenta. Amer. J. Obstetr. Gynecol. **102**:604–610, 1968.

Gujrati, V.R., Shanker, K., Vrat, S., Chandravati, M.S. and Parmar, S.S.: Novel appearance of placental nuclear monoamine oxidase: biochemical and histochemical evidence for hyperserotonomic state in preeclampsia-eclampsia. Amer. J. Obstet. Gynecol. **175**:1543–1550, 1996.

Gunther, R. and Harer, W.: Systemic scleroderma and pregnancy. Obstet. Gynecol. **23**:297–300, 1964.

Gusdon, J.P., Heise, E.R. and Herbst, G.A.: Studies of lymphocyte populations in pre-eclampsia-eclampsia. Amer. J. Obstetr. Gynecol. **129**:255–259, 1977.

Gusdon, J.P., Heise, E.R., Quinn, K.J. and Matthews, L.C.: Lymphocyte subpopulations in normal and preeclampsia pregnancies. Amer. J. Reprod. Immunol. **5**:28–31, 1984.

Haile, H.: Über Schädigung des Neugeborenen bei Eklampsie. Z. Geburtsh. Gynäkol. **120**:334–352, 1940.

Halberstadt, E., Schneider, D. und Gerber, E.: Über die vorzeitige Lösung der normal inserierten Placenta. Gynaecologia **167**:491–502, 1969.

Handin, R.I.: Neonatal immune thrombocytopenia—the doctor's dilemma. New Engl. J. Med. **305**:951–953, 1981.

Hanretti, K.P., Whittle, M.J. and Rubin, P.C.: Doppler uteroplacental waveforms in pregnancy-induced hypertension: a re-appraisal. Lancet **i**:850–852, 1988.

Haour, F. and Bertrand, J.: Insulin receptors in the plasma membranes of human placenta. J. Clin. Endocrinol. Metab. **38**:334–337, 1974.

Hardardottier, H., Kelly, K., Bork, M.D., Cusick, W., Campbell, W.A. and Rodis, J.: Atypical presentation of preeclampsia in high-order multifetal gestations. Obstet. Gynecol. **87**:370–374, 1996.

Harper, M.A., McVeigh, J.E., Thompson, W., Ardill, J.E.S. and Buchanan, K.D.: Successful pregnancy in association with Zollinger-Ellison syndrome. Amer. J. Obstet. Gynecol. **173**:863–864, 1995.

Harris, B.A., Gore, H. and Flowers, C.E.: Peripheral placental separation: a possible relationship to premature labor. Obstetr. Gynecol. **66**:774–778, 1985.

Haupt, H.: Über das Schocksyndrom des Neugeborenen nach vorzeitiger Plazentalösung. Münch. Med. Wchschr. **105**:441–449, 1963.

Haust, M.D.: Maternal diabetes mellitus—effects on the fetus and placenta. In, Perinatal Diseases. R.L. Naeye, J.M. Kissane and N. Kaufman eds., pp. 201–285. Williams & Wilkins, Baltimore, 1981.

Haust, M.D., Heras, J.L. and Harding, P.G.: Fat-containing uterine smooth muscle cells in "toxemia": possible relevance to atherosclerosis? Science **195**:1353–1354, 1977.

Hayes, G.W., Walsh, C.R. and d'Alessandro, E.E.: Scleroderma in pregnancy: report of a case. Obstet. Gynecol. **19**:273–274, 1962.

Haynes, D.M.: Experimental abruptio placentae in the rabbit. Amer. J. Obstetr. Gynecol. **85**:626–645, 1963.

Hayslett, J.P. and Reece, E.A.: Systemic lupus erythematosus in pregnancy. Clin. Perinatol. **12**:539–549, 1985.

Heite, H.-J. and Kaden, G.: Metastasierung bösartiger Tumoren, insbesondere des malignen Melanomas, in Plazenta und Kind. Münch. Med. Wochenschr. **114**:1909–1913, 1972.

Hefler, L., Jirecek, S., Heim, K., Grimm, C., Antensteiner, G., Zeillinger, R., Husslein, P. and Tempfer, C.: Genetic polymorphisms associated with thrombophilia and vascular disease in women with unexplained late intrauterine fetal death: a multicenter study. J. Soc. Gynecol. Invest. **11**:42–44, 2004.

Heller, D.S., Rush, D. and Baergen, R.N.: Subchorionic hematoma associated with thrombophilia: report of three cases. Pediatr. Developm. Pathol. **6**:261–264, 2003.

Hennessey, J.P. and Rottino, A.: Hodgkin's disease in pregnancy. Amer. J. Obstet. Gynecol. **87**:851–853, 1963.

Hertig, A.T.: Vascular pathology in hypertensive albuminuric toxemias of pregnancy. Clinics **4**:602–614, 1945.

Hibbard, B.M. and Hibbard, E.D.: Aetiological factors in abruptio placentae. Brit. Med. J. **ii**:1430–1436, 1963.

Hibbard, B.M. and Hibbard, E.D.: Folate metabolism and reproduction. Brit. Med. Bull. **24**:10–14, 1968.

Higgins, S.D. and Garite, T.J.: Late abruptio placenta in trauma patients: implications for monitoring. Obstetr. Gynecol. **63**:10S–12S, 1984.

Hill, J.G. and Brunton, F.J.: Arteriographic assessment of placental vascularity after antepartum haemorrhage. Brit. Med. J. **i**:25–26, 1968.

Himmelmann, A., Himmelmann, K., Svensson, A. and Hansson, L.: Glucose and insulin levels in young subjects with different maternal histories of hypertension: the hypertension in pregnancy offspring study. J. Int. Med. **241**:19–22, 1997.

Hochfeld, M., Druzin, M.L., Maia, D., Wright, J., Lambert, R.E. and McGuire, J.: Pregnancy complicated by primary antiphospholipid antibody syndrome. Obstet. Gynecol. **83**:804–805, 1994.

Hodari, A.A.: Chronic uterine ischemia and reversible experimental "toxemia of pregnancy." Amer. J. Obstetr. Gynecol. **97**:597–607, 1967.

Hoet, J.-P., Meyer, R. de and Meyer-Doyen, L. de: Hypothyroïdie et grossesse. Helv. Med. Acta **27**:178–195, 1960.

Hoff, C. and Bixler, C.: Maternofetal ABO antigenic dissimilarity and preeclampsia. Lancet **i**:729–730, 1984.

Holaday, W.J. and Castrow, F.F.: Placental metastasis from a fetal giant pigmented nevus. Arch. Dermatol. **98**:486–488, 1968.

Holland, E.: A case of transplacental metastasis of malignant melanoma from mother to foetus. J. Obstet. Gynaecol. Brit. Emp. **56**:529–538, 1949.

Hollister, M.C., Reid, D.L., Phernetton, T.M., Landauer, M. and Rankin, J.H.G.: Dose-response curves of the uterine and placental vascular beds to prostaglandin I₂. Amer. J. Obstetr. Gynecol. **159**:1372–1375, 1988.

Holmes, R.W.: Ablatio placentae. JAMA **51**:1845–1848, 1908.

Hölzl, M., Lüthje, D. und Seck-Ebersbach, K.: Placentaveränderungen bei EPH-Gestose. Morphologischer Befund und Schweregrad der Erkrankung. Arch. Gynäkol. **217**:315–334, 1974.

Honoré, L.H. and Brown, L.B.: Intervillous placental metastasis with maternal myeloid leukemia. Arch. Pathol. Lab. Med. **114**:450, 1990.

Horký, Z.: Angiolopathia myometrii bei Diabetes mellitus. Geburtsh. Frauenheilk. **28**:674–679, 1968.

Hörmann, G. and Lemtis, H.: Zur Frage der diaplazentaren Metastasierung maligner Blastome der Mutter. Z. Geburtsh. Gynäkol. **164**:1–8, 1965a.

Hörmann, G. and Lemtis, H.: Abwehrleistungen der "Einheit Fetus und Plazenta" gegenüber hämatogen verschleppten Zellverbänden maligner Blastome der Mutter. Z. Geburtsh. Gynäkol. **164**:129–142, 1965b.

Horn, J.T.v., Craven, C., Ward, K., Branch, D.W. and Silver, R.M.: Histologic features of placentas and abortion specimens from women with antiphospholipid and antiphospholipid-like syndromes. Placenta **25**:642–648, 2004.

Horn, L.C., Emmrich, P. and Rösch, A.: Intrauteriner Fruchttod bei mütterlichem Nikotinabusus? Verh. Dtsch. Ges. Pathol. **78**:580, 1994.

Horner, E.N.: Placental metastases: case report: maternal death from ovarian cancer. Obstet. Gynecol. **15**:566–572, 1960.

Hoskins, I.A., Friedman, D.M., Frieden, F.J., Ordorica, S.A. and Young, B.K.: Relationship between antepartum cocaine abuse, abnormal umbilical artery Doppler velocimetry, and placental abruption. Obstet. Gynecol. **78**:279–282, 1991.

Hou, S.: Pregnancy in women with chronic renal disease. NEJM **312**:836–839, 1985.

Houlton, M.C.C. and Jackson, M.B.A.: Gaucher's disease and pregnancy. Obstet. Gynecol. **51**:619–620, 1978.

Houwert-De Jong, M.H., Velde, E.R.te, Nefkens, M.J.J. and Schuurman, H.J.: Immune complexes in skin of patients with pre-eclamptic toxaemia. Lancet **ii**:387, 1982.

Howard, B.K. and Goodson, J.H.: Experimental placental abruption. Obstet. Gynecol. **2**:442–446, 1953.

Howard, R.B., Hosokawa, T. and Maguire, M.H.: Hypoxia-induced fetoplacental vasoconstriction in perfused human placental cotyledons. Amer. J. Obstetr. Gynecol. **157**:1261–1266, 1987.

Howley, H.E.A., Walker, M. and Rodger, M.A.: A systematic review of the association between factor V Leiden or prothrombin gene variant and intrauterine growth restriction. Amer. J. Obstet. Gynecol. **192**:694–708, 2005.

Huber, C.P., Carter, J.E. and Vellios, F.: Lesions of the circulatory system of the placenta. A study of 234 placentas with special reference to the development of infarcts. Amer. J. Obstetr. Gynecol. **81**:560–573, 1961.

Hulka, J.F.: Discussion of Grimes et al. in: Amer. J. Obstet. Gynecol. **153**:185, 1985.

Hulka, J.F. and Brinton, V.: Antibody to trophoblast during early postpartum period in toxemic pregnancies. Amer. J. Obstetr. Gynecol. **86**:130–134, 1963.

Hull, D., Binns, B.A.O. and Joyce, D.: Congenital heart block and widespread fibrosis due to maternal lupus erythematosus. Arch. Dis. Child. **41**:688–690, 1966.

Hunter, C.A., Howard, W.F. and McCormick, C.O.: Postpartum curettage effective in reducing hypertension of toxemia. Amer. J. Obstetr. Gynecol. **81**:884–889, 1961.

Huppertz, B. and Kingdon, J.C.P.: Apoptosis in the trophoblast—role of apoptosis in placental morphogenesis. J. Soc. Gynecol. Investig. **11**:353–362, 2004.

Iioka, H., Moriyama, I., Kyuma, M., Saitoh, M., Oku, M., Hino, K., Okamura, Y., Itani, Y. and Ichijo, M.: Nonezymatic glucosylation of human placental trophoblast basement membrane collagen. Relation to diabetic pathology. Acta Obstet. Gynaecol. Japon. **39**:400–404, 1987.

Iklé, A.: Trophoblastzellen im strömenden Blut. Schweiz. Med. Wchschr. **91**:943, 1961.

Iklé, F.A.: Dissemination von Syncytiotrophoblastzellen im mütterlichen Blut während der Gravidität. Bull. Schweiz. Akad. Med. Wiss. **20**:63–72, 1964.

Infante-Rivard, C., David, M., Gauthier, R. and Rivard, G.E.: Lupus anticoagulants, anticardiolipin antibodies, and fetal loss. A case-control study. NEJM **325**:1063–1066, 1991.

Infante-Rivard, C., Rivard, G.-E., Yotov, W.V., Génin, E., Guiguet, M., Weinberg, C., Gauthier, R. and Feoli-Fonseca, J.C.: Absence of association of thrombophilia polymorphisms with intrauterine growth restriction. NEJM **347**:19–25, 2002.

Isaksen, C.V., Austgulen, R., Chedwick, L., Romundstad, P., Vatten, L. and Craven, C.: Maternal smoking, intrauterine growth restriction, and placental apoptosis. Pediat. Developm. Pathol. **7**:433–442, 2004.

Ishihara, N., Matsuo, H., Murakoshi, H., Laoag-Fernandez, J.B., Samoto, T. and Maruo, T.: Increased apoptosis in the syncytiotrophoblast in human term placentas complicated by either preeclampsia or intrauterine growth retardation. Amer. J. Obstet. Gynceol. **186**:158–166, 2002.

Jäämeri, K.E.U., Koivuniemi, A.P. and Carpén, E.O.: Occurrence of trophoblasts in the blood of toxaemic patients. Gynaecologia **160**:315–320, 1965.

Jackson, M.R., Mayhew, T.M. and Haas, J.D.: Morphometric studies on villi in human term placentae and the effects of altitude, ethnic grouping and sex of newborn. Placenta **8**:487–495, 1987.

Jackson, M.R., Mayhew, T.M. and Haas, J.D.: Effects of high altitude on the vascularization of terminal villi in human placentae. In, Trophoblast Research, Vol. 3. P. Kaufmann and R.K. Miller, eds. pp. 351–360, Plenum, New York, 1988.

Jackson, R.: Discoid lupus in a newborn infant of a mother with lupus erythematosus. Pediatrics **33**:425–430, 1964.

Jácomo, K.H., Benedetti, W.L., Sala, M.A. and Alvarez, H.: Pathology of the trophoblast and fetal vessels of the placenta in maternal diabetes mellitus. Acta Diabetol. Lat. **13**:216–235, 1976.

James, R.F.: Snake bite in pregnancy. Lancet **2**:731, 1985.

Javert, C.T. and Reiss, C.: The origin and significance of macroscopic intervillous coagulation hematomas (red infarcts) of the human placenta. Surg. Gynecol. Obstet. **94**:257–269, 1952.

Jazayeri, A., Tsibris, J.C.M. and Spellacy, W.N.: Umbilical cord plasma erythropoietin levels in pregnancies complicated by maternal smoking. Amer. J. Obstet. Gynecol. **178**:433–435, 1998.

Jauniaux, E. and Burton, G.J.: The effect of smoking in pregnancy on early placental morphology. Obstet. Gynecol. **79**: 645–648, 1992.

Jauniaux, E., Hempstock, J., Greenwold, N. and Burton, G.J.: Trophoblast oxidative stress in relation to temporal and regional differences in maternal placental blood flow in normal and abnormal early pregnancies. Amer. J. Pathol. **162**:115–125, 2003.

Jeremy, J.Y., Barradas, M.A., Mikhailidis, D.P., Dandona, P.: Placental prostaglandin production in normal and toxemic pregnancies (letter). Amer. J. Obstet. Gynecol. **154**:212–214, 1986.

Johnson, F.D.: Pregnancy and concurrent chronic myelogenous leukemia. Amer. J. Obstet. Gynecol. **112**:640–644, 1972.

Johnson, P.M., Natvig, J.B., Ystehede, U.A. and Faulk, W.P.: Immunological studies on human placentae: The distribution and character of immunoglobulins in chorionic villi. Clin. Exper. Immunol. **30**:145–153, 1977.

Jones, C.J.P. and Desoye, G.: Glycogen distribution in the capillaries of the placental villus in normal, overt and gestational diabetic pregnancy. Placenta **14**:505–517, 1993.

Jones, C.J.P. and Fox, H.: Placental changes in gestational diabetes: an ultrastructural study. Obstet. Gynecol. **48**:274–280, 1976.

Jones, C.J.P. and Fox, H.: An ultrastructural and ultrahistochemical study of the human placenta in maternal pre-eclampsia. Placenta **1**:61–76, 1980.

Jones, D.C. and Hayslett, J.P.: Outcome of pregnancy in women with moderate or severe renal insufficiency. NEJM **335**:226–232, 1996.

Jones, E.M.: Placental metastases from bronchial carcinoma. Brit. Med. J. **1**:491–492, 1969.

Jones, K.L., Smith, D.W., Ulleland, C.N. and Streissguth, A.P.: Pattern of malformation in offspring of chronic alcoholic women. Lancet **1**:1267–1271, 1973.

Jones, T.G., Goldsmith, K.L.G. and Anderson, I.M.: Maternal and neonatal platelet antibodies in a case of congenital thrombocytopenia. Lancet **2**:1008–1009, 1961.

Jørgensen, K.R., Deckert, T., Pedersen, L.M. and Pedersen, J.: Insulin, insulin antibody and glucose in plasma of newborn infants of diabetic women. Acta Endocrinol. (Copenh.) **52**:154–167, 1966.

Jung, A.L., Roan, Y. and Temple, A.R.: Neonatal death associated with transplacental ethanol intoxication. Amer. J. Dis. Child. **134**:419–420, 1980.

Kåregård, M. and Gennser, G.: Incidence and recurrence rate of abruptio placentae in Sweden. Obstetr. Gynecol. **67**:523–528, 1986.

Kaibara, M., Kobayashi, T. and Matsumoto, S.: Idiopathic thrombocythemia and pregnancy: report of a case. Obstet. Gynecol. **65**:18S–19S, 1985.

Kalhan, S.C., Schwartz, R. and Adam, P.A.J.: Placental barrier to human insulin-I^{125} in insulin-dependent diabetic mothers. J. Clin. Endocrinol. Metab. **40**:139–142, 1975.

Kaminski, M., Rumeau-Rouquette, C. and Schwartz, D.: Effects of alcohol on the fetus. NEJM **298**:55–56, 1978.

Kaplan, M.M.: Acute fatty liver of pregnancy. NEJM **313**:367–370, 1985.

Kaplan, C., Daffos, F., Forestier, F., Tertian, G., Catherine, N., Pons, J.C. and Tchernia, G.: Fetal platelet counts in thrombocytopenic pregnancy. Lancet **336**:979–982, 1990.

Kaufmann, P. and Stark, J.: Ultrastruktur der Plazenta bei Diabetes, EPH-Gestose und Rh-Inkompatibilität. In, Neue Erkenntnisse über die Orthologie und Pathologie der Plazenta. J.J. Födisch, ed., pp. 53–62, 1977. Ferdinand Enke Verlag, Stuttgart.

Kaufmann, P., Kohnen, G. und Kosanke, G.: Wechselwirkungen zwischen Plazentamorphologie und fetaler Sauerstoffversorgung. Versuch einer zellbiologischen Interpretation pathohistologischer und experimenteller Befunde. Gynäkologe **26**:16–23, 1993.

Keith, J.C., Pijnenborg, R. and van Assche, F.A.: Placental syncytin expression in normal and preeclamptic pregnancies. Amer. J. Obstet. Gynecol. **187**:1122–1123, 2002 (reply to Knerr et al., 2002).

Kelemen, J.T. and Mandi, L.: Sarcoidose in der Placenta. Zentralbl. Allg. Pathol. **112**:18–21, 1969.

Kerber, I.J., Warr, O.S. and Richardson, C.: Pregnancy in a patient with a prosthetic mitral valve: associated with a fetal anomaly attributed to Warfarin sodium. JAMA **203**:223–225, 1968.

Khong, T.Y.: Immunohistologic study of the leukocytic infiltrate in maternal uterine tissues in normal and preeclamptic pregnancies at term. Amer. J. Reprod. Immunol. **15**:1–8, 1987.

Khong, T.Y. and Chambers, H.M.: Alternative method of sampling placentas for the assessment of uteroplacental vasculature. J. Clin. Pathol. **45**:925–927, 1992.

Khong, T.Y. and Hague, W.M.: The placenta is maternal hyperhomocysteinaemia. Placenta **18**:A33, 1997.

Khong, T.Y., Pearce, J.M. and Robertson, W.B.: Acute atherosis in preeclampsia: maternal determinants and fetal outcome in the presence of the lesion. Amer. J. Obstetr. Gynecol. **157**:360–363, 1987.

Khong, T.Y., Sawyer, I.H. and Heryet, A.: An immunohistologic study of endothelialization of uteroplacental vessels in human pregnancy—evidence that endothelium is focally disrupted by trophoblast in preeclampsia. Amer. J. Obstet. Gynecol. **167**:751–756, 1992.

Kilpatrick, D.C.: Immune mechanisms and pre-eclampsia. Lancet **ii**:1460–1461, 1987.

Kim, Y.M., Bujold, E., Chaiworapongsa, T., Gomez, R., Yoon, B.H., Thaler, H.T., Rotmensch, S. and Romero, R.: Failure of physiologic transformation of the spiral arteries in patients with preterm labor and intact membranes. Amer. J. Obstet. Gynceol. **189**:1063–1069, 2002.

Kimmerle, R. and Chantelau, E.A.: Transplacental passage of insulin. NEJM **324**:198–199, 1991.

Kirshon, B., Edwards, J. and Cotton, D.B.: Gordon's syndrome in pregnancy. Amer. J. Obstet. Gynecol. **156**:1110–1111, 1987.

Kitay, D.Z.: Folic acid in pregnancy. JAMA **204**:79, 1968.

Kitzmiller, J.L. and Benirschke, K.: Immunofluorescent study of placental bed vessels in pre-eclampsia of pregnancy. Amer. J. Obstetr. Gynecol. **115**:248–251, 1973.

Kitzmiller, J.L., Stoneburner, L., Yelenovsky, P.F. and Lucas, W.E.: Serum complement in normal pregnancy and pre-eclampsia. Amer. J. Obstetr. Gynecol. **117**:312–315, 1973.

Kitzmiller, J.L., Watt, N. and Driscoll, S.G.: Decidual arteriopathy in hypertension and diabetes in pregnancy: immunofluorescent studies. Amer. J. Obstetr. Gynecol. **141**:773–778, 1981.

Kjeldsen, J. and Pedersen, J.: Relation of residual placental blood-volume to onset of respiratory-distress syndrome in infants of diabetic and non-diabetic mothers. Lancet **1**:180–184, 1967.

Klebe, J.G. and Ingomar, C.J.: Placental transfusion in infants of diabetic mothers elucidated by placental residual blood volume. Acta Paediatr. Scand. **63**:59–64, 1974a.

Klebe, J.G. and Ingomar, C.J.: The influence of the method of delivery and the clamping technique on the red cell volume in infants of diabetic and non-diabetic mothers. Acta Paediatr. Scand. **63**:65–69, 1974b.

Kline, J., Stein, Z.A., Susser, M. and Warburton, D.: Smoking: a risk factor for spontaneous abortion. NEJM **297**:793–796, 1977.

Klippel, J.H., Grimley, P.M. and Decker, J.L.: Lymphocyte inclusions in newborns of mothers with systemic lupus erythematosus. NEJM **290**:96–97, 1974.

Klurfeld, D.M.: Identification of foam cells in human atherosclerotic lesions as macrophages using monoclonal antibodies. Arch. Pathol. **109**:445–449, 1985.

Knerr, I., Beinder, E. and Rascher, W.: Syncytin, a novel human endogenous retroviral gene in human placentae: evidence for its dysregulation in preeclampsia and HELLP syndrome. Amer. J. Obstet. Gynecol. **186**:210–213, 2002.

Knörr, K., Knörr-Gärtner, H. and Uebele-Kallhardt, B.: Zur Frage der Wirkung alkylierender Substanzen auf die Entwicklung der Frucht. Geburtsh. Frauenheilk. **29**:601–611, 1969.

Knox, G.E., Stagno, S., Volanakis, J.E. and Huddelston, J.F.: A search for antigen-antibody complexes in pre-eclampsia: further evidence against immunologic pathogenesis. Amer. J. Obstetr. Gynecol. **132**:87–89, 1978.

König, P.A.: Über Eklampsietod und Gefäßwandschaden bei Mutter und Kind. Z. Geburtsh. Gynäkol. **146**:292–307, 1956.

Koshy, M., Burd, L., Wallace, D., Moawad, A. and Baron, J.: Prophylactic red-cell transfusions in pregnant patients with sickle cell disease: a randomized cooperative study. NEJM **319**:1447–1451, 1988.

Kosova, L.A. and Schwartz, S.O.: Multiple myeloma and normal pregnancy: report of a case. Blood **28**:102–111, 1966.

Kowal-Vern, A., Fisher, S.G., Muraskas, J., Jandreski, M.A., Gianopoulos, J.G. and Husain, A.: Placental pathologic conditions in anticardiolipin antibody positive women whose infants had congenital heart defects. J. Perinatol. **16**:268–271, 1996.

Kramer, M.S., Usher, R.H., Pollack, R., Boyd, M. and Usher, S.: Etiologic determinants of abruptio placentae. Obstet. Gynecol. **89**:221–226, 1997.

Krayalcin, G., Imran, M. and Rosner, F.: "Blister cells": association with pregnancy, sickle cell disease, and pulmonary infarction. JAMA **219**:1727–1729, 1972.

Kuhnert, B.R., Kuhnert, P.M., Debanne, S. and Williams, T.G.: The relationship between cadmium, zinc, and birth weight in pregnant women who smoke. Amer. J. Obstet. Gynecol. **157**:1247–1251, 1987b.

Kuhnert, P.M., Kuhnert, B.R., Erhard, P., Brashear, W.T., Groh-Wargo, S.L. and Webster, S.: The effect of smoking on placental and fetal zinc status. Amer. J. Obstet. Gynecol. **157**:1241–1246, 1987a.

Kujovich, J.L.: Thrombophilia and pregnancy complications. Amer. J. Obstet. Gynecol. **191**:412–424, 2004.

Kupferminc, M.J., Lee, M.J., Green, D. and Peaceman, A.M.: Severe postpartum pulmonary, cardiac, and renal syndrome associated with antiphospholipid antibodies. Obstet. Gynecol. **83**:806–807, 1994.

Kupferminc, M.J., Eldor, A., Steinman, N., Many, A., Bar-Am, A., Jaffa, A. Fait, G. and Lessing, J.B.: Increased frequency of genetic thrombophilia in women with complications of pregnancy. NEJM **340**:9–13, 1999. (See also Editorial, pp. 50–51.)

Kutteh, W.H. and Franklin, R.D.: Assessing the variation in antiphospholipid antibody (APA) assays: Comparison of results from 10 centers. Amer. J. Obstet. Gynecol. **191**:440–448, 2004.

Labarrere, C.A.: Placental bed biopsy technique and vascular changes. Amer. J. Obstetr. Gynecol. **157**:1320–1322, 1987.

Labarrere, C.A. and Faulk, W.P.: Antigenic identification of cells in spiral artery trophoblastic invasion: validation of histologic studies by triple-antibody immunocytochemistry. Amer. J. Obstet. Gynecol. **171**:165–171, 1994.

Lacher, M.J. and Geller, W.: Cyclophosphamide and vinblastine sulfate in Hodgkin's disease during pregnancy. JAMA **195**:486–488, 1966.

Lakasing, L., Campa, J.S., Poston, R., Khamashta, M.A. and Poston, L.: Normal expression of tissue factor, thrombomodulin, and annexin V in placentas from women with antiphospholipid syndrome. Amer. J. Obstet. Gynecol. **181**:180–189, 1999.

Lao, T.T. and Wong, W.M.: Placental ratio—its relationship with mild anaemia. Placenta **18**:593–596, 1997.

Lau, H., Sackreuther, W., Bach, H.G., Grabberr, W. und Hundertmack, R.: Über die vorzeitige Lösung der normal sitzenden Placenta. Klinische Beobachtungen an 100 Fällen. Gynaecologia **157**:143–160, 1964.

Laureti, E., De Galateo, A. and Giorgino, F.: Ricerche quantitativa sultenore di idrossi prolina, di lipid e di esosi in placenta normali e diabeiche del 3° mese di gravidanza. Boll. Soc. Ital. Biol. Sper. **58**:702–707, 1982.

Laurini, R.N., Visser, G.H.A. and Ballegoodie, E. van: Morphological fetoplacental abnormalities despite well-controlled diabetic pregnancy. Lancet **1**:800, 1984.

Lazarchick, J. and Kizer, J.: The laboratory diagnosis of lupus anticoagulants. Arch Pathol. Lab. Med. **113**:177–180, 1989.

Leach, R.E., Romero, R., Kim, Y.M., Chaiworapongsa, T., Kilburn, B., Das, S.K., Dey, S.K., Johnson, A., Qureshi, F., Jacques, S. and Armant, D.R.: Pre-eclampsia and expression of heparin-like growth factor. Lancet **360**:1215–1219, 2002.

Lederman, R.P., Lederman, E., Work, B.A. and McCann, D.S.: The relationship of maternal anxiety, plasma catecholamines, and plasma cortisol to progress in labor. Amer. J. Obstet. Gynecol. **132**:495–500, 1978.

Lee, R.A., Johnson, C.E. and Hanlon, D.G.: Leukemia during pregnancy. Amer. J. Obstet. Gynecol. **84**:455–458, 1962.

Lemtis, H.: Über die vorzeitige Lösung der normal sitzenden Plazenta. Forschung, Praxis, Fortbildung **18**:231–237, 1967.

Lemtis, H. and Hörmann, G.: Über die sogenannten Plazentametastasen maligner Blastome der Mutter. In, Fortschritte der

Krebsforschung. C.G. Schmidt & O. Wetter, eds., pp. 521–527. F.K. Schattauer Verlag, Stuttgart, 1969.

Lentz, S.E., Coulson, C.C., Gocke, C.D. and Fantaskey, A.P.: Placental pathology in maternal and neonatal myeloproliferative disorders. Obstet. Gynecol. **91**:863, 1998.

Leone, G., Monetta, E., Paparatti, G. and Boni, P.: Von Willebrand's disease in pregnancy. NEJM **293**:456, 1975.

Leushner, J.R.A., Tevaarwerk, G.J.M., Clarson, C.L., Harding, P.G.R., Chance, G.W. and Haust, M.D.: Analysis of the collagens of diabetic placental villi. Cell. Molec. Biol. **32**:27–35. 1986.

Levine, J.S., Branch, D.W. and Rauch, J.: The antiphospholipid syndrome. NEJM **346**:752–763, 2002.

Levine, M.G. and Esser, D.: Total parenteral nutrition for the treatment of severe hyperemesis gravidarum: maternal nutritional effects and fetal outcome. Obstet. Gynecol. **72**:102–107, 1988.

Levine, R.J., Maynard, S.E., Qian, C., Lim, K.-H., England, L.J., Yu, K.F., Schisterman, E.F., Thadhani, R., Sachs, B.P., Epstein, F.H., Sibai, B.M., Sukhatme, V.P. and Karumanchi, S.A.: Circulating angiogenic factors and the risk of preeclampsia. NEJM **350**:672–683, 2004.

Li, M.C., Hertz, R. and Spencer, D.B.: Effects of methotrexate therapy upon choriocarcinomas and chorioadenomas. Proc. Soc. Exp. Biol. Med. **93**:361–366, 1956.

Lichtig, C., Deutsch, M. and Brandes, J.: Vascular changes of endometrium in early pregnancy. Amer. J. Clin. Pathol. **81**:702–707, 1984.

Liebhardt, M.: Tkanka Laczna lozysk pochodzacych z ciaz powiklanych prdzez cukrzyce matki. Ginecol Pol. **39**:1353–1362, 1968.

Lilford, R.J.: Classification of hypertensive disorders of pregnancy. Lancet **ii**:112–113, 1989.

Lin, S., Shimizu, I., Suehara, N., Nakayama, M. and Aono, T.: Uterine artery Doppler velocimetry in relation to trophoblast migration into the myometrium of the placental bed. Obstet. Gynecol. **85**:760–765, 1995.

Little, B.B., Snell, L.M., Klein, V.R. and Gilstrap III, L.C.: Cocaine abuse during pregnancy: maternal and fetal implications. Obstet. Gynecol. **73**:157–160, 1989.

Lockshin, M.D., Druzin, M.L. and Qamar, T.: Prednisone does not prevent recurrent fetal death in women with antiphospholipid antibody. Amer. J. Obstet. Gynecol. **160**:439–443, 1989.

Lockwood, C.J., Reece, E.A., Romero, R. and Hobbins, J.C.: Anti-phospholipid antibody and pregnancy wastage. Lancet **ii**:742–743, 1986.

Lockwood, C.J., Romero, R., Feinberg, R.F., Clyne, L.P., Coster, B. and Hobbins, J.C.: The prevalence and biologic significance of lupus anticoagulant and anticardiolipin antibodies in a general obstetric population. Amer. J. Obstet. Gynecol. **161**:369–373, 1989.

Loizoll, S., Byron, M.A., Englert, H.J., David, J., Hughes, G.R.V. and Walport, M.J.: Association of quantitative anticardiolipin antibody levels with fetal loss and time of loss in systemic lupus erythematosus. Quart. J. Med. **68**:525–531, 1988.

Long, E.G., Tsin, T.Y., Reinarz, J.A., Schnadig, V.J., McLucas, E. and Kelly, R.T.: "*Hydatoxi lualba*" identified. Amer. J. Obstet. Gynecol. **149**:462–463, 1984.

Lopez-Zeno, J.A., Carlo, W.A., O'Grady, J.P. and Fanaroff, A.A.: Infant survival following delayed postmortem cesarean delivery. Obstet. Gynecol. **76**:991–992, 1990.

Lotgering, F.K., Pijpers, L., Eijck, J.v. and Wallenburg, H.C.S.: Pregnancy in a patient with diffuse cavernous hemangioma of the uterus. Amer. J. Obstet. Gynecol. **160**:628–630, 1989.

Lubbe, W.F. and Liggins, G.C.: Lupus anticoagulant and pregnancy. Amer. J. Obstet. Gynecol. **153**:322–327, 1985.

Lubbe, W.F., Butler, W.S., Palmer, S.J. and Liggins, G.C.: Fetal survival after prednisone suppression of maternal lupus-anticoagulant. Lancet **i**:1361–1363, 1963.

Lueck, J., Brewer, J.I., Aladjem, S. and Novotny, M.: Observation of an organism found in patients with gestational trophoblastic disease and in patients with toxemia of pregnancy. Amer. J. Obstetr. Gynecol. **145**:15–26, 1983.

Lundberg, C., Marceau, F., Huey, R. and Hugli, T.E.: Anaphylatoxin C5a fails to promote prostacyclin release in cultured endothelial cells from human umbilical veins. Immunopharmacol. **12**:135–143, 1986.

Lyall, F., Bulmer, J.N., Duffie, E., Cousins, F., Theriault, A, and Robson, S.C.: Human trophoblast invasion and spiral artery transformation. The role of PECAM-1 in normal pregnancy, preeclampsia, and fetal growth restriction. Amer. J. Pathol. **158**:1713–1721, 2001.

Machin, G.A.: Maternal melanoma metastatic to the placenta. Pediatr. Pathol. **7**:490, 1987.

MacLean, M.A., Wilson, R., Thomson, J.A., Krishnamurthy, S. and Walker, J.J.: Immunological changes in normal pregnancy. Eur. J. Obstet. Gynecol. Reprod. Med. **43**:167–172, 1992.

MacLennan, A.H., Sharp, F. and Shaw-Dunn, J.: The ultrastructure of human trophoblast in spontaneous and induced hypoxia using a system of organ culture. A comparison with ultrastructural changes in pre-eclampsia and placental insufficiency. J. Obstetr. Gynaecol. Brit. Cwlth. **79**:113–121, 1972.

Magid, M.S., Kaplan, C., Sammaritano, L.R., Peterson, M., Druzin, M.L. and Lockshin, M.D.: Placental pathology in systemic lupus erythematosus: a prospective study. Amer. J. Obstet. Gynecol. **179**:226–234, 1998.

Mäkilä, U.-M., Viinikka, L. and Ylikorkala, O.: Evidence that prostacyclin deficiency is a specific feature in preeclampsia. Amer. J. Obstet. Gynecol. **148**:772–774, 1984.

Mäkilä, U.-M., Jouppila, P., Kirkinen, P., Viinikka, L. and Ylikorkala, O.: Placental thromboxane and prostacyclin in the regulation of placental blood flow. Obstet. Gynecol. **68**:537–540, 1986.

Many, A., Hubel, C.A., Fisher, S.J., Roberts, J.M. and Zhou, Y.: Invasive cytotrophoblasts manifest evidence of oxidative stress in preeclampsia. Amer. J. Pathol. **156**:321–331, 2000.

Maqueo, M., Azuela, J.C., Karchmer, S. and Arenas, J.C.: Placental morphology in pathologic gestations with or without toxemia: observations in cases of diabetes mellitus, hydrops fetalis, twin pregnancy, placenta previa, and hydatidiform mole. Obstet. Gynecol. **26**:184–191, 1965.

Marais, W.D.: Human decidual spiral arterial studies. Part II. A universal thesis on the pathogenesis of intraplacental fibrin deposits, layered thrombosis, red and white infarcts and toxic and non-toxic abruptio placentae. A microscopic study. J. Obstetr. Gynaecol. Brit. Cwlth. **69**:213–224, 1962a.

Marais, W.D.: Human decidual spiral arterial studies. Part III. Histological patterns and some clinical implications of decidual spiral arteriosclerosis. J. Obstetr. Gynaecol. Brit. Cwlth. **69**:225–233, 1962b.

Marais, W.D.: Human decidual spiral arterial studies. Part V. Pathogenetic patterns of intraplacental lesions. J. Obstetr. Gynaecol. Brit. Cwlth. **69**:944–955, 1962c.

Marais, W.D.: Human decidual spiral arterial studies. Part VI: Postmortem circulation studies on an in situ placenta. S. Afr. Med. J. **36**:678–681, 1962d.

Marais, W.D.: Human decidual spiral arterial studies. Part VII. The clinical evaluation of normal and abnormal spiral arterioles and of placental lesions. A statistical study. J. Obstetr. Gynaecol. **70**:777–786, 1963a.

Marais, W.D.: Human decidual spiral arterial studies. Part VIII. The aetiological relationship between toxaemia-hypertension of pregnancy and spiral arterial placental pathology. S. Afr. Med. J. **37**:117–120, 1963b.

Marbury, M.C., Linn, S., Monson, R., Schoenbaum, S., Stubblefield, P.G. and Ryan, K.J.: The association of alcohol consumption with outcome of pregnancy. Amer. J. Public Health **73**:1165–1168, 1983.

Marcuse, P.M.: Pulmonary syncytial giant cell embolism. Report of maternal death. Obstet. Gynecol. **3**:210–213, 1954.

Marks, F., Ordorica, S., Hoskins, I. and Young, B.K.: Congenital hereditary fructose intolerance and pregnancy. Amer. J. Obstet. Gynecol. **160**:362–363, 1989.

Marsh, R. de W. and Chu, N.M.: Placental metastasis from primary ocular melanoma: a case report. Amer. J. Obstet. Gynecol. **174**:1654–1655, 1996.

Martinelli, I., Taioli, E., Cetin, I., Marinoni, A., Gerosa, S., Villa, M.V., Bozzo, M. and Mannucci, P.M.: Mutations in coagulation factors in women with unexplained late fetal loss. NEJM **343**:1015–1018, 2000.

Martinez, A.E., Gonzalez, O.M., Quinones, G.A. and Ferrannini, E.: Hyperinsulinemia in glucose-tolerant women with pre-eclampsia. A controlled study. Amer. J. Hypertension **9**:610–614, 1996.

Martinez, C.R.J.: Foetus in maternal renal failure. Lancet **1**:504, 1967.

Maruko, K., Maeda, T., Kamitomo, M., Hatae, M. and Sueyoshi, K.: Transplacental transmission of maternal B-cell lymphoma. Amer. J. Obstet. Gynecol. **191**:380–381, 2004.

Massobrio, M., Benedetto, C., Bertini, E., Tetta, C. and Camussi, G.: Immune complexes in preeclampsia and normal pregnancy. Amer. J. Obstetr. Gynecol. **152**:578–583, 1985.

Matijevic, R., Meekins, J.W., Walkinshaw, S.A., Neilson, J.P. and McFadyen, I.R.: Spiral artery blood flow in the central and peripheral areas of the placental bed in the second trimester. Obstet. Gynecol. **86**:289–292, 1995.

Matos, A., Bernardes, J., Ayres-de-Campos, D. and Patricio, B.: Antepartum fetal cerebral hemorrhage not predicted by current surveillance methods in cholestasis of pregnancy. Obstet. Gynecol. **89**:803–804, 1997.

Maymon, R., Bahari, C. and Moroz, C.: Placental isoferritin: a new serum marker in toxemia of pregnancy. Amer. J. Obstet. Gynecol. **160**:681–684, 1989.

McCowan, L.M.E., Craigie, S., Taylor, R.S., Ward, C., McLintock, C. and North, R.A.: Inherited thrombophilias are not increased in "idiopathic" small-for-gestational-age pregnancies. Amer. J. Obstet. Gynecol. **188**:981–985, 2003.

McDonald, D.G., Kelehan, P., McMenamin, J.B., Gorman, W.A., Madden, D., Tobbia, I.N. and Mooney, E.E.: Placental fetal thrombotic vasculopathy is associated with neonatal encephalopathy. Hum. Pathol. **35**:875–880, 2004.

McFaul, P.B., Dornan, J.C., Lamki, H. and Boyle, D.: Pregnancy complicated by maternal heart disease: a review of 519 women. Brit. J. Obstet. Gynaecol. **95**:861–867, 1988.

McGlothlin, W.H., Sparkes, R.S. and Arnold, D.O.: Effect of LSD on human pregnancy. JAMA **212**:1483–1487, 1970.

McGowan, L.: Cancer and pregnancy. Obstet. Gynecol. Surv. **19**:285–307, 1964.

McFayden, I.R., Price, A.B. and Geirsson, R.T.: The relation of birthweight to histological appearances in vessels of the placental bed. Brit. J. Obstetr. Gynaecol. **93**:476–481, 1986.

McKay, D.G., Jewett, J.F. and Reid, D.E.: Endotoxin shock and the generalized Shwartzman reaction in pregnancy. Amer. J. Obstet. Gynecol. **78**:546–566, 1959.

McLaughlin, P.J., Stirrat, G.M., Redman, C.W.G. and Levinsky, R.J.: Immune complexes in normal and pre-eclamptic pregnancy. Lancet **i**:934–935, 1979.

McVerry, B.A., Machin, S.J., Parry, H. and Goldstone, A.H.: Reduced prostacyclin activity in systemic lupus erythematosus. Ann. Rheum. Dis. **39**:524–525, 1980.

Menon, R.K., Cohen, R.M., Sperling, M.A., Cutfield, W.S., Mimouni, F. and Khoury, J.C.: Transplacental passage of insulin in pregnant women with insulin-dependent diabetes mellitus. Its role in fetal macrosomia. NEJM **323**:309–315, 1990.

Mercado, A., Johnson, G., Calver, D. and Sokol, R.J.: Cocaine, pregnancy, and postpartum intracerebral hemorrhage. Obstet. Gynecol. **73**:467–468, 1989.

Mercer, B., Drouin, J., Jolly, E. and d'Anjou, G.: Primary thrombocythemia in pregnancy: a report of two cases. Amer. J. Obstet. Gynecol. **159**:127–128, 1988.

Messer, R.H.: Symposium on bleeding disorders in pregnancy: observations in pregnancy. Amer. J. Obstet. Gynecol. **156**: 1419–1425, 1987.

Metcalfe, J., Novy, M.J. and Peterson, E.N.: Reproduction at high altitude. In, Comparative Aspects of Reproductive Failure. K. Benirschke, ed., pp. 447–457. Springer-Verlag, New York, 1966.

Meyer, M.B. and Tonascia, J.A.: Maternal smoking, pregnancy complications, and perinatal mortality. Amer. J. Obstet. Gynecol. **128**:494–502, 1977.

Mijer, F. and Olsen, R.N.: Transplacental passage of L.E. factor. J. Pediatr. **52**:690–693, 1958.

Miller, J.M., Boudreaux, M.C. and Regan, F.A.: A case-control study of cocaine use in pregnancy. Amer. J. Obstet. Gynecol. **172**:180–185, 1995.

Mills, J.L., Simpson, J.L., Driscoll, S.G., Jovanovic-Peterson, L., Allen, M.V., Aarons, J.H., Metzger, B., Bieber, F.R., Knopp, R.H., Holmes, L.B., Peterson, C.M., Witham-Wilson, M., Brown, Z., Ober, C., Harley, E., MacPherson, T.A., Duckles, A., Mueller-Heubach, E., NICHD, and HD-DEPS: Incidence of spontaneous abortion among normal women and insulin-dependent diabetic women whose pregnancies were identified within 21 days of conception. NEJM **319**:1617–1623, 1988.

Milo, R., Neuman, M., Klein, C., Caspi, E. and Arlazoroff, A.: Acute intermittent porphyria in pregnancy. Obstet. Gynecol. **73**:450–452, 1989.

Miodovnik, M., Skillman, C., Holroyde, J.C., Butler, J.B., Wendel, J.S. and Siddiqi, T.A.: Elevated maternal glycohemoglobin in early pregnancy and spontaneous abortion among insulin-dependent diabetic women. Amer. J. Obstet. Gynecol. **153**:439–442, 1985.

Mirro, R. and Brown, D.R.: Edema, proteinuria, thrombocytopenia, and leukopenia in infants of preeclamptic mothers. Amer. J. Obstetr. Gynecol. **144**:851–852, 1982.

Moldenhauer, J.S., Stanek, J., Warshak, C., Khoury, J. and Sibai, B.: The frequency and severity of placental findings in women with preeclampsia are gestational age dependent. Amer. J. Obstet. Gynecol. **189**:1173–1177, 2003.

Mooney, E.E., Vaughan, J., Ryan, F., LaFont, A., McDonald, D., Gorman, W.A., Kelehan, P. and McMenamin, J.: Placental thrombotic vasculopathy is not associated with thrombophilic mutations. Modern Pathol. **16**:303A (abstract 1382), 2003.

Moore, T.R., Sorg, J., Miller, L., Key, T.C. and Resnik, R.: Hemodynamic effects of intravenous cocaine on the pregnant ewe and fetus. Amer. J. Obstet. Gynecol. **155**:883–888, 1986.

Morales, W.J. and Stroup, M.: Intracranial hemorrhage in utero due to isoimmune neonatal thrombocytopenia. Obstet. Gynecol. **65**:20S–24S, 1985.

Mordel, N., Birkenfeld, A., Goldfarb, A.N. and Rachmilewitz, E.A.: Successful full-term pregnancy in homozygous β-thalassemia major: case report and review of the literature. Obstet. Gynecol. **73**:837–840, 1989.

Morgan, M.A., Berkowitz, K.M., Thomas, S.J., Reimbold, P. and Quilligan, E.J.: Abruptio placentae: Perinatal outcome in normotensive and hypertensive patients. Amer. J. Obstet. Gynecol. **170**:1595–1599, 1994.

Morrow, R.J., Ritchie, J.W.K. and Bull, S.B.: Maternal cigarette smoking: the effects on umbilical and uterine blood flow velocity. Amer. J. Obstet. Gynecol. **159**:1069–1071, 1988.

Moses, E.K., Cooper, D.W. and Brennecke, S.P.: Genetic analysis of pre-eclampsia. IFPA meeting, abstract L8, 2002.

Mostello, D., Catlin, T.K., Roman, L., Holcomb, W.L. and Leet, T.: Preeclampsia in the parous woman: Who is at risk? Amer. J. Obstet. Gynecol. **187**:425–429, 2002.

Mueller-Eckhardt, C., Kiefel, V., Jovanovic, V., Künzel, W., Becker, T., Wolf, H. and Zeh, K.: Prenatal treatment of alloimmune thrombocytopenia. Lancet **2**:910, 1988.

Muller, G., Philippe, E., Lefakis, P., de Mot-Leclair, M., Dreyfus, J., Nusynowicz, G., Renaud, R. and et Gandar, R.: Les lésions placentaires de la gestose. Étude anatomo-clinique. Gynecol. Obstetr. **70**:309–316, 1971.

Mullinax, F.: Chimerism in scleroderma. Lancet **351**:1886, 1998.

Mund, A., Simson, J. and Rothfield, N.: Effect of pregnancy on course of systemic lupus erythematosus. JAMA **183**:917–920, 1963.

Murata, H., Nakauchi, H. and Sumida, T.: Microchimerism in Japanese women with systemic sclerosis. Lancet **354**:220, 1999.

Murphy, J.F., Mulcahy, R. and Drumm, J.E.: Smoking and the fetus. Lancet **2**:36, 1977.

Musci, T.J., Roberts, J.M., Rodgers, G.M. and Taylor, R.N.: Mitogenic activity is increased in the sera of preeclamptic women before birth. Amer. J. Obstetr. Gynecol. **159**:1446–1451, 1988.

Mvumbi, L., Manci, E.A., Ulmer, D. and Shah, A.K.: Glycogen levels in human term placental disks, umbilical cords, and membranes. Pediatr. Pathol. Lab Med. **16**:597–605, 1996.

Myatt, L., Eis, A.L.W., Brockman, D.E., Greer, I.A. and Lyall, F.: Endothelial nitric oxide synthase in placental villous tissue from normal, pre-eclamptic and intrauterine growth restricted pregnancies. Hum. Reprod. **12**:167–172, 1997.

Myers, R.E. and Fujikura, T.: Placental changes after experimental abruptio placentae and fetal vessel ligation of rhesus monkey placenta. Amer. J. Obstet. Gynecol. **100**:846–851, 1968.

Nadji, P. and Sommers, S.C.: Lesions of toxemia in first trimester pregnancies. Amer. J. Clin. Pathol. **59**:344–349, 1973.

Naeye, R.L.: Placental infarction leading to fetal or neonatal death. A prospective study. Obstetr. Gynecol. **50**:583–588, 1977.

Naeye, R.L.: Relationship of cigarette smoking to congenital anomalies and perinatal death: a prospective study. Amer. J. Pathol. **90**:289–294, 1978.

Naeye, R.L., Blanc, W., Leblanc, W. and Khatamee, M.A.: Fetal complications of maternal heroin addiction: abnormal growth, infections, and episodes of stress. J. Pediatr. **83**:1055–1061, 1973.

Naeye, R.L., Harkness, W.L. and Utts, J.: Abruptio placentae and perinatal death: a prospective study. Amer. J. Obstetr. Gynecol. **128**:740–746, 1977.

Nagey, D.A., Fortier, K.J. and Linder, J.: Pregnancy complicated by periarteritis nodosa: induced abortion as an alternative. Amer. J. Obstet. Gynecol. **147**:103–105, 1983.

Nelson, J.L.: Microchimerism and autoimmune disease. NEJM **338**:1224–1225, 1998.

Nelson, J.L.: Implications of fetal-maternal cell traffic for human health and disease. Placenta **25**:A3 (abstract K6), 2004.

Nelson, J.M., Furst, D.E., Maloney, S., Gooley, T., Evans, P.C., Smith, A., Bean, M.A., Ober, C. and Bianchi, D.W.: Microchimerism and HLA-compatible relationships of pregnancy in scleroderma. Lancet **351**:559–562, 1998.

Ness, P.M., Budzynski, A.Z., Olexa, S.A. and Rodvien, R.: Congenital hypofibrinogenemia and recurrent placental abruption. Obstetr. Gynecol. **61**:519–523, 1983.

Ness, R.B. and Roberts, J.M.: Heterogeneous causes constituting the single syndrome of preeclampsia: a hypothesis and its implications. Amer. J. Obstet. Gynecol. **175**:1365–1370, 1996 (and pp. 243–244, July, 1997).

Ness, R.B., Grisso, J.A., Hirschinger, N., Markovic, N., Shaw, L.M., Day, N.L. and Kline, J.: Cocaine and tobacco use and the risk of spontaneous abortion. NEJM **340**:333–339, 1999.

Nicholson, H.O.: Cytotoxic drugs in pregnancy. J. Obstet. Gynaecol. Brit. Commonw. **75**:307–312, 1968.

Nielsen, F.H., Jacobsen, B.B. and Rolschau, J.: Pregnancy complicated by extreme hyperlipaemia and foam-cell accumulation in placenta. Acta Obstet. Gynecol. Scand. **52**:83–89, 1973.

Nilsson, I.M., Astedt, B., Hedner, U. and Berezin, D.: Intrauterine death and circulating anticoagulant, "antithromboplastin." Acta Med. Scand. **197**:153–159, 1975.

Niswander, R.K. and Gordon, M.: The Women and their Pregnancies. W.B. Saunders, Philadelphia, 1972. p 43.

Nordlund, J.J., DeVita, V.T. and Carbone, P.P.: Severe vinblastine-induced leukopenia during late pregnancy with delivery of normal infant. Ann. Intern. Med. **69**:581–582, 1968.

Notelvitz, M., Bottoms, S.F., Dase, D.F. and Leichter, P.J.: Painless abruptio placentae. Obstetr. Gynecol. **53**:270–272, 1979.

Nummi, S., Koivisto, M. and Hakosalo, J.: Acute leukaemia in pregnancy with placental involvement. Ann. Chir. Gynaecol. Fenn. **62**:394–398, 1973.

Nuñez, J.A.C.: La placenta de las cardiacas. Rev. Esp. Obstet. Ginecol. **22**:129–134, 1963.

O'Brien, W.F., Knuppel, R.A., Saba, H.I., Angel, J.L., Benoit, R. and Bruce, A.: Platelet inhibitory activity in placentas from normal and abnormal pregnancies. Obstetr. Gynecol. **70**:597–600, 1987.

O'Brien, W.F., Knuppel, R.A., Saba, H.I., Angel, J.L., Benoit, R. and Bruce, A.: Serum prostacyclin binding and half-life in normal and hypertensive pregnant women. Obstetr. Gynecol. **73**:43–46, 1988.

O'Day, M.P., Nielsen, P., Al-Bozom, I. and Wilkins, I.A.: Orbital rhabdomyosarcoma metastatic to the placenta. Amer. J. Obstet. Gynecol. **171**:1382–1383, 1994.

Oga, M., Matsui, N., Anai, T., Yoshimatsu, J., Inoue, I. and Miyakawa, I.: Copper disposition of the fetus and placenta in a patient with untreated Wilson's disease. Amer. J. Obstet. Gynecol. **169**:196–198, 1993.

Ohba, T., Matsuo, I., Katabuchi, H., Nishimura, H., Fujisaki, S. and Okamura, H.: Adult T-cell leukemia/lymphoma in pregnancy. Obstet. Gynecol. **72**:445–447, 1988.

Okudaira, Y., Hirota, K., Cohen, S. and Strauss, L.: Ultrastructure of the human placenta in maternal diabetes mellitus. Lab. Invest. **15**:910–926, 1966.

O'Leary, J.A.: A continuing study of sarcoidosis and pregnancy. Amer. J. Obstet. Gynecol. **101**:610–613, 1968.

Ong, P.J.L. and Burton, G.J.: Thinning of the placental villous membrane during maintenance in hypoxic organ culture: structural adaptation or syncytial degeneration? Europ. J. Obstet. Gynecol. Reprod. Biol. **39**:103–110, 1991.

Ornoy, A., Yacobi, S., Matalon, S.T., Blank, M., Blumenfeld, Z., Miller, R.K. and Shoenfeld, Y.: The effects of antiphospholipid antibodies obtained from women with SLE/APS and associated pregnancy loss on rat embryos and placental explants in culture. Lupus **12**:573–578, 2003.

Orr, J.W., Grizzle, W.E. and Huddleston, J.F.: Squamous cell carcinoma metastatic to placenta and ovary. Obstet. Gynecol. **59**:81S–83S, 1982.

O'Shaugnessy, K.M., Ferraro, F., Fu, B., Downing, S. and Morris, N.H.: Identification of monozygotic twins that are concordant for preeclampsia. Amer. J. Obstet. Gynecol. **182**:1156–1157, 2000.

Oshiro, B.T., Silver, R.M., Scott, J.R., Yu, H. and Branch, W.: Antiphospholipid antibodies and fetal death. Amer. J. Obstet. Gynecol. **87**:489–493, 1996.

Out, H.J., Kooijman, C.D., Bruinse, H.W. and Derksen, R.H.W.M.: Histopathological findings in placentae from patients with intra-uterine fetal death and anti-phospholipid antibodies. Eur. J. Obstet. Gynecol. Reprod. Biol. **41**:179–186, 1991.

Out, H.J., Bruinse, H.W., Christiaens, G.C.M.L., Vliet, M.v., Groot, P.G.de, Nieuwenhuis, H.K. and Derksen, R.H.W.M.: A prospective, controlled multicenter study on the obstetric risks of pregnant women with antiphospholipid antibodies. Amer. J. Obstet. Gynecol. **167**:26–32, 1992.

Owen, J. and Hauth, J.C.: Polyarteritis nodosa in pregnancy: a case report and brief literature review. Amer. J. Obstet. Gynecol. **160**:606–607, 1989.

Padmanabhan, R., Al-Zuhair, A.G.H. and Ali, A.H.: Histopathological changes of the placenta in diabetes induced by maternal administration of streptozotocin during pregnancy in the rat. Congen. Anom. (Jpn.) **28**:1–15, 1988.

Page, D.V., Brady, K., Mitchell, J., Pehrson, J. and Wade, G.: The pathology of intrauterine thyrotoxicosis: two case reports. Obstet. Gynecol. **72**:479–481, 1988.

Page, D.V., Brady, K. and Ward, S.: The placental pathology of substance abuse. Modern Pathol. **2**(1):69A, 1989. (Abstract 410).

Page, K.R., Bush, P., Abramovich, D.R., Aggett, P.J., Burke, M.D. and Mayhew, T.M.: Effects of maternal smoking on placental structure and function. In, Placental Function and Fetal Nurtition. F.C. Battaglia, ed. Nestlé Nurtition Workshop Series, Vol. 39, pp. 247–249. Lippincott-Raven, Philadelphia, 1997.

Paidas, M.J., Berkowitz, R.L., Lynch, L., Lockwood, C.J., Lapinski, R., McFarland, J.G. and Bussel, J.B.: Alloimmune thrombocytopenia: fetal and neonatal losses related to cordocentesis. Amer. J. Obstet. Gynecol. **172**:475–479, 1995.

Palmer, A.E., London, W.T., Sly, D.L. and Rice, J.M.: Toxemia of pregnancy (preeclampsia, eclampsia, hypertensive disorders of pregnancy). In, Spontaneous Animal Models of Human Disease. Vol. I., E.J. Andrews, B.C. Ward and N.H. Altman, eds. pp. 213–215. Academic Press, New York, 1979.

Pampus, M.G.v., Dekker, G.A., Wolf, H., Huijgens, P.C., Koopman, M.M.W., Blomberg, M.E.v. and Büller, H.R.: High prevalence of hemostatic abnormalities in women with a history of severe preeclampsia. Amer. J. Obstet. Gynecol. **180**:1146–1150, 1999.

Pantanowitz, L., Schwartz, R. and Balogh, K.: The placenta in sickle cell disease. Arch. Pathol. Lab. Med. **124**:1565, 2000.

Parker, C.R., Illingworth, D.R., Bissonette, J. and Carr, B.R.: Endocrine changes during pregnancy in a patient with homozygous familial hypobetalipoproteinemia. NEJM **314**:557–560, 1986.

Pascoal, I.F., Lindheimer, M.D., Nalbantian-Brandt, C. and Umans, J.G.: Preeclampsia selectively impairs endothelium-dependent relaxation and leads to oscillatory activity in small omental arteries. J. Cin. Invest. **101**:464–470, 1998.

Pauer, H.-U., Neesen, J. and Hinney, B.: Factor V Leiden and its relevance in patients with recurrent abortions. Amer. J. Obstet. Gynecol. **178**:629, 1998.

Pavelka, M., Pavelka, R. and Gerstner, G.: Ultrastructure of the syncytiotrophoblast of the human term placenta in EPH-gestosis. Gynecol. Obstetr. Invest. **10**:177–185, 1979.

Payne, R.: Neonatal neutropenia and leukoagglutinins. Pediatrics **33**:194–204, 1964.

Payne, S.D., Resnik, R., Moore, T.R., Hedriana, H.L. and Kelly, T.F.: Maternal characteristics and risk of severe neonatal thrombocytopenia and intracranial hemorrhage in pregnancies complicated by autoimmune thrombocytopenia. Amer. J. Obstet. Gynecol. **177**:149–155, 1997.

Peaceman, A.M. and Rehnberg, K.A.: The effect of immunoglobulin G fractions from patients with lupus anticoagulant on placental prostacyclin and thromboxane production. Amer. J. Obstet. Gynecol. **169**:1403–1406, 1993.

Peaceman, A.M., Silver, R.K., MacGregor, S.N. and Socol, M.L.: Interlaboratory variation in antiphospholipid antibody testing. Amer. J. Obstet. Gynecol. **166**:1780–1787, 1992.

Pearce, J.M. and McParland, P.: Doppler uteroplacental waveforms. Lancet **i**:1287–1288, 1988.

Penn, I., Makowski, E.L. and Harris, P.: Parenthood following renal and hepatic transplantation. Transplantation **30**:397–400, 1980.

Pestelek, B. and Kapor, M.: Pheochromocytoma and abruptio placentae. Amer. J. Obstet. Gynecol. **85**:538–540, 1063.

Pfarrer, C., Macara, L., Leiser, R. and Kingdom, J.: Adaptive angiogenesis in placentas of heavy smokers. Lancet **354**:303, 1999.

Pijnenborg, R., Anthony, J., Davari, D.A., Rees, A., Tiltman, A., Vercruysse, L. and van Assche, A.: Placental bed spiral arteries in hypertensive disorders of pregnancy. Brit. J. Obstetr. Gynaecol. **98**:648–655, 1991.

Pijnenborg, R., Luyten, C., Vercruysse, L. and van Assche, F.A.: Attachment and differentiation in vitro of trophoblast from normal and preeclamptic human placentas. Amer. J. Obstet. Gynecol. **175**:30–36, 1996.

Pinette, M.G., Loftus-Brault, K., Nardi, D.A. and Rodis, J.F.: Maternal smoking and accelerated placental maturation. Obstet. Gynecol. **73**:379–382, 1989.

Pitkin, R.M., Plank, C.J. and Filer, L.J.: Fetal and placental composition in experimental maternal diabetes. Proc. Soc. Exp. Biol. Med. **138**:163–166, 1971.

Pittard III, W.B., Schleich, D.M., Geddes, K.M. and Sorensen, R.U.: Newborn lymphocyte subpopulations: The influence of labor. Amer. J. Obstetr. Gynecol. **160**:151–154, 1989.

Platt, H.S.: Effect of maternal sickle cell trait on perinatal mortality. Brit. Med. J. **2**:334–338, 1971.

Pober, J.S.: Cytokine-mediated activation of vascular endothelium. Physiology and pathology. Amer. J. Pathol. **133**:426–433, 1988.

Pollack, M.S., Kirkpatrick, D., Kapoor, N., Dupont, B. and O'Reilly, R.J.: The identification by HLA typing of intrauterine-derived maternal T cells in four patients with severe immunodeficiency. NEJM **307**:662–666, 1982.

Pollack, R.N., Pollack, M. and Rochon, L.: Pregnancy complicated by medulloblastoma with metastases to the placenta. Obstet. Gynecol. **81**:858–859, 1993.

Polzin, W.J., Kopelman, J.N., Robinson, R.D., Read, J.A. and Brady, K.: The association of antiphospholipid antibodies with pregnancies complicated by fetal growth restriction. Obstet. Gynecol. **78**:1108–1111, 1991.

Porter, K.B., Diebel, D. and Jazayeri, A.: Niemann-Pick disease type B in pregnancy. Obstet. Gynecol. **89**:860, 1997.

Potau, N., Riudor, E. and Ballabriga, A.: Insulin receptors in human placenta in relation to fetal weight and gestational age. Pediatr. Res. **15**:798–802, 1981.

Potter, J.F. and Schoeneman, M.: Metastasis of maternal cancer to the placenta and fetus. Cancer **25**:380–388, 1970.

Prentice, R.L., Gatenby, P.A., Loblay, R.H., Shearman, R.P., Kronenberg, H. and Basten, A.: Lupus anticoagulant in pregnancy. Lancet **ii**:464, 1984.

Preston, F.E., Rosendaal, F.R., Walker, I.D., Briet, E., Berntorp, E., Conard, J., Fontcuberta, J., Makris, M., Mariani, G., Noteboom, W., Pabinger, I., Legnani, C., Scharrer, I., Schulman, S. and Meer, F.J.M. van der: Increased fetal loss in women with heritable thrombophilia. Lancet **348**:913–916, 1996.

Priesel, A. and Winkelbauer, A.: Placentare Übertragung des Lymphogranuloms. Virchows Arch. [Pathol. Anat.] **262**:749–765, 1926.

Pritchard, J.A., Scott, D.E., Whalley, P.J. and Haling, R.F.: Infants of mothers with megaloblastic anemia due to folate deficiency. JAMA **211**:1982–1984, 1970.

Pritchard, M.H., Jessop, J.D., Trenchard, P.M. and Whiltaker, J.A.: Systemic lupus erythematosus, repeated abortions, and thrombocytopenia. Ann. Rheum. Dis. **37**:476–478, 1978.

Provost, T.T., Watson, R., Gammon, W.R., Radowsky, M., Harley, J.B. and Reichlin, M.: The neonatal lupus syndrome associated with U_1RNP (nRNP) antibodies. NEJM **316**:1135–1138, 1987.

Pulitzer, D.R., Collins, P.C. and Gold, R.G.: Embryonic implantation in carcinoma of the endometrium. Arch. Pathol. Lab. Med. **109**:1089–1092, 1985.

Ramahi, A.J., Lewkow, L.M., Dombrowski, M.P. and Bottoms, S.F.: Sickle cell E hemoglobinopathy and pregnancy. Obstet. Gynecol. **71**:493–495, 1988.

Rand, J.H., Wu, X.X., Andree, H.A.M., Lockwood, C.J., Guller, S., Scher, J. and Harpel, P.C.: Pregnancy loss in the antiphospholipid-antibody syndrome—a possible thrombogenic mechanism. NEJM **337**:154–160, 1997.

Rauramo, I. and Forss, M.: Effect of exercise on placental blood flow in pregnancies complicated by hypertension, diabetes or intrahepatic cholestasis. Acta Obstetr. Gynecol. Scand. **67**:15–20, 1988.

Raymond, E.G. and Mills, J.L.: Placental abruption. Maternal risk factors and associated fetal conditions. Acta Obstet. Gynecol. Scand. **72**:633–639, 1993.

Read, E.J. and Platzer, P.B.: Placental metastasis from maternal carcinoma of the lung. Obstet. Gynecol. **58**:387–391, 1981.

Redman, C.W.G. and Jefferies, M.: Revised definition of preeclampsia. Lancet **i**:809–812, 1988.

Redman, C.W.G., Bodmer, J.G., Bodmer, W.F., Beilin, L.J. and Bonnar, J.: HLA antigens in severe pre-eclampsia. Lancet **ii**:397–399, 1978.

Redman, C.W.G., Sacks, G.P. and Sargent, I.L.: Preeclampsia: an excessive maternal inflammatory response to pregnancy. Amer. J. Obstet. Gynecol. **180**:499–506, 1999.

Reece, E.A., Romero, R., Clyne, L.P., Kriz, N.S. and Hobbins, J.C.: Lupus-like anticoagulant in pregnancy. Lancet **i**:344–345, 1984.

Reece, E.A., Gabrielli, S., Cullen, M.T., Zheng, X.-Z., Hobbins, J.C. and Harris, E.N.: Recurrent adverse pregnancy outcome and antiphospholipid antibodies. Amer. J. Obstet. Gynecol. **163**:162–169, 1990.

Rees, D.C., Cox, M. and Clegg, J.B.: World distribution of factor V Leiden. Lancet **346**:1133–1134, 1995.

Reid, T.M.S.: Striking a balance in maternal immune response to infection. Lancet **351**:1670–1672, 1998.

Reiss, R.E., Kuwabara, T., Smith, M.L. and Gahl, W.A.: Successful pregnancy despite placental cystine crystals in a woman with nephropathic cystinosis. NEJM **319**:223–226, 1988.

Reshetnikova, O.S., Burton, G.J. and Teleshova, O.V.: Placental histomorphometry and morphometric diffusing capacity of the villous membrane in pregnancies complicated by maternal iron-deficiency anemia. Amer. J. Obstet. Gynecol. **173**:724–727, 1995.

Reshetnikova, O.S., Burton, G.J. and Milovanov, A.P.: Increased incidence of placental chorioangioma in high-altitude pregnancies: hypobaric hypoxia as a possible etiological factor. Amer. J. Obstet. Gynecol. **174**:557–561, 1996.

Retik, A.B., Sabesin, S.M., Hume, R., Malmgren, R.A. and Ketcham, A.S.: The experimental transmission of malignant melanoma cells through the placenta. Surg. Gynecol. Obstet. **114**:485–489, 1962.

Rewell, R.E. and Whitehouse, W.L.: Malignant metastasis to the placenta from carcinoma of the breast. J. Pathol. Bacteriol. **91**:255–256, 1966.

Rey, E., Kahn, S.R., David, M. and Shrier, I.: Thrombophilic disorders and fetal loss: a meta-analysis. Lancet **361**:901–908, 2003.

Reynolds, A.G.: Placental metastasis from malignant melanoma: report of a case. Obstet. Gynecol. **6**:205–209, 1955.

Rice, J.P., Kay, H.H. and Mahony, B.S.: The clinical significance of uterine leiomyomas in pregnancy. Amer. J. Obstet. Gynecol. **160**:1212–1216, 1989.

Richards, D.S., Wagman, A.J. and Cabaniss, M.L.: Ascites not due to congestive heart failure in a fetus with lupus-induced heart block. Obstet. Gynecol. **76**:957–959, 1990.

Ridker, P.M., Miletich, J.P., Stampfer, M.J., Goldhaber, S.Z., Lindpaintner, K. and Hennekens, C.H.: Factor V Leiden and risks of recurrent idiopathic venous thromboembolism. Circulation **92**:2800–2802, 1995.

Rigby, P.G., Hanson, T.A. and Smith, R.S.: Passage of leukemic cells across the placenta. NEJM **271**:124–127, 1964.

Rizzo, G., Arduini, D., Capponi, A. and Romanini, C.: Cardiac and venous blood flow in fetuses of insulin-dependent diabetic mothers: evidence of abnormal hemodynamics in early gestation. Amer. J. Obstet. Gynecol. **173**:1775–1781, 1995.

Robb, S.A. and Hytten, F.E.: Placental glycogen. Brit. J. Obstet. Gynaecol. **83**:43–53, 1976.

Robbins, P.G., Gorbach, A.G. and Reid, D.E.: Neurologic abnormalities at one year in infants delivered after late-pregnancy hemorrhage. Obstet. Gynecol. **29**:358–361, 1967.

Roberts, J.M.: Classification of hypertensive disorders of pregnancy. Lancet **ii**:112, 1989.

Roberts, J.M.: Pregnancy-related hypertension. In, Maternal-Fetal Medicine. Principles and Practice. R.K. Creasy and R. Resnik, eds. W.B. Saunders, Philadelphia, 1994.

Roberts, J.M. and Cooper, D.W.: Pathogenesis and genetics of pre-eclampsia. Lancet **357**:53–56, 2001.

Robertson, W.B., Brosens, I. and Dixon, H.G.: The pathological response of the vessels of the placental bed to hypertensive pregnancy. J. Pathol. Bacteriol. **93**:581–592, 1967.

Robertson, W.B., Khong, T.Y., Brosens, I., DeWolff, F., Sheppard, B.L. and Bonnar, J.: The placental bed biopsy: Review from three European centers. Amer. J. Obstetr. Gynecol. **155**:401–412, 1986.

Robillard, P.-Y., Hulsey, T.C., Périanin, Janky, E., Miri, E.H. and Papiernik, E.: Association of pregnancy-induced hypertension with duration of sexual cohabitation before conception. Lancet **344**:973–975, 1994.

Robinson, M.: Salt in pregnancy. Lancet **1**:178–181, 1958.

Robson, S.C., Simpson, H., Ball, E., Lyall, F. and Bulmer, J.N.: Punch biopsy of the human placental bed. Amer. J. Obstet. Gynecol. **187**:1349–1355, 2002.

Rodriguez, S.U., Leikin, S.L. and Hiller, M.C.: Neonatal thrombocytopenia associated with ante-partum administration of thiazide drugs. NEJM **270**:881–884, 1964.

Roe, D.A., Little, B.B., Bawdon, R.E. and Gilstrap, L.C.: Metabolism of cocaine by human placentas: Implications for fetal exposure. Amer. J. Obstet. Gynecol. **163**:715–718, 1990.

Roffman, B.Y. and Simons, M.: Syncytial trophoblastic embolism associated with placenta increta and pre-eclampsia. Amer. J. Obstetr. Gynecol. **104**:1218–1220, 1969.

Rojansky, N., Fasouliotis, S.J., Ariel, I. and Nadjari, M.: Extreme caudal agenesis. Possible drug-related etiology? J. Reprod. Med. **47**:241–245, 2002.

Rosenberg, A.M., Bingham, M.C. and Fong, K.C.: Antinuclear antibodies during pregnancy. Obstet. Gynecol. **68**:560–562, 1986.

Rosenfeld, C.R.: Preeclampsia: a review of the role of prostaglandins. Obstetr. Gynecol. **72**:284–285, 1988.

Rosenow, E.C. and Lee, R.A.: Cystic fibrosis and pregnancy. JAMA **203**:227–230, 1968.

Rosner, F., Soong, B.C., Krim, M. and Miller, S.P.: Normal pregnancy in a patient with multiple myeloma. Obstet. Gynecol. **31**:811–820, 1968.

Rosove, M.H., Tabsh, K., Wasserstrum, N., Howard, P., Hahn, B.H. and Kalunian, K.C.: Heparin therapy for pregnant women with lupus anticoagulant or anticardiolipin antibodies. Obstet. Gynecol. **75**:630–634, 1990.

Rote, N.S. and Caudle, M.R.: Circulating immune complexes in pregnancy, preeclampsia, and autoimmune diseases: evaluation of Raji cell enzyme-linked immunosorbent assay and polyethylene glycol precipitation methods. Amer. J. Obstetr. Gynecol. **147**:267–273, 1983.

Rote, N.S., Vogt, E. and Awaloei, H.: Antiphospholipid antibodies and preterm birth. Prenat. Neonat. Med. **3**:68–71, 1198.

Rothman, L.A., Cohen, C.J. and Astarloa, J.: Placental and fetal involvement by maternal malignancy: a report of rectal carcinoma and review of the literature. Amer. J. Obstet. Gynecol. **116**:1023–1034, 1973.

Rouget, J.P., Goudemand, J., Montreuil, G., Cosson, A. and Jaillard, J.: Lupus anticoagulant: a familial observation. Lancet **ii**:105, 1982.

Rubin, D.H., Krasilikoff, P.A., Leventhal, J.M., Weile, B. and Berget, A.: Effect of passive smoking on birth-weight. Lancet **2**:415–417, 1986.

Rushton, D.I.: Trophoblast cells in peripheral blood. Lancet **ii**:1153–1154, 1984.

Salafia, C.M. and Silberman, L.: Placental pathology and abnormal fetal heart rate patterns in gestational diabetes. Pediatr. Pathol. **9**:513–520, 1989.

Salafia, C.M., Pezzulo, J.C., López-Zeno, J.A., Simmens, S., Minior, V.K. and Vintzileos, A.M.: Placental pathologic features of preterm preeclampsia. Amer. J. Obstet. Gynecol. **173**:1097–1105, 1995.

Salamon, M.A., Sherer, D.M., Saller, D.N., Metlay, L.A. and Sickel, J.Z.: Placental metastases in a patient with recurrent breast carcinoma. Amer. J. Obstet. Gynecol. **171**:573–574, 1994.

Salmon, J.E., Girardi, G. and Holers, V.M.: Activation of complement mediates antiphospholipid antibody-induced pregnancy loss. Lupus **12**:535–538, 2003.

Samaan, N.A., Gallager, H.S., McRoberts, W.A. and Holt, B.: Differential evaluation of the fetoplacental unit in patients with diabetes. Amer. J. Obstet. Gynecol. **120**:825–832, 1974.

Sanerkin, N.G. and Evans, D.M.D.: Bilateral renal cortical necrosis in infants, associated with maternal antepartum haemorrhage. J. Pathol. Bacteriol. **90**:269–274, 1965.

Sanyal, M.K., Li, Y.-L., Biggers, W., Satish, J. and Barnea, E.R.: Augmentation of polynuclear aromatic hydrocarbon metabolism of human placental tissues of first-trimester pregnancy by cigarette smoke exposure. Amer. J. Obstet. Gynecol. **168**:1587–1597, 1993.

Sarig, G., Younis, J.S., Hoffman, R., Lanir, N., Blumenfeld, Z. and Brenner, B.: Thrombophilia is common in women with idiopathic pregnancy loss and is associated with late pregnancy wastage. Fertil. Steril **77**:342–347, 2002.

Sasseville, D., Wilkinson, R.D. and Schnader, J.Y.: Dermatoses of pregnancy. Int. J. Dermatol. **20**:223–241, 1981.

Schaffner, T., Taylor, K., Bartucci, E.J., Fischer-Dzoga, K., Beeson, J.H., Glasgo, S. and Wissler, R.W.: Arterial foam cells with distinctive immunomorphologic and histochemical features of macrophages. Amer. J. Pathol. **100**:57–80, 1980.

Schenker, J.G. and Polishuk, W.Z.: Idiopathic thrombocytopenia in pregnancy. Gynaecologia **165**:271–283, 1968.

Schenker, J.G., Segal, S. and Polishuk, W.Z.: Systemic lupus erythematosus in pregnancy. Harefuah **82**:1–4, 1972.

Schiff, E., Peleg, E., Goldenberg, M., Rosenthal, T., Ruppin, E., Tamarkin, M., Barkal, G., Ben-Baruch, G., Yahal, I., Blankstein, J., Goldman, B. and Mashiach, S.: The use of aspirin to prevent pregnancy-induced hypertension and lower the ratio of thromboxane A$_2$ to prostacyclin in relatively high risk pregnancies. NEJM **321**:351–356, 1989.

Schmidt, B.K., Muraji, T. and Zipursky, A.: Low antithrombin III in neonatal shock: DIC or non-specific protein depletion? Europ. J. Pediatr. **145**:500–503, 1986.

Schmidt, M.J., Cook, L. and Zhang, P.: Maternal vasculopathy and diagnosis of pre-eclampsia: Histologic analyses of placentas. Modern Pathol. **18** Suppl. 1: p. 306A, abstract 1416, 2005.

Schmorl, G.: Pathologisch-Anatomische Untersuchungen über Puerperale Eklampsie. F.C.W. Vogel, Leipzig, 1893.

Schneider, C.L.: "Fibrin embolism" (disseminated intravascular coagulation) with defibrination as one of the end results during placenta abruptio. Surg. Gynecol. Obstetr. **92**:27–34, 1951.

Schneider, C.L.: Abruptio placentae after fetal death in utero. Obstetr. Gynecol. **1**:321–326, 1953.

Schuhmann, R. und Geier, G.: Histomorphologische Placentabefunde bei EPH-Gestose. Ein Beitrag zur Morphologie der insuffizienten Placenta. Arch. Gynäkol. **213**:31–47, 1972.

Schuhmann, R. und Lehmann, W.D.: Beziehungen zwischen Placentamorphologie und biochemischen Befunden bei EPH-Gestose und Diabetes mellitus. Dehydroandrosteronb-

elastungstest, in vitro Umwandlungsrate von 4-^{14}C-Dehydroepiandrosteron in Oestrogene, Oestrogenausscheidung im 24 Std-Urin. Arch. Gynäkol. **215**:72–84, 1973.

Schultze, P.M., Stamm, C.A. and Roger, J.: Placental abruption and fetal death with airbag deployment in a motor vehicle accident. Obstet. Gynecol. **92**:719, 1998.

Scott, J.S.: Immunological diseases and pregnancy. Brit. Med. J. **1**:1559–1568, 1966.

Scott, J.R. and Beer, A.A.: Immunologic aspects of pre-eclampsia. Amer. J. Obstetr. Gynecol. **125**:418–427, 1976.

Scott, J.S. and Jenkins, D.M.: Review article. Immunogenetic factors in aetiology of pre-eclampsia/eclampsia (gestosis). J. Med. Genet. **13**:200–207, 1976.

Scott, J.S., Jenkins, D.M. and Need, J.A.: Immunology of pre-eclampsia. Lancet **i**:704–706, 1978.

Scott, J.R., Branch, D.W., Kochenour, N.K. and Ward, K.: Intravenous immunoglobulin treatment of pregnant patients with recurrent pregnancy loss caused by antiphospholipid antibodies and Rh immunization. Amer. J. Obstet. Gynecol. **159**:1055–1056, 1988.

Scully, R.E., Galdabini, J.J. and McNeely, B.U.: Cabot Case # 37–1976. NEJM **295**:608–614, 1976.

Seip, M.: Systemic lupus erythematosus in pregnancy with haemolytic anaemia, leucopenia and thrombocytopenia in the mother and her newborn infant. Arch. Dis. Child. **35**:364–366, 1960.

Shafrir, E. and Barash, V.: Placental glycogen metabolism in diabetic pregnancy. Israel J. Med. Sci. **27**:449–461, 1991.

Shanklin, D.R.: The human placenta with especial reference to infarction and toxemia. Obstetr. Gynecol. **13**:325–336, 1959.

Shanklin, D.R.: Clinicopathologic correlates in placentas from women with sickle cell disease. Amer. J. Pathol. **82**: abstract PPC-15, p. 5a, March, 1976.

Shanklin, D.R. and Sibai, B.M.: Ultrastructural aspects of pre-eclampsia. I. Placental bed and uterine boundary vessels. Amer. J. Obstetr. Gynecol. **161**:735–741, 1989.

Sharon, R. and Amar, A.: Maternal anti-HLA antibodies and neonatal thrombocytopenia. Lancet **1**:1313, 1981.

Shaw, E.B. and Rees, E.L.: Fetal damage due to aminopterin ingestion: follow-up at 17½ years of age. Amer. J. Dis. Child. **134**:1172, 1980.

Sheridan-Pereira, M., Porreco, R., Hays, T. and Burke, M.S.: Neonatal aortic thrombosis associated with the lupus anticoagulant. Obstet. Gynecol. **71**:1016–1018, 1988.

Shiono, P.H., Klebanoff, M.A., Nugent, R.P., Cotch, M.F., Wilkins, D.G., Rollins, D.E., Carey, J.C. and Behrman, R.E.: The impact of cocaine and marijuana use on low birth weight and preterm birth: a multicenter study. Amer. J. Obstet. Gynecol. **172**:19–27, 1995.

Sholl, J.S.: Abruptio placentae: clinical management in nonacute cases. Amer. J. Obstetr. Gynecol. **156**:40–51, 1987.

Sibai, B.M., Hauth, J., Caritis, S., Lindheimer, M.D., McPherson, C., Klebanoff, M., VanDorsten, J.P., Landon, M., Miodovnik, M., Paul, R., Meis, P., Thurnau, G., Dombrowski, M., Roberts, J. and McNellis, D.: Hypertensive disorders in twin versus singleton gestations. Amer. J. Obstet. Gynecol. **182**:938–942, 2000.

Sibai, B., Dekker, G. and Kupferminc, M.: Pre-eclampsia. Lancet **365**:785–799, 2005.

Siegel, P.: Beziehungen zwischen eklamptischen Placentarve-ränderungen und intrauterinem Fruchttod. Fortschr. Med. **80**:75–82, 1962.

Silver, M.M.: Massive placental infarction due to the lupus anticoagulant. Modern Pathol. **1**:abstract 508, 85A, 1988.

Silver, M.M., Laxer, R.M., Laskin, C.A., Smallhorn, J.F. and Gare, D.J.: Association of fetal heart block and massive placental infarction due to maternal autoantibodies. Pediatr. Pathol. **12**:131–139, 1992a.

Silver, R.K., MacGregor, S.N., Pasternak, J.F. and Neely, S.E.: Fetal stroke associated with elevated maternal anticardiolipin antibodies. Obstet. Gynecol. **80**:497–499, 1992b.

Silver, R.M., Pierangeli, S.S., Edwin, S.S., Umar, F., Harris, E.N., Scott, J.R. and Branch, D.W.: Pathogenic antibodies in women with obstetric features of antiphospholipid syndrome who have negative test results for lupus anticoagulant and anticardiolipin antibodies. Amer. J. Obstet. Gynecol. **176**:628–633, 1997a.

Silver, R.M., Smith, L.A., Edwin, S.S., Oshiro, B.T., Scott, J.R. and Branch, D.W.: Variable effects on murine pregnancy of immunoglobulin G fraction from women with antiphospholipid antibodies. Amer. J. Obstet. Gynecol. **177**:229–233, 1997b.

Silverstein, M.N., Aaro, L.A. and Kempers, R.D.: Evans' syndrome and pregnancy. Amer. J. Med. Sci. **252**:206–211, 1966.

Singer, D.B.: The placenta in pregnancies complicated by diabetes mellitus. Perspect. Pediatr. Pathol. **8**:199–212, 1984.

Sironi, M., Declich, P., Isimbaldi, G., Monguzzi, A. and Poggi, G.: Placental teratoma with three-germ layer differentiation. Teratology **50**:165–167, 1994.

Slate, W.G. and Graham, A.R.: Scleroderma and pregnancy. Amer. J. Obstet. Gynecol. **101**:335–341, 1968.

Sletnes, K.E., Wisloff, F., Moe, N. and Dale, P.O.: Antiphospholipid antibodies in pre-eclamptic women: relation to growth retardation and neonatal outcome. Acta Obstet. Gynecol. Scand. **71**:112–117, 1992.

Slukvin, I.I., Boyson, J.E., Watkins, D.I. and Golos, T.G.: The rhesus monkey analogue of human lymphocyte antigen-G is expressed primarily in villous syncytiotrophoblasts. Biol. Reprod. **58**:728–738, 1998.

Smith, J.A., Espeland, M., Bellevue, R., Bonds, D., Brown, A.K. and Koshy, M.: Pregnancy in sickle cell disease: experience of the cooperative study of sickle cell disease. Obstet. Gynecol. **87**:199–204, 1996.

Smith, M.L., Clark, K.F., Davis, S.E., Greene, A.A., Marcusson, E.G., Chen, Y.-J. and Schneider, J.A.: Diagnosis of cystinosis with use of placenta. NEJM **321**:397, 1989.

Smythe, A.R., Underwood, P.B. and Kreutner, A.: Metastatic placental tumors: report of three cases. Amer. J. Obstet. Gynecol. **125**:1149–1151, 1976.

Sokol, R.J., Hutchison, P., Cowan, D. and Reed, G.B.: Amelanotic melanoma metastatic to the placenta. Amer. J. Obstet. Gynecol. **124**:431–432, 1976.

Sokol, R.J., Miller, S.I. and Reed, G.: Alcohol abuse during pregnancy: an epidemiologic study: alcoholism. Clin. Exp. Res. **4**:135–145, 1980.

Soma, H., Yoshida, K., Mukaida, T. and Tabuchi, Y.: Morphologic changes in the hypertensive placenta. Contribut. Gynecol. Obstetr. **9**:58–75, 1982.

Sophian, J.: Antibodies to trophoblast post partum and toxemia. Amer. J. Obstet. Gynecol. **88**:280–281, 1964.

Sorensen, P.G., Mickley, H., Diederichsen, H. and Grunnert, N.: Maternal antibodies and neonatal thrombocytopenia. Lancet **1**:452, 1982.

Soyannwo, M.A.O., Armstrong, M.J. and McGeown, M.G.: Survival of the foetus in a patient in acute renal failure. Lancet **2**:1009–1011, 1966.

Spellacy, W.N.: Scleroderma and pregnancy: report of a case. Obstet. Gynecol. **23**:297–300, 1964.

Sprauve, M.E., Lindsay, M.K., Herbert, S. and Graves, W.: Adverse perinatal outcome in parturients who use crack cocaine. Obstet. Gynecol. **89**:674–678, 1997.

Sridama, V., Yang, S.L., Moawad, A. and De Groot, L.J.: T-cell subsets in patients with preeclampsia. Amer. J. Obstetr. Gynecol. **147**:566–569, 1983.

Srivatsa, B., Srivatsa, S., Johnson, K.L., Samura, O., Lee, S.L. and Bianchi, D.W.: Microchimerism of presumed fetal origin in thyroid specimens from women: a case-control study. Lancet **358**:2011–2012, 2001 (and **359**:1861–1862, 2002).

Stallmach, T., Hebisch, G., Meier, K., Dudenhausen, J.W. and Vogel, M.: Rescue by birth: defective maturation and late fetal mortality. Obstet. Gynecol. **97**:505–509, 2001.

Stark, J. und Kaufmann, P.: Infarktgenese in der Placenta. Arch. Gynäkol. **217**:189–208, 1974.

Steigrad, K.: Über die Beziehung von Plazentarinfarkten zur Schwangerschafts-Nephropathie. Zugleich ein Beitrag zur Pathologie der Plazenta. Gynaecologia **134**:273–322, 1952.

Steinke, J. and Driscoll, S.G.: The extractable insulin content of pancreas from fetuses and infants of diabetic and control mothers. Diabetes **14**:573–578, 1965.

Stephenson, H.E., Terry, C.W., Lukens, J.N., Shively, J.A., Busby, W.E., Stoeckle, H.E. and Esterly, J.A.: Immunologic factors in human melanoma "metastatic" to products of gestation (with exchange transfusion to mother). Surgery **69**:515–522, 1971.

Stormorken, H., Gjemdal, T. and Njoro, K.: Lupus anticoagulant: a unique case with lupus anticoagulant and habitual abortion together with antifactor II antibody and bleeding tendency. Gynecol. Obstet. Invest. **26**:83–88, 1988.

Streiff, R.R. and Little, A.B.: Folic acid deficiency in pregnancy. NEJM **276**:776–779, 1967.

Stuart, M.J., Clark, D.A., Sunderji, S.G., Allen, J.B., Yambo, T., Elrad, H. and Slott, J.H.: Decreased prostacyclin production: a characteristic of chronic placental insufficiency syndromes. Lancet **1**:1126–1128, 1981.

Susa, J.B., Neave, C., Sehgal, P., Singer, D.B., Zeller, W.P. and Schwartz, R.: Chronic hyperinsulinemia in the fetal rhesus monkey. Effects of physiologic hyperinsulinemia on fetal growth and composition. Diabetes **33**:656–660, 1984.

Sweeney, W.J. and Katz, V.L.: Recurrent pheochromocytoma during pregnancy. Obstet. Gynecol. **83**:820–822, 1994.

Tatum, H.J.: Placental abruption. Obstetr. Gynecol. **2**:447–453, 1953.

Taylor, R.N., Grimwood, J., Taylor, R.S., McMaster, M.T., Fisher, S.J. and North, R.A.: Longitudinal serum concentrations of placental growth factor: evidence for abnormal placental angiogenesis in pathologic pregnancies. Amer. J. Obstet. Gynecol. **188**:177–182, 2003.

Teasdale, F.: Histomorphometry of the placenta of the diabetic woman: class A diabetes mellitus. Placenta **2**:241–252, 1981.

Teasdale, F.: Histomorphometry of human placenta in class B diabetes mellitus. Placenta **4**:1–12, 1983.

Teasdale, F.: Histomorphometry of the human placenta in class C diabetes mellitus. Placenta **5**:69–86, 1984.

Teasdale, F.: Histomorphometry of the human placenta in maternal preeclampsia. Amer. J. Obstetr. Gynecol. **152**:25–31, 1985.

Teasdale, F. and Ghislaine, J.-J.: Morphological changes in the placentas of smoking mothers: a histomorphometric study. Biol. Neonate **55**:251–259, 1989.

Tedeschi, L.G. and Tedeschi, C.G.: Experimental trophoblastic embolism and hyperplasminemia. Arch. Pathol. **76**:387–397, 1963.

Tenney, B. and Parker, F.: The placenta in toxemia of pregnancy. Amer. J. Obstetr. Gynecol. **39**:1000–1005, 1940.

Thomas, K., Gasparo, M. de and Hoet, J.J.: Insulin levels in the umbilical vein and in the umbilical artery of newborns of normal and gestational diabetic mothers. Diabetes **3**:299–304, 1967.

Thomsen, K. and Lieschke, G.: Untersuchungen zur Placenta-morphologie bei Diabetes mellitus. Acta Endocrinol. (Copenh.) **29**:602–614, 1958.

Thornton, J.G. and Sampson, J.: Genetics of pre-eclampsia. Lancet **336**:1319–1320, 1990.

Thornton, J.P. and Onwoude, J.L.: Pre-eclampsia: discordance among identical twins. Brit. Med. J. **303**:1241–1242, 1991.

Thornton, Y.S., Birnbaum, S.J. and Lebowitz, N.: A viable pregnancy in a patient with myositis ossificans. Amer. J. Obstet. Gynecol. **156**:577–578, 1987.

Thorp, J.A., Walsh, S.W. and Brath, P.C.: Low-dose aspirin inhibits thromboxane, but not prostacyclin, production by human placental arteries. Amer. J. Obstetr. Gynecol. **159**:1381–1384, 1988.

Toder, V., Blank, M., Gleicher, N., Voljovich, I., Mashiah, S. and Nebel, L.: Activity of natural killer cells in normal pregnancy and edema-proteinuria-hypertension gestosis. Amer. J. Obstet. Gynecol. **145**:7–10, 1983.

Toivonen, S., Romppanen, E.L., Hiltunen, M., Helisalmi, S., Keski-Nisula, L., Punnonen, K. and Heinonen, S.: Low-activity haplotype of the microsomal epoxide hydrolase gene is protective against placental abruption. J. Soc. Gynecol. Invest. **11**:540–544, 2004.

Tominaga, T. and Page, E.W.: Accommodation of the human placenta to hypoxia. Amer. J. Obstet. Gynecol. **84**:679–691, 1966.

Torpin, R. and Swain, B.: Placental infarction in 1,000 cases correlated with the clinical findings. Amer. J. Obstetr. Gynecol. **94**:284–285, 1966.

Trauscht-Van Horn, J., Capeless, E., Bovill, E.G., Easterling, T.R. and Hermanson, B.: Pregnancy loss and thrombosis with protein C deficiency in pregnancy. Amer. J. Obstet. Gynecol. **166**:311 (abstract 114), 1992.

Triplett, D.A.: Antiphospholipid antibodies and recurrent pregnancy loss. Amer. J. Reprod. Immunol. **20**:52–67, 1989.

Triplett, D.A.: Antiphospholipid antibodies and thrombosis. A consequence, coincidence, or cause? Arch. Pathol. Lab. Med. **117**:78–88, 1993.

Triplett, D.A., Brandt, J.T. and Maas, R.L.: The laboratory heterogeneity of lupus anticoagulant. Arch. Pathol. Lab. Med. **109**:946–951, 1985.

Trudinger, B.J., Stewart, G.J., Cook, C.M., Connelly, A. and Exner, T.: Monitoring lupus anticoagulant-positive pregnancies with umbilical artery flow velocity waveforms. Obstet. Gynecol. **72**:215–218, 1988.

Tsujimura, T., Matsumoto, K. and Aozasa, K.: Placental involvement by maternal non-Hodgkin's lymphoma. Arch. Pathol. Lab. Med. **117**:325–327, 1993.

Unander, A.M., Norberg, R., Hahn, L. and Årfors, L.: Anticardiolipin antibodies and complement in ninety-nine women with habitual abortion. Amer. J. Obstet. Gynecol. **156**:114–119, 1987.

Uzan, S., Beaufils, M., Breart G., Bazin, B., Capitant, C. and Paris, J.: Prevention of fetal growth retardation with low-dose aspirin: findings of the EPREDA trial. Lancet **337**:1427–1431, 1991.

Vasquez-Escobosa, C., Perez-Medina, R. and Gomez-Estrada, H.: Circulating immune complexes in hypertensive disease of pregnancy. Obstet. Gynecol. **62**:45–48, 1982.

Vassalli, P., Morris, R.H. and McCluskey, R.T.: The pathogenic role of fibrin deposition in the glomerular lesions of toxemia of pregnancy. J. Exp. Med. **118**:467–478, 1963.

Vintzileos, A.M., Campbell, W.A., Nochimson, D.J. and Weinbaum, P.J.: Preterm premature rupture of the membranes: a risk factor for the development of abruptio placentae. Amer. J. Obstet. Gynecol. **156**:1235–1238, 1987.

Viscarello, R.R., Gennaro, N.J.de and Reece, E.A.: The fetus of the diabetic mother. In, The High-Risk Fetus. Pathophysiology, Diagnosis, Management. C.C. Lin, M.S. Verp. and R.E. Sabbagha, eds., pp. 396–427. Springer-Verlag, New York, 1993.

Vogel, J.J., Moerloose, P.A. de and Bounameaux, H.: Protein C deficiency and pregnancy: a case report. Obstet. Gynecol. **73**:455–456, 1989.

Vogel, M.: Plakopathia diabetica. Virchows Arch. [Pathol. Anat.] **343**:51–63, 1967.

Voigt, L.F., Hollenbach, K.A., Krohn, M.A., Daling, J.R. and Hickok, D.E.: The relationship of abruptio placentae with maternal smoking and small for gestational age infants. Obstet. Gynecol. **75**:771–774, 1990.

Vulsma, T., Gons, M.H. and de Vijlder, J.J.M.: Maternal-fetal transfer of thyroxine in congenital hypothyroidism due to a total organification defect or thyroid agenesis. NEJM **321**:13–16, 1989.

Waddington, H.K.: Fetal salvage in abruptio placentae. Amer. J. Obstetr. Gynecol. **73**:812–816, 1957.

Wagner, D.: Trophoblastic cells in the blood stream in normal and abnormal pregnancy. Acta Cytol. **12**:137–139, 1968.

Wagner, D., Schunck, R. und Isebarth, H.: Der Nachweis von Trophoblastzellen im strömenden Blut der Frau bei normaler und gestörter Gravidität. Gynaecologia **158**:175–192, 1964.

Walker, M., Garner, P., Keely, E. and Rock, G.: Changes in activated protein C resistance during pregnancy. Amer. J. Obstet. Gynecol. **176**: SPO abstract S189 #670, 1997.

Wallenburg, H.C.S.: Über den Zusammenhang zwischen Spätgestose und Placentarinfarkt. Arch. Gynäkol. **208**:80–90, 1969.

Wallenburg, H.C.S., Stolte, L.A.M. and Janssens, J.: The pathogenesis of placental infarction. I. A morphologic study in the human placenta. Amer. J. Obstetr. Gynecol. **116**:835–840, 1973a.

Wallenburg, H.C.S., Hutchinson, D.L., Schuler, H.M., Stolte, L.A.M. and Janssens, J.: The pathogenesis of placental infarction. II. An experimental study in the rhesus monkey placenta. Amer. J. Obstetr. Gynecol. 116:841–846, 1973b.

Walsh, S.W.: Preeclampsia: an imbalance in placental prostacyclin and thromboxane production. Amer. J. Obstetr. Gynecol. 152:335–340, 1985.

Walsh, S.W., Behr, M.J. and Allen, N.H.: Placental prostacyclin production in normal and toxemic pregnancies. Amer. J. Obstetr. Gynecol. 151:110–115, 1985.

Wang, J.X., Knottnerus, A.-M., Schuit, G., Norman, R.J., Chan, A. and Dekker, G.A.: Surgically obtained sperm, and risk of gestational hypertension and pre-eclampsia. Lancet 359:673–674, 2002.

Wapner, R.J., Cowchock, F.S. and Shapiro, S.S.: Successful treatment in two women with antiphospholipid antibodies and refractory pregnancy losses with intravenous immunoglobulin infusions. Amer. J. Obstet. Gynecol. 161:1271–1272, 1989.

Warrell, D.W. and Taylor, R.: Outcome for the foetus of mothers receiving prednisolone during pregnancy. Lancet i:117–118, 1968.

Warren, R.J., Rimoin, D.L. and Sly, W.S.: LSD exposure in utero. Pediatrics 45:466–469, 1970.

Watanabe, T., Minakami, H. and Sakata, Y.: Successful management of pregnancy in a patient with von Willebrand disease Normandy. Obstet. Gynecol. 89:859, 1997.

Watov, S.E. and De Sandre, R.: Gaucher's disease and pregnancy: report of one case involving four pregnancies. Obstet. Gynecol. 23:247–250, 1964.

Watson, W.J. and Fiegen, M.M.: Fetal thyrotoxicosis associated with nonimmune hydrops. Amer. J. Obstet. Gynecol. 172:1039–1040, 1995.

Wax, J.R., Eggleston, M.K. and Teague, K.E.: Pregnancy complicated by multiple endocrine neoplasia type IIA (Sipple's syndrome). Amer. J. Obstet. Gynecol. 177:461–462, 1997.

Weathers, W.T., Crane, M.M., Sauvain, K.J. and Blackhurst, D. W.: Cocaine use in women from a defined population: prevalence at delivery and effects on growth in infants. Pediatrics 91:350–354, 1993.

Weiner, C. and Keller, S.: Preeclampsia is not associated with excess fetal clotting. Obstet. Gynecol. 68:871–872, 1986.

Weir, P.E.: Immunofluorescent studies of the uteroplacental arteries in normal pregnancy. Brit. J. Obstetr. Gynaecol. 88: 301–307, 1981.

Wells, M. and Bulmer, J.N.: The human placental bed: histology, immunohistochemistry and pathology. Histopathology 13: 483–498, 1988.

Wen, S.W., Goldenberg, R.L., Cutter, G.R., Hoffman, H.J., Cliver, S.P., Davis, R.O. and DuBard, M.B.: Smoking, maternal age, fetal growth, and gestational age at delivery. Amer. J. Obstet. Gynecol. 162:53–58, 1990.

Werler, M.M.: Teratogen update: smoking and reproductive outcomes. Teratology 55:382–388, 1997.

Wentworth, P.: Placental infarction and toxemia of pregnancy. Amer. J. Obstetr. Gynecol. 99:318–326, 1967.

Whalley, P.J., Pritchard, J.A. and Richards, J.R.: Sickle cell trait and pregnancy. JAMA 186:1132–1135, 1963.

White, B.M. and Beischer, N.A.: Perinatal mortality in the infants of diabetic women. Austr. N. Z. J. Obstetr. Gynaecol. 30:323–326, 1990.

White, P.: Classification of obstetric diabetes. Amer. J. Obstet. Gynecol. 130:228–230, 1978.

Widmaier, G.: Zur Ultrastruktur menschlicher Placentazotten beim Diabetes mellitus. Arch. Gynäkol. 208:396–409, 1970.

Wieland, R.G., Shaffer, M.B. and Glove, R.P.: Cushing's syndrome complicating pregnancy: a case report. Obstet. Gynecol. 38:841–843, 1971.

Wielenga, G. and Willighagen, R.G.J.: Histochemical investigation of ischemic villi in the placenta. Amer. J. Obstet. Gynecol. 96:956–968, 1966.

Wiener-Megnagi, Z., Ben-Shlomo, I., Goldberg, Y. and Shalev, E.: Resistance to activated protein C and the Leiden mutation: high prevalence in patients with abruptio placentae. Amer. J. Obstet. Gynecol. 179:1565–1567, 1998.

Willems, J.: The etiology of preeclampsia. A hypothesis. Obstetr. Gynecol. 50:495–499, 1977.

Wingerd, J., Christianson, R., Lovitt, W.V. and Schoen, E.J.: Placental ratio in white and black women: relation to smoking and anemia. Amer. J. Obstet. Gynecol. 124:671–675, 1976.

Winick, M. and Noble, A.: Cellular growth in human placenta. II. Diabetes mellitus. Amer. J. Obstet. Gynecol. 71:216–219, 1967.

Winn, H.N., Setaro, J.F., Mazor, M., Reece, E.A., Black, H.R. and Hobbins, J.C.: Severe Takayasu's arteritis in pregnancy: the role of central hemodynamic monitoring. Amer. J. Obstet. Gynecol. 159:1135–1136, 1988.

Winston, H.G. and Mastroianni, L.: Sickle cell disease in pregnancy. Obstet. Gynecol. 2:73–77, 1953.

Wisot, A.L.: Silent abruptio placentae with marked hypofibrinogenemia. JAMA 207:557–558, 1969.

Wladimiroff, J.W., Barentsen, R., Wallenburg, H.C.S. and Drogendijk, A.C.: Fetal urine production in a case of diabetes associated with polyhydramnios. Obstet. Gynecol. 46:100–102, 1975.

Wolf, F. de, Robertson, W.B. and Brosens, I.: The ultrastructure of acute atherosis in hypertensive pregnancy. Amer. J. Obstet. Gynecol. 123:164–174, 1975.

Wolf, F. de, Carreras, L.O., Moerman, P., Vermylen, J., Assche, A.v. and Renaer, M.: Decidual vasculopathy and extensive placental infarction in a patient with repeated thromboembolic accidents, recurrent fetal loss, and lupus anticoagulant. Amer. J. Obstet. Gynecol. 142:829–834, 1982.

Wolf, H., Šabata, V., Frerichs, H. and Stubbe, P.: Evidence for the impermeability of the human placenta for insulin. Horm. Metab. Res. 1:274–275, 1969.

Woodhouse, S.: The lupus anticoagulant and the dilute Russell viper venom test. Pathologist, July: 432–433, 1984.

Woods, J.R., Plessinger, M.A. and Clark, K.E.: Effect of cocaine on uterine blood flow and fetal oxygenation. JAMA 257:857–961, 1987.

Wright, J.R., Samson, K.A., Cooper-Rosen, E. and Riddell, D. C.: Breus' mole: DNA shows massive subchorionic hematoma is maternal in origin. Pediatr. Pathol. Molec. Med. 18:151–156, 1999.

Wurzel, J.M.: TTP lesions in placenta but not fetus. NEJM 301:503–504, 1979.

Wynn, R.M.: The placenta in preeclampsia. Obstetr. Gynecol. Annual 6:191–196, 1977.

Xu, L., Chang, V., Murphy, A., Rock, J.A., Damewood, M., Schlaff, W. and Zacur, H.A.: Antinuclear antibodies in sera of patients with recurrent pregnancy wastage. Amer. J. Obstet. Gynecol. **163**:1493–1497, 1990. (For discussion see Amer. J. Obstet. Gynecol. **166**:1021–1022, 1992.)

Ylikorkala, O. and Mäkilä, U.-M.: Prostacyclin and thromboxane in gynecology and obstetrics. Amer. J. Obstet. Gynecol. **152**:318–329, 1985.

Yoon, B.H., Lee, C.M. and Kim, S.W.: An abnormal umbilical artery waveform: a strong and independent predictor of adverse perinatal outcome in patients with preeclampsia. Amer. J. Obstet. Gynecol. **171**:713–721, 1994.

Younis, J.S. and Samueloff, A.: Gestational vascular complications. Best Pract. Res. Clin. Haematol. **16**:135–151, 2003.

Younis, J.S., Brenner, B., Ohel, B., Tal, J., Lanir, N. and Ben-Ami, M.: Factor V Leiden mutation is associated with first as well as second trimester recurrent fetal loss. Amer. J. Reprod. Immunol. **43**:31–35, 2000a.

Younis, J.S., Ohel, B., Brenner, B., Haddad, S., Lanir, N. and Ben-Ami, M.: The effect of thromboprophylaxis on pregnancy outcome in patients with recurrent pregnancy loss associated with factor V Leiden mutation. Brit. J. Obstet. Gynaecol. **107**:415–419, 2000b.

Zacks, S. and Blazar, A.S.: Chorionic villi in normal pregnancy, pre-eclamptic toxemia, erythroblastosis, and diabetes mellitus. A light- and electron-microscope study. Obstetr. Gynecol. **22**:149–167, 1963.

Zeek, P.M. and Assali, N.S.: Vascular changes in the decidua associated with eclamptogenic toxemia of pregnancy. Amer. J. Clin. Pathol. **20**:1099–1109, 1950.

Zhou, Y., Chiu, K., Brescia, R.J., Combs, C.A., Katz, M.A., Kitzmiller, J.L., Heilbron, D.C. and Fisher, S.J.: Increased depth of trophoblast invasion after chronic constriction of the lower aorta in rhesus monkeys. Amer. J. Obstet. Gynecol. **169**:224–229, 1993.

Zhou, Y., Fisher, S.J., Janatpour, M., Genbacev, O., Dejana, E., Wheelock, M. and Damsky, C.H.: Human cytotrophoblasts adopt a vascular phenotype as they differentiate. A strategy for successful endovascular invasion? J. Clin. Invest. **99**:2139–2151, 1997.

Zipursky, A., Brown, E., Christensen, H., Sutherland, R. and Doyle, J.: Leukemia and/or myeloproliferative syndrome in neonates with Down syndrome. Semin. Perinatol. **21**:97–101, 1997.

Zugaib, M., Barros, A.C.S.D.de, Bittar, R.E., Burdmann, E. de A. and Neme, B.: Abruptio placentae following snake bite. Amer. J. Obstet. Gynecol. **151**:754–755, 1985.

20
Infectious Diseases

Prenatal infections are important aspects of placental pathology. They are common and varied. Their pathogenesis and related circumstances must be understood if the pathologic lesions are to be interpreted correctly. Many types of infection cause placental changes, but in some types the infection may be difficult to prove from placental examination. Ultrastructural studies are especially lacking in this area and might be helpful, particularly when virus infection is suspected. Infections may ascend from the endocervical canal, or they may reach the placenta hematogenously through the maternal blood. Rarely are they acquired by amniocentesis, chorionic villus sampling, amnioscopy (Horky & Amon, 1967), percutaneous umbilical blood sampling (PUBS; Wilkins et al., 1989), or intrauterine fetal transfusion (Goodlin, 1965; Scott & Henderson, 1972). Many infections cause gross and microscopic changes of the placenta, but others, for example, the Coxsackie virus infection, leave few characteristic or specifically recognizable traces. This is also the case with parvovirus B19 infection, which often leads to fetal hydrops but has no specific placental alteration other than perhaps intranuclear inclusions in nucleated red blood cell precursors and endothelium, as a report by Hartwick et al. (1989) showed. Samra et al. (1989) described villous necrosis and calcification in the placenta from a 20 weeks' gestation with hydrops due to this infection (see Chapter 16).

This chapter first covers chorioamnionitis, followed by infections with specific organisms that correlate with chorioamnionitis. Syphilis and necrotizing funisitis (inflammation of the umbilical cord) are next discussed, and then the virus infections and villitides are discussed. Finally, rare infectious diseases such as malaria and parasitic infections are covered. A complete review of the early literature, especially the European references, may be found in the work of Flamm (1959). The comprehensive text on infections of the fetus and newborn infant by Remington and Klein (1983) can also be consulted. Excellent and complete reviews of fetal and placental infections have been provided by Blanc (1981), Altshuler (1984, 1996), Carroll et al. (1996), and Wigglesworth (1996). Most recently, Hirsch and Wang (2005) have produced a mouse model for the study of banal infections and comprehensively reviewed the literature. They propose that the process begins with toll-like receptors (TRLs) and, once the cascade is established it is difficult to interrupt.

Chorioamnionitis

Macroscopic Appearance

Typically, the placenta of the amnionic sac infection syndrome is premature. It lacks the blue sheen of the normal immature organ, and the membranes are obscured by an inflammatory exudate of polymorphonuclear leukocytes (PMNLs, neutrophils) (Figs. 20.1 to 20.3). The surface becomes yellow when much leukocytic exudate has accumulated and when the process has been of long duration. The amnion may be roughened or have lost the luster it normally possesses. The placenta is also frequently malodorous, and the astute observer may identify the prevailing organism by the odor. Thus, the fecal odor of fusobacterial and *Bacteroides* infections, and the sweet odor of *Clostridium* and *Listeria* infections are useful identifiers. The membranes are typically more friable, and the decidua capsularis is frequently detached and hemorrhagic and may even be absent in the placental specimen having been left in the uterus to be later discharged as lochia. These prematurely delivered placentas are often accompanied by an acute marginal hemorrhage that undermines the edge of the placenta and that originates from deciduitis. Harris (1988) has described this in greater detail. Although this mimics abruptio placentae, this hemorrhagic process (Figs. 20.4 and 20.5) markedly differs from the typical abruptio placentae of preeclampsia, the *retroplacental* hematoma. Vintzileos et al. (1987) believed that true abruptio occurs after premature rupture of the membranes. They found an incidence of 6.3% (control 2.7%) of normally implanted placentas with "indentations in the placental substance." Unfortunately, they did not discuss inflammatory reactions. Gonen et al. (1989) also provided evidence that abruptio (loosely defined) is frequently preceded by prolonged rupture of membranes. Darby et al. (1989) compared severe preterm abruptions with control women requiring preterm delivery. The former group had significantly more frequently chorio-

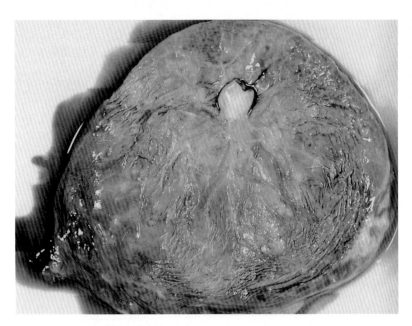

FIGURE 20.1. Near-term placenta with severe chorioamnionitis. Note the marginal hemorrhage at left, caused by deciduitis. The surface of the placenta is obscured by a whitish exudate that obscures the normal underlying blue color; the vasculature is also indistinct. Neonatal death.

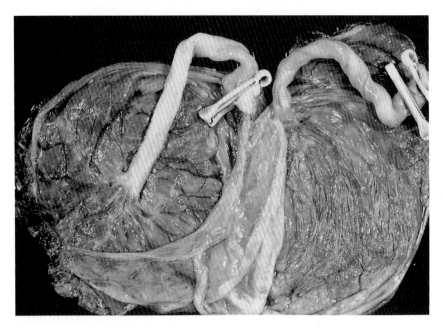

FIGURE 20.2. Immature diamnionic, dichorionic twin placenta from a cesarean section. Twin A (left, one cord clamp) was located higher in the uterus; twin B (right), with a marginally inserted cord, was near the lower uterine segment and had significant chorioamnionitis. Compare the luster of the normal placenta (left) with the indistinct features of the abnormal placenta (right), which are due to inflammation. Neonatal deaths.

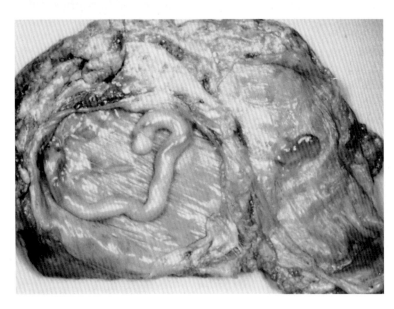

FIGURE 20.3. Immature twin placenta (19 weeks' gestation) from which twin A (right) had been delivered 1 week prior to twin B (left). Both twins had severe chorioamnionitis and fatal aspiration pneumonia. The placental surface was yellow, purulent, and malodorous.

FIGURE 20.4. Placenta at 21 weeks' gestation with massive chorioamnionitis and marked marginal/retroplacental hemorrhage caused by deciduitis.

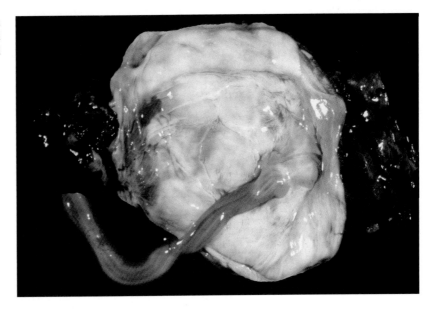

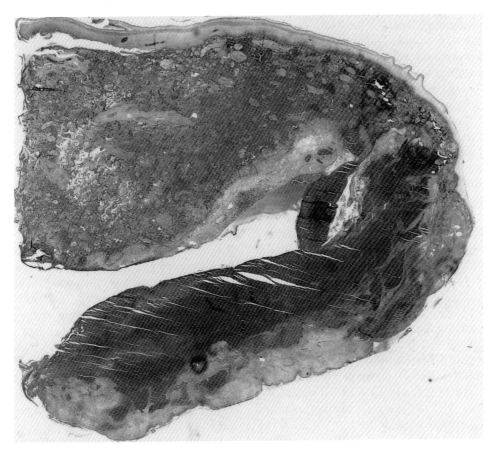

FIGURE 20.5. Margin of immature placenta at 23' weeks gestation with marked chorioamnionitis and abruptio. The abruption is represented by the dark marginal retromembranous hematoma which originates from marked deciduitis and its disrupted vessels. (H&E ×3.5).

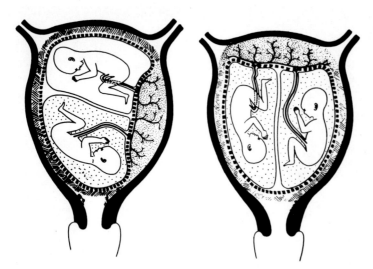

amnionitis and funisitis (41% versus 4%). They also believed that infection preceded abruptio, whereas Major et al. (1995) showed that rupture of membranes is often preceded by vaginal bleeding. This supports our notion that this decidual bleeding is secondary to deciduitis, and not the true abruptio placentae in the sense used in preeclampsia.

Touch preparations made from the fetal surface of placentas from women with prenatal infection may be used to identify the inflammatory exudate and the bacteria quickly, especially when the infection is due to *Listeria monocytogenes*. When chorioamnionitis is found in twin placentas, it is nearly invariably twin A whose cavity has inflammation or who has the more severely inflamed portion (Benirschke, 1960) (Fig. 20.6). We have considered this to mean that the amnionic sac infection is always ascending through the cervical canal. This correlation was questioned by Thiery et al. (1970), however, who found umbilical phlebitis in twin B as often as in twin A. These authors did not state how their twins were delivered, though, or how the twins were positively identified as to their intrauterine location. These specifications are crucial to the interpretation of such data.

Microscopic Appearance

Perhaps the earliest investigators to delineate chorioamnionitis were Wohlwill and Bock (1929), who described nine cases of "coccal" infection, some of which clearly followed attempted ("criminal") abortion. The reviews of Kückens (1938) and Müller (1956) made it clear that "round cell infiltration of the placenta" had been known before then. These authors suggested that infection of the fetus caused sepsis and then led to the placental inflammation. Wohlwill and Bock (1929) reviewed the placental inflammations that had been reported before their studies of chorioamnionitis (largely syphilis, tuberculosis, and

leprosy) and decided that the coccal infection they found was of a different character.

An extensive description of chorioamnionitis ("round cell infiltration") was authored by Kückens (1938). He found the literature to be contradictory and came to the following conclusions: The decidua has some round cell infiltration in 60% to 70% of normal placentas; villi never have such cellular infiltrates or abscesses; chorioamnionitis, with leukocytic origin from the intervillous space, and funisitis are common perinatal phenomena. Kückens suggested that an ascending origin of the infection was the most likely pathway, and this was supported by Knox and Hoerner (1950) as well. Kückens found that, with funisitis, the umbilical vein is the first vessel to be involved, with arterial inflammation to follow. He identified cocci in the lesions, found an incidence of 20.4% chorioamnionitis, and related it to the length of labor and rupture of membranes. Interestingly, a correlation with ophthalmia neonatorum from gonorrheal infection had already been suggested.

Blanc (1953, 1957, 1959, 1961a) described chorioamnionitis in many important contributions and in great detail; he also coined the descriptive term **amnionic sac infection syndrome**, which is now widely used. Blanc indicated methods for early diagnosis (gastric aspiration of the neonate, touch preparation from amnion), and he clearly explained that this was an ascending infection of the amnionic sac (see also Müller, 1956, and Pisarski et al., 1963, for references to the early European literature). There have been numerous pathologic and clinical studies of this important entity since then (reviewed by Altshuler, 1989; Carroll et al., 1996). It should be mentioned that Genest et al. (1998) introduced the term **pseudovasculitis** for lesions seen in early pregnancy that were, or might be, confused with real inflammation. The lesions described were degenerative in nature. It should be noted that virtually all of their cases were before 20 weeks' gestation, a time when funisitis is normally not a common feature because the fetus is still sluggish in leukocytic reaction. It goes without saying, then, that "funisitis" is the *fetal* response to infectious agents within the amnionic fluid compartment.

Hallman et al. (1989) have shown that high concentrations of ceramide lactoside are contained in the amnionic fluid of patients with chorioamnionitis. They suggested that the lipid derives from phagocytosing granulocytes. Kirshon et al. (1991) found that patients with prenatal infection had amnionic fluid glucose levels of less than 10 mg/dL. Romero et al. (1987b) showed that arachidonate lipoxygenase products are much elevated in this infection. In a later study, these authors (Romero et al., 1989b) identified as evidence of macrophage activation that infected amnionic fluid contained cachectin-tumor necrosis factor. Biggio et al. (2004) found that elevation of metalloproteinase-8 levels were strong predictors of subsequent prolonged premature rupture of membranes (PPROM). Many other intensive investigations have been published that clarify the role of amnionic sac infection in premature delivery. Importantly, Miyano et al. (1998) showed elevated fetal blood levels of a variety of complement components, lowered albumin, and other protein perturbations in chorioamnionitis. They then correlated these with "stages" of chorioamnionitis and necrotizing funisitis. The latter were thought to have "ended their initial active inflammatory states, but they still have subacute immune activation." Shim et al. (2004) correlated chorioamnionitis with PPROM and suggested that *inflammation* rather than *infection* should be used to designate the state of affairs because in only a limited percentage of their study, organisms were found in the fluid; it must be said, however, that not all possible organisms were attempted to be cultured either. In a subsequent contribution by Kim et al. (2004), specific changes in the expression of "pattern recognition markers," the Toll-like receptors 2 and 4 of amnionic epithelium were found. They suggested that these have a specific function of activating the immune system against very specific antigens. Interestingly, Akinbi et al. (2004) found that vernix caseosa and amnionic fluid normally contains numerous antimicrobial peptides in the absence of chorioamnionitis.

In our opinion, chorioamnionitis is *always* due to infection, and the work of Gibbs et al. (1992) and many others cited below support this notion. The speculations of Dominguez et al. (1960) are unfounded. They described umbilical cord inflammation (funisitis) in 10% of 1000 consecutively studied placentas and portrayed it as being "lymphocytic" (which it practically never is); they related funisitis to prolonged labor and meconium discharge. The complete absence of inflammation in most meconium-stained umbilical cords, the published negative findings of Fox and Langley (1971), and the personal experience of most placental pathologists negate the notion that the common funisitis is caused by hypoxia, as was suggested. Widholm et al. (1963) stated summarily that meconium causes funisitis. It is granted that meconium discharge and funisitis are occasionally combined, but meconium per se is not an inflammatory agent. Maudsley et al. (1966), who presented a good description of the amnionic sac infection syndrome, also insisted that the term be reserved for cases with verified infection. Some other authors have neglected the consideration that fastidious organisms may cause chorioamnionitis (e.g., Olding, 1970). There is thus still lingering doubt and confusion as to the nature of chorioamnionitis (Anonymous, 1989a), but when Arias and colleagues (1993) studied the problem of preterm labor in 105 women, they found that essentially two distinct subgroups exist: those with infection (*n* = 63) and those with decidual vasculopathy (*n* = 42). Moreover, Oyarzún et al. (1998) have shown a remarkable increase in identifying the presence of microorganisms in amnionic fluid (46%) when they employed the organisms by polymerase chain reaction than when they attempted culture (12%). They developed a technique to screen for 16 different organisms simultaneously that should be more useful for future studies.

Chorioamnionitis is an acute inflammatory reaction in which PMNLs principally participate. Eosinophils are found at times but only in protracted infections; and macrophages may participate to a variable extent. Plasma cells are generally absent in the membranes, however, except in some of the very chronic infections to be discussed below. The leukocytes come from two sources: the intervillous space (and are then maternal), and fetal surface blood vessels (Fig. 20.7). The emigration of leukocytes is always directional, toward the amnionic cavity, presumably toward an antigenic source. Pankuch and his colleagues (1989) studied this "amniotropism" of infected amnionic fluid. They found it to be a better indicator of infection than Gram stains, culture, or chromatography.

Recently, Fraser and Wright (2002) defined an additional entity. They found 12 cases of single-vessel inflammation **without** amniotropism, and in these cases eosinophils and T cells were the major components. They occurred in term infants without chorioamnionitis and were generally confined to single chorionic (rarely cord) vessels. The cause of this unusual inflammatory process is so far obscure.

In young gestations, especially those prior to the 20th week of gestation, the PMNLs are mainly of maternal origin. By midtrimester, the fetus begins to be capable of producing leukocytes that participate in the inflammatory response to leukotaxins (Müller, 1956). Sampson et al. (1997) found XY chromosomes in over 90% of leukocytes from amnionic fluid aspirates in four pregnancies with male fetuses. Interestingly, the membranes were all unruptured and bacteria were found on smears of the

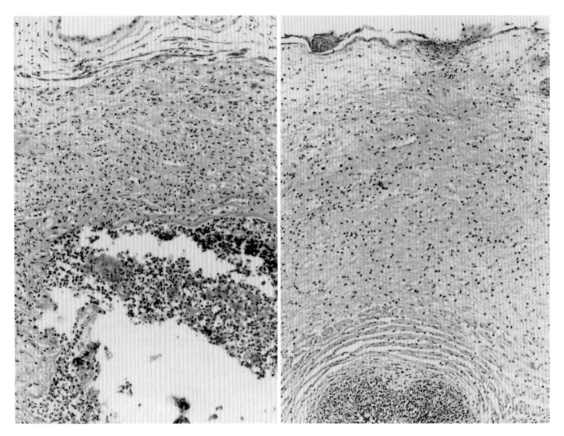

FIGURE 20.7. Placental surface in 30 weeks' gestation delivery. The patient had gonorrhea and her membranes had been ruptured for 40 hours. A 1200-g infant with pneumonia was delivered. Note the exudation of polymorphonuclear leukocytes (PMNLs) from the intervillous space (left), minimal vascular involvement (right), and amnion necrosis. H&E ×240 (left); ×160 (right).

aspirates in two cases. These investigators felt that emigration of leukocytes from maternal vessels was problematic, that emigration from cord vessels was hindered by the rapidity of blood flow, and suggested that leukodiapidesis may occur across fetal pulmonary membranes. That is contrary to the histopathologic findings of most perinatal pathologists. Neonates, when compared to adults, still have reduced leukocyte counts, and their PMNLs are also less capable of ingesting microbes. Premature infants, therefore, may be prone to developing sepsis (Cairo, 1989). We have seen, however, premature infants with white blood cell counts of over 100,000, presumably because of stimulation by specific organisms. The maturation of the fetal lymphocyte system was studied by Berry et al. (1992). Fetuses had significantly fewer CD57+ natural killer T cells, and other age-dependent changes are summarized in this study.

With funisitis, the inflammatory cells emigrate first from the umbilical vein and later from the arteries. They also migrate toward the amnionic surface, and only rarely toward the center of the cord. Many die during the migration. It has been suggested that they rarely reach the amnionic fluid but we believe that this suggestion is incorrect (Anonymous, 1989a). It is common, for instance, to find aspirated PMNLs in lung and stomach of neonates with chorioamnionitis, intermixed with squames. This pus is not produced in the fetal lung, as only late in the infectious process can one find an inflammatory accumulation within the alveolar tissue in response to infection. Pus can also, at times, be aspirated at amniocentesis. The dead inflammatory cells of the placental surface frequently accumulate in large quantities underneath the amnion in the potential space that exists between amnion and chorion (Fig. 20.8).

Experiments designed to identify the reason for the relatively slow permeation of the amnion by leukocytes have suggested that the type V collagen composition of the amnionic basal membrane prevents the ready transgression by PMNLs (Azzarelli & Lafuze, 1987). Some experimental evidence indicates that this amnionic sac infection reduces the strength of the chorion laeve (McGregor et al., 1987; Sbarra et al., 1987; Schoonmaker et al., 1989; Pressman et al., 2002). Sbarra et al. (1985) demonstrated that when membranes are incubated with lysolecithin or phospholipase A_2, their bursting pressure decreases. Membrane "stripping" alone causes the release

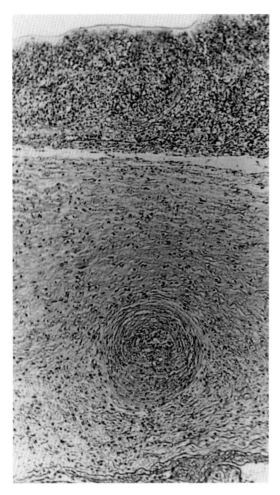

FIGURE 20.8. Massive chorioamnionitis in a stillborn at 23 weeks' gestation. Exudate is mostly necrotic and has accumulated in amnion. The placenta had a purulent surface and marked funisitis. Stillborn. H&E ×60.

of this enzyme (McColgin et al., 1993). It might parenthetically be pointed out that the term **amnionitis** is strictly speaking erroneous. The amnion has no blood vessels; thus inflammation, a vascular phenomenon, cannot take place in the amnion. It is only passively possible, by transmigration of leukocytes that originate elsewhere. Gleicher et al. (1979) have identified a blocking factor in the amnionic fluid that enhances leukocyte migration, presumably similar to the material that was studied by Schoonmaker et al. (1989).

The pus may reach the lung, stomach, and middle ears (Fig. 20.9). When chronic aspiration pneumonia occurs, the neonatal lung contains lymphocyte and plasma cell infiltrations. These result from an immunologic recognition of the antigen (Fig. 20.10). Benner (1940) found that 26% of stillborns had middle ear aspiration of pus. A strong correlation exists between chorioamnionitis and otitis. McLellan et al. (1962) found purulent exudate in 19 of 28 temporal bones of neonates weighing between 1000 and 1500 g. The widely patent eustachian tube of premature infants is believed to be a possible portal of entry of this aspirated infected amnionic fluid. Congenital pneumonia has been documented in numerous publications following Ballantyne's (1904) first description. It is correlated with chorioamnionitis and funisitis. Barter (1962) argued in favor of Dominguez' hypothesis of hypoxia as the cause of the inflammation (see letter from Osborn, 1962; see also Aherne & Davies, 1962; Browne, 1962). Anderson et al. (1962), Fujikura and Froehlich (1967), and Steiner et al. (1961), among many authors who studied the phenomenon, found that the "drowning in pus" correlates with chorioamnionitis, prematurity, and premature rupture of the membranes, and in long-standing infections, some plasma cell component may be found (Fig. 20.11). Some of the necrotic exudate underneath the amnion may ultimately calcify, but the fetus is usually delivered before this happens. Simon et al. (1989) undertook bacteriologic studies of infants born after premature rupture of membranes. They found that 26% had the same bacteria in placental arterial blood, ear swabs, and meconium, the predominant organisms being *Escherichia coli*, *Bacteroides fragilis*, and streptococci. A significant study of the nature of organisms that cause chorioamnionitis comes from Hillier et al. (1991). The organisms most frequently associated with preterm delivery and chorioamnionitis were group B *Streptococcus* and *Fusobacterium*; *Peptostreptococcus* was related only to preterm delivery, whereas *E. coli*, *Bacteroides*, and *Ureaplasma* were significantly related only to chorioamnionitis. Formerly considered to be a *Bacteroides* species, *Capnocytophaga* sp. is a newly recognized cause of severe chorioamnionitis. This gram-negative anaerobic organism is a common cause of periodontal disease and, not surprisingly, ascending infection leading to chorioamnionitis has followed oral sex (Edwards, et al., 1995; Hansen et al., 1995; Mikamo et al., 1996).

The fetal surface vessels partake in the inflammatory response to the leukotaxin, but generally little happens here before the 20th week of gestation. The maternal component of the leukocytic reaction originates in the intervillous space and in the maternal vessels of the decidua in the free membranes (Fig. 20.12). Even in dichorionic twin placentas, some exudate may be found in a part of the dividing membranes, where the PMNLs originate from persisting maternal vessels (Fig. 20.13). In this maternal response to amnionic sac infection, leukocytes first marginate beneath the fibrin under the chorionic plate. They then infiltrate the chorion and eventually the amnion. The subchorial accumulation has been designated "intervillositis," an unfortunate but often used term. It is true that other types of intervillositis occur (vide infra), but these are more chronic processes and they differ substantially from the acute infections. Infectious organisms are rarely seen in the intervillous space,

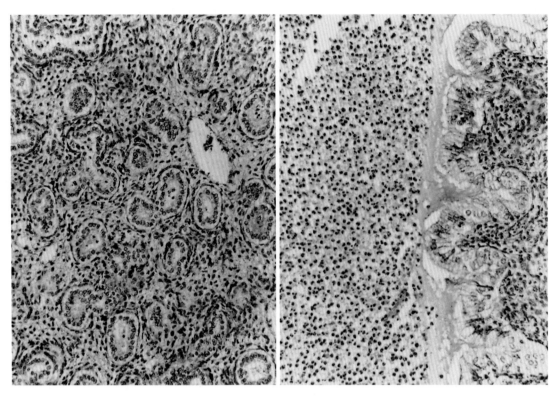

FIGURE 20.9. Aspiration of amnionic fluid pus in the still tubular alveolar spaces of a 16 weeks' gestation fetus (left) and stomach (right). H&E ×120.

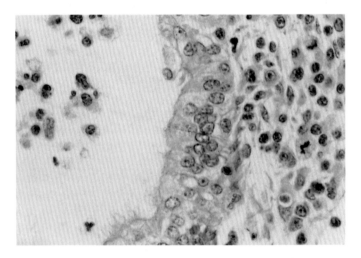

FIGURE 20.10. Chronic aspiration pneumonia in a stillborn. Note the pus in the bronchial lumen and plasma cells in the interstitial parenchyma. H&E ×160.

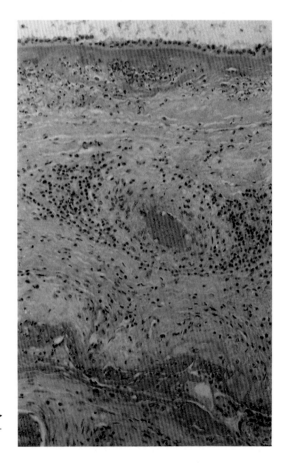

FIGURE 20.11. Placental surface at 28 weeks' gestation with chronic inflammation (plasma cells). H&E ×60.

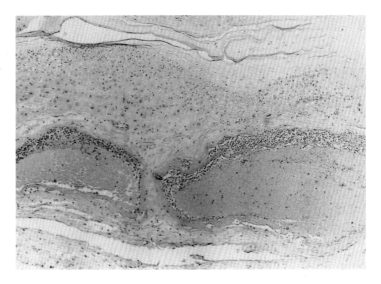

FIGURE 20.12. Placental membranes at term with early inflammation. Leukocytes are accumulating in maternal vessels, with direction toward the amnionic surface. Mural thrombosis is beginning. The patient was febrile, and funisitis was present. H&E ×60.

although toxins may accumulate here. In acute chorioamnionitis the leukocytes merely react to the leukotactic signal that has permeated through the placental surface; they then accumulate in the subchorial space and finally migrate. Abscess formation underneath the chorionic plate and dissemination of exudate between villous trunks are rare (Vernon & Gauthier, 1971). When it is present, one must consider congenital listeriosis and *Campylobacter* sp. infection first; other infections are much less frequently the cause. With listeriosis, villous and intervillous abscesses occur frequently (vide infra). Intervillous abscesses occur occasionally in maternal septicemias. We have seen them with maternal staphylococcal and *E. coli* infections. The mothers are usually so ill that labor and delivery occur before abscesses develop. Indeed, staphylococcal infection has only rarely been reported. Negishi et al. (1998), who described such a case, found only one previous report. Their patient was at 38 weeks and mild fever (37.8°C) was noted, but the membranes were intact.

She had been treated with chloramphenicol for bacterial vaginosis. The fetus died suddenly. Cord blood and placental surface grew *Staphylococcus aureus*, and there was chorioamnionitis. Levy (1981) believed that a placental abscess he discovered could be the cause of the maternal fever. This abscess occupied 25% to 39% of the placental surface in a term pregnancy, but no bacteria were isolated, and listeriosis was not ruled out. Another placental abscess was due to *Proteus mirabilis* infection in a febrile patient, gram-negative bacilli being present in sections (Ravid & Toaff, 1976). In another pregnant woman an intravenous line had been placed at 12 weeks' gestation as treatment for hyperemesis. She developed *Serratia* sepsis and was appropriately treated. When she delivered at 34 weeks, an old abscess without organisms was identified in the placenta. Bendon et al. (1998) reported on two fetal deaths due to placental abscesses from maternal *E. coli* sepsis with disseminated intravascular coagulation (DIC). There was focal infarction around the abscesses,

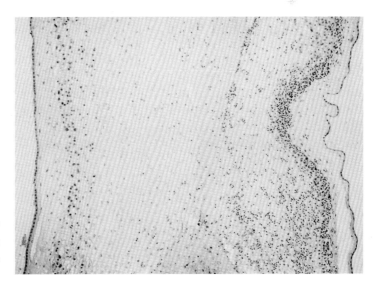

FIGURE 20.13. Dividing membranes of a diamnionic/dichorionic (DiDi) twin placenta with inflammation in the right sac. H&E ×25. (Courtesy of Dr. S.G. Driscoll, Boston.)

but chorioamnionitis was absent. **Villous** abscesses occur, as was reported, after intrauterine transfusion with infected blood (Scott & Henderson, 1972). The villi are otherwise almost never involved in common cases of chorioamnionitis, however severe that process may be. Subchorionic fibrin deposits are excellent sites from which to culture bacterial organisms, according to Aquino et al. (1984). These authors preferred to sample this site because it is not contaminated with vaginal organisms and because they experienced good recovery of bacteria from these specimens. They isolated group B hemolytic streptococci, anaerobic cocci, and "rods," organisms that commonly cause endometritis, pelvic infection, and neonatal sepsis.

The exudate in funisitis may occasionally be visible macroscopically (Fig. 20.14). It must be emphasized, however, that funisitis (umbilical vasculitis) does *not* signify the existence of fetal sepsis, as is often believed. It *does* signify the presence of a fetal inflammatory response, however. Blanc (1961a) has specified the possible means by which fetal sepsis can take place. It is a relatively late event in the course of prenatal infection with bacteria. Blanc opined that fetal sepsis may result from invasion of organisms through lung and intestinal tract.

Prior to the delineation of the amnionic sac infection syndrome, funisitis was thought to be primarily related to congenital syphilis, and spirochetes were usually sought from endothelial scrapings by darkfield examination. This association is now no longer held to be firm (reviewed by Beckmann & Zimmer, 1931). With funisitis, the leukocytes marginate first at the vascular intima and then begin to dissect among the muscle bundles of the umbilical vein and arteries, finally infiltrating Wharton's jelly (Fig. 20.15).

They also reach the cord's surface and may accumulate there in substantial numbers. The fetal PMNLs have the same fine-structural features as those from adults. When they emigrate through the umbilical vein wall, degeneration of its inner elastic components is observed (Fig. 20.16). With some infections, notably that with *Candida albicans*, small accumulations of PMNLs are seen on the cord surface. They are often visible macroscopically and have a typical, granular appearance. Old exudate in the cord may accumulate in concentric perivascular rings, giving the appearance of Ouchterlony immunodiffusion plates (Fig. 20.17). This old exudate is more prone to developing mineralization than is the exudate of the fetal surface of the placenta. In fact, this calcification may reach extraordinary proportions at times, so that the cord cannot be clamped readily (vide infra). It is then referred to as necrotizing funisitis.

The microorganisms that have caused the inflammatory response may be seen in many infected placentas, particularly in cases of listeriosis, candidiasis, fusobacterial infection, and some of the infections with common cocci. But many cases of chorioamnionitis result from infection with organisms that are not so readily demonstrated histologically or that are not commonly considered. Examples include *Chlamydia* (Andrews et al., 2000) and *Mycoplasma* and *Ureaplasma* (Lu et al., 2001; Yoon et al., 2003). Mural thrombosis in chorionic vessels is frequently present when the infection has been of longer duration (see also Arias et al., 1997). It begins at the intima of veins, usually toward the amnionic surface, and gradually increases (Fig. 20.18). The thrombi may be grossly apparent as yellow-white streaks, and eventually the villous tissue of the involved vessels atrophies. In the umbilical cord, thrombi have a less characteristic macro-

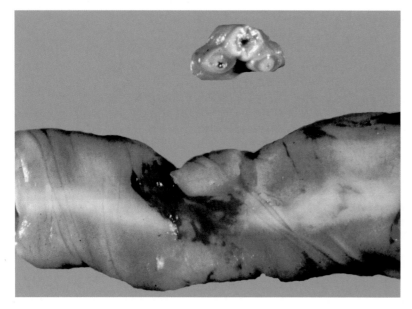

FIGURE 20.14. Longitudinal and cross section of an umbilical cord at 30 weeks' gestation. The patient had no fever. A yellow streak was seen along the umbilical vein, and the cord appeared brownish. There is a prominent white ring of acute inflammatory exudate around the umbilical vein.

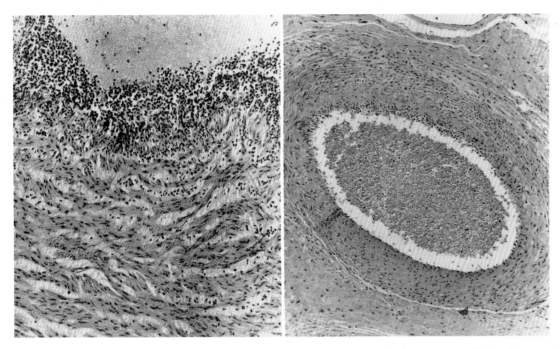

FIGURE 20.15. Umbilical phlebitis (left) and arteritis (right). Leukocytes are penetrating between muscle bundles toward the cord surface. H&E ×260.

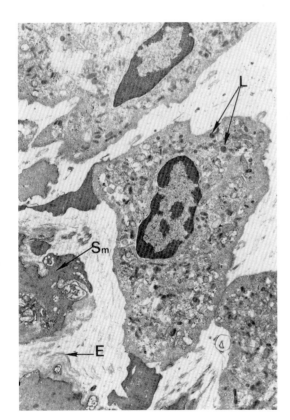

FIGURE 20.16. Electron micrograph of a polymorphonuclear leukocyte in the process of emigrating through an umbilical vein. Mature pregnancy, prolonged rupture of membranes. L, lysosomes; SM, smooth muscle cell; E, degenerating elastic membrane. ×9000. (Courtesy of Dr. G. Altshuler, Oklahoma City, Oklahoma.)

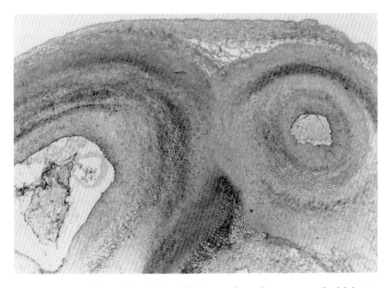

FIGURE 20.17. Chronic funisitis with rings of exudate, some of which are degenerated, around cord vessels. Small for gestational age (SGA) infant near term; no villitis. H&E ×40.

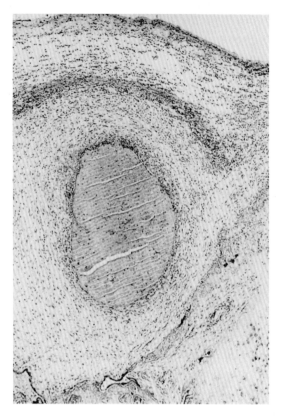

FIGURE 20.18. Long-standing chorioamnionitis and vasculitis of chorionic vessels at 26 weeks' pregnancy. The darker ring of exudate is degenerating, as is the amnionic epithelium. Early mural thrombosis is present at the surface of the vein. Malodorous placenta, 4 days premature rupture of membranes (PROM), 900-g infant. H&E ×20.

scopic appearance but may also involve arteries (Fig. 20.19). It is true, though, that most thromboses of large placental vessels have another etiology, mostly being secondary to obstruction of venous return. Finally, in the

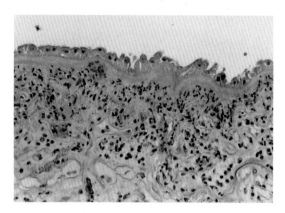

FIGURE 20.20. Chorioamnionitis associated with amnion necrosis. H&E ×160.

amnionic infection syndrome, the amnionic epithelium is frequently degenerated, especially in areas of severe inflammation (Fig. 20.20). Thrombosis of umbilical veins is rarely reported, and it is summarized by Wolfman et al. (1983), who saw it in a surviving neonate. It was associated with marked inflammation. These authors also review the sparse literature and draw attention to the greater frequency in diabetic gestations.

Chorioamnionitis is common. Fox and Langley (1971), for instance, found it in 24.4% of 1000 consecutive livebirths. A study of Salafia et al. (1989) showed that some degree of chorionitis was present in 4% of uncomplicated term deliveries; in 1.2% the chorioamnionitis was "clinically silent." Inflammation of membranes and cord is much commoner still in the immature organs of spontaneous, premature births and in patients with premature rupture of membranes. Hillier et al. (1988) found infection in 67% of preterm deliveries, compared with 21% of term gestations. Guzick and Winn (1985) did a prospective study of 2774 women and found the overall incidence

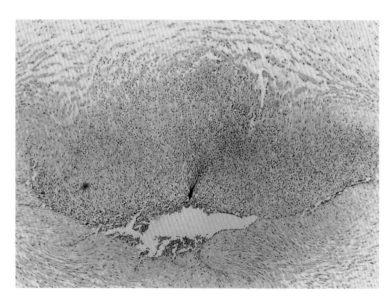

FIGURE 20.19. Organized, partially occlusive arterial thrombus in an umbilical artery, associated with arteritis. Infant developed cerebral palsy. H&E ×20.

of prematurity to be 5.4%. It was 11% when chorioamnionitis was present without membrane rupture, but 56.7% when premature rupture of membranes and chorioamnionitis coexisted. The authors concluded that 25% of premature deliveries were attributable to chorioamnionitis. Newton et al. (1989) showed in a large study that "duration of membrane rupture [was a] significant risk factor for intra-amniotic infection." The outcome of pregnancy in 59 patients with rupture of membranes before 26 weeks' gestation was studied by Bengtson et al. (1989). They ascertained chorioamnionitis in 45.8% (49.1% perinatal mortality) but also found that "there was a tendency for patients with extremely long latent periods to have lower rates of infection." Holcroft et al. (2004) found that chorioamnionitis and funisitis were not responsible for metabolic acidosis in preterm fetuses and that factors other than hypoxia (mostly culture positive infection) must be responsible for the frequent central nervous system (CNS) damage seen (see also Holcroft et al., 2004). Numerous other investigators have shown that chorioamnionitis is a significant risk factor for prematurity, CNS damage, fetal/neonatal sepsis, and fetal demise (deAraujo et al., 1999; Hansen & Leviton, 1999; Goldenberg et al., 2000; Yoon et al., 2001; Genen et al., 2002; Slattery & Morrison, 2002; Graham et al., 2004; Rouse et al., 2004). Duggan et al. (2001) showed that brain injury is more likely to occur in chorioamnionitis when fetal circulating levels of tumor necrosis factor-α (TNF-α) and interleukins (IL-1β, -6, and -10) as well as CD45RO$^+$T lymphocytes are elevated (see also Cooper & Nuovo, 2005). Patrick et al. (2004) have created a guinea pig model to study the CNS effects of chorioamnionitis. Quintero et al. (1998) sought to assess and "cure" premature rupture by endoscopic study. They identified the funnel-like site of rupture and unsuccessfully attempted "amniopatching" by application of platelets and cryoprecipitate. More recently, the same investigators placed a collagen membrane patch over the rupture site in a patient, thus prolonging the pregnancy by 2 weeks (Quintero et al., 2002).

Many attempts have been made to "grade" the inflammatory process, with the hypothesis that different severities of inflammation might correlate with neonatal outcome and possibly other parameters. This has been only minimally successful, but a study by Redline et al. (2003) showed reasonable reproducibility among a number of pathologists judging placental inflammatory lesions. Not taken into consideration was a study by Ohyama et al. (2002) that suggested the existence of a subacute form of chorioamnionitis, a form that is especially marked by amnion necrosis and that was an infection they felt to be of longer duration. These authors showed that the neonatal outcome was worse with this form of inflammation, especially from a chronic respiratory point of view. Several investigators have shown that

the effect of funisitis (arteritis and phlebitis has a greater impact when merely membranitis is present (Kim et al., 2001; Mittendorf et al., 2003). Miyano et al. (1998), who assessed the cord blood levels of various protein components, came closer to a useful means of subdividing the degree of inflammation. Then there are observations such as, for instance, a case of massive chorioamnionitis, funisitis with necrotizing features and severe edema, neonatal white blood cell count of 100,000 at 26 weeks' gestation, and an apparently healthy neonate who survived; conversely, minimal inflammation associated with group B streptococcal infection can be devastating. These and many similar experiences make us believe that the most important features of ascending infection are the type of infectious agent and perhaps the time of onset, but not the degree or the precise nature of the inflammatory response. *Trichomonas*, for instance, can be enormously leukotactic yet have little effect on neonatal morbidity, whereas it is associated with low birth weight and preterm delivery (Cotch et al., 1997). Conversely, group B streptococcus may prevent leukocyte migration and have a devastating effect on fetal/neonatal life. Thus, the extensive investigations on grading the inflammatory response by van Hoeven et al. (1996) and de Araujo et al. (1994), among other such studies, should be interpreted with this caution in mind.

The ascending nature of this infection is signaled by three pathologic findings, but is also supported by culture of intact sacs: (1) There is usually severe, acute deciduitis associated with the membranitis, and it often exceeds the degree of chorioamnionitis (Fig. 20.21). (2) When the intrauterine position of twins is known, including the location of the partition of their amnionic sacs, it is invariably twin A who has chorioamnionitis or whose membranes are more severely inflamed (see Figs. 20.2 and 20.3). (3) When membranes are rolled in such a manner as to have the point of spontaneous rupture on the inside, the degree of inflammation is most significant in the inner portions of the roll, that is, in the proximity of membrane rupture (Figs. 20.22 and 20.23) (Benirschke & Altshuler, 1971). It should be noted, however, that maternal fever **alone** is a poor indicator of the presence of chorioamnionitis, as many patients do not exhibit elevated temperature and others may have an intercurrent infection of other kinds.

It is well known that attempted abortion with nonsterile instruments is frequently followed by sepsis and chorioamnionitis (Studdiford & Douglas, 1956), but chorioamnionitis has also repeatedly been found with unruptured membranes (e.g., Miller et al., 1980b). A good example is the case of (amnionic fluid infection—"chorioamnionitis," according to the authors) with the uncommon organism *Eikenella corrodens* (Jeppson & Reimer, 1991). The 31-week gestation infant remained uninfected, perhaps because of prenatal antibiotic therapy when the

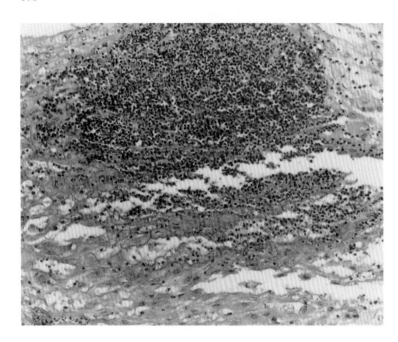

FIGURE 20.21. Acute and chronic deciduitis (decidua capsularis) in an immature placenta with chorioamnionitis. H&E ×160.

Gram-negative rods were identified by culture from amniocentesis. The association of prenatal infection with intact membranes is easiest to show with the relatively common *C. albicans* infection of the amnionic sac. Further, Gyr et al. (1994) showed that, experimentally, *E. coli* organisms could penetrate viable intact placental membranes, with simultaneous changes in glucose and lactate concentrations. Also, many cases have been described in which chorioamnionitis, with or without fetal pneumonia, existed in the presence of intact membranous sacs (en caul). Although this is an uncommon occurrence, it is an important finding for our understanding of the pathogenesis of infection (Royston & Geoghegan, 1985). The

general experience that inflamed membranes usually rupture prior to delivery does not argue against the fact that chorioamnionitis can exist with an intact sac. The loss of membrane integrity, resulting from inflammation, makes rupture a probability (Schoonmaker et al., 1989). Numerous reviews exist on this topic (Altshuler, 1984).

The predominant opinion now is that amnionic sac infection is a primary cause of premature rupture of membranes and premature labor, at least in those pregnancies that terminate spontaneously before 30 weeks' gestation (Garite & Freeman, 1982; Toth et al., 1988). This is also our opinion, and we believe that this is the most important unresolved problem in gestation, the reason

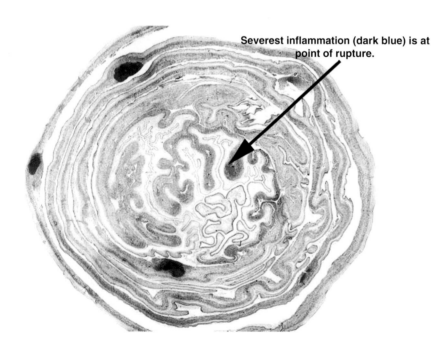

Severest inflammation (dark blue) is at point of rupture.

FIGURE 20.22. Membrane roll of placenta with marked chorioamnionitis. The edge of the spontaneous membrane rupture is in the center. Note the dark exudate in the decidua and chorion in the center. H&E ×12.

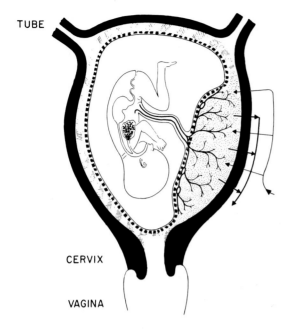

TUBE

CERVIX

VAGINA

FIGURE 20.23. Intrauterine position of fetus and placenta. Infectious organisms ascend through an opened endocervical canal. They first infect the membranes that cover the internal os and then penetrate into the amnionic cavity.

being that it not only is often recurrent (Mercer et al., 1999; Lee et al., 2003), but also leads to the most premature infant deliveries, of infants who are difficult to treat and many of whom develop cerebral palsy (Wood et al., 2000; Yoon et al., 2000; Kumazaki et al., 2002a). There is also evidence that these infections have an important role in the causation of stillbirths and neonatal deaths (Quinn et al., 1985). The formerly held idea that chorioamnionitis might protect the neonate against developing hyaline membrane disease by the attending stress was invalidated by the controlled clinicopathologic study of Dimmick et al. (1976).

To make the clinical diagnosis of chorioamnionitis may pose problems for the clinician, as only some gravidas experience fever, uterine tenderness, or fetal tachycardia with amnionic sac infection. Bobitt et al. (1981) aspirated amnionic fluid for culture from women in premature labor and found microorganisms in 25%. Seven of eight patients went into labor within 48 hours, and 75% of positive women had no fever. These authors also advocated Gram stains for rapid diagnosis of organisms, a method found to be helpful in the management of patients with premature rupture of membranes and chorioamnionitis (Broekhuizen et al., 1985). Others have advocated the use of gas-liquid chromatography for the early diagnosis of the amnionic sac infection syndrome (Gravett et al., 1982; Wagner et al., 1985; Romero et al., 1988b). This rationale was based on the detection of short-chain organic acids, which are the by-products of bacterial metabolism. Romero et al. (1989e) found that this method is insensi-

tive, especially when gram-negative organisms cause the infection, which is why Pankuch et al. (1989) suggested the use of leukotaxis studies. Maternal pyrexia and leukocytosis are also unreliable predictors, as has been found in numerous studies, and now fibronectin assays seem to be more profitable.

Hawrylyshyn et al. (1983) found that elevated C-reactive protein (CRP) levels correlated better with infection than did maternal fever. Elevation of CRP levels in maternal serum, advocated by Evans et al. (1980) as a means to predict chorioamnionitis, has also not been universally helpful. Farb et al. (1983) identified two patients with verified infection and normal levels; false-positive results were also obtained. Ernest et al. (1987) reported problems of both false-positive and false-negative levels. Watts and her colleagues (1993) found that elevated CRP levels were useful in deciding when to do cultures of amnionic fluid but they found poor correlation with chorioamnionitis. Other investigators, however, have found excellent correlation with CRP levels and chorioamnionitis and have advocated its use in the clinical setting (Romem & Artal, 1984; Ismail et al., 1985; Potkul et al., 1985).

Because of the importance of this ascending infection, investigators have sought new means of predicting the existence of chorioamnionitis before birth. Egley et al. (1988) suggested that amnionic fluid esterase levels (derived from PMNLs) have high specificity (100%) and sensitivity (81%). But, as in bacterial studies of cerebrospinal fluid (CSF), lactate, esterase, etc. are no more sensitive than looking for PMNLs from which they are derived. A Gram stain takes 5 minutes to perform and may be much more useful. Ohlsson and Wang (1990) reviewed 39 studies and concluded then that "an ideal test to predict chorioamnionitis or neonatal sepsis was not found."

Romero et al. (1987a, 1988a) and Cox et al. (1988) found that quantitation of the lipopolysaccharide component of Gram-negative organisms (endotoxin) might be used for identification of these infections. Both groups of investigators found elevated levels of endotoxin in specific infections with the *Limulus* test; and when the test was combined with Gram stains, a more adequate means of prenatal diagnosis seemed possible. A variety of kinins, especially IL-1 and TNF were next being investigated as possible prime movers in initiating uterine contraction (Romero et al., 1989a,b; see reviews by Mitchell et al., 1993; Oláh et al., 1996; Kayem et al., 2004). In one of the few studies of cervical mucus (which we consider to be of great importance in uterine defense mechanisms), Platz-Christensen et al. (1993) found that concentrations of endotoxin and IL-1α are significantly increased in vaginal fluid and cervical mucus of women with bacterial vaginosis. The primacy of cervical problems in ascending infection was related by Iams (1998), and Leppert (1998) sought cleavage of cross-linked collagen fibers as a possible early mechanism for cervical dilatation. We found markedly increased amounts of IL-1 and IL-1ra in several areas of placentas with chorioamnionitis (Baergen et al., 1994), indeed we believe that the principal problem is the absence of endocervical protective mucus. It is impressive to observe the quantity of this viscous mucus in the endocervical canal of hysterectomy specimens done for placenta percreta, and in animals that succumb during pregnancy at the San Diego Zoo from trauma or other unrelated causes. Moreover, Hein et al. (2001, 2002) in two excellent studies of the human endocervical mucus have shown its richness in defensive molecules and cells (Fig. 20.24). Genc et al. (2004) have measured the IL-1ra and IL-1β response in vaginal/cervical secretions and found that in women with various pathogens, the ratio of IL-1ra/IL-1β was decreased and was associated with preterm delivery. Similar observations of a decreased immune function of cervical secretions and subsequent chorioamnionitis were made by Simham et al. (2003).

Many other studies have since been conducted to further characterize the cytokine involvement of prenatal infection and premature labor (see review and new findings in Arntzen et al., 1998). Lockwood et al. (1994) found

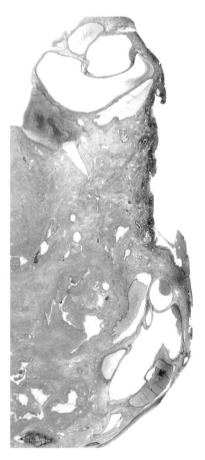

FIGURE 20.24. Endocervix of uterus from cesarean section for placenta percreta at 37 weeks' gestation. Thick purple mucus fills the canal and interdigitates with the mucus glands.

increased cervical IL-6 levels to be poor indicators of maternal infectious sequelae, whereas Coultrip et al. (1994), Andrews et al. (1995), and Yoon et al. (1995) described how amnionic fluid IL-6 levels are useful as rapid diagnostic tests to predict premature labor with intact membranes. Menon et al. (1995) determined that the amnion and chorion are the sites of inflammatory cytokine (IL-1 and IL-6) production when they sought these by messenger RNA detection (see also Reisenberger et al., 1998). In a later contribution, Yoon et al. (1997a,b) suggested that IL-6 and IL-1β or TNF-α may "play a role in the genesis of brain white matter lesions" in infants delivered with chorioamnionitis (see also Grether & Nelson, 1997). Stretching alone of the membranes was sufficient to release IL-8 and collagenase activity (Maradny et al., 1996). IL-8 and IL-10 were incriminated as participants in premature labor by Osmers et al. (1995) and Greig et al. (1995), whereas IL-1α was found to be elevated in studies by Dudley et al. (1996). Conflicting results concerning the cellular origin of many cytokines have been published. Thus, Reisenberger et al. (1998) found cultured amnion cells to produce IL-6 and IL-8 upon bacterial exposure; Steinborn et al. (1998) found the origin of TNF-α to be placental macrophages, whereas IL-1 and IL-6 came from placental endothelial cells. It is also of interest that women who had chorioamnionitis in an earlier gestation had significantly higher levels of TNF-α production after lipopolysaccharide stimulation than controls (Amory et al., 2001). It can thus be seen that the precise pathophysiology of the mechanism of premature labor and infection and the participation of various membranes and locales of cytokine production are under active study, without a final, agreed-upon resolution still forthcoming. Clearly, infection and inflammation are the most important aspects in the process. Most appealing to us, having long assumed that cervical/endocervical "competence" is an important aspect in preventing ascending infection, is the finding by Svinarich et al. (1997; also Quayle et al., 1998) that normally the endocervix is a rich source of defensin-5. This protein plays an important protective role against infection in other organs (bowel) and may become a significant player in the future. At present, the cervical/vaginal presence of elevated fibronectin levels seems to be the most practical way of monitoring progression of chorioamnionitis (Bartnicki et al., 1996; Garite et al., 1996; Rizzo et al., 1996; Goldenberg, 1997; Sennström et al., 1998). Simhan et al. (2004) have added elevated vaginal pH and neutrophils to this array of tests for PPROM, as it is now referred to. These tests have been commercially marketed and are highly successful in predicting delivery within a week (Peaceman et al., 1998). The fibronectin detected is thought to derive from the membranes.

Because labor is readily induced with prostaglandins, they have been studied as the possible main mediators of the preterm labor associated with chorioamnionitis. Although prostaglandins are well-known mediators of many aspects of disease, and they are also the chemicals that have proved to be useful in initiating labor, there are reservations about their primacy in the initiation of normal labor. While seeking a possible link between premature labor and placental inflammation, we found that arachidonic acid was consumed in the process of labor (Curbelo et al., 1981). The testing was done by chromatography of phospholipids from placental membrane extracts obtained from various types of delivery. Arachidonic acid appeared to be electively stored in the amnion. Later, a large number of microorganisms were tested for phospholipase activity because initiation of labor was believed to result from phospholipase A_2 activation and because of its association with infection. It was then found that many organisms contain this enzyme in considerable quantities (Bejar et al., 1981; McGregor et al., 1991). This observation led to the hypothesis that bacterially mediated enzymatic conversion of arachidonic acid may signal the onset of premature labor in pregnancies complicated by chorioamnionitis. Others have since studied many more organisms and found that phospholipase is liberated from a large number of microorganisms, with release of prostaglandin from amnion (Lamont et al., 1990). Bennett and Elder (1992) found that bacterial infection cannot initiate labor from "intrinsic biosynthesis and release of prostaglandins ... by the bacteria themselves." We now believe that there is an insufficient quantity of lipase to come from the usually relatively small number of bacteria to initiate and maintain labor. Rather, the enzyme is more likely being provided by the large number of leukocytes that are also known to possess phospholipase (Victor et al., 1981) and whose enzyme is activated by chemotactic peptides (Galbraith, 1988). The lipase also occurs in high concentrations in the placental membranes (review by Vadas & Pruzanski, 1986; Kredentser et al., 1995; Skannal et al., 1997). Okita et al. (1983) identified substantial stores of arachidonic acid in human amnion and concluded that it originates from amnionic fluid.

Lamont et al. (1985) also exposed amnion cells in culture to bacterial products and found prostaglandin E to rise markedly as a result. They thus affirmed that chorioamnionitis may cause premature labor. This finding was amplified by Bennett et al. (1987), who performed similar experiments. A correlation between chorioamnionitis and premature labor is additionally supported by findings of significantly elevated prostaglandin levels in infected amnionic fluid (Romero et al., 1986) and by the demonstration of markedly increased prostaglandin production from infected amnion (Lopez Bernal et al., 1987).

Despite these attractive findings of prostaglandin metabolism, attention has been paid to the increase of amnionic leukotriene concentrations during labor (Romero et al., 1988c) and to the decidual IL-1 production during premature labor (Romero et al., 1989a,f) as well as many other proteins. Deciduitis, decidual macrophage activation, and PMNL exudation, in particular, play an important role in the initiation of premature labor. It must be admitted, however, that although the evidence of infection as a primary cause of chorioamnionitis and of premature labor is no longer in doubt, the precise chemical cascade that ultimately leads to myometrial contractions is not yet elucidated. A multifactorial mechanism for preterm membrane rupture is advocated by Parry and Strauss (1998). They reviewed the large literature and paid special attention to the loss of strength of the placental membranes. Further, the primacy of infection is supported by the meta-analysis of seven studies on prophylactic antibiotic therapy in premature rupture of membranes (Egarter et al., 1996). It indicated reduced neonatal morbidity from infections in mothers with premature rupture of membranes (PROM) treated prenatally with different antibiotic regimens. A comprehensive review, especially concerning prevention and therapy of bacterial vaginosis, premature delivery and PROM comes from McGregor and French (1997). Regrettably, metronidazole treatment to prevent premature delivery in women with bacterial vaginosis did not reduce its occurrence, nor did this therapy prevent preterm delivery from trichomonas infections (Klebanoff et al., 2001).

Many investigators have graded the inflammatory infiltration (e.g., Thiery et al., 1970; Naeye et al., 1983) so as to perhaps correlate it with clinical findings, foe example, rupture of membranes and maternal fever. We have found this to be impractical for several reasons. For instance, there are severe prenatal infections with some types of organisms, in particular the group B streptococcus, that elicit little placental inflammatory reaction but that can produce devastating disease in the newborn. It is also likely that different organisms have differing ability to penetrate the membranes. This point was shown experimentally by Galask et al. (1984), who exposed membranes to bacterial cultures. They found that group B streptococci penetrated membranes more readily than did coliform bacilli and gonococci. We believe that the intensity of inflammation is more closely related to the nature of the organism, rather than to the chronicity of the infection. It seems also difficult to estimate how long the infection has been active. This uncertainty has hindered acceptance of the opinion that membrane rupture *follows* membranitis, rather than *causes* it (see Naeye & Peters, 1980). The prevailing view certainly is that membranes rupture first, to be followed by amnionitis.

The preponderance of chorioamnionitis in very immature pregnancies (20–30 weeks) is striking (Lahra & Jeffery, 2004). It has often been linked to the less effective bacteriostatic nature of amnionic fluid in immature pregnancies (Anonymous, 1989a). Thadepalli et al. (1978) showed that amnionic fluid of the first trimester is least inhibitory against anaerobic organisms. Schlievert et al. (1975, 1976a,b, 1977) had similar results using various organisms for analysis. Their studies showed that the inhibitory moiety of the amnionic fluid contains a zinc-dependent special peptide that develops mostly after 20 weeks' gestation. Others had identified immunoglobulins in amnionic fluid (Galsk & Snyder, 1970) and that the fluid from patients with chorioamnionitis had elevated immunoglobulin levels (Blanco et al., 1983). Specific inhibition against *Mycoplasma* and *Chlamydia* was demonstrated in amnionic fluid by Thomas et al. (1988), and Gray et al. (1987) concluded that even the small quantities of type-specific streptococcal antibodies in amnionic fluid that they demonstrated may protect the fetus against this infection. All of these points may explain why chorioamnionitis is much more common during early pregnancy than toward term. It is our view that the more important aspect of labor initiation resides with inflammation of the decidua, and that the bacteriostatic activity of amnionic fluid is not the primary event preventing labor and chorioamnionitis during later gestation.

GENERAL CONSIDERATIONS OF CHORIOAMNIONITIS

The amnionic sac infection syndrome develops from infection that commences in the endocervix and vagina and then ascends (Fig. 20.23). Abundant evidence supports this opinion, and there is also much evidence that prematurity is often caused by such an ascending prenatal infection. Premature rupture of the membranes (PROM) often results and is then a common accompaniment of infection. Garite (1985) labeled it the "enigma of the obstetrician" because of the controversial aspects of diagnosis and management. A further problem is the difficulty in predicting rupture of membranes and premature delivery. It has been suggested that assessment of vaginal fibronectin may provide such a clue (Lockwood et al., 1991; Iams et al., 1995), but Feinberg and Kliman (1992), and others have taken exception to this approach. Gibbs and Blanco (1982) found that PROM complicates 4.5% to 7.6% of all deliveries, and that 1% of all gestations have preterm delivery with PROM. This study reviewed the evidence favoring the notion that PROM is often the consequence of subclinical vaginal infection. They also gave detailed protocols for management. McDuffie et al. (1992) showed in an experimental model that intracervical administration of coliform bacilli in rabbits leads to rapid and marked elevation of the various mediators that are usually associated with labor. Elst et al. (1991) found elevated prostaglandins and leukocytes in amniotic fluids aspirated by fetuses from spontaneous premature labor and concluded that chorioamnionitis may initiate preterm labor. Lettieri and her colleagues (1993) suggested that "idiopathic" preterm labor can be explained in 96%. They incriminated faulty implantation in one half of cases, infection in 38%, immunologic factors in 30%, cervical incompetence in 16%, uterine factors in 14%, maternal factors in 10%, trauma (surgery) in 8%, and fetal anomalies in 6%. It is our impression that ascending infection is the most important cause of preterm labor and PROM, certainly so in the 20- to 30-week gestation group. There are now numerous studies that support this contention. Romero et al. (1989e) examined the amnionic fluid aspirated from 264 women with preterm labor and with intact membranes. They found positive cultures

in 91%; 42% delivered preterm neonates, 21.6% of which had positive amnionic fluid cultures. Preterm delivery was especially frequent when endotoxins were detected with the *Limulus* amebocyte lysate assay. The commonest organisms isolated were *Ureaplasma urealyticum, Fusobacterium* sp., and *Mycoplasma hominis*, but later studies have indicated a spectrum of other organisms (Romero et al., 1992a). Inflammatory lesions (chorioamnionitis, funisitis) are essentially present only when microbacterial contamination can be shown to exist in the amnionic cavity (Harger et al., 1991). This study also emphasized that antimicrobial therapy failed to prolong pregnancy when chorioamnionitis was extant.

There is now a very large body of investigations that incriminates all sorts of mediators in the initiation of labor during the process of ascending infection. Interleukin-1 was found elevated and championed by Taniguchi et al. (1991), but no elevation of levels of IL-1-receptor antagonists were identified (Romero et al., 1992b). In addition to IL-1, IL-6 was found to be increased in infections studied by Matsuzaki et al. (1991), but not in normal labor. Kelly et al. (1992) suggested that the "final common step of prostaglandin and antiprogestagen action in parturition was decidual release of IL-8." Hillier et al. (1992) found several cytokines and prostaglandin E_2 (PGE_2) to be elevated in amnionic fluid during preterm labor and suggested their usefulness in predicting labor. Tumor necrosis factor activates the cytokine machinery and may well be at the starting point of labor initiation by stimulating prostaglandin production from the decidua (Norwitz et al., 1992a,b; Romero et al., 1992c). Suffice it to say that the cytokine system is intimately involved in premature labor when it is caused by infection; absent inflammation, the kinin levels are not significantly elevated (Romero et al., 1993).

When membranes are ruptured and the endocervical mucus plug has disappeared, the amnionic cavity may be quickly colonized by organisms of the cervicovaginal tract (Miller et al., 1980a,b). Wahbeh et al. (1984) found that anaerobic organisms play an important role in PROM similar to the results of a study by Bobitt and Ledger (1977). When Pankuch et al. (1984) attempted the isolation of bacterial and chlamydial organisms from 75 placentas, they found that 72% of placentas with chorioamnionitis had bacteria (82% with clinical chorioamnionitis), whereas only 15% of uninflamed placentas contained organisms. Almost 50% were anaerobic organisms. When, as is frequently the case, no organisms are identified histologically by the pathologist one must consider that they are either histologically not recognized (e.g., mycoplasma, trichomonas, etc.) or that cytokines (chemokines: GRO-α and IL-8) may be the chemoattractants (Hsu et al., 1998). Johnson et al. (1981b) found in their large study of PROM that unless chorioamnionitis intervened, rapid delivery was not necessary. They cautioned that, with modern management, the risk to the fetus is primarily one of prematurity. Earlier studies of the same group had shown that neonatal infections were much more common in preterm than term infants, but that the risk of PROM alone was insignificant (Daikoku et al., 1981). Teppa and Roberts (2005) have now developed an enzymatic test for the apparently common asymptomatic bacteriuria in pregnancy but they do not correlate it with ascending infections. Many authors have suggested that maternal bacteriuria is specifically related to PROM and to prematurity (Naeye, 1979a), but it has not been confirmed by some well-controlled studies of maternal bacteriuria (Bryant et al., 1964). The relation of asymptomatic maternal bacteriuria to low birth weight and preterm delivery was reaffirmed by a meta-analysis of Romero et al. (1989d). They also believed that ascending infection was the mode for infection. An anamnestic lymphocyte response to the organism of maternal infection was demonstrated in some infants judged to be at high risk of dying (Wallach et al., 1969). Still somewhat controversial is whether ascending infection can truly be prevented by antibiotics and also whether treatment is beneficial (Christmas et al., 1992; Seo et al., 1992; Kirschbaum, 1993). Unresolved also is whether aggressive tocolysis is beneficial to prolonging the survival of neonates or prolonging pregnancy significantly. Thorp et al. (2002) saw a mixed outcome pattern in their meta-analysis of 14 reports, and Combes et al. (2004) found no benefit from tocolysis in PPROM before 34 weeks in 130 cases studied, and reported significant maternal complications. Dinsmoor et al. (2004) found some prolongation of gestation with expectant management, but poor outcome nevertheless. Gibbs (2002) advocated that this is a topic for prevention rather than therapy, with which we agree. His experimental studies (Gibbs et al., 2002) clearly showed that, in rabbits, antibiotic therapy was unable to eradicate organisms from amnionic fluid or the fetus.

Another presumed cause of PROM, abortion, and premature delivery has been the syndrome of "incompetent cervix," thought to have a congenital origin (review by Borglin, 1962). It has been suggested that 0.1% to 1% of pregnancies are thus complicated, and that up to 20% of midtrimester abortions result from an incompetent cervix (Anonymous, 1977b). Gans et al. (1966) suggested that trauma is the most common antecedent of an incompetent cervix, a notion with which we agree, especially when prior surgery is considered. They reported favorable surgical repairs of the defect. The alleged etiology of trauma is well supported by a review of the topic (Anonymous, 1983a). Hagen and Skjeldestad (1993) studied the outcome of cervical laser conization with a case-control approach. They reported an increased frequency (38% vs. 6%) of premature births in the operated cases and recommended that conization be done only in high-grade in situ neoplasia. Barford and Rosen (1984) were more cautious in their assessment of diagnosis and therapy, and Charles and Edwards (1981) listed the many serious infectious complications (e.g., puerperal sepsis, chorioamnionitis) that may ensue, particularly when the Shirodkar stitch is undertaken during the second trimester of pregnancy. Heinemann et al. (1977) and others (e.g., Dunn et al., 1959) have reported maternal sepsis after intraamnionic E. coli infection in such cases. Abundant bacillary growth was present in placental capillaries, but there was only minimal inflammation in the case of Heinemann et al. (1977). Romero et al. (1992d) advocated that amniocentesis with culture should be undertaken before a cerclage is placed in the midtrimester; they found a high frequency of bacterial invasion. In our opinion, it is not likely that incompetent cervix is frequently an inherited defect; rather, we believe that trauma and infection are more probable antecedents. The cervix, affected by severe chronic cervicitis, is often patulous and prone to premature dilatation, which may be the origin of many of the 20% incompetent cervices cited to be associated with PROM. Leveno et al. (1986) published a study of gravid cervical dilatation that supported this assumption. They found that dilated cervices tend to lead to premature delivery; recurrent PROM and premature delivery are then serious problems. Gomez et al. (2005) also suggested that a foreshortened cervix is a risk factor for microbial ascending infection and derived this finding from a study of women in premature labor. This premature labor, however, is quite likely to have been the cause of labor in the first place that subsequently shortened the measured endocervical length. Asrat et al. (1991) studied 255 pregnancies in 121 patients and identified a recurrence rate of PROM in about one third. Interestingly, Salafia et al. (1991) found about the same frequency of the amnionic sac infection syndrome in premature births. An abnormally short cervix, as ascertained by vaginal ultrasonography, was also found to be associated with preterm delivery (Iams et al., 1996). Papiernik et al. (1998) reported that cervical shortening or dilatation of the cervix is a prerequisite for ascending infection and premature delivery, but only when vaginal infection exists. They opined that a reduction of preterm delivery can only be hoped for when prophylactic antibiotic therapy is practiced. Seaward et al. (1998) found that chorioamnionitis and maternal colonization with group B streptococci were the most important predictors of subsequent neonatal infection. Since that summary, numerous additional studies on cerclage or indomethacin treatment for the prevention of prematurity have been published. A meta-analysis by Belej-Rak (2003) showed that cerclage has no benefit

for a sonographically identified short cervix, a finding subsequently confirmed by To et al. (2004). There are, however, different opinions on this very controversial and common dilemma faced by obstetricians. This is shown for instance by a series of papers that follow the one by Althuisius et al. (2000). Some authors find the Shirodkar operation to be a useful adjunct of therapy at the time of premature rupture of membranes, but others do not. Occasionally this treatment in the presence of active chorioamnionitis can have disastrous outcomes. This was shown in a set of twins of whom twin A died from Actinomyces sepsis after cerclage and treatment with various antibiotics; there was severe chorioamnionitis (Knee et al., 2004).

The presence of an intrauterine device (IUD) has been correlated with pelvic inflammatory disease (PID) in some studies (Lee et al., 1988). Other studies have been less convincing, and the large cooperative study published by Kessel (1989) asserted that the relation is mostly to the increased frequency of pelvic infections in general, noted since 1973, and not to IUD insertions. Generally, the device prevents pregnancy, but when it fails to do so (2% to 4%), premature labor and chorioamnionitis frequently ensue. The correlation of septic abortion and presence of an IUD has also been confirmed in the large study by Kessel (1989). In this context, Jewett (1973) reported a maternal death following E. coli infection at 22 weeks' gestation. Fatal maternal sepsis has also been reported as a complication of chorioamnionitis without an IUD (Webb, 1967). With cesarean section patients, myometritis is present in one third of asymptomatic patients whose inflamed membranes had ruptured for more than 6 hours (Azziz et al., 1988). An interesting association also exists between the occurrence of ectopic pregnancy and recurrent abortion (Fedele et al., 1989). It is likely that its basis is infection. Of parenthetical interest is the suggestion by Polunin (1958) that vaginal infection and birth practices in a North Bornean tribe (the Murut) caused sterility, and that it was the result of vaginal infection. In subsequent studies, an anaerobic coccal (probably streptococcal) infection was found to cause the vaginitis and PID found in this tribe (Hare & Polunin, 1960). Dinsmoor and Gibbs (1989) found that previous amnionic sac infection is not a risk factor for subsequent infection of the uterus.

Another topic of concern among the causes of premature labor, PROM, and fetal infections relates to the hypothesis that intercourse during late pregnancy may initiate premature delivery (Naeye, 1979b, 1980). Herbst (1979), in an editorial, reviewed evidence that meconium staining and risk of prematurity were greater when orgasm had been experienced during pregnancy. Naeye (1982) suggested that other causes of prematurity are smoking, parity, prior cervical surgery, and prior chorioamnionitis. There has been much criticism of these studies on coitus-related prematurity (e.g., Berg, 1980; Mills et al., 1981; Perkins, 1983), some of which has been answered by Naeye (1981, 1983, 1986). His finding of modal peaks of deliveries on certain days of presumed peak coital activity were used to further support a relation among coitus, infection, and premature labor. Klebanoff et al. (1984) could not accept this relation in their analysis of the same data, a study to which Naeye (1986) took exception. When Ekwo et al. (1993) studied coitus of late pregnancy to ascertain whether this bears risks for preterm rupture of membranes, they found that "most sexual positions and activities during late pregnancy are not associated with adverse outcomes." Neilson and Mutambira (1989) found no relationship of twin deliveries to coitus. Similarly, there was no relation to premature labor when frequent intercourse occurred in the patients studied by Read et al. (1993). This was so unless for some of those women who were already colonized with some specific organisms. Similarly, Kurki and Ylikorkala (1993) found that "in healthy nulliparous women, coitus during pregnancy is not related to bacterial vaginosis and does not predispose to preterm birth." The issue is currently not definitively decided, but additional data suggest that some relationship may exist between coitus and premature deliveries (Anonymous, 1984; Naeye, 1988a).

Specific Microorganisms

Neisseria gonorrhoeae is the organism responsible for gonorrhea, which occasionally complicates pregnancy. In a cervical culture study of 1309 antepartum patients, Kraus and Yen (1968) found a 5.73% asymptomatic infection rate during pregnancy, with 32% puerperal morbidity. They were then primarily concerned with ophthalmia neonatorum and did not address the possible risk posed by chorioamnionitis. This study and others indicated that active cervical infection with this organism does not necessarily lead to chorioamnionitis. Baddeley and Shardlow (1973) saw two patients with normal deliveries after gonococcal arthritis during pregnancy. Infection of the amnionic sac with gonococci has been reported by Nickerson (1973) and Rothbard et al. (1975). We have seen several cases as well, and they were similar to other types of acute chorioamnionitis. In Nickerson's case, the infection was not recognized until the gastric aspirate was cultured. The febrile patient was near term and had spontaneous rupture of membranes and a tender abdomen. The placenta was not studied.

Rothbard and colleagues (1975) probably reported the first case of antenatally diagnosed and treated gonorrheal chorioamnionitis. The aspirated amnionic fluid was purulent, and gram-negative diplococci (gonococci) were identified at 35 weeks' gestation. Cesarean section, performed after ampicillin therapy, led to the birth of a normal infant whose neonatal course was uneventful. The placenta was not described. Smith et al. (1989) reported a case of acute gonococcal chorioamnionitis with sepsis. Their patient had a dark red vaginal discharge at 32 weeks, emesis, chills, migratory arthralgia, and abdominal pain. The membranes were intact, and at amniocentesis, gonococci were demonstrated. The 1960-g infant did well. The placenta had acute chorioamnionitis.

Even acute gonococcal salpingitis has been described to complicate pregnancy (Genardy et al., 1976). Their patient was operated on for presumed appendicitis at 14 weeks' gestation; the fallopian tube had pus with gonococci identified therein, and the patient was successfully treated with cephalothin and kanamycin. At 37 weeks, she delivered a normal infant and a normal placenta. This event is rare, however, and when present, ascending infections involve the tube only early in gestation, before the decidua capsularis makes contact with the opposing uterine wall. We have seen only one placenta of a patient with a history of ruptured membranes for 4 weeks who, in addition to marked *E. coli* chorioamnionitis, had developed sepsis from acute unilateral salpingitis at 32 weeks' gestation. The inference in this patient was that the salpingitis developed after the chorioamnionitis, also by ascending means. Edwards and colleagues (1978) studied 178 patients with gonorrhea during pregnancy (2.75% of the pregnanies cared for), and reviewed the literature. They found chorioamnionitis in 26% (5% in controls). Premature rupture of membranes occurred significantly more often (63% versus 29%), a point that was denied by Amstey (1982).

Infections with **group B streptococci** (GBS) are important and frequent complications of the perinatal period, and we now differentiate between early- and late-onset neonatal infections because of their significant differences in outcome. This streptococcus is recognized to be one of the most virulent organisms during the perinatal period. Sepsis, pneumonia, and meningitis are common sequelae of this infection (Baker, 1977), and the organism emerged as the number two cause of neonatal meningitis (Anonymous, 1977a). Prematurity and premature rupture of membranes are strongly correlated with group B streptococcal infections. The diagnosis is often difficult unless it is actively pursued. Occult streptococcal infection is an important cause of fetal asphyxia, and stillbirths frequently occur with unruptured membranes (Naeye & Peters, 1978; Peevy & Chalhub, 1983). This important topic has been reviewed in some detail by Nizet and Rubens (2000) with special attention to the recently identified virulence factors. Pritzlaff et al. (2001) describe specific toxins of the streptococcal variants in a molecular publication and find a novel specific hemolysin and cytokinin and in yet another publication of these investigators (Doran et al., 2002a) the pathogenicity to the lung of various mutants is described. This organism has apparently specific toxicity to epithelial and also endothelial cells.

Novak and Platt (1985) described the placentas of 22 cases of early-onset group B streptococcal sepsis. They found that chorioamnionitis was present in 64%, 27% of patients had funisitis, and in 41% of these patients gram-positive organisms were found in the amnionic fluid. Importantly, though, some placentas showed no pathologic changes or had only villous edema. The authors were disappointed that, excepting neutropenia, the placental findings did not correlate well with fetal outcome. They also emphasized that the extensive colonization of amnion and the leukocytic response argued strongly against late acquisition of the organism by the fetus during fetal descent. They reviewed other studies that gave similar incidence figures and concluded that an important part of the fetal response is related to the specific enzymatic types of the individual organisms. In a study of autopsy files, de Paepe et al. (2004) found that GBS infection was diagnosed in 4.9% of neonatal autopsies (61 of 1236) and was the cause of death in 58 cases. Chorioamnionitis was found in 67% of preterm babies and only 33% of term infants. They concluded that "fetoplacental inflammation is a poor indicator of perinatal GBS infection." Importantly, when meconium is present, this apparently enhances the susceptibility of the neonate. Eidelman et al. (2002) found that meconium enhanced growth of streptococci in amnionic fluid, whereas *E. coli* growth was inhibited.

Altshuler (1984) stated, "There is no inflammation in the placentas of at least 75 percent of newborns in whom group B β-hemolytic streptococcus has been cultured." Our experience also indicates that many placentas of streptococcus-infected babies, even those with neonatal sepsis, have no inflammation. Only very careful search for bacteria will identify the cocci on the amnion. Vigorita and Parmley (1979), on the other hand, described focal abscesses underneath the amnion, areas of epithelial necrosis, and found an accumulation of bacterial colonies in a relevant case. Although we have also seen such abscesses, we have wondered if double infection may have been the cause, as this observation differs so much from previous reports.

Group B streptococci may actively grow in amnionic fluid alone. Abbasi and colleagues (1987) showed that virulent strains of streptococci grew as well in amnionic fluid as in optimal bacterial culture media, although some differences were found among various strains. The authors believed that this point is clinically significant. But when the clinical manifestations of those patients in whom amnionic contamination was proved are compared with those without positive cultures, no differences of clinical risk factors were ascertained (Silver et al., 1990). The differentiation and designation of the many different streptococcal bacteria may not be widely appreciated. Table 20.1 summarizes their designation and features.

Numerous studies have addressed the need for early diagnosis and rapid therapy of perinatal group B streptococcal infection. The most modern studies employ a DNA probe for rapid detection (Yancey et al., 1993), in part because previous methods (enzyme-linked immunosorbent assay and Gram stain) were inefficient for screening tests (Hagay et al., 1993). Thus there is by no means agreement just how best to screen for the colonization, or how to deal with it when colonization is recognized. Gibbs and Blanco (1981) investigated 48 patients with bacteremia, 31 of which resulted from group B organisms. Endometritis and chorioamnionitis were the most commonly diagnosed clinical features. Although fever was often present, few localizing signs appeared. The authors also discussed effective therapy but some studies have shown that even intrapartum administration of antibiotics often does not prevent neonatal sepsis (Ascher et al., 1993). This has changed in the recent past following introduction of more rigorous protocols. Thus, Schrag et al. (2000) and Wendel et al. (2002) described practical and successful regimens of intrapartum therapy for high-risk patients. Andrews et al. (2000) discovered no organisms that were resistant to penicillin while finding resistance to erythromycin and clindamycin, and Gilson et al. (2000) advocated screening and intrapartum antibiotic therapy with good success. Towers and Briggs (2002) also described the marked decrease in frequency of early-onset disease when chemoprophylaxis is provided.

A prospective study of colonization with this organism was undertaken by Regan et al. (1981). They found a significant increase in PROM and an association with prematurity. That was not the case in the study reported by Amstey (1982), however. Singer and Campognone (1983) found organisms in the blood of immature stillborns associated with villous edema and mild chorioamnionitis. Two placentas showed acute and chronic villitis, which suggested to them a transplacental (hematogenous) infection. It may well have been a dual infection also. They emphasized the high risk of colonization, particularly during the second trimester of pregnancy. Matorras et al. (1989) showed that maternal colonization (rectal or vaginal) carried a significant risk for PROM. Cervical colonization was especially deleterious. Fetal death from streptococcal sepsis has even been described after intrauterine funipuncture for karyotyping (McColgin et al., 1989).

That this organism does not necessarily arrive in the fetus via hematogenous means, though, was shown by M.A. Pass et al. (1980). They found a severely colonized dichorionic twin A whose co-twin (B) did not have the infection. They believed that twin pregnancies are particularly vulnerable. Doran et al. (2002b), however, described a set of monozygotic (MZ) twins with late-onset disease causing fulminant fatal meningitis in twin A, while twin B recovered completely. The twins had a monochorionic placenta but it was not further described. Forsnes et al. (1998a) described hydrops in one diamnionic/monochorionic (DiMo) twin from whose amnionic

TABLE 20.1. Classification of aerobic streptococci

Group	Designation of species	Blood agar reaction[a]
A	*S. pyogenes*	β-hemolytic
B	*S. agalactiae*	Usually β-hemolytic
C[b]	Several species	β-hemolytic
D (enterococci)	*S. faecalis, S. faecium*	α-, β- or nonhemolytic
E (nonenterococci)	*S. bovis*	α-, or nonhemolytic
F	*S. anginosus*	Small colony β[c]
G[b]	Many species	Usually β-hemolytic[c]
Viridans hemolytic species		α-hemolytic
Pneumococci	*S. pneumoniae*	α-hemolytic

[a] β reaction is clear, complete hemolysis; α reaction is green discoloration, partial hemolysis.

[b] Groups C and G, β-hemolytic streptococci.

[c] The British classify minute colonies of groups C, F, and G β-hemolytic streptococci and Lancefield-groupable, and capnophilic strains of α- and nonhemolytic *S. intermedius* and *S. constellatus* as *S. milleri*. The Centers for Disease Control uses the designation *S. anginosus* for minute colonies of β-streptococci and retains the designations *S. intermedius* and *S. constellatus* (C. Davies, personal communication, 1989).

Source: Modified from Gibbs & Blanco (1981).

fluid adenovirus was grown. Both twins died at 26 weeks and their cardiac size did not indicate the presence of twin transfusion syndrome. It was assumed that transplacental infection took place in only one twin. Anastomoses were not described. Iams and O'Shaughnessy (1982), who evaluated antenatal versus intrapartum screening, found no advantage in the former method, whereas Pass et al. (1982) correlated infection with puerperal fever and the finding of frequent chorioamnionitis in cases of perinatal infection. The attack rate in their study was two in 1000 deliveries. They recommended intrapartum antibiotic prophylaxis, as did Boyer and Gotoff (1986). Strickland et al. (1990) also suggested a frequency of two early-onset infections in 1000 births and found intrapartum screening for this infection to be cost-effective because of the severe handicaps that can result. Thomsen and colleagues (1987) found that urinary group B streptococcal infection correlated with preterm labor, and they also reported a beneficial effect from penicillin therapy. Dykes et al. (1985) investigated women who gave birth to infected babies. Chronic carriage in the urinary tract, without immunologic response, was therein apparent. Similar findings were reported by Moller et al. (1984). They also found an increased risk of ruptured membranes. Matorras et al. (1989) found that PROM was significantly correlated with vaginal or rectal carrier status. It has also been shown that successive group B streptococcal infection, with early-onset disease of neonates, can occur despite proper antibiotic therapy (Carstensen et al., 1988).

For all these reasons, rapid diagnosis of infection with group B streptococci is urgent, a point addressed in several studies (e.g., Morales et al., 1986; Morales & Lim, 1987). Morales et al. used coagglutination methods for identification; Sandy et al. (1988) tested Gram stains of cervicovaginal swabs; they found it to be an unreliable means for diagnosis. Of alternative methods explored in an editorial, most were considered to be unsatisfactory for routine use (Anonymous, 1986). Latex agglutination tests from swabs may be a useful means of rapid identification (Howe et al., 1987; Stiller et al., 1989). Baker et al. (1988) obtained promising results from immunization of pregnant women. In a large review of the possibility for immunization, Coleman et al. (1992) suggested that such vaccination is attainable and that studies in that direction be pursued; antigens such as cell wall polysaccharides and protein C are the most promising to be investigated.

The effect of this infection can be devastating to the newborn (and fetus), and its onset may be rapid. The neonatal diagnosis, manifestations, and therapy were lucidly discussed by McCracken (1976). Contrary to one's hopes, immediate penicillin therapy to the immature neonate does not prevent early-onset disease, nor does it reduce the excessive mortality (Pyati et al., 1983).

Of interest to the pathologist is the study of Katzenstein et al. (1976). Dissatisfied with the frequency of autopsy diagnosis of hyaline membrane disease in pregnancies at risk, they used immunofluorescence (on formalin-fixed tissue) to reexamine eight appropriate cases. They identified streptococci in the pulmonary hyaline membranes of five neonatal deaths. These structures were so numerous in one case that they appeared to make up the bulk of the fibrinous membrane. The deaths had previously been attributed to routine hyaline membrane disease at routine autopsy.

Hyde et al. (1989) have shown experimentally that extracts from cultures of this organism may cause isolated portions of umbilical vein wall to contract severely. They suggested that such effects may occur in vivo during intraamnionic infections, and that it may lead to reduced venous return from the placenta, causing fetal damage. Clinical investigations of this phenomenon are now commencing. Fleming et al. (1991) found a correlation of S/D (systolic/diastolic) ratios and biophysical profiles with chorioamnionitis, whereas Leo et al. (1992) did not. It must be pointed out, however, that the latter group did not study the placentas, and other problems exist with the protocol. It is too early to make decisions as to the possible value of predicting chorioamnionitis/funisitis with this methodology.

Group A β-hemolytic streptococci pose serious problems for mother and fetus (Swingler et al., 1988). Antenatal acquisition was shown by Monif (1975) in a febrile patient with a tender uterus at 34 weeks' gestation. The membranes were unruptured, and the cervix was closed. A depressed infant was born with leukocytosis, left shift of white blood cells, and positive cord blood culture. Placental histologic study was not undertaken. Other cases were reviewed by Lehtonen et al. (1984). The infection responds readily to penicillin or ampicillin, and the umbilical stump may be a reservoir for the organism. Puerperal infection with this organism, however, may pose serious risks (Silver et al., 1992). Both of their seriously ill patients required hysterectomy, but their pregnancies had ended uneventfully.

Fatal maternal and fetal infection with *Streptococcus pneumoniae* (type III) was reported by Tarpay et al. (1980); that placenta also was not studied. Duff and Gibbs (1983) identified two similar infections with *S. pneumoniae* demonstrable in amnionic fluid. They thought that ascending infection was unlikely because of the stringent pH requirements (pH 6.5 to 8.3) of the organism. They did not identify the source of infection and did not report on the placenta. Andreu et al. (1989), however, reported chorioamnionitis in the placentas of several infants, prenatally infected with this organism and having pneumonia.

Haemophilus influenzae was contracted prenatally in a premature infant reported by Barton et al. (1982). It had septicemia and recovered after ampicillin therapy. The membranes had ruptured 15 hours before delivery.

The placenta was not described. Gibson and Williams (1978) observed this infection in a 28-week gestation complicated by leukorrhea, abdominal pain, and fever. The amnionic fluid was opaque and contained the organisms on smears. The placenta had chorioamnionitis and funisitis. The infant died from hyaline membrane disease. There was no pneumonia. A study by Campognone and Singer (1986) of 19 patients with this infection drew attention to the serious nature of this disease. All of their cases had chorioamnionitis, and three had acute villitis in addition. Winn and Egley (1987) added another case with chorioamnionitis and funisitis. The patient had intact membranes. The organisms may be readily identified as gram-negative rods in smears. Rusan and her colleagues (1991) agree that this infection poses serious problems; they undertook a retrospective review and found 13 cases with chorioamnionitis or endometritis over a 10-year span. Of 23 infected neonates, 15 presented with sepsis or pneumonia.

Diplococcus pneumoniae (*Streptococcus pneumoniae*) was the cause of neonatal laryngitis in a term infant delivered to a febrile patient with positive amnion and cervical cultures (Hazard et al., 1964). It may here be mentioned that smears of the placental surface have been usefully employed by Nessmann-Emmanuelli et al. (1983) in establishing prenatal infection. Positive smears were obtained in 9% of a high-risk group (63% gram-positive, 17% gram-negative, and 20% mixed). It was especially useful for group B streptococcal and *E. coli* infections.

Gram-negative bacilli, in particular *E. coli*, frequently cause chorioamnionitis. Their association with neonatal meningitis is well known (Kagan et al., 1949; Watson, 1957; McCracken & Sarff, 1974). That this organism, especially the K1 type, is transmitted vertically has been firmly established by the large cooperative study of Sarff et al. (1975). These authors found a strong association with maternal rectal colonization of the organism and likened the acquisition to that of streptococcal infection. The investigators did not examine placentas. Their concept of pathogenesis included lung infection, intestinal infection, sepsis, and meningitis. We believe that the modus of transmission for neonatal meningitis is often through the aspirated amnionic fluid via the middle ear. DeSa (1974) has shown that squames, admixed with pus and organisms, are often found in the middle ears of stillborns and neonatal deaths.

Salmonella typhi and other salmonella organisms may cause meningitis of neonates. They may be transmitted vaginally. Pugh and Vakil (1952), Watson (1958), and Scialli and Rarick (1992) reported cases of congenital infection and some fetal deaths, and they also reviewed the literature. Infection by symptomatic women or carriers was also shown by Luder and Tomson (1963), and Freedman et al. (1970). The placenta is usually not mentioned. An exception is the case reported by Awadalla et al. (1985) of a patient with gastroenteritis at 26 weeks' gestation. A foul-smelling intact gestational sac containing cloudy amnionic fluid was delivered. Blood, stool, cervical specimens, and amnionic fluid yielded the organism. Despite these findings, the authors were of the opinion that transplacental, rather than ascending, infection took place. When Roll et al. (1996) saw a premature neonate die with *Salmonella enteritidis* infection, they cultured the organism from the infant and placenta, but there was no evidence of chorioamnionitis. Seoud et al. (1988) recorded the occurrence of typhoid fever during pregnancy in 13 patients. One infant died with pneumonia. The mothers were treated with chloramphenicol and did well.

Infection with *Shigella sonnei* caused septicemia and enterocolitis in a term infant reported by Kraybill and Controni (1968). Prenatal infection of this infant seemed likely, but the placenta was not studied.

Clostridium perfringens infection occasionally complicates pregnancy. Among anaerobic infections, this type has been particularly feared because of the postabortal sepsis and uterine gas gangrene that may be life-threatening for the gravida (Ramsey, 1949). Nash et al. (1963) described a patient at 35 weeks' gestation whose membranes had ruptured for 5 days, a tender uterus, fetal death, and abdominal crepitation from gas infiltration. They carefully described the placenta: It had a greenish amnionic surface and a putrefactive odor. The purulent exudate covered the membranes and fetal placental surface; it contained gram-positive rods. The maternal surface and villous tissue were not involved. A similar case is shown in Figure 20.25. Several reports of abortion due to *C. perfringens* infection have been published that emphasized the severity of this infection and the frequent lethal outcome (Decker & Hall, 1966; Pritchard & Whalley, 1971). Decker and Hall (1966) demonstrated that inflammatory exudate and necrosis of villous tissue may be found in septic cases, and the fetus may be invaded by organisms.

Diphtheroids or corynebacteria are frequent normal vaginal inhabitants and can often be cultured from placental surfaces. They have occasionally been shown to cause chorioamnionitis. Fitter et al. (1979) described a case of funisitis and chorioamnionitis due to *Corynebacterium kutscheri*. It occurred at 26 weeks of pregnancy in a grand multipara who delivered 24 hours after rupture of membranes. Gram-positive organisms were demonstrated and were grown in pure culture from cord, membranes, rectum, nose, throat, eye, and external ear. There was no sepsis in the 980-g premature infant who survived after ampicillin and gentamicin therapy. The placental surface was discolored and had gray-brown plaques. Similar plaques were present on the umbilical cord. The plaques were composed of organisms that also invaded the underlying tissue. Funisitis and chorioamnio-

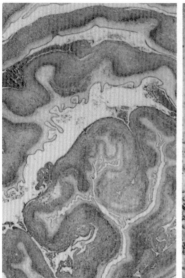 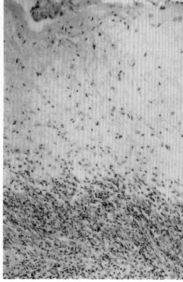 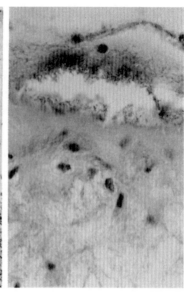

FIGURE 20.25. Clostridial chorioamnionitis at term. The membranes were friable and meconium-stained. The infant survived with antibiotic therapy. Membrane roll (left) shows intensive deciduitis and chorionitis. Note the umbilical arteritis (center, right) with a pocket of gram-positive rods underneath the amnion. Touch preparations were strongly positive. H&E ×16 (left); ×160 (center); ×640 (right).

nitis were pronounced. The case proves that not all diphtheroids isolated from the placenta or amnionic fluid are due to vaginal contamination at delivery. In this case, the infection must have occurred prior to membrane rupture.

Altshuler and Hyde (1985, 1988) have drawn attention to the importance of *Fusobacterium necrophorum* and *F. nucleatum* infections as significant complications of pregnancy. These pleomorphic, filamentous, gram-negative, anaerobic organisms were isolated from three of 297 placentas examined for various indications. These authors described in detail the fluorescent antibody identification, chromatography, and usefulness of the Warthin-Starry stain for identification on slides. Brown-Brenn stains were not so useful for demonstrating the bacteria, and in hematoxylin and eosin (H&E) preparations the organisms were even more difficult to identify microscopically. It is also important to note that Bouin's fixative makes their demonstration particularly difficult. Of 92 prematurely delivered placentas, 62 had chorioamnionitis, and of the latter, 11 (18%) had filamentous organisms in the membranes.

In the rat animal model developed by Altshuler and Hyde (1985), inflammation similar to chorioamnionitis was consistently produced. In a subsequent contribution (Altshuler & Hyde, 1988), these investigators reaffirmed the association of fusobacterial infection and prematurity. Among 586 placentas examined, they identified 14 with fusobacteria, and from their literature review, it is evident that as many as 30% of patients with occult chorioamnionitis may be infected with a *Fusobacterium* species. A typical case of fusobacterial chorioamnionitis is shown in Figure 20.26. It was associated with the scattered villous edema (Fig. 20.27) that Naeye et al. (1983) considered to be so important in causing prenatal hypoxia in association with chorioamnionitis and prematurity. Easterling and Garite (1985) reported three cases of fusobacterial infection and emphasized the importance of this rarely recognized organism as a cause of premature labor, and Romero et al. (1989e) found it commonly in prenatally obtained amnionic fluid with intact membranes. Cox et al. (1988) found bacterial endotoxin in the amnionic fluid of a patient with fusobacterial infection of a preterm delivery, reaffirming the suggestion by Altshuler and Hyde (1988) that these organisms are rich in lipopolysaccharide.

Bacteroides fragilis was found to be the cause of ascending infection in five of 15 patients with premature rupture of membranes reported by Evaldson et al. (1982). *Campylobacter (Vibrio) fetus*, a common enteric pathogen in humans and a common cause of venereally transmitted abortion in hoofstock, has been described to cause placentitis, infarcts, and fetal death (Gribble et al., 1981). Their patient had fever for 3 weeks and fetal death at 19 weeks. The amnionic fluid and placental surface were normal, but histologically there were areas of villous necrosis and "acute inflammation in the villous tissue." The organism was isolated from maternal blood, placenta and fetal spleen. These authors reviewed the few other cases reported with pregnancy; when described, the placentas were similar to their case. The route or source of infection was not identified in any of the cases, nor was

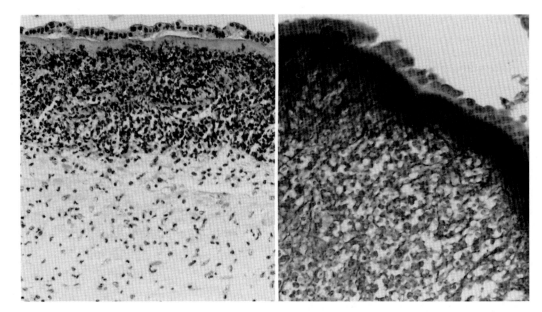

FIGURE 20.26. Chorioamnionitis due to fusobacteria in the placenta at 23 weeks' gestation. The placental surface was opaque. Fusobacteria were also found in the fetal lung. At left are Bouin-fixed membranes with inflammation; few indications exist of the massive bacterial growth seen with the silver stain at right. The dark filaments radiating from the amnionic basement membrane are easily identified as the filamentous organisms. H&E ×160 (left); GMS, ×240 (right).

venereal transmission verified. In the case described by Meyer et al. (1997), maternal colitis complicated a 22-week pregnancy, resulting in maternal sepsis, acute villitis, and fetal demise. The organism was identified genetically as well as by Warthin-Starry stain and occurred primarily within the immature villi. Some patients had recurrent abortions. Placental tropism has been suggested to exist in sheep. The earlier literature of infection with this organism was reviewed by White (1967).

Chorioamnionitis due to *Streptobacillus moniliformis*, the cause of rat-bite fever, was reported by Faro et al. (1980). The patient had cervical cerclage for repeated abortions, and with unruptured membranes, amniocentesis yielded pus and gram-negative rods. The placenta had a fetid odor. The patient's house was infested with rats. The organism also causes the Haverhill (milk) fever.

Gibbs et al. (1987) isolated the gram-variable organism *Gardnerella (Hemophilus, Corynebacterium) vaginalis* from 28% of 86 patients who had intraamnionic infection. Because controls had a similar frequency of isolation (21%), the authors suggested that this common vaginal organism is part of a microbial spectrum that does not cause PROM. We have isolated it occasionally from maternal and neonatal blood; it causes mild disease, but severe chorioamnionitis, premature delivery, and demise were reported by Pinar et al. (1998). Their description is

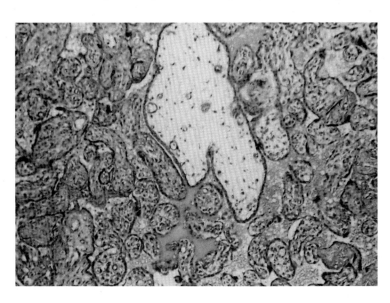

FIGURE 20.27. Villi of placenta in Figure 20.26, showing scattered villous edema. H&E ×160.

of further interest in that it depicted the turquoise staining of the umbilical cord secondary to amnionic injection of indigo carmine. Hillier et al. (1988), in a case-control study of chorioamnionitis, isolated *G. vaginalis* in 26% and *Ureaplasma urealyticum* in 47% of cases of prematurely delivered infants. They suggested that these organisms are etiologically important.

Tularemia is an uncommon disease, but the responsible organism (*Francisella tularensis*) had once been described as infecting placenta and fetus (Lide, 1947). The placenta of the macerated fetus showed granulomatous lesions with frequent central necrosis, and similar granulomas were found in the fetus. The patient had become infected while preparing rabbits for eating.

Brucellosis is caused by a variety of organisms belonging to the genus *Brucella*. Malta and Bang fevers, in humans, are due to infection with these organisms, but a wide variety of animal diseases are frequently caused by host-specific species of these organisms (Moore & Schnurrenberger, 1981). Among the animal diseases, abortion and placentitis are prominent findings. The placental lesions are frequently characteristic (Molello et al., 1963) and have been experimentally studied in goat by Anderson and his colleagues (1986a,b). Human infection with several of the *Brucella* species has been well documented. The infection may be fatal or lead to protracted disease; often it is self-limited, and the organism appears to be acquired from contact with animals or their products, especially raw milk and unpasteurized cheese (Anonymous, 1983b). Although human abortions have been described as being due to *Brucella abortus*, and the organism has been isolated from the fetus (Carpenter & Boak, 1931), it is an uncommon event. In cattle, the organisms are much enriched in placental cotyledons and allantoic fluid, and in mice this infection has provided an important model (Tobias et al., 1993). Meador and Deyoe (1989) depicted large numbers of these bacteria in the trophoblast of infected bovine placentas. Sarram et al. (1974) isolated *Brucella melitensis* from the placenta of abortion in a highly endemic area, and they suggested a causal relation to the abortion. The placentas were not described. The topic was completely reviewed by Porreco and Haverkamp (1974). They found little evidence of an increased abortion rate with this infection and cited only a few cases with positive isolation from the placenta or fetus. The patient they described had verified infection from fresh goat cheese during the 32nd week of gestation. She was treated with kanamycin and delivered a healthy infant at term. The placenta was normal. No characteristic lesions have been described in the human placenta with this disease. Salpingitis has often been reported with brucellosis, and sexual transmission was suggested in several studies (see Ruben et al., 1991). Mofleh et al. (1996) stated that, in endemic regions, infection commonly occurs from animals and their placentas.

Leprosy

Leprosy is due to *Mycobacterium leprae*. It is now relatively uncommon in the United States, but pregnancy-complicating leprosy has been investigated on many occasions. It has been reported that vertical transmission either usually is uncommon or does not occur, although Duncan et al. (1983) described two young children (12 and 17 months of age) with leprosy. Whether these children acquired the disease transplacentally or shortly after birth remains unknown. The authors examined sections of the placenta and failed to identify acid-fast bacilli. When they made concentrates of the 10 most "bacilliferous" patients' placentas, they found only scanty organisms or cell debris.

Maurus (1978) found no organisms in one placenta and gave up searching for organisms in the placenta following a report by King and Marks (1958) that said they were unable to identify placental organisms in treated leprosy. This statement contrasts with earlier reports, summarized by Duncan (1985), in which frequent abortion with bacterial isolation of organisms from placenta and cord blood was alleged.

For this reason, the detailed study of the human placenta in leprosy by Duncan et al. (1984) is of great value. In their review of the literature, there was one reported placenta with a granulomatous lepromatous lesion in villi; *M. leprae* was present in 66 of 172 placentas studied in the past. Duncan and colleagues (1984) reported a detailed investigation of 81 placentas from leprous women. No lepromatous lesions were detected histologically in the placentas by electron microscopy or immunologic study. Homogenates of placentas from two patients with active lepromatous leprosy yielded a few acid-fast bacilli. The previously recognized relatively small size of placentas in leprosy (Duncan, 1980) was reaffirmed. This "hypoplasia," however, was now held to be due to smaller placental cell sizes (rather than cell numbers) and not to an altered immune status. Patients with leprosy have depressed T-cell reactivity that is allegedly worse during pregnancy. For unknown reasons, these mothers excrete reduced amounts of estriol during pregnancy (Duncan & Oakey, 1982).

Nine-banded armadillos suffer leprosy frequently, and they can be infected with the human organism. When Job et al. (1987) studied the placentas of three pregnant nine-banded armadillos, they found acid-fast organisms in decidua, trophoblast, and villous cores, as well as in the spleens of some fetuses. Although focal villous necrosis was found, no granulomas were seen in the placentas. One animal had thrombosed cord vessels. In light of the occasional finding of organisms in placentas from leprous women, and because of some degree of similarity between armadillo and human placentas, vertical transmission remains a possibility, even though it may be uncommon.

Tuberculosis

In contrast to leprosy, congenital tuberculosis has been repeatedly demonstrated to occur, despite the fact that generalized tuberculosis is a frequent cause of sterility. In some cases there is doubt as to the timing of infection. Neonatal disease may have been acquired postpartum from milk or sputum of an infected mother. No epidemiologic doubt, however, exists about the disease in the macerated stillborn with the extrauterine pregnancy described by Nokes et al. (1957). This 23-cm crown–rump (CR) fetus, removed from an abdominal implantation, had multiple caseating pulmonary nodules and acid-fast bacilli in the liver, spleen, and kidneys. The placenta had many hard, white plaques that represented tubercles that contained acid-fast organisms. The patient had a partially tubally implanted pregnancy with tuberculous salpingitis, and miliary tuberculosis existed in most organs. The authors reviewed briefly 68 previously reported cases of extrauterine pregnancies complicated by tuberculosis.

Beitzke (1935) established criteria for the acceptance of congenital tuberculosis, which is now a rare and preventable disease of infants. These criteria included evidence of hematogenous infection via the umbilical vein. Beitzke also emphasized the need of separating the infant from the mother at birth. Nemir and O'Hare (1985) reviewed diagnostic criteria, reported the longest follow-up of a severely infected child, and gathered more than 200 cases from the literature. Their own case was criticized by Corrall (1986) as not fulfilling all of the established criteria. The discussion further elaborated on the difficulties of distinguishing truly transplacentally acquired tuberculosis from infection transmitted by inhalation of infected amnionic fluid and from neonatal disease acquired nosocomially.

The placenta has rarely been examined in putative cases of congenital tuberculosis. Schmorl and Kockel (1894) examined three patients who died with tuberculosis during pregnancy. The placentas appeared grossly normal. The fetuses were near term; all three associated placentas contained typical but rare granulomas with giant cells in the villous tissue. In two fetuses, tuberculous lesions were also found; the placental membranes were uniformly negative. Schmorl and Geipel (1904) found nine additional cases of placental tuberculosis among 20 new specimens. For some of these specimens, more than 2000 sections had to be prepared before tubercles were found. The authors insisted that acid-fast stains must be made, lest early lesions be overlooked. Even so, identification of acid-fast organisms required a prolonged search. Bacilli were frequently found in fetal vessels, intervillous fibrin, and septa. Warthin (1907) provided additional detailed descriptions of placental tuberculosis, with numerous tubercles and acid-fast bacilli identified. He found that the decidua contained areas of necrosis but no giant cells; there were many intervillous and villous granulomas, and the chorion was involved only sparsely. In a previous case, he also made thousands of sections to verify tuberculous infection. His initial opinion that the syncytium was resistant to infection was subsequently modified because he saw necrosis of trophoblast.

Boesaart (1959) also found tubercles in the placenta of an infected patient whose infant remained well. We saw a placenta membranacea at 35 weeks' gestation from a patient with tuberculous peritonitis. The placental floor had several tuberculous granulomas. The neonate was well and was treated prophylactically (Kaplan et al., 1980). In the same report we demonstrated numerous acid-fast bacilli in the therapeutically aborted villous tissue of a patient who had cavitary tuberculosis for which she was taking appropriate medication. There were neither necrosis nor a granulomatous reaction in this endometrium. Finding the organisms was unexpected. In other cases we have identified acute granulomas (consisting mostly of neutrophils) adjacent to villi and destroying the trophoblast and isolated giant cells in stem villi but without inflammation. We have also been impressed with the extensive and unusual necrosis at the decidua basalis and capsularis in patients with disseminated tuberculosis during pregnancy. The areas appeared bright yellow macroscopically and had a "cheesy" complexion microscopically, similar to what one expects in large granulomas.

Listeriosis

Listeriosis is caused by a gram-positive bacillus that is occasionally confused with diphtheroids. The disease occurs in a wide variety of mammals and birds, as well as in humans (Dennis, 1968). The literature suggests that the human disease is underdiagnosed (Bowmer et al., 1973). Most adults successfully eliminate the causative organism *Listeria monocytogenes*. Immunodeficiency of adults (Nieman & Lorber, 1980; Wetli et al., 1983), various chronic disease states (Boucher et al., 1984), and characteristically pregnancy may be complicated by significant disease (Gantz et al., 1975). Transmission from mother's milk has been recorded in neonates (Svabic-Vlahovic et al., 1988). Nosocomial infection occurs in nurseries (Nelson et al., 1985), and direct contact with infected animals has also caused infection (Anonymous, 1980). Southwick and Purich (1996) have reviewed the complex microbiology with this organism. Several serologic subtypes exist and specific antibodies are useful for diagnosis in otherwise difficult cases (Roberts, 1997).

Food-borne acquisition of the organism is the most common mode of infection (Gill, 1988; Lamont et al., 1988; Jones, 1990). Numerous epidemics have been reported, and the source of bacteria has been defined in some (Anonymous, 1985). Some of these epidemics have originated from pasteurized milk (D.W. Fleming et al.,

1985), Mexican-style cheese (Linnan et al., 1988), cabbage contaminated by sheep feces and made into coleslaw (Schlech et al., 1983), poorly cooked sausage and chicken (Schwartz et al., 1988), pâté (37 of 73 examined contained the organisms; Morris & Ribeiro, 1989), and other sources. At times, the precise source of an infection could not be defined, despite intensive search (Filice et al., 1978), but a gastrointestinal route appears to be the most likely mode of infection (Breer & Schopfer, 1988). The organism may survive moderate heat, and it thrives in chilled food (Kerr et al., 1988; Gilbert et al., 1989). Guidelines have thus been established for the food industry in order to avoid wide dissemination of this ubiquitous agent to susceptible people (Update, 1988).

The implication that livestock is the cause of transmission of this infection has been challenged, as the organism also occurs in the stool of many normal people and in the soil (Low & Donachie, 1989). Ortel (1975) investigated stools from a large population of normal people after a devastating outbreak occurred in Halle during 1968. Pregnant patients had a 24% rate of contamination (6.5% after delivery), meatpackers 3.6%, and nurse-midwives 9%; finally, the personnel of a laboratory had a 91.6% (!) rate of carriage.

The organism is a danger principally to pregnant women, newborns, and immunocompromised individuals. A 60% perinatal mortality has been ascribed to this infection (Barresi, 1980). We have seen congenital listeriosis in the offspring of a microbiology laboratory technician, suggesting that special vigilance is needed when such personnel are pregnant. Fortunately, the neonate was promptly treated and survived. In infants, listeriosis is known as granulomatosis infantiseptica. "Granulomatosis" is a misnomer because the visible lesions are truly abscesses, not granulomas (Seeliger, 1955). An autopsy report of seven children with perinatal listeriosis indicated that grossly visible microabscesses are relatively uncommon (Klatt et al., 1986). During an outbreak in Los Angeles, which originated from infected cheese, maternal pyrexia and a high index of suspicion were the most essential factors for the early diagnosis (Boucher & Yonekura, 1986). Neonatal meningitis is a serious complication of fetal infection with this organism (Ahlfors et al., 1977; Visintine et al., 1977; Laugier et al., 1978). A rash is often present in the neonate, and gastric aspirates as well as Gram stains (and culture) of skin rashes are helpful for identifying the organism (Halliday & Hirata, 1979). One case of nonimmune fetal hydrops has been attributed to listeriosis; the placenta and stillborn fetus had numerous abscesses (Gembruch et al., 1987). The diagnosis is easily established from cultures, when the infection is suspected. Berche et al. (1990) found that anti-listeriolysin O titers quickly develop after infection, and that they are useful for diagnosis. Despite the infrequency of listeriosis in Saudi Arabia, Boukhari et al.

(1999) described a term neonate with meningitis who was successfully treated, the first case in that country with early-onset disease. Benshushan et al. (2002) reviewed charts of neonates from a 10-year time span in Israel and found 11 pregnant patients with listeriosis in mother and infant. In the five placental examinations available, all had chorioamnionitis and abscesses. Plaza and Gilbert-Barness (2001) described a stillborn intrauterine growth restriction (IUGR) infant with listeriosis and superbly illustrated the placental lesions.

The placenta in listeriosis has the following characteristic lesions: villous abscesses, villous necrosis, necrotizing villitis, and an abundance of bacterial growth on the amnionic surface, usually accompanied by chorioamnionitis. Case reports with good descriptions of these lesions have been provided by Olding and Philipson (1960), Driscoll et al. (1962), Soma (1979), Roberts (1997) and many other pathologists. Yamazaki et al. (1977) found abscesses, chorioamnionitis, and funisitis in a stillborn with proved granulomatosis infantiseptica, but they were unable to demonstrate the organisms in the placenta. They referred to other authors with a similar experience. The development of unusual macroabscesses in congenital listeriosis was described by Steele and Jacobs (1979), and Topalovski et al. (1993) thought that the diagnosis could be made solely from a placental examination. They depicted the macroabscesses in the placenta and suggested that silver impregnation is a better means to demonstrate the organisms than a Gram stain. The diagnosis of listeriosis complicating pregnancy is important because prompt therapy with ampicillin rapidly cures the maternal and fetal infections. There is also good evidence that listeriosis is a common cause of abortion in France (Lallemand et al., 1992), and produces similar pathologic lesions. Forsnes et al. (1998b) observed an interesting diamnionic/dichorionic twin pregnancy in which the "higher" twin B had died in utero from listeriosis (culture proven), with twin A remaining healthy and delivered at 34 weeks. Areas of avascular villi and chorioamnionitis were found in the placenta of twin B. Another dichorionic twin gestation with congenital listeriosis comes from Beinder et al. (1999). Here, again, twin A was healthy but twin B died from the disease.

Aside from the usually opaque surface of the placenta, which is occasionally described as greenish, there are often typical abscesses visible in cross sections of the fresh placenta (Figs. 20.28 and 20.29). When smears of these yellowish lesions are stained with Gram solution, the organisms are often readily apparent. Microscopically, the abscess frequently has a central area of necrosis and is composed of a massive PMNL infiltration (Fig. 20.30). The chorioamnionitis is usually severe and often extends into the villous tissue; the amnion commonly contains a large number of organisms. There is no doubt that some of them have proliferated during cold storage

FIGURE 20.28. Numerous placental abscesses (white nodules at arrows) due to *Listeria* infection. Premature infant; immediate therapy with survival.

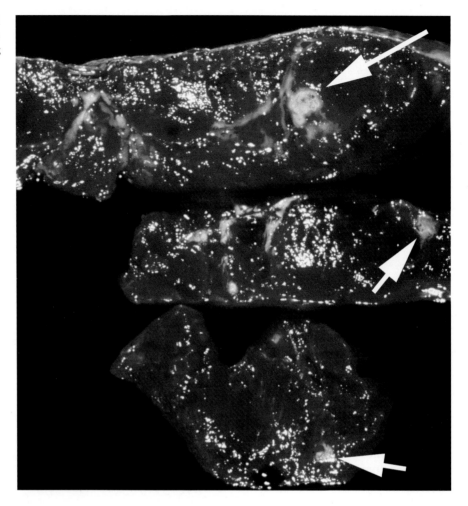

FIGURE 20.29. *Listeria* abscess in the placenta underneath the discolored chorionic plate at 37 weeks' gestation. Maternal fever was immediately diagnosed as due to listeriosis from the smears of the abscess. Ampicillin therapy of the neonate cured the infant who had a diffuse rash at birth.

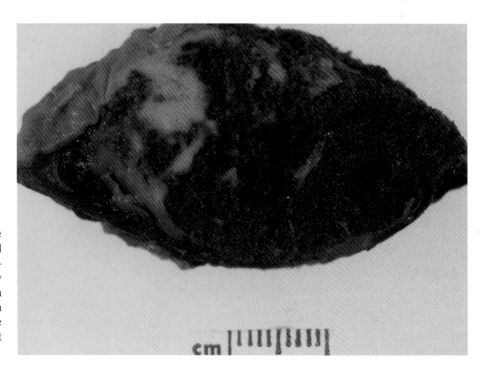

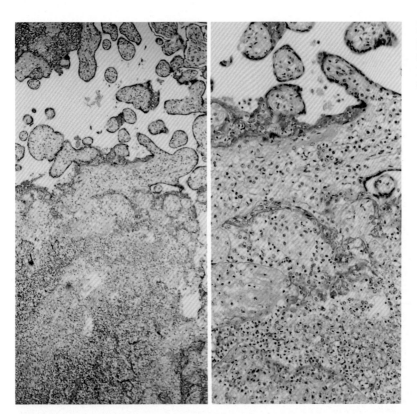

FIGURE 20.30. *Listeria* abscess in an immature placenta of stillborn twins. There is much necrosis of villi, fibrin deposition, and infiltration with PMNLs. Numerous organisms were found on Gram stain. H&E ×60 (left); ×240 (right).

of the placenta prior to examination (Fig. 20.31). The amnionic colonization is so prominent in utero, however, that amniocentesis for the differential diagnosis of febrile patients has been advocated (Petrilli et al., 1980).

When listeriosis is recognized during pregnancy and adequately treated, the placental abscesses undergo scarring. They are then sometimes still recognizable histologically as a former abscess. One must assume that abscesses in the fetus may have a similar fate. Effective therapy during pregnancy has been described by Zervoudakis and Cederqvist (1977) and A.D. Fleming et al. (1985). The latter authors presented another case and described meconium staining and chorioamnionitis. Koh et al. (1980) also saw meconium discharge and found many placental abscesses in a newborn who was severely ill; the infant recovered after ampicillin therapy, which had been commenced prenatally. A similar sporadic occurrence was related by Barresi (1980). The organisms were present in gastric aspirate and on body surfaces. Placental abscesses were present. In another case, treated at 13 weeks' gestation, the placenta and infant were normal when the patient delivered at term (Cruikshank & Warenski, 1989). Identical lesions of placenta and fetus have been described in nonhuman primates (McClure & Strozier, 1975).

Recurrence of listeriosis during subsequent pregnancies has occasionally been described (Rappaport et al., 1960; Dungal, 1961; Ruffolo et al., 1962). Such events and

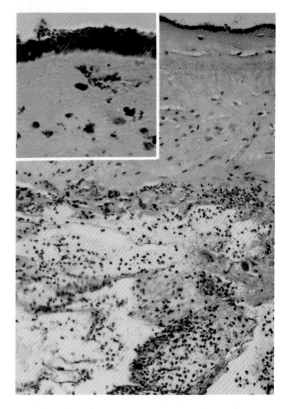

FIGURE 20.31. Listeriosis of the placenta in a stillborn. There is extensive subchorial infiltration with leukocytes, edema of membranes, and massive bacterial growth in amnion. H&E ×160. Inset: Gram stain. ×640.

the unexplained reason for the unusual frequency of severe listeriosis during pregnancy and in newborns have raised questions about the pathogenesis of this disease. Flamm (1959) experimented with rabbits and was of the opinion that septic transplacental infection causes the placental and fetal infection. This opinion is partly supported by the findings of typical abscesses in the placenta and the occasional finding of organisms within intact amnionic sacs. The presence of organisms in the vagina and in stool and the typically severe chorioamnionitis, however, suggest that an ascending mode of infection additionally occurs. Perhaps the placental abscesses form after fetal septicemia has taken place, similar to the abscesses in the fetus. Whether one or both of these modes of infection is the predominant way of fetal infection with listerial organisms is currently not known.

The susceptibility of immunodeficient and pregnant patients may result from their altered T-cell function. Schaffner et al. (1983) addressed this question experimentally by treating mice with cyclosporin A and cortisone, and by infecting nude mice. Their conclusion was that *Listeria* infection is biphasic: "Bacterial multiplication is controlled by nonspecific defense mechanisms in the early phase, and by acquired T-cell–dependent immunity in the second." This question was further explored in the work of Redline and Lu (1987), who found that local, decidual immune response regulated infection of the fetoplacental unit. They suggested an analogy to the nonrejection of the placental graft in regard to this immunologic interaction of *Listeria* and the decidua. In later studies, Redline et al. (1988) found that hormonal induction of deciduomas allows bacterial proliferation in the uterus, but that this endocrine manipulation does not influence the infection of peripheral organs of mice. It was also true when the mice were preimmunized. The investigators then studied the composition of the immune cells in the decidua and found that "increased bacterial titers were correlated with an inability of macrophages and T lymphocytes to reach [the] tissue *Listeria* [organisms] in discrete regions of deciduoma-bearing uteri." They further suggested that an antifetal (placental) immune response of the host was hindered by the same decidual mechanism that allows uncontrolled listerial growth locally (Redline & Lu, 1988). These findings suggested that the lack of recurrent listeriosis transmission by 74 women who had once delivered an infected child (Degen et al., 1970) is not the result of immunization. Bortolussi et al. (1989) found in rat experiments that neonatal interferon deficiency may be responsible for the susceptibility of infants.

Another organism that was reported to have caused the formation of placental abscesses is *Burkholderia pseudomallei*, the gram-negative bacillus causing **melioidosis** (Abbink et al., 2001). The mother had been treated with antibiotics for ulcerative colitis and a placenta previa

necessitated cesarean section. The neonate had sepsis and the organism was subsequently cultured from the cervix.

Actinomyces

Only three cases of placental inflammation due to this gram-positive anaerobic organism have been reported (Zakut et al., 1987; Abadi & Abadi, 1996). The infection observed by the latter authors occurred in an afebrile patient at 25 weeks' gestation of a dichorionic twin pregnancy with premature labor. Upon membrane rupture, foul-smelling fluid emerged. Both placentas had marked chorioamnionitis and histologically characteristic organisms. Zakut et al. (1987) had reported two cases with massive invasion by actinomycetes and necrotizing placentitis.

Mycoplasma Hominis *and* Ureaplasma Urealyticum

Mycoplasmas are a well-recognized group of pathogens of many animals. They cause infections of the urogenital tract, are responsible for respiratory and joint diseases, and are a frequent cause of epidemics in laboratory animal colonies (Tully & Whitcomb, 1979). Two organisms, *Mycoplasma hominis* and *Ureaplasma urealyticum* (also known as the "T strain" because the colonies are so tiny) are known urogenital pathogens for humans (Cassel & Cole, 1981); other *Mycoplasma* species affect different organ systems. *M. hominis* is a known cause of PID, febrile conditions during the postpartum period (Naessens et al., 1989), and possibly urinary tract infections. *U. urealyticum* (as well as *Chlamydia trachomatis*) is known to cause nongonococcal urethritis in men (Shepard, 1970; Taylor-Robinson & McCormack, 1980). The organism attaches itself to spermatozoa and may thus more readily penetrate the endocervical mucous barrier (see Fig. 20.24). It is also likely that combined infection with these two organisms is a cause of mucopurulent cervicitis in women (Paavonen et al., 1986). The available evidence suggests that these organisms are sexually transmitted (McCormack et al., 1972). Sterility in women is often secondary to PID, and much direct evidence exists that *U. urealyticum* infection of fallopian tubes is an important cause (e.g., Friberg, 1978). On the other hand, Gump et al. (1984) found that there is no relation between involuntary infertility and *Mycoplasma* infection. Yoon et al. (1998) showed the significant inflammatory reaction that follows infection with ureaplasma.

Kundsin et al. (1967) first suggested that infection with the T strain of *Mycoplasma* may cause chorioamnionitis and repeated abortion. They observed this new strain in cultures from decidua and aborted fetal membranes of a patient who had had four previous unsuccessful pregnancies. The fetal lung contained aspirated pus. Microorganisms were not identified histologically in the inflamed tissues. Additional specimens gave similar results. These observations suggested that this new strain (*U. urealyticum*) may be the cause of repetitive abortions, as well as of sterility. Premature rupture of membranes and premature delivery have recently been associated with both *Mycoplasma* and *U. urealyticum* (Perni et al., 2004). A case similar to that described by these investigators is depicted in Figure 20.32; it is a patient with four previous abortions. Severe chorioamnionitis in this abortus is evident from the opacity of the fetal surface. Subsequent treatment with antibiotics of this patient and her husband resulted in a healthy term pregnancy (Quinn et al., 1983).

Since the initial description of placental infection with *Mycoplasma*, there have been numerous clinical and pathologic studies that aimed to define the roles of these pathogens in reproductive failure of women, specifically attempting to relate them to PROM and chorioamnionitis. Some conflicting results have been obtained. The studies are hampered by the facts that these organisms have specific culture requirements and cannot be identified by routine microscopic examination of tissues. Prenatal infection of fetal tissues has been demonstrated microbiologically in many studies, but positive antepartum cultures do not predict outcome effectively (Carey et al., 1991). Furthermore, erythromycin treatment of infected women does not apparently prevent premature delivery (Eschenbach et al., 1991). Both organisms are a cause of neonatal meningitis (Waites et al., 1988); *M. hominis* has been the cause of neonatal lung abscess (Sacker et al., 1970), and *U. urealyticum* infection has been associated with chronic neonatal lung disease (Cassell et al., 1988; Sanchez & Regan, 1988; Wang et al., 1988).

Madan et al. (1988, 1989) made detailed microbiologic studies of autopsy and placental material; they found that "genital *Mycoplasma* were isolated from 36 cases (8.3%), and acute chorioamnionitis and funisitis were present significantly more often in cases with genital mycoplasmas." In their detailed study of perinatal deaths, including isolation of various pathogens from placenta and neonatal lung, they came to similar conclusions. One of their stillborns had myocardial calcifications, and some not only had aspirated pus in the lung but also an interstitial chronic inflammatory response, suggesting prolonged exposure to this mycoplasmal antigen. In this decisive pathologic study of perinatal infection with this organism, the authors were much impressed with the attending villous edema in the placenta.

The disease caused by these organisms is similar to that of other acute infections, except for the absence of demonstrable bacteria. The chorioamnionitis is similar as well. There have been some other suggestions that mycoplasmal infection causes villous alterations. Kundsin et al. (1967) found "unusual sclerosis of villi"; and Romano et al. (1971), who described aspiration bronchopneumonia in an aborted 19-week fetus with isolation of T-strain organisms, described degenerative changes of villous vessels, thrombosis, and villous edema. The illustration accompanying their article, however, depicted normal architecture. This study, as many others, was hampered by our current inability to demonstrate the organism microscopically in tissue sections. In the future it will require special techniques, such as study with immunofluorescence.

The relation of *Mycoplasma* to PROM, premature labor, and chorioamnionitis is still debated; Romero et al. (1989c,d; Romero, 1989) have critically reviewed 12 published studies to assess this relation. They criticized several of them as being indecisive and poorly designed. Their

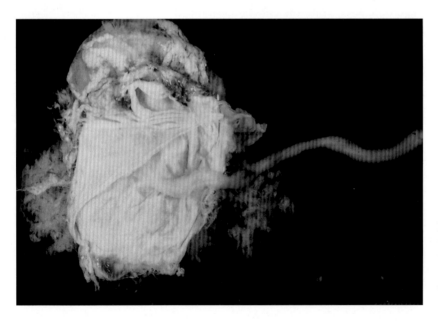

FIGURE 20.32. Placenta of spontaneous abortion due to *Ureaplasma urealyticum* infection. The patient had had four previous abortions with similar morphology. Note the creamy pus underneath amnionic surface, and fresh marginal hemorrhage.

opinions are that the association of cultured organisms and PROM "does not prove a cause-and-effect relationship," and when all studies were analyzed in detail, "it seems unlikely that genital colonization with *Mycoplasma* species without a failure of the host defense (fetal and/or maternal) leads to preterm delivery." This report was criticized by Kundsin and Horne (1989), and the reply must be read to appreciate the controversies, especially with respect to effective therapy.

In a prospective cohort study of 6500 women, no association of *U. urealyticum* infection with premature labor was found by Nugent et al. (1988). Pathologic and microbiologic studies on neonates from patients with and without chorioamnionitis by Quinn et al. (1987) established a strong correlation between *U. urealyticum* colonization and chorioamnionitis. Kundsin et al. (1996) found that prenatal infection with this organism increases significantly the longer the membranes have ruptured. They emphasized that eradication of the infection in a gravida should be attempted. Gauthier et al. (1994) felt that isolation of the organism would not lead automatically lead to delivery, and they treated women successfully with erythromycin. When maternal antibody response was taken into consideration, Gibbs et al. (1986) found a strong correlation of a pathogenic role of *M. hominis* infection. Considering the frequently mixed nature of infection, the high prevalence of some of these organisms, and the differences in the composition of the populations studied, it is presently impossible to come to a clear-cut decision. Our impression is that the genital mycoplasmas are pathogenic genital organisms, and that they are a frequent cause of chorioamnionitis and premature birth. In fact, several studies have shown that they are the principal organisms isolated from the placental surface and amnionic fluid of patients with PROM.

Chlamydia Trachomatis *and* C. Psittaci

The genus *Chlamydia* has several species (Peeling & Brunham, 1996). Of these, *Chlamydia psittaci* causes parrot fever (psittacosis), and *Chlamydia trachomatis* is responsible for the most common sexually transmitted disease in the United States (see also Gaydos et al., 1998; Peipert, 2003). It also causes trachoma, lymphogranuloma venereum, nongonococcal urethritis in men, and the diseases in women that will next be discussed. *Chlamydia pneumoniae* and *C. pecora* are now considered to be subdivisions of *C. psittaci* and have not yet been assigned as being gestational pathogens. It is estimated that between 10% and 20% of sexually active men and women are infected with one of these organisms (Saxer, 1989; Caul et al., 1997; Miller, 2005). Ryan et al. (1990) surveyed a large population of women by cervical culture and found that 21.08% were positive. They recommended routine culture for *Chlamydia*. Approximately half the infants born to infected mothers develop ophthalmia neonato-

rum ("inclusion body blenorrhoea"). Others develop pneumonitis. It is estimated that 3% to 4% of neonates have ophthalmia, and 1% to 2% have pneumonitis from infection with this organism (Harrison et al., 1978; Harrison, 1985).

The bacterium-like intracellular microbe can be visualized in the cytoplasm of infected cells by direct immunofluorescence study. *Chlamydia* has also been isolated from neonates, even from the pneumonia of stillborns infected through intact membranes (Thorp et al., 1989). Other than by culture, the infection can be diagnosed in infected tissues and amnionic fluid with the immunoperoxidase technique, as employed by Shurbaji et al. (1988), and by DNA sequences following polymerase chain reaction (PCR) amplification (Pao et al., 1991). The direct immunofluorescence technique has a sensitivity of approximately 89% (Binns et al., 1988), and fine-tuning allows some additional improvement (Pastorek et al., 1988). Livengood et al. (1988) investigated various staining methods and emphasized the diagnostic importance of having experience when reading the slides. An enzyme immunoassay was advocated by Binns et al. (1988) as being highly sensitive and therefore a good diagnostic test. Reports on the prevalence of the disease must be interpreted with these limitations in mind. But new, simple, and effective methods for detection (e.g., polymerase and ligase chain reactions) have been added to the armamentarium of epidemiologists (Pasternack et al., 1996; Andrews et al., 1997; Locksmith, 1997) that should much improve diagnosis and results from surveys. Thus, PCR from self-obtained samples of the introitus yielded excellent results (Wiesenfeld et al., 1996).

Chlamydia trachomatis infection of the cervix, where it causes mucopurulent cervicitis (Brunham et al., 1984, illustrated in color by Peipert, 2003), is also relatively easily demonstrated by the use of the direct fluorescence method (Graber et al., 1985). Brunham et al. (1984) provided impressive color photographs of the stained organisms. *C. trachomatis* is responsible for a significant number of cases of acute salpingitis (Magnusson et al., 1986), and it also causes chronic salpingitis and sterility (Guderian & Trobough, 1986; Moss et al., 1986). The effect of a *C. trachomatis* infection on pregnancy is still controversial. Sweet et al. (1987) reported that PROM was more likely to occur when infection had caused a maternal antibody response, but statistical significance was not reached. Alger et al. (1988) found that the organism was isolated from 44% of patients with PROM but only in 16% of controls. There are suggestions that PROM and perhaps chorioamnionitis are linked to this infection, but much more direct evidence needs to be marshaled before such a conclusion can be affirmed. The organism has not been isolated from the placenta, but has been demonstrated in amnionic fluid, and in the eye and nasopharynx of neonates (Thomas et al., 1990). It has also not yet been demonstrated conclusively to be a direct cause of chorioamnionitis, except in rat models (Rettig & Altshuler, 1981). Ryan and his colleagues (1990), however, accumulated data on the infection in pregnancy that suggested premature rupture of membranes to be much more likely when the infection was not treated. Other investigators support the notion that chlamydial infection in pregnancy should be treated with antibiotics (Forster et al., 1991; Crombleholme et al., 1990).

Chlamydia psittaci infection is rarely recognized as a cause of human abortion, although this infection commonly causes abortions in sheep and other domestic species. Initial infection is sheep is followed by a 30% abortion rate that later declines to 5% when the flock is thoroughly infected (Gunson, et al., 1983). Reports by Johnson et al. (1985) and Wong et al. (1985) indicated that sheep farmers and their wives have a high exposure to this pathogen. A pregnant wife of a farmer became infected and aborted at 28 weeks' gestation. Acute intervillositis was found in the grossly normal-appearing placenta. Syncytiotrophoblastic inclusions were present that showed numerous organisms by ultrastructural study and positive immunofluorescence. The fetus was also infected with organisms recovered from various organs. We have summarized the experience with such an infection (Hyde & Benirschke, 1997; Jorgensen, 1997). This abortion occurred following a febrile episode in a woman who had assisted with lambing. The sheep were later found to be chronically infected with this organism. Characteristically, the patient's DIC ceased after abortion of the infected placenta. In one instance, at least, the pregnant patient succumbed from the disease. The placenta had massive intervillous leukocyte accumulations, villous necroses, and the typical presence of masses of chlamydial organisms that appear to preferentially proliferate in the cytoplasm of the syncytiotrophoblast (Fig. 20.33A–D). Since that report another experience with abortion in pigs due to this agent has been published (Thoma et al., 1997).

Bacterial Vaginosis

Bacterial vaginosis has been defined by Westrom et al. (1985) as the "replacement of the lactobacilli of the vagina by characteristic groups of bacteria accompanied by changed properties of the vaginal fluid." The other bacterial species include *Bacteroides, Gardnerella vaginalis, Mycoplasma hominis, U. urealyticum,* and perhaps others. A relation to PROM and amnionic sac infection has been reported to exist (Gravett et al., 1986). Many authors since have suggested that bacterial vaginosis is a common cause of intraamnionic infection and premature birth (Silver et al., 1989; Hillier et al., 1995; Newton et al., 1997). Consideration of this entity, however, is beyond the scope of this chapter; suffice it to say that current opinion is that systemic antibiotic therapy is required and effective (Hauth et al., 1995; Joesoef et al., 1995; McGregor &

French, 1996). An extensive review has been provided by Martius and Eschenbach (1990) that considered the relation of vaginosis to chorioamnionitis, and numerous clinical publications have also considered this topic. A relation to preterm labor was shown by Subtil et al. (2002) and a meta-analysis by Leitich et al. (2003) showed it to be "a strong risk factor for preterm delivery and spontaneous abortion." Therapeutic trials of antibacterial treatment have been effective in reducing preterm births (Ugwumadu et al., 2003).

Syphilis

Infection with *Treponema pallidum* may occur at any time during pregnancy. The organism may pass to the fetus through the placenta during all stages of maternal syphilis infection. The responsible organism is a 4 to 10 μm long, 0.5 μm wide spirochete. According to Grossman (1977), "Most frequently, dissemination is associated with a placentitis arising from hematogenous spread of the spirochetes between the first and second stages of infection of the mother." The commonly held notion that the placenta is impermeable to spirochetes before the 20th week of pregnancy, because of the thickness of Langhans' cytotrophoblast layer (Fiumara, 1975), can no longer be accepted. Braunstein (1978) described a spontaneous abortus (12.8-cm CR length, approximately 4.5 months' gestation) with an abundance of spirochetes in the liver and other organs and marked placental changes. We had shown, by immunofluorescence and electron microscopic studies, that spirochetes can be demonstrated in fetuses as early as at 9 to 10 weeks' gestation (Harter & Benirschke, 1976). One reason why prior studies had failed to identify fetal syphilis is because the expression of the disease's features depends on the fetus's ability to react with antibody production to the spirochetal antigen. Histopathologic changes cannot be seen before that developmental time, and the disease is thus not diagnosed. Ohyama et al. (1990) have since demonstrated spirochetes in syphilitic placentas by the immunoperoxidase technique, and Nathan et al. (1997) also isolated spirochetes from early gestations and subsequently successfully treated the fetuses. Although spirochetes may be difficult to identify, a variety of new techniques are now available. The study of congenital syphilis by Guarner et al. (1999) describes histochemical means by which to demonstrate an abundance of spirochetal remnants in this disease, aside from complete spirochetes, thus making diagnosis considerably easier.

The relation of infection to disease was first clearly elucidated by Silverstein (1962) and Silverstein and Lukes (1962). They found congenital syphilis with attendant fetal plasma cell infiltration and reasoned that the inflammatory response was the cause of illness. Another reason for lack of recognition of early fetal infections is that it is

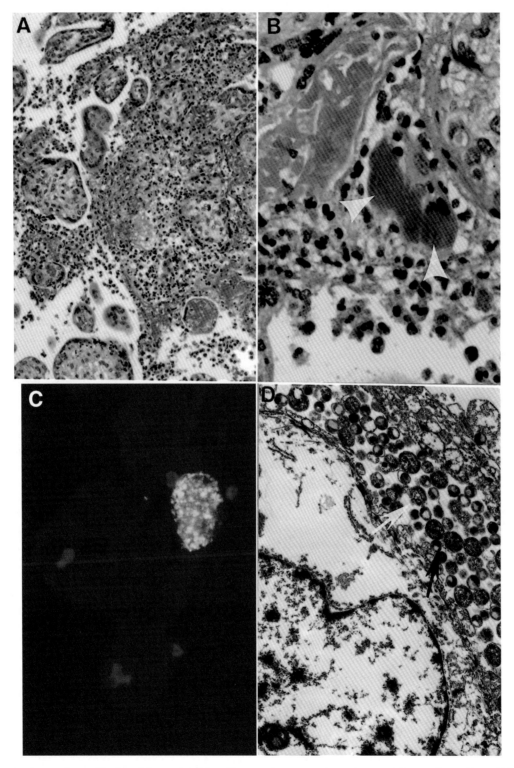

FIGURE 20.33. A: Acute intervillositis (abscess) with villous destruction in *Chlamydia psittaci* infection. B: Cluster of organisms in syncytial cytoplasm at arrowheads. C: Immunofluorescent localization of antigen. D: Electron microscopic (EM) demonstration of syncytial organisms. (A,B: H&E ×100, ×400; C: immunofluorescence ×400; D: EM ×1500) arrow at organism. (*Source:* Modified from Hyde & Benirschke, 1997.)

often difficult to demonstrate spirochetes histologically. Fetuses from such infections are often macerated, and radiographic study of long bones, often diagnostic of the infection, is frequently neglected. The disease may also appear as hydrops fetalis (Barton et al., 1992). The treponemes in macerated fetuses are most abundant in the liver; they are rare in the placenta and umbilical cord. Wendel et al. (1989, 1991) have shown that in gestations with fetal death from syphilis, darkfield examination of amnionic fluid always readily allows demonstration of treponemes. In addition to the conventional silver stains, it has been demonstrated that spirochetes may be stained with immunofluorescence in formalin-fixed tissue (Hunter et al., 1984). Thus Epstein and King (1985) demonstrated spirochetes in macerated liver tissue by immunofluorescence. Nevertheless, improved Warthin-Starry silver stains are probably the best means of identifying spirochetes in tissues (Kerr, 1938). It has now been established also that the organism can be identified in macerated fetuses with the Warthin-Starry stain (Young & Crocker, 1994).

A classic paper of the neonatal pathology in congenital syphilis was written by Oppenheimer and Hardy (1971). They confined their report to 16 neonatal deaths and did not consider the 31 macerated fetuses they saw during the same time. Hepatosplenomegaly was found in all, but after penicillin therapy spirochetes were not demonstrable with the Levaditi stain. The report does not include a consideration of placental lesions. Judge (1988) also provided an excellent review of congenital syphilis, with emphasis on the stage of pregnancy when the disease was acquired.

Many morphologic changes are found in the placenta and umbilical cord with congenital syphilis (Russell & Altshuler, 1974; Horn et al., 1992). By and large, the more severely the fetus is affected, the greater are the pathologic changes in the placenta. A macerated fetus with congenital syphilis may have a massively enlarged placenta with numerous pathologic features; a general increase in placental weight has been demonstrated by Malan et al. (1990). Most authors who have studied the placenta of congenital syphilis have concluded that there are no absolutely characteristic pathologic findings, but bulky villi and some other changes to be discussed should raise the suspicion. When suspicion of fetal syphilis exists, silver preparations for spirochetes are indicated. They may ultimately prove that lesions are due to syphilis when other means such as serology and radiographs of the fetus are not available. It must be cautioned, however, that the stains are not always easy to execute and that incomplete treatment with antibiotics may prevent identification of spirochetes. Fojaco et al. (1989) have claimed that necrotizing funisitis is a specific lesion of congenital syphilis and Knowles and Frost (1989) have expressed a similar view. Discussion of this fallacy is included in the

next section of this chapter. Because much of the informative literature on placental syphilis comes from an era when the other causes of banal types of chorioamnionitis and funisitis were not recognized, the early literature must be interpreted with caution.

When congenital syphilis was suspected in the past, physicians made scrapings of the umbilical venous intima for darkfield examination; and in the discussion of congenital syphilis by Ricci et al. (1989), beautiful silver preparations of this type were illustrated. They also showed the plasma cell villitis in such a case. Hörmann (1954) has reviewed this and other aspects of syphilis in great detail. Baniecki (1928) is one of many authors who sought treponemes in umbilical cords. He found inflammation in five of 14 living infants with syphilis; 12 of 17 stillborns had such inflammation, and five of 40 nonluetic infants had umbilical phlebitis. During the same year, Kaufmann (1928) found no placental lesions in two thirds of children with positive spirochetal infection. Beckmann and Zimmer (1931) made another detailed study of umbilical cords in syphilis. They had 420 cases, of which 392 were at term gestation, including nine stillborns; 28 were premature, including five stillborns. They found inflammation in 18.3% (77 cases; 25 only mild). Of these cases, only three infants had congenital syphilis. Conversely, 13 infants with congenital syphilis had no inflammation. They concluded that funisitis was not characteristic of syphilis but rather was a nonspecific inflammation that was perhaps caused "mechanically." Organisms are also readily identified in amnionic fluid (Wendel et al., 1989, 1991). In some cases of funisitis due to spirochetal infection we found the organisms only peripheral to the exudate and the necrosis, employing the Warthin-Starry stain.

The villous tissue has somewhat more characteristic changes with congenital syphilis. In Braunstein's (1978) 4 months' gestation fetus, the placenta had enlarged villi with endothelial and fibroblastic proliferation. Few mononuclear cells were present. The cellularity of the villi demonstrated in his photomicrographs, however, is impressive and is similar to that shown in Figure 20.34. McCord (1934) had described these features of villous "crowding" and enlargement of the placenta. Russell and Altshuler (1974) were also impressed with the placental enlargement, a feature already commented on by Hörmann (1954), who had referred to a case with a placental weight of 2500 g accompanied by a fetus weighing 2600 g. Russell and Altshuler's diagnostic features included relative villous immaturity, decidual plasma cell infiltration, perivascular fibrous tissue proliferation, and alterations of capillary endothelium. They also found plasma cell infiltrations in the enlarged villi of syphilitic placentas, a finding made repeatedly by us. These changes are all nonspecific. The nature of the infiltrating inflammatory cells within villi has been controversial. Most recently, they

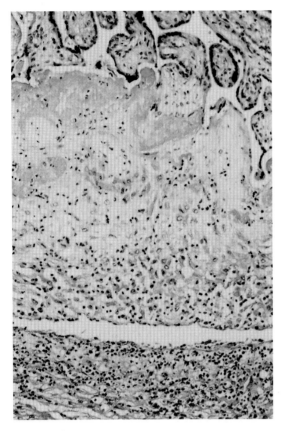

FIGURE 20.34. Plasma cell infiltration of decidua basalis in a placenta of 28 weeks' gestation and an infant afflicted with typical congenital syphilis. The placenta was large 580 gm. H&E ×160.

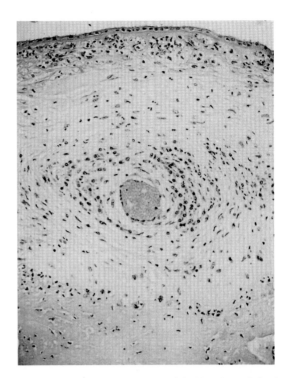

FIGURE 20.36. Perivascular plasma cell infiltration of chorion in congenital syphilis at 30 weeks' gestation. Mild chorioamnionitis is also present. H&E ×160.

were characterized by Kapur et al. (2004) and found to be largely (or exclusively?) of maternal origin. CD3 lymphocytes predominated in that study. Gummas or granulomas have never been reported in the placenta, but

Hörmann depicted villous abscesses that had also been seen in earlier studies. In our experience, the villous enlargement is often striking and there are frequent decidual infiltrations with plasma cells; foci of decidual necrosis are common (Fig. 20.35). Abscesses or villous necrosis is frequent in severe infections and chorioamnionitis may be present, but it is also often absent. When it is found, it may include plasma cells, which is an otherwise unusual finding in banal chorioamnionitis (Fig. 20.36). Spirochetes can be found, but often it requires a

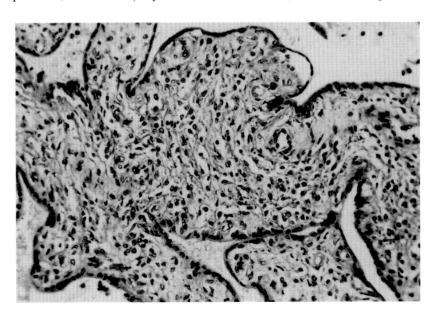

FIGURE 20.35. Villi of placenta in congenital syphilis (same case as in Figure 20.38). Villi are hypercellular, infiltrated with mononuclear cells. Note the focal necrosis and vascular obliteration. H&E ×240.

694   20. Infectious Diseases

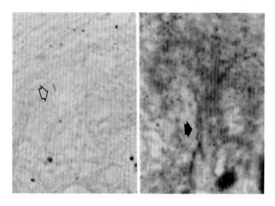

Figure 20.37. Spirochete (arrows) in the placenta of stillborn infant with congenital syphilis. Levaditi stain. ×1600.

prolonged search (Fig. 20.37). Moreover, and regrettably, the art of staining spirochetes in tissues is gradually being forgotten by histologists. There is a reported decrease of estriol production by the placenta in syphilis (Parker & Wendel, 1988), perhaps due to a possible decrease in fetal adrenal androgen precursors, rather than to a placental inability to aromatize androgens.

Necrotizing Funisitis

The term **subacute necrotizing funisitis** was introduced by Navarro and Blanc (1974) in a report of 16 cases. In the earlier literature this condition had been referred to as "phlegmonous funisitis" (see Hörmann, 1954). It is an infrequent and unusual type of a more chronic inflammation of the umbilical cord in which even calcification of the old exudate may occur. Calcifications of the umbilical cord had only rarely been reported before the descriptions by Navarro and Blanc. Eight of their cases were stillborn infants. With the exception of two isolations of *Candida* species, no pathogen was identified. Syphilis and other specific agents were carefully excluded by serology in that study. The umbilical cords of these infants had severe inflammation deposited in "successive waves." It was present in a ring-like fashion around the umbilical cord vessels. The exudate was often degenerated and had become calcific. Mural thrombosis was present in several vessels. Two infants had an uncommon presence of plasma cells in their umbilical cord. The nature of the exudate indicated that it is a chronic infection, as did similar inflammatory changes in the lungs of several stillborns. Other signs of chronic infection were found in the stillbirths, and they occurred during the neonatal life of survivors. Chorioamnionitis with frequent surface necrosis was invariably additionally present. In the opinion of Navarro and Blanc, the funisitis differed in severity and chronicity from the usual type of funisitis found in the amnionic sac infection syndrome. Miyano et al. (1998)

suggested that it represents the end of the infectious process, where only immune perturbations still exist.

Perrin and Bel (1965) had previously described three cases of cord calcification, one of which, however, may have originated in a hematoma. In one of these cases, there was difficulty in clamping the cord at delivery. An interesting aspect of this inflammation was the "neovascularization" of the exudate, with the origin of these capillaries being unknown. Schiff et al. (1976) described calcification of all three vessels in the cord and had even visualized it sonographically before birth. As in other cases, the calcifications followed the cord vessels, but they stopped before entering the abdomen of the infant. This observation is important, as it further clarifies the pathogenesis of chorioamnionitis and funisitis. It indicates the presence of antigen within the amnionic sac and negates the opinion that the umbilical vasculitis results from a systemic infection. No inflammation was described in their case, but the fetal growth restriction was thought to be secondary to the restriction of blood flow. Gille (1977) described a similar case and drew attention to the fact that granulation tissue was present in the vessels. The patient was a premature infant who did well. The exudate accompanied the vessels for the length of the cord, and a fresh thrombus was present within the vein. The accompanying photographs showed an impressive and uncommon amount of inflammation and "organization," which is otherwise rare in the placental vasculature. Knowles and Frost (1989) have added a case report of necrotizing funisitis in congenital syphilis with organisms plentiful in this lesion but sparse elsewhere.

Numerous cases of chronic, necrotizing funisitis have been seen by us. Some had calcifications, but others did not. In our view, they represent different stages in the evolution of funisitis. Figure 20.38 shows a cross section of umbilical cord in an immature placenta with necrotizing funisitis. Figure 20.39 shows the concentric rings of white exudate in a growth-retarded infant at 31 weeks; in contrast to the previous case, here the inflammatory reaction totally surrounds the vessels. In Figure 20.40, a radiograph shows the peripheral calcification that has formed in the old exudate. Numerous plasma cells were found in the inflammatory debris, but electron microscopic search for organisms was unrewarding. The mother had had a febrile illness during the first trimester, but otherwise mother and infant were entirely normal. In other cases, herpes virus II antigen could be localized to such cords with specific antibodies (Robb et al., 1986b).

Craver and Baldwin (1992) reviewed 60 cases of this necrotizing funisitis, 45 of which had clinical information. This is clearly the largest case collection of this lesion. It occurred in 0.1% of deliveries more than 20 weeks' gestation. Growth restriction (28%), stillbirths (18%), and necrotizing enterocolitis (22%) were prominently associated problems. These investigators did not find any single agent

FIGURE 20.38. Umbilical cord at 31 weeks' gestation with chronic inflammatory exudate (necrotizing funisitis). The exudate is concentrically deposited around the vessels; much old exudate is necrotic and beginning to calcify. A partially organized mural thrombus is present in the umbilical vein. The patient had rupture of the membranes for more than 12 hours, a circumvallate placenta, and massive chorioamnionitis. von Gieson. ×12.

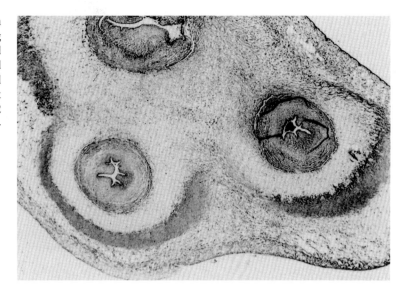

or maternal condition that caused chronic funisitis. Calcification was present in 47% of their cases and chorioamnionitis in 98%. The investigators suggested that a diffusible toxin in the amnionic cavity might cause this lesion because of its similarity to an Ouchterlony immunodiffusion plate. As stated earlier, Fojaco et al. (1989) suggested that necrotizing funisitis "permits a presumptive diagnosis of congenital syphilis at birth." They referred to the gross appearance as a "barber-pole cord" and found 16 cases of this association with congenital syphilis. All their cases of necrotizing funisitis were in luetic pregnancies, and spirochetes were found in four of 10 patients. Fojaco and her colleagues stated that information in the early literature suggests that necrotizing funisitis is diagnostic of syphilis. In fact, however, Hörmann (1954) had extensively studied syphilis and funisitis, and he did not find an absolute relation between these conditions. It is true that funisitis often occurs in syphilis, but not so regularly as suggested. Hörmann and other authors have also often found necrotizing funisitis in nonsyphilitic pregnancies. This point was well made by Craver and Baldwin (1992), with whom we agree. In some umbilical cords with

necrotizing funisitis, we have identified herpes antigen, to be discussed below. Thus, necrotizing funisitis is a chronic, severe inflammation of the cord, frequently associated with calcification, and caused by immune reaction to presumably several different antigens. Likewise, Jacques and Qureshi (1992) found this not to be a strong association, when they studied 45 cases. Like other investigators, they found *Candida, Streptococci,* and other bacteria to be responsible. The necrotizing funisitis is merely the manner by which the umbilical cord can express its chronic inflammatory damage, not being able to remove the debris efficiently that accumulates with chronic exudation. The connective tissue cells of the umbilical cord often degenerate completely with this reaction.

Other Spirochetal Diseases

Leptospirosis, an infection due to one of several species of *Leptospira,* has rarely been reported in pregnancy. Coghlan and Bain (1969) have gathered the few reports of abortion that were presumed to result from this infec-

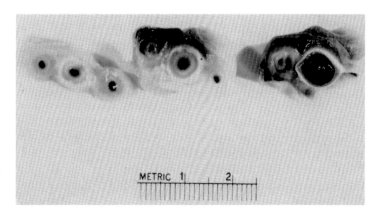

FIGURE 20.39. Concentric rings of perivascular exudate in necrotizing funisitis. There was marked chorioamnionitis in this 31-week pregnancy.

FIGURE 20.40. Radiographic appearance of calcific rings in a cord with necrotizing funisitis. A term, normal infant was delivered. There was no history of maternal problems except a febrile illness during the first trimester. (Courtesy of Dr. R.R. Oldham, Nashville, Tennessee.)

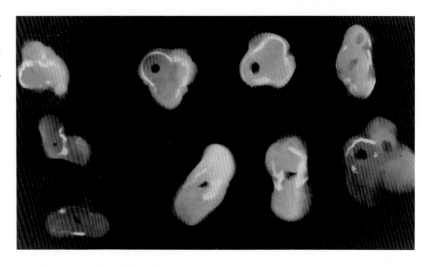

tion; they described the pregnancy of a patient who was infected with *L. canicola*, acquired from a pig. The mother delivered a macerated fetus. Organisms were not recovered from the fetus or from the placenta. Moreover, there were no histopathologic lesions. Abortion due to leptospirosis is said to be a common disease in China, with organisms having been recovered from the affected fetuses.

Borrelia, the spirochetal organism that causes relapsing fever, has been isolated from the blood of a febrile mother and her newborn infant who died shortly after birth (Fuchs & Oyama, 1969). The placenta was not described. The infection follows the bite of an infected tick and the disease is geographically widespread (e.g., Oregon: case just cited; Israel: Yagupsky & Moses, 1985). Shirts et al. (1983) reported a nonfatal case of congenital borreliosis in a febrile patient from Colorado. The spirochetes were depicted in the neonate's blood smear, placental villous capillaries, and umbilical artery. Placental lesions were not described.

Lyme disease (erythema migrans) is an emerging borreliosis of epidemic proportion in the northeastern United States (Athreya, 1989; Eichenfield, 1989; Lastavica et al., 1989; Steere, 1989). This infection, caused by *Borrelia burgdorferi*, has been encountered in other parts of the United States and Europe as well. Transplacental infection was reported in Wisconsin by Schlesinger et al. (1985) and in Utah by MacDonald et al. (1987). In the macerated stillborn of the latter case, the placenta was not enlarged and had "rare plasma cells in isolated villi." The specimen was grossly unremarkable. Spirochetes were identified in the fetus and placenta by special stains. The placental histology showed such excess of erythrocyte precursors (in the fetal circulation) that it could easily have been mistaken for erythroblastosis fetalis. In these two cases, the fetuses had congenital anomalies. Hemminki and Kyyrönen (1989) found an overrepresentation of gastrointestinal atresias in offspring from animal caretakers and forestry and agricultural workers. They suggested that

infection with *B. burgdorferi* may be an etiologic factor. The review of Steere (1989), however, suggested that there is no causal relation between this infection and anomalies. The same assertion was made by Strobino et al. (1993), who undertook a prospective study and found neither a definite increase of fetal anomalies nor adverse pregnancy outcomes.

Abramowsky et al. (1991) found nontreponemal spirochetes primarily in the intestines of four spontaneously aborted fetuses with chorioamnionitis, severe chronic villitis, and villous vasculitis in some. It was possible to rule out *Treponema*, *Borrelia*, *Leptospira*, and *Campylobacter*, and the precise nature of this organism remains to be determined. Infections with *Ehrlichia* have also been delineated, and are discussed below.

Fungus Infections

Candida albicans infection of the vagina is common during pregnancy. Oriel and colleagues (1972) estimated that 26% of women harbored yeast: *C. albicans* in 81%; *Torulopsis* (*Candida*) *glabrata* in 16%. The use of oral contraceptives increased the frequency. Peeters et al. (1972) reported similar results. They opined that an increased use of antibiotics, contraceptives, and trichomonacides may be responsible for this frequency. Bret and Coupe (1958) demonstrated that neonatal fungal infection (mostly candidiasis) can be traced to maternal vaginal infection in most cases. The organisms usually then disappear spontaneously for unknown reasons.

Prenatal infection of placenta, cord, and fetus has been reported in hundreds of cases since its first description (Benirschke & Raphael, 1958; Whyte et al., 1982; Qureshi et al., 1998). Figure 20.41 illustrates a classical case. The patient was a gravida VI, para I, who had had five consecutive abortions. The pregnancy terminated at 25 weeks with severe chorioamnionitis. The umbilical cord had

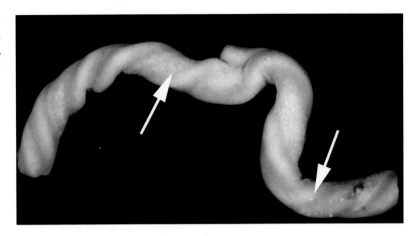

Figure 20.41. Umbilical cord from a patient with congenital candidiasis at 25 weeks' gestation. Note the numerous small, white plaques (arrows), representing abscesses ("granulomas"). Gravida VI, para I, abortus V.

numerous tiny plaques of white-yellow color. Histologically, these nodules consisted of infiltrates with acute inflammatory cells underneath areas of epithelial necrosis (Fig. 20.42). When one scrapes these small lesions and stains with periodic acid-Schiff (PAS) or silver methods, fungi are immediately recognized (Fig. 20.43). Hematoxylin an eosin (H&E) stains, on the other hand, hide the hyphae effectively. But fungal hyphae are also readily demonstrated with silver stains when they may be very difficult to identify in H&E preparations. Touch preparations from scraping cord lesions are diagnostic and thus helpful for neonatal therapy. Relative to the severity of the chorioamnionitis, the funisitis is generally only slight and it is often remarkably focal. The umbilical cord finding of surface granules with inflammatory cells and

fungi is characteristic of congenital candidiasis. Although *C. albicans* is the most common candidal organism, infection with *C. parapsilosis*, a common skin inhabitant, has also been reported (Kellogg et al., 1974). We have seen two cases of infection with *C. tropicalis*, and Nichols et al. (1995), who also reviewed the sparse literature, described a 25-week premature with this infection. The fetus had massive pneumonia and there was marked chorioamnionitis but no funisitis. The mother had an IUD in place. Other than for the lack of hyphae, the histologic findings of our case were generally similar (Fig. 20.44). In an immunosuppressed (bone marrow transplant) patient with diamnionic/dichorionic (DiDi) twins, vaginal bleeding led to amniocentesis and recovery of budding yeast, *Candida lusitaniae*. Three weeks' of amphotericin therapy

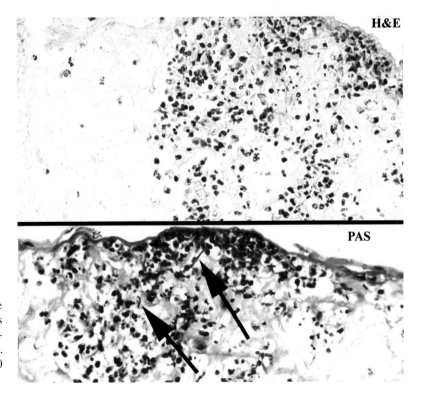

Figure 20.42. Candidiasis of umbilical cord. The lesions shown in Figure 20.41 are accumulations of inflammatory cells, debris, and hyphal organisms (arrows in PAS stain) of *Candida albicans*. Epithelial necrosis is striking at top H&E ×60 (top); ×240 (bottom).

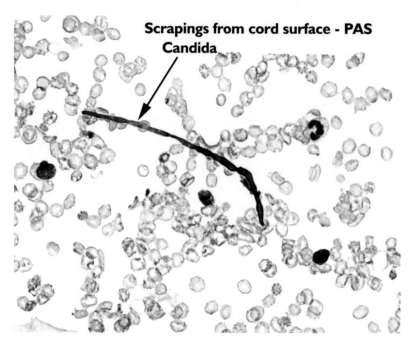

Scrapings from cord surface - PAS Candida

FIGURE 20.43. Scraping from one of the cord's surface nodules, stained with periodic acid-Schiff (PAS). Candidal organism at arrow.

apparently resolved the chorioamnionitis, although the placenta was not described (DiLorenzo et al., 1997).

A remarkable feature of congenital candidiasis is the frequency of its occurrence with unruptured membranes. We had postulated a silent, healed rupture in our original report. Our subsequent experience was that the organisms may readily penetrate the intact membranes. Why the placental infection is so uncommon, in comparison with the frequency of the vaginal infection, is unknown. It had been speculated that it results from fetal immunodeficiency, but findings of good plasma cell response to the congenital pulmonary infection negates this hypothesis (Hood et al., 1985). More likely is the efficiency of the endocervical mucus plug in preventing ascension. Neonatal candidiasis may be widespread, with skin rash,

dark red skin appearance, pneumonia (Emanuel et al., 1962), meningitis (Levin et al., 1978), sepsis, and frequent intestinal contamination (Taschdjan & Kozinn, 1957). It may cause death but has also been treated successfully on several occasions. Abortions have also been due to *Candida* infection (Buchanan & Sworn, 1979; Smith et al., 1988). We have seen elevations of neonatal WBC counts to 80,000 in congenital infection of a premature infant. There had been rupture of membranes for 3 days.

A well-studied case showed convincing evidence of antenatal septicemia (Bittencourt et al., 1984). In this case, a large fungal invasion into an umbilical vein was shown; moreover, there were many fetal and villous candidal lesions. The latter showed focal necrosis, chronic villitis, and intervillous abscesses. Congenital infection

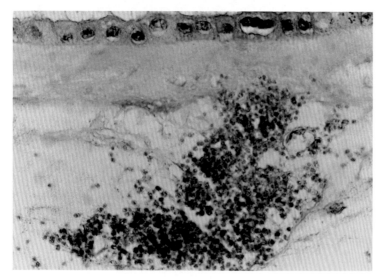

FIGURE 20.44. Subamnionic cluster of *Candida parapsilosis* in an infant with cutaneous congenital candidiasis (blisters) after prolonged rupture of membranes. The infant did well. Note the absence of hyphae and the intact amnionic epithelium. At other sites, chorioamnionitis was prominent. H&E ×600.

has been associated with a retained IUD on several occasions (Schweid & Hopkins, 1968; Ho & Aterman, 1970; Bittencourt et al., 1984; Spaun & Klünder, 1986; Smith et al., 1988; Elliott, 1989; Qureshi et al., 1998). Delaplane et al. (1983) believed that, in their case, the fungus may have been introduced by amniocentesis. Whyte et al. (1982) suggested that at least 30 cases had been reported, and they added 18 of their own. At least 10 additional cases can be added to this list, bringing the total to well over 50 congenital candidal infections, and Pradeepkumar et al. (1998) added five additional typical cases. Bader (1966) reported its occurrence in an anencephalus and depicted the extent of placental involvement. Rhatigan (1968) and Franciosi and Jarzynski (1970) each added a case. Nagata et al. (1981) described a fatal case of pulmonary mycosis and cited some cases from the Japanese literature. Johnson et al. (1981a) reported two cases and gave suggestions for therapy. Delprado et al. (1982) provided excellent illustrations in their report of three cases. They highlighted the association with unruptured membranes and a retained IUD. Shalev et al. (1994) delivered amphotericin transcervically when fungi were cultured from amniocentesis fluid. Rode et al. (2000) also administered amphotericin when, in serial amniocenteses for unexplained hydramnios, the organism was demonstrated and cultured. The neonate died from disseminated infection and the placenta was characteristic. Pera and associates (2002) deduced from chart review that neonatal candidiasis (*C. albicans* and *C. parapsilosis*) was more common in women receiving antibiotics and dexamethasone in pregnancy.

The case report by Levin et al. (1978) is of particular interest. It involved a set of DiMo twins delivered vaginally at approximately 30 weeks' gestation. The mother was febrile. The amniotomy of twin A resulted in meconium-stained fluid, but this infant did not have fungal infection at autopsy. Twin B, whose membranes had ruptured 9 days prior to delivery and whose amnionic sac was found to be dry at delivery, had cerebral candidiasis. In the placenta, a focus of candidal hyphae was found near the insertion of the umbilical cord from twin B, and chorioamnionitis was more severe.

A case of *Torulopsis (Candida) glabrata* infection of placenta and fetus in a patient with sickle cell anemia, was illustrated by Sander et al. (1983). They assumed that the maternal immune compromise may have rendered this infection more possible. The only previously described case was in a patient with a retained IUD. This widely distributed yeast has now been placed in the *Candida* genus; it lacks hyphae. In the two reported cases there was chorioamnionitis, but the umbilical cords had no lesions. In Sander's case, the patient had cerclage for repeated abortions; the stillborn twins had a fungal aspiration pneumonia. Infection had occurred before rupture of membranes, and marked deciduitis was present. The most remarkable feature of the lesion in the umbilical cord are the peripheral nodules with invading fungi. These nodules contain fungi but are compressed Wharton's jelly, perhaps from digestion of the mucopolysaccharides by the yeast. Few WBC are present in these nodules. Other comprehensive reviews are those by Johnson et al. (1981a), Gerberding et al. (1989), and Schwartz and Reef (1990).

Approximately 65 pregnant patients with **coccidioidomycosis** had been reported when VanBergen et al. (1976) reported a fatal case. The placenta had numerous infarcts with spherules of *Coccidioides immitis*, accompanied by inflammation, necrosis, and fibrin deposits. Figure 20.45 shows a cross section of a placenta with coccidioidomycosis. Figure 20.46 is a representative microscopic appearance of the lesions and the organisms. An acute inflammatory response around the fungal spherules is common, as is extensive fibrin deposition. Smale and Waechter (1970), in an analysis of 15 cases with disseminated infection, mentioned three with placental involvement and one presumed fetal infection. Most commonly, the organism remains confined to the placenta, where it produces infarctive necroses. This picture was first described by Vaughan and Ramirez (1951), who saw 33 cases of coccidioidomycosis complicating pregnancy.

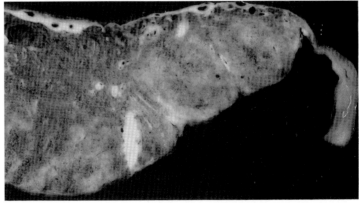

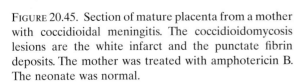

FIGURE 20.45. Section of mature placenta from a mother with coccidioidal meningitis. The coccidioidomycosis lesions are the white infarct and the punctate fibrin deposits. The mother was treated with amphotericin B. The neonate was normal.

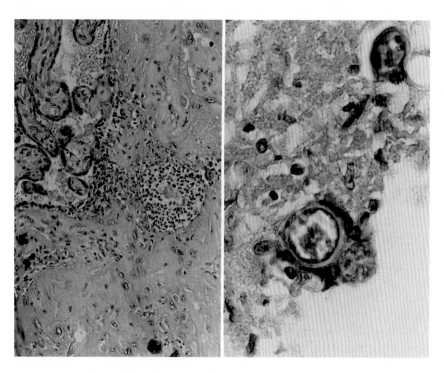

FIGURE 20.46. Microscopic view of coccidioidomycosis of the placenta (case in Fig. 20.45). Left: Note the spherule in the X-cell deposit with fibrin and an acute inflammatory reaction. Right: Several large spherules are engulfed in macrophages (right). H&E ×250 (left); ×640 (right).

Only one had lesions in the placenta. They were infarctive, necrotic lesions with "purulent filled centers, full of spherules." The premature infant delivered to that mother died at the age of 6 months but was free of the disease. The other infants also did not contract the infection transplacentally. Shafai (1978) described disseminated infection in a set of premature twins whose mother died soon after giving birth. They found no lesions in the placenta but still assumed that transplacental infection must have occurred. Bernstein et al. (1981) described another presumptive congenital infection, but they did not describe the placenta. Spark (1981) has critically reviewed all cases of congenital coccidioidomycosis and came to the conclusion that transplacental dissemination was unlikely for any of them. The mode of neonatal infection, he believed, was inhalation of infected material ("decidua") during delivery.

We have seen massive placental involvement with *Coccidioides* lesions unaccompanied by neonatal illness (McCaffree et al., 1978). In one patient in whom the disease was treated with amphotericin B during the entire gestation, the fetus was normal and the placenta merely showed old infarcts and fibrin deposits, without stainable organisms. Peterson et al. (1989) also described a patient with coccidioidal meningitis treated with amphotericin during two pregnancies in whose placentas there were no organisms. Walker et al. (1992) described maternal reactivation of coccidioidomycosis in pregnancy, positive neonatal cord titers, but a negative placenta. A pregnant patient with lymphadenopathy due to *Paracoccidioides brasiliensis* was described by Slevogt et al. (2004). The patient was treated successfully and a healthy infant was born.

Cryptococcosis of the placenta was found by Kida et al. (1989) in a patient with acquired immunodeficiency syndrome (AIDS). It had not invaded villi, and the infant did not develop lesions. The mother developed widespread cryptococcosis. Through the courtesy of Dr. G. Altshuler, we examined placental sections with cryptococcal abscesses of a patient with systemic lupus erythematosus (SLE). She suffered cryptococcal meningitis, presumably because of steroid therapy for SLE. In the intervillous spaces of the immature placenta there were large colonies of cryptococcal organisms; inflammation was scant and no invasion of the villi was found. The neonate (850 g) died and had no evidence of disease (Molnar-Nadasdy et al., 1994). We have also seen the slides of a patient who had been treated with ketoconazole for pulmonary **blastomycosis** 4 years earlier (Dr. E.G. Chadwick, Chicago, personal communication). The patient had been free of apparent disease but was initially infertile. A healthy term infant was eventually delivered. The placenta then appeared grossly peculiar as it had a nodular consistency, and numerous granulomas as well as chronic villitis at the maternal floor. Organisms were not identified. It remains unknown whether the lesions were due to endometrial blastomycosis or whether this is merely a case of villitis of unknown etiology (VUE).

Virus Infections and Villitides

Cytomegalovirus Infection

Congenital cytomegalovirus (CMV) infection is a common disease. Yow (1989) stated that 3000 to 4000 infants are born in the United States each year with symptomatic disease, and a large number of children suffer late-onset manifestations of the infection, including hearing loss, blindness, and retardation. Stagno et al. (1986) found that 1.6% of seronegative women of high-income groups converted CMV titers during pregnancy, whereas 3.7% of low-income group women did so. The writer of an editorial (Anonymous, 1989c) has found that the rate of transmission to the fetus after recent maternal infection is between 20% and 50%. Moreover, infection during the first half of pregnancy is more destructive to the fetus and it has now been found that infants also infected with HIV have a greater propensity to suffer CMV infection (Doyle et al., 1996). Symptomatic fetal infection can also occur from an immune mother when a new strain of virus is acquired (Boppana et al., 2001). Nigro et al. (1999) found discordant expression of CMV infection in dizygotic twins (one had hydropic change), and that the edema disappeared when the fetus was treated with hyperimmune globulin.

It is also now recognized that the virus is often acquired by sexual contact (Chretien et al., 1977). The widespread nature of this infection was first appreciated by Weller (1971), who had emphasized its protean clinical manifestations. Many virus infections are accompanied by severe inflammation of the placental villi ("villitis"). An excellent review of these lesions is found in the contribution by Altshuler and Russell (1975). Schwartz and his colleagues (1992) have characterized the inflammatory response in this villous infection. They found marked "hyperplasia of fetal-derived placental macrophages . . . lymphocytic villitis . . . characterized by positive staining with T-cell antibodies." Plasma cells staining for immunoglobulin G (IgG) and IgM secretion were present in the second trimester, but no IgA positivity was found. Van den Veyver et al. (1998) showed that the virus is readily identified in amnionic fluid, blood, pleural fluid, and tissues by employing PCR and showed a high frequency in samples of high-risk infants.

Infection with CMV is a major cause of chronic villitis. The fetal and neonatal disease has many manifestations, ranging from hydrops fetalis (Quagliarello et al., 1978; Fadel & Riedrich, 1988; Mazeron et al., 1994), obstructive uropathy (Symonds & Driscoll, 1974), meconium peritonitis (Pletcher et al., 1991), macerated stillbirth, and cerebral palsy, to minimal hearing loss (Saigal et al., 1982b) or severe CNS destruction (Schimmel et al., 2001). Moreover, some of these manifestations may be ascertained only years later (R.F. Pass et al., 1980; Williamson et al., 1982, 1990). Details of congenital CMV infection have been reported on many occasions (Embil et al., 1970; Krech et al., 1971). A very typical case of intrauterine CMV infection was described in detail as a Cabot case (Modlin et al., 2003).

Ahlfors and colleagues (1988) reviewed the literature of the infection in twins and reported two of their own cases that were discordant for manifestations of CMV infection. They postulated that monochorionic MZ twins were more likely to be concordant for CMV infection, but lamented that the information on placental and genetic status is too often missing from case reports to draw definitive conclusions. It was their suggestion that fetal (as well as maternal) immunologic response may be of importance in the expression of the prenatally acquired infection. They ruled out, from knowing the location of the twin placentas, that a CMV endocervicitis caused ascending fetal infection.

Congenital infection is perhaps also occasionally acquired from infected endometrium. The presence of CMV in endometrial glands was demonstrated in five of 59 spontaneous abortions by Dehner and Askin (1975). The CMV inclusions have also been found in endocervix (Wenckebach & Curry, 1976). The virus has often been cultured from seminal fluid (Lang & Kummer, 1972) and from amnionic fluid (Weiner and Grose, 1990). Stagno et al. (1982) showed that fetal infection is more serious when it occurs during a primary maternal infection than when it follows recurrent maternal disease. These cases are reasons to consider the benefit of a vaccine (Medearis, 1982). Neonates with this infection may excrete virus for years. They thus become a major source for infection of pregnant mothers and toddlers in day-care centers (Pass et al., 1987). In twin pregnancies, CMV infections have been seen in both twins (Saigal et al., 1982a) but occasionally also in only one twin (Eachempati & Woods, 1976; Stagno et al., 1982).

Fetal intracranial calcifications have been seen sonographically (Ghidini et al., 1989), and neonatal perivascular echogenic signals were demonstrated in their basal ganglia (Teele et al., 1988); the involvement of vessels is a hallmark of this infection. It has been suggested that it may be the cause of cerebral microgyria and other lesions (Dias et al., 1984). Other sonographic manifestations have been transient hydrops (Mazeron et al., 1994), abnormal triple-screen results and hyperechoic bowl (Peters et al., 1995), hydrocephaly, and growth retardation (Lipitz et al., 1997). Viral isolates can be obtained from amnionic fluid and fetal blood samples (Hagay et al., 1996). The virus may also be identified serologically, by immunofluorescence, PCR of DNA samples, or in situ hybridization (Ozono et al., 1997).

Fetal infection is undoubtedly most often acquired during primary maternal infection from maternal viremia and by the passage of virions through the destroyed trophoblast. This ability of CMV to infect and destroy the trophoblast has been shown in placental explants by Amirhessami-Aghili et al. (1987), and Chan et al. (2002) found this damage to be mediated by TNF-α. Interestingly, Pizzato et al. (2003) found by in vitro infection of cells that CMV infection downregulates the human leukocyte antigen (HLA)-G_1 expression. Despite this placental infection, no uniform **macroscopic** findings can identify CMV infection of the placenta; thus the selection

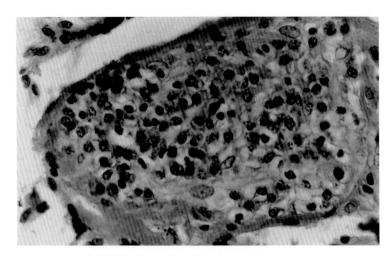

FIGURE 20.47. Congenital cytomegalovirus infection. Marked chronic villitis, composed almost entirely of plasma cells, is evident, as is focal necrosis of the trophoblast and capillary walls. The specimen is from a term gestation, and the mother reportedly had porphyria. H&E ×650.

of histologic material is difficult, although surface vessels are at times thrombosed and should arouse suspicion (Fig. 20.47). Small placentas with growth-restricted fetuses are common and thromboses may exist. A significant problem in understanding this infection is that some known prenatal infections (positive culture from amnionic fluid) may be followed by normal outcome (Weiner & Grose, 1990). We have also seen many cases of unsuspected CMV infection histologically when the placenta was sectioned for other reasons. For instance, in one case of maternal porphyria, typical CMV inclusions were found in the placenta and the neonate had hepatitis. The maternal disease was a manifestation of a primary infection with this virus and was misinterpreted as porphyria. In another case of a spontaneous abortus at 15 weeks' gestation with an unremarkable macerated fetus, there were widespread cytomegalic cells in the lung, spleen, skeletal muscle, and placenta. The mother had only had a minor "sore throat" 1 week prior. Remarkably, the placenta had extensive destructive villitis. Ultimately, either the virus has to be cultured, or inclusion body cells have to be identified. Although the classical histologic features

are not mistakable, they are often so widely scattered through the villous tissue that only extreme scrutiny of many sections allows the diagnosis from placental sections.

The **histologic** hallmark of CMV infection in the placenta are chronic lymphoplasmacytic villitis (Fig. 20.48), thrombosis of villous capillaries often with adjacent hemosiderin deposits, necrosis of villous tissue and trophoblast (Fig. 20.49), fibrosis of villous stroma (Fig. 20.50), and inclusion-bearing cytomegalic cells (Fig. 20.51). The inclusion bodies may be characteristic nuclear "owl-eye" cells, but are often also of cytoplasmic nature. They are commonly seen in villous capillary endothelium but are also found in the stromal cells of villi. Garcia et al. (1989), who provided an excellent study of placental changes in CMV infection, found owl-eye cells in decidua and amnion as well. They employed the fluorescent antibody technique for diagnosis (see also McCaffree & Altshuler, 1979) and suggested that some types of gross morphologic abnormalities are frequent. Mostoufi-Zadeh et al. (1984) depicted owl-eye cells in the epithelium of the umbilical cord. Saito et al. (1977) described an abortion

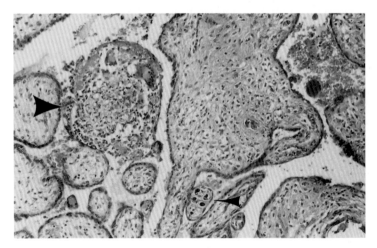

FIGURE 20.48. Destructive villitis (large arrowhead) in congenital cytomegalovirus (CMV) infection. Inclusion bodies, or owl-eye cells (small arrowhead), are also present in this 14 weeks' gestation. H&E ×150.

FIGURE 20.49. Evolution of fibrosis of the villi with a CMV infection. Left: A villus has plasma cell infiltration, trophoblast necrosis, vascular obliteration, and early fibrosis. Right: A completely hyalinized villus contains a focus of calcification and hemosiderin but no trace of CMV infection. H&E ×160 (left); ×260 (right).

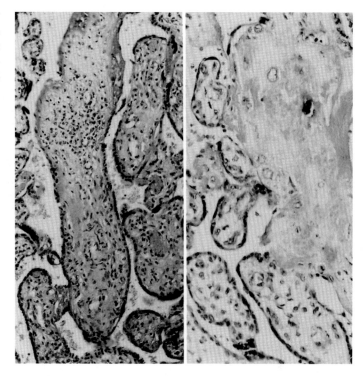

with a large number of villous inclusion bodies typical of CMV infection. They diagnosed it as herpes simplex infection, however. We believe they made an incorrect diagnosis caused by an error in the interpretation of the serologic results. The CMV titers were also rising. Their analysis included an excellent electron microscopic demonstration of the virus packets, typical of a herpes-type virus (see also Donnellan et al., 1966, for electron microscopy). Vasculitis of chorionic vessels (Fig. 20.52) may lead to thrombosis and calcification. Huikeshoven et al. (1982) as well as Grose and Weiner (1990) made the diagnosis of CMV infection by recovering the virus from amnionic fluid at amniocentesis, undoubtedly because of fetal renal involvement. The placental and neonatal features in the former study were typical of CMV infection. The virus can now be detected in histologic sections by in situ hybridization (Wolber & Lloyd, 1989). Sachdev et al. (1990) have used the hybridization technique to identify CMV infection in cases of chronic villitis. They found typical inclusions in three of eight cases of villitis and were able to diagnose three additional cases of CMV infection because of this technique. Mühlemann and her colleagues (1992) have provided an excellent immunocytochemical study of six CMV-infected placentas. They suggested that histologic features are often inconclusive in this congenital infection and found inclusion bodies in

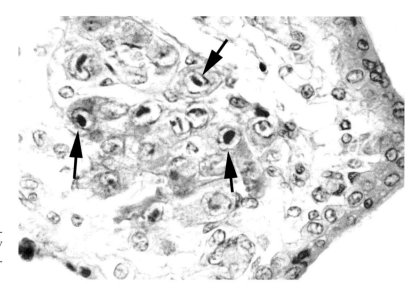

FIGURE 20.50. Owl-eye nuclei (arrows) of a cytomegalic cells in a villus of a patient with CMV placentitis. This cell also contains many cytoplasmic virus particles. H&E ×650.

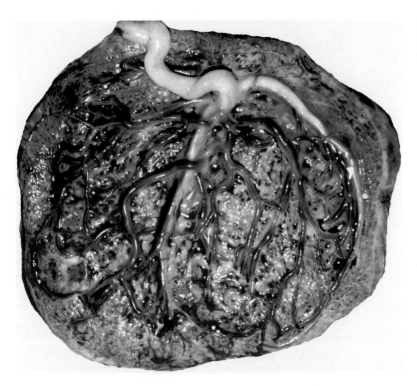

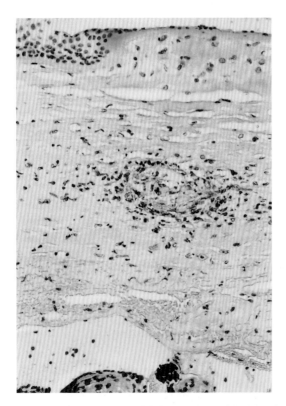

FIGURE 20.51. Term gestation of congenital CMV infection that led to calcified thrombosis of surface vessels (yellow streaks).

FIGURE 20.52. Chorionic vasculitis in a patient with CMV infection at term. There is more necrosis than inflammation. The placenta had marked chronic villitis. The fetus was stillborn. H&E ×160.

only one of six cases. Immunocytochemistry, on the other hand, revealed viral antigen in five of the six placentas. The antigen was found to be mostly in the villous stroma, once in the syncytiotrophoblast, and sometimes in endothelial cells as demonstrated by double-staining these cells. Kumazaki et al. (2002b) looked for CMV DNA in 254 placentas and correlated it with maternal serum status. Seronegative mothers had negative placentas; 30.5% of seropositive mothers' placenta had antigen in various locations.

The cellular response to this infection is characteristic. It is mononuclear; during the second half of gestation, it is typically accompanied by fetal plasma cells, but we have seen it as early as at 15 weeks' gestation in the placental villi. Here it is then a question of whether the plasma cells are of fetal or maternal origin. This question has not been satisfactorily answered as yet. Plasma cells are not expected to be produced by fetuses at 13 weeks' gestation. Hybridization studies with Y-chromosome probes in appropriate cases are indicated to rule out maternal B-cell immigration, an important consideration for the understanding of chronic VUE. Mostoufi-Zadeh et al. (1984) opined that the fetal infection is more severe when a plasmacellular, rather than a lymphocytic, response is found in the villi. The plasma cell infiltration and the cytomegalic cells in the placenta were first described by LePage and Schramm (1958) and subsequently by LeLong et al. (1960). Since then, there have been numerous observations substantiating and expanding on these findings (e.g., Rosenstein & Navarrete-Reyna, 1964; Monif & Dische, 1972). Blanc (1961b), in a thorough review of the placenta of prenatal infections, described the villous necrosis; Quan and Strauss (1962) discussed the differential diagnosis of CMV infection from erythroblastosis.

The findings of many other authors are summarized in our previous review (Benirschke et al., 1974). In that paper we described five cases, one of which is of particular interest. It was a therapeutic abortion at approximately 15 weeks' gestation. The patient had fever of unknown origin and antibody titers to CMV and toxoplasma. A double infection was suspected, but no toxoplasmosis was found in the abortus. At dissection, no macroscopic lesions were seen but viral inclusions were found in many organs histologically (Fig. 20.53). There was only a sparse inflammatory response. The villous infection and focal thrombosis in pulmonary vessels were particularly striking. A case of presumed double infection was described by De Zegher et al. (1988), in which *Toxoplasma* was definitely identified, and saliva and urine cultures yielded CMV. The alleged double infection illustrated by Demian et al. (1973), however, was not correctly identified. Only CMV was shown, the cytoplasmic granules representing virus, not *Toxoplasma* as was presumed.

It has often been asked just when the first fetal plasma cell response to CMV can be seen. This question is not yet resolved, as previously stated. Altshuler and McAdams (1971) clearly identified plasma cell villitis at 19 weeks' gestation, but it may commence as early as at 10 weeks, judging from Altshuler's (1973a) second case, seen at 13 weeks' gestation (Fig. 20.54). The owl-eye inclusions are characteristic of CMV infection, and the diagnosis can be made confidently on that basis alone. When only enlarged cells with cytoplasmic inclusions are present, however, the diagnosis of CMV infection is less secure. Serologic studies, virus isolation, and modern techniques of demonstrating the viral genome by hybridization are then

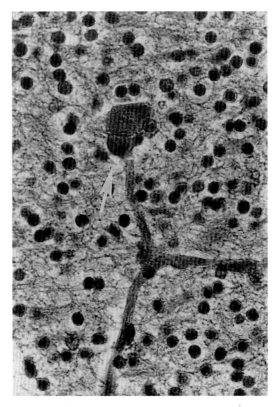

FIGURE 20.53. Fetal brain at 15 weeks' gestation with a CMV cell at the terminus of the capillary. There is no inflammation or destruction. Placenta had numerous CMV cells. H&E ×150. (*Source:* Benirschke et al., 1974, with permission.)

needed. When different strains of the virus were thus identified with endonuclease cleavage of viral DNA, "no common pattern could be associated with these eight strains (of congenitally acquired virus) in comparison with strains from postnatally infected children" (Grillner et al., 1987). Borisch et al. (1988) successfully identified the antigen in the nucleus and cytoplasm by in situ hybrid-

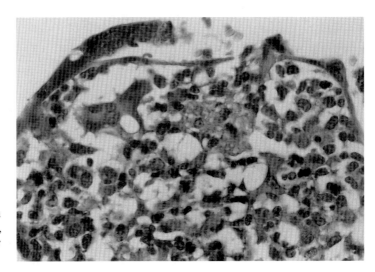

FIGURE 20.54. Cytomegalovirus infection of the placenta at 13 weeks' gestation, with plasma cell infiltration, edema, and trophoblast necrosis. H&E ×520. (Courtesy of Dr. G. Altshuler, Oklahoma City, Oklahoma.)

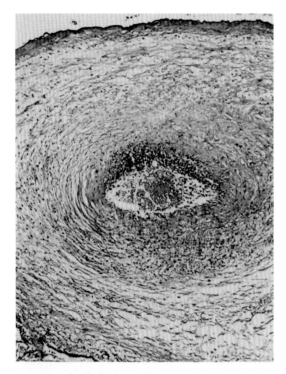

FIGURE 20.55. Chorionic vasculitis, necrosis, and early thrombosis with a congenital infection, presumably CMV, at 20 weeks' gestation. Outcome was a stillborn fetus. See Figure 20.56. H&E ×100.

ization, and Chehab et al. (1989) were able to do so with PCR of the DNA obtained from paraffin-embedded tissues. One can only hope that in the future the nature of such placental lesions, as depicted in Figures 20.55 and 20.56 will be resolved by these methods.

Herpes Simplex Virus Infection

Transplacental infection with herpes simplex virus (HSV) does occasionally occur. It is more serious for the fetus when primary, rather than recurrent, herpes virus infection occurs during pregnancy (Brown et al., 1987). But transplacental infection is uncommon, presumably because of the protective nature of transplacentally acquired maternal antibodies; most women become immune to HSV before reaching childbearing age (Nahmias et al., 1970). "The major problem in newborn infection then is one of natal transmission of HVH (*Herpesvirus hominis*) through recurrent type 2 infections of the maternal genital tract" (Alford et al., 1975). Why it is that fatal infections occur sometimes in utero, and not at other times, and what the reason is for recurrent and latent infections remain unresolved questions. Ideas about the latency of HSV were discussed in an editorial (Anonymous, 1989b), and a succinct review of the fetal infection with HSV has been provided by Baldwin and Whitley (1990). Johnson et al. (1989) found in a survey of 4201 serum samples that 16.4% of the U.S. population from 15 to 74 years of age was infected with HSV-2.

Herpes virus is silently shed by 2.3% of pregnant women (Wittek et al., 1984), although lower numbers (0.1–0.4%) have also been cited (Witlin et al., 1998). Yen et al. (1965) succinctly described and depicted the cervical and vaginal lesions of herpes virus infection and presented three infants with symptomatic mothers. Two newborns had an apparently congenital infection. Kell et al. (2000) suggested that neonates with disseminated herpes infection have acquired it in utero in 4%, natally in 86%, and postnatally in 10%; thus, prenatal infection

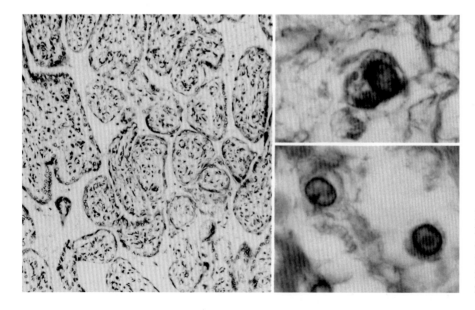

FIGURE 20.56. Same case as in Figure 20.55. Chronic villitis (left) with enlarged cells having some of the qualities of CMV cells. The inclusions are not typical, however. H&E ×160 (left); ×1600 (right).

is uncommon. In fact, it has led to intrauterine demise, as in the case described by Barefoot et al. (2002) with extensive facial necrosis demonstrates. Herpes virus has also been detected before delivery (of a healthy child) from aspirated amnionic fluid (Zervoudakis et al., 1980). Herpetic endometritis has been demonstrated with and without an IUD (Abraham, 1978; Schneider et al., 1982), and Altshuler (1974) presented evidence for prenatal infection with an involved placenta (vide infra). Another case of presumed ascending infection was presented by Hain et al. (1980). They described the premature birth of a 590-g infant with a rash; there was necrosis in various organs at autopsy. The placenta showed cloudy membranes due to "extensive necrosis of amnion without inflammation." Necrotic areas were also present in chorion, and a lymphoplasmacellular infiltration was evident, as in Altshuler's case. In their case, however, chorionic vessel thrombosis and many inclusion bodies as well as "ground-glass" nuclei were present. The mother had primary herpetic vulvitis 4 weeks before delivery. Hyde and Giacoia (1993) have described an important case of severe, destructive congenital HSV infection, delivered by cesarean section of a cervically infected patient. At those portions of the intact membranes that were closest to the cervix, they found immunologically HSV-positive cells in the subamnionic connective tissue, aside from a mild chronic funisitis. This case strongly supports an ascending infection, occurring even with intact membranes. Peng et al. (1996) also described a serious prenatal infection of a twin fetus, whose twin became infected with scalp lesion resulting after amniotomy for scalp electrode placement. Brown et al. (1997) found that when HSV is acquired during pregnancy near the time of delivery, congenital infection may be a sequel. Postpartum endometritis may also be a consequence of HSV infection (Hollier et al., 1997). Witlin et al. (1998) found only focal villous edema and sclerosis in the placenta of a clearly in utero infection.

The review of Baldwin and Whitley (1990) summarized 71 cases of presumed prenatal herpes virus infection. Many of these cases were not fully studied, and the placentas were examined in only a few. The early reports of fetal infection by Mitchell and McCall (1963), Zavoral et al. (1970), Torphy et al. (1970), and Monif et al. (1985) had no placental study. Witzleben and Driscoll (1965) were the first investigators to describe the placental changes in proved congenital herpes simplex infection, and they reviewed other fatal cases of neonatal herpes infections. The mother in their case suffered a primary disseminated infection 1 month before delivery. The neonate remained well until day 6 and then died from generalized disease. The placenta was grossly unremarkable but had many areas of villous necrosis. It included trophoblast and stroma. An inflammatory reaction was absent, but inclusions were found in the placenta and

fetus. Nakamura et al. (1985) demonstrated immunologic staining and, by electron microscopy, typical herpes particles in stromal cells of villi in a presumably hematogenously transplacental infection. Other cases with prenatal onset are those by Chatterjee et al. (2001) with placentitis, and 15-week monochorionic twins and bland villous necroses (Bedolla & Stanek, 2004).

Other excellent descriptions of the placenta in herpetic infection came from Altshuler (1974, 1984), who summarized the earlier-mentioned case in the context of other placental inflammations. There were no complications in the term pregnancy he described, and no herpetic lesions had been known or noted. The infant developed blisters on day 4, with isolation of HVH. He was treated and discharged but continued having skin lesions. The meconium-stained placenta had many areas of necrotizing deciduitis and amnionitis; chorionic vasculitis and funisitis were attended by superficial amnion necrosis. The exudate contained leukocytic and extensive plasmacellular infiltrates (Fig. 20.57). The villous tissue was not altered, and inclusion bodies were absent, but the prenatal acquisition of the infection is evident from the unusual plasmacellular funisitis, not known in banal infections. S. Hyde (personal communication) has also seen a case of neonatal herpes infection with extensive chronic villitis. In contrast to the usual cases of VUE, however, many villi showed an extensive acute necrosis. He examined the lymphocyte markers in this case, finding that 1% of villous inflammatory cells were CD45 Ro (B cells) marked, but no staining occurred in the necrotic villi; many positive CD45 Ro (T cells) and CD68 markers (macrophages) were present in the affected villi and the chorionic plate.

The role of molecular pathology in the diagnosis of transplacental herpes infection was described by Schwartz and Caldwell (1991). They reported the delivery of a neonate who remained well from a patient with suspicious genital lesions. Previously, HSV had been confirmed by culture. Microscopic sections of the placenta were grossly and microscopically normal. In situ hybridization with a biotinylated DNA probe for HSV was counterstained. Subchorionic tissue (maternal-derived tissue of the decidua capsularis) stained positively for the antigen. It is our opinion that these findings are not specific for herpes antigen but that they reflect the biotin content that was so well later defined in endometrium by Yokoyama et al. (1993). These investigators were aware of the similarity of apparent inclusions in endometrium with those of herpes infection; they showed, however, that these vacuoles contained biotin. Thus, extreme care should be exercised in the interpretation of such immunologic localizations employing biotinylated probes in the immunologic reaction.

Bendon et al. (1987) emphasized deciduitis associated with their two cases of intrauterine HVH infection. One

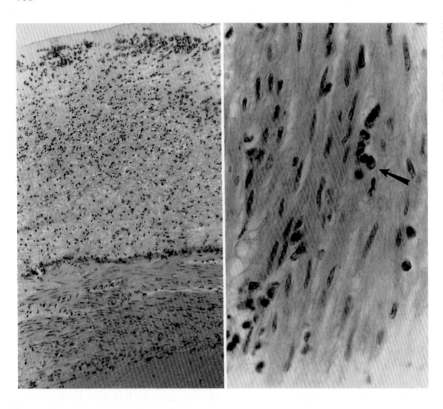

FIGURE 20.57. Congenital herpes virus infection of placenta. Note necrosis of the amnion, thickening of membranes, and intense plasma cell (arrow) infiltration. H&E ×160 (left); ×640 (right). (Courtesy of Dr. G. Altshuler, Oklahoma City, Oklahoma.)

was a stillborn 300-g abortus with macular skin lesions, and the other was a 3200-g neonate with blisters who was treated and survived. The authors were unable to detect antigen in cord or amnionic sac, by immunohistochemical reaction but found it at the decidual base of the placentas. For this reason, they suggested that infection may have been disseminated via neural fibers or through endometrial channels, rather than in an ascending manner. Berger et al. (1986) described a mother with herpetic encephalitis during pregnancy; a meconium-stained placenta and fetal infection occurred, despite acyclovir therapy. Gagnon (1968) recovered virus from the placenta but did not describe the organ. Dublin and Merten (1977) showed the severe cerebral necroses that occurred in discordantly affected DiMo twins at 29 weeks' gestation. They stated that the placenta was affected with hemorrhagic and fibrotic changes.

The differences in severity and types of placental and fetal reactions in prenatal herpes infection suggest that transplacental and ascending infection may both occur. Boué and Loffredo (1970) isolated herpes virus type 2 from abortion material and suggested that this infection may play a causal role in abortion. Naib et al. (1970) studied the outcome of pregnancy in women with herpes infection. When infection occurred during the first 4 months of pregnancy, abortions occurred significantly more frequently, suggesting a causal relation.

Two cases with undisputed congenital herpes infection have been seen by us. One was a stillborn without maternal illness or herpetic lesions. The placenta had necrotizing chorioamnionitis with true blisters (Figs. 20.58 and 20.59). Plasma cells were the most abundant cell type in the exudate. The unusual occurrence of plasma cells at this site cannot be overemphasized. The other case was

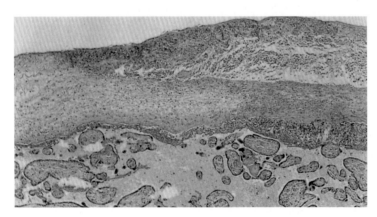

FIGURE 20.58. Congenital herpes simplex virus-2 (HSV-2) infection with stillbirth outcome. Note the subamnionic blister filled with plasma cells. Also present are chorionitis and amnion necrosis. H&E ×64.

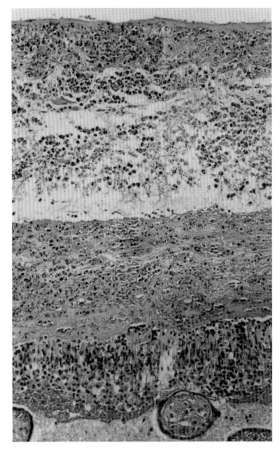

FIGURE 20.59. Congenital HSV-2 infection (same case as Fig. 20.58). The large collection of subamnionic plasma cells is unusual. H&E ×160.

reported by Herzen and Benirschke (1977). A cesarean section had been done for breech presentation; the membranes were intact. There was no maternal history of herpetic lesions, nor was the virus cultured from the mother. She had a titer of 1:32 that rose to 1:64 after birth, perhaps an insufficient criterion. The infant had severe disease and died. The placenta was circumvallate and had an unusually adherent amnion, and there were infarcts but no villitis. Inclusion bodies were found in the chorion. Severe plasma cell infiltration was present in the decidua; HSV-2 was isolated from fetal skin vesicles and the placental surface. Because of the absent villitis and the presence of chorioamnionitis, we speculated that it was an ascending infection. That opinion is supported by the absence of genital lesions in a large number of mothers with infected offspring.

This case raised further questions. In addition to the characteristic necrotic lesions found in neonatal herpes deaths (Hass, 1935), the autopsy findings included ocular, renal, and cerebral anomalies. The occasional association of congenital anomalies with HSV infection was discussed by Baldwin and Whitley (1989); some of these anomalies surely are the result of the virus infection. When this

infant died at 21 days of age, he had massive destructive disease of the brain, resembling hydranencephaly. Virus recovery was attempted by culture and electron microscopy. Because of this failure and the proved HSV-2 disease, we searched for antigen by immunohistologic procedures (Robb et al., 1986a). Characteristic staining was found with this technique in a variety of tissues from this infant. We then studied abortion specimens and other conditions with unresolved etiology for the presence of herpes antigens. In some of these cases, herpes viral DNA could be detected by hybridization study. The brain and placenta of the neonatal death just discussed also had a strong staining reaction (Robb et al., 1986b). Although we are aware that this method cannot prove the existence of local residual HSV antigen, it is presumptive evidence for this correlation. In the placenta the antigen was prominently found in a subamnionic location, as were the herpetic lesions. Strong antigen reactivity was seen in other cases as well, such as in necrotizing funisitis and many cases of "maternal floor infarction." Future studies must to be undertaken to interpret these findings. Finally, Altshuler (personal communication, 1992) sent us the placenta of a child with congenital herpes infection whose umbilical cord surface showed only extensive acellular necrosis, without any attending inflammatory response. Herman and Siegel (1994), who described another case of congenital HSV-2 infection, emphasized the many calcifications in the newborn's organs but did not discuss the placenta.

Varicella (Chickenpox)

Pregnancy complicated by chickenpox is fairly uncommon but it may have serious sequelae for fetus and mother (Katz et al., 1995). Despite the fact that most cases of adult chickenpox occur beyond the reproductive period (Stagno & Whitley, 1985), presumptive transplacental infection has been described several times. In a review of 18 maternal varicella pneumonias, Pickard (1968) noted that only three infants were without the disease; 38 neonatal cases of chickenpox had been described by then, with a 21% mortality. Sauerbrei and Wutzler (2000, 2001) review all of the clinical features and the length of incubation, and demonstrate the devastating nature of the illness when it is acquired in utero. Most interestingly, Bruder et al. (2000) observed a 33-week premature with anterior horn destruction, necrosis of one arm, and intestinal atresias that could be attributed to this viral infection. A chronic, necrotizing lesion was found in the placenta. Four other cases of major CNS lesions come from Mustonen et al. (2001) but without placental study. Purtilo et al. (1977) described numerous placental infarcts, without viral inclusions, in their report of a case of fatal varicella in a pregnant woman and newborn. Balducci and his colleagues (1992) identified in

a prospective study 40 patients with first trimester varicella. Three aborted, one was terminated, and the other
36 patients went to term. One had an omphalocele, and
the others were normal. From this information the authors
concluded that the risk of the congenital varicella syndrome is small. Enders and her coworkers (1994) did a
prospective study of 1373 women with varicella and 366
women who had herpes zoster during the first 36 weeks
of gestation. In this cohort, nine cases of congenital varicella syndrome were identified, all occurring when the
infection had taken place during the first 20 weeks of
gestation. A commentary with additional reports is to be
found in the editorial section of the journal (Liesnard et
al., 1994). Other reports attest to the uncommon association of fetal disease with varicella pneumonia (Qureshi
& Jaques, 1996; Chandra et al., 1998). When fetal disease
did occur, as in perhaps three of Qureshi's cases, the placenta showed basal chronic villitis with "occasional multinucleated giant cells." The congenital varicella syndrome
of cutaneous scars, limb hypoplasia, chorioretinitis, and
cataracts (see Williamson, 1975; Alkalay et al., 1987; Wigglesworth, 1996) was found in only one of 11 infants of
women with first-trimester varicella infection studied by
Paryani and Arvin (1986). According to these authors,
who comprehensively reviewed the topic, infection later
in gestation rarely has these fetal sequelae. Magliocco et
al. (1992) reported a severely malformed child with
numerous destructive lesions that are superbly illustrated.
The fetal infection dated from the 12th week of gestation.
The placenta showed only old infarcts and calcification.
In a 35-week neonate whose placenta we examined, tiny
dermal scars, hepatic calcification, chorioretinitis, and
CNS involvement were found; the mother had experienced varicella 4 months earlier (Benirschke et al., 1999).
At that time, the fetus developed hydrops that subsequently resolved gradually. The placenta had numerous
foci of marked VUE with occasional granulomatous
appearance. Immunohistochemically and by PCR, varicella (but not HSV) antigen was still present in the many
collapsed, occluded villous stem blood vessels. None was
found in the inflammatory regions. Many terminal villi
had atrophied, primarily those supplied by the occluded
stem vessels. This case, and a case of toxoplasmosis, would
ordinarily have been diagnosed as VUE, and the point is
made in that contribution that new studies need to search
more extensively for antigens as possible etiologic agents
in the otherwise still disputed nature of VUE. Jones and
his colleagues (1994) found only a small risk to the fetus
from first trimester varicella infection in their prospective
study. Paryani and Arvin (1986) and Brazin et al. (1979)
reported that herpes zoster–complicating pregnancy
usually has a benign prognosis. The fetus and placenta are
typically not affected, although some cases of fetal growth
retardation and blindness have occurred. Indeed, Higa et
al. (1987), who studied 52 infants of women with varicella

during pregnancy, found that 27 suffered anomalies due
to the infection when it occurred before 20 weeks' gestation. The placentas were not described. In their review of
zoster infections of pregnancy in women who had had
varicella in the past, the frequency of anomalies was
small. A comprehensive review of varicella infection in
pregnancy and the resulting fetal pathology, especially of
the nervous system, has been provided by Grose and
Itani (1989). Regrettably, they did not address possible
placental pathology of this infection. In fact, the placenta
of varicella infection in pregnancy has rarely been
described. Garcia (1963), who reported two congenital
cases, found scattered "firm areas, rice seed–like." He
depicted focal necroses. Garcia likened these lesions to
granulomas, with epithelioid cells and a giant cell component. Decidual cells contained inclusion bodies. No specific changes were encountered by Saito et al. (1989).
They described giant cell pneumonia in a small, prematurely delivered fetus who probably had varicella infection. Immunohistochemical staining of varicella antigens
was present on the giant cells in the neonatal lung, but
no such antigen was detected in the placenta. It showed
merely mild chorioamnionitis. We saw the placenta of a
baby with minimal cutaneous scars, chorioretinitis, and
seizures. The mother had suffered varicella infection 4
months earlier; then the fetus developed hydrops and
cardiac calcifications. They resolved. The placenta had
diffuse foci of severe chronic villitis (without plasma
cells) and many stem villous vessels were completely
obliterated. Immunohistochemistry identified antigen
only to the areas of former endothelium in the obliterated vessels. Giant cells were absent, and no inclusions
were present.

EPSTEIN-BARR VIRUS

Infection with the Epstein-Barr virus is uncommon during pregnancy. In
a few instances, however, congenital infection is believed to have produced congenital anomalies in fetuses. The topic has been reviewed
by Ornoy et al. (1982), who studied the induced abortuses of five such
pregnancies. They found lesions in all, consisting of deciduitis, villitis
with lymphoplasmacellular infiltration, trophoblastic necrosis, and endothelial damage to capillaries. Myocarditis was seen in two fetuses. The
cases are circumstantial in that the virus was not shown to be present,
but lesions as described are otherwise uncommon at that gestational
age. Thus at present one must assume that the virus can affect placenta
and fetus. Transplacental transfer of the Epstein-Barr virus to the fetus
has rarely been proved. In the few cases where it was shown (Joncas
et al., 1981), the placenta was not described. The child described by
these authors died from apparently simultaneous CMV infection.

Smallpox, Vaccinia, Alastrim, and Parvovirus B19

Fetal infection with smallpox virus has often been
depicted in early obstetrics texts. This virus can readily
pass the placenta and cause fetal death and abortion.

Prior to the eradication of smallpox, fetal and placental *vaccinia* occurred occasionally, primarily with primary vaccinations. Wentworth (1966) examined 65 placentas of women who were vaccinated during pregnancy; those mothers did not have an increased abortion rate. Histologic examination and the search for virus inclusions were negative.

Intrauterine infection was well described by Wielenga et al. (1961). The neonate died within a short time and had extensive skin lesions. There were numerous areas of villous and membrane necrosis, and a leukocytic response was present. The lesions were similar to a case we have seen (Fig. 20.60) in which there were extensive necrosis of trophoblast, intervillous fibrin deposits, and focal calcification, but no plasma cells were found. Killpack (1963) also found necrotic foci, "resembling miliary tubercles," and found scanty eosinophilic inclusions. Other descriptions came from Hood and McKinnon (1963) and Naidoo and Hirsch (1963). Garcia (1963) reported macerated stillborns affected with cutaneous *alastrim* (variola minor). Similar granulomatous areas of necrosis were depicted in the placentas accompanying these two fetuses. Guarnieri bodies were present in the decidua.

Infection with *parvovirus B19* is covered in Chapter 16. It is an apparently frequent cause of fetal anemia because of the preferential infection of erythrocyte precursors by this virus. Hartwick et al. (1989) have shown parvovirus B19 in a dot-blot hybridization study of a 9 weeks' gestation fetus. Considerable vascular endothelial damage was present in the embryo and placenta. In a portion of one umbilical artery the endothelium and muscle were partially destroyed, and in main stem vessels perivascular lymphocytic infiltration was seen. The lymphocytic infiltration was composed of cells belonging to the cytotoxic or suppressor T-cell variety. There is a provocative discussion of the origin of these inflammatory cells that bears relevance to the topic of "villitis of unknown origin" (vide infra). Despite the fact that, heretofore, the embryo was not believed to be capable of mounting an immunologic response at this stage of development, the authors gave cogent reasons for assuming that the T cells they identified were not of maternal origin. Interestingly, inclusions were absent in the red blood cell precursors of this embryo but were found in skeletal muscle cells. In an important study of presumed parvovirus B19 infection of the fetus, de Krijger et al. (1998) showed that the presence of putative inclusion bodies is not diagnostic of this infection. They uncovered many such inclusions as artifacts, and asserted that confirmation by PCR is mandatory. There is now excellent evidence that clinical outcome is correlated with the degree of trophoblastic apoptosis (Jordan & Butchko, 2002). These authors showed that the B19 receptor (globoside-containing) is present not only on red cells precursors but also on trophoblast, and that gestations with poor fetal outcome had a much greater degree of trophoblastic apoptosis than those with better results. The difficulty of making the correct diagnosis, especially in nonhydropic fetuses, is highlighted in a paper by Tolfvenstam et al. (2001). Only three of nine DNA-positive cases had erythroid inclusions; this led them to suggest that many more unresolved stillborn infants would have a diagnosis assigned if DNA study were added to the autopsy protocol. An additional problem in the diagnosis of parvovirus B19 diagnosis is the development, temporally different, of two distinct antibodies—linear and conformational (Jordan, 2002).

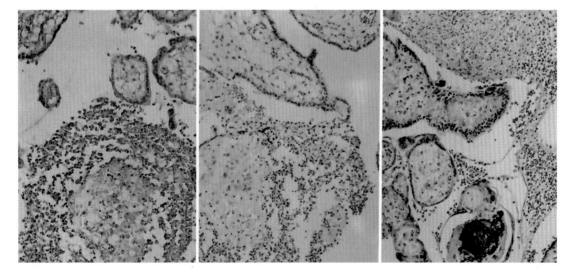

FIGURE 20.60. Vaccinia during pregnancy. Many villi are necrotic, and an intense inflammatory reaction is seen around their remnants. Note the focal calcification of the necrotic area at bottom right. H&E ×160. (Courtesy of Dr. B. Ivemark, Stockholm, Sweden.)

Samra et al. (1989) reviewed all reports on parvovirus infection of the fetus and concluded that the virus passes the placenta readily. They described a stillborn, hydropic fetus in whose placenta there were villous necrosis and calcifications. Infection with different species of parvoviruses has been shown to cause a wide spectrum of diseases in different animals, including congenital anomalies. The subject has been reviewed in detail by Margolis and Kilham (1975), who make reference to human conditions.

ENTEROVIRUSES

Transplacental *poliomyelitis* infection has been described, and the virus was isolated from the placenta in some of these cases (Barsky & Beale, 1957). No pathologic lesions of the placenta are known.

Infection with **enterocytopathogenic human orphan (ECHO)** and **Coxsackie** viruses occurs commonly during the neonatal period and may have serious consequences in neonates. When infection occurs during pregnancy, the fetus is usually spared, perhaps protected by maternal antibody transfer (Amstey et al., 1988). Amstey et al. also perfused two placentas with a mixture of viruses and found them not to transfer. Nevertheless, transplacental passage and fetal infection have occasionally been shown for ECHO viruses (Hughes et al., 1972; Modlin, 1986; C. Davis, personal communication, 1985), and for Coxsackie B virus (Kibrick & Benirschke, 1958; Sauerbrei et al., 2000). There is also speculation that such prenatal infection may be a cause of juvenile diabetes. The placentas of the few cases proved to have caused prenatal Coxsackie virus infection have shown occasional meconium staining, but other meaningful changes were usually absent. Fetal hydrops secondary to myocarditis has occurred with Coxsackie virus infection; placental lesions were not apparent in that abortus (Benirschke et al., 1986). Garcia et al. (1990) described three perinatal deaths from ECHO 33 and 27 infections with isolation of virus from placentas and fetal tissues. They described villitis and intervillositis in the placentas that may best be likened to VUE (vide infra). The same authors expanded on these findings in 1991. Interestingly, the viruses did not affect the fetus, while they were isolated from the placentas, many of which had typical chronic villitis. Some also suffered mural thromboses and vascular lesions in the umbilical cord. The electron microscopy is not convincing, but is also not expected to contribute in these RNA virus infections.

Batcup et al. (1985) reported villous necrosis and severe intervillositis in the placenta of a patient who had Coxsackie virus A9 meningitis at 33 weeks' gestation. A stillborn, macerated fetus was delivered 5 days later, and the virus was recovered from the placenta. Moreover, there were mild myocarditis and early meningitis in the fetus. Remarkably, the placenta had massive intervillous fibrin deposits, much as one sees in the *gitterinfarkts*, discussed in Chapter 9. Villous stem vessels had mural thrombi, and many aspects of the placenta showed features that are usually designated as VUE (vide infra). It is difficult to believe that the extensive placental alterations depicted in their report, could have arisen within this short time span, but further observations to investigate this possibility are clearly mandated.

Ogilvie and Tearne (1980) described three abortions during episodes of infection with Coxsackie A16 virus (hand, foot, and mouth disease) and recovered the virus from one placenta. The pathologic features of the placenta, however, were not discussed.

INFLUENZA, MUMPS, RABIES

Transplacental **influenza A2** (Hong Kong) infection was reported by Yawn et al. (1971). The virus was recovered from the fetus and amnionic fluid in the fatally ill gravida. Fetal tissues and placenta were found to be structurally normal. In an abortus delivered during the febrile period of parainfluenza-1 virus infection, Lavergne et al. (1969) observed a normal placenta. McGregor et al. (1984) recovered influenza A/Bangkok virus from maternal secretions and amnionic fluid of an acutely ill patient who appeared to have the amnionic fluid infection syndrome. The pregnancy continued, and a normal birth ensued. The placenta was not described, but transplacental infection was inferred. Conover and Roessmann (1990) reported the autopsy findings of a malformed infant in whose brain influenza virus was identified immunohistochemically. The placenta was not described.

Fetal **mumps** virus infection may occur, and it has been suggested that some congenital anomalies are due to this agent. Virus has been recovered from the placenta, but no histopathologic change has been described (Yamauchi et al., 1974). Herbst et al. (1970) found only ultrastructural changes in the placenta of a patient with mumps. Severe villous necrosis, simulating that of herpes simplex virus, was found in three cases of intrauterine mumps infection described by Garcia et al. (1980). They also reviewed the sparse and contradictory literature. Small cytoplasmic inclusion bodies were depicted in the decidua.

Transplacental **rabies** infection is not known to occur in women. Spence et al. (1975) observed two normal fetuses after maternal rabies complicated pregnancy. The placenta was not described.

Hepatitis

Transplacental infection with hepatitis viruses has been reported; the topic was reviewed by Altshuler and Russell (1975) and Snydman (1985). Because hepatitis A viremia is short and a carrier state does not occur, fetal infection with this virus is rare but is well documented. Leikin et al. (1996) described fetal ascites and subsequent meconium peritonitis in a fetus whose mother became infected at 20 weeks' gestation. The placenta was not described; other cases of fetal ascites are on record, and McDuffie and Bader (1999) attributed meconium peritonitis to transplacental infection. Asymptomatic hepatitis B infection, however, was found to occur in 0.66% of a low-risk population (Christian & Duff, 1989). Two studies have shown that the antigen passes the placenta (Wang & Zhu, 2000; Xu et al., 2001), and the latter publication traces the virus by fluorescence microscopy. Transmission of hepatitis C virus from chronically infected mothers to fetuses occurs but appears to be uncommon (Thaler et al., 1991; Wejstal et al., 1992; Silverman et al., 1993; Hunt et al., 1997). Gibb et al. (2000), in their review of 441 mother–child pairs, estimated the transmission rate as 6.7% and suggested that it was enhanced in HIV infection. Placentas from such cases of vertical transmission have not been described in the literature, but the ones we have seen have been entirely normal. Vertical transmission of the newly delineated hepatitis G virus has also been reported (Feucht et al., 1996; Inaba, 1997) without placental study. Lin et al. (1996) proposed that transplacental blood contamination may occur during labor.

In contrast to hepatitis A, the high carrier state of hepatitis B virus in adults is a potential hazard to many fetuses. It is generally agreed, however, that this virus is usually acquired enterically during birth or thereafter;

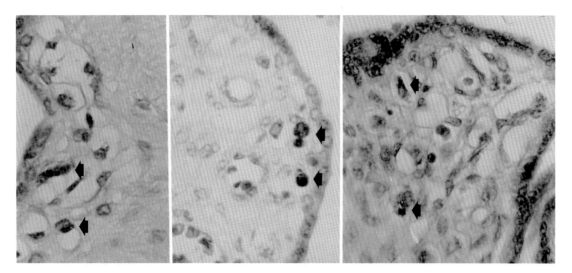

FIGURE 20.61. Placenta with hepatitis B. Pregnancy was interrupted at 20 weeks' gestation. Hofbauer cells are filled with bilirubin (arrows), but there was no inflammation. H&E ×240 (left, center); ×640 (right), red filter.

nevertheless, the transplacental acquisition of hepatitis B virus has occasionally been verified (Fawaz et al., 1975; Mulligan & Stiehm, 1994). Mitsuda et al. (1989) found positive cord blood once in 10 patients but showed that the antigen was present in colostrum of eight patients using the sensitive PCR method. Prospective studies of aborted fetuses from virus-carrying mothers showed that four of 48 fetuses (8%) were thus infected (Li et al., 1986).

The placenta has rarely been examined by pathologists. Altshuler and Russell (1975) stated that the placenta shows "relative immaturity." Buchholz et al. (1974) described the placenta of an infected infant delivered by cesarean section as showing "placental insufficiency." Studies with direct and indirect immunofluorescence indicated the presence of antigen, confined to the basement membranes of the (infantile part) of cells. The authors were uncertain that the placental insufficiency was caused by the infection.

Lucifora et al. (1988) studied the placentas of three asymptomatic hepatitis B surface antigen (HBsAg) carriers with immunohistochemistry. All showed strong reactivity of the Hofbauer cells and villous endothelium, but no pathologic changes were noted. Lucifora et al. (1990) then detected the hepatitis B core antigen (HBcAg) histochemically in all placentas of symptom-free carriers. It was again primarily localized in trophoblast and Hofbauer cells, but also found in fetal endothelium and fibroblasts. They suggested minor pathologic changes (edema, congestion) but are not convincing. We described the placentas of two patients with active hepatitis (Khudr & Benirschke, 1972). The only abnormal finding was the presence of large amounts of bilirubin in Hofbauer cells and chorionic membrane macrophages. There was neither degeneration nor inflammation. The pigment bleached readily when slides were exposed to light, apparently similar to that of meconium macrophages. We have seen the placenta and fetus of a patient who had a therapeutic abortion for hepatitis B. The patient was still icteric when the procedure was done. The fetus, umbilical cord, and membranes were entirely unstained and normal; however, the villous tissues were the color of marmalade, a deep yellow-green. Histologically, numerous deeply bilirubin-stained macrophages were present as villous Hofbauer cells (Fig. 20.61). Some syncytial trophoblastic cells and the membranes had relatively few stained cells. Focal syncytial cell necrosis was present, but there was no inflammation or obvious villous necrosis. There was intense enteritis of the fetus, with meconium deposits and eosinophilic leukocyte infiltration in the submucosa. Several intestinal ulcers were present, and in some areas the bowel was nearly perforated. We assumed that the fetus may have become infected by swallowing amnionic fluid. The case further indicates that bilirubin may traverse the placental barrier but that it then becomes trapped by villous Hofbauer cells.

Rubella (German Measles) and Other Viral Infections

The fetal rubella syndrome exemplifies transplacental fetal virus infection, but because of vaccination, rubella is now uncommon. Banatvala and Brown (2004) report an updated survey of the global infection rate and summarize the most recent diagnostic tools available. A variety of characteristic anomalies are produced in the fetus when infection occurs early, and the precise mechanism by which the degenerative changes responsible for the fetal rubella syndrome, such as cataracts, are generated has been a matter of intense investigation in the past.

Many investigators have detected the virus in the placenta, amnionic fluid, and abortus by virologic means (Alford et al., 1964; Thompson & Tobin, 1970; Catalano et al., 1971). When they isolated the virus from products of conception, Monif et al. (1965) suggested that many macerated fetuses died from placental, rather than fetal, infection. Töndury (1951, 1952a,b, 1964), in numerous contributions, has championed the idea that the fetal damage resulted from embolism of virus-damaged fetal (placental) endothelial cells. Others have suggested that the damage is due to chromosomal breakage.

Endothelial damage in villi of infected products of conception was confirmed in the large study conducted by Driscoll (1969) and by the finding of "endangitis obliterans" in about 40% of the stem villous vessels of infected cases seen by Horn and Becker (1992) and Horn et al. (1993). Driscoll further described sclerosing villous inflammation, which she interpreted to possibly be responsible for the growth retardation. Töndury and Smith (1966) observed focal trophoblastic necrosis and elaborated on their idea of extensive damage to the villous capillary endothelium in early embryos with rubella infection (Fig. 20.62). Selzer (1963, 1964) described basophilic inclusion bodies, but they have not been reported in other descriptions of placental lesions. Similar lesions have been described in a report of 45 cases interrupted because of gestational rubella infection (Ornoy et al., 1973). They discovered some placental lesions in all cases that resulted in malformed fetuses. Decidual perivascular round cell infiltration was prominent; in villi of early gestations, necrosis and fibrosis were found, and swollen Hofbauer cells were prominent. Vascular inflammation was also a prominent finding, similar to that reported earlier. These authors described inclusions in trophoblast and villous stroma but did not depict them, and other authors (Horn and Becker, 1992; Horn et al., 1993) were unable to identify inclusion bodies. It must be pointed out also that the endothelial abnormalities described are neither diagnostic nor present in all cases of virologically confirmed cases of rubella. Moreover, some of these changes are also observed in stillbirths unrelated to virus infections; thus, a degree of skepticism is needed in their interpretation.

The attenuated strain of rubella vaccine virus has been isolated from placentas and fetuses, but villous lesions have not been observed (Phillips et al., 1970; Vaheri et al., 1972). Only Larson et al. (1971) described "histologic changes in placenta or decidua consistent with rubella infection." The fetuses were normal, and apparently only decidual changes were detected.

Rubeola (Measles)

Measles in pregnancy has been very uncommon and its consequences have been described only rarely. There is,

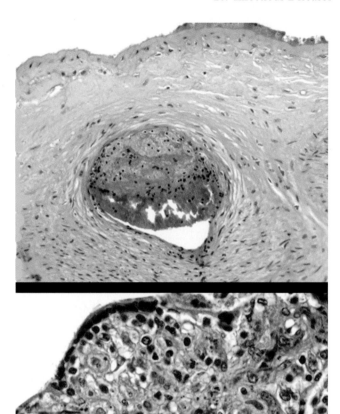

FIGURE 20.62. Sections of immature placenta from rubella-infected fetus. Note the mural thrombosis and nucleated red blood cells (NRBCs) in surface vessel (top) and round cell infiltration of villi (bottom).

however, an extensive database from the 1951 Greenland and the United States epidemics as to the effects of measles on pregnancy. The infection is apparently not teratogenic, and a significantly increased fetal mortality may relate primarily to fever. Access to this literature is provided by Stein and Greenspoon (1991). Placental disease has now been described, but congenital measles apparently does not exist (Eberhart-Phillips et al., 1993). The only report with identification of the antigen in the placenta is the case of Moroi et al. (1991). Their patient suffered fetal demise at 25 weeks after an acute infection, and the virus was detected in the decidua and syncytiotrophoblast by immunohistochemistry. It was not found in the fetus. The placenta was firm and infiltrated with an excessive amount of fibrin and mononuclear cells. Stein and Greenspoon (1991) described three cases: one had an unexplained intrauterine fetal demise (true knot of cord, 30% placental infarct), and the other two did well. Placental lesions were not described, and fetal infection was not apparent. However, Ohyama et al. (2001) described in detail the placenta and clinical findings of a monochorionic set of twins in which one was a macerated stillborn and the other survived without evidence of measles. The placenta of the stillborn had extensive fibrin deposits, and measles virus was definitively shown to be present in trophoblast (by electron microscopy and immunologically). The mother had become infected at 19 weeks and one twin died at 32 weeks. There were large surface inter-twin anastomoses present. It remains uncertain whether the fetus died from measles infection or because of MZ-twin vascular problems; nevertheless, the presence of inclusion bodies and their demonstration as virus in trophoblast is not doubted.

Human Immunodeficiency Virus Infection

Infection of the fetus with the human immunodeficiency virus (HIV) has frequently been reported (Berrebi et al., 1987; European Collaborative 1988; Sperling et al., 1989), but the exact time and mode of this vertical transmission is disputed. Moreover, perhaps because this transmission occurs often at the time of delivery, the treatment of HIV-positive mothers with azidothymidine (AZT) has led to a marked reduction of neonatal HIV infection. Pascual et al. (2000) found no virus transmission in early gestation; but other reports have differed. Therefore, the detailed review by Miller et al. (2000) is most helpful. It weighs the pros and cons of studies of this controversial topic; it discusses whether the immunologic stains of placental tissue are powerful enough to demonstrate the virus and, importantly, whether coexisting chorioamnionitis enhances virus transfer. But one result is universal: HIV infection of the placenta (if it occurs at all) leaves no specific lesions that can be diagnosed without equivocation. Indeed, experimental infection of trophoblast or placental lobules in vitro is usually impossible. The prevalence of HIV infection was studied in an obstetrical population by Barton et al. (1989). They found antibodies only in patients with risk factors (7.1%), whereas those without risk factors were negative. AIDS has occurred in some of the offspring, and the vertical transmission rate of HIV is estimated to be 24% (European Collaborative Study, 1988). Nevertheless, Katz and Wilfert (1989) were uncertain that the infection occurred transplacentally rather than during delivery. Their editorial discussed at length the reports of neonatal AIDS presented in the same journal issue. Fetal deaths and prematurity have been seen in women infected with HIV, but many of these patients had other problems that may have been responsible (Gloeb et al., 1988). Nevertheless, maternal HIV-1 infection is associated with prematurity and endometritis, whereas fetal growth retardation was not observed in the study conducted by Temmerman et al. (1994). These authors were also unable to identify histopathologic

abnormalities in the placentas. Monozygotic twins discordant for HIV infection and with a single placenta were reported by Menez-Bautista et al. (1986). The MZ twins had presumably been exposed to the agent only during fetal life. Alger et al. (1993) found no adverse effect upon pregnancy performance in women who are infected with HIV and showed that an HIV embryopathy does not exist.

The virus has been isolated from amnionic fluid (Mundy et al., 1987) and perhaps from the placenta (Hill et al., 1987). In the latter report, HIV was obtained from placenta but not from lochia, the infant, and cord blood. The infant was well; an electron micrograph of an infected T cell accompanied the report, presumably infected with virus from this placenta's culture, but the authors suggested that the isolation may reflect maternal blood infection. The report was criticized by Peuchmaur et al. (1989), who, subsequent to this report, failed to isolate HIV from placental samples. Greenspoon and Settlage (1989) also believed that the virus of this placenta was more likely contained within the maternal blood of the placenta; the child has remained well, now age 3 years. Since those reports, Soeiro et al. (1992) identified HIV-1 in 30% of fetal material from first trimester abortuses by PCR of HIV nucleic acid. Yet only one of eight infected abortuses showed positive in situ hybridization signals.

Brady et al. (1989) used immunoperoxidase stains on placentas of HIV-infected patients. They found positive staining, particularly in Hofbauer cells, and suggested that this presence of viral protein in placental macrophages might present a reservoir for perinatal infection. A morphologic study of the placentas of 49 HIV-infected patients was undertaken by Jauniaux et al. (1988). The light-microscopic findings were unremarkable. No significant alterations were seen, and the lesions were nonspecific. An ultrastructural study showed "retrovirus-like particles" in the syncytiotrophoblast of one induced abortus's placenta. Five other mature placentas showed isolated virus particles. They were similar to the C-type particles described formerly in many human placentas. Lewis et al. (1990) have demonstrated the presence of HIV by immunocytochemistry and in situ hybridization in maternal decidual leukocytes, trophoblast, Hofbauer cells, and embryonic blood cell precursors of aborted specimens (Fig. 20.63). Although the specific CD4 receptors were not identified on the trophoblastic surface, the authors referred to experiments with trophoblast culture that have demonstrated CD4 presence. It was suggested that transmission (around 30%) occurs directly, without transfer of maternal leukocytes being a prerequisite, as had been postulated. On the other hand, in a sizable prospective study of 44 patients with viremia, Ehrnst et al. (1991) found no transplacental HIV transmission to the 27 infants born. In only one of seven placentas was the virus identified. Andiman et al. (1990) similarly had a

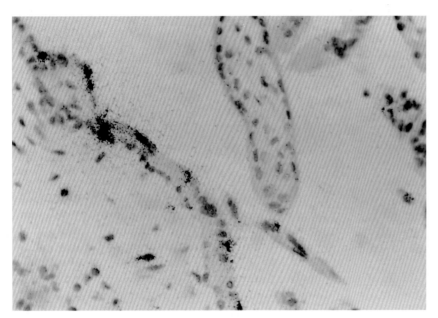

FIGURE 20.63. Eight weeks' gestation villi of HIV-1 infected mother. Specimen was hybridized with ^{35}S-labeled probe. Syncytium, Langhans' cells, and Hofbauer cells are labeled. Hematoxylin ×312. (Courtesy of Dr. S.H. Lewis, formerly of New York, New York.)

low vertical transmission rate but also did not examine the placentas. That placental explants can support growth of HIV was shown by Amirhessami-Aghili and Spector (1991). They cultured first-trimester villous tissue, infected it, and demonstrated the presence of the CD4 and HIV antigens; surprisingly, hCG and progesterone production rose in infected cultures. When Katz et al. (1997) sought markers for formalin-fixed placental localization of HIV, the nucleic acid was seen in syncytiotrophoblast by ^{35}S RNA in situ hybridization. The histopathologic findings, however, were unimpressive, with minor (nonspecific?) inflammatory reactions that are not truly diagnostic of infection. We have also not been able to detect histopathologic placental changes in patients with the infection. It has also been pointed out that unusual tumors metastatic to the placenta may signal HIV infection. Pollack et al. (1993) described a patient who had abdominal delivery for fetal distress. The grossly normal placenta (it had white granular areas on the maternal surface) had intervillous infiltrates by "sheets of small noncohesive, round tumor cells." This was diagnosed as non-Hodgkin's lymphoma. The mother developed further signs of AIDS, but the infant remained normal.

Kalter et al. (1973) had found **C-type particles** in four of six normal human placentas at the junction of syncytiotrophoblast and basement membrane. Their "budding" was more common in premature placentas. Other investigators have shown cross-reactivity of these particles to certain retroviruses (Sawyer et al., 1978; Maeda et al., 1983), and similar structures have been detected in many nonhuman primate placentas (Panem, 1979). C-type particles are nearly ubiquitous viruses, parasites, whose functions are presently unknown. Imamura et al. (1976) detected these RNA-virus–like structures in the placenta

of a patient with lupus but also in normal placentas, albeit in smaller numbers. They also described "tubuloreticular inclusions" in villous endothelium from patients with lupus erythematosus. Similar structures have been induced in Hofbauer cells by maternal interferon therapy in rhesus monkeys (Feldman et al., 1986).

The significance of all of these findings with respect to true viral infections remains uncertain, but congenital HIV infection occurs with certainty (see Goedert et al., 1989). Indeed, the neonatal mortality is significant, and most cases manifest during the first year of life (Scott et al., 1989).

Dengue virus transmission to the fetus has been described only a few times, but placental lesions are unknown. Boussemart et al. (2001) described two such neonates and summarized earlier reports. **West Nile Virus** transmission to the fetus has once been described (Alpert et al., 2003). The neonate had chorioretinal damage and CNS abnormalities, but the placenta was not described.

Toxoplasmosis

Toxoplasmosis is caused by the coccidian *Toxoplasma gondii*, a pan-global parasite of cats and other felids. In cats, a well-explored life cycle exists in the intestinal epithelium. Oocysts are shed in the stools of infected animals. Rodents and other animals ingest these oocysts and acquire the disease. Cats, preying on infected rodents, complete the cycle. The disease is also widespread in domestic animals.

There are several excellent reviews on congenital toxoplasmosis (Kirchhoff & Kräubig, 1966; Frenkel, 1973, 1974; Dubey, 1977; Dubey & Beattie, 1988; Sever et al.,

1988; Freij & Sever, 1996; Montoya & Liesenfeld, 2004). Frenkel (1971) presented a particularly good consideration of all aspects of this disease. The human infection is acquired in adults by two means: (1) contamination with oocysts from feces of infected cats; and (2) ingestion of cysts and tachyzoites in raw, infected meat—largely pork and mutton (Kean et al., 1969). Pregnant women should not eat undercooked or raw meat, and they should also avoid having contact with "wild" (i.e., hunting) cats. Heating to 150°F kills the organism. Cats raised solely on commercial diets are not infected; cats that hunt and are given raw meat may become infected. Emptying their litter box daily to prevent drying and dust-producing feces is recommended (Kimball et al., 1974). A thoughtful review of these aspects has been written by Swartzberg and Remington (1975). Of the Parisian human adult population, 84% have antibodies because of the frequency of raw meat consumption in France.

Transplacental toxoplasmosis is not uncommon. It has been well described to cause severe destructive disease in the offspring who are infected during early gestation. Minor degrees of damage are incurred when infection develops later in pregnancy. Chorioretinitis, encephalitis with hydrocephaly, and other organ involvement may nevertheless cause crippling disease. Wilson and Remington (1980) estimated that the lifetime support for the 3300 children born annually in the United States with toxoplasmosis is the staggering sum of over $200 million.

It is generally assumed that almost all, if not all, congenital *Toxoplasma* infections occur when a woman has her primary infection during pregnancy. Few reports exist that congenital toxoplasmosis occurs in successive pregnancies. It has also been assumed that the presence of maternal antibodies prevents fetal infection. That this is not so was shown by the important case detailed by Forther et al. (1991). They found a toxoplasma cyst in an abortion specimen from an immune patient who had contact with an infected cat that caused acute toxoplasmosis in her brother. Feldman (1963) has doubted that recurrent infection ever occurs. Desmonts and Couvreur (1974) have provided the most conclusive prospective study of toxoplasmosis in pregnancy. Almost 45% of Parisian women with primary infection during pregnancy had infants with congenital toxoplasmosis. The rate of infection increased with the gestational trimesters (17%, 25%, and 65%, respectively). Fetal destruction was the most severe during early, rather than late, gestation. The authors were skeptical that toxoplasmosis causes abortion and denied the occurrence of repeated congenital toxoplasmosis. Others have found *Toxoplasma* organisms in the placenta and uterus of infected, macerated fetuses (Mellgren et al., 1952) or have isolated it from spontaneously aborted products of conception (Remington et al., 1964; Forth et al., 1991). Stray-Pedersen and Lorentzen-Styr

(1977) studied endometrial biopsies of women with habitual abortion. Six of 96 women had tachyzoites in endometrium and menstrual blood, demonstrated by fluorescent antibody studies, but none was isolated in mouse inoculations. Treatment of these women abolished the organisms.

Because it is often difficult to positively identify the organism in routinely stained placental material, the method by which the organism is verified in tissues is of great importance. It is easiest to demonstrate toxoplasma by placing ground tissue samples into the peritoneal cavity of young mice or into appropriate tissue culture cell lines (Kaufman & Maloney, 1962). Handling this organism, however, is often avoided because of the hazards of infection. Immunologic means are generally preferred, although the results are often dubious. For positive identification in tissues, Dallenbach and Piekarski (1960) have advocated the fluorescence antibody technique. A similar methodology was used by Foulon et al. (1990a) in identifying the antigen from tissue cultures infected with chorionic villus sampling (CVS) specimens. The electron microscopic appearance of *Toxoplasma* cysts ("pseudocysts") is characteristic and has been well shown by Callaway et al. (1968). Detailed considerations of modern diagnostic tests for toxoplasmosis have been given in a review of all aspects of this disease by Koskiniemi et al. (1989). Savva and Hollman (1990) reviewed the PCR methodology that allows unequivocal detection of the toxoplasma DNA (see also Hohlfeld et al., 1994; Fricker-Hidalgo et al., 1998). The problems of prenatal diagnosis were considered by Foulon et al. (1990b), who had much success with amnionic fluid culture and funipuncture.

The organism has been isolated from amnionic fluid and placentas of infected pregnancies (Stray-Pedersen, 1980; Teutsch et al., 1980). The diagnosis of congenital infection was later made by fetal blood sampling, which led to beneficial prenatal therapy in some cases (Desmonts et al., 1985; Daffos et al., 1988). Foulon et al. (1999) found that fetal infection was best made with amnionic fluid PCR and culture, rather than by cordocentesis. Couvreur et al. (1976) described congenital toxoplasmosis in 14 twins. In two of these pairs, only one twin was affected. Although it is stated that these twins were dizygotic, one of the two had a DiMo placenta, and they thus must have been identical twins. The authors reviewed previous reports of discordant dizygotic (DZ) twins, whereas all MZ twins had been similarly affected. Cox et al. (1987) also reported two discordant twins when they assayed fetal blood during pregnancy for antibodies.

Evidence of congenital disease is at times difficult to find. It may require a long follow-up. Thus, the MZ twins reported by Glasser and Delta (1965) were judged to be normal at birth. Their placenta had many cysts in the membranes but no other pathologic features. The children first became symptomatic at 7 months of age. Another set of twins, described by Miller et al. (1971), also had late onset, and toxoplasmosis was not suspected until hydrocephaly developed. The mother had eaten ground beef during the pregnancy, the presumed source of infection. Late onset of symptomatology was further explored by Koppe et al. (1986), who showed that in children with congenital toxoplasmosis "new lesions continue to appear well after the age of 5 years, and the impairment can be severe." In other cases of apparent fetal well-being despite maternal infection during pregnancy, the maternal therapy may have prevented fetal disease (e.g., Hammer & Wegmann, 1966).

Placental infection with *Toxoplasma* has been well documented. It is presumably always produced by organisms circulating in the maternal blood, although the isolation of cysts from endometrium in chronic aborters makes direct infection from the endometrium possible (Werner et al., 1963). Altshuler (1973b), who described a fatal case with placental study, bemoaned that the placenta is not studied more often in this disease and suggested rapid means for identification of the organism. The case he studied was typical. The infant had hydranencephaly, a frequent feature of this disease (Larsen, 1977), hepatosplenomegaly, and hydrops. Hydrops in congenital toxoplasmosis has been described repeatedly. Typical cysts were present in the subamnionic/chorionic tissues, and they were unaccompanied by inflammation. It is only when the cysts rupture that a local plasmacellular reaction and necrosis take place. Altshuler found a marked increase in villous Hofbauer cells, erythroblasts in the fetal circulation, and vascular proliferation in placental villi. He also depicted a lymphocytic-plasmacellular villitis (Fig. 20.64).

Similar villitis, including necrosis and villous *Toxoplasma* cysts, were found by Elliott (1970) in the placenta of a 3-month macerated abortus. He described the placenta as being "shaggy." Becket and Flynn (1953) found the placenta in toxoplasmosis to be as pale as it is in cases of erythroblastosis. They depicted the cysts in villi in both of their cases. Driscoll noted that in most of her cases marked plasmacellular deciduitis was a pronounced feature (Benirschke & Driscoll, 1967). Excellent illustrations of cysts within villi, occurring apparently even within trophoblast, were provided by Werner et al. (1963). They considered it to be the result of transmission from infected endometrium. Edwina Popek (1992) described granulomatous villitis in an 18-week stillbirth with intensive chronic villitis; she also reviewed the literature on placental toxoplasma infection in this contribution. Popek found organisms in every section of her case and was able to stain them immunologically. Nevertheless, careful study identified the organisms without additional aid. There were no plasma cells in the villi.

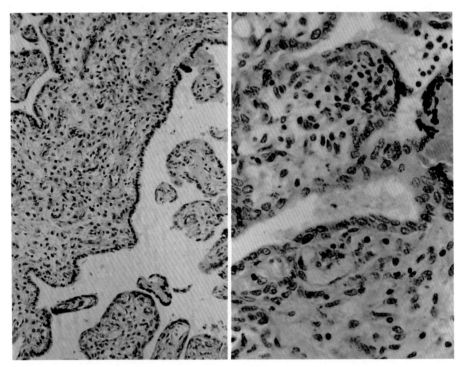

FIGURE 20.64. Villi in a patient with congenital toxoplasmosis. Left: Same case as in Figure 20.66. Right: Same case as in Figure 20.65. There is a diffuse lymphoplasmacytic infiltration, with sclerosis of the villi. H&E ×125 (left); ×240 (right). (Courtesy of Dr. G. Khodr, San Antonio, Texas, and Dr. J. Hustin, Loverval, Belgium.)

FIGURE 20.65. *Toxoplasma* cysts in amnion/chorion of a child with congenital infection and hydrocephaly at 31 weeks' gestation. Inset: Enlargement of a cyst. H&E ×640. Inset: H&E ×1200 (Case courtesy of Dr. Jean Hustin, Loverval, Belgium.)

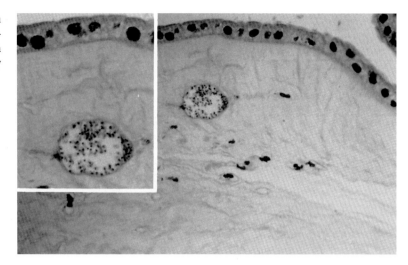

Although the cysts depicted by these authors are classical, care must be taken with the interpretation of *Toxoplasma* cysts in other publications. In consultation, we have seen several cases where cysts had been suspected; they were, however, degenerating syncytium. The photographs shown by Sarto et al. (1982) of syncytial nuclei in "endomitosis" simulate *Toxoplasma* cysts. They must not be mistaken for the organism. Janssen et al. (1970) have discussed these difficulties and urged that these problems must be borne in mind when toxoplasmosis is diagnosed from slides. As difficult as cyst identification is, the diagnosis of tachyzoites in histologic sections is impossible. Without fluorescent antibody staining or smears of infected tissue, they usually cannot be recognized with certainty. Dr. Jean Hustin (Belgium) has made available to us a case of a primary infection at 24 weeks' gestation that was treated with spiramycin. Despite this therapy, the fetus developed hydrocephaly and was aborted at 31 weeks. Numerous cysts were found in the chorion (Fig. 20.65), and plasmacellular infiltration, with necrosis and fibrosis, was found in villi. This maternal therapy is thus ineffective in combating the infection.

In toxoplasmosis, as in CMV infection, thrombosis of chorionic vessels occurs (see Fig. 20.67). The thrombi and vessel walls may be calcified, even vessels of the umbilical cord have been thus calcified (Khodr & Matossian, 1978). Pathologists are frequently challenged to provide a specific diagnosis when chronic villitis is found. They must then find cysts, proceed with antibody staining (Fig. 20.66), or, best, isolate the organism by injecting tissue homogenate into the peritoneal cavity of mice. Tissue culture methods of identification may also be used. Occasionally one may find cysts only in the umbilical cord, perhaps because they stand out better (Benirschke et al., 1999). But when calcified vessels of the placenta remain unexplained, especially when some chronic inflammation of villi is also encoun-tered, a detailed search for toxoplasma cysts needs to be undertaken.

The questions of whether recurrent toxoplasmosis occurs and with what frequency are not resolved. Kimball et al. (1971) conducted a prospective study of 5000 obstetrical patients and came to the conclusion that abortion is significantly associated with antibodies to *Toxoplasma*, but in none of their 260 abortion specimens could they show the organism. Moreover, habitual abortion was not due to toxoplasmosis in the mother. Feldman (1963) thought that recurrent toxoplasmosis does not occur. Others are dubious or believe that recurrent infection is most likely associated with immunosuppression. Langer (1963a,b) first suggested that toxoplasmosis may be a cause of spontaneous abortion. He inoculated mice with material from 70 repeat aborters and isolated organisms from 23 of them. However, he also obtained organisms

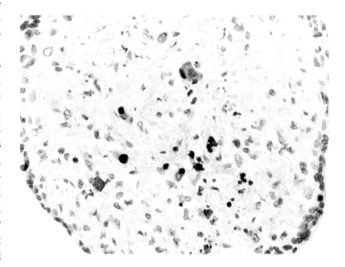

FIGURE 20.66. Villus in congenital toxoplasmosis, anti-toxo-plasma antibody staining (brown).

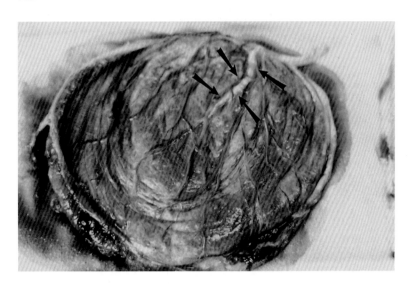

FIGURE 20.67. Placenta of a stillborn with hydranencephaly and other destructive features due to toxoplasmosis. Note the calcified venous thrombus at (arrows). (Courtesy of Dr. G. Khodr, San Antonio, Texas.)

from nine control specimens. Only 19 of the 23 patients had a positive serologic reaction. He isolated *Toxoplasma* from the brain of two successive abortuses. He also described another case with probable toxoplasmosis. In several cases, however, he required several passages for identification, an important aspect of his work.

Garcia (1968) observed a similar patient. This woman delivered a severely affected child who died within a day. Aside from many areas of typical destruction, organisms were shown to exist in several organs. The placenta had many cysts and villitis with conglutination of villi. Cysts were also found around the umbilical vein. A second pregnancy ended with a macerated abortus, also with typical histopathologic changes. Again, *Toxoplasma* organisms were identified; they were also present within the decidua, but they were much less well depicted there. Thus, some doubt of recurrent disease lingers. The suspicions that transplacental toxoplasma transmission may be enhanced in HIV-infected patients have not been supported by the study of Minkoff et al. (1997).

Kala-Azar

This visceral leishmaniasis is due to *Leishmania major* infection. It is endemic in parts of Africa, and placentas from infected pregnancies have rarely been observed, even though congenital infection is known to occur occasionally. Eltoum et al. (1992) described such a case, a 5 months abortus, as well as a transplacental infection. In the placenta of the abortus, numerous villous vessels were thrombosed and contained typical organisms, amastigotes, within and outside of macrophages. The organisms were confirmed by electron microscopy. There was no inflammation and only focal trophoblastic degeneration was observed.

Chagas' Disease

Chagas' disease (American trypanosomiasis) is caused by infection with *Trypanosoma cruzi*, an organism that is transmitted by the bite of an infected triatomid, the "kissing bug." The disease is largely limited to Brazil, Paraguay, Chile, and Argentina, but rare cases (also of organism and vector) have come from Mexico and the United States (Woody & Woody, 1974). Chagas' disease produces a wide variety of symptoms and is characterized by a frequently long latent period. Best known are myocarditis and esophagitis, but encephalitis, hepatosplenomegaly, and many other manifestations are well recorded. It is an important and frequent disease in northeastern Brazil. The disease is also known in Venezuela, from which the first congenitally acquired cases were described (Gavaller, 1953). Since then, numerous instances of congenital Chagas' disease have been published. Most have been from Salvador (Bahia, Brazil), but a mild transplacental infection in a Mexican patient was detailed by Gilson et al. (1995). The latter authors pointed out that with currently greater mobility of people, the infection should be more commonly suspected.

The extensive Brazilian literature on congenital and placental Chagas' disease has been reviewed in English by Bittencourt (1976), who is the major contributor to our knowledge of this disease in newborns. Her paper also described in detail the placental pathology. The (maternal) disease was often first identified by the autopsy of stillborn infants, whose organs contained large numbers of the organisms. When parasitemia exists in the mother, the trypanosomes gain access from the intervillous space by traversing the trophoblast as trypomastigotes. This step may occur during an acute infection but is most common in the chronic phase of the disease. In the villi, the organisms change character, becoming amastigotes, and remain

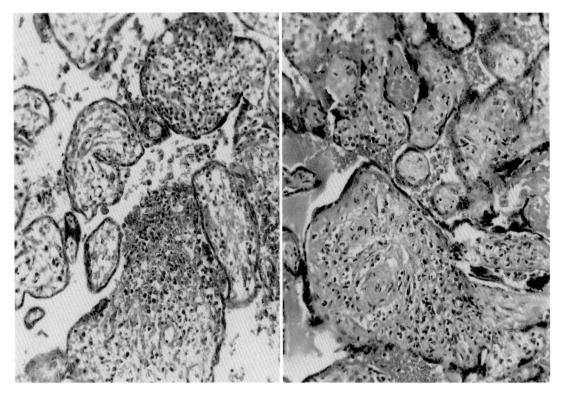

FIGURE 20.68. Chronic, destructive villitis due to Chagas' disease. Although many organisms are present, they cannot be seen at this magnification. The villi at top right are agglutinated; they have long been fibrosed and are functionless. H&E ×250. (Courtesy of Dr. Achiléa Lisboa Bittencourt, Bahia, Brazil.)

phagocytosed by Hofbauer cells. When they are released from these cells, they enter the fetal circulation as trypomastigotes. Not all placentas with Hofbauer cell infection cause congenital disease in the fetus. Most of the placentas studied by Bittencourt showed a massive parasitic load, chronic destructive villitis, and intervillous accumulation of fibrin and inflammatory cells (Fig. 20.68). Fibrosis and an occasional villous granuloma-like reaction were also seen. The amnionic epithelium and Hofbauer cells were the commonest place for amastigotes to be located, although in one case a massive accumulation was found in the syncytium (Fig. 20.69). In a later contribution, Bittencourt et al. (1981) beautifully depicted the amnionic amastigote infection, and showed that the umbilical cord also had surface and internal amastigote aggregates; she speculated that an important route of amnionic epithelial infection may be from infected fetal lung. The chorion also occasionally contained organisms.

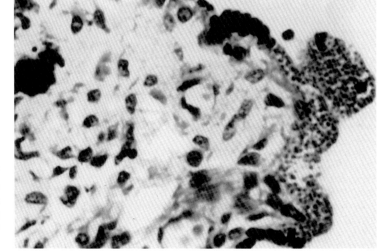

FIGURE 20.69. Placenta of a mother with Chagas' disease, showing amastigotes in the syncytiotrophoblast. This newborn was without overt disease, even though the placenta was infected during the acute phase of the maternal disease. H&E ×400. (Courtesy of Dr. Achiléa Lisboa Bittencourt, Bahia, Brazil.)

The placentas of many affected fetuses were markedly enlarged, pale, and disrupted. Drut and Araujo (2000) depicted unusually large cells in villous stroma and determined their hyperdiploid DNA content. Mezzano et al. (2005) described reduced expression of placental alkaline phosphatase in infected and in diabetic placentas and suggested a causal relation with the presence of trypanosomes in trophoblast. Perhaps, so they speculated, diabetic patients may be more susceptible. Mjihdi et al. (2002) induced placental and fetal lesions in experimental studies of mice using this organism, and Shippey et al. (2005) used trophoblast cell cultures and perfused cotyledons to investigate early infection with trypanosomes. The former mode of infection was more successful.

BABESIOSIS, TRICHOMONIASIS, RICKETTSIA, AND EHRLICHIA

Transplacental **babesiosis** has been described, but the placenta was not studied (Esernio-Jenssen et al., 1987). The mother had been bitten by a tick 1 week before delivery; the infant was treated successfully. The organism, *Babesia microti*, was identified in 5% of the child's red blood cells.

Trichomoniasis of the vagina, caused by *Trichomonas vaginalis*, frequently complicates pregnancy and is the most common sexually transmitted disease according to Stine (1993), and it has been suggested that it is a cause of premature delivery, especially because it may be associated with bacterial vaginosis (James et al., 1992; Cotch et al., 1997; Boon et al., 2002). Mason and Brown (1980), who studied 70 infected parturients and a control group of patients, found that there was no relation of premature delivery and vaginal trichomoniasis. Cotch et al. (1997) examined a large population of women. They ascertained that vaginal trichomoniasis in the middle trimester is associated with preterm delivery and low birth weight. They corrected for associated infections but were unable to correlate PROM with this trichomoniasis. These authors and Graves and Gardner (1993) considered the probable pathogenicity of this organism upon the endocervical canal and placental membranes. Neonatal infection of respiratory passages and pneumonia, presumably acquired at delivery, have been reported in a few newborns (Al-Salihi et al., 1974; McLaren et al., 1983; Smith et al., 2002; Hoffman et al., 2003). They were delivered vaginally; the placentas were not described. The organisms are difficult to identify histologically, and they would most likely be overlooked in routine examinations (see Lossick & Kent, 1991). Fetal and placental inflammatory lesions have been well delineated in bovine abortions due to a related flagellate (Rhyan et al., 1988), but detailed placental studies in humans have not been reported. They are desperately needed, as the light-microscopic examination of tissue sections is incapable of detecting this organism. Fortunately, new methods for identification have become available such as fluorescent DNA in situ hybridization (Muresu et al., 1994), and the sequence of the trichomonas adhesive protein has been identified (Rappelli et al., 1995). But it needs to be reemphasized that trichomoniasis is one of the most common (if not the most common) sexually transmitted diseases, and it has major sequelae that are in need of more decisive study (Soper, 2004).

Rickettsial disease (Rocky Mountain spotted fever) occurred during the pregnancy of a patient described by Markley et al. (1998). After chloramphenicol therapy the patient recovered; the placenta and infant were normal.

Ehrlichiosis is an infection with placental transmission identified in horses (Long et al., 1995). The infection causes abortion in sheep, cattle, and horses, and several different species of organisms have been delineated. There is one report of neonatal infection in humans, by Horowitz et al. (1998). The mother was infected, living in a tick-infested environment, and responded to doxycycline therapy. The neonate became clinically ill at age 7 days and had massive infection of granulocytes with the agent referred to as "human granulocytic ehrlichiosis." The placenta had not been examined, but circumstances suggested to the authors a prenatal, transplacental infection.

Malaria

Infection with one of the four species of malaria plasmodia is the commonest infectious disease in the world, but truly congenital infection has been described only rarely. Naeye (1988b) made the point that it is important to differentiate between malaria in endemic regions and malaria in areas where the disease is sporadic. The former have continuously new antigen presentation and different, enhanced immune reactions. He believed that this point may be important in the outcome of the disease and its possible transmission to the fetus. But the mechanism of fetal/neonatal infection is still uncertain, despite the prevalence of malaria.

Most authors have found that pregnancy substantially increases the severity of malaria. The disease is associated with premature births, and it reduces the weight of the fetus and placenta (references in Bruce-Chwatt, 1966; Wyler, 1983). There is also some evidence that malaria-infected erythrocytes may be "sequestered" in the intervillous space of pregnant patients (Bray & Sinden, 1979). This sequestration was explained by the expression of intercellular adhesion molecule-1 (ICAM-1) on monocytes in "chronic malaria infection" (Sugiyama et al., 2001). Muthusamy et al. (2004) showed that infected red cells adhere to trophoblast by a "low-sulfated chondroitin sulfate proteoglycan receptor." This attachment, so Crocker et al. (2004) suggested, leads to syncytiotrophoblastic degeneration, possibly thus relating to deficient fetal growth (see Nosten et al., 1999). The organisms have often been identified in the blood of the intervillous space (e.g., Jelliffe, 1968) and may be retained there because of the "sequestration" even after apparently adequate therapy (Procop et al., 2001). It is also stated that the placenta may be "diagnostically black at parturition" owing to malaria pigment (Anonymous, 1983c). This pigment ("haemozoin") has been quantitated by Sullivan et al. (2000), but its quantity was unrelated to fetal outcome. In a study that used polarization microscopy, Romagosa et al. (2004) have shown that this modality is superior in detecting the parasites, as well as the pigment, so long as the tissues were fixed in buffered formalin. Mount et al. (2004) showed that the impairment of humoral immunity to malaria surface antigens in pregnancy is occasionally the result of HIV infection, thus explaining the enhanced susceptibility in pregnancy to malaria.

Congenital infection with malarial organisms occurred in only one twin reported by Tanner and Hewlett (1935) and Balabat et al. (1995). The latter authors asserted that only 300 cases of congenital malaria have been described, and only five were in twin pregnancies. They also suggested that transplacental infection occurred most likely during delivery. Following an epidemic, Wickramasuriya (1935) described six cases of congenital malaria. He believed that congenital infection is much more common than was believed prior to his report. It included a review of previous statements that denied or assumed congenital infection to occur. The patients in his study were severely infected, and several died undelivered with fetus in utero. Parasites were found in umbilical cord blood of one patient, and in the brain and spleen of two. Five fetuses had malaria-pigmented spleens, and one placenta had many infarcts and an abruptio. Other reports of congenital malaria have been reviewed in case reports by Woods et al. (1974) and Thompson et al. (1977). A frequently cited report of Quinn et al. (1982) described four children who had their first febrile episode at 3 to 4 weeks of age. Their mothers had come to Seattle, Washington, from abroad, and the new infection is unlikely to have occurred in Seattle. The mothers had been febrile during labor or before; the placentas were not studied, and the mechanism of fetal infection is only surmised. It was suggested that perhaps antibodies or other proteins suppressed fever before the children finally became ill. In general, perhaps because of transferred immunity, symptomatic disease becomes evident only after several weeks in the neonate, as in the four infants just described. The disease is virtually never recognized at birth or it may be very difficult to diagnose (Hewson et al., 2003). That the transmission was prenatal (or occurred during delivery) in some of these cases is evidenced by reports of neonatal malaria in patients returning from abroad to the United States and delivering their infants here. Organisms have definitively identified in umbilical cord blood but is said to be more common when the fetus has had an opportunity to make IgM antibodies (Xi et al., 2003).

When it is stated in the literature, however, that the "placenta was infected," this usually refers to the demonstration of organisms in blood smears made from the placenta. Such organisms could have originated from the intervillous space, as was well demonstrated by the photograph in the studies by Miller and Telford (1997a,b) upon which Lane (1997) and Edwards (1997) commented. Histologic studies have usually not been done, or have been reported only infrequently. One such report, including ultrastructural study, came from Gabon (Walter et al., 1982). These investigators found placental parasites in smears from 33% of cases in an unselected population collected in an endemic area. Infected erythrocytes were frequent in the intervillous space, and there was an accumulation of associated macrophages (Fig. 20.70). An increased amount of intervillous fibrin was present; thickening of trophoblastic lamina was interpreted as possibly representing the results of an immune reaction. The authors suggested that syncytial damage may have occurred, and they found ample malaria pigment (a hemoglobin breakdown product) in fibrinoid, macrophages, and "free" in the intervillous space. In the authors' opinion, plasmodia cross the placenta infrequently, and in their study the event was not demonstrable. This opinion is different from that of Naeye (1988b), who quoted Reinhardt as having found parasites in the fetus as frequently as in 55% of cases.

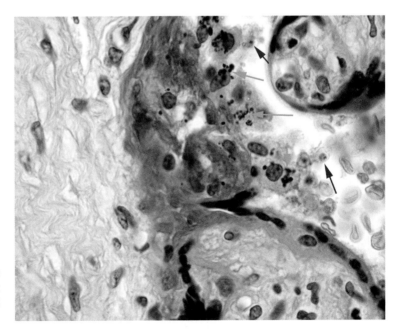

FIGURE 20.70. Malaria infected placenta with focus of syncytiotrophoblastic necrosis and pigment (hemozoin) at green arrows. Malaria parasites at red arrows.

The discrepancy is not resolved. The workers who have looked at the placentas histologically have not identified organisms in the fetal circulation. This is also our observation, based on studies of infected Vietnamese patients who have delivered at our hospital. Our present view is that the plasmodium does not cross by itself. When transplacental infection does occur, the parasites are probably transferred within red blood cells. Although maternal to fetal transfer of red blood cells is rare, it does occasionally happen (see Chapter 17). This concept accords with the original observations made by Wickramasuriya (1935) as well. He demonstrated organisms in some stillborns and in the umbilical cord blood of one fetus. His patients had unusually severe pregnancy complications, several having died before delivery. These complications may well have contributed to the enhanced transfer of infected red blood cells. Ordi et al. (1998) examined the placentas of a large cohort of patients in Tanzania and detected "massive chronic intervillositis" in 6.27% of their patients. Of 1179 placentas studied, 415 showed parasites as evidence of active infection, 475 had malaria pigment without parasites, 289 had no evidence of infection, and 74 had massive intervillositis. At least 75% of the intervillous space was involved with infiltration of mainly "monocytes and histiocytes" (CD68- and CD45-positive cells), and frequent fibrin deposits were also observed. Pigment was identified by polarized light study. Four cases had fetal vascular thromboses. The report has an extensive discussion of intervillositis of different origins, but fetal infection was not addressed by these authors (see also Chapter 21). The nature of the intervillous inflammatory cells was studied in greater detail by Ordi et al. (2001) in the same population. It was found that natural killer (NK) cells are conspicuously absent among the cells. Nebuloni et al. (2001) commented on this observation and presented a malaria patient with massive "intervillositis" (vide infra) and further identified the cell type (CD68, CD45RO–, few CD20+).

Coxiella burnetii is the organism that causes Q-fever, a zoonosis commonly contracted from domestic animals. Congenital infection with intrauterine fetal death was reported by Friedland et al. (1994). The placenta had a 40% involvement with severe necrotizing villitis with many organisms in the villi. Raoult and Stein (1994) reported another case and reviewed other cases from the abortion literature.

OTHER PARASITIC INFECTIONS

Kain and Keystone (1988) reported a patient with recurrent hydatid disease (*Echinococcus granulosus*) during pregnancy. A normal child was born; the placenta was not described. Invasion of the embryo by *Enterobius vermicularis* was described by Mendoza et al. (1987). They depicted a 2-cm embryo, with placenta, and showed the worm to reside within the abdomen of the embryo. The pregnancy was surgically aborted because of the presence of a dead embryo. There was no inflammatory reaction in the embryo or placenta. When Cort (1921) reviewed the topic of fetal worm infestation, he found only indisputable evidence for transmission of **hookworm** and *Schistosoma japonicum*. In dogs, sheep, and other animals, prenatal transmission of lung worm is well known. Sutherland et al. (1965) depicted placental infection with *Schistosoma haematobium* from a normal delivery. The organisms were located within decidua and villi, but no inflammatory reaction was described. In an addendum, additional cases were discovered. Several other references were made to a case of placental infection with different species of schistosomes. Thus, Bittencourt et al. (1980) found placental infection with *Schistosoma mansoni* in four cases. The gross morphology of the placenta showed no characteristic features, but microscopically granulomas around Schistosome eggs were present in fibrin and villi; occasional worms were also present and are illustrated. Although all four fetuses died, they had no evidence of infection by the worms. Presumably the rarity of this description relates to the paucity of placental studies. Pregnant women also suffer occasionally from disseminated **strongolydiasis**, but we are not aware of a report of placental pathology in this disease.

Villitis of Unknown Etiology

Chronic villitis occurs frequently. Rüschoff et al. (1985) found it in 6.6% of 1240 placentas studied, whereas Altshuler (personal communication, 1993) estimated a frequency of 5% to 10% in consecutive placentas. Labarrere et al. (1989, 1990), who referred to it as "villitis of unestablished origin" reviewed the incidence and found it to vary in studies from 6% to 33.8%. Villitis of unknown etiology (VUE) is especially frequent in the villi that are near the maternal floor of the placenta, and we have found it to be more commonly in placenta accreta at the implantation site (Fig. 20.71). At times, the etiology is apparent from the history (rubella) or the pathologic features (CMV infection). At other times, despite much effort, no specific etiology is elicited, often even when there are severe clinical abnormalities and autopsies are performed on the neonate. The entity has been termed **villitis of unknown etiology** since its original description (Gershon & Strauss, 1961; Benirschke & Altshuler, 1971; Altshuler, 1973c) and is now a well-recognized entity for placental pathologists. It remains a significant challenge to perinatal pathologists because of its frequency, its high recurrence rate, and the associated poor pregnancy outcome. Sporadic cases such as one we saw with maternal granulomatous disease do not assure a causal relation. No conclusive information on the etiology of VUE has been gained since it was first mentioned by Gershon and Strauss (1961). It is unfortunate that these authors misused the term *placental insufficiency* in this context, a designation to which we do not subscribe. In the literal sense, that term should be used only to represent a pathophysiologic state; it is not synonymous with specific morphologic abnormalities. In our view, few other well-defined lesions of the placenta exist (e.g., maternal floor infarct) for which a fetal or maternal cause cannot be assigned; the term *placental insufficiency* subtly implies that there

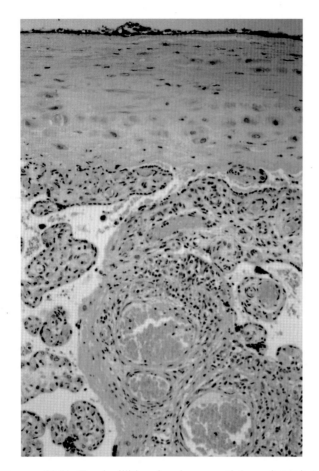

FIGURE 20.71. Focal villitis of unknown etiology (VUE) in anchoring villi at implantation site of a placenta percreta. The villi are attached to the connective tissue scar of previous cesarean section. H&E ×160.

is an intrinsic defect in placental function or its development. We believe the concept of placental insufficiency to be misleading and one that diverts attention from the search of pathogenetic mechanisms.

The pathologic findings of VUE have often been depicted since the initial emphasis on this entity's recognition (Benirschke & Altshuler, 1971), but there is evidence that the interpathologist diagnostic error of this diagnosis is considerable (Khong et al., 1993). The constituent lesions have a wide spectrum, from occasional villous involvement to extreme involvement wherein all villi have some pathologic reaction (Russell, 1980). Altshuler (1973c, 1984) summarized the salient features of VUE as follows: proliferative villitis; necrotizing villitis; granulomatous, cicatricial, reparative, evanescent villitis; fetal vasculopathy; avascular villi; placental dysmaturity; increase in nucleated red blood cells; hemosiderin; hemorrhagic vasculitis; necrotizing deciduitis; basal villitis; chorangiosis; and ischemia or infarction. All of these abnormalities may be found in cases of placental VUE, or only some of them may be present.

The similarity to known infectious causes of villitis, such as seen with CMV and rubella, is striking. Even though no infectious cause has been delineated for VUE, this entity is discussed here because of its presumed relation to congenital infection. It may well be proved in the future that VUE is not a single or uniform lesion, independent of host immune factors, but that it is composed of several etiologically distinct variants. It is a challenge for future investigation that has recently been taken up by several investigators.

One should also note that degenerative lesions, somewhat simulating VUE, occur peripheral to infarcts (subinfarctive villous degenerations). These lesions are not to be confused with typical VUE as here discussed. VUE is often associated with fetal growth restriction. Altshuler (1984) saw it in 33% of such cases, Dollmann and Schmitz-Moormann (1972) described it in their patient with recurrent abortions, and others found similar effects (Russell et al., 1980; Labarrere et al., 1982; Salafia et al., 1988). Rüschoff et al. (1985) described the placentas of VUE as "stiff," but a specific macroscopic delineation of VUE has not yet been possible. The placentas are occasionally smaller and have more fibrin content, but no other change allows macroscopic identification.

The frequency of VUE varies with the nature of the investigation, that is, the selection of the material. In general, one may expect VUE in approximately 5% to 8% of consecutively studied placentas. When those of complicated pregnancies, growth-restricted infants, or fetal deaths are studied, the incidence is much higher.

There is little doubt that VUE eliminates a considerable amount of placental parenchyma from nutrient transfer. Fetal growth restriction is thus not surprising. One must emphasize, however, that there is no absolute relation between the severity of VUE and the severity of fetal growth restriction. Attempts to show a relation to elevated fetal IgM levels have not been successful (Mortimer et al., 1985), nor have numerous attempts to identify specific organisms with a variety of serologic, cultural, or structural tools. When neonates survive even severe VUE, they have no detectable illness, and those who die show no lesions at autopsy.

Of greatest interest to us is the frequently recurrent nature of this lesion, so well described in the contribution by Dollmann and Schmitz-Moormann (1972). They saw a patient with two growth-restricted infants followed by three abortions, all with VUE as probable cause. They found that, in some instances, there was a marked intervillous accumulation of macrophages (intervillositis). These cells they determined to be of maternal origin, whereas most of the intravillous inflammatory cells could not be typed with sex chromatin but were thought to be of fetal origin. Jacques and Qureshi (1993) observed six cases of chronic intervillositis and determined the cells to be primarily histiocytes. They were unable to rule out

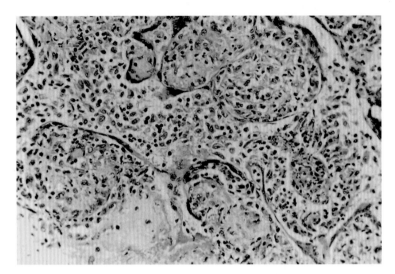

FIGURE 20.72. Placenta of 36 weeks' gestation stillborn with VUE. It was the second of three successive such events. Note the intense intervillositis with histiocytes and lymphocytes, villous infiltration, villous necroses, and vascular obliteration. H&E ×250.

infection, found an association with increased fibrin deposition, and identified some other pathologic features. Although the lesion had a poor prognosis, they were unable to define it more precisely or to identify an etiology. They favored an immunologic determination and next examined it in twin gestations (1994), as did Doss et al. (1995), who suggested a relation to recurrent abortion (see Chapter 21). Discordant involvement of twins was found in both DZ as well as MZ twins, and growth restriction was associated, as was also the case in Kaplan's description (2003) of a set of discordant MZ twins. They pointed out that both viral and immunologic hypotheses for the etiology of VUE are difficult to support when VUE affects the placental portion of only one of monochorionic MZ twins. The suggestion relating to VUE and for the adherence and possible penetration of maternal lymphocytes/monocytes to syncytial cells comes from the in vitro studies by Xiao et al. (1997). They showed that inflammatory cytokines of various types increases the avidity of monocyte-binding to syncytium through activation of surface ICAM-1. An immunologic pathogenesis of VUE with maternal cells infiltrating the villi has long been championed by Labarrere and his colleagues (1991). They had earlier first characterized the lesion of chronic intervillositis (Labarrere & Mullen, 1987) and now demonstrated the presence of tissue factor (an initiator of thrombosis through activation of factor VII) in normal villous stroma. In VUE, one often finds minor thromboses in villous capillaries and larger stem vessels. These investigators assume that these originated secondary to focal inflammation, thus releasing cytokines from locally activated helper T cells and macrophages. They envisaged that such reaction would locally engender thrombosis. Further discussion of intervillositis is to be found at the end of this section.

Another of the few attempts at determining the precise nature of the inflammatory cells in villitis is that of Hart-

wick et al. (1989) in a case of fetal parvovirus B19 infection. They found the cells to have a T-cell derivation and provided some support for the fetal origin in this admittedly different disease. Although most of the inflammation in VUE is apparently histiocytic/lymphocytic, plasma cells (B-cell derived) occur as well but much less commonly. We have reason to believe that, in CMV infection, the plasma cells are fetal in origin. Histologic considerations had led us also to believe that in many cases the inflammatory cells of VUE are of fetal origin, but recent studies now indicate that in many instances the majority of the infiltrating cells are maternal cells. In addition, it is apparent that frequently the major inflammatory component is located within the anchoring villi. Also, they are often associated with maternal plasma cell infiltration of the decidua basalis. Indeed, chronic villitis may be *limited* to anchoring villi. Here, the cellular components have a maternal origin, and a dual derivation of the histiocytes, therefore, cannot be excluded. Labarrere et al. (1982) and Russell (1980) have also emphasized the frequent decidual involvement with lymphocytic inflammation and have suggested that VUE may have a relation to chronic endometritis. Whether the recurrent VUE in a patient with recurrent herpes gestationis described by Baxi et al. (1991) has a causal relation will remain unknown until more cases are studied.

The possibility of chronic brucellosis was entertained in a patient of ours with three consecutive pregnancy failures and histologic VUE (Figs. 20.72 and 20.73). Detailed study, however, was negative. In a later pregnancy, the progress was monitored with estriol levels, and when they declined, an elective cesarean section was performed. The growth-restricted infant did well and has remained healthy during the 15 years since this occurrence. The placenta was so severely involved with villitis that one wonders how this infant could have been born alive (Figs. 20.74 and 20.75). The lesion of the first preg-

FIGURE 20.73. Same case of VUE as in Figure 20.72. The villous destruction and cellular infiltration are pronounced; occasional plasma cells are present. H&E ×640.

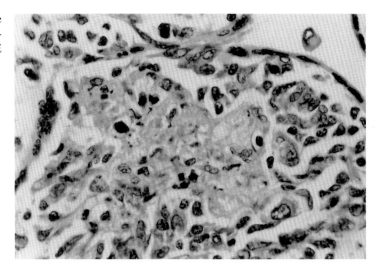

FIGURE 20.74. Placenta of the third pregnancy of a patient with recurrent losses and VUE (as in Figs. 20.72 and 20.73). Patient was also hypothyroid and on medication for this problem. When the amnionic fluid lecithin/sphingomyelin (L/S) ratio became more than 3:1, a cesarean section was done producing a viable fetus. Ten years later, the infant was well. Despite the extensive necrosis and inflammation, this infant weighed 2500 g at 37 weeks. The placenta was 510 g and had massive VUE with destruction of villi and trophoblast. H&E ×250.

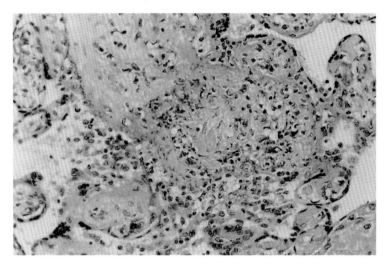

FIGURE 20.75. Same case as in Figure 20.74. Note the degeneration of the villous vessels. There is no trophoblast necrosis at this site, so the inflammatory cells are likely of fetal origin. H&E ×250.

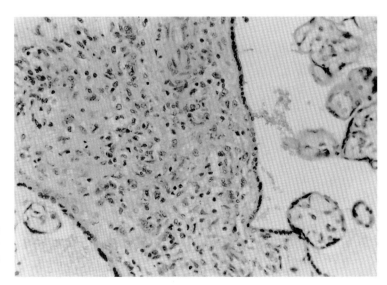

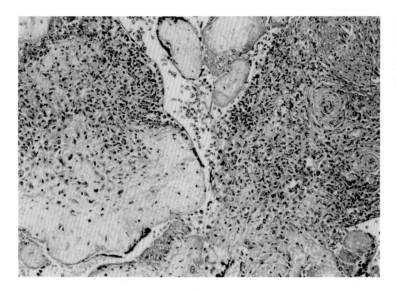

FIGURE 20.76. This placenta comes from the first still-born (at 37 weeks' gestation) of the patient with recurrent VUE (Figs. 20.72–20.75). There is even more necrosis and inflammation of villi than in the other pregnancies depicted. H&E ×100.

nancy was identical (Fig. 20.76). The severity and destructive nature of VUE is further exemplified in Figure 20.77, a stillborn, growth-restricted fetus. In yet another case, it was our opinion that the increased frequency of late decelerations during monitoring was caused by the placental lesions shown in Figure 20.78 (Benirschke, 1975). These inexplicable areas of villitis were scattered throughout the placenta. In the case of a severely compromised newborn, the placenta had many vascular occlusions and surface thrombi (Figs. 20.79 to 20.82). No virus infection was diagnosed. This picture is substantially different from the hemorrhagic endovasculitis (HEV) of Sander et al. (1986), which was discussed in Chapter 13.

The precise etiology of VUE is thus still unknown. In fact, we do not even know whether this is a uniform disease or one that, when it is better understood, falls into several etiologic categories. Altshuler and Hyde (1996) drew attention to the possible interaction of cytokines and ensuing fetal growth restriction. Infants can, however,

survive even severe placental villitis without showing subsequent impairment. Their long-term outcome requires much additional investigation. Three principal suggestions have been made with respect to the possible etiology of VUE:

1. It is an infectious (perhaps viral) disease, and due to an as yet unrecognized agent. That this concept has merit derives from the great histologic similarity of VUE to rubella and other known virus disorders that affect the placenta. Moreover, the discovery of parvovirus B19 infection and the similarity of placental response suggest that a viral agent must be sought in future studies. Furthermore, some of the common RNA viruses (Coxsackie, ECHO) are extremely difficult to recognize histologically or by electron microscopy. They also may cause few symptoms in the mother and may not be detected. The report by Garcia et al. (1991) brings this possibility into focus as well.

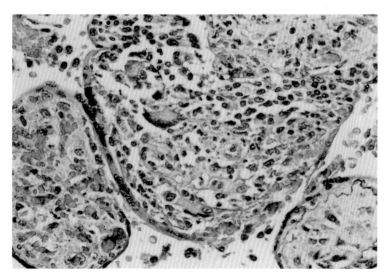

FIGURE 20.77. Villitis of unknown etiology in a stillborn fetus. The intense infiltration with lymphocytes, plasma cells, and histiocytes is widespread. Mineralization of the villous basement membrane is seen at bottom right. Several histiocytic giant cells are present in the central villus, whose trophoblast is degenerating focally. Vessels are obliterated. H&E ×640.

FIGURE 20.78. Mild chronic villitis in a 39-week pregnancy with good outcome. Late decelerations during labor were believed to be secondary to VUE. H&E ×250.

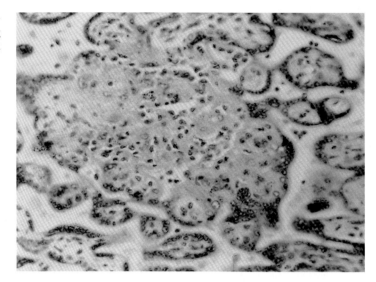

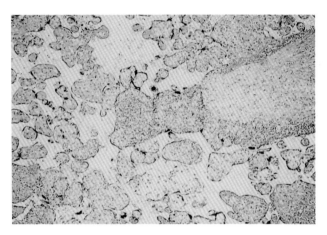

FIGURE 20.79. Severe chronic villitis in a premature infant with meconium aspiration. Extensive areas of villous destruction and inflammation are seen. H&E ×64.

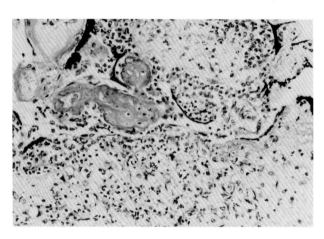

FIGURE 20.80. Same case as in Figure 20.79, showing the subtrophoblastic accumulation of lymphocytic infiltrate and villous necrosis. There were also chorionic vessel thrombi in this placenta. CMV and herpes infections were ruled out. H&E ×250.

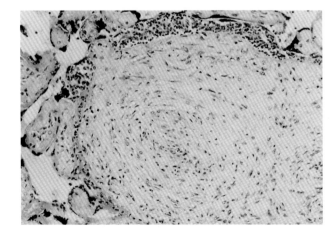

FIGURE 20.81. Same case as in Figures 20.79 and 20.80, again showing subtrophoblastic inflammatory cells and obliteration of villous stem vessel. H&E ×640.

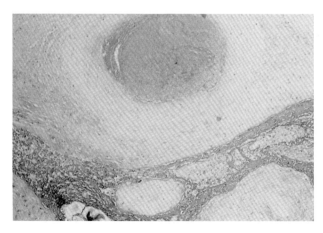

FIGURE 20.82. Same case as in Figures 20.79 to 20.81, showing an old thrombosis of a chorionic surface vessel in VUE. H&E ×64.

2. It is an immune reaction akin to placental "rejection" or even the graft-versus-host disease. Several investigators have raised this possibility, in particular because of the histiocytic predominance of the inflammatory reaction and the frequently recurrent episodes. At present, no new studies have conclusively shown or rejected this possibility. It is necessary to have more information on the "normal" fetomaternal immune interactions before this hypothesis can be rejected or affirmed. Moreover, professional immunologists need to be encouraged to become involved in the study of putative fetal antigen recognition. Redline and Abramowsky (1984) have commented on the possibility of the immune hypothesis. They found a 60% reproductive loss in patients with recurrent chronic villitis in contrast to a 37% loss in nonrecurrent villitis (Redline & Abramovsky, 1985). They suggested that VUE is much more common than heretofore believed; perhaps as many as 4% to 10% of placentas have some degree of VUE. They also suggested that "immunologic and structural abnormalities (uterine) in the host may play a role in its pathogenesis." Several of their patients had autoimmune diseases. Redline and Patterson (1993) found, with X-specific markers in male conceptuses' placentas, that approximately 60% of the infiltrating immunocytes of VUE represent maternal CD3 positive T-cells that have infiltrated from the intervillous space. This has now been proven. In studies conducted with a male fetus who succumbed in utero from this placental alteration was studied by colleagues of ours. They were able to show the fetal cells to lack the Y-chromosome marker conclusively, whereas it was present in all other villous and trophoblastic cells. The infiltrating cells were T cells and macrophages by immunocytochemistry, and of female gender. The reason for this response is presently unknown but is speculated upon in the contribution by Redline and Patterson. Essentially similar findings were made in the study by Kapur et al. (2004) and they found that essentially similar infiltrates of maternal origin characterized VUE as well as syphilitic villitis. One of our recent cases of VUE that led to fetal demise was also solely due to maternal infiltrates, as shown by Y-marker study. Greco and colleagues (1992) had also investigated the nature of villous stromal cells in VUE, syphilis, and CMV infection with a battery of antibodies and in situ hybridization. They concluded that these infiltrating elements had often markedly different phenotypes and that this was somewhat dependent on the nature of the underlying disease. They expressed an inability to decide about a possible immune reaction portrayed by this villitis (e.g., maternal cell invasion), but pointed out that "the expression of certain cellular markers for villous stromal cells is identical in both CMV and nonspecific villitis." For a review on the topic of placental nonrejection, see Hunt (1998). Labarrere et al. (1991) have championed this concept for

years, and much of their investigations are there summarized. From their evaluation of placentas derived from in vitro fertilizations, Styer et al. (2003) proposed that VUE is twice as common with donor eggs than native eggs and inferred an immunologic mechanism. This was confirmed more recently by Perni et al. (2005).

3. The disease has a relation to preeclampsia and infarcts. Most of the patients we have seen do not have signs of pregnancy toxemia, and the "villitis" that is associated with preeclampsia is different. It has much less inflammation and is mostly degenerative in nature and found adjacent to typical infarcts. Therefore, we prefer to reject this hypothesis.

Since the original description by Labarrere and Mullen (1987) that defined the entity, a large study of **chronic intervillositis** was undertaken by Boyd and Redline (2000). They studied 21 patients and showed it to be a major cause of IUGR, spontaneous abortion, and fetal death (77%). The recurrence rate was high (67%), and three patients were found to have fetal chromosomal errors. Moreover, there was much intervillous fibrin deposition and some placentas had infarcts. Autoimmune and allergic processes of different kinds were found in 52% of their patients. The cells composing this intervillous infiltrate were of the TH1-type response and included activated macrophages as well as a smattering of other cells. Although this condition is not very common, it does represent an important aspect of fetal demise and IUGR. The authors emphasized that malaria needs to be excluded, as was earlier suggested. This can only be done by careful search for intervillous erythrocytic parasites and hemozoin deposits. A representative example of chronic intervillositis is shown in Figures 20.83 to 20.85. The severely IUGR fetus of this gestation was stillborn at about 17 weeks' gestation and the mother had one earlier abortion and one normal child. There was excessive fibrin deposition in the entire placenta and massive infiltration of the intervillous space by macrophages (CD68 cells). There was no chronic villitis, however, and there was no significant X-cell proliferation as is seen in maternal floor infarction (MFI). The mother had no history or symptoms of autoimmune or allergic diseases. Interestingly, one large maternal vessel of the decidua basalis was thrombosed.

Chronic intervillositis and VUE are sometimes combined, but in our experience this is not really common and we consider the two histologic entities to be different. At this time, the only certain and common finding is that VUE is not the result of infection with common, known pathogens. No virus or other agent has been consistently identified. Moreover, the children who are born from such pregnancies, many of whom are small for gestational age (SGA), develop normally. The efforts of

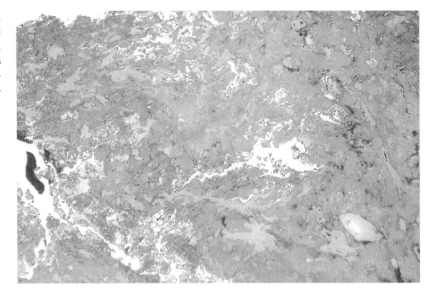

FIGURE 20.83. Low-power microphotograph of a typical case of chronic intervillositis. The entire placenta had this much fibrin deposition and collections of intervillous macrophages (dark blue). The intrauterine growth restriction (IUGR) fetus was stillborn but structurally normal.

several laboratories to identify the origin and nature of the inflammatory infiltrate suggest that a majority of the infiltrating cells is of maternal origin. Whether this is tantamount to an immune "rejection" phenomenon mounted by the mother against the placenta needs further investigation. The fact that the surviving infants of VUE placentas remain well and that the disease frequently recurs in families point in that direction. A recent comprehensive review of the frequency and relationship to IUGR and fetal demise has come from Becroft et al. (2005).

Likewise, chronic intervillositis has no definitive causal mechanism identified to date. It also may represent different end points of disease, such as malaria and maternal allergic conditions. Much more work is needed to unravel the complexity of these entities.

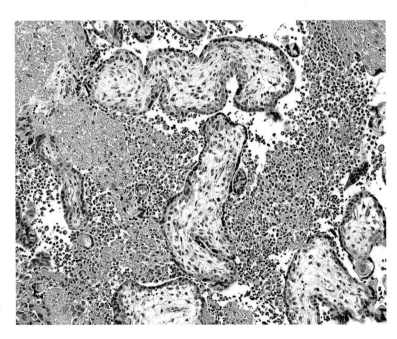

FIGURE 20.84. Chronic intervillositis at higher magnification with fibrin deposits and disuse infiltration of chronic inflammatory cells in the intervillous space.

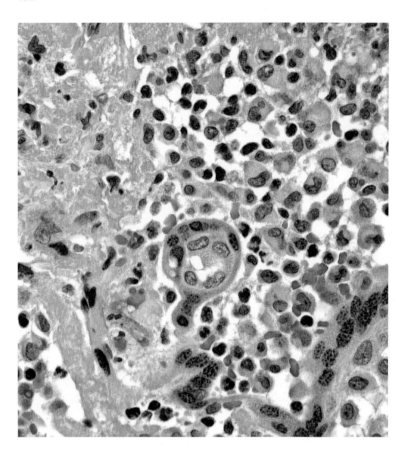

FIGURE 20.85. Still higher magnification of chronic intervillositis showing the chronic inflammatory cells (mostly activated macrophages), little villous erosion, and fibrin deposits.

References

Abadi, M.A. and Abadi, J.: *Actinomyces* chorioamnionitis and preterm labor in a twin pregnancy: a case report. Amer. J. Obstet. Gynecol. **175**:1391–1392, 1996.

Abbasi, I.A., Hemming, V.G., Eglinton, G.S. and Johnson, T.R.B.: Proliferation of group B streptococci in human amniotic fluid in vitro. Amer. J. Obstet. Gynecol. **156**:95–99, 1987.

Abbink, F.C., Orendi, J.M. and Beaufort, A.J. de: Mother-to-child transmission of *Burkholderia pseudomallei*. NEJM **344**:1171, 2001.

Abraham, A.A.: Herpesvirus hominis endometritis in a young woman wearing an intrauterine contraceptive device. Amer. J. Obstet. Gynecol. **131**:340–342, 1978.

Abramowsky, C., Beyer-Patterson, P. and Cortinas, E.: Non-syphilitic spirochetosis in second trimester fetuses. Pediatr. Pathol. **11**:827–838, 1991.

Aherne, W. and Davies, P.A.: Congenital pneumonia. Lancet **1**:275, 1962.

Ahlfors, C.E., Goetzman, B.W., Halsted, C.C., Sherman, M.P. and Wennberg, R.P.: Neonatal listeriosis. Amer. J. Dis. Child. **131**:405–408, 1977.

Ahlfors, K., Ivarsson, S.-A. and Nilsson, H.: On the unpredictable development of congenital cytomegalovirus infection: a study of twins. Early Hum. Dev. **18**:125–135, 1988.

Akinbi, H.T., Narendran, V., Pass, A.K., Markart, P. and Hoath, S.B.: Host defense proteins in vernix caseosa and amniotic fluid. Amer. J. Obstet. Gynecol. **191**:2090–2096, 2004.

Alford, C.A., Neva, F.A. and Weller, T.H.: Virologic and serologic studies on human products of conception after maternal rubella. NEJM **271**:1275–1281, 1964.

Alford, C.A., Stagno, S. and Reynolds, D.W.: Diagnosis of chronic perinatal infections. Amer. J. Dis. Child. **129**:455–463, 1975.

Alger, L.S., Lovchik, J.C., Hebel, J.R., Blackmon, L.R. and Crenshaw, M.C.: The association of Chlamydia trachomatis, Neisseria gonorrhoeae, and group B streptococci with premature rupture of the membranes and pregnancy outcome. Amer. J. Obstet. Gynecol. **159**:397–404, 1988.

Alger, L.S., Farley, J.J., Robinson, B.A., Hines, S.E., Berchin, J.M. and Johnson, J.P.: Interactions of human immunodeficiency virus infection and pregnancy. Obstet. Gynecol. **82**:787–796, 1993.

Alkalay, A.L., Pomerance, J.J. and Rimoin, D.L.: Fetal varicella syndrome. J. Pediatr. **111**:320–323, 1987.

Alpert, S.G., Fergerson, J. and Noel, L.P.: Intrauterine West Nile virus: ocular and systemic findings. Amer. J. Ophthalmol. **136**:733–735, 2003.

Al-Salihi, F.L., Curran, J.P. and Wang, J.-S.: Neonatal Trichomonas vaginalis: report of three cases and review of the literature. Pediatrics **53**:196–200, 1974.

Althuisius, S.M., Dekker, G.A., von Geijn, H.P., Bekedam, D.J. and Hummel, P.: Cervical incompetence prevention randomized cerclage trial (CIPRACT): Study design and preliminary results. Amer. J. Obstet. Gynecol. **183**:823–829, 2000.

Altshuler, G.: Implications of two cases of human placental plasma cells? Reports of cytomegalic inclusion disease in a thirteen week's fetus and of ascending herpes infection of the newborn. Amer. J. Pathol. **70**:18a, 1973a.

Altshuler, G.: Toxoplasmosis as a cause of hydranencephaly. Amer. J. Dis. Child. **125**:251–252, 1973b.

Altshuler, G.: Placental villitis of unknown etiology: harbinger of serious disease? A four months' experience of nine cases. J. Reprod. Med. **11**:215–222, 1973c.

Altshuler, G.: Pathogenesis of congenital herpesvirus infection: case report including a description of the placenta. Amer. J. Dis. Child. **127**:427–429, 1974.

Altshuler, G.: Placental infection, and inflammation. In, Pathology of the Placenta. E.V.D.K. Perrin, ed., pp.141–163. Churchill Livingstone, New York, 1984.

Altshuler, G.: The placenta. In, Diagnostic Surgical Pathology. S.S. Sternberg, ed., pp. 1503–1522. Raven Press, New York, 1989.

Altshuler, G.: Role of the placenta in perinatal pathology (revisited). Pediatr. Pathol. Lab. Med. **16**:207–233, 1996.

Altshuler, G. and Hyde, S.: Fusobacteria: an important cause of chorioamnionitis. Arch Pathol. Lab. Med. **109**:739–743, 1985.

Altshuler, G. and Hyde, S.: Clinicopathologic considerations of fusobacteria chorioamnionitis. Acta Obstet. Gynecol. Scand. **67**:513–517, 1988.

Altshuler, G. and Hyde, S.: Clinicopathologic implications of placental pathology. Clin. Obstet. Gynecol. **39**:549–570, 1996.

Altshuler, G. and McAdams, A.J.: Cytomegalic inclusion disease of a nineteen-week fetus: case report including a study of the placenta. Amer. J. Obstet. Gynecol. **111**:295–298, 1971.

Altshuler, G. and Russell, P.: The human villitides: A review of chronic intrauterine infection. Curr. Top. Pathol. **60**:63–112, 1975.

Amirhessami-Aghili, N., Manalo, P., Hall, M.R., Tibbitts, F.D., Ort, C.A. and Afsari, A.: Human cytomegalovirus infection of human placental explants in culture: histologic and immunohistochemical studies. Amer. J. Obstet. Gynecol. **156**:1365–1374, 1987.

Amirhessami-Aghili, N. and Spector, S.A.: Human immunodeficiency virus type 1 infection of human placenta: Potential route for fetal infection. J. Virol. **65**:2231–2236, 1991.

Amory, J.H., Hitti, J., Lawler, R. and Eschenbach, D.A.: Increased tumor necrosis factor-á production after lipopolysaccharide stimulation of whole blood in patients with previous preterm delivery complicated by intra-amniotic infection or inflammation. Amer. J. Obstet. Gynecol. **185**:1064–1067, 2001.

Amstey, M.S.: Group B streptococcus and premature rupture of membranes. Amer. J. Obstet. Gynecol. **143**:607–608, 1982.

Amstey, M.S., Miller, R.K., Menegus, M.A. and di Sant'Agnese, P.A.: Enterovirus in pregnant women and the perfused placenta. Amer. J. Obstet. Gynecol. **158**:775–782, 1988.

Anderson, G.S., Green, C.A., Neligan, G.A., Newell, D.J. and Russell, J.K.: Congenital bacterial pneumonia. Lancet **2**:585–587, 1962.

Anderson, T.D., Meador, V.P. and Cheville, N.F.: Pathogenesis of placentitis in the goat inoculated with *Brucella abortus*. I. Gross and histologic lesions. Vet. Pathol. **23**:219–226, 1986a.

Anderson, T.D., Meador, V.P. and Cheville, N.F.: Pathogenesis of placentitis in the goat inoculated with *Brucella abortus*. II. Ultrastructural studies. Vet. Pathol. **23**:227–239, 1986b.

Andiman, W.A., Simpson, J., Olson, B., Dember, L., Silva, T.J. and Miller, G.: Rate of transmission of human immunodefi-

ciency virus type 1 infection from mother to child and short-term outcome of neonatal infection. Amer. J. Dis. Child. **144**:758–766, 1990.

Andreu, A., Genover, E., Coira, A. and Farran, I.: Antepartum infection as a result of Streptococcus pneumoniae and sepsis in neonate. Amer. J. Obstet. Gynecol. **161**:1424–1425, 1989.

Andrews, W.W., Hauth, J.C., Goldenberg, R.L., Gomez, R., Romero, R. and Cassell, G.H.: Amniotic fluid interleukin-6: correlation with upper genital tract microbial colonization and gestational age in women delivered after spontaneous labor versus indicated delivery. Amer. J. Obstet. Gynecol. **173**:606–612, 1995.

Andrews, W.W., Lee, H.H., Roden, W.J. and Mott, C.W.: Detection of genitourinary tract *Chlamydia trachomatis* infection in pregnant women by ligase reaction assay. Obstet. Gynecol. **89**:556–560, 1997.

Andrews, W.W., Goldenberg, R.L., Mercer, B., Iams, J., Meis, P., Moawad, A., Das, A., VanDorsten, J.P., Caritis, S.N., Thurnau, G., Miodovnik, M., Roberts, J. and McNellis, D.: The preterm prediction study: Association of second-trimester genitourinary Chlamydia infection with subsequent spontaneous preterm birth. Amer. J. Obstet. Gynecol. **183**:662–668, 2000.

Anonymous: Group-B streptococci in the newborn. Lancet **1**:520–521, 1977a.

Anonymous: The Shirodkar stitch. Lancet **2**:691–692, 1977b.

Anonymous: Perinatal listeriosis. Lancet **1**:911, 1980.

Anonymous: Avoiding damage to the cervix. Lancet **2**:552–553, 1983a.

Anonymous: How does Brucella abortus infect human beings? Lancet **2**:1180, 1983b.

Anonymous: Malaria in pregnancy. Lancet **2**:84–85, 1983c.

Anonymous: Does coitus embarrass the fetus? Lancet **1**:374–375, 1984.

Anonymous: Listeriosis. Lancet **2**:364–365, 1985.

Anonymous: Rapid detection of beta haemolytic streptococci. Lancet **1**:247–248, 1986.

Anonymous: Chorioamnionitis: cause or effect? Lancet **1**:362, 1989a.

Anonymous: Herpes simplex virus latency. Lancet **1**:194–195, 1989b.

Anonymous: Screening for congenital CMV. Lancet **2**:599–600, 1989c.

Aquino, T.I., Zhang, J., Kraus, F.T., Knefel, R. and Taff, T.: Subchorionic fibrin cultures for bacteriologic study of the placenta. Amer. J. Clin. Pathol. **81**:482–486, 1984.

Araujo, M.C.K. de, Schultz, R., Vaz, F.A.C., Massad, E., Feferbaum, R., Araujo Ramos, J.L. de: A case-control study of histological chorioamnionitis and neonatal infection. Early Hum. Devel. **40**:51–58, 1994.

Araujo, M.C.K. de, Schultz, R., Latorre, M.do R.D de, Ramos, J.L.A. and Vaz, F.A.C.: A risk factor for early-onset infection in premature newborns: invasion of chorioamniotic tissues by leukocytes. Early Human Devel. **56**:1–15, 1999.

Arias, F., Rodriguez, L., Rayne, S.C. and Kraus, F.T.: Maternal placental vasculopathy and infection: Two distinct subgroups among patients with preterm labor and preterm ruptured membranes. Amer. J. Obstet. Gynecol. **168**:585–591, 1993.

Arias, F., Victoria, A., Cho, K. and Kraus, F.: Placental histology and clinical characteristics of patients with preterm premature rupture of membranes. Obstet. Gynecol. **89**:265–271, 1997.

Arntzen, K.J., Kjoellesdal, A.M., Halgunset, J., Vatten, L. and Austgulen, R.: TNF, IL-1, IL-6, IL-8 and soluble TNF receptors in relation to chorioamnionitis and premature labor. J. Perinat. Med. **26**:17–26, 1998.

Ascher, D.P., Becker, J.A., Yoder, B.A., Weisse, M., Waecker, N.J., Heroman, W.M., Davis, C., Fajardo, J.E. and Fischer, G.W.: Failure of intrapartum antibiotics to prevent culture-proved neonatal group B streptococcal sepsis. J. Perinatol. **13**:212–216, 1993.

Asrat, T., Lewis, D.F., Garite, T.J., Major, C.A., Nageotte, M.P., Towers, C.V., Montgomery, D.M. and Dorchester, W.A.: Rate of recurrence of preterm premature rupture of membranes in consecutive pregnancies. Amer. J. Obstet. Gynecol. **165**:1111–1115, 1991.

Awadalla, S.G., Mercer, L.J. and Brown, L.G.: Pregnancy complicated by intraamniotic infection by Salmonella typhi. Obstet. Gynecol. **65**:30S–31S, 1985.

Azzarelli, B. and Lafuze, J.: Amniotic basement membrane: a barrier to neutrophil invasion. Amer. J. Obstet. Gynecol. **156**:1130–1136, 1987.

Azziz, R., Cummings, J. and Naeye, R.: Acute myometritis and chorioamnionitis during cesarean section of asymptomatic women. Amer. J. Obstet. Gynecol. **159**:1137–1139, 1988.

Baddeley, P. and Shardlow, J.P.: Antenatal gonococcal arthritis. J. Obstet. Gynaecol. Br. Commonw. **80**:186–187, 1973.

Bader, G.: Beitrag zur Chorioamnionitis mycotica. Arch. Gynäkol. **203**:251–225, 1966.

Baergen, R., Benirschke, K. and Ulich, T.R.: Cytokine expression in the placenta. The role of interleukin 1 and interleukin 1 receptor antagonist expression in chorioamnionitis and parturition. Arch. Pathol. Lab. Med. **118**:52–55, 1994.

Baker, C.J.: Summary of workshop on perinatal infections due to Group B streptococcus. J. Infect. Dis. **136**:137–152, 1977.

Baker, C.J., Rench, M.A., Edwards, M.S., Carpenter, R.J., Hays, B.M. and Kasper, D.L.: Immunization of pregnant women with a polysaccharide vaccine of group B streptococcus. NEJM **319**:1180–1185, 1988.

Balabat, A.B.N., Jordan, G.W. and Halsted, C.: Congenital malaria in a nonidentical twin. Western Med. J. **162**:458–459, 1995.

Balducci, J., Rodis, J.F., Rosengren, S., Vintzileos, A.M., Spivey, G. and Vosseller, C.: Pregnancy outcome following first-trimester varicella infection. Obstet. Gynecol. **79**:5–6, 1992.

Baldwin, V. and Whitley, R.J.: Teratogen update: intrauterine herpes simplex virus infection. Teratology **39**:1–10, 1989.

Ballantyne, J.W.: Manual of Antenatal Pathology and Hygiene. The Embryo. Wm. Greene & Sons, Edinburgh, 1904.

Banatvala, J.E. and Brown, D.W.G.: Rubella. Lancet **363**:1127–1137, 2004.

Baniecki, H.: Über den Wert der histologischen Luesdiagnose der Nabelschnur. Z. Geburtsh. Gynäkol. **93**:313–315, 1928.

Barefoot, K.H., Little, G.A. and Ornvold, K.T.: Fetal demise due to herpes simplex virus: An illustrated case report. J. Perinatol. **22**:86–88, 2002.

Barford, D.A.G. and Rosen, M.G.: Cervical incompetence: diagnosis and outcome. Obstet. Gynecol. **64**:159–163, 1984.

Barresi, J.A.: Listeria monocytogenes: a cause of premature labor and neonatal sepsis. Amer. J. Obstet. Gynecol. **136**:410–411, 1980.

Barsky, P. and Beale, A.J.: The transplacental transmission of poliomyelitis. J. Pediatr. **51**:207–211, 1957.

Barter, R.A.: Congenital pneumonia. Lancet **1**:165, 1962.

Bartnicki, J., Casal, D., Kreadin, U.S., Saling, E. and Vetter, K.: Fetal fibronectin in vaginal specimens predict preterm delivery and very-low-birth-weight infants. Amer. J. Obstet. Gynecol. **174**:971–924, 1996.

Barton, J.J., O'Connor, T.M., Cannon, M.J. and Weldon-Linne, C.M.: Prevalence of human immunodeficiency virus in a general prenatal population. Amer. J. Obstet. Gynecol. **160**:1316–1324, 1989.

Barton, J.R., Thorpe, E.M., Shaver, D.C., Hager, W.D. and Sibai, B.M.: Nonimmune hydrops fetalis associated with maternal infection with syphilis. Amer. J. Obstet. Gynecol. **167**:56–58, 1992.

Barton, L.L., Cruz, R.D. and Walentik, C.: Neonatal Haemophilus influenzae type C sepsis. Amer. J. Dis. Child. **136**:463–464, 1982.

Batcup, G., Holt, P., Hambling, M.H., Gerlis, L.M. and Glass, M.R.: Placental and fetal pathology in Coxsackie virus A9 infection: a case report. Histopathology **9**:1227–1235, 1985.

Baxi, L.V., Kovilam, O.P., Collins, M.H. and Walther, R.R.: Recurrent herpes gestationis with postpartum flare: A case report. Amer. J. Obstet. Gynecol. **164**:778–780, 1991.

Becket, R.S. and Flynn, F.J.: Toxoplasmosis: report of two new cases, with a classification and with a demonstration of the organisms in human placenta. NEJM **249**:345–350, 1953.

Beckmann, S. and Zimmer, E.: Über die Bedeutung der "Nabelschnurentzündung." Arch. Gynäkol. **145**:194–218, 1931.

Becroft, D.M., Thompson, J.M. and Mitchell, E.A.: Placental villitis of unknown origin: Epidemiologic associations. Amer. J. Obstet. Gynecol. **192**:264–271, 2005.

Bedolla, G. and Stanek, J.: Intrauterine hematogenous herpetic infection. Arch. Pathol. Lab. Med. **128**:1189–1190, 2004.

Beinder, E., Lohoff, M., Rauch, R. and Volker, U.: Discrepant outcome of intrauterine listeria infection in dichorionic twins. Z. Geburtsh. Neonatol. **203** Suppl. **2**:12–15, 1999.

Beitzke, H.: Über die angeborene tuberkulöse Infection. Ergebn. Ges. Tuberk. Forsch. **7**:1–30, 1935.

Bejar, R., Curbelo, V., Davis, C. and Gluck, L.: Premature labor. II. Bacterial sources of phospholipase. Obstet. Gynecol. **57**:479–482, 1981.

Bendon, R.W., Perez, F. and Ray, M.B.: Herpes simplex virus: fetal and decidual infection. Pediatr. Pathol. **7**:63–70, 1987.

Bendon, R.W., Bornstein, S. and Faye-Petersen, O.M.: Two fetal deaths associated with maternal sepsis and with thrombosis of the intervillous space of the placenta. Placenta **19**:385–389, 1998.

Bengtson, J.M., VanMarter, L.J., Barss, V.A., Greene, M.F., Tuomala, R.E. and Epstein, M.F.: Pregnancy outcome after premature rupture of the membranes at or before 26 weeks' gestation. Obstet. Gynecol. **73**:921–927, 1989.

Benirschke, K.: Routes and types of infection in the fetus and the newborn. Amer. J. Dis. Child. **99**:714–721, 1960.

Benirschke, K.: Diseases of the placenta. Contemp. Obstet. Gynecol. **6**:17–20, 1975.

Benirschke, K. and Altshuler, G.: The future of perinatal physiopathology. In, Symposium on the Functional Physiopathology of the Fetus and Neonate. H. Abramson ed., pp. 158–168, Mosby, St. Louis, 1971.

Benirschke, K. and Driscoll, S.G.: The Pathology of the Human Placenta. Springer-Verlag, New York, 1967.

Benirschke, K. and Raphael, S.I.: Candida albicans infection of the amniotic sac. Amer. J. Obstet. Gynecol. **75**:200–202, 1958.

Benirschke, K., Mendoza, G.R. and Bazeley, P.L.: Placental and fetal manifestations of cytomegalovirus infection. Virchows Arch. [B] **16**:121–139, 1974.

Benirschke, K., Swartz, W.H., Leopold, G. and Sahn, D.: Hydrops due to myocarditis in a fetus. Amer. J. Cardiovasc. Pathol. **1**:131–133, 1986.

Benirschke, K., Coen, R., Patterson, B. and Key, T.: Villitis of known origin. Varicella and toxoplasma. Placenta **20**:395–399, 1999.

Benner, M.C.: Congenital infection of the lungs, middle ears and nasal accessory sinuses. Arch. Pathol. **29**:455–472, 1940.

Bennett, P.R. and Elder, M.G.: The mechanisms of preterm labor: common genital tract pathogens do not metabolize arachidonic acid to prostaglandins or to other eicosanoids. Amer. J. Obstet. Gynecol. **166**:1541–1545, 1992.

Bennett, P.R., Rose, M.P., Myatt, L. and Elder, M.G.: Preterm labor: stimulation of arachidonic acid metabolism in human amnion cells by bacterial products. Amer. J. Obstet. Gynecol. **156**:649–655, 1987.

Benshushan, A., Tsafrir, A., Arbel, R., Rahav, G., Ariel, I. and Rojansky, N.: Listeria infection during pregnancy: a 10 year experience. Isr. Med. Assoc. J. **4**:776–780, 2002.

Berche, P., Reich, K.A., Bonnichon, M., Beretti, J.-L., Geoffroy, C., Raveneau, J., Cossart, P., Gaillard, J.-L., Geslin, P., Kreis, H. and Veron, M.: Detection of anti-listeriolysin 0 for serodiagnosis of human listeriosis. Lancet **335**:624–627, 1990).

Berg, B.J.v.d.: Coitus and amniotic-fluid infections. NEJM **302**:632, 1980.

Berger, S.A., Weinberg, M., Treves, T., Sorkin, P., Geller, E., Yedwab, G., Tomer, A., Rabey, M. and Michaeli, D.: Herpes encephalitis during pregnancy: failure of acyclovir and adenine arabinoside to prevent neonatal herpes. Isr. J. Med. Sci. **22**:41–44, 1986.

Bernstein, D.I., Tipton, J.R., Schott, S.F. and Cherry, J.D.: Coccidioidomycosis in a neonate: maternal-infant transmission. J. Pediatr. **99**:752–754, 1981.

Berrebi, A., Puel, J., Federlin, M., Gayet, C., Kobuch, W.E., Monrozies, X. and Watrigant, M.P.: Transmission du HIV (human immunodeficiency virus) de la mère à l'enfant. Rev. Franç. Gynécol. Obstet. **82**:25–28, 1987.

Berry, S.M., Fine, N., Bichalski, J.A., Cotton, D.B., Dombrowski, M.P. and Kaplan, J.: Circulating lymphocyte subsets in second- and third-trimester fetuses: Comparison with newborns and adults. Amer. J. Obstet. Gynecol. **167**:895–900, 1992.

Biggio, J.R., Ramsey, P.S., Cliver, S.P., Lyon, M.D., Goldenberg, R.L. and Wenstrom, K.D.: Midtrimester amniotic fluid matrix metalloproteinase-8 (MMP-8) levels above the 90th percentile are a marker for subsequent preterm premature rupture of membranes. Amer. J. Obstet. Gynecol. **191**:109–113, 2004.

Binns, B., Williams, T., McDowell, J. and Brunham, R.C.: Screening for Chlamydia trachomatis infection in a pregnancy counseling clinic. Amer. J. Obstet. Gynecol. **159**:1144–1149, 1988.

Bittencourt, A.L.: Congenital Chagas disease. Amer. J. Dis. Child. **130**:97–103, 1976.

Bittencourt, A.L., Cardoso de Almeida, M.A., Iunes, M.A.F. and Casulari da Motta, L.D.C.: Placental involvement in schistosomiasis mansoni. Report of four cases. Amer. J. Trop. Med. Hyg. **29**:571–575, 1980.

Bittencourt, A.L., de Freitas, L.A.R., Galvao, M.O. and Jacomo, K.: Pneumonitis in congenital Chagas' disease: a study of ten cases. Amer. J. Trop. Med. Hyg. **30**:38–42, 1981.

Bittencourt, A.L., dos Santos, W.L.C. and de Oliveira, C.H.: Placental and fetal candidiasis: presentation of a case of an abortus. Mycopathologia **87**:181–187, 1984.

Blanc, W.A.: Infection amniotique et néonatale: diagnostic cytologique rapide. Gynaecologia **136**:101–110, 1953.

Blanc, W.A.: Role of the amniotic infection syndrome in perinatal pathology. Bull. Sloane Hosp. **3**:79–85, 1957.

Blanc, W.A.: Amniotic sac infection syndrome: pathogenesis, morphology and significance in circumnatal mortality. Clin. Obstet. Gynecol. **2**:705–734, 1959.

Blanc, W.A.: Amniotic infection syndrome: practical significance and quick diagnostic test. N.Y. State J. Med. **61**:1487–1492, 1961a.

Blanc, W.A.: Pathways of fetal and early neonatal infection: viral placentitis, bacterial and fungal chorioamnionitis. J. Pediatr. **59**:473–496, 1961b.

Blanc, W.A.: Pathology of the placenta, membranes, and umbilical cord in bacterial, fungal, and viral infections in man. In, Perinatal Diseases. R.L. Naeye, J.M. Kissane and N. Kaufman, eds., pp. 67–132. Williams & Wilkins, Baltimore, 1981.

Blanco, J.D., Gibbs, R.S. and Krebs, L.F.: A controlled study of amniotic fluid immunoglobulin levels in intraamniotic infection. Obstet. Gynecol. **61**:450–453, 1983.

Blej-Rak, T., Okun, N., Windrim, R., Ross, S. and Hannah, M.E.: Effectiveness of cervical cerclage for a sonographically shortened cervix: a systematic review and meta-analysis. Amer. J. Obstet. Gynecol. **189**:1679–1687, 2003.

Bobitt, J.R. and Ledger, W.J.: Unrecognized amnionitis and prematurity: a preliminary report. J. Reprod. Med. **19**:8–12, 1977.

Bobitt, J.R., Hayslip, C.C. and Damato, J.D.: Amniotic fluid infection as determined by transabdominal amniocentesis in patients with intact membranes in premature labor. Amer. J. Obstet. Gynecol. **140**:947–952, 1981.

Boesaart, J.W.: Een geval van placenta-tuberculose. Nederl. Tijdschr. Geneesk. **103**:1849–1852, 1959.

Boon, M.E., van Raavenswaay Claasen, H.H. and Kok, L.P.: Urbanization and baseline prevalence of genital infections including Candida, Trichomonas, and human papillomavirus and of a disturbed vaginal ecology as established in the Dutch cervical screening program. Amer. J. Obstet. Gynecol. **187**:365–369, 2002.

Boppana, S.B., Rivera, L.B., Fowler, K.B., Mach, M. and Britt, W.: Intrauterine transmission of cytomegalovirus to infants of women with preconceptional immunity. NEJM **344**:1366–1371, 2001.

Borglin, N.E.: Placental function in incompetence of the internal os of the cervix. Fertil. Steril. **13**:575–582, 1962.

Borisch, B., Jahn, G., Scholl, B.-C., Filger-Brillinger, J., Heymer, B., Fleckenstein, B. and Müller-Hermelink, H.K.: Detection of human cytomegalovirus DNA and viral antigens in tissues of different manifestations of CMV infection. Virchows Arch. [B] **55**:93–99, 1988.

Bortolussi, R., Issekutz, T., Burbridge, S. and Schellekens, H.: Neonatal host defense mechanisms against Listeria monocytogenes infection: the role of lipopolysaccharides and interferons. Pediatr. Res. **25**:311–315, 1989.

Boucher, M. and Yonekura, M.L.: Perinatal listeriosis (early-onset): correlation of antenatal manifestations and neonatal outcome. Obstet. Gynecol. **68**:593–597, 1986.

Boucher, M., Yonekura, M.L., Wallace, R.J. and Phelan, J.P.: Adult respiratory distress syndrome: a rare manifestation of Listeria monocytogenes infection in pregnancy. Amer. J. Obstet. Gynecol. **149**:686–688, 1984.

Boué, A. and Loffredo, V.: Avortement causé par le virus de l'herpès type II: isolement du virus à partir de tissus zygotiques. Presse Méd. **78**:103–106, 1970.

Boukhari, E., Mazroud, A.A., Zamil, F.A. and Kilani, R.A.: *Listeria monocytogenes* bacteremia and meningitis in a Saudi newborn. Ann. Saudi Med. **19**:539–540, 1999.

Boussemart, T., Babe, P., Sibille, G., Neyret, C. and Berchel, C.: Prenatal transmission of dengue: two new cases. J. Perinatol. **21**: 255–257, 2001

Bowmer, E.J., McKiel, J.A., Cockcroft, W.H., Schmitt, N. and Rappay, D.E.: Listeria monocytogenes infections in Canada. Can. Med. Assoc. J. **109**:125–135, 1973.

Boyd, T.K. and Redline, R.W.: Chronic histiocytic intervillositis: a placental lesion associated with recurrent reproductive loss. Hum. Pathol. **31**:1389–1396, 2000.

Boyer, K.M. and Gotoff, S.P.: Prevention of early-onset neonatal group B streptococcal disease with selective intrapartum chemoprophylaxis. NEJM **314**:1665–1669, 1986.

Brady, K., Martin, A., Page, D., Purdy, S. and Neiman, R.S.: Localization of human immunodeficiency virus in placental tissue. Mod. Pathol. **2**:11A, 1989 (abstract 63).

Braunstein, H.: Congenital syphilis in aborted second trimester fetus: diagnosis by histological study. J. Clin. Pathol. **31**:265–267, 1978.

Bray, R.S. and Sinden, R.E.: The sequestration of Plasmodium falciparum infected erythrocytes in the placenta. Trans. R. Soc. Trop. Med. Hyg. **73**:716–719, 1979.

Brazin, S.A., Simkovich, J.W. and Johnson, W.T.: Herpes zoster during pregnancy. Obstet. Gynecol. **53**:175–181, 1979.

Breer, C. and Schopfer, K.: Listeria and food. Lancet **2**:1022, 1988.

Bret, J. and Coupe, C.: Vaginites et infection neo-natale: étiologie des mycoses du nouveau-né. Presse Méd. **66**:937–938, 1958.

Broekhuizen, F.F., Gilman, M. and Hamilton, P.R.: Amniocentesis for Gram stain and culture in preterm premature rupture of the membranes. Obstet. Gynecol. **66**:316–321, 1985.

Brown, Z.A., Selke, S., Zeh, J., Kopelman, J., Maslow, A., Ashley, R.L., Watts, H., Berry, S., Herd, M. and Corey, L.: The acquisition of herpes simplex virus during pregnancy. NEJM **337**:509–515, 1997.

Brown, Z.A., Vontver, L.A., Benedetti, J., Critchlow, C.W., Sells, C.J., Berry, S. and Corey, L.: Effects on infants of a first episode of genital herpes during pregnancy. NEJM **317**:1246–1251, 1987.

Browne, F.J.: Congenital pneumonia. Lancet **1**:748, 1962.

Bruce-Chwatt, L.J.: Low birthweight. Lancet **1**:1161, 1966.

Bruder, E., Ersch, J., Hebisch, G., Ehrbar, T., Klimkait, T. and Stallmach, T.: Fetal varicella syndrome: disruption of neural development and persistent inflammation of non-neural tissues. Virchows Arch. **437**:440–444, 2000.

Brunham, R.C., Paavonen, J., Stevens, C.E., Kiviat, N., Kuo, C.-C., Critchlow, C.W. and Holmes, K.K.: Mucopurulent cervicitis—the ignored counterpart in women of urethritis in men. NEJM **311**:1–6, 1984.

Bryant, R.E., Windom, R.E., Vineyard, J.P., Sanford, J.P. and Mays, B.A.: Asymptomatic bacteriuria in pregnancy and its association with prematurity. J. Lab. Clin. Med. **63**:224–231, 1964.

Buchanan, R. and Sworn, M.J.: Abortion associated with intra-uterine infection by Candida albicans: case report. Br. J. Obstet. Gynaecol. **86**:741–744, 1979.

Buchholz, H.M., Frösner, G.G. and Ziegler, G.B.: HBAg carrier state in an infant delivered by cesarean section. Lancet **2**:343, 1974.

Cairo, M.S.: Neonatal neutrophil host defense: prospects for immunologic enhancement during neonatal sepsis. Amer. J. Dis. Child. **143**:40–46, 1989.

Callaway, C.S., Walls, K.W. and Hicklin, M.D.: Electron microscopic studies of Toxoplasma gondii in fresh and frozen tissue. Arch. Pathol. **86**:484–491, 1968.

Campognone P. and Singer, D.B.: Neonatal sepsis due to nontypable Haemophilus influenzae. Amer. J. Dis. Child. **140**:117–121, 1986.

Carey, J.C., Blackwelder, W.C., Nugent, R.P., Matteson, M.A., Rao, A.V., Eschenbach, D.A., Lee, M.L.F., Rettig, P.J., Regan, J.A., Geromanos, K.L., Martin, D.H., Pastorek, J.G., Gibbs, R.S., Lipscomb, K.A and the Vaginal Infections and Prematurity Study Group: Antepartum cultures for *Ureaplasma urealyticum* are not useful in predicting pregnancy outcome. Amer. J. Obstet. Gynecol. **164**:728–733, 1991.

Carey, J.C., Klebanoff, M.A., Hauth, J.C., Hillier, S.L., Thom, E.A., Ernest, J.M., Heine, R.P., Nugent, R.P., Fischer, M.L., Leveno, K.J., Wapner, R. and Varner, M.: Metronidazole to prevent preterm delivery in pregnant women with asymptomatic bacterial vaginosis. NEJM **342**:534–540, 2000.

Carpenter, C.M. and Boak, R.: Isolation of Brucella abortus from a human fetus. JAMA **96**:1212–1216, 1931.

Carroll, S.G., Sebire, N.J. and Nicolaides, K.H.: Preterm Prelabour Amniorrhexis. The Parthenon Publishing Group, New York, 1996.

Carstensen, H., Christensen, K.K., Grennert, L., Persson, K. and Polberger, S.: Early-onset neonatal group B streptococcal septicaemia in siblings. J. Infect. Dis. **17**:201–204, 1988.

Cassell, G.H. and Cole, B.C.: Mycoplasmas as agents of human disease. NEJM **304**:80–89, 1981.

Cassell, G.H., Waites, K.B., Crouse, D.T., Rudd, P.T., Canupp, K.C., Stagno, S. and Cutter, G.R.: Association of Ureaplasma urealyticum infection of lower respiratory tract with chronic lung disease and death in very-low-birth-weight infants. Lancet **2**:240–244, 1988.

Catalano, L.W., Fuccilo, D.A., Traub, R.G. and Sever, J.L.: Isolation of rubella virus from placentas and throat cultures of infants: a prospective study after the 1964–1965 epidemic. Obstet. Gynecol. **38**:6–14, 1971.

Caul, E.O., Horner, P.J., Leece, J., Crowley, T., Paul, I. and Davey-Smith, G.: Population-based screening programmes for *Chlamydia trachomatis*. Lancet **349**:1070–1071, 1997.

Chan, G., Hemmings, D.G., Yurochko, A.D. and Guilbert, L.J.: Human cytomegalovirus-caused damage to placental tropho-blasts mediated by immediate-early gene-induced tumor necrosis factor-á. Amer. J. Pathol. **161**:1371–1381, 2002.

Chandra, P.C., Patel, H., Schiavello, H.J. and Briggs, S.L.: Successful pregnancy outcome after complicated varicella pneumonia. Obstet. Gynecol. **92**:680–682, 1998.

Charles, D. and Edwards, W.R.: Infectious complications of cervical cerclage. Amer. J. Obstet. Gynecol. **141**:1065–1071, 1981.

Chatterjee, A., Chartrand, S.A., Harrison, C.J., Felty-Duckworth, A. and Bewtra, C.: Severe intrauterine herpes simplex disease with placentitis in a newborn of a mother with recurrent genital infection at delivery. J. Perinatol. **21**:559–564, 2001.

Chehab, F.F., Xiao, X., Kan, Y.W. and Yen, T.S.B.: Detection of cytomegalovirus infection in paraffin-embedded tissue specimens with the polymerase chain reaction. Mod. Pathol. **2**:75–78, 1989.

Chretien, J.H., McGinnis, C.G. and Muller, A.: Venereal causes of cytomegalovirus mononucleosis. JAMA **238**:1644–1645, 1977.

Christian, S.S. and Duff, P.: Is universal screening for hepatitis B infection warranted in all prenatal populations? Obstet. Gynecol. **74**:259–261, 1989.

Christmas, J.T., Cox, S.M., Andrews, W., Dax, J., Leveno, K.J. and Gilstrap, L.C.: Expectant management of preterm ruptured membranes: effects of antimicrobial therapy. Obstet. Gynecol. **80**:759–762, 1992.

Coghlan, J.D. and Bain, A.D.: Leptospirosis in human pregnancy followed by death of the foetus. Br. Med. J. **1**:228–230, 1969.

Coleman, R.T., Sherer, D.M. and Maniscalco, W.M.: Prevention of neonatal group B streptococcal infections: advances in maternal vaccine development. Obstet. Gynecol. **80**:301–309, 1992.

Combs, C.A., McCune, M., Clark, R. and Fishman, A.: Aggressive tocolysis does not prolong pregnancy or reduce neonatal morbidity after preterm premature rupture of the membranes. Amer. J. Obstet. Gynecol. **190**:1723–1731, 2004.

Conover, P.T. and Roesmann, U.: Malformed complex in an infant with intrauterine viral infection. Arch. Pathol. Lab. Med. **114**:535–538, 1990.

Cooper, L.D. and Nuovo, G.J.: Histologic and molecular correlates of neonatal mortality due to in utero infection. Modern Pathol. **18**:Suppl. 1, abstract 9, 2005.

Corrall, C.J.: Diagnostic criteria of congenital tuberculosis. Amer. J. Dis. Child. **140**:739–740, 1986.

Cort, W.W.: Prenatal infestation with parasitic worm. JAMA **76**:170–171, 1921.

Cotch, M.F., Pastorek, J.G., Nugent, R.P., Hillier, S.L., Gibbs, R.S., Martin, D.H., Eschenbach, D.A., Edelman, R., Carey, J.C., Regan, J.A., Krohn, M.A., Klebanoff, M.A., Rao, A.V., Rhoads, G.G. and the Vaginal Infections and Prematurity Study Group: Trichomonas vaginalis associated with low birth weight and preterm delivery. Sexually Transm. Dis. **24**:353–360, 1997.

Coultrip, L.L., Lien, J.M., Gomez, R., Kapernick, P., Khoury, A. and Grossman, J.H.: The value of amniotic fluid interleukin-6 determination in patients with preterm labor and intact membranes in the detection of microbial invasion of the amniotic cavity. Amer. J. Obstet. Gynecol. **171**:901–911, 1994.

Couvreur, J., Desmonts, G. and Girre, J.Y.: Congenital toxoplasmosis in twins: a series of 14 pairs of twins: absence of infection in one twin in two. J. Pediatr. **89**:235–240, 1976.

Cox, S.M., MacDonald, P.C. and Casey, M.L.: Assay of bacterial endotoxin (lipopolysaccharide) in human amniotic fluid: potential usefulness in diagnosis and management of preterm labor. Amer. J. Obstet. Gynecol. **159**:99–106, 1988.

Cox, W.L., Forestier, F., Capella-Pavlovsky, M. and Daffos, F.: Fetal blood sampling in twin pregnancies: prenatal diagnosis and management of 19 cases. Fetal Ther. **2**:101–108, 1987.

Craver, R.D. and Baldwin, V.: Necrotizing funisitis. Obstet. Gynecol. **79**:64–70, 1992.

Crocker, I.P., Tanner, O.M., Myers, J.E., Bulmer, J.N., Walraven, G. and Baker, P.N.: Syncytiotrophoblast degradation and the pathophysiology of the malaria-infected placenta. Placenta **25**:273–282, 2004.

Crombleholme, W.R., Schachter, J., Grossman, M., Landers, D.V. and Sweet, R.L.: Amoxicillin therapy for *Chlamydia trachomatis* in pregnancy. Obstet. Gynecol. **75**:752–756, 1990.

Cruikshank, D.P. and Warenski, J.C.: First-trimester maternal Listeria monocytogenes sepsis and chorioamnionitis with normal neonatal outcome. Obstet. Gynecol. **73**:469–471, 1989.

Curbelo, V., Bejar, R., Benirschke, K. and Gluck, L.: Premature labor. I. Prostaglandin precursors in human placental membranes. Obstet. Gynecol. **57**:473–478, 1981.

Daffos, F., Forester, F., Capella-Pavlovsky, M., Thulliez, P., Aufrant, C., Valenti, D. and Cox, W.L.: Prenatal management of 746 pregnancies at risk for congenital toxoplasmosis. NEJM **318**:271–275, 1988.

Daikoku, N.H., Kaltreider, D.F., Johnson, T.R.B., Johnson, J. W.C. and Simmons, M.A.: Premature rupture of membranes and preterm labor: neonatal infection and perinatal mortality risks. Obstet. Gynecol. **58**:417–425, 1981.

Dallenbach, F. und Piekarski, G.: Über den Nachweis von Toxoplasma gondii im Gewebe mit Hilfe markierter fluorescierender Antikörper (Methode nach Coons). Virchows Arch. [Pathol. Anat.] **333**:607–618, 1960.

Darby, M.J., Caritis, S.N. and Shen-Schwarz, S.: Placental abruption in the preterm gestation: an association with chorioamnionitis. Obstet. Gynecol. **74**:88–92, 1989.

Decker, W.H. and Hall, W.: Treatment of abortions infected with Clostridium welchii. Amer. J. Obstet. Gynecol. **95**:394–399, 1966.

Degen, R., Stimpel, E. and Morawietz, I.: Katamnestische Untersuchungen von 74 Frauen nach Geburt eines listeriosekranken Kindes. Wien. Klin. Wochenschr. **82**:875–880, 1970.

Dehner, L.P. and Askin, F.B.: Cytomegalovirus endometritis: report of a case associated with spontaneous abortion. Obstet. Gynecol. **45**:211–214, 1975.

De Krijger, R.R., van Elsacker-Niele, A.M.W., Mulder-Stapel, A., Salimans, M.M.M., Dreef, E., Weiland, H.T., van Krieken, J.H.J.M. and Vermeij-Keers, C.: Detection of parvovirus B 19 infection in first and second trimester fetal loss. Pediatr. Pathol. Lab. Med. **18**:23–34, 1998.

Delaplane, D., Wiringa, K.S., Shulman, S.T. and Yogev, R.: Congenital mucocutaneous candidiasis following diagnostic amniocentesis. Amer. J. Obstet. Gynecol. **147**:342–343, 1983.

Delprado, W.J., Baird, P.J. and Russell, P.: Placental candidiasis: report of three cases with a review of the literature. Pathology **14**:191–195, 1982.

Demian, S.D.E., Donnelly, W.H. and Monif, G.R.G.: Coexistent congenital cytomegalovirus and toxoplasmosis in a stillborn. Amer. J. Dis. Child. **125**:420–421, 1973.

Dennis, S.M.: Comparative aspects of infectious abortion: diseases common to animals and man. Int. J. Fertil. **13**:191–197, 1968.

De Paepe, M.E., Friedman, R.M., Gundogan, F., Pinar, H. and Oyer, C.E.: The histologic fetoplacental inflammatory response in fatal perinatal group B-streptococcal infection. J. Perinatol. **24**:441–445, 2004.

DeSa, D.J.: Infection and amniotic aspiration in the middle ears of stillbirths and newborn infants. Amer. J. Pathol. **74**:7a, 1974 (abstract 29).

Desmonts, G. and Couvreur, J.: Congenital toxoplasmosis: a prospective study of 378 pregnancies. NEJM **290**:1110–1116, 1974.

Desmonts, G., Daffos, F., Forestier, F., Capella-Pavlovsky, M., Thulliez, P. and Chartier, M.: Prenatal diagnosis of congenital toxoplasmosis. Lancet **1**:500–504, 1985.

De Zegher, F., Sluiters, J.F., Stuurman, P.M., van der Voort, E., Bos, A.P. and Neijens, H.J.: Concomitant cytomegalovirus infection and congenital toxoplasmosis in a newborn. Eur. J. Pediatr. **147**:424–425, 1988.

Dias, M.J.M., van Rijckevorsel, G.H., Landrieu, P. and Lyon, G.: Prenatal cytomegalovirus disease and cerebral microgyria: evidence for perfusion failure, not disturbance of histogenesis, as the major cause of fetal cytomegalovirus encephalopathy. Neuropediatrics **15**:18–24, 1984.

DiLorenzo, D.J., Wong, G. and Ludmir, J.: *Candida lusitaniae* chorioamnionitis in a bone marrow transplant patient. Obstet. Gynecol. **90**:702–703, 1997.

Dimmick, J., Mahmood, K. and Altshuler, G.: Antenatal infection: adequate protection against hyaline membrane disease? Obstet. Gynecol. **47**:56–62, 1976.

Dinsmoor, M.J. and Gibbs, R.S.: Previous intra-amniotic infection as a risk factor for subsequent peripartal uterine infections. Obstet. Gynecol. **74**:299–301, 1989.

Dinsmoor, M.J., Bachman, R., Haney, E.I., Goldstein, M. and MacKendrick, W.: Outcomes after expectant management of extremely preterm premature rupture of the membranes. Amer. J. Obstet. Gynecol. **190**:1830187, 2004.

Dollmann, A. and Schmitz-Moormann, P.: Rekurriende Plazentainsuffizienz durch villöse Plazentitis mit extremer fetaler Hypotrophie. (Geburtsgewicht 1030 g und 1000 g am Termin). Geburtsh. Frauenheilk. **32**:795–801, 1972.

Dominguez, R., Segal, A.J. and O'Sullivan, J.A.: Leukocytic infiltration of the umbilical cord: manifestation of fetal hypoxia due to reduction of blood flow in the cord. JAMA **173**:346–349, 1960.

Donnellan, W.L., Chantra-Umporn, S. and Kidd, J.M.: The cytomegalic inclusion cell: an electron microscopic study. Arch. Pathol. **82**:336–348, 1966.

Doran, K.S., Chang, J.C.W., Benoit, V.M., Eckmann, L. and Nizet, V.: Group B streptococcal β-hemolysin/cytolysin promotes invasion of human lung epithelial cells and the release of interleukin-8. J. Infect. Dis. **185**:196–203, 2002a.

Doran, K.S., Benoit, V.M., Gertz, R.E., Beall, B. and Nizet, V.: Late-onset group B streptococcal infection in identical twins:

Insight to disease pathogenesis. J. Perinatol. **22**:326–330, 2002b.

Doss, B.J., Greene, M.F., Hill, J., Heffner, L.J., Bieber, F.R. and Genest, D.R.: Massive chronic intervillositis associated with recurrent abortions. Hum. Pathol. **26**:1245–1251, 1995.

Doyle, M., Atkins, J.T. and Rivera-Matos, I.R.: Congenital cytomegalovirus infection in infants infected with human immunodeficiency virus type 1. Pediatr. Infect. Dis. J. **15**:1102–1106, 1996.

Driscoll, S.G.: Histopathology of gestational rubella. Amer. J. Dis. Child. **118**:49–53, 1969.

Driscoll, S.G., Gorbach, A. and Feldman, D.: Congenital listeriosis: diagnosis from placental studies. Obstet. Gynecol. **20**:216–220, 1962.

Drut, R. and Araujo, M.O.G.: Image analysis of nucleomegalic cells in Chagas' disease placentitis. Placenta **21**:280–282, 2000.

Dubey, J.P.: Toxoplasma, Hammondia, Besnoitia, Sarcocystis, and other tissue cyst-forming coccidia of man and animals. In, Parasitic Protozoa. Vol. III. J.P. Kreier, ed., pp. 101–237. Academic Press, New York, 1977.

Dubey, J.P. and Beattie, C.P.: Toxoplasmosis of Animals and Man. CRC Press, Boca Raton, 1988.

Dublin, A.B. and Merten, D.F.: Computed tomography in the evaluation of herpes simplex encephalitis. Radiology **125**:133–134, 1977.

Dudley, D.J., Hunter, C., Mitchell, M.D. and Varner, M.W.: Elevations of amniotic fluid macrophage inflammatory protein-1α concentrations in women during term and preterm labor. Obstet. Gynecol. **87**:94–98. 1996.

Duff, P. and Gibbs, R.S.: Acute intraamniotic infection due to Streptococcus pneumoniae. Obstet. Gynecol. **61**:25S–27S, 1983.

Duggan, P.J., Maalouf, E.F., Watts, T.L., Sullivan, M.H.F., Counsell, S.J., Allsop, J., Al-Nakib, L., Rutherford, M.A., Battin, M., Roberts, I. and Edwards, A.D.: Intrauterine T-cell activation and increased proinflammatory cytokine concentrations in preterm infants with cerebral lesions. Lancet **358**:1699–1700, 2001.

Duncan, M.E.: Babies of mothers with leprosy have small placentae, low birth weights and grow slowly. Br. J. Obstet. Gynaecol. **87**:471–479, 1980.

Duncan, M.E.: Perspectives in leprosy in mothers and children. In, Advances in International Maternal and Child Health. D.B. Jelliffe and E. Jelliffe, eds. Clarendon Press, Oxford. **5**:122–143, 1985.

Duncan, M.E. and Oakey, R.E.: Estrogen excretion in pregnant women with leprosy: evidence of diminished fetoplacental function. Obstet. Gynecol. **60**:82–86, 1982.

Duncan, M., Melsom, R., Pearson, J.M.H., Menzel, S. and Barnetson, R.St.C.: A clinical and immunological study of four babies of mothers with lepromatous leprosy, two of whom developed leprosy in infancy. Int. J. Leprosy **51**:7–17, 1983.

Duncan, M.E., Fox, H., Harkness, R.A. and Rees, R.J.W.: The placenta in leprosy. Placenta **5**:189–198, 1984.

Dungal, N.: Listeriosis in four siblings. Lancet **2**:513–516, 1961.

Dunn, L.J., Robinson, J.C. and Steer, C.M.: Maternal death following suture of incompetent cervix during pregnancy. Amer. J. Obstet. Gynecol. **78**:335–339, 1959.

Dykes, A.-K., Christensen, K.K. and Christensen, P.: Chronic carrier state in mothers of infants with group B streptococcus infections. Obstet. Gynecol. **66**:84–88, 1985.

Eachempati, U. and Woods, R.E.: Cytomegalic virus disease in pregnancy. Obstet. Gynecol. **47**:615–618, 1976.

Easterling, T.R. and Garite, T.J.: Fusobacterium: anaerobic occult amnionitis and premature labor. Obstet. Gynecol. **66**:825–828, 1985.

Eberhart-Phillips, J.E., Frederick, P.D., Baron, R.C. and Mascola, L.: Measles in pregnancy: a descriptive study of 58 cases. Obstet. Gynecol. **82**:797–801, 1993.

Edwards, B.: Congenital malaria. Letter to the editor. NEJM **336**:71, 1997.

Edwards, C., Yi, C.H. and Currie, J.L.: Chorioamnionitis caused by *Capnocytophaga*: Case report. Amer. J. Obstet. Gynecol. **173**:244–245, 1995.

Edwards, L.E., Barrada, M.I., Hamann, A.A. and Hakanson, E.Y.: Gonorrhea in pregnancy. Amer. J. Obstet. Gynecol. **132**:637–641, 1978.

Egarter, C., Leitich, H., Karas, H., Wieser, F., Husslein, P., Kaider, A. and Schemper, M.: Antibiotic treatment in preterm premature rupture of membranes and neonatal morbidity: a metaanalysis. Amer. J. Obstet. Gynecol. **174**:589–597, 1996.

Egley, C.C., Katz, V.L. and Herbert, W.N.P.: Leukocyte esterase: a simple bedside test for the detection of bacterial colonization of amniotic fluid. Amer. J. Obstet. Gynecol. **159**:120–122, 1988.

Ehrnst, A., Lindgren, S., Dictor, M., Johannson, B., Sönnborg, A., Czajkowski, J., Sundin, G. and Bohlin, A.-B.: HIV in pregnant women and their offspring: evidence for late transmission. Lancet **338**:203–207, 1991.

Eichenfield, A.H. and Athreya, B.H.: Lyme disease: of ticks and titers. J. Pediatr. **114**:328–333, 1989.

Eidelman, A.I., Nevet, A., Rudensky, B., Rabinovitz, R., Hammerman, C., Raveh, D. and Schimmel, M.S.: The effect of meconium staining of amniotic fluid on the growth of *Escherichia coli* and group B *Streptococcus*. J. Perinatol. **22**:467–471, 2002.

Ekwo, E.E., Gosselink, C.A., Woolson, R., Moawad, A. and Long, C.R.: Coitus late in pregnancy: Risk of preterm rupture of amniotic sac membranes. Amer. J. Obstet. Gynecol. **168**:22–31, 1993.

Elliott, J.P.: Candida warrants concern. Amer. J. Obstet. Gynecol. **161**:503, 1989.

Elliott, W.G.: Placental toxoplasmosis: report of a case. Amer. J. Clin. Pathol. **53**:413–417, 1970.

Elst, C.W. van der, Bernal, A.L. and Sinclair-Smith, C.C.: The role of chorioamnionitis and prostaglandins in preterm labor. Obstet. Gynecol. **77**:672–676, 1991.

Eltoum, I.A., Zulstra, E.E., Ali, M.S., Ghalib, H.W., Satti, M.M.H., Eltoum, B. and El-Hassam, A.M.: Congenital Kala-Azar and leishmaniasis in the placenta. Amer. J. Trop. Med. Hyg. **46**:57–62, 1992.

Emanuel, B., Lieberman, A.D., Goldin, M. and Sanson, J.: Pulmonary candidiasis in the neonatal period. J. Pediatr. **61**:44–52, 1962.

Embil, J.A., Ozere, R.L. and Haldane, E.V.: Congenital cytomegalovirus infection in two siblings from consecutive pregnancies. J. Pediatr. **77**:417–421, 1970.

Enders, G., Miller, E., Cradock-Watson, J., Bolley, I. and Ridehalgh, M.: Consequences of varicella and herpes zoster in pregnancy: prospective study of 1739 cases. Lancet **343**:1547–1550, 1994.

Epstein, H. and King, C.R.: Diagnosis of congenital syphilis by immunofluorescence following fetal death in utero. Amer. J. Obstet. Gynecol. **152**:689–690, 1985.

Ernest, J.M., Swain, M., Block, S.M., Nelson, L.H., Hatjis, C.G. and Meis, P.J.: C-reactive protein: a limited test for managing patients with preterm labor or preterm rupture of membranes? Amer. J. Obstet. Gynecol. **156**:449–454, 1987.

Eschenbach, D.A., Nugent, R.P., Rao, A.V., Cotch, M.F., Gibbs, R.S., Lipscomb, K.A., Martin, D.H., Pastorek, J.G., Rettig, P.J., Carey, J.C., Regan, J.A., Geromanos, K.L., Lee, M.L.F., Poole, W.K., Edelman, R. and the Vaginal Infections and Prematurity Study Group: A randomized placebo-controlled trial of erythromycin for the treatment of *Ureaplasma urealyticum* to prevent premature delivery. Amer. J. Obstet. Gynecol. **164**:734–742, 1991.

Esernio-Jenssen, D., Scimeca, P.G., Benach, J.L. and Tenenbaum, M.J.: Transplacental/perinatal babesiosis. J. Pediatr. **110**:570–572, 1987.

European Collaborative Study: Mother-to-child transmission of HIV infection. Lancet **2**:1039–1045, 1988.

Evaldson, G.R., Malmborg, A.S. and Nord, C.E.: Premature rupture of the membranes and ascending infection. Br. J. Obstet. Gynaecol. **89**:793–801, 1982.

Evans, M.I., Hajj, S.N., Devoe, L.D., Angerman, N.S. and Moawad, A.H.: C-reactive protein as a predictor of infectious morbidity with premature rupture of membranes and premature labor. Amer. J. Obstet. Gynecol. **138**:648–652, 1980.

Fadel, H.E. and Riedrich, D.A.: Intrauterine resolution of nonimmune hydrops associated with cytomegalovirus infection. Obstet. Gynecol. **71**:1003–1005, 1988.

Farb, H.F., Arnesen, M., Geistler, P. and Knox, G.E.: C-reactive protein with premature rupture of membranes and premature labor. Obstet. Gynecol. **62**:49–51, 1983.

Faro, S., Walker, C. and Pierson, R.L.: Amnionitis with intact amniotic membranes involving Streptobacillus moniliformis. Obstet. Gynecol. **55**:9S–11S, 1980.

Fawaz, K.A., Grady, G.F., Kaplan, M.M. and Gellis, S.S.: Repetitive maternal-fetal transmission of fatal hepatitis B. NEJM **293**:1357–1359, 1975.

Fedele, L., Acaia, B., Parazzini, F., Ricciardiello, O. and Candiani, G.B.: Ectopic pregnancy and recurrent spontaneous abortion: two associated reproductive failures. Obstet. Gynecol. **73**:206–208, 1989.

Feinberg, R.F. and Kliman, H.J.: Fetal fibronectin and preterm labor. NEJM **326**:708–709, 1992.

Feldman, D., Hoar, R.M., Niemann, W.H., Valentine, T., Cukierski, M. and Hendrickx, A.G.: Tubuloreticular inclusions in placental chorionic villi of rhesus monkeys after maternal treatment with interferon. Amer. J. Obstet. Gynecol. **155**:413–424, 1986.

Feldman, H.A.: Congenital toxoplasmosis. NEJM **269**:1212, 1963.

Feucht, H.H., Zöllner, B., Polywka, S. and Laufs, R.: Vertical transmission of hepatitis G. Lancet **347**:615–616, 1996.

Filice, G.A., Cantrell, F., Smith, A.B., Hayes, P.S., Feeley, J.C. and Fraser, D.W.: Listeria monocytogenes infection in neonates: investigation of an epidemic. J. Infect. Dis. **138**:17–23, 1978.

Fitter, W.F., DeSa, D.J. and Richardson, H.: Chorioamnionitis and funisitis due to Corynebacterium kutscheri. Arch. Dis. Child. **54**:710–712, 1979.

Fiumara, N.J.: Syphilis in newborn children. Clin. Obstet. Gynecol. **18**:183–189, 1975.

Flamm, H.: Die pränatalen Infektionen des Menschen. Unter besonderer Berücksichtigung von Pathogenese und Immunologie. Georg Thieme, Stuttgart, 1959.

Fleming, A.D., Ehrlich, D.W., Miller, N.A. and Monif, G.R.G.: Successful treatment of maternal septicemia due to Listeria monocytogenes at 26 weeks' gestation. Obstet. Gynecol. **66**:52S–53S, 1985.

Fleming, A.D., Salafia, C.M., Vintzileos, A.M., Rodis, J.F., Campbell, W.A. and Bantham, K.F.: The relationship among umbilical artery velocimetry, fetal biophysical profile, and placental inflammation in preterm premature rupture of the membranes. Amer. J. Obstet. Gynecol. **164**:38–41, 1991.

Fleming, D.W., Cochi, S.L., MacDonald, K.L., Brondum, J., Hayes, P.S., Plikaytis, B.D., Holmes, M.B., Audurier, A., Broome, C.V. and Reingold, A.L.: Pasteurized milk as a vehicle of infection in an outbreak of listeriosis. NEJM **312**:404–407, 1985.

Fojaco, R.M., Hensley, G.T. and Moskowitz, L.: Congenital syphilis and necrotizing funisitis. JAMA **261**:1788–1790, 1989.

Forsners, E.V., Eggleston, M.K. and Wax, J.R.: Differential transmission of adenovirus in a twin pregnancy. Obstet. Gynecol. **91**:817–818, 1998a.

Forsners, E.V., Heaton, J.O. and Bowen, E.: Intrauterine *Listeria* infection of the nonpresenting twin. Obstet. Gynecol. **92**:715, 1998b.

Forther, B., Aissi, E., Ajana, F., Dieusart, P., Denis, P., Lassalle, E.M. de, Lecomte-Houcke, M. and Vinatier, D.: Spontaneous abortion and reinfection by *Toxoplasma gondii*. Lancet **338**:444, 1991.

Foster, G.E., Estreich, S. and Hooi, Y.S.: Chlamydial infection and pregnancy outcome. Amer. J. Obstet. Gynecol. **164**:234, 1991.

Foulon, W., Naessens, A., Catte, L. de and Amy, J.-J.: Detection of congenital toxoplasmosis by chorionic villus sampling and early amniocentesis. Amer. J. Obstet. Gynecol. **163**:1511–1513, 1990a.

Foulon, W., Naessens, A., Mahler, T., Waele, M. de, Catte, L. de and Meuter, F. de: Prenatal diagnosis of congenital toxoplasmosis. Obstet. Gynecol. **76**:769–772, 1990b.

Foulon, W., Pinon, J.-M., Stray-Pedersen, B., Pollak, A., Lappalainen, M., Decoster, A., Villena, I., Jenum, P.A., Hayde, M. and Naessens, A.: Prenatal diagnosis of congenital toxoplasmosis: a multicenter evaluation of different diagnostic parameters. Amer. J. Obstet. Gynecol. **181**:843–847, 1999.

Fox, H. and Langley, F.A.: Leukocytic infiltration of the placenta and umbilical cord: a clinico-pathologic study. Obstet. Gynecol. **37**:451–458, 1971.

Franciosi, R.A. and Jarzynski, D.J.: Mycotic abortion in man: a case report. J. Reprod. Med. **4**:48–51, 1970.

Fraser, R.B. and Wright, J.R. Jr.: Eosinophilic/T-cell chorionic vasculitis. Pediatr. Developm. Pathol. **5**:350–355, 2002.

Freedman, M.L., Christopher, P., Boughton, C.R., Lucey, M., Freeman, R. and Hansman, D.: Typhoid carriage in pregnancy with infection of neonate. Lancet **1**:310–311, 1970.

Freij, B.J. and Sever, J.L.: What do we know about toxoplasmosis? Contemporary Ob/Gyn. **41**:41–69, 1996.

Frenkel, J.K.: Toxoplasmosis: mechanisms of infection, laboratory diagnosis and management. In, Current Topics of Pathology **54**:28–75, 1971.

Frenkel, J.K.: Toxoplasmosis: parasite life cycle, pathology and immunology. In, The Coccidia. D.M. Hammond and P.L. Long, eds., pp. 343–410. University Park Press, Baltimore, 1973.

Frenkel, J.K.: Pathology and pathogenesis of congenital toxoplasmosis. Bull. N.Y. Acad. Med. **50**:182–191, 1974.

Friberg, J.: Genital mycoplasma infections. Amer. J. Obstet. Gynecol. **132**:573–578, 1978.

Fricker-Hidalgo, H., Pelloux, H., Racinet, C., Grefenstette, I. Bost-Bru, C., Goullier-Fleuret, A. and Ambroise-Thomas, P.: Detection of *Toxoplasma gondii* in 94 placentae from infected women by polymerase chain reaction, in vivo, and in vitro cultures. Placenta **19**:545–549, 1998.

Friedland, J.S., Jeffrey, I., Griffin, G.E., Booker, M. and Courtenay-Evans, R.: Q fever and intrauterine death. Lancet **343**:288–289, 1994.

Fuchs, P.C. and Oyama, A.A.: Neonatal relapsing fever due to transplacental transmission of Borrelia. JAMA **208**:690–692, 1969.

Fujikura, T. and Froehlich, L.A.: Intrauterine pneumonia in relation to birth weight and race. Amer. J. Obstet. Gynecol. **97**:81–84, 1967.

Gagnon, R.A.: Transplacental inoculation of fetal herpes simplex in the newborn. Obstet. Gynecol. **31**:682–684, 1968.

Galask, R.P. and Snyder, I.S.: Antimicrobial factors in amniotic fluid. Amer. J. Obstet. Gynecol. **106**:59–65, 1970.

Galask, R.P., Varner, M.W., Petzold, C.R. and Wilbur, S.L.: Bacterial attachment to the chorioamniotic membranes. Amer. J. Obstet. Gynecol. **148**:915–928, 1984.

Galbraith, G.M.P.: Chemotactic peptide-induced arachidonic acid mobilization in human polymorphonuclear leukocytes. Amer. J. Pathol. **133**:347–354, 1988.

Gans, B., Eckerling, B. and Goldman, J.A.: Abortion due to incompetence of the internal os of the cervix: a report of 250 cases. Obstet. Gynecol. **27**:875–879, 1966.

Gantz, N., Myerowitz, R.L., Medeiros, A.A., Carrera, G.F., Wilson, R.E. and O'Brien, T.F.: Listeriosis in immunosuppressed patients. Amer. J. Med. **58**:637–643, 1975.

Garcia, A.G.P.: Fetal infection in chickenpox and alastrim, with histopathologic study of the placenta. Pediatrics **32**:895–901, 1963.

Garcia, A.G.P.: Congenital toxoplasmosis in two successive sibs. Arch. Dis. Child. **43**:705–710, 1968.

Garcia, A.G.P., Pereira, J.M.S., Vidigal, N., Lobato, Y.Y., Pegado, C.S. and Branco, J.P.C.: Intrauterine infection with mumps virus. Obstet. Gynecol. **56**:756–759, 1980.

Garcia, A.G.P., Fonseca, E.F., Marques, R.L. de, Lobato, Y.: Placental morphology in cytomegalovirus infection. Placenta **10**:1–18, 1989.

Garcia, A.G.P., Basso, N.G. daS., Fonseca, M.E.F. and Outanni, H.N.: Congenital ECHO virus infection—morphological and virological study of fetal and placental tissue. J. Pathol. **160**:123–127, 1990.

Garcia A.G.P., Da Silva, N.G., Fonseca, M.E.F., Zuardi, A.T. and Outanni, H.N.: Enteroviruses associated placental morphology: A light, virological, electron microscopic and immunologic study. Placenta **12**:533–547, 1991.

Garite, T.J.: Premature rupture of the membranes: the enigma of the obstetrician. Amer. J. Obstet. Gynecol. **151**:1001–1005, 1985.

Garite, T.J. and Freeman, R.K.: Chorioamnionitis in the preterm gestation. Obstet. Gynecol. **59**:539–545, 1982.

Garite, T.J., Casal, D., Garcia-Alonso, A., Kreaden, U., Jimenez, G., Ayala, J.A. and Reimbold, T.: Fetal fibronectin: A new tool for the prediction of successful induction of labor. Amer. J. Obstet. Gynecol. **175**:1516–1521, 1996.

Gauthier, D.W., Meyer, W.J. and Bieniarz, A.: Expectant management of premature rupture of membranes with amniotic fluid cultures positive for *Ureaplasma urealyticum* alone. Amer. J. Obstet. Gynecol. **170**:587–590, 1994.

Gavaller, B. de: Enfermedad de Chagas congénita: observacion anatomo-patologica en gemelos. Bol. Matern. Concepcion Palacios (Caracas) **4**:59–64,1953.

Gaydos, C.A., Howell, M.R., Pare, B., Clark, K.L., Ellis, D.A., Hendrix, R.M., Gaydos, J.C., McKee, K.T. and Quinn, T.C.: *Chlamydia trachomatis* infections in female military recruits. NEJM **339**:739–744, 1998.

Gembruch, U., Niesen, M., Hansmann, M. and Knöpfle, G.: Listeriosis: a cause of non-immune hydrops fetalis. Prenat. Diagn. **7**:277–282, 1987.

Genardy, R.R., Thompson, B.H. and Niebyl, J.R.: Gonococcal salpingitis in pregnancy. Amer. J. Obstet. Gynecol. **126**:512–514, 1976.

Genc, M.R., Witkin, S.S., DeLaney, M.L., Paraskevas, L.-R., Tuomala, R.E., Norwitz, E.R. and Onderdonk, A.B.: A disproportionate increase in IL-1β over IL-1ra in the cervicovaginal secretions of pregnant women with altered vaginal microflora correlates with preterm birth. Amer. J. Obstet. Gynecol. **190**:1191–1197, 2004.

Genen, L., Nuovo, G.J., Krilov, L. and Davis, J.M.: Correlation of in situ detection of infectious agents in the placenta with neonatal outcome. J. Pediatr. **144**:316–320, 2004.

Genest, D., Granter, S. and Pinkus, G.S.: Umbilical cord pseudovasculitis following second trimester fetal death: a clinicopathological and immunohistochemical study of 13 cases. Histopathology **30**:563–569, 1998.

Gerberding, K.M., Eisenhut, C.C., Engle, W.A. and Cohen, M.D.: Congenital candida pneumonia and sepsis: a case report and review of the literature. J. Perinatol. **135**:159–161, 1989.

Gershon, R. and Strauss, L.: Structural changes in human placentas associated with fetal inanition or growth arrest ("placental insufficiency syndrome"). Amer. J. Dis. Child. **102**:645–646, 1961.

Ghidini, A., Sirtori, M., Vergani, P., Mariani, S., Tucci, E. and Scola, G.C.: Fetal intracranial calcifications. Amer. J. Obstet. Gynecol. **160**:86–87, 1989.

Gibb, D.M., Goodall, R.L., Dunn, D.T., Healy, M., Neave, P., Cafferkey, M. and Butler, K.: Mother-to-child transmission of hepatitis C virus: evidence for preventable peripartum transmission. Lancet **356**:904–907, 2000.

Gibbs, R.S.: Management of clinical chorioamnionitis at term. Amer. J. Obstet. Gynecol. **191**:1–2, 2004.

Gibbs, R.S. and Blanco, J.D.: Streptococcal infections in pregnancy: a study of 48 bacteremias. Amer. J. Obstet. Gynecol. **140**:405–411, 1981.

Gibbs, R.S. and Blanco, J.D.: Premature rupture of the membranes. Obstet. Gynecol. **60**:671–679, 1982.

Gibbs, R.S., Cassell, G.H., Davis, J.K. and St. Clair, P.J.: Further studies on genital mycoplasms in intra-amniotic infection: blood cultures and serologic response. Amer. J. Obstet. Gynecol. **154**:717–726, 1986.

Gibbs, R.S., Weiner, M.H., Walmer, K. and St. Clair, P.J.: Microbiologic and serologic studies of Gardnerella vaginalis in intra-amniotic infection. Obstet. Gynecol. **70**:187–190, 1987.

Gibbs, R.S., Romero, R.S., Hillier, S.L., Eschenbach, D.A. and Sweet, R.L.: A review of premature birth and subclinical infection. Amer. J. Obstet. Gynecol. **166**:1515–1528, 1992.

Gibbs, R.S., Davies, J.K., McDuffier, R.S., Leslie, K.K., Sherman, M.P., Centretto, C.A. and Wolf, D.M.: Chronic intrauterine infection and inflammation in the preterm rabbit, despite antibiotic therapy. Amer. J. Obstet. Gynecol. **186**:234–239, 2002.

Gibson, M. and Williams, P.P.: Haemophilus influenzae amnionitis associated with prematurity and premature membrane rupture. Obstet. Gynecol. **52**:70S–72S, 1978.

Gilbert, R.J., Miller, K.L. and Roberts, D.: Listeria monocytogenes and chilled foods. Lancet **1**:383–384, 1989.

Gill, P.: Is listeriosis often a foodborne illness? J. Infect. **17**:1–6, 1988.

Gille, J.: Granulation tissue in the umbilical cord. J. Reprod. Med. **18**:35–37, 1977.

Gilson, G.J., Harner, K.A., Abrams, J., Izquierdo, L.A. and Curet, L.B.: Chagas disease in pregnancy. Obstet. Gynecol. **86**:646–647, 1995.

Gilson, G.J., Christensen, F., Romero, H., Bekes, K., Silva, L. and Qualls, C.R.: Prevention of group B streptococcus early-onset neonatal sepsis: comparison of the Center for Disease Control and Prevention Screening-based Protocol to a Risk-based Protocol in infants at greater than 37 weeks' gestation. J. Perinatol. **20**:491–495, 2000.

Glasser, L. and Delta, B.G.: Congenital toxoplasmosis with placental infection in monozygotic twins. Pediatrics **35**:276–283, 1965.

Gleicher, N., Cohen, C.J., Kerenyi, T.D. and Gusberg, S.B.: A blocking factor in amniotic fluid causing leukocyte migration enhancement. Amer. J. Obstet. Gynecol. **133**:386–390, 1979.

Gloeb, D.J., O'Sullivan, M.J. and Efantis, J.: Human immunodeficiency virus infection in women. I. The effects of human immunodeficiency virus on pregnancy. Amer. J. Obstet. Gynecol. **159**:756–761, 1988.

Goedert, J.J., Mendez, H., Drummond, J.E., Robert-Guroff, M., Minkoff, H.L., Holman, S., Stevens, R., Rubinstein, A., Blattner, W.A., Willoughby, A. and Landesman, S.H.: Mother-to-infant transmission of human immunodeficiency virus type 1: association with prematurity or low anti-gp120. Lancet **2**:1351–1354, 1989.

Goldenberg, R.L., Mercer, B.M., Iams, J.D., Moawad, A.H., Meis, P.J., Das, A., McNellis, D., Miodovnik, M., Menard, M.K., Caritis, S.N., Thurnau, G.R. and Bottoms, S.F.: The preterm prediction study: Patterns of cervicovaginal fetal fibronectin as predictors of spontaneous preterm delivery. Amer. J. Obstet. Gynecol. **177**:8–12, 1997.

Goldenberg, R.L., Hauth, J.C. and Andrews, W.W.: Intrauterine infection and preterm delivery. NEJM **342:**1500–1507, 2000.

Gomez, R., Romero, R., Nien, J.K., Chaiworapongsa, T., Medina, L., Kim, Y.M., Yoon, B.H., Carstens, M., Espinoza, J., Iams, J.D. and Gonzalez, R.: A short cervix in women with preterm labor and intact membranes: A risk factor for microbial invasion of the amniotic cavity. Amer. J. Obstet. Gynecol. **192**:678–689, 2005.

Gonen, R., Hannah, M.E. and Milligan, J.E.: Does prolonged preterm premature rupture of the membranes predispose to abruptio placentae? Obstet. Gynecol. **74**:347–350, 1989.

Goodlin, R.C.: Intrauterine transfusion complicated by amnionitis and maternal peritonitis: report of a case. Obstet. Gynecol. **26**:803, 1965.

Graber, C.D., Williamson, O., Pike, J. and Valicenti, J.: Detection of Chlamydia trachomatis infection in endocervical specimens using direct immunofluorescence. Obstet. Gynecol. **66**:727–730, 1985.

Graham, E.M., Holcroft, C.J., Rai, K.K., Donohue, P.K. and Allen, M.C.: Neonatal cerebral white matter injury in preterm infants is associated with culture positive infections and only rarely with metabolic acidosis. Amer. J. Obstet. Gynecol. **191**:1305–1310, 2004.

Graves, A. and Gardner, W.A.: Pathogenicity of *Trichomonas vaginalis*. Clin. Obstet. Gynecol. **36**:145–152, 1993.

Gravett, M.G., Eschenbach, D.A., Speigel-Brown, C.A. and Holmes, K.K.: Rapid diagnosis of amniotic-fluid infection by gas-liquid chromatography. NEJM **306**:725–728, 1982.

Gravett, M.G., Nelson, H.P., DeRouen, T., Critchlow, C., Eschenbach, D.A. and Holmes, K.K.: Independent association of bacterial vaginosis and Chlamydia trachomatis infection with adverse pregnancy outcome. JAMA **256**:1899–1903, 1986.

Gray, B.M., Springfield, J.D. and Dillon, H.C.: Type-specific streptococcal antibodies in amniotic fluid. Amer. J. Obstet. Gynecol. **156**:666–669, 1987.

Greco, M.A., Wieczorek, R., Sachdev, R., Kaplan, C., Nuovo, G.J. and Demopoulos, R.I.: Phenotype of villous stromal cells in placentas with cytomegalovirus, syphilis, and nonspecific villitis. Amer. J. Pathol. **141**:835–842, 1992.

Greenspoon, J.S. and Settlage, R.H.: Isolation of human immunodeficiency virus from the placenta or from maternal blood contaminating the placenta? Amer. J. Obstet. Gynecol. **161**:501–502, 1989.

Greig, P.C., Herbert, W.N.P., Robinette, B.L. and Teot, L.A.: Amniotic fluid interleukin-10 concentrations increase through pregnancy and are elevated in patients with preterm labor associated with intrauterine infection. Amer. J. Obstet. Gynecol. **173**:1223–1227, 1995.

Grether, J.K. and Nelson, K.B.: Maternal infection and cerebral palsy in infants of normal birth weight. JAMA **278**:207–211, 1997.

Gribble, M.J., Salit, I.E., Isaac-Renton, J. and Chow, A.W.: Campylobacter infections in pregnancy: case report and literature review. Amer. J. Obstet. Gynecol. **140**:423–426, 1981.

Grillner, L., Ahlfors, K., Ivarsson, S.-A., Harris, S. and Svanberg, L.: Endonuclease cleavage pattern of cytomegalovirus of strains isolated from congenitally infected infants with neurologic sequelae. Pediatrics **81**:27–30, 1987.

Grose, C. and Itani, O.: Pathogenesis of congenital infection with three diverse viruses: varicella-zoster virus, human parvovirus, and human immunodeficiency virus. Seminars Perinatol. **13**:278–293, 1989.

Grose, C. and Weiner, C.P.: Prenatal diagnosis of congenital cytomegalovirus infection: Two decades later. Amer. J. Obstet. Gynecol. **163**:447–450, 1990.

Grossman, J.: Congenital syphilis. Teratology **16**:217–224, 1977.

Guarner, J., Greer, P.W., Bartlett, J., Ferebee, T., Fears, M., Pope, V. and Zaki, S.R.: Congenital syphilis in a newborn: An immunopathologic study. Modern Pathol. **12**:82–87, 1999.

Guderian, A.M. and Trobough, G.E.: Residues of pelvic inflammatory disease in intrauterine device users: a result of the intrauterine device of Chlamydia trachomatis infection? Amer. J. Obstet. Gynecol. **154**:497–503, 1986.

Gump, D.W., Gibson, M. and Ashikaga, T.: Lack of association between genital mycoplasmas and infertility. NEJM **310**:937–941, 1984.

Gunson, D.E., Acland, H.M., Gillette, D.M. and Pearson, J.E.: Abortion and stillbirth with *Chlamydia psittaci* var *ovis* in dairy goats with high titers to *Toxoplasma gondii*. JAVMA **183**:1447–1450, 1983

Guzick, D.S. and Winn, K.: The association of chorioamnionitis with preterm delivery. Obstet. Gynecol. **65**:11–16, 1985.

Gyr, T.N., Malek, A., Mathez-Loic, F., Altermatt, H.J., Bodmer, T., Nicolaides, K. and Schneider, H.: Permeation of human chorioamniotic membranes by *Escherichia coli* in vitro. Amer. J. Obstet. Gynecol. **170**:223–227, 1994.

Hagay, Z.J., Miskin, A., Goldchmit, R., Federman, A., Matzkel, A. and Mogilner, B.M.: Evaluation of two rapid tests for detection of maternal endocervical group B streptococcus: Enzyme-linked immunosorbent assay and Gram stain. Obstet. Gynecol. **82**:84–87, 1993.

Hagay, Z.J., Biran, G., Ornoy, A. and Reece, E.A.: Congenital cytomegalovirus infection: A long-standing problem still seeking a solution. Amer. J. Obstet. Gynecol. **174**:241–245, 1996.

Hagen, B. and Skjeldestad, F.E.: The outcome of pregnancy after CO_2 laser conization of the cervix. Brit. J. Obstetr. Gynaecol. **100**:717–720, 1993.

Hain, J., Doshi, N. and Harger, J.H.: Ascending transcervical herpes simplex infection with intact fetal membranes. Obstet. Gynecol. **56**:106–109, 1980.

Halliday, H.L. and Hirata, T.: Perinatal listeriosis—a review of twelve patients. Amer. J. Obstet. Gynecol. **133**:405–410, 1979.

Hallman, M., Bry, K. and Pitkänen, O.: Ceramide lactoside in amniotic fluid: high concentration in chorioamnionitis and in preterm labor. Amer. J. Obstet. Gynecol. **161**:313–318, 1989.

Hammer, B. und Wegmann, T.: Toxoplasmose und Schwangerschaft. Geburt eines Kindes bei Lymphknotentoxoplasmose der Mutter in der Frühschwangerschaft. Schweiz. Med. Wochenschr. **96**:37–44, 1966.

Hansen, A. and Leviton, A.: Labor and delivery characteristics and risks of cranial ultrasonographic abnormalities among very-low-birth-weight infants. Amer. J. Obstet. Gynecol. **181**:997–1006, 1999.

Hansen, L.M., Dorsey, T.A., Batzer, F.A. and Donnefeld, A.E.: Capnoctyphaga chorioamnionitis after oral sex. Obstet. Gynecol. **88**:731, 1996.

Hare, R. and Polunin, I.: Anaerobic cocci in the vagina of native women in British North Borneo. J. Obstet. Gynaecol. Br. Emp. **67**:985–989, 1960.

Harger, J.H., Meyer, M.P., Amortegui, A., Macpherson, T., Kaplan, L. and Mueller-Heubach, E.: Low incidence of positive amnionic fluid cultures in preterm labor between 27–32 weeks in the absence of clinical evidence of chorioamnionitis. Obstet. Gynecol. **77**:228–234, 1991.

Harris, B.A. Jr.: Peripheral placental separation: a review. Obstet. Gynecol. Surv. **43**:577–581, 1988.

Harrison, H.R.: Chlamydial ophthalmia neonatorum: the dilemma of diagnosis and treatment. Amer. J. Dis. Child. **139**:550–551, 1985.

Harrison, H.R., English, M.G., Lee, C.K. and Alexander, E.R.: Chlamydia trachomatis infant pneumonitis: comparison with matched controls and other infant pneumonitis. NEJM **298**:702–708, 1978.

Harter, C.A. and Benirschke, K.: Fetal syphilis in the first trimester. Amer. J. Obstet. Gynecol. **124**:705–711, 1976.

Hartwick, N.G., Vermeij-Keers, C., van Elsacker-Niele, A.M.W. and Fleuren, G.J.: Embryonic malformations in a case of intrauterine parvovirus B 19 infection. Teratology **39**:295–302, 1989.

Hass, M.: Hepato-adrenal necrosis with intranuclear inclusion bodies; report of a case. Amer. J. Pathol. **11**:127–142, 1935.

Hauth, J.C., Goldenberg, R.L., Andrews, W.W., DuBard, M.B. and Copper, R.L.: Reduced incidence of preterm delivery with metronidazole and erythromycin in women with bacterial vaginosis. NEJM **333**:1732–1736, 1995.

Hawrylyshyn, P., Bernstein, P., Milligan, J.E., Soldin, S., Pollard, A. and Papsin, F.R.: Premature rupture of membranes: the role of C-reactive protein in the prediction of chorioamnionitis. Amer. J. Obstet. Gynecol. **147**:240–246, 1983.

Hazard, G.W., Porter, P.J. and Ingall, D.: Pneumococcal laryngitis in the newborn infant. NEJM **271**:361–362, 1964.

Hein, M., Helmig R.B., Schønheyder, H.C., Ganz, T. and Uldbjerg, N.: An in vitro study of antibacterial properties of the cervical mucus plug in pregnancy. Amer. J. Obstet. Gynecol. **185**:586–592, 2001.

Hein, M., Valore, E.V., Helmig, R.B., Uldbjerg, N. and Ganz, T.: Antimicrobial factors in the cervical mucus plug. Amer. J. Obstet. Gynecol. **187**:137–144, 2002.

Heinemann, M.-H., Tang, C.-K. and Kramer, E.E.: Placental bacteremia and maternal Shirodkar procedure. Amer. J. Obstet. Gynecol. **128**:226–228, 1977.

Hemminki, K. and Kyyrönen, P.: Gastrointestinal atresias and borreliosis. Lancet **1**:1395, 1989.

Herbst, A.L.: Coitus and the fetus. NEJM **301**:1235–1236, 1979.

Herbst, P., Multier, A.-M. and Jaluvka, V.: Morphologische Untersuchungen der Plazenta einer an Parotitis erkrankten Mutter. Z. Geburtshilfe Gynäkol. **174**:187–193, 1970.

Herman, T.E. and Siegel, M.J.: Special imaging casebook. J. Perinatol. **14**:80–82, 1994.

Herzen, J.L. v. and Benirschke, K.: Unexpected disseminated herpes simplex infection in a newborn. Obstet. Gynecol. **50**:728–730, 1977.

Hewson, M., Simmer, K. and Blackmore, T.: Congenital malaria in a preterm infant. J. Paediatr. Child Health **39**:713–315, 2003.

Higa, K., Dan, K. and Manabe, H.: Varicella-zoster virus infections during pregnancy: Hypothesis concerning mechanism of congenital malformations. Obstet. Gynecol. **69**:214–222, 1987.

Hill, W.C., Bolton, V. and Carlson, J.R.: Isolation of acquired immunodeficiency syndrome virus from the placenta. Amer. J. Obstet. Gynecol. **157**:10–11, 1987.

Hillier, S.L., Martius, J., Krohn, M., Kiviat, N., Holmes, K.K. and Eschenbach, D.A.: A case-control study of chorioamnionic infection and histologic chorioamnionitis in prematurity. NEJM **319**:972–978, 1988.

Hillier, S.L., Krohn, M.A., Kiviat, N.B., Watts, D.H. and Eschenbach, D.A.: Microbiologic causes and neonatal outcomes associated with chorioamnion infection. Amer. J. Obstet. Gynecol. **165**:955–961, 1991.

Hillier, S.L., Witkin, S.S., Krohn, M.A., Watts, D.H., Kiviat, N.B. and Eschenbach, D.A.: The relationship of amniotic fluid cytokines and preterm delivery, amniotic fluid infection, histologic chorioamnionitis, and chorioamnion infection. Obstet. Gynecol. **81**:941–948, 1993.

Hillier, S.H., Nugent, R.P., Eschenbach, D.A., Krohn, M.A., Gibbs, R.S., Martin, D.H., Cotch, M.F., Edelman, R., Pastorek, J.G., Rao, A.V., McNellis, D., Regan, J.A., Carey, J.C. and Klebanoff, M.A.: Association between bacterial vaginosis and preterm delivery of a low-birth-weight infant. NEJM **333**:1737–1742, 1995.

Hirsch, E. and Wang, H.: The molecular pathophysiology of bacterially induced preterm labor: Insights from the murine model. J. Soc. Gynecol. Inv. **12**:145–155, 2005.

Ho, C.-Y. and Aterman, K.: Infection of the fetus by Candida in a spontaneous abortion. Amer. J. Obstet. Gynecol. **106**:705–710, 1970.

Hoeven, K.H. van, Anyaegbunam, A., Hochster, H., Whitty, J.E., Distant, J., Crawford, C. and Factor, S.M.: Clinical significance of increasing histologic severity of acute inflammation in the fetal membranes and umbilical cord. Pediatr. Pathol. Lab. Med. **16**:731–744, 1996.

Hoffman, D.J., Brown, G.D., Wirth, F.H., Gebert, B.S., Bailey, C.L. and Anday, E.K.: Urinary tract infection with *Trichomonas vaginalis* in a premature newborn infant and the development of chronic lung disease. J. Perinatol. **23**:59–61, 2003.

Hohlfeld, P., Daffos, F., Costa, J.M., Thulliez, P., Forester, F. and Vidaud, M.: Prenatal diagnosis of congenital toxoplasmosis with a polymerase-chain-reaction test on amniotic fluid. NEJM **331**:695–696, 1994.

Holcroft, C.J., Askin, F.B., Patra, A., Allen, M.C., Blakemore, K.J. and Graham, E.M.: Are histopathologic chorioamnionitis and funisitis associated with metabolic acidosis in the preterm fetus? Amer. J. Obstet. Gynecol. **191**:2010–2014, 2004.

Hollier, L.M., Scott, L.L., Murphree, S.S. and Wendel, G.D.: Postpartum endometritis caused by herpes simplex virus. Obstet. Gynecol. **89**:836–838, 1997.

Hood, C.K. and McKinnon, G.E.: Prenatal vaccinia. Amer. J. Obstet. Gynecol. **85**:238–240, 1963.

Hood, I.C., Browning, D., DeSa, D.J. and Whyte, R.K.: Fetal inflammatory response in second trimester candidal chorioamnionitis. Early Hum. Dev. **11**:1–10, 1985.

Horky, Z. and Amon, K.: Rundzelluläre Infiltrationen der Eihäute nach Amnioskopie. Geburtshilfe Frauenheilk. **27**:1065–1074, 1967.

Hörmann, G.: Placenta und Lues: ein Beitrag zur Diagnose und Prognose konnataler Syphilis. Arch. Gynäkol. **184**:481–521, 1954.

Horn, L.-C. and Becker, V.: Morphologische Plazentabefunde bei klinisch-serologisch gesicherter und vermuteter Rötelninfektion in der zweiten Schwangerschaftshälfte. Z. Geburtsh. Perinatol. **196**:199–204, 1992.

Horn, L.-C., Emmrich, P. and Krugmann, J.: Plazentabefunde bei Lues connata. Pathologe **13**:146–151, 1992.

Horn, L.-C., Büttner, W. and Horn, E.: Rötelnbedingte Plazentaveränderungen. Perinatal Medizin **5**:5–10, 1993.

Horowitz, H.W., Kilchevsky, E., Haber, S., Aguero-Rosenfeld, M., Kranwinkel, R., James, E.K., Wong, S.J., Chu, F., Liveris, D. and Schwartz, I.: Perinatal transmission of the agent of human granulocytic Ehrlichiosis. NEJM **339**:375–378, 1998.

Howe, R.S., Voychehovski, T.H., Uraizee, F., Bentsen, C. and Spear, M.L.: Neonatal group B streptococcal disease. NEJM **316**:1163, 1987.

Hsu, C.D., Meaddough, E., Aversa, K. and Copel, J.A.: The role of amniotic fluid L-selectin, GRO-α, and interleukin-8 in the pathogenesis of intraamniotic infection. Amer. J. Obstet. Gynecol. **178**:428–432, 1998.

Hughes, J.R., Wilfert, C.M., Moore, M., Benirschke, K. and de Hoyos-Guevara, E.: Echovirus 14 infection associated with fatal neonatal hepatic necrosis. Amer. J. Dis. Child. **123**:61–67, 1972.

Huikeshoven, F.J.M., Wallenburg, H.C.S. and Jahoda, M.G.J.: Diagnosis of severe fetal cytomegalovirus infection from amniotic fluid in the third trimester of pregnancy. Amer. J. Obstet. Gynecol. **142**:1053–1054, 1982.

Hunt, C.M., Carson, K.L. and Sharara, A.I.: Hepatitis C in pregnancy. Obstet. Gynecol. **89**:883–890, 1997.

Hunt, J.S.: Immunobiology of the maternal-fetal interface. Prenat. Neonat. Med. **3**:72–75, 1998.

Hunter, E.F., Greer, P.W., Swisher, B.L., Simons, A.R., Farshy, C.E., Crawford, J.A. and Sulzer, K.R.: Immunofluorescent staining of Treponema in tissues fixed with formalin. Arch. Pathol. Lab. Med. **108**:878–880, 1984.

Hyde, S.R. and Benirschke, K.: Gestational psittacosis: case report and literature review. Modern Pathol. **10**:602–607, 1997.

Hyde, S.R. and Giacoia, G.P.: Congenital herpes infection: placental and umbilical cord findings. Obstet. Gynecol. **81**:852–855, 1993.

Hyde, S., Smotherman, J., Moore, J.I. and Altshuler, G.: A model of bacterially induced umbilical vein spasm, relevant to fetal hypoperfusion. Obstet. Gynecol. **73**:966–970, 1989.

Iams, J.D.: The cervix: an independent risk factor for preterm birth. Prenat. Neonat. Med. **3**:106–108, 1998.

Iams, J.D. and O'Shaughnessy, R.: Antepartum versus intrapartum selective screening for maternal group B streptococcal colonization. Amer. J. Obstet. Gynecol. **143**:153–156, 1982.

Iams, J.D., Casal, D., McGregor, J.A., Goodwin, T.M., Kreaden, U.S., Lowensohn, R. and Lockitch, G.: Fetal fibronectin improves the accuracy of diagnosis of preterm labor. Amer. J. Obstet. Gynecol. **173**:141–145, 1995.

Iams, J.D., Goldenberg, R.L., Meis, P.J., Mercer, B.M., Moawad, A., Das, A., Thom, E., McNellis, D., Copper, R.L., Johnson, F. and Roberts, J.M.: The length of the cervix and risk of spontaneous premature labor. NEJM **334**:567–572, 1996.

Imamura, M., Phillips, P.E. and Mellors, R.C.: The occurrence and frequency of type C virus-like particles in placentas from patients with systemic lupus erythematosus and from normal subjects. Amer. J. Pathol. **83**:383–394, 1976.

Inaba, N., Okajima, Y., Kang, X.S., Ishikawa, K. and Fukasawa, I.: Maternal-infant transmission of hepatitis G virus. Amer. J. Obstet. Gynecol. **177**:1537–1538, 1997.

Ismail, M.A., Zinaman, M.J., Lowensohn, R.I. and Moawed, A.H.: The significance of C-reactive protein levels in women with premature rupture of membranes. Amer. J. Obstet. Gynecol. **151**:541–544, 1985.

Jacques, S.M. and Qureshi, F.: Necrotizing funisitis: A study of 45 cases. Human Pathol. **23**:1278–1283, 1992.

Jacques, S.M. and Qureshi, F.: Chronic intervillositis of the placenta. Arch. Pathol. Lab. Med. **117**:1032–1035, 1993.

Jacques, S.M. and Qureshi, F.: Chronic villitis of unknown etiology in twin gestations. Pediatr. Pathol. **14**:575–584, 1994.

James, J.A., Thomason, J.L., Gelbart, S.M., Osypowski, P., Kaiser, P. and Hanson, L.: Is trichomoniasis often associated with bacterial vaginosis in pregnant adolescents? Amer. J. Obstet. Gynecol. **166**:859–863, 1992.

Janssen, P., Piekarski, G. and Korte, W.: Zum Problem des Abortes bei latenter Toxoplasma-Infektion der Frau. Klin. Wochenschr. **48**:25–30, 1970.

Jauniaux, E., Nessmann, C., Imbert, M.C., Meuris, S., Puissant, F. and Hustin, J.: Morphological aspects of the placenta in HIV pregnancies. Placenta **9**:633–642, 1988.

Jelliffe, E.F.P.: Low birth-weight and malarial infection of the placenta. Bull. W.H.O. **38**:69–78, 1968.

Jeppson, K.G. and Reimer, L.G.: *Eikenella corrodens* chorioamnionitis. Obstet. Gynecol. **78**:503–505, 1991.

Jewett, J.F.: Chorioamnionitis complicated by an intrauterine device. NEJM **289**:1251–1252, 1973.

Job, C.K., Sanchez, R.M. and Hastings, R.C.: Lepromatous placentitis and intrauterine fetal infection in lepromatous nine-banded armadillos (Dasypus novemcinctus). Lab. Invest. **56**:44–48, 1987.

Joesoef, M.R., Hillier, S.L., Wiknjosastro, G., Sumampouw, H., Linnan, M., Norojono, W., Idajadi, A. and Utomo, B.: Intravaginal clindamycin treatment for bacterial vaginosis: Effects on preterm delivery and low birth weight. Amer. J. Obstet. Gynecol. **173**:1527–1531, 1995.

Johnson, D.E., Thompson, T.R. and Ferrieri, P.: Congenital candidiasis. Amer. J. Dis. Child. **135**:273–275, 1981a.

Johnson, F.W.A., Matheson, B.A., Williams, H., Laing, A.G., Jandiel, V., Davidson-Lamb, R., Halliday, G.J., Hobson, D., Wong, S.Y., Hadley, K.M., Moffat, M.A.J. and Postlethwaite, R.: Abortion due to infection with Chlamydia psittaci in a sheep farmer's wife. Br. Med. J. **290**:592–594, 1985.

Johnson, J.W., Daikoku, N.H., Niebyl, J.R., Johnson, T.R.B., Khouzami, V.A. and Witter, F.R.: Premature rupture of the membranes and prolonged latency. Obstet. Gynecol. **57**:547–556, 1981b.

Johnson, R.E., Nahmias, A.J., Magder, L.S., Lee, F.K., Brooks, C.A. and Snowden, C.B.: A seroepidemiologic survey of the prevalence of herpes simplex virus type 2 infection in the United States. NEJM **321**:7–12, 1989.

Joncas, J.H., Alfieri, C., Leyritz-Wills, M., Brochu, P., Jasmin, G., Boldogh, I. and Huang, E.-S.: Simultaneous congenital infection with Epstein-Barr virus and cytomegalovirus. NEJM **304**:1399–1403, 1981.

Jones, D.: Foodborne listeriosis. Lancet **336**:1171–1174, 1990.

Jones, K.L., Johnson, K.A. and Chambers, C.D.: Offspring of women infected with varicella during pregnancy: A prospective study. Teratology **49**:29–32, 1994.

Jordan, J.A.: Appreciating the differences between immunoassays used to diagnose maternal parvovirus B19 infection: understanding the antigen before interpreting the results. Prim. Care Update Ob/Gyn **9**:154–159, 2002.

Jordan, J.A. and Butchko, A.R.: Apoptotic activity in villous trophoblast cells during B19 infection correlates with clinical outcome: assessment by caspase-related M30 CytoDeath antibody. Placenta 23:547–553, 2002.

Jorgensen, D.M.: Gestational psittacosis in a Montana sheep rancher. Emerging Infect. Dis. 3:191–194, 1997.

Judge, D.M.: Congenital syphilis. In, Transplacental Effects on Fetal Health. D.G. Scarpelli and G. Migaki, eds., pp. 87–106. Alan Liss, New York, 1988.

Kagan, B.M., Hess, B., Mirman, B. and Lundeen, E.: Meningitis in premature infants. Pediatrics 4:479–483, 1949.

Kain, K.C. and Keystone, J.S.: Recurrent hydatid disease during pregnancy. Amer. J. Obstet. Gynecol. 159:1216–1217, 1988.

Kalter, S.S., Helmke, R.J., Heberling, R.L., Panigel, M., Fowler, A.K., Strickland, J.E. and Hellman, A.: C-type particles in normal human placentas. J. Natl. Cancer Inst. 50:1081–1083, 1973.

Kaplan, C.G.: Massive perivillous histiocytosis in twins. Pediatr. Devel. Pathol. 6:592–594, 2003.

Kaplan, C., Benirschke, K. and Tarzy, B.: Placental tuberculosis in early and late pregnancy. Amer. J. Obstet. Gynecol. 137:858–860, 1980.

Kapur, P., Rakheja, D., Gomez, A.M., Sheffield, J., Sanchez, P. and Rogers, B.B.: Characterization of inflammation in syphilitic villitis and in villitis of unknown etiology. Pediat. Developm. Pathol. 7:453–458, 2004.

Katz, J.M., Fox, C.H., Eglinton, G.S., Meyers, W.A. and Queenan, J.T.: Relationship between human immunodeficiency virus-1 RNA identification in placenta and perinatal transmission. J. Perinatol. 17:119–124, 1997.

Katz, S.L. and Wilfert, C.M.: Human immunodeficiency virus infection of newborns. NEJM 320:1687–1689, 1989.

Katz V.L., Kuller, J.A., McMahon, M.J., Warren, M.A. and Wells, S.R.: Varicella during pregnancy. Maternal and fetal effects. Western Med. J. 163:446–450, 1995.

Katzenstein, A.-L., Davis, C. and Braude, A: Pulmonary changes in neonatal sepsis due to group B β-hemolytic Streptococcus: relation to hyaline membrane disease. J. Infect Dis. 133:430–435, 1976.

Kaufman, H.E. and Maloney, E.D.: Multiplication of three strains of Toxoplasma gondii in tissue culture. J. Parasitol. 48:358–361, 1962.

Kaufmann, K.: Zur histologischen Diagnostik luischer Plazenten. Z. Geburtshilfe Gynäkol. 93:306–313, 1928.

Kayem, G., Goffinet, F., Batteux, F., Jarreau, P.H., Weill, B. and Cabrol, D.: Detection of interleukin-6 in vaginal secretions of women with preterm premature rupture of membranes and its association with neonatal infection: A rapid immunochromatographic test. Amer. J. Obstet. Gynecol. 191:140–145, 2004.

Kean, B.H., Kimball, A.C. and Christenson, W.N.: An epidemic of acute toxoplasmosis. JAMA 208:1002–1004, 1969.

Kellogg, S.G., Davis, C. and Benirschke, K.: Candida parapsilosis: previously unknown cause of fetal infection: a report of two cases. J. Reprod. Med. 12:159–161, 1974.

Kelly, N.P., Raible, M.D. and Husain, A.N.: An 11-day-old boy with lethargy, jaundice, fever, and melena. Arch. Pathol. Lab. Med. 124:469–470, 2000.

Kelly, R.W., Leask, R. and Calder, A.A.: Choriodecidual production of interleukin-8 and mechanism of parturition. Lancet 339:776–777, 1992.

Kerr, D.A.: Improved Warthin-Starry method of staining spirochetes in tissue sections. Amer. J. Clin. Pathol. 8:63–67, 1938.

Kerr, K., Dealler, S.F. and Lacey, R.W.: Listeria in cook-chill food. Lancet 2:37–38, 1988.

Kessel, E.: Pelvic inflammatory disease with intrauterine device use: a reassessment. Fertil. Steril. 51:1–11, 1989.

Khodr, G. and Matossian, R.: Hydrops fetales and congenital toxoplasmosis: value of direct immunofluorescence test. Obstet. Gynecol. 51:74S–77S, 1978.

Khong, T.Y., Staples, A., Moore, L. and Byard, R.W.: Observer reliability in assessing villitis of unknown aetiology. J. Clin. Pathol. 46:208–210, 1993.

Khudr, G. and Benirschke, K.: Placental lesion in viral hepatitis. Amer. J. Obstet. Gynecol. 40:381–384, 1972.

Kibrick, S. and Benirschke, K.: Severe generalized disease (encephalohepatomyocarditis) occurring in the newborn period and due to infection with Coxsackie virus, group B: evidence of intrauterine infection with this agent. Pediatrics 22:857–875, 1958.

Kida, M., Abramowsky, C.R. and Santoscoy, C.: Cryptococcosis of the placenta in a woman with acquired immunodeficiency syndrome. Hum. Pathol. 20:920–921, 1989.

Killpack, W.S.: Prenatal vaccinia. Lancet 1:388, 1963.

Kim, C.J., Yoon, B.H., Romero, R., Moon, J.B., Kim, M., Park, S.-S. and Chi, J.G.: Umbilical arteritis and phlebitis mark different stages of the fetal inflammatory response. Amer. J. Obstet. Gynecol. 185:496–500, 2001.

Kim, Y.M., Romero, R., Chaiworapongsa, T., Kim, G.J., Kim, M.R., Kuivaniemi, H., Tromp, G., Espinoza, J., Bujold, E., Abrahams, V.M. and Mor, G.: Toll-like receptor-2 and -4 in the chorioamniotic membranes in spontaneous labor at term and in preterm parturition that are associated with chorioamnionitis. Amer. J. Obstet. Gynecol. 191:1346–1355, 2004.

Kimball, A.C., Kean, B.H. and Fuchs, F.: The role of toxoplasmosis in abortion. Amer. J. Obstet. Gynecol. 111:219–226, 1971.

Kimball, A.C., Kean, B.H. and Fuchs, F.: Toxoplasmosis: risk variations in New York City obstetrics patients. Amer. J. Obstet. Gynecol. 119:208–214, 1974.

King, J.A. and Marks, R.A.: Pregnancy and leprosy. Amer. J. Obstet. Gynecol. 76:438–442, 1958.

Kirchhoff, H. and Kräubig, H., eds.: Toxoplasmose: Praktische Fragen und Ergebnisse. Georg Thieme, Stuttgart, 1966.

Kirschbaum, T.: Antibiotics in the treatment of preterm labor. Amer. J. Obstet. Gynecol. 168:1239–1246, 1993.

Kirshon, B., Rosenfeld, B., Mari, G. and Belfort, M.: Amniotic fluid glucose and intraamniotic infection. Amer. J. Obstet. Gynecol. 164:818–820, 1991.

Klatt, E.C., Pavlova, Z., Teberg, A.J. and Yonekura, M.L.: Epidemic perinatal listeriosis at autopsy. Hum. Pathol. 17:1278–1281, 1986.

Klebanoff, M.A., Nugent, R.P. and Rhoads, G.G.: Coitus during pregnancy: is it safe? Lancet 2:914–917, 1984.

Klebanoff, M.A., Carey, J.C., Hauth, J.C., Hillier, S.L., Nugent, R.P., Thom, E.A., Ernest, J.M., Heine, R.P., Wapner, R.J., Trout, W., Moawad, A. and Leveno, K.J.: Failure of metranidazole to prevent preterm delivery among pregnant women with asymptomatic Trichomonas vaginalis infection. NEJM 345:487–493, 2001.

Knee, D.S., Christ, M.J., Gries, D.M. and Thompson, M.W.: *Actinomyces* species and cerclage placement in neonatal sepsis. A case report. J. Perinatol. **24**:389–391, 2004.

Knowles, S. and Frost, T.: Umbilical cord sclerosis as an indicator of congenital syphilis. J. Clin. Pathol. **42**:1157–1159, 1989.

Knox, I.C. and Hoerner, J.K.: Role of infection in premature rupture of membranes. Amer. J. Obstet. Gynecol. **59**:190–194, 1950.

Koh, K.S., Cole, T.L. and Orkin, A.J.: Listeria amnionitis as a cause of fetal distress. Amer. J. Obstet. Gynecol. **136**:261–263, 1980.

Koppe, J.G., Loewer-Sieger, D.H. and de Roever-Bonnet, H.: Results of 20-year follow-up of congenital toxoplasmosis. Lancet **1**:254–256, 1986.

Koskiniemi, M., Lappalainen, M. and Hedman, K.: Toxoplasmosis needs evaluation: an overview and proposals. Amer. J. Dis. Child. **143**:724–728, 1989.

Kraus, G.W. and Yen, S.S.C.: Gonorrhea during pregnancy. Obstet. Gynecol. **31**:258–260, 1968.

Kraybill, E.N. and Controni, G.: Septicemia and enterocolitis due to Shigella sonnei in a newborn infant. Pediatrics **42**:530–531, 1968.

Krech, U., Konjajev, Z. and Jung, M.: Congenital cytomegalovirus infection in siblings from consecutive pregnancies. Helv. Paediatr. Acta **26**:355–362, 1971.

Kredentser, J.V., Embree, J.E. and McCoshen, J.A.: Prostaglandin $F_{2\alpha}$ output by amnio-chorion-decidua: relationship with labor and prostaglandin E_2 concentration at the amniotic surface. Amer. J. Obstet. Gynecol. **173**:199–204, 1995.

Kückens, H.: Über Rundzelleninfiltrate in reifer Placenta mit Anhängen, sowie ihre Beziehungen zum Geburts- und Wochenbettverlauf. Arch. Gynäkol. **167**:564–621, 1938.

Kumazaki, K., Nakayama, M., Sumida, Y., Ozono, K., Mushiake, S., Suehara, N., Wada, Y. and Fujimura, M.: Placental features in preterm infants with periventricular leukomalacia. Pediatrics **109**:650–655, 2002a.

Kumazaki, K., Ozono, K., Yahara, T., Wada, Y., Suehara, N., Takeuchi, M. and Nakayama, M.: Detection of cytomegalovirus DNA in human placenta. J. Med. Virol. **68**:363–369, 2002b.

Kundsin, R.B. and Horne, H.W.: Is genital colonization with Mycoplasma hominis or Ureaplasma urealyticum associated with prematurity/low birth weight? Obstet. Gynecol. **74**:679, 1989.

Kundsin, R.B., Driscoll, S.G. and Ming, P.-M.L.: Strain of mycoplasma associated with human reproductive failure. Science **157**:1573–1574, 1967.

Kundsin, R.B., Leviton, A., Allred, E.N. and Poulin, S.A.: *Ureaplasma urealyticum* infection of the placenta in pregnancies that ended prematurely. Obstet. Gynecol. **87**:122–127, 1996.

Kurki, T. and Ylikorkala, O.: Coitus during pregnancy is not related to bacterial vaginosis or preterm birth. Amer. J. Obstet. Gynecol. **169**:1130–1134, 1993.

Labarrere, C.A. and Mullen, E.: Fibrinoid and trophoblastic necrosis with massive intervillositis: An extreme variant of villitis of unknown etiology. Amer. J. Reprod. Immunol. Microbiol. **12**:85–91, 1987.

Labarrere, C., Althabe, O. and Telenta, M.: Chronic villitis of unknown aetiology in placentae of idiopathic small for gestational age infants. Placenta **3**:309–318, 1982.

Labarrere, C.A., Faulk, W.P., McIntyre, J.A. and Althabe, O.H.: Materno-trophoblastic immunological balance. Amer. J. Reprod. Immunol. **21**:16–25, 1989.

Labarrere, C.A., McIntyre, J.A. and Faulk, W.P.: Immunohistologic evidence that villitis in human normal term placentas is an immunologic lesion. Amer. J. Obstet. Gynecol. **162**:515–522, 1990.

Labarrere, C.A., Carson, S.D. and Faulk, S.P.: Tissue factor in chronic villitis of unestablished etiology. J. Reprod. Immunol. **19**:225–235, 1991.

Lahra, M.M. and Jeffery, H.E.: A fetal response to chorioamnionitis is associated with early survival after preterm birth. Amer. J. Obstet. Gynecol. **190**:147–151, 2004.

Lallemand, A.V., Gaillard, D.A., Paradis, P.H. and Chippaux, C.G.: Fetal listeriosis during the second trimester of gestation. Pediatr. Pathol. **12**:665–671, 1992.

Lamont, R.F., Rose, M. and Elder, M.G.: Effect of bacterial products on prostaglandin E production by amnion cells. Lancet **2**:1331–1333, 1985.

Lamont, R.F., Anthony, F., Myatt, L., Booth, L., Furr, P.M. and Taylor-Robinson, D.: Production of prostaglandin E_2 by human amnion in vitro in response to addition of media conditioned by microorganisms associated with chorioamnionitis and preterm labor. Amer. J. Obstet. Gynecol. **162**:819–825, 1990.

Lamont, R.J., Postlethwhaite, R. and MacGowan, A.P.: Listeria monocytogenes and its role in human infection. J. Infection **17**:7–28, 1988.

Lane, R.B.: Congenital malaria. Letter to the editor. NEJM **336**:71, 1997.

Lang, D.J. and Kummer, J.F.: Demonstration of cytomegalovirus in semen. NEJM **287**:756–758, 1972.

Langer, H.: Intrauterine Toxoplasma-Infektion. Georg Thieme, Stuttgart, 1963a.

Langer, H.: Repeated congenital infection with Toxoplasma gondii. Obstet. Gynecol. **21**:318–329, 1963b.

Larsen, J.W.: Congenital toxoplasmosis. Teratology **15**:213–218, 1977.

Larson, H.E., Parkman, P.D., Davis, W.J., Hopps, H.E. and Meyer, H.M.: Inadvertent rubella virus vaccination during pregnancy. NEJM **284**:870–873, 1971.

Lastavica, C.C., Wilson, M.L., Berardi, V.P., Spielman, A. and Deblinger, R.D.: Rapid emergence of a focal epidemic of Lyme disease in coastal Massachusetts. NEJM **320**:133–137, 1989.

Laugier, J., Borderon, J.-C., Chantepie, A., Tabarly, J.-L. and Gold, F.: Meningite du nouveau-né a Listeria monocytogenes et contamination en maternité. Arch. Fr. Pédiatr. **35**:168–171, 1978.

Lavergne, E. de, Olive, D., Maurin, J. and Feugier, J.: Isolement d'une souche de "myxovirus parainfluenzae 1" chez un embryon humain, expulse au cours d'un avortement fébrile. Arch. Fr. Pédiatr. **26**:179–183, 1969.

Lee, N.C., Rubin, G.L. and Borucki, R.: The intrauterine device and pelvic inflammatory disease revisited: new results from the Women's Health Study. Obstet. Gynecol. **72**:1–6, 1988.

Lee, T., Carpenter, M.W., Heber, W.W. and Silver, H.M.: Preterm premature rupture of membranes: Risk of recurrent complications in the next pregnancy among a population-based sample of gravid women. Amer. J. Obstet. Gynecol. **188**:209–213, 2003.

Lehtonen, O.-P., Ruuskanen, O., Kero, P., Hollo, O., Erkkola, R. and Salmi, T.: Group-A streptococcal infection in the newborn. Lancet **2**:1473–1474, 1984.

Leikin, E., Lysikiewicz, A., Garry, D. and Tejani, N.: Intrauterine transmission of hepatitis A virus. Obstet. Gynecol. **88**:690–691, 1996.

Leitich, H., Bodner-Adler, B., Brunbauer, M., Kaider, A., Egarter, C. and Husslein, P.: Bacterial vaginosis as a risk factor for preterm delivery: a meta-analysis. Amer. J. Obstet. Gynecol. **189**:139–147, 2003.

LeLong, M., LePage, F., Vinh, L.T., Tournier, P. and Chany, C.: Le virus de la maladie des inclusions cytomégaliques. Arch. Fr. Pédiatr. **17**:1–14, 1960.

Leo, M.V., Skurnick, J.H., Ganesh, V.V., Adhate, A. and Apuzzio, J.J.: Clinical chorioamnionitis is not predicted by umbilical artery Doppler velocimetry in patients with premature rupture of the membranes. Obstet. Gynecol. **79**:916–918, 1992.

LePage, F. and Schramm, P.: Aspects histologiques du placenta et des membranes dans la maladies des inclusions cytomégaliques. Gynécol. Obstétr. **57**:273–279, 1958.

Leppert, P.C.: The biochemistry and physiology of the uterine cervix during gestation and parturition. Prenat. Neonat. Med. **3**:103–105, 1998.

Lettieri, L., Vintzileos, A.M., Rodis, J.F., Albini, S.M. and Salafia, C.M.: Does "idopathic" preterm labor resulting in preterm birth exist? Amer. J. Obstet. Gynecol. **168**:1480–1485, 1993.

Leveno, K.J., Cox, K. and Roark, M.L.: Cervical dilatation and prematurity revisited. Obstet. Gynecol. **68**:434–435, 1986.

Levin, S., Zaidel, L. and Bernstein, D.: Intrauterine infection of fetal brain. Amer. J. Obstet. Gynecol. **130**:597–599, 1978.

Levy, D.L.: Placental abscess as a cause of fever of unknown origin. Amer. J. Obstet. Gynecol. **140**:338–339, 1981.

Lewis, S.H., Reynolds-Kohler, C., Fox, H.E. and Nelson, J.A.: HIV-1 in trophoblastic and villous Hofbauer cells, and haematological precursors in eight-week fetuses. Lancet **335**:565–568, 1990.

Li, L., Sheng, M.-H., Tong, S.-P., Chen, H.-Z. and Wen, Y.-M.: Transplacental transmission of hepatitis B virus. Lancet **2**:872, 1986.

Lide, T.N.: Congenital tularemia. Arch. Pathol. **43**:165–169, 1947.

Liesnard, C., Donner, C., Brancart, F. and Rodesch, F.: Varicella in pregnancy. Lancet **344**:950–951, 1994.

Ling, H.H., Kao, J.H., Chen, P.J. and Chen, D.S.: Mechanism of vertical transmission of hepatitis G. Lancet **347**:1116, 1996.

Linnan, M.J., Mascola, L., Lou, X.D., Goulet, V., May, S., Salminen, C., Hird, D.W., Yonekura, L., Hayes, P., Weaver, R., Audurier, A., Plikaytis, B., Fannin, S.L., Kleks, A. and Broome, C.V.: Epidemic listeriosis associated with Mexican-style cheese. NEJM **319**:823–828, 1988.

Lipitz, S., Yagel, S., Shalev, E., Achiron, R., Mashiach, S. and Schiff, E.: Prenatal diagnosis of fetal primary cytomegalovirus infection. Obstet. Gynecol. **89**:763–767, 1997.

Livengood, C.H., Schmitt, J.W., Addison, W.A., Wrenn, J.W. and MacGruder-Habib, K.: Direct fluorescent antibody testing for endocervical Chlamydia trachomatis: factors affecting accuracy. Obstet. Gynecol. **72**:803–809, 1988.

Lockwood, C.J., Senyei, A.E., Dische, R., Casai, D., Shah, K.D., Thung, S.N., Jones, L., Deligdisch, L. and Garite, T.J.: Fetal fibronectin in cervical and vaginal secretions as a predictor of preterm delivery. NEJM **325**:669–674, 1991.

Lockwood, C.J., Ghidini, A., Wein, R., Lapinski, R., Casal, D. and Berkowitz, R.L.: Increased interleukin-6 concentrations in cervical secretions are associated with preterm delivery. Amer. J. Obstet. Gynecol. **171**:1097–1102, 1994.

Locksmith, G.J.: New diagnostic tests for gonorrhea and chlamydia. Prim. Care Update Ob/Gyn **4**:161–167, 1997.

Long, M.T., Goetz, T.E., Kakoma, I., Whiteley, H.E., Lock, T.E., Holland, C.J., Foreman, J.H. and Baker, G.J.: Evaluation of fetal infection and abortion in pregnant ponies experimentally infected with *Ehrlichia risticii*. Amer. J. Vet. Res. **56**:1307–1316, 1995.

Lopez Bernal, A., Hansell, D.J., Canete Soler, R., Keeling, J.W. and Turnbull, A.C.: Prostaglandins, chorioamnionitis and preterm labor. Br. J. Obstet. Gynaecol. **94**:1156–1158, 1987.

Lossick, J.G. and Kent, H.L.: Trichomoniasis: Trends in diagnosis and management. Amer. J. Obstet. Gynecol. **165**:1217–1222, 1991.

Low, J.C. and Donachie, W.: Listeria in food: a veterinary perspective. Lancet **1**:322, 1989.

Lu, G.C., Schwebke, J.R., Duffy, L.B., Cassell, G.H., Hauth, J.C., Andrews, W.W. and Goldenberg, R.L.: Midtrimester vaginal *Mycoplasma genitalium* in women with subsequent spontaneous preterm birth. Amer. J. Obstet. Gynecol. **185**:163–165, 2001.

Lucifora, G., Calabro, S., Carroccio, G. and Brigandi, A.: Immunocytochemical HBsAg evidence in placentas of asymptomatic carrier mothers. Amer. J. Obstet. Gynecol. **159**:839–842, 1988.

Lucifora, G., Martines, F., Calabro, S., Carroccio, G., Brigandi, A. and Pasquale, R. de: HbcAg identification in the placental cytotypes of symptom-free HBsAg-carrier mothers: A study with the immunoperoxidase method. Amer. J. Obstet. Gynecol. **163**:235–239, 1990.

Luder, J. and Tomson, P.R.V.: Salmonella meningitis in the newborn. Postgrad. Med. J. **39**:100–102, 1963.

MacDonald, A.B., Benach, J.L. and Birgdorfer, W.: Stillbirth following maternal Lyme disease. N.Y. State J. Med. **87**:615–616, 1987.

Madan, E., Meyer, M.P. and Amortegui, A.J.: Isolation of genital mycoplasmas and Chlamydia trachomatis in stillborn and neonatal autopsy material. Arch. Pathol. Lab. Med. **112**:749–751, 1988.

Madan, E., Meyers, M.P. and Amortegui, A.J.: Histologic manifestations of perinatal genital mycoplasmal infection. Arch. Pathol. Lab. Med. **113**:465–469, 1989.

Maeda, S., Mellors, R.C., Mellors, J.W., Jerabek, L.B. and Zervoudakis, I.A.: Immunohistologic detection of antigen related to primate type C retrovirus p30 in normal human placentas. Amer. J. Pathol. **112**:347–356, 1983.

Magliocco, A.M., Demetrick, D.J., Sarnat, H.B. and Hwang, W.S.: Varicella embryopathy. Arch. Pathol. Lab. Med. **116**:181–186, 1992.

Magnusson, S.S., Oskarsson, T., Geirsson, R.T., Sveinsson, B., Steingrimsson, O. and Thorarinsson, H.: Lower genital tract infection with Chlamydia trachomatis and Neisseria gonorrhoeae in Icelandic women with salpingitis. Amer. J. Obstet. Gynecol. **155**:602–607, 1986.

Major, C.A., Veciana, M. de, Lewis, D.F. and Morgan, M.A.: Preterm premature rupture of membranes and abruptio placentae: Is there an association between these pregnancy complications? Amer. J. Obstet. Gynecol. **172**:672–676, 1995.

Malan, A.F., Woods, D.L., v.d. Elst, C.W. and Meyer, M.P.: Relative placental weight in congenital syphilis. Placenta **11**:3–6, 1990.

Maradny, E.E., Kanayama, N., Halim, A., Machara, K. and Terao, T.: Stretching of fetal membranes increases the concentration of interleukin-8 and collagenase activity. Amer. J. Obstet. Gynecol. **174**:843–849, 1996.

Margolis, G. and Kilham, L.: Problems of human concern arising from animal models of intrauterine and neonatal infections due to viruses: a review. II. Pathological studies. Prog. Med. Virol. **20**:144–179, 1975.

Markley, K.C., Levine, A.B. and Chan, Y.: Rocky Mountain spotted fever in pregnancy. Obstet. Gynecol. **91**:860, 1998.

Martius, J. and Eschenbach, D.A.: The role of bacterial vaginosis as a cause of amniotic fluid infection, chorioamnionitis and prematurity—a review. Arch. Gynecol. Obstet. **247**:1–13, 1990.

Mason, P.R. and Brown, I.McL.: Trichomoniasis in pregnancy. Lancet **2**:1025–1026, 1980.

Matorras, R., Perea, A.G., Omenaca, F., Usandizaga, J.A., Nieto, A. and Herruzo, R.: Group B Streptococcus and premature rupture of membranes and preterm delivery. Gynecol. Obstet. Invest. **27**:14–18, 1989.

Matsuzaki, N., Taniguchi, T., Shimoya, K., Neki, R., Okada, T., Saji, F., Nakayama, M., Suehara, N. and Tanizawa, O.: Placental interleukin-6 production is enhanced in intrauterine infection but not in labor. Amer. J. Obstet. Gynecol. **168**:94–97, 1993.

Maudsley, R.F., Brix, G.A., Hinton, N.A., Robertson, E.M., Bryans, A.M. and Haust, M.D.: Placental inflammation and infection. Amer. J. Obstet. Gynecol. **95**:648–659, 1966.

Maurus, J.N.: Hansen's disease in pregnancy. Obstet. Gynecol. **52**:22–25, 1978.

Mazeron, M.C., Cordovi-Voulgaropoulos, L. and Péol, Y.: Transient hydrops fetalis associated with intrauterine cytomegalovirus infection: prenatal diagnosis. Obstet. Gynecol. **84**:692–694, 1994.

McCaffree, M.A. and Altshuler, G.: Placental fluorescent-antibody studies as test for congenital cytomegalovirus infection. Lancet **1**:1029–1030, 1979.

McCaffree, M.A., Altshuler, G. and Benirschke, K.: Placental coccidioidomycosis without fetal disease. Arch. Pathol. Lab. Med. **102**:512–514, 1978.

McClure, H.M. and Strozier, L.M.: Perinatal listeric septicemia in a Celebese black ape. J. Amer. Vet. Med. Assoc. **167**:637–638, 1975.

McColgin, S.W., Hess, L.W., Martin, R.W., Martin, J.N. and Morrison, J.C.: Group B streptococcal sepsis and death in utero following funipuncture. Obstet. Gynecol. **74**:464–465, 1989.

McColgin, S.W., Bennett, W.A., Roach, H., Cowan, B.D., Martin, J.N. and Morrison, J.C.: Parturitional factors associated with membrane stripping. Amer. J. Obstet. Gynecol. **169**:71–77, 1993.

McCord, J.R.: Syphilis of the placenta: the histologic examination of 1,085 placentas of mothers with strongly positive blood Wassermann reactions. Amer. J. Obstet. Gynecol. **28**:743–750, 1934.

McCormack, W.M., Almeida, P.C., Bailey, P.E., Grady, E.M. and Lee, Y.-H.: Sexual activity and vaginal colonization with genital mycoplasmas. JAMA **221**:1375–1377, 1972.

McCracken, G.H.: Neonatal septicemia and meningitis. Hosp. Pract. **11**:89–97, 1976.

McCracken, G.H. and Sarff, L.D.: Current status and therapy of neonatal E. coli meningitis. Hosp. Pract. **9**:57–64, 1974.

McDuffie, R.S. and Bader, T.: Fetal meconium peritonitis after maternal hepatitis. Amer. J. Obstet. Gynecol. **180**:1031–1032, 1999.

McDuffie, R.S., Sherman, M.P. and Gibbs, R.S.: Amniotic fluid tumor necrosis factor-α and interleukin-1 in a rabbit model of bacterially induced preterm pregnancy loss. Amer. J. Obstet. Gynecol. **167**:1538–1588, 1992.

McGregor, J.A. and French, J.I.: Bacterial vaginosis and preterm birth. NEJM **334**:1337–1338, 1996.

McGregor, J.A. and French, J.I.: Evidence-based prevention of preterm birth and rupture of membranes: infection and inflammation. J. Soc. Obstet. Gynaecol. Can. **19**:835–852, 1997.

McGregor, J.A., Burns, J.C., Levin, M.J., Burlington, B. and Meiklejohn, G.: Transplacental passage of influenza A/Bangkok (H_3N_2) mimicking amniotic fluid infection syndrome. Amer. J. Obstet. Gynecol. **149**:856–859, 1984.

McGregor, J.A., French, J.I., Lawellin, D., Franco-Buff, A., Smith, C. and Todd, J.K.: Bacterial protease-induced reduction of chorioamniotic membrane strength and elasticity. Obstet. Gynecol. **69**:167–174, 1987.

McGregor, J.A., Lawellin, D., Franco-Buff, A. and Todd, J.K.: Phospholipase C activity in microorganisms associated with reproductive tract infection. Amer. J. Obstet. Gynecol. **164**:682–686, 1991.

McLaren, L.C., Davis, L.E., Healy, G.R. and James, C.G.: Isolation of Trichomonas vaginalis from the respiratory tract of infants with respiratory disease. Pediatrics **71**:888–890, 1983.

McLellan, M.S., Strong, J.P., Johnson, Q.R. and Dent, J.H.: Otitis media in premature infants: a histopathologic study. J. Pediatr. **61**:53–57, 1962.

Meador, V.P. and Deyoe, B.L.: Intracellular localization of Brucella abortus in bovine placenta. Vet. Pathol. **26**:513–515, 1989.

Medearis, D.N.: CMV immunity: imperfect but protective. NEJM **306**:985–986, 1982.

Mellgren, J., Alm, L. and Kjessler, A.: The isolation of toxoplasma from the human placenta and uterus. Acta Pathol. Microbiol. Scand. **30**:59–67, 1952.

Mendoza, E., Jorda, M., Rafel, E., Simon, A. and Andrada, E.: Invasion of human embryo by Enterobius vermicularis. Arch. Pathol. Lab. Med. **111**:761–762, 1987.

Menez-Bautista, R., Fikrig, S.M., Pahwa, S., Sarangadharan, M.G. and Stoneburner, R.L.: Monozygotic twins discordant for the acquired immunodeficiency syndrome. Amer. J. Dis. Child. **140**:678–679, 1986.

Menon, R., Swan, K.F., Lyden, T.W., Rote, N.S. and Fortunato, S.J.: Expression of inflammatory cytokines (interleukin-1β and interleukin-6) in amniochorionic membranes. Amer. J. Obstet. Gynecol. **172**:493–500, 1995.

Mercer, B.M., Goldenberg, R.L., Moawad, A.H., Meis, P.J., Iams, J.D., Das, A.F., Caritis, S.N., Miodovnik, M., Menard, K., Thurnau, G.R., Dombrowski, M.P., Roberts, J.M. and McNellis, D.: The preterm prediction study: Effect of gestational age and cause of preterm birth on subsequent obstetric outcome. Amer. J. Obstet. Gynecol. 181:1216–1221, 1999.

Meyer, A., Stallmach, T., Goldenberger, D. and Altwegg, M.: Lethal maternal sepsis caused by *Campylobacter jejuni*: Pathologen preserved in placenta and identified by molecular methods. Mod. Pathol. 10:1253–1256, 1997.

Mezzano, L., Sartori, M.J., Lin, S., Repossi, G. and de Fabrio, S.P.: Placental alkaline phosphatase (PLAP) study in diabetic human placental villi infected with *Trypanosoma cruzi*. Placenta 26:85–92, 2005.

Mikamo, H., Kawazoe, K., Sato, Y., Izumi, K. and Tamaya, T.: Intra-amniotic infection caused by *Capnocytophaga* species. Infect. Dis. Obstet. Gynecol. 4:301–302, 1996.

Miller, I.J. and Telford, S.R. III: Placental malaria. NEJM 335:98, 1996.

Miller, I.J. and Telford, S.: Congenital malaria. NEJM 336:72, 1997.

Miller, J.M., Hill, G.B., Welt, S.I. and Pupkin, M.J.: Bacterial colonization of amniotic fluid in the presence of ruptured membranes. Amer. J. Obstet. Gynecol. 137:451–458, 1980a.

Miller, J.M., Pupkin, M.J. and Hill, G.B.: Bacterial colonization of premature labor. Amer. J. Obstet. Gynecol. 136:796–804, 1980b.

Miller, L.H., Reifsnyder, D.N. and Martinez, S.A.: Late onset of disease in congenital toxoplasmosis. Clin. Pediatr. 10:78–80, 1971.

Miller, R.K., Polliotti, B.M., Laughlin, T., Gnall, S., Iida, S., Carneiro, M., Lord, K., Ding, Y. and Sheikh, A.U.: Role of the placenta in fetal HIV infection. Teratology 61:391–394, 2000.

Miller, W.C.: Screening for chlamydial infection: are we doing enough? Lancet 365:456–457, 2005.

Mills, J.L., Harlap, S. and Harley, E.E.: Should coitus late in pregnancy be discouraged? Lancet 2:136–138, 1981.

Minkoff, H., Remington, J.S., Holman, S., Ramirez, R., Goodwin, S. and Landesman, S.: Vertical transmission of toxoplasma by human immunodeficiency virus-infected women. Amer. J. Obstet. Gynecol. 176:555–559, 1997.

Mitchell, J.E. and McCall, F.C.: Transplacental infection by herpes simplex virus. Amer. J. Dis. Child. 106:207–209, 1963.

Mitchell, M.D., Trautman, M.S. and Dudley, D.J.: Cytokine networking in the placenta. Placenta 14:249–275, 1993.

Mitsuda, T., Yokota, S., Mori, T., Ibe, M., Ookawa, N., Shimizu, H., Aihara, Y., Yoshida, N., Kosuge, K. and Matsuyama, S.: Demonstration of mother-to-infant transmission of hepatitis B virus by means of polymerase chain reaction. Lancet 2:886–888, 1989.

Mittendorf, R., Montag, A.G., MacMillan, W., Janeczek, S., Pryde, P.G., Besinger, R.E., Gianopoulos, J.G. and Roizen, N.: Components of the systemic fetal inflammatory response syndrome as predictors of impaired neurologic outcomes in children. Amer. J. Obstet. Gynecol. 188:1438–1446, 2003.

Miyamo, A., Miyamichi, T., Nakayama, M., Kitayima, H. and Shimizu, A.: Differences among acute, subacute, and chronic chorioamnionitis based on levels of inflammation-associated proteins in cord blood. Pediat. Development. Pathol. 1:513–521, 1998.

Mjihdi, A., Lambot, M.-A., Stewart, I.J., Detournay, O., Noë, J.-C., Carlier, Y. and Truyens, C.: Acute *Trypanosoma cruzi* infection in mouse induces infertility or placental parasite invasion and ischemic necrosis associated with massive fetal loss. Amer. J. Pathol. 161:673–680, 2002.

Modlin, J.F.: Perinatal echovirus infection: insight from a literature review of 61 cases of serious infection and 16 outbreaks in nurseries. Rev. Infect. Dis. 8:918–926, 1986.

Modlin, J.F., Grant, P.E., Makar, R.S., Roberts, D.J. and Krishnamoorthy, K.S.: Case 25–2003: A newborn boy with petechiae and thrombocytopenia. NEJM 349:691–700, 2003.

Mofleh, I.A.A., Aska, A.I.A., Sekait, M.A.A., Balla, S.R.A. and Nasser, A.N.A.: Brucellosis in Saudi Arabia: Epidemiology in the central region. Ann. Saudi Med. 16:349–352, 1996.

Molello, J.A., Jensen, R., Flint, J.C. and Collier, J.R.: Placental pathology. I. Placental lesions of sheep experimentally infected with Brucella ovis. Amer. J. Vet. Res. 24:897–904; 905–911; 915–922, 1963.

Moller, M., Thomsen, A.C., Borch, K., Dinesen, K. and Zdravkovic, M.: Rupture of fetal membranes and premature delivery associated with group B streptococci in urine of pregnant women. Lancet 2:69–70, 1984.

Molnar-Nadasdy, G., Haesly, I., Reed, J. and Altshuler, G.: Placental cryptococcus in a mother with systemic lupus erythematosus. Arch. Pathol. Lab. Med. 118:757–759, 1994.

Monif, G.R.G.: Antenatal group A streptococcal infection. Amer. J. Obstet. Gynecol. 123:213–214, 1975.

Monif, G.R.G. and Dische, R.: Viral placentitis in congenital cytomegalovirus infection. Amer. J. Clin. Pathol. 58:445–449, 1972.

Monif, G.R.G., Sever, J.L., Schiff, G.M. and Traub, R.G.: Isolation of rubella virus from products of conception. Amer. J. Obstet. Gynecol. 91:1143–1146, 1965.

Monif, G.R.G., Kellner, K.R. and Donnelly, W.H.: Congenital herpes simplex type II infection. Amer. J. Obstet. Gynecol. 152:1000–1002, 1985.

Montoya, J.G. and Liesenfeld, O.: Toxoplasmosis. Lancet 363:1965–1976, 2004.

Moore, C.G. and Schnurrenberger, P.R.: A review of naturally occurring Brucella abortus infections in wild mammals. JAVMA 179:1105–1122, 1981.

Morales, W.J. and Lim, D.: Reduction of group B streptococcal maternal and neonatal infections in preterm pregnancies with premature rupture of membranes through a rapid identification test. Amer. J. Obstet. Gynecol. 157:13–16, 1987.

Morales, W.J., Lim, D.V. and Walsh, A.F.: Prevention of neonatal group B streptococcal sepsis by use of rapid screening test and selective intrapartum chemoprophylaxis. Amer. J. Obstet. Gynecol. 155:979–983, 1986.

Moroi, K., Saito, S., Kurata, T., Sata, T. and Yanagida, M.: Fetal death associated with measles virus infection of the placenta. Amer. J. Obstet. Gynecol. 164:1107–1108, 1991.

Morris, I.J. and Ribeiro, C.D.: Listeria monocytogenes and pate. Lancet 2:1285–1286, 1989.

Mortimer, G., MacDonald, D.J. and Smeeth, A.: A pilot study of the frequency and significance of placental villitis. Br. J. Obstet. Gynaecol. 92:629–633, 1985.

Moss, T.R., Nicholls, A., Viercant, P., Gregson, S. and Hawkswell, J.: Chlamydia trachomatis and infertility. Lancet 2:281, 1986.

Mostoufi-Zadeh, M., Driscoll, S.G., Biano, S.A. and Kundsin, R.B.: Placental evidence of cytomegalovirus infection of the fetus and neonate. Arch. Pathol. Lab. Med. **108**:403–406, 1984.

Mount, A.M., Mwapasa, V., Elliott, S.R., Beeson, J.G., Tadesse, E., Lema, V.M., Molyneux, M.E., Meshnick, S.R. and Rogerson, S.J.: Impairment of humoral immunity to *Plasmodium falciparum* malaria in pregnancy by HIV infection. Lancet **363**:1860–1867, 2004.

Mühlemann, K., Miller, R.K., Metlay, L. and Menegus, M.A.: Cytomegalovirus infection of the human placenta: An immunocytochemical study. Hum. Pathol. **23**:1234–1237, 1992.

Müller, G.: Die primäre Fruchtwasserinfektion und die Möglichkeiten ihrer Entstehung. Virchows Arch. **328**:68–97, 1956.

Mulligan, M.J. and Stiehm, E.R.: Neonatal hepatitis B infection: Clinical and immunological considerations. J. Perinatol. **14**:2–9, 1994.

Mundy, D.C., Schinazi, R.F., Gerber, A.R., Nahmias, A.J. and Randall, H.W.: Human immunodeficiency virus isolated from amniotic fluid. Lancet **2**:459–460, 1987.

Muresu, R., Rubino, S., Rizzu, P., Baldini, A., Colombo, M. and Cappuccinelli, P.: A new fluorescent method for identification of Trichomonas vaginalis by fluorescent DNA in situ hybridization. J. Clin. Microbiol. **32**:1018–1022, 1994.

Mustonen, K., Mustakangas, P., Valanne, L., Professor, M.H. and Koskiniemi, M.: Congenital varicella-zoster virus infection after maternal subclinical infection: clinical and neuropathological findings. J. Perinatol. **21**:141–146, 2001.

Muthusamy, A., Achur, R.N., Bhavanandan, V.P., Fouda, G.G., Taylor, D.W. and Gowda, D.C.: *Plasmodium falciparum*-infected erythrocytes adhere both in the intervillous space and on the villous surface of human placenta by binding to the low-sulfated chondroitin sulfate proteoglycan receptor. Amer. J. Pathol. **164**:2013–2025, 2004.

Naessens, A., Foulon, W., Breynart, J. and Lauwers, S.: Postpartum bacteremia and placental colonization with genital mycoplasmas and pregnancy outcome. Amer. J. Obstet. Gynecol. **160**:647–650, 1989.

Naeye, R.L.: Causes of the excessive rates of perinatal mortality and prematurity in pregnancies complicated by maternal urinary-tract infections. NEJM **300**:819–823, 1979a.

Naeye, R.L.: Coitus and associated amniotic-fluid infections. NEJM **301**:1198–1200, 1979b.

Naeye, R.L.: Coitus and amniotic-fluid infections. NEJM **302**:633, 1980.

Naeye, R.L.: Safety of coitus in pregnancy. Lancet **2**:686, 1981.

Naeye, R.L.: Factors that predispose to premature rupture of fetal membranes. Obstet. Gynecol. **60**:93–98, 1982.

Naeye, R.L.: Adverse pregnancy outcome and coitus. Obstet. Gynecol. **62**:400, 1983.

Naeye, R.L.: Coitus and preterm delivery. Pediatr. Pathol. **5**:106–197, 1986.

Naeye, R.L.: Acute bacterial chorioamnionitis. In, Transplacental Effects on Fetal Health. D.G. Scarpelli and G. Migaki, eds., pp. 73–86. Alan Liss, New York, 1988a.

Naeye, R.L.: Antenatal malarial infection. In, Transplacental Effects on Fetal Health. D.G. Scarpelli and G. Migaki, eds., pp. 165–173. Alan Liss, New York, 1988b.

Naeye, R.L. and Peters, E.C.: Amniotic fluid infections with intact membranes leading to perinatal death: a prospective study. Pediatrics **61**:171–177, 1978.

Naeye, R.L. and Peters, E.C.: Causes and consequences of premature rupture of fetal membranes. Lancet **1**:192–194, 1980.

Naeye, R.L., Maisels, M.J., Lorenz, R.P. and Botti, J.J.: The clinical significance of placental villous edema. Pediatrics **71**:588–594, 1983.

Nagata, K., Nakamura, Y., Hosokawa, Y., Nakashima, T., Nagasue, N., Kabashima, K. and Hidaka, S.: Intrauterine Candida infection in premature baby. Acta Pathol. Jpn. **31**:695–699, 1981.

Nahmias, A.J., Alford, C.A. and Korones, S.B.: Infection of the newborn with herpes-virus. Adv. Pediatr. **17**:185–226, 1970.

Naib, Z.M., Nahmias, A.J., Josey, W.E. and Wheeler, J.H.: Association of maternal genital herpetic infection with spontaneous abortion. Obstet. Gynecol. **35**:260–263, 1970.

Naidoo, P. and Hirsch, H.: Prenatal vaccinia. Lancet **1**:196–197, 1963.

Nakamura, Y., Yamamoto, S., Tanaka, S., Yano, H., Nishimura, G., Saito, Y., Tanaka, T., Tanimura, A., Hirose, F., Fukuda, S., Shingu, M. and Hashimoto, T.: Herpes simplex viral infection in human neonates: an immunohistochemical and electron microscopic study. Human Pathol. **16**:1091–1097, 1985.

Nash, L., Janovski, N.A. and Bysshe, S.M.: Localized clostridial chorioamnionitis. Obstet. Gynecol. **21**:481–485, 1963.

Nathan, L., Bohman, V.R., Sanchez, P.J., Leos, N.K., Twickler, D.M. and Wendel, G.D.: *In utero* infection with *Treponema pallidum* in early pregnancy. Prenat. Diagn. **17**:119–123, 1997.

Navarro, C. and Blanc, W.A.: Subacute necrotizing funisitis: a variant of cord inflammation with a high rate of perinatal infection. J. Pediatr. **85**:689–697, 1974.

Nebuloni, M., Pallotti, F., Polizzotti, G., Pellegrinelli, A., Tosi, D. and Giordano, F.: Malaria placental infection with massive chronic intervillositis in a gravida 4 woman. Hum. Pathol. **32**:1022–1023, 2001.

Negishi, H., Matsuda, T., Okuyama, K., Sutoh, S., Fujioka, Y. and Fujimoto, S.: *Staphylococcus aureus* causing chorioamnionitis and fetal death with intact membranes at term. A case report. J. Reprod. Med. **43**:397–400, 1998.

Neilson, J.P. and Mutambira, M.: Coitus, twin pregnancy, and preterm labor. Amer. J. Obstet. Gynecol. **160**:416–418, 1989.

Nelson, K.E., Warren, D., Tomasi, A.M., Raju, T.N. and Vidyasagar, D.: Transmission of neonatal listeriosis in a delivery room. Amer. J. Dis. Child. **139**:903–905, 1985.

Nemir, R.L. and O'Hare, D.: Congenital tuberculosis: review and diagnostic criteria. Amer. J. Dis. Child. **139**:284–287, 1985; **140**:740–741, 1986.

Nessmann-Emmanuelli, C., Paul, G., Amiel-Tison, C., Goujard, J., Firtion, G., Henrion, R. and Sureau, C.: Frottis placentaires en maternité: intérêt pour le diagnostic précoce des infections bactériennes néonatales par contamination materno-foetale. J. Gynécol. Obstet. Biol. Rep. **12**:373–380, 1983.

Newton, E.R., Prihoda, T.J. and Gibbs, R.S.: Logistic regression analysis of risk factors for intra-amniotic infection. Obstet. Gynecol. **73**:571–575, 1989.

Newton, E.R., Piper, J. and Peairs, W.: Bacterial vaginosis and intraamniotic infection. Amer. J. Obstet. Gynecol. **176**:672–677, 1997.

Nichols, A., Khong, T.Y. and Crowther, C.A.: *Candida tropicalis* chorioamnionitis. Amer. J. Obstet. Gynecol. **172**:1045–1047, 1995.

Nickerson, C.W.: Gonorrhea amnionitis. Obstet. Gynecol. **42**:815–817, 1973.

Nieman, R.E. and Lorber, B.: Listeriosis in adults: a changing pattern; report of eight cases and review of the literature, 1968–1978. Rev. Infect. Dis. **2**:207–227, 1980.

Nigro, G., Torre, R.La, Anceschi, M.M., Mazzocco, M. and Cosmi, E.V.: Hyperimmunoglobulin therapy for a twin fetus with cytomegalovirus infection and growth restriction. Amer. J. Obstet. Gynecol. **180**:1222–1226, 1999.

Nizet, V. and Rubens, C.E.: Pathogenic mechanisms and virulence factors of group B streptococci. Chapter 13 (pp. 125–136) in: Gram-positive Pathogens. V.A. Fischetti ed., Amer. Soc. Microbiol., Washington, DC, 2000.

Nokes, J.M., Claiborne, H.A., Thornton, W.N. and Yiu-Tang, H.: Extrauterine pregnancy associated with tuberculous salpingitis and congenital tuberculosis in the fetus. Obstet. Gynecol. **9**:206–211, 1957.

Norwitz, E.R., Bernal, A.L. and Starkey, P.M.: Tumor necrosis factor-α selectively stimulates prostaglandin F$_{2\alpha}$ production by macrophages in human term decidua. Amer. J. Obstet. Gynecol. **167**:815–820, 1992a.

Norwitz, E.R., Starkey, P.M. and Bernal, A.L.: Prostaglandin D$_2$ production by term human decidua: cellular origins defined using flow cytometry. Obstet. Gynecol. **80**:440–445, 1992b.

Nosten, F., McGready, R., Simpson, J.A., Thwai, K.L., Balkan, S., Cho, T., Hkirijaroen, L., Looareesuwan, S. and White, N.J.: Effects of *Plasmodium vivax* malaria in pregnancy. Lancet **354**:546–549, 1999.

Novak, R.W. and Platt, M.S.: Significance of placental findings in early-onset group B streptococcal neonatal sepsis. Clin. Pediatr. **24**:256–258, 1985.

Nugent, R.P. [for the vaginal infection and pregnancy study]: Ureaplasma urealyticum and pregnancy outcome: results of an observational study and clinical trial. Amer. J. Epidemiol. **128**:929–930, 1988.

Ogilvie, M.M. and Tearne, C.F.: Spontaneous abortion after hand-foot-and-mouth disease caused by Coxsackie virus A 16. Br. Med. J. **281**:1527–1528, 1980.

Ohlsson, A. and Wang, E.: An analysis of antenatal tests to detect infection in preterm premature rupture of the membranes. Amer. J. Obstet. Gynecol. **162**:809–818, 1990.

Ohyama, M., Itani, Y., Tanaka, Y., Goto, A. and Sasaki, Y.: Syphilitic placentitis: demonstration of Treponema pallidum by immunoperoxidase staining. Virchows Arch. A Pathol. Anat. Histopathol. **417**:343–345, 1990.

Ohyama, M., Fukui, T., Tanaka, Y., Kato, K., Hoshino, R., Sugawara, T., Yamanaka, M., Ijiri, R., Sata, T. and Itani, Y.: Measles virus infection in the placenta of monozygotic twins. Modern Pathol. **14**:1300–1303, 2001.

Ohyama, M., Itani, Y., Yamanaka, M., Goto, A., Kato, K., Ijiri, R. and Tanaka, Y.: Re-evaluation of chorioamnionitis and funisitis with a special reference to subacute chorioamnionitis. Human Pathol. **33**:183–190, 2002.

Okita, J.R., Johnston, J.M. and MacDonald, P.C.: Source of prostaglandin precursor in human fetal membranes: arachidonic acid content of amnion and chorion laeve in diamnionic-dichorionic twin placentas. Amer. J. Obstet. Gynecol. **147**:477–482, 1983.

Oláh, K.S., Vince, G.S., Neilson, J.P., Deniz, G. and Johnson, P.M.: Interleukin-6, interferon-μ, interleukin-8, and granulo-cyte-macrophage colony stimulating factor levels in human amniotic fluid at term. J. Reprod. Immunol. **32**:89–98, 1996.

Olding, L.: Value of placentitis as a sign of intrauterine infection in human subjects. Acta Pathol. Microbiol. Scand. [A] **78**:256–264, 1970.

Olding, L. and Philipson, L.: Two cases of listeriosis in the newborn, associated with placental infection. Acta Pathol. Microbiol. Scand. **48**:24–30, 1960.

Oppenheimer, E.H. and Hardy, J.B.: Congenital syphilis in the newborn infant: clinical and pathological observations in recent cases. Johns Hopkins Med. J. **129**:63–82, 1971.

Ordi, J., Ismail, M.R., Ventura, P.J., Kahigwa, E., Hirt, R., Cardesa, A., Alonso, P.L. and Menendez, C.: Massive chronic intervillositis of the placenta associated with malaria infection. Amer. J. Surg. Pathol. **22**:1006–1011, 1998.

Ordi, J., Menendez, C., Ismail, M.R., Ventura, P.J., Palacin, A., Kahigwa, E., Ferrer, B., Cardesa, A. and Alonso, P.L.: Placental malaria is associated with cell-mediated inflammatory responses with selective absence of natural killer cells. J. Infect. Dis. **183**:1100–1107, 2001.

Oriel, J.D., Partridge, B.M., Denny, M.J. and Coleman, J.C.: Genital yeast infections. Br. Med. J. **4**:761–764, 1972.

Ornoy, A., Segal, S., Nishmi, M., Simcha, A. and Polishuk, W.Z.: Fetal and placental pathology in gestational rubella. Amer. J. Obstet. Gynecol. **116**:949–956, 1973.

Ornoy, A., Dudai, M. and Sadovsky, E.: Placental and fetal pathology in infectious mononucleosis: a possible indicator for Epstein-Barr virus teratogenicity. Diagn. Gynecol. Obstet. **4**:11–16, 1982.

Ortel, S.: Listerienausscheider und ihre epidemiologische Bedeutung. Münch. Med. Wochenschr. **117**:1145–1148, 1975.

Osborn, G.R.: Congenital pneumonia. Lancet **1**:275, 1962.

Osmers, R.G.W., Bläser, J., Kuhn, W. and Tschesche, H.: Interleukin-8 synthesis and the onset of labor. Obstet. Gynecol. **86**:223–229, 1995.

Oyarzún, E., Yamamoto, M., Kato, S. Gómez, R., Lizama, L. and Moenne, A.: Specific detection of 16 micro-organisms in amniotic fluid by polymerase chain reaction and its correlation with preterm delivery occurrence. Amer. J. Obstet. Gynecol. **179**:1115–1119, 1998.

Ozono, K., Mushiake, S., Takeshima, T. and Nakayama, M.: Diagnosis of congenital cytomegalovirus infection by examination of the placenta: application of polymerase chain reaction and in situ hybridization. Pediat. Pathol. Lab. Med. **17**:249–258, 1997.

Paavonen, J., Critchlow, C.W., DeRouen, T., Stevens, C.E., Kiviat, N., Brunham, R.C., Stamm, W.E., Kuo, C.-C., Hyde, K.E., Corey, L., Eschenbach, D.A. and Holmes, K.K.: Etiology of cervical inflammation. Amer. J. Obstet. Gynecol. **154**:556–564, 1986.

Panem, S.: C-type virus expression in the placenta. Curr. Top. Pathol. **66**:175–189, 1979.

Pankuch, G.A., Appelbaum, P.C., Lorenz, R.P., Botti, J.J., Schachter, J. and Naeye, R.L.: Placental microbiology and histology and the pathogenesis of chorioamnionitis. Obstet. Gynecol. **64**:802–806, 1984.

Pankuch, G.A., Cherouny, P.H., Botti, J.J. and Appelbaum, P.C.: Amniotic fluid leukotaxis assay as an early indicator of chorioamnionitis. Amer. J. Obstet. Gynecol. **161**:802–807, 1989.

Pao, C.C., Kao, S.-M., Wang, H.-C. and Lee, C.C.: Intraamniotic detection of *Chlamydia trachomatis* deoxyribonucleic acid sequences by polymerase chain reaction. Amer. J. Obstet. Gynecol. **164**:1295–1299, 1991.

Papiernik, E., Charlemain, C., Goffinet, F., Paul, G. and Keith, L.G.: Vaginal bacterial colonization, the uterine cervix and preterm births. Prenat. Neonat. Med. **3**:98–102, 1998.

Parker, C.R. and Wendel, G.D.: The effects of syphilis on endocrine function of the fetoplacental unit. Amer. J. Obstet. Gynecol. **159**:1327–1331, 1988.

Parry, S. and Strauss, J.F.: Premature rupture of the fetal membranes. NEJM **338**:663–670, 1998.

Paryani, S.G. and Arvin, A.M.: Intrauterine infection with varicella-zoster virus after maternal varicella. NEJM **314**:1542–1546, 1986.

Pascual, A., Bruna, I., Cerrolaza, J., Moreno, P., Ramos, J.T., Noriega, A.R. and Delgado, R.: Absence of maternal-fetal transmission of human immunodeficiency virus type 1 to second-trimester fetuses. Amer. J. Obstet. Gynecol. **183**:638–642, 2000.

Pass, M.A., Khare, S. and Dillon, H.C.: Twin pregnancies: incidence of group B streptococcal colonization and disease. J. Pediatr. **97**:635–637, 1980.

Pass, R.F., Stagno, S., Myers, G.J. and Alford, C.A.: Outcome of symptomatic congenital cytomegalovirus infection: results of long-term longitudinal follow-up. Pediatrics **66**:758–762, 1980.

Pass, M.A., Gray, B.M. and Dillon, H.C.: Puerperal and perinatal infections with group B streptococci. Amer. J. Obstet. Gynecol. **143**:147–152, 1982.

Pass, R.F., Little, E.A., Stagno, S., Britt, W.J. and Alford, C.A.: Young children as a probable source of maternal and congenital cytomegalovirus infection. NEJM **316**:1366–1370, 1987.

Pasternack, R., Mustila, A., Vuorinen, P., Heinonen, P.K. and Miettinen, A.: Polymerase chain reaction assay with urine specimens in the diagnosis of acute *Chlamydia trachomatis* infection in women. Infect. Dis. Obstet. Gynecol. **4**:276–280, 1996.

Pastorek, J.G., Mroczkowski, T.F. and Martin, D.H.: Fine-tuning the fluorescent antibody test for chlamydial infections in pregnancy. Obstet. Gynecol. **72**:957–960, 1988.

Patrick, L.A., Gaudet, L.M., Farley, A.E., Rossiter, J.P., Tomalty, L.L. and Smith, G.N.: Development of a guinea pig model of chorioamnionitis and fetal brain injury. Amer. J. Obstet. Gynecol. **191**:1205–1211, 2004.

Peaceman, A.M., Andrews, W.W., Thorp, J.M., Cliver, S.P., Lukes, A., Iams, J.D., Coultrip, L., Eriksen, N., Holbrook, R.H., Elliott, J., Ingardia, C. and Pietrantoni, M.: Fetal fibronectin as a predictor of preterm birth in patients with symptoms: A multicenter trial. Amer. J. Obstet. Gynecol. **177**:13–18, 1998.

Peeling, R.W. and Brunham, R.C.: Chlamydiae as pathogens: New species and new issues. Emerging Infect. Dis. **2**:307–319, 1996.

Peeters, F., Snauwaert, R., Segers, J., van Cutsem, J. and Amery, W.: Observations on candidal vaginitis: vaginal pH, microbiology, and cytology. Amer. J. Obstet. Gynecol. **112**:80–86, 1972.

Peevy, K.J. and Chalhub, E.G.: Occult group B streptococcal infection: an important cause of intrauterine asphyxia. Amer. J. Obstet. Gynecol. **146**:989–990, 1983.

Peipert, J.F.: Genital chlamydial infections. NEJM **349**:2424–2430, 2003.

Peng, J., Krause, P.J. and Kresch, M.: Neonatal herpes simplex virus infection after Cesarean section with intact amniotic membranes. J. Perinatol. **16**:397–399, 1996.

Pera, A., Byun, A., Gribar, S., Schwartz, R., Kumar, D. and Parimi, P.: Dexamethasone therapy and *Candida* sepsis in neonates less than 1250 grams. J. Perinatol. **22**:204–208, 2002.

Perkins, R.P.: Adverse pregnancy outcome and coitus. Obstet. Gynecol. **62**:399–400, 1983.

Perni, S.C., Vardhana, S., Korneeva, I. Tuttle, S.L., Paraskevas, L.R., Chasen, S.T., Kalish, R.B. and Witkin, S.: Mycoplasma hominis and Ureaplasma urealyticum in midtrimester amniotic fluid: association with amniotic fluid cytokine levels and pregnancy outcome. Amer. J. Obstet. Gynecol. **191**:1382–1386, 2004.

Perni, S.C., Cho, J.E. and Baergen, R.N.: Placental pathology and pregnancy outcomes in donor and non-donor oocyte in vitro fertilization pregnancies. J. Perinatal. Med. **33**:27–32, 2005.

Perrin, E.V.D. and Bel, J.K.-V.: Degeneration and calcification of the umbilical cord. Obstet. Gynecol. **26**:371–373, 1965.

Peters, M.T., Lowe, T.W., Carpenter, A. and Kole, S.: Prenatal diagnosis of congenital cytomegalovirus infection with abnormal triple-screen results and hyperechoic fetal bowel. Amer. J. Obstet. Gynecol. **173**:953–954, 1995.

Peterson, C.M., Johnson, S.L., Kelly, J.V. and Kelly, P.C.: Coccidial meningitis and pregnancy: a case report. Obstet. Gynecol. **73**:835–836, 1989.

Petrilli, E.S., D'Ablaing, G. and Ledger, W.J.: Listeria monocytogenes chorioamnionitis: diagnosis by transabdominal amniocentesis. Obstet. Gynecol. **55**:5S–8S, 1980.

Peuchmaur, M., Pons, J.C., Papiernik, E. and Delfraissy, J.F.: Isolation of acquired immunodeficiency syndrome virus from the placenta. Amer. J. Obstet. Gynecol. **160**:765, 1989.

Phillips, C.A., Maeck, J.V.S., Rogers, W.A. and Savel, H.: Intrauterine rubella infection following immunization with rubella vaccine. JAMA **213**:624–625, 1970.

Pickard, R.E.: Varicella pneumonia in pregnancy. Amer. J. Obstet. Gynecol. **101**:504–508, 1968.

Pinar, H., Sotomayor, E. and Singer, D.B.: Turquoise discoloration of the umbilical cord and membranes after intraamniotic injection of indigo carmine dye for premature rupture of membranes. Arch. Pediatr. Adolesc. Med. **152**:199–200, 1998.

Pisarski, T., Breborowicz, H. and Prybora, L.A.: Leucocytic infiltration in the placenta and membranes. Biol. Neonat. **5**:129–150, 1963.

Pizzato, N., Garmy-Susini, B., Bouteiller, P.Le and Lenfant, F.: Down-regulation of HLA-G1 surface expression in human cytomegalovirus infected cells. Amer. J. Reprod. Immunol. **50**:328–333, 2003.

Platz-Christensen, J.J., Mattsby-Baltzer, I., Thomsen, P. and Wiqvist, N.: Endotoxin and interleukin-1α in the cervical mucus and vaginal fluid of pregnant women with bacterial vaginosis. Amer. J. Obstet. Gynecol. **169**:1161–1166, 1993.

Plaza, M.C. and Gilbert-Barness, E.: Fetal death in utero secondary to *Listeria monocytogenes* placental infection. Pediat. Pathol. Molec. Med. **20**:433–437, 2001.

Pletcher, B.A., Williams, M.K., Mulivor, R.A., Barth, D., Linder, C. and Rawlinson, K.: Intrauterine cytomegalovirus infection presenting as fetal meconium peritonitis. Obstet. Gynecol. **78**:903–905, 1991.

Pollack, R.N., Sklarin, N.T., Rao, S. and Divon, M.Y.: Metastatic placental lymphoma associated with maternal human immunodeficiency virus infection. Obstet. Gynecol. **81**:856–857, 1993.

Polunin, I.: Infertility and depopulation: a study of the Murut tribes of North Borneo. Lancet **2**:1005–1008, 1958.

Popek, E.J.: Granulomatous villitis due to *Toxoplasma gondii*. Pediatr. Pathol. **12**:281–288, 1992.

Porreco, R.P. and Haverkamp, A.D.: Brucellosis in pregnancy. Obstet. Gynecol. **44**:597–602, 1974.

Potkul, R.K., Moawad, A.H. and Ponto, K.L.: The association of subclinical infection with preterm labor: the role of C-reactive protein. Amer. J. Obstet. Gynecol. **153**:642–645, 1985.

Pradeepkumar, V.K., Rajadurai, V.S. and Tan, K.W.: Congenital candidiasis: varied presentations. J. Perinatol. **18**:311–316, 1998.

Pressman, E.K., Cavanaugh, J.L. and Woods, J.R.: Physical properties of the chorioamnion throughout gestation. Amer. J. Obstet. Gynecol. **187**:672–675, 2002.

Pritchard, J.A. and Whalley, P.J.: Abortion complicated by Clostridium perfringens infection. Amer. J. Obstet. Gynecol. **111**:484–490, 1971.

Pritzlaff, C.A., Chang, J.C.W., Kuo, S.P., Tamura, G.S., Rubens, C.E. and Nizet, V.: Genetic basis for ß-haemolytic/cytolytic activity of group B *Streptococcus*. Molec. Microbiol. **39**:236–247, 2001.

Procop, G.W., Jessen, R., Hyde, S.R. and Scheck, D.N.: Persistence of *Plasmodium falciparum* in the placenta after apparently effective quinidine/clindamycin therapy. J. Perinatol. **21**:128–130, 2001.

Pugh, V.W. and Vakil, S.: Salmonella typhimurium meningitis in a premature infant during the neonatal period. Arch. Dis. Child. **27**:473–474, 1952.

Purtilo, D.T., Bhawan, J., Liao, S., Brutus, A., Yang, J.P.S. and Balogh, K.: Fatal varicella in a pregnant woman and a baby. Amer. J. Obstet. Gynecol. **127**:208–209, 1977.

Pyati, S.P., Pildes, R.S., Jacobs, N.M., Ramamurthy, R.S., Yeh, T.F., Raval, D.S., Lilien, L.D., Amma, P. and Metzger, W.I.: Penicillin in infants weighing two kilograms or less with early-onset group B streptococcal disease. NEJM **308**:1383–1389, 1983.

Quagliarello, J.R., Passalaqua, A.M., Greco, M.A., Zinberg, S. and Young, B.K.: Ballantyne's triple edema syndrome: prenatal diagnosis with ultrasound and maternal renal biopsy findings. Amer. J. Obstet. Gynecol. **132**:580–581, 1978.

Quan, A. and Strauss, L.: Congenital cytomegalic inclusion disease: observations in a macerated fetus with congenital defect, including study of the placenta. Amer. J. Obstet. Gynecol. **83**:1240–1247, 1962.

Quayle, A.J., Porter, E.M., Nussbaum, A.A., Wang, Y.M., Brabec, C., Yip, K.-P. and Mok, S.M.: Gene expression, immunolocalization, and secretion of human defensin-5 in human female reproductive tract. Amer. J. Pathol. **152**:1247–1258, 1998.

Quinn, P.A., Shewchuk, A.B., Shuber, J., Lie, K.I., Ryan, E., Chipman, M.L. and Bocilla, D.M.: Efficacy of antibiotic therapy in preventing spontaneous pregnancy loss among couples colonized with genital mycoplasmas. Amer. J. Obstet. Gynecol. **145**:239–250, 1983.

Quinn, P.A., Butany, J., Chipman, M., Taylor, J. and Hannah, W.: A prospective study of microbial infection in stillbirths and neonatal death. Amer. J. Obstet. Gynecol. **151**:238–249, 1985.

Quinn, P.A., Butany, J., Taylor, J. and Hannah, W.: Chorioamnionitis: its association with pregnancy outcome and microbial infection. Amer. J. Obstet. Gynecol. **156**:379–387, 1987.

Quinn, T.C., Jacobs, R.F., Mertz, G.J., Hook, E.W. and Locksley, R.M.: Congenital malaria: a report of four cases and a review. J. Pediatr. **101**:229–232, 1982.

Quintero, R.A., Morales, W.J., Kalter, C.S., Allen, M., Mendoza, G., Angel, J.L. and Romero, R.: Transabdominal intra-amniotic endoscopic assessment of previable premature rupture of membranes. Amer. J. Obstet. Gynecol. **179**:71–76, 1998.

Quintero, R.A., Morales, W.J., Bornick, P.W., Allen, M. and Garabelis, N.: Surgical treatment of spontaneous rupture of membranes: The amniograft—first experience. Amer. J. Obstet. Gynecol. **186**:155–157, 2002.

Qureshi, F. and Jacques, S.M.: Maternal varicella during pregnancy: correlation of maternal history and fetal outcome with placental histopathology. Hum. Pathol. **27**:191–195, 1996.

Qureshi, F., Jacques, S.M., Bendon, R.W., Faye-Peterson, O.M., Heifetz, S.A., Redline, R. and Sander, C.M.: *Candida* funisitis: a clinicopathologic study of 32 cases. Pediatr. Developm. Pathol. **1**:118–124, 1998.

Ramsey, A.M.: The significance of Clostridium welchii in the cervical swab and blood stream in post partum and post abortum sepsis. J. Obstet. Gynaecol. Br. Emp. **56**:247–258, 1949.

Raoult, D. and Stein, A.: Q fever during pregnancy—a risk for women, fetuses, and obstetricians. NEJM **330**:371, 1994.

Rappaport, F., Rabinovitz, M., Toaff, R. and Krochik, N.: Genital listeriosis as a cause of recurrent abortion. Lancet **1**:1273–1275, 1960.

Rappelli, P., Rocchigiani, A.M., Erre, G., Colombo, M.M., Cappuccinelli, P. and Fiori, P.: Sequence of cDNA coding for a 65 kDa adhesive protein for the specific detection of Trichomonas vaginalis by PCR. FEMS Microbiol. Lett. **129**:21–26, 1995.

Ravid, R. and Toaff, R.: Solitary abscess of the placenta in a pregnancy treated with cerclage. Int. Surg. **61**:553–554, 1976.

Read, J.S. and Klebanoff, M.A., for the Vaginal Infection and Prematurity Study Group: Sexual intercourse during pregnancy and preterm delivery: effects of vaginal microorganisms. Amer. J. Obstet. Gynecol. **168**:514–519, 1993.

Redline, R.W. and Abramowsky, C.R.: Clinical and pathological aspects of recurrent villitis. Lab. Invest. **50**:10P, 1984 (abstract).

Redline, R.W. and Abramowsky, C.R.: Clinical and pathological aspects of recurrent villitis. Hum. Pathol. **16**:727–731, 1985.

Redline, R.W. and Lu, C.Y.: Role of local immunosuppression in murine fetoplacental listeriosis. J. Clin. Invest. **79**:1234–1241, 1987.

Redline, R.W. and Lu, C.Y.: Specific defects in the anti-listerial immune response in discrete regions of the murine uterus and placenta account for susceptibility to infection. J. Immunol. **140**:3947–3955, 1988.

Redline, R.W. and Patterson, P.: Villitis of unknown etiology is associated with major infiltration of fetal tissues by maternal inflammatory cells. Amer. J. Pathol. **143**:473–479, 1993.

Redline, R.W., Shea, C.M., Papaionnou, V.E. and Lu, C.Y.: Defective anti-listerial responses in deciduoma of pseudo-pregnant mice. Amer. J. Pathol. **133**:485–497, 1988.

Redline, R.W., Faye-Petersen, O., Heller, D., Qureshi, F., Savell, V. and Vogler, C.: Amniotic infection syndrome: nosology and reproducibility of placental patterns. Pediatr. Devel. Pathol. **6**:435–448, 2003.

Regan, J.A., Chao, S. and James, L.S.: Premature rupture of membranes, preterm delivery, and group B streptococcal colonization of mothers. Amer. J. Obstet. Gynecol. **141**:184–186, 1981.

Reisenberger, K., Egarter, C., Knöfler, M., Schiebel, I., Gregor, H., Hirschl, A.M., Heinze, G. and Husslein, P.: Cytokine and prostaglandin production by amnion cells in response to the addition of different bacteria. Amer. J. Obstet. Gynecol. **178**:50–53, 1998.

Remington, J.S. and Klein, J.O., eds.: Infectious Diseases of the Fetus and Newborn Infant. 2nd Ed. Saunders, Philadelphia, 1983.

Remington, J.S., Newell, J.W. and Cavanaugh, E.: Spontaneous abortion and chronic toxoplasmosis: report of a case, with isolation of the parasite. Obstet. Gynecol. **24**:25–31, 1964.

Rettig, P.J. and Altshuler, G.: Rat model of prenatal Chlamydial trachomatis (Ct) infection. 21st Interscience Conference on Antimicrobial Agents and Chemotherapy. American Society of Microbiologists. Abstract 517, 1981.

Rhatigan, R.M.: Congenital cutaneous candidiasis. Amer. J. Dis. Child. **116**:545–546, 1968.

Rhyan, J.C., Stackhouse, L.L. and Quinn, W.J.: Fetal and placental lesions in bovine abortion due to Tritrichomonas foetus. Vet. Pathol. **25**:350–355, 1988.

Ricci, J.M., Fojaco, R.M. and O'Sullivan, M.J.: Congenital syphilis: the University of Miami/Jackson Memorial Medical Center experience, 1986–1988. Obstet. Gynecol. **74**:687–693, 1989.

Rizzo, G., Capponi, A., Arduini, D., Lorido, C. and Romanini, C.: The value of fetal fibronectin in cervical and vaginal secretions and of ultrasonographic examination of the uterine cervix in predicting premature delivery for patients with preterm labor and intact membranes. Amer. J. Obstet. Gynecol. **175**:1146–1151, 1996.

Robb, J.A., Benirschke, K. and Barmeyer, R.: Intrauterine latent herpes simplex virus infection. I. Spontaneous abortion. Hum. Pathol. **17**:1196–1209, 1986a.

Robb, J.A., Benirschke, K., Mannino, F. and Voland, J.: Intrauterine latent herpes simplex virus infection. II. Latent neonatal infection. Hum. Pathol. **17**:1210–1217, 1986b.

Roberts, D.J.: Case record # 15-1997. NEJM **336**:1439–1446, 1997.

Rode, M.E., Morgan, M.A., Ruchelli, E. and Forouzan, I.: *Candida* chorioamnionitis after serial therapeutic amniocenteses: a possible association. J. Perinatol. **5**:335–337, 2000.

Roll, C., Schmid, E.N., Menken, U. and Hanssler, L.: Fatal *Salmonella enteritidis* sepsis acquired prenatally in a premature infant. Obstet. Gynecol. **88**:692–693, 1996.

Romagosa, C., Menendez, C., Ismail, M.R., Quinto, L., Ferrer, B., Alonso, P.L. and Ordi, J.: Polarisation microscopy increases the sensitivity of hemozoin and Plasmodium detection in the histological assessment of placental malaria. Acta Trop. **90**:277–284, 2004.

Romano, N., Romano, F. and Carollo, F.: T-strain of mycoplasma in bronchopneumonic lungs of an aborted fetus. NEJM **285**:950–952, 1971.

Romem, Y. and Artal, R.: C-reactive protein as a predictor for chorioamnionitis in cases of premature rupture of the membranes. Amer. J. Obstet. Gynecol. **150**:546–550, 1984.

Romero, R.: Is genital colonization with Mycoplasma hominis or Ureaplasma urealyticum associated with prematurity/low birth weight? Obstet. Gynecol. **74**:679–680, 1989.

Romero, R., Emamian, M., Quintero, R., Wan, M., Hobbins, J.C. and Mitchell, M.D.: Amniotic fluid prostaglandin levels and intra-amniotic infections. Lancet **1**:1380, 1986.

Romero, R., Kadar, N., Hobbins, J.C. and Duff, G.W.: Infection and labor: the detection of endotoxin in amniotic fluid. Amer. J. Obstet. Gynecol. **157**:815–819, 1987a.

Romero, R., Quintero, R., Emamiam, M., Wan, M., Grzyboski, C.L.T., Hobbins, J.C. and Mitchell, M.D.: Arachidonate lipoxygenase metabolites in amniotic fluid of women with intra-amniotic infection and preterm labor. Amer. J. Obstet. Gynecol. **157**:1457–1460, 1987b.

Romero, R., Roslansky, P., Oyarzun, E., Wan, M., Emamian, M., Novitsky, T.J., Gould, M.J. and Hobbins, J.C.: II. Bacterial endotoxin in amniotic fluid and its relationship to the onset of preterm labor. Amer. J. Obstet. Gynecol. **158**:1044–1049, 1988a.

Romero, R., Scharf, K., Mazor, M., Emamian, M., Hobbins, J.C. and Ryan, J.L.: The clinical value of gas-liquid chromatography in the detection of intra-amniotic microbial invasion. Obstet. Gynecol. **72**:44–50, 1988b.

Romero, R., Wu, Y.K., Mazor, M., Hobbins, J.C. and Mitchell, M.D.: Increased amniotic fluid leukotriene C_4 concentration in term human parturition. Amer. J. Obstet. Gynecol. **159**:655–657, 1988c.

Romero, R., Brody, D.T., Oyarzun, E., Mazor, M., Wu, Y.K., Hobbins, J.C. and Durum, S.K.: Infection and labor. III. Interleukin-1: a signal for the onset of parturition. Amer. J. Obstet. Gynecol. **160**:1117–1123, 1989a.

Romero, R., Manogue, K.R., Mitchell, M.D., Wu, Y.K., Oyarzun, E., Hobbins, J.C. and Cerami, A.: Infection and labor. IV. Cachectin-tumor necrosis factor in the amniotic fluid of women with intraamniotic infection and preterm labor. Amer. J. Obstet. Gynecol. **161**:336–341, 1989b.

Romero, R., Mazor, M., Oyarzun, E., Sirtori, M., Wu, Y.K. and Hobbins, J.C.: Is genital colonization with Mycoplasma hominis or Ureaplasma urealyticum associated with prematurity/low birth weight? Obstet. Gynecol. **73**:532–536, 1989c.

Romero, R., Oyarzun, E., Mazor, M., Sirtori, M., Hobbins, J.C. and Bracken, M.: Meta-analysis of the relationship between asymptomatic bacteriuria and preterm delivery/low birth weight. Obstet. Gynecol. **73**:576–582, 1989d.

Romero, R., Sirtori, M., Oyarzun, E., Avila, C., Mazor, M., Callahan, R., Sabo, V., Athanassiadis, A.P. and Hobbins, J.C.: Infection and labor. V. Prevalence, microbiology, and clinical significance of intraamniotic infection in women with preterm labor and intact membranes. Amer. J. Obstet. Gynecol. **161**:817–824, 1989e.

Romero, R., Wu, Y.K., Brody, D.T., Oyarzun, E., Duff, G.W. and Durum, S.K.: Human decidua: a source of interleukin-1. Obstet. Gynecol. **73**:31–34, 1989f.

Romero, R., Salafia, C.M., Athanassiadis, A.P., Hanaoka, S., Mazor, M., Sepulveda, W. and Bracken, M.B.: The relationship between acute inflammatory lesions of the preterm placenta and amniotic fluid microbiology. Amer. J. Obstet. Gynecol. **166**:1382–1388, 1992a.

Romero, R., Sepulveda, W., Mazor, M., Brandt, F., Cotton, D.B., Dinarello, C.A. and Mitchell, M.D.: The natural interleukin-1 receptor antagonist in term and preterm parturition. Amer. J. Obstet. Gynecol. **167**:863–872, 1992b.

Romero, R., Mazor, M., Sepulveda, W., Avila, C., Copeland, D. and Williams, J.: Tumor necrosis factor in preterm and term labor. Amer. J. Obstet. Gynecol. **166**:1576–1587, 1992c.

Romero, R., Gonzalez, R., Sepulveda, W., Brandt, F., Ramirez, M., Sorokin, Y., Mazor, M., Treadwell, M.C. and Cotton, D.B.: Infection and labor. VIII. Microbial invasion of the amniotic cavity in patients with suspected cervical incompetence: Prevalence and clinical significance. Amer. J. Obstet. Gynecol. **167**:1086–1091, 1992d.

Romero, R., Baumann, P., Gomez, R., Salafia, C., Rittenhouse, L., Barberio, D., Behnke, E., Cotton, D.B. and Mitchell, M.D.: The relationship between spontaneous rupture of membranes, labor, and microbial invasion of the amniotic cavity and amniotic fluid concentrations of prostaglandins and thromboxane B_2 in term pregnancy. Amer. J. Obstet. Gynecol. **168**:1654–1668, 1993.

Rosenstein, D.L. and Navarrete-Reyna, A.: Cytomegalic inclusion disease. Amer. J. Obstet. Gynecol. **89**:220–224, 1964.

Rothbard, M.J., Gregory, T. and Salerno, L.J.: Intrapartum gonococcal amnionitis. Amer. J. Obstet. Gynecol. **121**:565–566, 1975.

Rouse, D.J., Landon, M., Leveno, K.J., Leindecker, S., Varner, M.W., Caritis, S.N., O'Sullivan, J., Wapner, R.J., Meis, P.J., Miodovnik, M., Sorokin, Y., Moawad, A.H., Mabie, W., Conway, D., Gabbe, S. and Spong, C.Y.: The maternal-fetal medicine units cesarean registry: chorioamnionitis at term and its duration—relationship to outcomes. Amer. J. Obstet. Gynecol. **191**:211–216, 2004.

Royston, D. and Geoghegan, F.: Amniotic fluid infection with intact membranes in relation to stillborns. Obstet. Gynecol. **65**:745–746, 1985.

Ruben, B., Band, J.D., Wong, P. and Colville, J.: Person-to-person transmission of *Brucella melitensis*. Lancet **337**:14–15, 1991.

Rüschoff, J., Böger, A. and Zwiens, G.: Chronic placentitis—a clinicopathological study. Arch. Gynecol. **237**:19–25, 1985.

Ruffolo, E.H., Wilson, R.B. and Lyle, W.A.: Listeria monocytogenes as a cause of pregnancy wastage. Obstet. Gynecol. **19**:533–536, 1962.

Rusan, P., Adam, R.D., Petersen, E.A., Ryan, K.J., Sinclair, N.A. and Weinstein, L.: *Haemophilus influenzae*: an important cause of maternal and neonatal infections. Obstet. Gynecol. **77**:92–96, 1991.

Russell, P.: Inflammatory lesions of the human placenta. III: The histopathology of villitis of unknown aetiology. Placenta **1**:227–244, 1980.

Russell, P. and Altshuler, G.: Placental abnormalities of congenital syphilis: a neglected aid to diagnosis. Amer. J. Dis. Child. **128**:160–163, 1974.

Russell, P., Atkinson, K. and Krishnan, L.: Recurrent reproductive failure due to severe placental villitis of unknown etiology. J. Reprod. Med. **24**:93–98, 1980.

Ryan Jr., G.M., Abdella, T.N., McNeeley, S.G., Baselski, V.S. and Drummond, D.E.: *Chlamydia trachomatis* infection in pregnancy and effect of treatment on outcome. Amer. J. Obstet. Gynecol. **162**:34–39, 1990.

Sachdev, R., Nuovo, G.J., Kaplan, C. and Greco, M.A.: In situ hybridization analysis for cytomegalovirus in chronic villitis. Pediatr. Pathol. **10**:909–917, 1990.

Sacker, I., Walker, M. and Brunell, P.A.: Abscess in newborn infants caused by mycoplasma. Pediatrics **46**:303–304, 1970.

Saigal, S., Eisele, W.A. and Chernesky, M.A.: Congenital cytomegalovirus infection in a pair of dizygotic twins. Amer. J. Dis. Child. **136**:1094–1095, 1982a.

Saigal, S., Lunyk, O., Bryce-Larhe, R.P. and Chernesky, M.A.: The outcome of children with congenital cytomegalovirus infection: a longitudinal follow-up study. Amer. J. Dis. Child. **136**:896–901, 1982b.

Saito, F., Yutani, C., Imakita, M., Ishibashi-Veda, H., Kanzaki, T. and Chiba, Y.: Giant cell pneumonia caused by varicella zoster virus in a neonate. Arch. Pathol. Lab. Med. **113**:201–203, 1989.

Saito, K., Koizumi, F. and Sumiyoshi, Y.: Viral placentitis—a case report. Acta Pathol. Jpn. **27**:275–282, 1977.

Salafia, C.M., Silberman, L., Herrera, N.E. and Mahoney, M.J.: Placental pathology at term associated with elevated midtrimester maternal serum α-fetoprotein concentration. Amer. J. Obstet. Gynecol. **158**:1064–1066, 1988.

Salafia, C.M., Weigl, C. and Silberman, L.: The prevalence and distribution of acute placental inflammation in uncomplicated term pregnancies. Obstet. Gynecol. **73**:383–389, 1989.

Salafia, C.M., Vogel, C.A., Vintzileos, A.M., Bantham, K.F., Pezzullo, J. and Silberman, L.: Placental pathologic findings in preterm birth. Amer. J. Obstet. Gynecol. **165**:934–938, 1991.

Sampson, J.E., Theve, R.P., Blatman, R.N., Shipp, T.D., Bianchi, D.W., Ward, B.E. and Jack, R.M.: Fetal origin of amniotic fluid polymorphonuclear leukocytes. Amer. J. Obstet. Gynecol. **176**:77–81, 1997.

Samra, J.S., Obhrai, M.S. and Constantine, G.: Parvovirus infection in pregnancy. Obstet. Gynecol. **73**:832–834, 1989.

Sanchez, P.J. and Regan, J.A.: Ureaplasma urealyticum colonization and chronic lung disease in low birth weight infants. Pediatr. Infect. Dis. J. **7**:542–546, 1988.

Sander, C.H., Martin, J.N., Rogers, A.L., Barr, M. and Heidelberger, K.P.: Perinatal infection with Torulopsis glabrata: a case associated with maternal sickle cell anemia. Obstet. Gynecol. **61**:21S–24S, 1983.

Sander, C.H., Kinnane, L., Stevens, N.G. and Echt, R.: Haemorrhagic endovasculitis of the placenta: a review with clinical correlation. Placenta **7**:551–574, 1986.

Sandy, E.A., Blumenfeld, M.L. and Iams, J.D.: Gram stain in the rapid determination of maternal colonization with group B beta-streptococcus. Obstet. Gynecol. **71**:796–798, 1988.

Sarff, L.D., McCracken, G.H., Schiffer, M.S., Glode, M.P., Robbins, J.B., Orskov, I. and Orskov, F.: Epidemiology of

Escherichia coli K1 in healthy and diseased newborns. Lancet **1**:1099–1104, 1975.

Sarram, M., Feiz, J., Foruzandeh, M. and Gazanfarpour, P.: Intrauterine fetal infection with Brucella melitensis as a possible cause of second-trimester abortion. Amer. J. Obstet. Gynecol. **119**:657–660, 1974.

Sarto, G.E., Stubblefield, P.A. and Therman, E.: Endomitosis in human trophoblast. Hum. Genet. **62**:228–232, 1982.

Sauerbrei, A. and Wutzler, P.: The congenital varicella syndrome. J. Perinatol. **20**:548–554, 2000.

Sauerbrei, A. and Wutzler, P.: Neonatal varicella. J. Perinatol. **21**:545–549, 2001.

Sauerbrei, A., Glück, B., Jung, K., Bittrich, H. and Wutzler, P.: Congenital skin lesions caused by intrauterine infection with coxsackievirus B3 infection **28**:326–328, 2000.

Savva, D. and Holliman, R.E.: PCR to detect toxoplasma. Lancet **336**:1325, 1990.

Sawyer, M.H., Nachlas, N.E. and Panem, S.: C-type viral antigen expression in human placenta. Nature **275**:62–64, 1978.

Saxer, J.J.: Chlamydia trachomatis genital infections in a community-based family practice clinic. J. Fam. Pract. **28**:41–47, 1989.

Sbarra, A.J., Selvaraj, R.J., Cetrulo, C.L., Feingold, M., Newton, E. and Thomas, G.B.: Infection and phagocytosis as possible mechanisms of rupture in premature rupture of the membranes. Amer. J. Obstet. Gynecol. **153**:38–43, 1985.

Sbarra, A.J., Thomas, G.B., Cetrulo, C.L., Shakr, C., Chaudhury, A. and Paul, B.: Effect of bacterial growth on the bursting pressure of fetal membranes in vitro. Obstet. Gynecol. **70**:107–110, 1987.

Schaffner, A., Douglas, H. and Davis, C.E.: Models of T cell deficiency in listeriosis: the effects of cortisone and cyclosporin A on normal and nude Balb/c mice. J. Immunol. **131**:450–453, 1983.

Schiff, I., Driscoll, S.G. and Naftolin, F.: Calcification of the umbilical cord. Amer. J. Obstet. Gynecol. **126**:1046–1048, 1976.

Schimmel, M.S., Fisher, D. and Schlesinger, Y.: Congenital cytomegalovirus infection. J. Perinatol. **21**:209–210, 2001.

Schlech, W.F., Lavigne, P.M., Bortolussi, R.A., Allen, A.C., Haldane, E.V., Wort, A.J., Hightower, A.W., Johnson, S.E., King, S.H., Nicholls, E.S. and Broome, C.V.: Epidemic listeriosis—evidence for transmission by food. NEJM **308**:203–206, 1983.

Schlesinger, P.A., Duray, P.H., Burke, B.A., Steere, A.C. and Stillman, M.T.: Maternal-fetal transmission of a Lyme disease spirochete Borrelia burgdorferi. Ann. Intern. Med. **103**:67–68, 1985.

Schlievert, P., Larsen, B., Johnson, W. and Galsk, R.P.: Bacterial growth inhibition by amniotic fluid. III. Demonstration of the variability of bacterial growth inhibition by amniotic fluid with a new plate-count technique. Amer. J. Obstet. Gynecol. **122**:809–813, 1975.

Schlievert, P., Johnson, W. and Galsk, R.P.: Bacterial growth inhibition by amniotic fluid. V. Phosphate-to-zinc ratio as a predictor of bacterial growth-inhibitory activity. Amer. J. Obstet. Gynecol. **125**:899–906, 1976a.

Schlievert, P., Johnson, W. and Galsk, R.P.: Bacterial growth inhibition by amniotic fluid. VI. Evidence for a zinc-peptide antibacterial system. Amer. J. Obstet. Gynecol. **125**:906–910, 1976b.

Schlievert, P., Johnson, W. and Galsk, R.P.: Bacterial growth inhibition by amniotic fluid. VII. The effect of zinc supplementation on bacterial inhibitory activity of amniotic fluids from gestation of 20 weeks. Amer. J. Obstet. Gynecol. **127**:603–608, 1977.

Schmorl, G. and Geipel, P.: Ueber die Tuberkulose der menschlichen Plazenta. Münch. Med. Wochenschr. **51**:1676–1679, 1904.

Schmorl, G. and Kockel: Die Tuberkulose der menschlichen Placenta und ihre Beziehung zur congenitalen Infection mit Tuberkulose. Beitr. Pathol. Anat. Pathol. **16**:313–339, 1894.

Schneider, V., Behm, F.G. and Mumaw, V.R.: Ascending herpetic endometritis. Obstet. Gynecol. **59**:259–262, 1982.

Schoonmaker, J.N., Lawellin, D.W., Lunt, B. and McGregor, J.A.: Bacteria and inflammatory cells reduce chorioamniotic membranes integrity and tensile strength. Obstet. Gynecol. **74**:590–596, 1989.

Schrag, S.J., Zywicki, S., Farley, M.M., Reingold, A.L., Harrison, L.H., Lefkowitz, L.B., Hadler, J.L., Danila, R., Cieslak, P.R. and Schuchat, A.: Group B streptococcal disease in the era of intrapartum antibiotic prophylaxis. NEJM **342**:15–20, 2000.

Schwartz, B., Ciesielski, C.A., Broome, C.V., Gaventa, S., Brown, G.R., Gellin, B.G., Hightower, A.W., Mascola, L. and the Listeriosis Study Group: association of sporadic listeriosis with consumption of uncooked hot dogs and undercooked chicken. Lancet **2**:779–782, 1988.

Schwartz, D.A. and Caldwell, E.: Herpes simplex virus infection of the placenta. Arch. Pathol. Lab. Med. **115**:1141–1144, 1991.

Schwartz, D.A. and Reef, S.: *Candida albicans* placentitis and funisitis: early diagnosis of congenital candidemia by histopathologic examination of umbilical cord vessel. Pediatr. Infect. Dis. J. **9**:661–665, 1990.

Schwartz, D.A., Khan, R. and Stoll, B.: Characterization of the fetal inflammatory response to cytomegalovirus placentitis. An immunohistochemical study. Arch. Pathol. Lab. Med. **116**:21–27, 1992.

Schweid, A.I. and Hopkins, G.B.: Monilial chorionitis associated with an intrauterine contraceptive device. Obstet. Gynecol. **31**:719–721, 1968.

Scialli, A.R. and Rarick, T.L.: Salmonella sepsis and second-trimester pregnancy loss. Obstet. Gynecol. **79**:820–821, 1992.

Scott, G.B., Hutto, C., Makuch, R.W., Mastrucci, M.T., O'Connor, T., Mitchell, C.D., Trapido, E.J. and Parks, W.P.: Survival of children with perinatally acquired human immunodeficiency virus type 1 infection. NEJM **321**:1791–1796, 1989.

Scott, J.M. and Henderson, A.: Acute villous inflammation in the placenta following intrauterine transfusion. J. Clin. Pathol. **25**:872–875, 1972.

Seaward, P.G., Hannah, M.E., Myhr, T.L., Farine, D., Ohlsson, A., Wang, E.E., Hodnett, E., Haque, K., Weston, J.A., Ohel, G. and Term PROM study group. Amer. J. Obstet. Gynecol. **179**:635–639, 1998.

Seeliger, H.: Listeriose. Barth, Leipzig, 1955.

Selzer, G.: Virus isolation, inclusion bodies, and chromosomes in a rubella-infected human embryo. Lancet **2**:336–337, 1963.

Selzer, G.: Rubella in pregnancy: virus isolation and inclusion bodies. South Afr. J. Obstet. Gynaecol. **2**:5–9, 1964.

Sennström, M.B., Granström, L.M., Lockwood, C.J., Omazic, B., Johansson, O., Malmström, A. and Ekman, G.E.: Cervical fetal fibronectin correlates with prostaglandin E₂–induced cervical ripening and can be identified in cervical tissue. Amer. J. Obstet. Gynecol. **178**:540–545, 1998.

Seo, K., McGregor, J.A. and French, J.I.: Preterm birth is associated with increased risk of maternal and neonatal infection. Obstet. Gynecol. **79**:75–80, 1992.

Seoud, M., Saade, G., Uwaydah, M. and Azoury, R.: Typhoid fever in pregnancy. Obstet. Gynecol. **71**:711–714, 1988.

Sever, J.L., Ellenberg, J.H., Ley, A.C., Madden, D.L., Fuccillo, D.A., Tzan, N.R. and Edmonds, D.M.: Toxoplasmosis: maternal and pediatric findings in 23,000 pregnancies. Pediatrics **82**:181–192, 1988.

Shafai, T.: Neonatal coccidioidomycosis in premature twins. Amer. J. Dis. Child. **132**:634, 1978.

Shalev, E., Battino, S., Romano, S., Blondhaim, O. and Ben-Ami, M.: Intraamniotic infection with *Candida albicans* successfully treated with transcervical amnioinfusion of amphotericin. Amer. J. Obstet. Gynecol. **170**:1271–1272, 1994.

Shepard, M.C.: Nongonococcal urethritis associated with human strains of "T" mycoplasmas. JAMA **211**:1335–1340, 1970.

Shim, S.-S., Romero, R., Hong, J.-S., Park, C.-W., Jun, J.K., Kim, B.I. and Yoon, B.Y.: Clinical significance of intra-amniotic inflammation in patients with preterm rupture of membranes. Amer. J. Obstet. Gynecol. **191**:1339–1345, 2004.

Shippey, S.H., Zahn, C.M., Cisar, M.M., Wu, T.J. and Satin, A.J.: Use of the placental perfusion model to evaluate transplacental passage of *Trypanosoma cruzi*. Amer. J. Obstet. Gynecol. **192**:586–591, 2005.

Shirts, S.R., Brown, M.S. and Bobitt, J.R.: Listeriosis and borreliosis as causes of antepartum fever. Obstet. Gynecol. **62**:256–261, 1983.

Shurbaji, M.S., Gupta, P.K. and Myers, J.: Immunohistochemical demonstration of chlamydial antigens in association with prostatitis. Mod. Pathol. **1**:348–351, 1988.

Silver, H.M., Sperling, R.S., St. Clair, P.J. and Gibbs, R.S.: Evidence relating bacterial vaginosis to intraamniotic infection. Amer. J. Obstet. Gynecol. **161**:808–812, 1989.

Silver, H.M., Gibbs, R.S., Gray, B.M. and Dillon, H.C.: Risk factors for perinatal group B streptococcal disease after amniotic fluid colonization. Amer. J. Obstet. Gynecol. **163**:19–25, 1990.

Silver, R.M., Heddleston, L.N., McGregor, J.A. and Gibbs, R.S.: Life-threatening puerperal infection due to group A streptococci. Obstet. Gynecol. **79**:894–896, 1992.

Silverman, N.S., Jenkin, B.K., Wu, C., McGillin, P. and Knee, G.: Hepatitis C virus in pregnancy: Seroprevalence and risk factors for infection. Amer. J. Obstet. Gynecol. **169**:583–587, 1993.

Silverstein, A.M.: Congenital syphilis and the timing of immunogenesis in the human foetus. Nature **194**:196–197, 1962.

Silverstein, A.M. and Lukes, R.: Fetal response to antigenic stimulus. I. Plasma cellular and lymphoid reactions in the human fetus to intrauterine infection. Lab. Invest. **11**:918–932, 1962.

Simham, H.N., Caritis, S.N., Krohn, M.A., de Tejada, B.M., Landers, D.V. and Hillier, S.L.: Decreased cervical proinflammatory cytokines permit subsequent upper genital tract infection during pregnancy. Amer. J. Obstet. Gynecol. **189**:560–567, 2003.

Simham, H.N., Caritis, S.N., Krohn, M.A. and Hillier, S.L.: The vaginal inflammatory milieu and the risk of early premature preterm rupture of membranes. Amer. J. Obstet. Gynecol. **191**:213–218, 2004.

Simon, C., Schröder, H., Weisner, D., Brück, M. and Krieg, U.: Bacteriological findings after premature rupture of the membranes. Arch. Gynecol. Obstet. **244**:69–74, 1989.

Singer, D.B. and Campognone, P.: Group B streptococcus: a hazard in the second trimester. Lab. Invest. **48**:13P–14P, 1983.

Skannal, D.G., Brockman, D.E., Eis, A.L.W., Xue, S., Siddiqi, T.A. and Myatt, L.: Changes in activity of cytosolic phospholipase A₂ in human amnion at parturition. Amer. J. Obstet. Gynecol. **177**:179–184, 1997.

Slattery, M.M. and Morrison, J.J.: Preterm delivery. Lancet **360**:1489–1497, 2002.

Slevogt, H., Tintelnot, K., Seybold, J. and Suttorp, N.: Lymphadenopathy in a pregnant woman from Brazil. Lancet **363**:1282, 2004.

Smale, L.E. and Waechter, K.G.: Dissemination of coccidioidomycosis in pregnancy. Amer. J. Obstet. Gynecol. **197**:356–361, 1970.

Smith, C.V., Horenstein, J. and Platt, L.D.: Intrauterine infection with Candida albicans associated with a retained intrauterine contraceptive device: a case report. Amer. J. Obstet. Gynecol. **159**:123–124, 1988.

Smith, L.G., Summers, P.R., Miles, R.W., Biswas, M.K. and Pernoll, M.L.: Gonococcal chorioamnionitis associated with sepsis: a case report. Amer. J. Obstet. Gynecol. **160**:573–574, 1989.

Smith, L.M., Wang, M., Zangwil, K. and Yeh, S.: *Trichomonas vaginalis* infection in a premature newborn. J. Perinatol. **22**:502–503, 2002.

Snydman, D.R.: Hepatitis in pregnancy. NEJM **313**:1398–1401, 1985.

Soeiro, R., Rubinstein, A., Rashbaum, W.K. and Lyman, W.D.: Maternofetal transmission of AIDS: Frequency of human immunodeficiency virus type 1 nucleic acid sequences in human fetal DNA. J. Infect. Dis. **166**:699–703, 1992.

Soma, H.: Feto-placental listeriosis as a model of intrauterine infection. Excerpta Med. Int. Cong. Ser. **512**:1020–1024, 1979.

Soper, D.: Trichomoniasis: under control or undercontrolled? Amer. J. Obstet. Gynecol. **190**:281–290, 2004.

Southwick, F.S. and Purich, D.L.: Intracellular pathogenesis of listeriosis. NEJM **334**:770–776, 1996.

Spark, R.P.: Does transplacental spread of coccidioidomycosis occur? Report of a neonatal fatality and review of the literature. Arch. Pathol. Lab. Med. **105**:347–350, 1981.

Spaun, E. and Klünder, K.: Candida chorioamnionitis and intra-uterine contraceptive device. Acta Obstet. Gynecol. Scand. **65**:183–184, 1986.

Spence, M.R., Davidson, D.E., Dill, G.S., Boonthal, P. and Sagartz, J.W.: Rabies exposure during pregnancy. Amer. J. Obstet. Gynecol. **123**:655–656, 1975.

Sperling, R.S., Sacks, H.S., Mayer, L., Joyner, M. and Berkowitz, R.L.: Umbilical cord blood serosurvey for human immunodeficiency virus in parturient women in a voluntary hospital in New York City. Obstet. Gynecol. **73**:179–181, 1989.

Stagno, S. and Whitley, R.J.: Herpesvirus infections of pregnancy. Part II. Herpes simplex virus and varicella-zoster virus infections. NEJM **313**:1327–1330, 1985.

Stagno, S., Pass, R.F., Dworsky, M.E., Henderson, R.E., Moore, E.G., Walton, P.D. and Alford, C.A.: Congenital cytomegalovirus infection: the relative importance of primary and recurrent maternal infection. NEJM **306**:945–949, 1982.

Stagno, S., Pass, R.F., Cloud, G., Britt, W.J., Henderson, R.E., Walton, P.D., Veren, D.A., Page, F. and Alford, C.A.: Primary cytomegalovirus infection in pregnancy: incidence, transmission to fetus, and clinical outcome. JAMA **256**:1904–1908, 1986.

Steele, P.E. and Jacobs, D.S.: Listeria monocytogenes macroabscesses of placenta. Obstet. Gynecol. **53**:124–127, 1979.

Steere, A.C.: Lyme disease. NEJM **321**:586–596, 1989.

Stein, S.J. and Greenspoon, J.S.: Rubeola during pregnancy. Obstet. Gynecol. **78**:925–929, 1991.

Steinborn, A., von Gall, C., Hildenbrand, R., Stutte, H.-J. and Kaufmann, M.: Identification of placental cytokine-producing cells in term and preterm labor. Obstet. Gynecol. **91**:329–335, 1998.

Steiner, B., Putnoky, G., Kovacs, K. and Földes, G.: Pneumonia in newborn infants. Acta Paediatr. Hung. **2**:227–236, 1961.

Stiller, R.J., Blair, E., Clark, P. and Tinghitella, T.: Rapid detection of vaginal colonization with group B streptococci by means of latex agglutination. Amer. J. Obstet. Gynecol. **160**:566–568, 1989.

Stine, G.J.: Acquired Immune Deficiency Syndrome: Biological, Medical, Social, and Legal Issues. Prentice-Hall, Englewood Cliffs, N.J., 1993.

Stray-Pedersen, B.: Infants potentially at risk for congenital toxoplasmosis: a prospective study. Amer. J. Dis. Child. **134**:638–642, 1980.

Stray-Pedersen, B. and Lorentzen-Styr, A.-M.: Uterine toxoplasma infections and repeated abortions. Amer. J. Obstet. Gynecol. **128**:716–721, 1977.

Strickland, D.M., Yeomans, E.R. and Hankins, G.D.V.: Cost-effectiveness of intrapartum screening and treatment for maternal group B streptococci colonization. Amer. J. Obstet. Gynecol. **163**:4–8, 1990.

Strobino, B.A., Williams, C.L., Abid, S., Chalson, R. and Spierling, P.: Lyme disease and pregnancy outcome: A prospective study of two thousand prenatal patients. Amer. J. Obstet. Gynecol. **169**:367–374, 1993.

Studdiford, W.E. and Douglas, G.W.: Placental bacteremia: a significant finding in septic abortion accompanied by vascular collapse. Amer. J. Obstet. Gynecol. **71**:842–858, 1956.

Styer, A.K., Parker, H.J., Roberts, D.J., Palmer-Toy, D., Toth, T.L. and Ecker, J.L.: Placental villitis of unclear etiology during ovum donor in vitro fertilization pregnancy. Amer. J. Obstet. Gynecol. **189**:1184–1186, 2003.

Subtil, D., Denoit, V., Goueff, F.L., Husson, M.O., Trivier, D. and Puech, F.: The role of bacterial vaginosis in preterm labor and preterm birth: a case-control study. Europ. J. Obstet. Gynecol. Reprod. Biol. **101**:41–46, 2002.

Sugiyama, T., Cuevas, L.E., Bailey, W., Makunde, R., Kawamura, K., Kobayashi, M., Masuda, H. and Hommel, M.: Expression of intercellular adhesion molecule 1 (ICAM-1) in *Plasmodium falciparum*-infected placenta. Placenta **22**:573–579, 2001.

Sullivan, A.D., Nyirenda, T., Cullinan, T., Taylor, T., Lau, A. and Meshnick, S.R.: Placental haemozoin and malaria in pregnancy. Placenta **21**:417–421, 2000.

Sutherland, J.C., Berry, A., Hynd, M. and Proctor, N.S.F.: Placental bilharziasis: report of a case. S. Afr. J. Obstet. Gynaecol. **3**:76–80, 1965.

Svabic-Vlahovic, M., Pantic, D., Pavicic, M. and Bryner, J.H.: Transmission of Listeria monocytogenes from mother's milk to her baby and to puppies. Lancet **2**:1201, 1988.

Svinarich, D.M., Wolf, N.A., Gomez, R., Gonik, B. and Romero, R.: Detection of human defensin 5 in reproductive tissues. Amer. J. Obstet. Gynecol. **176**:470–475, 1997.

Swartzberg, J.E. and Remington, J.S.: Transmission of Toxoplasma. Amer. J. Dis. Child. **129**:777–779, 1975.

Sweet, R.L., Landers, D.V., Walker, C. and Schachter, J.: Chlamydia trachomatis infection and pregnancy outcome. Amer. J. Obstet. Gynecol. **156**:824–833, 1987.

Swingler, G.R., Bigrigg, M.A., Hewitt, B.G. and McNulty, C.A.M.: Disseminated intravascular coagulation associated with group A streptococcal infection in pregnancy. Lancet **1**:1456–1457, 1988.

Symonds, D.A. and Driscoll, S.G.: Massive fetal ascites, urethral atresia, and cytomegalic inclusion disease. Amer. J. Dis. Child. **127**:895–897, 1974.

Taniguchi, T., Matsuzaki, N., Kameda, T., Shimoya, K., Jo, T., Saji, F. and Tanizawa, O.: The enhanced production of placental interleukin-1 during labor and intrauterine infection. Amer. J. Obstet. Gynecol. **165**:131–137, 1991.

Tanner, N.C. and Hewlett, R.F.L.: Congenital malaria with report in one of twins. Lancet **2**:369–370, 1935.

Tarpay, M.M., Turbeville, D.F. and Krous, H.F.: Fatal Streptococcus pneumoniae type III sepsis in mother and infant. Amer. J. Obstet. Gynecol. **136**:257–258, 1980.

Taschdjan, C.T. and Kozinn, P.J.: Laboratory and clinical studies on candidiasis in the newborn infant. J. Pediatr. **50**:426–433, 1957.

Taylor-Robinson, D. and McCormack, W.M.: The genital mycoplasmas. NEJM **302**:1003–1010; 1063–1067, 1980.

Teele, R.L., Hernanz-Schulman, M. and Sotrel, A.: Echogenic vasculature in the basal ganglia of neonates: a sonographic sign of vasculopathy. Radiology **169**:423–427, 1988.

Temmerman, M., Chomba, E.N., Ndinya-Achola, J., Plummer, F.A., Coppens, M. and Piot, P.: Maternal human immunodeficiency virus-1 infection and pregnancy outcome. Obstet. Gynecol. **83**:495–501, 1994.

Teppa, R.J. and Roberts, J.M.: The uriscreen test to detect significant bacteriuria during pregnancy. J. Soc. Gynecol. Investig. **12**:50–53, 2005.

Teutsch, S.M., Sulzer, A.J., Ramsey, J.E., Murray, W.A. and Juranek, D.D.: Toxoplasma gondii isolated from amniotic fluid. Obstet. Gynecol. **55**:2S–4S, 1980.

Thadepalli, H., Bach, V.T. and Davidson, E.C.: Antimicrobial effect of amniotic fluid. Obstet. Gynecol. **52**:198–204, 1978.

Thaler, M.M., Park, C.-K., Landers, D.V., Wara, D.W., Houghton, M., Veereman-Wauters, G., Sweet, R.L. and Han, J.H.: Vertical transmission of hepatitis C virus. Lancet **338**:17–18, 1991.

Thiery, M., le Sian, A.Y., Derom, R. and Boelaert, R.: Leukocytic infiltration of the umbilical cord in twins. Acta Genet. Med. Gemellol. **19**:92–95, 1970.

Thoma, R., Guscetti, F., Schiller, I., Schmeer, N., Corboz, L. and Pospischil, A.: Chlamydiae in porcine abortion. Vet. Pathol. **34**:467–469, 1997.

Thomas, G.B., Sbarra, A.J., Feingold, M., Cetrulo, C.L., Shakr, C., Newton, E. and Selvaraj, R.J.: Antimicrobial activity of amniotic fluid against Chlamydia trachomatis, Mycoplasma hominis, and Ureaplasma urealyticum. Amer. J. Obstet. Gynecol. **158**:16–22, 1988.

Thomas, G.B., Jones, J., Sbarra, A.J., Cetrulo, C. and Reisner, D.: Isolation of *Chlamydia trachomatis* from amniotic fluid. Obstet. Gynecol. **76**:519–520, 1990.

Thompson, D., Pegelow, C., Underman, A. and Powars, D.: Congenital malaria: a rare cause of splenomegaly and anemia in an American infant. Pediatrics **60**:209–212, 1977.

Thompson, K.M. and Tobin, J.O'H.: Isolation of rubella virus from abortion material. Br. Med. J. **2**:264–266, 1970.

Thomsen, A.C., Morup, L. and Hansen, K.B.: Antibiotic elimination of group-B streptococci in urine in prevention of preterm labour. Lancet **1**:591–593, 1987.

Thorp, J.M., Katz, V.L., Fowler, L.J., Kurtzman, J.T. and Bowles, W.A.: Fetal death from chlamydial infection across intact amniotic membranes. Amer. J. Obstet. Gynecol. **161**:1245–1246, 1989.

Thorp, J.M., Hartmann, K.E., Berkman, N.D., Carey, T.S., Lohr, K.N., Gavin, N.I. and Hasselblad, V.: Antibiotic therapy for the treatment of preterm labor: A review of the evidence. Amer. J. Obstet. Gynecol. **186**:587–592, 2002.

To, M.S., Alfirevic, Z., Heath, V.C.F., Cicero, S., Cacho, A.M., Williamson, P.R. and Nicolaides, K.H.: Cervical cerclage for prevention of preterm delivery in women with short cervix: randomized controlled trial. Lancet **363**:1849–1853, 2004.

Tobias, L., Cordes, D.O. and Schurig, G.G.: Placental pathology of the pregnant mouse inoculated with *Brucella abortus* strain 2308. Vet. Pathol. **30**:119–129, 1993.

Tolfvenstam, T., Papadogiannakis, N., Norbeck, O., Petersson, K. and Broliden, K.: Frequency of human parvovirus B19 infection in intrauterine fetal death. Lancet **357**:1494–1497, 2001.

Töndury, G.: Zum Problem der Embryopathia rubeolosa. Untersuchungen an menschlichen Keimlingen verschiedener Entwicklungsstadien. Bull. Schweiz. Akad. Med. Wiss. **7**:307–325, 1951.

Töndury, G.: Zur Wirkung des Erregers der Rubeolen auf den menschlichen Keimling. Helvet. Paediatr. Acta **7**:105–135, 1952a.

Töndury, G.: Zur Kenntnis der Embryopathia rubeolica, nebst Bemerkungen über die Wirkung anderer Viren auf den Keimling. Geburtsh. Frauenheilk. **12**:865–888, 1952b.

Töndury, G.: Über den Infektionsweg und die Pathogenese von Virusschädigung beim menschlichen Keimling. Bull. Schweiz. Akad. Med. Wiss. **20**:379–396, 1964.

Töndury, G. and Smith, D.W.: Fetal rubella pathology. J. Pediatr. **68**:867–879, 1966.

Topalovski, M., Yang, S.S. and Boonpasat, Y.: Listeriosis of the placenta: Clinicopathologic study of seven cases. Amer. J. Obstet. Gynecol. **169**:616–620, 1993.

Torphy, D.E., Ray, C.G., McAlister, R. and Du, J.N.H.: Herpes simplex virus infection in infants: a spectrum of disease. J. Pediatr. **76**:405–408, 1970.

Toth, M., Witkin, S.S., Ledger, W. and Thaler, H.: The role of infection in the etiology of preterm birth. Obstet. Gynecol. **71**:723–726, 1988; **73**:142–144, 1989.

Towers, C.V. and Briggs, G.G.: Antepartum use of antibiotics and early-onset neonatal sepsis: The next 4 years. Amer. J. Obstet. Gynecol. **187**:495–500, 2002.

Tully, J.G. and Whitcomb, R.F., eds.: The Mycoplasmas. Orlando: Academic Press, 1979.

Ugwumadu, A., Manyonda, I., Reid, F. and Hay, P.: Effect of early oral clindamycin on late miscarriage and preterm delivery in asymptomatic women with abnormal vaginal flora and bacterial vaginosis: a randomized controlled trial. Lancet **361**:983–988, 2003.

Update: Foodborne listeriosis. Bull. W.H.O. **66**:421–428, 1988.

Vadas, P. and Pruzanski, W.: Role of secretory phospholipases A_2 in the pathobiology of disease. Lab. Invest. **55**:391–404, 1986.

Vaheri, A., Vesikari, T., Oker-Bloom, N., Seppala, M., Parkman, P.D., Veronelli, J. and Robbins, F.C.: Isolation of attenuated rubella-vaccine virus from human products of conception and uterine cervix. NEJM **286**:1071–1074, 1972.

VanBergen, W.S., Fleury, F.J. and Cheatle, E.L.: Fatal maternal disseminated coccidioidomycosis in a nonendemic area. Amer. J. Obstet. Gynecol. **124**:661–664, 1976.

Vaughan, J.E. and Ramirez, H.: Coccidioidomycosis as a complication of pregnancy. Calif. Med. **74**:121–125, 1951.

Vernon, M. and Gauthier, C.: L'infection bactérienne du placenta dans les cas d'interruption spontanée de la grossesse: corrélation avec les lésions histologiques. Pathol. Biol. **19**:129–138, 1971.

Veyver, I.B. van den, Ni, J., Bowles, N., Carpenter, R.J. Jr., Weiner, C.P., Yankowitz, J., Moise, K.J., Henderson, J. and Towbin, J.A.: Detection of intrauterine viral infection using the polymerase chain reaction. Molec. Genet. Metabol. **63**:85–95, 1998.

Victor, M., Weiss, J., Klempner, M.S. and Elsbach, P.: Phospholipase A_2 activity in the plasma membrane of human polymorphonuclear leukocytes. FEBS Lett. **136**:298–300, 1981.

Vigorita, V.J. and Parmley, T.H.: Intramembranous localization of bacteria in β-hemolytic group B streptococcal chorioamnionitis. Obstet. Gynecol. **53**:13S–15S, 1979.

Vintzileos, A.M., Campbell, W.A., Nochimson, D.J. and Weinbaum, P.J.: Preterm premature rupture of the membranes: a risk factor for the development of abruptio placentae. Amer. J. Obstet. Gynecol. **156**:1235–1238, 1987.

Visintine, A.M., Oleske, J.M. and Nahmias, A.J.: Listeria monocytogenes infection in infants and children. Amer. J. Dis. Child. **131**:393–397, 1977.

Wagner, G.P., Hanley, L.S., Farb, H.F. and Knox, G.E.: Evaluation of gas-liquid chromatography for the rapid diagnosis of amniotic fluid infection: a preliminary report. Amer. J. Obstet. Gynecol. **152**:51–56, 1985.

Wahbeh, C.J., Hill, G.B., Eden, R.D. and Gall, S.A.: Intra-amniotic bacterial colonization in premature labor. Amer. J. Obstet. Gynecol. **148**:739–743, 1984.

Waites, K.B., Rudd, P.T., Crouse, D.T., Canupp, K.C., Nelson, K.G., Ramsey, C. and Cassell, G.H.: Chronic Ureaplasma urealyticum and Mycoplasma hominis infections of central nervous system in preterm infants. Lancet **1**:17–21, 1988.

Walker, M.P.R., Brody, C.Z. and Resnik, R.: Reactivation of coccidioidomycosis in pregnancy. Obstet. Gynecol. **79**:815–817, 1992.

Wallach, E.E., Brody, J.I. and Oski, F.A.: Fetal immunization as a consequence of bacilluria during pregnancy. Obstet. Gynecol. **33**:100–105, 1969.

Walter, P.R., Garin, Y. and Blot, P.: Placental pathologic changes in malaria: a histologic and ultrastructural study. Amer. J. Pathol. **109**:330–342, 1982.

Wang, E.E.L., Frayha, H., Watts, J., Hammerberg, O., Chernesky, M.A., Mahony, J.B. and Cassell, G.H.: Role of Ureaplasma urealyticum and other pathogens in the development of chronic lung disease of prematurity. Pediatr. Infect. Dis. J. **7**:547–551, 1988.

Wang, J.-S. and Zhu, Q.-R.: Infection of the fetus with hepatitis B e antigen via the placenta. Lancet **355**:989, 2000.

Warthin, A.S.: Tuberculosis of the placenta: a histological study with especial reference to the nature of the earliest lesions produced by the tubercle bacillus. J. Infect. Dis. **4**:347–398, 1907.

Watson, D.G.: Purulent neonatal meningitis: a study of forty-five cases. J. Pediatr. **50**:352–360, 1957.

Watson, K.C.: Salmonella meningitis. Arch. Dis. Child. **33**:171–175, 1958.

Watts, D.H., Krohn, M.A., Hillier, S.L., Wener, M.H., Kiviat, N.B. and Eschenbach, D.A.: Characteristics of women in preterm labor associated with elevated C-reactive protein levels. Obstet. Gynecol. **82**:509–514, 1993.

Webb, G.A.: Maternal death associated with premature rupture of the membranes. Amer. J. Obstet. Gynecol. **98**:594–601, 1967.

Weiner, C.P. and Grose, C.: Prenatal diagnosis of congenital cytomegalovirus infection by virus isolation from amniotic fluid. Amer. J. Obstet. Gynecol. **163**:1253–1255, 1990.

Wejstal, R., Widell, A., Mansson, A.-S., Hermodsson, S. and Norkrans, G.: Mother-to-infant transmission of hepatitis C virus. Ann. Intern. Med. **117**:887–890, 1992.

Weller, T.H.: The cytomegaloviruses: ubiquitous agents with protean manifestations. NEJM **285**:203–214; 262–274, 1971.

Wenckebach, G.F.C. and Curry, B.: Cytomegalovirus infection of the female genital tract: histologic findings in three cases and review of the literature. Arch. Pathol. Lab. Med. **100**:609–612, 1976.

Wendel, G.D., Maberry, M.C., Christmas, J.T., Goldberg, M.S. and Norgard, M.V.: Examination of amniotic fluid in diagnosing congenital syphilis with fetal death. Obstet. Gynecol. **74**:967–970, 1989.

Wendel, G.D., Sanchez, P.J., Peters, M.T., Harstad, T.W., Potter, L.L. and Norgard, M.V.: Identification of *Treponema pallidum* in amniotic fluid and fetal blood from pregnancies complicated by congenital syphilis. Obstet. Gynecol. **78**:890–895, 1991.

Wendel, G.D., Leveno, K.J., Sánchez, P.J., Jackson, G.L., McIntire, D.D. and Siegel, J.D.: Prevention of neonatal group B streptococcal disease: a combined intrapartum and neonatal protocol. Amer. J. Obstet. Gynecol. **196**:618–626, 2002.

Wentworth, P.: Studies on placentae and infants from women vaccinated for smallpox during pregnancy. J. Clin. Pathol. **19**:328–330, 1966.

Werner, H., Schmidtke, L. and Thomascheck, G.: Toxoplasmose-Infektion und Schwangerschaft: der histologische Nachweis des intrauterinen Infektionsweges. Klin. Wochenschr. **41**:96–101, 1963.

Westrom, L., Evaldson, G., Holmes, K.K., Meijden, W.v.d., Rylander, E. and Fredricksson, B.: Taxonomy of vaginosis; bacterial vaginosis—a definition. In, Bacterial Vaginosis. P.A. Mardh and D. Taylor-Robinson, eds., pp. 259–260. Almqvist & Wiksell, Stockholm, 1985.

Wetli, C.V., Roldan, E.O. and Fojaco, R.M.: Listeriosis as a cause of maternal death: an obstetric complication of the acquired immunodeficiency syndrome (AIDS). Amer. J. Obstet. Gynecol. **147**:7–9, 1983.

White, W.D.: Human vibriosis: indigenous cases in England. Br. Med. J. **1**:283–287, 1967.

Whyte, R.K., Hussain, Z. and DeSa, D.: Antenatal infections with Candida species. Arch. Dis. Child. **57**:528–535, 1982.

Wickramasuriya, G.A.W.: Some observations on malaria occurring in association with pregnancy: with special reference to the transplacental passage of parasites from the maternal to the fetal circulation. J. Obstet. Gynaecol. Br. Emp. **42**:816–834, 1935.

Widholm, O., Meyer, B. and Numers, C.v.: Inflammation of the umbilical cord in cases of foetal asphyxia of unknown clinical etiology. Gynaecologia **155**:385–399, 1963.

Wielenga, G., van Tongeren, H.A.E., Ferguson, A.H. and van Rijssel, T.G.: Prenatal infection with vaccinia virus. Lancet **1**:258–260, 1961.

Wiesenfeld, H.C., Heine, R.P., Rideout, A., Macio, I., DiBiasi, F. and Sweet, R.L.: The vaginal introitus: A novel site for *Chlamydia trachomatis* testing in women. Amer. J. Obstet. Gynecol. **174**:1542–1546, 1996.

Wigglesworth, J.S.: Perinatal Pathology. 2nd edition. W.B. Saunders, Philadelphia, 1996.

Wilkins, I., Mezrow, G., Lynch, L., Bottone, E.J. and Berkowitz, R.L.: Amnionitis and life-threatening respiratory distress after percutaneous umbilical blood sampling. Amer. J. Obstet. Gynecol. **160**:427–428, 1989.

Williamson, A.: The varicella zoster virus in the etiology of severe congenital defects. Clin. Pediatr. **14**:553–559, 1975.

Williamson, W.D., Desmond, M.M., LaFevers, N., Taber, L.H., Catlin, F.I. and Weaver, Y.G.: Symptomatic congenital cytomegalovirus: disorders of language, learning, and hearing. Amer. J. Dis. Child. **136**:902–905, 1982.

Williamson, W.D., Percy, A.K., Yow, M.D., Gerson, P., Catlin, F.I., Koppelman, M.L. and Thurber, S.: Asymptomatic congenital cytomegalovirus infection. Audiologic, neuroradiologic, and neurodevelopmental abnormalities during the first year. Amer. J. Dis. Child. **144**:1365–1368, 1990.

Wilson, C.B. and Remington, J.S.: What can be done to prevent congenital toxoplasmosis? Amer. J. Obstet. Gynecol. **138**:357–363, 1980.

Winn, H.N. and Egley, C.C.: Acute Haemophilus influenzae chorioamnionitis associated with intact amniotic membranes. Amer. J. Obstet. Gynecol. **156**:458–459, 1987.

Witlin, A.G., Olson, G.L., Gogola, J. and Hankins, G.D.V.: Disseminated neonatal herpes infection. Obstet. Gynecol. **92**:721, 1998.

Wittek, A.E., Yeager, A.S., Au, D.S. and Hensleigh, P.A.: Asymptomatic shedding of herpes simplex virus from the cervix and lesion site during pregnancy: correlation of antepartum shedding with shedding at delivery. Amer. J. Dis. Child. **138**:439–442, 1984.

Witzleben, C.L. and Driscoll, S.G.: Possible transplacental transmission of herpes simplex infection. Pediatrics **36**:192–199, 1965.

Wohlwill, F. and Bock, H.E.: Über Entzündungen der Placenta und fetale Sepsis. Arch. Gynäkol. **135**:271–319, 1929.

Wolber, R.A. and Lloyd, R.V.: Cytomegalovirus detection by nonisotopic in situ DNA hybridization and viral antigen immunostaining using a two-color technique. Hum. Pathol. **19**:736–741, 1989.

Wolfman, W.L., Purohit, D.M. and Self, S.E.: Umbilical vein thrombosis at 32 weeks' gestation with delivery of a living infant. Amer. J. Obstet. Gynecol. **146**:468–470, 1983.

Wong, S.Y., Gray, E.S., Buxton, D., Finlayson, J. and Johnson, F.A.H.: Acute placentitis and spontaneous abortion caused by Chlamydia psittaci in sheep origin: a histopathologic and ultrastructural study. J. Clin. Pathol. **38**:707–711, 1985.

Wood, N.S., Marlow, N., Costeloe, K., Gibson, A.T. and Wilkinson, A.R.: Neurologic and developmental disability after extremely preterm birth. NEJM **343**:378–384, 2000.

Woods, W.G., Mills, E. and Ferrieri, P.: Neonatal malaria due to Plasmodium vivax. J. Pediatr. **85**:669–671, 1974.

Woody, N.C. and Woody, H.B.: Possible Chagas's disease in United States. NEJM **290**:750–751, 1974.

Wyler, D.J.: Malaria—resurgence, resistance, and research. NEJM **308**:875–879, 1983.

Xi, G., Leke, R.G., Thuita, L.W., Zhou, A., Leke, R.J., Mbu, R. and Taylor, D.W.: Congenital exposure to Plasmodium falciparum antigens: prevalence and antigenic specificity of in utero-produced antimalarial immunoglobulin M antibodies. Infect. Immun. **71**:1242–1246, 2003.

Xiao, J., Garcia-Loret, M., Winkler-Lowen, B., Miller, R., Simpson, K. and Guilbert, L.J.: ICAM-1–mediated adhesion of peripheral blood monocytes to the maternal surface of placental syncytiotrophoblasts. Implications for placental villitis. Amer. J. Pathol. **150**:1845–1860, 1997.

Xu, D.-Z., Yan, Y.-P., Zou, S., Choi, B.C.K., Wang, S., Liu, P., Bai, G., Wang, X., Shi, M. and Wang, X.: Role of placental tissues in the intrauterine transmission of hepatitis B. virus. Amer. J. Obstet. Gynecol. **185**:981–987, 2001.

Yagupsky, P. and Moses, S.: Neonatal Borrelia species infection (relapsing fever). Amer. J. Dis. Child. **139**:74–76, 1985.

Yamauchi, T., Wilson, C. and St. Geme, J.W.: Transmission of live, attenuated mumps virus to the human placenta. NEJM **290**:710–712, 1974.

Yamazaki, K., Price, J.T. and Altshuler, G.: A placental view of the diagnosis and pathogenesis of congenital listeriosis. Amer. J. Obstet. Gynecol. **129**:703–705, 1977.

Yancey, M.K., Clark, P., Armer, T. and Duff, P.: Use of a DNA probe for the rapid detection of group B streptococci in obstetric patients. Obstet. Gynecol. **81**:635–640, 1993.

Yawn, D.H., Pyeatte, J.C., Joseph, J.M., Eichler, S.L. and Garcia-Bunuel, R.: Transplacental transfer of influenza virus. JAMA **216**:1022–1023, 1971.

Yen, S.S.C., Reagan, J.W. and Rosenthal, M.S.: Herpes simplex infection in female genital tract. Obstet. Gynecol. **25**:479–492, 1965.

Yokoyama, S., Kashima, K., Inoue, S., Daa, T., Nakayama, I. and Moriuchi, A.: Biotin-containing intranuclear inclusions in endometrial glands during gestation and puerperium. Amer. J. Clin. Pathol. **99**:13–17, 1993.

Yoon, B.H., Romero, R., Kim, C.J., Jun, J.K., Gomez, R., Choi, J.H. and Syn, H.C.: Amniotic fluid interleukin-6: A sensitive test for antenatal diagnosis of acute inflammatory lesions of preterm placenta and prediction of perinatal morbidity. Amer. J. Obstet. Gynecol. **172**:960–970, 1995.

Yoon, B.H., Jun, J.K., Romero, R., Park, K.H., Gomez, R., Choi, J.H. and Kim, I.O.: Amniotic fluid inflammatory cytokines (interleukin-6, interleukin-1β, and tumor necrosis factor-α), neonatal brain white matter lesions, and cerebral palsy. Amer. J. Obstet. Gynecol. **177**:19–26, 1997a.

Yoon, B.H., Romero, R., Kim, C.J., Koo, J.N., Choe, G., Syn, H.C. and Chi, J.G.: High expression of tumor necrosis factor-α and interleukin-6 in periventricular leukomalacia. Amer. J. Obstet. Gynecol. **177**:406–411, 1997b.

Yoon, B.H., Romero, R., Park, J.S., Chang, J.W., Kim, Y.A., Kim, J.C. and Kim, K.S.: Microbial invasion of the amniotic cavity with *Ureaplasma urealyticum* is associated with a robust host response in fetal, amniotic, and maternal compartments. Amer. J. Obstet. Gynecol. **179**:1254–1260, 1998.

Yoon, B.H., Romero, R., Park, J.S., Kim, C.J., Kim, S.H., Choi, J.-H. and Han, T.R.: Fetal exposure to an intra-amniotic inflammation and the development of cerebral palsy at the age of three years. Amer. J. Obstet. Gynecol. **182**:675–681, 2000.

Yoon, B.H., Romero, R., Moon, J.B., Shim, S.-S., Kim, M., Kim, G. and Jun, J.: Clinical significance of intra-amniotic inflammation in patients with preterm labor and intact membranes. Amer. J. Obstet. Gynecol. **185**:1130–1136, 2001.

Young, S.A. and Crocker, D.W.: Occult congenital syphilis in macerated stillborn fetuses. Arch. Pathol. Lab. Med. **118**:44–47, 1994.

Yow, M.D.: Congenital cytomegalovirus disease: a NOW problem. J. Infect. Dis. **159**:163–167, 1989.

Zakut, H., Achiron, R., Treschan, O. and Kutin, E.: *Actinomyces* invasion of placenta as possible cause of preterm delivery. Clin. Exp. Obstet. Gynecol. **2**:89–91, 1987.

Zavoral, J.H., Ray, W.L., Kinnard, P.G. and Nahmias, A.J.: Neonatal herpetic infection: a fatal consequence of penile herpes in a serviceman. JAMA **213**:1492–1493, 1970.

Zervoudakis, I.A. and Cederqvist, L.L.: Effect of Listeria monocytogenes septicemia during pregnancy on the offspring. Amer. J. Obstet. Gynecol. **129**:465–467, 1977.

Zervoudakis, I.A., Silverman, F., Senterfit, L.B., Strongin, M.J., Read, S. and Cederquist, L.L.: Herpes simplex in the amniotic fluid of an unaffected fetus. Obstet. Gynecol. **55**:16S–17S, 1980.

21
Abortion, Placentas of Trisomies, and Immunologic Considerations of Recurrent Reproductive Failure

For the present discussion, an abortion or miscarriage is designated a conceptus that is expelled before the 20th week of gestation. That is important to state at the outset, as the pathologic features of failed pregnancies differ markedly in specimens obtained later in gestation. In the United States, terminations before 20 weeks constitute abortions; later gestations are premature deliveries. A pregnancy of 20 weeks is legally at the dividing line; it is a gestation with an "embryo" (that may be treated as a surgical specimen); later it is a "fetus," whose examination constitutes an autopsy. The terminology employed in publications and statistics differs widely and it is not the same in different countries. For instance, Vogel in Germany (1969, 1992) considered an abortion to be an expelled fetus of less than 1000 g. He differentiated between embryonic and fetal (15–28 weeks) abortion. In many countries, legal viability is considered to be attained only at 28 weeks of gestation, when the fetus has attained approximately 1000 g in weight; but that is not so in the United States. Byrne et al. (1985), in a study of early fetal deaths, considered all specimens of less than 28 weeks' gestation. For these reasons it is difficult to place the studies of Vogel (1969, 1992) into context with current terminology. Hutchon (1998) reviewed the complex terminology of this topic and proposed (with concurrence of a British study group on terminology) that the term **abortion** be replaced with **miscarriage**, for all types under discussion. Most truly spontaneous abortions occur before 12 weeks of gestation and a majority is due to chromosomal errors in the conceptus. Relatively few really spontaneous abortions occur in the period from 12 to 20 week's gestation. Thereafter, between 20 and 30 weeks, another type of premature spontaneous termination becomes prevalent, that which is primarily due to ascending infection with chorioamnionitis. Infection is relatively uncommon before 20 weeks. These are fundamentally different processes with also vastly different pathologic findings.

Terms other than **spontaneous abortion** (involuntary) have been employed, and these have often confused the general abortion issue: "therapeutic abortion" (TAB; electively terminated), "missed" (retained for more than 8 weeks after embryonic death), "criminal" (illegally instrumented), "habitual," and "recurrent" abortions, and other terms designate specific entities. Not all of these definitions are universally accepted, and there is cogent argument that the term "missed abortion" should be abandoned (Pridjian & Moawad, 1989). It is best to clarify the specific nomenclature before one compares data from different institutions or countries. A useful method for categorization of abortion specimens was provided by Fujikura et al. (1966). They divided specimens into groups with and without embryos, those with ruptured and unruptured sacs, and included the degree of the completeness of the specimen. In their experience, 22% were classified as incomplete, and most (35.8%) had a normal embryo or fetus. An embryo may be considered to be a specimen with a crown–rump (CR) length of up to 30 mm (less than 9 weeks), and a fetus may be considered an unborn conceptus greater than 30 mm CR (Moore, 1982, 1994). When only incomplete specimens are available, it has been most practical to determine fetal age from measurements of fetal foot length. Other extensive considerations of classification and specimen examination are laid out in detail by Kalousek et al. (1990). Hern (1984) correlated various fetal measurements with gestational age in 1000 specimens and provided excellent tables from which reasonably exact age determination is possible. "Threatened abortions" are represented by those clinical cases in which vaginal bleeding occurs in the first trimester. Weiss et al. (2004) have reviewed a large study of this phenomenon and found that the amount of bleeding corresponds to different gestational entities such as preeclampsia, spontaneous abortion, abruptio, etc.

Spontaneous abortions are common. Despite this frequency, patients often do not understand its nature, and, especially when recurrent abortions occur, they find little comfort from consulting their physician. For that reason, Cohen (2005) has produced an excellent volume that comprises nearly all that needs to be known about the topic, especially for the parturient. The exact frequency with which pregnancy failure occurs spontaneously has been debated and our understanding of its pathogenesis has undergone remarkable changes in recent years. Its chromosomal causes are nicely reviewed by Cohen (2002), and Clouston et al. (2002) have examined the chromosomal errors in 438 human blastocysts. Of these, 3% were polyploidy (mostly tetraploid), 29% were diploid/tetraploid mosaics, and 68% were diploid and included a variety of trisomies. Trauma is no longer considered to be a common cause of abortion. Hertig and Sheldon (1943) found only one set of twins whose abortion was probably caused by external trauma among the 1000 miscarriages they studied. "Internal trauma" was incriminated in 22 cases. Published figures on the incidence of abortion depend largely on the method of sampling a population. When prospective studies of complete populations are done so as to include also all those pregnancies that give few or no clinical symptoms of pregnancy, it is found that nearly 50% of conceptions terminate in abortion spontaneously. For example, Miller et al. (1980) collected urine of 197 women who were wishing to conceive. They began the collection at ovulation to obtain the earliest evidence of pregnancy and investigated 623 menstrual cycles. Their diagnosis of pregnancy was made with sensitive radioimmunoassays for β-human chorionic gonadotropin (β-hCG). There were 152 conceptions, with a pregnancy loss of 43%; but only 14 of the abortions were recognized clinically as being pregnancies. The other 50 patients merely had a rise of urinary hCG level from which implantation was inferred. McLean (1987) reviewed other studies that arrived at similar figures. They cited that approximately 50% of implanted pregnancies aborted spontaneously, and most of them were clinically unrecognized. Additionally, there are probably conceptuses that vanish even before implantation. Wilcox et al. (1988) identified 31% spontaneous abortions of 707 cycles collected from 221 women. In a subsequent evaluation of early abortions, Wilcox et al. (1999) determined from hormone studies that optimal implantation occurs between days 8 and 10 after ovulation. Of 189 pregnancies, 75% went at least 6 weeks past last menses, 25% ended in early losses. Conversely, Regan and Rai (2000) indicated that 78% of fertilized ova fail to result in a live birth. They analyzed all aspects of miscarriage, especially recurrent abortion, and suggested that in the latter category, 50% occur by chance. They dedicated much space to a consideration of the antiphospholipid syndromes. Mills et al. (1988) found that diabetic women in good clinical control of their diabetes may expect similar rates of abortion and cited an incidence of 16% of clinically recognized gestations. Hertz-Picciotto and Samuels (1988) have criticized some of these results and gathered the following figures from four studies:

No. of losses		No. of recognized pregnancies	Risk of loss in recognized pregnancies
Subclinical	Clinical		
43	18	154	11.7
7	11	85	12.9
50	14	102	13.7
67	6	41	14.6

Most spontaneous abortions occur before 12 weeks of pregnancy, and chromosomal errors are their most prominent cause but the exact mechanism of the abortion event is still disputed. A recent review by Jauniaux and Burton (2005) suggested that oxidative stress may constitute an important aspect of spontaneous abortions. They argued that because trophoblastic ingrowth of maternal vessels is reduced in spontaneous abortion specimens, an earlier true perfusion of the intervillous space occurs that then results in trophoblastic damage. Numerous other factors are also evaluated in their comprehensive review. In a study of amniocentesis results over 20 years of women age 35 or more, Caron et al. (1999) found that 1.79% had chromosomal errors, with trisomies and structural rearrangements prominent findings. Stern and Coulam (1992) found in a study of recurrent abortions that the reduction in sonographic size of the "fetal pole" and differences in fetal heart rate activity at 6 weeks allowed great accuracy in anticipating an abortion. The hypoplasia of the placenta, so often observed and that presumably correlates with the decreased hCG secretion and hence progesterone support of the decidua, is an accepted possibility. A specific inquiry into the small gestational sac (sonographically) and other gestational parameters was undertaken by Dickey et al. (1992). They found small gestational sacs more often in chromosomally normal abortuses. It has recently been suggested that "illegal" blood flow into the intervillous space at an early gestational age may equally be of importance in causing spontaneous abortions (e.g., Jauniaux & Burton, 2005). Schaaps and Hustin (1988) and Hustin et al. (1988) had earlier reviewed the interesting evidence of early trophoblast invasion. From their findings they concluded that massive trophoblastic infiltration of uteroplacental arteries essentially occludes these vessels before 12 weeks' gestation. This trophoblastic proliferation, they suggested, permits only plasma filtrate to circulate in the intervillous space, at least in early gestation. It is apparently for this reason that chorionic villus sampling (CVS) specimens are usually bloodless. Sonographic and pathologic evidence suggest on the other hand that, in spontaneous abortuses, blood circulates in the intervillous space before the interruption of pregnancy. It is thus speculated that this may come about as the result of inadequate trophoblastic proliferation into the decidual arteries and that it affects normal nidation.

Increasing maternal age considerably increases the risk of spontaneous abortion, especially after the age of 35 (Stein, 1985), and it correlates with an enhanced risk of fetal trisomies. No such association could be made with respect to paternal age (Hatch et al., 1990). Moreover, Neuber et al. (1993) found that the frequency of monosomy X and of triploidy decreases with advancing maternal age. When triploids are observed in abortuses of older women, they tend to be more often the result of digyny, that is, maternal failure of producing a haploid gamete. Although this advanced maternal age phenomenon is clearly demonstrable from statistics and has been suggested to be the result of inadequate pairing at meiosis ("non-congression") by Hodges et al. (2002), the **actual age** of the oocyte, often suggested to be a causal mechanism especially in the frequency of Down syndrome, has been studied only once in humans. Simpson et al. (2002) did such a study of women in whose pregnancies the timing of conception could be deduced reasonably well. They found "no association between ageing gametes and major birth defects, including Down's syndrome." These and other studies have led to an inquiry into whether it is the nucleus or the oocyte cytoplasm that may be "at fault" in disturbed pregnancies. These are further discussed below (see Recurrent or Habitual Abortion).

Abortions due to chromosomal nondisjunction were lucidly detailed by Magenis (1988), who summarized especially well the paternal versus maternal nondisjunctional events in trisomies and X monosomy. Also, numerous investigators have commented on the apparent excess of male conceptuses among abortion specimens (reviewed by Shettles, 1964). Contradictory reports have been examined by Kellokumpu-Lehtinen and Pelliniemi (1984). They studied the sex ratio of 551 induced abortions by histologic examination of gonads or by sex chromatin. Early embryos had a sex ratio of 1.64, which became 1.17 in later fetal stages, presumably because of losses in early gestation. There is no convincing explanation for the disproportionately high loss of male embryos. Embryos also are often improperly sexed by pathologists. It has been our experience that male gender is often inaccurately assigned because of misinterpretation of the normally large clitoris in young female embryos. Kirby et al. (1967) have suggested immunologic reasons for the excess male wastage.

Clendenin and Benirschke (1963) and Carr (1965) were the first investigators to establish that spontaneous abortions principally result from chromosomal errors of the conceptus. Subsequent investigations from many countries have confirmed and extended these observations. Boué and Boué (1969) reported that 70% of spontaneous abortions occurring during the first 6 weeks of pregnancy had chromosomal errors, and 50% during the first 10 weeks. Trisomies constituted 56% of the errors, triploidy 18%, monosomy X 15%, and the remainder were double trisomies, tetraploidies, and individual chromosomal errors, such as rings, translocations, and mosaicism. Hassold et al. (1980), in a detailed study of 1000 spontaneous abortions, found 44.5% trisomies, 24.2% monosomy X, and 15.1% triploidy. Kajii et al. (1980) found 53% of their specimens to be chromosomally aberrant. Other studies, largely from cultured material, have produced approximately similar results (Kuliev, 1971; Creasy et al., 1976). Eiben and colleagues (1990) studied 750 spontaneous abortions with direct chromosome preparations (as opposed to preparations made from cultured cells). Roughly similar error rates were detected, but it was striking that there was a considerable excess of females in chromosomally normal abortions (sex ratio 0.71). The use of postmortem villus sampling after the specimen is delivered was advocated by Johnson et al. (1990). They not only found it to be more successful than skin biopsy and amniocentesis, but also discovered an unusually high error rate.

The pathologist is occasionally asked to provide material for chromosomal study from fetuses and placentas. In our experience, this is best done from embryonic tissue or from the chorionic surface when an embryo is not available. Although general sterile techniques are desirable when obtaining the material, Boué used tap-water–washed specimens with good results. Absolute sterility may not be needed, but it is preferable. When sampling the placenta, it is best to cleanse the fetal surface, peel the amnion away, and then to obtain chorionic tissue with sterile instruments, ideally to include some chorionic surface vessels. Geisler and Gropp (1967) have provided more detailed instructions for the explantation of this material.

Anatomic Findings

The evaluation of specimens from spontaneously aborted conceptions has greatly changed. The so-called *Windei* (blighted ovum) of early authors, the "pathologic ovum" (with its many subgroups), and many other designations used in the past have now become obsolete. Likewise, terms such as *nodular, cylindrical, stunted,* and *disorganized embryo* have little specific use in describing the nature of the embryonic abnormality (Fig. 21.1). For a better understanding of the pathogenesis of the many defects in aborted specimens, it is necessary to know their chromosomal constitution. It may not be reasonable to undertake complex cytogenetic studies of spontaneous abortion specimens on a routine basis because of the expense and because it adds little for management. This is disputed, however, by Wolf and Horger (1995), who presented cogent argument for such investigations.

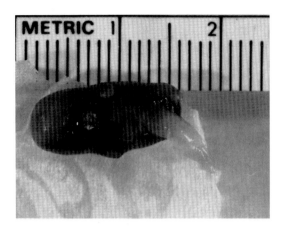

FIGURE 21.1. Cylindrical embryo of a spontaneous abortion at 9 weeks' gestation. Embryo is also growth-restricted (should be 2.5 cm) and hemorrhagic. It was undergoing autolysis on microscopic study; abortion is undoubtedly due to a chromosomal error.

Understanding the principles may be sufficient, but what to sample remains a personal choice. An excellent pictorial guide for the study of abortions is to be found in Kalousek et al. (1990). Salafia and her colleagues (1993) undertook a study to ascertain how the histopathologic findings can be used in making the diagnosis of chromosomally caused abortions. They devised scoring criteria and concluded that an intact fetal circulation, villous infarcts, decidual arteriopathy, and chronic "intervillositis" argued against cytogenetic error as the cause of an abortion (see also Doss et al., 1995). New methodology is evolving that will make it feasible to describe the genetic defects more accurately, such as DNA studies, the polymerase chain reaction (PCR), fluorescent in situ hybridization (FISH) of whole cells (e.g., Hogge et al., 1996; D'Alton et al., 1997; Bischoff et al., 1998; Clouston et al., 2002), and delineation of translocations by spectral color staining of chromosomes. Some of these tests are feasible even using fixed and selected individual cells from paraffin-embedded tissues (for reviews see Antonarakis, 1989; Kovacs et al., 1989; Kuchinka et al., 1995). The placental material also lends itself for paternity diagnosis (Strom et al., 1996). Horn and his colleagues (1991) suggested that abortion material be examined with a lens, so as to identify hydropic swelling and hypoplasia; histologically, few additional findings of importance are made.

Because hydropic villi are such a frequent finding in many placentas of spontaneous abortions, the differential diagnosis from moles and partial moles is often required and may present difficulty. To do so, we have advocated a much wider use of flow cytometry, the most rapid means for the delineation of diploidy and triploidy. The ploidy ($2n$ versus $3n$) of aborted specimens, particularly triploid "partial moles," are thus being differentiated from "true"

(complete) hydatidiform moles much more quickly (see Chapter 22). We also recommend that a mini-autopsy be performed on embryos when they are present, as its findings are often startling. Despite the frequent maceration of these embryos, an autopsy is easily done when running water over the dissected specimen is employed during the dissection. This allows easy identification of the presence of major structures. For comparison of gross and microscopic specimens, two excellent atlases by Chi et al. (1992) and Keeling (1994) are useful. How problematic it is to differentiate histologically between partial moles and placentas of spontaneous abortuses is well illustrated by the observation of Rakheja et al. (2004). Their abortion specimen had typical scalloping and syncytial "inclusions" that are usually seen primarily in partial hydatidiform moles. The karyotype of this specimen, however, was 46,XY, del 18q.

The youngest described abnormal specimens originated from the systematic studies of early human implantations. Hertig et al. (1959) summarized their extensive search for early conceptuses, which they conducted in 210 women. They described 34 early ova, 10 of which were abnormal. Histologic abnormalities included multinucleated blastomeres, necrotic blastomeres, lack of cavitation, hemorrhage, and deficient trophoblastic proliferation. These studies were done, however, before cytogenetic study was feasible. Harrison et al. (1966) depicted an abnormal 13-day ovum with unbranched villi and abnormal amnionic budding.

Most of the descriptions of aborted specimens come from systematic studies of spontaneous abortion. Kaeser (1949) presented an extensive study of the frequency, nature, and pathologic features of abortions, highlighting the "hydatidiform degeneration" of villi (Fig. 21.2). Huber et al. (1957) found in 76% of their specimens that the embryo was abnormal; 40% of the specimens had hydatid changes of villi. Sadovsky and Laufer (1961) emphasized the extensive decidual hemorrhage that is often regarded as being one cause of early abortions, especially those with intact villi (Fig. 21.3). Eckman and Carrow (1962) described the presence of extensive villous stromal collagenization as a prominent feature of their abortion specimens and found 29% to possess hydatid changes. The fibrosis of villi was considered to be secondary by Abaci and Aterman (1968), who studied 237 abortion specimens. They found changes of hydatidiform mole in 41.3% and subchorionic hematomas (Breus' mole) in 20.2% (Fig. 21.4).

The hydropic degeneration (hydatid change) of villi is a recurrent finding in all studies of abortion specimens (Fig. 21.5). This feature was reviewed by Ladefoged (1980), who compared 100 spontaneously aborted specimens with 160 therapeutic abortions. Whereas hydropic change was noted in as many as 81% of instrumented specimens (representing probably the normally edema-

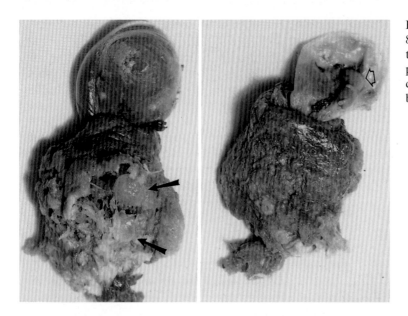

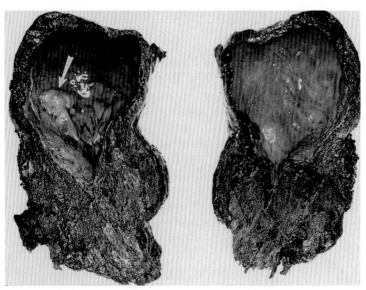

FIGURE 21.2. Spontaneous abortus at approximately 8 weeks' gestation. Note the opened sac at right with the nodular embryo (open arrow). The hypoplastic placenta with focal marked villous edema ("hydatid degeneration") is seen at the left (arrows). Decidua basalis is hemorrhagic.

FIGURE 21.3. Spontaneous abortus with a fragmented, macerated embryo (arrow). It would previously have been described as a "hematoma mole" (carneous mole). The specimen exhibits a common feature of many early abortions: The amnion is prematurely attached to the chorionic sac.

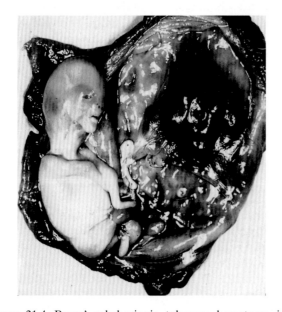

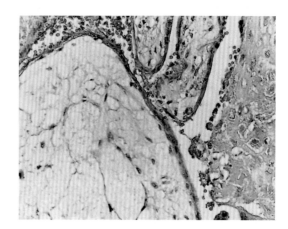

FIGURE 21.5. Hydatidiform swelling of a villus in a spontaneous abortus. Microcystic spaces develop in the distended villus. Note the trophoblastic hypoplasia and focal necrosis. H&E ×160.

FIGURE 21.4. Breus' subchorionic tuberous hematoma in a missed abortion at 6 months' gestation. Note the large hematoma to the right of the macerated fetus.

tous appearance of these villi), in only 6.9% was the hydatid change excessive, in contrast to the 41% found in spontaneously aborted specimens. Jurkovic and Muzelak (1970) observed focal hydatid changes in 21% of legal abortions, and in 2% it was diffusely distributed. Fibrosis was seen in 4.4%; other, nonspecific changes were less frequently identified. These authors emphasized that the frequency of pathologic findings demands more careful scrutiny of these specimens than is usually done. Abortions with hydatid changes had significantly more aneuploidies, as identified by flow cytometry, than was the case in nonhydropic abortuses (Fukunaga et al., 1993). A study of van Lijnschoten et al. (1994) sought to differentiate histologic features of induced from spontaneous abortions. The spontaneous abortuses had smaller villi with some hyalinization and fewer vessels. Moreover, the trophoblast was less hyperplastic. Because many villi are degenerating in specimens from spontaneous abortion, there is often much finely granular mineralization (calcification) along the trophoblastic basement membrane. We presume that it is accumulated because the usually avid calcium transport of trophoblast continues even after villous circulation has ceased.

Fujikura et al. (1971) also compared spontaneous with induced abortion specimens. They pointed out that the hydropic changes found in normal (induced) abortuses is primarily a feature of villi in the chorion laeve, where the villi are expected to undergo degenerative changes. Thus, the sampling site is of importance when such specimens are compared. In their analysis, the number of villi also did not differ in the two groups, and therefore reduced villous growth cannot be held responsible for abortion. The first ultrastructural studies of aborted specimens were presented by Herbst and Multier (1971). They depicted microvillous hypoplasia, lacunar spaces, and enlarged endoplasmic reticulum of the syncytium, as well as villous fibrosis. No specific and constant changes were described that characterized abortion specimens. The newer techniques to demonstrate programmed cell death (apoptosis) were employed to study placentas from patients with labor and in sectioned placentas by Thiet et al. (1995), and they were also used by Miller et al. (1996) and Lea et al. (1997b) to compare spontaneous and induced abortions. Although DNA laddering was observed in all specimens, there was no significant difference between the groups. Apoptosis occurs normally in trophoblast and stromal cells of the human placenta and it increases with gestational age (Smith et al., 1997a, 2000). It is also known, however, that apoptosis is much increased in the syncytiotrophoblast of placentas associated with intrauterine growth restriction (IUGR) (Smith et al., 1997b). Whether this is the result of hypoxia or a reason for the IUGR needs to be ascertained in the future; a beginning was made in the review by Jauniaux and Burton (2005).

All of the placental alterations described so far are relatively nonspecific. They are also not uniformly present, and many (e.g., the hydatid changes) may be the sequelae of embryonic death. The reason for the preponderance of hydatid change in aborted specimens is not fully understood. It is generally believed that, following fetal death, the trophoblast continues to transport water from the intervillous space into the villi, whence it cannot be removed by an absent fetal circulation; hence the villi enlarge. This explanation is probably too facile for a complex process, especially because fibrotic villi with intact trophoblastic cover also exist.

The comparison of chromosomally abnormal with euploid abortion material produced more insights. Singh and Carr (1967) made the first efforts to identify morphologic features of the aborted specimens and related them to cytogenetic findings, but Philippe (1986), collaborating with Boué (Philippe & Boué, 1969), has probably investigated this issue in more detail than most pathologists. These authors' observations and those by some other investigators (Honoré et al., 1976; Ornoy et al., 1981; Byrne et al., 1985; Göcke et al., 1985) allowed some subdivision of abortion specimens into major categories. Indeed, some of these investigators have gone so far as to suggest that many pathologic changes are so characteristic that they enable chromosomal diagnosis from the morphologic findings of the villous tissue alone. Others could not find a good correlation between cytogenetic findings and morphology (Rehder et al., 1989; Horn et al., 1991). Redline et al. (1998) examined the proliferative extent of trophoblast (and some other features) in specimens from spontaneous abortions that were also successfully karyotyped. An increase in trophoblastic proliferation was seen in trisomic abortuses, especially in trisomy 7 and 15. Much the same applies to molar or abortion material with significant hydatid change.

A group of investigators from Europe and Australia has analyzed the potential error in the diagnosis of molar (hydatid) specimens made by several observers (Howat et al., 1993). They took 50 molar abortion specimens of different types and sent them for independent assessment to seven colleagues, two with a special interest in gynecologic pathology. Interested readers can find the details in the article, but suffice it to say here that the experts and regular diagnostic pathologists were unable to specifically label a given microscopic appearance with confidence. Especially, they were not able to reliably distinguish complete moles from partial moles, and partial hydatidiform moles could not be reliably differentiated from nonmolar abortion material. The authors found that reliable histopathologic criteria do not exist for this differential diagnosis. We agree with this interpretation of their pathologic findings. Indeed, Rehder and her colleagues (1989) were unable to differentiate structural findings of aneuploid abortuses from those of euploid material. It is true that, generally, the placentas of spontaneous abortions are abnormally small and too thin. When examined by dissecting microscopy, their villous ramification is decreased and hydropic degeneration is visible in some (Honoré et al., 1989; Shepard et al., 1989b). More extensive data provided by Shepard et al. (1989c) showed that placentas of trisomy 18 fetuses were smaller, and some trisomy 13 placentas had low weights. In the placentas with triploidy, the placental weights correlated, in part at least, with their chromosomal contribution. In conformity with the findings of Jacobs et al. (1982), those triploids whose extra chromosome set was acquired from the mother were smaller, and when two paternal sets were present, the placentas were larger or hydropic. One might have postulated that anembryonic but nonmolar spontaneous abortion specimens have a genetic similarity to complete hydatidiform moles. A specific study directed to elucidate this point came from Henderson et al. (1991), who studied 14 such specimens with locus-specific minisatellite probes and showed that these anembryonic placentas possessed both maternal and paternal genomes. They were thus not androgenetic as are the hydatidiform moles. A succinct appraisal of the current dilemma in the differential diagnosis of general abortion material for histopathologists was provided by Fox (1993). He reviewed all the relevant publications and concluded that precise histopathologic classification is a "valueless exercise." Cytogenetic study and flow cytometry are now needed for more precision.

Summary of Placental Findings in Chromosomally Defined Abortions

Trisomies

For historical reasons only, the usage trisomy C, D, E, and so on is employed here. Because usually the exact chromosome involved in the trisomy is not immediately identified, we employ this grouping as merely indicating that these elements belong to the major subgroups of chromosomes so designated.

Trisomy E (16–18)

Trisomy 16 is one of the commonest cytogenetic anomalies found in spontaneous abortion material (Fig. 21.6). In general, the embryo is absent and the chorionic cavity is empty and small. Anembryonic gestations may be confused with other abnormal gestational products, and it is for that reason that, as mentioned earlier, Henderson et al. (1991) had examined the genetic makeup of anembryonic specimens. Trisomy 16 was one of the results. Importantly, these embryo-deficient abortuses had maternal and paternal genetic reasons for the extra chromosome. Most trisomy 16 abortuses constitute the typical blighted ovum, the *Windei* of the German literature. The villous growth is reduced, the trophoblast is hypoplastic, and the villi are usually avascular and some are hydropic (Vernof et al., 1992). Enlarged cytotrophoblastic giant cells (see

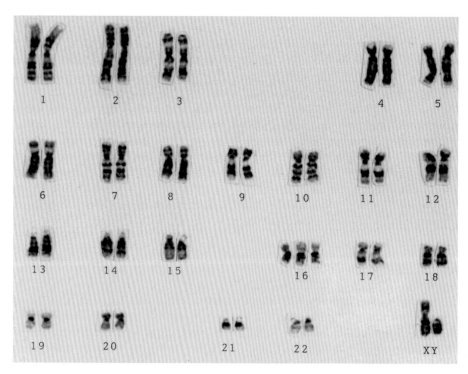

FIGURE 21.6. Trisomy 16, the commonest trisomy of spontaneous abortions. Giemsa-banded karyotype. (Courtesy of Dr. M. Bogart, Honolulu.)

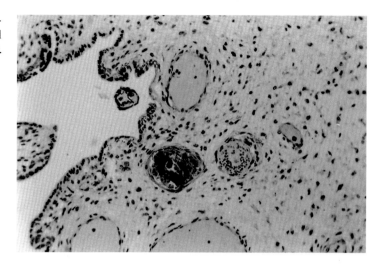

FIGURE 21.7. Spontaneous abortus at 17 weeks of 41-year-old woman, trisomy 13 (cleft lip, polydactyly, renal cysts). Scalloping of villi and trophoblastic inclusions. H&E ×250.

below) are found in the stroma of up to 30% of villi. Discrepancies of trisomy 16 are frequent in cytogenetic assessment of villi and amnionic fluid. Mosaicism is common. This topic was extensively reviewed by Benn (1998) but without further consideration of placental morphology. Sebire et al. (2000) found in ongoing gestations with trisomy 18 increased trophoblastic proliferation by using a specific antibody to the Ki-67 antigen, and they deduced from this an increased cell turnover.

Trisomy C (6–12)

Abortions with this genotype have a variable morphology, and the placenta is less mature than expected for gestational age. Giant villous trophoblast cells are found in 40%.

Trisomy D (13–15)

This chromosome anomaly exhibits variable placental maturation and reduced villous vasculature, and is also

reported to contain giant cytotrophoblast in 50% of villi. In our review, this is uncommon, however. Occasionally, markedly hydropic villi exist, and scalloping as well as trophoblastic inclusions may occur (Fig. 21.7). Although these changes are not invariable, they may be similar to what is often believed to be typical for partial moles (Fig. 21.8). The embryo frequently has facial and other anomalies.

Other Trisomies and Related Errors

There are even fewer characteristic patterns of the placentas of other trisomies; Zerres et al. (1988), however, described hydatid swelling of villi in four cases of trisomy 22. The villi also had vascularization. One of their cases was terminated at 36 weeks' gestation; it had fewer villous abnormalities. Honoré et al. (1974) described significant molar changes, including atypical trophoblastic proliferation in the placenta of trisomy 2, and trisomy 22 was found in the placenta of a severely growth-restricted infant by Stioui et al. (1989). Roberts et al. (2000) sug-

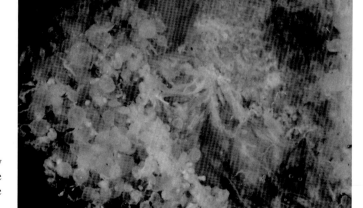

FIGURE 21.8. Partial hydatidiform mole in triploidy (69,XXX). Most villi have hydatid enlargement but are attached to a chorionic sac. A chorionic cavity would not be expected in a true mole.

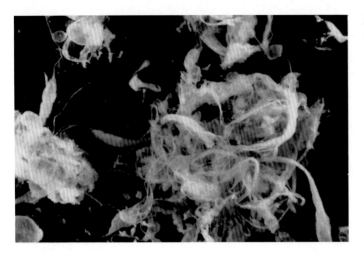

FIGURE 21.9. Partial molar degeneration in triploidy (69,XXY). Many villi are not hydropic.

gested that trisomy 21 placentas had more frequently two-layered trophoblastic surface, and more capillaries and nucleated red blood cells (NRBCs). In trisomy 18 and 13, more basophilic "stippling" (calcification) was found along the basement membrane. It may also be of interest to note that the first microarray study of placentas has been done. Gross et al. (2002) used samples of trisomy 21 placentas and controls for this analysis, and found that there is overexpression of two expressed sequence tags in this study when compared with normal controls. Rakheja et al. (2004) described scalloping of villi and "pseudoinclusions" of trophoblast in an abortus with a long arm deletion of chromosome 18.

Tetrasomy 12 is a well-recognized chromosomal error with usually lethal anomalies (e.g., Shivashankar et al., 1988). In a typical case we saw with similar malformations and neonatal demise to those in the case described in detail by these authors, the placenta was essentially normal. Because of associated preeclampsia there were

infarcts but neither placenta (450 g) nor neonate (3390 g) were growth-restricted. The villi were normally constructed, and the cord was 37 cm in length. In neonatal lymphocyte cultures the abnormal cells were quickly replaced by a population of 46,XX cells, whereas early fibroblast cultures were tetrasomic. Later cultures, again, began to be overgrown by 46,XX cells.

Polyploidies

Triploidy

The triploidy genotype is discussed in greater detail in the discussion of partial moles in Chapter 22. Macroscopically, the placentas of triploids are frequently at least partially molar (Figs. 21.8 and 21.9), but this depends largely on the origin of the extra set of chromosomes. It is the general finding that, when an extra **paternal** set is present, the placenta has molar change and a severely

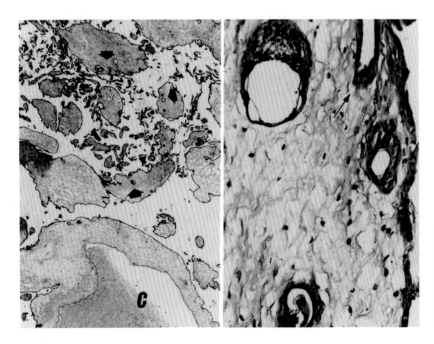

FIGURE 21.10. Triploid abortus with macrocystic villous hydropic change at bottom left (C) intermixed with small villi above. This picture is typical of a partial mole. Numerous trophoblastic inclusions are seen at arrows and at right. They come about by infolding, as seen at the white arrow. H&E ×64 (left); ×240 (right).

FIGURE 21.11. Two enlarged villi in a triploid abortus. One (left) is hypercellular, with faintly visible remnants of former fetal vessels; the other is hydropic. H&E ×160.

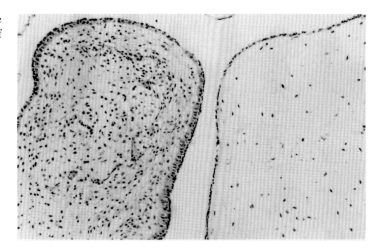

abnormal or absent embryo; when an extra **maternal** set is involved, then the embryo is better formed, has some characteristic anomalous features such as digital fusion, and the placenta is less molar or not at all hydropic. Also, the embryos, when present, are too small for the expected age. Some villi have microscopic cavities (lacunae) (Fig. 21.10), and others may be broken or they are compacted, with an increased cellularity (Fig. 21.11); the trophoblast is variably hypoplastic or moderately proliferated. There is characteristic "infolding" (scalloping) of trophoblast into the villi, with trophoblastic nests occurring seemingly isolated in the villous stroma (Fig. 21.10). A Breus' mole is occasionally found with triploid abortuses as well, although this is commoner in monosomy X. It is important for the pathologist to recognize that the villous edema disappears quickly when the specimen is stored. Numerous abnormalities, such as fusion of some digits or toes, have been described in the fetus of triploid conceptuses (Rehder & Gropp, 1971; Ornoy et al., 1978; Moen et al., 1984), but frequently the embryos are nodular and degenerating (Geisler et al., 1972). They may have a single umbilical artery (Kulazenko & Kulazenko, 1976), as is the case with many other spontaneous abortus specimens. Triploid fetuses rarely survive as long as the 10-month-old child described by Sherard et al. (1986). As expected, the extra set of chromosomes in that patient was of maternal origin. Digyny is much commoner in triploids than is diandry (McFadden et al., 1994) and was also present in the 2500-g triploid fetus who survived for 20 days (Puvabanditsin et al., 2004). The latter reviewed previous reports of live births, suggested a frequency of triploidy of 2%, and termination occurring usually before 24 weeks. Triploidy has even been described in an embryo pro-duced by in vitro fertilization (Rosenbusch et al., 1997).

Tetraploidy

Tetraploid abortuses have an empty cavity and voluminous, poorly vascularized villi. They frequently have severe decidual and villous hemorrhages, and their villi are invariably somewhat cystic. A specimen that we have recently seen had massive hydatid change, but, perhaps because one half of the placenta was supplying a normal diploid female neonate, many villi had normal, perfused blood vessels. We conjecture that this may have been a twin gestation. There is one report, however, of a liveborn tetraploid male at 37 weeks' gestation (Nakamura et al., 2003). The newborn weighed 1728g, had numerous congenital anomalies, and died shortly after birth. The placenta was small and not hydropic.

Monosomy X

Frequently, only a cord remnant is found in a cavity that is small for gestational age (Fig. 21.12). There are well-developed villous vessels. Intervillous thrombi of the so-called Breus' mole type are often present (Fig. 21.13). Occasionally, these specimens have a form of amnion nodosum (Fig. 21.14) that may be accompanied by hemosiderin deposits in the membranes. But often they appear to be relatively normal; there are no cystic villi, only villous fibrosis may exist. The embryo may have nuchal hygroma and severe hydrops (Fig. 21.15). Mostello et al. (1989) have reported spontaneous resolution of hygroma and hydrops in serial sonograms. Microscopic examination of the ovaries shows that they are nearly normal up to the second trimester; thereafter, they become depopulated of germinal cells. Of parenthetic interest is the recent study by Barr and Oman-Ganes (2002) that seeks to explain the cause of hydrops in Turner syndrome and the fetuses' frequent demise in mid-gestation. They examined in great detail the various hypotheses that had been advanced and concluded that hydrops may be related to or due to the myocardial hypoplasia, which they consider to be a primary defect.

The giant cytotrophoblastic cells in villi, discussed above, were initially described by Philippe and Boué (1969). Honoré et al. (1976) suggested that they were

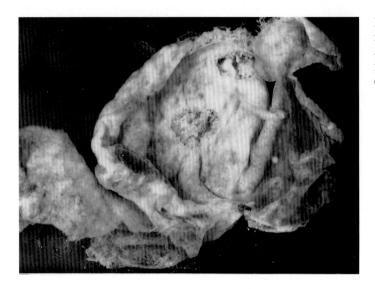

FIGURE 21.12. Monosomy X abortus, with only a cord remnant (arrowhead) present. A small yolk sac remnant is also found. The defects in the chorionic membranes are from cytogenetic sampling. This site is convenient for tissue culture material.

derived from internally delaminating cytotrophoblast. Ornoy et al. (1981) were more cautious in their interpretation of the origin of this cell type but apparently leaned toward the view that the cells are swollen (edematous) stromal cells; they suggested that the origin be clarified by ultrastructural study. We also believe that most of these cells are enlarged Hofbauer cells (Fig. 21.16).

Philippe (1986) suggested that a hallmark of many chromosomally aborted specimens is their growth restriction. Byrne et al. (1985) provided the most comprehensive correlation of fetal phenotype with chromosomal findings. Other studies of fetal morphology in spontaneous abortuses have been published by Bruyere et al. (1987) and Kalousek (1987). The latter investigator correlated chromosomal findings with embryonic phenotype. Ornoy et al. (1981) and Novak et al. (1988) found frequent inflammatory changes of the membranes and villi in their studies, changes not found by us or other investigators, and they are probably unrelated to the chromosomal aberrations. Shepard et al. (1989a) undertook a 20-year analysis of aborted specimens and found that 19% of fetuses had a localized defect. Neural tube defects existed in 3.6%, and recognizable abnormal phenotypes due to chromosomal errors were present in 2.7%. They encountered amnionic bands in four specimens, renal agenesis in two, and facial clefts in 30 of 214 abnormal embryos.

INDUCED ABORTIONS

Pregnancies may be terminated legally ("therapeutic" or "induced" abortion) or illegally ("criminal" abortion). There is little difference between the two from a pathologist's point of view, except that the latter

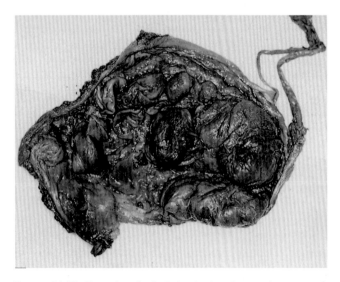

FIGURE 21.13. Breus' mole (subchorionic tuberous hematoma). No embryo is present. This finding is frequent in monosomy X.

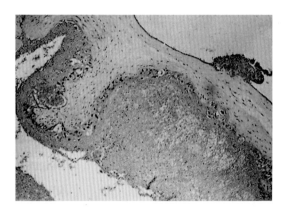

FIGURE 21.14. Microscopic appearance of Figure 21.14. There is old subchorionic, intervillous thrombus in pockets of bulging membranes. The amnion is focally defective and has attached debris. It has been considered as amnion nodosum, but the debris is not squames, as there is no embryo. Often seen with monosomy X. H&E ×40.

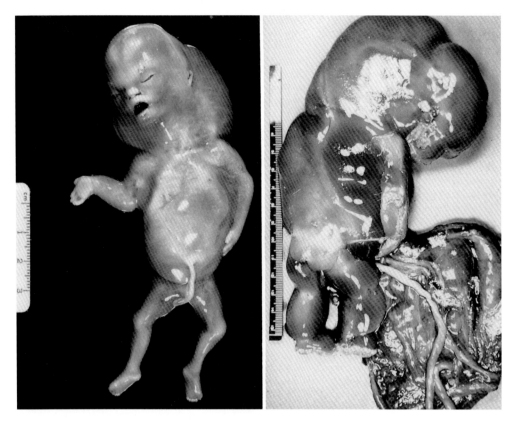

FIGURE 21.15. Two abortuses with monosomy X. The left embryo (10 weeks) has pronounced hygroma; that on the right is edematous and has hygroma as well. Note the hypoplastic placenta.

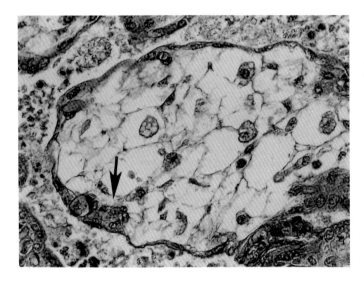

FIGURE 21.16. Villus with cytotrophoblastic giant cells in a spontaneous abortion. The much-enlarged cells in the villous core represent enlarged Hofbauer cells, although a suggestion of cytotrophoblast proliferation is seen (arrow). Cystic lacunae are developing in the villus. H&E ×400.

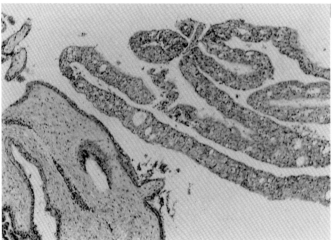

FIGURE 21.17. Yolk sac at 5 weeks' gestation, intermixed with primitive villi (left) from a therapeutic abortion. H&E ×64.

type is frequently followed by a uterine infection. Induced abortion has been a common cause of maternal mortality in the past, but since the legalization of abortion approximately one fourth of pregnancies in the United States are terminated. The safety of the procedure has increased dramatically, with a markedly reduced maternal mortality (approximately 1.5 in 100,000). A succinct review of legal abortion and its history was provided in an editorial (Anonymous, 1989). Induced abortions are performed by dilatation and curettage (D&C), the use of prostaglandins (with or without the use of cervical laminaria), intraamnionic injection of hypertonic saline or urea solutions, or other means (Palomaki & Little, 1972). The pathologic findings in the aborted fetal/placental specimen differ somewhat for each procedure. The study of therapeutic abortion material is often helpful for an understanding of the normal placental relations. A superb electron microscopic study was thus performed on a previllous ovum, 11 days old, one that had recently implanted (Knoth & Larsen, 1972). In such material, the pathologist may also find microscopic structures with which he or she is not familiar, particularly the early yolk sac. This normal feature of early gestation is shown in Figures 21.17 to 21.19. It is the probable initial site of α-fetoprotein (AFP) production and hematopoiesis, and may serve in early fetal nutrition (Luckett, 1972). When the pathologist examines histologic material from abortions, often the question is raised about the time of fetal demise. To determine this more accurately, Jacques et al. (2003) studied 36 placentas of known interval between the injection of KCl into the fetus and placental morphology. They concluded that these findings "cannot be used to accurately predict time of death."

When D&C or suction curettage is performed, instrumentation of the cervix and uterus have occasionally led to misplacement of fetal tissues as well as to sporadic uterine perforation (Kaali et al., 1989). Ayers et al. (1971) reported a 3-cm paracervical bony mass containing a fetal skeleton. The original suction curettage had been done 3 months earlier, when the mother was 10 weeks pregnant. (She had suffered symptoms of pulmonary embolism.) Placental and various other fetal tissues were present, including bone. Incompletely removed fetal tissues have been incriminated in causing infertility, as in the 11 cases of residual fetal bones reported by Moon et al. (1997). Dawood and Jarrett (1982) reported uterine retention of fetal bones for 6 years; the authors suggested that this material acted similar to an intrauterine device (IUD), perhaps by inducing endometrial synechiae. Melius and colleagues (1991) found bones in the uterus 13 years and 14 months after abortion. A similar case is shown in Figure 21.20. We have seen a case with maternal death following TAB at 20 weeks' gestation. The uterus was inadvertently perforated and massive intraabdominal hemorrhage occurred. The patient survived for 2 days and died with disseminated intravascular coagulation (DIC) and adult respiratory distress syndrome. Pulmonary emboli contained deported placental villi

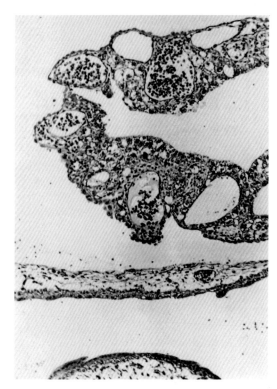

FIGURE 21.18. Yolk sac at 6 weeks' gestation with chorionic membrane, carrying a fetal vessel (below). Note the large sinusoids in the yolk sac epithelium filled with erythropoietic cells. H&E ×240.

enmeshed in fibrin coagulum (Fig. 21.21). Similarly deported villi are shown to be located in uterine veins (Fig. 21.22) in a patient whose uterus was removed when, during an abortion procedure, the uterus was perforated. Uterine perforations were the topic of a review by Darney et al. (1990). They suggested that errors in estimating the gestational age were common in such cases. Lawson et al. (1990) reviewed fatal pulmonary embolism after legal abortion. They found that 45 patients among 231 maternal deaths were caused by embolism with air, clot, or amnionic fluid. Disseminated intravascular coagulation occurred in 11 patients. But even in spontaneous deliveries, unexpected transport of tissues can take place. Thus, Baergen et al. (1997) found embolization of cerebellar material into lung and placental vessels in

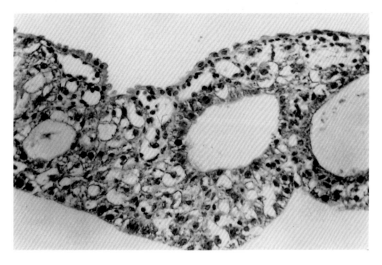

FIGURE 21.19. Same case as in Figure 21.18, yolk sac at 6 weeks' abortion. The tissue is rich in glycogen and has glandular spaces. Endodermal epithelium is inside (above). H&E ×640.

FIGURE 21.20. Retained, necrotic fetal bony lamellae in inactive endometrium that also shows mild chronic endometritis. They are remains of an abortion that took place several years ago. These fragments presumably acted as a contraceptive device; they were removed in 1987, and full term delivery ensued in 1989. H&E ×60. (Courtesy of Dr. W. Tench, San Diego.)

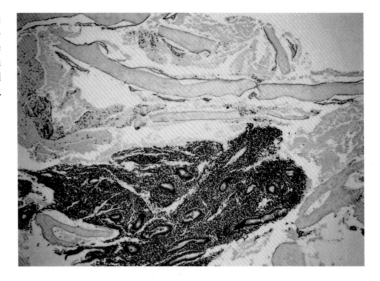

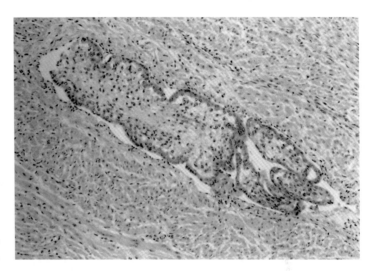

FIGURE 21.21. Deported villi in uterine vein; this happened during therapeutic abortion curettage. H&E ×160.

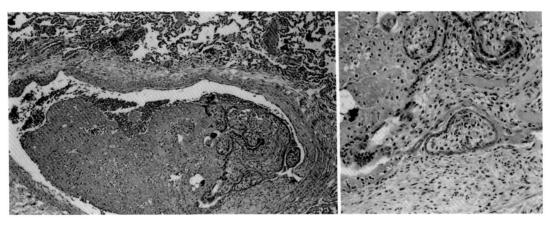

FIGURE 21.22. Pulmonary embolus following a therapeutic abortion complicated by fatal uterine perforation, abdominal hemorrhage, and disseminated intravascular coagulation. Immature villi are engulfed in a fibrin coagulum. H&E ×160 (left); ×240 (right).

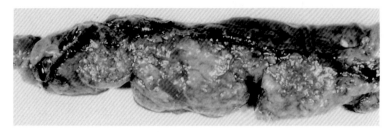

FIGURE 21.23. Macroscopic appearance of an immature placenta from a saline-induced abortion. Note the subchorionic hemorrhage and fibrin deposit, and pallor of the placenta. The superficial villi are necrotic; fetal blood is hemolyzed.

a spontaneous delivery at term and reviewed the sparse literature of similar events.

When bougies are used for termination of midtrimester pregnancies, the placentas were found to be entirely normal (Manabe et al., 1971). Suter et al. (1970) found that suction curettage in infected pregnancies was more difficult to complete; the reason was a presumably more adherent placenta.

There are severe placental changes when pregnancies are terminated with intrauterine installation of hypertonic saline, as extensive fetal ion fluxes occur promptly (Anderson & Turnbull, 1968; Frigoletto & Pokoly, 1971). When these are also reflected in the maternal circulation because of accidental injection into the maternal sinusoids, maternal hypernatremia and deaths have ensued (Schulman et al., 1971; Gustavii, 1972). Clostridial infection is another feared complication (Sehgal et al., 1972). Saline-induced terminations are now rarely done; they are performed without general anesthesia. Associated pathologic changes include amnion necrosis and fluid accumulation underneath the amnion. Most importantly, there are coagulation of intervillous blood and focal necrosis underneath the chorionic plate.

These changes were well illustrated in the study of Christie et al. (1966). A placenta from such a termination is shown in Figure 21.23. It has the characteristic band of hemorrhagic necrosis and coagulation underneath the chorionic plate. The villous tissue is typically pale owing to hemolysis of fetal blood. Another detailed study of the placental changes in saline terminations was reported in the dissertation of Gustavii (1973; see also Gustavii & Brunk, 1972). Other authors who have examined the effect of saline installation into the amnionic cavity are Bengtsson and Stormby (1962) and Jaffin et al. (1962). Gustavii found that saline installation into the extramembranous space quickly stripped the membranes from the uterine wall and led to marked sodium fluxes into the amnionic fluid. It caused decidual necrosis and lysis, whereas the trophoblast remained normal. Gustavii regarded the decidua as the "target" in the procedure. Steinberg et al. (1972) observed a febrile reaction after saline termination in about 20% of cases. From negative placental cultures, they deduced that it was rarely caused by infection.

Hospital admissions for septic abortion have decreased significantly since abortion became legal (Stewart & Goldstein, 1971; Seward et al., 1973). In the large Yugoslavian experience with legal abortion (D&C or suction), the maternal mortality was 0.02% and the morbidity 4.29% (Jurukovski, 1969). Similar reports have come from other countries. Kubatova and Trnka (1967) histologically examined the specimens of 100 legal abortions and found that myometrial admixture was more common in D&C (22%) than in suction curettage. Decidual necrosis and inflammation were common, but the villous tissue was usually normal.

The intentional termination of early pregnancies allows an insight into embryogenesis. Nishimura et al. (1968) thus studied the phenotype of 1213 "undamaged" fetuses from therapeutic terminations undertaken by D&C for psychosocial reasons. Fetal death had occurred in 2.39%, most commonly in women with genital bleeding and of slightly older age. The investigators found macroscopic anomalies in 1.15% of these embryos. It is also important to note that no hydatidiform moles were encountered by these investigators in this survey, even though this disease is so much more common in Japan than in this country. This

indicates to us that early moles are not recognized as such; only in their later evolution are the hydropic changes developed that makes the diagnosis feasible. Singh and Carr (1968) also described fetal specimens having anomalies but normal karyotypes; most common were omphaloceles. Several large studies have been undertaken to assess the karyotypes of legally aborted embryos. For instance, Sasaki et al. (1967) examined the chromosomes of 140 such abortion specimens, terminated at an average gestational age of 9.6 weeks of pregnancy. Of the 140 specimens, 133 were normal, three were mosaic, and four had other chromosomal errors (5%). The investigators additionally cited other published surveys. Yamamoto and Watanabe (1979) found a 6.4% incidence of chromosomal errors among 1661 legal abortions before the 12th week of gestation. Of interest again is the therein reported absence of hydatidiform moles, despite the prevalence of moles.

Jewett (1973) reported maternal deaths when saline had been instilled illicitly, and Monrozies (1971), who studied 426 "criminal" abortions, found that 55 (13%) had serious complications, including uterine hemorrhages, perforations, DIC, and life-threatening infections.

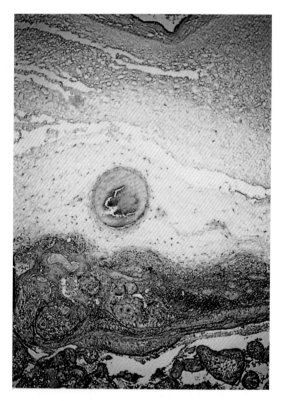

FIGURE 21.24. Placental surface in urea termination at 19 weeks' gestation. The large chorionic, fetal vessel is thrombosed, there is much edema in the membranes, and underneath the chorionic plate is a dense accumulation of fibrin, blood clot and some polymorphonuclear leukocytes. H&E ×40.

FIGURE 21.25. Placental site from curettings of an incomplete spontaneous abortion. There are foci of decidual necrosis, lymphocyte and macrophage infiltration, and fibrin deposition throughout this former placental implantation site. H&E ×64.

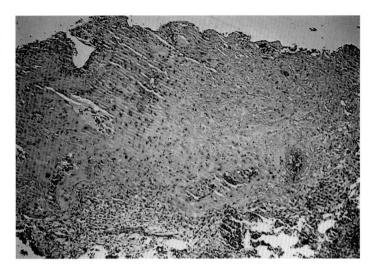

In placentas of septic abortions, Studdiford and Douglas (1956) found acute villitis, intervillositis, and bacterial colonies filling the fetal villous capillaries. Because they had elicited no inflammatory reaction in some of the cases, the colonies doubtless grew postmortem, although sepsis must have preceded the deaths.

Segal et al. (1976) studied the placental changes associated with infusion of hypertonic urea solution. They examined 52 placentas and found subchorionic fibrin deposits (similar to those of saline infusion) and swollen Hofbauer cells. These authors indicated that no placental changes occur with hypertonic glucose instillation. It should be cautioned, however, that swollen Hofbauer cells have also been observed in the usual abortions and may thus be nonspecific activation of these macrophages (Matsubara et al., 1998). In our experience, the changes seen in the subchorionic space following urea termination are usually much less severe than when hypertonic saline solutions are used. Accumulations of polymorphonuclear leukocytes are frequent in the subchorionic space as well but not in the fetal vasculature. In other cases there is chorionic vascular obliteration and much the same subchorionic thrombosis as is seen with hypertonic saline (Fig. 21.24). A detailed study of these changes was reported by Babaknia and colleagues (1979).

Incomplete Abortion

Pathologists are often expected to make the definitive diagnosis of intrauterine pregnancy from curettings of women who are presumed to have sustained an abortion. When villi or syncytiotrophoblast are seen, the diagnosis is obvious, but frequently these elements are not present in the decidual debris that is intermixed with fibrin and hemorrhagic material. The diagnosis of pregnancy is then more difficult and depends on the pathologist's ability to differentiate degenerating decidual changes (which could result from an ectopic pregnancy) from those of intrauterine implantation sites. The decidua basalis at the placental implantation site undergoes characteristic morphologic changes that should be identified in curettings, even in the absence of villi and syncytium, and that serve as a diagnostic clue. These changes include infiltration with fibrin, alterations of decidual blood vessels (physiologic changes; see Chapter 9), and most characteristically, the decidua basalis contains X cells (extravillous trophoblast) at the implantation site. These cells are usually easily recognized in spontaneous abortions, and their presence establishes the presence of placentation at this site. They are larger than decidual cells, do not possess the silver-impregnable cell borders of decidua, have an amphophilic cytoplasm, and are mostly uninucleate. They stain with cytokeratin and antibodies to major basic protein (MPB). In addition, there are frequently some decidual degeneration and inflammatory cell infiltration. The principal microscopic indicators of a placental site are shown in Figures 21.25 and 21.26.

Lichtig et al. (1988) described the vascular component of this decidual change. They believed that it is a pathologic change, and thus they differ from the many authors who have considered the vascular invasion by extravillous trophoblast as physiological. They cited these authors but still preferred a different interpretation. What is important in their contribution is that they addressed the dilemma often faced by the practicing pathologist, and they provided valuable and practical suggestions for the differential diagnosis.

The term **placental polyp** is occasionally applied. It refers to the residuum of placental tissue, either from abortion or, more often, following term pregnancy. A placental polyp is frequently embedded in degenerating blood clot. Its cause may have been a placenta accreta or incompletely aborted placental tissue. Placental remnants can now also be accurately identified by sonography (Tal et al., 1997). This condition is more fully discussed in Chapter 10.

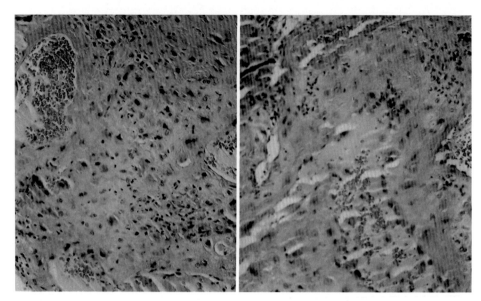

FIGURE 21.26. Placental site of spontaneous abortion, curettings. Note the infiltration with fibrinoid and large placental site giant cells. They are X cells (intermediate trophoblast) and have infiltrated and altered the blood vessel wall at right. Despite the absence of villi and syncytium, this histologic picture suffices for the diagnosis of placental site. H&E ×260.

Placenta in Chorionic Villus Sampling

Alvarez (1966) first used placental biopsy for differential diagnosis of hydatidiform mole and later for assessment of villous morphology in erythroblastosis, syphilis, and other disorders. Chorionic villus sampling (CVS) was subsequently used to determine fetal sex (Anonymous, 1975), and Kazy et al. (1982) applied chorionic villus sampling to determine fetal genetic disorders. Chorionic villus sampling is now widely used for the prenatal diagnosis of chromosomal and genetic disorders and is undertaken during the first trimester. Some clinicians prefer this method because it allows access to the fetal genotype before performing an amniocentesis is feasible. Chieri and Aldini (1989) used CVS also during the second trimester, and encountered one abortion in 220 patients. Others have preferred early amniocentesis with generally good results (for discussion see Eiben et al., 1997). Similarly, Daniel et al. (1998) found that early amniocentesis is safe and a good alternative to CVS.

Although CVS is generally a safe procedure, it has occasionally caused placental complications, including fetal bleeding (Shulman et al., 1990). Cashner et al. (1987) suggested that great difficulties exist in the precise risk evaluation from CVS because of the general risk of spontaneous abortion in this gestational age group. With a live fetus from an 8- to 12-week gestation, the risk of spontaneous abortion was 2% in their analysis, and it was greater in older women, who are more likely to be sampled. Lippman et al. (1984) estimated the associated spontaneous abortion rates, and were not convinced that CVS is a significant cause of fetal loss. The complications of CVS were followed by sonographic surveillance in 714 patients studied by Wade and Young (1989). They had a 4.1% "unintended" abortion rate by 20 weeks' gestation, and it was higher when repeated catheter insertion was necessary. Subchorionic bleeding was witnessed in one patient, with abortion following in 48 hours. Late abortions were "more likely to have in utero death or premature rupture of the membranes." During CVS, Pozniak et al. (1988) noted sonographically the rapid development of a retromembranous hematoma that formed from a venous lake. Its expansion ceased spontaneously. Facial hemorrhages in the fetus were demonstrated by fetoscopy during CVS by Quintero et al. (1993).

Occasional cases of septic abortion have followed CVS. Brambati and Varotto (1985), who found bacterial cultures from the cervix of CVS patients to be positive in a large percentage of cases, performed 700 CVS procedures and found acute infection twice. Barela et al. (1986) reported septic shock and renal failure 4 days after CVS at 11.5 weeks' gestation. Associated endomyometritis ultimately necessitated hysterectomy. Muggah et al. (1987) found degenerated villi with transcervical CVS at 73 days' gestation. Chorionic villus sampling was repeated 4 days later. The patient experienced fever that disappeared at 12 weeks' gestation. She miscarried at 16 weeks and was treated for septic shock. Coliform organisms were cultured from the placenta and fetal parts but not from amnionic fluid. Marini et al. (1988) reported septic abortion 10 weeks following CVS. The placenta (at 20 weeks) showed acute chorioamnionitis, but it is doubtful that this event was causally related to the CVS.

In general, CVS does not usually have serious placental sequelae. When we have examined the placentas of patients who have had CVS during the first trimester, no abnormal findings were apparent. Similar results came from a large multicenter study of 2278 CVS procedures; the findings were compared with the results of amniocentesis in 617 patients. There was only a 0.8% increase of fetal loss in the CVS group (Rhoads et al., 1989). Concern has been expressed over the finding that limb-reduction defects may follow CVS (Firth et al., 1991; Burton et al., 1992). Letters to the editor (1991) in *Lancet* have subsequently examined the issue. In some of these letters, "organized thrombi" were found in fetal stem vessels (Scott, 1991); a vascular etiology was also suggested by Burton et al. (1992). Other reports of a correlation of fetal age at CVS and limb defects comes from Firth et al. (1994) and a collaborative American study (Olney et al., 1994; see also Botto et al., 1996). It is currently felt that the relation may exist principally in the gestationally earlier CVS that has been practiced in Europe, although contrary opinions have been reported (Froster & Jackson, 1996). No limb-reduction defects were identified in the large series by Williams et al. (1992) when CVS was done after 9 weeks.

Most concern about prenatal diagnosis relates to discrepancies of chromosomal findings among results obtained from CVS, amniocentesis, and fetal blood culture. Often the cause is real mosaicism and even chimerism; at other times, pseudomosaicism exists. The differentiation between mosaicism and other causes is important and may be difficult. It was readily accomplished by Falik-Borenstein et al. (1994) because of the presence of XX and XY+9 cells, but they were confined to the placenta and probably represented a vanished twin from superovulation. Some authors have attributed this to the usage of the Chang tissue culture medium (Krawczun et al., 1989); contamination with maternal tissue is another possible cause. The finding of mosaic cell lines has caused much concern in the fetal prenatal assessment, and discrepant results are not always easy to explain. They may reflect the differing origin of cells from the inner cell mass (fetus) or its shell (placental trophoblast), as well as nondisjunctional events taking place in the sometimes prolonged tissue culture. It is essential to understand the handling of the materials from this procedure. Chromosome preparations are feasible from the **direct** analysis of cells that happen to be in division (largely cytotrophoblast) or from cells cultured for several days, representing primarily the connective tissue compartment of the villi. The former cells derive from the "shell" of the blastocyst and, as we will see, mosaic preimplantation embryos have now been identified; these trophoblast cells may not accurately reflect the **fetal** cytogenetic constitution. We have presented elsewhere (Chapter 11) what is known of the derivation of the connective tissue of villi. They are clearly **fetal** cells, rather than **placental** elements, as the placental connective tissue derives from the epiblast of embryo, not the trophoblastic shell (Enders & King, 1988; Bianchi et al., 1993). Thus, one must know which cells are found to be chromosomally abnormal when CVS is done in order

to infer probable fetal genotype. Griffin et al. (1997) analyzed the topic appropriately. They analyzed 691 spontaneous abortions by long-term culture, and 177 with additional short-term mitotic study. Success rates were 82% and 76%, respectively. They believed also that the cultures have had a significant maternal (decidual) contamination, because many more 46,XX cells were found than expected. They caution that results need careful interpretation. An additional aspect of this complex array of prenatal diagnostic measures is that one must be aware of "imprinting" occurring on fetal and placental tissues, and that numerous cases of uniparental disomy are now known to complicate confined placental mosaicism. Imprinting, that is, the transcriptional silencing of a portion of one parental genome, is a reality affecting placentation and many disease states (Tycko, 1994). Presumably it is accomplished by DNA methylation of specific genes (Zuccotti & Monk, 1996). Good evidence has been accumulated that some paternal genes are silenced during embryonic development, whereas maternal genes are silenced in placental development (paternal imprinting). It is an important feature in understanding triploidy and the development of partial hydatidiform moles. The genetic consequences and possible phylogenetic advantages of parental imprinting have been critically examined by Wilkins and Haig (2003), although not from a placentation point of view. Uniparental disomy (UPD), that is, the presence of two chromosomes from one parent, is an occasional finding in growth-restricted newborns (Moore et al., 1997) and appears to be linked to confined placental mosaicism (Bennett et al., 1992). It is postulated to take its origin from a trisomic conceptus with the loss of one trisomic chromosome during cell division, and this may be an additional cause of abortion. A systematic search for UPD in spontaneous abortions by Shaffer et al. (1998) failed to identify any cases.

One of the most interesting cases in this respect has been the finding of trisomy 16 confined to villi, with the ultimate finding of a normal fetal karyotype. Verp et al. (1989) reported such a case; there was a grossly and histologically normal placenta, but it was associated with a growth-restricted fetus. They also referred to a report with a normal stillborn fetus described earlier. These investigators cautioned that the presence of a fetus with an otherwise lethal karyotype in CVS should alert one to the possible confinement of aneuploidy to the placenta. Perhaps the aneuploid placenta functioned less efficiently than a normal organ would. This might have produced the fetal growth restriction they observed. Another interesting case addresses a similar problem. Nonmosaic trisomy 16 was observed by CVS in a pregnancy associated with an apparently normal fetus by Tharapel et al. (1989). Fetus and placenta were found to be normal 46,XX at delivery, but a placental nodule had 46,XX/47,XX,+16 mosaicism. It was inferred that this represented a vanished twin gestation. Regrettably, a histologic study of the nodule was not undertaken. A similar case of pure trisomy 16 in placenta and normal 46,XY fetus was observed by Vernof et al. (1992) in a severely preeclamptic woman. The neonate was growth restricted but normal. At other times, placenta and fetus were found chromosomally and structurally normal after a nonmosaic trisomy 16 diagnosis from CVS (Sundberg & Smidt-Jensen, 1991). In the large study reported by Rhoads et al. (1989), 1.8% of the samples were correctly diagnosed as being aneuploid. Reports of two specimens (tetraploidy and trisomy 22) were later proved to be false. A study by Stavropoulos et al. (1998) described a molecular study using FISH in a fetus with trisomy 16 placental mosaicism. Cultured placental stroma showed disomy and trisomy 16; amnion was disomic, whereas high levels of trisomy 16 were found in trophoblast and chorion. Only disomy was present in fetal kidney, brain, lung, and cord blood. Remarkably, 26% of fetal oocytes were trisomic, and uniparental maternal disomy was found in fetal lung and adrenal gland. This remarkable finding has profound implications for our future understanding of CVS results and prenatal diagnosis in general.

Not all aneuploidies are due to meiotic errors. Kalousek and Dill (1983) have produced the first good evidence that chromosomal mosaicism is often confined to the placenta (confined placental mosaicism, CPM); they have expanded this concept in many subsequent contributions to the literature. Handyside (1996) reviewed the evidence now accumulating that many preimplantation embryos have a mosaic chromosomal constitution, caused by mitotic nondisjunction. In a relevant review, Kalousek and Barrett (1994; Kalousek, 2001) found it most likely that, in many cases, the embryo had originally been trisomic as well. Regrettably, there is not yet much direct correlation with placental phenotype (e.g., pathologic features) in the various types of CPM that have been described. DeLozier-Blanchet et al. (1993) suggested that the chromosomally abnormal areas of villous biopsies show structural pathologic features, but have not yet elaborated further. It would appear, however, that CPM is found more frequently in unexplained stillbirths. Its elucidation has certainly made the interpretation of some chromosomal errors in CVS more difficult. Phillips et al. (1996) found that approximately 10% of gestations with CPM have fetal cytogenetic abnormalities. As indicated earlier, Falik-Borenstein et al. (1994) found two cells lines in CVS, and because of their different sex chromosomes (46,XX and 47,XT,+9) interpreted this as confined placental chimerism. In a study of CPM of growth-restricted fetuses and placentas, Wilkins-Haug et al. (1995) found it three times more commonly with IUGR. All neonates had normal blood karyotypes, their placentas were smaller but not histologically abnormal. Breed et al. (1986) found a deletion of chromosome 16 in a CVS specimen but a normal fetal karyotype. The chorionic tissue was later found to be mosaic. Brandenburg et al. (1996) found nonmosaic trisomy 16 in CVS (euploid

fetuses) and found all pregnancies to have bad outcomes. Verjaal et al. (1987) reported six discrepant results and cited many other such inconsistencies from the literature. Schulze et al. (1987) found two cases of CVS with mosaic trisomic cells in which the aborted fetuses were euploid, and Vernof et al. (1992) had another. Cheung et al. (1987) suggested that direct preparations of extended chromosomes be made from multiple villi in order to ascertain mosaicism that is confined to the placenta. Some investigators have argued that such mosaicism, detected at CVS and amnionic fluid study, should be followed by fetal blood karyotyping. They have suggested that it usually would reveal fetal euploidy, but Kaffe et al. (1988) confirmed the mosaicism found earlier in amnionic fluid cells. Thus, mosaicism is not always confined to the placenta. It is of interest here that Kalousek and McGillivray (1987) found that all surviving fetuses with trisomy 13 and trisomy 18 had placental karyotype mosaicism. Subsequently, this finding was extended to terminated pregnancies with these trisomies (Kalousek et al., 1989). The mosaicism was confined to cytotrophoblast and was not found in villous stroma, chorion, or amnion. Moreover, no such mosaicism was found in fetuses with trisomy 21. The suggestion is that trisomics with mosaic (aneuploid/diploid) placentas have a better chance of reaching maturity than those with truly trisomic placentas. A large review of the San Francisco experience with CVS comes from Goldberg and Wohlferd (1997). They found an incidence of 1.3%, and in 20% it was confirmed in the fetus, but neonatal outcome was normal for all fetuses with mosaic placentas.

Villous tissue is useful for structural and genetic studies. Besley et al. (1988) diagnosed Gaucher's disease (and trisomy 21) from deficiency of β-glucosidase in aspirated villi. We had the opportunity to examine tissues of a fetus that was diagnosed by amnionic fluid analysis as having Hunter's syndrome (mucopolysaccharidosis II, iduronate sulfatase deficiency). Although some inclusions were present in the liver, the spinal cord showed striking abnormalities. Ultrastructural analysis of the placenta was normal. Further discussion of the identification of fetal storage disorders with CVS is found in Chapter 18.

Cytogenetic analysis is also now feasible from trophoblast shed into the cervical canal. These are collected by cytobrush (Kingdom et al., 1995) or by irrigation (Bahado-Singh et al., 1995). The cells recovered are mainly syncytiotrophoblast from which DNA can be recovered or on which FISH can be done for specific chromosomes. Adinolfi et al. (1993) diagnosed trisomy 18 in nucleated cells from cervical flushes.

Fetal cells may enter the maternal circulation in sufficient numbers to allow chromosomal diagnosis by aspiration of maternal blood. Lo et al. (1990) identified Y-specific sequences, but Holzgreve et al. (1990) as well as Gänshirt-Ahlert et al. (1992) were not convinced. Kao et al. (1992) were more successful in positively identifying Y-chromosome–specific genes; Elias et al. (1992) used hybridization with chromosome 21–specific probes to identify fetal trisomy 21, and Sekizawa et al. (1996) were able to determine fetal RhD genotype from a single NRBC so recovered. The fetal cells in the maternal circulation were tentatively identified by Suzumori et al. (1992) as being red blood cells contaminating the maternal blood. This new method is still under study to enhance a less invasive fetal diagnosis. It relies on sorting fetal cells with flow cytometry, using antibodies and studying the DNA after the use of PCR. Enrichment of the sample is variably handled, but magnetic sorting seems to be the least destructive method for the cells (e.g., van Wijk et al., 1996). Others (Takabayashi et al., 1995) used micromanipulators successfully for isolation of fetal NRBCs from maternal blood. A symposium held to address these issues should be consulted for details (Simpson and Elias, 1994). Fetal chromosome determination from these cells, employing FISH for five different chromosomes, has been elegantly demonstrated by Bischoff et al. (1998). The most current studies employ circulating DNA in maternal blood from which Y-sequences from male fetuses can be recovered (Lo et al., 1997). Although one might think that this signal comes from perhaps degrading and deported syncytial cells, Smid et al. (1997) found the amount of free fetal DNA to decrease with advancing gestation, and suggested its derivation from NRBCs. Fetal RhD typing from free DNA in maternal plasma was demonstrated in the report by Gautier et al. (2005), but Moise in an editorial of the same journal emphasized that it is not routinely used in the United States, although it is commonly done in Europe.

Trisomic Placentas

There are few specific findings that truly characterize a delivered placenta with trisomy, but many types of abnormality have been found sporadically. Thus, the incidence of single umbilical artery (SUA) is higher. Hecht (1963) reported five cases of trisomy 18 and found that the associated placentas were unusually small. Histologically, one of his specimens showed markedly increased fibrin deposits, syncytial knotting, and infarcts. Similar findings were reported by Matayoshi et al. (1977). Rochelson and colleagues (1990) studied the placentas of 18 trisomic fetuses with quantitative morphometry, using appropriate controls. Doppler analysis of umbilical arterial blood flow had been performed in 10 of them. They found that the placentas had a "significant reduction in small muscular artery count and small muscular artery/villus ratio," which correlated with abnormal Doppler waveforms. A quantitative study of normal and chromosomally abnormal placentas between 18 and 23 weeks' gestation was reported by Kuhlmann et al. (1990). They found no differences in fetal and placental weights but a significant decrease in small muscular arteries and total vessel counts was seen in the aneuploids. Aside from smaller size, we have noted an increase in syncytial knots in trisomy 18 (Fig. 21.27), increased cellularity of villous stroma (Fig. 21.28), or vascular abnormalities. The latter were either old occlusions or fresh thromboses of surface and umbilical cord vessels (see Fig. 21.30). Villitis of unknown etiology (VUE; Chapter 20) was found in another case, but its relation to trisomy 18 may be spurious. In one case of trisomy 18 associated with many abnormalities of fetal development, the small placenta had numerous cysts scattered throughout. They were composed of large villi with cisternae (see Fig. 21.31). Although this appearance was very different from that of the partial moles in triploidy, this morphology certainly is not characteristic for or diagnostic of trisomy 18. In trisomy 13, the placenta is also frequently smaller and more often has SUA; the villi are frequently dysmature and sometimes had trophoblastic inclusions (Figs. 21.29 and 21.32). We have the impression that the villi may also have deficient capillarization. The relation of SUA to

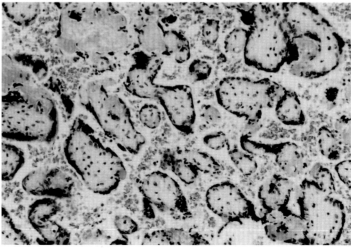

FIGURE 21.27. Villi of immature placenta (28 weeks' gestation) of a growth-restricted (370-g) stillborn fetus with trisomy 18. There is markedly increased syncytial knotting despite the absence of preeclampsia. Villi lack fetal vessels because of fetal demise, but many have hyalinized centers. H&E ×64.

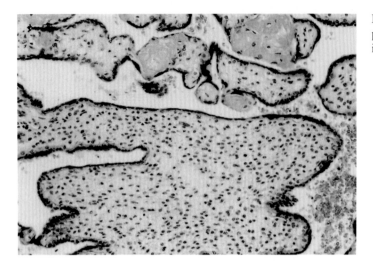

FIGURE 21.28. Other areas of the trisomy 18 premature placenta shown in Figure 21.27. Note the marked increase in villous stromal cells. H&E ×160.

chromosome errors has been explored by Saller et al. (1990) in 109 chromosomally abnormal pregnancies, with 53 cords identified. Six single umbilical arteries were found (two of nine trisomy 18; two of six with trisomy 13; two in other cytogenetic errors). Quantitative studies, especially combined with assessment of SUA, have not been done. Trisomy 21 is not accompanied by characteristic pathologic changes in the placenta. Kouvalainen and Österlund (1967) found a somewhat enlarged placental weight in trisomy 21 and suggested that it may "be a reflection of an immunologic reaction of the mother against her incompatible fetus." Qureshi et al. (1994) found an increased number of irregular villi ("dysmature

villi") and some villous hypovascularity in trisomy 21 placentas.

CHEMICAL MARKERS AND TRISOMY

Steier et al. (1986) evaluated the amount of hCG in the blood and uterine contents of women with legal abortions, spontaneous abortions, and ectopic pregnancies. They found identical values in the first group, but in the other two groups the uterine levels were significantly higher than those obtained from the peripheral circulation. When Bogart et al. (1987) measured hCG, the α-subunit levels of hCG, and AFP in serum of pregnancies with chromosomally normal and abnormal conceptuses, they found that 56% of the abnormal gestations had elevated gonadotropin levels beyond 18 weeks' gestation (1.35% of normals). Elevated α-subunit levels were found in 28% of abnormal pregnancies

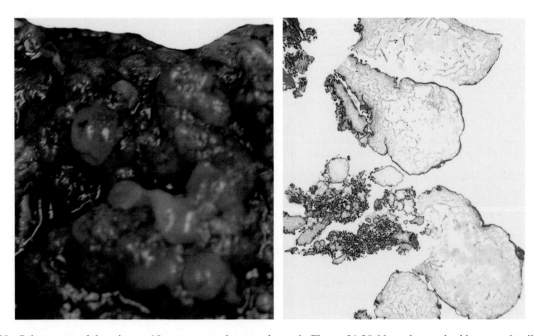

FIGURE 21.29. Other areas of the trisomy 18 premature placenta shown in Figure 21.28. Note the marked increase in villous stromal cells. H&E ×160.

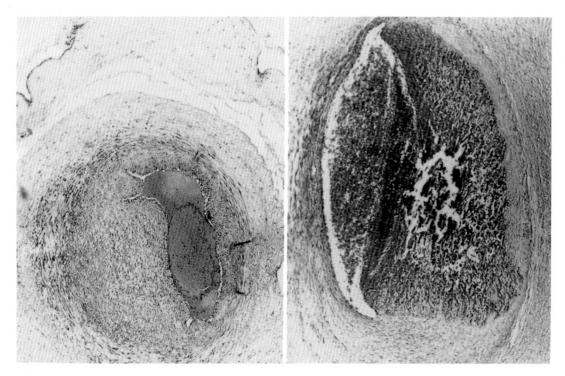

FIGURE 21.30. Umbilical vessels of a placenta with trisomy 18, showing thrombosis, hemorrhage into the vascular wall, and irregular thickening of the vessel wall. H&E ×60.

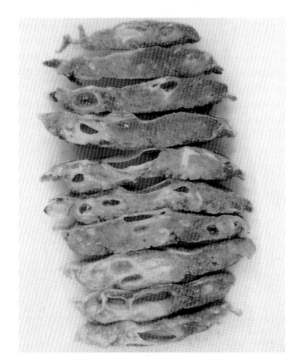

FIGURE 21.31. Cross sections through placenta of trisomy 18 stillbirth. The cysts are composed of enlarged villi; the fetus had numerous anomalies, aside from growth retardation.

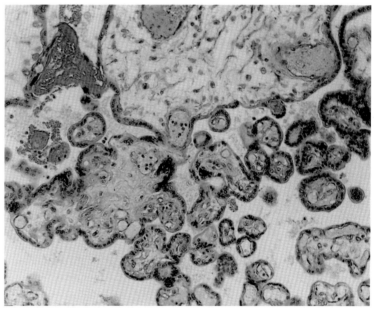

FIGURE 21.32. Placental villi in trisomy 13 at 27 weeks' gestation. Villi are irregularly matured. Some are edematous, with capillary ectasia, and others are excessively small with deficient vascularization. H&E ×160.

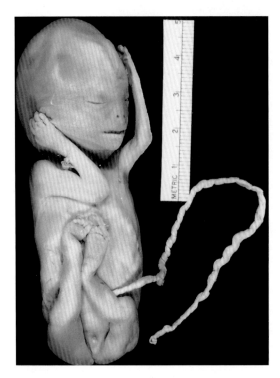

FIGURE 21.33. Fetal demise due to a tight, true knot in the umbilical cord, followed by abortion at 10 weeks' gestation.

and in none of the normals. The authors then suggested that these findings may be useful for screening procedures; they are now universally undertaken. In a later study, Bogart et al. (1989) examined maternal sera for these hormones in earlier pregnancies and found that aneuploid fetuses did not deviate from the normal controls, and their earlier findings were confirmed. There is still no satisfactory explanation for these and other deranged chemical markers, such as free β-hCG and dimeric inhibin A (Wenstrom et al., 1997). The importance of adequate monitoring was highlighted by the danger of overlooking an ectopic abortion when a therapeutic abortion is undertaken; three fatal cases of this complication were reported by Li and Smialek (1993).

Other Findings

There are many other causes of spontaneous abortion than the genetic abnormalities just described. Among these there are amnionic adhesions (Chapter 11), infections (Chapter 20), knots in the umbilical cord (Fig. 21.33) and excessive umbilical cord twists (Chapter 12). The pathologist is urged to undertake microscopic study of even macerated fetuses. Frequently unexpected features are found, for example, cytomegalovirus infection that cannot be anticipated from the history or gross morphology. Fetal and maternal deaths are more likely to occur in women using IUDs, especially the formerly used Dalkon Shield (Cates et al., 1976). We have found in the placenta of a spontaneous abortion specimen large numbers of Hofbauer cells whose cytoplasm contained granular accumulations that resembled Russell bodies, but they were not plasma cells (Fig. 21.34). Their presence remains an unresolved mystery.

Recurrent or Habitual Abortion

Habitual abortion has been variously defined. Wall and Hertig (1948) considered it a "condition in which a woman had two or more consecutive abortions." They examined 100 such patients and observed that the same pathologic findings were made in 58% of their cases. Of them, 43% were considered to result from ovular factors and 15% from other maternal factors. A comprehensive review of this topic has been made by Gant (1989). He lamented not only that this entity has been differently defined but also that other aspects of nomenclature hinder precise analysis. Stirrat (1990a), in an extensive analysis of recurrent abortion, felt that the definition should be three or more spontaneous abortions because after two mishaps the chance of successful pregnancy was 80%. As indicated earlier, some recent insights have been gained into oocyte maturation and possible reasons for recurrent spontaneous abortions. For instance, because of the labo-

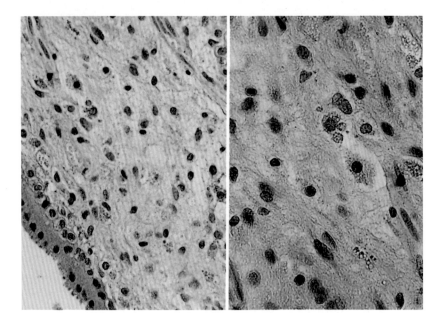

FIGURE 21.34. Villi of a spontaneous abortion with accumulation of a large number of granular, proteinaceous Hofbauer cell inclusions, whose origin remained obscure. H&E ×160 (left); ×600 (right).

rious efforts involved in routine karyotyping, Daniely et al. (1998) have shown that by genomic hybridization study, they were able to detect trisomies, translocations, and monosomies; 48% of their samples from recurrent abortions were abnormal. In a later study, however, the same group used cytogenetics and banding for this purpose and found 29% chromosomal errors (Carp et al., 2001). They then studied the mothers and found an increased frequency of aneuploid cell that suggested to them "mitotic instability" that remained unexplained (Daniely et al., 2001). An interesting editorial by Lockwood (2000) reviews much additional investigation (e.g., cannabis metabolism in spontaneous abortion) and draws attention to a study by Zhang et al. (1999). These investigators transferred the germinal vesicles of oocytes from older women into enucleated eggs of younger age and found that the maturation proceeded more successfully than when no transfer was done. Related studies of chromosomes obtained from in vitro fertilization studies by Simon et al. (1998) had shown that those obtained from older patients had more chromosomal errors. These are probably some of the reasons for the recently more widely practiced preimplantation genetics, which seeks to avoid implanting chromosomally abnormal embryos or those afflicted with single gene mutations. The topic has been reviewed by Sermon et al. (2004) and Sampson et al. (2004); it is beyond the scope of this chapter. The prenatal diagnosis of X-linked diseases by the study of male cells from maternal blood is currently under active study (Costa et al., 2002; Béroud et al., 2003; Kilpatric et al., 2004).

Several distinct types of recurrent abortion exist, the known etiologies vary widely, and many causes are either poorly understood or overrated (Stirrat, 1990b). Infectious causes are discussed in Chapter 20; chronic debilitating disease, for example, lupus erythematosus, maternal heart disease, endocrine disorders, and nephritis, are discussed in Chapter 19; recurrent villitis of unknown etiology (VUE; Chapter 20), and maternal floor infarction (MFI; Chapter 9), constitute another group. The relation of substance abuse to spontaneous abortion and to abruptio placentae is difficult to evaluate, especially the possible contribution of maternal smoking. Many patients who smoke or use various toxic substances additionally consume alcohol, have various infections, and are prone to suffer misuse and trauma. Although they probably do not make up a large segment of repetitive abortions, they form a substantial aspect of polemics in medicine. Direct studies are few; most are epidemiologic correlations that seem to establish a connection between these agencies and abortion (Ness et al., 1999). Studies suggest that increased levels of tumor necrosis factor (TNF) may play an etiologic role (Mallmann et al., 1991; Shaarawy and Nagui, 1997). Lea et al. (1997a), however, found that recurrent abortions are characterized by a decrease in the expression of TNF-α in syncytiotrophoblast, in contrast to its normal expression in random spontaneous abortion specimens. Doss and colleagues (1995) reported on 10 cases of recurrent abortions with massive, repetitive chronic intervillositis and excess fibrin deposits. Chronic villitis was present in some, but not all, of these placentas. The intervillous cellular infiltrate consisted of predominantly leukocyte common antigen (LCA) and CD68-positive cells, suggesting an immunologic origin of the abortive event.

Parental chromosome aberrations and some immunologic errors associated with placentation are other well-studied causes of recurrent abortion and they need special consideration here. Occasionally, a balanced chromosomal translocations of one parent has been the cause of habitual abortion. Granat et al. (1981) described a 22/22 translocation in a man whose wife had had six consecutive abortions. All of the specimens had been early, partially necrotic, and incomplete missed abortions. As is usual, the presumably aneuploid conceptuses were not studied chromosomally. The authors reviewed previous studies of similar case material but with different cytogenetic errors. Their experience led them to urge physicians that, in couples with recurrent abortions, the mother *and* her husband be examined cytogenetically. Simpson et al. (1989), who studied 342 women and 297 men with more than one first-trimester miscarriage, found that parental translocations were not a common cause of recurrent spontaneous abortions. Such chromosomal errors were more frequent only when anomalies and other reproductive failures were combined. Smith and Gaha (1990) found an appreciable incidence of translocation carriers in a large study of recurrent abortion families. There were 15 balanced reciprocal translocations and 9 Robertsonian fusions in that population. Table 21.1 reviews some of the large cytogenetic studies of recurrent abortions. There are

TABLE 21.1. Cytogenetic studies of recurrent abortions

Source	Year	No. of families	Error rate (%)	Types of errors
Rosenmann et al.	1977	12	38.4	Variants
Mennuti et al.	1978	34	14.7	Translocations (T)
Heritage et al.	1978	37	8.1	2 T; 1 XXX
Neu et al.	1979	30	3.3	Translocation
Turleau et al.	1979	413	2.3	T, inversion (I), others
Ward et al.	1980	100	6.0	I, variants
Sachs et al.	1985	500	10.0	20 T, mosaics, I, deletions
Castle & Bernstein	1988	688	6.83	XXX, XYY, mosaics, T, I
Portnoi et al.	1988	1,142	4.8	T, I, others
Hussain et al.	2000	193	7.7	11 T, 2 inversion 2 mosaic
Hogge et al.	2003	517 (28 no growth)	6.2	Not specified, inherited

a number of reasons why studies of this kind are difficult to compare: The methods of analysis differ, the interpretation of chromosomal "variants" is problematic, and aneuploidy is usually only inferred to be the reason for spontaneous abortion as the aborted specimen is virtually never karyotyped. Some recurrent abortions then are caused by parental chromosomal errors; others are due to increasing maternal age with its increased chance of aneuploidy. The morphology of the specimens does not differ from those of other spontaneous abortions. The pathologist can make a contribution to a better understanding of the etiology by requesting cytogenetic evaluation of aborted specimens from recurrent aborters. Lanasa et al. (2001) examined six families with unexplained recurrent abortions, and of these, four had a "highly skewed X inactivation pattern" with selective loss of male conceptions. A novel insight into unexplained recurrent abortions was gained by the study of Lissak et al. (1999). They studied 41 patients with recurrent losses and found in both anembryonic and embryonic gestational specimens a high prevalence of nucleotide substitution (methylenetetrahydrofolate reductase nucleotide 677—cytosine to thymine). Although I (K.B.) have been skeptical of the causative relationship of this enzymatic defect and fetal demise, a recent case makes me reconsider this possibility. This patient with tetrahydrofolate reductase deficiency produced an extremely premature and growth-restricted infant who soon succumbed. Remarkably, the placental surface had large thrombi for which no other explanation could be found. Moreover, one thrombus had central calcifications, testifying to its age.

There is not only considerable disagreement as to whether immunologic disturbances cause abortion, there is even more controversy as to the management of such mothers. Because autoimmune diseases, such as lupus erythematosus, have such a deleterious effect on pregnancy (Scott et al., 1987), it has been suggested that an immunologic mechanism may also be responsible for rejection of the fetal genotype. These considerations could involve specific antibodies, whose actions may be evident in arterial lesions; but such has not often been shown to be the case with the usual habitual abortions. That there are changes in a variety of immune parameters with pregnancy, and perhaps especially with abortions, has been shown by MacLean et al. (1991), who described alterations in T-cell counts (down), WBC (up), mitogen response (up), and interleukin-2 receptors (marked increase in abortion). Parazzini and colleagues (1991) studied 220 women with recurrent abortion and found lupus anticoagulant in 17 and none in the controls. Increased anticardiolipins were present in 19, and they suggested that in at least a portion of such patients immunologic causes may be operative. They did not describe the associated placentas. Kwak et al. (1992) made similar

observations but warned that "what constitutes an autoimmune abnormality in women with recurrent spontaneous abortion is not yet defined or agreed on." Bahar et al. (1993) studied 103 patients with unexplained recurrent abortions in Kuwait and found anticardiolipin antibodies significantly more frequently in this population. It must be noted, however, that antiphospholipid antibodies normally rise in pregnancy, even with in vitro fertilization (Rai & Regan, 1997), and that other studies (Gleicher, 1997) have failed to confirm a definite causal relation to abortion. Bizzaro et al. (2005) have evaluated the prevalence of antiphospholipid and other antibodies in patients with systemic lupus erythematosus (SLE) and in recurrent miscarriages. Their results suggested that elevated anti–annexin V constitutes a definite risk in recurrent pregnancy losses. Other investigators have studied a possible relation of activated protein C resistance to abortion, finding none (Balasch et al., 1997). The complexity of this problem, **thrombophilia**, and the lack of our understanding of fetal/maternal immunologic interactions is further discussed extensively in letters to the editor (1992) of the *New England Journal of Medicine* that address the case-control study of Infante-Rivard et al. (1992). It can also be illustrated by the existence of several large texts that attempt to summarize relevant data (Edwards et al., 1975; Beer & Billingham, 1976; Wegmann et al., 1983; Gill et al., 1987). Despite the large body of investigative data, there are still many areas of uncertainty. It would be inappropriate to itemize all of these findings in a text of placental pathology. Central to the problem is our deficient understanding of the failure by the mother to reject the placental graft. The physiology of this adaptation has been a topic of intense study for many years, and resolution of this paradox is yet to occur. Of the many approaches, the following main positions have been investigated:

1. The mother does not "recognize" the placenta as a foreign genotype perhaps because the trophoblast does not present histocompatibility antigens. Recent studies have examined the differences in major histocompatibility complex (MHC) antigen structure with identification of the human leukocyte antigen (HLA)-G, expressed by young human trophoblast (Kovats et al., 1990; review by Yokoyama, 1997). A complex interaction exists with decidual natural killer (NK) cells that is under investigation and may provide the answer to the nonrejection of placental trophoblast. Suffice it to say that recurrent abortion is not influenced by HLA presentation (Eroglu et al., 1992; see also Hill et al., 1995). From studies of monkey histocompatibility antigens Knapp et al. (1996) concluded that sharing of class I MHC antigens significantly (72%) predicted pregnancy losses.

2. Maternal immune recognition (and rejection) may be intact but thwarted by local (decidual) regulators. The

presence of large numbers of NK cells in the decidua is currently unexplained.

3. Maternal immune cells, normally endowed with properties to reject allogeneic grafts (T-lymphocytes, macrophages) cannot reach the target (because of decidual barriers). Michel et al. (1989) have suggested that the decidual "granular cells" contained smaller granules in repetitive abortion material. For further consideration, see Chapter 9.

Cogent evidence has been provided by immunologic studies that placentation proceeds more advantageously when fetus and mother have maximal histocompatibility differences. It is admitted, however, that inbred lines of mice, having no such dissimilarity, have successful gestations. This species, however, does not possess HLA-G. These studies showed that the circulation of maternal blocking antibodies to paternal (placenta present) antigens prevent rejection. These antibodies can be assayed; they are present in normal pregnancies. Other antibodies (against fetal leukocytes, for instance) can also be detected in maternal sera. That fetal proteins interact with maternal lymphocytes in vitro (suppressing their proliferation) has long been recognized (Olding et al., 1974). Whether this interaction has sequelae in vivo is undecided. Proteins from embryos ("early pregnancy factor") have been shown to modulate immunosuppressive properties (Bose et al., 1989). Most recently, extensive studies on 300 couples with recurrent abortion and 30 control women have shown that a large proportion of the former possess factors in their circulation that are directly toxic to trophoblast and/or embryonic tissues. These authors suggested that this newly recognized cause of recurrent abortion may "involve the 18kd, heat-labile, T-lymphocyte cytokinin interferon gamma" (Hill et al., 1992). The delicate balance between fetal antigens and maternal recognition is further discussed in the comments by Reid (1998), especially with reference to unusual infections that are more common during pregnancy.

Vincent et al. (1998) demonstrated that women with recurrent miscarriage generate increased amounts of thrombin. They found in a study of 86 women with history of recurrent abortion that the thrombin-antithrombin (ATA) complexes were significantly raised and concluded that "thrombosis . . . plays a pivotal role in recurrent miscarriage." Debus and colleagues (1998) investigated the relation of the common factor V Leiden mutation to congenital porencephaly. The resistance to anticoagulation by activated protein C is usually the result of an Arg-to-Gln point mutation in the factor V gene. They found that of 24 patients, 13 had genetic risk factors for thrombosis: Leiden, three; protein C deficiency type I, six; increased lipoprotein a (Lpa), three; protein S deficiency, one. Other papers suggesting a strong relation of thrombophilia to recurrent abortion were reviewed by Younis

(1998). Suffice it to state at this time that hypercoagulability of various inherited types is presumably responsible in a major way for recurrent miscarriage and for fetal thrombotic states. These are only now being investigated with greater efficiency, and the future is likely to bring many new insights.

Because of the desperate wish for children, parents with habitual abortions have tried many immunologic therapeutic interventions, including transfusion and immunization with paternal cells (e.g., Mowbray et al., 1985; McIntyre et al., 1986; Cauchi et al., 1987). Fraser et al. (1993) who reviewed the topic in some detail felt that immunization for recurrent pregnancy loss should be abandoned. Treatment with polyvalent intravenous immunoglobin has been advocated with some seemingly good result by Mueller-Eckhardt et al. (1991), and intravenous infusion of trophoblast plasma membranes isolated from term placentas was undertaken by Johnson et al. (1988). Some of the many studies have been summarized in the cited reference texts and by Stirrat (1990b). In an effort to circumvent possible cryptic endometrial herpes virus infection, Kundsin et al. (1987) have used acyclovir to treat women with habitual abortions. It was moderately successful in the small number of cases treated.

Other than the placentas of patients with lupus erythematosus, those of habitual aborters have no distinctive pathologic features. Most emphatically, they do not possess histologic changes of rejection, as seen in other transplanted tissues. Salafia and Burns (1989) have found decidual vasculitis in some such specimens and suggested that it may signal pregnancy loss on an immunologic basis. Still, it is sobering to read that, despite all these new insights, the study of Plouffe et al. (1992) failed to show any improvement of outcome with varied therapy when they compared recurrent abortions in two widely separated time spans (1968–1977 and 1987–1991). Aksel (1992) who reviewed all aspects of reproductive immunologic disease is also cautious in advocating immunotherapy for recurrent abortion.

References

Abaci, F. and Aterman, K.: Changes of the placenta and embryo in early spontaneous abortion. Amer. J. Obstet. Gynecol. **102**:252–263, 1968.

Adinolfi, M., Davies, A., Sharif, S., Soothill, P. and Rodeck, C.: Detection of trisomy 18 and Y-derived sequences in fetal nucleated cells obtained by transcervical flushing. Lancet **342**:403–404, 1993.

Aksel, S.: Immunologic aspects of reproductive disease. JAMA **268**:2930–2934, 1992.

Alvarez, H.: Diagnosis of hydatidiform mole by transabdominal placental biopsy. Amer. J. Obstet. Gynecol. **95**:538–541, 1966.

Anderson, A.B.M. and Turnbull, A.C.: Changes in amniotic fluid, serum and urine following the intra-amniotic injection of hypertonic saline. Acta Obstet. Gynecol. Scand. **47**:1–21, 1968.

Anonymous: Anshan department of obstetrics and gynecology: fetal sex prediction by sex chromatin of chorionic villi cells during early pregnancy. Chin. Med. J. **1**:117–126, 1975.

Anonymous: Abortion USA. Lancet **1**:879–880, 1989.

Antonarakis, S.E.: Diagnosis of genetic disorders at the DNA level. NEJM **320**:153–163, 1989.

Ayers, L.R., Drosman, S. and Saltzstein, S.L.: Iatrogenic para-cervical implantation of fetal tissue during therapeutic abortion: a case report. Obstet. Gynecol. **37**:755–760, 1971.

Babaknia, A., Parmley, T.H., Burkman, R.T., Atienza, M.F. and King, T.M.: Placental histopathology of midtrimester termination. Obstet. Gynecol. **53**:583–586, 1979.

Baergen, R.N., Castillo, M.M., Mario-Singh, B., Stehly, A.J. and Benirschke, K.: Embolism of fetal brain tissue to the lungs and the placenta. Pediatr. Pathol. Lab. Med. **17**:159–167, 1997.

Bahado-Singh, R.O., Kliman, H., Feng, T.Y., Hobbins, J., Copel, J.A. and Mahoney, M.J.: First-trimester endocervical irrigation: feasibility of obtaining trophoblast cells for prenatal diagnosis. Obstet. Gynecol. **85**:461–464, 1995.

Bahar, A.M., Alkarmi, T., Kamel, A.S. and Sljivic, V.: Anticardio-lipin and antinuclear antibodies in patients with unexplained recurrent abortions. Ann. Saudi Med. **13**:535–540, 1993.

Balasch, J., Reverter, J.C., Fábregues, Tàssies, D., Rafel, M., Creus, M. and Vanrell, J.A.: First-trimester repeated abortion is not associated with activated protein C resistance. Human Reprod. **12**:1094–1097, 1997.

Barela, A.I., Kleinman, G.E., Golditch, I.M., Menke, D.J., Hogge, W.A. and Golbus, M.S.: Septic shock with renal failure after chorionic villus sampling. Amer. J. Obstet. Gynecol. **154**:1100–1102, 1986.

Barr, M. and Oman-Ganes, L.: Turner syndrome morphology and morphometrics: Cardiac hypoplasia as a cause of mid-gestation death. Teratology **66**:65–72, 2002.

Beer, A.E. and Billingham, R.E.: The Immunobiology of Mammalian Reproduction. Prentice Hall, Englewood Cliffs, N.J., 1976.

Bengtsson, L.P. and Stormby, N.: The effect of intraamniotic injection of hypertonic sodium chloride in human mid-pregnancy. Acta Obstet. Gynecol. Scand. **41**:115–123, 1962.

Benn, P.: Trisomy 16 and trisomy 16 mosaicism: a review. Amer. J. Med. Genet. **79**:121–133, 1998.

Bennett, P., Vaughan, J., Henderson, D., Loughna, S. and Moore, G.: Association between confined placental trisomy, fetal uni-parental disomy, and early intrauterine growth retardation. Lancet **340**:1284–1285, 1992.

Béroud, C., Karliova, M., Bonnefont, J.P., Benachi, A., Munnich, A., Dumez, Y., Lacour, B. and Paterlini- Bréchot, P.: Prenatal diagnosis of spinal muscular atrophy by genetic analysis of circulating fetal cells. Lancet **361**:1013–1014, 2003.

Besley, G.T.N., Ferguson-Smith, M.E., Frew, C., Morris, A. and Gilmore, D.H.: First trimester diagnosis of Gaucher disease in a fetus with trisomy 21. Prenat. Diagn. **8**:471–474, 1988.

Bianchi, D.W., Wilkins-Haug, L.E., Enders, A.C. and Hay, E.D.: Origin of extraembryonic mesoderm in experimental animals: Relevance to chorionic mosaicism in humans. Amer. J. Med. Genet. **46**:542–550, 1993.

Bischoff, F.Z., Lewis, D.E., Nguyen, D.D., Murrell, S., Schober, W., Scott, J., Simpson, J.L. and Elias, S.: Prenatal diagnosis with use of fetal cells isolated from maternal blood: Five-color fluorescent in situ hybridization analysis on flow-sorted cells for chromosomes X,Y,13,18, and 21. Amer. J. Obstet. Gynecol. **179**:203–209, 1998.

Bizzaro, N., Tonutti, E., Villalta, D., Tampoia, M. and Tozzoli, R.: Prevalence and clinical correlation of anti-phospholipid-binding protein antibodies in anticardiolipin-negative patients with systemic lupus erythematosus and women with unexplained recurrent miscarriages. Arch. Pathol. Lab. Med. **129**:61–68, 2005.

Bogart, M.H., Pandian, M.R. and Jones, O.W.: Abnormal maternal serum chorionic gonadotropin levels in pregnancies with fetal chromosome abnormalities. Prenat. Diagn. **7**:623–630, 1987.

Bogart, M.H., Golbus, M.S., Sorg, N.D. and Jones, O.W.: Human chorionic gonadotropin levels in pregnancies with aneuploid fetuses. Prenat. Diagn. **9**:379–384, 1989.

Bose, R., Cheng, H., Sabbadini, E., McCoshen, J., Mahadevan, M.M. and Fleetham, J.: Purified human early pregnancy factor from preimplantation embryo possesses immunosuppressive properties. Amer. J. Obstet. Gynecol. **160**:954–960, 1989.

Botto, L.D., Olney, R.S., Mastroiacovo, P., Khoury, M.J., Moore, C.A., Alo, C.J., Costa, P., Edmonds, L.D., Flood, T.J., Harris, J.A., Howe, H.L., Olsen, C.L., Panny, S.R. and Shaw, G.M.: Chorionic villus sampling and transverse digital deficiencies: Evidence for anatomic and gestational-age specificity of the digital deficiencies in two studies. Amer. J. Med. Genet. **62**:173–178, 1996.

Boué, J.G. and Boué, A.: Fréquence des aberrations chromoso-miques dans les avortements spontanés humains. C. R. Acad. Sci. Paris **269**:283–288, 1969.

Brambati, B. and Varotto, F.: Infection and chorionic villus sampling. Lancet **2**:609, 1985.

Brandenburg, H., Los, F.J. and Veld, P.I.: Clinical significance of placenta-confined nonmosaic trisomy 16. Amer. J. Obstet. Gynecol. **174**:1663–1664, 1996.

Breed, A., Mantingh, A., Govaerts, L., Booger, A., Anders, G. and Laurini, R.: Abnormal karyotype in the chorion, not confirmed in a subsequently aborted fetus. Prenat. Diagn. **6**:375–377, 1986.

Bruyere, H.J., Arya, S., Kozel, J.S., Gilbert, E.F., Fitzgerald, J.M., Reynolds, J.F., Lewin, S.O. and Opitz, J.M.: The value of examining spontaneously aborted human embryos and placenta. Birth Defects **23**:169–178, 1987.

Burton, B.K., Schulz, C.J. and Burd, L.I.: Limb anomalies associated with chorionic villus sampling. Obstet. Gynecol. **79**:726–730, 1992.

Byrne, J., Warburton, D., Kline, J., Blanc, W. and Stein, Z.: Morphology of early fetal deaths and their chromosomal characteristics. Teratology **32**:297–315, 1985.

Caron, L., Tihy, F. and Dallaire, L.: Frequencies of chromosomal abnormalities at amniocentesis: Over 20 years of cytogenetic analyses in one laboratory. Amer. J. Med. Genet. **82**:149–154, 1999.

Carp, H., Toder, V., Aviram, A., Daniely, M., Mashiach, S. and Barkai, G.: Karyotype of the abortus in recurrent miscarriage. Fertil. Steril. **75**:678–682, 2001.

Carr, D.H.: Chromosomal studies in spontaneous abortions. Obstet. Gynecol. **26**:308–326, 1965.

Cashner, K.A., Christopher, C.R. and Dysert, G.A.: Spontaneous fetal loss after demonstration of a live fetus in the first trimester. Obstet. Gynecol. **70**:827–830, 1987.

Castle, D. and Bernstein, R.: Cytogenetic analysis of 688 couples experiencing multiple spontaneous abortions. Amer. J. Med. Genet. **29**:549–556, 1988.

Cates, W., Ory, H.W., Rochat, R.W. and Tyler, C.W.: The intrauterine device and deaths from spontaneous abortion. NEJM **295**:1155–1159, 1976.

Cauchi, M.N., Koh, S.H., Tait, B., Mraz, G., Kloss, M. and Pepperell, R.J.: Immunogenetic studies in habitual abortion. Aust. N.Z.J. Obstet. Gynaecol. **27**:52–54, 1987.

Cheung, S.W., Crane, J.P., Kyine, M. and Cui, M.Y.: Direct chromosome preparations from chorionic villi: a method for obtaining extended chromosomes and recognizing mosaicism confined to the placenta. Cytogenet. Cell Genet. **45**:118–120, 1987.

Chi, J.G., Lee, S.K., Suh, Y.L. and Park, S.H.: Sequential Atlas of Human Development. Korea Medical Publishing Co., Seoul, Korea, 1992.

Chieri, P.R. and Aldini, A.J.R.: Feasibility of placental biopsy in the second trimester for fetal diagnosis. Amer. J. Obstet. Gynecol. **160**:581–583, 1989.

Christie, J.L., Anderson, A.B.M., Turnbull, A.C. and Beck, J.S.: The human placenta and membranes: a histological and immunofluorescent study of the effects of intra-amniotic injection of hypertonic saline. J. Obstet. Gynaecol. Br. Commonw. **73**:399–409, 1966.

Clendenin, T.M. and Benirschke, K.: Chromosome studies in abortions. Lab. Invest. **12**:1281–1292, 1963.

Clouston, H.J., Herbert, M., Fenwick, J., Murdoch, A.P. and Wolstenholme, J.: Cytogenetic analysis of human blastocysts. Prenat. Diagn. **22**:1143–1152, 2002.

Cohen, J.: Sorting out chromosome errors. Science **296**:2164–2166, 2002.

Cohen, J.: Coming to Term. Uncovering the Truth about Miscarriage. Houghton Mifflin Company, Boston & New York, 2005.

Costa, J.-M., Benachi, A. and Gautier, E.: New strategy for prenatal diagnosis of X-linked disorders. NEJM **346**:1502, 2002.

Creasy, M.R., Crolla, J.A. and Alberman, E.D.: A cytogenetic study of human spontaneous abortions using banding techniques. Hum. Genet. **31**:177–196, 1976.

D'Alton, M.E., Malone, F.D., Chelmov, D., Ward, B.E. and Bianchi, D.W.: Defining the role of fluorescence in situ hybridization on uncultured amniocytes for prenatal diagnosis. Amer. J. Obstet. Gynecol. **176**:769–776, 1997.

Daniel, A., Ng, A., Kuah, K.B., Reiha, S. and Malafiej, P.: A study of early amniocentesis for prenatal cytogenetic diagnosis. Prenat. Diagn. **18**:21–28, 1998.

Daniely, M., Aviram-Goldring, A., Barkai, G. and Goldman, B.: Detection of chromosomal aberration in fetuses arising from recurrent abortion by comparative genomic hybridization. Hum. Reprod. **13**:805–809, 1998.

Daniely, M., Aviram, A., Carp, H.J., Shaki, R. and Barkai, G.: The association between sporadic somatic parental aneuploidy and chromosomally abnormal placentae in habitual abortions. Early Pregnancy **5**:153–163, 2001.

Darney, P.D., Atkinson, E. and Hirabayashi, K.: Uterine perforation during second-trimester abortion by cervical dilation and instrumental extraction: a review of 15 cases. Obstet. Gynecol. **75**:441–444, 1990.

Dawood, M.Y. and Jarrett, J.C.: Prolonged intrauterine retention of fetal bones after abortion causing infertility. Amer. J. Obstet. Gynecol. **143**:715–717, 1982.

Debus, O., Koch, H.G., Kurlemann, G., Sträter, R., Vielhaber, H., Weber, P. and Nowak-Göttle, U.: Factor V Leiden and genetic defects of thrombophilia in childhood porencephaly. Arch. Dis. Child. Fetal Neonatal Ed. **78**:F121–F124, 1998.

DeLozier-Blanchet, C., Francipane, L., Ebener, J., Cox, J. and Extermann, P.: Cytogenetic discrepancies between fetus and placenta: a frequent cause of reproductive pathologies? Placenta **14**:(abstract), p. A.14, 1993.

Dickey, R.P., Olar, T.T., Taylor, S.N., Curole, D.N. and Matulich, E.M.: Relationship of small gestational sac-crown-rump length differences to abortion and abortus karyotypes. Obstet. Gynecol. **79**:554–557, 1992.

Doss, B.J., Greene, M.F., Hill, J., Heffner, L.J., Bieber, F.R. and Genest, D.R.: Massive chronic intervillositis associated with recurrent abortions. Hum. Pathol. **26**:1245–1251, 1995.

Eckman, T.R. and Carrow, L.A.: Placental lesions in spontaneous abortion. Amer. J. Obstet. Gynecol. **84**:222–228, 1962.

Edwards, R.G., Howe, C.W.S. and Johnson, M.H.: Immunobiology of Trophoblast. Cambridge University Press, Cambridge, 1975.

Eiben, B., Bartels, I., Bähr-Porsch, S., Borgmann, S., Gatz, G., Gellert, G., Goebel, R., Hammans, W., Hentemann, M., Osmers, R., Rauskolb, R. and Hansmann, I.: Cytogenetic analysis of 750 spontaneous abortions with the direct-preparation method of chorionic villi and its implications for studying genetic causes of pregnancy wastage. Amer. J. Hum. Genet. **47**:656–663, 1990.

Eiben, B., Hammans, W. and Goebel, R.: Chorionic villus sampling versus early amniocentesis. Lancet **350**:1253–1254, 1997.

Elias, S., Price, J., Dockter, M., Wachtel, S., Tharapel, A., Simpson, J.L. and Klinger, K.W.: First trimester prenatal diagnosis of trisomy 21 in fetal cells from maternal blood. Lancet **340**:1033, 1992.

Enders, A.C. and King, B.F.: Formation and differentiation of extraembryonic mesoderm in the rhesus monkey. Amer. J. Anat. **181**:327–340, 1988.

Eroglu, G., Betz, G. and Torregano, C.: Impact of histocompatibility antigens on pregnancy outcome. Amer. J. Obstet. Gynecol. **166**:1364, 1369, 1992.

Falik-Borenstein, T.C., Korenberg, J.R. and Schreck, R.R.: Confined placental mosaicism: Prenatal and postnatal cytogenetic and molecular analysis, and pregnancy outcome. Amer. J. Med. Genet. **50**:51–56, 1994.

Firth, H.V., Boyd, P.A., Chamberlain, P., MacKenzie, I.Z., Lindenbaum, R.H. and Huson, S.M.: Severe limb abnormalities after chorion villus sampling at 56–66 days' gestation. Lancet **337**:762–763, 1992.

Firth, H.V., Boyd, P.A., Chamberlain, P.F., MacKenzie, I.Z., Morris-Kay, G.M. and Huson, S.M.: Analysis of limb reduction defects in babies exposed to chorionic villus sampling. Lancet **343**:1069–1071, 1994.

Fox, H.: Histological classification of tissue from spontaneous abortions: a valueless exercise? Histopathology **22**:599–600, 1993.

Fraser, E.J., Grimes, D.A. and Schulz, K.F.: Immunization as therapy for recurrent spontaneous abortion: A review and meta-analysis. Obstet. Gynecol. **82**:854–859, 1993.

Frigoletto, F.D. and Pokoly, T.B.: Electrolyte dynamics in hypertonic saline-induced abortions. Obstet. Gynecol. **38**:647–652, 1971.

Frost, U.G. and Jackson, L.: Limb defects and chorionic villus sampling: Results from an international registry, 1992–1994. Lancet **347**:489–494, 1996.

Fujikura, T., Froehlich, L.A. and Driscoll, S.G.: A simplified anatomic classification of abortions. Amer. J. Obstet. Gynecol. **95**:902–905, 1966.

Fujikura, T., Ezaki, K. and Nishimura, H.: Chorionic villi and syncytial sprouts in spontaneous and induced abortions. Amer. J. Obstet. Gynecol. **110**:547–555, 1971.

Fukunaga, M., Ushigome, S. and Fukunaga, M.: Spontaneous abortions and DNA ploidy. An application of flow cytometric DNA analysis in detection of non-diploidy in early abortions. Modern Pathol. **6**:619–624, 1993.

Gänshirt-Ahlert, D., Burschyk, M., Garritsen, H.S.P., Helmer, L., Miny, P., Horst, J., Schneider, H.P.G. and Holzgreve, W.: Magnetic cell sorting and the transferrin receptor as potential means of prenatal diagnosis from maternal blood. Amer. J. Obstet. Gynecol. **166**:1350–1355, 1992.

Gant, N.F.: Recurrent spontaneous abortion. Supplement 21 to Williams Obstetrics. J.A. Pritchard, P.C. MacDonald and N.F. Gant, eds., pp. 1–11. Appleton & Lange, East Norwalk, CN, 1989.

Gautier, E., Benachi, A., Giovangrandi, Y., Ernault, P., Olivi, M., Gaillon, T. and Costa, J.-M.: Fetal RhD genotyping by maternal serum analysis: a two-year experience. Amer. J. Obstet. Gynecol. **192**:666–669, 2005.

Geisler, M. and Gropp, A.: Zur Methode der Züchtung von Abortmaterial für Chromosomenuntersuchungen. (Zugleich Mitteilung über die Beobachtung einer B-Trisomie bei Abortus). Geburtsh. Frauenheilk. **27**:113–126, 1967.

Geisler, M., Kleinebrecht, J. and Degenhardt, K.-H.: Histologische Analysen von triploiden Spontanaborten. Humangenetik **16**:283–294, 1972.

Gill, T.J., Wegmann, T.G. and Nisbet-Brown, E.: Immunoregulation and Fetal Survival. Oxford University Press, New York, 1987.

Gleicher, N.: Antiphospholipid antibodies and reproductive failure: what they do and what they do not do; how to, and how not to treat! Human Reprod. **12**:13–16, 1997.

Göcke, H., Schwanitz, G., Muradow, I. and Zerres, K.: Pathomorphologie und Genetik in der Frühschwangerschaft. Pathologe **6**:249–259, 1985.

Goldberg, J.D. and Wohlferd, M.M.: Incidence and outcome of chromosomal mosaicism found at the time of chorionic villus sampling. Amer. J. Obstet. Gynecol. **176**:1349–1353, 1997.

Granat, M., Aloni, T., Makler, A. and Dar, H.: Autosomal translocation in an apparently normospermic male as a cause of habitual abortion. J. Reprod. Med. **26**:52–55, 1981.

Griffin, D.K., Millie, E.A., Redline, R.W., Hassold, T.J. and Zaragoza, M.V.: Cytogenetic analysis of spontaneous abortions: Comparison of techniques and assessment of the incidence of confined placental mosaicism. Amer. J. Med. Genet. **72**:297–301, 1997.

Gross, S.J., Ferreira, J.C., Morrow, B., Dar, P., Funke, B., Khabele, D. and Merkatz, I.: Gene expression profile of trisomy 21 placentas: a potential approach for designing noninvasive techniques of prenatal diagnosis. Amer. J. Obstet. Gynecol. **187**:457–462, 2003.

Gustavii, B.: Studies on accidental intravascular injection in extra-amniotic saline induced abortion and a method for reducing this risk. J. Reprod. Med. **8**:70–74, 1972.

Gustavii, B.: Studies on the mode of action of intra-amniotically and extra-amniotically injected hypertonic saline in therapeutic abortion. Acta Obstet. Gynecol. Scand. [Suppl.] **25**:1–22, 1973.

Gustavii, B. and Brunk, U.: A histological study of the effect on the placenta of intra-amniotically and extra-amniotically injected hypertonic saline in therapeutic abortion. Acta Obstet. Gynecol. Scand. **51**:121–125, 1972.

Handyside, A.H.: Moisaicism in the human preimplantation embryo. Reprod. Nutr. Dev. **36**:643–649, 1996.

Harrison, R.G., Jones, C.H. and Jones, E.P.: A pathological presomite human embryo. J. Pathol. Bacteriol. **92**:583–584, 1966.

Hassold, T., Chen, N., Funkhouser, J., Jooss, T., Manuel, B., Matsuura, J., Matsuyama, A., Wilson, C., Yamana, J.A. and Jacobs, P.A.: A cytogenetic study of 1000 spontaneous abortions. Ann. Hum. Genet. **44**:151–178, 1980.

Hatch, M., Kline, J., Levin, B., Hutzler, M. and Warburton, D.: Paternal age and trisomy among spontaneous abortions. Hum. Genet. **85**:355–361, 1990.

Hecht, F.: The placenta in trisomy 18 syndrome: report of 2 cases. Obstet. Gynecol. **22**:147–148, 1963.

Henderson, D.J., Bennett, P.R., Rodeck, C.H., Gau, G.S., Blunt, S. and Moore, G.E.: Trophoblast from anembryonic pregnancy has both a maternal and paternal contribution to its genome. Amer. J. Obstet. Gynecol. **165**:98–102, 1991.

Herbst, R. and Multier, A.-M.: Structures pathologiques du placenta examinées au microscope électronique: premières observations des villosités de l'oef abortif humain. Gynécol. Obstet. (Paris) **70**:369–376, 1971.

Heritage, D.W., English, S.C., Young, R.B. and Chen, A.T.L.: Cytogenetics of recurrent abortions. Fertil. Steril. **29**:414–417, 1978.

Hern, W.M.: Correlation of fetal age and measurements between 10 and 26 weeks of gestation. Obstet. Gynecol. **63**:26–32, 1984.

Hertig, A.T. and Sheldon, W.H.: Minimal criteria required to prove prima facie case of traumatic abortion or miscarriage: an analysis of 1000 spontaneous abortions. Ann. Surg. **117**:596–606, 1943.

Hertig, A.T., Rock, J., Adams, E.C. and Menkin, M.C.: Thirty-four fertilized human ova, good, bad and indifferent, recovered from 210 women of known fertility: a study of biologic wastage in early human pregnancy. Pediatrics **23**:202–211, 1959.

Hertz-Picciotto, I. and Samuels, S.J.: Incidence of early loss of pregnancy. NEJM **319**:1483–1484, 1988.

Hill, J.A., Polgar, K., Harlow, B.L. and Anderson, D.J.: Evidence of embryo- and trophoblast-toxic cellular immune response(s) in women with recurrent spontaneous abortion. Amer. J. Obstet. Gynecol. **166**:1044–1052, 1992.

Hill, J.A., Melling, G.C. and Johnson, P.M.: Immunohistochemical studies of human uteroplacental tissues from first-trimester spontaneous abortion. Amer. J. Obstet. Gynecol. **173**:90–96, 1995.

Hodges, C.A., Ilagan, A., Jennings, D., Keri, R., Nilson, J. and Hunt, P.A.: Experimental evidence that changes in oocyte growth influence meiotic chromosome segregation. Hum. Reprodut. **17**:1171–1180, 2002.

Hogge, W.A., Surti, U., Kochmar, S.J., Mowery-Rushton, P. and Cumbie, K.: Molecular cytogenetics: An essential component of modern prenatal diagnosis. Amer. J. Obstet. Gynecol. **175**:352–357, 1996.

Hogge, W.A., Byrnes, A.L., Lanasa, M.C. and Surti, U.: The clinical use of karyotyping spontaneous abortions. Amer. J. Obstet. Gynecol. **189**:397–402, 2003.

Holzgreve, W., Gänshirt-Ahlert, D., Burschyk, M., Horst, J., Miny, P., Gal, A. and Pohlschmidt, M.: Detection of fetal DNA in maternal blood by PCR. Lancet **335**:1220–1221, 1990.

Honoré, L.H., Dill, F.J. and Poland, B.J.: The association of hydatidiform mole and trisomy 2. Obstet. Gynecol. **43**:232–237, 1974.

Honoré, L.H., Dill, F.J. and Poland, B.J.: Placental morphology in spontaneous humans abortuses with normal and abnormal karyotypes. Teratology **14**:151–166, 1976.

Honoré, L.H., Lin, C.C. and Bamforth, J.S.: Spontaneous abortion with uncommon forms of trisomy: a clinicopathologic study of fifteen cases. (Abstract P41.) Five cases of trisomy 15 in first trimester spontaneous abortion: gross and microscopic pathology. (Abstract P42.) Teratology **37**:458–459, 1989.

Horn, L.-C., Rosenkranz, M. and Bilek, K.: Wertigkeit der Plazentahistologie für die Erkennung genetisch bedinger Aborte. Z. Geburtsh. Perinatol. **195**:47–53, 1991.

Howat, A.J., Beck, S., Fox, H., Harris, S.C., Hill, A.S., Nicholson, C.M. and Williams, R.A.: Can histopathologists reliably diagnose molar pregnancy? J. Clin. Pathol. **46**:599–602, 1993.

Huber, C.P., Melin, J.R. and Vellios, F.: Changes in chorionic tissue of aborted pregnancy. Amer. J. Obstet. Gynecol. **73**:569–578, 1957.

Hussain, M.A., Al-Nuaim, L., Talib, Z.A. and Zaki, O.K.: Cytogenetic study in cases with recurrent abortion in Saudi Arabia. Ann. Saudi Med. **20**:233–236, 2000.

Hustin, J., Schaaps, J.P. and Lambotte, R.: Anatomical studies of the utero-placental vascularization in the first trimester of pregnancy. Trophoblast Res. **3**:49–67, 1988.

Hutchon, D.J.R.: Understanding miscarriage or insensitive abortion: Time for more defined terminology. Amer. J. Obstet. Gynecol. **179**:397–398, 1998.

Infante-Rivard, C., David, M., Gauthier, R. and Rivard, G.-E.: Lupus anticoagulants, anticardiolipin antibodies, and fetal loss. NEJM **325**:1063–1066, 1992.

Jacobs, P.A., Szulman, A.E., Funkhouser, J., Matsuura, J.S. and Wilson, C.C.: Human triploidy: relationship between parental origin of the additional haploid complement and development of partial hydatidiform mole. Ann. Hum. Genet. **46**:223–231, 1982.

Jacques, S.M., Qureshi, F., Johnson, A., Alkatib, A.A. and Kmak, D.C.: Estimation of time of fetal death in the second trimester by placental histopathological examination. Pediatr. Developm. Pathol. **6**:226–232, 2003.

Jaffin, H., Kerenyi, T. and Wood, E.C.: Termination of missed abortion and the induction of labor in midtrimester pregnancy. Amer. J. Obstet. Gynecol. **84**:602–608, 1962.

Jauniaux, E. and Burton, G.J.: Pathophysiology of histological changes in early pregnancy loss. Placenta **26**:116–123, 2005.

Jewett, J.F.: Two deaths from mid-trimester abortion. NEJM **288**:47–48, 1973.

Johnson, M.P., Drugan, A., Koppitch, F.C., Uhlmann, W.R. and Evans, M.I.: Postmortem chorionic villus sampling is a better method for cytogenetic evaluation of early fetal loss than culture of abortus material. Amer. J. Obstet. Gynecol. **163**:1505–1510, 1990.

Johnson, P.M., Chia, K.V., Hart, C.A., Griffith, H.B. and Francis, W.J.A.: Trophoblast membrane infusion for unexplained recurrent miscarriage. Br. J. Obstet. Gynaecol. **95**:342–347, 1988.

Jurkovic, I. and Muzelak, R.: Frequency of pathologic changes in the young human chorion in therapeutic abortions of normal pregnancies: a report of 500 cases studied histologically. Amer. J. Obstet. Gynecol. **108**:382–386, 1970.

Jurukovski, J.N.: Complications following legal abortions. Proc. R. Soc. Med. **62**:830–831, 1969.

Kaali, S.G., Szigetvari, I.A. and Bartfai, G.S.: The frequency and management of uterine perforations during first-trimester abortions. Amer. J. Obstet. Gynecol. **161**:406–408, 1989.

Kaeser, O.: Studien an menschlichen Aborteiern mit besonderer Berücksichtigung der frühen Fehlbildungen und ihrer Ursachen. Schweiz. Med. Wochenschr. **79**:509–515; 780–785; 803–805; 1050–1056; 1979–1084, 1949.

Kaffe, S., Benn, P.A. and Hsu, L.Y.F.: Fetal blood sampling in investigation of chromosome mosaicism in amniotic fluid cell culture. Lancet **2**:284, 1988.

Kajii, T., Ferrier, A., Niikawa, N., Takahara, H., Ohama, K. and Avirachan, S.: Anatomic and chromosomal anomalies in 639 spontaneous abortuses. Hum. Genet. **55**:87–98, 1980.

Kalousek, D.K.: Anatomic and chromosome anomalies in specimens of early spontaneous abortion—7 year experience. Birth Defects **23**:153–168, 1987.

Kalousek, D.K.: Clinical effect of confined placental mosaicism. Pediatr. Devel. Pathol. **4**:313 (abstract), 2001.

Kalousek, D.K. and Barrett, I.: Confined placental mosaicism and stillbirth. Pediatr. Pathol. **14**:151–159, 1994.

Kalousek, D.K. and Dill, F.J.: Chromosomal mosaicism confined to the placenta in human conceptions. Science **221**:665–667, 1983.

Kalousek, D. and McGillivray, B.: Confined placental mosaicism and intrauterine survival of trisomy 13 and 18. Amer. J. Hum. Genet. **41**:A278, 1987 (abstract 828).

Kalousek, D.K., Barrett, I.J. and McGillivray, B.C.: Placental mosaicism and intrauterine survival of trisomies 13 and 18. Amer. J. Hum. Genet. **44**:338–343, 1989.

Kalousek, D.K., Fitch, N. and Paradice, B.A.: Pathology of the Human Embryo and Previable Fetus. An Atlas. Springer-Verlag, New York, 1990.

Kao, S.-M., Tang, G.-C., Hsieh, T.-T., Young, K.-C., Wang, H.-C. and Pao, C.C.: Analysis of peripheral blood of pregnant women for the presence of fetal Y chromosome-specific ZFY gene deoxyribonucleic acid sequences. Amer. J. Obstet. Gynecol. **166**:1013–1019, 1992.

Kazy, Z., Rozovsky, I.S. and Bakharev, V.A.: Chorion biopsy in early pregnancy: a method for early prenatal diagnosis for inherited disorders. Prenat. Diagn. **2**:39–45, 1982.

Keeling, J.W.: Fetal Pathology. Churchill Livingstone, Edinburgh. 1994.

Kellokumpu-Lehtinen, P. and Pelliniemi, L.J.: Sex ratio of human conceptuses. Obstet. Gynecol. **64**:220–222, 1984.

Kilpatrick, M.W., Tafas, T., Evans, M.I., Jackson, L.G., Antsaklis, A., Brambati, B. and Tsipouras, P.: Automated detection of rare fetal cells in maternal blood: eliminating the false-positive XY signals in XX pregnancies. Amer. J. Obstet. Gynecol. **190**:1571–1581, 2004.

Kingdom, J., Sherlock, J., Rodeck, C. and Adinolfi, M.: Detection of trophoblast cells in transcervical samples collected by lavage or cytobrush. Obstet. Gynecol. **86**:283–288, 1995.

Kirby, D.R.S., McWhirter, K.G., Teitelbaum, M.S. and Darlington, C.D.: A possible immunological influence on sex ratio. Lancet **2**:139–140, 1967.

Knapp, L.A., Ha, J.C. and Sackett, G.P.: Parental MHC antigen sharing and pregnancy wastage in captive pigtailed macaques. J. Reprod. Immunol. **32**:73–88, 1996.

Knoth, M. and Larsen, J.F.: Ultrastructure of a human implantation site. Acta Obstet. Gynecol. Scand. **51**:385–393, 1972.

Kouvalainen, K. and Österlund, K.: Placental weights in Down's syndrome. Ann. Med. Exp. Fenn. **45**:320–322, 1967.

Kovacs, B.W., Shahbahrami, B. and Comings, D.E.: Studies of human germinal mutations by deoxyribonucleic acid hybridization. Amer. J. Obstet. Gynecol. **160**:798–804, 1989.

Kovats, S., Main, E.K., Librach, C., Stubblebine, M., Fisher, S.J. and DeMars, R.: A class I antigen, HLA-G, expressed in human trophoblast. Science **248**:220–223, 1990.

Krawczun, M.S., Jenkins, E.C., Masia, A., Kunaporn, S., Stark, S.L., Duncan, C.J., Sklower, S.L. and Rudelli, R.D.: Chromosomal abnormalities in amniotic fluid cell cultures: a comparison of apparent pseudomosaicism in Chang and RPMI-1640 media. Clin. Genet. **35**:139–145, 1989.

Kubatova, A. and Trnka, V.: Induced abortions of 8 to 12 weeks pregnancy: evaluation of methods and histological findings in decidua and chorionic villi. Acta Univ. Carol. Med. (Prague) **13**:483–491, 1967.

Kuchinka, B.D., Kalousek, D.K., Lomax, B.L., Harrison, K.J. and Barrett, I.J.: Interphase cytogenetic analysis of single cell suspension prepared from previously formalin-fixed and paraffin-embedded tissues. Modern Pathol. **8**:183–186, 1995.

Kuhlmann, R.S., Werner, A.L., Abramowicz, J., Warsof, S.L., Arrington, J. and Levy, D.L.: Placental histology in fetuses between 18 and 23 weeks' gestation with abnormal karyotype. Amer. J. Obstet. Gynecol. **163**:1264–1270, 1990.

Kulazenko, V.P. and Kulazenko, L.G.: Pathomorphological changes in an early spontaneous abortus with triploidy (69, XXX). Hum. Genet. **32**:211–215, 1976.

Kuliev, A.M.: Cytogenetic investigation of spontaneous abortions. Humangenetik **12**:275–283, 1971.

Kundsin, R.B., Falk, L., Hertig, A.T. and Horne, H.W.: Acyclovir treatment of twelve unexplained infertile couples. Int. J. Fertil. **32**:200–204, 1987.

Kwak, J.Y.H., Gilman-Sachs, A. and Beaman, K.D.: Reproductive outcome in women with recurrent spontaneous abortions

of alloimmune and autoimmune causes: preconception versus postconception treatment. Amer. J. Obstet. Gynecol. **166**:1787–1798, 1992.

Ladefoged, C.: Hydropic degeneration: a histopathological investigation of 260 early abortions. Acta Obstet. Gynecol. Scand. **59**:509–512, 1980.

Lanasa, M.C., Hogge, A., Kubik, C.J., Ness, R.B., Harger, J., Nagel, T., Prosen, T., Markovic, N. and Hoffman, E.P.: A novel X chromosome-linked genetic cause of recurrent spontaneous abortion. Amer. J. Obstet. Gynecol. **185**:563–568, 2001.

Lawson, H.W., Atrash, H.K. and Franks, A.L.: Fatal pulmonary embolism during legal induced abortion in the United States from 1972 to 1985. Amer. J. Obstet. Gynecol. **162**:986–990, 1990.

Lea, R.G., Al-Sharekh, N., Tulppala, M. and Critchley, H.O.D.: The immunolocalization of bcl-2 at the maternal-fetal interface in healthy and failing pregnancies. Human Reprod. **12**:153–158, 1997a.

Lea, R.G., Tulppala, M. and Critchley, H.O.D.: Deficient syncytiotrophoblast tumor necrosis factor-α characterizes failing first trimester pregnancies in a subgroup of recurrent miscarriage patients. Human Reprod. **12**:1313–1320, 1997b.

Letters to the Editor. Lancet **337**:1091–1092, 1991.

Letters to the Editor: Antiphospholipid antibodies and fetal loss. NEJM **326**:951–954, 1992.

Li, L. and Smialek, J.E.: Sudden death due to rupture of ectopic pregnancy concurrent with therapeutic abortion. Arch. Pathol. Lab. Med. **117**:698–700, 1993.

Lichtig, C., Korat, A., Deutch, M. and Brandes, J.M.: Decidual vascular changes in early pregnancy as a marker for intrauterine pregnancy. Amer. J. Clin. Pathol. **90**:284–288, 1988.

Lijnschoten, G. van, Arends, J.W. and Geraedts, J.P.M.: Comparison of histological features in early spontaneous and induced trisomic abortions. Placenta **15**:765–773, 1994.

Lippman, A., Vekemans, M.J.J. and Perry, T.B.: Fetal mortality at the time of chorionic villi sampling. Hum. Genet. **68**:337–339, 1984.

Lissak, A., Sharon, A., Fruchter, O., Kassel, A., Sanderovitz, J. and Abramovici, H.: Polymorphism for mutation of cytosine to thymine at location 677 in the methylenetetrahydrofolate reductase gene is associated with recurrent early fetal loss. Amer. J. Obstet. Gynecol. **181**:126–130, 1999.

Lo, Y.M.D., Patel, P., Sampietro, M., Gillmer, M.D.G., Fleming, K.A. and Wainscoat, J.S.: Detection of single-copy fetal DNA sequence from maternal blood. Lancet **335**:1463–1464, 1990.

Lo, Y.M.D., Corbetta, N., Chamberlain, P.F., Rai, V., Sargent, I.L., Redman, C.W.G. and Wainscoat, J.S.: Presence of fetal DNA in maternal plasma and serum. Lancet **350**:485–487, 1997.

Lockwood, C.J.: Prediction of pregnancy loss. Lancet **355**:1292–1293, 2000.

Luckett, W.P.: The development of the yolk sac during the first three weeks of gestation in the human and rhesus monkey. Anat. Rec. **172**:358, 1972.

MacLean, M.A., Wilson, R., Thomson, J.A., Krishnamurthy, S. and Walker, J.J.: Changes in immunologic parameters in normal pregnancy and spontaneous abortion. Amer. J. Obstet. Gynecol. **165**:890–895, 1991.

Magenis, R.E.: On the origin of chromosomal anomaly. Amer. J. Hum. Genet. **42**:529–533, 1988.

Mallmann, P., Mallmann R. and Krebs, D.: Determination of tumor necrosis factor alpha (TNF alpha) and interleukin 2 (IL 2) in women with idiopathic recurrent miscarriage. Arch. Gynecol. Obstet. **249**:73–78, 1991.

Manabe, Y., Okamura, H. and Yoshida, Y.: Bougie-induced abortion at mid-pregnancy and placental function: histological and histochemical study of the placenta. Endokrinologie **57**:389–394, 1971.

Marini, A., Suma, V., Baccichetti, C. and Lenzini, E.: A case of septic miscarriage, a probable complication of chorion villus sampling. Prenat. Diagn. **8**:399–400, 1988.

Matayoshi, K., Yoshida, K., Soma, H., Miyabara, S. and Okamoto, N.: Placental pathology associated with chromosomal anomalies of the human neonate: a survey of seven cases. Congen. Anom. (Japan) **17**:507–512, 1977.

Matsubara, S., Minakami, H., Yamada, T., Koike, T., Izumi, A., Takizawa, T., Saito, T. and Sato, I.: Stimulated Hofbauer cells in the placental villi from patients with second-trimester abortions. Acta Histochem. Cytochem. **31**:447–452, 1998.

McFadden, D.E., Pantzer, J.T. and Langlois, S.: Parental origin of triploidy—digyny, not diandry. Modern Pathol. **7**:abstract 28, p. 5P, 1994.

McIntyre, J.A., Faulk, W.P., Nichols-Johnson, V.R. and Taylor, C.G.: Immunologic testing and immunotherapy in recurrent spontaneous abortion. Obstet. Gynecol. **67**:169–174, 1986.

McLean, J.M.: Early embryo loss. Lancet **1**:1033–1034, 1987.

Melius, F.A., Julian, T.M. and Nagel, T.C.: Prolonged retention of intrauterine bones. Obstet. Gynecol. **78**:919–921, 1991.

Mennuti, M.T., Jingeleski, S., Schwarz, R.H. and Mellman, W.J.: An evaluation of cytogenetic analysis as a primary tool in the assessment of recurrent pregnancy wastage. Obstet. Gynecol. **52**:308–313, 1978.

Michel, M., Underwood, J., Clark, D.A., Mowbray, J.F. and Beard, R.W.: Histologic and immunologic study of uterine biopsy tissue of women with incipient abortion. Amer. J. Obstet. Gynecol. **161**:409–414, 1989.

Miller, J.F., Williamson, E., Glue, J., Gordon, Y.B., Grudzinskas, J.G. and Sykes, A.: Fetal loss after implantation: a prospective study. Lancet **2**:554–556, 1980.

Miller, K., Metze, V., Wang, R., Lin, X. and Rehder, H.: Proliferation kinetics of chorionic villi in chromosomally normal and abnormal spontaneous abortions analyzed by premature chromosome condensation and northern blot. Annal. Genét. **39**:159–167, 1996.

Mills, J.L., Simpson, J.L., Driscoll, S.G., Jovanovic-Peterson, L., van Allen, M., Aarons, J.H., Metzger, B., Bieber, F.R., Knopp, R.H., Holmes, L.B., Peterson, C.M., Witham-Wilson, M., Brown, Z., Ober, C., Harley, E., MacPherson, T.A., Duckles, A., Mueller-Heubach, E. and National Institute of Child Health: Incidence of spontaneous abortion among normal women and insulin-dependent diabetic women whose pregnancies were identified within 21 days of conception. NEJM **319**:1617–1623, 1988.

Moen, D.W., Werner, J.K. and Bersu, E.T.: Analysis of gross anatomical variations in human triploidy. Amer. J. Med. Genet. **18**:345–356, 1984.

Moise, K.J.: Fetal RhD typing with free DNA in maternal plasma. Editorial. Amer. J. Obstet. Gynecol. **192**:663–665, 2005.

Monrozies, M.: La gravité actuelle de l'avortement provoqué. Gynécol. Obstet. (Paris) **70**:79–94, 1971.

Moon, H.S., Park, Y.H., Kwon, H.Y., Hong, S.H. and Kim, S.K.: Iatrogenic secondary infertility caused by residual intrauterine bone after midtrimester abortion. Amer. J. Obstet. Gynecol. **176**:369–370, 1997.

Moore, G.E., Ali, Z., Khan, R.U., Blunt, S., Bennett, P.R. and Vaughan, J.I.: The incidence of uniparental disomy associated with intrauterine growth retardation in a cohort of thirty-five severely affected babies. Amer. J. Obstet. Gynecol. **176**:294–299, 1997.

Moore, K.L.: The Developing Human: Clinically Oriented Embryology. 3rd Ed. W.B. Saunders, Philadelphia, 1982.

Moore, K.L., Persaud, T.V.N. and Shiota, K.: Color Atlas of Clinical Embryology. W.B. Saunders, Philadelphia, 1994.

Mostello, D.J., Bofinger, M.K. and Siddiqi, T.A.: Spontaneous resolution of fetal cystic hygroma and hydrops in Turner syndrome. Obstet. Gynecol. **73**:862–865, 1989.

Mowbray, J.F., Gibbings, C., Liddell, H., Reginald, P.W., Underwood, J.L. and Beard, R.W.: Controlled trial of treatment of recurrent spontaneous abortion by immunisation with paternal cells. Lancet **1**:941–944, 1985.

Mueller-Eckhardt, G., Heine, O. and Polten, B.: IVIG to prevent recurrent spontaneous abortion. Lancet **337**:424–425, 1991.

Muggah, H.F., D'Alton, M.E. and Hunter, A.G.W.: Chorionic villus sampling followed by genetic amniocentesis and septic shock. Lancet **1**:867–868, 1987.

Nakamura, Y., Takaira, M., Sato, E., Kawano, K., Miyoshi, O. and Niikawa, N.: A tetraploid liveborn neonate. Cytogenetic and autopsy findings. Arch. Pathol. Lab. Med. **127**:1612–1614, 2003.

Ness, R.B., Grisso, J.A., Hirschinger, N., Markovic, N., Shaw, L.M., Day, N.L. and Kline, J.: Cocaine and tobacco use and the risk of spontaneous abortion. NEJM **340**:333–339, 1999.

Neu, R.L., Entes, K. and Bannerman, R.M.: Chromosome analysis in cases with repeated spontaneous abortions. Obstet. Gynecol. **53**:373–375, 1979.

Neuber, M., Rehder, H., Zuther, C., Lettau, R. and Schwinger, E.: Polyploidies in abortion material decreases with maternal age. Hum. Genet. **41**:563–566, 1993.

Nishimura, H., Takano, K., Tanimura, T. and Yasuda, M.: Normal and abnormal development of human embryos: first report of the analysis of 1,213 intact embryos. Teratology **1**:281–290, 1968.

Novak, R., Agamanolis, D., Dasu, S., Igel, H., Platt, M., Robinson, H. and Shehata, B.: Histologic analysis of placental tissue in first trimester abortions. Pediatr. Pathol. **8**:477–482, 1988.

Olding, L., Benirschke, K. and Oldstone, M.B.A.: Inhibition of mitosis of lymphocytes from human adults by lymphocytes from newborns. Clin. Immun. Immunopathol. **3**:79–89, 1974.

Olney, R.S., Khoury, M.J., Alo, C.J., Costa, P., Edmonds, L.D., Flood, T.J., Harris, J.A., Howe, H.L., Moore, C.A., Olsen, C.L., Panny, S.R. and Shaw, G.M.: Increased risk for transverse digital deficiency after chorionic villus sampling: Results of the United States multistate case-control study, 1988–1992. Teratology **51**:20–29, 1995.

Ornoy, A., Kohn, G., Zur, Z.B., Weinstein, D. and Cohen, M.M.: Triploidy in human abortions. Teratology **18**:315–320, 1978.

Ornoy, A., Salamon-Arnon, J., Ben-Zur, Z. and Kohn, G.: Placental findings in spontaneous abortions and stillbirths. Teratology **24**:243–252, 1981.

Palomaki, J.F. and Little, A.B.: Surgical management of abortion. NEJM **287**:752–754, 1972.

Parazzini, F., Acacia, B., Faden, D., Lovotti, M., Marelli, G. and Cortelazzo, S.: Antiphospholipid antibodies and recurrent abortion. Obstet. Gynecol. **77**:854–858, 1991.

Philippe, E.: Pathologie Foeto-Placentaire. Masson, Paris, 1986.

Philippe, E. and Boué, E.: Le placenta des aberrations chromosomiques létales. Ann. Anat. Pathol. (Paris) **14**:249–266, 1969.

Phillips, O.W., Tharapel, A.T., Lerner, J.L., Park, V.M., Wachtel, S.S. and Shulman, L.P.: Risk of fetal mosaicism when placental mosaicism is diagnosed by chorionic villus sampling. Amer. J. Obstet. Gynecol. **174**:850–855, 1996.

Plouffe, L., White, E.W., Tho, S.P., Sweet, C.S., Layman, L.C., Whitman, G.F. and McDonough, P.G.: Etiologic factors of recurrent abortion and subsequent reproductive performance of couples: Have we made any progress in the past 10 years? Amer. J. Obstet. Gynecol. **167**:313–321, 1992.

Portnoi, M.-F., Joye, N., van den Akker, J., Morlier, G. and Taillemite, J.-L.: Karyotypes of 1142 couples with recurrent abortion. Obstet. Gynecol. **72**:31–34, 1988.

Pozniak, M.A., Cullenward, M.J., Zickuhr, D. and Curet, L.B.: Venous lake bleeding: a complication of chorionic villous sampling. J. Ultrasound Med. **7**:297–299, 1988.

Pridjian, G. and Moawad, A.H.: Missed abortion: still appropriate terminology? Amer. J. Obstet. Gynecol. **161**:261–262, 1989.

Puvabanditsin, S., Garrow, E., Rabi, F.A., Titapiwatanakun, R. and Kuniyoshi, K.M.: A live birth with triploidy syndrome (69,XXY): a case report and review of the literature. Neonat. Intens. Care **16**:19–21, 2004.

Quintero, R.A., Romero, R., Mahoney, M.J., Abuhamad, A., Vecchio, M., Holden, J. and Hobbins, J.C.: Embryoscopic demonstration of hemorrhagic lesions on the human embryo after placental trauma. Amer. J. Obstet. Gynecol. **168**:756–759, 1993.

Qureshi, F., Jacques, S.M., Johnson, M.P. and Evans, M.I.: Histopathologic and growth characteristics of trisomy 21 placentas. Modern Pathol. **7**:abstract 40, p. 7P, 1994.

Rai, R. and Regan, L.: Antiphospholipid antibodies in women undergoing in-vitro fertilization. Human Reprod. **12**:197–199, 1997.

Rakheja, D., Wilson, K.S. and Rogers, B.B.: Dysmorphic villi mimicking partial mole in a case with del (18) (q21). Pediat. Developm. Pathol. **7**:546–548, 2004.

Redline, R.W., Hassold, T. and Zaragoza, M.: Determinants of villous trophoblastic hyperplasia in spontaneous abortions. Modern Pathol. **11**:762–768, 1998.

Regan, L. and Rai, R.: Epidemiology and the medical causes of miscarriage. Best Pract. Res. Clin. Obstet. Gynaecol. Vol. **14**:839–854, 2000.

Rehder, H. and Gropp, A.: Triploidie als Ursache fötoplacentarer Fehlbildung bei Abortus. Verh. Dtsch. Ges. Pathol. **55**:525–529, 1971.

Rehder, H., Coerdt, W., Eggers, R., Klink, F. and Schwinger, E.: Is there a correlation between morphological and cytogenetic findings in placental tissue from early missed abortions? Hum. Genet. **82**:377–385, 1989.

Reid, T.M.S.: Striking a balance in maternal immune response to infection. Lancet **351**:1670–1672, 1998.

Rhoads, G.G., Jackson, L.G., Schlesselman, S.E., de la Cruz, F.F., Desnick, R.J., Golbus, M.S., Ledbetter, D.H., Lubs, H.A.,

Mahoney, M.J., Pergament, E., Simpson, J.L., Carpenter, R.J., Elias, S., Ginsberg, N.A., Goldberg, J.D., Hobbins, J.C., Lynch, L., Shiono, P.H., Wapner, R.J. and Zachary, J.M.: The safety and efficacy of chorionic villus sampling for early prenatal diagnosis of cytogenetic abnormalities. NEJM **320**:609–617, 1989.

Roberts, L., Sebire, N.J., Fowler, D. and Nicolaides, K.H.: Histomorphological features of chorionic villi at 10–14 weeks of gestation in trisomic and chromosomally normal pregnancies. Placenta **21**:678–683, 2000.

Rochelson, B., Kaplan, C., Guzman, E., Arato, M., Hansen, K. and Trunca, C.: A quantitative analysis of placental vasculature in the third-trimester fetus with autosomal trisomy. Obstet. Gynecol. **75**:59–63, 1990.

Rosenbusch, B., Schneider, M. and Sterzik, K.: Triploidy caused by endoreduplication in a human zygote obtained after in-vitro fertilization. Human Reprod. **12**:1059–1061, 1997.

Rosenmann, A., Palti, Z., Segal, S. and Cohen, M.M.: Chromosomes in familial primary sterility and in couples with recurrent abortions and stillbirths. Isr. J. Med. Sci. **13**:1131–1133, 1977.

Sachs, E.S., Jahoda, M.G.J., van Hemel, J.O., Hoogeboom, A.J.M. and Sandkuyl, L.A.: Chromosome studies of 500 couples with two or more abortions. Obstet. Gynecol. **65**:375–378, 1985.

Sadovsky, A. and Laufer, A.: Placental changes in early spontaneous abortion. Obstet. Gynecol. **17**:678–683, 1961.

Salafia, C.M. and Burns, J.P.: The correlation of placental and decidual histology with karyotype and fetal viability. Teratology **39**:478 (P37), 1989.

Salafia, C., Maier, D., Vogel, C., Pezzullo, J., Burns, J. and Silberman, L.: Placental and decidual histology in spontaneous abortion: Detailed description and correlations with chromosome number. Obstet. Gynecol. **82**:295–303, 1993.

Saller, D.N., Keene, C.L., Sun, C.-C.J. and Schwartz, S.: The association of single umbilical artery with cytogenetically abnormal pregnancies. Amer. J. Obstet. Gynecol. **163**:922–925, 1990.

Sampson, J.E., Ouhibi, N., Lawce, H., Patton, P.E., Battaglia, D.A., Burry, K.A. and Olson, S.B.: The role for preimplantation genetic diagnosis in balanced translocation carriers. Amer. J. Obstet. Gynecol. **190**:1707–1713, 2001.

Sasaki, M., Makino, S., Muramoto, J.-I., Ikeuchi, T. and Shimba, H.: A chromosome survey of induced abortuses in a Japanese population. Chromosoma **20**:267–283, 1967.

Schaaps, J.P. and Hustin, J.: In vivo aspect of the maternal-trophoblastic border during the first trimester of gestation. Trophoblast Res. **3**:39–48, 1988.

Schulman, H., Kaiser, I.H. and Randolph, G.: Outpatient saline abortion. Obstet. Gynecol. **37**:521–526, 1971.

Schulze, B., Schlesinger, C. and Miller, K.: Chromosomal mosaicism confined to chorionic tissue. Prenat. Diagn. **7**:451–453, 1987.

Scott, J.R., Rote, N.S. and Branch, D.W.: Immunologic aspects of recurrent abortion and fetal death. Obstet. Gynecol. **70**:645–656, 1987.

Scott, R.: Limb abnormalities after chorionic villus sampling. Lancet **337**:1038–1039, 1991.

Sebire, N.J., Fowler, D., Roberts, L., Mahmood, S. and Nicolaides, K.H.: Trophoblast proliferation is increased in chorionic villi from pregnancies with fetal trisomy 18. Placenta **21**:584–586, 2000.

Segal, S., Ornoy, A., Bercovici, B., Antebi, S.O. and Polishuk, W.Z.: Placental pathology in midtrimester pregnancies interrupted by intra-amniotic injection of hypertonic urea. Br. J. Obstet. Gynaecol. **83**:156–159, 1976.

Sehgal, N., Parr, M. and Haslett, E.: Clostridium infection after intra-amniotic hypertonic saline injection for induced abortion. J. Reprod. Med. **8**:67–69, 1972.

Sekizawa, A., Watanabe, A., Kimura, T., Saito, H., Yanaihara, T. and Sato, T.: Prenatal diagnosis of the fetal RhD blood type using a single fetal nucleated erythrocyte from maternal blood. Obstet. Gynecol. **87**:501–505, 1996.

Sermon, K., Steirteghem, A. van and Liebars, I.: Preimplantation genetic diagnosis. Lancet **363**:1633–1641, 2004.

Seward, P.N., Ballard, C.A. and Ulene, A.L.: The effect of legal abortion on the rate of septic abortion at a large county hospital. Amer. J. Obstet. Gynecol. **115**:335–338, 1973.

Shaarawy, M. and Nagui, A.R.: Enhanced expression of cytokines may play a fundamental role in the mechanisms of immunologically mediated recurrent spontaneous abortion. Acta Obstet. Gynecol. Scand. **76**:205–211, 1997.

Shaffer, L.G., McCaskill, C., Adkins, K. and Hassold, T.J. Systematic search for uniparental disomy in early fetal losses: the results and a review of the literature. Amer. J. Med. Genet. **79**:366–372, 1998.

Shepard, T.H., Fantel, A.G. and Fitzsimmons, J.: Congenital defect rates among spontaneous abortuses: twenty years of monitoring. Teratology **39**:325–331, 1989a.

Shepard, T.H., Fitzsimmons, J.M., Fantel, A.G. and Pascoe-Mason, J.: Placental weights of normal and aneuploid early human fetuses. Teratology **39**:481 (P54), 1989b.

Shepard, T.H., Fitzsimmons, J.M., Fantel, A.G. and Pascoe-Mason, J.: Placental weights of normal and aneuploid early human fetuses. Pediatr. Pathol. **9**:425–431, 1989c.

Sherard, J., Bean, C., Bove, B., DelDuca, V., Esterly, K.L., Karcsh, H.J., Munshi, G., Reamer, J.F., Suazo, G., Wilmoth, D., Dahlke, M.B., Weiss, C. and Borgaonkar, S.: Long survival in a 69,XXY triploid male. Amer. J. Med. Genet. **25**:307–312, 1986.

Shettles, L.: The great preponderance of human males conceived. Amer. J. Obstet. Gynecol. **89**:130–133, 1964.

Shivashankar, L., Whitney, E., Colmorgen, G., Young, T., Munshi, G., Wilmoth, D., Byrne, K., Reeves, G., Borgoankar, D.S., Picciano, S.R. and Martin-Deleon, P.A.: Prenatal diagnosis of tetrasomy 47,XY,+i(12p) confirmed by *in situ* hybridization. Prenat. Diagn. **8**:85–91, 1988.

Shulman, L.P., Meyers, C.M., Simpson, J.L., Andersen, R.N., Tolley, E.A. and Elias, S.: Fetomaternal transfusion depends on amount of chorionic villi aspirated but not on method of chorionic villus sampling. Amer. J. Obstet. Gynecol. **162**:1185–1188, 1990.

Simon, C., Rubio, C., Vidal, F., Gimenez, C., Moreno, C., Parrilla, J.J. and Pellier, A.: Increased chromosome abnormalities in human preimplantation embryos after in-vitro fertilization in patients with recurrent miscarriage. Reprod. Fertil. Dev. **10**:87–92, 1998.

Simpson, J.L. and Elias, S.: Fetal Cells in Maternal Blood. Annals N.Y. Academy of Sciences **731**:1–270, 1994.

Simpson, J.L., Meyers, C.M., Martin, A.O., Elias, S. and Ober, C.: Translocations are infrequent among couples having repeated

spontaneous abortions but no other abnormal pregnancies. Fertil. Steril. **51**:811–814, 1989.

Simpson, J.L., Gray, R., Perez, A., Mena, P., Queenan, J.T., Barbato, M., Pardo, F., Kambic, R. and Jennings, V.: Fertilisation involving ageing gametes, major birth defects, and Down's syndrome. Lancet **359**:1670–1671, 2002.

Singh, R.P. and Carr, D.H.: Anatomic findings in human abortions of known chromosomal constitution. Obstet. Gynecol. **29**:806–818, 1967.

Singh, R.P. and Carr, D.H.: Congenital anomalies in embryos with normal chromosomes. Biol. Neonat. **13**:121–128, 1968.

Smid, M., Lagona, F., Papasergio, N., Ferrari, A., Ferrari, M. and Cremonesi, L.: Influence of gestational age on fetal deoxyribonucleic acid retrieval in maternal peripheral blood. Amer. J. Obstet. Gynecol. **177**:1517–1522, 1997.

Smith, A. and Gaha, T.J.: Data on families of chromosome translocation carriers ascertained because of habitual abortion. Austr. N.Z.J. Obstet. Gynaecol. **30**:57–62, 1990.

Smith, S.C., Baker, P.N. and Symonds, E.M.: Placental apoptosis in normal human pregnancy. Amer. J. Obstet. Gynecol. **177**:57–65, 1997a.

Smith, S.C., Baker, P.N. and Symonds, E.M.: Increased placental apoptosis in intrauterine growth restriction. Amer. J. Obstet. Gynecol. **177**:1395–1401, 1997b.

Smith, S.C., Leung, T.N., To, K.F. and Baker, P.N.: Apoptosis is a rare event in first-trimester placental tissue. Amer. J. Obstet. Gynecol. **183**:697–699, 2000.

Stavropoulos, D.J., Bick, D. and Kalousek, D.K.: Molecular cytogenetic detection of confined gonadal mosaicism in a conceptus with trisomy 16 placental mosaicism. Amer. J. Hum. Genet. **63**:1912–1914, 1998.

Steier, J.A., Sandvei, R. and Myking, O.L.: Human chorionic gonadotropin in early normal and pathological pregnancy: discordant levels in peripheral maternal blood and blood from the uterine and abdominal cavities. Amer. J. Obstet. Gynecol. **154**:1091–1094, 1986.

Stein, Z.A.: A woman's age: childbearing and child rearing. Amer. J. Epidemiol. **121**:327–342, 1985.

Steinberg, C.R., Berkowitz, R.L., Merkatz, I.R. and Roberts, R.B.: Fever and bacteremia associated with hypertonic saline abortion. Obstet. Gynecol. **39**:673–678, 1972.

Stern, J.J. and Coulam, C.B.: Mechanism of recurrent spontaneous abortion. I. Ultrasonographic findings. Amer. J. Obstet. Gynecol. **166**:1844–1852, 1992.

Stewart, G.K. and Goldstein, P.J.: Therapeutic abortion in California. Effects on septic abortion and maternal mortality. Obstet. Gynecol. **37**:510–514, 1971.

Stioui, S., de Silvestris, M., Molinari, A., Stripparo, L., Ghisoni, L. and Simoni, G.: Trisomic 22 placenta in a case of severe intrauterine growth retardation. Prenat. Diagn. **9**:673–676, 1989.

Stirrat, G.M.: Recurrent miscarriage I: definition and epidemiology. Lancet **336**:673–675, 1990a.

Stirrat, G.M.: Recurrent miscarriage II: clinical associations, causes, and management. Lancet **336**:728–733, 1990b.

Strom, C.M., Rechitsky, S., Ginsberg, N., Verlinsky, O. and Verlinsky, Y.: Prenatal paternity testing with deoxyribonucleic acid technique. Amer. J. Obstet. Gynecol. **174**:1849–1854, 1996.

Studdiford, W.E. and Douglas, G.W.: Placental bacteremia: a significant finding in septic abortion accompanied by vascular collapse. Amer. J. Obstet. Gynecol. **71**:842–858, 1956.

Sundberg, K. and Smidt-Jensen, S.: Non-mosaic trisomy 16 on chorionic villus sampling but normal placenta and fetus after termination. Lancet **337**:1233–1234, 1991.

Suter, P.E.N., Chatfield, W.R. and Kotonya, A.O.: The use of suction curettage in incomplete abortion. J. Obstet. Gynaecol. Br. Commonw. **77**:464–466, 1970.

Suzumori, K., Adachi, R., Okada, S., Narukawa, T., Yagami, Y. and Sonta, S.: Fetal cells in the maternal circulation: Detection of Y-sequence by gene amplification. Obstet. Gynecol. **80**:150–154, 1992.

Takabayashi, H., Kuwabara, S., Ukita, T., Ikawa, K., Yamafuji, K. and Igarashi, T.: Development of non-invasive fetal DNA diagnosis from maternal blood. Prenat. Diagn. **15**:74–77, 1995.

Tal, J., Timor-Tritsch, I. and Degani, S.: Accurate diagnosis of postabortal placental remnant by sonohysterography and color Doppler sonographic studies. Gynecol. Obstet. Invest. **43**:131–134, 1997.

Tharapel, A.T., Elias, S., Shulman, L.P., Seely, L., Emerson, D.S. and Simpson, J.L.: Resorbed co-twin as an explanation for discrepant chorionic villus results: non-mosaic 47,XX,+16 in villi (direct and culture) with normal (46,XX) amniotic fluid and neonatal blood. Prenat. Diagn. **9**:467–472, 1989.

Thiet, M.P., Suwanvanichkij, V., Kwok, C. and Yeh, J.: DNA laddering, consistent with programmed cell death, is a normal finding in human placentas. Amer. J. Obstet. Gynecol. **172**:272 (abstract 47), 1995.

Turleau, C., Chavin-Colin, F. and de Grouchy, J.: Cytogenetic investigation in 413 couples with spontaneous abortions. Eur. J. Obstet. Gynecol. Reprod. Biol. **9**:65–74, 1979.

Tycko, B.: Genomic imprinting: mechanism and role in human pathology. Amer. J. Pathol. **144**:431–443, 1994.

Verjaal, M., Leschot, N.J., Wolf, H. and Treffers, P.E.: Karyotypic differences between cells from placenta and other fetal tissues. Prenat. Diagn. **7**:343–348, 1987.

Vernof, K.K., Ney, J.A. and Dewald, G.W.: Pure placental trisomy 16 associated with a 46,XY infant and severe preeclampsia: a case report. Amer. J. Obstet. Gynecol. **166**:434 (abstract), 1992.

Verp, M.S., Rosinsky, B., Sheikh, Z. and Amarose, A.P.: Non-mosaic trisomy 16 confined to villi. Lancet **2**:915–916, 1989.

Vincent, T., Rai, R., Regan, L. and Cohen, H.: Increased thrombin generation in women with recurrent miscarriage. Lancet **352**:116, 1998.

Vogel, M.: Placentabefunde beim Abort: ein Beitrag zur Patho-Morphologie placentarer Entwicklungsstörungen. Virchows Arch. [A] **346**:212–223, 1969.

Vogel, M.: Atlas der Morphologischen Plazentadiagnostik. Springer-Verlag, Berlin, 1992.

Wade, R.V. and Young, S.R.: Analysis of fetal loss after transcervical chorionic villus Sampling—A review of 719 patients. Amer. J. Obstet. Gynecol. **161**:513–519, 1989.

Wall, R.L. and Hertig, A.T.: Habitual abortion. Amer. J. Obstet. Gynecol. **56**:1127–1133, 1948.

Ward, B.E., Henry, G.P. and Robinson, A.: Cytogenetic studies in 100 couples with recurrent spontaneous abortions. Amer. J. Hum. Genet. **32**:549–554, 1980.

Wegmann, T.G., Gill, T.J., Cumming, C.D. and Nisbet-Brown, E., eds.: Immunology of Reproduction. Oxford University Press, New York, 1983.

Weiss, J.L., Malone, F.D., Vidaver, J., Ball, R.H., Nyberg, D.A., Comstock, C.H., Hankins, G.D., Berkowitz, R.L., Gross, S.J., Dugoff, L., Timor-Tritsch, I.E., D'Alton, M.E. and the FASTER Consortium: Threatened abortion: A risk factor for poor pregnancy outcome, a population-based screening study. Amer. J. Obstet. Gynecol. **190**:745–750, 2004.

Wenstrom K.D., Owen, J., Chu, D.C. and Boots, L.: α-fetoprotein, free β-human chorionic gonadotropin, and dimeric inhibin A produce the best results in a three-analyte, multiple marker screening test for fetal Down syndrome. Amer. J. Obstet. Gynecol. **177**:987–991, 1997.

Wijk, I.J. van, Vugt, J.M.G. van, Mulders, M.A.M., Könst, A.A.M., Weima, S.M. and Oudemjans, C.B.M.: Enrichment of fetal trophoblast cells from maternal peripheral blood followed by detection of fetal deoxyribonucleic acid with a nested X/Y polymerase chain reaction. Amer. J. Obstet. Gynecol. **174**:871–876, 1996.

Wilcox, A.J., Weinberg, C.R., O'Connor, J.F., Baird, D.D., Schlatterer, J.P., Canfield, R.E., Armstrong, E.G. and Nisula, B.C.: Incidence of early loss of pregnancy. NEJM **319**:189–194, 1988.

Wilcox, A.J., Baird, D.D. and Weinberg, C.R.: Time of implantation of the conceptus and loss of pregnancy. NEJM **340**:1796–1799, 1999.

Wilkins, J.F. and Haig, D.: What good is genomic imprinting: The function of parent-specific gene expression. Nature Rev. Genet. **4**:359–368, 2003.

Wilkins-Haug, L., Roberts, D.J. and Morton, C.C.: Confined placental mosaicism and intrauterine growth retardation: a case-control analysis of placentas at delivery. Amer. J. Obstet. Gynecol. **172**:44–50, 1995.

Williams, J., Wang, B.T., Rubin, C.H. and Aiken-Hunting, D.: Chorionic villus sampling: Experience with 3016 cases performed by a single operator. Obstet. Gynecol. **80**:1023–1029, 1992.

Wolf, G.C. and Horger, E.O.: Indications for examination of spontaneous abortion: a reassessment. Amer. J. Obstet. Gynecol. **173**:1364–1368, 1995.

Yamamoto, M. and Watanabe, G.: Epidemiology of gross chromosomal anomalies at early embryonic stage of pregnancy. Contrib. Epidemiol. Biostatist. **1**:101–106, 1979.

Yokoyama, W.M.: The mother-child union: The case of missing-self and protection of the fetus. Proc. Natl. Acad. Sci. **94**:5998–6000, 1997.

Younis, J.S.: Factor V Leiden—a novel etiology of the longstanding thrombosis theory for recurrent pregnancy loss. Amer. J. Obstet. Gynecol. **178**:1107–1108, 1998.

Zerres, K., Niesen, M., Schwanitz, G. and Hansmann, M.: Trisomie 22—Pränatale Befunde unterschiedlicher Entwicklungsstadien. Geburtsh. Frauenheilk. **48**:720–723, 1988.

Zhang, J., Wang, C.W., Krey, L., Liu, H., Meng, L., Blaszczyk, A., Adler, A. and Grifo, L.: In vitro maturation of human preovulatory oocytes reconstructed by germinal vesicle transfer. Fertil Steril. **71**:726–731, 1999.

Zuccotti, M. and Monk, M.: The mouse *Xist* gene: a model for studying the gametic imprinting phenomenon. Acta Genet. Med. Gemellol. **45**:199–204, 1996.

22
Molar Pregnancies

Hydatidiform Moles and Partial Moles

The term **gestational trophoblastic neoplasia** (GTN) has become popular in recent years, although it comprises entities that are clearly not neoplastic, such as triploid "partial" moles. Others commonly now refer to these entities as gestational trophoblastic disease (GTD). Driscoll (1981), in an excellent review of the morphology of these diseases, strongly favored abandonment of the time-honored term **hydatidiform mole**. Fox (1989) has added fuel to the fire by suggesting the following: "Is it, in fact, justifiable to continue distinguishing complete from partial moles in routine histopathologic practice?" He based this opinion primarily on the exceptional finding of a single case of choriocarcinoma said to have followed a partial hydatidiform mole (PHM) (Looi & Sivanesratnam, 1981). Persisting trophoblastic disease has also been described by Rice et al. (1990). Fox (1997), in analyzing the histologic differences between complete hydatidiform mole (CHM) and PHM, concluded that a degree of subjectivity accompanies these decisions, an opinion with which we strongly agree. Malinowski et al. (1995) go even further by suggesting a continuum to exist from molar degeneration to choriocarcinoma when they suggested the existence of the "sad fetus syndrome," the association of a fetus with molar or neoplastic conditions. This view is not ours, however. After all, choriocarcinoma is also an occasional sequela of an apparently "normal" gestation, as Fox readily conceded in which there may have been a choriocarcinomatous cell line *ab initio*.

This chapter discusses the typical hydatidiform mole (the CHM), syncytial endometritis, invasive moles (chorioadenoma destruens), "benign metastasizing mole," the PHM with or without fetus, and ectopic moles. Their terminology is often confusing and imprecisely used, but we do not favor abandonment of the term **hydatidiform mole**. Rather, we implore that it be used more precisely. Choriocarcinoma is discussed in Chapter 23.

Hydatidiform moles are excessively edematous immature placentas, characterized by massive fluid accumulation within the villous parenchyma; this fluid characteristically leads to the formation of microcysts (cisternae or lacunae) within the villi. In general, there is also an absence of fetal blood vessels. When all villi are thus changed, we speak of a "true" or "complete" mole. When only some villi are involved macroscopically, with large portions of the placenta being grossly more or less normal, then the process is called a "partial" mole. The distinction is often difficult, and strict morphologic guidelines are not easily established. This definition rests, however, on the **macroscopic** features alone. It can be supported by subsequent study or not; the gross description defines the denominational entity. To confuse even more, the distinction is often blurred at early gestational ages, during the evolution of the altered placenta. Because choriocarcinoma (chorionepithelioma) so frequently follows the occurrence of a complete hydatidiform mole, all of these entities are now often encompassed by the term **gestational trophoblastic disease**. Several comprehensive books have discussed this group of placental diseases (Smalbraak, 1957; Holland & Hreshchyshyn, 1967; Park, 1971; Goldstein & Berkowitz, 1982; Szulman & Buchsbaum, 1987; as well as the November 1997 issue of *General Diagnostic Pathology*). These volumes discuss the evolution of our understanding of the genetic derivation of moles, the frequently confusing terminology, the clinical features, and the therapy of these entities.

Hydatidiform Moles

The CHM is a diffusely edematous and enlarged placenta in which the macroscopically enlarged villi generally lack blood vessels and have cistern-like fluid-filled cavities. The villi are connected to one another by thin strands of connective tissue, the former mainstem villi. Intervillous thrombi occur frequently. Although there is usually no embryo or identifiable chorionic cavity in CHM, a few exceptions have been described (Baergen et al., 1996). The CHM may also occasionally coexist with a normal twin and even triplet pregnancy, but this does not make it a "partial mole." It can be differentiated genetically as well as macroscopically.

The PHM, which is discussed below in greater detail, is macroscopically composed of normal and distended villi, and it is also more often associated with an embryo or remnants thereof. The trophoblast of complete moles is usually, but not always, more abundant than it is in PHM and in normal placentas. In the CHM there is also frequently much nuclear pleomorphism and anaplasia. These cellular abnormalities have given rise to several grading classifications, some of which have endeavored to assign prognostic values. Thus, a hydatidiform mole of grade V was considered to have a greater malignant potential than one to which a grade II designation was attached. Hydatidiform moles usually occur as uterine pregnancies, but they are occasionally also present as ectopics in the fallopian tube (Depypere et al., 1993) and ovary. The trophoblast of moles invades the uterus, much like it does in a placenta increta. When hydatid villi and their trophoblast invade the uterus and destroy a portion of it in the process, then this entity is designated an invasive mole or a chorioadenoma destruens.

Moles have occasionally been observed to occur repetitively, and Parazzini et al. (1991) found that this was much more likely to be the case in patients with CHM. Sand et al. (1984), who reviewed this literature, suggested that it occurred in 0.60% to 2.57% of patients. There were no differences in outcome. Hsu et al. (1963) described five cases of two moles in the same patient; one patient suffered three moles. Johnson (1966) observed a patient with four consecutive moles. We have seen a young African-American woman who had three consecutive complete moles; the last developed into a fatal choriocarcinoma. It is of further interest that this patient conceived these moles with two different husbands. Kronfol et al. (1969) described five patients with repetitive moles and commented on the greater frequency of the condition in the Lebanese population. Patek and Johnson (1978) and Endres (1961) each had a patient with five consecutive hydatidiform moles and no children. Wu (1973) observed a patient with nine consecutive molar pregnancies. Remarkably, all of the moles in the last case lacked Barr bodies, and one was karyotyped as being 46,XY. Although the author speculated on a paternal cause for this repetitive event, normal paternal and maternal karyotypes were found. Semen analysis was refused. Ambrani et al. (1980) reported familial moles in three family trees, but the possible genetic cause was not determined. Parazzini et al. (1984) found two sisters, one with three CHMs and the other with one. La Vecchia et al. (1982) described monozygotic twins, each with molar pregnancy. Most recently, Slim et al. (2005) have analyzed familial moles genetically. They studied a family in which five women had seven moles, three miscarriages, and three children. Their conclusion was that a previously linked locus to 19q13.4 was not responsible and that other factors modulate the occurrence of moles. An important genetic study of the origin of two choriocarcinomas was undertaken by Osada et al. (1991). They examined the restriction fragment length (RFL) polymorphism of the moles and preceding pregnancies in two patients. In one family the choriocarcinoma could be traced to a previous complete, androgenetic hydatidiform mole, not the two normal pregnancies. In the other patient, however, the tumor derived from the third of three normal pregnancies and carried both parental chromosomal markers. The publication does not provide details whether one or the other genome had a better prognosis. The few similar reports in the literature are referred to by these authors. Since then, Seoud et al. (1995) evaluated the familial recurrent moles (13 moles in the pedigree) of two sisters with moles and found a high degree of unusual lymphocyte antigen histocompatibility. Studies of this kind should probably now be employed to better understand the genetic reasons for molar gestations and to correlate choriocarcinoma with putative precursors. Such an effort is especially important when long time spans separate pregnancy and tumor, or when primary choriocarcinomas of presumably nongestational types are observed, for example, the cervical lesion reported by Ben-Chetrit et al. (1990). We have seen a placenta of a near-term gestation with surviving, normal female infant and a sharp division between a molar portion and normal placental tissue (Fig. 22.1). Flow cytometry on the molar portion showed it to be uniformly tetraploid, and the normal tissue was diploid. DNA was isolated from paraffin-embedded tissue and polymerase chain reaction (PCR) studies were then undertaken. Employing five different markers, all RFLs were uniform, assuring with highest probability the identical genotype of the tissues. There was one chorionic sac and no second cavity or embryonic remnant. Remarkably, many hydatid, tetraploid villi had fetal blood vessels, some atrophied, and others well circulated by the living infant. We interpreted this specimen as having one of two possible origins. Either a focus of placental tissue underwent polyploidization (unlikely), or a monozygotic, monochorionic twin developed as tetraploid fetus (and died), leaving behind the mole. Meanwhile, the other twin's circulation kept perfusing some of the molar villous tissue. Although the gross impression was initially of a partial mole, the studies ruled this out, as did the presence of a normal surviving infant. Follow-up study showed no untoward sequelae (Benirschke et al., 2000). Higashino et al. (1999) described triplets, two normal fetuses (46,XX and 46,XY) and normal placentas and a typical androgenetic mole (46,XY), that were followed by persistent trophoblastic disease. They were totally separate placentas, however, in contrast to the case described by us.

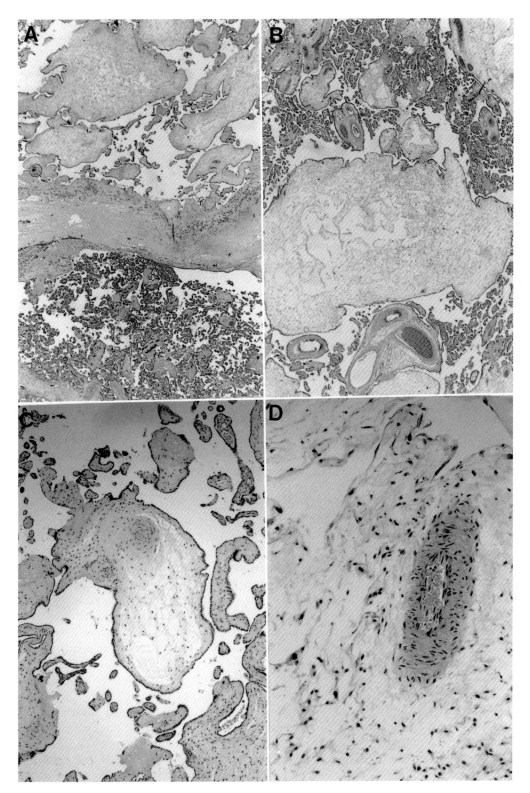

FIGURE 22.1. A: Sharp division of molar (top) and normal placental tissue (bottom) in presumed monozygotic (MZ) twin. Molar tissue is tetraploid, diploid female infant survived. B: Focal intermingling of molar with normal villi. C: Molar vesicle with atrophying blood vessel. D: Molar villus with intact, perfused fetal blood vessel. Note tetraploid connective tissue of mole. H&E ×16 (A), ×16 (B), ×64 (C), ×160 (D).

The natural history of recurrent molar disease was discussed by Federschneider et al. (1980) in their presentation of seven patients. They also reviewed the literature and stated that their recurrent cases were more malignant and more often required treatment for residual disease than nonrecurrent moles (see also Rice et al., 1989). Mor-Joseph and his colleagues (1985) reported four recurrent moles following three spontaneous abortions. The moles occurred after clomiphene therapy, as was previously described by Schneider and Waxman (1972). These experiences support the finding by Parazzini et al. (1985) that moles are significantly more common with increasing numbers of spontaneous abortion. An interesting case with three recurrent CHMs was described by Fisher et al. (2000a). All three were biparental (not androgenetic), yet CHMs; moreover, the male partners were two different individuals and two moles were XX, one was XY. This finding has implications for possible in vitro fertilization (IVF) efforts in patients with recurrent moles. Helwani et al. (1999) had also described CHM with biparental origin in the seven (!) moles from two Lebanese sisters. The authors suggested the existence of an autosomal-recessive gene that was responsible. In a subsequent publication, Moglabey et al. (1999) studied members of these two families and identified an aberrant gene on 19q. Most interestingly, Sensi et al. (2000) found in an unrelated Italian family with recurrent moles of biparental nature (!) an abnormality of 19q in two sisters. Fisher et al. (2004b) reviewed the entire topic of recurrent moles (152 pregnancies) and stated that the sequelae were similar to the usual CHMs. It is thought that this abnormal gene is involved in imprinting and thus suppresses the usual influence of the maternal gene, causing enhanced expression of the paternal allele. In this way, a molar phenotype would be expressed even though the mole was biparental. Not only is the genetic derivation of complete moles unusual (most have only paternal chromosomes, that is, are "androgenetic"), but there is great variation in the prevalence of moles in different populations. Asian women, especially Japanese and Filipinas, suffer a much-increased frequency of molar pregnancies. It is further remarkable that hydatidiform moles have been observed only in human pregnancies; only one other primate has exhibited this pathology despite extensive breeding records. This was a mole occurring in a chimpanzee reported by Debyser et al. (1993). This *Pan troglodytes*, while pregnant, died from massive genital hemorrhage and ovarian torsion. The entire uterus was filled with a PHM that had commonly accepted histologic features. Its DNA content was hyperdiploid, possibly triploid, and a degenerated fetus was present. There are rare reports of moles in cows (Folger, 1934), and Drieux and Thiéry (1948) reviewed rare cases described in a cat and dog. These are truly exceptional circumstances and their analogy to human CHM is uncertain. This was the case

until Meinecke et al. (2002) presented their specimen of a typical hydatidiform mole in cattle that was associated with a stillborn male calf. They also reviewed the few previously reported cases of moles in animals. For the first time it was conclusively shown that the 60,XX molar tissue was indeed androgenetic and the co-twin calf was 60,XY. There were rare chimeric cells in the two tissues that derived most likely from the formerly present placental anastomoses, but the term (that includes freemartin) is strictly speaking incorrect, as the normal fetus was male. Apparently there were no sequelae to the cow that delivered the twins. Choriocarcinoma is also exceptionally uncommon in animals, although it has been reported in a rhesus monkeys (Chapter 23).

Incidence

The exact incidence of hydatidiform moles varies in different populations and it is impossible to ascertain it exactly. An estimate of 1 per 2000 pregnancies is generally cited for the United States (Hertig, 1950). When Grimes (1984) undertook an extensive epidemiologic study of many different populations he found an CHM incidence of 1 in 1000 pregnancies for the general U.S. population. Etiologic factors were not obtained from his investigation. In part, the inability to ascertain a precise incidence is due to the probable confusion of CHM with PHMs, the presumed triploid conceptuses. Undoubtedly also, PHMs have often been counted as CHMs (the presumed androgenetic moles), especially when one reviews the early literature. We know from personal experience that this is still the case. The methodologic problems in ascertaining a true incidence have been dealt with particularly well by Buckley (1987), and the later contribution by di Cintio et al. (1997) is relevant. In their review of the epidemiology of gestational trophoblastic disease they found that the incidence in the U.S. is 108/100,000 pregnancies, whereas in Northern Italy it was only 62/100,000. In Indonesia it was 993/100,000, whereas in China it was 667/100,000 pregnancies. There is then little doubt that vast differences in frequency of CHM and other GTDs exist; CHM is especially common in the populations of Hawaii, the Philippines, and Japan. Table 22.1 summarizes incidence figures derived from several relevant studies. Other tables may be found in these publications and in the books cited. Several authors have provided additional reviews of early incidence figures that add little important information. There is thus a general agreement that the incidence of moles is, at least partially, racially influenced. This phenomenon is not completely explicable by the higher parity and older age of Asian gravidas (Iverson et al., 1959). Das (1938) found moles more commonly in the Indian than the Caucasian population. In an inquiry that distinguishes environmental from racial causes, Natoli and Rashad (1972) observed

TABLE 22.1. Incidence of complete hydatidiform moles in various populations

Country	Author	Year	Time span of the study	Incidence/term gestation
India	Das	1938	108,951 gestations	1:502
Mexico	Márquez-Monter	1963	1961 gestations	1:200
Hong Kong	Chun et al.	1964	1953–1961 gestations	1:242
Sweden	Ringertz	1970	1958–1965 gestations	1:1560
Singapore	Teoh	1971	1963–1965 gestations	1:823
Israel	Matalon	1972	1950–1965 gestations	1:1300
Hawaii	Natoli	1972	1950–1970 gestations	1:977
Paraguay	Rolon	1977	1960–1969 gestations	1:4369
Paraguay	Rolon et al.	1990	1970–1982 gestations	1:3906
Netherlands	Franke	1983a	1978–1980 gestations	1:2270
Italy	Mazzanti	1986	1979–1982 gestations	1:1510
England	Bagshawe	1986	1973–1983 gestations	1:1000 to 1.54:1000

moles much more often in the Japanese and Hawaiian stock, than in Chinese and Caucasian residents of Hawaii; many other examples of racial influences can be found in the cited publications. It must also be recognized that postmenopausal women are not necessarily free from the possibility of conceiving a molar gestation. Over 100 cases of moles past age 50 have been described, and Garcia et al. (2004), who reviewed the topic, even found a 61-year-old woman with this disease. She recovered after evacuation.

These reports all found that the incidence of CHM correlated with race rather than with geography. A review of molar pregnancy suggested also that the traditional clinical picture presented by patients with moles has changed, but that persistent trophoblastic disease has become more common (Soto-Wright et al., 1995). Bracken (1987) undertook a special study of these features and found that the incidence of CHM in Japanese was inexplicably twofold higher than that of Caucasians and Chinese. He stated, "Maternal age is the most consistently demonstrated risk factor; teenagers and, especially, women over age 35 being at increased risk" (see also Bandy et al., 1984).

Maudsley and Robertson (1965), who described the development of a mole in a 52-year-old woman, reviewed the literature of approximately 60 similar cases in older women. Mathieu (1939) made a thorough review of moles and choriocarcinomas and found a 55-year-old woman, emphasizing the dependency on maternal age. Clearly, older maternal age (and somewhat also extremely young age) predisposes to GTDs (di Cintio et al., 1997). The possible influence of the father's age has also been studied. No relationship was ascertained in most studies, except in that undertaken by La Vecchia et al. (1984), who found a higher incidence in fathers over 45 years, and this predilection was compounded by smoking. Other investigators have not identified smoking as a risk factor. The possible and disputed etiologic role of herbicides is unlikely to be resolved, according to Bracken (1987).

McCorriston (1968) evaluated possible reasons for the higher incidence in particular racial groups of Hawaii and stated that their different food preferences are unlikely etiologic antecedents. This point was further examined in a case-control study from China where no relation to diet was identified by Brinton et al. (1989). Berkowitz et al. (1985a) suggested that vitamin A deficiency may be causally related to molar gestations, and suggested carotene supplements for prevention. There have been no other meaningful concepts that explain the racial differences of CHMs. Indeed, the possibility has been studied that the marked ethnic differences in molar incidence reflect different diets, and possibly other environmental factors might disappear upon immigration to other countries. A key question thus is whether the incidence of CHM in Asians who emigrated to San Francisco and then lived Western lifestyles differs from that of Caucasians. Overstreet (personal communication, 1963) ascertained that, in the immigrant Asian population of San Francisco, the incidence of CHM is 1 per 2000 deliveries, much the same as in Caucasian women. Atrash et al. (1986) similarly ascertained molar pregnancies among 84,318 abortions from different institutions. The incidence of moles was 7.5 per 10,000 pregnancies (1 per 1333). Bracken (1988), however, has criticized this result on methodologic grounds and as being a gross underestimate. Although more moles were found in Chinese, this difference was not significant. African Americans had the same incidence as whites. The only significant correlation occurred with maternal age.

A number of **classifications** of GTDs should be mentioned. The World Health Organization (WHO) recognizes the following scheme (Tavasolli & Devilee, 2003):

Hydatidiform mole
  Complete mole
  Partial mole
  Invasive mole
  Metastatic mole

Trophoblastic neoplasms
   Choriocarcinoma
   Placental site trophoblastic tumor
   Epithelioid trophoblastic tumor
Nonneoplastic, nonmolar trophoblastic lesions
   Placental site nodule and plaque
   Exaggerated placental site

The International Federation of Gynecology and Obstetrics (FIGO) and the National Institutes of Health (NIH) use different systems for classification, and prognostic scores were assigned by the classification issued from the WHO. These aspects and histologic criteria are well covered by Horn and Bilek (1997).

Genetics

Ever since Park's early studies (1957), cytogeneticists have known that sex determination of trophoblastic tumors appeared to be impossible. Shorofsky (1960), applying cytometrics, found that nuclei of molar trophoblast had the same parameters as normal trophoblast. Márquez-Monter (1966), using radioautography, showed that the syncytium of molar trophoblast originates from cytotrophoblastic precursors, just as it does in normal villi. With the discovery of the sex chromatin, it became known that most moles possess a Barr body (sex chromatin: the inactivated X chromosome of females) (see Tominaga & Page, 1966; Baggish et al., 1968; Loke, 1969). Early systematic studies by Sasaki et al. (1962) had also shown that most hydatidiform moles possessed an apparently normal female or occasionally male diploid complement. Bourgoin et al. (1965a,b) also found male and female karyotypes but further observed some aneuploidy in their specimens. They encountered methodologic difficulties in making cell preparations, however. Sajiri Makino and his colleagues in Japan (1964, 1965) ascertained that some apparent hydatidiform moles, now referred to as partial moles, have a triploid chromosomal constitution, an observation that was soon confirmed by Carr (1969). It is now known that triploidy is the karyotype of most PHMs.

The major breakthrough in our understanding of molar pregnancies came when Kajii and Ohama (1977) showed that hydatidiform moles are "androgenetic," that is to say, all molar chromosomes are paternally derived. It is easiest to envisage that this occurs as the result of fertilization of an "empty egg," with subsequent duplication of the haploid spermatozoal complement. That mechanism also explains why moles are almost always 46,XX. If a male-determining spermatozoon with Y chromosome were to fertilize an empty egg, a karyotype of 46,YY would result from such sperm duplication, and this is apparently a lethal cellular condition. It must be mentioned, however, that nobody has shown an "empty egg" as yet in ovaries

or ovulated follicles. Thus, it may be possible that chromosomal or other nuclear abnormalities predispose to the female component's regression. The theoretical aspects of this vexing problem have been discussed at great length by Golubovsky (2003), a paper worth reading as it also attempts to explain twins and chimeras in these products of gestation. Kajii and Ohama karyotyped 20 moles and determined the disposition of the chromosomal Q- and R-band polymorphism. There is sufficient heterogeneity in the normal human chromosome structures that this polymorphism allowed them to ascertain with confidence that, in CHM, these markers were exclusively paternal (Fig. 22.2). These findings were quickly confirmed by Wake et al. (1978a) and Jacobs et al. (1978), and Azuma et al. (1991) showed that the molar mitochondrial DNA has a maternal origin. Many markers are now available for chromosome identification. They extend from the Q and R bands to C bands, shown by fluorescent in situ hybridization (FISH), and they also include the identification of inversions, translocations, and other minor varieties, as shown in Figure 22.2. Since this original description of androgenicity, not only has the concept been amply confirmed, but androgenesis has also been verified by genetic markers, such as homozygosity of polymorphic enzymes (Jacobs et al., 1980) and human leukocyte antigen (HLA) markers (Wake et al., 1978b; Couillin et al., 1985; Goldman-Whol et al., 2001). Interestingly, two of the mothers studied by Kajii and Ohama (1977) had reciprocal translocations of different chromosomes. Similar findings were then made in the later studies of Lawler et al. (1979) and Vejerslev et al. (1987d). This apparent frequency of translocations might initially be assumed to have possible etiologic significance for the creation of an empty egg, but subsequent studies have negated this possibility. Vejerslev et al. (1987d) karyotyped 237 mothers and 217 fathers of CHM as well as 125 mothers and 106 fathers of PHM. "No significant increase in the frequency of translocations . . . was found."

To explain the genesis of moles, it is further hypothesized that molar transformation of the conceptus results from the homozygous concentration of some lethal genes. It is commonly estimated that four or five lethal genes are regularly carried (in the heterozygous state) in normal individuals. When they become homozygous (as they would be in CHM), the duplication of lethal genes causes embryonic death; only the placenta survives, to be transformed into molar vesicles. The notion of an empty egg with fertilization by a 23,X sperm and subsequent chromosomal duplication was supported by the genetic studies of Jacobs et al. (1980). Moreover, experimental investigations in mice indicated that maternal and paternal genomes are essential for normal embryonic and placental development. Paternal genes are apparently especially important for normal placenta formation. It was found that embryos from two female pronuclei (gynogenesis)

FIGURE 22.2. Normal human diploid karyotype, 46,XY, Q-banded (Q = quinacrine). In the normal karyotype, chromosomes may be banded by different techniques. Here, a normal male set is banded with quinacrine stain (Q bands), which allows precise comparison between elements (maternal and paternal). Note that in this male there are differences between the banding pattern of several elements. Various segments do not "match"; they represent normal variations in our chromosomes that are inherited. The following chromosomes differ in this karyotype: No. 1, the right element has additional heterochromatin at the centromere; No. 9, the left element has additional centromeric heterochromatin, and the right chromosome has an inversion; No. 14, there are prominent satellites; No. 15, the right chromosome has a centromeric variant; No. 16, the right chromosome has additional centromeric material; No. 22, the left chromosome has prominent satellites, and the right chromosome has a centromeric variant. It has been possible to show that, in the typical complete hydatidiform mole (CHM), there is only the banding profile of the paternal chromosome set, both elements are exactly alike (Kajii & Ohama, 1977). (Courtesy of Dr. Mark Bogart, Honolulu.)

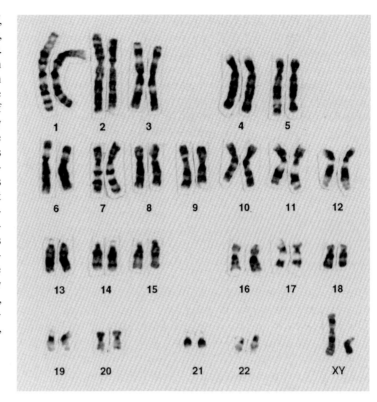

developed poorly, and particularly their placental membranes were abnormal. The embryos derived from two male pronuclei died very early, but their placentas were reasonably well formed (Surani & Barton, 1983; Barton et al., 1984; Ho et al., 1984). Irregular X-chromosome inactivation inexplicably also occurs in placental membranes of female conceptuses. There is preferential female X-chromosome activity in a variety of cells of the placenta of female fetuses (Tagaki & Sasaki, 1975; Roper et al., 1978; Harrison & Warburton, 1986; Harrison, 1989).

After this definition of androgenesis as the cause of molar development had been clarified, many cytogenetic studies were performed on CHMs and PHMs to further delineate the possible relations of chromosome sets and the possible impact on the prognosis of the various molar conceptions. Tsuji et al. (1981) determined that there is a higher frequency of aneuploidy ($2n = >46$) in the moles from older women, and also in invasive moles and in choriocarcinomas. They suggested that it may have prognostic significance. Jacobs et al. (1978) had also observed an apparently malignant mole with aneuploidy and hypotetraploidy but with a paternal origin of all chromosomes. When trophoblastic cells are separated from molar tissue and then cultured, Habibian and Surti (1987) found that these cells exhibit a 2.8 times greater frequency of polyploidy when compared to normal trophoblast. Chromosomal breakage was also much more common. The X-chromosomal replication pattern of diploid, androgenetic molar cells, however, was normal (Tsukahara &

Kajii, 1985). A useful review may be found in the paper of Lindor et al. (1992). The participation of imprinting and of telomerase activity in moles was reviewed by Li et al. (2002). Castrillo et al. (2001) had shown that the imprinted gene product p57[KIP2] is paternally imprinted, and that it was absent or markedly underexpressed in cytotrophoblast and mesenchyme of CHMs because of their paternal derivation, while decidua, PHMs, and normal placentas had good expression. This proves to be a potentially useful additional means of differentiation between the moles, and an immunohistochemical stain has been developed and used successfully (Jun et al., 2003). In a later study, however, Fisher et al. (2004b) showed paradoxical gene expression due to retention of a maternal copy of chromosome 11 (plus two paternal copies) in a case of CHM, thus explaining the rare abnormal expression of this gene in marker studies for p57[KIP2]. Fukunaga (2004) found aberrant expression of p57[KIP2] in two tetraploid (92,XXYY) moles. This suggests derivation from two sets of chromosomes, paternal and maternal. Saxena et al. (2003) showed that the *IPL* gene (also imprinted) is absent from the syncytium in moles. It is also of interest to note that N.J. Sebire et al. (2004), employing this stain on choriocarcinomas, were unable to infer their origin.

As more moles were investigated genetically, exceptions to the early findings have come to light. The existence of 46,XY moles was then first recognized (Surti et al., 1979; Ohama et al., 1981; Pattillo et al., 1981; Surti et al., 1982). Fisher and Lawler (1984) found three 46,XY moles and determined that they derived from dispermy. It now appears that about 8% of CHMs are the result of fusion of two male pronuclei following dispermic fertilization (Ford et al., 1986). In addition to the XY moles, occasional heterozygous 46,XX moles were found (approximately 5% to 10% of moles are now known to be heterozygous and androgenetic). Wake et al. (1981) suggested that these moles may have a greater malignant potential. Kajii et al. (1984) studied nine XY moles and compared the clinical outcome with 16 normal XX moles. Their study showed dispermy as the causal mechanism in the XY moles. Three of eight XY moles and five of 15 XX moles had a delayed decrease in human chorionic gonadotropin (hCG) titers. Mutter et al. (1993) were unable to show that an increased risk for metastasis exists in the XY moles that they studied with PCR. They found 7.7% of the moles with metastatic consequence and 9.1% of the metastatic group in their large sample of moles studied possessed a Y chromosome. In the experience of Fisher and Lawler (1984), patients with heterozygous moles needed further treatment of trophoblastic tumor in 31%. In a subsequent study of this important observation, Lawler and Fisher (1987) examined 163 moles, 38 (23%) of which were PMHs and 125 were CHMs. All of the PHM were either triploid or hypertriploid, with most having arisen by dispermic fertilization; they had no untoward sequelae. Of the CHM, whose genetic study was informative, 10% were heterozygous diploid moles. Of these heterozygous moles, 25% required subsequent chemotherapy, in contrast to 17.6% of the CHMs with homozygous constitution, a result that was not statistically significant.

Hitchcock et al. (1991) addressed the difficult differential diagnosis between CHM and PHM when they undertook an important retrospective flow cytometric study of molar specimens diagnosed at the Armed Forces Institute of Pathology (AFIP). Their diagnosis of CHM differed from that of the submitting pathologist in 78%, and in the diagnosis of PHM in 57% of cases. Howat et al. (1993) evaluated the pathologist's ability to reliably distinguish between these conditions and provided specific criteria. The findings of an evaluation of 50 molar pregnancies by seven competent pathologists gave no assurance of a correct diagnosis. Fukunaga et al. (1996) found by employing flow cytometry on paraffin-embedded tissues of 35 hydropic villi that 25 were complete hydatidiform moles, while 10 were hydropic abortions; none were partial moles. Ten hydropic abortions were of maternal and paternal contributions, with two being tetraploid. Two tetraploid moles developed invasive lesions, one a choriocarcinoma. They suggested that tetraploid moles require special follow-up and strongly advocated the use of DNA determination of moles (see also Fukunaga et al., 1993). Lage (1991) deter-

mined that one course of single-agent chemotherapy caused complete remission in all triploid PHMs, and more were required in the two diploid PHM they studied. Later, these authors examined 142 hydropic placentas (Lage et al., 1992) and found 38% CHM, 35% PHM, and 26% hydropic abortuses, the majority of the latter being near diploid; only 11% were triploid. "Persistent tumor" was seen in 33% of CHM and 12% of PHM. Additional insight has been gained through the publications by van de Kaa and her colleagues (1991, 1993, 1997), who are strong advocates for a genetic/ploidy study to objectively differentiate CHM from PHM and hydropic abortuses. Berezowsky et al. (1995) found a high proportion (42%) of nonmolar and molar (47%) conceptuses in their DNA study, while most partial moles (89%) were triploid. They suggested that tetraploid moles derive from diploid conceptions with subsequent polyploidization.

From these studies, then, it appears that it is not yet possible to reliably diagnose the molar pregnancies by hematoxylin and eosin (H&E) histologic study alone, let alone assign a prognosis on the basis of a CHM karyotype. Others have come to the same conclusion and strongly urge cytometry to be part of the evaluation (Conran et al., 1993). The most important decision to be made when encountering a mole is to differentiate between triploidy and diploidy, for which flow cytometry is the most important methodology whose usage should be more widely employed. The patients with PHMs never experienced metastatic disease. Only rarely have such patients required chemotherapy for persistent trophoblast, and we doubt that it was needed in many cases; moreover, the diagnosis may be in error or is poorly supported, as was the case in the patient recorded by Gardner and Lage (1992). Bae and Kim (1999) showed that the possession of telomerase activity of CHM is more likely to eventuate in persistent trophoblastic disease. In recent years, however, pathologists have added new tools to their armamentarium in order to distinguish CHMs from PHMs and hydropic abortuses. This was especially well accomplished by antibody staining for p57.

Although the gross morphology alone of PHM is often persuasive, difficult cases do arise, especially when twin pregnancies are admixed with moles. The existence of confined placental mosaicism (CPM) has been evoked to explain unusual cases. Thus, Sarno et al. (1993) described a partial mole (69,XXX) associated with a surviving diploid premature girl. We saw the placental material from a triploid conceptus born at 33 weeks and who survived for some time without anomalies (C. Kaplan, personal communication). The placenta of this 2050-g boy was a 1000-g placenta with chorangiosis but without hydatid changes. As has been alluded to earlier, because cytogenetic studies are not feasible for all laboratories, it has been strongly advocated that ploidy of moles be determined by the rapid method of flow cytometry

(Anonymous, 1987; Benirschke, 1989). Fisher et al. (1987) showed early on that this technique unequivocally distinguishes the two molar entities. The same method was employed by Hemming et al. (1987), who demonstrated that CHMs more often had hyperdiploid cells. Lage et al. (1988) also produced similarly good results in separating CHMs from PHMs with this method (Fig. 22.3). It is noteworthy that paraffin-embedded material can be used for retrospective flow cytometric studies. Bell et al. (1989, 1998) recommended such studies and PCR for more difficult cases. Moreover, because flow cytometry easily distinguishes diploid complete moles from triploid partial moles, it is important to note that occasional and unexpected findings occur that further mandate employment of this methodology. As an example, Lage et al. (1989) found three tetraploid moles. One of them, a 92,XXXX mole, was a CHM. Another specimen had a complement of 92,XXYY (two paternal and two maternal genomes), and one was diploid/triploid mosaic (69,XXY/90,XXXY).

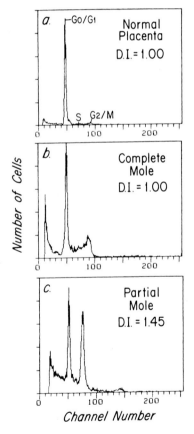

FIGURE 22.3. DNA histogram of normal placenta (above), a complete mole (center), and a triploid partial mole (below). The vertical axis is the number of cells; the horizontal axis is fluorescence and indicates DNA content. There is a single diploid peak in the normal placenta, a large diploid peak in the CHM with a minor peak at tetraploidy, and a large peak of triploid cells (arrow) in the partial mole. (*Source:* Lage et al., 1988, with permission.)

After evacuation, none of these moles had recurrent trophoblastic disease. Martin et al. (1989) also determined the ploidy of various moles from paraffin blocks, as in the study of Hitchcock et al. (1991) reviewed above. The outcome for the patients following delivery of the moles was known. It was found that moles with an aneuploid population of cells had a significantly higher incidence of gestational neoplastic sequelae than did those with diploid (euploid) moles. Although these malignant" moles also had a higher proliferative index, this was not statistically significant. A retrospective study of 13 complete moles by Bewtra et al. (1997) identified eight (61.5%) as being tetraploid, and diploid moles often had tetraploid cells as well. None developed sequelae and no histologic differences were found in these populations. Tetraploid moles tended to occur in older patients and were accompanied by higher β-hCG levels. Newer technology employs DNA fingerprinting from very small samples to differentiate these conditions (Nobunaga et al., 1990; Ko et al., 1991); also, PCR is advocated for rapid diagnosis (Fisher & Newlands, 1993). Ishii et al. (1998) advocated the use of short tandem repeat-derived DNA polymorphism for the differential diagnosis of twins with moles and partial moles with fetus. Lai et al. (2004) had to reclassify some specimens when they examined moles by fluorescent microsatellite genotyping and ploidy study by in situ hybridization. They found that the diagnosis of CHM was more readily done histologically than that of PHM. Three PHMs developed GTDs, but the authors did not define their nature.

Mixed populations of cells with different karyotypes occur in the occasional exceptional CHM. Takagi et al. (1969) described a triploid/diploid "mosaic" XX mole without providing further relevant information. Ford et al. (1986) found an avascular, androgenetic diploid CHM (608 g) that was mosaic for normally fertilized cells. Interestingly, there was a reciprocal translocation in one population that enhanced the ease of analysis of the chromosomal origins. To explain their finding, the authors suggested that the fusion of dizygotic (DZ) twins was unlikely; they favored an origin from the abnormal fertilization of a single egg. In our interpretation, fusion of two DZ twins (a chimera) remains a strong possibility. The case also argues strongly against the perhaps overly simplistic notion that moles result from fertilization of an empty egg. The authors urged that other diploid moles be examined for possible differentiation of mosaicism/chimerism. Vejerslev et al. (1987a) found two homozygous moles with second cell lines that also suggested twin gestations. Other possible admixtures of fraternal twins, one a mole and the other normal, are discussed below. Vejerslev et al. (1987c) have summarized all unusual karyotypes of CHM, diploid PHM, and the hyperdiploid CHM. In recent studies of our own service, a PHM was found in a specimen whose amniocentesis showed uniform trisomy 3 and whose aborted fetus had the characteristic features of this trisomy.

Among other exceptional karyotypes there are exist the tetraploid specimens. Vejerslev et al. (1987b) found one tetraploid mole with three paternal contributions and one maternal contribution among 29 molar conceptuses, 24 of which were dispermic triploids. This tetraploid specimen was, in principle, similar to the PHM but did not have the clinical presentation of that entity. Lage et al. (1989) identified three tetraploid moles. One of them, a CHM, had 92,XXXX; the two PHMs had 92,XXYY and 90,XXXY,-11,-13/69,XXY, respectively, reason for these authors to strongly advocate the use of flow cytometry for identification of unusual specimens. It now appears that most diploid moles have also some tetraploid peaks at flow cytometric study; those with diploid genomes occurred in younger women (Bewtra et al., 1997). The newer diagnostic methods of genetic analysis already referred to may be just as rapid in appropriately equipped laboratories, and they are decisive. Saji et al. (1989) showed elegantly by DNA fingerprinting that CHMs have only paternal genes. The advantage of such a study with restriction fragment length polymorphism (RFLP) is that only minute samples are required. When RFLP studies of trophoblast and corresponding fetuses were compared in 50 samples, four pairs showed differences in DNA content (Butler et al., 1988). This unexpected finding has not yet been fully explained, but it is likely to be important.

Morphology

A "hydatidiform mole is defined as a conceptus, usually devoid of an intact fetus, in which all or many of the chorionic villi show (1) gross nodular swelling culminating in cyst formation, (2) disintegration of blood vessels, and (3) variable proliferation of trophoblast" (Edmonds, 1959). This must be regarded as the swelling of most or all of the villi in a placenta that may once have been more normal. When moles are diagnosed in the course of a pregnancy, the molar tissue fills most of the uterine cavity (Fig. 22.4). Intervillous coagula are common because of the aberrant intervillous circulation, and it may be associated with vaginal bleeding. Moles occasionally present with the clinical picture of abruptio placentae, according to Sauter (1965). The uterus may be markedly distended and may even rupture, especially when it is stimulated to contract (Lee & Siegel, 1965). Ovarian theca lutein cysts are often present (Fig. 22.4) because of the ovarian overstimulation by the excessive hCG production. Because the ovarian cysts regress spontaneously after evacuation of the mole, the ovaries do not need to be removed when hysterectomy is performed for molar sequelae.

The molar villi are fairly uniformly distended by fluid. McKay et al. (1955a,b) have analyzed this fluid biochemically and found its osmolality to be lower than that of maternal serum. The authors suggested that later gestational trophoblast has different capacities, which they explained as a reason why villi atrophy rather than expand when fetal death occurs in later fetal life. Jauniaux et al. (1998), who also reviewed subsequent studies, compared the content of molar vesicles with nuchal fluid, amnionic fluid, and maternal serum. They found significantly lower urea content and determined that the vesicle fluid α-fetoprotein was more yolk sac–like, whereas nuchal fluid was more liver-like. When molar tissue is floated in water (Fig. 22.5), the translucent nature of the distended terminal villi is evident. The protein content of the fluid is apparent when such villi are first fixed and then floated (Fig. 22.6). The connections to a possible former chorionic

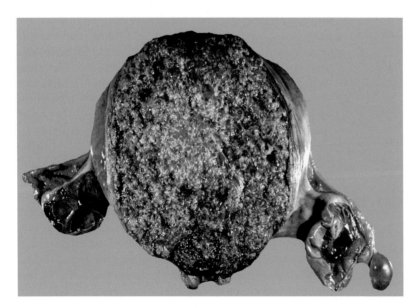

FIGURE 22.4. Hydatidiform mole in situ. Note the distention of the uterus and bilateral theca lutein cysts of ovaries. The vesicular nature of molar villi is apparent.

FIGURE 22.5. Hydatidiform molar villi photographed under water. Note the bulbous swelling of terminal villi and the slender nature of mainstem villi.

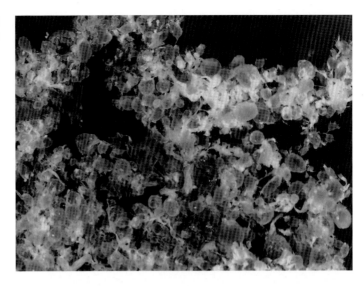

sac also then become evident. The swelling is primarily one of the terminal villi and can be construed to result from the continued water transport by trophoblast. The syncytium has this singular transport function. In the absence of fetal vessels to remove the transported fluid, the villi expand, and enlarged cisternae develop in the villi and vacuoles in the syncytial cytoplasm. The absence of a fetus, the lack of a chorionic cavity, and deficiency of chorionic vasculature are characteristic of CHM. Nevertheless, a few cases with tiny embryos have been described.

Thus, Hertig (1968) depicted a chorionic cavity in the center of an apparently complete mole that was fixed in situ within a uterus (his Figure 196). This chorionic sac contained a deformed, stunted embryo with this mole (his Figure 199). Because an embryo was associated with the specimen, it may be argued in retrospect that the specimen was a PHM. This consideration is invalidated by the case shown in Figure 22.7. In this patient, a tiny embryo was present within a typical hydatidiform mole (the patient's third). This pregnancy was followed by fatal, disseminated choriocarcinoma. Baergen et al. (1996) showed that a hydatidiform mole (androgenetic) had a "fetal pole" and a gestational sac at early sonography. In fact, Weaver et al. (2000) even showed that the occasional amnion that can thus be found in verified CHM has an androgenetic pattern. Several authors have found that fetal red blood cells and other fetal structures occur in verified CHMs and that the usually avascular villi may possess capillaries early in development (Fisher et al., 1997; Paradinas et al., 1997; Qiao et al., 1997; Zaragoza et al., 1997; Neudeck et al., 2003). Thus, occasional embryos accompany moles, especially perhaps during their earliest development. This is an important point as pathologists often rely solely on microscopic features for the differential diagnosis and these do not necessarily conform to the teaching they received. This point should have been evident from the presence of connective tissue in the villi alone. As was discussed in some detail in Chapter 12, the connective tissue of the placenta has an *embryonic* derivation; it does not come from the trophoblastic shell, as was formerly thought. That the differential diagnosis

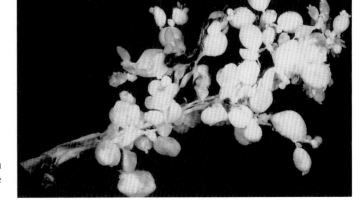

FIGURE 22.6. Same villi as in Figure 22.5 but after fixation in Bouin's fixative. The protein has precipitated, making the villi opaque. The connecting stalks are obvious.

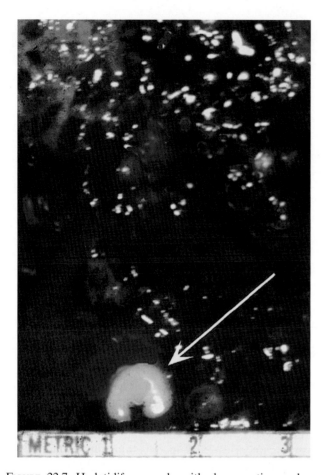

FIGURE 22.7. Hydatidiform mole with degenerating embryo. There were no vessels in this "malignant" mole. It was the third consecutive CHM and was followed by fatal choriocarcinoma. The tiny embryo is visible above the 1.0- to 1.5-cm portion of the ruler. The choriocarcinoma of this pregnancy is shown in Chapter 23.

between the three categories—hydropic abortus, PHM, and CHM—is difficult on histologic grounds alone was well demonstrated by Gschwendtner et al. (1998). They studied, retrospectively, their "molar" specimens with ploidy analysis. This was done after the stricter criteria proposed by Paradinas (1994) had been applied. Despite this special care, ploidy study necessitated reclassification in many cases. This aspect has also been studied by Genest (2001). Agreement was found in histology and ploidy results with CHM, and in 79% of PHM and triploidy. Their discussion indicates, however, that completely reliable histologic features do not exist that allow accurate categorization; ploidy study is required, especially in gestationally young specimens.

Moles are now typically removed by suction curettage. Because the specimens are usually markedly disrupted and accompanied by much clot, it is not surprising that possible chorionic sacs and embryos are not found more often. The stalks from which the hydatid villi emanate, however, also indicate that a more normal structure must have preceded the typical CHM configuration. Also, in younger CHMs, there is generally less villous swelling, and the connections to a possible chorionic sac by stem villi are more visible (Fig. 22.8). Kajii et al. (1984), moreover, found that younger moles had smaller, elliptic or club-shaped villi and poorly delineated cisternae, whereas older moles had more globular villi (see also Keep et al., 1996). The latter also had more trophoblastic hyperplasia and fewer remnants of capillaries; no significant morphologic differences were found between XY and XX moles.

It is of historical interest to cite the invasive mole described by Jarotzky and Waldeyer (1868). They observed a chorionic cavity in the center of this typical invasive mole whence all the hydropic villi emanated. One may thus ask: What would a CHM, usually delivered between 15 and 20 weeks' gestation, have looked like at 6 weeks'

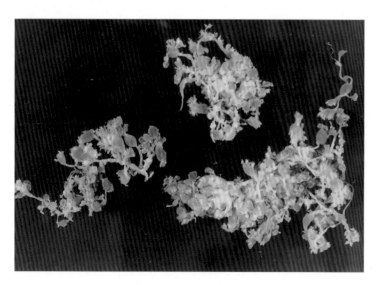

FIGURE 22.8. Hydropic villi of "early" CHM at 10 weeks' gestation. Note that only some villi are bulbous and that the connecting mainstem villi are still prominent. (*Source:* Benirschke, 1981, with permission.)

gestation? The answer is unknown, but the observations by Sasaki et al. (1967) and Nishimura et al. (1968) suggested that typical hydatidiform moles might not be recognized in such young developmental age groups. For that reason these investigators examined a large number of therapeutic abortions in Japan and found no CHMs, although many would have been expected in that population. Early CHMs might also contain fetal blood vessels, similar to the occasional embryos that have been seen with CHM just enumerated. Blood vessels in the placenta disappear rapidly after fetal death. Their absence from a CHM does not ensure that there never were villous capillaries. We suggest then that in transitional stages, the differential diagnosis may be difficult to make by morphology alone. It is here that flow cytometry and DNA fingerprinting have become useful adjuncts.

Edmonds (1959) employed the term **transitional mole**. Whether it applied to the transition from a more normal young placenta or to what is now known as a partial mole remains unknown. For these reasons, we prefer not to use this terminology. It would be much better if we identified these abortions as diploid androgenetic, triploid, or diploid-triploid moles, if distinctions are needed. The availability of more precise techniques now demands this precision from pathologists. Cohen et al. (1979) suggested that eight of their 4829 elective first-trimester abortion specimens were molar. In our opinion, however, the criteria for their diagnosis of CHM and their photomicrographs are not convincing.

Microscopically, moles are characterized by swollen villi with apparently empty cisternae. The cisternae result from the dissociation of loose villous connective tissue; transitional stages are frequently observed (Fig. 22.9). Characteristically, there are no blood vessels or recognizable vascular remnants, with the exception of the cases

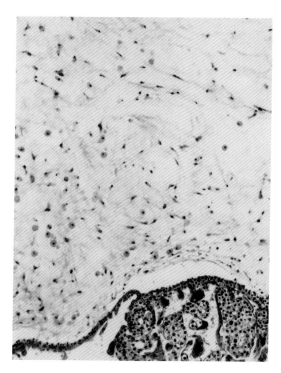

FIGURE 22.9. Microscopic appearance of the villous surface in CHM. The villous core lacks fetal capillaries; it shows marked edema and early cisterna formation at right. There are many Hofbauer cells. The villous surface has normal epithelium at left and markedly hyperplastic trophoblast on the right. H&E ×100.

alluded to above. An abundance of Hofbauer cells is frequent, as it is in PHM. The trophoblastic covering of CHM varies enormously from mole to mole. It may even vary within a mole (Fig. 22.10). Occasionally, the trophoblast is degenerated or enmeshed in fibrin. Hertig and

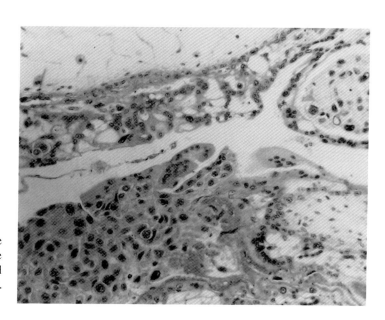

FIGURE 22.10. Surface of molar villus with greater degree of trophoblastic proliferation than that seen in Figure 22.9. Note the aneuploidy of many syncytial nuclei and the syncytial cisternae (dilated transport vesicles) at top. H&E ×160.

Sheldon (1947) paid particular attention to the nature and abundance of trophoblast. Using this feature, they subdivided moles into groups I to VI (later revised to three groups), from benign to malignant, and sought a correlation with subsequent development of choriocarcinoma and other sequelae. Hertig (1950), however, later stated, "It is well nigh impossible to predict accurately which mole will be followed by this most rapidly malignant of all cancers." Although Douglas (1962) affirmed this relation between graded moles and choriocarcinoma, most other pathologists have had difficulty with so rigorously classifying moles, and their results have not allowed a perfect correlation with outcome (Novak, 1950; Hunt et al., 1953; Javey et al., 1979; Genest et al., 1991). A detailed study by Messerli et al. (1987) showed that the classification of moles and related entities had poor correlation among different observers. A quantitative study of nuclear dimensions of trophoblastic cells in CHM by Franke et al. (1985) also failed to use such parameters as predictors of outcome. Benign moles are said to have been followed by pulmonary metastases of choriocarcinoma (e.g., Bonnar & Tennent, 1962), and choriocarcinoma has even followed normal pregnancy and abortion. For these reasons and because clinical follow-up with hCG titers is efficient, this scheme of classifying moles into groups with histologic differences is no longer followed. A variety of histochemical studies on molar villi have added little useful information regarding pathogenesis and prognosis (Bur et al., 1962; Lauslahti, 1969).

Several **ultrastructural studies** of CHM have been undertaken. They also have yielded little additional information to our understanding of the biology of these placental errors. Wynn and Davies (1964) showed especially clearly the spectrum of cells that are transitional between cytotrophoblast and syncytium. They also pointed to the fluid imbibition by the syncytium, which is often clearly seen light microscopically as empty spaces (vacuolation) in syncytial cytoplasm (Fig. 22.10; see also Fig. 22.26). They found a correlation between hCG levels and the abundance of syncytium, but not with that of cytotrophoblast. Essentially similar findings were reported by González-Angulo et al. (1966) and Okudaira and Strauss (1967). Merkow et al. (1971), who studied a mole that progressed to choriocarcinoma, were impressed by the lipid inclusions in the syncytiotrophoblast. Ockleford et al. (1989) undertook a scanning electron microscopic study of 31 CHMs and 12 placentas. They observed peculiar and novel surface organelles in several moles. These structures are absent from normal trophoblast, especially the reticular organization of the surface that betrays the underlying cytoskeletal architecture of villi.

Several studies have attempted to localize various markers and antigens to molar trophoblast. Thus, to better understand possible immunologic interactions with the mother, HLA antigen characterization of moles has been done. Lawler et al. (1974) found HLA antibodies against husband's antigens in women with persistent trophoblastic disease, and Berkowitz et al. (1983a) showed that monoclonal anti-HLA antibodies stained villous stroma but not the trophoblast of CHM. Using the peroxidase antibody technique, Sunderland et al. (1985) showed that class II antigens are not present on molar trophoblast. They detected class I histocompatibility antigens, however, on "proliferating extravillous trophoblast and on villous stromal cells, but not on quiescent villous trophoblast." This finding is similar to those in normal first-trimester placentas. When Yamashita et al. (1979) compared the HLA types of parents with those of the molar tissue, they identified the molar antigen as paternal. Berkowitz et al. (1985b) also detected transferrin receptors in the villous trophoblastic surface, similar to those that occur in normal tissue. These investigators localized trophoblast-leukocyte common antigens on normal and molar villous surfaces (Berkowitz et al., 1983a, 1986). $Rh_0(D)$ antigens were demonstrated on the malignant trophoblast of a D-negative patient who became sensitized by a choriocarcinoma, which had developed after the delivery of a D-positive child (Fischer et al., 1985). Goto et al. (1980) had previously demonstrated that trophoblast may contain the D antigen, and Tomoda et al. (1981) subsequently suggested that the racial disparity of incidence in gestational neoplastic disease may be secondary to the irregular distribution of the D antigen. Sarkar et al. (1986) found an expression of c-myc and c-ras oncogenes in early trophoblast, CHM, and malignant trophoblast cell lines. This pattern was absent from an 11-week conceptus. The expression of merosin, a novel basement membrane protein, was found in normal and malignant trophoblast (Leivo et al., 1989). Remarkably, this antigen was present only in intermediate trophoblast (X cells: extravillous trophoblast). It was not in the syncytium or Langhans' cells. This observation further suggests that the X cells represent a distinct and separate lineage of chorionic cells. Minami et al. (1993) demonstrated with antibody staining methodology that molar trophoblast contains inhibin-activin subunits, after having shown earlier their presence in normal placentas. Certain moieties are found in syncytium and cytotrophoblast, others in extravillous trophoblast. But, like the localization of various other placental hormones to different trophoblastic components (Sasagawa et al., 1987), the immunologic localization does not necessarily prove that these cells are the production sites. Trophoblastic production of hormones was further elucidated by studies of moles. Thus, Sagawa et al. (1997) found leptin production in molar pregnancy. Petit et al. (1996) showed an alteration of the elaboration of G proteins in moles and related it to placental lactogen and hCG production. An excessive production of plasminogen activator inhibitor-1 (PAI-1) was established by Estellés et al. (1996) and related to the increased incidence of PIH in molar gestations. Various other histochemical stains were employed by Olvera et al. (2001) without adding really useful new tools to our armamentarium, however.

The **prenatal diagnosis** of CHM moles is now usually possible with sonography. Ultrasonography identifies the lack of a fetus and displays the multiple echogenic signals, the "speckled" or "snowstorm" appearance of the molar placental tissue. Additionally, in PHMs a fetus may be visualized (Harper & MacVicar, 1963). Despite general knowledge of molar gestations, physicians make the diagnosis infrequently at the first antenatal visit (Ringertz, 1970), probably because in early gestation the villous swelling is only minimal. Other physicians who have made similar observations have also pointed to the frequent difficulty of early diagnosis (e.g., Stroup, 1956). The sonographic differentiation from missed abortions was further refined by the studies of Fine et al. (1989). Gynecologists have had the experience, however, that sonography during early pregnancy fails to make the diagnosis consistently (e.g., Woodward et al., 1980). Romero et al. (1985), therefore, correlated hCG levels with sonography. They set the hCG level of 82,350 mIU/mL as a diagnostic criterion, in addition to absent heart movement seen by ultrasonography. The diagnostic accuracy of recognizing moles thereby increased from 41.6% to 88.8%. Amniography has also been utilized (Gerber, 1970), as has arteriography (Hendrickse et al., 1964; Borell et al., 1966; Breit & Schedel, 1970). It is of special interest that ultrasonographic examination of first trimester pregnancies that eventuated in CHM did not show alterations that could be used to anticipate molar development (Woodward et al., 1980).

OTHER ATTRIBUTES

Maternal hyperthyroidism often accompanies hydatidiform moles (Hershman & Higgins, 1971; Sanchez & Sanchez, 1998), and sometimes it causes pulmonary edema. Both disappear promptly after evacuation. The nature of the thyroid-stimulating agent that is presumably released from the placental tissue is controversial. Some findings have suggested that it is identical to placental hCG (Nisula & Taliafouros, 1980). Amir et al. (1984) conducted a detailed study to identify this agent and concluded that it was unlikely to be hCG, but that it must represent another protein moiety released from the trophoblast of moles. Gunasegaram et al. (1986) suggested that it was a thyroid-stimulating hormone (TSH)-like protein, distinct from the hCG and the luteinizing hormone (LH) that they identified in molar vesicles. Other alterations of enzymes and proteins have been described in molar gestations. Thus α-fetoprotein is consistently absent in choriocarcinoma patients. It is rarely found in moles and then only in low concentration (Ishiguro, 1975). Yoshimatsu et al. (1987) immunologically examined tissues of various types of abortuses for the presence of α-fetoprotein. Molar fluid and trophoblast were consistently negative, but the protein was found in villi of PHM. Elevated serum glutamic oxaloacetic transaminase (SGOT) levels, found in some moles by Tobin (1963), were believed to result from cellular degeneration. Borek et al. (1983) suggested that urinary levels of DNA breakdown products after molar evacuation may be a useful adjunctive measure to indicate successful therapy. They found nucleosides and some DNA-derived enzymes to be elevated when active trophoblast remained after therapy. The disappearance especially of β-aminoisobutyric acid from the urine, even in the presence of persisting hCG levels, forecasts a good prognosis. Lee et al. (1981) found that circulating levels of the pregnancy-specific β_1-glycoprotein (SP-1) and placental protein 5 (PP5) were markedly reduced in patients with untreated CHM and choriocarcinoma. They suggested that this measurement was a decisive means for differentiating benign and malignant trophoblast.

The usual means for following patients with CHM is the serial determination of serum hCG levels or its β-subunits. This hormone is concentrated in molar villi, according to the studies of Sciarra (1970). He found mean values of 1524 mIU/mL in the fluid of small vesicles, and 1202 mIU/mL in the larger villi. Normal values of all hormones and secretory products of neoplastic trophoblast have been ably summarized by Clayton et al. (1981). Yedema and colleagues (1993) have constructed a gonadotropin regression curve from 130 patients with no trophoblastic sequelae after the evacuation of a molar pregnancy. They found that 71 of 77 patients with persistent trophoblastic disease could be identified from their elevated hCG levels, and in more than 50% it was possible to achieve this diagnosis within 6 weeks of operation. Khazaeli et al. (1986) suggested that the determination of a ratio between β-hCG and hCG has prognostic significance. The more malignant moles apparently produce significantly more free β-hCG units

(Khazaeli et al., 1989). Ozturk et al. (1988) found that the ratio of β-hCG to hCG fairly reliably distinguishes between normal pregnancy and CHM, and between CHM and choriocarcinoma. Presumably the hCG secretion, known to be of syncytial origin (Yorde et al., 1979; Bonduelle et al., 1988), reflects the increased quantity of syncytium in moles, rather than a qualitative change in its secretion pattern, although abnormal trophoblast appears to produce an excessive amount of β-hCG subunits. The rate of decline in β-hCG levels following delivery of moles was also summarized by Yuen (1983), a study that also included data on prolactin and estradiol secretion. In general, the β-hCG levels fall rapidly to zero within 8 weeks after evacuation. Bagshawe et al. (1986) stated that in 42% of women with CHM serum, hCG was undetectable 56 days after evacuation; none of the patients required chemotherapy. Franke et al. (1983b) determined that the average disappearance time of serum hCG after CHM was 99.3 days, after PHM 58.9 days, and after hydatid degeneration in abortuses 50.7 days. They recommended that, provided there is a continued decrease in the levels, therapy not commence before day 100 after evacuation. Human placental lactogen (hPL) levels correlated poorly with hCG levels of moles and choriocarcinomas; they were generally low (Ehnholm et al., 1967). This finding suggests that chorionepithelium is not the principal source of hPL, and that its cellular source, the X cell, has undergone little proliferation during molar development, which is borne out histologically. The interpretation of enhanced hCG secretion by moles because of increased villous (and hence trophoblastic) surface may be an oversimplification. The suggestion has been made that it relates to the expression of paternal genes. Goshen and Hochberg (1994), commenting on a paper by Fejgin et al. (1993) that studied placental hormone secretion, made these interesting comments. They suggested that high hCG values are expected in CHM because of paternal disomy 19 (the hCG locus is on that chromosome); low levels are expected (and found) in triploid PHM with **maternal** contribution of the extra haploid set.

Numerous studies have examined how the **implantation site** of moles might differ from that of normal gestation. The reader is referred to the section on X cells (see Chapter 9). In CHMs the site of implantation often shows exuberant trophoblast and, especially, placental site giant cells. They are mostly X cells (extravillous trophoblast), but syncytiotrophoblast is also present. The amount of trophoblast at the placental site may be confusing, and there may be difficulty in differentiating it from invasive choriocarcinoma. King (1956) paid special attention to the borderline lesions of gestational trophoblastic neoplasia. These lesions encompass (1) residual mole and syncytial endometritis, and (2) invasive mole (chorioadenoma destruens). To minimize the problem of recurrent disease, King advocated routine curettage after removal of a CHM.

Syncytial endometritis is not a neoplasm. It represents "a residuum of trophoblastic cells after a normal pregnancy, abortion, or hydatidiform mole" (Novak & Seah, 1954). Strictly speaking, syncytial endometritis does not contain molar villi. Also, there are no solid areas of pure trophoblast that might indicate the presence of choriocarcinoma. The placental floor in syncytial endometritis is composed of trophoblast and this is intermingled with decidual cells, with a few inflammatory cells also admixed. Its cellular composition is highly variable. This lesion is now termed exaggerated placental site. Berkowitz et al. (1982) examined the composition of the maternal floor in 11 CHM cases, specifically looking for deposits of immunoglobulins (Igs) and complement. Immunofluorescent deposits of IgG, IgM, and C3 were confined to the spiral arterioles. The authors thus concluded that CHM does not evoke "a vigorous host humoral immune response." In a later study, Kabawat et al. (1985) showed the presence of increased numbers of inflammatory cells at molar implantation sites, especially T cells with predominance of T4[+] cells. They speculated that this infiltrate relates to the development of a delayed hypersensitivity reaction, participating in rejection. In the peripheral circulation of patients with trophoblastic tumors, however, there is a significant reduction of T cells and other immunocytes (Ho et al., 1986). Ho and his colleagues discussed the immunologic significance of these findings.

Because there is no accompanying fetus in CHMs, they also lack the fetal adrenal precursors for estriol formation. They have therefore an extremely low E_3 content (Chamberlain et al., 1968). Incubation studies with dehydroisoandrosterone and other androgenic precursors indicate, however, that moles and choriocarcinoma do possess the ability to convert this steroid to estriol (MacDonald & Siiteri, 1966; Houtzager et al., 1970). From their in vivo studies with the appropriate precursors, Barlow et al. (1967) suggested that the low E_3 production may be useful for differentiating moles from normal early pregnancies.

Moles and partial moles are also frequently associated with preeclampsia. Llewellyn-Jones (1967) related this to uterine size. Eclampsia was seen at 17 weeks in a triploid pregnancy with partial molar transformation of the placenta by Slattery et al. (1993) and by Ramsey et al. (1998) at 14 weeks gestation. The existence of pregnancy-induced hypertension (PIH), however, is not a useful differential diagnostic feature for clinical differentiation between CHM and PHM. Scott (1958) reviewed this subject in context with the frequent PIH that is found in hydrops and hydramnios. He concluded that similar hormonal disturbances must exist to evoke PIH. Fatal eclampsia has occurred with molar pregnancy. Lee (1965) described a mother with a mole and severe PIH at 13 weeks' gestation. Sicuranza and Tisdall (1976) found eclampsia associated with what was apparently a PHM and with a live fetus of 125 g. Their report was similar to the case earlier described by Lloyd (1921). An increase of syncytiotrophoblastic glycogen content was observed by Arkwright et al. (1993) to exist in molar and PIH-related trophoblast. Choriocarcinomatous cells contain the most glycogen. The authors suggested that this accumulation may be a marker of "immaturity" of this cell. We have earlier alluded to the finding of altered PAI-1 expression in mole and its possible relation to PIH (Estellés et al., 1996). The relation to PIH was one of increased syncytial turnover in PIH that was observed by Chua et al. (1991).

Deportation

Molar tissue, as is true of the normal syncytium, may be transported to the lung. This deportation may occur spontaneously and during the evacuation of a molar uterus. It may cause acute pulmonary hypertension, edema, and even death. In other cases, such vascular deportation has been associated with disseminated intravascular coagulation (DIC). Benign molar tissue has even been observed to grow in the lung; hence the term **benign metastasizing mole**. This term was coined by Ring (1972), who observed two patients with isolated pulmonary nodules associated with invasive moles. Both lesions pursued a benign course. Leeder (1964) had previously described a molar pregnancy with metastatic molar tissue in lung, vagina, and vulva. All regressed spontaneously. The patient described by Johnson et al. (1979) suffered hemothorax from a pleural mole that improved only after chemotherapy. Meyer (1966) also reported a pulmonary nodule composed of molar tissue. The patient had a typical CHM with considerable trophoblastic pleomorphism. She developed the lung lesion and had persistent uterine trophoblast 7 weeks after delivery of the mole. There was an intense lymphoplasmacellular reaction at the pulmonary site. Reed et al. (1959) reported similar cases, and Bardawil et al. (1957) described a case with spontaneous regression of pulmonary metastases developing months after evacuation of a mole. They considered an immunologic rejection to have been the most likely mechanism for this regression. Mark and Moel (1961) discussed the radiologic differential diagnosis, and Hsu et al. (1962) found that deported molar metastases occurred most commonly in the pudendal tissues. These entities all fall into the broader category of invasive mole. Clinical follow-up and therapy do not differ from those of CHM that remains confined to the uterus. Although deportation of complete molar villous tissue can readily produce radiologic pulmonary lesions, the events described by Cohle and Petty (1985) and Lipp et al. (1962) are more difficult to understand. They found extensive pulmonary capillary plugging by syncytial cells and suggested that it was the cause of fatal embolism.

Syncytium normally reaches the lung of pregnant patients (Schmorl, 1905; Lee et al., 1986; see also discussion by Pool et al., 1987; Chua et al., 1991; see also Chapter 17); presumably this dissemination occurs even more readily in molar gestations (Figs. 22.11 and 22.12). Hankins et al. (1987) studied this problem with pulmonary artery catheters during mole evacuation. They found multinucleated giant cells (probable syncytium) but no villi. Moreover, there was no change in pulmonary arterial pressures or lung perfusion. Tanimura et al. (1985) identified deported trophoblast in pulmonary capillaries in nine of 10 patients who died after abortion or delivery. That this deportation of cells can be massive enough so as to occlude the pulmonary circulation remains to be shown. It is more likely that DIC occurred in these cases, as similar instances have been observed repeatedly (Beyth, 1973; Egley et al., 1975; Orr et al., 1980). Paren-

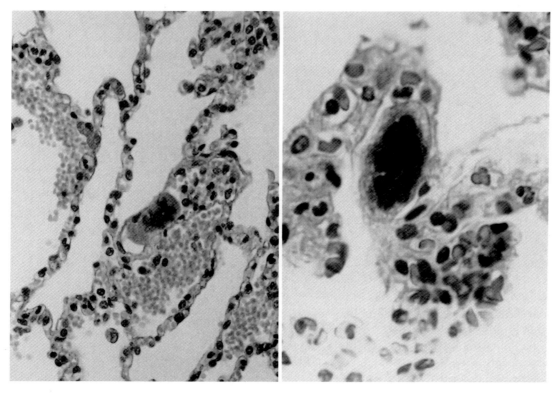

FIGURE 22.11. Syncytial trophoblast in pulmonary capillaries of maternal death at 16 weeks' gestation. H&E ×100 (left); ×260 (right).

thetically, it might be mentioned that intrauterine instillation of hypertonic saline (for attempted pregnancy termination) may be fatal to patients with hydatidiform mole (Frost, 1968). Even normal villi are deported on occasion. Figure 22.13 shows the presence of immature villi, enmeshed in coagulum, within a pulmonary artery. This was discovered at autopsy of a woman who died after traumatic disruption of the uterus during therapeutic abortion.

Chorioadenoma Destruens (Invasive Mole)

Invasive mole is a malignant neoplasm composed of infiltrating trophoblast and molar villi. The tumor invades the uterus and often the adjacent structures. It overlaps the aforementioned condition of benign metastasizing mole and the pseudotumor, later renamed placental site trophoblastic tumor (discussed in Chapter 23). Invasive mole is differentiated from true choriocarcinoma only by

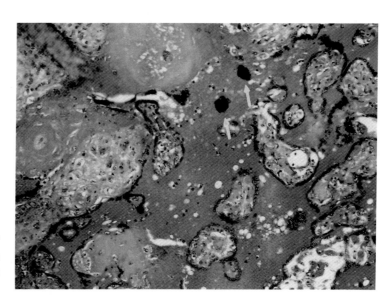

FIGURE 22.12. Term placenta with syncytial "knots" (arrows) having detached and being swept into the maternal intervillous circulation, whence they reach the maternal lung. H&E ×160.

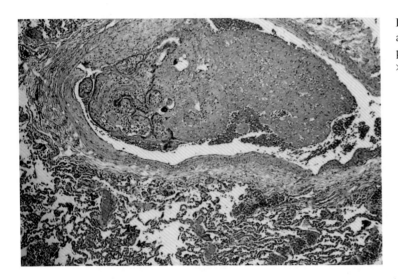

FIGURE 22.13. Pulmonary artery filled with thrombus and immature villi. They were deported during therapeutic abortion, when the uterus was perforated. H&E ×60.

the presence of villi scattered among the trophoblast. Its behavior often is also similar to that of choriocarcinoma, and usually it requires similar therapy. Perhaps it is unwise to retain this category. King (1956) placed it into his category of borderline conditions. An invasive mole is nothing more than the molar equivalent of placenta increta, and it may be as destructive. The term was coined by Ewing (1910). King distinguished three types: simple invasive mole, invasive mole with regression, and invasive mole with signs of progression. The terms speak for themselves. The prognosis is conditional on the initial nature of the mole and the efficacy of its primary removal. Figure 22.14 shows a typical case of invasive mole. The molar villi, including exuberant trophoblast, have deeply invaded the myometrium. Often this picture is combined with much more hemorrhage than is demonstrated by this particular case. Invasive moles often present challenging diagnostic and therapeutic problems. The following case illustrates it well.

A 34-year-old gravida III had vaginal bleeding at 3 months; sonographic studies at 14 weeks were suspicious but not diagnostic of mole. An amniogram at 16 weeks showed CHM, which was evacuated by suction after a single dose of methotrexate (5 mg) had been administered. The molar tissue showed much trophoblastic exuberance (Figs. 22.15 and 22.16). Methotrexate was continued for 5 more days, causing the development of oral lesions and leukopenia. The patient had serial hCG titers shown in Figure 22.17. Two pulmonary metastases were diagnosed radiologically, 2.5 months after evacuation. After five additional courses of methotrexate and two courses of actinomycin D therapy, the lung lesions faded. Six months after evacuation, the hCG levels had still not returned to normal. Three additional courses of actinomycin D were given. Arteriography was performed and found to be negative. Hysterectomy was done at this time. Serial slicing of the uterus showed a single hemorrhagic cavity (Fig. 22.18) that contained a small group of degenerated villi (Fig. 22.19), adjacent to which was intramuscular viable trophoblast with positive fluorescence by anti-hCG antibodies. The patient remained well thereafter.

Similar cases abound in the literature. Invasive moles are also known to produce late pulmonary metastases.

Such cases are well illustrated and discussed by Spademan and Tuttle (1964) and many other authors. Conservative therapy was advocated by Rubin (1964) because many of these "tumors" have an innate benign potential. There is even a report of uterine perforation by a destructive mole (Kyodo et al., 1988), but this patient also had an apparently normal fetus. It is not clear from the report, however, whether the mole was a partial molar triploid pregnancy or a twin gestation. Thiele and de Alvarez (1962) described two patients with CHM and metastases.

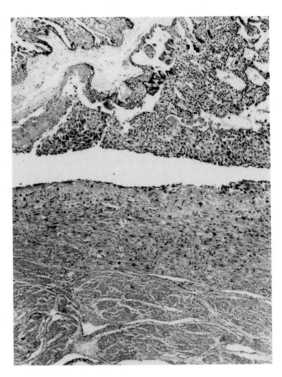

FIGURE 22.14. Invasive mole (chorioadenoma destruens) in the myometrial wall (below), showing marked trophoblastic hyperplasia. H&E ×40.

FIGURE 22.15. Molar villous surface of a patient with the invasive mole shown in Figures 22.16 to 22.18. There is moderate trophoblastic hyperplasia in an otherwise typical CHM. H&E ×100.

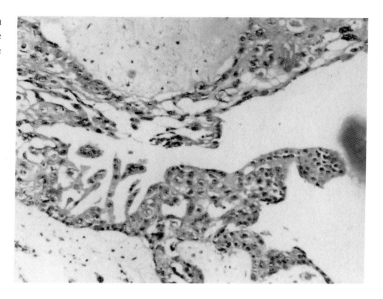

They reviewed the literature on invasive moles and secondary implants, and Thatcher et al. (1989) described the tubal equivalent of such a lesion. Most tubal pregnancies are accretas and, when they rupture, they resemble placenta percreta. The implantation of trophoblast outside the tube is therefore not surprising. These authors saw secondary peritoneal implants of trophoblast after laparoscopic salpingostomy (see also Cataldo et al., 1990). The nodules were excised and proved to be normal trophoblast; the patient recovered. Ultrastructurally, invasive moles are similar to normal placenta, CHM, and choriocarcinoma (Wynn & Harris, 1967), but the chromosomes of invasive chorionic lesions have rarely been studied. Makino et al. (1963) found invasive moles to have hyperdiploid and aneuploid chromosome numbers more frequently than CHM; choriocarcinoma was even more aneuploid.

THERAPY

The treatment of trophoblastic neoplasms has changed drastically with the introduction of methotrexate therapy in 1956 (Li et al., 1956). Li et al. recognized the specific toxicity of this agent to trophoblastic and embryonic cells because of its folic acid–inhibiting quality. It has effects in vitro as well (Sand et al., 1986) and comprises the well-known leucovorin rescue that is often used during therapy. Detailed protocols for the various trophoblastic disorders have been provided in the contributions to the Symposium on Gestational Trophoblastic Neoplasms (Goldstein & Berkowitz, 1981). This area is beyond the scope of this book. As Acosta-Sison (1964) so aptly stated already, there are changing attitudes to the management of moles, and this continues today. Early and complete evacuation is perhaps the most important aspect of successful therapy (Mathieu, 1939). When properly done, the new therapeutic regimens are nearly uniformly effective (Lurain et al., 1983; Schlaerth et al., 1988). Some patients require no therapy, and it has repeatedly been noted that metastatic lesions may disappear spontaneously. There is continued controversy as to the wisdom of prophylactic therapy for all patients with CHM (Goldstein, 1971; Kim et al., 1986). Hertz et al. (1963) showed that rigorous treatment with methotrexate

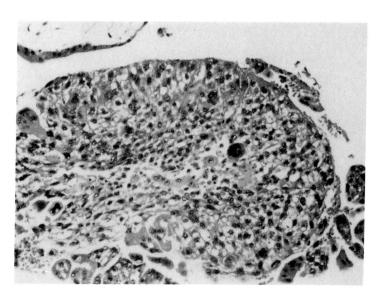

FIGURE 22.16. Same case as in Figure 22.15; invasive mole. Note the markedly "anaplastic" area of trophoblast. H&E ×100.

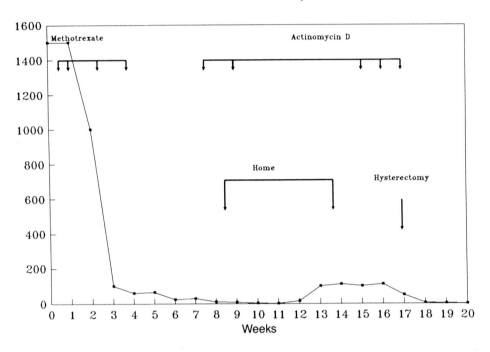

FIGURE 22.17. Course of a patient who developed pulmonary metastases and invasive mole after evacuation of an intrauterine mole (see text). The mole is shown in Figures 22.15 and 22.16 and the chorioadenoma destruens in Figures 22.18 and 22.19.

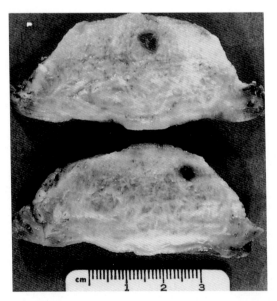

FIGURE 22.18. Same patient as in Figures 22.15 to 22.17. The hysterectomy specimen shown here had a small subendometrial hemorrhagic cavity containing molar tissue.

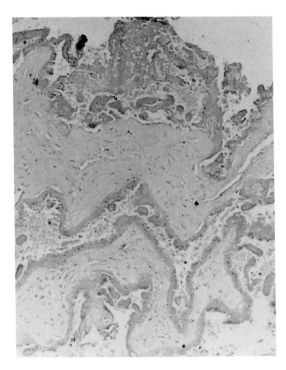

FIGURE 22.19. Invasive mole of the patient in Figures 22.15 to 22.18. Note the largely degenerated villi and trophoblast. H&E ×40.

and actinomycin D is generally completely successful when metastases develop. Kashimura et al. (1986) suggested that the recurrence rate of trophoblastic disease is between 5.7% and 26.0%. These investigators followed 420 patients with CHM, 293 of whom were given prophylactic methotrexate (10mg for 7 days). There was a significant improvement of those receiving therapy (7.5% versus 18.1%), and it was more marked in older patients.

The surveillance of molar cases after evacuation with serial hCG levels is a convenient way to ensure success. It must be reemphasized, however, that the exclusion of PHM cases from therapeutic regimens is mandatory. Such patients are most easily identified with routine flow cytometry on the initial specimen. Hysterectomy is now rarely necessary. Moreover, appropriate chemotherapy is compatible with future fertility (Song et al., 1988). What has been controversial, though, is which pregnancies should be screened for possible GTD sequelae. Because early CHM cannot be diagnosed reliably and because 15% of CHMs and 0.5% of PHMs are followed by neoplasias, M.J. Sebire et al. (2004) have suggested that all pregnancy terminations (for whatever reason) should be screened for possible GTDs.

Ectopic Moles

The occurrence of moles in the fallopian tube and ovary has been described and it includes tubal rupture (Westerhout, 1964); indeed the occurrence of placental site nodules has been reported in the fallopian tube (Muto et al., 1991; Nayer et al., 1996). Data from the older literature are not necessarily convincing, however, because of the possible presence of a PHM among these reports. Pettit (1941) reviewed 42 cases of tubal moles and choriocarcinomas and reported a new case with good outcome. Sze et al. (1988) described a patient who had an intrauterine "molar pregnancy" 2 months after salpingostomy for tubal ectopic pregnancy. The mole was accompanied by a malformed fetus. It was a partial mole, most likely a triploid conceptus. The authors believed this report to be the first description of such a combination of implantations. The case is important because it highlights the care one must exercise when reviewing the topic. Although listed as "molar" pregnancy, the text clearly described it to be a PHM. It is also acknowledged that the excessive levels of hCG in this patient (467,000mIU/mL) are not helpful in the differential diagnosis between CHM and PHM. Other examples of triploid PHM in the tube abound in the literature, as for instance the case of Montgomery et al. (1993).

On rare occasions, a hydatidiform mole is believed to have originated in the ovary. Jock et al. (1981) described the sixth such reported case and estimated that this condition occurs perhaps only once in 50 million pregnancies. They also reviewed the literature. Their patient, a 27-year-old primigravida, was admitted for evacuation of a sonographically evident intrauterine mole at 12 weeks' gestation. The uterus, however, was found to be empty. The mole was present within a 14-cm ovarian mass. No postoperative chemotherapy was needed. Of interest was the extensive pseudodecidual change found on the omental surface. The case described by Stanhope et al.

(1983) resulted in a benign outcome following local resection. Yenen et al. (1965), who described and illustrated a similar case, removed the uterus. In retrospect, this surgery seems to have been unnecessary.

Partial Hydatidiform Mole

Macroscopically, the usual CHM has an almost uniform distribution of hydatid villi, the placenta is much enlarged and remnants of fetal capillaries or other embryonic remnants are exceptionally rare. There are, however, molar specimens in which only a portion of the placenta is hydropically altered, the so-called PHM. These moles are also more often associated with fetuses. Atkin and Klinger (1962) were the first to correlate triploidy with this type of molar change. Sporadic reports followed (Schlegel et al., 1966). It was Carr (1971), however, who first established that "85% of triploid and hypertriploid embryos showed hydatidiform degeneration or mole." Subsequently, Vassilakos et al. (1977) drew sharp attention to the entity that we now know as PHM. They clearly distinguished it from the CHM. In a series of 811 spontaneous and 1097 induced abortions, they found 75 placentas with gross villous swelling, most of which showed chromosomal anomalies, primarily triploidy and trisomy 16. None had marked trophoblastic dysplasia, and all had a good outcome. The diagnosis of PHM is not always correctly established by pathologic criteria, as the studies with flow cytometry and DNA fingerprinting have shown (see Takahashi et al., 1990). Therefore, one must be cautious in interpreting the data from many series that have been published in the past. Moreover, there are numerous exceptional cases, mosaics, and chimeras, and also theoretical considerations of the unusual centrosome behavior of triploids that warrant better explanations for these errors of fertilization. They are cogently discussed in a large contribution by Golubovsky (2003) that needs to be studied in detail. He states, "Dispermic zygotes, in contrast to digynic ones, are characterized by (a) cytogenetic phenomenon described here as postzygotic diploidization of triploids (PDT)," and he then produces examples that would explain the mixoploids and other unusual findings that have been reported in the past. One such aberrant case was studied by Zhang et al. (2000). A normal male fetus (46,XY) was associated with a placenta that was admixed (diploid/triploid) in whose hydropic villi fetal blood was circulating. Genetic study showed that this was not a chimera, as both diploid and triploid markers were identical. Makrydimas et al. (2002) also described an unusual mole. This term female singleton gestation also had a placenta with diffusely intermixed hydropic villi. Amazingly, the genetic study showed that all cells had a monospermic origin, and the neonate was diploid and biparental, but the hydatid villi were androgenetic and monospermic. The authors referred to this as confined placental mosaicism.

Vassilakos and Kajii (1976) coined the phrase "hyda-tidiform mole, two entities." This observation was immediately confirmed, and PHM is now well established as a distinct entity. Szulman and Surti (1978a,b) have made many contributions to delineate this placental abnormality. All but three of their initial 12 cases had an associated fetus. There was often a striking elevation of hCG levels, but these levels dropped rapidly after delivery. These authors emphatically stated that there is no transition between mole types and that the older term *transitional mole* is inappropriate. One of their cases of PHM with 46,XX and fetal parts is of interest. Its true nature remains unknown, but it served to caution that these designations are not watertight syndromes. It should be pointed out that not all triploid conceptuses have elevated hCG titers. Fejgin et al. (1992) suggested that placental insufficiency may be one cause of such low levels, and Morrish et al. (1992) felt that PHMs have an impaired facility of hormone production in response to stimulants.

The **morphology of PHM** is variable, and it is also dependent on the genotype. The villi of PHM are much more irregularly swollen than those of CHM, and many normal villi may intervene among grossly molar tissue. Cisternae may be present but they are also generally less common than is true for CHM. The more important feature for the differential diagnosis is the very frequent presence of villous capillary remnants (Fig. 22.20). Many of these contain fetal red blood cells, even though the fetus may have died or was not recognized in the specimen received. There is generally much less, and usually only focal, trophoblastic hyperplasia. The villous covering is frequently scalloped, and villous inclusions of tropho-blast (tangentially cut surfaces) are common (Fig. 22.21). Most investigators have suggested that these trophoblas-tic inclusions are found only in triploids, but that is somewhat contrary to our experience. We find trophoblastic

inclusions occasionally even in normal immature placentas and certainly in other chromosomally abnormal abortuses (see also Novak et al., 1988, and Chapter 21). Therefore, we do no use this criterion as an important feature for the diagnosis of PHM. These inclusions are sometimes quite large and have been beautifully demonstrated in color pictures by Kliman and Segel (2003). They suggested that the included trophoblast derives by cytotrophoblast absorption and provided a theoretical model. A particularly useful review contribution by Sebire et al. (2002a) describes the morphologic characteristics of the two types of moles and hydatid changes in abortion specimens. Although the authors suggested that the differential diagnosis of the nature of the lesion can usually be made by morphologic criteria alone, the use of ancillary techniques in questionable cases is advocated (Genest, 2001). Szulman et al. (1981) reviewed cytogenetically verified triploid abortuses and found that 86% of them had placentas that could be classified as PHM. Their fetuses tended to have died by the eighth week of pregnancy, but uterine retention was commonly longer than for other chromosomally aberrant conceptuses.

Szulman and Surti (1982) estimated from a hospital population that CHM occurs in 1 of 1330 pregnancies and PHM in 1 of 1730 pregnancies. All types of triploidy arise in approximately 1% of recognized human pregnancies for as yet unknown reasons. Berkowitz et al. (1995) recognized that it occurred more often in women with irregular cycles and oral contraceptive usage, and that dietary factors played no role in the etiology of PHM. Jacobs et al. (1982) reported that most triploids are due to the fertilization with two paternal genomes (dispermy). Only 1% to 3% eventuate in a molar pregnancy (Lawler et al., 1979). The analysis of 106 triploid specimens by Jacobs et al. (1982) is especially interesting. The extra haploid set of chromosomes was of paternal origin (androgenetic)

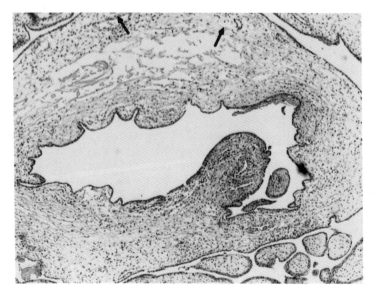

FIGURE 22.20. Histologic appearance of villi of triploid partial hydatidiform mole (PHM) at 12 weeks' gestation. Note the irregular size of the villi and the minimal amount of trophoblast. Remnants of atrophying fetal capillaries are present (arrows). There is early cisterna formation of villi between arrows and prominent infolding (scalloping) of villi. H&E ×65.

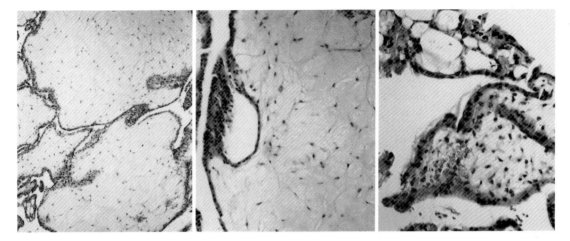

FIGURE 22.21. Partial (triploid) hydatidiform mole with extensive edema and prominent infolding (scalloping) of the minimally hyperplastic trophoblast. This infolding leads to the histologic appearance of trophoblast islands within edematous villi. There is much syncytial cisterna dilatation at right. H&E ×60 (left); ×120 (center); ×260 (right).

in 51 cases; it was maternally derived (gynogenetic) in 15. The former gestations lasted longer (122 days) than the latter (74 days). This difference may explain, in part, why paternally derived triploid conceptuses are concentrated among the PHMs, as it takes time for grossly visible villous swelling to come about. The studies of Uchida and Freeman (1985) gave similar results. There is evidence that molar villous swelling only gradually takes place and makes early sonographic diagnosis, for instance, difficult (Jauniaux et al., 1997). For that reason, most triploid abortions escape detection unless cytogenetic analysis is done. Ohama and his collaborators (1986) investigated the chromosome status of 56 partial moles. They found that 46 were triploid, and nine were diploid. The diploid moles lacked trophoblastic hyperplasia and stromal inclusions (Fig. 22.22). Importantly, four of these nine diploid PHMs had chromosomal heteromorphisms. In other words, they were not androgenetic, as is typical for the diploid CHM. Although most partial moles are triploid, a few are not. McFadden et al. (1994) found different origins of the extra set of chromosomes. They identified more cases of digyni rather than the former prevalent diandry. All PHM were diandric triploids, whereas only one of four diandrics developed PHM. Similarly, in a large study by Zaragoza et al. (2000), most PHMs were found to have a diandric origin; but the authors caution

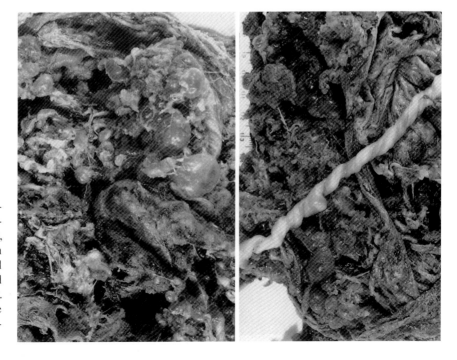

FIGURE 22.22. Possible partial hydatidiform mole with diploid, 46,XX, and homozygous karyotype on C banding. A 720–g, 24 weeks' gestation, female infant with renal dysplasia resulted with neonatal death. The placenta weighed 1460 g and had scattered molar vesicles throughout. The umbilical cord was normal, and there was virtually no trophoblastic proliferation. Maternal outcome was good.

that only a small portion of triploid conceptuses eventuates in PHMs, indicating that the mere presence of two paternal genomes is not sufficient for molar development. Of parenthetic interest is that Hasegawa et al. (1999) described a digynic nonmosaic female triploid infant who survived for 46 days. The small immature neonate had numerous congenital anomalies, including the characteristic digital fusions. Of four previous survivors they summarized, only one was diandric. Philipp et al. (2004) studied the embryos of triploids by embryoscopy and showed their early marked developmental abnormalities when associated with partial moles.

The important question arises whether there is a possibly different prognosis for these groups. Davis et al. (1987), who analyzed ploidy by flow cytometry in 35 assumed PHMs, unexpectedly found that six (17%) were triploid and 29 (83%) were diploid. These investigators did not find any complications in the triploid group, but five (17%) of the diploid cases had nonfatal sequelae. Examples of these complications included the need for recurettage and chemotherapy. Teng and Ballon (1984) described three patients with mole and a coexisting fetus. The patients had persistent hCG elevations and two required chemotherapy. This report has been criticized by Szulman and Surti (1985), who considered these cases to be DZ twin gestations and urged that stricter criteria be employed in reporting these conditions.

Some reports have emphasized the existence of preeclampsia with PHM, and that ovarian theca lutein cysts may complicate PHM (Lewis & Cefalo, 1979). These cystic changes of molar and partial molar placentas have been recognized sonographically (Harper & MacVicar, 1963; Bendon et al., 1988; Jauniaux et al., 1996). Several investigators have studied hCG levels in CHMs and compared them with those in PHMs. Smith et al. (1984) found that, after evacuation of the uterus, the hCG levels disappeared similarly quickly, but that the levels found immediately after evacuation were significantly higher in CHM. Berkowitz et al. (1989), in a detailed analysis of the various gonadotropin moieties, found the following in maternal serum: CHMs had higher levels of β-hCG than PHMs, but the latter had higher α-hCG levels; both moles had higher levels of both subunit levels than did comparable normal pregnancies (see also Khazaeli et al., 1986). Markedly elevated α-fetoprotein levels were present in two patients with PHM and triploidy (Kazazian et al., 1989), something that does not happen in CHM.

The **natural history of PHM** has been evaluated by several authors, especially with emphasis on possible malignant sequelae. Czernobilsky et al. (1982) found no untoward outcome in 25 PHMs. Berkowitz et al. (1983b) followed 81 patients with PHM. Serum hCG levels exceeded 100,000 mIU/mL in only two patients. Eight of their patients (9.9%) developed nonmetastatic trophoblastic disease that was successfully treated with metho-

trexate. In six of eight patients, residual molar tissue was found on curettage; there were no choriocarcinomas. One possible exception in the large experience with partial moles is the case of Looi and Sivanesaratnam (1981). The patient in their study was said to have developed a choriocarcinoma following a partial mole. Kohorn (1986) has questioned the need for this (premature) intervention with chemotherapy. There are very few reports that have verified true trophoblastic neoplasia to occur following partial moles, an important point made in the report by Heifetz and Czaja (1992). Their 69,XXX gestation with fetus had a nodule of what would appear to be choriocarcinoma in situ. But the postpartum course was entirely benign. Szulman et al. (1981) did a retrospective study of 13 PHM patients from Hong Kong. One, a case of invasive (partial) mole, required chemotherapy. In our opinion, the case was one of placenta increta of a triploid specimen, not true trophoblastic neoplasia. Gaber et al. (1986) reported a similar case. PHM may recur (Honoré, 1987; Honoré et al., 1988). We believe that when the diagnosis of triploidy is truly established for a PHM, then a complete evacuation generally cures the patient. Bagshawe and his colleagues (1990) undertook a study of 11 patients whose condition had been originally diagnosed as PHM and whose course was complicated by gestational trophoblastic tumor. DNA analysis led to revision of PHM to CHM in four cases, and two cases had been incorrectly diagnosed as complete moles but were not. These authors suggested that four patients required chemotherapy, although their last pregnancy was a triploid PHM. No proof is provided, however, that these lesions were choriocarcinomas, and it was also not discussed how far the GTD had spread. Little doubt, however, can be expressed when the study of Seckl et al. (2000) is read. They reviewed 3000 patients with partial moles of whom 15 required chemotherapy for persisting GTD; three eventuated in choriocarcinomas. Lawler et al. (1991), who studied 202 molar specimens (51 PHM with 44 triploids; 149 CHM with 105 diploid, one haploid[!], one triploid), saw no need for chemotherapy in any of their PHMs. Other reports should be consulted concerning the persistence of trophoblastic disease after partial moles, such as Rice et al. (1990) and Muto et al. (1991). Forrester and Merz (2003) did a survey of triploidy in a population from Hawaii (1986–1999) and identified 38 cases. Of these, 31 were early fetal deaths; 39% were XXX, 58% XXY, and 3% XYY. The maternal consequences were not detailed and advanced maternal age was found, contrary to earlier reports, but the authors admitted a possible bias for chromosome studies at that age group.

Differential Diagnosis

Distinguishing the various entities discussed here constitutes a continuous challenge for the practicing pathologist. Thus, it must first be stated that completely satisfactory methods do not exist, but some practical steps are possible. The pathologist must recognize that even CHMs may start out as small placentas with an appearance of spontaneous abortuses that possess hydatid changes; they may even have diminutive embryos. Further, partial moles are not all triploid and some chromosomally abnormal (trisomics, not triploid) and aborted specimens may have some cystic, molar villi. How then to proceed?

Our suggestion is to proceed as follows, if the tools are available: If a fetus is present with a mole, examine its fingers for possible fusions (suggesting triploidy with imprinting). Stain the slides with antibodies to the commercially available p57: Normal specimens (abortions) show expression by strong nuclear staining of trophoblast and mesenchymal tissue. Complete moles show no expression, whereas PHMs may show minimal to moderate expression (Jun et al., 2003; Romaguera et al., 2004). If the results are not completely satisfactory, perform flow cytometry for ploidy; this can even be done from paraffin-embedded tissues. Ideally, chromosome preparations are made for complete resolution of the diagnosis; this is most helpful in cases with possible mosaicism or twinning, but it requires fresh tissue and considerable effort.

Mesenchymal Dysplasia

This entity is only marginally related to PHMs, but it needs discussion and bears some connection to partial moles with which it may be confused, especially sonographically. Moscoso et al. (1991) and then Jaunieux et al. (1997) described the entity perhaps first as representing placentas that were markedly enlarged with what appeared to be an excess of mesenchyma, although they then referred to somewhat similar cases from the older literature. A most typical case was described by Ohyama and colleagues (2000) of a 26-year-old Japanese gravida I whose 46,XX fetus died at 34 weeks with growth restriction (1516 g). The placenta was large (1050 g) and was mostly composed of enlarged villi with a "myxoid stroma" and decreased, occasionally obliterated fetal blood vessels. Thrombi were found in some surface vessels but the trophoblast appeared to be normal and the term **pseudo-partial mole with angiomatous proliferation** was coined. Remarkably, some of the surface vessels were massively enlarged and "noodle-like," and many were thrombosed. The authors gathered 17 cases of similar nature from the literature and added 15 cases of placentas associated with the Beckwith-Wiedemann syndrome (BWS) because there are significant similarities at least in the placental manifestations (Chapter 24). This is especially true because in some areas there was significant vascular proliferation that bordered on chorangiomas. The vascular abnormalities, also described as "cirsoid aneurysms" (Chapter 12), resemble two placentas

described by Zhang and Benirschke (2000; see Fig. 22.27). Their fetal karyotypes were also diploid and similar histologic placental features were then described. Paradinas et al. (2001) identified 15 cases in their database, and cautioned that some had been labeled partial moles, which was incorrect. The same is true of a case described by Matsui et al. (2003) in which the BWS was specifically excluded. The most recent description of a case of mesenchymal dysplasia is by Gibson et al. (2004), also with normal 46,XY karyotype. Prenatally, cysts had been seen in the placenta; the 3250-g infant delivered at 39 weeks, and the placenta weighed 1258 g and had numerous cysts, normal villi, and intervillous thrombi. Interestingly, the neonate had a vascular hamartoma of the face and ptosis. The combination of fetal angioma and chorangioma is common; perhaps these placentas then relate mostly to an angiomatous malformation. Their vascular growth factors thus need to be studied. The precise pathogenesis of this seemingly specific placental abnormality needs much further study, especially with a genetic evaluation of the chromosomal region that defines BWS (11p15.5) and its possibly altered methylation status. It should be emphasized, though, that these cases in no way relate to the so-called association of Breus' mole in PHM as was described by Kim et al. (2002). We believe that their interpretation is correct, namely that the subchorionic tuberous hematomas, which they found to be composed of mostly maternal blood, were the result of sluggish intervillous blood return and that they antedated fetal demise.

Complete Mole and Fetus

There have been numerous reports of molar pregnancies with associated fetuses, and Malinowski et al. (1995) referred to this as the "sad-fetus syndrome," implying that there exists a continuum of moles to choriocarcinoma. Care must be exercised in the differential diagnosis of this condition. Although it is often assumed that the coexistence of a fetus with a molar placenta implies the diagnosis of partial mole, DNA analysis negates this often. Thus, Choi-Hong et al. (1995) studied nine pregnancies of this kind and found in eight cases normal placentas with FISH study for X and Y chromosomes; four had Y signals in the normal tissue and X signals in the moles, implying dizygosity and CHM in at least these rare cases. Popek (1994) who studied 10 cases of CHM with a twin fetus indicated the incidence to be 1:10,000 gestations, the majority being triploid specimens. But CHM with a twin fetus does exist and was estimated to be as uncommon as 1:250,000. Such fetuses occasionally survive, and the situation warrants answers to the following precise questions: Are these truly triploid gestations, or are they DZ twins with one being a CHM or a PHM, and the other a normal conceptus (Fig. 22.23)? The differential diagno-

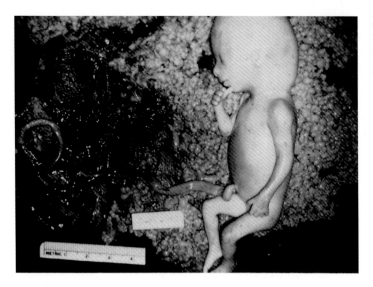

FIGURE 22.23. Mole with "living coexisting fetus." It is most likely a triploid conceptus: a male fetus, 9-cm crown–rump (CR) length, nearly completely molar change of placenta.

sis of these cases is often uncertain from macroscopic review alone, and frequently it cannot be reconstructed from the published reports. Moreover, is it possible that such gestations will become more common as artificial reproductive technology (ART) is practiced commonly now in older women? The case presented by Wax et al. (2003) suggests this possibility. It was the product of IVF with sperm donation in a 41-year-old woman; and Amr et al. (2000) found a triplet gestation from ART with normal male and female newborns plus a complete, androgenetic mole. Another unsuccessful usage of IVF/ART in a patient with habitual abortion and two triploid conceptuses was related by Bar-Ami et al. (2003). Abnormal ova and sperm as well as fertilization products were identified in this relatively young couple (30 and 29 years). The largest series of CHM with DZ twin comes from Sebire et al. (2002b), who had 77 cases in their registry. (Interestingly, there is a United Kingdom Web site for mole: www.hmole-chorio.org.uk). According to their data, 60% of women who decided not to terminate the gestation lost the fetus in utero or had a complete pregnancy loss; 19% developed GTDs, not an increased frequency over that of the usual CHMs (16%). The natural history of eight well-documented cases of apparent CHM and coexisting fetus was described by Steller et al. (1994). These authors also analyzed the literature of this topic and found that the presence of a fetus often led to the sonographic (mis)diagnosis of PHM. They performed flow cytometry and found that five of these eight patients developed persistent trophoblastic disease that required chemotherapy. In other cases, the characteristic pattern of fetal anomalies allows identification of triploidy, especially the digital fusions. Not only is there a rich literature on the frequency of triploidy in spontaneous abortuses, but numerous cases have delineated the various anomalies occurring in liveborn infants with triploidy (e.g. Uher

et al., 1963; Beischer et al., 1967; Goecke, 1967; Butler et al., 1969; Schmickel et al., 1971; deGrouchy et al., 1974; Niebuhr, 1974; Fraikor et al., 1980; Graham et al., 1989). In some of these cases, the infant was living (Crooij et al., 1985) and the outcome was otherwise not complicated by trophoblastic sequelae. It is noteworthy that the placenta of some large triploid fetuses has not included hydatid changes. Fetus and placenta are also often growth-retarded, and a single umbilical artery is common. Absent umbilical artery diastolic flow has been reported in them (Sherer et al., 1993). It would be interesting to correlate the phenotypes of placentas with paternal/maternal sets of chromosomal contributions. The present belief is that, with triploidy, two paternal chromosome sets more often lead to PHM than do two maternal sets of chromosomes, which is more characterized by malformed fetuses. Some cases of PHM with fetus have been diploid, with a normal heterozygotic chromosome set (Kubo et al., 1986). Feinberg et al. (1988) reported such a case (46,XX) that was diagnosed sonographically. The fetus was hydropic but did not have any congenital anomalies. Urbanski et al. (1996) reported a normal diploid twin pregnancy associated with a tetraploid hydatidiform mole. Following the spontaneous passage of molar tissue, premature delivery was accomplished by cesarean section; the patient developed no persistent trophoblastic disease. A normal male embryo (25 g) was found associated with a CHM, reported by Al-Takroni et al. (1994). Following delivery the mother developed a choriocarcinoma, successfully treated with methotrexate. In a study of six patients with molar pregnancy and fetus or embryo studied by van de Kaa et al. (1995), two patients developed persistent disease, which led the authors to recommend special vigilance in their follow-up. They employed DNA probes for specific chromosomal regions to make the differential diagnosis and found frequent polyploidy and trophoblastic hyperplasia in the molar components of the placentas. In four of their well-described six cases the 46,XY constitution of the fetuses declared dizygosity.

We described above a relevant case, diagnosed as partially hydropic placenta sonographically. The pregnancy ended with a normal female surviving infant. Approximately half of the enlarged placenta (see Fig. 22.1) was molar and the other half was normal. Flow cytometry indicated tetraploidy of the molar portion, and diploidy of the normal, and PCR done on paraffin-embedded tissue showed similar DNA constitution of the two components; thus, the genomic origin of the two components was the same. The vascular tissue of these tetraploid villi was diploid. Of the two interpretations, we prefer to think that this was a monozygotic twin with tetraploidization of one, followed by fetal demise. The perfusion by one twin's blood vessels would thus not be unusual, as anastomoses between monochorionic twins is common. Assuredly, these were not DZ twins with one being triploid, and this was not a partial mole in the usual sense. Gonadotropin titers remained normal in mother and neonate.

Partial Hydatidiform Mole with Twin Gestation

The occurrence of a macroscopically PHM with a fetus always raises the question of triploidy; alternatively, there is a possibility of a twin pregnancy when not the entire placenta shows hydatidiform changes. The complex topic is discussed in some detail by Vejerslev et al. (1991), who described five pregnancies in a woman who had four consecutive molar pregnancies. The one that was associated with the fetus was a biparental diploid mole, which they considered to constitute a distinct and separate entity. Most cases turn out to be singleton pregnancies. There are many reports, however, in which one normal placenta and fetus was present with a molar placenta. The assumption is often made that all of the cases are DZ gestations. The fact that some of them were later complicated by choriocarcinoma (Hohe et al., 1971) indicates that at least some of the moles may have been typical CHM. Table 22.2 summarizes the major reports describing such twin gestations, and a typical case is shown in Figures 22.24 to 22.26. Beischer and Fortune (1968) used the sex chromatin method (Barr bodies) to approach the nature of karyotypes in their early studies of this phenomenon. They delineated a number of twin gestations, wherein one was normal and the other molar. Important summaries of large series of moles with coexisting fetuses are those by Beischer (1966) and Vejerslev et al. (1986). They contain several cases of verified twin gestations and can be consulted for details. Nugent and his colleagues (1996) reported on a twin pregnancy, one a normal 46,XX and with a normal placenta, the other 69, XXY with PHM. Selective termination of the triploid fetus at 15 weeks was followed by the development of severe preeclampsia that necessitated termination at 19 weeks. They made the point that placental growth and PIH are not prevented by elimination of the triploid embryo. How complex such cases can be is shown in the case reported by us (Benirschke et al., 2000). The placenta was sharply divided into a normal organ (with normal, surviving fetus) and a typical CHM, which, however, had still perfused vessels. DNA analysis showed tetraploidy of the molar connective tissue, but euploidy of the perfusing vessels. This indicated to us that a formerly normal monozygotic (MZ) twin gestation was changed into this con-

TABLE 22.2. Twin pregnancies, one a molar gestation

Author	Year	Fetus	Mole	Outcome
Krone	1955	3200 g, ♀, live	Separate	Twin family; good; review
Logan	1957	16 weeks	Separate	Good
Beischer	1961	36 weeks, ♂, live	Separate	Good
		39 weeks, ♀, live	Separate	Good; 13 cases diffuse
Chamberlain	1963	18 weeks, ♂	Separate, ♀	Good
Hohe et al.	1971	1975 g, ♂, live	Attached, separate	Choriocarcinoma
Jones & Lauersen	1975	2900 g, ♀	Fused	Good
		13 weeks, ♀	?Fused	Needed chemotherapy
Suzuki et al.	1980	1425 g, ♀	Separate	Good; review of cases
Yee et al.	1982	910 g, ♂ died	Separate	Needed chemotherapy
Block & Merrill	1982	1850 g, ♂, live	Separate	Barr body-negative mole
		2020 g, ♂, live	Fused	Barr body-negative mole
Sande & Eyjolfsson	1985	22 weeks, ♂	Separate	Good
		Dead fetus	Separate	Good
Khoo et al.	1986	2000 g, ♂, live	Fused	Review of 23 cases
Vejerslev et al.	1986	22 weeks, ♀, dead	Separate	Mole androgenetic; review
Benirschke et al.	1999	Resorbed	Fused	Good
Wax et al.	2003	2520 g, 36 weeks, ♂	Separate	Good
Gul et al.	2004	2 diagn. @ 11 and 14 weeks	Abstract only	Good

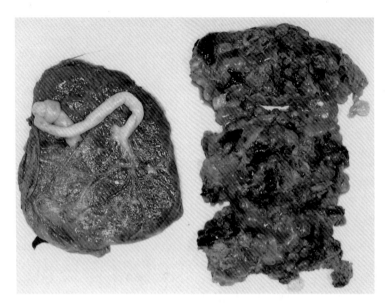

FIGURE 22.24. Twin with mole. The patient was a 24–year-old woman who had had three pregnancies, one ending in abortion. Her course was benign until 32 weeks, when she delivered a 1900-g boy who did well. There was a normal 330-g placenta and separate 780-g complete, Barr body-positive hydatidiform mole (see Fig. 22.25).

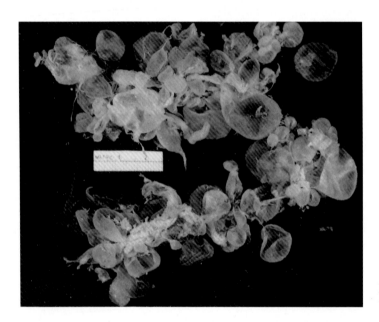

FIGURE 22.25. Molar villi of Figure 22.24 show typical, uniform villous swelling.

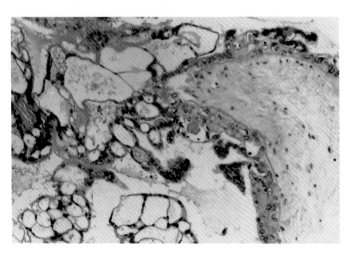

FIGURE 22.26. Histologic appearance of twin's mole in Figures 22.24 and 22.25. There is moderate trophoblastic hyperplasia and, especially, proliferation of cytotrophoblast, rarely seen in PHM. H&E ×400.

FIGURE 22.27. This is another example of a placenta with apparently molar transformation of one third of its villi. The reason for the latter, however, was extensive aneurysmal dilatation with thrombosis and infarction of surface vessels (see text).

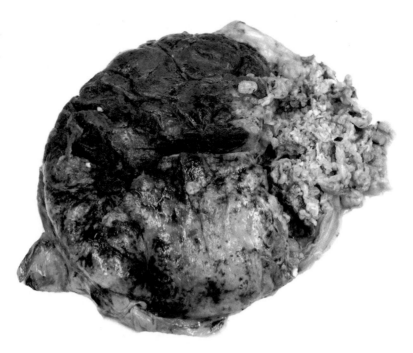

figuration by polyploidization of one embryo (who was then lost) but whose placenta had already developed anastomoses to the surviving twin (see Fig. 22.1). Another observation of a placenta with apparently fused molar mass indicates how complex the differential diagnosis may be. Figure 22.27 shows a placenta from a severely growth-restricted fetus (1300 g at 31 weeks' gestation) whose problems were due to extensive aneurysmal distentions with thrombosis of surface vessels ("cirsoid aneurysms"). Portions of the villous tissue showed typical molar changes but were genetically found to be of the fetus' origin (Zhang & Benirschke, 2000). Thus, a twin pregnancy was excluded.

References

Acosta-Sison, H.: Changing attitudes in the management of hydatidiform mole. Amer. J. Obstet. Gynecol. **88**:634–636, 1964.

Al-Takroni, A.M., Mendis, K.B.L. and Agrawal, S.: Twin pregnancy consisting of a complete hydatidiform mole and a fetus. Ann. Saudi Med. **14**:519–520, 1994.

Ambrani, L.M., Vaidya, R.A., Rao, C.S., Daftary, S.D. and Motashaw, N.D.: Familial occurrence of trophoblastic disease—report of recurrent molar pregnancies in sisters in three families. Clin. Genet. **18**:27–29, 1980.

Amir, S.M., Osathanondh, R., Berkowitz, R.S. and Goldstein, D.P.: Human chorionic gonadotropin and thyroid function in patients with hydatidiform mole. Amer. J. Obstet. Gynecol. **150**:723–728, 1984.

Amr, M.F., Fisher, R.A., Foskett, M.A. and Paradinas, F.J.: Triplet pregnancy with hydatidiform mole. Intern. J. Gynecol. Cancer **10**:76–81, 2000.

Anonymous: Editorial: flow cytometry and gestational trophoblastic disease. Lancet **2**:950, 1987.

Arkwright, P.D., Rademacher, T.W., Dwek, R.A. and Redman, C.W.G.: Pre-eclampsia is associated with an increase in trophoblast glycogen content and glycogen synthase activity, similar to that found in hydatidiform moles. J. Clin. Invest. **91**:2744–2753, 1993.

Atkin, N.B. and Klinger, H.P.: The superfemale mole. Lancet **2**:727, 1962.

Atrash, H.K., Hogue, C.J.R. and Grimes, D.A.: Epidemiology of hydatidiform mole during early gestation. Amer. J. Obstet. Gynecol. **154**:906–909, 1986.

Azuma, C., Saji, F., Tokugawa, Y., Kimura, T., Nobunaga, T., Takemura, M., Kameda, T. and Tanizawa, O.: Application of gene amplification by polymerase chain reaction to genetic analysis of molar mitochondrial DNA: the detection of anuclear empty ovum as the cause of complete mole. Gynecol. Oncol. **40**:29–33, 1991.

Bae, S.N., Kim, S.J.: Telomerase activity in complete hydatidiform mole. Amer. J. Obstet. Gynecol. **180**:328–333, 1999.

Baergen, R.N., Kelly, T., McGinnis, M.J., Jones, O.W. and Benirschke, K.: Complete hydatidiform mole with a coexisting embryo. Hum. Pathol. **27**:731–734, 1996.

Baggish, M.S., Woodruff, J.D., Tow, S.H. and Jones, H.W.: Sex chromatin pattern in hydatidiform mole. Amer. J. Obstet. Gynecol. **102**:362–370, 1968.

Bagshawe, K.D., Dent, J. and Webb, J.: Hydatidiform mole in England and Wales 1973–1983. Lancet **2**:673–677, 1986.

Bagshawe, K.D., Lawler, S.D., Paradinas, F.J., Dent, J., Brown, P. and Boxer, G.M.: Gestational trophoblastic tumours following initial diagnosis of partial hydatidiform mole. Lancet **335**:1074–1076, 1990.

Bandy, L.C., Clarke-Pearson, D.L. and Hammond, C.B.: Malignant potential of gestational trophoblastic disease at the extreme ages of reproductive life. Obstet. Gynecol. **64**:395–399, 1984.

Bar-Ami, S., Seibel, M.M., Pierce, K.E. and Zilberstein, M.: Pre-implantation genetic diagnosis for a couple with recurrent pregnancy loss and triploidy. Birth Def. Res. **67A**:946–950, 2003.

Bardawil, W.A., Hertig, A.T. and Velardo, J.T.: Regression of trophoblast. I. Hydatidiform mole; a case of unusual features, possibly metastasis and regression; review of literature. Obstet. Gynecol. **10**:614–625, 1957.

Barlow, J.J., Goldstein, D.P. and Reid, D.E.: A study of in vivo estrogen biosynthesis and production rates in normal pregnancy, hydatidiform mole and choriocarcinoma. J. Clin. Endocrinol. Metab. **27**:1028–1034, 1967.

Barton, S.C., Surani, M.A.H. and Norris, M.L.: Role of paternal and maternal genomes in mouse development. Nature **311**: 374–376, 1984.

Beischer, N.A.: Hydatidiform mole with co-existent foetus. J. Obstet. Gynaecol. Brit. Commonw. **68**:231–237, 1961.

Beischer, N.A.: Hydatidiform mole with coexistent foetus. Aust. N.Z. J. Obstet. Gynaecol. **6**:127–141, 1966.

Beischer, N.A. and Fortune, D.W.: Significance of chromatin patterns in cases of hydatidiform mole with an associated fetus. Amer. J. Obstet. Gynecol. **100**:276–282, 1968.

Beischer, N.A., Fortune, D.W. and Fitzgerald, M.G.: Hydatidiform mole and coexisting foetus, both with triploid chromosome constitution. Brit. Med. J. **2**:476–478, 1967.

Bell, D.A., Flotte, T.J., Pastel-Levy, C., Ware, A., Preffer, F. and Colvin, R.B.: Flow cytometric analysis of DNA-ploidy in partial hydatidiform moles (PHM) utilizing paraffin-embedded material. Mod. Pathol. **2**:8A, 1989 (abstract No. 44).

Bell, K.A., van Deerlin, V.M.D., Addya, K, Clevenger, C.V., van Deerlin, P.G. and Leonard, D.G.B.: Molecular genetic testing from paraffin embedded tissue distinguishes non-molar hydropic abortion from hydatidiform moles. Modern Pathol. **11**:100A (abstract 579), 1998.

Ben-Chetrit, A., Yagel, S., Ariel, I., Zacut, D., Shimonovitz, S. and Celnikier-Hochner, D.: Successful conservative management of primary nonmetastatic cervical choriocarcinoma. Amer. J. Obstet. Gynecol. **163**:1161–1163, 1990.

Bendon, R.W., Siddiqi, T., Soukup, S. and Srivastava, A.: Prenatal detection of triploidy. J. Pediatr. **112**:149–153, 1988.

Benirschke, K.: Abortions and moles. In, Perinatal Diseases. R.L. Naeye, J.M. Kissane and N. Kaufman, eds., pp. 23–48. Williams & Wilkins, Baltimore, 1981.

Benirschke, K.: Editorial: flow cytometry for ALL mole-like abortion specimens. Hum. Pathol. **20**:403–404, 1989.

Benirschke, K., Spinosa, J.C., McGinnis, M.J., Marchevsky, A. and Sanchez, J.: Partial molar transformation of the placenta of presumably monozygotic twins. Pediat. Development. Pathol. **3**:95–100, 2000.

Berezowsky, J., Zbieranowski, I., Demers, J. and Murray, D.: DNA ploidy of hydatidiform moles and nonmolar conceptuses: a study using flow and tissue section image cytometry. Mod. Pathol. **8**:775–781, 1995.

Berkowitz, R.S., Mostoufizadeh, M., Kabawat, S.E., Goldstein, D.P. and Driscoll, S.G.: Immunopathologic study of the implantation site in molar pregnancy. Amer. J. Obstet. Gynecol. **144**:925–930, 1982.

Berkowitz, R.S., Anderson, D.J., Hunter, N.J. and Goldstein, D. P.: Distribution of major histocompatibility (HLA) antigens in chorionic villi of molar pregnancy. Amer. J. Obstet. Gynecol. **146**:221–220, 1983a.

Berkowitz, R.S., Goldstein, D.P. and Bernstein, M.R.: Natural history of partial molar pregnancy. Obstet. Gynecol. **66**:677–681, 1983b.

Berkowitz, R.S., Cramer, D.W., Bernstein, M.R., Cassells, S., Driscoll, S.G. and Goldstein, D.P.: Risk factors for complete molar pregnancy from a case-control study. Amer. J. Obstet. Gynecol. **152**:1016–1020, 1985a.

Berkowitz, R.S., Dubey, D.P, Goldstein, D.P. and Anderson, D. J.: Localization of transferrin receptor in the chorionic villi of complete molar pregnancy. Amer. J. Obstet. Gynecol. **151**:128–129, 1985b.

Berkowitz, R.S., Umpierre, S.A., Johnson, P.M., McIntyre, J.A. and Anderson, D.J.: Expression of trophoblast-leukocyte common antigens and placental-type alkaline phosphatase in complete molar pregnancy. Amer. J. Obstet. Gynecol. **155**:443–446, 1986.

Berkowitz, R., Ozturk, M., Goldstein, D., Bernstein, M., Hill, L. and Wands, J.R.: Human chorionic gonadotropin and free subunits' serum levels in patients with partial and complete hydatidiform moles. Obstet. Gynecol. **74**:212–216, 1989.

Berkowitz, R.S., Bernstein, M.R., Harlow, B.L., Rice, L.W., Lage, J.M., Goldstein, D.P. and Cramer, D.W.: Case-control study of risk factors for partial molar pregnancy. Amer. J. Obstet. Gynecol. **173**:788–794, 1995.

Bewtra, C., Frankforter, S. and Marcus, J.: Clinicopathologic differences between diploid and tetraploid complete hydatidiform moles. Intern. J. Gynec. Pathol. **16**:239–244, 1997.

Beyth, Y.: Hypofibrinogenemia in hydatidiform mole. J. Reprod. Med. **11**:223–224, 1973.

Block, M.F. and Merrill, J.A.: Hydatidiform mole with coexisting fetus. Obstet. Gynecol. **60**:129–134, 1982.

Bonduelle, M.-L., Dodd, R., Liebaers, I., van Steirteghem, A., Williamson, R. and Akhurst, R.: Chorionic gonadotrophin-β mRNA, a trophoblast marker, is expressed in human 8-cell embryos derived from tripronucleate zygotes. Hum. Reprod. **3**:909–914, 1988.

Bonnar, J. and Tennent, R.A.: Benign hydatidiform mole followed by late pulmonary choriocarcinoma. J. Obstet. Gynaecol. Brit. Commonw. **69**:999–1005, 1962.

Borek, E., Sharma, O.K. and Brewer, J.I.: Urinary nucleic acid breakdown products as markers for trophoblastic diseases. Amer. J. Obstet. Gynecol. **146**:906–910, 1983.

Borell, U., Fernström, I., Moberger, G. and Ohlson, L.: The Diagnosis of Hydatidiform Mole, Malignant Hydatidiform Mole and Choriocarcinoma with Special Reference to the Diagnostic Value of Pelvic Arteriography. Charles C Thomas, Springfield, IL, 1966.

Bourgoin, P., Baylet, R. and Ballon, C.: Études des chromosomes de la grossesse molaire. C. R. Soc. Biol. **159**:957, 1965a.

Bourgoin, P., Baylet, R. and Grattepanche, H.: Exploration d'une hypothèse sur l'étiopathogénie des môles hydatiformes: étude chromosomique. Rev. Fr. Gynécol. Obstétr. **60**:673–684, 1965b.

Bracken, M.B.: Incidence and aetiology of hydatidiform mole: an epidemiological review. Brit. J. Obstet. Gynaecol. **94**:1123–1135, 1987.

Bracken, M.B.: Incidence of hydatidiform mole. Amer. J. Obstet. Gynecol. **158**:1016–1017, 1988 (letter to the editor).

Breit, A. and Schedel, E.: Ergebnisse der Beckenarteriographie bei Plazentatumoren. Fortschr. Geb. Roentgenstr. Nuklearmed. **112**:431–439, 1970.

Brinton, L.A., Wu, B.-Z., Wang, W., Ershow, A.G., Song, H.-Z., Li, J.-Y., Bracken, M.B. and Blot, W.J.: Gestational trophoblastic disease: a case-control study from the People's Republic of China. Amer. J. Obstet. Gynecol. **161**:121–127, 1989.

Buckley, J.: Epidemiology of gestational trophoblastic diseases. In, A.E. Szulman and H.J. Buchsbaum eds., pp. 8–26. Gestational Trophoblastic Disease. Springer-Verlag, New York, 1987.

Bur, G.E., Hertig, A.T., McKay, D.G. and Adams, E.C.: Histochemical aspects of hydatidiform mole and choriocarcinoma. Obstet. Gynecol. **19**:156–182, 1962.

Butler, L.J., Chantler, C., France, N.E. and Keith, C.G.: A liveborn infant with complete triploidy (69,XXX). J. Med. Genet. **6**:413–421, 1969.

Butler, W.J., Schwartz, C.E., Sauer, S.M., Wilson, J.T. and McDonough, P.G.: Discordance in deoxyribonucleic acid analysis of fetus and trophoblast. Amer. J. Obstet. Gynecol. **158**:642–645, 1988.

Carr, D.H.: Cytogenetics and the pathology of hydatidiform degeneration. Obstet. Gynecol. **33**:333–342, 1969.

Carr, D.H.: Chromosome studies in selected spontaneous abortions: polyploidy in man. J. Med. Genet. **8**:164–174, 1971.

Castrillon, D.H., Sun, D., Weremowicz, S., Fisher, R.A., Crum, C.P. and Genest, D.R.: Discrimination of complete hydatidiform mole from its mimics by immunohistochemistry of the paternally imprinted gene product p57^{KIP2}. Amer. J. Surg. Pathol. **25**:1225–1230, 2001.

Cataldo, N.A., Nicholson, M. and Bihrle, D.: Uterine serosal trophoblastic implant after linear salpingostomy for ectopic pregnancy at laparotomy. Obstet. Gynecol. **76**:523–525, 1990.

Chamberlain, G.: Hydatidiform mole in twin pregnancy. Amer. J. Obstet. Gynecol. **87**:140–142, 1963.

Chamberlain, J., Morris, N.F. and Smith, N.C.: Steroids of hydatidiform moles. J. Endocrinol. **41**:289–290, 1968.

Choi-Hong, S.R., Genest, D., Crum, C.P., Berkowitz, R., Goldstein, D. and Schofield, D.: Evaluation of X- and Y-chromosomal content in twin pregnancies with complete hydatidiform mole and coexisting fetus using fluorescent in situ hybridization (FISH). Med. Pathol. **8**:87A (abstract 500), 1995.

Chua, S., Wilkins, T., Sargent, I. and Redman, C.: Trophoblast deportation in pre-eclamptic pregnancy. Brit. J. Obstetr. Gynaecol. **98**:973–979, 1991.

Chun, D., Braga, C., Chow, C. and Lok, L.: Clinical observations on some aspects of hydatidiform mole. J. Obstet. Gynaecol. Brit. Commonw. **71**:180–184, 1964.

Cintio, E. di, Parazzini, F., Rosa, C., Chatenoud, L. and Benzi, G.: The epidemiology of gestational trophoblastic disease. Gen. Diagn. Pathol. **143**:103–108, 1997.

Clayton, L.A., Tyrey, L., Weed, J.C. and Hammond, C.B.: Endocrine aspects of trophoblastic neoplasia. J. Reprod. Med. **26**:192–199, 1981.

Cohen, B.A., Burkman, R.T., Rosenshein, N.B., Atienza, M.F., King, T.M. and Parmley, T.H.: Gestational trophoblastic disease within an elective abortion population. Amer. J. Obstet. Gynecol. **135**:452–454, 1979.

Cohle, S.D. and Petty, C.S.: Sudden death caused by embolization of trophoblast from hydatidiform mole. J. Forensic Sci. **30**:1279–1283, 1985.

Conran, R.M., Hitchcock, C.L., Popek, E.J., Norris, H.J., Griffin, J.L., Geissel, A. and McCarthy, W.F.: Diagnostic considerations in molar gestations. Hum. Pathol. **24**:41–48, 1993.

Couillin, P., Afoutou, J.M., Faye, O., Correa, P. and Boué, A.: Androgenetic origin of African complete hydatidiform moles demonstrated by HLA markers. Hum. Genet. **71**:113–116, 1985.

Crooij, M.J., van der Harten, J.J., Puyenbroek, J.I., van Geijn, H.P. and Arts, N.F.: A partial hydatidiform mole, dispersed throughout the placenta, coexisting with a normal living fetus: case report. Brit. J. Obstet. Gynaecol. **92**:104–106, 1985.

Czernobilsky, B., Barash, A. and Lancet, M.: Partial moles: a clinicopathologic study of 25 cases. Obstet. Gynecol. **59**:75–77, 1982.

Das, P.C.: Hydatidiform mole: a statistical and clinical study. J. Obstet. Gynaecol. Brit. Emp. **45**:265–280, 1938.

Davis, J.R., Kerrigan, D.P., Way, D.L. and Weiner, S.A.: Partial hydatidiform moles: deoxyribonucleic acid content and course. Amer. J. Obstet. Gynecol. **157**:969–973, 1987.

Debyser, I.W.J., Soma, H. and Zwart, P.: Partial hydatidiform mole in a pregnant chimpanzee (*Pan troglodytes*). Zoo Biol. **12**:299–305, 1993.

De Grouchy, J., Roubin, M., Risse, J.-C. and Sarrut, S.: Enfant triploide (69,XXX) ayant vécu neuf jours. Ann. Génét. (Paris) **17**:283–286, 1974.

Depypere, H.T., Dhont, M., Verschraegen-Spae, M.R. and Coppens, M.: Tubal hydatidiform mole. Amer. J. Obstet. Gynecol. **169**:209–210, 1993.

Douglas, G.W.: Malignant changes in trophoblastic tumors. Amer. J. Obstet. Gynecol. **84**:884–894, 1962.

Drieux, H. and Thiéry, G.: Les tumeurs du placenta chez les animaux domestiques. Rev. Pathol. Comp. **48**:445–451, 1948.

Driscoll, S.G.: Trophoblastic growths: morphologic aspects and taxonomy. J. Reprod. Med. **26**:181–191, 1981.

Edmonds, H.W.: Genesis of hydatidiform mole: old and new concepts. Ann. N.Y. Acad. Sci. **80**:86–104, 1959.

Egley, C.C., Simon, L.R. and Haddox, T.: Hydatidiform mole and disseminated intravascular coagulation. Amer. J. Obstet. Gynecol. **121**:1122–1123, 1975.

Ehnholm, C., Seppälä, M., Tallberg, T. and Widholm, O.: Immunological studies in human placental lactogen hormone in chorionepithelioma and hydatidiform mole. Ann. Med. Exp. Fenn. **45**:318–319, 1967.

Endres, R.J.: Hydatidiform mole: report of a patient with 5 consecutive hydatidiform moles. Amer. J. Obstet. Gynecol. **81**:711–714, 1961.

Estellés, A., Grancha, S., Gilabert, J., Thinnes, T., Chirivella, M., España, F., Aznar, J. and Loskutoff, D.J.: Abnormal expression of plasminogen activator inhibitor in patients with gestational trophoblastic disease. Amer. J. Pathol. **149**:1229–1239, 1996.

Ewing, J.: Chorioma: a clinical and pathological study. Surg. Gynecol. Obstet. **10**:366–392, 1910.

Federschneider, J.M., Goldstein, D.P., Berkowitz, R.S., Marean, A.R. and Bernstein, M.R.: Natural history of recurrent molar pregnancy. Obstet. Gynecol. **55**:457–459, 1980.

Feinberg, R.F., Lockwood, C.J., Salafia, C. and Hobbins, J.C.: Sonographic diagnosis of a pregnancy with a diffuse hydatidiform mole and coexisting 46,XX fetus: a case report. Obstet. Gynecol. **72**:485–488, 1988.

Fejgin, M.D., Amiel, A., Goldberger, S., Barnes, I., Zer, T. and Kohn, G.: Placental insufficiency as a possible cause of low maternal serum human gonadotropin and low maternal serum unconjugated estriol levels in triploidy. Amer. J. Obstet. Gynecol. 167:766–767, 1992.

Fine, C., Bundy, A.L., Berkowitz, R.S., Boswell, S.B., Berezin, A.F. and Doubilet, P.M.: Sonographic diagnosis of partial hydatidiform mole. Obstet. Gynecol. 73:414–418, 1989.

Fischer, H.E., Lichtiger, B. and Cox, I.: Expression of $Rh_0(D)$ antigen in choriocarcinoma of the uterus in an $Rh_0(D)$-negative patient: report of a case. Human Pathol. 16:1165–1167, 1985.

Fisher, R.A. and Lawler, S.D.: Heterozygous complete hydatidiform moles: do they have a worse prognosis than homozygous complete moles? Lancet 2:51, 1984.

Fisher, R.A. and Newlands, E.S.: Rapid diagnosis and classification of hydatidiform moles with polymerase chain reaction. Amer. J. Obstet. Gynecol. 168:563–569, 1993.

Fisher, R.A., Lawler, S.D., Ormerod, M.G., Imrie, P.R. and Povey, S.: Flow cytometry used to distinguish between complete and partial hydatidiform moles. Placenta 8:249–256, 1987.

Fisher, R.A., Paradinas, F.J., Soteriou, B.A., Foskett, M. and Newlands, E.S.: Diploid hydatidiform moles with fetal red blood cells in molar villi. 2—genetics. J. Pathol. 181:189–195, 1997.

Fisher, R.A., Khatoon, R., Paradinas, F.J., Roberts, A.P. and Newlands, E.S.: Repetitive complete hydatidiform mole can be biparental in origin and either male or female. Human Reprod. 15:594–598, 2000.

Fisher, R.A., Hodges, M.D. and Newlands, E.S.: Familial recurrent hydatidiform mole: a review. J. Reprod. Med. 49:595–601, 2004a.

Fisher, R.A., Nucci, M.R., Thaker, H.M., Weremowicz, S., Genest, D.R. and Castrillon, D.H.: Complete hydatidiform mole retaining a chromosome 11 of maternal origin: molecular genetic analysis of a case. Modern Pathol. 17:1155–1160, 2004b.

Folger, A.F.: Über die Blasenmole beim Rinde. Acta Pathol. Microbiol. Scand. [Suppl.] 18:104–128, 1934.

Ford, J.H., Brown, J.K., Lew, W.Y. and Peters, G.B.: Diploid complete hydatidiform mole, mosaic for normally fertilized cells and androgenetic homozygous cells: case report. Brit. J. Obstet. Gynaecol. 93:1181–1186, 1986.

Forrester, M.B. and Merz, R.D.: Epidemiology of triploidy in a population-based birth defects registry, Hawaii, 1986–1999. Amer. J. Med. Genet. 119A:319–323, 2003.

Fox, H.: Hydatidiform moles: editorial. Virchows Arch. [A] 415:387–389, 1989.

Fox, H.: Differential diagnosis of hydatidiform moles. Gen. Diagn. Pathol. 143:117–125, 1997.

Fraikor, A.L., Vigneswaran, R. and Honeyfield, P.: Live-born triploid. Amer. J. Dis. Child. 134:988–989, 1980.

Franke, H.R., Risse, E.K.J., Kenemans, P., Vooijs, G.P. and Stolk, J.G.: Epidemiologic features of hydatidiform mole in The Netherlands. Obstet. Gynecol. 62:613–616, 1983a.

Franke, H.R., Risse, E.K.J., Kenemans, P., Houx, P.C.W., Solk, J.G. and Vooijs, G.P.: Plasma human chorionic gonadotropin disappearance in hydatidiform mole: a central registry report from the Netherlands. Obstet. Gynecol. 62:467–473, 1983b.

Franke, H.R., Alons, C.L., Caron, F.J.M., Boog, M.C., Oort, J. and Stolk, J.G.: Quantitative morphology: a study of the trophoblast. Virchows Arch. [Pathol. Anat.] 406:323–331, 1985.

Frost, A.C.G.: Death following intrauterine injection of hypertonic saline solution with hydatidiform mole. Amer. J. Obstet. Gynecol. 101:342–344, 1968.

Fukunaga, M.: Immunohistochemical characterization of $p57^{KIP2}$ expression in tetraploid hydropic placentas. Arch. Pathol. Lab. Med. 128:897–900, 2004.

Fukunaga, M., Ushigome, S., Fukunaga, M. and Sugishita, M.: Application of flow cytometry in diagnosis of hydatidiform moles. Mod. Pathol. 6:353–359, 1993.

Fukunaga, M., Endo, M. and Ushigome, S.: Clinicopathologic study of tetraploid hydropic villous tissue. Arch. Pathol. Lab. Med. 120:569–572, 1996.

Gaber, L.W., Redline, R.W., Mostoufi-Zadeh, M. and Driscoll, S.G.: Invasive partial mole. Amer. J. Clin. Pathol. 85:722–724, 1986.

Garcia, M., Romaguera, R.L. and Gomez-Fernandez, C.: A hydatidiform mole in a postmenopausal woman. A case report and review of the literature. Arch. Pathol. Lab. Med. 128:1039–1042, 2004.

Gardner, H.A.R. and Lage, J.M.: Choriocarcinoma following a partial hydatidiform mole. A case report. Human Pathol. 23:468–471, 1992.

Genest, D.R.: Partial hydatidiform mole: Clinicopathologic features, differential diagnosis, ploidy and molecular studies, and gold standards for diagnosis. Int. J. Gynecol. Pathol. 20:315–322, 2001.

Genest, D.R., Laborde, O., Berkowitz, R.S., Goldstein, D.P., Bernstein, M.R. and Lage, J.: A clinicopathologic study of 153 cases of complete hydatidiform mole (1980–1990): histologic grade lacks prognostic significance. Obstet. Gynecol. 78:402–409, 1991.

Gerber, A.H.: Amniographic diagnosis of trophoblastic disease. JAMA 212:630, 1970.

Gibson, B.R., Muir-Padilla, J., Champeaux, A. and Suarez, E.S.: Mesenchymal dysplasia of the placenta. Placenta 25:671–672, 2004.

Goecke, C.: Partielle Blasenmole und fötale Mißbildungen. Z. Geburtsh. Gynäkol. 166:201–210, 1967.

Goldman-Wohl, D., Ariel, I., Greenfield, C., Hochner-Celnikier, D., Lavy, Y. and Yagel, S.: A study of human leukocyte antigen G expression in hydatidiform moles. Amer. J. Obstet. Gynecol. 185:476–480, 2001.

Goldstein, D.P.: Prophylactic chemotherapy of patients with molar pregnancy. Obstet. Gynecol. 38:817–822, 1971.

Goldstein, D.P. and Berkowitz, R.S.: Gestational trophoblastic neoplasms: an invitational symposium. J. Reprod. Med. 26:179–229, 1981.

Goldstein, D.P. and Berkowitz, R.S.: Gestational Trophoblastic Neoplasms. Clinical Principles of Diagnosis and Management. Saunders, Philadelphia, 1982.

Golubovsky, M.D.: Postzygotic diploidization of triploids as a source of unusual cases of mosaicism, chimerism and twinning. Human Reprod. 18:236–242, 2003.

Gonzalez-Angulo, A., Márquez-Monter, H., Zavala, B.J., Yabur, E. and Salazar, H.: Electron microscopic observations in hydatidiform mole. Obstet. Gynecol. 27:455–467, 1966.

Goshen, R. and Hochberg, A.A.: The genomic basis of the β-subunit of human chorionic gonadotropin diversity in triploidy. Amer. J. Obstet. Gynecol. **170**:700–701, 1994.

Goto, S., Nishi, H. and Tomoda, Y.: Blood group Rh-D factor in human trophoblast determined by immunofluorescent method. Amer. J. Obstet. Gynecol. **137**:707–712, 1980.

Graham, J.M., Rawnsley, E.F., Simmons, G.M., Wurster-Hill, D.H., Park, J.P., Marin-Padilla, M. and Crow, H.C.: Triploidy: pregnancy complications and clinical findings. in seven cases. Prenat. Diagn. **9**:409–419, 1989.

Grimes, D.A.: Epidemiology of gestational trophoblastic disease. Amer. J. Obstet. Gynecol. **150**:309–318, 1984.

Gschwendtner, A., Neher, A., Kreczy, A., Müller-Holzner, E., Volgger, B. and Mairinger, T.: DNA ploidy determination of early molar pregnancies by image analysis. Comparison to histologic classification. Arch. Pathol. Lab. Med. **122**:1000–1004, 1998.

Gul, A., Agrali, G., Ulker, V., Numanoglu, C., Aslan, H. and Tekirdag, A.I.: Complete hydatidiform mole and coexisting live fetus in dichorionic twin pregnancy; report of two cases. Twin Res. **7**(4):Abstract, 2004.

Gunasegaram, R., Peh, K.L., Loganath, A., Kottegoda, S.R. and Ratnam, S.S.: Elevated intravesicular fluid thyroid-stimulating hormone concentration in hydatidiform mole. Intern. J. Gynaecol. Obstet. **24**:177–181, 1986.

Habibian, R. and Surti, U.: Cytogenetics of trophoblasts from complete hydatidiform moles. Cancer Genet. Cytogenet. **29**:271–287, 1987.

Hankins, G.D.V., Wendel, G.D., Snyder, R.R. and Cunningham, F.G.: Trophoblastic embolization during molar evacuation—central hemodynamic observations. Obstet. Gynecol. **69**:368–372, 1987.

Harper, W.F. and MacVicar, J.: Hydatidiform mole and pregnancy diagnosed by sonar. Brit. Med. J. **2**:1178–1179, 1963.

Harrison, K.B.: X-chromosome inactivation in the human cytotrophoblast. Cytogenet. Cell Genet. **52**:37–41, 1989.

Harrison, K.B. and Warburton, D.: Preferential X-chromosome activity in human female placental tissues. Cytogenet. Cell Genet. **41**:163–168, 1986.

Hasegawa, T., Harada, N., Ikeda, K., Ishii, T., Hokuto, I., Kasai, K., Tanaka, M., Fukuzawa, R., Niikawa, N. and Matsuo, N.: Digynic triploid surviving for 46 days. Amer. J. Med. Genet. **87**:306–310, 1999.

Heifetz, S.A. and Czaja, J.: In situ choriocarcinoma arising in partial hydatidiform mole: Implications for the risk of persistent trophoblastic disease. Pediatr. Pathol. **12**:601–611, 1992.

Helwani, M.N., Seoud, M., Zahed, L., Zaatari, G., Khalil, A. and Slim, R.: A familial case of recurrent hydatidiform molar pregnancies with biparental genomic contribution. Human Genet. **105**:112–115, 1999.

Hemming, J.D., Quirke, P., Womack, C., Wells, M., Elston, C.W. and Bird, C.C.: Diagnosis of molar pregnancy and persistent trophoblastic disease by flow cytometry. J. Clin. Pathol. **40**:615–620, 1987.

Hendrickse, J.P.de V., Cockshott, W.P., Evans, K.T.E. and Barton, C.J.: Pelvic angiography in the diagnosis of malignant trophoblastic disease. NEJM **271**:859–866, 1964.

Hershman, J.M. and Higgins, H.P.: Hydatidiform mole—a cause of clinical hyperthyroidism: report of two cases with evidence that molar tissue secreted a thyroid stimulator. NEJM **284**:573–577, 1971.

Hertig, A.T.: Hydatidiform mole and chorionepithelioma. In, Progress in Gynecology, Vol. II. J.V. Meigs and S.H. Sturgis, eds., pp. 372–394. Grune & Stratton, New York, 1950.

Hertig, A.T.: Human Trophoblast. Charles C. Thomas, Springfield, IL, 1968.

Hertig, A.T. and Sheldon, W.H.: Hydatidiform mole—a pathologico-clinical correlation of 200 cases. Amer. J. Obstet. Gynecol. **53**:1–36, 1947.

Hertz, R., Ross, G.T. and Lipsett, M.B.: Primary chemotherapy of nonmetastatic trophoblastic disease in women. Amer. J. Obstet. Gynecol. **86**:808–814, 1963.

Higashino, M., Harad, N., Hataya, I., Nishimura, N., Kato, M. and Niikawa, N.: Trizygotic pregnancy consisting of two fetuses and a complete hydatidiform mole with dispermic androgenesis. Amer. J. Med. Genet. **82**:67–69, 1999.

Hitchcock, C.L., Conran, R.M. and Griffin, J.L.: Hydatidiform moles and the use of flow cytometry in their diagnosis. In, Pediatric Molecular Pathology. Garvin, A.J., O'Leary, T.J., Bernstein, J. and Rosenberg, H.S. eds. Perspective Pediatr. Pathol. **15**:117–141, 1991, Karger, Basel.

Ho, P.-C., Wong, L.C., Lawton, J.W.M. and Ma, H.K.: Mixed lymphocyte reaction in hydatidiform mole. Amer. J. Reprod. Immunol. **6**:25–27, 1984.

Ho, P.-C., Lawton, J.W.M., Wong, L.-C. and Ma, H.-K.: T-cell subsets and natural killer cell activity in patients with gestational trophoblastic neoplasia. Amer. J. Obstet. Gynecol. **155**:330–334, 1986.

Hohe, P.T., Cochrane, C.R., Gmelich, J.T. and Austin, J.A.: Coexisting trophoblastic tumor and viable pregnancy. Obstet. Gynecol. **38**:899–904, 1971.

Holland, J.F. and Hreshchyshyn, M.M., eds.: Choriocarcinoma. Springer-Verlag, Heidelberg, 1967.

Honoré, L.H.: Recurrent partial hydatidiform mole: report of a case. Amer. J. Obstet. Gynecol. **156**:922–924, 1987.

Honoré, L.H., Lin, E.C. and Morrish, D.W.: Recurrent partial mole. Amer. J. Obstet. Gynecol. **158**:442, 1988.

Horn, L.-C. and Bilek, K.: Histologic classification and staging of gestational trophoblastic disease. Gen. Diagn. Pathol. **143**:87–101, 1997.

Houtzager, H.L., van Leusden, H.A. and Siemerink, M.: Conversion of androgens into oestrogens by hydatidiform moles in vitro. Acta Endocrinol. (Copenh.) **64**:17–37, 1970.

Howat, A.J., Beck, S., Fox, H., Harris, S.C., Hill, A.S., Nicholson, C.M. and Williams, R.A.: Can histopathologists reliably diagnose molar pregnancy? J. Clin. Pathol. **46**:599–602, 1993.

Hsu, C.-T., Huang, L.-C. and Chen, T.-Y.: Metastases in benign hydatidiform mole and chorioadenoma destruens. Amer. J. Obstet. Gynecol. **84**:1412–1424, 1962.

Hsu, C.-T., Lai, C.H., Chanchien, C.-L. and Changchien, B.-C.: Repeat hydatidiform moles. Amer. J. Obstet. Gynecol. **87**:543–547, 1963.

Hunt, W., Dockerty, M.B. and Randall, L.M.: Hydatidiform mole: a clinicopathologic study "grading" as a measure of possible malignant change. Obstet. Gynecol. **1**:593–609, 1953.

Ishiguro, T.: Serum α-fetoprotein in hydatidiform mole, choriocarcinoma, and twin pregnancy. Amer. J. Obstet. Gynecol. **12**:539–541, 1975.

Ishii, J., Iitsuka, Y., Takano, H., Matsui, H., Osada, H. and Sekiya, S.: Genetic differentiation of complete hydatidiform moles coexisting with normal fetuses by short tandem repeat-derived deoxyribonucleic acid polymorphism analysis. Amer. J. Obstet. Gynecol. **179**:628–634, 1998.

Iverson, L. and the Joint Project Investigators: Geographic variation in the occurrence of hydatidiform mole and chorio-carcinoma. Ann. N.Y. Acad. Sci. **80**:178–195, 1959.

Jacobs, P.A., Hassold, T.J., Matsuyama, A.M. and Newlands, I.M.: Chromosome constitution of gestational trophoblastic disease. Lancet **2**:49, 1978.

Jacobs, P.A., Wilson, C.M., Sprenkle, J.A., Rosenheim, N.B. and Migeon, B.R.: Mechanism of complete hydatidiform moles. Nature **286**:714–716, 1980.

Jacobs, P.A., Szulman, A.E., Funkhouser, J., Matsuura, J.S. and Wilson, C.C.: Human triploidy: relationship between parental origin of the additional haploid complement and development of partial hydatidiform mole. Ann. Hum. Genet. **46**:223–231, 1982.

Jarotzky, v. and Waldeyer: Traubenmole in Verbindung mit dem Uterus: intraparietale und intravasculäre Weiterentwicklung der Chorionzotten. Arch. Pathol. Anat. Physiol. Klin. Med. **44**:88–94, 1868.

Jauniaux, E., Kadri, R. and Hustin, J.: Partial mole and triploidy: screening patients with first-trimester spontaneous abortion. Obstet. Gynecol. **88**:616–619, 1996.

Jauniaux, E., Brown, R., Snijders, R.J.M., Noble P. and Nicolaides, K.H.: Early prenatal diagnosis of triploidy. Amer. J. Obstet. Gynecol. **176**:550–554, 1997.

Jauniaux, E., Gulbis, B., Hyett, J. and Nicolaides, K.H.: Biochemical analyses of mesenchymal fluid in early pregnancy. Amer. J. Obstet. Gynecol. **178**:765–769, 1998.

Javey, H., Borazjani, G., Behnard, S. and Langley, F.A.: Discrepancies in the diagnosis of hydatidiform mole. Brit. J. Obstet. Gynaecol. **86**:480–483, 1979.

Jock, D.E., Schwartz, P.E. and Portnoy, L.: Primary ovarian hydatidiform mole: addition of a sixth case to the literature. Obstet. Gynecol. **58**:657–660, 1981.

Johnson, F.L.: Recurrent hydatidiform mole. Can. Med. Assoc. J. **94**:344, 1966.

Johnson, T.R., Comstock, C.H. and Anderson, D.G.: Benign gestational trophoblastic disease metastatic to pleura: unusual cause of hemothorax. Obstet. Gynecol. **53**:509–511, 1979.

Jones, W.B. and Lauersen, N.H.: Hydatidiform mole with coexisting fetus. Amer. J. Obstet. Gynecol. **122**:267–272, 1975.

Jun, S.Y., Ro, J.Y. and Kim, K.R.: p57kip2 is useful in the classification and differential diagnosis of complete and partial hydatidiform moles. Histopathol. **43**:17–25, 2003.

Kabawat, S.E., Mostoufi-Zadeh, M., Berkowitz, R.S., Driscoll, S.G., Goldstein, D.P. and Bhan, A.K.: Implantation site in complete molar pregnancy: a study of immunologically competent cells with monoclonal antibodies. Amer. J. Obstet. Gynecol. **152**:97–99, 1985.

Kajii, T. and Ohama, K.: Androgenetic origin of hydatidiform mole. Nature **268**:633–634, 1977.

Kajii, T., Kurashige, H., Ohama, K. and Uchino, F.: XY and XX complete moles: clinical and morphological correlations. Amer. J. Obstet. Gynecol. **150**:57–64, 1984.

Kashimura, Y., Kashimura, M., Sugimori, H., Tsukamoto, N., Matsuyama, T., Matsukuma, K., Kamura, T., Saito, T., Kawano,

D., Nose, R., Nose, Y., Nakano, H. and Taki, I.: Prophylactic chemotherapy for hydatidiform mole: five to 15 years follow-up. Cancer **58**:624–629, 1986.

Kazazian, L.C., Baramki, T.A. and Thomas, R.L.: Triploid fetus: an important consideration in the evaluation of very high maternal serum alpha-fetoprotein. Prenat. Diagn. **9**:27–30, 1989.

Keep, D., Zaragoza, M.V., Hassold, T. and Redline, R.W.: Very early complete hydatidiform mole. Hum. Pathol. **27**:708–713, 1996.

Khazaeli, M.B., Hedayat, M.M., Hatch, K.D., To, A.C.W., Soong, S.-J., Shingleton, H.M., Boots, L.R. and LoBuglio, A.F.: Radio-immunoassay of free β-subunit of human chorionic gonado-tropin as a prognostic test for persistent trophoblastic disease in molar pregnancy. Amer. J. Obstet. Gynecol. **155**:320–324, 1986.

Khazaeli, M.B., Buchina, E.S., Pattillo, R.A., Soon, S.-J. and Hatch, K.D.: Radioimmunoassay of free β-unit of human chorionic gonadotropin in diagnosis of high-risk and low-risk gestational trophoblastic disease. Amer. J. Obstet. Gynecol. **160**:444–449, 1989.

Khoo, S.K., Monks, P.L. and Davies, N.T.: Hydatidiform mole coexisting with a live fetus: a dilemma of management. Aust. N.Z. J. Obstet. Gynaecol. **26**:129–135, 1986.

Kim, D.S., Moon, H., Kim, K.T., Moon, Y.J. and Hwang, Y.Y.: Effects of prophylactic chemotherapy for persistent tropho-blastic disease in patients with complete hydatidiform mole. Obstet. Gynecol. **67**:690–694, 1986.

Kim, D.T., Riddell, D.C., Welch, J.P., Scott, H., Fraser, R.B. and Wright, J.R.Jr.: Association between Breus' mole and partial hydatidiform mole: chance or can hydropic villi precipitate placental massive subchorionic thrombosis? Pediat. Pathol. Molec. Med. **21**:451–459, 2002.

King, G.: Hydatidiform mole and chorion-epithelioma—the problem of the borderline case. Proc. R. Soc. Med. **49**:381–390, 1956.

Kliman, H.J. and Segel, L.: The placenta may predict the baby. J. Theoret. Biol. **225**:143–145, 2003.

Ko, T.-M., Hsieh, C.-Y, Ho, H.-N., Hsieh, F.-J and Lee, T.-Y.: Restriction fragments length polymorphism analysis to study the genetic origin of complete hydatidiform mole. Amer. J. Obstet. Gynecol. **164**:901–906, 1991.

Kohorn, E.I.: Natural history of partial molar pregnancy. Obstet. Gynecol. **68**:731–732, 1986.

Krone, H.A.: Blasenmole mit einem ausgetragenen lebenden Kind. Zentralbl. Gynäkol. **77**:1391–1395, 1955.

Kronfol, N.M., Iliya, F.A. and Hajj, S.N.: Recurrent hydatidiform mole: a report of five cases with review of the literature. Lebanese Med. J. **22**:507–520, 1969.

Kubo, H., Abe, Y., Shimada, M., Katayama, S. and Date, R.: Two cases of hydatidiform mole with a surviving coexisting fetus. Congen. Anomal. **26**:256, 1986.

Kyodo, Y., Inatomi, K., Abe, T. and Kudo, K.: A case report of destructive mole after uterine rupture. Amer. J. Obstet. Gynecol. **158**:1182–1183, 1988.

Lage, J.M., Driscoll, S.G., Yavner, D.L., Olivier, A.P., Mark, S.D. and Weinberg, D.S.: Hydatidiform moles: application of flow cytometry in diagnosis. Amer. J. Clin. Pathol. **89**:596–600, 1988.

Lage, J.M., Weinberg, D.S., Yavner, D.L. and Bieber, F.R.: The biology of tetraploid hydatidiform moles: histopathology, cytogenetics, and flow cytometry. Hum. Pathol. **20**:419–425, 1989.

Lage, J.M., Berkowitz, R.S., Rice, L.W., Goldstein, D.P., Bernstein, M.R. and Weinberg, D.S.: Flow cytometric analysis of DNA content in partial hydatidiform moles with persistent gestational trophoblastic tumor. Obstet. Gynecol. **77**:111–115, 1991.

Lage, J.M., Mark, S.D., Roberts, D.J., Goldstein, D.P., Bernstein, M.R. and Berkowitz, R.S.: A flow cytometric study of 137 fresh hydropic placentas: correlation between types of hydatidiform moles and nuclear DNA ploidy. Obstet. Gynecol. **79**:403–410, 1992.

Lai, C.Y.L., Chan, K.Y.K., Khoo, U.-S., Ngan, H.Y.S., Xue, W.-C., Chiu, P.M., Tsao, S.-W. and Cheung, A.N.Y.: Analysis of gestational trophoblastic disease by genotyping and chromosome *in situ* hybridization. Modern Pathol. **17**:40–48, 2004.

Lauslahti, K.: A histological and histochemical study of trophoblastic disease in a Finnish material 1958–1962. Acta Pathol. Microbiol. Scand. [Suppl.] **201**:1–71, 1969.

La Vecchia, C., Franceschi, S., Fasoli, M. and Mangioni, C.: Gestational trophoblastic neoplasms in homozygous twins. Obstet. Gynecol. **60**:250–252, 1982.

La Vecchia, C.L., Parazzini, F., Decarli, A., Franceschi, S., Fasoli, M., Favalli, G., Negri, E. and Pampallona, S.: Age of parents and risk of gestational trophoblastic disease. J. Natl. Cancer Inst. **73**:639–642, 1984.

Lawler, S.D. and Fisher, R.A.: Genetic studies in hydatidiform mole with clinical correlations. Placenta **8**:77–88, 1987.

Lawler, S.D., Kloudas, P.T. and Bagshawe, K.D.: Immunogenicity of molar pregnancies in the HL-A system. Amer. J. Obstet. Gynecol. **120**:857–861, 1974.

Lawler, S.D., Pickthall, V.J., Fisher, R.A., Povey, S., Evans, M.W. and Szulman, A.E.: Genetic studies of complete and partial hydatidiform moles. Lancet **2**:580, 1979.

Lawler, S.D., Fisher, R.A. and Dent, J.: A prospective genetic study of complete and partial hydatidiform moles. Amer. J. Obstet. Gynecol. **164**:1270–1277, 1991.

Lee, A.T.C. and Siegel, I.: Hydatidiform mole with rupture of the uterus: report of a case. Obstet. Gynecol. **26**:133–134, 1965.

Lee, E.E.: Gross early enlargement of a hydatidiform mole with severe pre-eclampsia. Can. Med. Assoc. J. **93**:79–80, 1965.

Lee, J.N., Salem, H.T., Al-Ani, A.T.M., Huang, S.C., Ouyang, P.C., Wei, P.Y. and Seppälä, M.: Circulating concentrations of specific placental proteins (human chorionic gonadotropin, pregnancy-specific beta-1 glycoprotein, and placental protein 5) in untreated gestational trophoblastic tumors. Amer. J. Obstet. Gynecol. **139**:702–704, 1981.

Lee, W., Ginsburg, K.A., Cotton, D.B. and Kaufman, R.H.: Squamous and trophoblastic cells in the maternal pulmonary circulation identified by invasive hemodynamic monitoring during the peripartum period. Amer. J. Obstet. Gynecol. **155**:999–1001, 1986.

Leeder, J.R.: Metastasizing hydatidiform mole. Amer. J. Obstet. Gynecol. **88**:833–835, 1964.

Leivo, I., Laurila, P., Wahlström, T. and Engvall, E.: Expression of merosin, a tissue-specific basement membrane protein, in the intermediate trophoblast cells of choriocarcinoma and placenta. Lab. Invest. **60**:783–790, 1989.

Lewis, P.E. and Cefalo, R.C.: Triploidy syndrome with theca lutein cysts and severe pre-eclampsia. Amer. J. Obstet. Gynecol. **133**:110–111, 1979.

Li, M.C., Hertz, R. and Spencer, D.B.: Effect of methotrexate therapy upon choriocarcinoma and chorioadenomas. Proc. Soc. Exp. Biol. Med. **93**:361–366, 1956.

Lindor, N.M., Ney, J.A., Gaffey, T.A., Jenkins, R.B., Thibodeau, S.N. and Dewald, G.W.: A genetic review of complete and partial hydatidiform moles and nonmolar triploidy. Mayo Clin. Proceed. **67**:791–799, 1992.

Lipp, R.G., Kindshi, J.D. and Schmitz, R.: Death from pulmonary embolism associated with hydatidiform mole. Amer. J. Obstet. Gynecol. **83**:1644–1647, 1962.

Llewellyn-Jones, D.: Relation of pregnancy toxaemia to trophoblastic tumours. Brit. Med. J. **2**:720, 1967.

Lloyd, C.E.: A case of hydatidiform mole associated with toxaemia. J. Obstet. Gynaecol. Brit. Emp. **28**:307–310, 1921.

Logan, B.J.: Occurrence of a hydatidiform mole in twin pregnancy: case report. Amer. J. Obstet. Gynecol. **73**:911–913, 1957.

Loke, Y.W.: Sex chromatin of hydatidiform moles. J. Med. Genet. **6**:22–25, 1969.

Looi, L.M. and Sivanesaratnam, V.: Malignant evolution with fatal outcome in a patient with partial hydatidiform mole. Aust. N.Z. J. Obstet. Gynaecol. **21**:51–52, 1981.

Lurain, J.R., Brewer, J.I., Torok, E.E. and Halpern, B.: Natural history of hydatidiform mole after primary evacuation. Amer. J. Obstet. Gynecol. **145**:591–595, 1983.

MacDonald, P.C. and Siiteri, P.K.: The in vivo mechanisms of origin of estrogen in subjects with trophoblastic tumors. Steroids **8**:589–603, 1966.

Makino, S., Sasaki, M.S. and Fukuschima, T.: Preliminary notes on the chromosomes of human chorionic lesions. Proc. Jpn. Acad. **39**:54–58, 1963.

Makino, S., Sasaki, M.S. and Fukuschima, T.: Triploid chromosome constitution in human chorionic lesions. Lancet **2**:1273–1275, 1964.

Makino, S., Sasaki, M.S. and Fukuschima, T.: Cytologic studies of tumors. XLI. Chromosomal instability in human chorionic lesions. Okajimas Fol. Anat. Jpn. **40**:439–465, 1965.

Makrydimas, G., Sebire, N.J., Thornton, S.E., Zagorianakou, N., Lolis, D. and Fisher, R.A.: Complete hydatidiform mole and normal live birth: a novel case of confined placental mosaicism: case report. Human Reprod. **17**:2459–2463, 2002.

Malinowski, W., Biskup, I. and Dec, W.: Sad fetus syndrome—gestational disease concurrent with a living fetus or fetuses. Acta Genet. Med. Gemollol. **44**:193–202, 1995.

Mark, L.K. and Moel, M.: Pulmonary metastasis from trophoblastic tumors. Radiology **76**:601–605, 1961.

Márquez-Monter, H.: Deoxyribonucleic acid synthesis of hydatidiform moles in organ culture: an autoradiographic investigation. Nature **209**:1037–1038, 1966.

Márquez-Monter, H., de la Vega, G.A., Robles, M. and Bolio-Cicero, A.: Epidemiology and pathology of hydatidiform mole in the general hospital in Mexico. Amer. J. Obstet. Gynecol. **85**:856–864, 1963.

Martin, D.A., Sutton, G.P., Ulbright, T.M., Sledge, G.W., Stehman, F.B. and Ehrlich, C.E.: DNA content as a prognostic index in gestational trophoblastic neoplasia. Gynecol. Oncol. **34**:383–388, 1989.

Matalon, M. and Modan, B.: Epidemiologic aspects of hydatidiform mole in Israel. Amer. J. Obstet. Gynecol. **112**:107–112, 1972.

Mathieu, A.: Hydatidiform mole and chorio-epithelioma: collective review of the literature for the years 1935, 1936 and 1937. Surg. Gynecol. Obstet. **68**:52–70; 181–198, 1939.

Matsui, H., Iitsuka, Y., Yamazawa, K., Tanaka, N., Mitsuhashi, A., Seki, K. and Skiya, S.: Placental mesenchymal dysplasia initially diagnosed as partial mole. Pathol. Int. **53**:810–813, 2003.

Maudsley, R.F. and Robertson, E.M.: Hydatidiform mole in a woman over 52 years old: report of a case. Obstet. Gynecol. **26**:542–543, 1965.

Mazzanti, P., La Vecchia, C., Parazzini, F. and Bolis, G.: Frequency of hydatidiform mole in Lombardy, Northern Italy. Gynecol. Oncol. **24**:337–342, 1986.

McCorriston, C.C.: Racial incidence of hydatidiform mole. Amer. J. Obstet. Gynecol. **101**:377–382, 1968.

McFadden, D.E., Pantzer, J.T. and Langlois, S.: Parental origin of triploidy—digyny, not diandry. Modern Pathol. **7**:abstract 28, p. 5P, 1994.

McKay, D.G., Roby, C.C., Hertig, A.T. and Richardson, M.V.: Studies of the function of early human trophoblast. I. Observations on the chemical composition of the fluid of hydatidiform moles. Amer. J. Obstet. Gynecol. **69**:722–734, 1955a.

McKay, D.G., Richardson, M.V. and Hertig, A.T.: Studies of the function of early human trophoblast. III. A study of the protein structure of mole fluid, chorionic and amniotic fluids by paper electrophoresis. Amer. J. Obstet. Gynecol. **75**:699–707, 1955b.

Meinecke, B., Kuiper, H., Drögemüller, C., Leeb, T. and Meinecke-Tillmann, S.: A mola hydatidosa coexistent with a foetus in a bovine freemartin pregnancy. Placenta **24**:107–112, 2002.

Merkow, L.P., Acevedo, H.F., Gilmore, J. and Pardo, M.: Trophoblastic disease: a correlative ultrastructural and biochemical study. Obstet. Gynecol. **37**:348–357, 1971.

Messerli, M.L., Parmley, T., Woodruff, J.D., Lilienfeld, A.M., Bevilacqua, L. and Rosenshein, N.B.: Inter- and intra-pathologist variability in the diagnosis of gestational trophoblastic neoplasia. Obstet. Gynecol. **69**:622–626, 1987.

Meyer, J.S.: Benign pulmonary metastasis from hydatidiform mole: report of a case. Obstet. Gynecol. **28**:826–829, 1966.

Minami, S., Yamoto, M. and Nakano R.: Immunohistochemical localization of inhibin-activin subunits in hydatidiform mole and invasive mole. Obstet. Gynecol. **82**:414–418, 1993.

Moglabey, Y.B., Kircheisen, R., Seoud, M., Mogharbel, N.E., van den Veyver, I. and Slim, R.: Genetic mapping of a maternal locus responsible for familial hydatidiform moles. Human Molec. Genet. **8**:667–671, 1999.

Montgomery, E.A., Roberts, E.F., Conran, R.M. and Hitchcock, C.L.: Triploid abortus presenting as an ectopic pregnancy. Arch. Pathol. Lab. Med. **117**:652–653, 1993.

Mor-Joseph, S., Anteby, S.O., Granat, M., Brzezinsky, A. and Evron, S.: Recurrent molar pregnancies associated with clomiphene citrate and human gonadotropins. Amer. J. Obstet. Gynecol. **151**:1085–1086, 1985.

Morrish, D.W., Honoré, L.H. and Bhardwaj, D.: Partial hydatidiform moles have impaired differentiated function (human chorionic gonadotropin and human placental lactogen secretion) in response to epidermal growth factor and 8–bromocyclic adenosine monophosphate. Amer. J. Obstet. Gynecol. **166**:160–166, 1992.

Moscoso, G., Jauniaux, E. and Hustin, J.: Placental vascular anomaly with diffuse mesenchymal stem villous hyperplasia. A new clinico-pathologic entity? Pathol. Res. Practice **187**:324–328, 1991.

Muto, M.G., Lage, J.M., Berkowitz, R.S., Goldstein, D.P. and Bernstein, M.R.: Gestational trophoblastic disease of the fallopian tube. J. Reprod. Med. **36**:57–60, 1991.

Mutter, G.L., Pomponio, R.J., Berkowitz, R.S. and Genest, D.R.: Sex chromosome composition of complete hydatidiform moles: relationship to metastasis. Amer. J. Obstet. Gynecol. **168**:1547–1551, 1993.

Natoli, W.J. and Rashad, M.N.: Hawaiian moles. Amer. J. Roentgenol. Radium Ther. Nucl. Med. **114**:142–144, 1972.

Nayer, R., Silverberg, S.G., Snell, J. and Lage, J.M.: Placental site nodule occurring in a fallopian tube. Hum. Pathol. **27**:1243–1245, 1996.

Neudeck, H., Kronenberger, C. and Vogel, M.: Detection of villous blood vessels by CD34 in complete hydatidiform mole and hydropic abortion. Placenta **24**(10):abstract P105, 2003.

Niebuhr, E.: Triploidy in man: cytogenetical and clinical aspects. Humangenetik **21**:103–125, 1974.

Nishimura, H., Takano, K., Tanimura, T. and Yasuda, M.: Normal and abnormal development of human embryos: first report of an analysis of 1,213 intact embryos. Teratology **1**:281–290, 1968.

Nisula, B.C. and Taliafouros, G.S.: Thyroid function in gestational trophoblastic neoplasia: evidence that the thyrotropic activity of chorionic gonadotropin mediates the thyrotoxicosis of choriocarcinoma. Amer. J. Obstet. Gynecol. **138**:77–85, 1980.

Nobunaga, T., Azuma, C., Kimura, T., Tokugawa, Y., Takemura, M., Kamiura, S., Saji, F. and Tanizawa, O.: Differential diagnostic between complete mole and hydropic abortus by deoxyribonucleic acid fingerprint. Amer. J. Obstet. Gynecol. **163**:634–638, 1990.

Novak, E.: Pathological aspects of hydatidiform mole and choriocarcinoma. Amer. J. Obstet. Gynecol. **59**:1355–1372, 1950.

Novak, E. and Seah, C.S.: Benign trophoblastic lesions in the Mathieu Chorionepithelioma Registry (hydatidiform mole, syncytial endometritis). Amer. J. Obstet. Gynecol. **68**:376–390, 1954.

Novak, R., Agamanolis, D., Dasu, S., Igel, H., Platt, M., Robinson, H. and Shehata, B.: Histologic analysis of placental tissue in first trimester abortions. Pediat. Pathol. **8**:477–482, 1988.

Nugent, C.E., Punch, M.R., Barr, M., LeBlanc, L., Johnson, M.P. and Evans, M.I.: Persistence of partial molar placenta and severe preeclampsia after selective termination in a twin pregnancy. Obstet. Gynecol. **87**:829–831, 1996.

Ockleford, C., Barker, C., Griffiths, J., McTurk, G., Fisher, R. and Lawler, S.: Hydatidiform mole: an ultrastructural analysis of syncytiotrophoblast surface organization. Placenta **10**:195–212, 1989.

Ohama, K., Kajii, T., Okamoto, E., Fukuda, Y., Imaizumi, K., Tsukahara, M., Kobayashi, K. and Hagiwara, K.: Dispermic origin of XY hydatidiform moles. Nature **292**:551–552, 1981.

Ohama, K., Ueda, K., Okamoto, E., Takenaka, M. and Fujiwara, A.: Cytogenetic and clinicopathologic studies of partial moles. Obstet. Gynecol. **68**:259–262, 1986.

Ohyama, M., Kojyo, T., Godota, H., Sato, T., Ijiri, R. and Tanaka, Y.: Mesenchymal dysplasia of the placenta. Pathol. Intern. **50**:759–764, 2000.

Okudaira, Y. and Strauss, L.: Ultrastructure of molar trophoblast: observations on hydatidiform mole and choriocarcinoma destruens. Obstet. Gynecol. **30**:172–187, 1967.

Olvera, M., Harris, S., Amezcua, C.A., McCourty, A., Rezk, S., Koo, C., Felix, J.C. and Brynes, R.K.: Immunohistochemical expression of cell cycle proteins E2F-1, Cdk-2, Cyclin E, p27kip, and Ki-67 in normal placenta and gestational trophoblastic disease. Modern Pathol. **14**:1036–1042, 2001.

Orr, J.W., Austin, J.M., Hatch, K.D., Shingleton, H.M., Younger, J.B. and Boots, L.R.: Acute pulmonary edema associated with molar pregnancies: a high-risk factor for development of persistent trophoblastic disease. Amer. J. Obstet. Gynecol. **136**:412–415, 1980.

Osada, H., Kawata, M., Yamada, M., Okumura, K. and Takamizawa, H.: Genetic identification of pregnancies responsible for choriocarcinomas after multiple pregnancies by restriction fragment length polymorphism analysis. Amer. J. Obstet. Gynecol. **165**:682–688, 1991.

Ozturk, M., Berkowitz, R., Goldstein, D., Bellet, D. and Wands, J.R.: Differential production of human chorionic gonadotropin and free subunits in gestational trophoblastic disease. Amer. J. Obstet. Gynecol. **158**:193–198, 1988.

Paradinas, F.J.: The histologic diagnosis of hydatidiform moles. Curr. Diagn. Pathol. **1**:24–32, 1994.

Paradinas, F.J., Fisher, R.A., Browne, P. and Newlands, E.S.: Diploid hydatidiform moles with fetal red blood cells in molar villi. 1—pathology, incidence, and prognosis. J. Pathol. **181**:183–188, 1997.

Paradinas, F.J., Sebire, N.J., Fisher, R.A., Rees, H.C., Foskett, M., Seckl, M.J. and Newlands, E.S.: Pseudo-partial moles: placental stem vessel hydrops and the association with Beckwith-Wiedemann syndrome and complete moles. Histopathology **39**:447–454, 2001.

Parazzini, F., La Vecchia, C., Franceschi, S. and Mangili, G.: Familial trophoblastic disease: case report. Amer. J. Obstet. Gynecol. **149**:382–383, 1984.

Parazzini, F., La Vecchia, C., Pampallona, S. and Franceschi, S.: Reproductive patterns and the risk of gestational trophoblastic disease. Amer. J. Obstet. Gynecol. **152**:866–870, 1985.

Parazzini, F., Mangili, G., La Vecchia, C., Negri, E., Bocciolone, L. and Fasoli, M.: Risk factors for gestational trophoblastic disease: a separate analysis of complete and partial hydatidiform moles. Obstet. Gynecol. **78**:1039–1045, 1991.

Park, W.W.: The occurrence of sex chromatin in chorionepitheliomas, and hydatidiform moles. J. Pathol. Bacteriol. **74**:197–206, 1957.

Park, W.W.: Choriocarcinoma: A Study of Its Pathology. Davis, Philadelphia, 1971.

Patek, E. and Johnson, P.: Recurrent hydatidiform mole: report of a case with five recurrences. Acta Obstet. Gynecol. Scand. **57**:381–383, 1978.

Pattillo, R.A., Sasaki, S., Katayama, K.P., Roesler, M. and Mattingly, R.F.: Genesis of 46,XY hydatidiform mole. Amer. J. Obstet. Gynecol. **141**:104–105, 1981.

Petit, A., Geoffroy, P., Bessette, P. and Bélisle, S.: Expression of G proteins in human placentae from molar pregnancies. Placenta **17**:337–343, 1996.

Pettit, M.D.W.: Hydatidiform mole following tubal pregnancy. Amer. J. Obstet. Gynecol. **42**:1057–1060, 1941.

Philipp, T., Grillenberger, K., Separovic, E.R., Philipp, K. and Kalousek, D.K.: Effect of triploidy on early human development. Prenat. Diagn. **24**:276–281, 2004.

Pool, C., Aplin, J.D., Taylor, G.M. and Boyd, R.D.H.: Trophoblast cells and maternal blood. Lancet **1**:804–805, 1987.

Popek, E.J.: Complete hydatidiform mole with coexisting twin: 10 cases. Modern Pathol. **7**:abstract 39, p. 7P, 1994.

Qiao, S., Nagasaka, T. and Nakashima, N.: Numerous vessels detected by CD34 in the villous stroma of complete hydatidiform moles. Intern. J. Gynecol. Pathol. **16**:233–238, 1997.

Ramsey, P.S., Winter, J.T.v., Gaffey, T.A. and Ramin, K.D.: Eclampsia complicating hydatidiform molar pregnancy with coexisting, viable fetus. A case report. J. Reprod. Med. **43**:456–458, 1998.

Reed, S., Coe, J.I. and Bergquist, J.: Invasive hydatidiform mole metastatic to the lung. Obstet. Gynecol. **13**:749–753, 1959.

Rice, L.W., Lage, J.M., Berkowitz, R.S., Goldstein, D.P. and Bernstein, M.R.: Repetitive complete and partial hydatidiform mole. Obstet. Gynecol. **74**:217–219, 1989.

Rice, L.W., Berkowitz, R.S., Lage, J.M., Goldstein, D.P. and Bernstein, M.R.: Persistent gestational trophoblastic tumor after partial hydatidiform mole. Gynecol. Oncol. **36**:358–362, 1990.

Ring, A.M.: The concept of benign metastasizing hydatidiform moles. Amer. J. Clin. Pathol. **58**:111–117, 1972.

Ringertz, N.: Hydatidiform mole, invasive mole and choriocarcinoma in Sweden 1958–1965. Acta Obstet. Gynecol. Scand. **49**:195–203, 1970.

Rolon, P.A. and de Lopez, B.H.: Epidemiological aspects of hydatidiform mole in the Republic of Paraguay (South America). Brit. J. Obstet. Gynaecol. **84**:862–864, 1977.

Rolon, P.A., Hochsztajn, B. and Llamosas, F.: Epidemiology of complete hydatidiform mole in Paraguay. J. Reprod. Med. **35**:15–18, 1990.

Romaguera, R.L., Rodriguez, M.M., Bruce, J.H., Zuluaga, T., Viciana, A., Penalver, M.A. and Nadji, M.: Molar gestations and hydropic abortions differentiated by p57 immunostaining. Fetal Pediat. Pathol. **23**:181–190, 2004.

Romero, R., Horgan, G., Kohorn, E.I., Kadar, N., Taylor, K.J.W. and Hobbins, J.C.: New criteria for the diagnosis of gestational trophoblastic disease. Obstet. Gynecol. **66**:553–558, 1985.

Roper, H.H., Wolff, G. and Hitzeroth, H.W.: Preferential X-inactivation in human placenta membranes: is the paternal X-inactive in early embryonic development of female mammals? Hum. Genet. **43**:265–273, 1978.

Rubin, N.W.: Chorioadenoma destruens—perforation, resection, and subsequent pregnancy. Amer. J. Obstet. Gynecol. **89**:536–538, 1964.

Sagawa, N., Mori, T., Masuzaki, H., Ogawa, Y. and Nakao, K.: Leptin production by hydatidiform mole. Lancet **350**:1518–1519, 1997.

Saji, F., Tokugawa, Y., Kimura, T., Nobunaga, T., Azuma, C. and Tanizawa, O.: A new approach using DNA fingerprinting for the determination of androgenesis as a cause of hydatidiform mole. Placenta **10**:399–405, 1989.

Sanchez, J.C. and Sanchez, J.E.: Hyperthyroidism with a hydatidiform mole. Pathological case of the month. Arch. Pediat. Adolesc. Med. **152**:827–828, 1998.

Sand, P.K., Lurain, J.R. and Brewer, J.I.: Repeat gestational trophoblastic disease. Obstet. Gynecol. **63**:140–144, 1984.

Sand, P.K., Stubblefield, P.A. and Orvy, S.J.: Methotrexate inhibition of normal trophoblast in vitro. Amer. J. Obstet. Gynecol. **155**:324–329, 1986.

Sande, H.A. and Eyjolfsson, O.: Case report: hydatidiform mole with a coexisting fetus. Acta Obstet. Gynecol. Scand. **64**:353–355, 1985.

Sarkar, S., Kacinski, B.M., Kohorn, E.I., Merino, M.J., Carter, D. and Blakemore, K.J.: Demonstration of myc and ras oncogene expression by hybridization in situ in hydatidiform mole and in the BeWo choriocarcinoma cell line. Amer. J. Obstet. Gynecol. **154**:390–393, 1986.

Sarno, A.P., Moorman, A.J. and Kalousek, D.K.: Partial molar pregnancy with fetal survival: An unusual example of confined placental mosaicism. Obstet. Gynecol. **82**:716–719, 1993.

Sasagawa, M., Yamazaki, T., Sudo, Y., Kanazawa, K. and Takeuchi S.: Immunohistochemical localization of hCGα, hCGβ CTP, hPL and SP1 on villous and extravillous trophoblasts in normal human pregnancy. Acta Obstetr. Gynaecol. Jpn. **39**:1073–1079, 1987.

Sasaki, M., Fukushima, T. and Makino, S.: Some aspects of the chromosome constitution of hydatidiform moles and normal chorionic villi. Gann **53**:101–106, 1962.

Sasaki, M., Makino, S., Muramoto, J.-I., Ikeuchi, T. and Shimba, H.: A chromosome survey of induced abortuses in a Japanese population. Chromosoma **20**:267–283, 1967.

Sauter, H.: Uteroplazentare Apoplexie bei Blasenmole. Gynaecologia **159**:296–300, 1965.

Saxena, A., Frank, D., Panichkul, P., van den Veyver, I.B., Tycko, B. and Thaker, H.: The product of the imprinted gen *IPL* marks human villous cytotrophoblast and is lost in complete hydatidiform mole. Placenta **24**:835–842, 2003.

Schlaerth, J.B., Morrow, C.P., Montz, F.J. and d'Ablaing, G.: Initial management of hydatidiform mole. Amer. J. Obstet. Gynecol. **158**:1299–1306, 1988.

Schlegel, R.J., Neu, R.L., Leao, J.C., Farias, E., Aspillaga, M.J. and Gardner, L.I.: Observations on the chromosomal, cytological and anatomical characteristics of 75 conceptuses: including euploid, triploid XXX, triploid XYY and mosaic triploid XXY/diploid XY cases. Cytogenetics **5**:430–446, 1966.

Schmickel, R.D., Silverman, E.M., Floyd, A.D., Payne, F.E., Pooley, J.M. and Beck, M.L.: A live-born infant with 69 chromosomes. J. Pediatr. **79**:97–103, 1971.

Schmorl, G.: Über das Schicksal embolisch verschleppter Plazentarzellen. Verh. Dtsch. Pathol. Gesellsch. **8**:39–46, 1905.

Schneider, C.I. and Waxman, B.: Clomid therapy and subsequent hydatidiform mole formation: a case report. Obstet. Gynecol. **39**:787–788, 1972.

Sciarra, N.: Human chorionic gonadotrophin in hydatidiform moles. J. Obstet. Gynaecol. Brit. Commonw. **77**:420–423, 1970.

Scott, J.S.: Pregnancy toxaemia associated with hydrops foetalis, hydatidiform mole and hydramnios. J. Obstet. Gynaecol. Brit. Emp. **65**:689–701,1958.

Sebire, M.J., Gillmore, R., Foskett, M., Sebire, N.J., Rees, H. and Newlands, E.S.: Routine terminations of pregnancy—should we screen for gestational trophoblastic neoplasia? Lancet **364**:705–707, 2004 (and comment by B. Piura, pp. 645–646).

Sebire, N.J., Fisher, R.A. and Rees, H.C.: Histopathological diagnosis of partial and complete hydatidiform mole in the first trimester of pregnancy. Pediatr. Developm. Pathol. **6**:69–77, 2002a.

Sebire, N.J., Foskett, M., Paradinas, F.J., Fisher, R.A., Francis, R.J., Short, D., Newlands, E.S. and Seckl, M.: Outcome of twin pregnancies with complete hydatidiform mole and healthy co-twin. Lancet **359**:2165–2166, 2002b.

Sebire, N.J., Rees, H.C., Peston, D., Seckl, M.J., Newlands, E.S. and Fisher, R.A.: p57[KIP2] immunohistochemical staining of gestational trophoblastic tumours does not identify the type of the causative pregnancy. Histopathol. **45**:135–141, 2004.

Seckl, M.J., Fisher, R.A., Salerno, G., Rees, H., Paradinas, F.J., Foskett, M. and Newlands, E.S.: Choriocarcinoma and partial hydatidiform moles. Lancet **356**:1443–1444, 2000.

Sensi, A., Gualandi, F., Pittalis, M.C., Calabrese, O., Falciano, F., Maestri, I., Bovicelli, L. and Calzolarri, E.: Mole maker phenotype: possible narrowing of the candidate region. Eur. J. Human Genet. **8**:641–644, 2000.

Seoud, M., Khalil, A., Frangieh, A., Zahed, L., Azar, G. and Nuwayri-Salti, N.: Recurrent molar pregnancies in a family with extensive intermarriage: report of a family and review of the literature. Obstet. Gynecol. **86**:692–695, 1995.

Sherer, D.M., Glantz, J.C., Metlay, L.A. and Saller, D.N.: Absent umbilical artery diastolic flow in a fetus with a partial mole at 18 weeks' gestation. Amer. J. Obstet. Gynecol. **169**:1167–1168, 1993.

Shorofsky, M.: A karyometric comparison of the normal human chorion with that of the hydatidiform mole. Acta Anat. (Basel) **41**:45–56, 1960.

Sicuranza, B.J. and Tisdall, L.H.: Hydatidiform mole and eclampsia with coexistent living fetus in the second trimester of pregnancy. Amer. J. Obstet. Gynecol. **126**:513–514, 1976.

Slattery, M.A., Khong, T.Y., Dawkins, R.R., Pridmore, B.R. and Hague, W.M.: Eclampsia in association with partial molar pregnancy and congenital abnormalities. Amer. J. Obstet. Gynecol. **169**:1625–1627, 1993.

Slim, R., Fallahian, M., Rivière, J.-B. and Zali, M.R.: Evidence of a genetic heterogeneity of familial hydatidiform moles. Placenta **26**:5–9, 2005.

Smalbraak, J.: Trophoblastic Growths. A Clinical, Hormonal and Histopathological Study of Hydatidiform Mole and Chorionepithelioma. Elsevier, Amsterdam, 1957.

Smith, E.B., Szulman, A.E., Hinshaw, W., Tyrey, L., Surti, U. and Hammond, C.B.: Human chorionic gonadotropin levels in complete and partial hydatidiform moles and in nonmolar abortuses. Amer. J. Obstet. Gynecol. **149**:129–132, 1984.

Song, H.-Z., Wu, P.-C., Wang, Y.-E., Yang, X.-Y. and Dong, S.-Y.: Pregnancy outcomes after successful chemotherapy for choriocarcinoma and invasive mole: long-term follow-up. Amer. J. Obstet. Gynecol. **158**:538–545, 1988.

Soto-Wright, V., Bernstein, M., Goldstein, D.P. and Berkowitz, R.S.: The changing clinical presentation of complete molar pregnancy. Obstet. Gynecol. **86**:775–779, 1995.

Spademan, L.C. and Tuttle, W.M.: Chorioadenoma destruens. Amer. J. Obstet. Gynecol. **88**:549–550, 1964.

Stanhope, C.R., Stuart, G.C.E. and Curtis, K.L.: Primary ovarian hydatidiform mole: review of the literature and report of a case. Amer. J. Obstet. Gynecol. **145**:886–888, 1983.

Steller, M.A., Genest, D.R., Bernstein, M.R., Lage, J.M., Goldstein, D.P. and Berkowitz, R.S.: Natural history of twin pregnancy with complete hydatidiform mole and coexisting fetus. Obstet. Gynecol. **83**:35–42, 1994.

Stroup, P.E.: A study of thirty-eight cases of hydatidiform mole at the Pennsylvania hospital. Amer. J. Obstet. Gynecol. **72**:294–303, 1956.

Sunderland, C.A., Redman, C.W.G. and Stirrat, G.M.: Characterization and localization of HLA antigens on hydatidiform mole. Amer. J. Obstet. Gynecol. **151**:130–135, 1985.

Surani, M.A.H. and Barton, S.C.: Development of gynogenetic eggs in the mouse: implications for parthenogenetic embryos. Science **222**:1034–1036, 1983.

Surti, U., Szulman, A.E. and O'Brien, S.: Complete (classic) hydatidiform mole with 46,XY karyotype of paternal origin. Hum. Genet. **51**:153–155, 1979.

Surti, U., Szulman, A.E. and O'Brien, S.: Dispermic origin and clinical outcome of three complete hydatidiform moles with 46,XY karyotype. Amer. J. Obstet. Gynecol. **144**:84–87, 1982.

Suzuki, M., Matsunobu, A., Wakita, K., Nishijima, M. and Osanai, K.: Hydatidiform mole with a surviving coexisting fetus. Obstet. Gynecol. **56**:384–386, 1980.

Sze, E.H.M., Adelson, M.D., Baggish, M.S. and Contente, N.: Combined tubal and molar pregnancy: case report. Amer. J. Obstet. Gynecol. **159**:1217–1219, 1988.

Szulman, A.E. and Buchsbaum, H.J., eds.: Gestational Trophoblastic Disease. Springer-Verlag, New York, 1987.

Szulman, A.E. and Surti, U.: The syndromes of hydatidiform mole. I. Cytogenetic and morphologic correlations. Amer. J. Obstet. Gynecol. **131**:665–671, 1978a.

Szulman, A.E. and Surti, U.: The syndromes of hydatidiform mole. II. Morphologic evolution of the complete and partial mole. Amer. J. Obstet. Gynecol. **132**:20–27, 1978b.

Szulman, A.E. and Surti, U.: The clinicopathologic profile of the partial hydatidiform mole. Obstet. Gynecol. **59**:597–602, 1982.

Szulman, A.E. and Surti, U.: Strict clinicopathologic criteria in the diagnosis of partial hydatidiform mole: a plea renewed. Amer. J. Obstet. Gynecol. **152**:1107–1108, 1985.

Szulman, A.E., Ma, H.-K., Wong, L.C. and Hsu, C.: Residual trophoblastic disease in association with partial hydatidiform mole. Obstet. Gynecol. **57**:392–394, 1981.

Takagi, N. and Sasaki, M.: Preferential inactivation of the paternally derived X chromosome in the extraembryonic membranes of the mouse. Nature **256**:640–652, 1975.

Takagi, N., Asano, S.-I., Fujisawa, M. and Ichinoe, K.: A possible triploid/diploid case of hydatidiform mole. Chromos. Inform. Serv. **10**:21–22, 1969.

Takahashi, H., Kanazawa, K., Ikarashi, T., Sudo, N. and Tanaka, K.: Discrepancy in the diagnoses of hydatidiform mole by macroscopic and microscopic findings and the deoxyribonucleic acid fingerprint method. Amer. J. Obstet. Gynecol. **163**:112–113, 1990.

Tanimura, A., Natsuyama, H., Kawano, M., Tanimura, Y., Tanaka, T. and Kitazono, M.: Primary choriocarcinoma of the lung. Hum. Pathol. **16**:1281–1284, 1985.

Tavassoli, F.A. and Devilee, P.: World Health Organization Classification of Tumours: Pathology and Genetics. Tumours of the Breast and Female Genital Organs. Lyon, France. IARC Press, 2003.

Teng, N.N.H. and Ballon, S.C.: Partial hydatidiform mole with diploid karyotype: report of three cases. Amer. J. Obstet. Gynecol. **150**:961–964, 1984.

Teoh, E.S., Dawood, M.Y. and Ratnam, S.S.: Epidemiology of hydatidiform mole in Singapore. Amer. J. Obstet. Gynecol. **110**:415–420, 1971.

Thatcher, S.S., Grainger, D.A., True, L.D. and de Cherney, A.H.: Pelvic trophoblastic implants after laparoscopic removal of a tubal pregnancy. Obstet. Gynecol. **74**:514–515, 1989.

Thiele, R.A. and de Alvarez, R.R.: Metastasizing benign trophoblastic tumors. Amer. J. Obstet. Gynecol. **84**:1395–1406, 1962.

Tobin, S.M.: A further aid in the diagnosis of hydatidiform mole—the serum glutamic oxalacetic transaminase. Amer. J. Obstet. Gynecol. **87**:213–217, 1963.

Tominaga, T. and Page, E.W.: Sex chromatin of trophoblastic tumors. Amer. J. Obstet. Gynecol. **96**:305–309, 1966.

Tomoda, Y., Kaseki, S., Goto, S., Nishi, H., Hara, T. and Naruki, M.: Rh-D factor in trophoblastic tumors: a possible cause of the high incidence in Asia. Amer. J. Obstet. Gynecol. **139**:742–743, 1981.

Tsuji, K., Yagi, S. and Nakano, R.: Increased risk of malignant transformation of hydatidiform moles in older gravidas: a cytogenetic study. Obstet. Gynecol. **58**:351–355, 1981.

Tsukahara, M. and Kajii, T.: Replication of X chromosomes in complete moles. Hum. Genet. **71**:7–10, 1985.

Uchida, I.A. and Freeman, V.C.: Triploidy and chromosomes. Amer. J. Obstet. Gynecol. **151**:65–69, 1985.

Uher, J., Jirasek, J.E. and Sima, A.: Histochemische Studie von Blasenmole und Plazenta eines fünf Monate alten Fetus. Zentralbl. Gynäkol. **85**:477–482, 1963.

Urbanski, T.K., Higgins, P.G., Murray, M.L. and Joffe, G.: Hydatid mole with a coexisting pregnancy. J. Perinatol. **16**:478–480, 1996.

Van de Kaa, C.A., Nelson, K.A.M., Ramaekers, F.C.S., Vooijs, P.G. and Hopman, A.H.N.: Interphase cytogenetics in paraffin sections of routinely processed hydatidiform moles and hydropic abortions. J. Pathol. **165**:281–287, 1991.

Van de Kaa, C.A., Hanselaar, A.G.J.M., Hopman, A.H.N., Nelson, K.A.M., Peperkamp, A.R., Gemmink, J.H., Beck, J.L.M., Wilde, P.C.M. de, Ramaekers, F.C.S. and Vooijs, G.P.: DNA cytometric and interphase cytogenetic analyses of paraffin-embedded hydatidiform moles and hydropic abortions. J. Pathol. **170**:229–238, 1993.

Van de Kaa, C.A., Robben, J.C.M., Hopman, A.H.N. and Hanselaar, A.G.J.M.: Complete hydatidiform mole in twin pregnancy: differentiation from partial mole with interphase cytogenetic and DNA cytometric analyses on paraffin embedded tissues. Histopathology **26**:123–129, 1995.

Van de Kaa, C.A., Schijf, C.P.T., Wilde, P.C.M. de, Hanselaar, A.G.J.M. and Vooijs, P.G.: The role of deoxyribonucleic acid image cytometric and interphase cytogenetic analyses in the differential diagnosis, prognosis, and clinical follow-up of hydatidiform moles. A report from the central molar registration in the Netherlands. Amer. J. Obstet. Gynecol. **177**:1219–1229, 1997.

Vassilakos, P. and Kajii, T.: Hydatidiform mole: two entities. Lancet **1**:259, 1976. (See Stone, M. and Bagshawe, K.D.: Lancet **1**:535–536, 1976.)

Vassilakos, P., Riotton, G. and Kajii, T.: Hydatidiform mole: two entities. A morphologic and cytogenetic study with some clinical considerations. Amer. J. Obstet. Gynecol. **127**:167–170, 1977.

Vejerslev, L.O., Dueholm, M. and Nielsen, F.H.: Hydatidiform mole: cytogenetic marker analysis in twin gestation. Amer. J. Obstet. Gynecol. **155**:614–617, 1986.

Vejerslev, L.O., Dissing, J., Hansen, H.E. and Poulsen, H.: Hydatidiform mole: genetic markers in diploid abortuses with macroscopic villous enlargement. Cancer Genet. Cytogenet. **26**:143–155, 1987a.

Vejerslev, L.O., Dissing, J., Hansen, H.E. and Poulsen, H.: Hydatidiform mole: genetic origin in polyploid conceptuses. Hum. Genet. **76**:11–19, 1987b.

Vejerslev, L.O., Fisher, R.A., Surti, U. and Wake, N.: Hydatidiform mole: cytogenetically unusual cases and their implications for the present classification. Amer. J. Obstet. Gynecol. **157**:180–184, 1987c.

Vejerslev, L.O., Fisher, R.A., Surti, U. and Wake, N.: Hydatidiform mole: parental chromosome aberrations in partial and complete moles. J. Med. Genet. **24**:613–615, 1987d.

Vejerslev, L.O., Sunde, L., Hansen, B.F., Larsen, J.K., Christensen, I.J. and Larsen, G.: Hydatidiform mole and fetus with normal karyotype: support of a separate entity. Obstet. Gynecol. **77**:868–874, 1991.

Wake, N., Takagi, N. and Sasaki, M.: Androgenesis as a cause of hydatidiform mole. J. Natl. Cancer Inst. **60**:51–57, 1978a.

Wake, N., Shiina, Y. and Ichinoe, K.: A further cytogenetic study of hydatidiform mole, with reference to its androgenetic origin. Proc. Jpn. Acad. **54**:533–537, 1978b.

Wake, N., Tanaka, K., Chapman, V., Matsui, S. and Sandberg, A.A.: Chromosomes and cellular origin of choriocarcinoma. Cancer Res. **41**:3137–3143, 1981.

Wax, J.R., Pinette, M.G., Chard, R., Blackstone, J. and Cartin, A.: Prenatal diagnosis by DNA polymorphism analysis of complete mole with coexisting twin. Amer. J. Obstet, Gynecol. **188**:1105–1106, 2003.

Weaver, D.T., Fisher, R.A., Newlands, E.S. and Paradinas, F.J.: Amniotic tissue in complete hydatidiform moles can be androgenetic. J. Pathol. **191**:67–70, 2000.

Westerhout, F.C.: Ruptured tubal hydatidiform mole: report of a case. Obstet. Gynecol. **23**:138–139, 1964.

Woodward, R.M., Filly, R.A. and Callen, P.W.: First trimester molar pregnancy: nonspecific Ultrasonographic appearance. Obstet. Gynecol. **55**:31S–33S, 1980.

Wu, F.Y.W.: Recurrent hydatidiform mole: a case report of nine consecutive molar pregnancies. Obstet. Gynecol. **41**:200–204, 1973.

Wynn, R.M. and Davies, J.: Ultrastructure of hydatidiform mole: correlative electron microscopic and functional aspects. Amer. J. Obstet. Gynecol. **90**:293–307, 1964.

Wynn, R.M. and Harris, J.A.: Ultrastructure of trophoblast and endometrium in invasive hydatidiform mole (chorioadenoma destruens). Amer. J. Obstet. Gynecol. **99**:1125–1135, 1967.

Yamashita, L., Wake, N., Araki, T., Ichinoe, K. and Makoto, K.: Human lymphocyte antigen expression in hydatidiform mole: androgenesis following fertilization by a haploid sperm. Amer. J. Obstet. Gynecol. **135**:597–600, 1979.

Yedema, K.A., Verheijen, R.H., Kenemans, P., Schijf, C.P., Borm, G.F., Segers, M.F. and Thomas, C.M.: Identification of patients with persistent trophoblastic disease by means of a normal human chorionic gonadotropin regression curve. Amer. J. Obstet. Gynecol. **168**:787–792, 1993.

Yee, B., Tu, B. and Platt, L.D.: Coexisting hydatidiform mole with a live fetus presenting as a placenta previa on ultrasound. Amer. J. Obstet. Gynecol. **144**:726–728, 1982.

Yenen, E., Inanc, F.A. and Babuna, C.: Primary ovarian hydatidiform mole: report of a case. Obstet. Gynecol. **26**:721–724, 1965.

Yorde, D.E., Hussa, R.O., Garancis, J.C. and Pattillo, R.A.: Immunocytochemical localization of human choriogonadotropin in human malignant trophoblast: model for human choriogonadotropin secretion. Lab. Invest. **40**:391–398, 1979.

Yoshimatsu, N., Hoshi, K., Sato, A., Munakata, S. and Fukushima, T.: The significance of alpha-fetoprotein-negativity in the interstitial area of total hydatidiform mole tissue. Nippon Sanka Fujinka Gakkai Zasshi **39**:918–924, 1987 [Japanese].

Yuen, B.H.: Relationship of prolactin and estradiol to human chorionic gonadotropin following molar gestation. Amer. J. Obstet. Gynecol. **145**:618–620, 1983.

Zaragoza, M.V., Keep, D., Genest, D.R., Hassold, T. and Redline, R.W.: Early complete hydatidiform moles contain inner cell mass derivatives. Amer. J. Med. Genet. **70**:273–277, 1997.

Zaragoza, M.V., Surti, U., Redline, R.W., Millie, E., Chakravarti, A. and Hassold, T.J.: Parental origin and phenotype of triploidy in spontaneous abortions: Predominance of diandry and association with the partial hydatidiform mole. Amer. J. Hum. Genet. **66**:1807–1820, 2000.

Zhang, P. and Benirschke, K.: Placental Pathology Casebook. J. Perinatol. **1**:63–65, 2000.

Zhang, P., McGinnis, M.J., Sawai, S. and Benirschke, K.: Diploid/triploid mosaic placenta with fetus. Towards a better understanding of 'partial moles'. Early Human Develop. **60**:1–11, 2000.

23
Trophoblastic Neoplasms

Among trophoblastic neoplasms, choriocarcinoma is the most well known. The classification of gestational trophoblastic disease (GTD) has been alluded to in the previous chapter, and Soper et al. (1994), who evaluated 454 tumors according to three classifications, found the prognostic aspects to be fairly similar among these otherwise divergent classifications. Perhaps the clinical staging provided the best prognostication. An excellent and concise review of chorionic tumors has summarized the progress made in understanding these lesions and prescribing therapy for them (Berkowitz & Goldstein, 1996). A checklist for the characterization of trophoblastic malignancies has been provided by Lage (1999), and several other noteworthy reviews among many others are those by Silverberg and Kurman (1992), Baergen (1997), and Baergen and Rutgers (1997). The classification of GTD, recently endorsed by the World Health Organization (WHO) (Tavassoli et al., 2003), is the most widely used and is shown in Table 23.1.

Choriocarcinoma

Choriocarcinoma is a malignant neoplasm composed exclusively of cytotrophoblast and syncytiotrophoblast. If villi are associated with such invasive tumors, then the lesion is referred to as "invasive mole" or chorioadenoma destruens (Chapter 22). The nature of choriocarcinoma was first correctly identified by Marchand (1895). Teacher's detailed observations in 1903 followed Marchand's description. The early history of this tumor, the "deciduoma" as it was first known, has been admirably recounted by Ober and Fass (1961). Until the neoplastic elements of choriocarcinoma were ultimately shown to be derived from the embryonic as opposed to maternal cells, their derivation had been in dispute. Ewing (1910) was the first investigator to differentiate between the various types of trophoblastic neoplasms. He introduced or used terms such as **invasive mole**, **syncytial endometritis**, and **syncy-**

tioma. Some of these terms are still in use, even though the latter two have been replaced as greater knowledge of the biology has been accumulating.

In the United States, gestation-related choriocarcinoma is said to occur with a frequency of about 1 per 40,000 pregnancies (Hertig & Mansell, 1956). In their oft-depicted diagram (Fig. 23.1), Hertig and Mansell estimated that the lesion was preceded by a complete hydatidiform mole (CHM) in 50%, an abortion in 25%, a normal pregnancy in 22.5%, and an ectopic pregnancy in 2.5%. There is wide geographic variation in its incidence as it is in that of its precursors. In a study of choriocarcinoma from Japan, five of eight choriocarcinomas followed complete moles, one followed a term pregnancy (the only patient who died), and two followed abortions (Fukunaga & Ushigome, 1993a). All were diploid by flow cytometry.

The tumor consists of solid sheets of cytotrophoblast and syncytium. Choriocarcinoma has the great propensity of vascular invasion (Fig. 23.2) and, consequently, many choriocarcinomas are hemorrhagic and friable (Figs. 23.3 and 23.4). So much blood may be present in some choriocarcinoma metastases that one may have to search long for the tumor cells (Fig. 23.5). Characteristically, broad sheets of cytotrophoblast form the central portion of the tumor, the periphery being syncytium. Nuclear pleomorphism is common, but mitoses are confined to the cytotrophoblast. Wolf and Michalopoulos (1992) studied the distribution of nuclear antigen in normal placentas and trophoblastic tumors. Its presence correlated with mitotic, reproductive activity and, in placentas, it was also confined to the cytotrophoblast, where it was strongly expressed. The same was true in CHM and choriocarcinomas; the cytotrophoblast and extravillous trophoblast (X cells) stained, but not the syncytium. Several studies have shown that many intermediate trophoblastic cells are present in choriocarcinoma, even though they are not the hallmark of the lesion. These are the cells truly intermediate between cytotrophoblast and syncytium and are not

TABLE 23.1. World Health Organization classification of gestational trophoblastic disease

Hydatidiform mole
  Complete mole
  Partial mole
  Invasive mole
  Metastatic mole
Trophoblastic neoplasms
  Choriocarcinoma
  Placental site trophoblastic tumor
  Epithelioid trophoblastic tumor
Nonneoplastic, nonmolar trophoblastic lesions
  Placental site nodule and plaque
  Exaggerated placental site

Source: Tavassoli et al., 2003.

the intermediate trophoblastic cells described in lesions of extravillous trophoblast (vide infra). They are especially readily identified by electron microscopy (Pierce & Midgley, 1963; Wynn & Davies, 1964) (Fig. 23.6). The X cells, the other major line of trophoblastic elements, the extravillous trophoblast, were identified with certainty in choriocarcinoma-like lesions; they are also not a striking feature of hydatidiform moles. Because of its dilated cytoplasmic cisternae, the syncytium of choriocarcinomas is frequently vacuolated. This vacuolation may obscure the true nature of the cells. Much glycogen may also be contained in this tissue (Arkwright et al., 1993). When Crescimanno et al. (1996) cloned BeWo choriocarcinoma cells (human choriocarcinoma cell lines) and identified two separate lines of cells, they found different behavioral expression in these two lines. One was rapidly invasive and produced tumors and metastases in nude mice, and the other did not. The invasive line produced much greater quantities of gelatinase A (and less gelatinase B), and this activity was found to be stimulated by laminin and matrigel. This is a first approach for understanding the com-

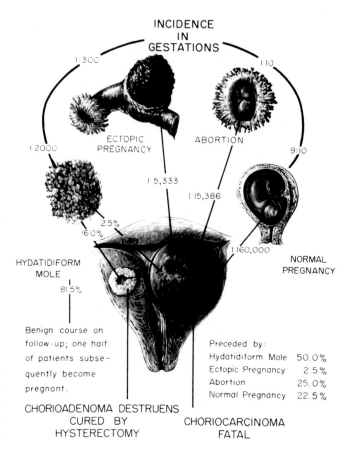

FIGURE 23.1. Frequency relations of choriocarcinoma to its various precursors. (*Source:* Hertig & Mansell, 1956, with permission.)

plexity of invasion of the placenta into the decidua at implantation, as well as for understanding the invasive properties of some trophoblastic tumors, but not others.

It is usually difficult to assign a prognosis from the histologic picture of a choriocarcinoma. Some choriocar-

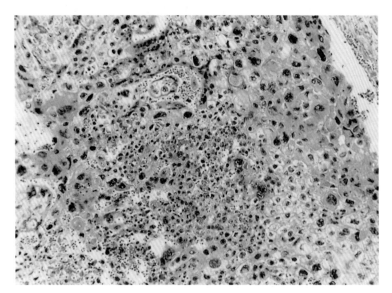

FIGURE 23.2. Choriocarcinoma of the uterus. Solid sheets of neoplastic cytotrophoblast with much nuclear pleomorphism and syncytium are intermixed with blood. H&E × 160.

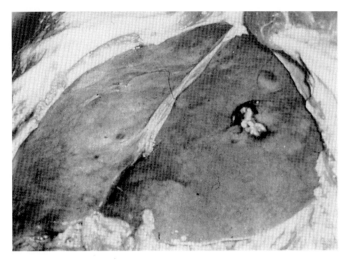

FIGURE 23.3. Liver metastases of choriocarcinoma following a third hydatidiform mole. There was no tumor in the uterus.

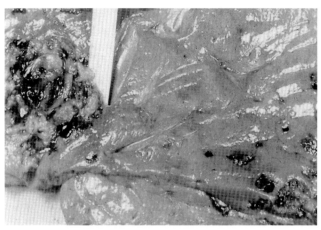

FIGURE 23.4. Same patient as in Figure 23.3. Numerous friable, hemorrhagic tumor nodules have caused massive enlargement of liver. The ruler is placed underneath a large tumor growth within a hepatic vein.

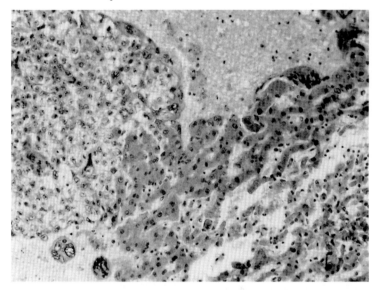

FIGURE 23.5. Same patient as Figures 23.3 and 23.4. Metastatic choriocarcinoma is in the liver following hydatidiform mole. Cords of disrupted liver cells are seen at right; a large tumor mass is at left and consists primarily of cytotrophoblast, with some syncytial surface. H&E × 160.

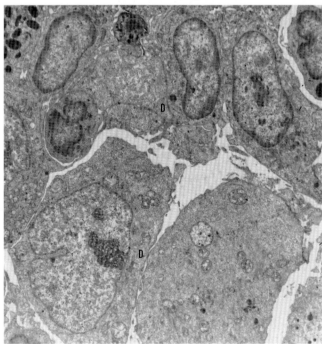

FIGURE 23.6. Electron micrograph of two types of cytotrophoblast. At top are uniform oval nuclei and abundant ribosomes, but few other cytoplasmic constituents. Below are two large cells with irregular nuclei and many more mitochondria. Desmosomes (D) are seen in both. (*Source:* Wynn & Davies, 1964, with permission.)

cinomas (even metastatic lung lesions) have regressed spontaneously (see Bardawil & Toy, 1959; Rauter, 1968). Deligdisch and her coworkers (1978) suggested that solid tumor nests, with high pleomorphism and mitotic activity, have the worst prognosis. Fibrin deposits at the interface between tumor and host tissues are of good prognostic value. Another feature that bespeaks a better prognosis is a significant cellular "reaction" around the tumor (Elston, 1969). Sebire et al. (2004) have endeavored to use immunohistochemistry staining for p57^{KIP2}, a maternally expressed gene *CDKN1C* to differentiate choriocarcinoma derived from moles or nonmolar pregnancies. They found, however, that this marker does not provide a sufficiently accurate means.

To be inclusive it must also be mentioned that nongestational choriocarcinomas have been described on rare occasion. Thus, Liu et al. (2001) presented a gastric choriocarcinoma that was associated with an adenocarcinoma. It secreted large quantities of gonadotropin, which decreased after initially successful therapy. But the tumor recurred, with elevation of gonadotropins, and eventually led to the patient's demise. Although she had three pregnancies in the past, no connection to these could be established, and the authors considered "dedifferentiation" as a possible mechanism of formation. Interestingly, in their literature review of extrauterine primary choriocarcinomas, the authors found that they are more frequent in the Japanese population.

Choriocarcinoma **metastases** occur most commonly in the lung and in the brain, but many other organs may be involved. The distribution of metastases was well recorded by Ober et al. (1971). That presentation also excelled in the description of the macroscopic lesions and in the microscopic appearance of choriocarcinoma. Vaginal secondaries and metastases to the cervix occur relatively frequently (Marquez-Monter & Velasco, 1967; Martin et al., 1983). Acosta-Sison (1958), who studied primary metastases in 32 patients, found the lung to be involved in 44% and the vagina in 31%. Eventually, the lungs were the site of metastases in 94% and the vagina in 44%; other organs were much less often involved. A relatively uncommon site is the kidney, although isolated cases have been reported (Jarrett & Pratt-Thomas, 1984; Soper et al., 1988). Some patients have been successfully treated, despite large tumor burdens. A patient whose third hydatidiform mole (Fig. 23.3) proved fatal had extensive metastases in the liver, but she died from an exsanguinating hemorrhage that originated in a duodenal lesion. This location is otherwise a relatively uncommon site of metastasis.

Pulmonary dissemination of molar tissue occurs often, but such vascular tumor deportation may lie dormant for many years. Figures 23.7 to 23.10 illustrate the lung of a patient who died from pulmonary hypertension 4 years after delivery of a hydatidiform mole. Her pulmonary arteries had thrombi and numerous masses of pure trophoblast. Neoplastic tissue was present in many vessels, but it did not completely traverse the vascular wall. There was an intense chronic inflammatory reaction at these sites, suggesting a barrier to invasion (Fig. 23.10). Similar patients have been described by Seckl et al. (1991) but they were successfully treated. The hypertensive effects of tumor embolization to the lung in general have been discussed in detail by Veinot and colleagues (1992), who believed this to be an important and often unrecognized problem.

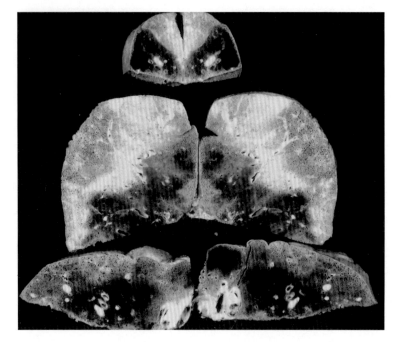

FIGURE 23.7. Lung sections from a patient with pulmonary hypertension and infarction 4 years after hydatidiform mole. Throughout this lung the arteries were obstructed by choriocarcinoma and thrombi. (Courtesy of Dr. A.T. Hertig. Patient discussed by Bardawil & Toy, 1959.)

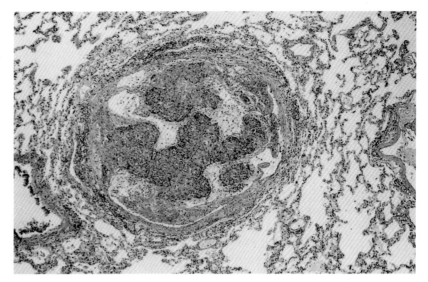

FIGURE 23.8. Same patient as in Figure 23.7. Pulmonary artery is filled with solid choriocarcinoma metastasis. There is an inflammatory reaction in the vascular wall at the point of invasion. H&E × 40.

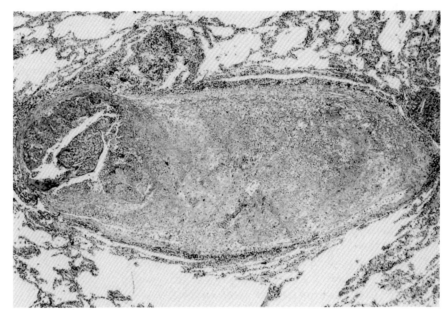

FIGURE 23.9. Same patient as in Figures 23.7 and 23.8. A small amount of viable tumor is present at left, the remainder of the artery is filled with thrombus. H&E × 40.

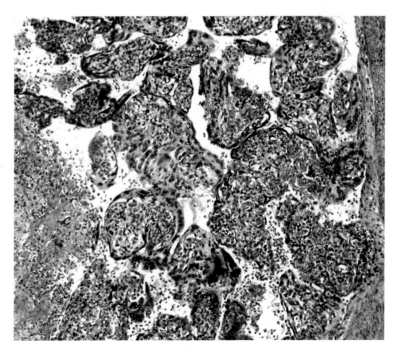

FIGURE 23.10. Same patient as Figures 23.7 to 23.9. Choriocarcinoma fills the artery and is enmeshed in thrombus. At points of invasion there is much chronic inflammation, including many plasma cells. No "villous stroma" is produced. H&E × 100.

The cellular response to choriocarcinoma has been studied in some detail by Elston (1969). He found variable degrees of lymphocytic, histiocytic, and plasmacellular reactions in response to invading tumor cells and correlated this with outcome. Patients with tumors that had the most intense reaction fared best with chemotherapeutic treatment. Elston also saw in the maternal cellular response an attempt of the host to "reject" the neoplasm. This pulmonary complication of latent vascular tumor growth is apparently not uncommon. Fahrner et al. (1959) described a patient who died with cor pulmonale and endarterial tumor growth 5 years after delivery of a mole. Spiegel (1964) had a similar case and reviewed 10 others from the literature. Excellent preservation of neoplastic tissue resulted from the ability of the neoplasm to grow within blood. Other cases have come from Dyke and Fink (1967); and Bagshawe and Nobel (1966) discussed the various types of pulmonary metastasis in some detail. They paid special attention to the radiologic and cardiac aspects. The latter authors and Evans and Hendrickse (1965) accumulated large series of this intraarterial pulmonary tumor spread. Many of the cases were associated with acute pulmonary hypertension and cor pulmonale.

Diagnostic curettage for the treatment of moles may be the mechanism of dissemination of malignant trophoblast with villous tissue. Indeed, villi are occasionally present in such embolic lesions. Bagshawe (1964) pointed out that the presence of villi in trophoblastic lesions "cannot be taken as a guarantee that it will remain benign indefinitely." We strongly agree with this statement but recognize the difficulty experienced by the practicing pathologist and the dilemma of diagnostic semantics. Often an absolute diagnosis of chorionic malignancy cannot be made from curettings alone, especially when villi are present. Optimal care requires follow-up with serial gonadotropin titer determinations. Carlson and his colleagues (1984) described a patient who developed fatal pulmonary lesions immediately after normal pregnancy, despite chemotherapy. Bagshawe (1988) is incorrect, however, to state that the pulmonary lesions occur only in London, and that they have not been recognized during life. They are rarely considered, to be sure, unless preceded by a recent CHM.

Choriocarcinoma most commonly follows CHM and invasive moles. Hertig and Mansell (1956) estimated that only 18.5% of CHM terminate with choriocarcinoma. Most patients pursue a benign course once the uterus has been evacuated. As Figure 23.1 shows, choriocarcinoma may also follow normal gestations. The neoplasm has then occasionally been found within otherwise normal placentas and is then designated choriocarcinoma in situ. Thus, Fukunaga et al. (1995, 1996) observed two cases in the placentas of spontaneous abortuses, clearly arising from stem villi. Other cases of choriocarcinoma in situ are described below. Other origins of choriocarcinoma include gonadal teratomas and, rarely, teratomas at other

sites, but they are then not GTDs. It is unusual for choriocarcinoma to arise without a known antecedent neoplasm. Suzuki et al. (1993) were able to determine the origin of their choriocarcinomas with DNA analysis. Two cases followed complete hydatidiform moles and had androgenetic profiles, whereas another had parental DNA and followed a full-term pregnancy. They concluded from nine cases that polymerase chain reaction (PCR) study of the DNA of these tumors allows determination of the androgenetic origin. Seckl et al. (2000) made an important contribution when they studied the outcome of 3000 patients with partial hydatidiform mole (PHM). Having verified the true triploidy in the PHMs studied, they found that 15 had required chemotherapy for persisting trophoblastic disease, and three of these women developed choriocarcinoma. It was the authors' point to emphasize that PHMs also need serial follow-up in order to prevent this serious consequence.

Choriocarcinoma has no villi, in contrast to **chorioadenoma destruens** (invasive mole), in which villi are present. This arbitrary designation of the two lesions does not signify any significant difference in their biologic behavior, as chorioadenoma destruens may be significantly invasive and destructive (Fig. 23.11). Indeed, the

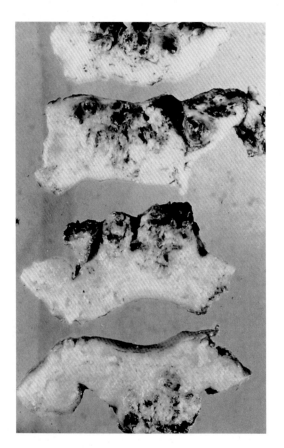

FIGURE 23.11. Invasive mole (chorioadenoma destruens). Slices of uterus show the invasive, hemorrhagic mass of tissue. It is composed of mostly solid trophoblast with a few villous remnants.

two lesions are behaviorally essentially identical. Choriocarcinomas have also been reported in some experimental animals, but their commonest antecedent, the CHM, has not been observed in nonhuman primate pregnancies. It is unknown if these animal choriocarcinomas have the same unusual genetic background as some of the human gestational choriocarcinomas. There are several large reviews that discuss the major aspects of choriocarcinoma, including its historical perspectives, diagnosis, and treatment (Bagshawe, 1969; Ober et al., 1971; Park, 1971; Goldstein & Berkowitz, 1982; Silverberg & Kurman, 1992).

Choriocarcinoma In Situ and Choriocarcinoma Coincident with Pregnancy

Driscoll (1963) described an incidental "choriocarcinoma" in the mature, circumvallate placenta of a normal pregnancy (Figs. 23.12 and 23.13). The mother and child did well. A small "infarct"-like lesion was sampled for histology and found to be a typical choriocarcinoma. The tumor invaded adjacent villi but not their vessels. Now that placentas are more often examined routinely, such tumors have been detected more commonly, and are always detected as infarcts on macroscopic study. Perhaps they should now be called placental choriocarcinoma. Brewer and Gerbie (1966) had two cases of choriocarcinoma developing within otherwise normal placentas. These authors paid special attention to the earliest formation of this proliferative lesion and described the degenerative changes that occur within it. The degenerative process, they thought, may lead to detachment and deportation of tumor fragments. We have seen similar cases, three of which were the cause of massive transplacental fetal hemorrhage, and in one of them hydrops and fetal death (Santamaria et al., 1987) (Fig. 23.14). In another case, the anemic neonate had bled 250 mL into the maternal circulation, but survived. Mother and child had normal postpartum human chorionic gonadotropin (hCG) titers and remained well. The lesion appeared to be an infarct on gross examination and was sampled only because of the neonatal anemia. In yet another patient the mother developed central nervous system (CNS) and pulmonary metastases 1 month after delivery; the neonate had anemia and elevated hCG levels but remained well. In a case published by Lele et al. (1999), the 2 cm × 1.5 cm incidental choriocarcinoma in a mature placenta led to disseminated metastases that were successfully treated. It appeared as a typical infarct but was histologically a typical choriocarcinoma that had invaded adjacent normal villi. Metastatic choriocarcinomas identified during pregnancy have been seen more often. In a description of a pertinent case, Barnes et al. (1982) found 18 cases described before 1970, and reviewed the literature at that time. Their patient, a gravida II (routine spontaneous abortion 13 months earlier and with normal histology), suffered a metastatic choriocarcinoma in brain and lung in the second trimester. The fetus died and was devoid of metastases. The 270-g placenta contained a

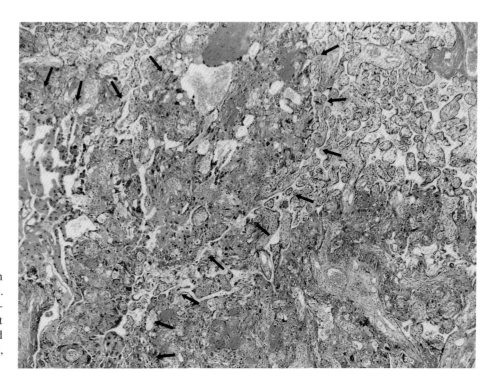

FIGURE 23.12. Mature placenta with choriocarcinoma in situ (arrows). This lesion was accidentally discovered and thought to be an infarct macroscopically. The patient did well. H&E × 76. (*Source:* Driscoll, 1963, with permission.)

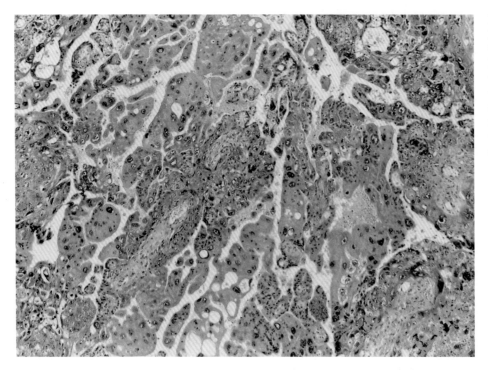

FIGURE 23.13. Same case as in Figure 23.12, but a higher power view of the tumorous elements. Note the obvious pleomorphism of tumor cells that surround the central villus. There is more syncytium than is usually present in choriocarcinoma. The dilated cisternae of the syncytium are obvious (bottom, center). H&E × 200. (*Source:* Driscoll, 1963, with permission.)

6 × 6 × 4 cm choriocarcinoma that had not metastasized to the stillborn fetus. Following chemotherapy and irradiation, the woman had two normal pregnancies but suffered a glioblastoma from which she died 7½ years after the original tumor. Fox and Laurini (1988) found two additional cases of placental choriocarcinoma. In one, the fetus was stillborn, but the other did well. The placental lesion had the macroscopic appearance of an infarct. A particularly interesting case is that of Lage and Roberts (1993). Many white nodules in the placenta were diagnosed as choriocarcinoma, and pulmonary metastases ensued that responded to therapy. Placental villi had not been invaded. The 46,XX neonate remained normal. Further, this publication brings together all of the literature on choriocarcinoma in situ. It may be argued that these histologically identified lesions are not "malignant" but, rather, in the sense used by Huber (1969), represent benign lesions, which he described as "chorionepitheliosis interna." It may be so, except that not all such cases eventuated without causing metastases. The concept of choriocarcinoma in situ is variably interpreted, and more must be learned from future biologic studies of early lesions. They are probably much more common than recognized and fall, in a way, into the spectrum of confined

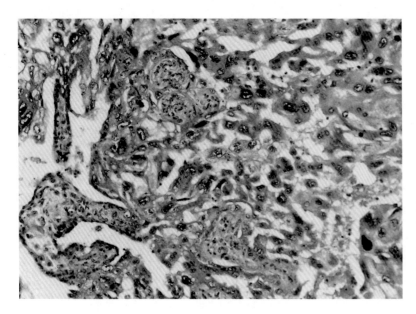

FIGURE 23.14. Choriocarcinoma in situ in an otherwise normal placenta. Solid nests of partially anaplastic tumor cells surround degenerating villi; note also the invaded villi (arrow). Fetus was hydropic and stillborn due to transplacental hemorrhage. H&E × 125. (*Source:* Santamaria et al., 1987, with permission.)

placental mosaicism. A relevant case is shown in Figure 23.15. This was a normal placenta, and random section disclosed this unusual villus with multiple layers of trophoblast and several mitoses. It is possible that such a lesion eventuates into a choriocarcinoma. The important case described by Heifetz and Czaja (1992) emphasized this. In their 69,XXX triploid PHM with fetus, a small nodule of truly malignant-appearing trophoblastic growth was found. Despite this, the woman pursued a normal postpartum course; the report also summarized the 10 or so choriocarcinomas in situ reported to 1992. Additional cases with fetomaternal hemorrhage or with a rise of α-fetoprotein (AFP) levels and benign subsequent course were presented by Duleba et al. (1992) and Ollendorff et al. (1990). Duleba et al., as did several others, treated their patient "expectantly" and showed in photographs that the lesion appeared grossly as an infarct. Ollendorff's patient with elevated maternal serum AFP (MSAFP) and a placental choriocarcinoma had rising hCG titers and developed a pulmonary nodule. The discussion following this paper (Hustin & Jauniaux, 1991) proves that the lesion differed from their chorioangiocarcinoma (vide infra). Jacques et al. (1998) described five cases of intraplacental choriocarcinoma identified in a 5-year period. In two women, pulmonary metastases were present, but none of the fetuses suffered disease, although two were premature and one had anemia. In situ hybridization for Y chromosomes was positive in the two gestations with male fetuses. The lesions had the gross appearances of infarcts. These authors also suggested that this intraplacental neoplasm may be more common than heretofore recognized.

Schopper and Pliess (1949) used the term **chorionepitheliosis** for borderline cases in a lengthy discussion of trophoblastic properties. They were especially concerned with spontaneous cures of alleged choriocarcinomas and with ectopic chorionepitheliomatous growths. They described a woman with a vulvar trophoblastic tumor

that had developed during normal pregnancy. Benson et al. (1962) described massive fetomaternal hemorrhage in a patient who subsequently developed uterine choriocarcinoma with pulmonary metastases. Blackburn (1976) and Feldman (1977) reported similar cases. In four additional patients with small placental choriocarcinomas reported by Brewer and Mazur (1981), disseminated maternal lesions were found. The infants did not have tumors, but three were stillborn.

Hertig and Mansell (1956) indicated that choriocarcinoma follows (in the United States) normal pregnancies in a 1 per 160,000 incidence. It is thus not surprising that choriocarcinoma should also be found occasionally coincident with pregnancy and abortions (Fig. 23.1). Relevant cases are those by Heller and Householder (1952), Driscoll (1983), Miller et al. (1979), and Olive et al. (1984). It is apparent from reviewing these reports that the choriocarcinoma that follows normal term pregnancy has a much poorer prognosis than that which follows CHM. Patients with this complication of pregnancy also have often much earlier metastatic disease (Hutchison et al., 1968; Greene & McCue, 1978; Miller et al., 1979). In occasional cases of neonates with tumors, the placental choriocarcinoma was not detected or the placenta had not been examined. This was the case with cerebral choriocarcinoma metastases that caused death in a 1-month-old child described by Chandra et al. (1990). The mother had no untoward sequelae and delivered another child, with normal placenta.

There are many other reports of choriocarcinoma that occur simultaneously in mother and infant or fetus. Buckell and Owen (1954) described the death of a 7-week-old infant from chorionepitheliomatous metastases; the mother needed a hysterectomy because she suffered postpartum choriocarcinoma. The authors referred to a similar case described by Emery in 1952. Mercer et al. (1958) found a fatal choriocarcinoma in a 3-month-old infant whose mother died from dissemi-

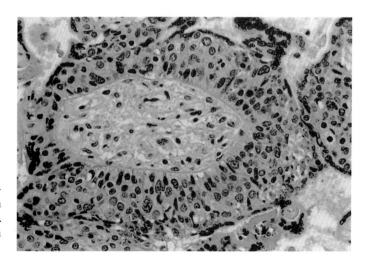

Figure 23.15. A single villus within a term placenta, randomly sectioned, shows proliferation of trophoblast with several mitoses and hyperdiploidy, as judged by nuclear size. Perhaps this is the precursor lesion of choriocarcinoma in situ. H&E × 400.

nated disease. Another case, fatal for mother and infant, was reported by Daamen and colleagues (1961). Witzleben and Bruninga (1968), who reported a case, suggested that these findings constituted a specific syndrome. In their case, the mother had no obvious disease initially but later died from disseminated choriocarcinoma. Metastatic choriocarcinoma was the cause of fetal death in the report from Kruseman et al. (1977). The hydropic fetus had bled transplacentally. The mother developed metastatic disease and was successfully treated.

Chorangiocarcinoma

Yet another new tumor type was reported by Jauniaux and colleagues (1988). They called this lesion chorangiocarcinoma. It was described as a "missing link," but they still believed that "it is a true malignant neoplasm or a voluminous chorangioma covered by extreme trophoblastic hyperplasia" (Hustin & Jauniaux, 1991). The unique lesion they described appeared to be a solitary chorioangioma with extensive trophoblastic hyperplasia at its borders. The authors also concluded that chorangiomas are not hamartomas but true neoplasms. Trask et al. (1994) published a second case of chorangiocarcinoma, a choriocarcinoma in situ with accompanying chorangiosis, occurring in a twin pregnancy. The other twin's placenta was normal and the mother did well. The lesion appeared to be an infarct macroscopically, as most other similar lesions have been. It introduces the question as to whether one should routinely sample all infarcts for histologic study, a practice that we have thus far avoided. The third case was described by Guschmann et al. (2003), again an incidental finding without deleterious consequences. Even the angiogenetic factors that they studied in this case were normal; they postulated this to be a "collision tumor," at least as being one possibility for the genesis of the tumor.

Exaggerated Placental Site: Placental Site Nodule, Placental Site Trophoblastic Tumor, and Epithelioid Trophoblastic Tumor

Kurman et al. (1976) introduced the term **trophoblastic pseudotumor** to designate a trophoblastic lesion they saw in 12 patients that behaved in a benign manner. The lesion tended to occur in young women, usually after pregnancy or abortion. The authors considered this entity to be "an exaggerated form" of the older entity syncytial endometritis. These placental site lesions were usually treated successfully by curettage. The trophoblastic *pseudotumor*, however, also formed occasional hemorrhagic nodules in the myometrium. This entity, we believe, is equivalent to the concept of chorionepitheliosis, which was discussed at

length by Schopper and Pliess (1949). It also probably encompasses the chorioma of Ewing (1910) and perhaps the syncytioma and other vague designations of borderline trophoblastic lesions discussed in the past. These entities are not uncommon but were infrequently reported. As better delineation became available, more cases were described, and a good survey is provided by Baergen and Rutgers (1997). The designation of these lesions depends much on the interpretation by individual pathologists and on the clinical behavior (see Fig. 23.19).

Because of the superficial resemblance to choriocarcinoma, it thus came as no surprise that metastatic consequences were later observed, despite the earlier belief that the trophoblastic pseudotumor was a benign growth. Because several patients with apparently malignant lesions have since been identified, this led Scully and Young (1981) to introduce yet another term, the **placental site trophoblastic tumor** (PSTT), which is characterized by mononuclear extravillous trophoblast that infiltrates within the uterus and its vessels. Only rarely, are villi present. The absence of cytotrophoblastic cell masses and the usual absence of syncytiotrophoblast differentiates the entity from choriocarcinoma. The lesion is largely composed of placental site cells (extravillous trophoblast, or X cells) and blends with placental site nodules and plaques as well as exaggerated placental site (vide infra). Such a lesion is shown in Figures 23.16 to 23.18. Here it is a nodule of trophoblast that had perforated the uterus 18 months after a normal term pregnancy. After hysterectomy, the patient thrived. There were no metastases. Finkler and his colleagues (1988) treated seven patients with PSTTs and included a detailed review. One case followed a CHM, and the others occurred after abortion or premature delivery, in contrast to choriocarcinoma, which more commonly follows a CHM. All but one that followed an abortion pursued a benign course. Despite chemotherapy, this exceptional patient had metastatic disease in pelvic nodes. Although the authors did not publish any photomicrographs, they did describe an unprecedented high mitotic count. This point is particularly noteworthy because placental site cells (X-cells or extravillous trophoblast) are not usually very mitotic.

In the relatively short time since the description of PSTT, a large number of cases have been reported, in spite of the fact that it is the rarest proliferative lesion of trophoblast. An interesting study of this lesion was undertaken by Eckstein et al. (1985), who also reviewed the literature most competently. In their view, differentiation from choriocarcinoma should be easy because the lesion is a "well-circumscribed yellowish mass in which hemorrhage and necrosis are less conspicuous than in choriocarcinoma." The histology is more like a placental site than like choriocarcinoma. The tumor in the aforementioned patient followed an apparently normal pregnancy but was eventually fatal with widespread metastases. It

FIGURE 23.16. Placental site trophoblastic tumor that had penetrated the uterus 18 months after a normal, term delivery. Hysterectomy alone cured this patient. The "malignant" cells are pleomorphic placental site giant cells (largely X cells). There are no solid sheets of cytotrophoblast and few syncytial cells. There are no mitoses. H&E × 100.

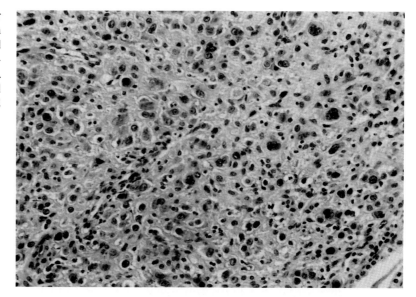

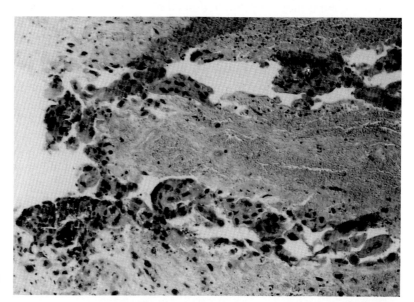

FIGURE 23.17. Placental site trophoblastic tumor; same case as in Figure 23.16. H&E × 160.

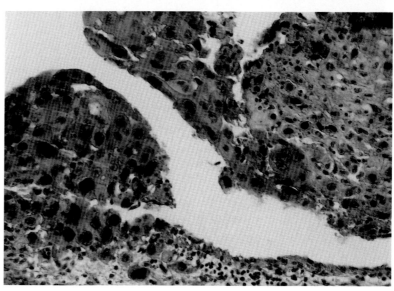

FIGURE 23.18. Placental site trophoblastic tumor. H&E × 250.

had a diploid DNA content, and biopsies were easily transplanted into nude mice. Unlike other lesions of this type, the tumor cells did not have a high mitotic rate. Fukunaga and Ushigome (1993a,b) reviewed the entire topic comprehensively and added three cases of PSTT to the literature. One of their patients died with widespread metastases. That patient had a term delivery and returned 9 months later with uterine, vaginal, bladder, and lung tumors that resisted chemotherapy. Of the three cases they reported, two recovered, all had diploid flow cytometric DNA values, and all were of pregnancies with female babies. Characteristically, many fewer mitoses were seen in these lesions than in typical choriocarcinomas, and histochemically they showed significantly less hCG production, and more human placental lactogen (hPL) staining despite their epithelioid appearance (Rhoton-Vlasak et al., 1998). As in eight other cases described, their fatal case had associated nephrotic syndrome, a complication not reported in choriocarcinoma. They estimated that perhaps 10% of PSTTs behave in a malignant manner.

Although histologic and clinical features of the tumor, such as tumor stage, advanced age, interval from previous pregnancy of greater than 2 years, previous term pregnancy, clear cytoplasm, tumor necrosis, mitotic rate, and myometrial invasion, have been shown to be of prognostic value, no specific feature or features can predict benign versus malignant behavior (Rutgers et al., 1995, Baergen & Rutgers 1997). Furthermore, high mitotic rates have been identified in patients who ultimately pursued a benign course and low mitotic rates have been seen in patients with metastatic or even fatal disease (Fig. 23.19).

Rosenheim et al. (1980), who described a patient with uterine hemorrhage after abortion, decided that this diagnosis can be made only on a hysterectomy specimen. The uterus they studied showed an endometrial polyp that was composed of clot, with masses of atypical trophoblast interspersed. Villi had earlier been obtained by curettage from this patient. The tissue was like that of a CHM. The trophoblast invaded 30% of the myometrium. After its removal, the patient experienced full recovery. Nagelberg and Rosen (1985) described other interesting biologic features in a patient following a normal pregnancy. They performed many endocrine studies, because the tumor was accompanied by virilization due to testosterone production, possibly secondary to ovarian theca cell stimulation. It was also relatively resistant to chemotherapy, a characteristic that distinguishes PSTT from choriocarcinoma. After an eventual hysterectomy, the pathologist found a solitary 2-cm mass of tumor cells. This report provided much insight into other endocrine parameters of this condition. The prolonged production of hPL by the X cells of such a lesion was held to be responsible for the erythrocytosis in a patient reported by Brewer et al. (1992). After hysterectomy the symptoms disappeared; the lesion was a 6-cm hemorrhagic mass that infiltrated the myometrium but was primarily composed of X cells. The difficulty of differential diagnosis was also highlighted by Horn et al. (1997). They described a patient in whom a uterine lesion was initially mistaken for a cervical carcinoma. Radical hysterectomy proved to have been unnecessary; indeed, the lesion may merely have been an exaggerated placental site rather than a PSTT. Caution and experience are necessary in the diagnosis before critical therapy is instituted. Another large cervical GTD (presumably a choriocarcinoma) was treated only with chemotherapy and disappeared (Sohn et al., 1996). The only

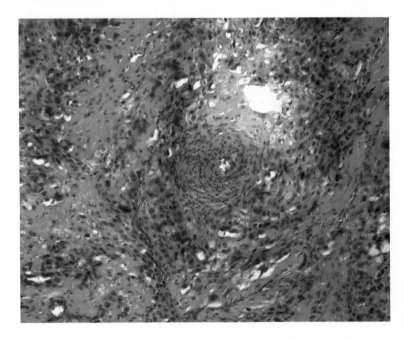

FIGURE 23.19. Placental site trophoblastic tumor with epithelioid appearance and numerous mitoses. H&E × 400.

guides were hormone levels and the postgestational history of the lesion.

Fukunaga and Ushigome (1993a) believed that intermediate forms of these tumors exist. The case described by Hopkins et al. (1985) would thus perhaps still best be considered a choriocarcinoma following normal pregnancy, rather than a placental site tumor. Its histologic composition most conformed to cytotrophoblast and syncytium, rather than to extravillous trophoblast. More precise methods to differentiate among these various lesions are desirable. Horn et al. (1996) presented differential diagnostic criteria for these lesions. Such efforts may be accomplished by the use of histochemistry, as performed by Wells and Bulmer (1988) and Fukunaga and Ushigome (1993a,b). These authors found in one such lesion the existence of a few tumor cells with hCG markers; more cells contained hPL antigen (see also Rhoton-Vlasak et al., 1998). Duncan and Mazur (1989) compared the ultrastructure of one such tumor (following normal pregnancy) with that of nine choriocarcinomas. The findings included an absence of cytotrophoblastic nests in the placental site tumor. The cellularity was composed primarily of intermediate trophoblast (extravillous trophoblast, X cells), with occasional interspersed syncytium. The authors found by immunohistochemistry that some of the neoplastic X cells contained hPL as well as hCG, which is not usually the case in normal cells. The cells in PSTT also stain positively for α-inhibin, Mel-CAM CD 146, a cell surface adhesion molecule and placental alkaline phosphatase (Shih & Kurman, 1998b).

The most recently described neoplastic lesion of trophoblast is the **epithelioid trophoblastic tumor**. Shih and Kurman (1998b) described 14 cases of this unusual lesion that is characterized by sheets of large mononuclear cells that resemble epithelial carcinoma. The infiltrative neoplasm is thought to derive from a specialized lineage of extravillous trophoblast and has a behavior more similar to that of migratory extravillous trophoblast, such as exist in the chorionic plate and extraplacental membranes. Several patients have had metastases and some died from wide dissemination, but this tumor appears to have a similar behavior and prognosis as the usual type of placental site trophoblastic tumor.

Syncytial endometritis is an ancient term that reflects the presence of many trophoblastic giant cells in the floor of the placenta. Others might have used the term **chorionepitheliosis** to describe this morphology. This lesion is considered to be nonneoplastic and merely an exaggeration of a normal physiologic process. It is common in molar implantations. It has no relation to any inflammatory or infectious lesion, and the term has been abandoned in favor of exaggerated placental site (Tavassoli et al., 2003). In reality, though, it is often impossible to distinguish this lesion from normal placental sites. One must also remember that few normal placental sites ever come to be

observed by pathologists, as they are rarely curetted and death is uncommon at that stage of development (Dallenbach-Hellweg, 1981). Therefore, the pathologist may be unduly alarmed by the appearance of a normal postpartum placental site. A relevant example is shown in Figures 23.20 and 21.21. It came from the curettage of a placental bed in an 8-week gestation and had no adverse consequences. But the exuberance of normal trophoblast at this site is apparent. Figure 23.22 illustrates another exaggerated placental site. A cytogenetic NISH (nonradioactive in situ hybridization) study done by Faul et al. (1994) in cases of exaggerated placental site trophoblast indicated that the often-bizarre nuclei found in these lesions are polyploid or aneuploid, perhaps arising by cell fusion or by endoreduplication of chromosomes. Two cases of chorionepitheliosis were published by Van Bogaert and Staquet (1977), presumably representing the same entity. The authors also considered the lesion to be a benign proliferation of trophoblastic elements. To clarify the differential diagnosis, these authors developed a scheme for differential diagnosis which has been adapted in Table 23.2.

Yet another lesion of extravillous trophoblast that has been described is the **placental site nodule**, which is a benign, nonneoplastic lesion that may be diagnosed many years after the preceding pregnancy. Nickels et al. (1978) described such a lesion in a 52-year-old woman whose last pregnancy was 20 years earlier. According to them, the lesion was "a normal anatomic event at the placental site after miscarriage or full-term pregnancy." A review of 20 cases of placental site nodules and plaques was undertaken by Young and colleagues (1990), and 40 cases were

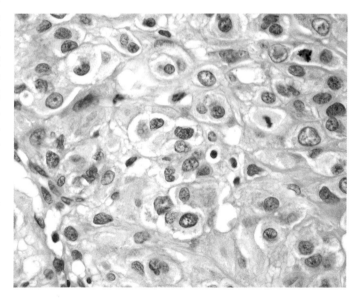

FIGURE 23.20. Exaggerated placental site at 8 weeks. The infiltrating cells split myometrial bundles and are composed of uni- or multinuclear extravillous trophoblast. This is a benign, normal placental floor but histologically may easily be confused with a placental site trophoblastic tumor. H&E × 160.

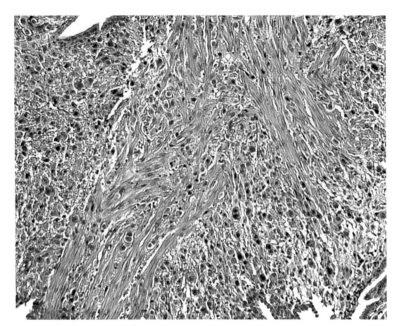

FIGURE 23.21. Exaggerated placental site following fetal demise at 8 weeks. Endometrial glands are surrounded by extravillous trophoblast and these are admixed with multinucleated giant cells. H&E × 250.

reviewed by Huetter and Gersell (1993). Most of the cells stained with antibodies to hPL and cytokeratin; all lesions were either incidental findings or followed with a benign course. There is now agreement that these nodules represent retained placental sites in which much hyalinization and degenerative change are found. A useful marker for the identification of the proliferating cells is the presence of major basic protein (MBP), and less useful is placental lactogen. Rhoton-Vlasak et al. (1998) found 100% of exaggerated placental site nodules to be positive for MBP, and 78% of PSTTs. Tsang et al. (1993) identified Mallory bodies in two cases, representing high molecular weight cytokeratins. Shih et al. (1999) were able to differentiate the cells composing these lesions of extravillous trophoblast into distinct types—those presumably arising from the membranous extravillous trophoblast (mild proliferation, smaller, glycogen-rich) and those from the intervillous/placental floor spaces (more eosinophilic, larger, and pleomorphic). We found a nodule like this 5 years after the last pregnancy when a patient had hysterectomy for cervical carcinoma.

It is difficult to define these lesions precisely, especially when the diagnosis depends on tissue obtained at curettage (see also Horn et al., 1996; Horn & Bilek, 1997). A

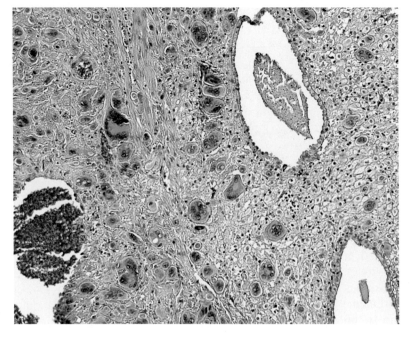

FIGURE 23.22. Curettings after normal pregnancy. There was postpartum bleeding of this 35-year-old woman who had had eight pregnancies, with two live births. The lesion was interpreted as choriocarcinoma, but the patient had an uneventful course without chemotherapy. It is best interpreted as exaggerated placental site. The cells are placental site giant cells (largely X cells). No solid sheets of cytotrophoblast are present, and there are no mitoses. H&E × 260.

TABLE 23.2. Diagnostic differences between trophoblastic pseudotumor and other diseases

Signs	PSTT	Exaggerated placental site	Choriocarcinoma	Mole
Blood vessel invasion	+	–	+	–
Placental villi	–	+	–	+
Necrosis	+/–	+/–	+	–
Trophoblastic invasion	+	+	+	+
Syncytial trophoblast	+/–	+	+	+
Cytotrophoblast	–	+	+	+
Hemorrhage	+/–	–	+	–

PSTT, placental site trophoblastic tumor.

detailed review with illustrations and prognostic predictions has been provided by Baergen and Rutgers (1997), but it remains a difficult topic for most pathologists. The hope of differentiating a potential malignancy among these placental site lesions by an assessment of ploidy or DNA has been disappointing. Most lesions have been diploid or tetraploid, as summarized by Lage and Sheikh (1997). To ascertain whether one could anticipate the development of persistent trophoblastic lesions, de Kaa et al. (1996) performed DNA analyses and cytogenetics. They found this of limited value and also concluded that nuclear pleomorphism of CHM was of no prognostic significance.

Detailed study of genes by comparative genomic hybridization of four archival cases of PSTT undertaken by Hui et al. (2004) has shown chromosomal gain in two cases, no chromosomal losses, and neither gain nor loss in the remaining two cases. Initial results of studies by Shih and Kurman (1998a), who have been most interested in defining these lesions, showed that double immunohistology using Ki-67 and Mel-CAM antibodies allows some differentiation of exaggerated placental site, PSTT, and choriocarcinoma.

Interesting attempts at the differential diagnosis have been published in the intervening years since the last edition of this book. First, in an exhaustive study, Oldt et al. (2002) showed with numerous markers that the cells that compose these gestational trophoblastic neoplasias (GTNs) (other than the choriocarcinoma) have fetal genetic and chromosomal markers; they are thus not maternal neoplasms. Further, all of these 42 tumors studied had heterozygous SNIPS (single nuclear polymorphisms) and were thus different from the androgenetic moles and choriocarcinomas. It has been possible for Shih et al. (2004) to assign some of these lesions to different categories from a study of certain isoforms of the expression patterns of the *p63* gene, and thus to assign putative ancestors among the trophoblast lineages, the

membranous vs. placental extravillous cytotrophoblast. This has led to improved understanding of the otherwise confusing histopathology. In essence, then, this contribution has confirmed their earlier deduction of the specific origin of these lesions (Shih & Kurman, 2001).

Ultrastructure of Trophoblastic Tumors

Wynn and Davies (1964) studied the fine structure of trophoblastic neoplasms that were transplanted to hamster cheek pouches. They combined their morphologic study with an endocrine assessment; they were unable to demonstrate estrogenic activity. Except for excessive dilatation of syncytial cytoplasmic channels, the tumor resembled early human trophoblast. Larsen et al. (1967) made similar observations and showed that syncytial cells performed phagocytosis. Other electron microscopy (EM) studies were carried out directly on human choriocarcinomas that had not been transplanted (Inferrera et al., 1967; Knoth et al., 1969a; Arai et al., 1976; Duncan & Mazur, 1989). The various investigators made the same observations. Several of the descriptions included cells that are truly intermediate between cytotrophoblast and syncytium ("transitional" cells) (see Fig. 23.16), which was also shown in the choriocarcinomatous cell lines maintained in vitro by Knoth and colleagues (1969b).

ANTIGENIC STUDIES OF TROPHOBLASTIC TUMORS

Most choriocarcinomas have at least some paternal genome. Perhaps most (at least those derived from hydatidiform moles) have only paternal chromosomes. It is therefore possible that the tumor's antigenic determinants may engender immunologic rejection. This assumption was an important explanation for their frequently favorable prognosis. Elston (1969), though, described variably intense cellular reactions to the invading trophoblastic neoplasm and related it to outcome. Observations such as this one have led to the study of immune interactions of the tumors with the host and to the determination of human leukocyte antigens (HLAs) in choriocarcinoma.

Mogensen and Kissmeyer-Nielsen (1968) studied HLA types in mothers, fathers, and their children in conjunction with placenta-associated choriocarcinoma. Despite antigenic differences between father and mother, most of the children were histocompatible with the mother. This compatibility, the authors suggested, made the tumors capable of growing in the uterus, rather than being rejected. Tomoda and his colleagues (1976) investigated HLAs and ABO antigens in patients with gestational trophoblastic neoplasia and their husbands. ABO types had no correlation, but patients with choriocarcinoma were "frequently incompatible" at various HLA types. Nevertheless, patients with choriocarcinoma were more frequently histocompatible with their husbands than those having invasive moles. Rudolph and Thomas (1971) had found significantly different HLAs in the mother and child of a patient who developed choriocarcinoma. The authors thereby refuted the notion that the tumors develop because of a failure of trophoblast to be rejected. Lawler et al. (1971) found that there was no increased histocompatibility between mothers and children in choriocarcinoma cases. There was a suggestion that major incompatibilities of HLA and ABO types protected the mother from disseminated disease. This aspect was further supported by findings of Mogensen and Kissmeyer-Nielsen (1971). Ivaskova and her colleagues (1969) found lymphocytotoxic antibodies against HLAs in 12 of 13 patients with choriocarcinoma or moles and speculated that these antigens may be important in tumor rejection. Differences in the population of the HLA_2 membrane attack complex of complement (MAC) did not exist from controls in a French population of choriocarcinoma patients (Amiel & Lebovici, 1970). Ho et al. (1989) found that whites did not share HLAs, whereas Chinese with choriocarcinomas did. Yamashita et al. (1984) performed direct tissue studies to ascertain the possible presence of histocompatibility antigens on choriocarcinoma cells. By this method, normal villi, hydatidiform moles, and two choriocarcinomas did not have any apparent class I and II antigens. Differences in responsiveness to class I and II antigens were concisely reviewed by Nepom (1989).

When ABO blood group antigens were studied in a Lebanese population, families with trophoblastic disease had a normal distribution, as controls (Iliya et al., 1969). Bagshawe et al. (1971) observed that blood group A women married to blood group O husbands have the highest risk of trophoblastic neoplasia; those married to blood group A husbands have the lowest risk. Blood group AB patients have tumors that metastasized widely and were least affected by chemotherapy. The investigators considered that these effects show immunologic modulation of the tumor.

Because Rh(D) antigen is said to be expressed on trophoblastic surfaces, Tomoda et al. (1981) suggested that hydatidiform moles [with Rh(D)] would be rejected by the Rh(d) host (see also Fischer et al., 1985), and that the difference in Rh antigens of Orientals could explain their high incidence of trophoblastic disease. Support for this idea has also come from the early studies by Scott (1962, 1968).

It is not yet certain that biologic trophoblast-specific antigen expression exists. Cheng and Johnson (1988) endeavored to produce antibodies to such possible antigens. When the antibodies were carefully absorbed, these authors found a low incidence (3.6%) of corresponding antibodies in serum samples of infertile women. These investigators suggested that the earlier results of Grimmer and colleagues (1988) were erroneous, those that suggested a possible relation of these antibodies to lupus-like disorders. Srivannaboon (1971) found, in immunologic studies with a trophoblast line, that choriocarcinoma contained an antigen that was not shared by normal trophoblast. The nature of this antigen was not identified.

There have also been attempts to treat gestational trophoblastic neoplasia with immunologic methods. Doniach et al. (1958) immunized a patient with choriocarcinoma by injecting her husband's cells. Hackett and Beech (1961) injected concentrates of the husband's leukocytes intradermally without inciting a reaction. They also employed Freund's adjuvant therapy and noted a gradual diminution in metastatic tumor nodules. Final tumor resolution, however, occurred only after chemotherapy. The conclusion of these authors was that choriocarcinoma is not antigenic in the usual sense. Others have not agreed with this conclusion. Cinader et al. (1961) thought that their patient was successfully treated with leukocytes but were unable to rule out spontaneous remission. Although some spontaneous remissions of choriocarcinoma are well documented (Brewer et al., 1961), this is not a common event and certainly spontaneous remission cannot be reliably anticipated in clinical management. Ewing (1941), in fact, did not accept such lesions that regressed as having been true choriocarcinomas.

The immunologic tolerance of the husband's skin graft was explored in two patients with choriocarcinoma by Robinson et al. (1963), and Mathé et al. (1964) found variable skin graft survival in some patients with choriocarcinoma. There is no doubt that some GTNs elicit a cellular and immunologic response and that this may be related to survival (see Ober, 1969). It is also the presumed explanation for the poorer response to chemotherapeutic agents of the testicular choriocarcinomas in men because they lack foreign antigens. Until the precise mechanism of graft rejection is understood and we know more about the tolerance afforded to normal placental trophoblast, it is useless to engage in further speculation. The reader is referred to the numerous papers from symposia that have dealt with this question (Edwards et al., 1975; Beer & Billingham, 1976; Wegmann & Gill, 1983; Gill et al., 1987).

As with hydatidiform moles, the frequency of choriocarcinoma is irregularly distributed in different populations. It is also difficult to enumerate precisely because malignant moles are often included with choriocarcinoma. Nevertheless, there are major differences in prevalence. For instance, Ho et al. (1989) found the prevalence of GTN to be lowest in whites (3/100,000 to 6/100,000) and highest in Chinese (68/100,000 to 202/100,000). They studied cellular antigens and found that Chinese had significant HLA sharing; whites did not. This finding suggested to them that genetic and nongenetic factors are of etiologic importance, and that this may also explain the generally better prognosis in whites. Rolon and Lopez (1979) summarized much of the epidemiologic aspects; their data and those of others are summarized in Table 23.3.

The higher incidence of choriocarcinoma in older women is also apparent in most of these studies. Oettle (1961) made the point that, despite the frequency of choriocarcinoma in Bantu women, there is no increased frequency of hydatidiform moles in that population. They believed that the higher incidence of choriocarcinoma in that population may result from higher ages at childbearing. In a study of Lebanese patients, Iliya et al. (1967) hypothesized that consanguinity is an important cause of choriocarcinoma. Parazzini et al. (1988a) adduced some data in favor of specific dietary deficiencies (e.g., vitamin A) in gestational trophoblastic neoplasia; "however, the limitation of available evidence still introduces serious uncertainties in the interpretation of these findings."

Endocrine Aspects of Gestational Trophoblastic Neoplasia

The most important endocrine consideration of choriocarcinoma is its production of hCG or subunits thereof (see also Chapter 22). Follow-up of patients with CHM and choriocarcinomas is effectively done by assay of this hormone in serum (Delfs, 1959). Urine hCG values above 100,000 IU/24 hours (or serum levels of β-subunits measured by radioimmunoassay) strongly suggest the presence of a hydatidiform mole or malignant GTN. Conventionally, patients are monitored with weekly determination of hCG levels until none is detected for 3 consecutive weeks after the initial treatment of complete moles. In the usual case, hCG becomes undetectable within 8 to 173 days (Yuen et al., 1977). Chorionic gonadotropin is cleared by renal mechanisms, with a half-life of 35 hours (Midgley & Jaffe, 1968). Hammond et al. (1981) suggested that, after the titers have disappeared, hCG should be monitored for 1 year after evacuation of a mole. Even so, late recurrences have been reported and they have frequently occurred despite adherence to this regimen (e.g., Kirk, 1965; Vaughn et al., 1980). The observations by Rotmensch and Cole (2000) in the treatment of possible GTNs on the basis of elevated hCG titers should be appreciated. These authors showed clearly that elevated hCG titers, by themselves, are not a reliable indication of trophoblastic tumors. This is due to the variable nature of antibodies against hCG used commercially and perhaps also to the possible binding of preexisting antibodies to mouse immunoglobulin G (IgG). Inasmuch as this elevation of titers had led to the inappropriate therapy

TABLE 23.3. Frequency of choriocarcinoma and chorioadenoma destruens among number of pregnancies

Authors	Region	Choriocarcinoma	Chorioadenoma destruens
Hertig & Mansell (1956)	US	43,000	
Wei & Cuyang (1963)	India	912	
Mills (1964)	England	70,000	
Tow (1965)	Singapore	5,000	
Acosta-Sison (1966)	Philippines	1,382–2,229	
Kolstad & Hognestad (1965)	Norway	20,000	
Aranda & Martinez (1968)	Puerto Rico	32,460	
Yen & MacMahon (1968)	Rhode Island	40,000	
Reddy & Rao (1969)	Taiwan	496	
Mogensen & Olsen (1972)	Denmark	49,000	126,000
Matalon et al. (1972)	Israel	15,000	
Baltazar (1976)	Philippines	5,747	
Rolon & Lopez (1979)	Paraguay	43,489	70,252

Source: Modified from Rolon & Lopez (1979).

of 12 patients, they recommended greater scrutiny in the face of such laboratory findings. A possible improvement of monitoring cases with GTN is perhaps feasible with the determination of β-subunits of hCG in urine by radio-immunoassay (Wehmann et al., 1981). Through simultaneous measurements of serum and spinal fluid β-hCG levels, studies suggested that it may be possible to anticipate cerebral metastases (Soma et al., 1980).

Yazaki et al. (1980) compared isoelectric homogeneity of serum hCG in various types of normal and abnormal pregnancies. They found that normal gestations, CHM, and invasive moles had "normal" isoelectric peaks, whereas additional peaks were detected in sera of patients with choriocarcinoma. A variety of studies have shown that the hCG originates from the syncytial component of the choriocarcinoma. When Dawood (1975) measured progesterone levels in patients with choriocarcinoma, he found that it correlated with hCG. He believed that the elevated progesterone levels resulted from its production by the hCG-stimulated ovaries, as many patients experience theca lutein cysts with this neoplasm (Kohorn, 1983), rather than the trophoblast. Lacking appropriate fetal adrenal precursors, estrogen production is sparse in choriocarcinoma patients, and its determination is not useful. It is different in men with choriocarcinoma. They have excessive estrogen production and often suffer gynecomastia (Martin & Carden, 1963), presumably because of Leydig cell stimulation. Follow-up with hPL, MBP, and other trophoblastic proteins has either not been undertaken or has not been useful for therapeutic and management purposes.

Occasionally, choriocarcinoma is associated with excessive androgen production. These rare reports have been competently reviewed by Nagelberg and Rosen (1985). The origin of the androgens is still in dispute, although some in vitro work suggested a trophoblast origin. Searle et al. (1978) measured a placenta-specific β₁-glycoprotein in the serum of patients with GTN and found a moderate elevation in CHM and choriocarcinoma patients—much

less than that of hCG, however. They were not enthusiastic about the use of this marker in the management of patients. Nisbet et al. (1982) localized another placenta protein marker (PP5) to syncytium of placentas and its tumors. Serum levels, however, were not sufficiently elevated for its clinical use.

PSTTs are also associated with increased production of hormones, specifically hCG. Serum levels of hCG, however, are only moderately elevated, usually up to only 10,000 IU, as opposed to the extremely high levels seen in choriocarcinoma. In addition, only about 75% to 80% of patients show any elevation at all (Baergen & Rutgers, 1997).

Ectopic Choriocarcinomas; Tumors in Men

Aside from the truly gestational choriocarcinoma that most commonly follows a complete hydatidiform mole, choriocarcinoma has occasionally been reported in the fallopian tube, ovary, and other locations. These lesions may then be referred to as heterotopic chorioepithelioma (Nanke, 1959). Nanke, however, discovered such a tumor after hysterectomy was performed for hydatidiform mole, and it is most likely that the CHM was the tumor's antecedent of the cerebral, renal, and pulmonary metastases. The author opined that the tumor arose from deportation of benign trophoblast that subsequently dedifferentiated. He termed it "chorioepitheliosis." As detailed in Chapter 22, such uncertainties can now be resolved when genetic markers are studied. Three rare cases of choriocarcinoma in tubal pregnancies were the topic of a publication by Horn et al. (1994). All were successfully treated and metastases did not occur.

The primary choriocarcinoma in the lung of a patient without any other lesions, reported by Tanimura et al. (1985), most likely resulted from a prior therapeutic abortion. To support such a proposal, the authors examined the lungs of 10 patients dying after delivery or abortion and found pulmonary trophoblast in nine. Tubal choriocarcinoma was reported by Madden (1950) following tubal abortion, as did most of the 48 other cases reviewed by the author. Other reports on tubal choriocarcinoma have come from Riggs et al. (1964) and Lurain et al. (1986). A comprehensive review was published by Ober and Maier (1981), who found 93 cases in the entire literature, deemed 58 to be acceptable, and added 18 of their own. These investigators indicated that small tumors are difficult to distinguish from ectopic pregnancy. They found two cases that still contained villi and thus should not be called choriocarcinoma. Some patients were cured by simple hysterectomy, whereas others (94%) responded well to chemotherapy.

Ectopic lesions of extravillous trophoblast have rarely been reported. Baergen et al. (2003) added seven new cases to the previous 12 descriptions in the literature of extrauterine lesions of intermediate trophoblastic proliferation. Follow-up was benign and an origin from ectopic pregnancies was postulated. The fact that trophoblast is so highly susceptible to methotrexate has led to many trials of the medical treatment of ectopic pregnancies with this agent (Ory et al., 1986; Carson et al., 1989). Five of six patients had no further need for therapy; one required subsequent salpingectomy. As described earlier, Barnes et al. (1982) reported the successful treatment of a placental choriocarcinoma, metastatic to the brain and lung. Following two normal pregnancies, however, this was followed by a primary lethal brain glioblastoma 7½ years after the choriocarcinoma, a lesion that was perhaps secondary to irradiation. Creinin et al. (1998) studied the action of methotrexate in early pregnancy and concluded that its main result is the disruption of the change from cytotrophoblast to syncytium—cytotrophoblast syncytialization as they called it.

Some choriocarcinomas occur without known antecedent pregnancy (Acosta-Sison, 1957). Benjamin and Rorat (1978) reported ovarian choriocarcinomas as "primary." Their patient developed the fatal ovarian (and hepatic) tumor apparently spontaneously. The uterine cavity contained only necrotic debris. The authors found six previous cases similar to theirs in the literature. Turner et al. (1964) reported on a successfully treated patient with an apparently primary ovarian choriocarcinoma. No antecedent or coincident pregnancy was found, although the authors called the tumor gestational. Cunanan et al. (1980) reported an ovarian choriocarcinoma that was associated with a normal uterine pregnancy delivered by hysterotomy several weeks after resection of the mass. The patient did well on chemotherapy; the infant and placenta were normal. This report included a review of 24 additional choriocarcinomas coexisting with pregnancy. In 10, the tumor was found in the placenta, in five it was absent, and in the remaining 10 cases there was a lack of information. Axe et al. (1985) found six similar cases in their Registry of Ovarian Tumors. One of those patients died.

Manivel et al. (1987) reviewed the extensive literature of trophoblastic differentiation from germ cell tumors. This tumor is outside the scope of the present book. Suffice it to say that these investigators paid special attention to the presence of intermediate trophoblast in these germinal tumors. The cells were designated large mononuclear cells with a variety of immunologic characteristics that had led Kurman et al. (1984) to call them intermediate trophoblast. They should now be studied with more specific markers, such as MBP, and the designation "extravillous trophoblast" is more appropriate. Choriocarcinoma may differentiate from primary germ cell tumors of testis and mediastinum, and from teratocarcinomas. Fine et al. (1962) reviewed this topic adequately and reported a fatal case in which the tumor arose in the mediastinum, and paid special attention to the endocrine aspects of the neoplasm.

Wenger et al. (1968) reported a mediastinal choriocarcinoma in a man. This tumor is unusual. They had seen only 17 choriocarcinomas in men at the Mayo Clinic. Chemotherapy is significantly less effective in men than for trophoblastic neoplasms, which has been assumed to be due to the assistance of immunologic rejection mechanisms in the gestational tumor. Soma et al. (1973), who studied the chromosomes of a man with gastric choriocarcinoma, identified fluorescent Y bodies in this hyperdiploid cell line. Fukunaga and Ushigome (1993a) found their eight tumors to be diploid and reviewed the evidence that suggested that chromosomes of these tumors are normally diploid. A primary choriocarcinoma without antecedent lesion was described in the lung of a 51-year-old man (Sullivan, 1989). A pulmonary choriocarcinoma was also reported in a 60-year-old woman (15 years after menopause). Because of her age, it is unlikely that it had derived from a preceding gestation (Pushchak & Farhi, 1987). Pushchak and Farhi speculated that it came from epithelial metaplasia, as she (and the patient of Sullivan) had been heavy smokers.

These cases must all be interpreted with caution, however, especially when one knows of the remarkable patient described by Dougherty et al. (1978): an 86-year-old woman with fatal pulmonary and cerebral metastases whose uterus had choriocarcinoma with degenerated villi. The inference was that the villi and trophoblast had existed since her last pregnancy, 34 years earlier. She had been amenorrheic after that pregnancy. This case is truly exceptional. Another remarkable case is that reported by Lathrop et al. (1978) of a choriocarcinoma that developed 14 years after tubal ligation.

THERAPY OF GESTATIONAL TROPHOBLASTIC NEOPLASIA

Aside from the attempts at immunotherapy discussed previously, surgery and chemotherapy are used for the treatment of choriocarcinoma and its precursors. Initially, only surgical excision, perhaps prophylactic hysterectomy, was available for eradication of residual trophoblast after evacuation of hydatidiform moles. The survival rate after hysterectomy was only 31.9% with uncomplicated choriocarcinoma; when metastases were present, it was 19.2% (Brewer et al., 1963). Some patients with metastases had spontaneous regression, a surprising observation then. A complete review of various therapeutic modalities, including new chemotherapeutic agents and modern methods of detection, has been provided by Seckl and Newlands (1997). An important aspect of therapy is to determine the best time to commence therapy when a choriocarcinoma is suspected. This can be important, for instance, in the follow-up of patients with choriocarcinoma in situ, accidentally discovered in the placenta. Because such patients are followed by serial determination of hCG levels, knowledge of the disappearance rate of gonadotropin levels following normal delivery is essential. Korhonen et al. (1997) studied this in some detail in six women following normal delivery. From levels of around 35,000 IU/mL at the end of pregnancy, rapid decline leads to virtual elimination (5 IU/mL) by 21 days after delivery, hCG-α having a much more rapid decline than hCG-β.

Much more rapid progress was made after the discovery that the folic acid antagonist methotrexate produced beneficial results (Li et al., 1956). The historical developments that followed were succinctly recalled by Hertz (1972) and Li (1972); in a larger thesis, Hertz (1978) provided a complete overview. So effective is methotrexate against proliferating trophoblast that it was even used for therapeutic abortion (Thiersch, 1952) and it is now often employed in the treatment of ectopic pregnancies (Ory et al., 1986). Others have employed this agent to cause the involution of residual trophoblast in abdominal implantations (St. Clair et al., 1969; Rahman et al., 1982). This method of therapy has improved patient survival remarkably (Brewer et al., 1964; Lewis et al., 1966; Goldstein, 1972). Many contributions have been published since these early studies and are aptly summarized in books by Goldstein and Berkowitz (1982) and Szulman and Buchsbaum (1987). Individual reports have established that immunologic interactions occur when metastatic disease is treated chemotherapeutically in incompatible situations (Gallmeier et al., 1970). Even the feared cerebral metastases have a 50% remission rate when treated vigorously with chemotherapy and radiation (Weed & Hammond, 1980).

Despite these excellent results from methotrexate, actinomycin D, and other newer agents, there remains the problem of early diagnosis. This point is important. Delays and repeat chemotherapeutic treatment after a symptom-free interval often result in resistant metastases. Parazzini et al. (1988b) found that patients over age 40, with AB blood group, and with a history of complete mole had an especially poor outlook. Surwit et al. (1984) provided suggestions for aggressive therapy in other categories of poor-prognosis GTDs. Interestingly, students of this disease still disagree as to whether patients with hydatidiform moles should receive prophylactic chemotherapy in an effort to prevent the occurrence of choriocarcinoma. Bagshawe et al. (1969) believed it to be contraindicated. It is the experience of some physicians, however, that such a prophylactic regimen is not only safe but also useful (Homesley et al., 1988). These considerations require a correct, precise diagnosis. We believe that patients with triploid, partial moles should be exempted from this consideration of prophylactic chemotherapy because only very rarely do choriocarcinomas follow such moles. A most readable review of the progress made in the therapy of this tumor comes from Walter Jones (1990), who paid special tribute to Kenneth Bagshawe as having initiated a new age in the therapy of GTN.

Because of the relative frequency (approximately 10%) of neoplastic sequelae when a placental site trophoblastic tumor is diagnosed, hysterectomy is usually advised and is considered the mainstay of treatment. That complete excision may be feasible and followed by normal gestations was shown by Leiserowitz and Wenn (1996). The tumor they saw was typical for a PSTT; it was visible sonographically and, after simple excision, the patient had three pregnancies. Patients are usually treated successfully by surgery when the tumor is confined to the uterus; however, when metastases are present, chemotherapy is advocated.

Unfortunately, the success of chemotherapeutic treatment in choriocarcinoma is not shared by the PSTT. Occasionally, patients with single metastases have been treated successfully with resection of the metastatic lesion, but additional chemotherapy is usually necessary, and even then success is not assured. The overall management of GTDs has been summarized in an American College of Obstetricians and Gynecologists (1993) technical bulletin.

It has often been asked if the multiple chemotherapeutic agents that are used to treat this neoplasm have an adverse effect on ovarian follicles. Several prospective studies have affirmed that normal pregnancy is subsequently possible (Patterson, 1956; van Thiel et al., 1970; Walden & Bagshawe, 1976; Garner et al., 2003). Despite experimental evidence that alkylating agents damage rodent ova, there is no reported increase in congenital anomalies and chromosomal anomalies of future offspring. Occasional life-threatening hemorrhage may occur during the evolution of choriocarcinoma; Pearl and Braga (1992) were able to treat two such patients by local embolization. Roberts and Lurain (1996) reported good success in low-risk GTD with single-agent therapy. All their 92 patients were cured, employing methotrexate, actinomycin D, or a combination of both. Only one patient needed multiple-agent therapy. However, 22 patients also had hysterectomy. The agent Taxol (a derivative of yew tree bark) had potent effect in choriocarcinomatous cell culture and is a future agent for therapy (Marth et al., 1995; Osborne et al., 2005).

Choriocarcinoma in Animals

Although there have been very few reports of true hydatidiform moles in animals, especially nonhuman primates, spontaneous choriocarcinoma has been observed a few times in several species. Lindsey et al. (1969) reported the first spontaneous choriocarcinoma in a rhesus monkey. The primary lesion was in the uterus and there were widespread pulmonary metastases. Pregnancy had been confirmed by rectal palpation, no known abortion had taken place, and the tumor was unequivocally a choriocarcinoma by histologic study. Madarame et al. (1989) found a localized hemorrhagic tumor in the uterus of a DDD (Inbred mouse strain) mouse at age 601 days. Histologically, the pathology was clearly choriocarcinoma with appropriate immunochemical and electron microscopic characteristics. Experimental choriocarcinoma has often been produced in rats (Stein-Werblowsky, 1960; Shintani et al., 1966; Miyamoto, 1971), the nine-banded armadillo (Marin-Padilla & Benirschke, 1963), and the rabbit (Kushima et al., 1967). More recently, Fleetwood et al. (2004) described a placental site trophoblastic tumor in a cynomolgus monkey that had an ovarian origin and behaved in a benign manner. Vascular invasion and few mitoses were identified nevertheless. The tumor was positive for hPL but only few cells reacted with hCG antibodies. Farman et al. (2005) described a choriocarcinoma in a rhesus monkey that had elevated hCG levels.

Choriocarcinoma in Cell Lines and Genetics

It has long been possible to transplant trophoblastic neoplasms into the cheek pouches of Syrian hamsters (Galton et al., 1963). The transplanted tumor grows to a large size. This experimental system has been useful to determine susceptibility to chemotherapeutic agents and to study tumor biology and its cytogenetics. Immunologic rejection processes could also be studied with this model. Apparently, the cheek pouch is an immunologically "privileged" site, and metastases do not occur in Syrian hamsters unless the neoplasm is transplanted to other sites (Ehrman & Gliserman, 1964). Chromosome numbers of such transplanted tumors are hyperdiploid ($2n \approx 80$) and they increase with time. This finding coincides with the DNA studies of trophoblastic tumors by Makino et al. (1963) and Goldfarb et al. (1971). The latter investigators found mostly hyperdiploid (often tetraploid) values for choriocarcinomas, chorioadenoma destruens, and some moles, including values obtained for cytotrophoblastic cells (see also Atkin, 1965). Park (1957), who studied the Barr body content of the tumors, found that they were equally aggressive whether coming from a male or female pregnancy. In cytogenetic studies, some choriocarcinomas have been shown to have chromosomal polymorphisms, heterozygosity, and many are aneuploid (Wake et al., 1981; Sheppard et al., 1985). The few other decisive modern chromosome and DNA studies carried out on choriocarcinoma are referred to in Chapter 22. Shih et al. (2002) reported on the creation of cell lines from extravillous trophoblast. They created these lines from PSTTs and CHMs by employing genes from the human papilloma virus. The former line had paternal and maternal genes, the latter only paternal chromosomes. These cells did not establish tumors when injected into nude athymic mice.

Transplantation of choriocarcinoma into rhesus monkey brain was also successful, but not all implantations into the lung yielded tumor growth (Lewis et al., 1968). This finding suggested that immunologic factors are involved in the rejection of such neoplasms. Carr (1979) found that when mouse trophoblast was transplanted into the lungs of mice, it was accepted only by neonatal mice; adults failed to support trophoblast growth. Carr reviewed the well-known deportation of chinchilla trophoblast to the lung of normal gestation. Kato et al. (1982) made the interesting observation that when tissue from 21 hydatidiform moles and 10 invasive moles (chorioadenoma destruens) was transplanted into nude mice or immunosuppressed hamsters, it was not accepted. Only seven of nine cases of choriocarcinoma could be successfully transplanted. Kato et al., therefore, concluded that choriocarcinoma is a true neoplasm, but moles are not. Izhar et al. (1986) observed the development of trophoblast from human teratocarcinoma cell lines.

References

Acosta-Sison, H.: Apparent metastatic chorioepithelioma without demonstrable primary chorionic malignancy in the uterus: report of 3 cases; a new possible explanation of its occurrence. Obstet. Gynecol. **10**:165–168, 1957.

Acosta-Sison, H.: The relative frequency of various anatomic sites as the point of first metastasis in 32 cases of chorionepithelioma. Amer. J. Obstet. Gynecol. **75**:1149–1152, 1958.

Acosta-Sison, H.: Choriocarcinoma from July 4, 1963 to June 30, 1965. Philippine J. Surg. **21**:41–42, 1966.

American College of Obstetricians and Gynecologists: Technical Bulletin No. 178. Management of Gestational Trophoblastic Disease. March, 1993.

Amiel, J.-L. and Lebovici, S.: Choriocarcinoma and the HL-A$_2$ antigen (MAC). Rev. Eur. Étud. Clin. Biol. **15**:191–192, 1970.

Arai, K., Soma, H. and Hokano, M.: Ultrastructure of trophoblastic tumor cells. J. Clin. Electron Microsc. **9**:5–6, 1976.

Aranda, J.M. and Martinez, I.: Incidence of choriocarcinoma in Puerto Rico: a 15-year study. Cancer **23**:506–507, 1969.

Arkwright, P.D., Rademacher, T.W., Dwek, R.A. and Redman, C.W.G.: Pre-eclampsia is associated with an increase in trophoblast glycogen content and glycogen synthase activity, similar to that found in hydatidiform moles. J. Clin. Invest. **91**:2744–2753, 1993.

Atkin, N.B.: Sex chromosome studies on trophoblast. In, The Early Conceptus, Normal and Abnormal. pp. 130–134. University Court of the University of St. Andrews, Scotland, 1965.

Axe, S.R., Klein, V.R. and Woodruff, J.D.: Choriocarcinoma of the ovary. Obstet. Gynecol. **66**:111–114, 1985.

Baergen, R.N.: Gestational choriocarcinoma. Gen. Diagn. Pathol. **143**:127–141, 1997.

Baergen, R.N. and Rutgers, J.L.: Trophoblastic lesions of the placental site. Gen. Diagn. Pathol. **143**:143–158, 1997.

Baergen, R.N., Rutgers, J. and Young, R.H.: Extrauterine lesions of intermediate trophoblast. Int. J. Gynecol. Pathol. **22**:362–367, 2003.

Bagshawe, K.D.: Hydatidiform mole and chorioncarcinoma. Brit. Med. J. **1**:1509–1510, 1964.

Bagshawe, K.D.: Choriocarcinoma. The Clinical Biology of the Trophoblast and Its Tumors. Williams & Wilkins, Baltimore, 1969.

Bagshawe, K.D.: Pulmonary hypertension in gestational choriocarcinoma: a West London syndrome? Lancet **2**:223, 1988.

Bagshawe, K.D. and Noble, M.I.M.: Cardio-respiratory aspects of trophoblastic tumors. Q. J. Med. **35**:39–54, 1966.

Bagshawe, K.D., Golding, P.R. and Orr, A.H.: Choriocarcinoma after hydatidiform mole: studies related to effectiveness of follow-up practice after hydatidiform mole. Brit. Med. J. **2**:733–737, 1969.

Bagshawe, K.D., Rawlins, G., Pike, M.C. and Lawler, S.D.: ABO blood-groups in trophoblastic neoplasia. Lancet **1**:553–557, 1971.

Baltazar, J.C.: Epidemiological features of choriocarcinoma. Bull. W.H.O. **54**:523–532, 1976.

Bardawil, W.A. and Toy, B.L.: The natural history of choriocarcinoma: problems of immunity and spontaneous regression. Ann. N.Y. Acad. Sci. **80**:197–261, 1959.

Barnes, A.E., Liwnicz, B.H., Schellhaus, H.F., Altshuler, G., Aron, B.S. and Lippert, W.A.: Successful treatment of placental choriocarcinoma metastatic to brain followed by primary brain glioblastoma. Gynecol. Oncol. **13**:108–114, 1982.

Beer, A.E. and Billingham, R.E.: The Immunobiology of Mammalian Reproduction. Prentice-Hall, Englewood Cliffs, NJ, 1976.

Benjamin, F. and Rorat, E.: Primary gestational choriocarcinoma of the ovary. Amer. J. Obstet. Gynecol. **131**:343–345, 1978.

Benson, P.F., Goldsmith, L.L.G. and Rankin, G.L.S.: Massive foetal haemorrhage into maternal circulation as a complication of choriocarcinoma. Brit. Med. J. **1**:841–842, 1962.

Berkowitz, R.S. and Goldstein, D.P.: Chorionic tumors. NEJM **335**:1740–1748, 1996.

Blackburn, G.K.: Massive fetomaternal hemorrhage due to choriocarcinoma of the uterus. J. Pediatr. **89**:680–681, 1976.

Brewer, J.I. and Gerbie, A.B.: Early development of choriocarcinoma. Amer. J. Obstet. Gynecol. **94**:692–705, 1966.

Brewer, J.I. and Mazur, M.T.: Gestational choriocarcinoma: its origin in the placenta during seemingly normal pregnancy. Amer. J. Surg. Pathol. **5**:267–277, 1981.

Brewer, J.I., Rinehart, J.J. and Dunbar, R.W.: Choriocarcinoma. Amer. J. Obstet. Gynecol. **81**:574–583, 1961.

Brewer, J.I., Smith, R.T. and Pratt, G.B.: Choriocarcinoma. Absolute 5 year survival rates of 122 patients treated by hysterectomy. Amer. J. Obstet. Gynecol. **85**:841–843, 1963.

Brewer, J.I., Gerbie, A.B., Dolkart, R.E., Skom, J.H., Nagle, R.G. and Torok, E.E.: Chemotherapy in trophoblastic diseases. Amer. J. Obstet. Gynecol. **90**:566–578, 1964.

Brewer, C.A., Adelson, M.D. and Elder, R.C.: Erythrocytosis associated with a placental-site trophoblastic tumor. Obstet. Gynecol. **79**:846–849, 1992.

Buckell, E.W.C. and Owen, T.K.: Chorionepithelioma in mother and infant. J. Obstet. Gynaecol. Brit. Emp. **61**:329–330, 1954.

Carlson, J.A., Day, T.G., Kuhns, J.G., Howell, R.S. and Masterson, B.J.: Endoarterial pulmonary metastasis of malignant trophoblast associated with a term intrauterine pregnancy. Gynecol. Oncol. **17**:241–248, 1984.

Carr, D.H.: Trophoblast growth in the lungs of mice. Obstet. Gynecol. **54**:461–466, 1979.

Carson, S.A., Stovall, T., Umstot, E., Andersen, R., Ling, F. and Buster, J.E.: Rising human chorionic somatomammotropin predicts ectopic pregnancy rupture following methotrexate chemotherapy. Fertil. Steril. **51**:593–597, 1989.

Chandra, S.A., Gilbert, E.F., Viseskul, C., Strother, C.M., Haning, R.V. and Javid, M.J.: Neonatal intracranial choriocarcinoma. Arch. Pathol. Lab. Med. **114**:1079–1082, 1990.

Cheng, H.-M. and Johnson, P.M.: Specificity of trophoblast-reactive antibodies in human pregnancy. Arch. Pathol. Lab. Med. **112**:1081, 1988.

Cinader, B., Hayley, M.A., Rider, W.D. and Warwick, O.H.: Immunotherapy of a patient with choriocarcinoma. Can. Med. Assoc. J. **84**:306–309, 1961.

Creinin, M.D., Stewart-Akers, A.M. and DeLoia, J.A.: Methotrexate effects on trophoblast and the corpus luteum in early pregnancy. Amer. J. Obstet. Gynecol. **179**:604–609, 1998.

Crescimanno, C., Foidart, J.-M., Noel, A., Polette, M., Maquoi, E., Birembaut, P., Baramova, E., Kaufmann, P. and Castellucci, M.: Cloning of choriocarcinoma cells shows that invasion correlates with expression and activation of gelatinase A. Exp. Cell Res. **227**:240–251, 1996.

Cunanan, R.G., Lippes, J. and Tancinco, P.A.: Choriocarcinoma of the ovary with coexisting normal pregnancy. Obstet. Gynecol. **55**:669–672, 1980.

Daamen, C.B.F. and Bloem, G.W.D.: Chorioepithelioma in mother and child. Ned. Tid. Geneesk. **105**:651–656, 1961; J. Obstet. Gynaecol. Brit. Commonw. **68**:144–149, 1961.

Dallenbach-Hellweg, G.: Histopathology of the Endometrium. Springer-Verlag, N.Y. 1981.

Dawood, M.Y.: Serum progesterone and serum human chorionic gonadotropin in gestational and nongestational choriocarcinoma. Amer. J. Obstet. Gynecol. **123**:762–765, 1975.

de Kaa, C.A. van, Schijf, C.P.T., de Wilde, P.C.M., de Leeuw, H., Gemmink, J.H., Robben, J.C.M. and Vooijs, P.G.: Persistent gestational trophoblastic disease: DNA image cytometry and interphase cytogenetics have limited predictive value. Modern Pathol. **9**:1007–1014, 1996.

Delfs, E.: Chorionic gonadotrophin determinations in patients with hydatidiform mole and choriocarcinoma. Ann. N.Y. Acad. Sci. **80**:125–142, 1959.

Deligdisch, L., Driscoll, S.G. and Goldstein, D.P.: Gestational trophoblastic neoplasms: morphologic correlates of therapeutic response. Amer. J. Obstet. Gynecol. **130**:801–806, 1978.

Doniach, I., Crookston, J.H. and Cope, T.I.: Attempted treatment of a patient with choriocarcinoma by immunization with her husband's cells. J. Obstet. Gynaecol. Brit. Emp. **65**:553–556, 1958.

Dougherty, C.M., Cunningham, C. and Mickal, A.: Choriocarcinoma with metastasis in a postmenopausal woman. Amer. J. Obstet. Gynecol. **132**:700–701, 1978.

Driscoll, S.G.: Choriocarcinoma: an "incidental finding" within a term placenta. Obstet. Gynecol. **21**:96–101, 1963.

Driscoll, S.G.: Choriocarcinoma following delivery. Lab. Med. **48**:21A, 1983.

Duleba, A.J., Miller, D., Taylor, G. and Effer, S.: Expectant management of choriocarcinoma limited to placenta. Gynecol. Oncol. **44**:277–280, 1992.

Duncan, D.A. and Mazur, M.T.: Trophoblastic tumors: ultrastructural comparison of choriocarcinoma and placental-site trophoblastic tumor. Hum. Pathol. **20**:370–381, 1989.

Dyke, P.C. and Fink, L.M.: Latent choriocarcinoma. Cancer **20**:150–154, 1967.

Eckstein, R.P., Russell, P., Friedlaender, M., Tattersall, M.H.N. and Bradfield, A.: Metastasizing placental site trophoblastic tumor: a case study. Hum. Pathol. **16**:632–636, 1985.

Edwards, R.G., Howe, C.W.S. and Johnson, M.H., eds.: Immunobiology of Trophoblast. Cambridge University Press, Cambridge, 1975.

Ehrman, R.L. and Gliserman, L.E.: Choriocarcinoma: growth patterns in hamster tissues. Nature **202**:404–406, 1964.

Elston, C.W.: Cellular reaction to choriocarcinoma. J. Pathol. **97**:261–268, 1969.

Emery, J.L.: Chorionepithelioma in a new-born male child with hyperplasia of the interstitial cells of the testis. J. Pathol. Bacteriol. **64**:735–739, 1952.

Evans, K.T. and Hendrickse, P. de V.: Pulmonary changes in malignant trophoblastic disease. Brit. J. Radiol. **38**:161–171, 1965.

Ewing, J.: Chorioma. Surg. Gynecol. Obstet. **10**:366–392, 1910.

Ewing, J.R.: Neoplastic Diseases. 4th ed. Saunders, Philadelphia, 1941.

Fahrner, R.J., McQueeney, A.J., Mosely, J.M. and Petersen, R.W.: Trophoblastic pulmonary thrombosis with cor pulmonale: report of a case due to malignant hydatidiform mole of five years' duration. JAMA **170**:1898–1901, 1959.

Farman, C.A., Benirschke, K., Horner, M. and Lappin, P.: Ovarian choriocarcinoma in a rhesus monkey associated with elevated serum chorionic gonadotropin levels. Vet. Pathol. **42**:226–229, 2005.

Faul, P., Kelehan, P. and Dervan, P.: Interphase cytogenetic study of exaggerated placental site trophoblast using a biotin-labelled peroxidase method. Modern Pathol. **7**:88A (abstract 503), 1994.

Feldman, K.: Choriocarcinoma with neonatal anemia. NEJM **296**:880, 1977.

Fine, G., Smith, R.W. and Pachter, M.R.: Primary extragenital choriocarcinoma in the male subject: case report and review of the literature. Amer. J. Med. **32**:776–794, 1962.

Finkler, N.J., Berkowitz, R.S., Driscoll, S.G., Goldstein, D.P. and Bernstein, M.R.: Clinical experience with placental site trophoblastic tumors at the New England Trophoblastic Disease Center. Obstet. Gynecol. **71**:854–857, 1988.

Fischer, H.E., Lichtiger, B. and Cox, I.: Expression of $Rh_0(D)$ antigen in choriocarcinoma of the uterus in an $Rh_0(D)$-negative patient: report of a case. Hum. Pathol. **16**:1165–1167, 1985.

Fleetwood, M., Dunn, D.G., Stamatakos, M.D., McGill, L.D. and Lass, T.P.: Ovarian placental site trophoblastic tumor in a cynomolgus monkey (*Macaca fascicularis*). Vet. Pathol. **41**(5):582 (abstract 148), 2004.

Fox, H. and Laurini, R.N.: Intraplacental choriocarcinoma: report of two cases. J. Clin. Pathol. **41**:1085–1088, 1988.

Fukunaga, M. and Ushigome, S.: Malignant trophoblastic tumors: immunohistochemical and flow cytometric comparison of choriocarcinoma and placental site trophoblastic tumors. Human Pathol. **24**:1098–1106, 1993a.

Fukunaga, M. and Ushigome, S.: Metastasizing placental site trophoblastic tumor. An immunohistochemical and flow cytometric study of two cases. Amer. J. Surg. Pathol. **17**:1003–1010, 1993b.

Fukunaga, M., Ushigome, S. and Ishikawa, E.: Choriocarcinoma in situ: a case at an early gestational age. Histopathol. **27**:473–476, 1995.

Fukunaga, M., Nomura, K. and Ushigome, S.: Choriocarcinoma in situ at a first trimester. Report of two cases indicating an origin of trophoblast of stem villus. Virchows Archiv **429**:185–188, 1996.

Gallmeier, W.M., Bertrams, J., Kuwert, E. and Schmidt, C.G.: Regression des Chorionepithelioms: Zytostatikawirkung und/oder Immunreaktion? Dtsch. Med. Wochenschr. **95**:1810–1815, 1970.

Galton, M., Goldman, P.B. and Holt, S.F.: Karyotypic and morphologic characterization of a serially transplanted human choriocarcinoma. J. Natl. Cancer Inst. **31**:1019–1035, 1963.

Garner, E., Goldstein, D.P., Berkowitz, R.S. and Wenzel, L.: Psychosocial and reproductive outcomes of gestational trophoblastic diseases. Best Pract. Res. Clin. Obstet. Gynaecol. **17**:959–968, 2003.

Gill, T.J., Wegmann, G. and Nisbet-Brown, E.: Immunoregulation and Fetal Survival. Oxford University Press, New York, 1987.

Goldfarb, S., Richart, R.M. and Okagaki, T.: A cytophotometric study of nuclear DNA content of cyto- and syncytiotrophoblast in trophoblastic disease. Cancer **27**:83–92, 1971.

Goldstein, D.P.: The chemotherapy of gestational trophoblastic disease. Principles of clinical management. JAMA **220**:209–213, 1972.

Goldstein, D.P. and Berkowitz, R.S., eds.: Trophoblastic Neoplasms. Clinical Principles of Diagnosis and Management. Saunders, Philadelphia, 1982.

Greene, J.B. and McCue, S.A.: Choriocarcinoma with cerebral metastases coexistent with a first pregnancy. Amer. J. Obstet. Gynecol. **131**:253–254, 1978.

Grimmer, D., Landas, S. and Kemp, J.D.: IgM antitrophoblast antibodies in a patient with a pregnancy-associated lupuslike disorder, vasculitis, and recurrent intrauterine fetal demise. Arch. Pathol. Lab. Med. **112**:191–193, 1988.

Guschmann, M., Schulz-Bischof, K. and Vogel, M.: Incidental chorangiocarcinoma. Case report, immunohistochemistry and theories of possible histogenesis. Pathologe **24**:124–127, 2003 (in German).

Hackett, E. and Beech, M.: Immunologic treatment of a case of choriocarcinoma. Brit. Med. J. **2**:1123–1126, 1961.

Hammond, C.B., Weed, J.C., Barnard, D.E. and Tyrey, L.: Gestational trophoblastic neoplasia. CA **31**:322–332, 1981.

Heifetz, S.A. and Czaja, J.: In situ choriocarcinoma arising in partial hydatidiform mole: Implications for the risk of persistent trophoblastic disease. Pediatr. Pathol. **12**:601–611, 1992.

Heller, E.L. and Householder, J.M.: Clinicopathologic conference. Amer. J. Clin. Pathol. **22**:883–889, 1952.

Hertig, A.T. and Mansell, H.: Tumors of the female sex organs. Part I. Hydatidiform mole and choriocarcinoma. In, Atlas of Tumor Pathology. Sect. IX, Fasc. 33. Armed Forces of Pathology, Washington, DC, 1956.

Hertz, R.: Quantitative monitoring of chemotherapy of endocrine tumors by hormone assay. JAMA **222**:1163, 1972.

Hertz, R.: Choriocarcinoma and Related Gestational Trophoblastic Tumors in Women. Raven Press, New York, 1978.

Ho, H.-N., Gill, T.J., Klionsky, B., Ouyang, P.-C., Hsieh, C.-Y. and Kunschner, A.: Differences between white and Chinese populations in human leukocyte antigen sharing and gestational trophoblastic tumors. Amer. J. Obstet. Gynecol. **161**:942–948, 1989.

Homesley, H.D., Blessing, J.A., Rettenmaier, M., Capizzi, R.L., Major, F.J. and Twiggs, L.B.: Weekly intramuscular methotrexate for nonmetastatic gestational trophoblastic disease. Obstet. Gynecol. **72**:413–418, 1988.

Hopkins, M., Nunez, C., Murphy, J.R. and Wentz, W.B.: Malignant placental site trophoblastic tumor. Obstet. Gynecol. **66**:95S-100S, 1985.

Horn, L.-C. and Bilek, K.: Histologic classification and staging of gestational trophoblastic disease. Gen. Diagn. Pathol. **143**:87–101, 1997.

Horn, L.-C., Bilek, K., Pretzsch, G. and Baier, D.: Chorionkarzinom bei tubarer Extrauteringravidität. Geburtsh. Frauenheilk. **54**:375–377, 1994.

Horn, L.-C., Emmrich, P., Bilek, K. and Bruder, E.: Der frühe Trophoblast. II. Tumorförmige Störungen der trophoblastären Entwicklung. Zbl. Gynäkol. **118**:591–597, 1996.

Horn, L.-C., Göretzlehner, U. and Dirnhofer, S.: Placental site trophoblastic tumor (PSTT) initially misdiagnosed as cervical carcinoma. Pathol. Res. Pract. **193**:225–230, 1997.

Huber, H.: Das Chorionepitheliom. Arch. Gynäkol. **207**:187–201, 1969.

Huetter, P.C. and Gersell, D.J.: Placental site nodule: an analysis of 40 cases. Modern Pathol. **4**:74A; abstract 422, 1993.

Hui, P., Riba, A., Pejovic, T., Johnson, T., Baergen, R.N. and Ward, D.: Comparative genomic hybridization study of placental site trophoblastic tumour: a report of four cases. Modern Pathol. **17**:248–251, 2004.

Hustin, J. and Jauniaux, E.: Markedly elevated maternal serum alpha-fetoprotein associated with a normal fetus and choriocarcinoma of the placenta. Obstet. Gynecol. **77**:329–330, 1991.

Hutchison, J.R., Peterson, E.P. and Zimmermann, E.A.: Coexisting metastatic choriocarcinoma and normal pregnancy: therapy during gestation with maternal remission and fetal survival. Obstet. Gynecol. **31**:331–336, 1968.

Iliya, F.A., Williamson, S. and Azar, H.A.: Choriocarcinoma in the Near East. Consanguinity as a possible etiologic factor. Cancer **20**:144–149, 1967.

Iliya, F.A., Khuri, F.P. and Khuri, S.F.: Multisystem blood group study in trophoblastic disease. Lebanese Med. J. **22**:707–711, 1969.

Inferrera, C., Pulle, C., Rigano, A. and Palmara, D.: Aspetti ultrastrutturali e citochimici del coriocarcinoma uterino. Arch. Ostetr. Ginecol. **72**:707–744, 1967.

Ivaskova, E., Jakoubkova, J., Zavadil, M., Schneid, V., Koldovsky, P. and Ivanyi, P.: HL-A antigens and choriocarcinoma. Transplant. Proc. **1**:80–81, 1969.

Izhar, M., Siebert, P.D., Oshima, R.G., DeWolf, W.C. and Fukuda, M.N.: Trophoblastic differentiation of human teratocarcinoma cell line HT-H[1]. Dev. Biol. **116**:510–518, 1986.

Jacques, S.M., Qureshi, F., Doss, B.J. and Munkarah, A.: Intraplacental choriocarcinoma associated with viable pregnancy: pathologic features and implications for the mother and infant. Pediat. Development. Pathol. **1**:380–387, 1998.

Jarrett, D.D. and Pratt-Thomas, H.R.: Metastatic choriocarcinoma appearing as a unilateral renal mass. Arch. Pathol. Lab. Med. **108**:356–357, 1984.

Jauniaux, E., Zucker, M., Meuris, S., Verherst, A., Wilkin, P. and Hustin, J.: Chorangiocarcinoma: an unusual tumour of the placenta; the missing link? Placenta **9**:607–613, 1988.

Jones, W.B.: Gestational trophoblastic disease: What have we learned in the past decade? Amer. J. Obstet. Gynecol. **162**:1286–1295, 1990.

Kato, M., Tanaka, K. and Takeuchi, S.: The nature of trophoblastic disease initiated by transplantation into immunosuppressed animals. Amer. J. Obstet. Gynecol. **142**:497–505, 1982.

Kirk, J.A.: Persistence of abnormal trophoblast. Amer. J. Obstet. Gynecol. **92**:667–669, 1965.

Knoth, M., Hesseldahl, H. and Larsen, J.F.: Ultrastructure of human choriocarcinoma. Acta Obstet. Gynecol. **48**:100–118, 1969a.

Knoth, M., Pattillo, R.A., Garancis, J.C., Gey, G.O., Ruckert, A.C.F. and Mattingly, R.F.: Ultrastructure and hormone synthesis of choriocarcinoma. Amer. J. Pathol. **54**:479–488, 1969b.

Kohorn, E.I.: Theca lutein ovarian cyst may be pathognomonic for trophoblastic neoplasia. Obstet. Gynecol. **62**:80S–81S, 1983.

Kolstad, P. and Hognestad, J.: Trophoblastic tumours in Norway. Acta Obstet. Gynecol. Scand. **44**:80–88, 1965.

Korhonen, J., Alfthan, H., Ylöstalo, P., Veldhuis, J. and Stenman, U.-H.: Disappearance of human chorionic gonadotropin and its α- and β-subunits after term pregnancy. Clin. Chem. **43**:2155–2163, 1997.

Kruseman, A.C.N., van Lent, M., Blom, A.H. and Lauw, G.P.: Choriocarcinoma in mother and child, identified by immunoenzyme histochemistry. Amer. J. Clin. Pathol. **67**:279–283, 1977.

Kurman, R.J., Scully, R.E. and Norris, N.J.: Trophoblastic pseudotumor of the uterus: an exaggerated form of "syncytial endometritis" simulating a malignant tumor. Cancer **38**:1214–1226, 1976.

Kurman, R.J., Main, C.S. and Chen, H.-C.: Intermediate trophoblast: a distinctive form of trophoblast with specific morpho-

logical, biochemical and functional features. Placenta **5**:349–370, 1984.

Kushima, K., Noda, K. and Makita, M.: Experimental production of chorionic tumor in rabbits. Tohoku J. Exp. Med. **91**:209–214, 1967.

Lage, J.M.: Protocols for the examination of specimens from patients with gestational trophoblastic malignancies. A basis for checklists. Arch. Pathol. Lab. Med. **123**:50–54, 1999.

Lage, J.M. and Roberts, D.J.: Choriocarcinoma in a term placenta: Pathologic diagnosis of tumor in an asymptomatic patient with metastatic disease. Intern. J. Gynecol. Pathol. **12**:80–85, 1993.

Lage, J.M. and Sheikh, S.S.: Genetic aspects of gestational trophoblastic diseases: A general overview with emphasis on new approaches in determining genetic composition. Gen. Diagn. Pathol. **143**:109–115, 1997.

Larsen, J.F., Ehrman, R.L. and Bierring, F.: Electron microscopy of human choriocarcinoma transplanted into hamster liver. Amer. J. Obstet. Gynecol. **99**:1109–1124, 1967.

Lathrop, J.C., Wachtel, T.J. and Meissner, G.F.: Uterine choriocarcinoma fourteen years following bilateral tubal ligation. Obstet. Gynecol. **51**:477–482, 1978.

Lawler, S.D., Klouda, P.T. and Bagshawe, K.D.: HL-A system in trophoblastic neoplasia. Lancet **2**:834–837, 1971.

Leiserowitz, G.S. and Webb, M.J.: Treatment of placental site trophoblastic tumor with hysterotomy and uterine reconstruction. Obstet. Gynecol. **88**:696–699, 1996.

Lele, S.M., Crowder, S.E. and Grafe, M.R.: Asymptomatic intraplacental choriocarcinoma diagnosed on routine placental examination. J. Perinatol. **19**:244–247, 1999.

Lewis, J., Gore, H., Hertig, A.T. and Goss, D.A.: Treatment of trophoblastic disease. Amer. J. Obstet. Gynecol. **86**:710–722, 1966.

Lewis, J.L., Brown, W.E., Hertz, R., Davis, R.C. and Johnson, R.H.: Heterotransplantation of human choriocarcinoma in monkeys. Cancer Res. **28**:2032–2038, 1968.

Li, M.C.: Chemotherapeutic and immunological aspects of choriocarcinoma. JAMA **222**:1163–1164, 1972.

Li, M.C., Hertz, R. and Spencer, D.B. Effect of methotrexate therapy upon choriocarcinoma and chorioadenoma. Proc. Soc. Exp. Biol. Med. **93**:361–366, 1956.

Lindsey, J.R., Wharton, L.R., Woodruff, J.D. and Baker, H.J.: Intrauterine choriocarcinoma in a rhesus monkey. Pathol. Vet. **6**:378–384, 1969.

Liu, Z., Mira, J.L. and Cruz-Caudillo, C.: Primary gastric choriocarcinoma. A case report and review of the literature. Arch. Pathol. Lab. Med. **125**:1601–1604, 2001.

Lurain, J.R., Sand, P.K. and Brewer, J.I.: Choriocarcinoma associated with ectopic pregnancy. Obstet. Gynecol. **68**:286–287, 1986.

Madarame, H., Sakurai, H. and Konno, S.: Choriocarcinoma in a DDD mouse: a case report with immunohistochemical and ultrastructural studies. Lab. Anim. Sci. **39**:255–258, 1989.

Madden, S.: Chorionepithelioma of the fallopian tube. J. Obstet. Gynaecol. Brit. Emp. **57**:68–70, 1950.

Makino, S., Sasaki, M.S. and Fukushima, T.: Preliminary notes on the chromosomes of human chorionic lesions. Proc. Jpn. Acad. **39**:54–58, 1963.

Manivel, J.C., Niehans, G., Wick, M.R. and Dehner, L.P.: Intermediate trophoblast in germ cell neoplasms. Amer. J. Surg. Pathol. **11**:693–701, 1987.

Marchand, F.J.: Über die sogenannten "decidualen" Geschwülste im Anschluss an normale Geburt, Abort, Blasenmole und Extrauterinschwangerschaft. Monatsschr. Geburtsh. Gynäkol. **1**:419–438; 513–560, 1895.

Marin-Padilla, M. and Benirschke, K.: Thalidomide induced alterations in the blastocyst and placenta of the armadillo, Dasypus novemcinctus mexicanus, including a choriocarcinoma. Amer. J. Pathol. **43**:999–1016, 1963.

Marquez Monter, H. and Velasco, A.F.: Patologia de los tumores trofoblasticos. Bol. Asoc. Mex. Patol. **5**:11–16, 1967.

Marth, C., Lang, T., Widschwendter, M., Müller-Holzner, E. and Daxenbichler, G.: Effects of taxol on choriocarcinoma cells. Amer. J. Obstet. Gynecol. **173**:1835–1842, 1995.

Martin, B.R., Orr, J.W. and Austin, J.M.: Cervical choriocarcinoma associated with an intrauterine contraceptive device: a case report. Amer. J. Obstet. Gynecol. **147**:343–344, 1983.

Martin, F.I.R. and Carden, A.B.G.: Gynaecomastia in chorionepithelioma—oestrogen levels and probable pathogenesis. Acta Endocrinol. (Copenh.) **43**:203–212, 1963.

Matalon, M., Paz, B., Modan, M. and Modan, B.: Malignant trophoblastic disorders: epidemiologic aspects and relationship to hydatidiform mole. Amer. J. Obstet. Gynecol. **112**:101–106, 1972.

Mathé, G., Dausset, J., Hervet, E., Amiel, J.L., Colombani, J. and Brule, G.: Immunological studies in patients with placental choriocarcinoma. J. Natl. Cancer Inst. **33**:193–208, 1964.

Mercer, R.D., Lammert, A.C., Anderson, R. and Hazard, J.B.: Choriocarcinoma in mother and infant. JAMA **166**:482–483, 1958.

Midgley, A.R. and Jaffe, R.B.: Regulation of human gonadotropins: II. Disappearance of human chorionic gonadotropin following delivery. J. Clin. Endocrinol. **28**:1712–1718, 1968.

Miller, J.M., Surwit, E.A. and Hammond, C.B.: Choriocarcinoma following term pregnancy. Obstet. Gynecol. **53**:207–212, 1979.

Mills, W.: Chorion-carcinoma in the midlands. Clin. Radiol. **15**:260–262, 1964.

Miyamoto, M.: Experimental induction of choriocarcinoma in rats. Gann **62**:55–56, 1971.

Mogensen, B. and Kissmeyer-Nielsen, F.: Histocompatibility antigens on the HL-A locus in generalised gestational choriocarcinoma: a family study. Lancet **1**:721–724, 1968.

Mogensen, B. and Kissmeyer-Nielsen, F.: Current data on HL-A and ABO typing in gestational choriocarcinoma and invasive mole. Transplant. Proc. **3**:1267–1269, 1971.

Mogensen, B. and Olsen, S.: Gestational choriocarcinoma in Denmark 1940–1969: a reappraisal based on modern histologic criteria. Acta Obstet. Gynecol. Scand. **51**:63–69, 1972.

Nagelberg, S.B. and Rosen, S.W.: Clinical and laboratory investigation of a virilized woman with placental-site trophoblastic tumor. Obstet. Gynecol. **65**:527–534, 1985.

Nanke, E.: Über primär heterotopes (ektopisches) Chorionepitheliom und Chorionepitheliosis. Geburtsh. Frauenheilk. **19**:523–531, 1959.

Nepom, G.T.: The effects of variations in human immune-response genes. NEJM **321**:751–752, 1989.

Nickels, J., Risberg, B. and Melander, S.: Trophoblastic pseudo-tumour of the uterus. Acta Pathol. Microbiol. Scand. [A] **86**:14–16, 1978.

Nisbet, A.D., Brehmer, R.D., Horne, C.H.W., Brooker, D., Twiggs, L.B. and Okagaki, T.: Placental protein 5 in gesta-

tional trophoblastic disease: localization and circulating levels. Amer. J. Obstet. Gynecol. **144**:396–401, 1982.

Ober, W.B.: Gestational choriocarcinoma: immunological aspects, diagnosis and treatment. Excerpta Medica Int. Congr. Ser. **203**:304–315, 1969.

Ober, W.B. and Fass, R.O.: The early history of choriocarcinoma. J. Hist. Med. Allied Sci. **16**:49–73, 1961.

Ober, W.B. and Maier, R.C.: Gestational choriocarcinoma of the fallopian tube. Diagn. Gynecol. Obstet. **3**:213–231, 1981.

Ober, W.B., Edgcomb, J.H. and Price, E.B.: The pathology of choriocarcinoma. Ann. N.Y. Acad. Sci. **172**:299–426, 1971.

Oettle, A.G.: Malignant neoplasms of the uterus in the white, "coloured," Indian and Bantu races of the Union of South Africa. Acta Uni. Int. Contra Canc. **17**:915–933, 1961.

Oldt, R.J., Kurman, R.J. and Shih, L.-M.: Molecular genetic analysis of placental site trophoblastic tumors and epithelioid trophoblastic tumors confirms their trophoblastic origin. Amer. J. Pathol. **161**:1033–1037, 2002.

Ollendorff, D.A., Goldberg, J.M., Abu-Jawdeh, G.M. and Lurain, J.R.: Markedly elevated maternal serum alpha-fetoprotein associated with a normal fetus and choriocarcinoma of the placenta. Obstet. Gynecol. **76**:494–497, 1990.

Olive, D.L., Lurain, J.R. and Brewer, J.I.: Choriocarcinoma associated with term gestation. Amer. J. Obstet. Gynecol. **148**:711–716, 1984.

Ory, S.J., Villanueva, A.L., Sand, P.K. and Tamura, R.K.: Conservative treatment of ectopic pregnancy with methotrexate. Amer. J. Obstet. Gynecol. **154**:1299–1306, 1986.

Osborne, R., Covens, A., Mirchandani, D. and Gerulath, S.: Successful salvage of relapsed high-risk gestational trophoblastic neoplasia patients using a novel paclitaxel-containing doublet. J. Reprod. Med. **49**:655–661, 2004. [Erratum: **50**:376, 2005]

Parazzini, F., La Vecchia, C., Mangili, G., Caminiti, C., Negri, E., Cecchetti, G. and Fasoli, M.: Dietary factors and risk of trophoblastic disease. Amer. J. Obstet. Gynecol. **158**:93–100, 1988a.

Parazzini, F., Mangili, G., Belloni, C., La Vecchia, C., Liati, P. and Marabini, R.: The problem of identification of prognostic factors for persistent trophoblastic disease. Gynecol. Oncol. **30**:57–62, 1988b.

Park, W.W.: The occurrence of sex chromatin in chorionepitheliomas and hydatidiform moles. J. Pathol. Bacteriol. **74**:197–206, 1957.

Park, W.W.: Choriocarcinoma: A Study of Its Pathology. Davis, Philadelphia, 1971.

Patterson, W.B.: Normal pregnancy after recovery from metastatic choriocarcinoma. Amer. J. Obstet. Gynecol. **72**:183–187, 1956.

Pearl, M.L. and Braga, C.A.: Percutaneous transcatheter embolization for control of life-threatening pelvic hemorrhage from gestational trophoblastic disease. Obstet. Gynecol. **80**:571–574, 1992.

Pierce, G.B. and Midgley, A.R.: The origin and function of human syncytiotrophoblastic giant cells. Amer. J. Pathol. **43**:153–173, 1963.

Pushchak, M.J. and Farhi, D.C.: Primary choriocarcinoma of the lung. Arch. Pathol. Lab. Med. **111**:477–479, 1987.

Rahman, M.S., Al-Suleiman, S.A., Rahman, J. and Al-Sibai, M.H.: Advanced abdominal pregnancy—Observations in 10 cases Obstet. Gynecol. **59**:366–372, 1982.

Rauter, B.: Zum Problem des Chorionepithelioms. Wien. Klin. Wochenschr. **80**:634–636, 1968.

Reddy, D.B. and Rao, N.: Trophoblastic tumors: II. Choriocarcinoma: a review of 50 cases. Indian J. Med. **23**:532–537, 1969.

Rhoton-Vlasak, A., Wagner, J.M., Rutgers, J.L., Baergen, R.N., Young, R.H., Roche, P.C., Plummer, T.B. and Gleich, G.J.: Placental site trophoblastic tumor: human placental lactogen and pregnancy-associated major basic protein as immunohistologic markers. Human Pathol. **29**:280–288, 1998.

Riggs, J.A., Wainer, A.S., Hahn, G.A. and Farell, D.M.: Extrauterine tubal choriocarcinoma. Amer. J. Obstet. Gynecol. **88**:637–641, 1964.

Roberts, J.P. and Lurain, J.R.: Treatment of low-risk metastatic gestational trophoblastic tumors with single-agent chemotherapy. Amer. J. Obstet. Gynecol. **174**:1917–1924, 1996.

Robinson, E., Shulman, J., Ben-Hur, N., Zuckerman, H. and Neuman, Z.: Immunological studies and behaviour of husband and foreign homografts in patients with chorionepithelioma. Lancet **1**:300–302, 1963.

Rolon, P.A. and Lopez, B.H. de: Malignant trophoblastic disease in Paraguay. J. Reprod. Med. **23**:94–96, 1979.

Rosenheim, N.B., Wijnen, H. and Woodruff, J.D.: Clinical importance of the diagnosis of trophoblastic pseudotumors. Amer. J. Obstet. Gynecol. **136**:635–638, 1980.

Rotmensch, S. and Cole, L.A.: False diagnosis and needless therapy of presumed malignant disease in women with false-positive human chorionic gonadotropin concentrations. Lancet **355**:712–715, 2000.

Rudolph, R.H. and Thomas, E.D.: HL-A antigens and choriocarcinoma. Lancet **2**:408–409, 1971.

Rutgers, J.L., Baergen, R.N., Young, R.H. and Scully, R.E.: Placental site trophoblastic tumor: clinicopathologic study of 64 cases. Mod. Pathol. **8**:96A, 1995.

Santamaria, M., Benirschke, K., Carpenter, P.M., Baldwin, V.J. and Pritchard, J.A.: Transplacental hemorrhage associated with placental neoplasms. Pediatr. Pathol. **7**:601–615, 1987.

Schopper, W. and Pliess, G.: Über Chorionepitheliosis: ein Beitrag zur Genese, Diagnostik und Bedeutung ektopischer chorionepithelialer Wucherungen. Virchows Arch. **317**:347–384, 1949.

Scott, J.S.: Choriocarcinoma. Amer. J. Obstet. Gynecol. **83**:185–193, 1962.

Scott, J.S.: Histocompatibility antigens in choriocarcinoma. Lancet **1**:865–866, 1968.

Scully, R.E. and Young, R.H.: Trophoblastic pseudotumor: a reappraisal. Amer. J. Surg. Pathol. **5**:75–76, 1981.

Searle, F., Leake, B.A., Bagshawe, K.D. and Dent, J.: Serum-SP$_1$-pregnancy-specific-β-glycoprotein in choriocarcinoma and other neoplastic disease. Lancet **1**:579–581, 1978.

Sebire, N.J., Rees, H.C., Peston, D., Seckl, M.J., Newlands, E.S. and Fisher, R.A.: p57^{KIP2} immunohistochemical staining of gestational trophoblastic tumours does not identify the type of the causative pregnancy. Histopathol. **45**:135–141, 2004.

Seckl, M.J., Rustin, G.J.S., Newlands, E.S., Gwyther, S.J. and Bomanji, J.: Pulmonary embolism, pulmonary hypertension, and choriocarcinoma. Lancet **338**:1313–1315, 1991.

Seckl, M.J. and Newlands, E.S.: Treatment of gestational trophoblastic disease. Gen. Diagn. Pathol. **143**:159–171, 1997.

Seckl, M.J., Fisher, R.A., Salerno, G., Rees, H., Paradinas, F.J., Foskett, M. and Newlands, E.S.: Choriocarcinoma and partial hydatidiform moles. Lancet **356**:11443–1444, 2000.

Sheppard, D.M., Fisher, R.A. and Lawler, S.D.: Karyotypic analysis and chromosome polymorphisms in four choriocarcinoma cell lines. Cancer Genet. Cytogenet. **16**:251–258, 1985.

Shih, I.M. and Kurman, R.J.: Ki-67 labeling index in the differential diagnosis of exaggerated placental site, placental site trophoblastic tumor, and choriocarcinoma: a double immunohistochemical staining technique using Ki-67 and Mel-CAM antibodies. Human Pathol. **29**:27–33, 1998a.

Shih, I.-M. and Kurman, R.J.: Epithelioid trophoblastic tumor. A neoplasm distinct from choriocarcinoma and placental site trophoblastic tumor simulating carcinoma. Amer. J. Surg. Pathol. **22**:1393–1403, 1998b.

Shih, I.M. and Kurman, R.J.: The pathology of intermediate trophoblastic tumors and tumor-like lesions. Int. J. Gynecol. Pathol. **20**:31–47, 2001.

Shih, I.M. and Kurman, R.J.: p63 expression is useful in the distinction of epithelioid trophoblastic and placental site trophoblastic tumors by profiling trophoblastic subpopulations. Amer. J. Surg. Pathol. **28**:1177–1183, 2004.

Shih, I.M., Seidman, J.D. and Kurman, R.J.: Placental site nodule and characterization of distinctive types of intermediate trophoblast. Human Pathol. **30**:687–694, 1999.

Shih, I.-M., Singer, G. and Kurman, R.J.: Establishment of intermediate trophoblastic cell lines from PSTT and complete hydatidiform mole. Modern Pathol. **15**:p210A, abstract 880, 2002.

Shintani, S., Glass, L.E. and Page, E.W.: Studies of induced malignant tumors of placental and uterine origin in the rat. I. Survival of placental tissue following fetectomy. II. Induced tumors and their pathogenesis with special reference to choriocarcinoma. III. Identification of experimentally induced choriocarcinoma by detection of placental hormone. Amer. J. Obstet. Gynecol. **95**:542–549; 550–558; 559–563, 1966.

Silverberg S.G. and Kurman, R.J.: Tumors of the uterine corpus and gestational trophoblastic disease. Atlas of Tumor Pathology, Third Series, Fascicle 3, AFIP, Washington, D.C. 1992.

Sohn, N., Chen, S. and Kalra, J.: Nonmetastatic trophoblastic neoplasia of the cervix following termination of a cervical pregnancy. Obstet. Gynecol. **88**:733, 1996.

Soma, H., Kiyokawa, T., Akaeda, T., Miyashita, T. and Matayoshi, K.: The chromosomes of a human choriocarcinoma cell line in vitro with special reference to the presence of Y chromosome. Acta Obstet. Gynaecol. Jpn. **20**:239–242, 1973.

Soma, H., Takayama, M., Tokoro, K., Kikuchi, T., Kikuchi, K. and Saegusa, H.: Radioimmunoassay of hCG as an early diagnosis of cerebral metastases in choriocarcinoma patients. Acta Obstet. Gynecol. Scand. **59**:445–448, 1980.

Soper, J.T., Mutch, D.G., Chin, N., Clarke-Pearson, D.L. and Hammond, C.B.: Renal metastases of gestational trophoblastic disease: a report of eight cases. Obstet. Gynecol. **72**:796–798, 1988.

Soper, J.T., Evans, A.C., Conaway, M.R., Clarke-Pearson, D.L., Berchuck, A. and Hammond, C.B.: Evaluation of prognostic factors and staging in gestational trophoblastic tumor. Obstet. Gynecol. **84**:969–973, 1994.

Spiegel, J.A.: Endoarterial choriocarcinoma of the lung: report of a case and review of the literature. Obstet. Gynecol. **24**:740–748, 1964.

Srivannaboon, S.: Antigenicity of human choriocarcinoma. Intern. J. Fertil. **16**:36–41, 1971.

St. Clair, J.T., Wheeler, D.A. and Fish, S.A.: Methotrexate in abdominal pregnancy JAMA **208**:529–531, 1969.

Stein-Werblowsky, T.: Induction of a chorion-epitheliomatous tumour in the rat. Nature **186**:980, 1960.

Sullivan, L.G.: Primary choriocarcinoma of the lung in a man. Arch. Pathol. Lab. Med. **113**:82–83, 1989.

Surwit, E.A., Alberts, D.S., Christian, C.D. and Graham, V.E.: Poor-prognosis gestational trophoblastic disease: an update. Obstet. Gynecol. **64**:21–26, 1984.

Suzuki, T., Goto, S., Nawa, A., Kurauchi, O., Saito, M. and Tomoda, Y.: Identification of the pregnancy responsible for gestational trophoblastic disease by DNA analysis. Obstet. Gynecol. **82**:629–634, 1993.

Szulman, A.E. and Buchsbaum, H.J., eds.: Gestational Trophoblastic Disease. Springer-Verlag, New York, 1987.

Tanimura, A., Natsuyama, H., Kawano, M., Tanimura, Y., Tanaka, T. and Kitazono, M.: Primary choriocarcinoma of the lung. Hum. Pathol. **16**:1281–1284, 1985.

Tavassoli, F.A. and Devilee, P.: World Health Organization Classification of Tumours: Pathology and Genetics. Tumours of the Breast and Female Genital Organs. Lyon, France: IARC Press, 2003.

Teacher, J.H.: On chorionepithelioma and the occurrence of chorionepitheliomatous and hydatidiform mole-like structures in teratomata: a pathological and clinical study. J. Obstet. Gynaecol. Brit. Emp. **4**:1–64, 145–199, 1903.

Thiersch, J.B.: Therapeutic abortions with a folic acid antagonist, 4-minopteroylglutamic acid (4-amino P.G.A.) administered by the oral route. Amer. J. Obstet. Gynecol. **63**:1298–1304, 1952.

Tomoda, Y., Fuma, M., Saiki, N., Ishizuka, N. and Akaza, T.: Immunologic studies in patients with trophoblastic neoplasia. Amer. J. Obstet. Gynecol. **126**:661–667, 1976.

Tomoda, Y., Kaseki, S., Goto, S., Nishi, H., Hara, T. and Naruki, M.: Rh-D factor in trophoblastic tumors: a possible cause of the high incidence in Asia. Amer. J. Obstet. Gynecol. **139**:742–743, 1981.

Tow, S.H.: Choriocarcinoma: a review of current concepts based on the Singapore experience. Singapore Med. J. **6**:117–126, 1965.

Trask, C., Lage, J.M. and Roberts, D.J.: A second case of "chorangiocarcinoma" presenting in a term asymptomatic twin pregnancy: choriocarcinoma in situ with associated villous vascular proliferation. Intern. J. Gynecol. Pathol. **13**:87–91, 1994.

Tsang, W.Y.W., Chum, N.P.Y., Tang, S.K., Tse, C.C.H. and Chan, J.K.C.: Mallory's bodies in placental site nodule. Arch. Pathol. Lab. Med. **117**:547–550, 1993.

Turner, H.B., Douglas, W.M. and Gladding, T.C.: Choriocarcinoma of the ovary. Obstet. Gynecol. **24**:918–920, 1964.

Van Bogaert, L.-J. and Staquet, J.-P.: Chorionepitheliosis: a rare benign trophoblastic disease. Acta Obstet. Gynecol. Scand. **56**:69–73, 1977.

Van Thiel, D.H., Ross, G.T. and Lipsett, M.B.: Pregnancies after chemotherapy of trophoblastic neoplasms. Science **169**:1326–1327, 1970.

Vaughn, T.C., Surwit, E.A. and Hammond, C.B.: Late recurrences of gestational trophoblastic neoplasia. Amer. J. Obstet. Gynecol. **138**:73–76, 1980.

Veinot, J.P., Ford, S.E. and Price, R.G.: Subacute cor pulmonale due to tumor embolization. Arch. Pathol. Lab. Med. **116**:131–134, 1992.

Wake, N., Tanaka, K., Chapman, V., Matsui, S. and Sandberg, A.A.: Chromosomes and cellular origin of choriocarcinoma. Cancer Res. **41**:3137–3143, 1981.

Walden, P.A.M. and Bagshawe, K.D.: Reproductive performance of women successfully treated for gestational trophoblastic tumors. Amer. J. Obstet. Gynecol. **125**:1108–1114, 1976.

Weed, J.C. and Hammond, C.B.: Cerebral metastatic choriocarcinoma: intensive therapy and prognosis. Obstet. Gynecol. **55**:89–94, 1980.

Wegmann, T.G. and Gill, T.J.: Immunology of Reproduction. Oxford University Press, New York, 1983.

Wehmann, R.E., Ayala, A.R., Birken, S., Canfield, R.E. and Nisula, B.C.: Improved monitoring of gestational trophoblastic neoplasia using a highly sensitive assay for urinary human chorionic gonadotropin. Amer. J. Obstet. Gynecol. **140**:753–757, 1981.

Wei, P.Y. and Cuyang, P.C.: Trophoblastic disease in Taiwan: a review of 157 cases in a 10 year period. Amer. J. Obstet. Gynecol. **85**:844–849, 1963.

Wells, M. and Bulmer, J.N.: The human placental bed: histology, immunohistochemistry and pathology. Histopathology **13**:483–498, 1988.

Wenger, M.E., Dines, D.E., Ahmann, D.L. and Good, C.A.: Primary mediastinal choriocarcinoma. Mayo Clin. Proc. **43**:570–575, 1968.

Witzleben, C.L. and Bruninga, G.: Infantile choriocarcinoma: a characteristic syndrome. J. Pediatr. **73**:374–378, 1968.

Wolf, H.K. and Michalopoulos, G.K.: Proliferating cell nuclear antigen in human placenta and trophoblastic disease. Pediatr. Pathol. **12**:147–154, 1992.

Wynn, R.M. and Davies, J.: Ultrastructure of transplanted choriocarcinoma and its endocrine implications. Amer. J. Obstet. Gynecol. **88**:618–633, 1964.

Yamashita, K., Nakamura, T. and Shimizu, T.: Absence of major histocompatibility complex antigens in choriocarcinoma. Amer. J. Obstet. Gynecol. **150**:896–897, 1984.

Yazaki, K., Yazaki, C., Wakabayashi, K. and Igarashi, M.: Isoelectric heterogeneity of human chorionic gonadotropin: presence of choriocarcinoma specific components. Amer. J. Obstet. Gynecol. **138**:189–194, 1980.

Yen, S. and MacMahon, B.: Epidemiologic features of trophoblastic disease. Amer. J. Obstet. Gynecol. **101**:126–132, 1968.

Young, R.H., Kurman, R.J. and Scully, R.E.: Placental site nodules and plaques. A clinicopathologic analysis of 20 cases. Amer. J. Surg. Pathol. **14**:1001–1009, 1990.

Yuen, B.H., Cannon, W., Benedet, J.L. and Boyes, D.A.: Plasma ß-subunit human chorionic gonadotropin assay in molar pregnancy and choriocarcinoma. Amer. J. Obstet. Gynecol. **127**:711–712, 1977.

24
Benign Tumors and Chorangiosis

Angiomas

With rare exceptions, vascular tumors are the only benign tumors of the placenta. Tumors designated chorioangiomas, chorangiomas, fibroangiomyxomas, fibromas, and the many other names that have been applied in the past are essentially similar, relatively common neoplasms of the placenta. Three large reviews have been published that bring together most of the literature. DeCosta et al. (1956) found about 250 case reports and listed all the synonyms applied previously. They also made reference to the frequency of hydramnios and associated fetal angiomas. Fox (1967), who also reviewed the often confusing nomenclature, indicated that Clarke described the first such tumor in 1798. Since then, the review by Siddall (1924) encompassed 130 cases, that by Marchetti (1939) comprised 209 cases, and Fox traced another 127 cases. Fox accounted for 344 published cases and gave incidence figures of 1 in 9000 to 1 in 50,000 placentas. When careful study of placentas is undertaken, the real prevalence may be as high as 1 in 100 pregnancies, according to some authors, although in our experience this number is somewhat excessive. Wallenburg (1971) provided 13 new cases and summarized publications between 1939 and 1970. His reported incidence in consecutively collected placentas was 1 in 117. These authors provided an extensive literature documentation that would be redundant to repeat. Bashiri et al. (2002) found a significant risk of preterm delivery in patients with chorangiomas. Soma et al. (1991) found that the tumor existed in 0.2% of placentas in Japanese women but was more common (2.5–7.6%) in the high-altitude population of Nepal (Soma, 2001). This is similar to the higher frequency of chorioangioma observed in placentas of women living at altitude by Reshetnikova et al. (1996). We have seen chorioangiomas associated with chronic vascular thrombi and elevated nucleated red blood cells (NRBCs) in the fetal circulation. Thus, an hypoxic stimulus is inferred to lead to excessive villous capillary proliferative stimula-

tion. Although still speculative, such angiogenesis may well be regulated by such vascular growth factors as demonstrated to occur in the placenta by Jackson et al. (1994). A more detailed consideration of the placental villous adaptation to hypoxia can be found in the contribution by Kaufmann et al. (1993), and Kadyrov et al. (1998) provided information on how anemic women produce increased placental angiogenesis in early development. The control of angiogenesis is complex, but it is an essential aspect of placentation and regulation during anemia, preeclampsia, and other pathologic states in pregnancy. There are numerous factors now being explored and many have significant impact on the villous vascularization. A detailed review was provided by Sherer and Abulafia (2001) that is too complex, however, for the brief consideration possible in this chapter. Guschmann (2002, 2003) and his colleagues in Berlin (Guschmann et al., 2003a) have described various angiogenesis factors in chorangiomas. It was their experience that high expression of angiopoietin-1 and -2 and their receptors was demonstrated in chorangiomas, whereas vascular endothelial growth factor (VEGF) was uniform with the normal villi, but variability existed. Further remarkable in their series was that 72% of accompanying babies were of female gender, and tumors occurred much more commonly in the first pregnancy. North et al. (2001) studied immunoreactivity for a variety of antigens in chorangiomas and juvenile angiomas. Thus, FcgammaRII, Lewis Y antigen, merosin, and glucose transporter-1 (GLUT1) were found to be highly expressed in the small placental vessels and angiomas, but not in control blood vessels or those of granulomas etc.

The typical chorioangioma is composed of fetal blood vessels that are usually supported by only scant connective tissue. The tumors often bulge on the fetal surface of the placenta (Fig. 24.1). When they are embedded in the villous tissue, they are located closer to the fetal surface (Fig. 24.2). The vessels comprising this tumor may be capillary or sinusoidal (Fig. 24.3). Frequently, the stromal

863

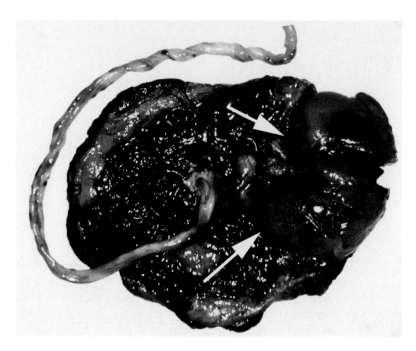

FIGURE 24.1. Typical chorioangioma (left), bulging on the fetal surface. Fetus and pregnancy were normal; there is slight circumvallation of the placenta at right.

component is abundant, and the lesion resembles a fibroma (Fig. 24.4). When Wharton's jelly–like material participates in the formation of the tumor, the appearance is that of a myxomatous neoplasm. The latter is particularly frequent when a chorioangioma arises near the base of the umbilical cord (see Chapter 12, Figs. 12.68 and 12.69). In such cases, a mucicarmine stain reveals the presence of mucus (Dunn, 1959). Chorioangiomas are invariably covered by trophoblast; one may envisage them to be the proliferation of fetal capillaries of a villus whose surface thus expands (Figs. 24.5 and 24.6). Ogino and Redline (2000) suggest that chorangiomas derive specifically from stem villi rather than terminal villi. The

tumors often have degenerative changes, calcification, infarcts, and thromboses, which may leave hemosiderin behind (Dunn, 1959). At times, thrombosis and infarction are clinically manifest with cessation of maternal symptomatology, such as the frequent hydramnios that is associated with these lesions. Chazotte et al. (1990) observed such a lesion sonographically in a fetus that also had meconium peritonitis; when the chorangioma shrank there was some improvement of the hydramnios. The 5-cm chorangioma in the 620-g placenta had focal infarcts. Hsieh and Soong (1992) challenged this report and presented a larger lesion with hydrops. It is now also possible to laser-fulgurate the vessels that supply symptomatic chorioangiomas and thus treat the hydrops fetalis at

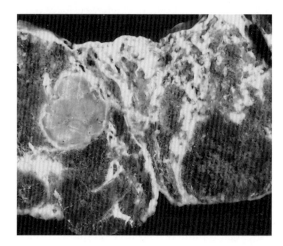

FIGURE 24.2. Partially infarcted 1-cm chorioangioma underneath the chorionic surface of an otherwise normal, mature placenta. It had a golden-yellow appearance and could easily have been mistaken for an infarct.

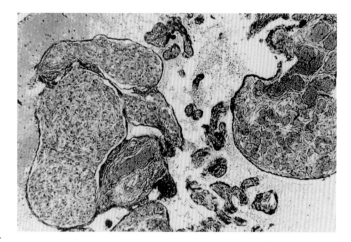

FIGURE 24.3. Multiple chorioangiomas in mature placenta, some of capillary type and others of more cavernous type. H&E ×50.

FIGURE 24.4. Chorioangioma with primarily fibromatous appearance. It measured 2.5 cm and occurred in a 29 weeks' gestation placenta. The cellularity of this lesion has suggested that such tumors may represent sarcomas. H&E ×170.

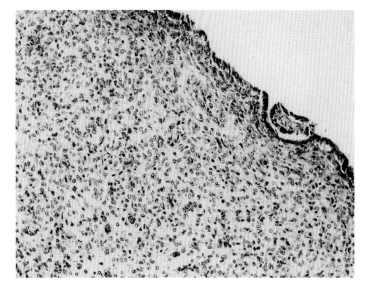

its root cause. Another modality of therapy, the injection with alcohol, has been suggested by Nicolini et al. (1999). These authors injected 1 mL of absolute alcohol into the veins centrally in two patients' large tumors (5 and 6 cm) whose pregnancy was complicated by hydramnios. It was followed by immediate cessation of blood flow; a second injection was necessary in both patients. Both eventually delivered normal infants; the state of the tumors at delivery, however, was not described. A case similar to this was treated by colleagues in Wisconsin (courtesy of R. Franciosi, 2002) and eventuated with a large placental infarct.

Macroscopically, chorioangiomas may be small and multiple (Fig. 24.7); alternatively, they may constitute large masses that displace villous tissue and bulge on the fetal surface. They are fleshy, dark, often congested, and invariably benign. Previous authors, impressed with mitoses and the great cellularity of some tumors, suggested that occasional chorioangiomas represent sarco-

mas. Metastases and true invasion, however, have never been seen. Cary (1914) considered his case of "sarcoma" to be "well authenticated," but he did not provide photographs. Moreover, mother and infant did not suffer any known deleterious consequences from the 6.5 × 4.0 × 3.0 cm, focally calcified tumor. Similar observations were made by Mesia et al. (1999), who described an atypical case that was "mitotically active." Despite this feature and their review of the other rare cases described with similar findings, invasion or metastases did not take place. Another unusual case comes from Guschmann et al. (2003b), who described the lesion they found as "chorangiocarcinoma" (the world's third case), even though mother and fetus did well. The possibility of a "collision tumor" and "reactive lesion" were considered but not resolved. Expressions of angiogenic factors were not increased, but the markers for trophoblast were strongly expressed.

The tumors labeled haemangioendothelioblastomas by Williams (1921) were apparently benign. Variability of

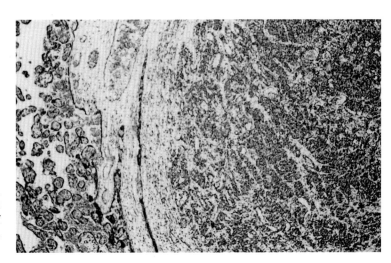

FIGURE 24.5. Chorioangioma that was associated with fetal transplacental exsanguination. The congested capillaries of the tumor are evident. The convexity of the tumor is covered by syncytiotrophoblast. H&E ×160.

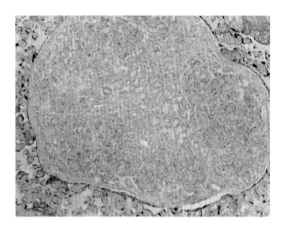

FIGURE 24.6. This chorioangioma displays the feature of over-grown capillaries in an enlarged villus covered by syncytium. H&E ×40.

the histologic appearance, often within the same tumor, has confused many authors. Capillary, cavernous, endo-theliomatous, fibrosing, and fibromatous tumors have been included in the nomenclature suggested by Schulz-Hetzel (1978). We believe that such precision is unwar-ranted because the clinical outcome is almost always the same, and it depends more on the size of the mass(es) than on the composition of the tumor(s). One may regard these tumors as hemangiomas or as hamartomas. The latter designation, however, probably is unwarranted as other placental elements (e.g., trophoblast) never partici-pate in their composition. This would be expected if the designation hamartoma were to apply, a point amply dis-cussed by Marchetti (1939). This nomenclature was also examined in some detail by Barry et al. (1951) in a discus-sion of angiomas of cord and placenta. They ruled out that the lesions represent hamartomas and supported a neoplastic etiology.

It is theoretically possible to differentiate between a neoplasm and malformation-like tumor (hamartoma)

with some precision. Linder and Gartler (1965) found that when they investigated leiomyomas of the uterus using glucose-6-phosphate dehydrogenase (G-6-PD) variants as markers in the frequently (15%) heterozygous African-American population, a single-cell origin was the rule for these neoplasms. The same was found to be true for most other tumors. Congenital tumors such as neuro-fibromas, on the other hand, had multiple cell derivation. These tumors represent a malformation or hamartoma-like type of lesion. A study of chorioangiomas using this simple technique could be decisive in differentiating hamartoma from "true" neoplasm in females with G-6-PD heterozygosity.

The relation of chorioangioma to hydramnios has been known at least since Siddall's extensive review in 1924. He observed that hydramnios was particularly associated with large tumors, but that the prognosis for the gravida was otherwise excellent. Marchetti (1939), who gathered 209 cases and added eight of his own, drew attention to the much commoner location of chorioangiomas near the fetal surface. He also suggested their subdivision into three types and debated whether it represented a true tumor (he thought not) or a malformation, perhaps a hamartoma. The association with hydramnios was of par-ticular interest to McInroy and Kelsey (1954). They saw a pregnancy from whose amnionic cavity 3400mL amni-onic fluid was withdrawn. The placental tumor weighed 454g, measured 10.5cm in greatest dimension, and had its own vascular pedicle. They suggested that the tumor represented "dead space" and was therefore responsible for fluid exudation. Such a large tumor, associated with a stillborn fetus that had cardiomegaly, is shown in Figure 24.8. In an extensive consideration of this tumor, Kühnel (1933) opined that the tumor would have to cause venous obstruction before it could cause hydramnios.

Klaften (1929), who observed a patient with 6000mL of hydramnios and a 1700-g stillbirth, found a fist-sized tumor bulging on the fetal surface of the placenta. He

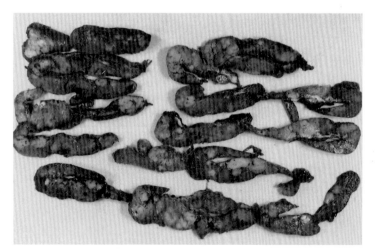

FIGURE 24.7. Chorioangiomatosis of the placenta. The nodular, pale lesions represent chorioangiomas, which comprise approximately 50% of the placenta. The lesions could easily have been mistaken for infarcts. The pla-centa weighed 430g and was accompanied by a 3200-g infant with cardiomegaly, anemia (hematocrit 40%), and thrombocytopenia at birth. Chromosomes were normal. (Courtesy of Dr. P. Bromburger, Kaiser Hospital, San Diego.)

FIGURE 24.8. Exceptionally large (400 g) chorioangioma shelled out from its placenta. The infant was stillborn and had cardiomegaly.

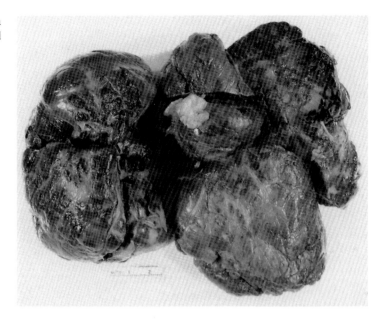

discounted previous opinions that hydramnios was caused by the enlargement of amnionic surface from the bulging tumor mass. Rather, he believed that the tumor caused increased vascular resistance with transudation ensuing. A different mechanism for fetal hydrops was suggested by the case described in detail by Hirata et al. (1993). They discovered the 8.8-cm placental mass by Doppler and color flow mapping sonographically, and when hydrops developed, fetal blood sampling identified a hematocrit of only 17%. The hydrops improved after intrauterine transfusion. The anemia was attributed to microangiopathic hemolytic anemia, but a Kleihauer-Betke test was not done on maternal blood. This might have shown transplacental bleeding as has been observed in other cases of placental chorangiomas. Large chorangiomas may also affect the fetal circulation directly as was probably the case in the patient with a 7-cm tumor whose premature neonate had periventricular leukomalacia (Harigaya et al., 2002).

Numerous large angiomas have been described (e.g., Lopez and Kristoffersen, 1989). These authors saw a patient with placenta previa at mid-gestation with sonographically recognized tumor. They suggested that placenta previa is one of several recognized complications with chorioangioma. The fetus was growth-restricted (899 g), and the placental tumor weighed 503 g. There are many other reports of large chorioangiomas associated with hydramnios, hydrops fetalis, and fetal death. The placenta may be edematous and large in such cases. For instance, Knoth et al. (1976) found a 1150-g placenta with multiple chorioangiomas throughout the placenta, associated with a 3250-g stillborn fetus. Other cases of fetal hydrops with large chorioangiomas were reported by Mandelbaum et al. (1969), Sweet et al. (1973), and Imakita

et al. (1988). Size alone, however, may not be the decisive factor. In Figure 24.9 we show the 900-g chorangioma (14 × 13 × 10 cm) on a 950-g placenta in a neonate with virtually no problems who survived. The umbilical cord was massively edematous (110 g) and the neonate had normal platelet counts, 14 NRBCs/100 white blood cells (WBCs) and mild hepatic enlargement and minimal edema. There had been no hydramnios, and the cesarean section done for breech presentation was the time when the neoplasm was discovered. The large artery supplying this tumor was four-fifths occluded by old thrombus with calcification. This presumably was the reason for the infarction of four fifths of the tumor. The villous tissue was edematous, and there was certainly impending cardiac failure, although the cardiac size was normal. Dorman and Cardwell (1995) were the first authors to present a description of the Ballantyne syndrome with a large chorioangioma. This syndrome (also referred to as maternal hydrops syndrome, pseudotoxemia, triple edema, mirror syndrome) occasionally exists in a variety of conditions, such as non-immune hydrops, moles, teratoma, etc. The patient described by these authors had severe hypertension, proteinuria, and edema with an hydropic fetus due to a 9 × 6 × 8 cm chorangioma at 19 weeks gestation. After delivery, the placenta was found to have numerous infarcts in addition to the chorangioma. Ideally, such tumors will be treated in utero with laser vascular ablation in future.

The hearts of these newborns are often enlarged. The neonates may also be severely anemic, and we believe that hydrops usually develops because of fetal heart failure (Nuutinen et al., 1988). Similar observations are made when large fetal angiomas or arteriovenous fistulas cause hydrops (Cohen & Sinclair, 1963; Cooper & Bolande, 1965; Daniel & Cassady, 1968; Murray et al., 1969). Cardiomeg-

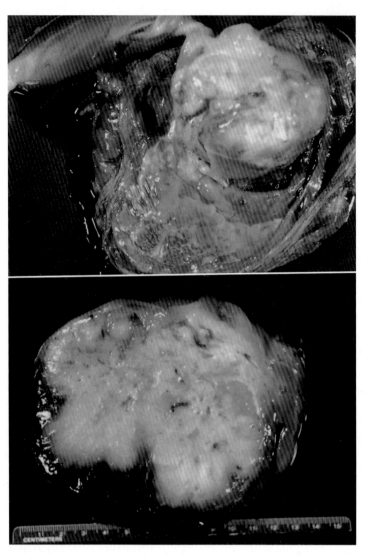

FIGURE 24.9. A 900-g subchorionic chorangioma with marked edema of the umbilical cord and thrombosis of the nourishing chorionic artery. Four fifths of the tumor was infarcted, and there was villous edema and minimal neonatal cardiac failure. The infant did well.

aly alone was reported with the chorangioma described by Benson and Joseph (1961). That neoplasm measured $16 \times 10 \times 6$ cm and weighed 542 g. High output cardiac failure and hydramnios occurred with a $9 \times 8 \times 8$ cm mass studied sonographically by Eldar-Geva et al. (1988).

Thrombocytopenia is also often observed in the newborns whose placentas have chorioangiomas. It may be associated with heart failure and disseminated intravascular coagulation (Greene & Iams, 1984). Froehlich and Housler (1971) and Froehlich et al. (1971) described thrombocytopenia. The latter authors found the tumors to occur more frequently in white than in African-American mothers, more often with twins, and also more often with malformed neonates. They mentioned an association with fetal angiomas, as did Leblanc and Carrier (1979) and Bakaris et al. (2004). We have seen several neonates with hemangiomas whose placentas contained chorioangiomas, perhaps further supporting the notion that this tumor, as fetal angiomas, represents in reality some form

of congenital malformation, rather than a true neoplasm. Many authors have posed the same question. Bakaris et al. (2004) presented a case associated with neonatal hemangiomatosis and infantile angioma of the liver. Drut et al. (1992) reported the presence of hemangioendotheliomas and multiple chorioangiomas in the Beckwith-Wiedemann syndrome (BWS) (Fig. 24.10) and referred to a few case descriptions of similar combinations. Additional consideration of the BWS will be found below and in Chapter 22. The notion of "hamartosis" was also inconclusively discussed. Demonstration of factor VIII within the neoplastic cells suggested to Majlessi and coauthors (1983) that the origin of the large and unusually cellular tumor (327 g) they observed was endothelial. Sieracki et al. (1975), in a description of six cases, found one tumor that resembled pericytes. Accordingly, they suggested the diagnosis of pericytoma. Hydropic bovine fetuses have been associated with chorioangiomas (Corcoran & Murphy, 1965), and Kirkbride et al. (1973) found an

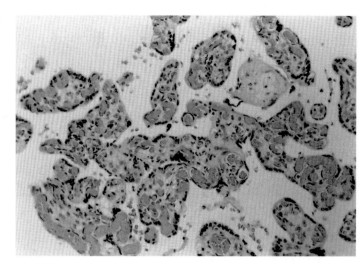

aborted calf with dermal, oral, and placental angiomas. We saw a stillborn bongo (*Tragelaphus eurycerus*) with four huge chorangiomas (weighing up to 975 g) in which some smooth muscle fibers were frequent; also, bizarre multinucleated cells were found whose origin remains obscure. Limaye and Tchabo (1989) observed maternal thrombocytopenia during the course of a pregnancy that was complicated by a 5-cm chorioangioma. They believed that the thrombocytopenia was the result of necrosis in the angioma.

Several authors have noted that chorioangiomas were associated with preeclampsia (e.g., Heggtveit et al., 1965). Stiller and Skafish (1986) found fetomaternal hemorrhage with a placenta that had eight chorioangiomas. Santamaria et al. (1987) saw fetal exsanguination result from such tumors. Perhaps the significantly increased fetal circulation caused by large tumors produces fetal growth restriction (Müller & Rieckert, 1967; Mahmood, 1977; King & Lovrien, 1978). In a series of seven chorioangiomas, Philippe et al. (1969) found four underdeveloped fetuses. Adducci (1975) reported fetal distress resultant from a large chorangioma. Aside from hydramnios, it is frequently reported that premature delivery and placenta previa are associated with chorioangiomas. Asadourian and Taylor (1968) described the occurrence of abruptio placentae with this placental tumor. Premature separation was also seen by Sulman and Sulman (1949), who additionally reported elevated maternal human chorionic gonadotropin (hCG) titers. Others have also found altered levels of pregnancy hormones with large chorioangiomas.

Giant chorioangiomas have been alluded to in several publications (e.g., 570 g in Burrows et al., 1973); the record is probably held by the 1500-g (30 × 20 × 5 cm) tumor described by Arodi et al. (1985). It was associated with breech presentation, placenta previa, hydramnios, preeclampsia, and abruptio placentae. The 32 weeks' gesta-tion fetus weighed 1000 g and died from anemia and asphyxia.

Placental chorioangiomas present other challenging pathologic features. Although placentomegaly, often with typical hydropic villi, is probably directly related to cardiac failure, anemia, and hypoproteinemia, there is no good explanation for an associated umbilical artery thrombosis as described by Sen (1970). Perhaps it is easiest to explain the anemia by the proliferative response that has been identified by Kosanke et al. (1998). These investigators showed that the hypoxia resulting from anemia increased the proliferation of trophoblast and mesenchymal cells of the human placenta. Reiner and Fries (1965) found arteriovenous fistulas in their injection study of a chorioangioma; the neonate experienced rapidly disappearing cardiomegaly. Repetitive multiple chorioangiomas were noted by Battaglia and Woolever (1968), who speculated that sequestration of plasma proteins into the interstices of the lesion may have accounted for the associated hypoproteinemia and edema of their case. Other cases of recurrence have been described and were reviewed by Benirschke (1999). Ludighausen and Sahiri (1983) described a woman who's first and third gestation placentas had multiple chorangiomas. They were the presumed cause of fetal demise in both. Likewise, Chan and Leung (1988) found recurrence of multiple chorioangiomas, both eventuating in fetal demise. We have observed a case of recurrent chorangiomatosis. The 2205-g boy was born after 39 weeks' gestation to a 17-year-old gravida II. He had Apgar scores of 9/9 and did well. The 430-g placenta had numerous typical chorangiomatous nodules (Fig. 24.11), was markedly congested, and had numerous NRBCs in the fetal circulation. Sonographically, "unusual notching of the umbilical vein" had been reported. A previous pregnancy, 1 year earlier, was also complicated by multiple placental chorangiomas. Thus, in all four families summarized here the recur-

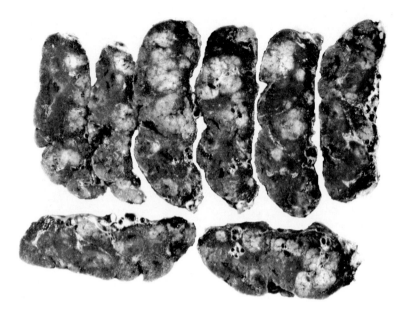

rent chorangiomas were composed of multiple lesions, perhaps best defined as chorangiomatosis. Whether isolated chorangiomas can occur repetitively is unknown. Earn and Penner (1950) depicted a chorioangioma that was separate from the placenta; it was attached by a long vascular pedicle whose vein was diffusely calcified. The macerated fetus associated with this placenta was hydropic. Sonographic diagnosis has repeatedly been made of chorioangiomas and was well described by Dao et al. (1981), who found two large tumors (see also Hirata et al., 1993).

Because we had previously found a severely retarded fraternal twin that had a chromosomal error [46, XX t (2q–; 15q+)], with angiomatous masses in the placenta (Wurster et al., 1969) (Fig. 24.12), we later studied a single chorangioma cytogenetically; it was normal (Kim et al., 1971). Ultrastructural studies done at the same time showed normal endothelial cells and capillaries. Subsequent electron microscopic studies of chorioangiomas were performed by Cash and Powell (1980); they revealed no major additional features. Soma et al. (1991) also studied the tumors electron microscopically and found them to be composed of angioblastic proliferation. The few other cases of chorangioma in twin gestations have been commented upon by Benirschke (1999); they are uncommon, although Wallenburg (1971) and Froehlich et al. (1971) thought otherwise. They are also more common in triplet gestations.

One publication suggested that a "missing link" might have been found between chorioangiomas and choriocarcinomas. Jauniaux et al. (1988) described a lesion they termed "chorangiocarcinoma." The placenta of this 35 weeks' pregnancy contained a solitary small nodule fairly typical of a chorioangioma. Its surface, however, was covered by apparently proliferated trophoblastic epithelium. The mother and child did well; there was no other chemical or cytochemical evidence of choriocarcinoma. Electron microscopy also was no more decisive in suggesting that it was a combination of the two disparate tumors (see Chapter 23).

OTHER BENIGN TUMORS

Some benign tumors of the placenta have been discussed in Chapters 11, 12, and 25. There are, for instance, rare teratomas (Castaldo et al., 1972; Fox, 1978), possibly representing twins. The partial hydatidiform moles, not representing true tumors, are covered in Chapters 21 and 22. Heterotopic tissues, such as adrenal gland, have occasionally occurred in the placenta. They were never neoplastic, but they have occasionally been associated with a growth-restricted infant (Cox & Chavrier, 1980). Fox (1978) had suggested that acceptable placental teratomas should reside on the fetal surface of the placenta.

The report by Chen et al. (1986) presented a novel type of placental tumor. It was a presumed **hepatocellular adenoma**. The authors observed a small-for-gestational-age (1781 g at 37 weeks) infant with a 530-g placenta that contained a 7.0 × 4.2 × 2.7 cm firm mass. The tumor was tan-white, sharply delimited, and composed of polyhedral cells that had the appearance of hepatocytes. There was no bile pigment, but the cells contained glycogen, and some reacted with antibodies to α-fetoprotein and α₁-antitrypsin. Study by electron microscopy showed structures that strongly resembled bile canaliculi. The authors believed that the lesion was a "monodermal teratoma," although it was not on the placental surface. The fetus and mother had an entirely benign course. Four additional hepatic adenomas were described in some detail by Khalifa et al. (1998). They were benign as well, and two had an intravillous and two a subchorionic location. Their histology and special staining characteristics were similar to those in the previous case, but hematopoiesis was a consistent finding. These authors believed that an origin from displaced yolk sac structures was the most likely. Guschmann et al. (2000) described a 2-mm nodule in the twin placenta of a mosaic Turner syndrome patient and interpreted

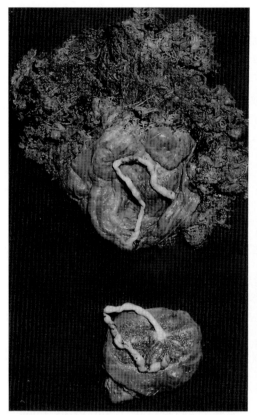
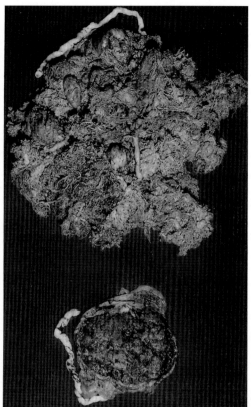

FIGURE 24.12. Placentas of dizygotic (DZ) twins at term. The mother had five pregnancies, was 34 years old, and suffered hydramnios at 36 weeks in this gestation. Twin A was a normal girl (2585 g); the placenta weighed 420 g. Twin B was a boy (1642 g), with a placenta weighing 3600 g. It was interpreted as a "mole." Microscopically, there was primarily angiomatous change of the entire placenta, and the fetus had a translocation with duplication. (*Source:* Wurster et al., 1969, with permission.)

it as a heterotopic adrenal lesion. The entire literature of benign, unusual placental tumors is here also competently reviewed. Doss and her colleagues (1998) reported on a hydropic neonate with hepatoblastoma of the liver whose placental vessels were crowded with metastatic hepatoblastoma cells.

Chorangiosis and Chorangiomatosis

The terminology for chorangiosis and chorangiomatosis is poorly defined; indeed, Marchetti (1939) considered that this lesion was merely a diffuse ectasia of placental villous capillaries. One may possibly think of chorangiomatosis as representing multiple chorioangiomas, but chorangiosis is most certainly not a neoplastic condition. Because of its histologic similarity to some aspects of chorioangioma, it may as well be discussed here, although it has a decidedly different pathogenesis. Meyenburg (1922) had considered this lesion as "diffuse hemangiomatosis of the placenta," but it was Hörmann (1958) who coined the term **chorioangiosis**. Later authors suggested that it results from abnormal maturation of villi and hypoxia. In particular, the differentiation from the con-

gestion of diabetic mothers' placentas has caused confusion in the literature. It must also be cautioned that removal of blood from capillaries renders villi relatively bloodless and thus to appear as being without vessels, whereas infusion distends the capillaries and may produce pictures like chorangiosis. Care must be taken in interpreting the lesion properly.

Caldwell et al. (1977) considered this lesion to be a "vascular anomaly of the placental villi with increased capillarity of their stroma." They saw a 3100-g infant whose mother had received isoxsuprine over 5 months for vaginal bleeding and uterine contractions. The infant had thrombocytopenia and petechiae. Also present were hydramnios and a circumvallate placenta that weighed 1770 g and measured 24 × 23 × 6.5 cm. It was unusually thick. The villi had hugely distended vessels that were numerically increased. As is true with chorioangiomas, the depressed platelet count was probably the result of sequestration in the placental capillaries.

It was not until Altshuler (1984) considered this entity in considerable detail that some clarity resulted about the nature of chorangiosis. He diagnosed the condition principally by low-power lens inspection of histologic sections (stained with hematoxylin and eosin, H&E): "Chorangiosis was diagnosed when inspection with a ×10 objective, showed ten villi, each with ten or more vascular channels in ten or more noninfarcted and nonischemic zones of at least three different placental areas." He graded chorangiosis from grade 1 to 3, depending on the profusion of vessels within villi. He found an overall incidence of 5.5% among 1350 placentas and distinguished it clearly from congestion. Because of the frequency and importance of this condition, refinements of the numerical assessment have been made. Perhaps the most important observation is that by Mutema and Stanek (1998). They found that, when counting is done on slides stained with CD34 immunohistochemistry (endothelial marker), more vessels were counted in nonchorangiomatous villi (eight to 15), and thus when H&E staining only is performed, the frequency of chorangiosis may be overestimated.

Chorangiosis is not common but may have an ominous connotation (Benirschke, 1994a). Altshuler saw it associated with high frequency in stillbirths and many perinatal circumstances that suggested to him long-standing hypoxia. Thus, it is more commonly observed in the placentas of babies who develop cerebral palsy. We find it more often with cord problems of one kind or another (Benirschke, 1994b). The increase in capillary lumen cross sections seen in this lesion comes about, we believe, through endothelial proliferation. It thus takes time to develop. Perhaps it takes as much as weeks to develop full-blown, marked chorangiosis. Its presence betrays a deleterious intrauterine environment for the fetus, and we see in its manifestation an attempt (teleologically speaking) of the placenta to enlarge its diffusional surface. It is thus not surprising to note that somewhat similar observations were made in placentas from high altitude when they were quantitatively compared with those of lower strata (Jackson et al., 1987; Reshetnikova et al., 1993, 1994, 1996; and many others). When Ali (1997) compared stereologically the villous structure of placentas from high altitude (3000 m) with those at sea level, his main finding was an increase in the number of cytotrophoblast at altitude. Birth weights, placental weights, and placental index were all lower at altitude. The increased recruitment of cytotrophoblast was thought to result from relative hypoxia and increased syncytial turnover. Although not discussed, the microscopic picture of villi shown suggests an increase in capillaries as well.

Placental villous congestion is particularly prominent with uncontrolled diabetes and, in our experience it may mask this lesion (chorangiosis) if one is not careful (Fig. 24.13). In chorangiosis, there is an obvious numerical increase of the vessels per villus (Fig. 24.14); with congestion, the vessels are merely distended. Chorangiosis correlated significantly with perinatal deaths (39%) (e.g., Keenan & Altshuler, 1975) and congenital anomalies (27%) and was thus deemed to be an important signal for scrutiny, particularly in placentomegaly. Its final etiology, if a specific one really exists, remains to be elucidated. It must be cautioned, however, that not all infants whose placenta shows diffuse chorangiosis are significantly affected. Thus, the case reported by de la Ossa et al. (2001) had as the only complication severe preeclampsia that necessitated a cesarean section. Despite the chorangiosis, the infant developed normally, and no other features that might have induced chorangiosis were known.

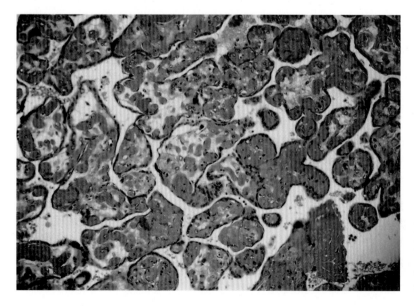

FIGURE 24.13. Severe villous congestion in mature placenta of trisomy 21. This picture is difficult to distinguish from that of chorangiosis. Quantitative measurements and vessel counts are necessary to make a clear distinction. H&E ×160.

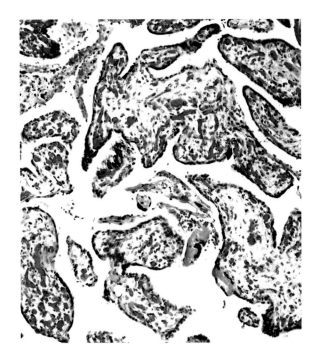

FIGURE 24.14. Chorangiosis of villi in a placenta of severely growth-restricted neonate. The cause of chorangiosis in this case was not ascertained. H&E ×160.

Mesenchymal Dysplasia and the Beckwith-Wiedemann Syndrome

Chapter 22 discussed aspects of mesenchymal dysplasia because the morphology exhibited by this lesion is so often mimicked by features of partial hydatidiform moles. These considerations will not be repeated here. It is necessary, however, to draw attention to the overlaps with BWS and chorangiomas, as they are often very similar in morphologic expression. Indeed, a clear definition of mesenchymal dysplasia that separates these entities is still forthcoming. The recent cases of Paradinas et al. (2001) and Matsui et al. (2003) were cited because of such overlaps. Drut et al. (1992) had described a case of BWS and chorangioma that was also associated with abnormal kidneys and liver angiomas. Thus, clearly difficulties exist for a clean separation of these three entities. The photograph of the placenta in one of our cases with BWS (Fig. 24-10) exemplifies the chorangiosis in this condition. How can progress be made in this area of confusion? First it must be recognized that the BWS has many anomalies that are often minor and may not be recognized in the immediate neonatal period. Thus, it is uncommon that in the placental lesions here summarized, appropriate genetic studies are undertaken to rule out the syndrome. It is a syndrome whose gene appears to be located on 11p15 and has variability with respect to imprinting domains and mutations of p57(KIP2) (see

Niemitz et al., 2004). Deletions had not been recognized until their case was described; thus refined genetic scrutiny would be in order also for the chorangiomas, which, after all, also represent a form of neoplastic tendency as is the case with BWS. It just might be that some of the recurrent chorioangiomas thus find an explanation. Other recent studies of the molecular defect are those by Du et al. (2004) and Le Caignec et al. (2004), whose contributions should be consulted. Mesenchymal dysplasia is often associated with "cirsoid aneurysms" of the placental surface, and the vascular abnormality may extend into stem vessels. Moreover, often one also finds some degree of chorangiosis. In addition, cases with an admixture of abnormal and dysplastic tissues should be studied chromosomally, as they may well be of chimeric nature. In any event, such studies, and the pursuit of angiogenic factor expression or their possible abnormalities may be of interest in the clarification of these dysplasias.

References

Adducci, J.E.: Chorioangioma of the placenta: causing fetal distress. Minn. Med. **58**:820–821, 1975.

Ali, K.Z.M.: Stereological study of the effect of altitude on the trophoblast cell populations of human term placental villi. Placenta **18**:447–450, 1997.

Altshuler, G.: Chorangiosis: an important placental sign of neonatal morbidity and mortality. Arch. Pathol. Lab. Med. **108**:71–74, 1984.

Arodi, J., Auslender, R., Atad, J. and Abramovici, H.: Case report: giant chorioangioma of the placenta. Acta Obstet. Gynecol. Scand. **64**:91–92, 1985.

Asadourian, L.A. and Taylor, H.B.: Clinical significance of placental hemangiomas. Obstet. Gynecol. **31**:551–555, 1968.

Bakaris, S., Karabiber, H., Yuksel, M., Parmaksiz, G. and Kiran, H.: Case of large placental chorangioma associated with diffuse neonatal hemangiomatosis. Pediatr. Developm. Pathol. **7**:258–261, 2004.

Barry, F.E., McCoy, C.P. and Callahan, W.P.: Hemangioma of the umbilical cord. Amer. J. Obstet. Gynecol. **62**:675–680, 1951.

Bashiri, A., Furman, B., Erez, O., Wiznitzer, A., Holcberg, G. and Mazor, M.: Twelve cases of placental chorioangioma. Pregnancy outcome and clinical significance. Arch. Gynecol. Obstet. **266**:53–55, 2002.

Battaglia, F.C. and Woolever, C.A.: Fetal and neonatal complications associated with recurrent chorioangiomas. Pediatrics **41**:62–66, 1968.

Benirschke, K.: Placenta pathology questions to the perinatologist. J. Perinatol. **14**:371–375, 1994a.

Benirschke, K.: Obstetrically important lesions of the umbilical cord. J. Reprod. Med. **39**:262–272, 1994b.

Benirschke, K.: Recent trends in chorangiomas, especially those of multiple and recurrent chorioangiomas. Pediatr. Developm. Pathol. **2**:264–269, 1999.

Benson, P.F. and Joseph, M.C.: Cardiomegaly in a newborn due to placental chorioangioma. Brit. Med. J. **1**:102–105, 1961.

Burrows, S., Gaines, J.L. and Hughes, F.J.: Giant chorioangioma. Amer. J. Obstet. Gynecol. **115**:579–580, 1973.

Caldwell, C., Purohit, D.M., Levkoff, A.H., Garvin, A.J., Williamson, H.O. and Horger III, E.O.: Chorangiosis of the placenta with persistent transitional circulation. Amer. J. Obstet. Gynecol. 127:435–436, 1977.

Cary, W.H.: Report of a well-authenticated case of sarcoma of the placenta. Amer. J. Obstet. 69:658–664, 1914.

Cash, J.B. and Powell, D.E.: Placental chorioangioma: presentation of a case with electron-microscopic and immunochemical studies. Amer. J. Surg. Pathol. 4:87–92, 1980.

Castaldo, F., Guariglia, L., Lanzone, A., Marana, R. and Plotti, G.: Tumori non trofoblastici della placenta. I: Tumori primitivi. Recenti Prog. Med. 70:445–456, 1981.

Chan, K.W. and Leung, C.Y.: Recurrent multiple chorangiomas and intrauterine death. Pathology 20:77–78, 1988.

Chazotte, C., Girz, B., Koenigsberg, M. and Cohen, W.R.: Spontaneous infarction of placental chorioangioma and associated regression of hydrops fetalis. Amer. J. Obstet. Gynecol. 163:1180–1181, 1990.

Chen, K.T.K., Ma, C.K. and Kassel, S.H.: Hepatocellular adenoma of the placenta. Amer. J. Surg. Pathol. 10:436–440, 1986.

Cohen, M.I. and Sinclair, J.C.: Neonatal death from congestive heart failure associated with large cutaneous cavernous hemangioma. Pediatrics 32:924–925, 1963.

Cooper, A.G. and Bolande, R.P.: Multiple hemangiomas in an infant with cardiac hypertrophy: postmortem angiographic demonstration of the arteriovenous fistulae. Pediatrics 35:27–35, 1965.

Corcoran, C.J. and Murphy, E.C.: Rare bovine placental tumour—a case report. Vet. Rec. 77:1234–1235, 1965.

Cox, J.N. and Chavrier, F.: Heterotopic adrenocortical tissue within a placenta. Placenta 1:131–133, 1980.

Daniel, S.J. and Cassady, G.: Non-immunologic hydrops fetalis associated with a large hemangioendothelioma. Pediatrics 42:829–833, 1968.

Dao, A.H., Rogers, C.W. and Wong, S.W.: Chorioangioma of the placenta: report of 2 cases with ultrasound study in 1. Obstet. Gynecol. 57:46S–49S, 1981.

DeCosta, E.J., Gerbie, A.B., Andresen, R.H. and Gallanis, T.C.: Placental tumors: Hemangiomas. With special reference to an associated clinical syndrome. Obstet. Gynecol. 7:249–259, 1956.

De la Ossa, M.M., Cabello-Inchausti, B. and Robinson, M.J.: Placental chorangiosis. Arch. Pathol. Lab. Med. 125:1258, 2001.

Dorman, S.L. and Cardwell, M.S.: Ballantyne syndrome caused by a large placental chorioangioma. Amer. J. Obstet. Gynecol. 173:1632–1633, 1995.

Doss, B.J., Vicari, J., Jacques, S.M. and Qureshi, F.: Placental involvement in congenital hepatoblastoma. Pediat. Development. Pathol. 1:538–542, 1998.

Drut, R., Drut, R.M. and Toulouse, J.C.: Hepatic hemangioendotheliomas, placental chorioangiomas, and dysmorphic kidneys in Beckwith-Wiedemann syndrome. Pediatr. Pathol. 12:197–203, 1992.

Du, M., Zhou, W., Beatty, L.G., Weksberg, R. and Sadowski, P.D.: The KCNQ1OT1 promoter, a key regulatory of genomic imprinting in human chromosome 11p15.5. Genomics 84:288–300, 2004.

Dunn, R.I.S.: Haemangioma of the placenta (chorio-angioma). J. Obstet. Gynaecol. Brit. Emp. 66:51–57, 1959.

Earn, A.A. and Penner, D.W.: Five cases of chorioangioma. J. Obstet. Gynaecol. Brit. Emp. 57:442–444, 1950.

Eldar-Geva, T., Hochner-Celnikier, D., Ariel, I., Ron, M. and Yagel, S.: Fetal high output cardiac failure and acute hydramnios caused by large placental chorioangioma: case report. Brit. J. Obstet. Gynaecol. 95:1200–1203, 1988.

Fox, H.: Vascular tumors of the placenta. Obstet. Gynecol. Surv. 22:697–711, 1967.

Fox, H.: Pathology of the Placenta. Saunders, London, 1978.

Froehlich, L.A. and Housler, M.: Neonatal thrombocytopenia and chorangioma. J. Pediatr. 78:516–519, 1971.

Froehlich, L.A., Fujikura, T. and Fisher, P.: Chorioangiomas and their clinical implications. Obstet. Gynecol. 37:51–59, 1971.

Greene, E.E. and Iams, J.D.: Chorioangioma: a case presentation. Amer. J. Obstet. Gynecol. 148:1146–1148, 1984.

Guschmann, M.: Growth factors and apoptosis rate in an unusual chorangioma. Pathologe 23:389–391, 2002 (in German).

Guschmann, M.: Solitary and multiple chorangiomas—clinical consequences, expression of growth factors and differences in the growth rate. Z. Geburtsh. Neonatol. 207:6–11, 2003.

Guschmann, M., Vogel, M. and Urban, M.: Adrenal tissue in the placenta: a heterotopia caused by migration and embolism? Placenta 21:427–431, 2000.

Guschmann, M., Henrich, W. and Dudenhausen, J.W.: Chorioangiomas—new insights into a well-known problem. II. An immuno-histochemical investigation of 136 cases. J. Perinat. Med. 31:170–175, 2003a.

Guschmann, M., Schulz-Bischof, K. and Vogel, M.: Incidental choriangiocarcinoma. Case report, immunohistochemistry and theories of possible histogenesis. Pathologe 24:124–127, 2003b (in German).

Harigaya, A., Nako, Y., Morikawa, A., Okano, H. and Takagi, T.: Premature infant with severe periventricular leukomalacia associated with a large placental chorioangioma: A case report. J. Perinatol. 22:252–254, 2002.

Heggtveit, H.A., de Carvalho R. and Nuyens, A.J.: Chorioangioma and toxemia of pregnancy. Amer. J. Obstet. Gynecol. 91:291–292, 1965.

Hirata, G.I., Masaki, D.I., O'Toole, M., Medearis, A.L. and Platt, L.D.: Color flow mapping and Doppler velocimetry in the diagnosis and management of a placental chorioangioma associated with nonimmune fetal hydrops. Obstet. Gynecol. 81:850–852, 1993.

Hsieh, C.-C. and Soong, Y.-K: Infarction of placental chorioangioma and associated regression of hydrops fetalis. Amer. J. Obstet. Gynecol. 166:1306, 1992.

Hörmann, G.: Zur Systematik einer Pathologie der menschlichen Plazenta. Arch. Gynäkol. 191:297–344, 1958.

Imakita, M., Yutani, C., Ishibashi-Ueda, H., Murakami, M. and Chiba, Y.: A case of hydrops fetalis due to placental chorioangioma. Acta Pathol. Jpn. 38:941–945, 1988.

Jackson, M.R., Mayhew, T.M. and Haas, J.D.: Morphometric studies on villi in human term placentae and the effects of altitude, ethnic grouping and sex of newborn. Placenta 8:487–495, 1987.

Jackson, M.R., Carney, E.W., Lye, S.J. and Knox Ritchie, J.W.: Localization of two angiogenic growth factors (PDECGF and VEGF) in human placentae throughout gestation. Placenta 15:341–353, 1994.

Jauniaux, E., Zucker, M., Meuris, S., Verherst, A., Wilkin, P. and Hustin, J.: Chorangiocarcinoma: an unusual tumour of the placenta: the missing link? Placenta 9:607–613, 1988.

Kadyrov, M., Kosanke, G., Kingdom, J. and Kaufmann, P.: Increased fetoplacental angiogenesis during first trimester in anaemic women. Lancet 352:1747–1749, 1998.

Kaufmann, P., Kohnen, G. and Kosanke, G.: Wechselwirkungen zwischen Plazentamorphologie und fetaler Sauerstoffversorgung. Gynäkologe 26:16–23, 1993.

Keenan, W.J. and Altshuler, G.: Massive pulmonary hemorrhage in a neonate. J. Pediatr. 86:466–471, 1975.

Khalifa, M.A., Gersell, D.J., Hansen, C.H. and Lage, J.M.: Hepatic (hepatocellular) adenoma of the placenta: A study of four cases. Intern. J. Gynecol. Pathol. 17:241–244, 1998.

Kim, C.K., Benirschke, K. and Connolly, K.S.: Chorangioma of the placenta: chromosomal and electron microscopic studies. Obstet. Gynecol. 37:372–376, 1971.

King, C.R. and Lovrien, E.W.: Chorioangioma of the placenta and intrauterine growth failure. J. Pediatr. 93:1027–1028, 1978.

Kirkbride, C.A., Bicknell, E.J. and Robl, M.G.: Hemangioma of a bovine fetus with a chorioangioma of the placenta. Vet. Pathol. 10:238–240, 1973.

Klaften, E.: Chorionhaemangioma placentae. Z. Geburtshilfe Gynäkol. 95:426–437, 1929.

Knoth, M., Rygaard, J. and Hesseldahl, H.: Chorioangioma with hydramnios and intra-uterine fetal death. Acta Obstet. Gynecol. Scand. 55:279–281, 1976.

Kosanke, G., Kadyrov, M., Korr, H. and Kaufmann, P.: Maternal anemia results in increased proliferation in human placental villi. Trophobl. Res. 11:339–357, 1998.

Kühnel, P.: Placental chorangioma. Acta Obstet. Gynecol. Scand. 13:143–194, 1933.

Leblanc, A. and Carrier, C.: Chorio-angiome placentaire, angiomes cutanes et cholestase néonatale. Arch. Fr. Pédiatr. 36:484–486, 1979.

Le Caignec, C., Gicquel, C., Gruber, M.C., Guyot, C., You, M.C., Laurent, A., Joubert, M., Winer, N., David, A. and Rival, J.M.: Sonographic findings in Beckwith-Wiedemann syndrome related to H19 hypermethylation. Prenat. Diagn. 24:165–168, 2004.

Limaye, N.S. and Tchabo, J.-G.: Asymptomatic thrombocytopenia associated with chorioangioma of placenta. Amer. J. Obstet. Gynecol. 161:76–77, 1989.

Linder, D. and Gartler, S.M.: Glucose-6-phosphate dehydrogenase mosaicism: utilization as a cell marker in the study of leiomyomas. Science 150:67–69, 1965.

Lopez, H.B.B. and Kristoffersen, S.E.: Chorioangioma of the placenta. Gynecol. Obstet. Invest. 28:108–110, 1989.

Ludighausen, M.V. and Sahiri, I.: Chorangiome der Plazenten als Ursache wiederholter Totgeburten. Geburtsh. Frauenh. 43:233–235, 1983.

Mahmood, K.: Small chorioangiomas and small-for-gestational age baby. Amer. J. Obstet. Gynecol. 127:440–442, 1977.

Majlessi, H.F., Wagner, K.M. and Brooks, J.J.: Atypical cellular chorangioma of the placenta. Int. J. Gynecol. Pathol. 1:403–408, 1983.

Mandelbaum, B., Ross, M. and Riddle, C.B.: Hemangioma of the placenta associated with fetal anemia and edema: report of a case. Obstet. Gynecol. 34:335–338, 1969.

Marchetti, A.A.: A consideration of certain types of benign tumors of the placenta. Surg. Gynecol. Obstet. 68:733–743, 1939.

Matsui, H., Iitsuka, Y., Yamazawa, K., Tanaka, N., Mitsuhashi, A., Seki, K. and Sekiya, S.: Placental mesenchymal dysplasia initially diagnosed as partial mole. Pathol. Int. 53:810–813, 2003.

McInroy, R.A. and Kelsey, H.A.: Chorio-angioma (haemangioma of placenta) associated with acute hydramnios. J. Pathol. Bacteriol. 68:519–523, 1954.

Mesia, A.F., Mo, P. and Ylagan, L.R.: Atypical cellular chorangioma. A mitotically active tumor of the placenta. Arch. Pathol. Lab. Med. 123:536–538, 1999.

Meyenburg, H.V.: Über Hämangiomatosis diffusa placentae. Beitr. Pathol. Anat. Allg. Pathol. 70:510–512, 1922.

Müller, G. and Rieckert, H.: Beitrag zur Frage der Placentarinsuffizienz an Hand eines diffusen Chorangioms. Arch. Gynäkol. 204:78–88, 1967.

Murray, D.E., Meyerowitz, B.R. and Hutter, J.J.: Congenital arteriovenous fistula causing congestive heart failure in the newborn. JAMA 209:770–771, 1969.

Mutema, G. and Stanek, J.: Numerical criteria for the diagnosis of placental chorangiosis using CD34 immunostaining. Placenta 19:A-39, 1998 (abstract).

Nicolini, U., Zuliani, G., Caravelli, E., Fogliani, R., Poblete, A. and Roberts, A.: Alcohol injection: a new method of treating placental chorangiomas. Lancet 353:1674–1675, 1999.

Niemitz, E.L., DeBaun, M.R., Fallon, J., Murakami, K., Kugoh, H., Oshimura, M. and Feinberg, A.P.: Microdeletion of LIT1 in familial Beckwith-Wiedemann syndrome. Amer. J. Human Genet. 75:844–849, 2004.

North, P.E., Waner, M., Mizeracki, A., Mrak, R.E., Nicholas, R., Kincannon, J., Suen, J.Y. and Mihm, M.C.Jr.: A unique microvascular phenotype shared by juvenile hemangiomas and human placenta. Arch Dermatol. 137:559–570, 2001.

Nuutinen, E.W., Puistola, U., Herva, R. and Koivisto, M.: Two cases of large placental chorioangioma with fetal and neonatal complications. Europ. J. Obstetr. Gynecol. Reprod. Biol. 29:315–320, 1988.

Ogino, S. and Redline, R.W.: Villous capillary lesions of the placenta: distinctions between chorangioma, chorangiomatosis, and chorangiosis. Hum. Pathol 31:945–954, 2000.

Paradinas, F.J., Sebire, N.J., Fisher, R.A., Rees, H.C., Foskett, M., Seckl, M.J. and Newlands, E.S.: Pseudo-partial moles: placental stem vessel hydrops and the association with Beckwith-Wiedemann syndrome and complete moles. Histopathology 39:447–454, 2001.

Philippe, E., Muller, G., Dehalleux, J.-M., Lefakis, P. and Gandar, R.: Le chorio-angiome et ses complications foeto-maternelles. Rev. Fr. Gynécol. 64:335–341, 1969.

Reiner, L. and Fries, E.: Chorangioma associated with arteriovenous aneurysm. Amer. J. Obstet. Gynecol. 93:58–64, 1965.

Reshetnikova, O.S., Burton, G.J. and Milovanov, A.P.: Hypoxia at altitude and villous vascularisation in the mature human placenta. Placenta 14:A62, 1993 (abstract).

Reshetnikova, O.S., Burton, G.J. and Milovanov, A.P.: Effects of hypobaric hypoxia on the fetoplacental unit: The morphometric diffusing capacity of the villous membrane at high altitude. Amer. J. Obstet. Gynecol. 171:1560–1565, 1994.

Reshetnikova, O.S., Burton, G.J. and Milovanov, A.P.: Increased incidence of placental chorioangioma in high-altitude pregnancies: hypobaric hypoxia as a possible etiological factor. Amer. J. Obstet. Gynecol. **174**:557–561, 1996.

Santamaria, M., Benirschke, K., Carpenter, P.M., Baldwin, V.J. and Pritchard, J.A.: Transplacental hemorrhage associated with placental neoplasms. Pediatr. Pathol. **7**:601–615, 1987.

Schulz-Hetzel, I.: Über das Chorioangiom. Arch. Gynäkol. **225**:131–146, 1978.

Sen, D.K.: Placental hypertrophy associated with chorangioma. Amer. J. Obstet. Gynecol. **107**:652–654, 1970.

Sherer, D.M. and Abulafia, O.: Angiogenesis during implantation, and placental and early embryonic development. Placenta **22**:1–13, 2001.

Siddall, R.S.: Chorioangiofibroma (chorioangioma). Amer. J. Obstet. Gynecol. **8**:430–456; 554–568, 1924.

Sieracki, J.C., Panke, T.W., Horvat, B.L., Perrin, E.V. and Nanda, B.: Chorioangiomas. Obstet. Gynecol. **46**:155–159, 1975.

Soma, H.: Lesson from Nepalese Placenta. Based on 20 years' Pathological Studies. Industrial Publ. & Consulting, Inc. Tokyo, Japan, 2001 (http://www.ipij.com).

Soma, H., Satoh, M., Higashi, S., Ogura, H., Horikiri, H. and Hata, T.: Ultrastructure of choriocarcinoma. J. Clin. Electron Microscopy **24**:5–6, 1991.

Stiller, A.G. and Skafish, P.R.: Placental chorangioma: a rare cause of fetomaternal transfusion with maternal hemolysis and fetal distress. Obstet. Gynecol. **67**:296–298, 1986.

Sulman, F.G. and Sulman, E.: Increased gonadotrophin production in a case of detachment of placenta due to placental haemangioma. J. Obstet. Gynaecol. Br. Emp. **56**:1033–1034, 1949.

Sweet, L., Reid, W.D. and Robertson, N.R.C.: Hydrops fetalis in association with chorioangioma of the placenta. J. Pediatr. **82**:91–94, 1973.

Wallenburg, H.C.S.: Chorioangioma of the placenta: thirteen new cases and a review of the literature from 1939–1970 with special reference to the clinical complications. Obstet. Gynecol. Surv. **26**:411–425, 1971.

Williams, J.T.: Angioma of the placenta: with pathological report and microphotography by Dr. Frank B. Mallory. Surg. Gynecol. Obstet. **32**:523–526, 1921.

Wurster, D.H., Hoefnagel, D., Benirschke, K. and Allen, F.H.: Placental chorangiomata and mental deficiency in a child with 2/15 translocation; 46XX; t(2q−; 15q+). Cytogenetics **8**:389–399, 1969.

25
Multiple Pregnancies

In a remarkable paper that correlates prenatal events and discordance of twins with postnatal outcome, Price (1950) emphasized the importance of "prenatal biases." He was much concerned with the influence of placentation upon twin development, an aspect that had not often been considered in twin studies. Similar ideas were echoed by Phillips (1993), who emphasized the influence of the proximity of twin placentas on their ability to support fetal growth. But it was Galton (1875), cousin of Charles Darwin, and after whom the Galton Institute of Genetics in London is named, who was probably the first to suggest that twins, if properly studied, would yield information that might allow us to discriminate between the effects of heredity and those of the environment—his famous "nature vs. nurture" concept. The extensive studies conducted by Friedrich Schatz at about the same time, suggested that prenatal influences among twins found reflection in the ultimate the outcome of the twins. He was instrumental in clarifying that placental study is essential for this understanding. His extensive work is annotated in a bibliographic oddity (Schatz, 1900). It summarized all of his papers and citations therein. Some of his numerous contributions were partially translated for the book on twin placentation by Strong and Corney (1967). A concise review of the biologic aspects of the human twinning process was published by Benirschke and Kim (1973), and *Twinning and Twins*, by MacGillivray and his colleagues (1988), summarizes most relevant aspects of this interesting phenomenon of nature. Baldwin (1994) produced a remarkable volume that contains all relevant aspects of placentation of multiple pregnancies and it is well illustrated. Finally, Gall (1996) summarized all practical aspects of multiple gestations, especially the clinical manifestations and therapy. Several cases of hydatidiform mole in twin gestations have been reported (e. g., Chu et al., 2004). These are discussed in more detail in Chapter 22.

No doubt, the complexity of human twinning cannot be understood without knowledge of the placentation of twins. Moreover, despite all the benefits reaped from animal studies, the placentation of most relevant species is often very dissimilar from that of humans. Thus, conclusions drawn from animal multiple pregnancies must be interpreted with great care. In recent years, ultrasonographic studies have added materially to our knowledge of prenatal events in twinning and its placentation. Of interest, for instance, are the remarkable observations by Arabin et al. (1996) of extensive inter-twin physical interactions. They were observed to occur earlier in monochorionic twins than in those with a dichorionic twin placenta.

ZYGOSITY

There are "fraternal" (better named dizygotic, DZ) and "identical" (monozygotic, MZ) twins. In higher multiple births, these may be admixed. That such different classes of twins exist derives from several observations. Fraternal twins may be of different or like sex. A hypothesis is herein helpful: if all twins were DZ, then one would expect a similar sex ratio to be found as that for singletons, that is, approximately 50% MF, 25% MM, and 25% FF. This is not the case. When large statistics of infants' sex at birth are examined, it is found that there is an excess of like-sex twins. This excess is presumed to result from the number of MZ (identical) twins. By subtracting these from the total number of twins, we have an estimate for the distribution of MZ and DZ twins in a population. This is the so-called Weinberg rule (1901). [Hrubec and Robinette (1984) pointed out that the basis for this rule had previously been published by Bertillon (1874).] Weinberg's "differential method" can be stated with the following formula:

$$MZ\,twins = All\,twins - \frac{Unlike\text{-}sex\,twins}{2pq}$$

where p is the frequency of male births, and q is the frequency of female births in a population.

Weinberg's formula should be taken as providing estimates, with considerable errors if it were taken literally. This is particularly understandable when one considers the frequencies of different classes of twins as they exist at the time of conception; for there is much evidence that MZ twins have a higher prenatal death rate than do DZ twins. The Weinberg method cannot correct for losses of only one twin in a gestation, information that is also usually not recorded in birth statistics. It is, therefore, not surprising that the method has often been criticized (e.g., Renkonen, 1967, and reply by Cannings, 1969; James, 1971, 1984; Keith, 1974). Nevertheless, it is a unique and valuable tool to assess the approximate frequency of DZ vs. MZ twins in a population. Moreover, a prospective study that attempted to validate the method found that the results agree well with findings from placentation and known zygosity of twins (Vlietinck et al., 1988). An interesting observation by James (1971) is that, among DZ twins, there is an excess of like-sex pairs. This observation is based on small samples of twins whose zygosity was ascertained by blood grouping. It has so far remained unexplained, but some additional data (James, 1977a,b) show an even more marked excess of females among monoamnionic/monochorionic (MoMo) twins, and perhaps in twins with acardiacs. More light has been shed on this phenomenon by the large study of Derom et al. (1988), who provided data from the Belgian prospective twin study that included zygosity diagnosis and placental assessment. Not only was the proportion of males reduced in MZ twins (irrespective of chorion status), but also there was a marked reduction of male MoMo twins from what might be expected if this form of twinning occurred at random. The sex proportion of all MZ twins was 0.487, and that of MoMo was 0.231, whereas the DZ twins had a proportion of 0.518. Although no large data sets are yet available, the authors cited evidence that conjoined twins at term are more commonly females, whereas those of abortuses may be more often males. Of the two possibilities to explain this unexpected observation—greater frequency of late twinning in female conceptuses and greater abortion rate of male MoMo conceptuses—the authors favored the former. They referred to the suggestion made by Burn et al. (1986) that "unequal lyonization" of X chromosomes may be a cause of late twinning, and that feature is unique to females. But Goodship et al. (1996) found no support for this hypothesis when they examined X-inactivation patterns of umbilical cords of various types of twins. Monteiro et al. (1998a) studied this a little further by comparing X-inactivation patterns of lymphocytes and buccal cells of monochorionic (MC)-MZ and dichorionic (DC)-MZ twins. They assumed from earlier studies that lyonization occurs when there are 10 to 20 cells in the embryo and deduced from modeling that "MC-MZ twinning occurs three or four rounds of replication *after* X inactivation, whereas DC-MZ twinning event occurs earlier, before or around the time of X inactivation." The apparent excess of female acardiacs is possibly further confirmation (James, 1977) of this phenomenon. The largest prospective survey of twins comes from Belgium (Loos et al., 1999), which encompassed 5089 twins, 158 triplets, and 14 quadruplets or higher multiples. In this survey, zygosity was established by sex, placentation, and genetic markers in over 95%. Dizygotic twins had the same sex proportions as singletons, whereas MZ twins had an excess of females.

Considerations of the MZ twinning rates come from Allen and Hrubec (1987), who proposed that a slight suggestion exists of a relationship of the MZ twinning rate to maternal age, as is very certain for DZ twins. These "constants," of DZ to MZ twin frequencies, identified from various statistical considerations, however, are still considered to be arbitrary, and they also appear to differ among various populations.

Other reasons for considering that a proportion of twins are identical, or monozygotic, come from the numerous reports on genetic identity, as well as the physical similarity exhibited by some twins. Twin research has traditionally involved ascertainment of zygosity by assessment of likeness. Dermatoglyphics (Newman, 1931a; Allen, 1968; Brismar, 1968; Herrlin et al., 1970; Reed et al., 1975), and blood grouping (Robertson, 1969; Selvin, 1970) are some of many parameters that have been employed. But these methods have not always been decisive in assigning the zygosity for an individual set of twins, although their general reliability is high. For that reason, methods such as mixed leukocyte stimulation (Jarvik et al., 1969), skin exchange graft survival (Stranc, 1966), and repeated blood group study (Osborne, 1958) have been advocated. Analysis of banded chromosomes, C-bands and Q-

bands, has also been used to ascertain monozygosity (Neurath et al., 1972; McCracken et al., 1978; Morton et al., 1981; Pedrosa et al., 1983). Until recently, this has been the most reliable methodology. These methods established mostly probabilities of twins' zygosity, and they were often somewhat imprecise. The mathematical aspects of phenotypic likeness studies have been treated by Meulepas et al. (1988). New methods have now been developed that are more decisive. How important they can be is manifest from the report by St. Clair et al. (1998). Unlike-appearing twins, thought to be dizygotic, had successful inter-twin renal transplant because of mushroom poisoning to one twin. DNA fingerprinting found them later to be monozygotic, whereupon the immunosuppressive therapy was successfully discontinued.

The techniques for the direct comparison of DNA variants have much to be recommended as primary tools. They determine the restriction fragment length polymorphism (RFLP) of twins, and cogent reasons for routinely employing this methodology have been advanced by Machin (1994). These methods of comparing fragments of DNA are quick and decisive, and can be executed on placental tissue, blood, and other tissues (Derom et al., 1985; Hill & Jeffreys, 1985). Importantly, the quantities of tissue needed for this study can be quite small when combined with polymerase chain reaction (PCR). Microsatellites have also proven to be useful and rapid in the definitive differential diagnosis of MZ vs. DZ twins (Erdmann et al., 1993; Becker et al., 1997). Thus, antenatal samples may readily be processed by this and related modern techniques for accurate determination of twin zygosity (Kovacs et al., 1988) and they have been decisively used to identify the genetic relationships between twins and triplets (Motomura et al., 1987; Azuma et al., 1989). It is of further interest that this method can also be used to identify DNA patterns of macerated stillborn fetuses (Derom et al., 1991). Neuman and her colleagues (1990) have proved with RFLPs the dizygosity of aborted tubal twins and suggested that the alleged common monozygosity of ectopic twins may be in error. Norton et al. (1997) advocated the use of DNA diagnostic study of discordant multiple gestational products when chorionic status is indeterminate or not helpful.

The least decisive method for the identification of the zygosity of twins, the likeness assessment, however, is also the most widely practiced. It is the easiest method to execute and it correctly asserts that physical characteristics are more alike in MZ twins than they are in DZ twins (e.g., tooth morphology: Lundström, 1963; skin color: Collins et al., 1966; cardiac findings: Preis & Srubarova, 1966; immunoglobulin levels: Sowards & Monif, 1972; cholesterol levels: Corey et al., 1975; etc.). A fairly reliable accuracy of zygosity diagnosis is said to be achieved with other simple tests, including the use of questionnaires (Cederlöf et al., 1961; Nichols & Bilbro, 1966). These oversimplifications, however, have also led to many misconceptions. Moreover, they have confused neonatologists who care for often markedly discordant twins in the neonatal period and who need better guidelines for care than are generally available.

It is now certain that MZ twins are frequently discordant in development; some of this discordance can be secondary to unique placental vascular relations between twins (Schatz, 1886; Verschuer, 1927; Price, 1950), others have their cause in abnormal placentation. Discordance for congenital anomalies is higher in MZ twins than in DZ twins, a feature that has been critically analyzed by Boklage (1987a), Mastroiacovo and Botto (1994), and Hall (1996). There are also other fascinating problems to be resolved; for instance, Zaw and Stone (2002) reported caudal regression syndrome in a set of monozygotic but dichorionic twins. Is that due to growth disparity of the twins or to the possibility that only one of the twins was exposed to the abnormalities of glucose imbalance of the MZ twins at the time of putative exposure? Some such questions can potentially be resolved by the twin methodology, and Hobbs et al. (2002) drew attention to this in their review of the genetic aspects of congenital anomalies. Twins, in general, have also been found to have higher hematocrits and somewhat elevated levels of nucleated red blood cell counts, irrespective of prenatal hypoxia or intrauterine growth restriction (IUGR) (Sheffer-Mimouni et al., 2004). Triplets share this feature, according to Suslak et al. (1987). Melnick and Myrianthopoulos (1979) found that the twofold increase of anomalies in MZ twins cannot be validly ascribed to the monochorionic placental status that is so prevalent in MZ twins. An exception to this are acardiacs and the destructive results from prenatal disseminated intravascular coagulation (DIC) or acute blood loss, which may depend in their origin from the monochorionic status of their twin placenta. These authors suggested as a possible explanation, that the "impetus" for MZ twinning may be similar to that which is the cause of the developmental anomalies. In recent years, Steinman (2001a–c, 2002a,b, 2003) has proposed that the possible reason for MZ twinning is the deficiency of cellular adhesion between embryonic cells, mediated perhaps by calcium-dependent adhesion molecules. Some support for this hypothesis is afforded by the occurrence of MZ twins among assisted reproductive technology (ART)-derived multiples since the blastocysts are often cultured in ethylenediaminetetraacetic acid (EDTA)-chelating media for several days. The relative frequency of anomalies in MZ twins (6–9%, with 80% discordance) has important implications with respect to prenatal diagnosis of early embryos (Jarmulowicz, 1989). It has been suggested that, with the new methodology of PCR of DNA amplification, single blastomeres might be sexed and that they could then be genetically defined in the future. It is unknown at this time whether such loss of blastomeres could result in anomalies, and whether the discordant anomalies of MZ twins are perhaps caused by an unequal splitting of the morula. Also, monozygotic twins with discordance of organ laterality in ciliary dyskinesia (Kartagener syndrome) has important connotations for an explanation of this disorder (Noone et al., 1999). Similarly, the concordance of truncus arteriosus in MZ twins has implications for that anomaly (Mas et al., 1999). These and similar considerations are important questions for future research. Similarly, the monochorionic twins with significant phenotypic differences described by Gringras (1999) cannot presently be explained, but they need to be borne in mind when discussing identical twins. The PCR fingerprints of these twins were identical.

Twin studies, as advocated by Galton (1875), endeavor to distinguish between genetic and environmental influences on fetal development. To be successful, they require accurate zygosity determination of the probands. Walker (1957) stated this requirement emphatically. Moreover, it has been found that if the linkage of genetic traits is not taken into consideration in the zygosity assignment, the probability of monozygosity is overestimated (Sorensen & Fenger, 1974). Kempthorne and Osborne (1961) and Allen and Hrubec (1978) have developed models to undertake such analyses. Allen (1965) proposed excellent guidelines for the design of twin studies that should be consulted. Kruyer et al. (1994) used this sort of knowledge in ascertainment when the full implementation of the fragile X syndrome mutation is attained—postzygotically, as it turns out.

The Placenta in the Study of Zygosity

To derive any benefit from placental studies for twin research, it is mandatory that the umbilical cords be labeled in the order the twins are delivered, for positive identification of the infants. This is best done by placing one or more ties or clamps around the placental cut ends of the cords. Examination of twin placentas (and those of higher multiple births) may then contribute to the determination of zygosity and an understanding of abnormal events. It is also mandatory that a placental record be made. This is needed for an understanding of possible discordant development of twins, and for our understanding of many other pathologic features that twins present. The proposition that **all** monochorionic placentas belong to MZ twins (but that **not all** MZ twins have monochorial placentas) was first clearly stated in the seminal contribution of Curtius (1930). He then called for a detailed reexamination of the understanding of placentation in humans. In general, this proposition has been amply confirmed, for instance in the placental study of 182 like-sexed live-born twins by Ramos-Arroyo et al. (1988). But there are a few well-proven exceptions that are discussed below. The correlation of prematurity, twin development (growth and growth restriction), and placental causes of disturbances has been evaluated by Bleker and his colleagues (1979, 1988, 1995, 1997). Not surprisingly it was found that monochorial twins were delivered earlier and that they had a higher mortality than dichorionic twins. Abnormal cord insertion occurred more commonly in multiple gestations and was related to smaller fetal weights. The authors expressed the notion that placental weight importantly influences and often restricts fetal growth in multiple pregnancies. Min et al. (2000) compared the weights of a larger number of twins (according to chorionicity and sex as well) with those of singletons and provided an excellent reference table. They concluded that "well-grown twins and singletons do not differ as much as previously believed." Cooperstock et al. (2000) demonstrated that significant growth differences (40% before 32 weeks) among twins constitute a risk factor for premature birth.

In principle, there are two types of twin placentation: monochorionic and dichorionic. In higher multiple births, these may be admixed, or one or the other types may be present. Monochorionic placentas, so we believe, virtually **always** come from MZ (identical) twins. The reason for this assumption is that no verified monochorial human placenta has been associated with twins of unlike sex (there are only the rarest exceptions). Furthermore, when genetic markers are studied in monochorionic twins, they are always identical (Corney et al., 1968; the rare exceptions are discussed below). Dichorionic placentas, however, may be associated with both DZ and MZ twins; most are associated with DZ twins. A decisive study of this topic is that of Cameron (1968). He examined the placentas of 668 twin pairs and determined their zygosity with studies of blood groups and placental enzymes. From the fetal sex and the structure of the placental membranes alone, the zygosity could be ascribed accurately in 55%. Genotyping was necessary in the remaining 45%. His analysis gave the following results:

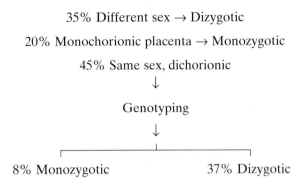

35% Different sex → Dizygotic

20% Monochorionic placenta → Monozygotic

45% Same sex, dichorionic

↓

Genotyping

↓

8% Monozygotic   37% Dizygotic

Of his 668 pairs, 80% had diamnionic/dichorionic (DiDi) placentas; and of these pairs, 90% were DZ. There were 20% monochorionic (and therefore monozygotic) twins. With the improved methodology of modern sonographic equipment, it is now usually possible to make the diagnosis of chorionic status before birth; however, discussion continues as to the sonographic accuracy and as to criteria to be employed at specific gestational ages. Irrespective of numerous papers urging that this diagnosis of chorionicity be made at birth in all multiple deliveries, Cleary-Goldman et al. (2004) found in their survey that this means of assessing some twins' zygosity is unknown to many obstetricians.

The sonographic appearance of the "diving membranes" is now reasonably securely established by competent ultrasonographic studies. The development of the techniques employed and references to the findings made after 1985 are competently summarized by Tutschek et al. (1998). Thus, D'Alton and Dudley (1989) made the correct diagnosis in 68 of 69 prospectively studied cases using ultrasound and counting the layers of the dividing membranes. Winn et al. (1989) suggested sonographic criteria for assessing the width of "dividing membranes." When amniocentesis was done for genetic reasons, the thickness of this dividing membrane was measured in 32 patients. The cutoff point was 2mm. An accuracy of 82% was said to be achieved by this means. This method may be helpful in the future management of twin gestations. Finberg (1992) found that the "twin peak sign" was diagnostic of dichorionic twinning. He showed that a triangular projection of membranes can be seen above the placental surface in dichorionic twins or triplets; Wood et al. (1996) agreed with that in their study. Monteagudo and her colleagues (1994) asserted from their large experience that transvaginal sonography before 14 weeks' gestation easily establishes the nature of the partitioning layers in multiple pregnancies. Sepulveda et al. (1996) nearly always succeeded sonographically to make a correct diagnosis by analysis of the so-called Ipsilon zone (the Y-shaped area of conjunction of sacs in triplets). Vayssière et al. (1996) succeeded to a high degree of accuracy by counting layers of the dividing membranes in the second and third trimesters, whereas Stagiannis

et al. (1995) asserted that the method has a high intra- and interobserver variability. At least once, in a pregnancy with discordant twin growth and absent twin peak sign, monochorionicity was established by the injection of Levovist, a microbubble contrast enhancement agent. After injection into one twin's intrahepatic vein, the contrast agent later appeared in the other twin's heart (Denbow et al., 1997), thus confirming vascular anastomoses and, thereby, monochorionic status. Malinowski (1997) was able to reliably differentiate the twin membrane layers by transvaginal sonography as follows: DiDi at 4 weeks; diamnionic/monochorionic (DiMo) at 5 weeks; and MoMo vs. DiMo at 7 weeks of gestation.

Monochorionic twin placentas virtually always present as single disks. It is most unusual for monochorionic twin placentas to possess separate placental masses; and often they are then connected with small bridges. Nevertheless, Altshuler and Hyde (1993) have described such an exceptional case in which two completely separate disks were connected by a thin bridge. Underneath the chorion of this bridge was atrophied villous tissue. Rare observations of two disks in monochorionic twins have also been made in conjoined twins (see below). Monochorionic twin placentas fall into two categories: (1) the MoMo twin placentas, in which the twins are in the same sac; and (2) the DiMo placenta. The MoMo placenta is the less common. It is also associated with the highest perinatal mortality of twins because of cord entanglement. The higher mortality and complication rate for monozygotic twins has been critically examined by Kovacs et al. (1989). Multiple births not only have higher perinatal mortality but also have greater morbidity. Because of the inordinate contribution to adverse outcomes, Powers and Kiely (1994) provided ultrasound (US)-based population figures that suggested that "to lower the rates of adverse outcomes in twin pregnancies should become a major public health priority." Heyborne et al. (2005) have shown that much improved perinatal survival can be expected when mothers with known MoMo twins undergo early hospitalization for surveillance.

Dichorionic (DiDi) twin placentas may be fused into one mass (DiDi fused), or they may be separated (DiDi separate) organs (Benirschke, 1958). From a practical consideration of the analysis of the placentation of individual twins, it is important to first examine these membrane relations. It is most reliably done by making a cross section of the "dividing membranes," that is, the partition between the two sacs. By excising and rolling a square of these dividing membranes, the two types can then be differentiated (Fig. 25.1). As an alternative method, one may take for histologic study a section from the site where the membranes insert on the placental surface; two "T sections" are seen in Figure 25.2. This method has been particularly well illustrated by Allen and Turner (1971). Either of these methods for taking sections preserves a

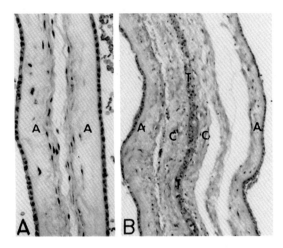

FIGURE 25.1. A: Diamnionic (monochorionic) "dividing membranes" of identical (monozygotic, MZ) twins. There is always a space between the two amnions. The amnion consists of epithelial cells and connective tissue. B: Diamnionic/dichorionic (DiDi) dividing membranes. The right amnion is dislodged from the underlying chorion, a frequent artifact. The central trophoblastic remnants have fused. A, amnion; C, chorion; T, trophoblast. H&E ×100.

permanent record. For the experienced placentologist, it is just as effective to make the diagnosis of DiMo versus DiDi twin placentation by macroscopic inspection.

The dividing membranes of DiMo placentas are usually translucent (Fig. 25.3). They are thin and not opaque, and there are no blood vessel remnants within them. When

one separates the two amnions and comes to their insertion on the placental surface, one may continue to strip the amnions off a DiMo placenta, away from the chorionic plate (Fig. 25.4). In addition, the fetal surface does not show a ridge of fibrin, present as a slightly raised white ridge that is present in DiDi placentas. Bleisch (1964) emphasized this point effectively. DiDi membrane partitions are considerably more opaque (Fig. 25.5). They have remnants of villi and vessels in their four layers and when, by separating the two layers of each placental component, one comes to the chorionic plate, further dissection is impossible (Fig. 25.6). If one attempts to further cleave them, the surface of the placenta is disrupted.

As already stated, the advancements in sonographic equipment have made it possible to distinguish the thickness of the dividing membranes long before birth (Barss et al., 1985; Mahony et al., 1985; Hertzberg et al., 1987; Finberg, 1992). This diagnostic modality is particularly helpful in the diagnosis of MoMo twins who are at risk of cord entanglement. Belfort and his colleagues (1993) demonstrated, by color flow Doppler sonography, such cord entanglement in three sets of MoMo twins. They identified obstruction of flow in the umbilical vein by this means and made the point that this diagnosis can lead to improved outcome of these problematic gestations. It is the practice in our hospital now to hospitalize such patients for possible rapid intervention when problems arise.

The other important point to be made is that monochorionic twin placentas usually have blood vessel

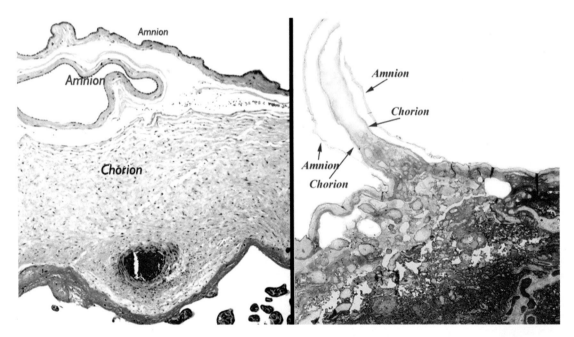

FIGURE 25.2. Left: T-section of dividing membranes of monochorionic/diamnionic twins. Note the contiguity of the chorion over the surface of the placenta at bottom and the separation of amnions. Right: T-section of diamnionic/dichorionic twin placenta. There are atrophic villi and trophoblastic remnants extending between the two chorionic membranes. H&E ×40.

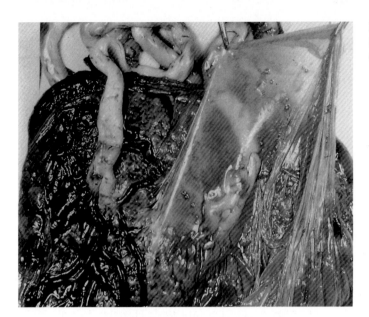

Figure 25.3. Diamnionic/monochorionic twin placenta. The dividing membranes are held up, to disclose their transparency. (See Figure 25.5 for contrast with DiDi placenta.)

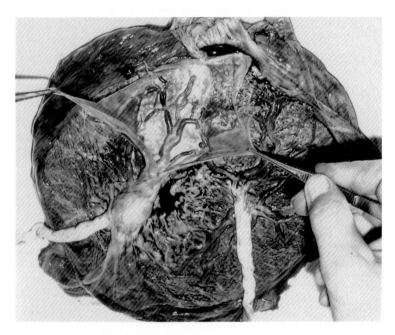

Figure 25.4. Diamnionic/monochorionic twin placenta. The dividing membranes are being separated; at their base they are easily peeled off the chorionic surface. The vascular communications between the two fetal vascular beds are thus disclosed.

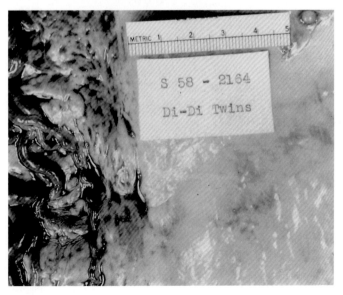

Figure 25.5. Dividing membranes of diamnionic/dichorionic twins are characteristically opaque. They are only rarely translucent.

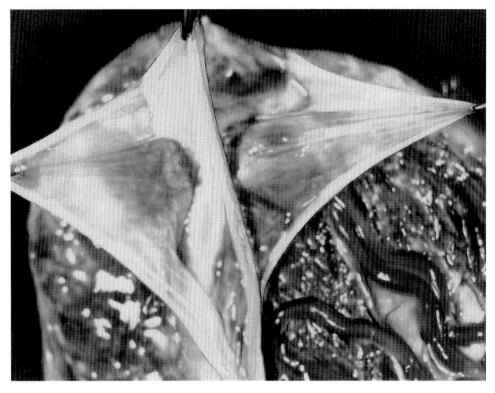

FIGURE 25.6. Diamnionic/dichorionic twin placenta. The two amnions are being peeled off the central two chorionic leaves. The latter cannot be completely stripped off the placental mass without disrupting it.

connections between the fetal circulations; they are not generally present in dichorionic twin placentas. These anastomoses are discussed in greater detail later in this chapter. Note also that not all authorities have concurred with the ease of distinction between DiMo and DiDi placentas just elaborated. Thus, the famous gemellologist H.H. Newman (1931a) believed that one could easily mistake a DiMo for a fused DiDi placenta. This is certainly not the case in experienced hands, but it points to the desirability of examining histologic sections for affirmation. Moreover, it must be recognized that blood group studies in twins have the problem that fetal blood is commonly admixed because of the frequent blood vessel anastomoses in the monochorionic group. It then follows that if DZ twins were associated with a monochorionic placenta in which anastomoses existed, their different blood antigens would permanently mingle. Only a highly sophisticated analysis of their blood groups would ascertain the presence of "blood chimerism." The unusually high frequency (approximately 8%) of blood chimerism reported by van Dijk et al. (1996) remains puzzling and needs verification before it can be accepted as proven. On the other hand, Quintero et al. (2003b) reported a well-studied case of a DiMo twin placenta with discordant sex and unsuccessfully treated twin-to-twin transfusion syndrome, clearly a great exception. Also, the genital development of the twins was normal despite the blood

chimerism, unlike that found in Artiodactyla (freemartins) and similar to what is found to be so in marmosets (vide infra).

In this connection it is important to mention that Mortimer (1987) has challenged the concept that monochorionic placentas are diagnostic of MZ twins on the basis of blood studies. Cord blood grouping studies were conducted on 12 sets of monochorionic twins for 16 red blood cell antigens. In three sets, there were discrepancies between the antigens, despite the presence of artery-to-artery and vein-to-vein anastomoses. These discrepancies always involved single and minor blood groups. How such antigenic difference can come about is difficult to understand, as the anastomoses should have guaranteed complete mixing, as is the case in the few blood chimeras to be considered later. In our view, this study is insufficient evidence for Mortimer's proposition that 25% of the monochorionic twins studied were dizygotic. If this were so, there should be many more boy/girl twins found with monochorionic placentas, and it is not the case. Only two, perhaps three, such examples can be cited, and they were not well studied. The use of the DNA methods (with DNA to be obtained from solid tissues!) discussed earlier will dispel any doubt in the future if twins with such apparent discrepancies come to light.

After it was recognized that monochorionic placentation is useful for the identification of at least two thirds

TABLE 25.1. Distribution of placental types in twins

Source	DiDi (%)	DiMo (%)	MoMo (% or ?)
Szendi (1938)	66	34	0
Vermelin & Ribon (1949)	45 (like sex) 32 (unlike sex)	23	
Benirschke (1961)	68.5	30	1.5
Potter (1963)	76	21	3?
Cameron (1968)	80	20	
Corney et al. (1968)	41 (like sex) 37 (unlike sex)	21.8	
Fujikura & Froehlich (1971)	73	24	2.4
Nylander (1970)	76 (Aberdeen) 92 (Yoruba-Nigeria)	19 5	5? 3?
Derom et al. (1988)	72	27	0.9
Barss (1988)	74.2	24.2	1.7

of MZ twins, several larger series of twin placentas were published. They are summarized in Table 25.1. Note that marked differences exist in the distribution of the different twin groups in these reports. Thus, the frequency of monochorial (MZ) twins is much lower in Nigeria, where the incidence of twinning is especially high, owing to the high frequency of DZ twins in the Yoruba tribe. Knox and Morley (1960) found Western Nigerian Yoruba twin frequency as high as 5.3%, with 91% being DZ. The converse is true of some Oriental populations. Sekiya and Hafez (1977) determined the type of placentation in 84 sets of Japanese twins. They found that 40 were dichorionic [26 fused (31.0%), 14 separate (16.7%)]; 41 were DiMo (48.8%), and three were MoMo (3.6%) (Fig. 25.7).

The placental relations of DiMo and DiDi twins are easiest to identify in very young pregnancies (Fig. 25.8). The youngest implantation sites of DiDi twins (10 to 12 days) have been illustrated by Meyer and Meyer (1981). They featured tiny blastocysts that had implanted far away from one another in the uterine fundus. Parenthetically, it should be mentioned that Ohel et al. (1987) suggested that, as seen by ultrasonographic "grading" methods (calcifications), the placentas of twins exhibit advanced maturation compared to age-matched singleton placentas.

Twin placentas differ in many other respects from those of singletons (Table 25.2). The frequency of marginal and velamentous cord insertion has great relevance in interpreting birth weights and mortality. Succenturiate lobes are much more common, perhaps because of focal areas of placental atrophy, and they are more often immature structurally because of early delivery. It was surprising, though, to note less commonly a finding of meconium staining and villous infarcts, the reason for these differences being less clear.

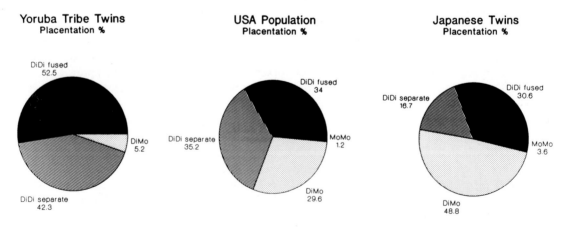

FIGURE 25.7. Twin placentation in three racial populations. The figures for the Yoruba (left) are from MacGillivray et al. (1975); those for the U.S. population come from Benirschke and Driscoll (1967); those for the Japanese population come from Sekiya and Hafez (1977).

FIGURE 25.8. Left: Uterus with diamnionic/monochorionic (DiMo) (identical, MZ) twins at 8 weeks' gestation. Note the two delicate amnions enclosed in a single chorion. Two yolk sacs are present at the arrow. Right: Uterus with diamnionic/dichorionic twin implantation. The uterus has been opened laterally, and the cervical halves are seen at top and bottom. The two separate placental membranes are easily seen. If these placentas later expand, they will certainly collide and fuse.

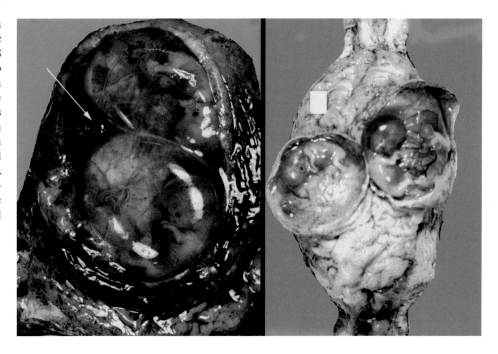

Causes and Incidence of Multiple Births

A fundamental difference exists in the respective etiologies of DZ and MZ twins. DZ twins (and many higher multiples) are the result of polyovulation. It may be hereditary; it is certainly age-related and it can be induced by the administration of gonadotropins and other hormones. The strongest evidence that hormones (gonadotropins) are responsible for multiple ovulations comes from their therapeutic use in infertility patients. Intentional induction of multiple ovulations with gonadotropins is regularly employed in the livestock industry (e.g., Chupin et al., 1976), and is well studied in laboratory animals and, more recently, in during the practice of ART.

Milham (1964), therefore, hypothesized that spontaneous DZ twinning in humans may be explained by a maternal increase in pituitary gonadotropin production. He

TABLE 25.2. Cord insertions and other pathologic features of 7090 consecutive placentas of which 143 were multiple births (1985–1986)

	Singletons (%)	Multiple gestations (%)
Marginal insertion of cord	8.9	28.7
Velamentous insertion of cord	1.1	16.1
Meconium staining	14.9	4.9
Succenturiate lobe	7.6	37
Immaturity	7.8	37.8
Abruptio placentae	4.9	2.8
Infarcts	20.7	11.2

based this idea on the increase in pituitary size with advancing age, the larger pituitaries found in African Americans, and the increase in size of the hypophysis after repeated pregnancies. These features correlate with an increase in DZ twinning rates. Numerous studies have since been undertaken to verify this hypothesis. In humans, there is now good evidence that the recruitment of follicles for ovulation is controlled by follicle-stimulating hormone (FSH) (Vermesh & Kletzky, 1987). Marshall (1970) reviewed the findings following ovulation induction by gonadotropic hormones and clomiphene. The administration of clomiphene led to a 6% incidence of twins, and gonadotropin administration was followed by a 5% to 50% incidence of twins. These variable frequencies were found to be dose-related. Nylander (1973) determined that Nigerian women of the Yoruba tribe, known to have very high rates of DZ twins, also had elevated levels of FSH and luteinizing hormone (LH), when compared with whites. Soma et al. (1975), noting the lower frequency of DZ twins in Japanese when compared to other populations, measured the FSH and LH levels in 10 Japanese women. They found significantly lower values for both hormones than are present in Nigerian women. The values were also lower than those reported for the American populations (Fig. 25.9). Because these two sets of data came from women near the time of expected ovulation, the validity of the results was questioned and the thesis then reexamined. Presumably, recruitment of follicles for the next ovulation takes place around the time of menstruation. For that reason, Martin et al. (1984a,b) undertook a study of various hormonal levels in women during the first 4 days of their menstrual cycles. They compared women who had at least one set of DZ twins with

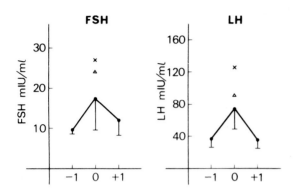

FIGURE 25.9. Follicle-stimulating hormone (FSH) and luteinizing hormone (LH) levels in women around the time of ovulation. ×, peak value in Yoruba tribe women of Africa; Δ, peak value in U.S. Whites; solid line, 10 Japanese women. (*Source:* Soma et al., 1975, with permission.)

those who had no twins. They also found that FSH and LH (less so) were elevated in twin-bearing mothers. Estradiol was also elevated. Spellacy et al. (1982) attempted to ascertain if the pituitaries of twin-bearing women were more responsive to the injection of gonadotropin-releasing hormone (GnRH). It proved not to be the case. It must be cautioned, however, that Spellacy's studies were undertaken during the luteal phase of the cycle and may thus not reflect the natural effect on FSH production needed for follicle recruitment. Lambalk and Boomsma (1998) determined that in twin-prone women the elevated FSH levels are "entirely related to an increase in number of FSH pulses." The elevated FSH levels of older women, they argue, results from a decrease of ovarian inhibin production.

The aforementioned hormone studies supported the notion that the genesis of DZ twins is indeed the result of excess production of FSH. Milham (1964) had suggested that the higher gonadotropin production he assumed to be the basis for DZ twinning is a racial characteristic of the hypophysis. This idea was challenged by Eriksson (1964), who pointed out that in some countries the DZ twinning rate has recently declined and that it could not be explained by an assumed lowering of the age of pregnant women and by differences in racial composition. His point was that DZ twinning is a "genetic trait." We believe that the gene responsible for higher FSH levels must now be considered to be the principal agent in familial twinning. The hormonal assays from many sources all point in this direction. Whether the effect of increased FSH production is the sequel of more pituitary cells or more GnRH production, or is also due to greater follicle sensitivity, needs to be studied. A further investigation supports the genetic nature of the multiple ovulation event. When women who had delivered DZ twins were followed sonographically, it was found that

they had considerably more ovulatory activity than controls (Martin et al., 1991).

In addition to inducing twin gestations, hormonal induction of ovulation is often followed by the birth of triplets and higher multiples. Schenker et al. (1981) reviewed this topic in detail, including the complications that arise from such pregnancies. They also made recommendations as to the prevention and management of multiple births. Although it is true that multiple births are generally multizygotic, it has long been noted that, among such multiple offspring, there is often an admixture of DZ and MZ infants. For instance, Atlay and Pennington (1971) reported on quadruplets born after pituitary gonadotropin stimulation; two of the infants were monoamnionic and thus MZ twins. Whether the incidence of twinning rises following the discontinuation of chemical contraception ("the pill") is controversial. Rice-Wray et al. (1971) found no such increase in their study of 516 women, whereas Rothman (1977) and Bracken (1979) found that twinning was about doubled when pregnancy occurred within 1 to 2 months after cessation of oral contraception. The increase was found to be due to DZ twins in both of these studies. Bracken inferred that it results from pituitary response to oral contraceptives. An interesting discussion followed Bracken's paper (Honoré, 1979; James, 1979), which suggested that after oral contraception pituitary gonadotropin release may in fact lead to DZ twinning. Whether it is also responsible for an increase in embryonic aneuploidy (particularly the occurrence of triploidy as has also been suggested) awaits further study. It has been hinted that currently a general rise in MZ twinning rates is occurring, and that this is perhaps related to the use of oral contraceptives (Bressers et al., 1987). Possible other environmental agents, however, could not be excluded by these investigators.

As had been noted by Weinberg (1909), twinning may be familial. Weinberg asserted that DZ twinning is inherited; however, it was believed that hereditary factors played no role for MZ twinning. Hamamy et al. (2004) have now shown in a remarkable family that five generations had apparently MZ twinning (13 pairs in 2035 members interviewed) inherited by what they assumed to be an autosomal-dominant gene. Shapiro et al. (1978), who had already brought some similar, albeit smaller, pedigrees together, also assumed a possible autosomal gene, and advanced the view that one might look upon MZ twins as "altered morphogenesis." The situation in DZ twinning tendency differs. Such a possible genetic effect can be manifested only by a woman with the genetic background for twinning, not by the father of twins. He may pass on this gene to his offspring, but only double ovulation in women can **prove** the existence of the gene. It is thus sex-limited. The finding by Bulmer (1960) that increased twinning among relatives of fathers of twins is due to underreporting of singletons does not seem to alter the inheritance of presumably higher FSH levels. These aspects are further elaborated by White and Wyshak (1964).

In our opinion, familial and racial predisposition to DZ twinning results from enhanced production of FSH. Montgomery et al. (2000, 2001, 2003; Duffy et al. 2001) have searched for possible gene linkage, finding none so far. It may be relevant, however, that McNatty et al. (2001) found an X–chromosomal mutation that leads to multiple ovulation and is dose-dependent, and Galloway et al. (2000) had similar findings in human families. Busjahn et al. (2000) suggested that a gene on chromosome 3 relates to DZ twinning; obviously more work will be done in the future and a more conclusive result can be anticipated. Others suggested that there may be an altered FSH receptor gene mutation, but that has not been firmly established either. Now, Montgomery et al. (2004) studied families with DZ twinning frequency and identified a deletion mutation in *GDF9* (on chromosome 5q31.1), much as had been seen in sheep. The racial relation to DZ twinning is most impressively shown by comparing the frequency in Nigerian women from the Yoruba tribe with Oriental women (Nylander & Corney, 1969; Nylander, 1971a). Nylander et al. observed that monochorial twins were rare in Nigerian women of the Yoruba tribe, and that zygosity determinations indicated a vast preponderance of DZ twins. The frequency of MZ twins was the same as that found in whites (4.5 per 1000). In the north of Nigeria, the twinning rate was 21 per 1000, in the midregion 31 per 1000, and in the west and east 45 per 1000. These data contrast with reports from Japan, where the overall twinning rate is 6.1 per 1000, with a 1.65 : 1.00 ratio of MZ/DZ twins (Inouye, 1957). Similar rates have been reported from Taiwan (Wei & Lin, 1967). In Europe there tends to be a "progressive decrease in the frequency of twins from north to south" (Eriksson, 1962).

The known higher frequency of DZ twins in older mothers may then also be due to their enhanced FSH secretion. There is a steady rise in DZ twinning to the maternal age of 35; after that age, there is a sharp decline in DZ twinning. Although longitudinal studies of FSH secretion have not been published for individual women, some data exist to indicate that FSH levels rise steadily with maternal age (Albert et al., 1956). This finding supports the notion that the increased DZ twinning frequency observed with advanced maternal age is due to enhanced FSH excretion by older women's pituitaries, but it does not prove it. The FSH levels are much higher still in postmenopausal women. Longitudinal studies are needed. Lawrence et al. (2004) tested the hypothesis that food fortification with folic acid might affect the twinning rate but found this not to be so.

The interesting question has been raised as to whether the higher gonadotropin secretion of individuals with the genetic trait to produce twins is also manifest in men. For sheep and other domestic animal species, some evidence exists that, in individual races, there are differences in the frequency of DZ twinning (Land et al., 1973). It has also been suggested that the testicular weights from such animals is greater in males that carry the gene for twinning (Land, 1973; Islam et al., 1976). To study this aspect further, Short (1984) reported ethnic variations of testicular size in men and found that Orientals have smaller testes than Europeans. There are no data yet from Yoruba men, but racially different testosterone levels have been reported by Ross et al. (1986). They tend to support the same principle and are viewed as being in support of the marked differences in prostatic cancer (Gittes, 1991). These and related aspects were considered in some detail in Diamond's stimulating editorial (1986). The differences of placentation in three well-studied racial groups are depicted in Figure 25.7, which displays graphically how meaningfully different the placentas of twins are constructed when their zygosity is so variable.

The **cause of MZ twinning** is not fully understood. Whereas DZ twins (and multiples) derive from the fertilization of more than one ovum, MZ twins must originate from the spontaneous separation of blastomeres. Although this process occurs in all animals species with approximately the same frequency as that observed in humans, there are two nearly similar species in which this polyembryony occurs with regularity: the two *Dasypus* species of armadillo—*Dasypus novemcinctus* (nine-banded armadillo) and *Dasypus septemcinctus al. hybridus* (seven-banded armadillos; mulita) (Fernandez, 1909; Newman & Patterson, 1910; Hamlett, 1933). The precise understanding of the mechanism of their polyembryony eludes us. Hamlett (1933) was critical of the statements made by Newman, who had inferred that it was the delayed implantation of armadillos that leads to impoverished nutrition and deficient oxygenation of the blastocyst, and it was thus the cause of polyembryony. It is of additional relevance that other species with delayed implantation do not share this phenomenon of polyembryony. Hamlett advocated that segregation of blastomeres is determined by genetic factors. Loughry et al. (1998) advanced the notion that this feature resulted from the small implantation site in a unique uterus, but they cautioned that this needs further analysis. They were the first, however, to show clearly the monozygosity of the litters by their finding complete identity of DNA microsatellites.

The nine-banded armadillo, ranging from Texas to Uruguay, always has identical quadruplets; the mulita may produce seven to 12 male or female identical offspring. Although the mulita is much smaller, the two species are closely related and possess, for instance, identical chromosomes. The mulita is a common animal in Uruguay and Argentina; it has a single blastocyst (and corpus luteum) in a pregnancy that is also characterized by delayed implantation. Immediately after implantation, the embryonic mass separates into multiple offspring. Whether it is by "fission or budding" was a hotly contended point of the discussions between Newman and Hamlett. In contrast to the monozygotic twinning in other mammals, the production of multiple births of these two armadillo species is so well regulated that anomalies, such as conjoined twins, acardiacs, and most other abnormal events occurring in human MZ twins, have not been observed (Hamlett, 1933). We deduced that one reason for these discrepancies may be that, in these species, the splitting of blastomeres is a precisely timed event. Also, placental anastomoses do not occur in armadillos (Anderson & Benirschke, 1963), possibly because of the different timing of their placentation. Perhaps it is the reason for their relative freedom from placental problems.

Other mammals, those that have approximately similar rates of MZ twinning as humans, have no precisely timed MZ twinning period. In them and in humans, the splitting of the embryonic mass appears to occur at random during the early embryonic period. It has also been observed that MZ twins commonly occur after surgical transfer of single bovine blastocysts into pseudopregnant cattle recipients (Moyaert et al., 1982; Kraay et al., 1983). Paulson et al. (1988) reported that triplets were born after the transfer of two previously frozen human embryos. Surprisingly, after assisted reproductive help, monochorionic, even monoamnionic multiple pregnancies have repeatedly been reported, by Edwards et al. (1986) and by Salat-Baroux et al. (1994). Massip et al. (1983) observed cinematographically the atypical hatching of a cow blastocyst *in vitro* and suggested that it may be the mechanism by which dichorionic MZ twins take their origin. They observed partial protrusion of blastomeres from a zona; and after the "hatching" was complete, the two-cell masses were connected only by a diminutive bridge. That hatched blastocysts are capable of twinning was demonstrated by surgical division of sheep embryos (Willadsen, 1979) as well as in mice (Tsunoda & McLaren, 1983), horses (Allen & Pashen, 1984), goats (Tsunoda et al., 1985), pigs (Nagashima et al., 1989), and other animals. In many such experiments implantation led to normal development of these split embryos. Nevertheless, a prospective study by Blickstein et al. (1999) came to different conclusions. They studied the outcome of human in vitro fertilization (IVF) results with those of single sperm injection fertilization. Although the former procedure had a 12 times the expected MZ twinning rate, the latter technique (although presumably more destructive to the zona pellucida) produced no twins. Their conclusion was that it is perhaps the handling of eggs during in vitro fertilization that results in the splitting. Steinman (2001a–c, 2002a,b, 2003) incriminated the adverse role of ethylenediamonetetraacetic acid (EDTA) (calcium-depleting) in the culture media. The true cause remains elusive, however.

It is necessary to recognize that there are many temporal differences in the development of the inner cell mass and the setting aside of the trophectoderm in animals. Thus, when different species are compared, it is difficult to draw precise analogies to human development, especially to placental growth. Thus, the mouse segregates embryo from trophectoderm at the fourth cleavage stage (about 12 to 16 cells). The peripheral cells develop tight junctions and form the future placenta (Ziomek & Johnson, 1982), an event taking place much later in the sheep and cow. In humans, similar to the mouse, the event occurs at about the fifth division of cells. In 1% of cultured mouse embryos, spontaneous separation of blastomeres into MZ twins takes place, analogous to what would be expected of the process that leads to conjoined twins (Hsu & Gonda, 1980). Runner (1984) observed two inner cell masses in a mouse blastocyst at the stage of proamnion cavitation, which suggested to him late division of the embryonic mass and development of mirror imagery, which is also more commonly seen in MZ human twins. Experimental fission of quail embryos has also produced conjoined twins (Lutz & Lutz-Ostertag, 1963). The production of MZ twins in sea urchins was demonstrated by the isolation of first-cleavage blastomeres (Driesch, 1891). These embryos were rarely normal. Marcus (1979) showed that by shaking fertilized sea urchin eggs to remove their envelope and with subsequent exposure to hypertonic water, he was able to promote separation of blastomeres. Many of these MZ twins were also underdeveloped. It is particularly interesting to note that there were many inter-twin morphologic differences. Ludwig (1927) had commented on the irregular division of "hereditary material" in MZ twins, but did not believe that blastomeres were capable of separating. He thought twinning to be a late event and also expected that MZ twins would often be different.

When pregnant mice were exposed to low doses of vincristine on days 7 and 8, unexpectedly many MZ twins developed, some being monoamnionic (Kaufman & O'Shea, 1978). Kaufman and O'Shea cited the few other reports of conjoined twins produced by experimental teratogens. Perhaps best known are the experiments of Witschi (1934), in which he produced twins in the frog by fertilizing eggs that were 3 to 5 days overripe. Witschi observed the development of several blastopores and gastrulation. Other sporadic observations of MZ animal twins have been cited by Corner (1955). He reviewed the few available specimens of early human MZ twin embryos, which are not dissimilar from those observed in experimental animals. Corner also cited the interesting observation of frequent admixture of MZ and DZ twins, to which we previously alluded.

The results of statistical surveys suggest that multiple ovulation due to hormonal stimulation is not the sole cause of enhanced multiple gestations. Derom et al. (1987)

observed that MZ twinning (1.2%) is significantly higher than would be expected from random births (0.45%). Boklage (1987a) has in fact gone so far as to ascribe the causes of MZ twinning to factors that differ little from those that induce DZ twins. When all evidence is taken together, it must be said that spontaneous MZ twinning is still a poorly understood phenomenon. Boklage (1981) takes exception to the notion of embryonic "splitting" as the etiology of MZ twinning. He pointed out that the high embryonic mortality that occurred in the early experimental studies makes splitting an unlikely cause of MZ twins. There is no doubt any longer, however, that splitting can take place in mammals and it can definitely be done experimentally. Boklage also stated that none of the many experimental chimeras that have been produced in mice experimentally had resulted in MZ twins. This, in itself, however, is insufficient proof against splitting, it seems to us. Few mice eventuate in MZ twins in the first place, and not many offspring of experimental chimeras have been sufficiently studied to identify their possible monozygotic derivation. The arguments on this topic are not unlike the controversy of "splitting versus budding" of the past, and these are well denominated as being a "skirmish in semantics" by Hamlett (1933).

To explain MZ twinning, Boklage conceived that forces responsible for organizing a field or gradient in early embryos may be the reason for the MZ twinning event. He opined that a "weakness in the enforcement of that directive might allow a second such organizing center to induce a second developmental scheme." He was particularly concerned with understanding neural symmetry and with mirroring in twins. McManus (2002) produced an interesting book on the mirroring aspect of twinning and other events of asymmetry.

In our opinion, the armadillo is the best animal from which to gain a better understanding of this puzzling yet frequent event of embryonic duplication. It is to be regretted that they are difficult to breed in captivity, which makes it difficult to accumulate the relevant observations. Other than for the pregnancy outcome, there is no good evidence that heredity in some way controls the MZ twinning event (other than in armadillos). The incidence of MZ twinning is nearly the same throughout the world and it is not significantly influenced by maternal age or the environment. It appears to be a sporadic event. Because of the nature of the fetal placental membrane relation in human MZ twins, one assumes that MZ twinning can occur at any time during the first 2 weeks of development. It then appears to be randomly distributed.

For lack of a better term and better insight into the etiology of MZ twinning, we have referred to the cause as the "twinning impetus." We make further inference that this impetus affects the developing embryos at random and that, because of this randomness of the timing, the different placental membrane relations shown in Figure 25.10 come about. We believe this impetus to be effective from days 1 to 14 of embryonic development. Our hypothesis further assumes that it is impossible for the impetus to split an already formed embryonic cavity such as the yolk sac, chorionic cavity, or amnion. The monozygotic twinning process, then, is a biologic continuum during this early period.

The phenomenon was discussed by Gould (1982) in an entertaining thesis on the not-so-trivial question as to whether conjoined twins are one or two persons. Finally, an interesting result, with experimentally derived MZ mouse twins, has been published by Gärtner and Baunack (1981). They produced MZ twins at the eight-cell stage

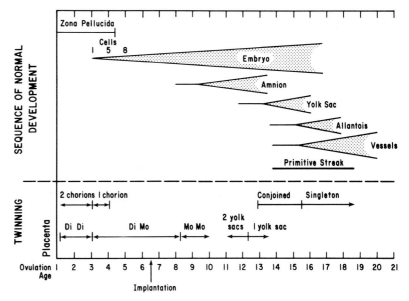

FIGURE 25.10. Interpretation of early events in the MZ twinning event. The earliest observed embryonic events of various are depicted in the upper portion. The bottom portion suggests that certain placental structures result if twinning occurs at certain times. Note that the DiDi/DiMo frequencies correspond roughly to the observed 1:3 ratio. It is also assumed that with later development (after day 8) MZ twinning becomes ever more difficult because of the enlarging embryonic/placental masses. Once the primitive streak is formed, conjoined twins may develop at first. Soon, however, the presumed twinning "impetus" is ineffective.

and compared their growth with that of DZ twins in the same strain of mice. Despite the fact that they worked with an isogenic strain, the DZ twins differed more from each other in a variety of characteristics than did the MZ twins. The cause of this unexpected finding is not yet understood.

THIRD TYPE OF TWIN

The possibility of the existence of a "third type of twin" is occasionally considered in discussions of the twinning events. It proposes that MZ twins do not consist solely of identical" twins, but that nonidentical twins, arising from a single ovulation event, make up part of the spectrum. It may amount to some 1% of twins who would usually be classed as DZ twins because of some dissimilarities of their genotypes. This concept envisages that polar body fertilization may occur. Thus, the twins would then come from a single maternal, but two paternal, genomes. They would be intermediate in their genetic configuration between MZ and DZ twins. Such a possibility is supported by the occasional finding of polar bodies that have a similar size as the normal oocyte. This is especially so in some bat species. Furthermore, there are some theoretical considerations detailed by Mijsberg (1957) that suggest the existence of "third twins." In fact, the fertilization and further development of polar bodies has been observed. Dixon (1927) has described human polar bodies in mitosis, synchronous with the oocyte mitosis. It is also noteworthy that, in humans and in a variety of animals, binucleated ova are observed. They may produce such twins or even result in the development of chimeras. Binucleated eggs have been described repeatedly in the ovaries of a variety of animals, in women (Kennedy & Donahue, 1969) (Fig. 25.11), and in children. Manivel et al. (1988) found binucleated oocytes in 19%, and binovular follicles

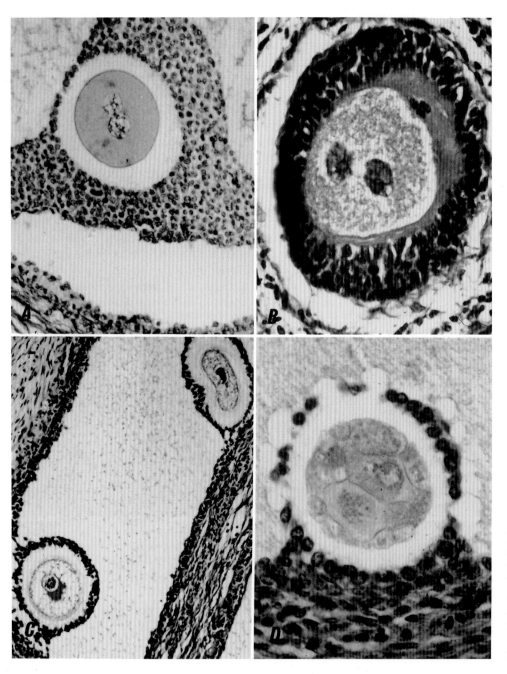

FIGURE 25.11. Four Graafian follicles with abnormal ova whose future potential cannot be anticipated. A,B: Binucleate ova in Graafian follicles. C: Binovular follicle. D: Segmenting ovum within graafian follicle. H&E ×100 (A); ×160 (B); ×80 (C); ×100 (D).

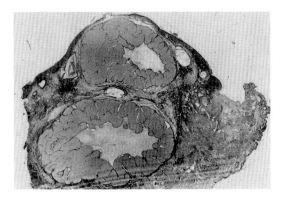

FIGURE 25.12. Cross section of an ovary at 8 weeks' gestation with two corpora lutea of pregnancy. One is hidden from external view because of its position, so only one would have been recognized by inspection. This specimen is from the diamnionic/monochorionic (hence assumed to be MZ) twin gestation shown in Figure 25.8. H&E ×4.

in 52% of their pediatric autopsy material. The fertilization of such abnormal ova has been observed by Zeilmaker and colleagues (1983).

The occurrence of "third twins" would explain the occasional finding of a single corpus luteum associated with fertilizations that were diagnosed to be DZ twins. The concept has been considered in some detail by Elston and Boklage (1978). Later, Boklage (1987b) suggested the term **tertiary oocyte**, rather than **polar body fertilization**, and critiqued the acceptance of the Weinberg formula in assigning zygosity, in particular for discordant twins. He also favored the notion that over-ripe ova may be responsible for some of these abnormal fertilization products. It must be cautioned, however, that mere inspection of ovaries (at operation) is insufficient evidence for the presence of a solitary corpus luteum only. A second corpus luteum may be present and found buried underneath another, as is shown in Figure 25.12. The macroscopic inspection of the ovary in this case would have been misleading. Further complicating the resolution of the question is that two normal ova may reside in a single antrum (Fig. 25.11). Such a graafian follicle would result in a single corpus luteum and yet possibly produce fraternal twins. Finally, it can be said that a possible instance of polar body twins, one an acardiac fetus with triploid chromosome constitution and the other diploid, has been studied in detail described by Bieber et al. (1981). On the other hand, employing molecular methodologies, Fisk et al. (1996) were able to rule out polar body fertilization in nine sets of twins with acardiac gestations. This subject is discussed in greater detail below (see Acardiac Twins).

Twinning Incidence

The incidence of multiple pregnancies has been the topic of numerous investigations. This aspect was particularly well covered by Bulmer (1970) in his classical book on twinning in humans. It has also been the topic of several discussions, published in the third issue of the *Acta Geneticae Medicae et Gemellologiae* (Vol. 36, 1987). The rate for dizygotic twinning in various populations has been summarized by Diamond (1986), whose data are shown in the table below.

Ethnic group and locality	DZ twinning rate (per 1,000 births)
Asians	
Japanese	
Hawaii	2.2
Japan	2.3
Chinese	
Formosa	1.4
Hawaii	2.1
Malaya	2.8
Singapore	4.1
Hong Kong	6.8
Malays	
Hawaii	2.2
Manila	2.7
Malaya	5.2
Hawaiians	
Hawaii	3.9
Koreans	
Korea	5.1
Korea	5.8
Korea	7.9
Indians	
Bombay	6.8
Bangalore	7.3
Calcutta	8.1
Caucasians	
Europeans	
Spain	5.9
France	7.1
Switzerland	8.1
Holland	8.1
West Germany	8.2
Norway	8.3
Sweden	8.6
Britain	8.9
African blacks	
Bantu	
Johannesburg	16.0
Leopoldville	19.0
Yoruba	
Ibadan	40.0
Ilesha	49.0

These data impressively show that DZ twinning has a profound racial variation. In contrast, the MZ twinning rate "is nearly constant at about three and a half per thousand in all races" (Bulmer, 1970). Eriksson (1962) has drawn attention to the decline of twinning rates from north to south in Europe, which is due to variations of DZ twinning rates. The twinning rates and outcomes for a large U.S. population have been analyzed by Myrianthopoulos (1970a,b). He reviewed the data of the United States Multicenter Collaborative Study, which analyzed 56,249 pregnancies with known outcome. It contained 615 twins (1 per 91.5 births). The differences in the ethnic background of that U.S. population and its relation to multiple pregnancies can be seen in the following data from his report:

Group	Twins (No.)	Population (No.)	DZ twins (No./births)
Whites	259	25,991	1/100.3
Blacks	331	26,080	1/78.8
Puerto Ricans	25	4,178	1/167.1

The zygosity of 508 of these twins was examined as best as then possible, but a large number of twins remained unclassified. The results were as follows:

MZ = 29.6%
DZ = 51.4%
?Z = 19%

The profound influence of maternal age is well documented in these reports. The incidence of DZ twinning rises until, at 35 years maternal age, there is an abrupt fall in the incidence. A greater frequency of twins in the U.S. black population had also been noted in the large database summarized by Guttmacher (1953). He reported on the frequency of triplets and higher multiple births at a time that preceded the use of fertility drugs. Over a 22-year period, viable twin births occurred in 1 per 92.4 (whites) and 1 per 73.8 (blacks); triplets occurred in 1 per 9828 (whites) and 1 per 5631 (blacks).

The occurrence of higher multiple births, such as triplets, quadruplets, has commonly been estimated by the Hellin-Zeleny hypothesis: If twins occur with $1/n$, then triplets occur with $(1/n)^2$ and quadruplets with $(1/n)^3$. This method is merely an approximation and is subject to maternal age, medical therapy, race, and other factors.

Multiple pregnancies showed a progressive decline from 1938 to 1949; later declines in the twinning rate have been studied by a number of investigators. Akesson et al. (1970) showed that the incidence of twinning in Sweden fell from 1.4% in 1871 to 1.1% in 1960. This change was due to fluctuations in the number of DZ twins born. Changes in maternal age were considered but they were not deemed to be the cause of this decline. Reports from the United States, Canada, Australia, and other countries have been similar (Elwood, 1973; James, 1973). The decrease in twin births in Holland was believed to be secondary to a decrease in maternal age at conception (Hoogendoorn, 1973). James (1975) suggested that either the decline may relate to exogenous agents or it is secondary to voluntary birth control. That the latter effect may have some significance is borne out by the apparent cessation of the DZ twinning decline in Canada (Elwood, 1983) and Hungary (Métneki & Czeizel, 1983); but James (1983) was not convinced. Allen (1987) provided data to show that there was no decline in U.S. twin births from 1964 to 1983. Imaizumi (1998) has summarized the twinning and triplet rates for 16 countries from 1972 to 1996 and indicated that most countries have a slightly **rising** rate of multiples.

In recent years, however, there has been a remarkable increase in multiple gestations and much of it appears to be the result of ART. It is the case also in other developed countries; in the U.S. the frequency of multiple births is now 1:30, perhaps as a result of this practice (Martin et al., 2003). Interestingly, only certain regions and populations are so affected but the results are startling. Thus, a review by the March of Dimes (MOD) Foundation (2003) states, "Fewer than 1% of live births result from IVF, they account for about one third of all twin births and more than 40% of triplets or higher-order births in the US." There has been much discussion as to the value and nature of ART; because superovulation so often leads to an uncontrolled number of fertilized eggs (and the frequent need for fetal "reduction"), Vidaeff et al. (2000) thus suggested that blastocyst transfer by ART may be more appropriate for infertile couples. Gleicher et al. (2000) examined the risk of higher numbers of conceptuses by superovulation and suggested that a smaller amount of gonadotropins needs to be employed than was then used. But this still does not really control the process, which is what is hoped for. The practice of ART is also changing over time; it consists of IVF, intracytoplasmic sperm injection (ICSI), blastocyst development by culture in vitro for up to 7 days (see Sills et al., 2003; also many different culture media are used), and transfer of a variable number of blastocysts to the recipient uterus. Rijnders and Jansen (1998b) stated that not all fertilized ova developed normally in vitro, which, in part at least, may be responsible for some of the abnormal outcomes that are observed, especially in implantation and placental development. The ova to be fertilized are obtained following superovulation by hormonal means.

Additionally, there are other modalities employed such as transfer into a surrogate uterus and employment of donated sperm and eggs, and other practices are under development. Small wonder, then, that the outcome varies as to the number of embryos resulting (often depending on how many blastocysts are transferred), sacrifice (reduction) of one or more embryos depending on the numbers conceived, and frequently abnormal placentation. Daniel et al. (1999) even found that singleton placentas of pregnancies conceived by ART are abnormal (slightly larger and thicker, abnormal cord insertion). The highest numbers of successfully transferred embryos we have seen are sextuplets delivered from a compound placenta at 28 weeks' gestation. Most remarkable has been the frequency of the development of more than the number of transferred blastocysts by the splitting of one or more blastocysts (Rijnders and Jansen, 1998a; Behr et al., 2000; Lancaster, 2004). Platt et al. (2001) estimated that 15.7% of ART twins are monozygotic, and that monochorionic twins are more problematic is well demonstrated by Dubé et al. (2002). Sills et al. (2000) impressively discussed the possible mechanisms by which monochorionic placentas can develop in such manipulations, perhaps by alteration of the zona pellucida, a concept to be discussed more fully below. Daniel et al. (2000) found among the twin pregnancies so conceived that they were more commonly undertaken in older mothers, that they more often were prematurely delivered, and that they were associated with pregnancy-induced hypertension (PIH) and various other complications of pregnancy. Later (2001) they described the abnormality of placental development in such nonreduced twin gestations; they found mostly DiDi placentas that were thinner, more infarcted, and had anomalous cord insertions.

The economic impact and other aspects are discussed by Nkemayim et al. (2000), who also present suggestions for the limitation of he blastocysts transferred, now lawful in several European countries (see also Ozturk & Templeton, 2002, who suggest limiting transfer to two blastocysts). Templeton (2004), Nunley (2004), and an editorial in *Lancet* (2003) addressed the problems attending ART and the social implications faced by its practitioners. Jain et al. (2004a) summarized these trends of transferring fewer ova in recent years, concomitant with a greater survival of the ART gestations. Most recently, Thurin et al. (2004) compared single- vs. double-embryo transfer in women younger than 36 years in order to reduce the number of multiples. Blickstein (2005) reviewed in detail the frequencies of MZ splitting in ART and its various forms of embryo culture and comes to the conclusion that exact genetic diagnosis of such multiples is necessary. Finally, it must be mentioned that the neonatal outcome is often suboptimal, aside from their prematurity and number. Some of these concerns have been reviewed by Schieve et al. (2002) and Strömberg et al. (2002). The latter paper led to intensive discussion (Akande & Murphy, 2002; Leviton et al., 2002; Davies & Norman, 2003).

The incidence of DZ twinning has also been shown to have a seasonal relation. Timonen and Carpen (1968), who observed this phenomenon in the Finnish population, deduced that this results from the continuous light stimulation, which induces enhanced gonadotropin release. The peak of twin births occurred during early spring and summer. Elwood (1978) found the peak for a Canadian population to be in October, whereas Edwards (1938) had reported two peaks for conceptions (February and August) in a British population. The effect was more pronounced with twins than with singletons. Harlap et al. (1985) raised the possibility that an increase in DZ twins results from the development of overripe ova.

SUPERFETATION AND SUPERFECUNDATION

Twins may have different fathers through the process known as **superfecundation** (two ova are fertilized by spermatozoa from different fathers). That the concept is valid was proved by finding human leukocyte antigen (HLA) differences in the twins studied by Terasaki et al. (1978). In the accompanying editorial, Ryan (1978) referred to other cases and to its occurrence in "test-tube babies." Another report, with one white and one black twin, was forthcoming from Harris (1982). This report is most remarkable because the fertilizations apparently occurred 1 week apart. Verma et al. (1992) proved superfecundation by two different fathers with cytogenetic markers but were refused DNA fingerprinting. Harris (1982) also referred to a case of **superfetation** with twins of apparently different gestational ages (34 and 37 weeks). Rhine and Nance (1976) described the pedigree of a relevant family. They suggested that superfetation was the basis for the repeated dissimilarities of twins. They assumed it to be inherited as a dominant trait and expressed through a putative placental inability to suppress new ovulation after conception.

Vascular Anatomy of Twin Placentas

One of the most important observations to be made in the study of twin placentas is the accurate determination of the nature of fetal surface blood vessels. Their relation to one another is perhaps the single most important determinant for the outcome of many twin pregnancies. These aspects were first clearly demonstrated by Friedrich Schatz, whose numerous contributions have been summarized in English by Strong and Corney (1967). Price (1950) considered the various vascular anastomoses of monochorionic twin placentas to be the most important determinants for the frequently discordant development of MZ twins. This notion dates back more than a hundred years, and many observers since then have reached similar conclusions that anastomoses have a profound influence on outcome.

The demonstration of anastomoses is relatively simple. Once the anatomy of the placental vascular architecture is learned, injection studies are rarely necessary, they aid, however, in delineating the patterns for the novice and should be performed routinely. A simple method for the detection of anastomoses has been described by Coen and Sutherland (1970). They used milk for injection because it is so readily available and demonstrative, but other liquids are equally useful. For the purposes of injection it is best to cut the umbilical cords near their placental surface, so as to reduce vascular resistance. One should also have stripped the amnion from the chorionic surface, which exposes the fetal surface vessels well (Fig. 25.13). The general examination of the placenta should have been completed, but samples for histologic study should be taken only after the injection has been done. For optimal results, several tools are desirable and they are depicted in Figure 25.14. It must be admitted, however, that a simple syringe and water are usually adequate. One must inspect the surface of the placenta carefully, follow major vessels to their ends, and determine, visually at first, which vessels are likely to have communications between the two fetal circulations. In the normal placenta, the fetal

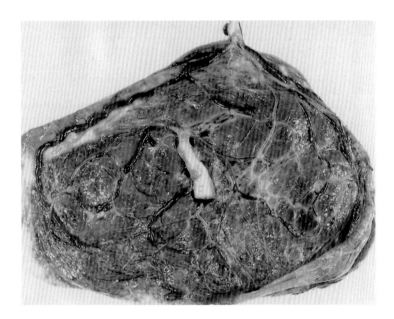

FIGURE 25.13. Diamnionic/monochorionic twin placenta (26 weeks' gestation) with velamentous insertion of one cord. This twin had a much smaller portion of placental tissue and died.

arteries terminate in the periphery, dip into the villous tissue, and emerge nearby as veins, which then course back toward the same umbilical cord. The arteries are recognized as those vessels that cross *over* veins, particularly those of a larger caliber. A 1:1 relationship is usually found in the final vascular ramifications: one artery to one vein. Bajoria et al. (1995) demonstrated that the likelihood of the presence of the typical twin-to-twin transfusion syndrome (TTTS) is greater when fewer anastomoses are present.

When no returning vein can be identified to accompany a peripheral arterial branch in a twin placenta, an artery-to-vein (AV) communication may exist from one twin to the other. This area then becomes important for the exploration of a so-called deep anastomosis. These AV anastomoses perfuse a common (or shared) cotyledon and form the basis for the transfusion syndrome, discussed below. They are common and constitute the "third circulation" of twin placentas. Most frequent are artery-to-artery anastomoses (AA shunts); vein-to-vein (VV) communications are the least frequent types of anastomoses, as found by Schatz in 1875 and more extensively in 1886. He believed that AA anastomoses are more common because of the higher blood pressure existing in arteries; therefore VV anastomoses are rare, and they were thought to obliterate more commonly before birth.

To document the presence of a direct AA or VV anastomosis, it is often sufficient to stroke blood back and forth through a major shunt. If one wishes to demonstrate

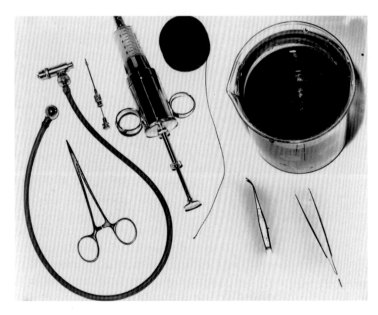

FIGURE 25.14. Ideal set of tools to inject twin placentas: syringe with beaded needle, string to tie needle in place, colored liquid (e.g., milk), clamps, and forceps.

FIGURE 25.15. Injection of DiDi twin placenta. A potential anastomotic area has been isolated, the amnion is stripped, and a needle is inserted and tied in place.

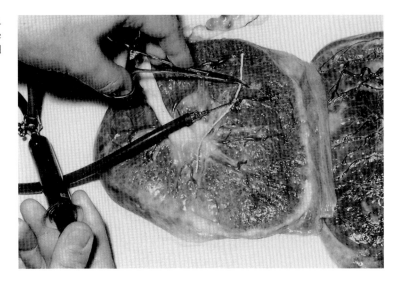

it conclusively, injection of milk, colored water, or similar solution is feasible. To do so, one inserts a needle near the point of presumed anastomosis and then gently injects the liquid, which usually readily passes to the other side of the twin placenta (Figs. 25.15 to 25.16). The injection of as little as 5 to 10 mL of fluid is usually sufficient. Note from Figure 25.15 that it may help to have a needle with a bead and to tie it into the vessels to allow more pressure to be exerted during injection. Usually, grasping the end of the needle in the vessel with the thumb and index finger of the other hand is sufficient to allow injection of fluid with some pressure. It is also important to recognize that one should not attempt to inject the entire placental bed from the vessels near the cord insertion. This measure requires so much volume of injection fluid that pressures are generally insufficient to demonstrate finer anastomoses (Fig. 25.17). Moreover, the villous tissue of twin placentas is often damaged during delivery, and the placenta then leaks when injected from the umbilical cord. This frequent disruption can make adequate demonstration of anastomoses difficult.

The identification of AV shunts is usually the most difficult. It is best to inspect the surface carefully to identify possible areas of AV shunts and then inject them successively. It is immaterial here whether one fills them from the arterial or the venous end. When the fluid is injected slowly under some pressure, one sees an area of placenta distend and increase in thickness. After a short while, the fluid emerges from the other side, and it can then be traced to a larger vessel where its nature (artery or vein) can be ascertained. The delineation, direction, and number of these shunts are especially important if one wishes to understand the basis for the transfusion syndrome. Finally, it is recommended that a drawing of the entire vascular relation is made for the record at the end of the procedure. Figures 25.18 and 25.19 show various types of anas-

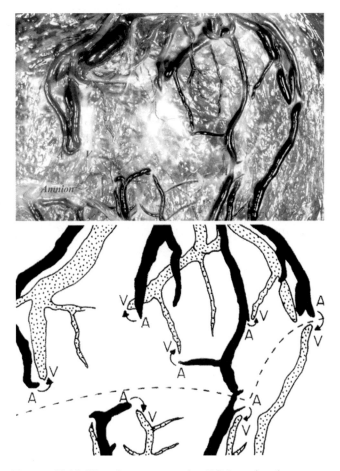

FIGURE 25.16. Vascular equator of a DiMo twin placenta to show artery-to-artery (AA) and artery-to-vein (AV) anastomoses, as well as the normal cotyledonary supply. The diagram (bottom) is self-explanatory.

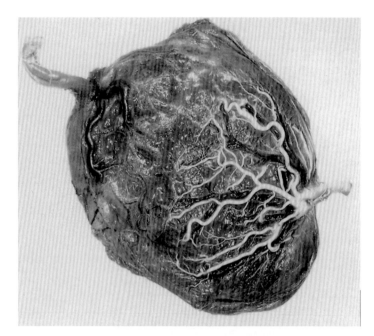

FIGURE 25.17. A DiMo twin placenta with amnion stripped off; the right side has been injected with barium sulfate through one umbilical artery. There are no anastomoses. Both cords have a marginal insertion; arteries cross over veins. This method failed to disclose two small AV shunts (bottom) because of the lack of sufficient pressure exerted when the entire tree is filled. (Courtesy of Dr. S. Romney, New York, New York.)

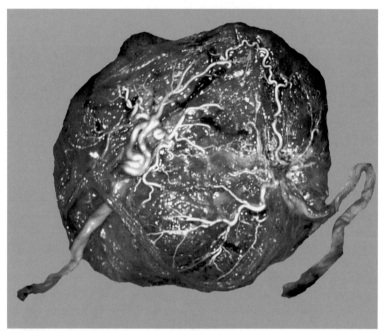

FIGURE 25.18. A DiMo twin placenta with single large AA anastomosis (A) at top left. It has also been injected with barium. Finer AV areas have not been filled.

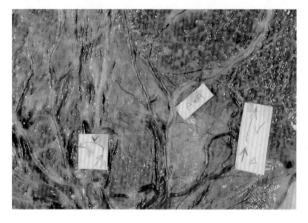

FIGURE 25.19. A DiMo twin placenta, vascular equator. The amnions have been removed and the various types of anastomosis are delineated on pieces of paper.

FIGURE 25.20. A DiMo twin placenta that has been injected with colored plastics and then made into a corrosion cast. A pink vessel, injected from the left half can be seen over the yellow injected vessels on the right. The possible presence of "shared cotyledons" is impossible to identify.

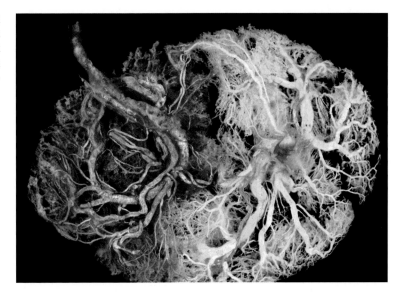

tomoses in two monochorionic twin placentas at their "vascular equators."

If one wishes to make injections of the placental vasculature with plastics for later corrosion, special procedures are necessary. The placenta must be intact. It must first be washed out with warm dextran to open all vessels and to remove the fetal blood. Saline has been found to be less satisfactory (Robertson & Neer, 1983). After the specimen has been flushed, one can then achieve gradual filling with plastics solutions in different colors and with ever-increasing strengths (see Torretta & Cobellis, 1966). A DiMo twin placenta, thus prepared, is shown in Figure 25.20. As will be seen, there is slight filling of a (pink) arterial branch over the yellow-injected placenta, but only exhaustive examination of such a specimen allows one to identify the possible presence of shared cotyle-

dons. By and large, these preparations are more beautiful than they are useful. Only experienced observers such as Hyrtl (1870) have profited from their preparation.

One might suspect that the proximity of cord insertions in twin placentas may influence the frequency and type of anastomoses, but that has not been our experience. Although it is true that in placentas with cords next to each other, as depicted for instance in Figure 25.21 (also see Figs. 25.26, and 25.38), large communications often exist whose injection is scarcely needed, they cannot be assumed a priori. Many MoMo placentas have no communications, irrespective of their cords' proximity. This point was well made in the study by Wenner (1956). He was surprised to find no anastomoses in the placental vascular ramifications of a thoracopagus. The demonstration of anastomoses is most difficult when one fetus has

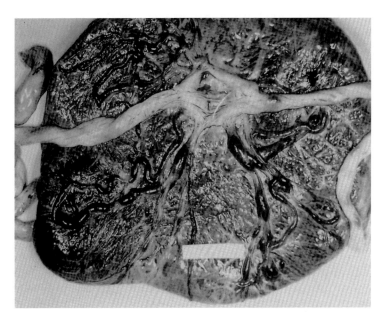

FIGURE 25.21. A monoamnionic/monochorionic (MoMo) twin placenta with amnions removed. The cords insert next to each other, adjacent to major anastomoses.

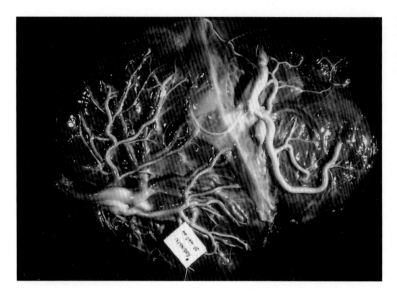

FIGURE 25.22. A DiDi twin placenta with minute anastomosis coursing over the dividing membranes. The associated like-sex twins were MZ. (*Source:* Cameron, 1968, Figure 5, with permission.)

died before birth. It is thus often impossible to demonstrate vascular connections in DiMo placentas with a fetus papyraceus and also when the placenta has been fixed in formalin beforehand.

Despite numerous injection attempts, we have never seen anastomoses between blood vessels of dichorionic twin placentas. That they may exist in rare cases is not doubted. The finding of rare blood chimeras (vide infra) and occasional reports of such connections by competent observers (Fig. 25.22) (Cameron, 1968; see his Figure 5) make them a reality of great interest. In contrast, anastomoses occur frequently in the DZ twins of some other species, such as marmosets, monkeys, and cattle. This aspect is discussed further below.

The observed frequency of inter-twin blood vessel anastomoses in human MZ twins is difficult to assess because of the differences in techniques employed for their demonstration. We previously reported the following relationships of anastomoses in 60 injected monochorionic twin placentas (Benirschke & Driscoll, 1967):

Type of anastomosis	Total found	Infant survival (No).
AA (one or more)	17	12
AA + AV	17	14
AA + VV	5	3
VV	3	2
AV	7	3
AV + VA	2	1
None	9	6

Similar findings have been published by others. Robertson and Neer (1983) reported on 278 twin placentas (of 23,810 births; incidence 1/86; seven triplets). They used dextran and heparin for injection, cannulated the

vessels, and injected 100 mL over 30 minutes. The vessels were then infused with warmed solutions of dyes in colloid suspension. India ink did not work well. Nineteen placentas were damaged and excluded; 97 placentas were separate masses. Of 162 successfully injected fused placentas, 96 (59%) were DiDi; the remainder were monochorionic. Of 56 monochorionic twin placentas studied, all but one had demonstrable anastomoses. The one placenta without anastomoses had an infarcted area that had produced a separation between the two halves. There may have been a communication in the past, as obliteration of such anastomoses is not uncommon. In one dichorionic placenta, the injection material exchanged between the two sides through a tiny villous area. The long-term outcome of these twins is not known, as is true for Cameron's case (Fig. 25.22). These twins had identical blood groups, even though the pair was dichorionic. As we indicated above, identical blood groups should be expected when vascular shunts exist in the placenta of twins. Four cases of the typical transfusion syndrome were found in the study by Robertson and Neer (1983).

The topic of DZ twins having a monochorionic placenta and vascular inter-twin anastomoses is somewhat controversial. Scipiades and Burg (1930) first described anastomoses in two boy/girl twin placentas. Lassen (1931) and Tüscher (1936) each added a rare case of MZ dichorial twins with fine anastomoses. It must be emphasized, however, that some of these cases are not well supported by pictorial or other conclusive evidence. Even Lassen (1931), who performed stereoradiography on a placenta, was not absolutely certain of the connections he demonstrated. The technique of stereoradiography is not very satisfactory, as the findings in seven placentas from DZ twins with anastomoses have shown (Pérez et al., 1947). Szendi (1938) admitted this lack clearly in his discussion of the stereoscopic analysis in four of 20 dichorial placentas with putative anastomoses. Bleisch (1964) found arterial anastomoses in all 18 monochorionic, but in none of 42 dichorionic, twin placentas. He also succinctly explained why one should not accept the diagnosis of MoMo placentation in the boy/girl twin placenta reported by Pickering (1946). Wenner (1956) reemphasized Schatz's point of the rarity of VV anastomoses. He found only three such cases among the perhaps 100 placentas that were studied. He suggested that this type of connection may have lethal consequences because "one fetus aspirates blood through these anastomoses from the other," a point to which we return later. In a later study, Bleisch (1965) found that all of his 75 monochorionic twin placentas had anastomoses. In all but one case the anastomoses were grossly identifiable, and the sizes of anastomoses were partially related to the distance of the cord insertions. He was unable to identify any specific reasons for the directions of flow, but death of one twin was associated with thrombosis. Only one VV anastomosis was found, and Bleisch hypothesized first that the possibility exists for large blood shifts through large anastomoses, particularly given different intrauterine pressures, a point that is especially relevant when intrauterine demise of one monochorionic twin occurs. No connections were found between the circulations of dichorionic twins.

Twin placentas have other vascular peculiarities. Bhargava et al. (1971) made a detailed study of the vessels in the chorionic plate of 166 placentas from twins and triplets. They found many more placentas with arterial and venous tortuosities, "arteriovenous dissociations," and reversal of arteriovenous relations when they compared twin placentas with 167 singleton placentas. Their conclusion was that these vascular abnormalities are determined "mainly under the influence of the functional demands of the corresponding foetus." Identification of these anomalies may enhance our understanding of prenatal development.

The frequency of abnormal insertion of the umbilical cords in multiple gestations is particularly important, as was demonstrated in Chapter 12, Table 12.3. Kobak and Cohen (1939) described the incidence of velamentous insertion of one cord as being nine times higher in twins (routinely in triplets, according to De Lee, as quoted by Kobak and Cohen) than the 1% or so found in singleton placentas. Similar results were reported by Englert et al. (1987), when they observed abnormal placental shapes and cord insertions in multiple pregnancies after IVF. Eberle et al. (1993), who investigated the placental pathology of weight-discordant twins, found that discordant placental lesions were correlated more with dichorionic than monochorionic twins, rather than this discordance being correlated with placental weight. Feldman et al. (2002) found that velamentous cord insertion in triplets correlated significantly with fetal growth restriction. Likewise, in the searching review of placental lesions with

abnormal growth in twins, Redline et al. (2001) found that peripheral cord insertion and, less significantly, avascular villi and evidence of reduced maternal perfusion are associated. Further, Benirschke and Masliah (2001) have reviewed the issue of discordant placental development in DiMo and DiDi placentas and considered the "competition for space" as one possible reason for the differences occurring in the placental development of multiples conceived by ART. Abnormal cord insertions are of concern to the perinatologist because of the possibly greater frequency of vasa previa in twins. Kobak and Cohen (1939) described the stillbirth of a twin following vaginal bleeding that had resulted from disrupted vasa previa. Two similar cases of DiMo placentas and vasa previa were described by Whitehouse and Kohler (1960). Three of their six reported infants died from exsanguination. When this problem is anticipated, Kleihauer stains of the vaginal blood disclose the presence of fetal blood. We have seen several similar cases. In one, the fetal blood loss was recognized, and immediate neonatal transfusion with 100 mL of maternal blood saved the infant. A similar case has been described by Duenhoelter (1989). In another case we saw, vasa previa were present in the dividing membranes of DiDi twins. They ruptured, and fatal exsanguination occurred within 3 minutes of the second sac's rupture (Figs. 25.23 to 25.25). Because there are often large anastomoses between DiMo twins, rapid exsanguination of the second twin may also occur when vasa previa are ruptured in the first twin. It can also occur through an untied umbilical cord after delivery of the first twin. This potential exsanguination of a second twin is allegedly the reason for routine clamping of the placental end of the umbilical cord, lest an undiagnosed twin bleed

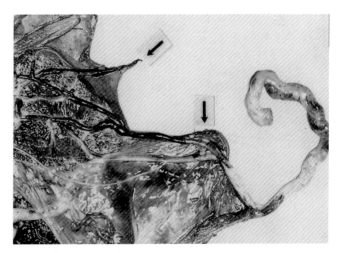

FIGURE 25.23. A DiDi twin placenta with velamentous insertion of the cord from twin B. He exsanguinated within 3 minutes after rupture of the second sac. There was disruption of the velamentous vessels (arrows).

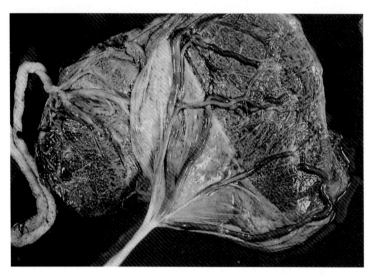

FIGURE 25.24. A DiDi fused twin placenta with large vessels of twin A coursing over the dividing membranes. Twin A has a single umbilical artery. These twins delivered at 34 weeks' gestation. The superficial chorionic veins of twin B (right) were nearly completely thrombosed. The infants survived.

from the cut end of the first-born. Velamentous vessels of twins may thrombose before birth, or they may atrophy. Rarely are they of vitelline origin and then of no importance (Fig. 25.26).

Antoine et al. (1982) grossly underestimated the reported frequency of vasa previa in twin placentas, when they cited only eight cases. They described a case in which sinusoidal fetal heart rate patterns initiated appropriate fetal studies, for example, amnioscopy and examination of the blood. Despite these efforts, both DiMo twins exsanguinated. Ramos-Arroyo et al. (1988) have also found that abnormal cord insertion was higher in twin gestations. Velamentous or marginal cords were found in 27.4% of monochorionic placentas, compared with 13.8% in dichorionic organs. They considered this as evidence in favor of trophotropism (see Chapter 7). Conversely,

Gavriil et al. (1993), who studied the placentas of IVF, interpreted the more frequently eccentric insertion in twins as resulting from "oblique orientation of the blastocyst at the nidation" but provide no further explanation why this should happen. The excess frequency of velamentous cords in DiMo twin placentas has significant correlation with the transfusion syndrome. Fries et al. (1993) found that one third of DiMo twin placentas had such abnormal cord insertions and that 64% were involved with transfusion syndrome cases and delivered significantly earlier. They thus sought an etiologic role for this abnormal insertion. It may also be considered that velamentous insertion is so common in this syndrome because normal placental development failed to take place.

Bruner et al. (1995) found a similarly high frequency of velamentous cord insertions of the donor twins, and

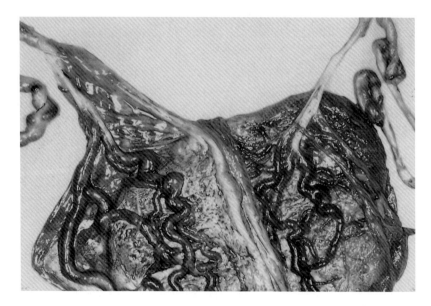

FIGURE 25.25. A DiDi fused twin placenta with velamentous cord insertion of the left cord. Its fetal vessels are markedly dilated and course over the membranes at left. Note that the major vessels of these twins do not approach the dividing membranes.

FIGURE 25.26. Immature DiMo twin placenta whose translucency of the dividing membranes is apparent. The cords seem to arise at the same spot but are nevertheless in separate amnionic compartments. Note the remains of a single yolk sac (arrow), whence omphalomesenteric vessels course toward the cords.

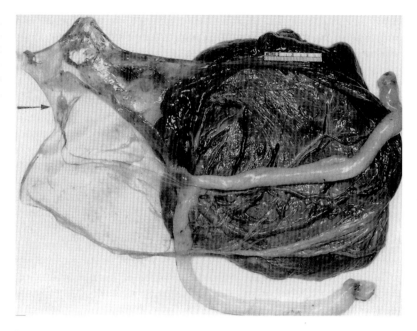

Mari et al. (1995, 1998) also felt that it may have an etiologic role in causing the imbalance that leads to the transfusion syndrome. We believe this to be possible because of the constant slight drainage of blood that occurs from the placenta with the velamentous cord into the other twin. Therefore, this placenta with reduced pressure may not have grown as avidly and centrifugally as it should have. The primacy of the vascular component in villous capillary development was addressed by Giles et al. (1993). These authors studied sonographically abnormal umbilical artery waveforms [systolic/diastolic (S/D) ratios] in twins and correlated these with villous vasculature. They found that "microvascular disease" of villi (reduction) correlates with growth restriction and abnormal S/Ds. Velamentous cord insertion was found as frequently as in 45% of monochorionic twin placentas by Machin (1997). He opined that it was an added risk factor of the twinning phenomenon and found growth discrepancies more commonly in central/velamentous cord insertions of monochorionic twins. Also, AV anastomoses were more common in this situation.

There is a wide spectrum of vascular relations in twin placentas. How do they come about, and what is so different in other species? In marmosets the assuredly DZ twins always have placental anastomoses; in Artiodactyla (especially *Bos* but also *Sus, Ovis, Bubalus,* and others) DZ twins often have fused placentas, and blood traverses from one fetus to the other. In marmosets it leads invariably to blood chimerism, but, other than for an occasional fetus papyraceus, the anastomoses cause no known complications. With Artiodactyla, however, in addition to the blood chimerism, the female twin becomes a freemartin (v.i.) when she is connected to a male's placental circulation.

This is not the case in humans, where dichorionic twins rarely have anastomoses, but where they have clearly occurred because of blood chimerism. Heterosexual blood chimerism is rare and it is not associated with sterility, that is, freemartinism in women (see Quintero et al., 2003b).

The reason for the differences must be found in the early embryologic development of the embryo and placenta. In marmosets, fusion of chorions occurs very early (Benirschke & Layton, 1969), but in human DZ twins no such fusion of chorionic circulations occurs. Here, the placentas may become intimately fused, but they do not develop interplacental vascular anastomoses. Indeed, despite numerous suggestions to the contrary, villi do not fuse in the human placenta, however closely they may become approximated. When sections of India-ink–injected, intimately fused dichorionic twin placentas are prepared, one observes that the villi may intermingle, but they do not connect with one another. No blood vessels traverse from the villi of one fraternal twin to those of the co-twin.

To understand the vascular commonality of monochorionic twin placentas, it is easiest with a review of their early embryology (Fig. 25.10). We suggest with this diagram that, in human placental development, the single chorionic sac has long since formed when vessels develop from the yolk sac or in situ, on about the 13th day. One must envisage that these primitive vascular precursors sprout all over the inner surface of the primitive chorionic membrane and, when the fetal heart gradually begins to pump, these fine vascular precursors begin to fill with blood. The vessels undoubtedly link with one another at this early time. The type of anastomosis that ultimately develops is probably a matter of chance. Whether the vessels become arteries or veins is determined by the direction of blood flow and its pressure. Some of the anastomoses are kept open, and others atrophy, depending on the velocity of flow. It may also be presumed that MZ twins often derive from embryonic splits with unequal cell numbers; it is therefore possible that one heart beats sooner or stronger, and that this influences the direction of flow in the anastomoses.

Monoamnionic/Monochorionic Twin Placenta

The MoMo twin placenta is the least common type. It occurs in approximately one or two of 100 sets of twins in the U.S. population but has now a nearly 40% perinatal mortality. Barss (1988) found that fetal demise occurred mostly before 24 weeks, when enough room for fetal motions and entanglement was still available in utero; Carr et al. (1990) found that after 30 weeks no further deaths occurred. Similarly, Tessen and Zlatnik (1991), who reviewed 21 sets of MoMo twins, found that fetal death did not occur after 32 weeks. Double survival used to be so uncommon that many papers were published with the title "MoMo Twins with Double Survival." The classical paper on MoMo twins is that by Quigley (1935), who believed the condition to occur only once in 60,000 pregnancies. Quigley found only one case report in the preceding 12 years. Altogether perhaps 110 cases had been reported at the time of his review. More recent papers give an incidence of 1:10,000 to 16,000 pregnancies. Quigley found double survival in only 15.6% and an overall fetal mortality of 68%.

Most commonly, fetal death is due to entangling of umbilical cords because of fetal movements. This knotting of cords is unpredictable and is often found in very young pregnancies, with abortion ensuing. It can now be visualized sonographically before birth, and management of such cases is changing. Thus, Belfort et al. (1993) identified not only cord entanglement but also venous obstruction by color Doppler flow study. This diagnosis led to successful interruption of an otherwise endangered pregnancy. More surprising is the case described by Krause and Goh (1998). Their twins had clearly entangled cord with compromise of the circulation, but a monochorionic placenta with diamnionic membranes was found. There must have been a window in the dividing membranes of this DiMo twin placenta for the entanglement to have occurred. Shahabi et al. (1997) were unable to save one twin despite making the diagnosis at 20 weeks; such cases are the reason why in our hospital these twins are hospitalized early, so that we can intervene quickly when flow compromise is diagnosed. Tabsh (1990a) suggested that the diagnosis of monoamnionic twin placentation is easily

made at amniocentesis by injection of indigo carmine, but the sonographic demonstrations by Belfort and his colleagues (1993) indicated that this new modality is superior to previous studies. They found cord entanglement and venous obstruction with Doppler flow studies that led to better management of their three pregnant patients. Abuhamad and his colleagues (1995) reported similar findings in two MoMo twin pregnancies. Rodis et al. (1997) studied 13 MoMo twin pregnancies with 26 liveborns (two died neonatally for other reasons) and deduced that their early diagnosis and appropriate management improved perinatal survival. Cord entanglement was noted in eight of their twins, and two sets had the transfusion syndrome. These authors found 96 publications on the topic, with 202 sets of MoMo twins. Other complications occur in MoMo pregnancies, such as prenatal coagulation, exsanguination through placental anastomoses, or bleeding from one twin into the other through anastomoses, and congenital malformations. Westover et al. (1994) found rare nuchal cords by Doppler imaging in MoMo twins that allowed appropriate management at delivery. Quintero et al. (1997) successfully ligated one of the umbilical cords in MoMo twin pregnancies when one twin was diagnosed as being nonviable.

Other obstetricians have also hoped, as did Belfort et al. (1993), that through early prenatal diagnosis (Dunnihoo & Harris, 1966; Sutter et al., 1986) the chances of MoMo twin survival can be improved. Rodis et al. (1987) managed three sets of twins successfully despite severely knotted cords; they also made suggestions for management. They identified one of these twins as having the typical transfusion syndrome. Driscoll (personal communication, 1970) has also seen the transfusion syndrome in MoMo twins. To find the transfusion syndrome in MoMo twins is otherwise uncommon (Wharton et al., 1968).

Table 25.3 presents a summary of some of the relevant literature on MoMo twin survival. Of 169 sets of MoMo twins, only 202 infants (60%) survived. The causes of death were predominantly cord entanglement [with stillbirth (Fig. 25.27; also see Fig. 25.35) or neonatal death], prematurity, and congenital anomalies. The aim of prenatal surveillance is to prevent the knots or entanglements of the cords becoming fatal. It is not known when knots first form, but because it requires considerable fetal mobility to produce knots, they are frequently found early in pregnancy, when more fluid exists (e.g., Fig. 25.27). On the other hand, it must be noted that term neonatal MoMo twins can have extensive knotting without compromise of the umbilical circulation. One assumes that space limitations in the uterine cavity prevented the formation of new knots with advancing gestation, which may also be the reason why such knotting is uncommon in triplets. Only knots that are already present from an earlier gestation may have the potential to compromise the fetus.

TABLE 25.3. Reports of monoamnionic twin pregnancies (incomplete)

Source	Year	Sets of MoMo twins	No. of survivors	Remarks
Quigley	1935	1	1	Review of 109 cases
Litt & Strauss	1935	1	0	Knots, one anencephalic
Parks & Epstein	1940	1	2	Knot, no anastomoses
Coulton et al.	1947	2	4	No entangling
Wilson	1955	5	4	Anencephaly, CHD, knots, tangles, anastomoses, fold
Whitehouse	1955	1	1	1 Papyraceus, knots, anastomoses
Craig	1957	1	2	Entangling; 166 cases cited
Librach & Terrin	1957	3	6	One knotted
Walters & Whitehead	1957	2	2	Both knotted
Sinykin	1958	1	3	First triplets, entangling
Pickhardt & Breen	1958	1	2	No knots; anastomoses
Semmens	1958	1	0	(1) Anemia, RDS; (2) CHD. No knots
Green et al.	1960	1	2	Knot, entangling
Zuckerman & Brzezinski	1960	2	1	2 sets macerated, knots; other knots; 1 lived, 1 macerated
Tafeen et al.	1960	3	4	2 knotted
Raphael	1961	5	5	2 anomalies; 4 knot/entangling
Wensinger & Daly	1962	3	5	3 knots/entangling
Timmons & Alvarez	1963	4	4	3 knots; 1 CNS damage; 1 fold
Goplerud	1964	1	2	No knots/entangling
Benirschke & Driscoll	1967	3	3	Knots
Dunnihoo & Harris	1966	1	2	No knots
Simonsen	1966	2	2	1 Knots
Wharton et al.	1968	18	24	1 CHD, 1 palsy, anastomoses
Larson et al.	1969a	1	0	Forked cord
Larson et al.	1969b	1	1	Both anomalies; no knots
Moestrup	1970	2	2	1 SUA (third case); no knots
Israelstam	1973	1	0	Knotting
Chapman	1974	3	2	Knotting
Mauer et al.	1974	1	1	Both discordant anomalies
Averback & Wigglesworth	1977	1	1	No knots
Litschgi & Stucki	1980	1	1	Macerated, entangling
McLeod & McCoy	1981	1	2	Cord of No. 2 around neck of No. 1, cut during delivery, both velamentous, IUD
Colburn & Pasquale	1982	1	2	Entangling
Colgan & Luk	1982	1	1	Torsion & thrombi of cord
Berry et al.	1984	1	1	SUA, severe anomalies; knots
Lumme & Saarikoski	1986	23	13	4 anomalies; knots, entangling
Sutter et al.	1986	1	2	Knots
Rodis et al.	1987	3	6	3 knotted
Barss	1988	5	9	Knots in 1; transfusion syndrome; anomaly; twinning in 1/87 pregnancies, after 20 weeks
Lee et al.	1988	59	77	Review of prenatally diagnosed MoMo twins
Tessen & Zlatnik	1991	21	28	Controlled study; no deaths after 32 weeks
Tabsh	1990	2	4	Method for diagnosis *in utero*
Total		192 (384 twins) 100%	234 Survivors (60%)	150 Dead (40%)

RDS, respiratory distress syndrome; CHD, congenital heart disease; IUD, intrauterine death; CNS, central nervous syndrome.

Lee et al. (1988) endeavored to ascertain the best mode of pregnancy management when MoMo placentation is diagnosed sonographically. They surveyed perinatologists and ascertained 59 pregnancies with an overall perinatal mortality of 34.7%. A much higher mortality was found when the diagnosis was made before 25 weeks' gestation than later. Although entangling of cords was an important cause of late deaths, there was an astonishing frequency of transfusion syndrome fatalities during earlier gestation. Frequent nonstress tests were recommended as the principal strategy for supervising these gestations.

The proximity of cord insertion is apparently not the principal determinant of knotting. We have seen extensive knotting in cords that were inserted at opposite margins of the placenta and no knots in some placentas whose cords arose next to one another (see Fig. 25.20). When a cord is obstructed for long periods, it may become very thin (Fig. 25.28), a condition described in several

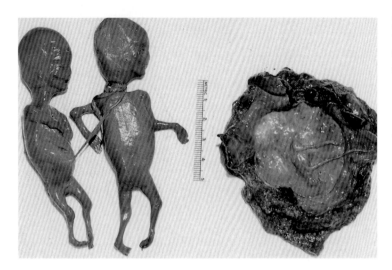

FIGURE 25.27. Macerated monoamnionic twins (12 weeks) with extensive knotting and entangling of cords. Fetal movements must have been extensive at an early embryonic age.

papers (Table 25.3). But the long-standing obstruction that can occur when MoMo twins' cords entangle is often evidenced by thromboses in placental surface veins (Fig. 25.29). Even when these twins survive, defects may have been caused by such hypoxic states. One complication of MoMo twinning is that the accoucheur may inadvertently cut the wrong umbilical cord during delivery. Donald (1964) described such a case, and a similar set of MoMo twins was observed by McLeod and McCoy (1981). When the first twin could not be delivered because the cord was extensively entwined about the infant's neck, the cord was severed. Only after the fetus was fully extracted was

it realized that a mistake had been made. After rapid delivery of the second twin, both twins survived.

The placental surface of MoMo twin placentas usually has a continuous sheet of amnion without folds between the cord insertions. However, there have been four observations of the existence of folds. Timmons and de Alvarez (1963), in their report of four cases of MoMo twins, found "a short fold of what was thought to be membrane ... present in the midportion of the fetal surface but [it] did not extend between the origins of the umbilical cords." Another plica ("fringe") was described in one of the five MoMo twins reported by Wilson (1955). It inserted

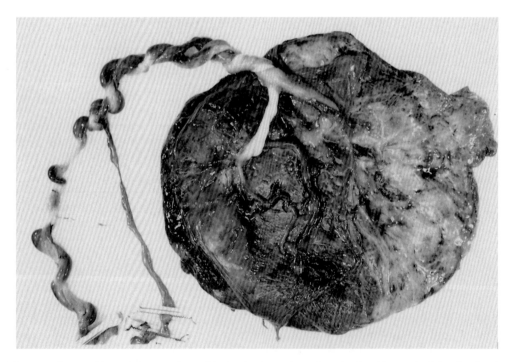

FIGURE 25.28. MoMo twins at 38 weeks' gestation with fetal death of one at 23 weeks (20-cm crown–rump length, 400-g macerated). Survivor is alive and well. Note the entangling and knotting of cords, the thin cord of the dead twin, and the extensive infarction of the right placental half. Anastomoses cannot be demonstrated this late after fetal death.

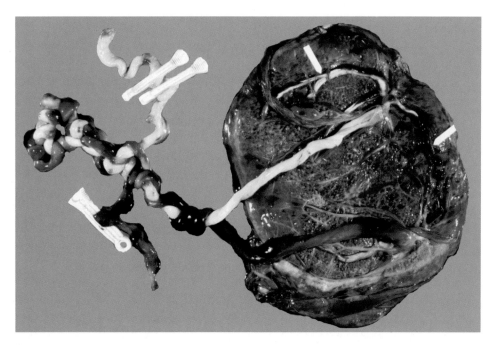

FIGURE 25.29. Monoamnionic twin pregnancy with extensive entangling of umbilical cords. One (dark) twin was stillborn, the other died with extensive areas of cerebral necrosis. Note the calcified veins in the liveborn twin (top) and more recent thrombi (right, at white arrow).

between the two cords of a set of MoMo macerated twins born with a surviving DZ triplet. A similar case has been described by Wolf (1920), and another is shown in Figures 25.30 and 25.31. One of these twins had the Klippel-Feil anomaly and died during the neonatal period. The cords arose from a single point and had six vessels that merged into three (arrow in Fig. 25.30) at their base. A thin, fal-ciform plica extended from the cords to the margin of the placenta. The tip of this plica, which consisted of two fused amnions, showed degenerative changes and scar-ring (Fig. 25.31). It is possible that disruption of the divid-ing membranes of two former amnionic cavities had occurred. It is also possible that the twinning took place just about at the time (7 days) when the amnion is first

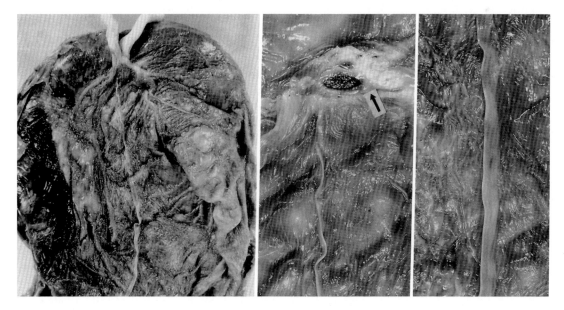

FIGURE 25.30. A MoMo twin placenta; one twin had Klippel-Feil syndrome. The two cords arise from the same spot, where vessels merge (arrow). Thin plica, composed of two amnions, extends from cord insertion to the margin. It is presumably the remains of an early attempt at formation of two amnionic cavi-ties, interrupted by the twinning event.

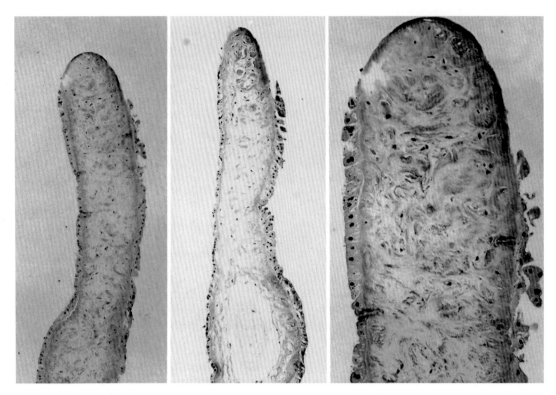

FIGURE 25.31. Sections through the tip of the plica shown in Figure 25.30. Note the degeneration of amnionic epithelium and the scarring of underlying connective tissue. H&E ×260.

set aside, thus preventing the formation of two complete amnionic sacs. It is difficult to conceive that an apparently single cavity could form from the spontaneous breakdown of the dividing membranes in a DiDi placenta, although this was assumed by Pickering (1946) in his description of boy/girl twins with a MoMo placenta. Nylander and Osunkoya (1970) also described "heterosexual twins with monochorionic placenta." They depicted a ridge with DiDi configuration present in one part and a DiMo relation in another portion of the placenta. Another unexplained case of monochorial placenta with fraternal twins was recorded by Van Verschuer (1925). He relied on the placental diagnosis of an assistant, and the dizygosity was based only on some physical differences (e.g., hair color). Gilbert and his colleagues (1991) not only identified several new cases of twins with rupture of the dividing membrane occurring in utero ("pseudomonoamniotic," according to Megory et al., 1991), but also highlighted the morbidity that may ensue, such as entangling of extremities in bands and entangling of cords. Diamnionic placentas can also be transformed into MoMo organs by amniocentesis and funipuncture (Magyar et al., 1991; Feldman et al., 1998) and spontaneously, perhaps by fetal activity. In tracing the history of MoMo twinning one step further, one may postulate that the placenta of Figure 25.32 was determined shortly after that which yielded the plica. Here the two cords, arising

nearly one from the other, are bound together by a delicate amnionic membrane.

We have observed a placenta from a set of MoMo twins with unusual findings that are relevant to the understanding of prenatal injury. One of the twins had cerebral atrophy that was attributed to the entwining of the umbilical cords. There was focal amnion necrosis, but this was confined to the regions directly above the fetal surface blood vessels; elsewhere the amnion was intact. This finding and the observation that the nodules of amnion nodosum are generally absent on cord and free membranes and that they occur primarily in amnion between the surface vessels led us to speculate that the amnion maintenance depends on the oxygen supplied from different sources. Oxygen tension in amnionic fluid is low (Jauniaux et al., 2003), and it is possible that it is augmented by oxygen from fetal surface vessels, the decidua capsularis, and the vessels in the umbilical cord. Further evidence for this surmise is that partial necrosis of thrombosed vessel walls can be seen in some cases with occluded cord vessels (see Chapter 12). Thus, in the present case with cord entanglement, we hypothesize that the entanglement led to reduced flow of one twin's vasculature (hence the cerebral atrophy of that twin) and the necrosis of the surface vasculature's amnion.

Anastomoses of fetal blood vessels appear to occur even more commonly in MoMo placentas than in DiMo

FIGURE 25.32. A MoMo twin placenta at term with extensive interfetal vascular anastomoses. The nearly commonly arising cords are bound within an amnionic fold. This stage presumably arises shortly after the placenta shown in Figures 25.30 and 25.31.

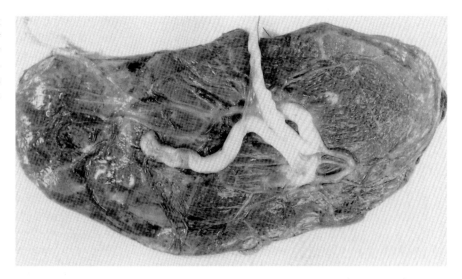

twin placentas when injection studies are made (Bajoria, 1998), this perhaps being the reason for the rarity of the twin transfusion syndrome in MoMo twins. Umur et al. (2003a) came to the same conclusions in their review of 24 MoMo vs. 200 DiMo twin placentations. The proximity of the cord insertion may be one determinant, as the cords are more often centrally located. Of great importance also is that, when large inter-twin communications exist, the cell and blood traffic between the two fetuses may have greater influence on the fetal well-being. The example depicted in Figure 25.33 features the placenta of a macerated MoMo twin and a co-twin who expired soon after birth (Benirschke, 1961). This case has aroused much interest subsequent to its occurrence. The initially surviving infant died within 62 hours. Bilateral renal cortical necrosis, cerebral liquefaction, and other degenerative changes, including thrombi and focal mineralization (Fig. 25.34), were present. These findings are descriptive of the sequelae from DIC. We then postulated that thromboplastin from the macerating twin had entered the survivor's bloodstream via interplacental anastomoses prior to birth and had thus initiated DIC. The development of DIC, as resulting from thromboplastins liberated by the dead twin, now seems to us to be far-fetched, because the fetus is dead and cannot contribute much to the survivor's circulation. But, there have been several other reports of neonatal deaths with findings of DIC (Table 25.4). During the past few years we have been consulted with many similar cases, where the medicolegal question arose as to possible preventive cesarean section after the death of one twin. Many of the descriptions in the literature are also similar to the case here shown, but conclusive proof of prenatal DIC with definitive coagulation studies has been difficult to obtain. In a case of macerated MoMo twin with a term liveborn co-twin, Bulla et al. (1987) found neonatal platelet counts of 67,000/mm^3 that later rose to

300,000/mm^3. The infant died on day 10 with bilateral renal, splenic, and central nervous system (CNS) necroses. Patten et al. (1989b), who examined five co-twins with one fetus having died prenatally and who used the term **twin embolization syndrome** (TES), identified active consumptive thrombocytopenia in one of their cases with renal and CNS defects. Microcephaly and various other CNS abnor-

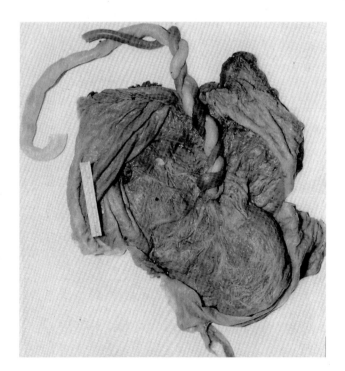

FIGURE 25.33. A MoMo twin placenta with one macerated fetus (dark cord). The survivor, who had disseminated intravascular coagulation, died at age 62 hours (see Fig. 25.34) (*Source:* Benirschke, 1961, with permission.)

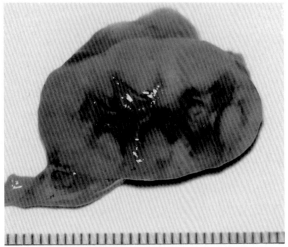

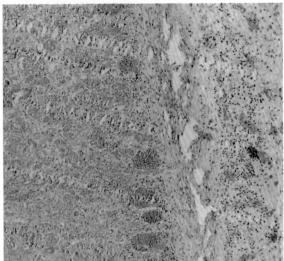

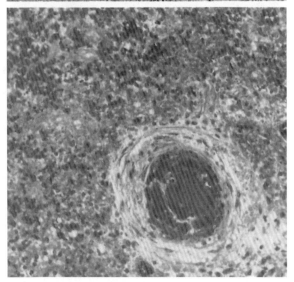

FIGURE 25.34. Organs of a premature neonate whose placenta is shown in Figure 25.33. There were bilateral renal cortical necrosis and widespread thrombosis when this infant died at 62 hours (left). The kidney had diffuse, yellow, cortical infarction. Center: Microscopic appearance of renal cortical necrosis. Right: Splenic thrombus.

malities, in addition to intestinal, peritoneal, and renal destructive lesions, were the focus of their observations. They urged prenatal sonographic studies of such pregnancies. As to the evidence of consumptive coagulopathy, diligent study of some other cases ruled out their existence when fetal demise of one twin had occurred (Hanna & Hill, 1984). Okamura et al. (1994) did funipuncture in seven surviving twins following the demise of the co-twin. Coagulation parameters were not abnormal, although three infants suffered cerebral abnormalities. This was seen as strong evidence for the primacy of acute anemia due to presumed acute hypotension (shunting through anastomoses) as the cause of the cerebral destruction, rather than DIC or embolization. This is further discussed subsequently and was eloquently shown to be correct by prenatal blood sampling (Nicolini et al., 1998).

This is a complex issue of great importance. Many investigators have tried to answer the many questions that arise from these observations. Litschgi and Stucki (1980) reviewed their twin material and found that in 13 cases of 191 twin pregnancies (6.8%; 0.07% of all births) a macerated fetus was delivered with a live twin. They found one MoMo, seven DiMo, and five DiDi cases, and suggested that immediate delivery is not advisable when one twin has died. In view of the distribution of deaths in relation to ultimate delivery, they recommended that all such pregnancies be terminated by 39 weeks. This aspect is discussed further in the section on fetus papyraceus as this pathologic feature is not limited to MoMo placentation but affects all monochorial twins. Because the probability of thromboplastin infusion from a dead twin is actually highly unlikely (because its circulation has stopped), alternative explanations have been sought. They are completely summarized in a large paper by Liu et al. (1992) and are further discussed later in this chapter. Specifically, Liu et al. suggested that acute hypotensive events occur in the surviving twin immediately after one twin dies because of the common placental vasculature. Jou et al. (1993) even observed sonographically the reversal of blood flow in the umbilical cord after fetal death of one twin. Less decisive flow disturbances after demise of one twin were recorded by Malinowski et al. (1996). That such an event may occur is also evident from the detailed postmortem description of the original Siamese twins Chang and Eng Bunker (Kormann, 1869). After the death of Chang, Eng complained of chest tightness and expired within 2 hours. Large anastomoses were present in their xiphoid connections at autopsy through which exsanguination of Eng presumably occurred, and autopsy indicated exsanguination of Eng into Chang. An important case report has been published by Sherer et al. (1993), who showed the rapid development of the cerebral consequences of such fetal demise. They followed a twin transfusion set of twins with fetal death of one at 23 weeks, followed by spontaneous resolution of hydrops.

TABLE 25.4. Summary of twins with prenatal damage perhaps due to vascular transport of coagulation products or acute blood loss

Source	Year	Placenta	Remarks
Benirschke	1961	MoMo	Macerated twin; survivor with renal cortical necrosis, porencephaly; presumed DIC (Figures 25.33 and 25.34)
Figure 25.35	1959	MoMo	Macerated twin, thrombi in umbilical vessels; survivor died with extensive cerebral palsy
Figures 25.39 and 25.40	1986	MoMo	32 weeks; stillborn 1800 g, survivor 2400 g died with hydrops (? due to cord tangles); AA, AV anastomoses, arthrogryposis, CNS atrophy
Figure 25.41	1986	DiMo	Fetus papyraceus, velamentous cord; survivor has porencephaly; **mother** had DIC after delivery; transfusion syndrome
Timmons & Alvarez	1963	MoMo	Case 4 had cerebral palsy from "embarrassed circulation"
Rosenquist	1963	DiMo	Adrenal, pulmonary, renal calcifications in donor of transfusion syndrome
Moore et al.	1969	DiMo	(1) Singleton with velamentous cord and DIC. (2) Monochorionic, macerated; survivor developed DIC and died; blood studies were normal; (3) DiMo, one macerated stillborn, other had anemia and bilateral renal cortical necrosis, but survived
Dimmick et al.	1971	DiMo	Velamentous cord, CNS and renal necroses; unable to identify anastomoses; secondary to cord insertion?
Thomas	1974	Tri?Di	Male had intraventricular hemorrhage (IVH) and coagulation disorder; one female macerated, one with mild coagulation disorder
Durkin et al.	1976		Review of 8 cases; monochorionics at highest risk
Mannino et al.	1977	DiMo	Fetus papyraceus with aplasia cutis in survivor; review
Melnick	1977	?	Macerated twin; CNS damage in survivor who died with CNS necrosis; review of Collaborative Study and risk assessment
Yoshioka et al.	1979	?, MZ	Three sets of twins had porencephaly and macerated stillborn; thrombosis of cerebral artery; authors considered emboli as cause
Jung et al.	1984	?	Review of hydranencephaly and porencephaly; 11% had twins, most were macerated
Barth & Harten	1985	DiMo	Term with macerated twin (death at 13–16 weeks); gastroschisis, CNS damage
Nakayama et al.	1986	DiMo	Macerated fetuses with infarcts of CNS, kidney, spleen, liver; reviewed 14 twins, only monochorionics had poor prognosis
Hughes & Miskin	1986	DiMo?	Fetal death at 20 weeks, following which prenatally diagnosed CNS cysts developed, microcephaly, renal dysplasia
Yoshida & Soma	1986	DiMo	Review; macerated with cerebral palsy in survivor; skin defects in male; macerated female co-twin
Szymonowicz et al.	1986	? DiMo	Six cases with survivors having CNS deficits; other infarcts; review of total literature (53 cases)
Bulla et al.	1987	MoMo	Renal and CNS necroses; other was a macerated fetus AA and VV anastomoses
Leidig et al.	1988	?	Two of four cases with prenatal IVH were twins
Jones	1988	?	Hydranencephaly; 30 cm fetus papyraceus
Patten et al.	1989b	DiMo	5 cases with various brain, kidney, and intestinal defects
Fisher & Siongco	1989	DiMo	Massive porencephaly; renal splenic infarcts
Cherouny et al.	1989	MoMo	20 cases; one MoMo twin developed brain cysts, prenatal evaluation was reassuring
Anderson et al.	1990	DiMo	Four cases, second trimester fetal deaths, CNS lesions GI lesion in 2
Larroche et al.	1990	DiMo	15 monochorionics, vascular "instability"
Fusi et al.	1991	DiMo	CNS and renal necroses, no coagulation defect, transfusion
Margono et al.	1992	DiMo	Foot necrosis before birth
Liu et al.	1992	DiDi/DiMo/MoMo	38 twins, 3 triplets; damage in 19 offspring (72% monochorionics)
Grafe	1993	DiMo	CNS necroses in both twins

They were able to demonstrate sonographically that echogenic changes had become prominent in the brain of the survivor within 48 hours already. The authors considered these to be hemorrhages that eventuated into a severely microcephalic anomaly. Death of one MZ twin was observed at 27 weeks by Lander et al. (1993). Doppler sonographic observations within 24 hours after the death showed "remarkable variability in flow velocity waveforms in the umbilical artery of the surviving fetus.

Changes from reversed to normal end-diastolic flow velocities were recorded within 6 minutes."

These are simplistic hemodynamic explanations for a very complex dynamic state that exists in utero of ill-defined vascular communications. Because hemodynamic results of these anastomoses have been largely inaccessible to us until the event of Doppler flow studies, relatively little hard information is available at this time, and it is common to oversimplify from our incomplete knowledge.

That the situation is much more complex in utero is to be inferred from the case report of Grafe (1993). She described DiMo liveborn premature twins, both with antenatal white matter necrosis; they died subsequently. Aside from a velamentous insertion of twin A's umbilical cord, there were AA and VV anastomoses. We assume that irregular flow back and forth through these anastomoses was responsible for the cerebral destruction. Perhaps such variable blood exchange occurs often in monochorionic twins.

At this point, it is important to understand the possible fates of placental tissue when one twin dies. If there are large interfetal vascular communications, the placental half of the dead fetus may continue to be perfused by the survivor. If, on the other hand, the anastomoses are small, the placenta of the dead fetus gradually atrophies and eventually appears as though infarcted. It is much the same as what happened to placental tissue when experimental fetal removal was practiced in rhesus monkeys. There is gradual atrophy of placenta, with much deposition of intervillous fibrin.

The problem of **maternal** DIC with a dead fetus is often discussed under the heading "dead-fetus syndrome" (Strauss et al., 1978). Although it has been described in some cases where one twin had died in utero (Skelly et al., 1982; Romero et al., 1984), in other patients it did not develop (Wittmann et al., 1986; Cherouny et al., 1989). The reason for the differences is not clear. When Zorlu et al. (1997) examined what happened to maternal coagulation parameters in 25 women with one dead twin, they found that coagulation parameters were temporarily abnormal in two, but rectified by delivery. They felt that, for the mother's health, no undue concern needs to be had. This complex aspect is not treated further in this text.

To explain some cases of prenatal damage observed in twins after the death of the co-twin, it has also been postulated that thrombi in the fetal circulation embolize via the interfetal anastomoses, from the dead to the living twin. Although it is true that thrombi from fetal vascular occlusions can embolize to the fetus (Wolf et al., 1985), the lesions usually seen in the survivors of pregnancies with a macerated co-twin, however, are not typical of those caused by emboli. Yoshioka et al. (1979) postulated that the CNS damage of the twins they examined, which had macerated co-twins, resulted from occlusion of large vessels. They believed that emboli from macerated co-twins were the most reasonable explanation for the damage. In support of this hypothesis, they cited a case by Clark and Linell (1954), who described an erythroblastotic stillborn whose mother had been treated with cortisone and had an occlusion of the internal carotid artery and cerebral vessels. The authors suggested that, because the thrombus did not look like loose clot, it probably originated from an embolus; and they opined that it represented embolized "placental tissue." This assumption cannot be the case, for there were no villous remains in the clot. Admittedly, it contained erythroblasts, but degenerating placental tissue never embolizes to the fetus. Clots could embolize from venous vessels, which have occasionally been shown to be thrombosed. Such an event is shown in the fetal vessels in Figure 25.35.

Massive plethora in a macerating twin masqueraded as the recipient of the twin transfusion syndrome in several cases. The transfusion syndrome could be ruled out, however, because the twins were of the same size and had similar-sized hearts, and there were large placental anastomoses. We assumed that the plethoric twin had recently received large quantities of blood from the survivor via large vascular communications in the placenta. This acute transplacental fetus-to-fetus bleeding, with resulting plethora of one twin, was first mentioned by Lehndorff (1961) and was also described by Cameron (1968). Lehndorff correctly hypothesized that marked shifts may occur through large anastomoses during, or even before,

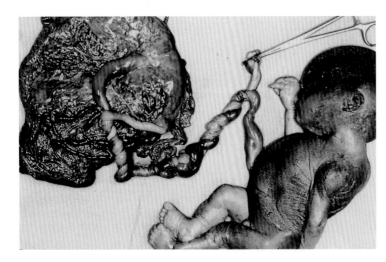

FIGURE 25.35. Macerated stillborn MoMo twin with extensive knotting of cords. The surviving infant died 3 months later with extensive brain necroses.

delivery. Later, Bleisch (1965) had the same thought. This phenomenon is different from the typical transfusion syndrome, which constitutes a specific entity and is discussed below, and it should not be labeled as such.

All these cases have assumed great importance in the legal realm because cerebral palsy is so common in twins (Durkin et al., 1976; Scheller & Nelson, 1992). Eastman et al. (1962) estimated it to be five times more common than in controls and assigned as the chief cause the prematurity of twins and an unfavorable intrauterine environment. This higher incidence of cerebral palsy (and of mental deficiency) affects primarily monozygotic twins (Berg & Kirman, 1960; Russell, 1961). Furthermore, a characteristic type of skin defect that is secondary to prenatal dermal necrosis (aplasia cutis) is also primarily associated with DiMo placentation and fetus papyraceus (Mannino et al., 1977). It is thus challenging to better understand what causes these prenatal insults. Moreover, as stated, there has been much litigation in cases of twins with cerebral palsy. In these legal suits it is commonly assumed that the obstetrician must be at fault when brain damage occurs in one twin because, according to these suits, this damage would not have occurred had a quick cesarean section been done. It must be pointed out in this context that Bejar et al. (1990) have shown that porencephaly may already be present at birth, and that it correlates best with one of two circumstances: (1) fetal infection (chorioamnionitis, funisitis); or (2) MZ twins having placental vascular anastomoses. Leviton and Paneth (1990) reviewed the possible causes of CNS white matter necrosis. They concluded, as did Larroche et al. (1990), that circulatory phenomena were important aspects in the causation of cerebral palsy. Fusi and colleagues (1991) found no coagulation disorder but observed acute twin–twin transfusion as the cause of brain damage. They were emphatic that intervention would have to take place before fetal death occurred if CNS sequelae were to be prevented. Norman (1980, 1982) made somewhat similar observations on prenatal brain necrosis in DiMo twins. A large retrospective review of brain damage in twins was undertaken in Sweden by Rydhstroem (1995). He found no difference in relation to birth order and like-sex vs. unlike-sex status, but there was an increase of cerebral damage in the heavier of twins. Interestingly, Maier et al. (1995), who assessed degrees of hypoxia in twins, found that the smaller twin has higher concentrations of erythropoietin. The principal reason for CNS damage was seen to be the increased prematurity of multiple gestations, with cystic periventricular cystic white matter necrosis following (Allan et al., 1994). The outcome is not significantly different from that of singleton premature infants (Kilpatrick et al., 1996; Nielsen et al., 1997) when matched for gestational age.

For all these reasons it is of future importance that we delineate more precisely the pathogenesis that leads to this prenatal CNS damage, so that it may be anticipated

and prevented, if possible. Hurst and Abbitt (1989) observed that encephalomalacia and intraventricular CNS hemorrhage developed prenatally in a set of twins with the classical transfusion syndrome. In the case described by Hughes and Miskin (1986), bleeding complicated a known twin pregnancy at 20 weeks, and subsequently one twin became macerated. In the survivor, brain cyst development could be followed sonographically after 30 weeks and was found in the newborn after cesarean section at 37 weeks. Interestingly, the kidneys of this microcephalic and porencephalic infant had cystic changes, which we assume stemmed from former focal areas of necrosis. Nakayama et al. (1986) studied 14 liveborn twins with macerated co-twins. Among the three with neonatal death, CNS, renal, splenic, and liver necroses were found. Several other relevant contributions have been forthcoming (Dudley & D'Alton, 1986; Liu et al., 1992), but a consensus as to the best management of monochorionic and monoamnionic twin pregnancies has not yet emerged (Hagay et al., 1985). Melnick (1977) estimated that some 3% of near-term monozygotic twins have a dead co-twin. Furthermore, one third of the survivors, or possibly 1% of MZ twin births, have severe brain defects as a consequence of putative DIC (Jones, 1988).

These considerations are especially important in view of the evolving practice of intentional fetal elimination when discordant anomalies of twins are found, when too many multiples are conceived, during the therapy of the prenatally diagnosed transfusion syndrome, and for prenatally diagnosed genetic disorders (Åberg et al., 1978). In these situations, it must be recognized that there are possible consequences for the second twin when one is eliminated and the status of anastomoses not ascertained (Wittmann et al., 1986). Yamagishi et al. (1998) reported on the discordance of male MZ twins with deletion of a chromosomal band in No. 22 (22q11.2). The twins had the TTTS, and one twin (the donor), but not the other, had tetralogy of Fallot. Prenatal cardiovascular adjustment to the TTTS was considered to be the reason for the major discordance. Discordance for some diseases may also be the sequel of the TTTS. Thus, Lazda (1998) recorded the occurrence of endocardial fibroelastosis in the larger of two recipients of this unequal blood sharing of twins prenatally. Other unusual features may occur. We draw attention to the fetal demise due to hydrops from parvovirus 19 infection in a DiDi twin placenta in which the other fetus survived and did not have the infection (Foster & Allen, 2004). Remarkably, the gravida developed DIC 4 weeks after fetal demise.

The possibility of DIC developing in the remaining living twin, after one had died, led Cox et al., (1987) to sample the fetal vasculature of 19 twins. This evolving technique of fetal blood sampling promises much insight into the prenatal vascular relations among twins. It is for these complex reasons that we have summarized relevant case information in twin pregnancies with fetal death in one twin (Table 25.4). Other large tables may be found in Liu et al. (1992), where all relevant literature is also discussed. As will be seen, there is a good possibility that the survivor in cases of prenatal twin death experiences significant acute blood loss through superficial, large interplacental anastomoses. One can envisage that when one twin dies the other bleeds into this vascular bed, now devoid of counterpressure. Indeed, paradoxical plethora has been seen in discordant twins, in which the smaller (earlier dead) twin is plethoric. Modern studies with Doppler sonography have come closer to an understanding of the redistributional changes of blood in twin placentation (Gaziano et al., 1998). These authors found a much more important and more frequent effect of the vascular anastomoses in DiMo placentas than originally anticipated and discuss eloquently the impact of these on cerebral arterial perfusion in the fetus.

To accumulate relevant prenatal information of such occurrences, Toubas et al. (1981) studied the fetal response to acute hemorrhage (15%) in the lamb. The arterial blood pressure, pH, and heart rate of the fetus fell significantly, and the cardiac output decreased. The blood flow in the fetus (kidneys, gastrointestinal tract, and lungs) and to the placenta were markedly reduced. Toubas et al. did not report any structural changes of these organs due to the hemorrhage. It will be necessary in future cases of prenatal death of one MZ twin to accumulate information on neonatal hematologic parameters. Measurements of hematocrit, deformed red blood cells (schistocytes), split fibrin degradation products, platelet changes, and nucleated red blood cells can provide some of the information needed for better understanding this entity.

MoMo twins presumably arise at approximately days 8 to 10 of fertilization age and are next to last in the spectrum of the MZ twinning events (Coulton et al., 1947). This type of placenta is also nearly always found with conjoined twins, only one exception having been published (Weston et al., 1990). Monoamnionic twins may have a single or a forked umbilical cord (Fig. 25.36; see also Fraser et al., 1997, who reported liveborn twins), or there may be two separate cords. Forked cords are occasionally found also in completely separate MoMo twins (Fig. 25.36). In other MoMo twins, the cords originate close to each other on the placental surface, as in the cephalopagous conjoined twins whose placenta is shown

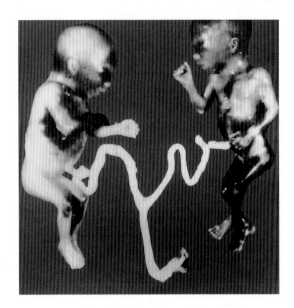

FIGURE 25.36. Forked umbilical cord of MoMo twin abortuses at 17 weeks' gestation. The smaller twin (right) had a single umbilical artery but no other anomalies. (Courtesy of Dr. Marilyn Jones, San Diego, California.)

in Figure 25.37. Forked cords have been described by Larson et al. (1969a) in a set of macerated abortuses. MoMo twins often have extensive vascular anastomoses between the fetal circulations, particularly when the cords are in close apposition (Figs. 25.38 to 24.40). The impact that the cord position may have on the outcome of the surviving MoMo twin (after fetal death of one) is further documented in Table 25.4. When velamentous insertion of one cord complicates placentation in such cases, growth restriction and fetal death are especially common (Fig.

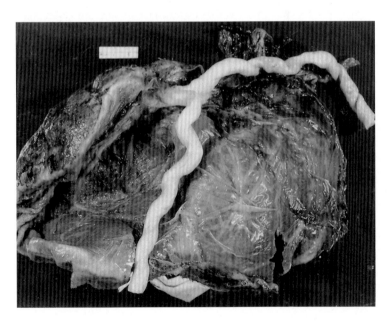

FIGURE 25.37. Forked umbilical cord of MoMo cephalopagous conjoined twins. (Courtesy of Dr. S. Romanski, Los Angeles, California.)

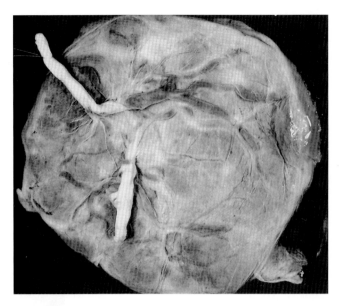

FIGURE 25.38. Term MoMo twin placenta. Note the extensive vascular anastomoses on the fetal surface.

25.41). Monoamnionic twins, as other MZ twins, may have remarkably different development, as was true of the case described by Larson et al. (1969a). Discordant anomalies are particularly common. Observations on MoMo twins have led to a better understanding of some types of congenital anomaly. Thus, the occurrence of renal agenesis in one of MoMo twins (unilateral agenesis in the other, who survived) was not associated with the Potter syndrome, as expected. Rather, the adequate production of amnionic fluid by the more normal twin prevented this phenotype and indicated that lung development depends purely on the volume of amnionic fluid present (Mauer et al., 1974). The anomalous twin also had normal respiratory function. It died of uremia at 12 days of age. Similar observations were later made of MoMo twins, where one had sirenomelia.

Monoamnionic placentation has also been observed in MZ triplets. Sinykin (1958) described the triple survival of MoMo triplets whose placenta is shown in Figure 25.42. We have observed a monoamnionic triplet placenta of stillborns. The pregnancy was terminated with prostaglandins at 27 weeks when fetal death had become evident. One was a tiny acardiac fetus, one was an anencephalic, and the third was a normal macerated fetus

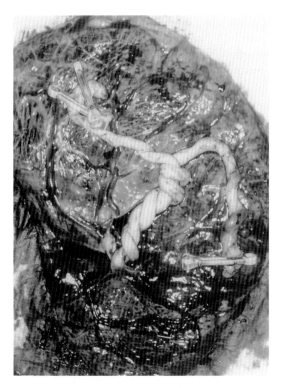

FIGURE 25.39. A MoMo twin placenta with entangling of umbilical cords. Twin B (top left) died from nonimmune hydrops. At autopsy no cause was found for the hydrops. It was assumed to be the result of interference with venous return from the placenta. Figure 25.40 shows the large anastomoses after the cords have been untangled.

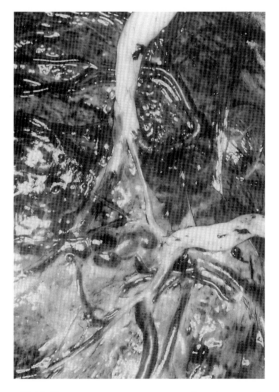

FIGURE 25.40. Large anastomoses are seen between cord vessels of the MoMo twin placenta in Figure 25.39.

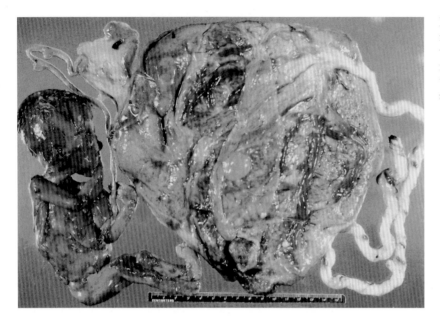

FIGURE 25.41. A DiMo twin placenta with macerated fetus papyraceus at left, having velamentous insertion of its cord. The surviving fetus had porencephaly and was presumed to be the recipient in a transfusion syndrome.

(Fig. 25.43). The long-standing nature of thrombotic events in such twins is evident from the frequent mineralizations found in their placental vessels (Fig. 25.44).

It would be expected that MoMo twins, who are probably determined between days 8 to 10 of development (see Fig. 25.10), may differ in the number of yolk sacs they possess. Figure 25.45 shows two early gestations of MoMo twins with an only partially divided yolk sac. It is considered to be the product of splitting on day 11 if the developmental table shown is precise enough for such inference. In another set of stillborn MoMo twins (with a dichorial triplet) we have seen two yolk sacs; that placenta also had two velamentous cords and presumably had its embryologic origin prior to the placenta with partially divided yolk sac.

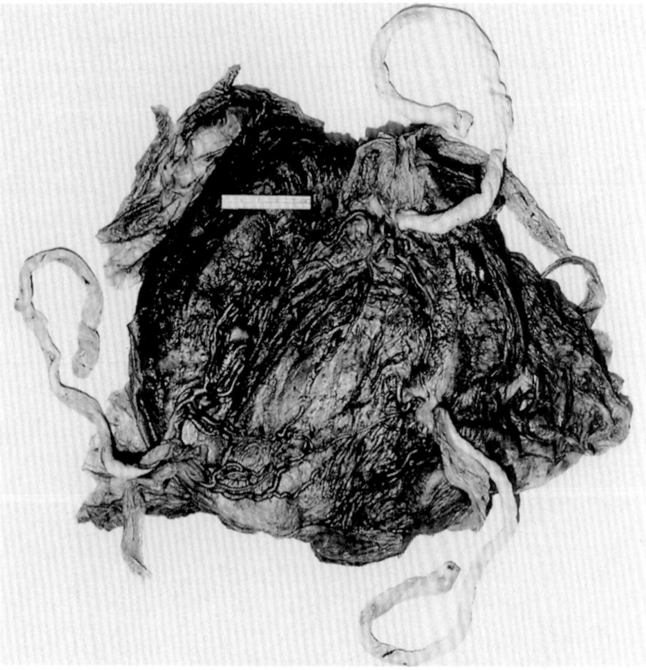

FIGURE 25.42. A MoMo triplet placenta at term. There were anastomoses among all circulations and no entangling of cords. The triplets survived. (Courtesy of Dr. M.B. Sinykin, San Antonio, Texas.)

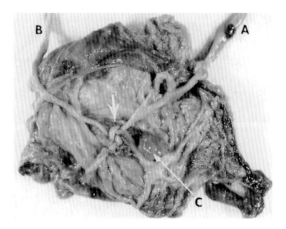

FIGURE 25.43. Monoamnionic triplets, all of whom were macerated. Labor was induced at 27 weeks. Triplet A was structurally normal; B was anencephalic; C was a diminutive acardiac fetus. Note the extensive knotting (large arrow).

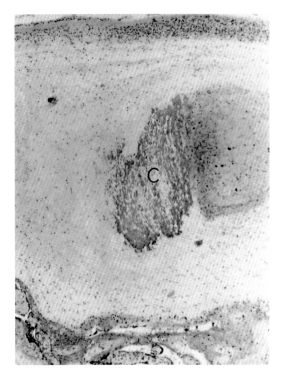

FIGURE 25.44. Calcification of the vascular wall and an old thrombus in the placental surface vessel of one of MoMo twins that was macerated.

Diamnionic/Monochorionic Twin Placenta

The DiMo twin placenta is the commonest form of placentation of identical or monozygotic twins. Each twin is enclosed in its own amnionic sac, and the dividing membranes are composed of two amnions only (see Figs. 25.1 to 25.4). As will be seen in these photomicrographs, the amnion possesses epithelium and connective tissue. The presence of a layer of connective tissue has occasionally been mistaken, regrettably, as being diagnostic of chorion; that is the reason for being so adamant about the identification of these dividing membranes. These amnionic membranes can be moved freely over the chorionic surface. Because they are often moved before birth, it is not unusual to find the dividing membranes at a place that does not correspond with the vascular equator of the two twins' placental halves (Fig. 25.46). DiMo placentas usually have two yolk sacs, and virtually all of them have vascular anastomoses, as was delineated earlier in this chapter. The cord insertion, as in all twin placentas, is more often marginal or velamentous than that of singletons. Single umbilical artery (SUA) is also commoner in one or both of these twins (Thomas, 1961). Yoshida (1998) found that SUA occurred in 3% of twin gestations, whereas it was found in 0.53% of singletons. Because the amnion does not have its own blood vessels, the dividing membranes must survive on the nutrients and oxygen contained within the amnionic fluid. This notion is supported by the finding of amnion necrosis in cases of fetal death, or amnion nodosum when one of the twins is oligohydramneic (Fig. 25.47). In such cases, only the amnionic epithelium degenerates. The underlying connective tissue is generally preserved. In cases of prenatal infection, the inflammation is also lacking in these dividing membranes, and meconium pigmentation is sparse when it is found elsewhere in the amnionic cavity. What has been surprising with the increasing practice of ART is the fact that MZ twinning is often superimposed upon multiple embryo transfers and that the placentation of these twins is then usually (or always?) a DiMo placenta. This does not jibe with the notion that MZ twinning is perhaps due to improper handling of the blastocysts and disruption of the zona pellucida before implantation, as this would be expected to have led to DiDi MZ twins. Jain et al. (2004b) have examined some aspects of this topic and found that MZ twinning was higher when blastocysts were directly transferred than when 3-day embryos were implanted. At present the mechanism that leads to MZ twinning in ART is not fully understood.

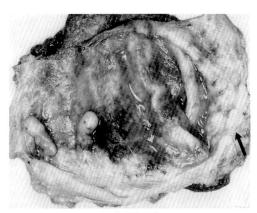

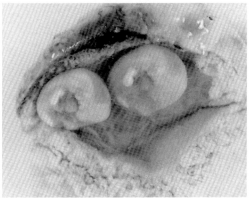

FIGURE 25.45. Monoamnionic twin abortuses, structurally normal (top). Note the partially duplicated, bean-shaped yolk sac (arrow). Therapeutic abortion of DiMo twins was done at 33 days' gestation (bottom).

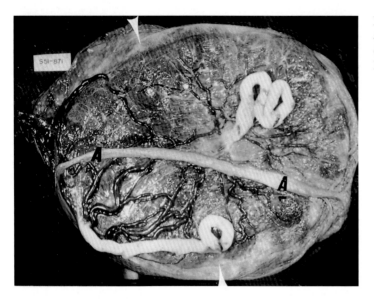

FIGURE 25.46. A DiMo twin placenta with apposing amnions (A, A) meeting at angles to the vascular equator (arrowheads). Note the marginal insertion of the cord at left.

The lack of intersac transfer of solutes is illustrated by the results from injection of hypertonic saline when abortion is intended. Kovacs et al. (1972) injected 200 mL of a 20% NaCl solution into one sac after having removed 380 mL of amnionic fluid at 22 weeks. Cardiac activity stopped in 2 hours in one twin, and labor commenced 20 hours later. The DiMo twins weighed 300 g each; the injected fetus was macerated, but the other was alive at delivery. Only the amnion of the injected side was necrotic. Hoch et al. (1972) made similar observations in a dichorionic twin pregnancy, but in this placentation it is more expected that solute transfer does not occur between the two sacs. Finally, a most unusual DiMo twin placenta, sent to us in consultation, is illustrated in Figure 25.48. This placenta shows one amnionic sac contained within the other; the twins differed appreciably in size.

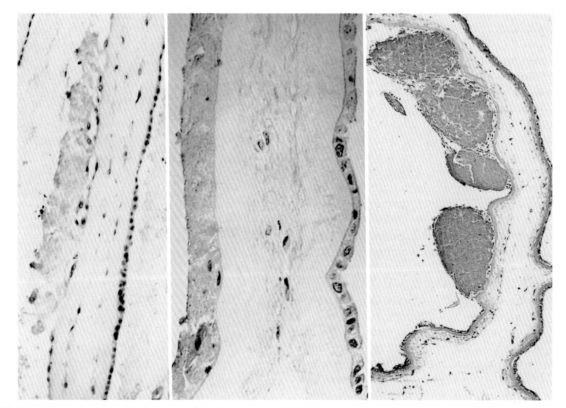

FIGURE 25.47. Various degenerative features of the left amnion of dividing membranes in cases of DiMo placentas with one fetus dead (center, right) and amnion nodosum (left).

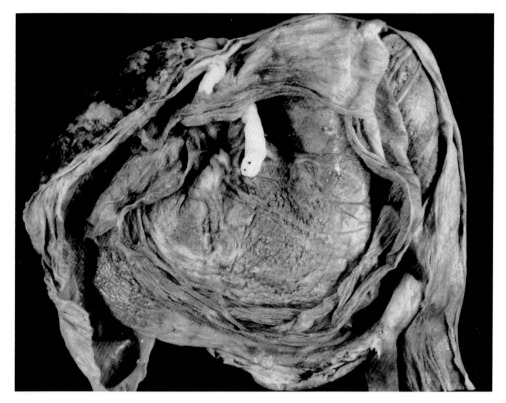

FIGURE 25.48. A DiMo twin placenta (550 g) of MZ twins. One amnionic sac is enclosed by the other. The outer sac contained a smaller fetus with velamentous insertion of the cord. (Courtesy of Drs. V. Anderson and Z. Weinraub, Martin Luther King Hospital, Los Angeles, California.)

Diamnionic/Dichorionic Twin Placenta

The DiDi twin placenta may be composed of separate disks, or the two placental portions may be intimately fused. It is the most common type of twin placentation and shares with the other types an increased frequency of marginal and velamentous insertion of umbilical cords. The fused placentas present the appearance seen in Figure 25.49. When the fetal vessels are injected, there is no exchange of the injection fluid between the two fetuses.

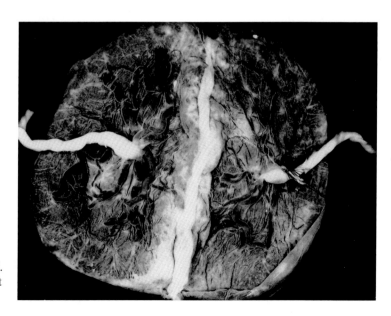

FIGURE 25.49. A DiDi twin placenta, intimately fused. Left cord has a single umbilical artery (SUA); right cord is being injected without transfer of fluids.

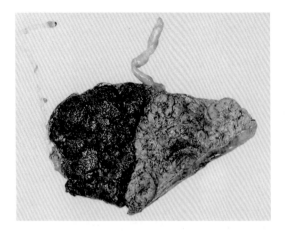

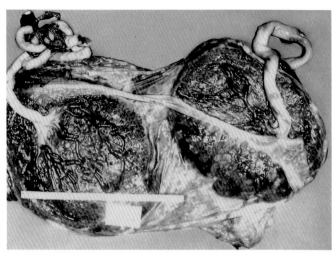

FIGURE 25.50. A DiDi fused twin placenta, maternal surface. Twin at left is Rh-negative and living; twin at right is Rh-positive and macerated. There were two corpora lutea at delivery. Note the clear dividing line between the two placentas.

FIGURE 25.51. A DiDi twin placenta with irregular chorionic fusion. The chorion laeve of the left placenta overlaps one third of the placenta at right. There is no vascular fusion.

This finding is also borne out by a sharp line that divides the placentas, easily seen when one twin has died before birth (Fig. 25.50). A frequent and unusual feature of DiDi twin placentas is the phenomenon of irregular chorionic fusion, a feature well shown in Figure 25.51. In such placentas, the membranes do not meet over the areas perfused by the individual fetuses; in fact, the placentas may be separated, and a portion of one may be covered by the membranes of the other. This phenomenon is best explained by assuming that the intraamnionic fluid pressure of one cavity gradually expands its sac, pushing the other away (Fig. 25.52). It is not unlike the process of lifting the marginal chorion in cases of circumvallate placentation. It has no influence on the well-being of the fetuses, and no vascular fusion takes place in the areas of overlap.

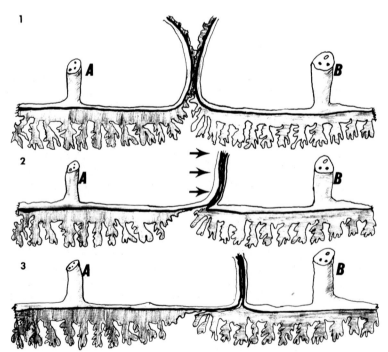

FIGURE 25.52. Presumed mechanism that leads to irregular chorionic fusion as in Figure 25.51.

When the fetal outcome of fused DiDi twin placentas is compared with that of separated DiDi placentas, Buzzard et al. (1983) found that there is a greater difference in birth weights with fused placentas. The inference is that placental proximity has a prenatal influence on fetal development, perhaps because of competition for space during placental expansion. On occasion, prenatal diagnosis mistakes the membrane relations and other features of consequence to fetal survival. Thus, Baergen et al. (1995) described a placenta after recurrent leakage and hemorrhage, also with SUA; the placentas were fused but one twin had died because of being born within an extramembranous gestational condition.

Vanishing Twin Phenomenon

It is not uncommon that one twin dies long before birth. If the pregnancy continues undisturbed, this fetus may disappear when it is very young. It may become flattened (fetus compressus, fetus papyraceus), or when it is large, it may macerate, lose much of its fluid, and become misshapen. Although fetus papyraceus has long been known, the phenomenon of a "vanishing twin" is a more recent addition to our nomenclature. The term should be reserved for multiple pregnancies that are identified sonographically during the first 15 weeks of pregnancy and that have, as their outcome, a single fetus. It must be appreciated, however, that the rate of occurrence will always be underestimated. For instance, we have seen many placentas from ART practices where we know that several blastocysts were placed and implanted but in whose placentas there was no morphologic evidence of a vanished twin.

The seminal report on the vanishing twin was that of Levi (1976), who repeatedly studied sonographically 6690 early pregnancies. Of 118 patients identified to have twins, only 86 sets of twins were delivered. When the diagnosis of twins was made prior to 10 weeks, the disappearance rate was 71%. When the diagnosis was made between 10 and 15 weeks, the disappearance rate was 62%. When twins were first diagnosed after 15 weeks, none disappeared. Similar figures of twin resorption (70%) were reported by Robinson and Caines (1977).

The vanishing twin is thus a feature of early pregnancy; its diagnosis is made by the ultrasonographic finding of two echogenic "rings" denoting the presence of two sacs. Although the existence of vanishing twins is not doubted, the possibility of error in the diagnosis of twin gestations was mentioned by Levi. It was expanded upon in greater detail by Landy et al. (1982), who reviewed the literature and wrote a letter of inquiry to colleagues. It is possible

that a yolk sac or amnionic sac that is still separate from the chorion or other features of early embryonic life are occasionally mistaken for twin cavities (e.g., Green & Hobbins, 1988). Moreover, only rare reports of placental examination have accompanied these studies. Even more rarely have empty sacs or old hemorrhages been identified. An exception is the report by Jauniaux and his colleagues (1988). They reported the placental findings of 10 such cases, five of which came from IVF, and five were spontaneous. First trimester bleeding was the only clinical evidence of this occurrence. In five cases, the vanished twins were identified as "well delineated plaques of perivillous fibrin deposition, associated in one case with embryonic remnants." There are other reports of frequent early vaginal bleeding episodes in these patients. Those events may represent the spontaneous abortions of twins. If the reported cases are applicable to the general population, the excessively high frequency of calculated twin gestations is surprising.

The term *vanishing twin* was perhaps first used by Jeanty et al. (1981). It is now an established entity in obstetrics, and more careful study of the placenta is needed to secure its place. When such a twin is found sonographically or only a remnant of a second sac is identified, every attempt should be made to obtain some karyotype information from the chorionic sac at birth. The results from such studies may eventually indicate whether these vanishing twins are chromosomally abnormal. Additionally, RFLP should define zygosity readily.

Such fetuses would perhaps have been aborted were it not for the presence of a normal twin in the same uterus. Gruenwald (1970) described three such specimens, two of which, however, are best considered to be fetus papyracei. One specimen consisted of a local thickening in the membranes that, when sectioned, disclosed ribs and other fetal tissues. We have seen numerous placentas with vanished twins enclosed in the membranes, but their presence had not been detected sonographically or was not anticipated. Figures 25.53 to 25.56 show what their appearance may be. In all of these specimens, clear evidence of a second sac existed. In two of these cases and in several others we have observed, tiny embryos could be identified. Those embryos had surely died before 8 weeks' gestation. The fact that they were still recognizable suggests that when a vanished twin cannot be detected in the term placenta, the diagnosis must have been either erroneous, or an empty sac of a "blighted" ovum had been present and aborted. It is surprising in the embryos shown here how long an embryonic structure can coexist with a normally developing twin. A similar early, vanished embryo was first shown by Bergman et al. (1961) in their description of a "blighted" fetus. The tiny embryo, also present in the membranes, was essentially similar to the one shown in Figure 25.54. The empty-sac feature was further

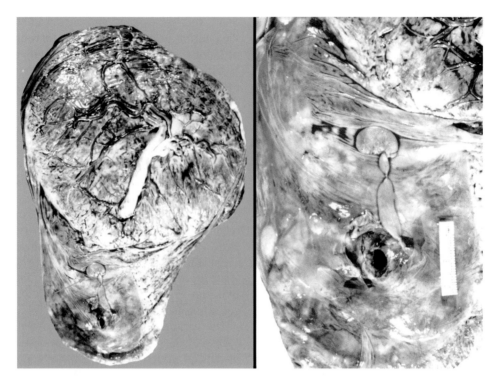

FIGURE 25.53. A DiDi separated twin placenta at term. The patient presented with alleged "abruption." A normal term twin was delivered; a second placenta with a tiny (2 cm) embryo was found in the membranes. When its sac was opened (right), a yellow embryo of the opposite sex was attached to a swollen umbilical cord.

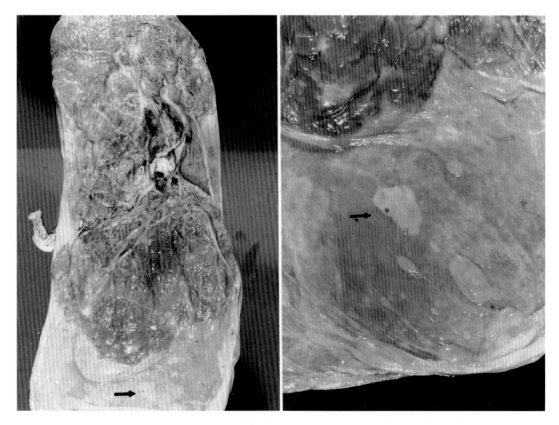

FIGURE 25.54. A term placenta with a separate embryo in the membranes (arrows). This embryo is similar to that shown by Bergman et al. (1961). The ocular pigment is readily seen. No placental remains were seen.

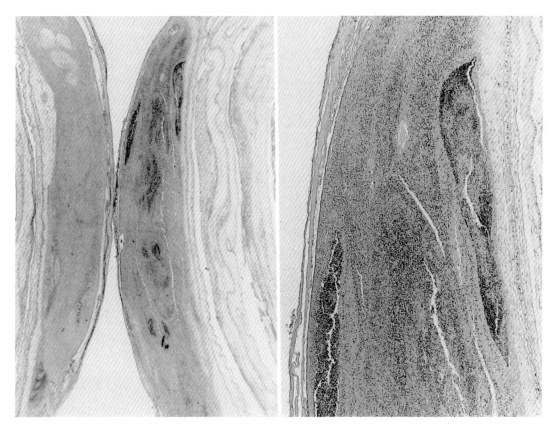

FIGURE 25.55. Membrane roll with embryo of Figure 25.54. Macerated embryonic structures are visible. H&E ×16 (left); ×60 (right).

discussed in the prospective study of 1000 pregnancies by Landy et al. (1986). The authors calculated a minimum twinning incidence from this material as 3.29%, if not 5.39%. This is very much higher than the currently esti- mated twinning frequency of the general population. These authors suggested that vanishing twins may possi- bly be the source of rhesus sensitization. In view of the small quantities of blood potentially present to stimulate

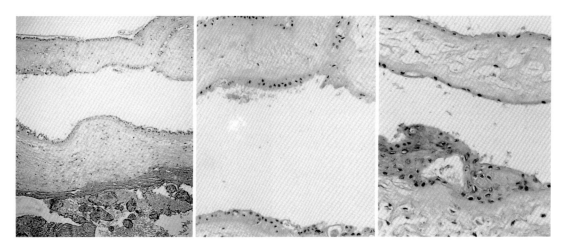

FIGURE 25.56. Mature placenta with vanished twin. A subamni- onic sac containing debris is the remnant of a DiMo placenta. Note the squamous metaplasia (right), vacuolation (center), and amnion nodosum-like degeneration (left top). H&E ×16 (left); ×40 (center); ×60 (right).

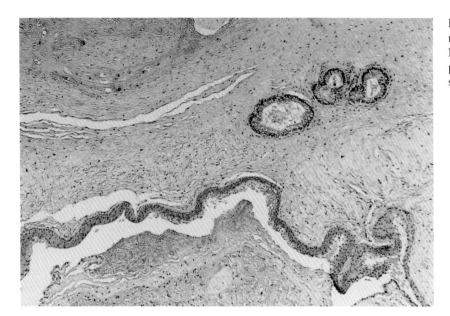

FIGURE 25.57. Remnant of a triplet in the membranes of a term DiMo twin placenta. Note the inclusion of columnar, mucus-producing epithelium and a cyst with squamous lining in the chorion. H&E ×60.

the mother, this proposal seems to represent an unduly pessimistic concern. Sulak and Dodson (1986) have presented evidence for two vanished triplets by demonstrating an empty chorionic sac. When the placental sac of the surviving singleton was studied, it was found to be filled with debris. Kapur et al. (1991) found an empty cavity of a former twin associated with a sirenomelic co-twin whose pregnancy was terminated at 18 weeks. Triplets had been diagnosed sonographically 4 weeks after conception by IVF. It is more difficult to be certain that such structures as are shown in Figure 25.57 are the remains of vanished embryos, in this case a triplet, although we prefer to believe this view rather than ascribing these rests to be teratomas. In their study of 189 sonographically studied twin pregnancies, Yoshida and Soma (1986) found that 21 twins died. Nine qualified for the term *vanishing twin*. The association with prenatal bleeding was also emphasized by these observers. Sebire et al. (1997c) identified 102 monochorionic and 365 dichorionic twins between 10 and 14 weeks; they found a higher fetal loss rate in the former (12.2% vs. 1.8%) before 28 weeks. Perinatal mortality and prematurity were also significantly higher in monochorionic twins.

In the differential diagnosis, it must be cautioned that retromembranous hemorrhages may occur after amniocentesis and they can also occur spontaneously, that is, without our knowing the cause. Such hemorrhages must not be mistaken for vanished twins. The typical sonographic appearance of a small vanishing twin with normal co-twin at 14 weeks is shown in Figure 25.58.

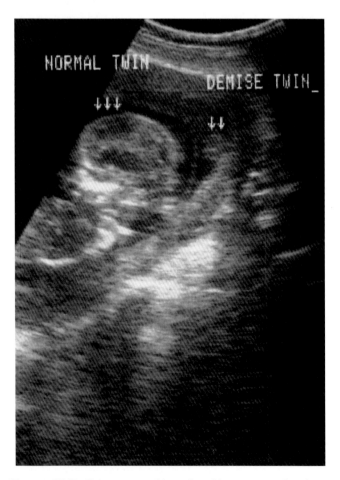

FIGURE 25.58. Sonogram at 14 weeks with one normal and one dead ("vanishing") twin. The latter still has a separate cavity and measures 1.7cm. (Courtesy of Dr. J.D. Stephens, San Jose, California.)

FIGURE 25.59. Diminutive fetus papyraceus in the membranes of a normal twin's placenta (arrows). Its dichorionic placenta was a flattened mass of fibrin.

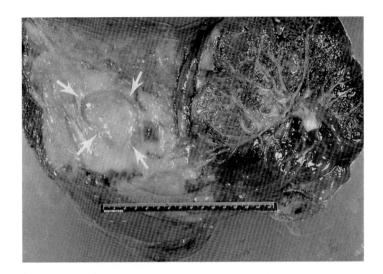

The presence of vanished twins or of a fetus papyraceus has posed other difficult clinical problems. It has thus been reported that the maternal α-fetoprotein (AFP) may be significantly elevated in pregnancies complicated by a vanishing twin (Lange et al., 1979). The finding of high AFP and acetylcholinesterase levels has led to therapeutic abortion, the vanished twin not having been diagnosed (Winsor et al., 1987). There may also be an elevation of the amnionic fluid acetylcholinesterase levels. In the case described by Cruikshank and Granados (1988), this elevation was blamed on coexisting aplasia cutis. It goes without saying that such gestations also are not recorded as twin gestations in most hospital statistics.

Fetus Papyraceus

A fetus papyraceus forms when one of twins or higher multiple pregnancies dies during gestation and becomes compressed as pregnancy continues. There is no clear distinction between the vanishing twin and a fetus compressus or papyraceus. Although such fetuses exist fairly frequently, they are often overlooked. They may be so compressed that small ones are found only when a careful inspection of the placenta and its membranes is made (Fig. 25.59). We recommend that radiographs be obtained when such areas of thickened membranes are found and that the area be dissected carefully. The case shown in Figures 25.60 to 25.63 is a typical circumstance

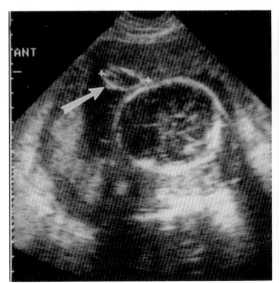

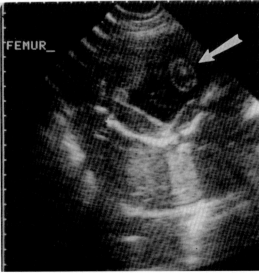

FIGURE 25.60. Sonogram of twin pregnancy with fetus papyraceus. The skull is seen at the arrows; the normal twin's skull is next to it (left); femora are at the bottom. (Courtesy of Dr. G.R. Leopold, San Diego, California.)

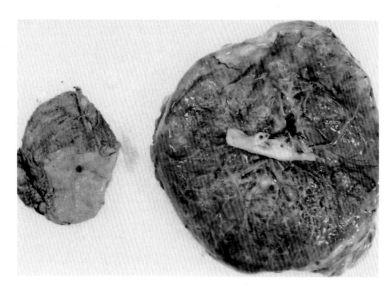

FIGURE 25.61. The specimen at term shown in Figure 25.60. The fetus papyraceus was in a separate mass at left.

(Jackson & Benirschke, 1989). Sonographically, a typical fetus compressus was demonstrated (Fig. 25.60); at delivery it was a separate mass of fibrin compressed in the membranes of the normal twin's placenta (Fig. 25.61). Careful peeling of the DiDi membranes showed the fetus compressus with umbilical cord (Fig. 25.62), whose skeleton was normal by radiography (Fig. 25.63). The fetus compressus of Figure 25.64, on the other hand, was enclosed in a separate amnion. It was an acardiac twin with SUA and had six toes. The frequency of finding a fetus papyraceus has increased substantially in recent years. This is mostly the result of intentional reduction of fetuses in ART patients in whose pregnancies too many embryos existed, where premature birth was anticipated, or in whom a smaller number of infants was requested. This ablation is commonly undertaken by intracardiac injection of 1 ml KCl and example is shown later (see Fig. 25.98). It is advantageous to take radiographs of such fetuses because these occasionally disclose unknown anomalies; in this case, an encephalocele was discovered. Yaron et al. (1999) incisively discussed this issue in their study of 143 triplets (12 controls) that were reduced to twins. It lowered the frequency of prematurity and IUGR.

Several of these compressed fetuses had living co-twins with skin defects (Fig. 25.65). Some have well defined, infarcted placentas (Figs. 25.50 and 25.65). In others, one can demonstrate that twisting of the umbilical cord at its fetal insertion was the presumed cause of demise. The cause of death, however, is not always discerned. Thus, when the donor in the transfusion syndrome dies, its placenta may be so atrophied or infarcted that the causative

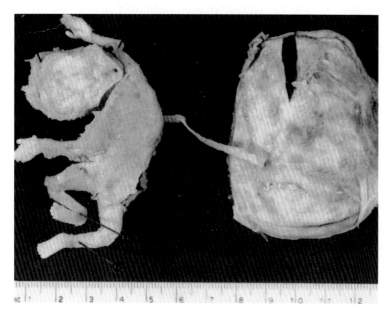

FIGURE 25.62. Same case as in Figures 25.60 and 25.61. The dissected fetus is attached to a short umbilical cord.

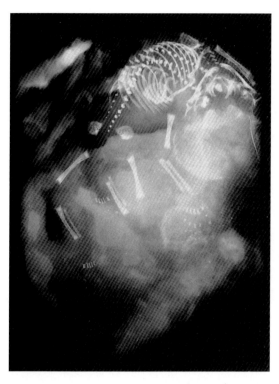

FIGURE 25.63. Radiograph of the specimen in Figure 25.62, showing a normal skeleton.

vascular anastomoses can no longer be verified. Chromosome preparations of the macerated twin are rarely feasible because of the advanced state of maceration. Cytogenetic examination may be possible, however, from samples of the chorionic membranes, as would be an RFLP study, which should be attempted. At least once, such a study of the DNA of a fetus papyraceus showed it to have a dizygotic relation to the living twin (Lemke et al., 1993). Acardiac fetuses are readily distinguished radiologically and by dissection from the normal, usual fetus papyraceus. A careful study of these vanished twins is doubtlessly worth the effort. Although it seems useless to dissect a fetus papyraceus, it proves to be quite feasible when it is done in a continuous stream of water. It has been suggested that vanishing twins may be associated with the CNS defects of cerebral palsy in the survivor (Pharoah & Cooke, 1997), but their later systematic inquiry (Newton et al., 2003) showed this not to be the case. Moreover, the detailed study of Hargitai et al. (2003) of placentas in patients with cerebral palsy found no vanished twins. When fetal demise occurs later in the gestation of monochorionic twins with vascular anastomoses (and then usually with larger fetuses), however, cerebral palsy (CP) in the survivor is a distinct possibility, as Liu et al. (1992) determined (see also Glinianaia et al., 2002). A thoughtful comment on the (small) prevalence of CP in twins vs. the overall CP problem needs to be considered; this is important so that in larger prospective series zygosity, ART and chorionicity can be individually dissected for their individual relevance to the origin of CP in multiples (Blickstein, 2004). Other investigators have weighed in on the possible neurodevelopmental sequelae of TTTS. Thus, Cincotta et al. (2000) followed 23 children and found that 22% had significant abnormalities. Banek et al. (2003) studied outcomes after laser ablation and identified minor abnormalities in 11%; major CNS deficits were found in another 11% of cases. The ensuing letters by de Lia and Worthington (2003) and the replies need to be read for a complete assessment, regarding not only the complex methods of surgery but also the difficulty of correct evaluation. When no laser ablation is

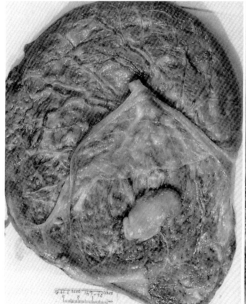

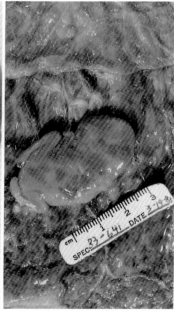

FIGURE 25.64. Fetus papyraceus in a separate amnion (DiMo placenta). It had SUA and six toes, and was an acardiac upon dissection.

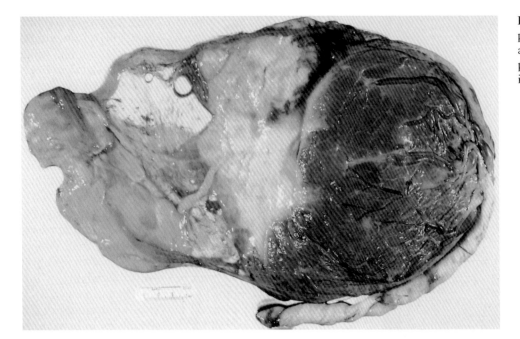

FIGURE 25.65. Typical fetus papyraceus with cord visibly attached to the infarcted twin placenta (DiMo). The surviving twin had scalp defects.

undertaken, the CNS morbidity is even higher (Lopriore et al., 2003). It might also be mentioned that, on very rare occasion, after demise of the recipient twin, the donor (!) may develop acutely hydrops fetalis (Ries et al., 1999). Wataganara et al. (2005) showed that laser ablation in TTTS leads to a persistent elevation of circulating fetal DNA levels in the maternal circulation.

When maceration is advanced, the fetus may have the appearance of a **lithopedion** (Fig. 25.66). This feature is more commonly found when a fetus is retained for months beyond the expected gestation; indeed, it need not even be a twin (e.g., El-Sherbini, 1963). The formation of a lithopedion is particularly commonly described in retained fetuses of nonhuman primates (e.g., Mueller-Heubach & Battelli, 1981; Swindle et al., 1981). Miller and Dillon (1989), who cited relevant literature on the frequency of lithopedion, estimated that perhaps 400 cases had been described. They presented the case of a 94-year-old woman with lithopedion that had been present for probably 61 years without doing harm. One of the most unusual placentas of a presumed former twin in our collection is depicted in Figure 25.67. It is the placenta of a normal infant at term, with marginal insertion of the cord. In the center of the larger placental mass was what appeared to have been the site of insertion of another cord, with fetal vessels radiating to it. No twin was found, as was also the case with Moshiri et al. (1996), who found 16 cases of lithopedion reported in the literature. They added another case, occurring in an 86-year-old woman and presumably having originated 44 years earlier. Not to be outdone, Speiser and Brezina (1995) found a lithopedion in a 92-year-old woman that had been present

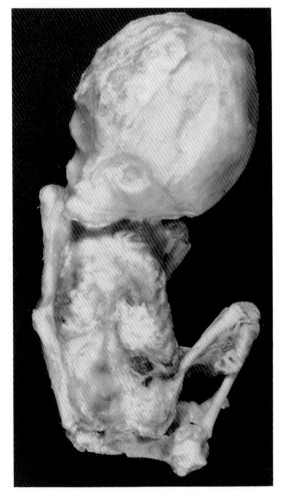

FIGURE 25.66. Fetus papyraceus with the appearance of a lithopedion.

FIGURE 25.67. Term placenta with near-marginal insertion of the cord. At the arrow is a structure that has the appearance of a second cord, with fetal vessels radiating toward it. No twin was found.

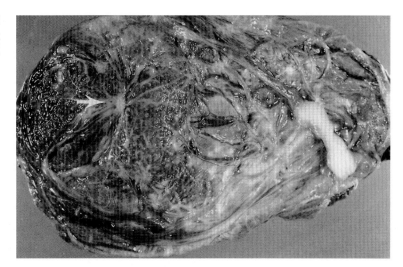

presumably for 60 years. It had the size of a 31-week-gestation fetus.

On occasion, a large fetus papyraceus presents with dystocia at delivery (Leppert et al., 1979). A fetus papyraceus may also be one of triplets (Roos et al., 1957; Benelli, 1962) (see Fig. 25.43). It has also been reported to us that a triplet placenta was associated with two fetus papyracei (Shih, personal communication, 1986; see also Esposito, 1963). They may be of monochorionic or dichorionic gestations; congenital anomalies other than acardia have been occasionally identified on dissection. The co-twin of a fetus papyraceus may also have anomalies, such as microcephaly, absent ear (Roos et al., 1957), gastroschisis (Weiss et al., 1976), ileal atresia (Saier et al., 1975), or pulmonic stenosis (Baker & Doering, 1982; reviewed by Szymonowicz et al., 1986). In a discussion of a case of ileal atresia, Sander (1983) drew attention to the possible cause of these anomalies. He suggested that they may have a prenatal thrombotic etiology, in analogy with the phenomenon of DIC discussed above. Whether the occasional scalp lesions in co-twins of fetus papyracei are analogous to the aplasia cutis described by Mannino et al. (1977) is not clear. Demmel (1975), who reviewed all types of neonatal skin defect, does not mention the occurrence of macerated co-twins with these cases, but then the placenta was probably not examined in his somewhat older case population. A case similar to that of Mannino et al. (1977) was presented by McCrossin and Roberton (1989). Although their case was complicated by toxoplasmosis, the extensive skin defects of this neonate were essentially similar to the aplasia cutis described by Mannino et al. They were also in the process of healing at birth, and as early as 18 weeks' gestation a macerated, much smaller twin was demonstrated sonographically. Lemke and colleagues (1993) described extensive aplasia cutis in a twin associated with a dizygotic fetus papyraceus; regrettably the placenta was not studied.

Innumerable reports of fetus papyracei have been published in the literature. The bulk of these cases from the older literature may be found in the comprehensive review by Kindred (1944) and publications of the material from the clinics of Litschgi and Stucki (1980), Yoshida and Soma (1986), and Johnson et al. (1986). Kindred reviewed 150 cases that had been published up to 1944. Of the 141 cases with adequate information given, 66% were dichorionic twins and three cases were MoMo twins. Mills (1949) was critical of many of Kindred's concepts. He reported three sets of monochorial twins, one of which was macerated. He wanted to distinguish mummified from compressed fetuses when many authors make no such distinction. In our opinion, that question is moot. Litschgi and Stucki (1980) observed five dichorial and eight monochorial (one MoMo) twins. They suggested that when a macerated twin is recognized, delivery should occur by the 39th week. That this advice is not uniformly accepted was mentioned earlier in the chapter.

For unknown reasons, death of the other twin may follow when a fetus papyraceus is present (Camiel, 1967; Yoshida & Soma, 1986). Forman (1956), who described a case with dichorionic placenta, stated that fetus papyraceus was first mentioned by Pliny (70 A.D.). Johnson et al. (1986) attempted to ascertain the incidence of fetus papyracei in 34,677 deliveries from their hospital. A total of 515 twins were observed, of which 27 (5%) had a single intrauterine fetal death; 16 of 25 (64%) liveborn co-twins survived. The placenta was monochorial in 70%. One survivor had multiple infarcts, another had a gangrenous leg at birth, and several had thrombi. Puckett (1988) discussed the management of pregnancies when a second trimester twin dies, and Chescheir and Seeds (1988b) observed the spontaneous disappearance of hypofibrinogenemia following in utero death of a twin. They suggested that prophylactic heparin therapy is not warranted when one of twins dies. Enbom (1985), who reported two cases of antenatal death of one of DiMo twins, was also fearful of this thrombotic complication and reviewed the literature. The survivors did not show sequelae of DIC. Foot necrosis and thrombosis of placental vessels were recorded in the survivor after fetal death of one twin by Margono et al. (1992). That this can occur in the living recipient twin of TTTS was shown by Hecher et al. (1994b). They observed necrosis of digits while the donor twin was still living and attributed it to both the recipient's high hematocrit and "steal" because of the presence of a single umbilical artery. Bass et al. (1986) observed persistently elevated amnionic fluid AFP and acetylcholinesterase levels after death of one twin, findings supported by Streit et al. (1989).

Carlson and Towers (1989) also found that in the 17 multiple gestations with fetal death of one twin they studied, there was significant risk to the survivor. Their review suggested that fetal death of one twin occurs as often as in 2.6% of multiple gestations and three times more often in monochorionic than dichorionic twins. This occurrence is the reason why Cox et al. (1987) have used fetal blood sampling in the surveillance of such surviving twins.

Szymoniwicz et al. (1986) reported six cases of a monozygotic twin surviving with CNS defects after the death of a co-twin 1 to 11 weeks before delivery. They also reviewed the 16 reports in the literature (with a total of 53 such cases) and concluded that delivery should be seriously considered when one twin dies in utero. In their survey of these cases, 72% had CNS defects, 19% had gastrointestinal (including liver and spleen) defects, 15% had renal lesions, and 8% had pulmonary lesions. Anderson et al. (1990) found not only CNS necrosis but saw also bowel injury in two of four cases with prenatal demise of a monochorionic twin. Szymoniwicz et al. described placental thrombi in some of their cases and continuing hematuria that lasted 2 weeks in such a survivor, suggesting a continuing process that was initiated before birth. Their vascular disruption hypothesis suggested infusion of thromboplastins, but they gave no account of the placental vascular anastomoses of their cases. The report by Liu et al. (1992) of 41 cases with one prenatal death gave similar findings and suggested that exsanguination is the primary cause of injury to the survivor. Other aspects of intrauterine death of one twin are discussed in some detail by D'Alton and Simpson (1995).

Twin-to-Twin Transfusion Syndrome

The twin-to-twin transfusion syndrome (TTTS) is considered to be a specific entity in twins, caused by the unidirectional, prenatal transfusion of blood through AV anastomoses in the monochorionic twin placenta. It occurs in approximately 10% of monochorionic twins with dismal prognosis (Gul et al., 2003). One twin is the "donor" and the other is the "recipient." Its severity totally depends on the nature and direction of the anastomotic circulation. The syndrome was first clearly delineated by Schatz (1882, 1886), when he observed a set of monochorial twins with gross discordance in size and development. One was edematous and urinated many times before dying at 12 hours of age; the other was a hypotrophic twin who never urinated and who had an empty bladder at death (53 hours). The atrophic twin had decubiti of the knees and ankles, much like the aplasia cutis described by Mannino et al. (1977). Schatz (1882) had already suggested that the fetal vessels were anastomotic through a "third circulation," which he was subsequently able to demonstrate clearly by injection of the DiMo placenta. He hypothesized also that the anastomoses were the cause of the fetus papyracei. In fact, he had described the "stuck twin" from clinical observations alone. This "third" circulation was then clearly perceived as proceeding from one of the donor's superficial (terminal) arteries into a shared cotyledon, whence it drained into the venous circulation of the recipient (Fig. 25.68). This anastomosis is thus a capillary one. It is not always easy to demonstrate unless careful injections are made with thin liquids of selected areas in the placenta. It is highly speculative just how it is that such complex anastomoses of twin placental vascular beds develop and why they are so variable. Gaziano et al. (2000) produced a diagram of the hypothetical implantation of such twin blastocysts and suggested that the monochorionic monozygotic "twin blastocyst has an intrinsic polarity

Twin-to-Twin Transfusion Syndrome (TTTS)

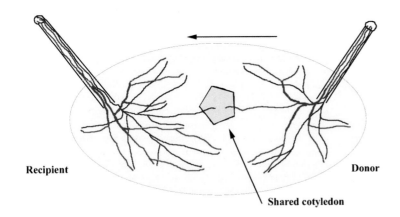

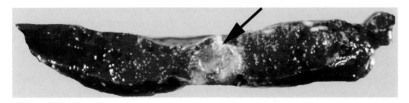

Recipient   Donor

Shared cotyledon

FIGURE 25.68. Top: Principal vasculature connection that causes the transfusion syndrome of MZ twins. Bottom: The shared cotyledon here was injected with water; it appears blanched. Note that the right half of this placenta is paler than the recipient's left half.

defect at implantation." This is difficult to comprehend, and, naturally, it lacks anatomic support at this time. Perhaps the embryo splits with different cell numbers and hence the onset of cardiac perfusion of placental villi differs. All is speculation at this time, and the only new insight that we can foresee about how new data can become available is by descriptions of really early stages of DiMo twin specimens. With the advent of successful therapy by laser ablation of the connecting vessels by De Lia et al. (1985a), there has been a veritable flood of publications, some of which are discussed here in some detail. Insight has come from four or five different center in Europe and the U.S., centers that have dominated in the practice of laser therapy. Often they have also differed in their approaches, the results, interpretation of the fluid mechanics of this syndrome, and other aspects that pertain to interpreting the TTTS. Moreover, De Lia et al. (2000) stated that the syndrome is influenced by aberrations of the maternal metabolism and that these need to be corrected in order to optimize fetal survival.

Because AV anastomoses may be multiple and of varying size, and they may also proceed in opposite directions, the syndrome is variable in its consequences. This point has been elegantly shown with Doppler ultrasonographic studies of pregnancies complicated with this syndrome (Pretorius et al., 1988a). Pretorius et al. found it easy to demonstrate greater placental vascular resistance in one fetus, findings that were also shown in the therapeutic intervention in this syndrome by De Lia and Cruikshank (1989). Pretorius et al. (1988a) were unable to predict from their studies which was the donor, and they were also unable to anticipate the outcome. They confirmed that "the transfusion syndrome is an extremely complex dynamic physiologic state." Hecher et al. (1994a) delineated the Doppler signals of AA anastomoses and later described the various anastomoses as they were identified during surgery (Diehl et al., 2001). In 126 cases of severe TTTS they saw AV anastomoses in all, 31% also had AA, and 12% had VV connections. Denbow et al. (2000) as well as Umur et al. (2002) found that AA anastomoses largely protected against the severe forms of the TTTS, whereas VV connections reduced perinatal survival. Denbow et al. (2004) were able to determine modest flow rates in AA anastomoses by Doppler waveform analysis. Similarly, Tan et al. (2004) demonstrated the flow and concluded that "detection of A-A anastomosis predicts higher perinatal and double survival in TTTS, independently of disease stage." In an interesting case report, Tan et al. (2004) showed the acute first onset of TTTS in a twin gestation in which a previously patent AA anastomosis became obliterated. A somewhat oversimplified classification (A to D) was proposed for monochorionic placental anastomoses by Bermúdez et al. (2002). Nevertheless, it demonstrated that, in general,

only the "deep" AV anastomoses are the critical ones. But other problems with this system as well as the method of demonstrating anastomoses for this classification were pointed out by Taylor et al. (2003). This reply to the paper addresses primarily the method of demonstration of anastomoses and the protective effect of large direct surface AA connections. Needless to say, these points are critical for understanding TTTS and, especially, for appropriate therapy. To anticipate more adequately the timing and method of therapy, Quintero et al. (1999, 2003a) introduced a method of staging the TTTS (stages I–IV). It has also allowed better follow-up of the results and is now being widely employed, albeit with modifications (Fisk et al., 2004). De Lia and Cruikshank (1989) found markedly greater vascular resistance in the donor. Bromley et al. (1992) suggested from their experience with 12 sets that, when clinical manifestations were clear-cut at 20 weeks, the prognosis with conservative therapy was poorer than when the syndrome was diagnosed later in gestation. In general, TTTS has a poor prognosis if it remains untreated. A later review of the sonographic techniques, especially the findings at Doppler study and others employed in this differential diagnosis, is to be found in the publication by Plath and Hansmann (1998). Taylor et al. (2000a) attempted to predict the outcome of TTTS by prenatal sonographic features; absent AA anastomosis, abnormal venous pulsatility, and reversed end-diastolic flow in the donor's artery had poor prognosis. Later (2000b) they were able to detect AA anastomoses (better in later gestation) and mapped sonographically also the AV connections (2000c). Ishii et al. (2004) have since shown that excessive flow in the umbilical vein of the recipient changes after laser surgery. But there is still much controversy over the presence of AA anastomoses in stage III TTTS, as can be seen in the contribution by Taylor et al. (2004) and the detailed criticism by Van Gemert et al. (2004). Indeed, what is observed endoscopically as specific color or pulsatility may not reflect in what is seen by injection studies later. Actually very few publications discuss injected placentas from the postlaser studies, and these show that some AV areas were missed at surgery (De Paepe et al., 2004). As indicated above, Bermúdez et al. (2002) have proposed a categorization of TTTS placental types: A, no anastomoses (0%); B, only deep anastomoses (100%); C, only superficial anastomoses (5.6%); and D, deep and superficial anastomoses (79.12%). They recommended this classification for the purposes of adjudicating results from laser surgery and thereby suggested also that, despite direct superficial connections, TTTS may still occur.

It is important to realize that the precise angioarchitecture of cotyledonary perfusion has not been sufficiently delineated, and that this is extremely difficult to do. The focal injections with milk, water, air, etc. do not provide a permanent record that can be scrutinized minutely. Therefore, plastic injections have been performed such as shown in Figure 25.21. Even when these are handled with a delicate digestion procedure, they are hard to interpret. The situation is worse when a placenta has had laser surgery and is perhaps weeks after the procedure. Wee et al. (2005) have attempted to correct this in a plastic injection procedure that is detailed and followed by acid corrosion of monochorionic placentas (one with TTTS). Their findings contradict what has been generally assumed to be the case for "shared cotyledons." They suggest from their study that intercotyledonary fine anastomoses exist below the chorionic plate that cannot be seen externally by inspection. When examining the color pictures in some detail, we conclude that this possibility cannot be completely ruled out but also that these putative anastomoses are hard to characterize because the acid digestion has also removed the chorionic plate. If these subchorionic anastomoses truly exist (and their mechanism of formation is hard to envisage), then this would make selection of shared cotyledons for laser ablation even more difficult than it already is. But also, the success with most ablations becomes more difficult to understand. More work of this type is needed.

Clinically, the transfusion syndrome is typically first recognized by acute hydramnios that develops around mid-gestation. Many authors have made crucial observations since Schatz's description (e.g., Wurzbach & Bunkin, 1949), and a summarizing review comes from Lopriore et al. (1995). When sonograms or radiographs are obtained after the hydramnios appears, the presence of a twin pregnancy is often recognized for the first time, although the sizes of the twins may already be significantly different (Schneider et al., 1985; Brown et al., 1989). In these cases, the placenta is later almost always found to be monochorial. The occurrence of acute hydramnios is considered to foreshadow a somber prognosis (Weir et al., 1979); one twin may show edema, best recognized sonographically in the scalp (Wittmann et al., 1981). The amounts of amnionic fluid vary enormously. Thus, we have learned of a remarkable case of DiMo twins with severe hydramnios; at 20 weeks' gestation, the amount of amnionic fluid was 5000 mL (withdrawn); another estimated 2000 mL was left unaspirated (K.L. Staisch, personal communication, 1976).

Not all authors agree with the concept that anastomoses may be the ultimate cause of the hydramnios in monochorionic twin pregnancies (Krauer, 1964). Perhaps the first to voice his opposition to Schatz's notion of excessive urination of the recipient twin was Forssell (1912). He incorrectly interpreted that the placentas had "endarteritis" in their main-stem vessels, and that the cause of the hydramnios was a degenerative amnionic epithelial change. These changes are clearly secondary. There is so much variation in the clinical expression of the transfusion syndrome that care must be exercised before making the diagnosis on clinical grounds alone (Wenstrom et al., 1992). Magnetic resonance imaging (MRI) has been usefully employed for the differential diagnosis (Brown & Weinreb, 1988). Not all hydramnios with twins, particularly chronic hydramnios, is due to the transfusion syndrome (Dorros, 1976). Accurate sonographic differentiation of the dividing membranes, therefore, should be attempted (Mahony et al., 1985; Townsend et al., 1988; D'Alton & Dudley, 1989). When acute hydramnios is found in a twin pregnancy, the second twin often has little or no amnionic fluid (oligohydramnios). This twin may move much less than the recipient, so the term *stuck twin* has been applied to this feature (Hashimoto et al., 1986; Brown et al., 1989; Patten et al., 1989a; Mahony et al., 1990). When Berry et al. (1995) evaluated hematologic and chemical parameters in such twins by cordocentesis, they found that all stuck twins had a minimally 2.4 g/dL less hemoglobin concentration. On rare occasion a stuck twin may result from triploidy (Wax et al., 1998).

To better explain the mechanism of hydramnios in this syndrome, Nageotte et al. (1989) proposed involvement of the atrial natriuretic peptide (atriopeptin) in the pathogenesis. In two cases they found markedly elevated atriopeptide levels in the recipient and lower levels in the donor of this syndrome (2251 vs. 43 pg/mL, and 134 versus 79 pg/mL). They suggested that the hormone is released because of the recipient's hypervolemia, and that its elevated levels may be responsible for the renal effects. Talbert et al. (1996), as well as Bajoria et al. (2002, 2003), found elevated atrial natriuretic peptide and endothelin-1 levels in the recipient twin and inferred it to be a sequel of failing heart in the recipient, perhaps also being important for amnionic fluid regulation.

This prenatal unidirectional exchange of blood results in deprivation of nutrients from one twin and excessive development of the other. The twins may be remarkably discordant, as seen in the classical example shown in Figures 25.69 to 25.71 (also see Fig. 25.73). One twin was dehydrated and anemic, and possessed organs that were significantly smaller than expected for the stage of development. The recipient was plethoric and had much enlarged organs and higher mean arterial blood pressure after birth that quickly became normal (Cordero & Johnson, 2002; Cordero et al., 2003). The discrepancy was particularly striking in the heart, but other organs were similarly affected. Lazda (1998) believed that the discordance of fibroelastosis occurring in two recipient twins were the ultimate result. In the absence of AA anastomoses, the hydramnios leads to very premature labor or to rupture of the membranes, with delivery before the 30th week of gestation. Alternatively, one twin may die

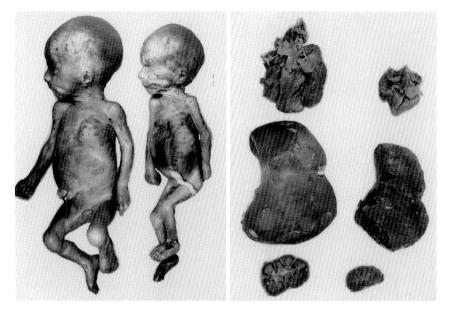

FIGURE 25.69. Twins with the typical transfusion syndrome. MZ twins at 27 weeks, delivered after two amniocenteses (4000 and 3000 mL) had partially relieved the hydramnios. Recipient (left): 540 g, edema, heart 12.5 g, liver and one kidney less severely hypertrophied. Donor (right): 410 g, heart 2.7 g.

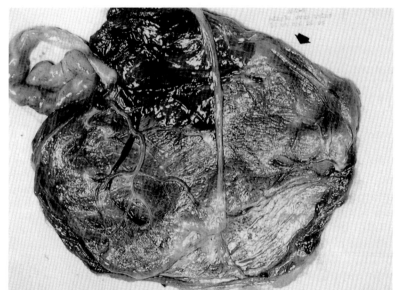

FIGURE 25.70. The placenta of the DiMo twins in Figure 25.69. Recipient had an edematous cord (left). The cord of the donor (right) is torn and was marginal. Note the area of common villous district (arrow; see also Figure 25.71).

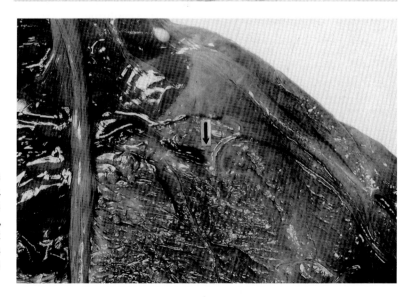

FIGURE 25.71. Common villous district of the case in Figures 25.69 and 25.70 is shown at the arrow. An artery from the donor (at right) dips into the placental tissue and emerges as a congested vein, coursing to the recipient (at left). The oval body at top is the remains of the yolk sac (single); there is also slight amnion nodosum in this cavity of the donor, who had oligohydramnios.

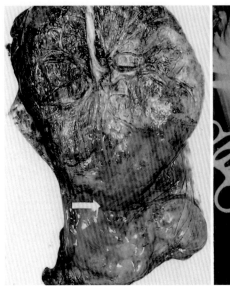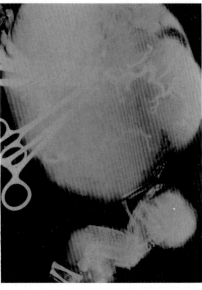

FIGURE 25.72. A DiMo twin placenta with fetus papyraceus. Severe hydramnios at 20 weeks abated spontaneously. One twin died at that time: The pregnancy normalized, and a normal twin was delivered at term with this fetus compressus. Its placental portion was completely infarcted.

and become a fetus papyraceus (Fig. 25.72). In that case, the hydramnios ceases nearly immediately and the pregnancy may reach term. The same is true when the anastomoses are obliterated by laser therapy (De Lia et al., 1990, 1993). Another alternative of the development of TTTS was described in some detail by Nikkels et al. (2002). They found acute onset of TTTS at 25 weeks following spontaneous thrombosis of a venous connecting branch.

The development of intracranial hemorrhage in the recipient has been witnessed to occur already in utero, and periventricular encephalomalacia in the donor of this syndrome may also take place (Hurst & Abbitt, 1989). Other pathophysiologic consequences of the syndrome have occasionally been recorded when prompt neonatal studies were undertaken. The set of DiMo twins with the transfusion syndrome whose data are shown next were delivered at 27 weeks' gestation and they were studied unusually well. The mother had preeclampsia, hydramnios, and placenta previa, and she had required a cesarean section. Both twins developed hyaline membrane disease and intraventricular hemorrhage. Their data were made available to me by colleagues from Minnesota. Because the results are so impressive they are shown here:

Parameter	Donor twin	Recipient twin
Age at death (hours)	25	28
Birth weight (g)	732	1100
Head circumference (cm)	23.5	26
Initial hemoglobin (g/dL)	3.2	22.4
Initial hematocrit (%)	12	70.5
Blood pressure (mm Hg)	20	50
Liver at autopsy (g)	42.4	32.2
Pancreas (g)	1.5	2.1
Kidneys, two (g)	7.7	13.8
Adrenal glands, two (g)	3.9	3.1

Some other cases in which clinical values are given are listed as follows (weight in grams, hemoglobin in grams per deciliter, hematocrit in percent):

Source	Donor	Recipient
Klingberg et al. (1955)		
Weight (g)	1770	2690
Hemoglobin (g/dL)	3.7	25.2
Hematocrit (%)		87
Sacks (1959)		
Weight	1431	2084
Hemoglobin	5.5	24
Weight	1424	1843
Hemoglobin	18	30
Hematocrit	58	75
Weight	2041	2523
Hemoglobin	12.8	33
Hematocrit	93	
Weight	1021	1162
Hemoglobin	15	27
Hematocrit	41	80
Kresky (1964)		
Weight	1900	2600
Hemoglobin	11.3	22.1
Hematocrit	42	77
Bolens et al. (1968)		
Weight	2410	2510
Hemoglobin	25.9	13
Hematocrit	90	47

Many other reports of blood values at birth have been published, with wide variations. At times, the hematocrits reached astounding values. In a case referred to us, the plethoric newborn had necrosis of one leg due to arterial thrombosis. The other extremities infarcted shortly thereafter (Dr. J. Pritchard, personal communication). Partial necrosis of the left foot of a recipient twin was seen by Hecher et al. (1994b) at fetoscopic laser surgery of a case

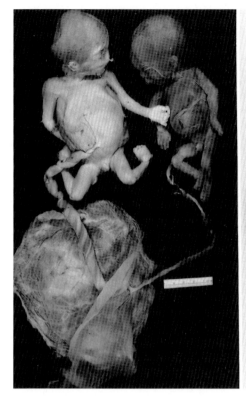
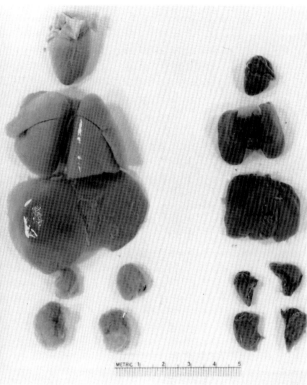

FIGURE 25.73. Macerated DiMo twins with the transfusion syndrome at 28 weeks' gestation. The donor (B) is plethoric, the recipient (A) is edematous and pale. A: 285 g; 15-cm crown–rump (CR) length; heart 3 g; lungs 10 g; liver 17.5 g; kidneys 1.5 g.

B: 189 g; 13-cm CR length; heart 0.7 g; lungs 3 g; liver 4 g; kidneys 1 g. The plethora of twin B is thought to be due to this twin's earlier death, with exsanguination of A into B.

of TTTS. The fetus had an absent right umbilical artery, and vascular "steal" was assumed to be the etiology. Polycythemia was believed to have been the cause of necrosis of the lower extremity in a recipient twin reported by Scott and Evans (1995). Similarly, Dawkins et al. (1995) found a foot necrosis due to hyperviscosity of a recipient twin whose TTTS had been managed aggressively with amniocenteses. Skin necrosis on the thigh, resembling aplasia cutis, was observed in the survivor of a transfusion syndrome case with laser surgery at 16 weeks (Stone et al., 1998). It is not certain how this defect occurred; it healed quickly after birth at 31 weeks. Some of the reports contain expressive color photographs of the twins (Becker & Glass, 1963). There is no correlation between the infants' size, the length of gestation, and the degree of plethora observed at birth. Moreover, the plethoric twin may be the smaller of the two, as seen in Figure 25.73. This discrepancy can be explained only when the anastomoses are carefully delineated, and the circumstances of birth are known. This topic was especially well discussed in the case reports by Donnenfeld et al. (1989), and Bendon and Siddiqi (1989). An equally striking case is shown in Figures 25.74 and 25.75. The DiMo twins were both stillborn, but histologic preservation was better in the anemic twin, and it is assumed that it died last. The

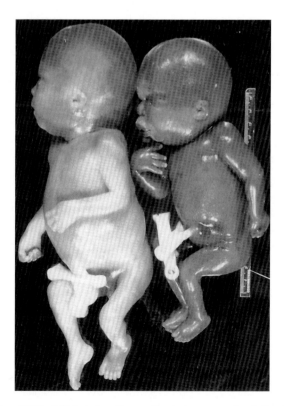

FIGURE 25.74. DiMo twins, the smaller being severely plethoric. The smaller size of the twin at right is due to the velamentous insertion of the umbilical cord.

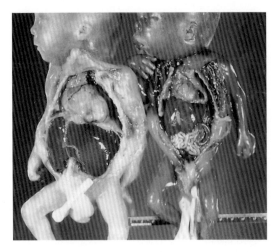

FIGURE 25.75. Same twins as in Figure 25.74. Note the smaller heart in the smaller and plethoric twin (right). See text.

weights of such twins (Figs. 25.74 to 25.76) are important and are as follows:

Organs	Anemic twin	Plethoric twin
Body (g)	550	410
CR length (cm)	20	17.5
Heart (g)	11.3	3
Lung (g)	11.9	5
Spleen (g)	1	0.5
Liver (g)	37.2	8.3
Adrenals (g)	2.3	1.4
Kidneys (g)	4.9	2
Thymus (g)	0.9	0.2
Brain (g)	0	40

The smaller twin was growth-restricted because of its velamentous insertion of the cord. This case does not represent a twin transfusion syndrome. The plethora was caused by reverse flow from the now-anemic twin, occurring through the large AA anastomosis (demonstrated with milk injection) because of his longer survival. In several other cases of discordant twins that we autopsied,

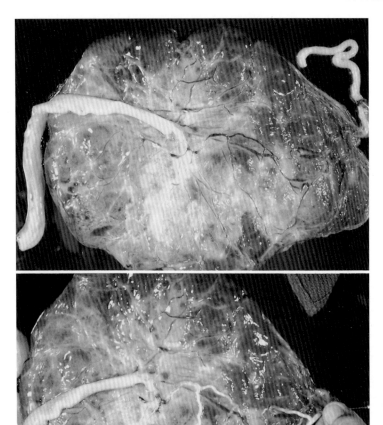

FIGURE 25.76. Placenta of twins in Figures 25.74 and 25.75. One large AA anastomosis exists. Through this anastomosis, the larger twin, who died last, must have exsanguinated into the plethoric twin. This situation is not the transfusion syndrome.

the donor was plethoric. Clinical information and sonography indicated in each case that the plethoric twin had died first; the anemic recipient died later (in one case from listeriosis). Autopsy confirmed the transfusion syndrome from the marked discordance of cardiac size (Benirschke, 1992, 1993; Benirschke & Masliah, 2001). Indeed, it is our opinion that discordance of relative cardiac size is the most important means for the diagnosis of the transfusion syndrome. The fact that after birth of one twin (and after demise as well) rapid blood shifts may occur between the twins often negates the usefulness of hematologic values; furthermore, the placenta is frequently too damaged for accurate analysis of anastomoses. This is forcefully supported by the studies on fetal organ growth of Naeye (1964a,b), Pridjian et al. (1991), and Barr (1996). Moreover, Lachapelle et al. (1997) found in all recipient twins they studied echocardiographically thickened ventricular walls, and Simpson et al. (1997) reported common cardiac dysfunction in the recipient twins, as did Bajoria et al. (2002). A thoughtful review of the diagnostic pitfalls comes from Weiner and Ludomirski (1994), who diagnosed the disease by finding divergent hematologic values from prenatal cordocentesis. They also showed that amniocentesis did not alter the degree of blood shunting between the twins.

Several authors have addressed similar unusual findings. Lehndorff (1961), who also reviewed the relevant literature, assumed that in most cases the transfusion takes place during the terminal periods of delivery, when pressure changes occur because of uterine contractions. Klebe and Ingomar (1972) also believed that much of the transfer occurs during labor. With variable cord clamping practices, it may occur immediately after birth. We have seen a pertinent case. New term twins with significant birth weights had hematocrits of 32% and 63%, respectively. The smaller twin was plethoric and had no problems; the larger twin was anemic and required transfusion. The smaller twin had velamentous insertion of his umbilical cord, with much old retromembranous hemorrhage behind the cord insertion. Injection of the DiMo placenta showed that two large AA anastomoses existed, in addition to AV shunts. The villous blood content appeared similar, but the smaller twin's placental portion was much smaller. Our interpretation is that the growth-restricted twin (because of the velamentous cord insertion) was eventually unable to withstand the pressure column exerted from the larger twin that took place through the AA anastomoses; he thus became plethoric, perhaps during the terminal stages of labor. No cardiac hypertrophy was found in the larger twin, there was no hydramnios, and the fact that this pregnancy went to term suggested that it was not the classic twin transfusion syndrome. Features of long-term circulatory aberrations include cardiac hypertrophy, thromboses, and the presence of nucleated red blood cells. These findings bespeak the prolonged prenatal problem of adjustment to different circulatory phenomena.

The youngest specimens that we have observed to have signs of a well-established circulatory imbalance were a set of DiMo twin abortuses of about 10 to 12 weeks' gestation (Fig. 25.77). Although those twins were still similar in size, their hearts were already grossly discordant. In another specimen of stillborn twins at 15 weeks, the plethora of the recipient was evident and the cardiac hypertrophy already well expressed (2.28g vs. 0.67g). Despite this marked discrepancy, the bodies were virtually identical in their sizes and weights. The differences of fetal size commence later in gestation, usually after 25 weeks

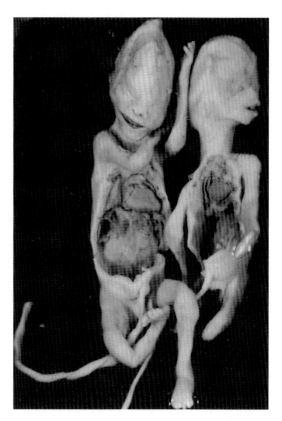

FIGURE 25.77. DiMo twin abortuses with the transfusion syndrome, at about 11 weeks' gestation, weighted 31 and 20g; 8 and 7cm CR length; and the hearts weighed 440 and 193mg. This picture is the earliest evidence of the transfusion syndrome, with marked cardiac enlargement but relatively few bodily differences as yet.

(see also Benirschke & Masliah, 2001). Aherne et al. (1968) and Arts and Lohman (1971) reported that the anastomoses in typical transfusion syndrome twins are usually transvillous and do not involve the larger surface vessels. It must be reemphasized that the mere plethora of one twin and anemia of the other do not necessarily signify the existence of the transfusion syndrome. To make the diagnosis of the transfusion syndrome it is important that the twins be of different size; and as minimal criteria they should have different heart sizes as well. It is clearly possible that large AA or VV anastomoses allow rapid transfer of blood when pressure relations change during parturition, and that the anastomoses can result in anemia or polycythemia, but differences in blood values alone do not justify the term *transfusion syndrome*. Indeed, there is much argument as to what clinical parameters to use when designating a set of twins as having the transfusion syndrome. In some opinions, it is a hemoglobin difference of more than 5g/dL; others also wish to include a coincident weight difference of more than 20%. These aspects were discussed by Danskin and Neilson (1989), who studied 178 consecutive twin pregnancies with a variety of parameters. They concluded that generally acceptable guidelines are not yet available, as dichorionic twins with such differences were found in their series who clearly did not have the syndrome.

Quantitative placental studies have rarely been undertaken on the placentas of the transfusion syndrome. Sala and Matheus (1989) addressed this issue with a relevant case. They found that the plethoric recipient had thinned trophoblastic villous covering and that the villous vessels were markedly distended. In contrast, the anemic "donor" had thick trophoblast and frequently "empty" villous capillaries. They also undertook a stereologic study of the villous architecture and provided quantitative data of differences in villous development. Their case is unusual in several ways. The hydramnios that one might have expected was apparently not present; it was presumably absent because the pregnancy came to near term. That is distinctly unusual for the untreated transfusion syndrome. Although there was the expected marked difference in neonatal sizes (2470 vs. 1920 g), hemoglobin levels (29.3 vs. 10.0 g/dl), and hematocrit val ues (75% vs. 24%), the placenta had an AA anastomosis. The smaller twin had velamentous insertion of the cord. The fact that there was an AA anastomosis and that the pregnancy was carried to 36 weeks' gestation makes this observation less typical, and the data may not fit the usual cases of the immature gestation with the classical syndrome. Bendon (1995) made a thorough study of 21 monochorionic placentas with injection of different colors. His findings indicated that the placental features are complex in the TTTS and that placental weight correlated with fetal weight, whereas hematologic values were often erroneous. Because of this remarkable complexity Van Gemert and Sterenborg (1998), and Van Gemert et al. (1997, 1998a,b) and Talbert et al. (1996) have constructed dynamic computerized models in order to understand the contribution of different types of anastomoses to the TTTS. They help in understanding the intricacies of the "third circulation" and must be read in the original because of their complexity. It is likely that through greater accuracy of

Doppler flow observations in the placental surface vessels of monochorionic twins (see Gaziano et al., 1998) and such physical models, we will learn more precisely what pathologic alterations of blood flow are most responsible for the syndrome. This will also help the laser surgeon in the elimination of the offending vessels, and Van Gemert et al. (1998c) have suggested how therapy based on knowledge influences outcome. Because the umbilical cord coiling index (Chapter 12) in the recipient twin of three cases studied was twice that of the donor, Strong (1997) suggested that this "pump" may have implications in the etiology of TTTS. How best to demonstrate the third circulation (i.e., shared cotyledons) is shown in Figure 25.78. The always available milk was used to inject specific suspicious shared cotyledons. They are thus clearly distinguished.

The frequency of the transfusion syndrome is difficult to estimate, but observations suggest that it is more common than is usually cited (Shah & Chaffin, 1989; see also Lopriore et al., 1995). Urig et al. (1990) reviewed their cases of all twins and found the transfusion syndrome to have occurred in one of 30 twin pregnancies. They also emphasized that there is wide spectrum of severely affected twin pregnancies and less severe cases; thus, assigning a precise frequency, and accurately assessing therapeutic efficacy, is difficult. For unknown reasons the syndrome has been reported to be very much more common in female twins (Nores et al., 1997). Bebbington and Wittmann (1989) found 25 cases in their series of 595 multiple pregnancies, that is, approximately 4% of twin gestations, which perhaps involves 5% to 10% of twins with monochorial placentas. Reviews of the syndrome are to be found in papers by Kloosterman (1963), de Marco

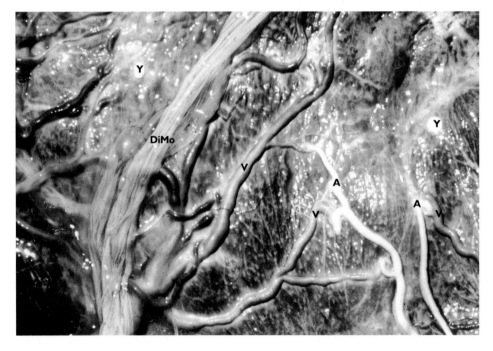

FIGURE 25.78. DiMo twin placenta whose arteries were injected with milk. The "shared cotyledons" can be identified by the color change as the milk returns from the villous capillaries and is pink. A, artery; V, vein.

(1964), Rausen et al. (1965), and Corney and Aherne (1965) and in more recent textbooks, but agreement about the precise criteria is not easily obtained among the many points of view (Bruner & Rosemond, 1993). Single cases from different countries make other literature available: Littlewood (1963), Van der Kolk (1964), Verger et al. (1963), Tojo et al. (1971), Koranyi and Kovacs (1975), Tuncer (1970), Sekiya and Hafez (1977), and others too numerous to cite. When the condition is diagnosed before 28 weeks of gestation, the overall survival rate was found to be only 21% (Gonsoulin et al., 1990b). Hydrops correlated with poor survival in this study, but decompression by amniocentesis was not beneficial in the outcome. The condition has also been described in one of triplets and higher multiple births, as for instance in the triplets described by Sekiya et al. (1973), another by Chasen et al. (2002), and yet an additional case reported by Baschat et al. (2003). Berg et al. (2002) reported onset of TTTS at 11 weeks in an ART-conceived quadruplet gestation with quadramnionic, trichorionic placenta. The most remarkable and exceptional case of TTTS was reported by Quintero et al. (2003b), who described a male/female set of twins with monochorionic placentation and anastomoses.

Aside from differences in weights and blood values, the transfusion syndrome has many other consequences. For instance, hyperbilirubinemia is often seen in the recipient (Conway, 1964), and Reisner et al. (1965) found symptomatic hypoglycemia in the donor to be a frequent neonatal complication. They speculated that it may be an etiologic factor for "mental subnormality" in the twin's future. Falkner (1965) challenged this idea on the basis that the investigators had inadequate data. Reduced placental perfusion in the territory of the donor was held to be responsible for the marked differences seen during placental examination of these twins (Aherne et al., 1968). They suggested that the small placental volume may also have consequences related to reduced nutrient retrieval from the placenta, which they deduced would lead to fetal malnutrition. Conversely, one may speculate that the presumably lower blood pressure of the donor circulation prevents a normal placental expansion and that it may relate to the high incidence of velamentous cord insertion. The constant loss of blood proteins into the recipient twin through the arteriovenous shunt may be another important factor for poor fetal growth. Oberg et al. (1999) for instance showed remarkably different development of the renal tubular apparatus. They interpreted this to general hypoperfusion of the donor twin. Abraham (1967) has shown dramatic differences in the villous structure of the two twins' placental villi. He suggested that the term *parabiotic circulation*, as used for experimental animal studies (Linke & Kuni, 1969) and sometimes applied to this syndrome, is not an appropriate designation. The term was popular at a time when immunologic phenomena were first studied in depth, but it should no longer be used for twins. Abraham (1967) showed the lack of uniform concordance of hemoglobins with birth weights of 53 pairs in an interesting way:

Twin	No. with low hemoglobin	No. with high hemoglobin
Big	6	24
Small	19	4

The remarkable anemia of one twin's placental portion and polycythemia of the other's placenta was studied by Michaels (1967), and Aherne et al. (1968). Not only are the macroscopic features striking in their color difference, but the histologic structure of villi can differ substantially as well (Figs. 25.79 and 25.80). The discordant organ development in twins with the transfusion syn-

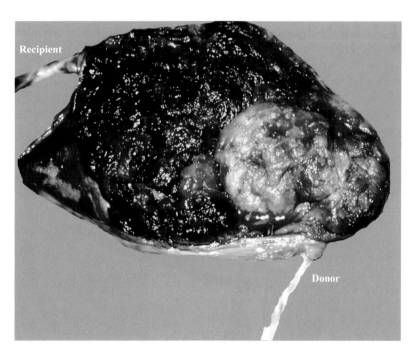

FIGURE 25.79. A DiMo twin placenta at 34 weeks. Recipient had congestive heart failure (2160 g, hyperbilirubinemia, blood pressure 70 mm Hg). Its placental portion (left) is plethoric and thicker. The donor (anemic, thin portion of placenta at right) weighed 940 g and died neonatally. (Courtesy of Dr. S. Kassel, Fresno, California.)

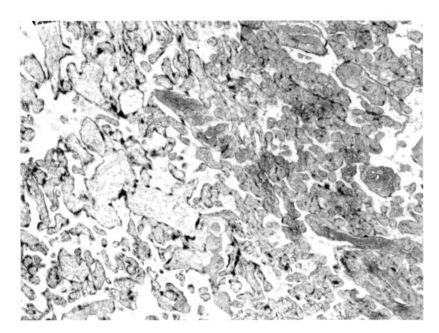

FIGURE 25.80. Histologic appearance of the two twins' placental portions. The donor's placenta (left) is much more immature in appearance than the villi of the recipient (left), which are smaller and congested. H&E ×160.

drome has been variously studied by several authors. Thomas (1962) found not only hypertrophy of cardiac muscle fibers in the plethoric twin but also that hyperplastic changes existed. Fesslova et al. (1998) observed echocardiographically features of cardiac hypertrophy in this condition, judged to be reversible. Barrea et al. (2005) studied the cardiovascular response of TTTS in more detail and with sophisticated methods. Their conclusion was that the recipient more commonly suffers damage and has cardiac hypertrophy and predominantly ventricular dysfunction, and that despite amnioreduction, the cardiovascular dysfunction persists. Naeye (1964a,b, 1965; Naeye & Letts, 1964) undertook the most comprehensive organ analyses. Within this framework he was much concerned with hypoglycemia. By quantitative studies of tissue components, he found that the donor had significantly reduced, and the recipient had significantly increased, cytoplasmic material. Differences of nuclear size and composition were less striking. He likened the findings to malnutrition in the donor and was particularly concerned with the reduction of brain weight. Studies of fetal growth parameters in various categories of twins (grouped according to placental type) confirm the essential findings of Naeye (Pridjian et al., 1991). DiMo twins were found to "have a high degree of brain-sparing growth restriction in the smaller twin and cardiac hyperplasia in the larger twin, most likely caused by hemodynamic inequalities." When Chauhan et al. (2004) studied the chorionicity of 126 sets of twins sonographically in an effort to determine if IUGR related to the type of placentation, they found that monochorionic twins had twice as much discordance in growth when compared with dichorionic placentation. Winner (1963) asserted that the different development was perhaps due to unequal

genetic contribution from unequal splitting of the twins. That opinion does not bear in mind the complex nature of the syndrome. It is an ill-founded criticism. Naeye correctly retorted (1963), for example, that the presumed erythropoietin production by the donor would be equally distributed between the twins, and that the already plethoric twin would be stimulated to even greater hematopoiesis by infusion of blood from the anemic co-twin. Schwartz et al. (1984) described subcutaneous erythropoiesis in the donor twin, akin to the familiar "blueberrymuffin spots" of newborns with cytomegalovirus and rubella virus infections.

Marx (1956) described the glomerular hyperplasia of the recipient twin's kidney in a report of a hydropic triplet with the transfusion syndrome. He conjectured that the increased perfusion of the kidney, under higher pressure, was responsible for this enhancement of glomerular development. He deduced, as did Schatz, that this situation led to the increased urination and hydramnios. The urine output (Kirshon, 1989) and pathophysiology of the syndrome were further elaborated on by Achiron et al. (1987), but the direct cause of this glomerular hyperplasia remains unresolved. Studies in patients with polycythemia (Corrin, 1961) have shown that it is not the cause. Glomerular hyperplasia has been observed in patients with tetralogy of Fallot (Bauer & Rosenberg, 1960) and cor pulmonale (Ellis, 1961). In these situations, hypoxia was thought to be the most important etiologic factor. In addition to changes in glomerular structure, Naeye and Blanc (1972) found dilatation of renal tubules. They deduced that excessive urination was the cause of the hydramnios. That the recipient urinates excessively had been decisively demonstrated by Schatz (1882). In the interesting discussion that followed that paper, Schatz expressed the opinion that the donor may have some amnionic fluid remaining because of sweating. Shah and Chaffin (1989) found a 55% overall mortality due to this syndrome. An interesting observation was reported by Popek et al. (1993). They found three monochorionic twins with prenatal calcification of the pulmonary artery in the absence of valvular anomalies. Two twins were "pump" twins of an acardiac fetus, the other the "recipient" of the transfusion syndrome. The authors speculated that this complication was due to increased prenatal cardiac output (see also Samon et al., 1995).

Mahieu-Caputo et al. (2000) and Kilby et al. (2001) studied the renin-angiotensin system in the kidneys of donor and recipient twins and found overexpression of renin in the donor's glomeruli. Various renal sequelae were found and discussed extensively such as tubular apoptosis (De Paepe et al., 2003). They are secondary phenomena, however, not primary features of the TTTS. It should also be mentioned that Bajoria et al. (2000), finding significantly amino acid concentrations in the two twins, believed that this is an indication that the severe growth restriction of the donor may not be due primarily to the anastomotic loss of blood but that it is the possible result of impaired transplacental transport of amino acids. We differ with this interpretation.

We have twice attempted to re-create the transfusion syndrome in sheep, pregnant with fraternal twins (Resnik & Benirschke, unpublished). Having inserted intravascular catheters, we transferred daily 10 mL of blood from the female to the male twin over 17 days. Our findings included the following male/female weights: total, 3600/3375 g; hearts, 24.5/23.5 g; livers, 96.5/86.0 g; spleens, 10.5/5.2 g; kidneys, 27/22 g; and cotyledon, 440/370 g. The second experiment, done closer to term, gave similar results. Thus, one can simulate the transfusion syndrome experimentally and perhaps better understand the adaptations that occur subsequent to the twin transfusion. Wilson (1979) studied the postnatal growth of dissimilar twins and concluded that "monozygotic twins become progressively more concordant with age . . . while dizygotic twins became less concordant."

It was earlier stated that the recognition of twin-related hydramnios during early pregnancy has a bad outcome unless one twin dies. The transfusion then stops, and often the survivor is delivered near term and is normal (Fig. 25.72). At the other end of the spectrum, various management schemes have been proposed for the twins after their birth, for example, that by Shorland (1971), which sought to correct the anemia, hypoglycemia, polycythemia, and hyperbilirubinemia. Before birth, incisive treatment is more difficult and controversial. The thoughtful review by Blickstein (1990) puts the various diagnostic modalities and treatment regimes into an unbiased perspective. Temporizing for a month by repeated amniocentesis and withdrawal of fluid is sometimes feasible for a while (Figs. 25.69 to 25.71) but not for long (Feingold et al., 1986; Vetter & Schneider, 1988; Lange et al., 1989; Elliott et al., 1991; Elliott, 1992; Reisner et al., 1993). There is a large literature on this topic, and the results are not uniform. Nevertheless, when an international trial of amniocentesis vs. laser ablation was conducted, it was stopped prematurely because the results were infinitely better with laser therapy (Senat et al., 2004). That publication (and two publications by Ropacka et al., 2002, and Odibo & Macones, 2002) reviewed many of the prior publications of various techniques (corticoids, amnioreduction, septostomy), and it was followed by a succinct editorial by Fisk and Galea (2004). At present, then, careful sonographic evaluation, followed by laser ablation of the offending anastomoses would seem to be the best means of treating TTTS. Presumably then, the results of therapy depend on the nature of the anastomoses and on the timing of onset of hydramnios. Gary et al. (1996) have shown significant pressure differences in TTTS. Some authors strongly advocate amniocentesis as therapy

(Mahony et al., 1990; Urig et al., 1990; Elliott et al., 1991; Saunders et al., 1992; Dickinson, 1995; Dennis & Winkler, 1997), whereas Gonsoulin et al. (1990a) showed in a careful study that the 21% overall survival rate was not improved by amniocentesis when the syndrome is diagnosed before 28 weeks. Pinette et al. (1993) also showed that early aggressive amniocentesis is an effective therapy, but prolongation of gestation was minimal. Bromley and colleagues (1992) found only a 25% survival rate when the diagnosis was made before 20 weeks, which was higher when the diagnosis was made later and when conservative therapy was instituted. Grischke and colleagues (1990) were similarly skeptical, and one wonders why the therapy is still being used at all. Bebbington and Wittmann (1989) found that gestational outcome depends mostly on age at delivery and that amniocentesis may be beneficial. In a pregnancy in which hydrops and hydramnios had developed, Trespidi et al. (1997) were also more reserved, although their results are fairly encouraging. Smith et al. (1997) provided some Doppler study evidence of "improved hemodynamics" after many amnioreductions. Despite this, there were many dysmorphic findings in the still small donor at delivery. Garry et al. (1998) measured intramnionic pressures in TTTS, before and after amniocentesis. It was significantly higher than in normal gestations and was reduced to normal levels by amniocentesis, findings similar to those obtained by Meagher et al. (1995). In the editorial comments preceding this paper, however, cautionary words are introduced that do not correspond with our views. It was suggested that hemoglobin differences in TTTS were not necessarily correlated with hydramnios, but the fact that exchange of blood through anastomoses at the time of delivery can obscure such data was not considered. The accumulation of fluid is primarily the result of fetal urination, and this has been examined and modeled in great detail by several investigators (Umur et al., 2001a,b, 2002). It is too complex for consideration here. The developing hydramnios is the primary cause of premature delivery in untreated TTTS; rarely, it can also lead to uterine rupture. Tutschek et al. (2004) reported such a case where rupture occurred at 19 weeks, presumably because of previous uterine scarring. De Lia et al. (1985a) treated the mother of a TTTS in utero with digoxin at 27 weeks. They observed reversal of fetal cardiac failure in the recipient twin. The fetuses survived after cesarean section, which was done at 34 weeks. It is worth mentioning that these authors estimated that 2200 fetuses succumb annually in the U.S. from this syndrome alone. Moise (1991) and Jones et al. (1993) failed to arrest the syndrome in three pregnancies by administering indomethacin, whereas Al-Takroni et al. (1995) seem to have more success in their case. Another means of therapy is to divide the intervening amnionic membranes. Saade et al. (1995) did this in two cases with instant filling of the stuck twin's sac; they did not report the outcomes, however. In the nine cases done by Berry et al. (1997), no cord entanglement occurred; there was a change in arterial flow, but no real impact on survival seems to have occurred.

Wittmann et al. (1986) chose to sacrifice the donor of a severe transfusion syndrome case at 25 weeks' gestation. They inserted a needle into the heart under sonographic guidance. After the fetus died, the hydramnios disappeared and the pregnancy stabilized. No obvious maternal coagulopathy developed, and the healthy 2890-g survivor was born at 37 weeks. The fetus papyraceus weighed 180 g. The placenta was DiMo. Subsequently, Baldwin and Wittmann (1990) summarized their favorable experience with this procedure in three cases of the transfusion syndrome. Weiner (1987) had earlier reported a similar experience. In the days that long preceded sonography, we had unsuccessfully attempted a similar procedure (Benirschke & Driscoll, 1967). Another failure was reported by Chescheir and Seeds (1988a). They filled the pleural space of the donor with fluid until there was cessation of cardiac activity. This maneuver normalized the urine output of the survivor, but the hydramnios did not abate. Infection terminated the pregnancy prematurely. One certain way of preventing CNS damage of one of the twins is cord ligation, as was practiced by Crombleholme et al. (1996) in the abnormal MZ twin affected by congenital heart disease.

Under ideal circumstances, it may become possible in the future to obliterate the interfetal vascular connections, which should then lead to complete normalization of the pregnancy. Schatz (1886) already proposed that some vessels may thrombose and thus compromise further blood exchange. De Lia et al. (1985b, 1989) began experimentation with the obliteration of selected fetal surface vessels in experimental animals by treatment with neodymium:yttrium-aluminum-garnet (Nd:YAG) laser. They were successful with this procedure in sheep and rhesus monkeys and then successfully treated three patients with the transfusion syndrome (De Lia & Cruikshank, 1989). Delivery occurred several months after the vascular obliteration, and marked improvement of urination in the donor, with expansion of its amnionic sac, occurred immediately. The placentas showed the scarred cotyledons supplied by the coagulated vessels. Such therapy has now been tried in many cases of the transfusion syndrome. De Lia et al. (1990, 1996) have published much greater details of their experience, including a set of triplets in other articles. These publications also provide additional insight into the instrumentation, methodology, and vascular findings in the twin placentas. In the meantime, De Lia has done more than 100 cases (personal communication, 1998). The results have improved over time, and now at least 80% of patients can take one healthy child home after this therapy. The procedure is now referred to as fetoscopic laser occlusion of chorioangipagous vessels (FLOC). In one case, the authors pursued

the vessels across a tear made in the dividing membranes. This disruption of dividing membranes may not be without hazard. As indicated earlier, amnionic bands may form or the MoMo twins resulting may entangle cords. The prenatal therapy by laser obliteration of vessels has since been practiced successfully by other teams (Natori et al., 1992; Ville et al., 1992, 1995, 1998). It is now even possible to undertake the ablation when anterior placentas are present and, with the exception of the complexity and the need for instrumentation, it is clearly the most decisive therapy for the transfusion syndrome. There is evidence that laser surgery executed by competent surgeons yields better results than repetitive amniocentesis (Ville et al., 1998). An unexplained finding in the transfusion syndrome is the recognition that the recipient has much higher levels of proteins, but that immunoglobulin G (IgG) levels were much out of line in a study by Bryan and Slavin (1974). On occasion the laser ablation fails; this may be the result of failure to recognize all arteriovenous shunts or due to unusual connections. Thus, Poch et al. (2005) have described such a failure and attributed it to the existence of a direct arteriovenous fistula in the donor twin's vascular bed. Only once or twice before have such *direct* AV connections been reported to exist in singletons. They are clearly exceptional. As mentioned earlier, TTTS can occur in triplet or higher number gestations as well. That they are also accessible to fetoscopic ablation was detailed by Sepulveda et al. (2005).

This chapter is not the place to review in detail the ultimate outcome of twin pregnancies. One aspect, nevertheless, is noteworthy. Because monozygosity largely eliminates genetic effects, the transfusion syndrome has served as a model to analyze aspects of the etiology of mental retardation. Several investigators have found that the smaller of MZ twins has a slightly lower IQ than the larger twin (Kaelber & Pugh, 1969; Hohenauer, 1971; Babson & Phillips, 1973). The larger the twins' size difference was at birth, the greater were the effects. Record et al. (1970) did not confirm these results using the data from the Birmingham Twin Study; they pointed out that the differences are postnatal in origin, rather than due to monozygosity and placentation. Likewise, Fujikura and Froehlich (1974) and Buckler and Robinson (1974) studied the postnatal equilibration of MZ twins who had been born with marked natal differences. They found only "negligible differences in . . . intelligence and educational attainment." The complexity of the problem is exemplified by reanalyses of the various data published by Munsinger (1977) and his critic Kamin (1978). The former believed that prenatal influences can be shown to have this deleterious effect; the latter did not. Both affirmed that future studies of this vexing question must include placental data. Denbow and colleagues (1998) found CNS damage in both the donor and recipient of the TTTS and called for more detailed follow-up studies as well. The criticism of former studies is echoed by O'Brien and Hay (1987) in an incisive analysis. These authors found differences when male co-twin development was compared with that of female co-twins. They also studied the effect of placentation on handedness. Left-handedness is known to be more frequent in "birth-stressed" individuals, and it may be for that reason that left-handedness is more frequent among twins (Coren, 1994). A good example of left/right-handedness of MZ twins is shown by Frothingham (1997/8) in twins, one of whom suffered adrenal insufficiency, but the twins were also opposite-handed and cut their hair on opposite sides. This topic, however, is most complex as was decisively reviewed by McManus (2002) in an excellent book.

Acardiac Twins

Acardiac twins are the most severely malformed fetuses that one can imagine. They range from small, teratoma-like masses to large fetuses with a great variety of anomalies. The absence of a heart is not obligatory to the diagnosis of this entity, as a severely malformed heart is occasionally present. Schatz has used the terms *hemicardia* and *hemiacardius* to referred to these twins, but Frutiger (1969) pointed out that these terms are incorrect. He proposed the term **pseudoacardius** for those cases in which remnants of cardiac structures are found. A wide variety of names have been applied to this spectrum of acardiac fetuses; a veritable taxonomy was created, as in Schwalbe's and Schatz's writings. The most comprehensive treatise that encompasses all these attributes is the seminal book of Schatz (1898), who made the major contribution to our understanding of acardiacs. A total of 88 cases from Japan were summarized by Sato et al. (1984), and we have reviewed 49 acardiac pregnancies (Moore et al., 1990).

A human acardiac fetus is one of MZ twins or higher multiple births whose development is severely disturbed, and who usually has no cardiac remnants. There is good evidence that acardiacs are more common in higher multiple births than in twins (James, 1977b). That an acardiac can develop at all is due to the presence of two anastomoses in the monochorial placenta. An AA anastomosis brings blood from an usually normal co-twin to the "monster," and a VV anastomosis returns the blood. The normal twin provides the cardiac flow to the monster but in a reversed fashion. The reversal of blood flow has been proved to exist with the use of Doppler sonography (Pretorius et al., 1988b; Zucchini et al., 1993; Quintero et al., 1994; Coulam, 1996). One interesting exception to the nature of the twin placenta has been published by French et al. (1998), who found a typical acardiac amorphous with anastomoses to a normal twin in a verified DiDi placenta and determined by genetic studies that the twins were monozygotic as well. This challenges our understanding of how the chorionic vascularization in early placentation is accomplished. Schatz observed that the frequent presence of omphaloceles in acardiacs is an important obstruction to venous return, and he believed in an etiologic role. Later studies have not borne out this finding, as many acardiacs lack an omphalocele. Schatz believed that this kind of obstruction could be the cause of many such anomalous infants. We believe that the presence of the two types of placental anastomoses is the fundamental cause of the acardiac dysmorphism and it is just possible that an absent Hyrtl anastomosis contributes. Dichorionic (and DZ) human twins cannot develop into acardiacs as they lack the placental communications, but very rare exceptions have been recorded in which the two placentas have vascular fusions. No blood would be circulated through fetal vessels if a spontaneous acardia were to exist in a DiDi twin, and such an embryo would vanish early. The fact, however, that such placental communications do exist among many fraternal (DZ) twins of some other species was already recognized by Schatz, who discussed the acardiacs found in ruminants and carnivores.

The wide spectrum of the appearance of acardiacs that one can observe is illustrated in Figures 25.81 to 25.85. One of these fetuses had the appearance of a teratoma, turned inside out (see also Jamal, 1999), another had remnants of a face and arms, and the third is unusual in that it had an exceptionally long umbilical cord. Despite

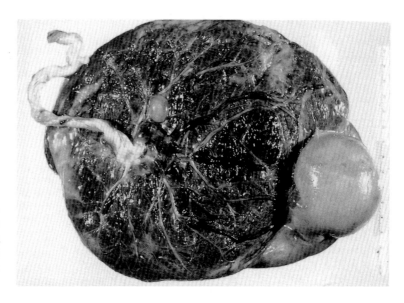

FIGURE 25.81. Acardiac twin, having the appearance of a teratoma. The normal twin was 2910 g, the acardiac ("holoacardius amorphous") weighed 40 g, had a diminutive cord, and was in a MoMo placenta with large anastomoses. (Courtesy of the late Dr. N.J. Eastman, Baltimore, Maryland.)

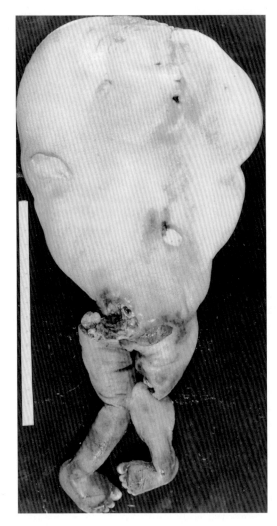

FIGURE 25.82. Well-formed 1210-g male acardiac delivered at 28 weeks. Co-twin died neonatally and had aortic hypoplasia. The acardiac had a skull, remnants of brain, a small spinal cord, and many other organ remnants. (Courtesy of Dr. J.D. Wilkes, New York, New York.)

mation, DiMo placentation was found in 22 cases and MoMo in eight cases (Moore et al., 1990).

Dissection of the fetuses shows many gradations, ranging from a total absence of most organs to well-differentiated structures of others, including gonads. Only liver tissue has never been observed by us. Schatz has written of the same experience. More recently, however, Giménez-Scherer and Davies (2003) demonstrated some liver tissue (with degenerative changes) in three of 18 acardiac fetuses they dissected. Upper limb anomalies were the most prominent findings. Driggers et al. (2002) found a small liver in an interesting acardiac anomaly. It was extremely hydropic and possessed a "severely malformed, almost nonexistent heart." They suggested that at one time in early gestation there had been a TTTS but, because of the cardiac anomaly, twin reversed arterial perfusion (TRAP) developed and caused the edema and other abnormalities. This is a novel way of interpreting the genesis of these complex anomalous twins. A female sex preponderance of acardiacs has been noted by James (1977b). For the study of acardiacs, it is usually best to

the absence of any cerebral structures, the last-mentioned acardiac was sonographically witnessed to move actively. Also well shown in this fetus was the plethora, frequently observed in acardiacs. We believe it represents stagnation of blood, transfused by the pale, normal co-twin. The increased resistance to perfusion has been demonstrated by prenatal Doppler velocimetry (Sherer et al., 1989). The fetal mobility of an acardiac may be so great on occasion that they die because of cord entanglement (Fig. 25.84). In all of the twins shown, the placenta was MoMo but many others have been described with a DiMo placenta. In such cases, there is usually amnion nodosum of the acardiac's cavity because of its deficient or absent urine production. Sonographic examination of such cases then discovers a "stuck twin." Among the 30 acardiac twin pregnancies we studied and that had enough infor-

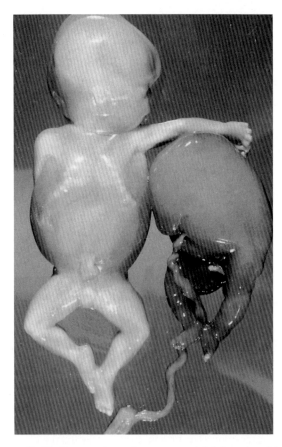

FIGURE 25.83. Exsanguinated premature MoMo twin with plethoric acardiac fetus. This specimen is unusual because of the long umbilical cord. The fetus had been seen to move at sonography; it had no brain but a normal spinal cord.

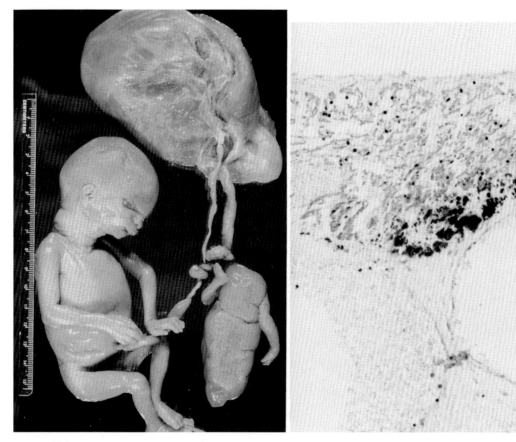

FIGURE 25.84. Macerated MoMo twins, one an acardiac (150 and 20 g). The twins died because of entangling of cords. Note the single umbilical artery of the cord and large AA and VV anastomoses. The acardiac had a remnant of heart with calcification in the remaining muscle fibers. H&E ×160. (Courtesy of Dr. S. Kassel, Fresno, California.)

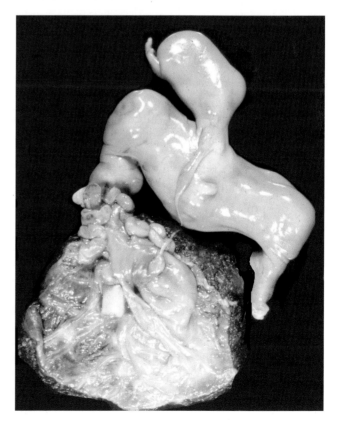

FIGURE 25.85. Unusual acardiac twin whose abdominal contents were embedded on the placental surface (Emery et al., 2004).

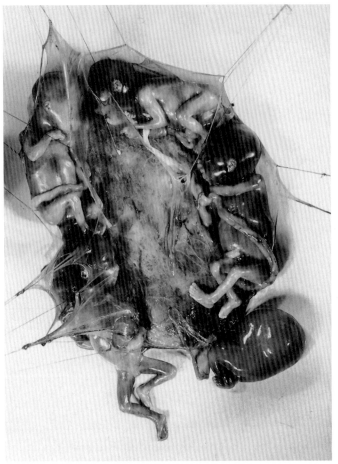

FIGURE 25.86. Acardiac quintuplet in monochorial placenta with five amnionic sacs (bottom right). Note its plethora. Three yolk sacs were identified. (*Source:* Hamblen et al., 1937, with permission.)

obtain a radiograph of the specimen before dissection, as it gives some idea of the complexity of the abnormality, enables better classification, and delineates if a skull is present (Dicker et al., 1983; Bhatnagar et al., 1986).

Most acardiac fetuses have only a single umbilical artery. The absence of one umbilical artery, though, cannot be held responsible for the development of the anomaly because it is not invariable. In contrast to Schatz's ideas, an omphalocele has been absent in at least half of the cases we have seen. One of the few hemiacardiacs we dissected possessed a two-chambered heart (Benirschke, 1970a). This heart and that of another hemiacardiac exhibited endocardial fibrosis. The first twin shown here also had a fairly well formed head with a brain and a bilateral cleft palate. One of monochorionic quintuplets with five amnions was an acardiac fetus (Hamblen et al., 1937) (Fig. 25.86), and we described triplets with one acardiac in the previous edition of this book; many other triplets, one being an acardiac, are recorded in the literature (e.g., Sanjaghsaz et al., 1998). They may be MZ trip-

lets (Ross, 1951; Landy et al., 1988) or multizygotic (Stoeckel, 1945; Wylin, 1971; Kirkland, 1982). The acardiacs described by Amatuzio and Gorlin (1981) were conjoined and associated with a MoMo triplet in heart failure. Parenthetically it may be mentioned that some pregnancies complicated by an acardiac (as in fetus papyraceus, discussed earlier) have unexplained high levels of α-fetoprotein and acetylcholinesterase in their amnionic fluid (Winsor et al., 1987; Entezami et al., 1997). Kaplan (1994; see her Figs. 6 to 12) depicted monochorionic triplets, two of whom had the TTTS, and a third was acardiac.

One of the most remarkable specimens is that described by Fujikura and Wellings (1964) and shown in Figure 25.87. This malformed specimen was attached to the chorionic surface 1.5 cm from the insertion of the umbilical cord of a larger fetus. This more normal twin had amelia of the right arm, phocomelia of the right leg, hydrocephaly, and myelomeningocele; his right umbilical artery was absent. The acardiac was described as a teratoma-like mass. Another description of what we consider to be more likely to have been an acardiac fetus rather than a teratoma is the case discussed by Sironi et al. (1994). We have previously expressed our reservation about chori-

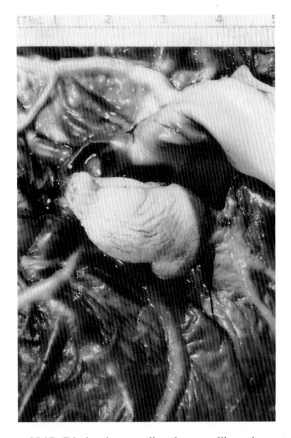

FIGURE 25.87. Diminutive acardiac that was likened to a teratoma. It is 1.5 cm from the cord insertion of a malformed twin with single umbilical artery (SUA). Large vessels led to the mass. (Courtesy of Dr. T. Fujikura, Portland.)

onic teratomas and prefer to think of this specimen as acardiacs who lacked the development of a defined umbilical cord. The presence of a cord is usually a prerequisite for the diagnosis of "acardiac fetus" (e.g., Joseph & Vogt, 1973), although the length of umbilical cords of acardiacs varies from 0 cm as in Figure 25.81 (see also Frutiger, 1969) to 53 cm as in Figure 25.83. The "lack of organization," as emphasized by Fox and Butler-Manuel (1964) in a similar case, is not a strong argument that these masses are teratomas. Such disorganization occurs often in small "holoacardii amorphi" with good umbilical cords. Holoacardii amorphi are not true neoplasms ("teratomas"); they are part of the wide spectrum of acardiac twinning. Kreyberg (1958) reported a similar case and had the same opinion. The differential diagnosis (acardiac or teratoma) was further considered by Stephens et al. (1989), who reviewed 96 cases and presented an additional bovine acardiac fetus. It was their opinion that the presence or absence of an umbilical cord was insufficient evidence for diagnosis, and they relied more heavily on the finding of an axial skeleton. Emery et al. (2004) reported another most unusual case of acardiac twin in a MoMo gestation. Completely separated from the macerated acardiac was its intestinal content enclosed in a sac on the surface of the placenta (Fig. 25.85). It was conjectured that the phenomenon arose from a "detached" omphalocele. As stated earlier, Schatz had even suggested that the omphalocele was the cause of acardiac twin formation; thus this may not be so surprising after all. An excellent example of such large omphalocele was provided by Chmait and Hull (2001).

The **incidence** of acardiac pregnancies is difficult to ascertain, as most are not reported. Gillim and Hendricks (1953) estimated it to be 1 per 34,600 births, or approximately 1 in 100 MZ twin pregnancies. This finding agrees with that derived by Napolitani and Schreiber (1960). Bhatnagar et al. (1986) based their estimate of 1 per 48,000 births on data from a variety of studies. They admitted the probability of a gross underestimate and we agree with this, especially because the advent of ablation by various means of cord obliteration has led to a flood of publications. Most acardiacs are probably not reported in the literature. Well over 600 cases have been reported, and there are probably hundreds that go unpublished. Our own series now exceeds 50 cases, and many of these cases will remain undescribed.

Acardiacs often develop hydrops, and the pregnancy is thus frequently complicated by hydramnios. Hydropic acardiacs may then become much larger than the normal co-twin. The hydropic acardiac described by Pavlica (1967) was such a case. It weighed 2150 g, whereas the co-twin was only 850 g. It was further remarkable that its umbilical cord forked from that of the normal co-twin. Markavy and Scanlon (1978) described additional hydropic acardiacs with hydramnios and considered that

this problem may result from hypoproteinemia. They also observed thrombosis of one umbilical artery in one of these acardiac fetuses.

Because the hydramnios may be severe and the large acardiac may present problems with dystocia (Loughead & Halbert, 1969), Platt et al. (1983) proposed that a ligature be placed around its umbilical cord through an amnioscope. Simpson et al. (1983) were successful in treating a pregnancy with a hydropic acardiac by digitalization. The mechanism of hydramnios and congestive heart failure is complex. It is likely related to the size of the acardiac fetus, but suggestions in the literature allude to a correlation with the presence of renal tissue in the acardiac (Moore et al., 1990). Prospective studies, with ascertainment of urination by the acardiac, are needed. Sullivan et al. (2003) recommended a conservative approach to the treatment. Nevertheless, they lost one "pump" twin of the 10 cases studied.

Another way of treating an acardiac pregnancy is by selective removal of the anomalous twin. Intervention in acardiac pregnancies has been advocated by Healey (1994), who reviewed the outcome of 184 such gestations. He found that 35% of the "pump" twins died (45% in triplets), mainly from prematurity. He also ascertained other risk factors associated with acardiac gestations, such as SUA and MoMo placentation. Selective removal of the acardiac has been successfully accomplished by Robie et al. (1989), who removed a sonographically identified acardiac fetus at 22.5 weeks' gestation that weighed 710 g. A normal twin was subsequently delivered at 33 weeks' gestation. Ash and colleagues (1990) successfully managed such a pregnancy with indomethacin. It led to marked reduction of amnionic fluid volume so that a normal fetus (and 785-g acardiac) were delivered at 34 weeks. Porreco et al. (1991) occluded the umbilical artery of an acardiac fetus in utero with a metal coil. It stopped the reversed flow and led to normal delivery at 39 weeks. Rodeck et al. (1998) successfully thermocoagulated identified connecting vessels in four acardiac gestations. The short cords of most acardiacs was one reason for choosing this new methodology of therapy. McCurdy et al. (1993) endoscopically attempted to ligate the umbilical cord of an acardiac fetus at 18 weeks. Both twins died. Quintero et al. (1994) succeeded with ligating the umbilical cord near mid-gestation through a fetoscopic approach and salvaged the normal twin. The acardiac weighed 31 g at birth. Johnson et al. (2001) provided evidence that the cord can be effectively obliterated by bipolar cauterization in acardiacs as well as the TTTS (Taylor et al., 2002), and Porreco (2004) used percutaneous sonographically guided injection of alcohol successfully. In a DiMo twin with one twin having Turner's syndrome, Tsao et al. (2002) and Shevell et al. (2004) used radiofrequency obliteration of cord vessels successfully. Tan and Sepulveda (2003) reviewed the outcome of 74 acardiac twin pregnancies that were treated by different, minimally invasive methods. These included alcohol injection, monopolar diathermy, and interstitial laser and radiofrequency ablations. Their conclusion was that "intrafetal ablation is the treatment of choice ... because it is simpler, safer and more effective when compared with the cord occlusion techniques." Selective removal of an acardiac fetus was undertaken at 23 weeks after her death in utero by Ginsberg et al. (1992), with the normal twin proceeding normally to 39 weeks. Interestingly, the two cords branched one from another at their marginal insertion on the placenta and both fetuses as well as normal members of the family had a chromosomal inversion [46,XX,inv (10)(p12q25)]. Wenstrom (1993) felt that elective removal of this acardiac was unnecessary. Chitkara et al. (1989) reported on selective termination of 17 anomalous twins, 14 of which were aneuploid, but not acardiac fetuses. They emphasized the need for operator skill in this procedure, and had much better success later on in their series. Intracardiac injection of potassium chloride was the most effective means to accomplish the feticide. Neither the mothers nor the surviving twins suffered DIC. Other cases were reviewed by Donnenfeld and his colleagues (1989). They attempted to ascertain the presence of inter-twin anastomoses by prenatal angiography because of hydrocephaly in one twin. Complications led to fetal death and exsanguination of the normal twin into the abnormal fetus. Large AA anastomoses were found in the monochorionic placenta. Holzgreve and his colleagues (1994) injected through a spinal needle multiple pieces of ethanol-soaked suture material into the umbilical cord of an acardiac, with immediate cessation of blood flow. Hydramnios disappeared and a healthy twin was born. Sepulveda et al. (1995) succeeded by injecting alcohol into the abdominal portion of the umbilical artery at 23 weeks' gestation. Again, hydramnios and heart failure abated promptly. Foley et al. (1995) ligated the umbilical cord of an acardiac fetus with a special device, followed by rapid resolution of hydramnios. These results all support the notion that hydramnios in such pregnancies results from cardiac failure of the "pump" twin. It was therefore of interest to Martinez-Poyer et al. (1997) to follow the redistribution of blood in the survivor after cord ligation in five sets of twins (four pump twins survived), done by Doppler flow studies. They concluded that ligation was not associated with an increased impedance to the blood flow of the survivor, although a significant influence on venous flow was seen. Coincidentally, in several of these reports normal karyotypes were observed. Arias et al. (1998) successfully used endoscopic laser coagulation to stop the reversed perfusion.

Another acardiac fetus with forked cord ("funiculopagus") has been described by Averback and Wigglesworth (1978), who also reviewed the literature of this uncommon event. Their acardius was in a separate amnionic sac and

was rather well developed. The umbilical arteries, derived from the umbilical cords that had joined close to the placental surface, fused and provided a completely common circulation. It is interesting that this could occur at all because of the presence of umbilical cord furcation, and in a DiMo placenta. When we ascertained the frequency of SUA in acardiacs, we found that SUA occurred 16 times in 29 cases; 13 had normal cords. Of 27 normal co-twins, four had SUA and 23 were normal (Moore et al., 1990).

Not only are the acardiac twins malformed, but many of the co-twins also have congenital anomalies. Schinzel et al. (1979) suggested that about 10% of the co-twins are malformed. It is important to note that, with one possible exception, the sex of human acardiacs has been the same as that of the co-twin, providing it was accurately ascertained by, at least, a sex chromatin study (Benirschke, 1959), morphologic identification of gonads (Kappelman, 1944), or cytogenetic analysis. Only Buxbaum and Wachsman (1938) described an aberrant case, that of a female twin with an apparently male acardiac co-twin. The sex of the latter was assessed by finding "a structure that closely resembled a penis." That this finding is insufficient evidence for its male gender has been demonstrated to us. We saw an acardiac with a sonographically identified penile structure that was subsequently delivered with a normal female co-twin. On dissection, this penile structure was an enlarged clitoris, and normal ovaries were present. The reason for the clitoral enlargement remained obscure. C. Kaplan (in letters) found an anomalous pump twin with encephalocele, including imperforate anus, an absent kidney, and many other anomalies in 46,XY twins. The acardiac had a single-chambered heart and SUA. Baldwin (1993) has made similar observations.

The most controversial aspect of acardiacs is their pathogenesis and etiology. Frutiger (1969), who described five acardiac cases, believed that the absence of the heart was secondary to the acardiac suffering a deficient oxygen and nutrient supply, a suggestion that had previously been made popular by Loeschke (1948). He had the idea that the acardiac twin suffered malnutrition and hypoxia because it developed in the decidua capsularis, which, however, is clearly often not the case. Alderman (1973) challenged this notion and proposed a "primary failure of organ development." Köhn (1953) and Dahm (1955) also favored primary developmental problems. They suggested that "pathologic division" of the embryo and perhaps extraneous factors were responsible for acardiac development. They entertained the possibility of heritable causes. Gruenwald (1942) described a young, partially duplicated human embryo that might well have become an acardiac twin. He considered the two principal and opposing theories: (1) primary maldevelopment, and (2) vascular reversal leading to suppression of cardiac development. His statement, "an anomaly, anatomical or functional, intra-embryonic or extraembryonic, may turn one twin into an acardius if its circulation becomes dependent on that of the other embryo," probably best reflects our current thinking about the nature of these monsters. Lachman et al. (1980) have also presented reasonable theories of etiology in their discussion of a relevant case.

That vascular reversal nourishes the acardiac is without question. Much of the failure of organ systems to develop at all, or to do so in a diminutive fashion, is due to a deficient circulation. The circulating blood not only is deoxygenated but also arrives at a reduced pressure. The fact that the lower limbs of acardiacs are usually better formed than the arms has been considered to result from preferential perfusion of the legs as they are closest to the incoming reversed arterial flow. The fact that the central nervous tissue is often reasonably well developed contradicts some notions that unimpaired neural development guarantees limb development, an area that has been summarized by Boulgakow (1926).

An important etiologic consideration for the development of acardiacs is that these anomalies may occur in one of dizygotic twins of certain animals. Some species, in contrast to human twins, share anastomoses between fraternal twins. This situation is best known from the freemartin condition of cattle (Lillie, 1917). Here, the male twin is responsible for atrophy of the female genitalia of the co-twin, with which he is vascularly connected, the basis of freemartinism. These connections also lead to permanent blood chimerism. Similar anastomoses are regularly present in the twins of marmosets and tamarins (Benirschke et al., 1962). In these species, however, sexual disturbances

do not occur. Schatz (1898) had remarked that there are many ruminant acardiacs. Occasionally, they are found in carnivores but not in horses. Figure 25.88 shows a bovine acardiac monster, and such a twin from a goat is seen in Figure 25.89. Table 25.5 summarizes some of the literature of animal acardiacs. They are a crucial component in the consideration of the genesis of these anomalies. One may speculate that these fraternal twins were originally normal but that, because of happenstance chorionic anastomoses, they became anomalous by virtue of circulatory reversal. This speculation is supported by the hypothesis of original normality, first enunciated by Claudius (1859) and later by Ahlfeld (1879). Schwalbe (1907) sided with Schatz, in that he assumed a primary inequality of the twins, and that secondary alterations (macrocardia, microcardia, SUA, omphalocele) determine its ultimate outcome.

Evidence for a primary anomaly of at least some acardiacs has been gathered from cytogenetic studies. In a few acardiac monsters, investigators have found abnormal karyotypes that were different from those of the co-twin. Other acardiacs have had normal chromosomal complements identical with those of the normal co-twin, as in the example shown in Figure 25.90. These interesting findings are summarized in Table 25.6. One must caution, however, that only those studies in which the chromosome analysis was undertaken from the solid tissues of the acardiac specimens can be considered valid. The lymphocyte populations would be admixed a priori, and thus their karyotypic analysis is not helpful. Moreover, it is known that the lymphocyte contribution of the acardiac,

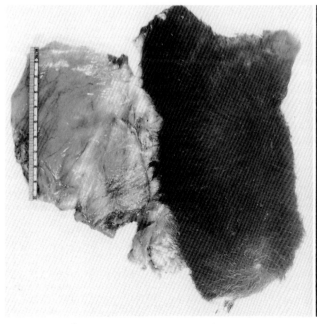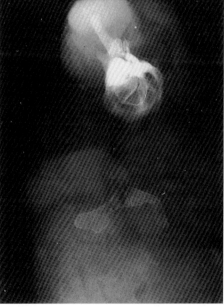

FIGURE 25.88. Bovine acardiac monster attached to remnants of membranes. This 600-g elongated structure had a semblance of pelvis (bottom right) and even more ossified cranial struc-tures (top right). Karyotype was 60,XX. (*Source:* Benirschke, 1970b, with permission.)

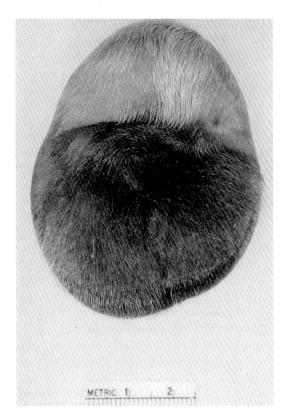

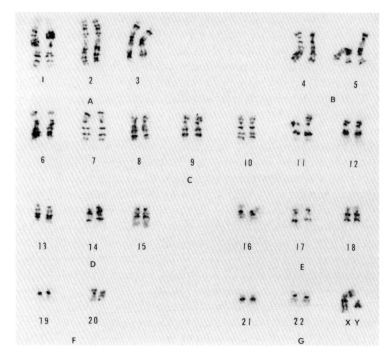

FIGURE 25.90. Normal male karyotype from skin of the acardiac shown in Figure 25.82. Giemsa banding.

FIGURE 25.89. "Amorphus globosus" from quadruplet pregnancy of a goat (♂♂;♀), weighing 20 g. It had a short cord with two vessels and a small amount of cartilage and muscle amid fat.

TABLE 25.5. Karyotypic studies in animal acardiacs

Source	Year	Species	Sex	Remarks
Sutton	1899	Cattle		Anidian monster
Simonds & Gowen	1925	Cattle		13 amorphi
		Sheep/goat		3 cases
		Bird		1 case; extensive literature
Cole & Craft	1945	Sheep	Female	
Roberts	1956	Horse		
		Cattle		
Dunn et al.	1967	Cattle	Female	60,XX; 61,XX (??mosaic)
			Male	co-twin 60,XY
Neal & Wilcox	1967	Cattle		2 amorphous twins, 1 heifer
Dennis & Leipold	1968	Sheep		1 holoacardius acephalus
Herzog & Rieck	1969	Cattle	Female	60,XX misinterpreted
Benirschke	1970b	Cattle	Female	60,XX, normal co-twin
Dunn & Roberts	1972	Sheep	Male	54,XY (co-twin); 54,XY/53,XY
Crossman & Dickens	1974	Horse		Mass (500 g)
Höfliger	1974	Horse		Review
		Cattle		Acormus (head only)
Hein et al.	1985	Monkey	Female	DiMo; AA anastomosis

TABLE 25.6. Karyotypic studies of human acardiac fetuses

Source	Year	Donor	Acardiac	Placenta Remarks
Richart & Benirschke	1963	ND	46,XY (F)	DiMo
Rashad & Kerr	1966	46,XY (F)	46,XY (L)	DiMo
		47,XY (F)	Extra C element	
Turpin et al.	1967	46,XX (F)	46,XX (F)	MoMo
			47,XX (L)	
			Extra minute element	
Scott & Ferguson-Smith	1973	46,XY (L,F)	46,XY (L)	DiMo
		46,XY (L)	Failed	DiMo
Machin	1974	46,XX (F)	46,XX (F)	?Triplets, 46,XX
Benirschke & Harper	1977	ND	46,XY (F) MoMo	See Figure 25.90
Rehder et al.	1978	47,XXY (F)	47,XXY (F)	?
Kaplan & Benirschke	1979	46,XX (F,L)	46,XX (F)	DiMo
		46,XX (F,L)	46,XX (F)	DiMo
Deacon et al.	1980	45,X (F)	46,XX (F,L)	?
Bieber et al.	1981	46,XY (L)	69,XXX(F)	DiMo
		Genetic studies indicated acardiac to derive from polar body		
Gewolb et al.	1983	46,XY (?)	46,XY (?)	DiMo Authors stated DiDi, but depicted DiMo
Van Allen et al.	1983	46,XX (?)	45,XX t(4;21)del(4p)	DiMo
		Nature of hromosome study unknown;		
Shapiro et al.	1986	46,XX (?)	46,XX	
		47,XX +11 (F)	?	
Moore et al.	1987	47,XXY (?)	92,XXXXYY (?)?	Review of the 11 previous acardiacs with karyotype
Bhatnagar etc.	1986	47,XX,tri 18	ND	?Mo
Moore et al.	1987	47,XXY (L)	47,XXY (L)	DiMo
		47,XXY (L)	92,XXXXYY (F,L)	DiMo
Landy et al.	1988	45,X/46,XX (A)	46,XX (A,L,F)	TriMo Triplets; mosaic fetus was normal female
			TriMo Triplets; mosaic fetus was normal female	
Wolf et al.	1991	46,XX	46,X,i(Xp)	DiMo Hydropic 3720 g
Ginsberg et al.	1992	46,XX,inv10	46,XX,inv10	MoMo Normal members with same inversion
Benirschke, K.	1992	46,XX	46,XX	Two normal acardiacs
Bolaji et al.	1992	46,XX	46,XX + 4n, +6n	TriMoTriplets, well-formed acardiac, Hyperdiploid cells from "lymphoid aggregate" of acardiac

A, amnionic fluid cells; F, fibroblast; L, lymphocytes; ND, not done.

who also usually lacks a thymus, may be minimal (Nigro, 1977). Therefore, the new molecular studies by Fisk et al. (1996) are of importance. These authors studied the DNA of placental and fetal solid tissues in acardiacs and their placentas, to find evidence of the monozygotic derivation of these unusual gestational products. Finally it is of interest that at least two "normal" co-twins of acardiacs have had an abnormal chromosomal constitution (Table 25.6). Thus, the cytogenetic picture is complex and does not lend itself to a resolution of the question of which event is primary in the etiology of acardiacs. Acardiac twins may be observed at young gestations and then already

have all the characteristic stigmata (Fig. 25.91). We have concluded that, whatever happens to their anatomic development, it is an early process. Our own concept is that the reversal of circulations is the cause of the anomaly.

The characteristic vascular arrangement pertaining to most acardiacs is illustrated in Figure 25.92. It mirrors many descriptions of former authors. The term TRAP has been applied to this syndrome (Van Allen et al., 1983). In this paper, which presents 14 acardiac cases, the spectrum of anomalies is well delineated. They described an additional specimen with chromosomal error. We have

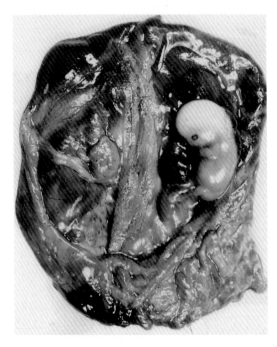

FIGURE 25.91. A DiMo twin abortus at approximately 9 weeks' gestation. At left is a degenerating acardiac. Note that it has a large amnionic cavity.

recently karyotyped two new acardiacs and their co-twins and found both to have normal chromosome complements in solid tissues. An excellent review of the origin of acardiac twins and TRAP can be found by Malinowski and Wierzba (1998). They also gave frequency figures for the various anomalies of acardiac fetuses. That acardiac fetuses may even have a more developed cephalic portion

was presented by Mohanty et al. (2000); likewise, Sergi and Schmitt (2000) presented an acardiac with microcephaly and discussed various CNS anomalies found in such cases. Petersen et al. (2001) even reported the relative normality of development in an edematous acardiac that was thought to have been dead sonographically.

Conjoined Twins

Incompletely separated twins (conjoined, Siamese, x-pagi, double monsters) presumably take their origin after day 13 of embryogenesis. Because it has been most seriously questioned whether conjoined twins are one person or two, the reader is directed to the searching review of this topic by Gould (1982), who concluded that this question is not answerable, and perhaps it may even be an erroneous inquiry. The MZ twinning process is a continuum, and sharp divisions do not exist, as is often the case in biologic phenomena. It is even more problematic to make clear decisions as to the classification of whole-body chimerae, as we will see below. Moreover, the precise manner of the formation of conjoined twins is uncertain. Opposing views suggest incomplete splitting and partial fusion of embryonic precursors. The reader is referred to the searching reviews of over 1000 cases by Spencer (1992, 2000, 2003), who has clearly had the greatest experience with this topic. Spencer's special interest has been the embryologic development of conjoined twins, and she posits as her basic tenet that fusion (rather than incomplete splitting) is the principal mechanism of their formation. The reason for her view is primarily that many cases of conjoined twins cannot possibly be

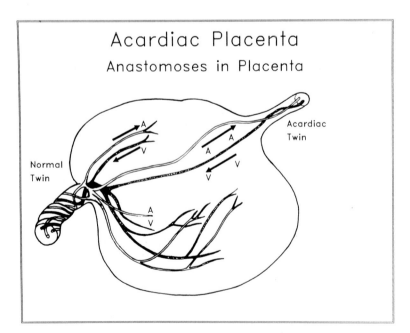

FIGURE 25.92. Usual vascular relations (anastomoses) among an acardiac and co-twin.

explained by a fission event although she begins the evolution of conjoined twinning by assuming a primary MZ splitting event (see also the review by Kaufman, 2004). The reader is led to believe that, because the MZ twins are oriented on either an amnionic "bubble" or large yolk sac, their potential proximity leads to this fusion. It must be pointed out, though, that to the best of our knowledge, all conjoined twins have been of the same sex, which one might not expect if fusion were the principal mechanism. In another contribution, Spencer (2001) suggested that conjoined twins, fetus in fetu, parasitic twins, and acardiacs really form a spectrum and that the primary abnormality is a cardiac malformation; it is of further interest that she also supported the abundance of female conceptuses and that there is often a history of familial twinning. Another detailed study from the same author discusses the rare occurrence of rachipagous conjoined twins (Spencer, 1995). In addition, an encyclopedic review book was published by Quigley (2003) that addresses many of the ethical and social issues confronted by these twins; another book by Dreger (2004) is perhaps more directed to the lay public but it discusses some serious scientific issues. Even more provocative is the observation by Logroño et al. (1997). They reported a "heteropagous" conjoined twin with male pelvis and lower extremities attached to the chest of a male autosite and inferred from a fluorescent in situ hybridization (FISH) genetic study of the dizygosity of these joined parts. The autosite also had a cardiac anomaly, but the placenta was not described. The unequal craniopagi reported by Aquino et al. (1997) had two umbilical cords with velamentous insertion, one being diminutive and with a single artery. There were surface placental anastomoses. We have observed exactly the same features in one of the many acardiac pregnancies sent to us.

Most fused twins are joined at the chest (thoracopagus), but all sorts of unions have been described (Harper et al., 1980). Numerous triplets have included conjoined twins (Koontz et al., 1985; Seo et al., 1985; Gardeil et al., 1998). In triplets, the placentas may be monochorionic (Tan et al., 1971b), with the conjoints living in their separate amnionic cavity, or they may be dichorionic (Vestergaard, 1972). We have observed term thoraco-omphalopagous girls with a monochorionic (diamnionic) normal female co-twin. The umbilical cord to the conjoined triplets was split (two arms with artery and vein each) at the placental surface, which then joined to produce a cord with two arteries and two veins. Another of these rare diamnionic twin placentas with omphalopagous conjoined twins has been described by Weston and colleagues (1990). The typical placenta of conjoined twins, however, is a monoamnionic/monochorionic one. The former speculations that fusion of fraternal twins may be a mechanism of conjoint twinning is no longer tenable. For instance, chromosome studies of the twins have always been identical (Kreutner et al., 1963; Kim et al., 1971). In one case, the twins and their mother had a pericentric inversion of one chromosome 9 (Delprado & Baird, 1984) and all have been of the same sex. Mackenzie et al. (2002) studied the natural history of 14 conjoined twins diagnosed prenatally; the frequency of serious anomalies thus identified allows more definitive decision regarding potential viability. This is an important consideration for the possible future treatment of conjoined twins in whom perhaps survival of one is unlikely and where decisions of surgery are paramount. The intervention by the courts and the problems arising from this decision to seek its advice are highlighted in an excellent article by Annas (2001). Surprisingly, approximately 70% of conjoined twins are females (James, 1980). Burn et al. (1986) used this fact to support their hypothesis that unequal lyonization is associated with MoMo twinning. MacKenzie et al. (2004) have contributed another most unusual set of conjoined twins, a fetus with a partial twin joined on the abdomen, and differentiated it from TRAP sonographically. Incompletely separated twins have been described in a wide variety of species, for example, rat (Levinsky, 1973; Mutinelli et al., 1992), swine (Selby et al., 1973), turtle (Szabuniewicz & McCrady, 1967; Lewis et al., 1992), and Cetacea (Kawamura, 1969; Kawamura & Kashita, 1971). We have seen several California king snakes, calves, kittens, and other animals with double heads. Even in plants this event occurs with some frequency (Ahmad et al., 1977) (see also Fig. 25.93) and is there referred to as fasciation. It is remarkable and not yet fully understood why MZ bird twins have all been female. Conjoined chicken twins, described by Munro (1965), shared the single yolk sac.

Conjoined twins occur in approximately 1 of 50,000 births (Schmidt et al., 1981), or in 1 of 600 twins. The figures vary substantially among surveys (Tan et al., 1971a; Bankole et al., 1972; Harper et al., 1980; Castilla et al., 1988). They are reported to be much higher in the Japanese population (Miyabara et al., 1973). Reports have also indicated that this anomaly occurs more commonly in Nigeria, and Bhettay et al. (1975) suggested a much higher rate to exist in South Africa. This statement, however, has been criticized by Hanson (1975). Difficulty of ascertainment is further discussed by Viljoen et al. (1983) in a large series of conjoined twins from Southern Africa; contrary to earlier reports, these authors found no skewing in favor of the black population. Milham (1966) analyzed 22 sets and suggested local clustering of this anomaly. That suggestion was supported by Viljoen et al. (1983). The ultrasonographic diagnosis of conjoined twins can now be made as early as at 8 weeks' gestation (Lam et al., 1997, 1998), and three-dimensional sonography is helpful in further diagnosis of their anomalies (Maymon et al., 1998). This is also important for the selective termination of such anomalous conceptuses.

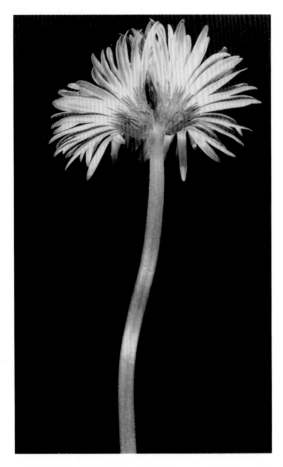

FIGURE 25.93. Conjoined "twin" Transvaal daisy (*Gerbera jamesonii*). The stem is fused; the flowers, with their identical number of petals (55/55), are separate.

The **etiology** of conjoined twinning remains unknown. Sporadic reports have suggested that it is due to teratogen exposure (e.g., griseofulvin) (Rosa et al., 1987), and that its prevalence may include seasonal fluctuation. The relation of conjoined twinning to griseofulvin intake was disputed by the large data collected by Knudsen (1987), however. Ingalls (1969), who applied heat and hypoxia to zebra fish, was able to observe eight conjoined fish among 5000 specimens; he described an "epidemic" in trout. Ferm (1969, 1978) found four conjoined hamsters whose mothers were subjected to teratogens. When Kao et al. (1986) injected solutions of lithium chloride into a blastomere of 32-cell-stage *Xenopus* eggs, a second head developed. Wan et al. (1982) observed conjoined twins in 0.4% of Swiss-Webster mice and in 0.06% of triplets. Treatment with vincristine or other manipulations did not increase the yield. Whether these data are relevant to the human condition has not been decided. It is known, however, that conjoined twins frequently have other congenital anomalies, including cleft palate, anencephaly, and particularly congenital heart disease (Noonan, 1978; Marin-Padilla et al., 1981; Seo et al., 1985). Newman

(1931b) noted marked differences in the development of various structures. Finally, arguing against the notion that fusion is the principal mechanism of conjoined twinning, the complex case of Bannykh et al. (2001) (and other similar complex instances) needs to be reviewed. This (male) singleton had two sets of external genitalia, portions of bowel, meningomyelocele and cardiac isomerism that can hardly be explained by a fusion event.

Keeler (1929) suggested that **mirror imagery** existed in 77% of conjoined twins, compared with 22% in monozygotic, separate twins. It must be cautioned, though, that situs inversus and mirroring are complex problems (see McManus, 2002). Torgersen (1949) identified it to occur in 0.01% of a large population of Norwegians studied by mass radiography. Its incidence paralleled that of twinning, and he found that it was "not much higher" in MZ twins and was "rare" in DZ twins. For further insight into situs inversus and related aspects, see Layton (1976) and McManus (2002). Hydramnios is said to occur in about half of conjoined twins (Wedberg et al., 1979). The frequencies of various types of conjoined twins has been given by Edmonds and Layde (1982), with thoracoomphalopagus (28%) being the commonest form.

The placenta of conjoined twins is usually a single disk with MoMo membranes. The structure of the umbilical cords, however, varies widely, approximately 6% having two cords (Spencer, 1992). This fact much supports her view of fusion. The umbilical cord in Figure 25.94 was

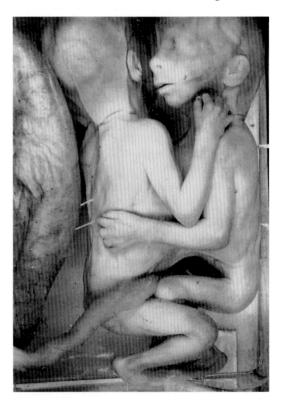

FIGURE 25.94. Thoracoabdominopagous twins with monoamnionic placenta and a single umbilical cord.

single and contained two arteries and a vein. It is similar to those described by Kreutner et al. (1963), de Leon (1974), and Itoh et al. (1974), who observed that the co-twins had a fused subdiaphragmatic aorta whence the umbilical arteries originated. Gilbert et al. (1972) and Tan et al. (1971b) described thoracopagi with one artery coming from one twin and the other from the second twin, who also received the single vein. The twins in Figure 25.95 had a single umbilical artery and a velamentous insertion of the umbilical cord. An SUA was also found in four of seven conjoined twins reported by Miyabara et al. (1973). Kim et al. (1971) described thoracopagi with a single cord that possessed six vessels—four arteries and two veins. Mitrani (1968) saw one conjoined set of twins with six arteries and two veins. In the cases reported by Seo et al. (1985), two placentas had single cords with four arteries and one vein, one had three arteries and two veins, and three had normal cords with two arteries and one vein. Two placentas, however, were separate disks; one of them had a fused cord. Delprado and Baird (1984) reported cephalothoracopagi with two cords. One was thick, ran in the membranes, and contained one artery and one vein; the smaller cord contained only one vessel. Another thoracopagous set of twins was reported

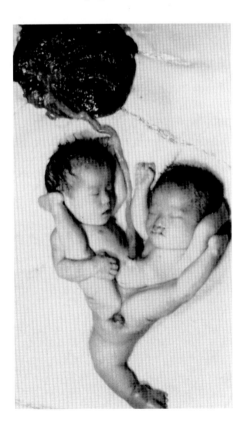

FIGURE 25.95. Conjoined twins (ischiopagi) with a MoMo placenta, a single velamentous umbilical cord, and SUA. They were delivered at 40 weeks' gestation. One had a cleft face and microcardia. There were two female genital tracts. (Courtesy of Dr. S. Sekiya, Tokyo, Japan.)

by Freedman et al. (1962). They had two separate cords that inserted 1.5 cm apart and fused 13 cm from the placental surface. The fused structure contained three arteries and two veins; the placenta was DiMo and contained a triplet of the same sex. Wiegenstein and Iozzo (1980) found two separated cords (11 cm apart) in a conjoined twin. The cords fused after having entangled in the placental portion and ran in a tented segment of amnion. A case with similarly fused, but separately originating cords was described with a dicephalus, dibrachius (Beischer & Fortune, 1968). In the thoracopagi examined by Marin-Padilla et al. (1981), the single cord split 9 cm before reaching the placental surface. One branch contained two arteries; the other cord had a velamentous insertion and contained the single vein. An interesting set of vessels was found in the umbilical cord of a thoracopagus studied by Chaurasia (1975). The smaller twin had a rudimentary heart, a large left and diminutive right umbilical artery, and no vein; the larger twin had a single large artery and vein. Reversal of circulation in the smaller twin was considered.

There is thus great variety in the spectrum of cord vasculature and structure, and no clear relations emerge as to the associated type of conjoined twin. One might expect that embryonic splitting at slightly different times produces different fusion anomalies and different cord structures and insertions. Future correlations may uncover these as yet unknown parameters. It is especially noteworthy that not all MoMo placentas of conjoined twins with two umbilical cords have vascular anastomoses on the placental surface. Finally, there exist anomalous fetuses with diminutive parasitic "twins" presenting as inclusions or appendages. They represent transitions to the next topic. Four such cases were described in some detail by Drut and colleagues (1992). Because they have no relation to placental pathology, they will not be discussed further.

Sacrococcygeal Teratoma and Epignathus

Sacrococcygeal teratoma and epignathus are, in our opinion, malformed twins that represent a part of the spectrum of the monozygotic twinning continuum, and Spencer (2001) has a similar opinion. Some may take exception to this concept; nevertheless, findings of perfectly formed extremities, digits, and other structures favor this view. These are occasionally combined with more disorganized tumors (Cousins et al., 1980; Tokunaga et al., 1986). Schwalbe (1907) and Willis (1958) extensively discussed this aspect with illustrative material that also supports this notion. Exelby (1972) reviewed the origin and therapy of these tumors and found them to be

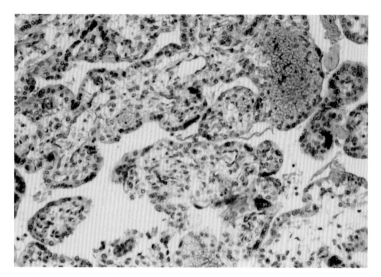

FIGURE 25.96. Villi of immature placenta in a patient with a large sacrococcygeal teratoma. Placenta weighed 880 g at 31 weeks. The neonate died with extensive cerebral necroses. The villi are irregular and patchily edematous, and have distended fetal capillaries. There is focal hemorrhage, and numerous nucleated red blood cells are present. The cytotrophoblast is more prominent than expected at this age. H&E ×160.

much commoner in females (4 F : 1 M); they also indicated that there is frequently a strong family history of twinning. In one parturient whose child had a large sacrococcygeal teratoma, an ovarian teratoma was found simultaneously (Rayburn & Barr, 1982). These authors emphasized that genetic study had shown that these neoplasms have different genetic backgrounds.

There are also frequent concurrent anomalies in children with these tumors. Most of the neoplasms are benign, which is different from the rare teratomas of other sites, in which prenatal metastases have been reported (Semchyshyn et al., 1982). At times, however, an apparently benign sacrococcygeal teratoma eventuates in a malignancy. Lack et al. (1993) found an eventually fatal adenocarcinoma in a man 40 years after a sacrococcygeal teratoma had been incompletely removed at age 2 months. An alternate etiologic point of view is that sacrococcygeal tumors and epignathi derive from misplaced germ cells. In a study of obstetrical complications with sacral tumors, Spitzer (1932) commented on the female sex preponderance and noted that the tumors are often complicated by hydramnios during pregnancy. That point has been reiterated in other publications about the prenatal diagnoses of these lesions (Horger & McCarter, 1979; Hallgrimsson, 1981).

Placentomegaly has often been described to be a complication of sacrococcygeal teratomas (Cousins et al., 1980; Gergely et al., 1980; Kohga et al., 1980; Feige et al., 1982). The same is true of the placenta in epignathi (Kaplan et al., 1980; Chervenak et al., 1985), and yet other teratomas may be associated with hydramnios and fetal hydrops (Rosenfeld et al., 1979; Banfield et al., 1980; Semchyshyn et al., 1982; Mostoufi-Zadeh et al., 1985). The placental enlargement may be striking, and it is then usually exceptionally pale. There is severe edema of villi, which often appear to be excessively cellular, contain numerous Hofbauer cells, and are severely congested

(Fig. 25.96). One often finds numerous nucleated red blood cells in the fetal placental vessels. Ultrastructural examination of such specimens was first undertaken by Arai et al. (1977; see also Soma et al., 1979). It showed marked alterations of the syncytium, with distention of the transport vesicles (Fig. 25.97), and unusually dense mitochondria. We believe that placental enlargement is the result of high output failure of the fetus and that it is similar to that found with large chorangiomas. This concept finds confirmation in the frequently present fetal cardiac enlargement. In effect, the teratoma acts as an arteriovenous fistula. This is further supported by the experience of Langer et al. (1989). They resected one of the tumors at 24 weeks and returned the fetus to the uterus (of three cases described). Hydrops improved and Doppler study showed a decrease in cardiac output. Nakayama et al. (1991) made similar observations when they resected the tumor in a newborn. Feige et al. (1982)

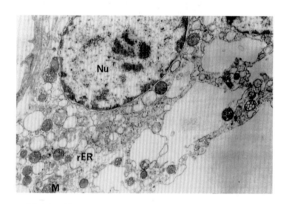

FIGURE 25.97. Ultrastructural view of villi in a sacrococcygeal teratoma, showing hugely distended syncytial transport vesicles. Data: 28 weeks' gestation, hydramnios; elevated human chorionic gonadotropin (hCG) levels (9,830,400 IU/L), 680 g placenta. ×5600. NU, nucleus; rER, rough endoplasmic reticulum. (Courtesy of Dr. H. Soma, Tokyo, Japan.)

unreasonably claimed that the placentomegaly represents an attempt by the placenta to compensate for the increased needs of the fetal tumor. Whenever karyotypic analysis has been done, the chromosomes of the tumors have been normal and identical to those of the host (Kaplan et al., 1979; Cousins et al., 1980). An interesting question remains regarding the "hairy polyp" removed from the throat of occasional patients (Isaacs, 2002). Should it be regarded as an epignathus or teratoma? We have seen such an anomaly in a newborn with respiratory distress. The polyp impinged upon the defective soft palate. After removal, it was found to have a lanugo-covered skin and, internally, it was composed of fat, cartilage, nerve, and skin remnants.

CONGENITAL ANOMALIES

Twins have congenital anomalies more often than do singletons. Hendricks (1966) evaluated the outcome of 438 multiple pregnancies and found not only that their perinatal mortality rate is "startlingly high" (14%) but also that anomalies occurred with a frequency of 10.6% (approximately three times that of singletons). In a review of anomalies of Swedish twins, Källén (1986) noted that some anomalies (posthemorrhagic hydrocephalus?, patent ductus) are undoubtedly an effect of the prematurity of many twins. Other anomalies, notably those referred to as the VACTERL association [vertebral, anal, cardiac, tracheal, esophageal, renal, and limb anomalies, a variant of the VATER (vertebral, anal, tracheal, esophageal, and renal) association] and anencephaly were overrepresented in twins. A new international study of malformations in twins was authored by Mastroiacovo et al. (1999). Of 260,865 twins, 5572 malformations were identified, affecting virtually all organ systems. The associations previously already known to exist were confirmed, although higher rates were found. James (1976) found that anencephaly occurs in DZ twins with the same frequency as in singletons, but that its incidence is increased in one or both of MZ twins. When it occurs in dichorionic twins, expectant management is advocated (Lipitz et al. (1995), although hydramnios may occur. In contrast, when it is found in monochorionic twins, "expectant management is associated with a high rate of intrauterine lethality of the normal twin" (Sebire et al., 1997a). Of 11 such pregnancies, these authors observed fetal demise of both twins in three pregnancies.

Schinzel et al. (1979) studied the structural defects of MZ twins in greater detail. They considered that some of these anomalies are related to the MZ twinning process per se. This concept is certainly true for the acardiacs, the conjoined twins, and probably also for those defects that arise as the result of vascular anastomoses (e.g., porencephaly, intestinal occlusions). When twin abortuses were studied, it was found that the incidence of twinning, particularly MZ twinning, is much higher than expected (1 in 35 abortions). The rate of associated anomalies was not significantly different from the rate in the total population (Livingston & Poland, 1980). Livingston and Poland (1980) found that 35 of 53 pairs were monochorionic MZ, two were opposite sex (DZ), and 16 were same sex and dichorionic. Uchida et al. (1983) found seven of 15 to be opposite sex. In other situations, MZ twins apparently react differently to environmental teratogens, as was the case of the MoMo twins of Reitnauer et al. (1997).

A striking increase in twinning was found in infants with sirenomelia (symmelia). Usually, only one of the twins had that anomaly. Only rarely have both of MZ twins been concordantly affected by anomalies in general and symmelia in particular (Roberge, 1963). Davies et al. (1971) gathered 327 cases of sirenomelia from the literature and found that there is a 100-fold increase of this anomaly in MZ twins when compared with singletons. We have previously discussed how the

hypoplasia of sirenomelics' lungs, the Potter syndrome features, and amnion nodosum are prevented by the presence of the normal amnionic environment, guaranteed by a normal co-twin. This idea is beautifully demonstrated in the case described by Kohler (1972), and McNamara et al. (1995) added two more cases. Klinger et al. (1997) found additional support for this idea. They reported absence of "Potter" features in a MoMo twin with absent kidneys, genitalia, anal atresia, and SUA. Kapur et al. (1991) described sirenomalia in one twin, the other (dichorionic) having vanished.

Discordance for major anomalies in MZ twins seems to be the unexplained rule rather than the exception. It has been the topic of numerous publications (e.g., Fogel et al., 1965; Benirschke & Masliah, 2001). Machin (1996) has summarized all known or hypothesized facts and theories of such unusual cases. Imaizumi (1989a) found that concordance of congenital hydrocephalus in Japan was only 15% for all twins (21% in like-sex twins), but that the corresponding figures from the literature were 4.6% and 7.8%, respectively. They also saw two like-sex sets with anencephaly and hydrocephaly. Hernandez-Johnstone and Benirschke (1976) cited much of the relevant literature. This concept, however, has been considered to be a "tautology" (Boklage, 1987b). Boklage suggested that most surveys of anomalies in twins employ the Weinberg formula for the assignments of zygosity. We cannot agree with this statement. In numerous studies, the chorionic status was the method that decided the presence of MZ twins. Boklage was also critical of the concept that MZ twinning and anomalies are related processes; he favored the interpretation that, because such features as non–right-handedness and familial twinning are overrepresented in these anomalous twins, the relation between MZ twinning and anomalies does not hold. His concept was that many such twins derive from "polar body" fertilization, which he considered to be tertiary oocytes. That twinning and cardiovascular anomalies may have common origins was detailed in a large study by Berg et al. (1989). Most remarkably, Hamasaki et al. (1998) found discordance of the expression of the mutated prion that leads to Gerstmann-Sträussler-Scheinker disease in identical twins. Both had the mutation, but only one twin expressed the symptomatology.

In some cases, major disruptions of fetal structures can be explained by amnionic bands or adhesions of fetus to large sheets of amnion (Khudr & Benirschke, 1972; Donnenfeld et al., 1985). Boulot and colleagues (1990) proposed that the anencephaly-like anomaly they observed may have resulted from injury at "embryonic reduction." It is of parenthetic interest to point out that the presence of placental anastomoses in DiMo twins, one being anencephalic, has served to better understand the regulation of fetal adrenal development (Kohler & MacDonald, 1972).

In most of these anomalies, there is no evidence of a genetic component. It is perhaps even more surprising to learn that anomalies with a strong genetic etiology, for example, cleft lip and cleft palate, are frequently discordant in MZ twins. Metrakos et al. (1958) reviewed 108 twin pairs and found the concordance in MZ twins to be 31%; in DZ twins it was 6.3%. These authors and others proved monozygosity for some pairs by means of exchange skin grafts. Discordance of facial clefts is unusually common in MZ twins. Their evidence and that from many other studies clearly indicates a familial disposition of cleft lip/palate. Murray et al. (2004) searched for gene abnormalities in twins discordant for clefts and detected none. They concluded that this "supports the hypothesis that non-etiologic post-twinning mutations are rare." Studies of twins for other defects (e.g., club foot, dislocated hip) have led to the concept of causation by "polygenic genetic predisposition interacting with additional unknown intrauterine environmental triggers" (Carter, 1968). This concept of a quasicontinuous variation or a threshold character with anomalies of multifactorial etiology (Fraser, 1970) is currently the best way to interpret these seemingly contradictory findings. It remains to be elucidated as to what the prenatal factors are that place the affected twin beyond the critical threshold. It could be adverse placentation (e.g., velamentous insertion of cord or SUA), as

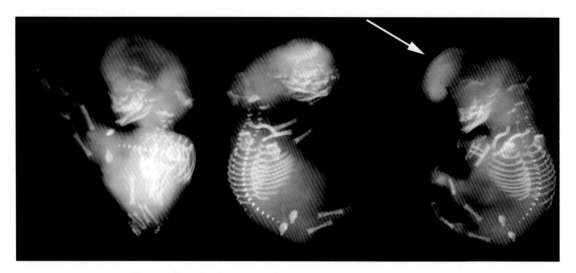

FIGURE 25.98. Triplet fetus papyracei from assisted reproductive technology (ART) gestation. The triplet at right has an encephalocele that was not recognized macroscopically. The radiograph shows the value of taking x-rays of such fetuses.

we have championed, or it could be one of many, as yet undetermined, other factors. It may relate to unequal splitting. Too little is known of the placental conformation of most such twins to allow us to come to any definitive conclusion. More data must be collected on the precise placentation of twins with discordance for defects. The relative frequency of intestinal atresias reported may have a more direct relation to monochorionic twinning as they are overrepresented in like-sex twins. Perhaps it is caused by periods of hypotension, so-called vascular disruptions (Cragan et al., 1994). Discordance of twins, one with the Beckwith-Wiedemann syndrome (BWS), is definitely more frequent in monochorionic twins. In one relevant case that we observed there were calcified thrombi in superficial placental veins of both twins, aside from massive enlargement of the affected twin's umbilical cord. Other MZ twins with discordant BWS were reported by Weksberg et al. (2002), who suggested that this imprinting abnormality (on chromosome 11p13–15) perhaps predisposes to MZ twinning. Much other work on the imprinting abnormality in BWS and Angelman's syndrome has recently been conducted, and at least some findings suggest that there is a higher incidence when ART is performed for conception (Fig. 25.98) (DeBaun et al., 2003; Gicquel et al., 2003; Maher et al., 2003).

Two major reviews of discordant anomalies in twins were undertaken in an effort to delineate the prognosis of such gestations (Malone et al., 1996; Alexander et al., 1997). Both groups of authors came to the conclusion that this constellation significantly increases the risk of premature delivery. Malinowski and Biskup (1997) found two sets of monochorionic twins in whom the survivors had gastroschisis, and they related this anomaly to possible ischemia of the abdominal wall occurring at the time of fetal demise of their co-twins.

Cytogenetics and Heterokaryotypic Monozygotic Twins

Twins may have the same chromosomal errors as singletons. Rohmer et al. (1971) described a set of DZ twins with Down syndrome and collected 200 cases of trisomy 21 in the twin literature. One of these twins was a pure trisomic; the other had a small, subsequently diminishing population of trisomic cells; it had a normal phenotype. The authors speculated that blood chimerism might exist but were unable to verify it; the DiDi placenta contained no anastomoses. Most commonly, MZ twins are concordant for a particular aneuploidy (e.g., 48,XXXY in Simpson et al., 1974). Mosaicism has been observed on occasion, as in the MZ twins with trisomy 21 described by Shapiro and Farnsworth (1972).

A number of unusual, so-called heterokaryotypic twins have been reported. They were monozygotic by various criteria, but their chromosome number differed. The list of these heterokaryotypic MZ twins reported has become so large that it is impractical to summarize all the reports here. Reasonably complete reviews may be found in the contributions by Dallapiccola et al. (1985) and Machin (1996). The former authors described a heterokaryotypic triplet and summarized, in table form, the 25 cases reported prior to their publication. Monteiro et al. (1998b) investigated the X-inactivation of the X chromosome in twin girls and found that different inactivation pattern occurred only in dichorionic twins. From a comparison of blood and buccal cell X-inactivation patterns they reason that splitting of the MZ twins occurs **after** the timing of this chromosomal inactivation, around day 4 (see also Goodship et al., 1996; Machin, 1996). Cantú et al. (1998) did an interesting study of the segregation of X-chromosomal variants of the fragile-X gene in a set of MZ triplets. The **paternal** gene was identical in all, but the **maternal** gene was different in all three triplets. This effectively eliminated their prior hypothesis of a single chromatid mutation **before** ovulation but also indicated that, despite physical similarity of these MZ triplets, their genetic disposition was different. The authors went so far as to state: "Genomically speaking, there are no identical twins."

The commonest chromosomal variant is discordance associated with the Turner syndrome. The 45,X genotype is prone to abort during early gestation. Of the relatively few survivors, most had mosaicism for cells composed of 45,X and 46,XX (or XY) genotypes. Mosaicism results from the simultaneous occurrence of twinning and somatic nondisjunction of chromosomes. If the Y chromosome of a 46,XY embryo is lost by nondisjunction during early development, male and female (45,X) MZ twins may be the outcome (e.g., Schmid et al., 2000; Wachtel et al., 2000). This formerly inexplicable situation, MZ twins of different sex, has in fact been recorded in several instances to have resulted in this fashion, as for instance by Gonsoulin et al. (1990a). The 45,X MZ twin of their report was additionally hydropic. Shevell et al. (2004) ablated such an abnormal MZ twin with 45,X by using radiofrequency obliteration of the umbilical cord. Investigators have more often documented MZ twins with various degrees and types of mosaicism, of X, XX, and XXX, or Y chromosomes. There is a wide spectrum. Kurosawa et al. (1992) have reported a set of MZ twins who were mosaic for two populations of cells, 45,X and 47,XYY, in lymphocytes and fibroblasts. One twin had a greater proportion of male-determining cells and had a male phenotype, and the other had a female phenotype. The fact that often both twins are mosaic may betray the influence of monochorionic placentation with anastomoses (when the mosaicism is confined to lymphocytes). Alternatively, when the fibroblasts of only one twin are mosaic or have a different complement from the karyotype of the co-twin, it may suggest the loss of one chromosome in one twin after splitting has occurred. Such is likely to have occurred in the two sets of mosaic monozygotic twins (45,X/46,XY) reported by Costa et al. (1998), who also reviewed the entire literature of this unusual phenomenon. Most of the placentas associated with this phenomenon have been DiMo, but an occasional twin has had a MoMo placenta. Precise studies of placenta and of lymphocyte, fibroblast, and chorionic karyotypes will enhance our knowledge as to the timing of this unusual event.

Prenatal diagnosis of such errors was once difficult because the intentional sampling of individual amnionic cavities was impractical. Young et al. (1974) introduced a feasible method to sample the individual cavities for the surveillance of Rh-sensitized pregnancies. It has now been reported to be successfully accomplished for 79%, 94%, and 98% of cases, respectively (Librach et al., 1984; Taylor et al., 1984; Tabsh et al., 1985). This methodology has not only allowed precise diagnosis but has led to fetal transfusions, now practiced routinely (Bowman, 1985; Pijpers et al., 1988). An alternative method for aspirating the two cavities was advocated by Jeanty et al. (1990). They were nearly uniformly successful but the possibility of destruction of the dividing membranes exists with this technique. Selective feticide can then be undertaken when fetal trisomy is diagnosed by any of these techniques (Kerenyi & Chitkara, 1981; Chitkara et al., 1989; see also Donnenfeld et al., 1989). Pijpers et al. (1988) studied 83 pregnancies and obtained karyotypes of both twins in 77 cases (93%). They found elevated AFP levels (in both sacs) in two cases that were due to renal abnormalities. This finding suggested to them that AFP diffuses through the membranous partition. Unfortunately, the types of placenta present in these cases were not recorded. Franke and Estel (1978) had previously found that AFP permeates the membranes.

Chimerism and Mosaicism

It is not uncommon in cytogenetic studies to identify cell lines with different chromosome number or different complements. This has most recently become a problem in amniocentesis and placental cell cultures. The latter aspects were considered in Chapter 21; here it is essential to make the differential diagnosis of mosaicism and chimerism. Whole-body chimerism may develop when, in very early stages of development, dizygotic twin embryos fuse to form a single individual. The resulting genetic chimera, a "whole-body chimera" is an individual composed of two populations of cells whose origin are two genetically completely different fertilization products. In addition to this mechanism, the possibility exists that two spermatozoa fertilize an ovum and a polar body, and that these structures then make up a single embryo. This second explanation is the mechanism that is favored by most investigators for the production of chimeras. Chimeras differ from mosaics and they should be clearly distinguished.

Mosaics are individuals composed of different cell lines but derived from a single embryonic precursor. Because of the process of "lyonization," all females are considered to be mosaics. Not only may mosaics have different cell lines with different chromosome numbers but, because of mutations, they may also have lines of cells with different phenotypic expression. An individual with cancer, for instance, could be a mosaic; one line of cells would be the normal body constituents, the other would be those cells that form the neoplasm. Healey et al. (2001) examined lyonization in MZ twins genetically and deduced from their findings of 20 discordant female twins that adult height was not correlated with different lyonization patterns. It is convenient and important to distinguish two pathogenetically different types of chimeras: (1) blood chimeras (also called "twin chimeras" by Tippett, 1984); and (2) whole-body chimeras ("dispermic chimeras").

Blood chimeras have been long been known to occur in cattle. In bovine fetuses the placentas often fuse, the fetal blood vessels join, and blood is exchanged between the embryonic twins. Because embryonic blood is largely like bone marrow, there is seeding of the other twin's marrow space with genotypically different hematopoietic elements and lymphocytes. It results in a lifelong admixture because these cells are not rejected by the immunologically impotent embryo; the foreign cells are subsequently regarded as "self." When male and female bovine fetuses are thus joined, it is easy to identify clones of male lymphocytes in the female and vice versa. This phenomenon is restricted to motile hematopoietic system cells. The fixed tissue cells do not participate.

The fact that chimerism first was recognized in cattle results from the masculinization of the female twin in heterosexual bovine co-twins. The female becomes a "freemartin" (Lillie, 1917), an animal that has external masculinization, an absent uterus, atrophied ovaries, and female genotype. The degree of masculinization does not depend on the percentage of chimeric male hemopoietic cells (Herzog, 1969). Complex chimerism may be detected when triplets or quadruplets are thus admixed (Basrur et al., 1970). Although long known, the virilization of female artiodactyl twins has not yet been satisfactorily explained. Lillie (1917) and most subsequent investigators have assumed that it was the result of embryonic hormone action, secreted by the male gonads. Such an obvious hypothesis proved facile when it was discovered that marmoset monkeys of South America not only always have DZ twins but also regularly have fused placentas, and that they are all blood-chimeric. Although 50% are XX/XY chimeric, the females are not sterilized in analogy with the freemartin effect (Benirschke, 1971; Gengozian, 1971). Currently, no rational explanation exists for this discrepancy among species. One might speculate that there are differences in the müllerian inhibiting substance or the receptor because they are not subject to hormonal influences. We have always assumed that these are analogous in different taxa, but perhaps it is an error to make such an assumption. Niku et al. (2004) showed that among the hematopoietic precursors are some remarkably multipotent cells that are irregularly distributed throughout the body and that become especially prominent in granulation tissue. From the same laboratory comes evidence of the variable percentage of B and T cells. These systems are currently of particular interest as the role of circulating stem cells is central to our understanding of chimerism (Pessa-Morikawa et al., 2004). Freemartinism occurs in other artiodactyla, in birds, and in a few other species. We used to believe that some primitive germ cells might also travel through embryonic inter-twin anastomoses to take up residence in the opposite-sex host; findings by Gengozian et al. (1980), however, have made this unlikely. In addition, many investigations have addressed issues of immunologic tolerance in chimerism (Porter & Gengozian, 1969; Tippett, 1984).

In contrast to marmosets and cattle, anastomoses between DZ twin placentas of humans are rare indeed.

One dichorionic twin placenta with an anastomosis has been described by Cameron (1968) and is depicted in Figure 25.22. Genetic study of the twins, however, showed them to be MZ. Lage et al. (1989) presented a dichorionic twin placenta with anastomoses that was also accompanied by a mild form of the transfusion syndrome. The hematocrits of the twins were 43% and 59%, respectively. Molnar-Nadasdy and Altshuler (1996) saw a similar case at autopsy of macerated immature fetuses. The female stillborns possessed dichorionic dividing membranes (with velamentous cords) and had marked discrepancy in heart weights and coloration. Another unusual set of twins is that recorded by King et al. (1995). These presumably MZ twins had DiDi placentation, with ink-injection confirmed anastomoses. Although blood exchange had occurred, the typical TTTS was absent; one fetus had died with hydrocephaly before the other was aborted. More recently, Souter et al. (2003) reviewed the topic and presented a set of monochorionic, heterosexual twins conceived by IVF and who also had blood chimerism. The chimerism must have resulted from the "fine arterial-to-arterial anastomoses" that were identified by fluid injection. Redline (2003), who made editorial comments on the case, reviewed the development of twin embryos and also entertained the possibility that the IVF manipulation could have been a factor in the genesis of these unusual twins. As has been indicated earlier, the occurrence of monochorionic twins after IVF and embryo transfer is not uncommon now, and the dogma that monochorionic twins *must be* MZ twins is no longer tenable. To prove the existence of such unusual placentas, it is necessary that injection of the vessels be done. Therefore, another report, of anastomoses in a dichorionic twin placenta of twins with CMV infection, is more difficult to interpret (Foschini et al., 2003). The anastomotic arrangement was suggested only by stereomicroscopy of formalin-fixed placentas and described as being subchorial. Because there are generally never any subchorial anastomoses in any placenta, we reserve judgment on this case. More challenging still is the report by Quintero et al. (2003b) on a set of heterosexual twins with TTTS (unsuccessfully treated with laser ablation of AV anastomoses) and DiMo placenta; this is truly exceptional but points to the need for full genetic and pathologic study.

These cases are truly exceptional. In addition to these observations it must be recorded that spontaneous "blood chimerae" have been observed in a few other occasional human fraternal twins. They have had no sexual abnormalities and are like marmosets in that respect. When their *fixed* tissue has been studied, it was not found to be admixed. The chimerae, therefore, must have received the foreign clone of blood cells either through placental anastomoses or, less likely, transplacentally. Kadowaki et al. (1965) reported the transfer of maternal lymphocytes to the fetus. They described a phenotypically normal male with XY/XX blood chimerism and apparent graft-versus-host rejection disease. Such transplacental exchange of lymphocytes, however, must be uncommon (Olding, 1972). Only on rare occasions have prospective studies shown minor transplacental lymphocyte chimerism. This transplacental traffic of cells was discussed in Chapter 17; it may affect singletons as well as twins and has recently been of great interest because the resulting microchimerism of blood and stem cells finds correlation with maternal autoimmune diseases (Johnson et al., 2001; Nelson, 2001; Srivatsa et al., 2001; Adams & Nelson, 2004).

The occurrence of blood chimerism in human DZ twins was first demonstrated by Dunsford et al. (1953). Since then, more than 30 cases have been described (Tippett, 1984). They are usually detected when blood group tests have peculiar results that necessitate full genetic investigation; it usually happens long after birth. The associated placenta of such a chimera has been fully studied only in the case of Nylander and Osunkoya (1970). Hartemann et al. (1963) suggested that placental study of twin placentas would more often identify anastomoses among fraternal twins. This has not been our experience, despite the fact that we have tried on many occasions to verify anastomoses among DiDi twins by the use of dye injections. Anastomoses that become apparent by radiographic examination of injected twin placentas and those discovered by corrosion casts made following plastics injection (Scipiades & Burg, 1930; Pérez et al., 1947), give unreliable results. Crookston et al. (1970) described the unusual and complex immunologic breakdown of tolerance that rarely occurs in such twins. On occasion, most unusual situations are encountered with chimerism; thus, O'Donnell et al. (2004) found blood chimerism for 47,XY and 47,XY+21 in a monochorionic set of twins that was naturally conceived. Genetic analysis revealed monozygosity; how the trisomy then developed in a DiMo placenta is a bit speculative. "Trisomy rescue" is often assumed but not easily compatible with a DiMo placentation.

Whole-Body Chimerism

In whole-body chimeras, the entire body consists of cells with two or more genetic lineages that are derived from separate fertilization products. Most common among them is probably the fertilization of an ovum and a polar body by two spermatozoa, with the maternal contribution being similar. Such individuals represent, genetically speaking, fraternal twins fused into one body. They are not necessarily clinically manifest and may be fertile, even when XX and XY lineages coexist. The topic was discussed in great detail by Yu et al. (2002) because of the discovery of a fertile 46/XX/46,XX woman who was tested for transplantation antigen. It is accompanied by excellent drawings and discussion. Most total body chimerae, however, are discovered when the two populations of cells have different sex chromosomes (XX/XY), which frequently results in gonadal abnormalities, most common among which is true hermaphroditism (see also Kim et al., 2002). The diagnosis was initially made by amniocentesis in a detailed report by Lawce (1985). The male neonate was entirely normal and had an overall 48/98 XX/XY cell admixture. Remarkably, the ratio was 40:8 in placental membranes but 1:39 in placental tissue. Other cytogenetic errors with multiple karyotypes are also known (Moreno & Sánchez, 1971). Whole-body chimeras may also be discovered during routine blood grouping tests. Still others may be found because of unusual phenotypic features, such as heterochromia (eyes of different color). Some such cases may even possess "striping" of skin, or they may have abnormal patches of the skin, resulting from the irregular distribution of melanocyte precursors that are derived from different genotypes (Zuelzer et al., 1964; Corey et al., 1967). An especially striking case of chimerism was reported by Karam and Baker (2004). The neonate had a vertical pigment difference, right-sided male genitals, and left-sided female genitals, and was 46,XX/46,XY on karyotyping. This skin coloration is particularly obvious in the rare male tricolored (tortoiseshell) cats because the colors black and orange are allelic on the X chromosome in felines. Tricolored cats must all be female, or else they have chimerism (rarely are they endowed with 39,XXY chromosomes) as the basis for their abnormal coloration (Centerwall & Benirschke, 1975). It is thus important to clearly distinguish between mosaicism and chimerism, something often not duly considered in the literature. The placentas of these individuals never seem to have been examined but then there is no reason to believe that they would be unusual.

The question of how spontaneous whole-body chimerism originates is not yet completely answered. It is readily achieved experimentally by fusing morulae of experimental animals after their zonae pellucidae have been removed (Tarkowski, 1961). How this happens in vivo is speculative. The finding of diploid/triploid chimeras (e.g., Van de Berghe & Verresen, 1970) was taken as evidence that fertilization of a large polar body (common in mice) produced such abnormal individuals (dispermic chimeras). Other proposed mechanisms, such as secondary nondisjunction of whole haploid sets (Jenkins et al., 1971), are much less likely. De la Chapelle et al. (1974) suggested, as did other investigators, that early fusion of two embryos may be the way that whole-body chimeras are produced spontaneously, much as in the experimental model. This idea has subsequently been disputed because of the paucity of markers available. These concepts and the wide complexity of chimerism and hermaphroditism are topics of the review by Tippett (1984). Finally, an interesting true hermaphrodite (46,XX/46,XY) was described by Strain et al. (1998). It resulted most likely from fusion of two early fertilized ova and was the result of IVF and implantation of three fertilized ova; a male singleton resulted in an inguinal hernia that contained an ovary tube and uterine horn. Whole-body chimerism was elegantly proved by DNA study, and the occurrence suggests that manipulation of early ova may have such undesirable result. Since that report, other cases of abnormal blastocyst behavior following IVF have been reported, especially the increased frequency of MZ twins among multiples, when smaller numbers of ova were transferred than babies born.

Triplets and Higher Multiple Births

The frequency of spontaneously conceived higher multiple births is customarily estimated with the help of Hellin's rule, which was discussed earlier. Because of ovulation induction with hormones, many higher multiple births have occurred; nonatuplets hold the record, but they did not survive. Survival of septuplets was first observed in the U.S. in 1997, and surviving, prematurely delivered octatuplets were delivered in Houston in 1998. For reasons of widespread hormone usage in assisted reproduction, it is presently difficult to ascertain the real and spontaneous occurrence of higher multiple births in any population. Many excessive numbers are reported in the newspapers, and they are usually artificially induced. The patient who aborted the nonatuplets during the 12th week of pregnancy was not further described. Octuplets, born prematurely to a Mexican woman who had taken contraceptives until 8 months earlier, all died from complications of prematurity (Anonymous, 1967). The frequency of higher multiple births has increased significantly in recent years because of the practice of "assisted reproduction." Thus, Collins and Bleyl (1990) were able to summarize results of 71 quadruplet pregnancies. They advocated delivery by the 34th week of pregnancy because of the growth deficit occurring thereafter. Elliott and Radin (1992) reviewed their own 10 quadruplet pregnancies and made specific management recommendations. They had no bad outcomes, even though their gestations terminated at about 32.5 weeks. Interestingly, the older the mothers of quadruplets and quintuplets, the better were the outcomes (Salihu et al., 2004a). Kiely et al. (1992) surveyed the trends of higher-order multiple births from 1972 to 1989. There had occurred a 113% increase among white and a 22% increase among African-American mothers, with a 50% reduction in perinatal mortality. We have recently had surviving sextuplets (six chorions) at 28 weeks with three separated placentas on each anterior and posterior portions of the uterus. They were conceived after hormonal superovulation and survived. At the same time sextuplets were born at 32

weeks in Pennsylvania, also after hormonal medication usage.

When Allen (1960) applied the Weinberg formula to higher multiple offspring, he observed for triplets that the proportion of MZ/DZ/trizygotic (TZ) was 1:3:2 among African Americans, and 1:2:1 among whites; quadruplet whites were 2:6:5:4. In Japan, with different rates of multiple births, the ratios for triplets were more like 2.5:1:1, reflecting the lower DZ twinning rate of this genetically different population (Imaizumi & Inouye, 1980). The high DZ rate of Nigerians is reflected in their distribution of zygosity in triplets, approximately 1:4:6 (Nylander, 1971b). The frequent admixture of MZ and DZ twins in plural births is well reflected in their placentation. They may all be monochorionic or they have mono-, di-, and trichorionic placentation. Nylander and Corney (1971) found in the Yoruba population of triplets one monochorionic, 10 dichorionic, and 29 trichorionic specimens. Most other reports are of single gestations or are from smaller series than those collected by Nylander and Corney. Boyd and Hamilton (1970) had the following placentation in their eight triplet pregnancies: four monochorionic, three dichorionic, and one trichorionic. They were thus different from that in African women, which reflects the different causes of twinning in the populations studied. Not all dichorionic triplets are polyzygotic. Thus, the dichorionic triplets described by Komai and Fukuoka (1931) were shown to be monozygotic.

Triplets and higher plural births not only are smaller than expected for their gestational age (McKeown & Record, 1952) but also commonly deliver much earlier than twins or singletons. The perinatal mortality of 59 triplet pregnancies was 23% in the study of Itzkowic (1979). This investigator emphasized that "cervical incompetence" was not a significant factor in their premature deliveries. Others (Gabos, 1972) reported that cervical failure may require surgical intervention in these higher multiple gestations. O'Sullivan (1968) even advocated it routinely in multiple pregnancies with hydramnios. Michlewitz et al. (1981) found a perinatal mortality of 13% past 20 weeks and 7% when 15 triplet pregnancies past 28 weeks were studied. A very large experience of the outcome of assisted reproduction from Norfolk (Seoud et al., 1992) found that there was the expected progressive increase of perinatal complications and prematurity with higher-order births. Keith et al. (2002) edited a book on all aspects of triplet deliveries.

Lipitz and his colleagues (1989) showed that the outcome of triplet pregnancies was improving. They studied 78 triplet pregnancies between 1975 and 1988, with 88% occurring after ovulation induction. Their finding was that elective cerclage neither improved fetal loss nor enhanced the length of gestation. Of the babies they were able to follow, 10.5% had severe neurologic handicaps. Some triplets have been delivered with long time intervals. Simpson et al. (1984) had the first infant born at 23 weeks' gestation (neonatal death with 505 g weight, congenital infection), and 99 days later (with Shirodkar stitch, antibiotics, and isoxsuprine) a cesarean section was done at 37 weeks. One triplet was macerated, and the other lived (2580 g); the placenta was a fused TriTri organ. Cardwell et al. (1988) described the survival of one triplet, with the first being born at 23 weeks (hyaline membrane disease); the second was born 4 days later and died with hyaline membrane disease. The third triplet delivered 16 days after the first and survived. Chorioamnionitis complicated this pregnancy as it does in many plural pregnancies. A pregnancy with one triplet aborting during the 16th week of pregnancy and the other triplets surviving to delivery at 35 weeks was reported by Banchi (1984). The aborted triplet had a separate chorionic sac; the survivors had a DiMo placenta. A most remarkable case of triplets in a uterus didelphys was described by Mashiach et al. (1981). The clomiphene-induced pregnancy resulted in triplets: two in one horn and one in the other. One was found dead at 22 weeks; and at 27 weeks, uterine contractions expelled a macerated triplet from the right horn, but cesarean section was done to deliver its co-twin who later died. The left horn did not go into labor. At 37 weeks, a normal triplet was delivered by cesarean section. R. Gonen et al. (1990a) reported on five triplet gestations with fetal death of one or two fetuses. Four of these were monochorionic and delivery took place 30 (±26) days after the diagnosis of fetal death. Blickstein et al. (2003) found frequently large discrepancies in birth weight and implied "exhaustion of fetal growth potential." Salihu et al. (2004b) compared survival of triplets in white and black populations, finding substantially higher mortality in the black population, being highest postnatally. Al-Kouatly et al. (2003) commented on the high frequency of thrombocytopenia in triplets and inferred that its commonest cause was pre-eclampsia. Luke et al. (2002) found that the outcome of 178 sets of triplets was most favorable when there was a prior gestation with good outcome, adequate weight gain, and greater length of gestation.

The various types of triplet placentations are shown in Figures 25.99 to 25.103. In addition to these three variants, the placentas of DiDi triplets may be separate. This is relatively uncommon, however, as the uterine surface area available for the implantation of multiple placentas is not large enough for them to remain separate. The liveborn monozygotic triplets whose placenta is shown in Figure 25.99 were monoamnionic and monochorionic (Sinykin, 1958). Triplet pregnancy does not always prevent entangling of cords when they are monoamnionic, as in the case shown in Figure 25.104, although entangling is less common in triplets than in twins. In this case, one anencephalic and a tiny acardiac fetus were associated with a normal triplet. All were aborted because of cord entanglements. Kohler and MacDonald (1972) reported triplets, one of whom was anencephalic and who had a normal DiMo co-twin. There was a normal separate chorionic triplet. The DiMo twins of the TriDi placenta shown in Figure 25.100 had suffered the typical transfusion syndrome, with A being the runted donor and B the recipient who died neonatally. All were females, with C represent-

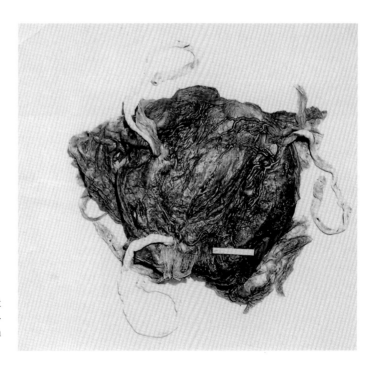

FIGURE 25.99. A MoMo triplet term placenta, without entangling of cords but anastomoses among all circulations. The triplets survived. (*Source:* Sinykin, 1958, with permission.)

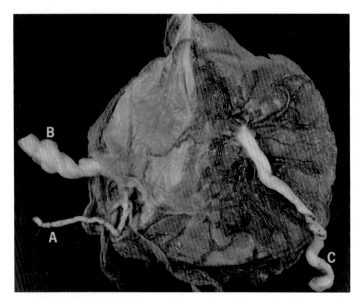

FIGURE 25.100. Triamnionic/dichorionic triplets, all females. A is the donor of the transfusion syndrome, and B is the recipient in a DiMo placenta. C has a separate amnion and chorion, and blood groups different from those the twins. (Blood groups courtesy of Dr. F.H. Allen, New York, New York.)

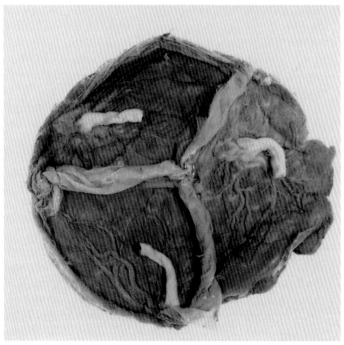

FIGURE 25.101. Triamnionic/monochorionic triplet placenta at term. Many large anastomoses are present.

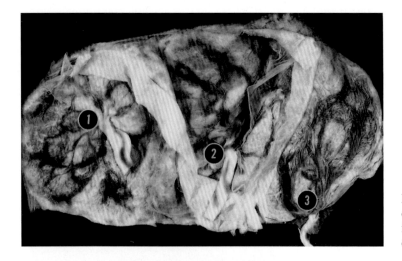

FIGURE 25.102. Triamnionic/trichorionic term placenta. There are no anastomoses and, despite intimate fusion, no blood chimerism. Note the velamentous cord insertion of No. 3.

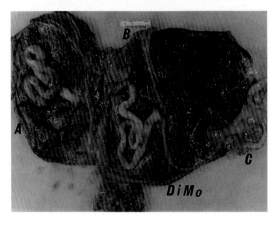

FIGURE 25.103. Triamnionic/dichorionic triplet placenta at 36 weeks' gestation, all males. The diamnionic set of twins are at right with a single AV anastomosis from C to B. All survived. The slightly separated dichorionic placenta of triplet A (at left) has an area of circummargination at top, where the membranes of the right triplets pushed its membranes away.

FIGURE 25.104. A MoMo triplet placenta from a spontaneous abortion. Note the entangling of all umbilical cords. One was a normal fetus, and one an anencephalic; the small fetus, placed separately on the piece of paper, was an acardiac.

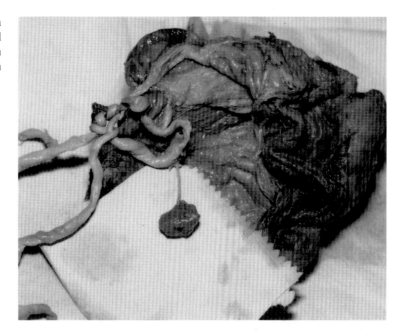

ing a separate zygote, as established by blood grouping (courtesy of Dr. F.H. Allen, New York, New York). Another TriDi set of triplets is seen in Figure 25.103.

It has long been known that an admixture of MZ and DZ multiple births is more common than would be expected by chance, but the reason is not clear. In addition to these examples, we have seen a DiMo triplet pregnancy abort with two monoamnionic pygopagous twins, a term DiMo triplet placenta with one set of thoracopagi, as well as a TriTri triplet pregnancy with two fetus papyracei, the other fetus coming to term and being normal. The prenatal death of the two fetuses may therein have been due to their velamentous cord insertions. A triplet pregnancy produced by IVF was reported in Chapter 6. Five ova had been transferred, three implanted, and one became a placenta percreta that had to be removed from its interstitial implantation during the second month of pregnancy. The two remaining fetuses were delivered by cesarean section near term, one having amnionic bands. We have witnessed yet another triplet placenta percreta. Thus plural pregnancies can present multiple problems with many anomalies of placentation alone.

It has often been asked how triplets or quintuplets (e.g., the famous Dionne quintuplets) can be MZ, as one might expect even numbers to result. Uneven numbers of monozygotic multiples may be explained by assuming that, on occasion, one embryo may not have survived or that "one division may set back development of the daughter products so that secondary division can occur at the same stage or even an earlier stage than did the primary division ... or ... three or more embryonic centers might arise simultaneously instead of two" (Allen, 1960). Allen presented a graphic demonstration of the genesis of multiple embryos, assuming binary divisions as

the principal modus operandi. Monochorionic, tetraamnionic quadruplet girls have been recorded by Steinman (1998); born by cesarean section, they weighed between 940 and 1440 g and did well.

Quadruplets and quintuplets have also become more common in recent years. Whereas in the past most had not been induced by hormone administration, such treatment is clearly now a factor. We have met a diabetic patient who had three sets of fraternal triplets and then a set of fraternal twins, and her uterus finally had to be removed when it ruptured with a quadruplet pregnancy. Sinclair (1940) depicted the QuaTri placenta of a set of surviving quadruplets. A similar placenta from three-egg quadruplets was described by Ryan and Wislocki (1954). Hamilton et al. (1959) reported the quadrichorial placenta depicted in Figure 25.105. They found in the 16 cases of the English-language literature that "every possible combination of ovulation had occurred except for double monozygous, often stated never to appear." Diddle and Burford (1935), however, described just such a case in stillborns. Atlay and Pennington (1971) observed a quadruplet pregnancy after ovulation induction with pituitary gonadotropins. It was composed of a set of monoamnionic twins, the others all having their separate amnion, and they were of different sex. The 30 weeks' gestation quadruplets had a good outcome. In this contribution, Atlay and Pennington provided much hormonal data that may be helpful in the surveillance of plural pregnancies. McFee et al. (1974) reported on two sets of quadruplets, among which only one of the eight premature newborns succumbed. The authors gave detailed and helpful instructions as to preparations needed by staff and family for the anticipated delivery of plural births. Williams (1926) described the quadruplet pregnancy of a 38-year-old woman whose

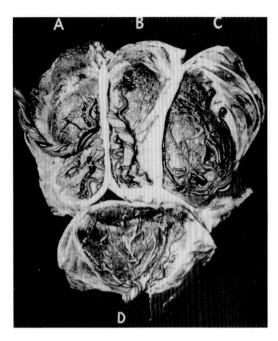

FIGURE 25.105. Quadruplet placenta with four chorionic sacs, all surviving. (*Source:* Hamilton et al., 1959, with permission.)

offspring all died. The placenta was TriTri and fused. He also reported on the fact \that 24% of the 280 sets of twins observed at the Johns Hopkins Hospital were monochorionic; of four triplets, three were TriDi and one was TriTri. We have seen several quadruplet placentas with four chorions and one with four amnions and three chorions (Fig. 25.106). Imaizumi (1989b) reported on 16 sets of quintuplets from Japan. Three sets were liveborn, eight were stillborn, and five were live- and stillborn, with 51 of 80 offspring being stillborn. The mean weight of 40 quintuplets was 1048 g.

Nichols (1954) published a list of 17 quintuplet births in the United States and two in Canada, as well as five sextuplets in the United States. An editorial (Anonymous, 1968) estimated spontaneous quintuplets to occur as rarely as 1 in 8 million to 54 million births. The combined weights for four surviving sets were 10.61, 14.08, 12.11, and 23.52 pounds. We have seen surviving quintichorial quintuplets, conceived after clomiphene citrate (Clomid) induction and delivered at 31 weeks. Their combined weight was 8200 g (1420 to 1820 g). Three of the umbilical cords had marginal insertions. As can be imagined, such enormous uterine distention gives rise to maternal dyspnea, hydramnios(?), excessive weight gain, preeclampsia, edema, varices, and cardiac failure. In another

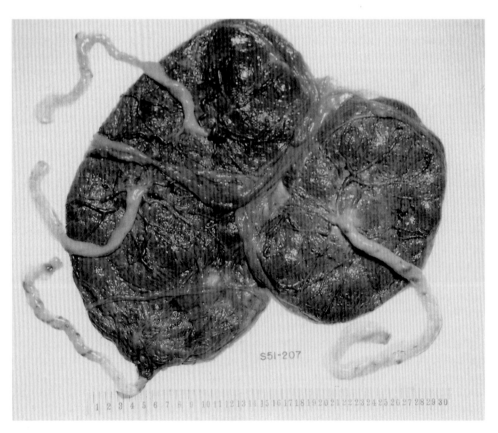

FIGURE 25.106. Quadruplet placenta (QuaTri), with DiMo MZ twins at bottom left, one having marginal insertion of the umbilical cord (35 weeks, 920 g).

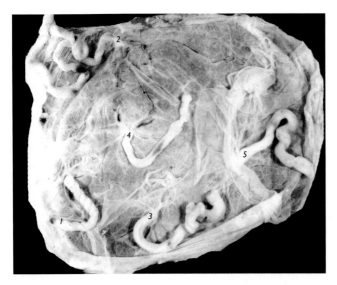

FIGURE 25.107. Monochorionic (quint-amnionic) quintuplet placenta, immature. All infants died from hyaline membrane disease; No. 5 had SUA. Large anastomoses are present. (*Source:* Gibbs et al., 1960, and Neubecker et al., 1962, with permission.)

editorial (Anonymous, 1963a), 50 sets of quintuplets were listed as having been reported in the entire medical literature. It is interesting to note that several of the well-described quintuplet placentas were diagnostic of MZ quintuplets, as were the Dionne quintuplets. The fact that one of the latter gave birth to a set of male twins is presumably a random occurrence.

A monozygotic quintuplet placenta was superbly studied by Gibbs et al. (1960); it is depicted in Figure 25.107. This placenta had a single chorion and five amnions. There were many vascular anastomoses on the chorionic surface; several cords inserted marginally, and that of No. 5 had a single umbilical artery. All these extremely immature infants succumbed from hyaline membrane disease. The placenta was redescribed by Neubecker et al. (1962). Quintuplets reported by Berbos et al. (1964) were QuiQua (quint-amnionic; quadrichorial); a quintuplet pregnancy induced with gonadotropins and studied by Aubert (1960) resulted in three male and two female infants, with QuiQua placenta, and the successful quintuplet pregnancy reported by Liggins and Ibbertson (1966) had five chorionic sacs (QuiQui). Bender and Brandt (1974) studied a quintuplet placenta by morphometry. It was induced by hormones and had QuiQui membranes. These authors drew attention to the irregular chorionic fusion of the dividing membranes, discussed earlier and depicted in Figures 25.51 and 25.52. Altshuler (personal communication, 1975) also observed a QuiQui placenta that, when injected with milk, exhibited no anastomoses. Finally, the monochorionic quintuplets (QuiMo) with one acardiac fetus reported by Hamblen et al. (1937) are shown in Figure 25.86.

No sextuplet placentas had been described as far as we can ascertain from the literature, and few sextuplets have been reported to have occurred. Figure 25.108 shows such a specimen from a patient treated with fertility drugs that was provided by Dr. M.A. Fletcher from a delivery

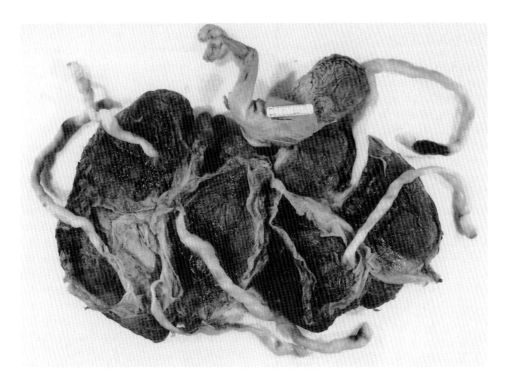

FIGURE 25.108. Sextuplet placenta with six chorionic sacs and a male fetus papyraceus. (Courtesy of Dr. M.A. Fletcher, Washington, D.C.)

in Washington, D.C., in 1983. It was a fused placenta with six amnions and six chorions. It also contained a fetus papyraceus, estimated to have died at 20 weeks' gestation. That fetus had a normal skeleton, but its cord had velamentous insertion, and this insertion was the presumed reason for his demise. Three other fetuses had marginal cord insertion. Two cords had a left, and three a right, spiral; that of the fetus papyraceus was not spiraled at all. One specimen of a septuplet pregnancy, induced by gonadotropins and prematurely delivered (Turksoy et al., 1967) was depicted by Boyd and Hamilton (1970). The sacs each had their own chorion and amnion; one was separated, and the others were fused. The cords were mostly marginal and one had SUA.

Because plural gestations generally have poor outcomes, their early diagnosis and selective reduction of some cases is currently being advocated. By ultrasonography, Campbell and Dewhurst (1970) diagnosed hormone-induced quintuplets as early as at 19 weeks' gestation. The pregnancy went to 31 weeks. Labor ensued and the healthy quintuplets were delivered by cesarean section. Kanhai et al. (1986) punctured the hearts of three quintuplets at 10 weeks' gestation (one was repeated at 11 weeks). The mother subsequently delivered full-term healthy twin girls. The placenta had only one 2.5-cm embryonic rest. Various authors have addressed fetal reduction of multiple gestations in recent years, primarily, we believe, because of the poorer outcome of multiples and because so many more large "litters" are being produced. Thus, Miller et al. (2000) addressed the fiscal aspects of hospitalization and those occurring in later life. Stone et al. (2002) found that additional fetal losses occurred mostly in sextuplets, less so with other multiples, and found an overall loss rate of 5.4% in 1000 (!) consecutive cases. Fetocide was performed for a variety of reasons, and its frequency had been steadily increasing in these authors' experience, with more mothers now opting to retain a singleton rather than twins. The authors' previous publications on this topic are referred to in this paper as well, and the rate is compared to the findings of other institutions. In the second paper of this institution (Eddleman et al., 2002), the authors reviewed 200 terminations for anomalous multiples and caution that dichorionicity needs to be established sonographically before an attempt at potassium chloride injection is done. It is also interesting to note that, when Dickey et al. (2002) studied the *spontaneous* reductions of multiples, they found that more than 50% of triplets had intrauterine fetal deaths (IUFDs) before 12 weeks (36% of twins, 53% of triplets, 65% of quadruplets). Similar findings come from La Sala et al. (2004). Heyborne and Porreco (2004) used reduction in three cases of severe preeclampsia complicating twin gestations with discordance and found that PIH resolved in all three and allowed lengthening of gestation.

Most commonly, this reduction is accomplished by cardiac injection of KCl, but on occasion this is dangerous, as the maternal cardiac arrest (resolved) in a patient reported by Coke et al. (2004) describes. They reviewed the usage of KCl injection in general. Another hormone-induced quintuplet pregnancy was managed by Farquharson et al. (1988). At 9 weeks two embryos had intracardiac injection of hypertonic saline. Five days later the procedure was repeated with another embryo. The maternal serum human chorionic gonadotropin levels declined substantially and, at 37 weeks, heterosexual twins were delivered vaginally. Their placenta was DiDi. In the membranes, a plaque of atrophied villi and a cavity (but no fetuses) were found.

Evans and colleagues (1988) presented four such cases of therapeutic intervention. They also discussed the legal and other implications that attend this novel therapy. Their first case had nine gestational sacs at 7 weeks. Three fetuses were "needled" at 8 weeks and three additional ones at 9 weeks. The patient delivered two healthy males at 35 weeks. Their second case was a hormone-induced quadruplet pregnancy with elimination of two sacs by cardiac puncture at 10 weeks. Two healthy children delivered at 36 weeks. In the third case, IVF led to implantation of four embryos; two embryos were eliminated at 10 weeks. One remaining fetus was then found to have Potter's syndrome. The other died in utero. In their fourth case, four fetuses had been induced with hormones, and two were eliminated at 11 weeks. The remaining twins were aborted because of "cervical incompetence." They delivered, despite cerclage, at 19 weeks; the placentas were not described by these authors. They emphasized ethical issues and the need for regulated hormone induction of pregnancy for infertile patients, an aspect that was further elaborated on in discussion by Weiner (1988). It might be mentioned parenthetically that there has been much discussion as to whether cerclage is indicated in multiple pregnancy because of the frequently observed cervical dilatation. Michaels et al. (1991) recommend that it not be used routinely; they used ultrasonic criteria to select those patients who might benefit from this operation. Their results suggest that some patients' twin pregnancy is lengthened when cerclage is done. Berkowitz et al. (1988) reported their experience with selective embryocide in 12 multifetal pregnancies (2 in sextuplets; 1 in quintuplets; 5 in quadruplets; 4 in triplets). They reduced the number to two fetuses in 11 pregnancies and to three fetuses in one pregnancy. The surgery was undertaken between 9 and 13 weeks. Seven healthy twins were born. One produced a healthy singleton, and four had only fetal deaths. Later, these authors reported on 200 multifetal reductions (Berkowitz et al., 1993), and Boulot et al. (1993) concluded that the reduction reduces but does not prevent preterm labor. The difficulty and rationale for the procedure were highlighted in an editorial by

Hobbins (1988). One problem is the development of unforeseen complications in the survivor. Mahone et al. (1993) had such an experience. They described a twin transfusion syndrome at 23 weeks' gestation where the selective feticide of the hydropic recipient was followed quickly by hydrops in the remaining donor. They speculated that perhaps one mechanism of cardiac failure in the donor was the additional blood loss into the plethoric donor. Their photograph of the twins supports this notion. It also suggests to us that the best therapy for this ominous syndrome is the interruption of the anastomosing vessels, as practice by De Lia (see below).

Since these earlier reports on embryo reduction, there have been numerous reports that should be consulted. Thus Wapner et al. (1990) reviewed 46 cases with 80 fetuses remaining; 94% of these survived. Lynch et al. (1990) discussed 28 triplet, 47 quadruplet, four quintuplet, four sextuplet, one septuplet, and one nonatuplet pregnancies with reductions, usually to twins. Their outcomes were excellent. Tabsh (1990b) reviewed 40 cases, and Melgar et al. (1991) suggested that their results from the reduction of quadruplets indicated marked improvement in outcome, whereas that for triplets remains controversial. The intentional delivery of a 710-g acardiac fetus at 22 weeks' gestation by Robie et al. (1989) is also relevant in this regard. It was followed by delivery of a normal girl. The case is of special interest because the acardiac had a penile structure, yet possessed ovaries. She also had a normal female karyotype, and the co-twin was a normal girl. Itskovitz et al. (1989) and Gonen et al. (1990b,c) elected to use a transvaginal ultrasound approach for selective embryo reduction. The latter authors used intrathoracic KCl injection and had one case of chorioamnionitis follow the procedure. They considered the procedure to be not without significant risk. Tabsh (1993) reported the result of 131 transabdominal reductions done by one practitioner, with 103 deliveries ensuing. He had a 7% pregnancy loss rate from the intervention that occurred within 4 weeks and concluded that this is a safe procedure. Macones et al. (1993) showed that reducing triplets to twins markedly improves fetal survival. A large international experience was summarized by Evans et al. (1994), with the majority of infants being born after 33 weeks when reduction had been done. The procedure was judged to be safe. Other studies to be consulted are those by Lipitz et al. (1994, 1997), Berkowitz (1996), Haning et al. (1996), Lynch et al. (1996), and Smith-Levitin (1996). Sebire et al. (1997b) reported less fortunate results when reducing triplets to twin pregnancies, whereas Albrecht and Tomich (1996) and Lipitz et al. (1996) suggested they had better successes. Finally, Evans et al. (1995) reported that, despite increased triplet and quadruplet pregnancies, higher multiple conceptions have declined because of better management of the superovulation techniques.

Twins in Abortion and Ectopic Pregnancy

Multiple pregnancies occur also as abortions and in ectopic gestations, but they are not often reported or perhaps they are frequently overlooked. Many specimens from spontaneous abortions do not contain an embryo, many are chromosomally abnormal, and many are fragmented when they are observed in the laboratory. Javert (1957) reviewed most of the relevant literature. He found citations of twin frequencies ranging from 6% to 20%. In his own material of 2000 abortuses, he had an incidence of only 1.2%. Our own observations have yielded a still lower figure (0.3%) (Benirschke & Driscoll, 1967). There is general agreement, however, that monochorial twins are overrepresented in abortion material. Numerous MoMo twins, for instance, vanish during early development (Figs. 25.43 and 25.84); and still other twins succumb from the transfusion syndrome or because they are acardiacs (Fig. 25.91). It is impossible to give accurate figures. The great student of twinning, Guttmacher (1937), believed that twins were twice as common in abortions as in births (1 in 37 versus 1 in 86.5), and the investigations of Livingston and Poland (1980) and Uchida et al. (1983) pointed in the same direction.

It should be easier to identify ectopic twin gestations, as they are generally better preserved. Indeed, many such cases are on record (e.g., Starks, 1980). The exceptional case of a tubal triplet gestation was reported by Forbes and Natale (1968), who believed it to be only the fourth case published. It was TriMo, and only a single corpus luteum cyst was found. Fujii et al. (1981) described a unilateral tubal quadruplet pregnancy with QuaMo placenta and unequal development of the embryos. Twin ectopics have been seen more often. Considering the frequencies of ectopic pregnancy and twinning, it is surprising that Storch and Petrie (1976) found only 87 reported cases of ectopic twins. More astonishing still is the fact that most tubal ectopics are monochorionic. This finding is much out of proportion to the general distribution of twin placentation, and the topic is discussed in detail by Neuman et al. (1990). They proved with RFLPs the dizygosity of tubal aborted twins, and suggested that the alleged common monozygosity of ectopic twins may be in error. Arey (1923a,b) was the first to report that ectopic twins have a 15 times greater frequency of monochorionic placentation than do intrauterine gestations. He reported MoMo twins, quintuplets, three triplets, and one thoracopagus and, in an earlier publication (Arey, 1922), suggested that these findings argued in favor of chorionic fusion. The proof of this contention, the occurrence of monochorial heterosexual twins, has not been reported. Later, Arey considered the possibility of an environmental insult that produced MZ twins in this abnormal location. It is our opinion that most case reports are incomplete and too superficial; thus, usually they do not allow a clear decision on this interesting point. Perhaps monochorial gestational sacs are larger ab initio, and have more difficulty passing through the tube. Even less commonly described are twin ovarian ectopic pregnancies. Kalfayan and Gundersen (1980) reported a case of DiDi ovarian gestational sacs in a patient wearing an intrauterine device. They found three other reported cases.

"Heterotopic pregnancy is defined as a coexisting, intrauterine and extrauterine pregnancy" (Goodno & Gentry, 1962). It is apparently more common than is usually assumed. Gamberdella and Marrs (1989), who described a much higher frequency in ART, considered heterotopic pregnancies to occur 1 per 30,000 pregnancies. It often involves an interstitial (cornual) and an intrauterine gestation. Sotrel et al. (1976) suggested that more than 600 cases had been reported in the literature. They identified a case that occurred after ovulation induction. These pregnancies are often complicated by placenta accreta/increta (Starks, 1980) and they are usually dichorionic. Because they were able to make the diagnosis early, Porreco et al. (1990) electively eliminated the ectopic fetus and allowed the intrauterine gestation to proceed to term. Laband et al. (1988), who reported four such cases, suggested that the incidence of this unusual, dangerous gestational complication may be greater than 1 in 30,000. Payne et al. (1971) have seen triplets in this situation after ovulation induction. A similar case is reported in Chapter 6 with interstitial placenta percreta, removed during the second month, with twins remaining in the uterus.

It is also surprising how many cases of twin gestation have been described in uterus didelphys and how frequently they have been delivered at different times. Laird et al. (1957) reported on a miscarriage from one side, 6 months before the delivery of a normal twin from the other. Dawson and Ainslee (1958) saw premature twins delivering from a bicornuate uterus in short succession. Kennedy (1959) delivered an asphyxiated infant from one side, and 3 weeks later the other twin was born from the other uterus. Mingeot and Keirse (1971) delivered such twins within 9 hours of each other. Brown and Nelson (1967) reported that a patient with completely split genital tracts intentionally became pregnant on separate occasions in each uterus, with live infants resulting. A complex case was seen by Zervoudakis et al. (1976) in which curettage emptied an aborting pregnancy, but the patient remained pregnant in a blind uterine horn. Six weeks later, the horn was surgically emptied when a chemical interruption failed. There were no apparent connections, although Loendersloot (1977) later suggested that a perforation may have been present from first curettage. Nhân and Huisjes (1983) induced the second uterine horn after delivery of a normal child from one horn. Finally, Ahram et al. (1984) delivered twins

from both horns of a bicornuate uterus. They, as many before, had to initiate labor of the second horn before delivery could be effected. In most of these cases the placenta is not described. When it is discussed, the twins are usually considered to be binovular.

In a review of the obstetrical performance of 150 cases with uterine anomalies (with 325 pregnancies), Jones (1957) noted that twinning was not more common in these women. It may also be noted that delivery of twins at different times has been described in women with normal uteri. Thomsen (1978) reported a case where the first twin was delivered at 27 weeks and the second at 31 weeks. We have seen twins deliver 4 weeks apart, with the placenta of the first twin remaining in utero and becoming atrophied. The second twin survived. Previously, the maximum interval of 65 days was reported by Drucker et al. (1960), but Feichtinger et al. (1989) described an even longer interval: The patient delivered one twin at 21 weeks' gestation, followed by tocolysis and cerclage. She delivered a healthy 1750-g twin 12 weeks later; the placenta was dichorionic and had an infarcted portion. The survivor had a velamentous cord insertion. There was no inflammation. Another recent report on delayed delivery of second twins comes from Vancouver (Wittmann et al., 1992). The authors observed four cases with delivery intervals ranging from 41 to 143 days, and then reviewed 21 cases from the literature. The overall salvage rate was 84%; careful management protocols are suggested by these authors.

Morbidity and Mortality

An abundant obstetrical literature discusses the causes of the excessive mortality of twins and the frequent obstetrical complications encountered during their delivery. Relatively rare but easy to understand is the phenomenon of "locked twins." Khunda (1972) discussed 37 such cases and estimated that it occurs with a frequency of 1 in 1000 twin deliveries, and that it has a high stillbirth rate. Breech/vertex presentation of twins is the commonest factor; also common are primigravidity and large pelves. Cohen et al. (1965) had previously reported similar figures. In their experience, interlocking was present once in 817 twin deliveries and once in 87 breech/vertex presentations of twins. It is a particularly serious event when it occurs at or below the pelvic inlet, with death of twin A quickly ensuing. Amniotic sac dystocia has been described once, by Nickerson (1967). The membranes from the second twin then prolapsed in front of the first delivering twin. This abnormality was easily corrected, and delivery accomplished.

Of the numerous maternal complications that attend multiple gestations, Seski and Miller (1963) listed in descending order of frequency: premature delivery, preeclampsia, hydramnios, placenta previa, abruptio placentae, cord prolapse, uterine inertia, and postpartum hemorrhage. Placental abnormalities often mirror these events. Hydramnios in twin pregnancies is most commonly due to the transfusion syndrome; good evidence exists that the amnionic fluid index of normal twin gestations is the same as in singletons (Hill et al., 2000). Next most frequently, hydramnios results from fetal or placental anomalies. It has been debated as to whether pre-eclampsia is commoner with DZ twins than with MZ twins; that it is more frequent in twin gestations is not disputed. We have seen numerous dizygotic twin placentas in which only one placental half was affected with infarcts and decidual atherosis. It suggests that fetal and maternal interactions of respective genotypes are critical in the determination of PIH and preeclampsia. Campbell et al. (1977) studied this subject in greater detail and reviewed the literature. They analyzed 343 twin pregnancies, with exact zygosity determination, and found that DZ and MZ twin pregnancies had the same incidence of mild and severe toxemia of pregnancy. Skupski et al. (1996) found that the rate of PIH is higher in triplet gestations conceived by IVF than if conceived spontaneously and when reduced to twins. Maxwell et al. (2001) found no difference in the risk for PIH with twin zygosity.

Perhaps the most debated topic in the management of twins is the manner in which the second twin is to be delivered and how rapidly it must be accomplished. Increased fetal mortality for the second twin has often been suggested but was also frequently not confirmed by studies in detail (Adam et al., 1991). In almost all respects (e.g., Apgar score, pH, and weight) twin A is said to be favored (Young et al., 1985). The higher mortality of twin B was particularly evident in Spurway's report on the management of twin deliveries (1962). Others have not found such dramatic differences, particularly when cases in which prenatal deaths (macerated stillborns, acardiacs) and infants weighing less than 1500 g were excluded from such analyses (Thompson & Johnson, 1966; Rayburn et al., 1984; Adam et al., 1991). Nevertheless, the mortality of twins is much greater than that of singletons, and reports from the American, European, and African literature are summarized in the thoughtful review by Powers (1973). Those reports are listed in Table 25.7, as are later surveys. In general, the perinatal mortality of twins hovers around 10%, but the statistics are largely influenced by the inclusion or exclusion of twins from early gestations and also depend on the date of the study, as marked improvements have been achieved. Thus, in a case-control study of Spellacy et al. (1990), the overall mortality of twins more than 500 g in weight now was 4.88% for twin A, and 6.41% for twin B. As in this study, there is little doubt that prematurity, often the result of hydramnios, is the most important factor in determining outcome. Rouse et al. (1993) related fundal height measurement to preterm delivery. They decided that single measurement excessive fundal height does not predict premature labor. This was to be expected, as excessive size alone cannot be the trigger for labor; rather, it is the rapidity of increase in uterine size (as occurs in hydramnios from the transfusion syndrome) that has this effect. At times, preterm labor is heavily influenced by the presence of the amnionic fluid infection syndrome (chorioamnionitis). Thus, Naeye et al. (1978), who recorded a 13.8% twin perinatal mortality, found that infection was the cause of twin deaths in 2.3%, in contrast to 0.6% in singletons. It was much higher (13.0% versus 1.8%) in Ethiopia. Premature rupture of membranes occurred more commonly in twins than singletons, but its outcome (latency to labor, infection) did not differ from singleton pregnancies (Mercer et al., 1993). These authors remarked on the paucity of abruptio occurring in multiple gestations. No significant differences between twins were found in the occurrence of the respiratory distress syndrome (Arnold et al., 1987) or cerebral hemorrhages (Pearlman & Batton, 1988). Most impressive, however, is the difference of perinatal mortality between monochorial and dichorial twins. Monochorionic twins have a significantly higher mortality, and that of monoamnionic twins is the highest (Benirschke, 1961; Cameron, 1968; Fujikura & Froehlich, 1971). On occasion it may be necessary to delay delivery of a second twin after premature birth of one. This topic was addressed by Arias (1994), who found it possible to occasionally significantly delay the birth of a second twin with cerclage and other modalities.

Early bed rest has been proposed to improve twin survival (Anonymous, 1963b). The cost of this measure is formidable (Powers & Miller, 1979), however, and careful appraisal with random trials has shown that it is inefficacious. In fact, with early admission and bed rest, the prematurity rate is increased. Robertson (1964b) who had earlier sought statistical improvement from early admission and did not find it, thought that random trials would be unethical. One study of the possible benefits comes from Rydhstrom (1988). Pregnancy outcome for 78 twin-bearing women who were prescribed prophylactic leave of absence from work to prevent preterm delivery was compared with a group of 78 twin-pregnant controls who did not take prophylactic leave. Gestational duration and birth weight did not differ between the two groups. The results indicated that prophylactic leave of absence from work did not improve the outcome of a twin pregnancy. Crowther et al. (1989) and MacLennan et al. (1990) also found that bed rest had no beneficial outcome in twin survivals. Indeed, "evidence is accumulating that rest may even increase premature labour" (Thornton & Rout, 1990; see also Andrews et al., 1991). Although cesarean section rates had increased from 3% (1963–1972) to 51% (1978–1984), Bell et al. (1986) were unable to show that even this modality of care improved the condition of

TABLE 25.7. Perinatal mortality of twins

Source	Year	No. of twins	Toxemia (%)	Breech (%)	Mortality (%)
Powers	1973 (review)	794	33		18.8
Europe and		2,012	25	18.4	12
Africa		98	20.4	30	16
		944	24		11
		706	35.4	36.8	12.2
		510	24.4	32	18.8
		210	31		6
		992	32	20	14
		2,000	10.1	32.1	16.1
		412	26.2	24.5	10.9
		358	34		12.3
		3,152			9.5
Tow	1959	408			12.3
Paepe	1959	108			8.8
Farrell	1964	1,000			16.1
Scholtes	1971	200			11.8
Bleker et al.	1979	1,655			14
Powers	1973 (review)	666	21.3	26.6	13.8
U.S. and Canada		270	16	30.5	28.6
		750	5	33	18.5
		504	21	28.3	15.6
		384	29.2		14
		1,000	28.2	21.2	9.8
		834			9.2
		384	27	31.3	14.1
		406	10.8	33	10.1
		17,168			9.9
		2,654	4.9	29.9	13.3
		986	37.5	24.4	9.9
		1,744	5	9.8	14.4
		2,798	14		11.8
		206	4.8	25	10.3
		1,046	16.5	31	10.8
		758			14
		1,054			13.4
		104			17.3
Ferguson	1964	3,238			9.3
Robertson	1964a	496	32		12.2
Myrianthopoulos	1970a	1,230			17.3
Ho & Wu	1975	177			10.7
Medearis et al.	1979	3,594			11.7
Keith et al.	1980	588			14.6
Hawrylyshyn et al.	1982	177			13.2
Laros & Dattel	1988	206			13.3
Fowler et al.	1991	41,554 white			4.71
		10,062 African American			7.93

twins at birth (see also Saunders et al., 1985, and Greig et al., 1992). Only attendance at prenatal twin care clinics seemed to have had a beneficial effect on outcome (Ellings et al., 1993).

The excessive mortality of multiple offspring has been given as one reason for selective reduction during early pregnancy. Layzer (1988) noted that a 16% perinatal mortality exists in triplets, and another 15% do not

survive infancy. The figures for quadruplets and quintuplets are 21% and 22%, respectively; for sextuplets the respective figures are 41% and 50%. At the other end of this spectrum, large twins have also been recorded. Leonard (1957) has reviewed this topic and reported twins weighing 4075 and 5180g (20.4 pounds together). They were dichorionic (male/female) and are the largest recorded in the literature.

HORMONES IN TWIN PREGNANCY

In efforts to predict twin pregnancies, various serologic parameters have been studied for better surveillance. Halpin (1970) found excessively high human chorionic gonadotropin (hCG) titers in a twin pregnancy, and Thiery et al. (1976) determined that hCG titers in twins were 2.5 times higher than in singletons. This increase was confirmed by studies of Jovanovic et al. (1977). Thiery et al. (1976) also reviewed the literature on the elevation of chorionic gonadotropin levels in pregnancy and simultaneously studied the human placental lactogen (hPL) levels. The latter were found to be 1.5 times higher than in singleton pregnancies. Other investigators have made similar observations (Gennser et al., 1975; Grennert et al., 1976a; Mägiste et al., 1976; Daw, 1977). In general, the values are 1 standard deviation above those for singletons, and when one twin dies, a noticeable fall has been recorded (Kenney et al., 1976). It has also been shown that, following elective embryocide, there is a marked fall in chorionic gonadotropin levels, but that progesterone and estradiol levels remain stable (O'Keane et al., 1988). α-Fetoprotein was found to be elevated in seven of 10 twin pregnancies reported by Ishiguro (1973), as was the level of cystylaminopeptidase (Einerh & Jacobsson, 1976). Because of the considerable scatter of hPL values in pregnancy, Dhont et al. (1976) suggested that simultaneous determination of hCG and hPL values gives more reliable results in the anticipation of twins (see reply by Grennert et al., 1976b).

References

Åberg, A., Mitelman, F., Cantz, M. and Gehler, J.: Cardiac puncture of fetus with Hurler's disease avoiding abortion of unaffected co-twin. Lancet 2:990–991, 1978.

Abraham, J.M.: Intrauterine feto-fetal transfusion syndrome: clinical observations and speculations on pathogenesis. Clin. Pediatr. 6:405–410, 1967.

Abuhamad, A.Z., Mari, G., Copel, J.A., Cantwell, C.J. and Evans, A.T.: Umbilical artery flow velocity waveforms in monoamniotic twins with cord entanglement. Obstet. Gynecol. 86:674–677, 1995.

Achiron, R., Rosen, N. and Zakut, H.: Pathophysiologic mechanism of hydramnios development in twin transfusion syndrome. J. Reprod. Med. 32:305–308, 1987.

Adam, C., Allen, A.C. and Baskett, T.F.: Twin delivery: Influence of the presentation and method of delivery on the second twin. Amer. J. Obstet. Gynecol. 165:23–27, 1991.

Adams, K.M. and Nelson, J.L.: Microchimerism: an investigative frontier in autoimmunity and transplantation. JAMA 291:1127–1131, 2004.

Aherne, W., Strong, S.J. and Corney, G.: The structure of the placenta in the twin transfusion syndrome. Biol. Neonat. 12:121–135, 1968.

Ahlfeld, F.: Beiträge zur Lehre von den Zwillingen. VI. Die Entstehung der Acardiaci. Arch. Gynäkol. 14:321–360, 1879.

Ahmad, Q.N., Britten, E.J. and Byth, D.E.: Haploid soybeans a rare occurrence in twin seedlings. J. Hered. 68:67, 1977.

Ahram, J.A., Toaff, M.E., Chandra, P., Laffey, P. and Chawla, H.S.: Successful outcome of a twin gestation in both horns of a bicornuate uterus. Amer. J. Obstet. Gynecol. 150:323–324, 1984.

Akande, V. and Murphy, D.J.: Neurological sequelae in in-vitro fertilization babies. Lancet 360:718–719, 2002.

Akesson, H.O., Smith, G.F. and Thrybom, B.R.: Twinning and associated stillbirth in Sweden, 1871–1960. Hereditas 64:193–198, 1970.

Albert, A., Randall, R.V., Smith, R.A. and Johnson, C.E.: The urinary excretion of gonadotrophin as a function of age. In, Hormones and the Ageing rocess. E.T. Engle and G. Pincus, eds., Academic Press, Orlando, pp. 49–62. 1956.

Albrecht, J.L. and Tomich, P.G.: The maternal and neonatal outcome of triplet gestations. Amer. J. Obstet. Gynecol. 174:1551–1556, 1996.

Alderman, B.: Foetus acardius amorphus. Postgrad. Med. J. 49:102–105, 1973.

Alexander, J.M., Ramus, R., Cox, S.M. and Gilstrap, L.C.: Outcome of twin gestations with a single anomalous fetus. Amer. J. Obstet. Gynecol. 177:849–852, 1997.

Al-Kouatly, H.B., Chasen, S.T., Kalish, R.B. and Chervenak, F.A.: Causes of thrombocytopenia in triplet gestations. Amer. J. Obstet. Gynecol. 189:177–180, 2003.

Allan, W.C., Dransfield, D.A. and Kessler, D.L.: Cerebral palsy in preterm infants. Lancet 343:1048, 1994.

Allen, G.: A differential method for estimation of type frequencies in triplets and quadruplets. Amer. J. Hum. Genet. 12:210–224, 1960.

Allen, G.: Twin research: Problems and prospects. Prog. Med. Genet. 4:242–269, 1965.

Allen, G.: Diagnostic efficiency of fingerprint and blood group differences in a series of twins. Acta Genet. Med. Gemellol. 17:359–374, 1968.

Allen, G.: The non-decline in U.S. twin birth rates, 1964–1983. Acta Genet. Med. Gemellol. 36:313–323, 1987.

Allen, G. and Hrubec, Z.: Twin concordance: a more general model. Acta Genet. Med. Gemellol. 28:3–13, 1979.

Allen, G. and Hrubec, Z.: The monozygotic twinning rate: Is it really constant? Acta Genet. Med. Gemellol. 36:389–396, 1987.

Allen, M.S. and Turner, U.G.: Twin birth—identical or fraternal twins? Obstet. Gynecol. 37:538–542, 1971.

Allen, W.R. and Pashen, R.L.: Production of monozygotic (identical) horse twins by embryo micromanipulation. J. Reprod. Fertil. 71:607–613, 1984.

Al-Takroni, A.M., Medis, K.B.L., Reddy, I. and Agrawal, S.: Indomethacin for treatment of fetofetal transfusion syndrome. Ann. Saudi. Med. 15:284–285, 1995.

Altshuler, G. and Hyde, S.: Placental Pathology Case Book: a bidiscoid, monochorionic placenta. J. Perinatol. 13:492–493, 1993.

Amatuzio, J.C. and Gorlin, R.J.: Conjoined acardiac monsters. Arch. Pathol. Lab. Med. 105:253–255, 1981.

Anderson, J.M. and Benirschke, K.: Fetal circulations in the placenta of Dasypus novemcinctus Linn. and their significance in tissue transplantation. Transplantation 1:306–310, 1963.

Anderson, R.L., Golbus, M.S., Curry, C.J.R., Callen, P.W. and Hastrup, W.H.: Central nervous system damage and other anomalies in surviving fetus following second trimester antenatal death of co-twin: report of four cases and literature review. Prenat. Diagn. 10:513–518, 1990.

Andrews, W.W., Leveno, K.J., Sherman, M.L., Mutz, J., Gilstrap, L.C. and Whalley, P.J.: Elective hospitalization in the management of twin pregnancies. Obstet. Gynecol. 77:826–831, 1991.

Annas, G.J.: Conjoined twins—the limits of law at the limits of life. NEJM 344:1104–1108, 2001.

Anonymous: Quintuplet births. AMA News. Nov. 25:3, 1963a.

Anonymous: Twin pregnancy. Lancet **2**:79–80, 1963b.

Anonymous: Mexico City octuplets succumb within 13 hours. Med. World News, March 31, 1967.

Anonymous: Quintuplets. Br. Med. J. **1**:534, 1968.

Antoine, C., Young, B.K., Silverman, F., Greco, M.A. and Alvarez, S.P.: Sinusoidal fetal heart rate pattern with vasa previa in twin pregnancy. J. Reprod. Med. **27**:295–300, 1982.

Aquino, D.B., Timmons, C., Burns, D. and Lowichik, A.: Craniopagus parasiticus: a case illustrating its relationship to craniopagus conjoined twinning. Pediat. Pathol. Lab. Med. **17**:939–944, 1997.

Arabin, B., Bos, R., Rijlaarsdam, R., Mohnhaupt, A. and van Eyck, J.: The onset of inter-human contacts: longitudinal ultrasound observations in early twin pregnancies. Ultrasound Obstet. Gynecol. **8**:166–173, 1996.

Arai, K., Soma, H. and Hokano, M.: Ultrastructure of human placental villi in abortion, premature birth and stillbirth. J. Clin. Electron Microsc. **10**:5–6, 1977.

Arey, L.B.: Chorionic fusion and augmented twinning in the human tube. Anat. Rec. **23**:253–262, 1922.

Arey, L.B.: Two embryologically important specimens of tubal twins. Surg. Gynecol. Obstet. **36**:407–415, 1923a.

Arey, L.B.: Tubal twins and tubal pregnancy. Surg. Gynecol. Obstet. **36**:803–810, 1923b.

Arias, F.: Delayed delivery of multifetal pregnancies with premature rupture of membranes in the second trimester. Amer. J. Obstet. Gynecol. **170**:1233–1237, 1994.

Arias, F., Sunderji, S., Gimpelson, R. and Colton, E.: Treatment of acardiac twinning. Obstet. Gynecol. **91**:818–821, 1998.

Arnold, C., McLean, F.H., Kramer, M.S. and Usher, R.H.: Respiratory distress syndrome in second-born versus first-born twins: a matched case-control analysis. NEJM **317**:1121–1125, 1987.

Arts, N.F.T. and Lohman, A.H.M.: The vascular anatomy of monochorionic diamniotic twin placentas and the transfusion syndrome. Eur. J. Obstet. Gynecol. **3**:85–93, 1971.

Ash, K., Harman, C.R. and Gritter, H.: TRAP sequence–successful outcome with indomethacin treatment. Obstet. Gynecol. **76**:960–962, 1990.

Atlay, R.D. and Pennington, G.W.: The use of clomiphene citrate and pituitary gonadotropin in successive pregnancies: the Sheffield quadruplets. Amer. J. Obstet. Gynecol. **109**:402–407, 1971.

Aubert, L.: Développement aigu d'un kyste de l'ovaire et grossesse quintuple chez une femme ayant reçu successivement des gonadotrophines sériques et chorioniques. Ann. Endocrinol. (Paris) **21**:176–182, 1960.

Averback, P. and Wigglesworth, F.W.: Monochorionic, monoamniotic, double-battledore placenta with stillbirth and postpartum cerebellar syndrome. Amer. J. Obstet. Gynecol. **128**:697–699, 1977.

Averback, P. and Wigglesworth, F.W.: Congenital absence of the heart: observation of human funiculopagous twinning with insertio funiculi furcata, fusion, forking, and interpositio velamentosa. Teratology **17**:143–150, 1978.

Azuma, C., Kamiura, S., Nobunaga, T., Negoro, T., Saji, F. and Tanizawa, O.: Zygosity determination of multiple pregnancy by deoxyribonucleic acid fingerprints. Amer. J. Obstet. Gynecol. **160**:734–736, 1989.

Babson, S.G. and Phillips, D.S.: Growth and development of twins dissimilar in size at birth. N. Engl. J. Med. **289**: 937–940, 1973. (see also the editorial: pp. 973–974 by J.B. Hardy).

Baergen, R.N., Boué, D.R. and Mannino, F.: Liveborn twin of an Extramembranous pregnancy. J. Perinatol. **15**:510–513, 1995.

Bajoria, R.: Abundant vascular anastomoses in monoamniotic vs. diamniotic monochorionic placentas. Amer. J. Obstet. Gynecol. **179**:788–793, 1998.

Bajoria, R., Wigglesworth, J. and Fisk, N.M. Angioarchitecture of monochorionic placentas in relation to the twin-twin transfusion syndrome. Amer. J. Obstet. Gynecol. **172**:856–863, 1995.

Bajoria, R., Hancock, M., Ward, S., D'Souza, S.W. and Sooranna, S.R.: Discordant amino acid profiles in monochorionic twins with twin-twin transfusion syndrome. Pediatr. Res. **48**:821–828, 2000.

Bajoria, R., Ward, S. and Chatterjee, R.: Natriuretic peptides in the pathogenesis of cardiac dysfunction in the recipient fetus of twin-twin transfusion syndrome. Amer. J. Obstet. Gynecol. **186**:121–127, 2002.

Bajoria, R., Ward, S. and Chatterjee, R.: Brain natriuretic peptide and endothelin-1 in the pathogenesis of polyhydramnios-oligohydramnios in monochorionic twins. Amer. J. Obstet. Gynecol. **189**:189–194, 2003.

Baker, V.V. and Doering, M.C.: Fetus papyraceus: an unreported congenital anomaly of the surviving infant. Amer. J. Obstet. Gynecol. **143**:234, 1982.

Baldwin, V.J.: Pathology of Multiple Pregnancy. Springer-Verlag, New York, 1994.

Baldwin, V.J. and Wittmann, B.K.: Pathology of intragestational intervention in twin-to-twin transfusion syndrome. Pediatr. Pathol. **10**:79–93, 1990.

Banchi, M.T.: Triplet pregnancy with second trimester abortion and delivery of twins at 35 weeks' gestation. Obstet. Gynecol. **63**:728–730, 1984.

Banek, C.S., Hecher, K., Hackeloer, B.J. and Bartmann, P.: Long-term neurodevelopmental outcome after intrauterine laser treatment for severe twin-twin transfusion syndrome. Amer. J. Obstetr. Gynecol. **188**:876–880, 2003.

Banfield, F., Dick, M., Behrendt, D.M., Rosenthal, A., Pescheria, A. and Scott, W.: Intracardial teratoma: a new and treatable cause of hydrops fetalis. Amer. J. Dis. Child. **134**:1174–1175, 1980.

Bankole, M.A., Oduntan, S.A., Oluwasanmi, J.O., Itayemi, S.O. and Khwaja, S.: The conjoined twins of Warri, Ibadan. Arch. Surg. **104**:294–301, 1972.

Bannykh, S.I., Bannykh, G.L., Mannino, F.L., Jones, K.L., Hansen, L., Benirschke, K. and Masliah, E.: Partial caudal duplication in a newborn associated with meningomyelocele and complex heart anomaly. Teratology **63**:94–99, 2001.

Barr, M.: Twin growth profiles and identification of twin-twin transfusion in midgestation. In, Proceedings Greenwood Genetics Center, R.A. Saul and M.C. Phelan, eds. **15**:151–152, 1996.

Barrea, C., Alkazaleh, F., Ryan, G., McCrindle, B.W., Roberts, A., Bigras, J.-L., Barrett, J., Seaward, G.P., Smallhorn, J.F. and Hornberger, L.K.: Prenatal cardiovascular manifestations in the twin-to-twin transfusion syndrome recipients and the impact of therapeutic amnioreduction. Amer. J. Obstet. Gynecol. **192**:892–902, 2005.

Barss, V.A.: Monoamniotic twin pregnancy. In, Abstracts of the Society of Perinatal Obstetricians, Las Vegas, February 1988. [Cited with the author's permission.]

Barss, V.A., Benacerraf, B.R. and Frigoletto, F.D.: Ultrasonographic determination of chorion type in twin gestation. Obstet. Gynecol. **66**:779–783, 1985.

Barth, P.G. and Harten, J.J. van der: Parabiotic twin syndrome with topical isocortical disruption and gastroschisis. Acta Neuropathol. (Basel) **67**:345–349, 1985.

Baschat, A.A., Muench, M.V., Mighty, H.E. and Harman, C.R.: Successful intrauterine management of severe feto-fetal transfusion in a monochorionic triplet pregnancy using bipolar umbilical cord coagulation. Fetal. Diagn. Ther. **18**:397–400, 2003.

Basrur, P.K., Kosaka, S. and Kanagawa, H.: Blood cell chimerism and freemartinism in heterosexual bovine quadruplets. J. Hered. **61**:15–18, 1970.

Bass, H.N., Oliver, J.B., Srinivasan, M., Petrucha, R., Ng, W. and Lee, J.O.S.: Persistently elevated AFP and AChE in amniotic fluid from a normal fetus following demise of its twin. Prenat. Diagn. **6**:33–35, 1986.

Bauer, W.C. and Rosenberg, B.F.: Quantitative study of glomerular enlargement in children with tetralogy of Fallot: condition of glomerular enlargement without increase in renal mass. Amer. J. Pathol. **37**:695–772, 1960.

Bebbington, M.W. and Wittmann, B.K.: Fetal transfusion syndrome: antenatal factors predicting outcome. Amer. J. Obstet. Gynecol. **160**:913–915, 1989.

Becker, A.H. and Glass, H.: The twin-to-twin transfusion syndrome. Amer. J. Dis. Child. **106**:624–629, 1963.

Becker, A., Busjahn, A., Faulhaber, H.D., Bähring, S., Robertson, J., Schuster, H. and Luft, F.C.: Twin zygosity. Automated determination with microsatellites. J. Prod. Med. **42**:260–266, 1997.

Behr, B., Fisch, J.D., Racowsky, C., Miller, K., Pool, T.B. and Milki, A.A.: Blastocyst-ET and monozygotic twinning. J. Assist. Reprod. Genet. **17**:349–351, 2000.

Beischer, N.A. and Fortune, D.W.: Double monsters. Obstet. Gynecol. **32**:158–170, 1968.

Bejar, R., Vigliocco, G., Gramajo, H., Solana, C., Benirschke, K., Berry, C., Coen, R. and Resnik, R.: Antenatal origin of neurologic damage in newborn infants. Part II. Multiple gestations. Amer. J. Obstet. Gynecol. **162**:1230–1236, 1990.

Belfort, M.A., Moise, K.J., Kirshon, B. and Saade, G.: The use of color flow Doppler ultrasonography to diagnose umbilical cord entanglement in monoamniotic twin gestation. Amer. J. Obstet. Gynecol. **168**:601–604, 1993.

Bell, D., Johansson, D., McLean, F.H. and Usher, R.H.: Birth asphyxia, trauma, and mortality in twins: has cesarean section improved outcome? Amer. J. Obstet. Gynecol. **154**:235–239, 1986.

Bender, H.G. and Brandt, G.: Morphologie und Morphometrie der Fünflings-Placenta. Arch. Gynäkol. **216**:61–72, 1974.

Bendon, R.W.: Twin transfusion syndrome: Pathological studies of the monochorionic placenta in liveborn twins and of the perinatal autopsy in monochorionic twin pairs. Pediat. Pathol. Lab. Med. **15**:363–376, 1995.

Bendon, R.W. and Siddiqi, T.: Clinical pathological conference: acute twin-to-twin in utero transfusion. Pediatr. Pathol. **9**:591–598, 1989.

Benelli, A.: Gravidanza trigemina con trasformazione papiracea di un feto. Clin. Ostetr. Gynecol. (Roma) **64**:663–670, 1962.

Benirschke, K.: Placental membranes in twins. Obstet. Gynecol. Survey **13**:88–91, 1958.

Benirschke, K.: Nuclear sex of holoacardii amorphi. Obstet. Gynecol. **14**:72–78, 1959.

Benirschke, K.: Twin placenta in perinatal mortality. N.Y. State J. Med. **61**:1499–1508, 1961.

Benirschke, K.: Discordance for genetic defects in monozygous twins: a pathogenetic concept. Acta Facult. Med. Zagreb. [Suppl.1] **18**:15–24, 1970a.

Benirschke, K.: Spontaneous chimerism in mammals: a critical review. Curr. Top. Pathol. **51**:1–61, 1970b.

Benirschke, K.: Chimerism, mosaicism and hybrids. In: Human Genetics, Proceedings Fourth International Congress Human Genetics, Paris, pp. 212–231, Excerpta Medica, Amsterdam, 1971.

Benirschke, K.: The contribution of placental anastomoses to prenatal twin damage. Human Pathol. **23**:1319–1320, 1992.

Benirschke, K.: Intrauterine death of a twin: Mechanisms, implications for surviving twin, and placental pathology. In, Seminars in Diagnostic Pathology, W.B. Saunders, Co. **10**:222–231, 1993.

Benirschke, K. and Driscoll, S.G.: The Pathology of the Human Placenta. Springer-Verlag, New York 1967.

Benirschke, K. and Harper, V.D.R.: The acardiac anomaly. Teratology **15**:311–316, 1977.

Benirschke, K. and Kim, C.K.: Multiple pregnancy. NEJM **288**:1276–1284, 1329–1336, 1973.

Benirschke, K. and Layton, W.: An early twin blastocyst of the golden lion marmoset, *Leontocebus rosalia* L. Folia Primatol. **10**:131–138, 1969.

Benirschke, K. and Masliah, E.: The placenta in multiple pregnancy: outstanding issues. Reprod. Fertil. **13**:615–622, 2001.

Benirschke, K., Anderson, J.M. and Brownhill, L.E.: Marrow chimerism in marmosets. Science **138**:513–515, 1962.

Berbos, J.N., King, B.F. and Janusz, A.: Quintuple pregnancy: report of a case. JAMA **188**:813–816, 1964.

Berg, C., Baschat, A.A., Geipel, A., Germer, U., Smrcek, J., Krapp, M. and Gembruch, U.: First trimester twin-to-twin transfusion syndrome in a trichorionic quadruplet pregnancy—a diagnostic challenge. Fetal Diagn. Ther. **17**:357–361, 2002.

Berg, J.M. and Kirman, B.H.: The mentally defective twin. Br. Med. J. **1**:1911–1917, 1960.

Berg, K.A., Astemborski, J.A., Boughman, J.A. and Ferencz, C.: Congenital cardiovascular malformations in twins and triplets from a population-based study. Amer. J. Dis. Child. **143**:1461–1463, 1989.

Bergman, P., Lundin, P. and Malmstrom, T.: Twin pregnancy with early blighted fetus. Obstet. Gynecol. **18**:348–351, 1961.

Berkowitz, R.L., Lynch, L., Chitkara, U., Wilkins, I.A., Mehalek, K.E. and Alvarez, E.: Selective reduction of multifetal pregnancies in the first trimester. NEJM **318**:1043–1047, 1988.

Berkowitz, R.L., Lynch, L., Lapinski, R. and Bergh, P.: First-trimester transabdominal multifetal pregnancy reduction: A report of two hundred completed cases. Amer. J. Obstet. Gynecol. **169**:17–21, 1993.

Berkowitz, R.L., Lynch, L., Stone, J. and Alvarez, M.: The current status of multifetal pregnancy reduction. Amer. J. Obstet. Gynecol. **174**:1265–1272, 1996.

Bermúdez, C., Becerra, C.H., Bornick, P.W., Allen, M.H., Arroyo, J. and Quintero, R.A.: Placental types and twin-twin transfusion syndrome. Amer. J. Obstet. Gynecol. **187**:489–494, 2002.

Berry, D., Montgomery, L., Johnson, A., Saade, G. and Moise, K.: Amniotic septostomy for the treatment of the stuck twin sequence. Amer. J. Obstet. Gynecol. **176**:S19 (abstract 44), 1997.

Berry, S.A., Johnson, D.E. and Thompson, T.R.: Agenesis of the penis, scrotal raphe, and anus in one of monoamniotic twins. Teratology **29**:173–176, 1984.

Berry, S.M., Puder, K.S., Bottoms, S.F., Uckele, J.E., Romero, R. and Cotton, S.B.: Comparison of intrauterine hematologic and biochemical values between twin pairs with and without stuck twin syndrome. Amer. J. Obstet. Gynecol. **172**:1403–1410, 1995.

Bertillon, M.: Des combinaisons de sexe dans les grossesses gémellaires (doubles ou triples), de leur cause et de leur caractère ethnique. Bull. Soc. Anthropol. **9**:267–290, 1874.

Bhargava, I., Chakravarty, A. and Raja, P.T.K.: An anatomical study of the fetal blood vessels on the chorial surface of the human placenta. III. Multiple pregnancies. Acta Anat. (Basel) **80**:465–479, 1971.

Bhatnagar, K.P., Sharma, S.C. and Bisker, J.: The holoacardius: a correlative computerized tomographic, radiologic, and ultrasonographic investigation of a new case with review of literature. Acta Genet. Med. Gemellol. **35**:77–89, 1986.

Bhettay, E., Nelson, M.M. and Beighton, P.: Epidemic of conjoined twins in Southern Africa? Lancet **2**:741–743, 1975.

Bieber, F.R., Nance, W.E., Morton, C.C., Brown, J.A., Redwine, F.O., Jordan, R.L. and Mohanakumar, T.: Genetic studies of an acardiac monster: evidence of polar body twinning in man. Science **213**:775–777, 1981.

Bleisch, V.R.: Diagnosis of monochorionic twin placentation. Amer. J. Clin. Pathol. **42**:277–284, 1964.

Bleisch, V.R.: Placental circulation of human twins. Amer. J. Obstet. Gynecol. **91**:862–869, 1965.

Bleker, O.P. and Oosting, J.: Term and postterm twin gestations. Placental cause of perinatal mortality. J. Reprod. Med. **42**:715–718, 1997.

Bleker, O.P., Breur, W. and Huidekoper, B.L.: A study of birth weight, placental weight and mortality of twins as compared to singletons. Br. J. Obstet. Gynaecol. **86**:111–118, 1979.

Bleker, O.P., Oosting, J. and Hemrika, D.J.: On the cause of the retardation of fetal growth in multiple gestations. Acta Genet. Med. Gemellol. **37**:41–46, 1988.

Bleker, O.P., Wolf, H. and Oosting, J.: The placental cause of fetal growth retardation in twin gestations. Acta Genet. Med. Gemellol. **44**:103–106, 1995.

Blickstein, I.: The twin-twin transfusion syndrome. Review. Obstet. Gynecol. **76**:714–722, 1990.

Blickstein, I.: Letter to the editor. Amer. J. Obstet. Gynecol. **190**:383–384, 2004.

Blickstein, I.: Estimation of iatrogenic monozygotic twinning rate following assisted reproduction: Pitfalls and caveats. Amer. J. Obstet. Gynecol. **192**:365–368, 2005.

Blickstein, I., Verhoeven, H.C. and Keith, L.G.: Zygotic splitting after assisted reproduction. NEJM **340**:738–739, 1999.

Blickstein, I., Jacques, D.L. and Keith, L.G.: A novel approach to intertriplet birth weight discordance. Amer. J. Obstet. Gynecol. **188**:1026–1030, 2003.

Boklage, C.E.: On the timing of monozygotic twinning events. In, Twin Research 3. Part A: Twin Biology and Multiple Pregnancy. L. Gedda, P. Parisi and W.E. Nance, eds., pp. 155–165. Alan R. Liss, New York, 1981.

Boklage, G.E.: Race, zygosity, and mortality among twins: interaction of myth and method. Acta Genet. Med. Gemellol. **36**:275–288, 1987a.

Boklage, C.E.: Twinning, nonrighthandedness, and fusion malformations: evidence for heritable causal elements held in common. Amer. J. Med. Genet. **28**:67–84, 1987b.

Bolaji, I.I., Mortimer, G., Meehan, F.P., England, S. and Greally, M.: Acardius in a triplet pregnancy: Cytogenetic and morphological profile. Acta Genet. Med. Gemellol. **41**:27–32, 1992. (Errata **41**:365, 1992.)

Bolens, M., Lacourt, G. and Mottu, T.H.E.: Un nouveau cas de transfusion interfoetale: surcharge ventriculaire droite et hypocoagulabilité chez la jumelle pléthorique; atteinte neurologique chez la jumelle anémique. Schweiz. Med. Wochenschr. **98**:412–417, 1968.

Boulgakow, B.: Arrest of development of an embryo: a case of acephalus holoacardius showing arrest of development of all tissues in embryonic period. J. Anat. Physiol. **61**:68–93, 1926.

Boulot, P., Hedon, B., Deschamps, F., Laffargue, F., Viala, J.L., Humeau, C. and Arnal, F.: Anencephaly-like malformation in surviving twin after embryonic reduction. Lancet **335**:1155–1156, 1990.

Boulot, P., Hedon, B., Pelliccia, G., Lefort, G., Deschamps, F., Arnal, F., Humeau, C., Laffargue, F. and Viala, J.L.: Multifetal pregnancy reduction: a consecutive series of 61 cases. Brit. J. Obstetr. Gynaecol. **100**:63–68, 1993.

Bowman, J.M.: Alloimmunization in twin pregnancies. Amer. J. Obstet. Gynecol. **153**:7–13, 1985.

Boyd, J.D. and Hamilton, W.J.: The Human Placenta. W. Heffer & Sons, Cambridge, 1970.

Bracken, M.J.: Oral contraception and twinning: an epidemiologic study. Amer. J. Obstet. Gynecol. **133**:432–434, 1979.

Bressers, W.M.A., Eriksson, A.W., Konstense, P.J. and Parisi, P.: Increasing trend in the monozygotic twinning rate. Acta Genet. Med. Gemellol. **36**:397–408, 1987.

Brismar, B.: Dermatoglyphics of twins: a study based on a new systematics. Acta Genet. Med. Gemellol. **17**:375–380, 1968.

Bromley, B., Frigoletto, F.D., Estroff, J.A. and Benacerraf, B.R.: The natural history of oligohydramnios/polyhydramnios sequence in monochorionic diamniotic twins. Ultrasound Obstet. Gynecol. **2**:317–320, 1992.

Brown, C.E.L. and Weinreb, J.C.: Magnetic resonance imaging appearance of growth retardation in a twin pregnancy. Obstet. Gynecol. **71**:987–988, 1988.

Brown, D.C. and Nelson, R.F.: Uterus didelphys and double vagina with delivery of a normal infant from each uterus. Can. Med. Assoc. J. **96**:675–677, 1967.

Brown, D.L., Benson, C.B., Driscoll, S.G. and Doubilet, P.M.: Twin-twin transfusion syndrome: sonographic findings. Radiology **170**:61–63, 1989.

Bruner, J.P. and Rosemond, R.L.: Twin-to-twin transfusion syndrome: a subset of the twin oligohydramnios-polyhydramnios sequence. Amer. J. Obstet. Gynecol. **169**:925–930, 1993.

Bruner, J., Anderson, T. and Rosemond, R.: Twin-to-twin transfusion syndrome: the real problem is poor placentation. Amer. J. Obstet. Gynecol. **172**:311 (abstract 183), 1995.

Bryan, E. and Slavin, B.: Serum IgG levels in feto-fetal transfusion syndrome. Arch. Dis. Child. **49**:908–910, 1974.

Buckler, J.M.H. and Robinson, A.: Matched development of a pair of monozygous twins of grossly different size at birth. Arch. Dis. Child. **49**:472–76, 1974.

Bulla, M., von Lilien, T., Goecke, H., Roth, B., Ortmann, M. and Heising, J.: Renal and cerebral necrosis in survivor after in utero death of co-twin. Arch. Gynecol. **240**:119–124, 1987.

Bulmer, M.G.: The familial incidence of twinning. Ann. Hum. Genet. **24**:1–3, 1960.

Bulmer, M.G.: The Biology of Twinning in Man. Oxford University Press, London, 1970.

Burn, J., Povey, S., Boyd, Y., Munro, E.A., West, L., Harper, K. and Thomas, D.: Duchenne muscular dystrophy in one of monozygotic twin girls. J. Med. Genet. **23**:494–500, 1986.

Busjahn, A., Knoblauch, H., Faulhaber, H.-D., Aydin, A., Uhlmann, R., Tuomilehto, J., Kaprio, J., Jedrusik, P., Januszewicz, A., Strelau, J., Schuster, H., Luft, F.C. and Müller-Myshok, B.: A region on chromosome 3 is linked to dizygotic twinning. Nature Genet. **26**:398–399, 2000.

Buxbaum, H. and Wachsman, D.V.: A case of acephalus holoacardius. Amer. J. Obstet. Gynecol. **36**:1055–1057, 1938.

Buzzard, I.M., Uchida, I.A., Norton, J.A. and Christian, J.C.: Birth weight and placental proximity in like-sexed twins. Amer. J. Hum. Genet. **35**:318–323, 1983.

Cameron, A.H.: The Birmingham twin survey. Proc. R. Soc. Med. **61**:229–234, 1968.

Camiel, M.R.: Fetus papyraceus with intrauterine sibling death. JAMA **202**:247, 1967.

Campbell, D.M., MacGillivray, I. and Thompson, B.: Twin zygosity and pre-eclampsia. Lancet **2**:97, 1977.

Campbell, S. and Dewhurst, C.J.: Quintuplet pregnancy diagnosed and assessed by ultrasonic compound scanning. Lancet **1**:101–103, 1970.

Cannings, C.: A discussion of Weinberg's rule on the zygosity of twins. Ann. Hum. Genet. **32**:403–405, 1969.

Cantú, J.M., Diaz-Gallardo, M.Y., Barros-Núñez, P. and Figuera, L.E.: Heteroallelic monozygotic twins and triplets. Amer. J. Med. Genet. **77**:166–167, 1998.

Cardwell, M.S., Caple, P. and Baker, L.C.: Triplet pregnancy on three separate days. Obstet. Gynecol. **71**:448–449, 1988.

Carlson, N.J. and Towers, C.V.: Multiple gestation complicated by the death of one fetus. Obstet. Gynecol. **73**:685–689, 1989.

Carr, S.R., Aronson, M.P. and Coustan, D.R.: Survival rates of monoamniotic twins do not decrease after 30 weeks' gestation. Amer. J. Obstet. Gynecol. **163**:719–722, 1990.

Carter, C.O.: Congenital defects. Proc. R. Soc. Med. **61**:991–995, 1968.

Castilla, E.E., Lopez-Camelo, J.S., Orioli, I.M., Sanchez, O. and Paz, J.E.: The epidemiology of conjoined twins in Latin America. Acta Genet. Med. Gemellol. **37**:111–118, 1988.

Cederlöf, R., Friberg, L., Jonsson, E. and Kaij, L.: Studies on similarity diagnosis in twins with the aid of mailed questionnaires. Acta Genet. (Basel) **11**:338–362, 1961.

Centerwall, W.R. and Benirschke, K.: An animal model for the XXY Klinefelter syndrome in man: tortoiseshell and calico male cats. Amer. J. Vet. Res. **36**:1275–1280, 1975.

Chapman, K.: Monoamniotic twins. Lancet **2**:1456, 1974.

Chasen, S.T., Al-Kouatly, H.B., Ballabh, P., Skupski, D.W. and Chervenak, F.A.: Outcomes of dichorionic triplet pregnancies. Amer. J. Obstet. Gynecol. **186**:765–767, 2002.

Chauhan, S.P., Shields, D., Parker, D., Sanderson, M., Scardo, J.A. and Magann, E.F.: Detecting fetal growth restriction or discordant growth in twin gestations stratified by placental chorionicity. J. Reprod. Med. **49**:279–284, 2004.

Chaurasia, B.D.: Abnormal umbilical vessels and systemic circulatory reversal in thoracopagus twins. Acta Genet. Med. Gemellol. **24**:261–268, 1975.

Cherouny, P.H., Hoskins, I.A., Johnson, T.R.B. and Niebyl, J.R.: Multiple pregnancy with late death of one fetus. Obstet. Gynecol. **74**:318–320, 1989.

Chervenak, F.A., Isaacson, G., Touloukian, R., Tortora, M., Berkowitz, R.L. and Hobbins, J.C.: Diagnosis and management of fetal teratomas. Obstet. Gynecol. **66**:666–671, 1985.

Chescheir, N.C. and Seeds, J.W.: Polyhydramnios and oligohydramnios in twin gestations. Amer. J. Obstet. Gynecol. **71**:882–884, 1988a.

Chescheir, N.C. and Seeds, J.W.: Spontaneous resolution of hypofibrinogenemia associated with death of a twin in utero: a case report. Amer. J. Obstet. Gynecol. **159**:1183–1184, 1988b.

Chitkara, U., Berkowitz, R.L., Wilkins, I.A., Lynch, L., Mehalek, K.E. and Alvarez, M.: Selective second-trimester termination of the anomalous fetus in twin pregnancies. Obstet. Gynecol. **73**:690–694, 1989.

Chmait, R. and Hull, A.: Placental Pathology Casebook. J. Perinatol. **21**:150–152, 2001.

Chu, W., Chapman, J., Persons, D.L. and Fan, F.: Twin pregnancy with partial hydatidiform mole and coexisting fetus. Arch. Pathol. Lab. Med. **128**:1305–1306, 2004.

Chupin, D., Huy, N.N., Azan, M., Mauléon, P. and Ortavant, R.: Induction hormonale de naissance gémellaires: principales conséquences sur les performances zootechniques. Ann. Zootech. **25**:79–94, 1976.

Cincotta, R.B., Gray, P.H., Phythian, G., Rogers, Y.M. and Chan, F.Y.: Long term outcome of twin-twin transfusion syndrome. Arch. Dis. Child. Fetal Neonatal Ed. **83**:F171–176, 2000.

Clark, M. and Linell, E.A.: Case report: prenatal occlusion of the internal carotid artery. J. Neurol. Neurosurg. Psychiatry **17**:295–297, 1954.

Claudius, M.: Die Entwicklung der Herzlosen Migeburten. Schwers, Kiel, 1859.

Cleary-Goldman, J., Morgan, M.A., Robinson, J.N., d'Alton, M.E. and Schulkin, J.: Multiple pregnancy: knowledge and practice patterns of obstetricians and gynecologists. Obstet. Gynecol. **104**:232–237, 2004.

Coen, R.W. and Sutherland, J.M.: Placental vascular communications between twin fetuses. Amer. J. Dis. Child. **120**:332, 1970.

Cohen, M., Kohl, S.G. and Rosenthal, A.H.: Fetal interlocking complicating twin gestation. Amer. J. Obstet. Gynecol. **91**:407–412, 1965.

Coke, G.A., Baschat, A.A., Mighty, H.E. and Malinow, A.M.: Maternal cardiac arrest associated with attempted fetal injection of potassium chloride. Int. J. Obstet. Anesth. **13**:287–290, 2004.

Colburn, D.W. and Pasquale, S.A.: Monoamniotic twin pregnancy. J. Reprod. Med. **27**:165–168, 1982.

Cole, L.J. and Craft, W.A.: An acephalic lamb monster in sheep. J. Hered. **36**:29–32, 1945.

Colgan, T.J. and Luk, S.C.: Umbilical-cord torsion, thrombosis, and intrauterine death of a twin fetus. Arch. Pathol. Lab. Med. **106**:101, 1982.

Collins, M.S. and Bleyl, J.A.: Seventy-one quadruplet pregnancies: management and outcome. Amer. J. Obstet. Gynecol. **162**:1384–1392, 1990.

Collins, R.N., Lerner, A.B. and McGuire, J.S.: The relationship of skin color to zygosity in twins. J. Invest. Dermatol. **47**:78–82, 1966.

Conway, C.F.: Transfusion syndrome in multiple pregnancy. Obstet. Gynecol. **23**:745–751, 1964.

Cooperstock, M.S., Tummaru, R., Bakewell, J. and Schramm, W.: Twin birth weight discordance and risk of preterm birth. Amer. J. Obstet. Gynecol. **183**:63–67, 2000.

Cordero, L. and Johnson, J.R.: Mean arterial pressure in extremely low birth weight concordant and discordant twins during the first day of life. J. Perinatol. **22**:526–534, 2002.

Cordero, L., Giannone, P.J. and Rich, J.T.: Mean arterial pressure in very low birth weight (801 to 1500 g) concordant and discordant twins during the first day of life. J. Perinatol. **23**:545–551, 2003.

Coren, S.: Twinning is associated with an increased risk of left-handedness and inverted writing hand posture. Early Hum. Devel. **40**:23–27, 1994.

Corey, L.A., Harris, R.E., Kang, K.W., Christian, J.C. and Nance, W.E.: Variability of total cholesterol in monochorionic and dichorionic MZ twins. Amer. J. Hum. Genet. **27**:28A, 1975.

Corey, M.J., Miller, J.R., MacLean, R. and Chown, B.: A case of XX/XY mosaicism. Amer. J. Hum. Genet. **19**:378–387, 1967.

Corner, G.W.: The observed embryology of human single-ovum twins and other multiple births. Amer. J. Obstet. Gynecol. **70**:933–951, 1955.

Corney, G. and Aherne, W.: The placental transfusion syndrome in monozygous twins. Arch. Dis. Child. **40**:264–270, 1965.

Corney, G., Robson, E.B. and Strong, S.J.: Twin zygosity and placentation. Ann. Hum. Genet. **32**:89–96, 1968.

Corrin, B.: Glomerular size in polycythemia. J. Pathol. Bacteriol. **82**:534–535, 1961.

Costa, T., Lambert, M., Teshima, I., Ray, P.N., Richer, C.L. and Dallaire, L.: Monozygotic twins with 45X,46,XY mosaicism discordant for phenotypic sex. Amer. J. Med. Genet. **75**:40–44, 1998.

Coulam, C.B.: First trimester diagnosis of acardiac twins. Obstet. Gynecol. **88**:729, 1996.

Coulton, D., Hertig, A.T. and Long, W.N.: Monoamniotic twins. Amer. J. Obstet. Gynecol. **54**:119–123, 1947.

Cousins, L., Benirschke, K., Porreco, R. and Resnik, R.: Placentomegaly due to fetal congestive failure in a pregnancy with a sacrococcygeal teratoma. J. Reprod. Med. **25**:142–144, 1980.

Cox, W.L., Forestier, F., Capella-Pavlovsky, M. and Daffos, F.: Fetal blood sampling in twin pregnancies: prenatal diagnosis and management of 19 cases. Fetal Ther. **2**:101–108, 1987.

Cragan, J.D., Martin, L., Waters, G.D. and Khoury, M.J.: Increased risk of small intestinal atresia among twins in the United States. Arch. Pediatr. Adolesc. Med. **148**:733–739, 1994.

Craig, I.T.: Monoamniotic twins with double survival. Amer. J. Obstet. Gynecol. **73**:202–205, 1957.

Crombleholme, T.M., Robertson, F., Marx, G., Yarnell, R. and D'Alton, M.E.: Fetoscopic cord ligation to prevent neurologic injury in monozygous twins. Lancet **348**:191, 1996.

Crookston, M.C., Tilley, C.A. and Crookston, J.H.: Human blood chimaera with seeming breakdown of immune tolerance. Lancet **2**:1110–1112, 1970. (**1**:396, 1971).

Crossman, P.J. and Dickens, P.S.E.M.: Amorphus globosus in the mare. Vet. Rec. **95**:22, 1974.

Crowther, C.A., Neilson, J.P., Verkuyl, D.A.A., Bannerman, C. and Ashurst, H.M.: Preterm labour in twin pregnancies: can it be prevented by hospital admission? Br. J. Obstet. Gynaecol. **96**:850–853, 1989.

Cruikshank, S.H. and Granados, J.L.: Increased amniotic acetylcholinesterase activity with a fetus papyraceus and aplasia cutis congenita. Obstet. Gynecol. **71**:997–999, 1988.

Curtius, F.: Nachgeburtsbefunde bei Zwillingen und Ähnlichkeitsdiagnose. Arch. Gynäkol. **140**:361–366, 1930.

Dahm, K.: Über zwei Beobachtungen von Akardie und zur Frage ihrer Genese. Zentralbl. Allg. Pathol. Pathol. Anat. **93**:41–50, 1955.

Dallapiccola, B., Stomeo, C., Ferranti, G., Di Lecci, A. and Purpura, M.: Discordant sex in one of three monozygotic triplets. J. Med. Genet. **22**:6–11, 1985.

D'Alton, M.E. and Dudley, D.K.: The ultrasonographic prediction of chorionicity in twin gestation. Amer. J. Obstet. Gynecol. **160**:557–561, 1989.

D'Alton, M.E. and Simpson, L.L.: Syndromes in twins. Seminars in Perinatol. **19**:375–386, 1995.

Daniel, Y., Schreiber, Y., Geva, E., Amit, A., Pausner, D., Kupferminc, M.J. and Lessing, J.B.: Do placentae of term singleton pregnancies obtained by assisted reproductive technologies differ from those of spontaneously conceived pregnancies? Human Reprod. **14**:1107–1110, 1999.

Daniel, Y., Ochshorn, Y., Fait, G., Geva, E., Bar-Am, A. and Lessing, J.B.: Analysis of 104 twin pregnancies conceived with assisted reproductive technologies and 193 spontaneously conceived twin pregnancies. Fertil. Steril. **74**:683–689, 2000.

Daniel, Y., Schreiber, L., Geva, E., Lessing, J.B., Bar-Am, A. and Amit, A.: Morphologic and histopathologic characteristics of placentas from twin pregnancies spontaneously conceived and from reduced and nonreduced assisted reproductive technologies. J. Reprod. Med. **46**:735–742, 2001.

Danskin, F.H. and Neilson, J.P.: Twin-to-twin transfusion syndrome: what are appropriate diagnostic criteria? Amer. J. Obstet. Gynecol. **161**:365–369, 1989.

Davies, J., Chazen, E. and Nance, W.E.: Symmelia in one of monozygotic twins. Teratology **4**:367–378, 1971.

Davies, M. and Norman, R.: Neurological sequelae in in-vitro fertilization babies. Lancet **360**:718–719, 2002.

Daw, E.: Human placental lactogen and twin pregnancy. Lancet **2**:299–300, 1977.

Dawkins, R.R., Marshall, T.L. and Rogers, M.S.: Prenatal gangrene in association with twin-twin transfusion syndrome. Amer. J. Obstet. Gynecol. **172**:1055–1057, 1995.

Dawson, W.M. and Ainslie, W.H.: Twin pregnancy in a uterus didelphys: a case report. J. Med. Soc. N.J. **55**:649, 1958.

Deacon, J.S., Machin, G.A., Martin, J.M.E., Nicholson, S., Nwanko, D.C. and Wintemute, R.: Investigation of acephalus. Amer. J. Med. Genet. **5**:85–99, 1980.

DeBaun, M.R., Niemitz, E.L. and Feinberg, A.P.: Association of in vitro fertilization with Beckwith-Wiedemann syndrome and epigenetic alterations of *LIT1* and *H19*. Amer. J. Human. Genet. **72**:156–160, 2003.

De la Chapelle, A., Schröder, J., Rantanen, P., Thomasson, B., Niemi, M., Tilikainen, A., Sanger, R. and Robson, E.B.: Early fusion of two human embryos? Ann. Hum. Genet. **38**:63–75, 1974.

De Leon, F.: Siamesische Zwillinge mit differenten Herzmimildungen. Virchows Arch. [A] **362**:51–57, 1974.

De Lia, J.E.: Surgery of the placenta and umbilical cord. Clin. Obstet. Gynecol. **39**:607–625, 1996.

De Lia, J.E. and Cruikshank, D.P.: Fetoscopic laser occlusion of chorioangiopagus in severe twin transfusion syndrome. Acta Genet. Med. Gemellol. **38**:218, 1989 (abstract).

De Lia, J.E. and Worthington, D.: Long-term neurodevelopmental outcome after intrauterine laser treatment for twin-twin transfusion syndrome (TTTS). Amer. J. Obstetr. Gynecol. **190**:1170–1172, 2004.

De Lia, J.E., Emery, M.G., Sheafor, S.A. and Jennison, T.A.: Twin transfusion syndrome: successful in utero treatment with digoxin. Int. J. Gynaecol. Obstet. **23**:197–201, 1985a.

De Lia, J.E., Rogers, J.G. and Dixon, J.A.: Treatment of placental vasculature with a neodymium-yttrium-aluminum-garnet laser via fetoscopy. Amer. J. Obstet. Gynecol. **151**:1126–1127, 1985b.

De Lia, J.E., Cukierski, M.A., Lundergan, D.K. and Kochenour, N.K.: Neodymium:yttrium-aluminum-garnet laser occlusion of rhesus placental vasculature via fetoscopy. Amer. J. Obstet. Gynecol. **160**:485–489, 1989.

De Lia, J.E., Cruikshank, D.P. and Keye, W.R.: Fetoscopic neodymium:Yag laser occlusion of placental vessels in severe twin-twin transfusion syndrome. Obstet. Gynecol. **75**:1046–1953, 1990.

De Lia, J.E., Kuhlmann, R.S., Cruikshank, D.P. and O'Bee, L.R.: Current topic: placental surgery: a new frontier. Placenta **14**:477–485, 1993.

De Lia, J.E., Kuhlmann, R.S., Harstad, T.W. and Cruikshank, D.P.: Fetoscopic laser ablation of placental vessels in severe previable twin-twin transfusion syndrome. Amer. J. Obstet. Gynecol. **172**:1202–1211, 1995.

De Lia, J.E., Kuhlmann, R.S. and Emery, M.G.: Maternal metabolic abnormalities in twin-to-twin transfusion syndrome at mid-pregnancy. Twin Res. **3**:113–117, 2000.

Delprado, W.J. and Baird, P.J.: Cephalothoracopagus syncephalus: a case report with previously unreported anatomical abnormalities and chromosomal analysis. Teratology **29**:1–9, 1984.

De Marco, P.G.: Feto-fetal transfusions in monozygotic twins: review of the literature and report of two cases. Clin. Pediatr. **3**:709–713, 1964.

Demmel, U.: Clinical aspects of congenital skin defects. Eur. J. Pediatr. **121**:21–50, 1975.

Denbow, M.L., Blomley, M.J.K., Cosgrove, D.O. and Fisk, N.M.: Ultrasound microbubble contrast angiography in monochorionic twin fetuses. Lancet **349**:773, 1997.

Denbow, M.L., Battin, M.R., Cowan, F., Azzopardi, D., Edwards, A.D. and Fisk, N.M.: Neonatal cranial ultrasonographic findings in preterm twins complicated by severe fetofetal transfusion syndrome. Amer. J. Obstet. Gynecol. **178**:479–483, 1998.

Denbow, M.L., Cox, P., Taylor, M., Hammal, D.M. and Fisk, N.M.: Placental angioarchitecture in monochorionic twin pregnancies: relationship to fetal growth, fetofetal transfusion syndrome, and pregnancy outcome. Amer. J. Obstet. Gynecol. **182**:417–426, 2000.

Denbow, M.L., Taylor, M. and Fisk, N.M.: Derivation of rate of arterio-arterial anastomotic transfusion between monochorionic twin fetuses by Doppler waveform analysis. Placenta **25**:664–670, 2004.

Dennis, L.G. and Winkler, C.L.: Twin-to-twin transfusion syndrome: aggressive therapeutic amniocentesis. Amer. J. Obstet. Gynecol. **177**:342–349, 1997.

Dennis, S.M. and Leipold, H.W.: Congenital cardiac defects in lambs. Amer. J. Vet. Res. **29**:2337–2340, 1968.

De Paepe, M.E., Stopa, E., Huang, C., Hansen, K. and Luks, F.I.: Renal tubular apoptosis in twin-to-twin transfusion syndrome. Pediatr. Developm. Pathol. **6**:215–225, 2003.

De Paepe, M.E., Friedman, R.M., Poch, M., Hansen, K., Carr, S.R. and Luks, F.I.: Placental findings after laser ablation of communicating vessels in twin-to-twin transfusion syndrome. Pediatr. Devel. Pathol. **7**:159–165, 2004.

Derom, C., Bakker, E., Vlietninck, R., Derom, R., van den Berghe, H., Thiery, M. and Pearson, P.: Zygosity determination in newborn twins using DNA variants. J. Med. Genet. **22**:279–282, 1985.

Derom, C., Vlietinck, R., Derom, R., van den Berghe, H. and Thiery, M.: Increased monozygotic twinning rate after ovulation induction. Lancet **1**:1236–1238, 1987.

Derom, C., Vlietinck, R., Derom, R., van den Berghe, H. and Thiery, M.: Population-based study of sex proportion in monoamniotic twins. NEJM **319**:119–120, 1988.

Derom, C., Vlietinck, R., Derom, R., Boklage, C., Thiery, M. and van den Berghe, H.: Genotyping of macerated stillborn fetuses. Amer. J. Obstet. Gynecol. **164**:797–800, 1991.

Dhont, M., Thiery, M. and Vandekerckhove, D.: Hormonal screening for detection of twin pregnancies. Lancet **2**:861, 1976.

Diamond, J.M.: Variation in human testis size: ethnic differences. Nature **320**:488–489, 1986.

Dicker, D., Peleg, D., Samuel, N., Feldberg, D. and Goldman, J.A.: Holoacardius: radiologic investigation. Early Hum. Devel. **9**:59–65, 1983.

Dickey, R.P., Taylor, S.N., Lu, P.Y., Sartor, B.M., Storment, J.M., Rye, P.H., Pelletier, W.D., Zender, J.L. and Matulich, E.M.: Spontaneous reduction of multiple pregnancy: incidence and effect on outcome. Amer. J. Obstet. Gynecol. **186**:77–83, 2002.

Dickinson, J.E.: Severe twin-twin transfusion syndrome: current management concepts. Aust. N.Z. J. Obstet. Gynaecol. **35**:1–16, 1995.

Diddle, A.W. and Burford, T.H.: Study of set of quadruplets. Anat. Rec. **61**:281–293, 1935.

Diehl, W., Hecher, K., Zikulnig, L., Vetter, M. and Hackelöer, B.-J.: Placental vascular anastomoses visualized during fetoscopic laser surgery in severe mid-trimester twin-twin transfusion syndrome. Placenta: **22**:876–881, 2001.

Dijk, B.A. van, Boomsma, D.I. and de Man, A.J.M.: Blood group chimerism in human multiple births is not rare. Amer. J. Med. Genet. **61**:264–268, 1996.

Dimmick, J.E., Hardwick, D.F. and Ho-Yuen, B.: A case of renal necrosis, and fibrosis in the immediate newborn period: association with the twin-to-twin transfusion syndrome. Amer. J. Dis. Child. **122**:345–347, 1971.

Dixon, A.F.: Human oocyte showing first polar body, and second polar body in metaphase. C. R. Assoc. Anat. **22**:265–266, 1927.

Donald, J.G.: Unusual twin pregnancy. Br. Med. J. **ii**:1330, 1964.

Donnenfeld, A.E., Dunn, L.K. and Rose, N.C.: Discordant amniotic band sequence in monozygotic twins. Amer. J. Med. Genet. **20**:685–694, 1985.

Donnenfeld, A.E., Glazerman, L.R., Cutillo, D.M., Librizzi, R.J. and Weiner, S.: Fetal exsanguination following intrauterine angiographic assessment and selective termination of a hydrocephalic, monozygotic co-twin. Prenat. Diagn. **9**: 301–308, 1989.

Dorros, G.: The prenatal diagnosis of intrauterine growth retardation in one fetus of a twin gestation. Obstet. Gynecol. **48**:46s–48s, 1976.

Dreger, A.D.: One of Us: Conjoined Twins and the Future of Normal. Harvard University Press, Cambridge, 2004.

Driesch, H.: Entwicklungs-mechanische Studien. I. Der Werth der beiden ersten Furchungszellen in der Echinodermentwicklung: experimentelle Erzeugung von Theil-und Doppelbildungen. Z. Wiss. Zool. **53**:160–184, 1891.

Driggers, R.W., Blakemore, K.J., Bird, C., Ackerman, K.E. and Hutchins, G.M.: Pathogenesis of acardiac twinning: clues from an almost acardiac twin. Fetal Diagn. Ther. **17**:185–187, 2002.

Drucker, P., Finkel, J. and Savel, L.E.: Sixty-five-day interval between the births of twins. Amer. J. Obstet. Gynecol. **80**: 761–762, 1960.

Drut, R., Garcia, C. and Drut, R.M.: Poorly organized parasitic conjoined twins: Report of four cases. Pediatr. Pathol. **12**:691–700, 1992.

Dubé, J., Dodds, L. and Armson, B.A.: Does chorionicity or zygosity predict adverse perinatal outcomes in twins. Amer. J. Obstet. Gynecol. **186**:579–583, 2002.

Dudley, D.K.L. and D'Alton, M.E.: Single fetal death in twin gestation. Semin. Perinatol. **10**:65–72, 1986.

Duenhoelter, J.H.: Survival of twins after acute fetal hemorrhage from ruptured vasa previa. Obstet. Gynecol. **73**:866–867, 1989.

Duffy, D.L., Montgomery, G.W., Hall, J., Mayne, C., Healey, S.C., Brown, J., Boomsma, D.I. and Martin, N.G.: Human twinning is not linked to the region of chromosome 4 syntenic with sheep twinning gene FecB. Amer. J. Med. Genet. **100**:182–186, 2001.

Dunn, H.O. and Roberts, S.J.: Chromosome studies of an ovine acephalic-acardiac monster. Cornell Vet. **62**:425–431, 1972.

Dunn, H.O., Lein, H. and Kenney, R.M.: The cytological sex of a bovine anidian (amorphous) twin monster. Cytogenetics **6**:412–419, 1967.

Dunnihoo, D.R. and Harris, R.E.: The diagnosis of monoamniotic twinning by amniography. Amer. J. Obstet. Gynecol. **96**:894–895, 1966.

Dunsford, I., Bowley, C.C., Hutchison, A.M., Thompson, J.S., Sanger, R. and Race, R.R.: A human blood group chimera. Br. Med. J. **2**:81, 1953.

Durkin, M.V., Kaveggia, E.G., Pendleton, E., Neuhaeser, G. and Opitz, J.M.: Analysis of etiologic factors in cerebral palsy with severe mental retardation. I. Analysis of gestational, parturitional and neonatal data. Eur. J. Pediatr. **123**:67–81, 1976.

Eastman, N.J., Kohl, S.G., Maisel, J.E. and Kavaler, F.: The obstetrical background of 753 cases of cerebral palsy. Obstet. Gynecol. Surv. **17**:459–500, 1962.

Eberle, A.M., Levesque, D., Vintzileos, A.M., Tsapanos, V. and Salafia, C.M.: Placental pathology in discordant twins. Amer. J. Obstet. Gynecol. **169**:931–935, 1993.

Eddleman, K.A., Stone, J.L., Lynch, L. and Berkowitz, R.L.: Selective termination of anomalous fetuses in multifetal pregnancies: two hundred cases at a single center. Amer. J. Obstet. Gynecol. **187**:1168–1172, 2002.

Editorial: Eggs shared, given, and sold. Lancet **362**:413, 2003.

Edmonds, L.D. and Layde, P.M.: Conjoined twins in the United States. Teratology **25**:301–308, 1982.

Edwards, J.: Season and rate of conception. Nature **142**:357, 1938.

Edwards, R.G., Mettler, L.E. and Walters, D.E.: Identical twins and in vitro fertilization. J. In Vitro Fertil. Embryo Transfer **3**:114–117, 1986.

Einerh, Y. and Jacobsson, K.: Screening for early detection of twin pregnancies. Lancet **1**:745, 1976.

Ellings, J.M., Newman, R.B., Hulsey, T.C., Bivins, H.A. and Keenan, A.: Reduction in very low birth weight deliveries and perinatal mortality in a specialized, multidisciplinary twin clinic. Obstet. Gynecol. **81**:387–391.

Elliott, J.P.: Amniocentesis for twin-twin transfusion syndrome. Contemporary Ob/Gyn 30–42, August 1992.

Elliott, J.P. and Radin, T.G.: Quadruplet pregnancy: contemporary management and outcome. Obstet. Gynecol. **80**:421–424, 1992.

Elliott, J.P., Urig, M.A. and Clewell, W.H.: Aggressive therapeutic amniocentesis for treatment of twin-twin transfusion syndrome. Obstet. Gynecol. **77**:537–540, 1991.

Ellis, P.A.: Renal enlargement in chronic cor pulmonale. J. Clin. Pathol. **14**:552–556, 1961.

El-Sherbini, R.: Retention of an 8–month foetus in utero for two and a half years. J. Obstet. Gynaecol. Br. Commonw. **70**:514–516, 1963.

Elston, R.C. and Boklage, C.E.: An examination of fundamental assumptions of the twin method. In, Twin Research: Psychology and Methodology, W.E. Nance, ed., pp. 189–199, Alan R. Liss, New York, 1978.

Elwood, J.M.: Decline in dizygotic twinning. NEJM **289**:486, 1973.

Elwood, J.M.: Maternal and environmental factors affecting twin births in Canadian cities. Br. J. Obstet. Gynaecol. **85**:351–358, 1978.

Elwood, J.M.: The end of the drop in twinning rates? Lancet **1**:470, 1983.

Emery, S.C., Vaux, K.K., Pretorius, D., Masliah, E. and Benirschke, K.: Acardiac twin with externalized intestine adherent to placenta: unusual manifestation of omphalocele. Pediat. Developm. Pathol. **7**:81–85, 2004.

Enbom, J.A.: Twin pregnancy with intrauterine death of one twin. Amer. J. Obstet. Gynecol. **152**:424–429, 1985.

Englert, Y., Imbert, M.C., van Rosendael, E., Belaisch, J., Segal, L., Feichtinger, W., Wilkin, P., Frydman, R. and Leroy, F.: Morphological anomalies in the placentae of IVF pregnancies: preliminary report of a multicentric study. Hum. Reprod. **2**:155–157, 1987.

Entezami, M., Runkel, S., Sarioglu, N., Hese, S. and Weitzel, H.K.: Diagnostic dilemma with elevated level of α-fetoprotein in an undiagnosed twin pregnancy with a small discordant holoacardius acephalus. Amer. J. Obstet. Gynecol. **177**:466–468, 1997.

Erdmann, J., Nöthen, M.M., Stratmann, M., Fimmers, R., Franzek, E. and Propping, P.: The use of microsatellites in zygosity diagnosis of twins. Acta Genet. Med. Gemellol. **42**:45–51, 1993.

Eriksson, A.: Variations in the human twinning rate. Acta Genet. (Basel) **12**:242–250, 1962.

Eriksson, A.W.: Pituitary gonadotrophin and dizygotic twinning. Lancet **2**:1298–1299, 1964.

Esposito, A.: Singolare caso di gravidanza trigemina con due feti mummeficati. Clin. Obstet. Gynecol. (Roma) **75**:537–544, 1963.

Evans, M.I., Fletcher, J.C., Zador, I.E., Newton, B.W., Quigg, M.H. and Struyk, C.D.: Selective first-trimester termination in octuplet and quadruplet pregnancies: clinical and ethical issues. Obstet. Gynecol. **71**:289–296, 1988.

Evans, M.I., Dommergues, M., Timor-Tritsch, I., Zador, I.E., Wapner, R.J., Lynch, L., Dumez, Y., Goldberg, J.D., Nicolaides, K.H., Johnson, M.P., Golbus, M.S., Boulot, P., Aknin, A.J., Monteagudo, A. and Berkovitz, R.L.: Transabdominal versus transcervical and transvaginal multifetal pregnancy reduction: international collaborative experience of more than one thousand cases. Amer. J. Obstet. Gynecol. **170**:902–909, 1994.

Evans, M.I., Littmann, L., Louis, L.St., LeBlanc, L., Addis, J., Johnson, M.P. and Moghissi, K.S.: Evolving patterns of iatrogenic multifetal pregnancy generation: implications for aggressiveness of infertility treatments. Amer. J. Obstet. Gynecol. **172**:1750–1755, 1995.

Exelby, P.R.: Sacrococcygeal teratomas in children. CA **22**:202–208, 1972.

Falkner, F.: The smaller of twins and hypoglycaemia. Lancet **1**:869, 1965.

Farquharson, D.F., Wittmann, B.K., Hansmann, M., Yuen, B.H.Y., Baldwin, V.J. and Lindahl, S.: Management of quintuplet pregnancy by selective embryocide. Amer. J. Obstet. Gynecol. **158**:413–416, 1988.

Farrell, A.G.W.: Twin pregnancy: a study of 1,000 cases. S. Afr. J. Obstet. Gynaecol. **2**:35–41, 1964.

Feichtinger, W., Breitenecker, G. and Fröhlich, H.: Prolongation of pregnancy and survival of twin B after loss of twin A at 21 weeks' gestation. Amer. J. Obstet. Gynecol. **161**:891–893, 1989.

Feige, A., Gille, J., v. Maillot, K. and Mulz, D.L.: Pränatale Diagnostik eines Steißbeinteratoms mit Hypertrophie der Plazenta. Geburtsh. Frauenheilk. **42**:20–24, 1982.

Feingold, M., Cetrulo, C.L., Newton, E.R., Weiss, J., Shakr, C. and Shmoys, S.: Serial amniocenteses in the treatment of twin to twin transfusion complicated with acute hydramnios. Acta Genet. Med. Gemellol. **35**:107–113, 1986.

Feldman, D.M., Odibo, A., Campbell, W.A. and Rodis, J.F.: Iatrogenic monoamniotic twins as a complication of therapeutic amniocentesis. Obstet. Gynecol. **91**:815–816, 1998.

Feldman, D.M., Borgida, A.F., Trymbulak, W.P., Barsoom, M.J., Sanders, M.M. and Rodis, J.F.: Clinical implications of velamentous cord insertion in triplet gestations. Amer. J. Obstet. Gynecol. **186**:809–811, 2002.

Ferguson, W.F.: Perinatal mortality in multiple gestations: a review of perinatal deaths from 1609 multiple gestations. Obstet. Gynecol. **23**:861–870, 1964.

Ferm, V.H.: Conjoined twinning in mammalian teratology. Arch. Environ. Health **19**:353–357, 1969.

Ferm, V.H.: Cranio-dirachischisis totalis in cephalothoracopagus twins. Teratology **17**:159–164, 1978.

Fernandez, M.: Beiträge zur Embryologie der Gürteltiere. I. Zur Keimblätterinversion und spezifischen Polyembryonie der Mulita (*Tatusia hybrida* Desm.) Morphol. Jahrb. **39**:302–333, 1909.

Fesslova, V., Villa, L., Nava, S., Mosca, F. and Nicolini, U.: Fetal and neonatal echocardiographic findings in twin-twin transfusion syndrome. Amer. J. Obstet. Gynecol. **179**:1056–1062, 1998.

Finberg, H.J.: The "twin peak" sign: reliable evidence of dichorionic twinning. J. Ultrasound Med. **11**:571–577, 1992.

Fisher, J.E. and Siongco, A.: Case 3: complications from in utero death of a monozygous co-twin. Pediatr. Pathol. **9**:765–771, 1989.

Fisk, N.M. and Galea, P.: Twin-twin transfusion—as good as it gets? NEJM **351**:182–184, 2004.

Fisk, N.M., Ware, M., Stanier, P., Moore, G. and Bennett, P.: Molecular genetic etiology of twin reversed arterial perfusion sequence. Amer. J. Obstet. Gynecol. **174**:891–894, 1996.

Fisk, N.M., Tan, T.Y.T. and Taylor, M.J.O.: Re: Stage-based treatment of twin-twin transfusion syndrome Amer. J. Obstet. Gynecol. **190**:1491–1492, 1810–1811, 2004.

Fogel, B.J., Nitowsky, H.M. and Gruenwald, P.: Discordant abnormalities in monozygotic twins. Amer. J. Obstet. Gynecol. **66**:64–72, 1965.

Foley, M.R., Clewell, W.H., Finberg, H.J. and Mills, M.D.: Use of Foley cordostat grasping device for selective ligation of the umbilical cord of an acardiac twin: a case report. Amer. J. Obstet. Gynecol. **172**:212–214, 1995.

Forbes, D.A. and Natale, A.: Unilateral tubal triplet pregnancy: report of a case. Obstet. Gynecol. **31**:360–362, 1968.

Forman, R.C.: Twin pregnancy with one twin blighted. Amer. J. Obstet. Gynecol. **72**:1180–1181, 1956.

Forssell, O.H.: Zur Kenntnis des Amnionepithels in normalem und pathologischem Zustande. Arch. Gynäkol. **96**:436–460, 1912.

Foschini, M.P., Gabrielli, L., Dorji, T., Kos, M., Lazzarotto, T., Lanari, M. and Landini, M.P.: Vascular anastomoses in dichorionic diamniotic-fused placentas. Int. J. Gynecol. Pathol. **22**:359–361, 2003.

Foster, R.T. and Allen, S.R.: Differential transmission of parvovirus B19 in a twin gestation: a case report. Twin Res. **7**:412–414, 2004.

Fowler, M.G., Kleinman, J.C., Kiely, J.L. and Kessel, S.S.: Amer. J. Obstet. Gynecol. **165**:L15–22, 1991.

Fox, H. and Butler-Manuel, R.: A teratoma of the placenta. J. Pathol. Bacteriol. **88**:137–140, 1964.

Franke, H. and Estel, C.: Untersuchungen über die Ultrastruktur und Permeabilität des Amnions unter besonderer Berücksichtigung mikrofilamentärer und mikrotubulärer Strukturen. Arch. Gynecol. **225**:319–338, 1978.

Fraser, F.C.: The genetics of cleft lip and cleft palate. Amer. J. Hum. Genet. **22**:336–352, 1970.

Fraser, R.B., Liston, R.M., Thompson, D.L. and Wright, J.R.: Monoamniotic twins delivered liveborn with a forked umbilical cord. Pediat. Pathol. Lab. Med. **17**:639–644, 1997.

Freedman, H.L., Tafeen, C.H. and Harris, H.: Conjoined thoracopagous twins: case report. Amer. J. Obstet. Gynecol. **84**:1904–1909, 1962.

French, C.A., Bieber, F.R., Bing, D.H. and Genest, D.R.: Twins, placentas, and genetics: acardiac twinning in a dichorionic, diamniotic, monozygotic twin gestation. Human Pathol. **29**:1028–1031, 1998.

Fries, M.H., Goldstein, R.B., Kilpatrick, S.J., Golbus, M.S., Callen, P.W. and Filly, R.A.: The role of velamentous cord insertion in the etiology of twin-twin transfusion syndrome. Obstet. Gynecol. **81**:569–574, 1993.

Frothingham, R.: A medical mystery. NEJM **337**:1666, 1997; **338**:266–267, 1998.

Frutiger, P.: Zum Problem der Akardie. Acta Anat. (Basel) **74**:505–531, 1969.

Fujii, S., Ban, C., Okamura, H. and Nishimura, T.: Unilateral tubal quadruplet pregnancy. Amer. J. Obstet. Gynecol. **141**:840–842, 1981.

Fujikura, T. and Froehlich, L.A.: Twin placentation and zygosity. Obstet. Gynecol. **37**:34–43, 1971.

Fujikura, T. and Froehlich, L.A.: Mental and motor development in monozygotic co-twins with dissimilar birth weights. Pediatrics **53**:884–889, 1974.

Fujikura, T. and Wellings, S.R.: A teratoma-like mass on the placenta of a malformed infant. Amer. J. Obstet. Gynecol. **89**:824–825, 1964.

Fusi, L., McParland, P., Fisk, N., Nicolini, U. and Wigglesworth, J.: Acute twin-twin transfusion: a possible mechanism for brain-damaged survivors after intrauterine death of a monochorionic twin. Obstet. Gynecol. **78**:517–520, 1991.

Gabos, P.: Triplet pregnancy and cervical incompetence: a case report. Fertil. Steril. **23**:940–942, 1972.

Gärtner, K. and Baunack, E.: Is the similarity of monozygotic twins due to genetic factors alone? Nature **292**:646–647, 1981.

Gall, S.A.: Multiple Pregnancy and Delivery. Mosby, St. Louis, 1996.

Galloway, S.M., McNatty, K.P., Cambridge, L.M., Laitinen, M.P.E., Juengel, J.L., Jokiranta, S., McLaren, R.J., Luiro, K., Dodds, K.G., Montgomery, G.W., Beattie, A.E., Davis, G.H. and Ritvos, O.: Mutations in an oocyte-derived growth factor gene (*BMP15*) cause increased ovulation rate and infertility

in a dosage-sensitive manner. Nature Genet. **25**:279–283, 2000.

Galton, F.: The history of twins as a criterion of the relative powers of nature, and nurture. J. Br. Anthropol. Inst. **5**:391–406, 1875.

Gamberdella, F.R. and Marrs, R.P.: Heterotopic pregnancy associated with assisted reproductive technology. Amer. J. Obstet. Gynecol. **160**:1520–1524, 1989.

Gardeil, F., Greene, R., NiScanaill, S. and Skinner, J.: Conjoined twins in a triplet pregnancy. Obstet. Gynecol. **92**:716, 1998.

Garry, D., Lysikiewicz, A., Mays, J., Canterino, J. and Tejani, N.: Intra-amniotic pressure reduction in twin-twin transfusion syndrome. J. Perinatol. **18**:284–286, 1998.

Gärtner, K. and Baunack, E.: Is the similarity of monozygotic twins due to genetic factors alone? Nature **292**:646–647, 1981.

Gavriil, P., Jauniaux, E. and Leroy, F.: Pathologic examination of placentas from singleton and twin pregnancies obtained after in vitro fertilization and embryo transfer. Pediatr. Pathol. **13**:453–462, 1993.

Gaziano, E., Gaziano, C. and Brandt, D.: Doppler velocimetry determined redistribution of fetal blood flow: correlation with growth restriction in diamniotic monochorionic and dizygotic twins. Amer. J. Obstet. Gynecol. **178**:1359–1367, 1998.

Gaziano, E.P., De Lia, J.E. and Kuhlman, R.S.: Diamnionic monochorionic twin gestations: an overview. J. Maternal-Fetal Med. **9**:89–96, 2000.

Gengozian, N.: Male and female cell populations in the chimeric marmoset. In, Medical Primatology, pp. 926–938, Karger, New York, 1971.

Gengozian, N., Brewen, J.G., Preston, R.J. and Batson, J.S.: Presumptive evidence for the absence of functional germ cell chimerism in the marmoset. J. Med. Primatol. **9**:9–27, 1980.

Gennser, G., Grennert, L., Kullander, S., Persson, P.H. and Wingerup, L.: Human placental lactogen in screening for multiple pregnancies. Lancet **1**:274, 1975.

Gergely, R.Z., Eden, R., Schifrin, B.S. and Wade, M.E.: Antenatal diagnosis of congenital sacral teratoma. J. Reprod. Med. **24**:229–231, 1980.

Gewolb, I.H., Freedman, R.M., Kleinman, C.S. and Hobbins, J.C.: Prenatal diagnosis of a human pseudoacardiac anomaly. Obstet. Gynecol. **61**:657–662, 1983.

Gibbs, C.E., Boldt, J.W., Daly, J.W. and Morgan, H.C.: A quintuplet gestation. Obstet. Gynecol. **16**:464–468, 1960.

Gicquel, C., Gaston, V., Mandelbaum, J., Siffroi, J.-P., Flahault, A. and Le Bouc, Y.: Amer. J. Human Genet. **72**:1338–1341, 2003.

Gilbert, E.F., Suzuki, H., Kimmel, D.L., Klingberg, W.G. and Lancaster, J.R.: A case of thoracopagus: conjoined twins. Teratology **6**:197–200, 1972.

Gilbert, W.M., Davis, S.E., Kaplan, C., Pretorius, D., Merritt, T.A. and Benirschke, K.: Morbidity associated with prenatal disruption of the dividing membrane in twin gestations. Obstet. Gynecol. **78**:623–630, 1991.

Giles, W., Trudinger, B., Cook, C. and Connelly, A.: Placental microvascular changes in twin pregnancies with abnormal umbilical artery waveforms. Obstet. Gynecol. **81**:556–559, 1993.

Gillim, D.L. and Hendricks, C.H.: Holoacardius: review of the literature and case report. Obstet. Gynecol. **2**:647–653, 1953.

Giménez-Scherer, J.A. & Davies, B.R.: Malformations in acardiac twins are consistent with reversed blood flow: liver as a clue to their pathogenesis. Pediatr. Devel. Pathol. **6**:520–530, 2003.

Ginsberg, N.A., Applebaum, M., Rabin, S.A., Caffarelli, M.A., Kuuspalu, M., Daskal, J.L., Verlinsky, Y., Strom, C.M. and Barton, J.J.: Term birth after midtrimester hysterotomy and selective delivery of an acardiac twin. Amer. J. Obstet. Gynecol. **167**:33–37, 1992.

Gittes, R.F.: Carcinoma of the prostate. NEJM **324**:236–245, 1991.

Gleicher, N., Oleske, D.M., Tur-Kaspa, I., Vidali, A. and Karande, V.: Reducing the risk of high-order multiple pregnancy after ovarian stimulation with gonadotropins. NEJM **343**:2–7, 2000.

Glinianaia, S.V., Pharoah, P.O., Wright, C., Rankin, J.M., Northern Region Perinatal Mortality Survey Steering Group: Arch. Dis. Child Fetal Neonatal Ed. **86**:F9–15, 2002.

Gonen, R., Heyman, E., Asztalos, E. and Milligan, J.E.: The outcome of triplet gestations complicated by fetal death. Obstet. Gynecol. **75**:175–178, 1990a.

Gonen, R., Heyman, E., Asztalos, E., Ohlsson, A., Pitson, L.C., Shennan, A.T. and Milligan, J.E.: The outcome of triplet, quadruplet, and quintuplet pregnancies managed in a perinatal unit: Obstetric, neonatal, and follow-up data. Amer. J. Obstet. Gynecol. **162**:454–459, 1990b.

Gonen, Y., Blankier, J. and Casper, R.F.: Transvaginal ultrasound in selective embryo reduction for multiple pregnancy. Obstet. Gynecol. **75**:720–721, 1990c.

Gonsoulin, W., Copeland, K.L., Carpenter, R.J., Hughes, M.R. and Elder, F.B.: Fetal blood sampling demonstrating chimerism in monozygotic twins discordant for sex and tissue karyotype (46, XY and 45, X). Prenat. Diagn. **10**:25–28, 1990a.

Gonsoulin, W., Moise, K.J., Kirshon, B., Cotton, D.B., Wheeler, J.M. and Carpenter, R.J.: Outcome of twin-twin transfusion diagnosed before 28 weeks of gestation. Obstet. Gynecol. **75**:214–216, 1990b.

Goodno, J.A. and Gentry, W.: Coexistent interstitial and intra-uterine pregnancy: a case report. JAMA **179**:295–296, 1962.

Goodship,. J., Carter, J. and Burn, J.: X-inactivation patterns in monozygotic and dizygotic twins. Amer. J. Med. Genet. **22**:205–208, 1996.

Goplerud, C.P.: Monoamniotic twins with double survival: report of a case. Obstet. Gynecol. **23**:289–290, 1964.

Gould, S.J.: Living with connections: are Siamese twins one person or two? Natural Hist. **91**:18–22, 1982.

Grafe, M.R.: Antenatal cerebral necrosis in monochorionic twins. Pediatr. Pathol. **13**:15–19, 1993.

Green, J.J. and Hobbins, J.C.: Abdominal ultrasound examination of the first-trimester fetus. Amer. J. Obstet. Gynecol. **159**:165–175, 1988.

Green, Q.L., Jackson, J. and Miller, A.: Monoamniotic twins: report of a case with surviving normal infants. Amer. J. Obstet. Gynecol. **79**:1082–1084, 1960.

Greig, P.C., Veille, J.-C., Morgan, T. and Henderson, L.: The effect of presentation and mode of delivery on neonatal outcome in the second twin. Amer. J. Obstet. Gynecol. **167**:901–906, 1992.

Grennert, L., Persson, P.-H., Gennser, G. and Kullander, S.: Ultrasound and human-placental-lactogen screening for early detection of twin pregnancies. Lancet **1**:4–6, 1976a.

Grennert, L., Persson, P.-H., Gennser, G., Kullander, S. and Thorell, J.: Hormonal screening for twin pregnancies. Lancet **2**:1257–1258, 1976b.

Gringras, P.: Identical differences. Lancet **353**:562, 1999.

Grischke, E.M., Boos, R., Schmidt W. and Bastert, G.: Twin pregnancies with fetofetal transfusion syndrome. Z. Geburtsh. Perinatol. **194**:17–21, 1990.

Gruenwald, P.: Early human twins with peculiar relations to each other and the chorion. Anat. Rec. **83**:267–279, 1942.

Gruenwald, P.: Environmental influences on twins apparent at birth: a preliminary study. Biol. Neonat. **15**:79–93, 1970.

Gul, A., Aslan, H., Polat, I., Cebeci, A., Bulut, H., Sahin, O. and Ceylan, Y.: Natural history of 11 cases of twin-twin transfusion syndrome without intervention. Twin Res. **6**:263–266, 2003.

Guttmacher, A.F.: An analysis of 521 cases of twin pregnancy. I. Differences in single ovum and double ovum twinning. Amer. J. Obstet. Gynecol. **34**:76–84, 1937.

Guttmacher, A.F.: The incidence of multiple births in man and some of the other unipara. Obstet. Gynecol. **2**:22–35, 1953.

Hagay, Z.J., Mazor, M. and Leiberman, J.R.: Multiple pregnancy complicated by a single intrauterine fetal death. Obstet. Gynecol. **66**:837–838, 1985.

Hall, J.G.: Twinning: mechanisms and genetic implications. Current Opinion in Genet. Devel. **6**:343–347, 1996.

Hallgrimsson, J.T.: Sacro-coccygeal teratoma with acute hydramnios. Acta Obstet. Gynecol. Scand. **60**:517–518, 1981.

Halpin, T.F.: Human chorionic gonadotropin titers in twin pregnancies. Amer. J. Obstet. Gynecol. **106**:317–318, 1970.

Hamamy, H.A., Ajlouni, H.K. and Ajlouni, K.M.: Familial monozygotic twinning: Report of an extended multigeneration family. Twin Res. **7**:219–222, 2004.

Hamasaki, S., Shirabe, S., Tsuda, R., Yoshimura, T., Nakamura, T. and Eguchi, K.: Discordant Gerstmann-Sträussler-Scheinker disease in monozygotic twins. Lancet **352**: 1358–1359, 1998.

Hamblen, E.C., Baker, R.D. and Derieux, G.D.: Roentgenographic diagnosis and anatomic studies of a quintuple pregnancy. JAMA **109**:10–12, 1937.

Hamilton, W.J., Brown, D. and Spiers, B.G.: Another case of quadruplets. J. Obstet. Gynaecol. Br. Emp. **66**:409–412, 1959.

Hamlett, G.W.: Polyembryony in the armadillo: genetic or physiological ? Q. Rev. Biol. **8**:348–358, 1933.

Haning, R.V., Seifer, D.B., Wheeler, C.A., Frishman, G.N., Silver, H. and Pierce, D.J.: Effects of fetal number and multifetal reduction on length of in vitro fertilization pregnancies. Obstet. Gynecol. **87**:964–968, 1996.

Hanna, J.H. and Hill, J.M.: Single intrauterine fetal demise in multiple gestation. Obstet. Gynecol. **63**:126–130, 1984.

Hanson, J.W.: Incidence of conjoined twinning. Lancet **2**:1257, 1975.

Hargitai, B., Porter, H., Cziniel, M., Sheriff, A., Edmond, A., Golding, J. and Berry, P.J.: Cerebral palsy and the vanishing twin phenomenon: a histopathologic study. Pediatr. Devel. Pathol. **6**:193–192 (abstract), 2003.

Harlap, S., Shahar, S. and Baras, M.: Overripe ova and twinning. Amer. J. Hum. Genet. **37**:1206–1215, 1985.

Harper, R.G., Kenigsberg, K., Sia, C.G., Horn, D., Stern, D. and Bongiovi, V.: Xiphopagus conjoined twins: a 300-year review of the obstetric, morphopathologic, neonatal, and surgical parameters. Amer. J. Obstet. Gynecol. **137**:617–629, 1980.

Harris, D.W.: Letter to the editor. J. Reprod. Med. **27**:39, 1982.

Hartemann, J., Peters, A., Dellestable, P., Duprez, A. and Touati, E.: Les transfusions foeto-foetales lors des grossesses biovulaires existent-elles? Gynecol. Obstet. (Paris) **62**:663–668, 1963.

Hashimoto, B., Caallen, P.W., Filly, R.A. and Laros, R.K.: Ultrasound evaluation of polyhydramnios and twin pregnancy. Amer. J. Obstet. Gynecol. **154**:1069–1072, 1986.

Hawrylyshyn, P.A., Barkin, M., Bernstein, A. and Papsin, F.R.: Twin pregnancies—a continuing perinatal challenge. Obstet. Gynecol. **59**:463–466, 1982.

Healey, M.G.: Acardia: predictive risk factors for the co-twin's survival. Teratology **50**:205–213, 1994.

Healey, S.C., Kirk, K.M., Hyland, V.J., Munns, C.F., Henders, A.K., Batch, J.A., Heath, A.C., Martin, N.G. and Glass, I.A.: Height discordance in monozygotic females is not attributable to discordant inactivation of X-linked stature determining genes. Twin Res. **4**:19–24, 2001.

Hecher, K., Jauniaux, E., Campbell, S., Deane, C. and Nicolaides, K.: Artery-to-artery anastomosis in monochorionic twins. Amer. J. Obstet. Gynecol. **171**:570–572, 1994a.

Hecher, K., Ville, Y. and Nicolaides, K.: Umbilical artery steal syndrome and distal gangrene in a case of twin-twin transfusion syndrome. Obstet. Gynecol. **83**:862–865, 1994b.

Hein, P.R., van Groeninhen, J.C. and Puts, J.J.G.: A case of acardiac anomaly in the cynomolgus monkey (*Macaca fascicularis*): a complication of monozygotic monochorial twinning. J. Med. Primatol. **14**:133–142, 1985.

Hendricks, C.H.: Twinning in relation to birth weight, mortality, and congenital anomalies. Obstet. Gynecol. **27**:47–53, 1966.

Hernandez-Johnstone, B. and Benirschke, K.: Monozygotic twins discordant for urinary tract anomalies and presenting as hydramnios. Obstet. Gynecol. **47**:610–615, 1976.

Herrlin, K.-M., Hauge, M. and Eriksson, S.A.: Finger print patterns in an unselected series of triplets. Hum. Hered. **20**:336–355, 1970.

Hertzberg, B.S., Kurtz, A.B., Choi, H.Y, Kaczmarczyl, J.M., Warren, W., Wapner, R.J., Needleman, R.J., Baltarowich, O.H., Pasto, M.E., Rifkin, M.D., Pennell, R.G. and Goldberg, B.B.: Significance of membrane thickness in the sonographic evaluation of twin gestations. A.J.R. **148**:151–153, 1987.

Herzog, A.: Korrelieren die pathologisch-anatomischen Befunde an den Geschlechtsorganen von Rinderzwicken mit den quantitativen Relationen des Gonosomenchimärismus [XX/XY] in Blutzellen? Zuchthygiene **4**:156–159, 1969.

Herzog, A. and Rieck, G.W.: Chromosomenanomalie bei einem Acardius (Amorphus globosus). Zuchthygiene **4**:57–60, 1969.

Heyborne, K.D. and Porreco, R.P.: Selective fetocide reverses preeclampsia in discordant twins. Amer. J. Obstet. Gynecol. **191**:477–480, 2004.

Heyborne, K.D., Porreco, R.P., Garite, T.J., Phair, K. and Abril, D.: Improved perinatal survival of monoamniotic twins with intensive inpatient monitoring. Amer. J. Obstet. Gynecol. **192**:96–101, 2005.

Hill, A.V.S. and Jeffreys, A.J.: Use of minisatellite DNA probes for determination of twin zygosity at birth. Lancet **2**:1394–1395, 1985.

Hill, L.M., Krohn, M., Lazebnik, N., Tush, B., Boyles, D. and Ursiny, J.J.: The amniotic fluid index in normal twin pregnancies. Amer. J. Obstet. Gynecol. **182**:950–954, 2000.

Ho, S.K. and Wu, P.Y.K.: Perinatal factors and neonatal morbidity in twin pregnancy. Amer. J. Obstet. Gynecol. **122**:979–987, 1975.

Hobbins, J.C.: Selective reduction-a perinatal necessity? N. Engl. J. Med. **318**:1062–1063, 1988.

Hobbs, C.A., Cleves, M.A. and Simmons, C.J.: Genetic epidemiology and congenital malformations. From chromosomes to the crib. Arch Pediatr. Adolesc. Med. **156**:315–320, 2002.

Hoch, Z., Peretz, B.A., Brandes, J.M. and Peretz, A.: Intraamniotic hypertonic saline treatment in a case of dizygotic twin pregnancy. Int. J. Gynaecol. Obstet. **10**:156–160, 1972.

Höfliger, H.: Beitrag zur Kenntnis der Akardier. Schweiz. Arch. Tierheilk. **116**:629–644, 1974. [Extensive review]

Hohenauer, L.: Prenatal nutrition and subsequent development. Lancet **1**:644–645, 1971.

Holzgreve, W., Tercanli, S., Krings, W. and Schuierer, G.: A simpler technique for umbilical-cord blockade of an acardiac twin. NEJM **331**:56–57, 1994.

Honoré, L.H.: Twinning in postpill spontaneous abortions. Amer. J. Obstet. Gynecol. **135**:700–700, 1979.

Hoogendoorn, D.: Daling van het aantal meerlinggeboorten. Nederl. Tijdschr. Geneesk. **117**:805–807, 1973.

Horger, E.O. and McCarter, L.M.: Prenatal diagnosis of sacrococcygeal teratoma. Amer. J. Obstet. Gynecol. **134**:228–229, 1979.

Hrubec, Z. and Robinette, C.D.: The study of human twins in medical research. NEJM **310**:435–441, 1984.

Hsu, J. and Gonda, M.A.: Monozygotic twin formation in mouse embryos in vitro. Science **209**:605–606, 1980.

Hughes, H.E. and Miskin, M.: Congenital microcephaly due to vascular disruption: in utero documentation. Pediatrics **78**:85–87, 1986.

Hurst, R.W. and Abbitt, P.L.: Fetal intracranial hemorrhage and periventricular leukomalacia: complications of twin-twin transfusion syndrome. Amer. J. Neurol. Res. **10**:S62–S63, 1989.

Hyrtl, J.: Die Blutgefäße der Menschlichen Nachgeburt in normalen und abnormen Verhältnissen. Braumüller, Vienna, 1870.

Imaizumi, Y.: Concordance and discordance of congenital hydrocephalus in 107 twin pairs in Japan. Teratology **40**:1010–103, 1989a.

Imaizumi, Y.: Stillbirth rate and weight at birth of quintuplets in Japan. Acta Genet. Med. Gemellol. **38**:65–69, 1989b.

Imaizumi, Y.: A comparative study of twinning and triplet rates in 17 countries, 1972–1996. Acta Genet. Med. Gemell. **47**:101–114, 1998.

Imaizumi, Y. and Inouye, E.: Analysis of multiple birth rates in Japan. III. Secular trend, maternal age effect and geographical variation in triplet rates. Jpn. J. Hum. Genet. **25**:73–81, 1980.

Ingalls, T.H.: Conjoined twins in zebra fish. Arch. Environ. Health **19**:344–352, 1969.

Inouye, E.: Frequency of multiple birth in three cities of Japan. Amer. J. Hum. Genet. **9**:317–320, 1957.

Isaacs, H. Jr.: Tumors of the Fetus and Infant. An Atlas. Springer-Verlag, N.Y., 2002.

Ishiguro, T.: Alpha-fetoprotein in twin pregnancy. Lancet **2**:1214, 1973.

Ishii, K., Chmait, R.H., Martinez, J.M., Nakata, M. and Quintero, R.A.: Ultrasound assessment of venous blood flow before and after laser therapy: approach to understanding the pathophysiology of twin-twin transfusion syndrome. Ultrasound Obstetr. Gynecol. **24**:164–168, 2004.

Islam, A.B.M., Hill, W.G. and Land, R.B.: Ovulation rates in lines of mice selected for testis weight. Genet. Res. **27**:23–32, 1976.

Israelstam, D.M.: Mono-amniotic twin pregnancy: a case report. S. Afr. Med. J. (Suppl. S. Afr. J. Obstet. Gynaecol.) **47**:2026–2027, 1973.

Itoh, H., Kambe, S., Maeba, Y. and Hirai, T.: A case of duplicitas lateralis superior. Congen. Anom. (Jpn.) **14**:1–11, 1974.

Itskovitz, J., Boldes, R., Thaler, I., Bronstein, M., Erlik, Y. and Brandes, J.M.: Transvaginal ultrasonography-guided aspiration of gestational sacs for selective abortion in multiple pregnancy. Amer. J. Obstet. Gynecol. **160**:215–217, 1989.

Itzkowic, D.: A survey of 59 triplet pregnancies. Br. J. Obstet. Gynaecol. **86**:23–28, 1979.

Jackson, J. and Benirschke, K.: The recognition and significance of the vanishing twin. J. Amer. Board Fam. Pract. **2**:58–63, 1989.

Jain, J.K., Boostanfar, R., Slater, C.C., Francis, M.M. and Paulson, R.J.: Monozygotic twins and triplets in association with blastocyst transfer. J. Assist. Reprod. Genet. **21**:103–107, 2004b.

Jain, T., Missmer, S.A. and Hornstein, M.D.: Trends in embryo-transfer practice and in outcomes of the use of assisted reproductive technology in the United States. NEJM **350**:1639–1945, 2004a.

Jamal, A.A.: Placental teratoma: a case report and review of the literature. Ann. Saudi Med. **19**:359–361, 1999.

James, W.H.: Excess of like sexed pairs of dizygotic twins. Nature **232**:277–278, 1971.

James, W.H.: Decline in dizygotic twinning (cont.) NEJM **289**:1204–1205, 1973.

James, W.H.: The declines in dizygotic twinning rates and in birth rates. Ann. Hum. Biol. **2**:81–84, 1975.

James, W.H.: Twinning and anencephaly. Ann. Hum. Biol. **3**:401–409, 1976.

James, W.H.: The sex ratio of monoamniotic twin pairs. Ann. Hum. Biol. **4**:143–153, 1977a.

James, W.H.: A note on the epidemiology of acardiac monsters. Teratology **16**:211–216, 1977b.

James, W.H.: Sex ratio and placentation of twins. Ann. Hum. Biol. **7**:273–276, 1980.

James, W.H.: Twinning rates. Lancet **1**:934–935, 1983.

James, W.H.: Zygosity and Weinberg's rule. J. Reprod. Med. **13**:197–199, 1984.

James, W.H., Bracken, M.B. and Honore, L.H.: Letters to the editor on: twinning rates and the "pill." Amer. J. Obstet. Gynecol. **135**:699–701, 1979.

Jarmulowicz, M.: Embryo biopsy. Lancet **1**:547, 1989.

Jarvik, L.F., Falek, A., Schmidt, R. and Platt, M.: The mixed leukocyte reaction as a possible test of zygosity in twins. Hum. Hered. **19**:668–673, 1969.

Jauniaux, E., Elkazen, N., Leroy, F., Wilkin, P., Rodesch, F. and Hustin, J.: Clinical and morphologic aspects of the vanishing twin phenomenon. Obstet. Gynecol. **72**:577–581, 1988.

Jauniaux, E., Gulbis, B. and Burton, G.J.: Physiological implications of the materno-fetal oxygen gradient in human early pregnancy. Reprod. BioMedicine Online: www.rbmonline.com/Article/871. **7**:250–253, 2003.

Javert, C.T.: Spontaneous and Habitual Abortion. Blakiston, New York, 1957.

Jeanty, P., Rodesch, F., Verhoogen, C. and Struyven, J.: The vanishing twin. Ultrasonics **2**:25–31, 1981.

Jeanty, P., Shah, D. and Roussis, P.: Single-needle insertion in twin amniocentesis. J. Ultrasound Med. **9**:511–517, 1990.

Jenkins, M.E., Eisen, J. and Seguin, F.: Congenital asymmetry and diploid-triploid mosaicism. Amer. J. Dis. Child. **122**:80–84, 1971.

Johnson, M., Crombleholme, T.M., Hedrick, H.L., King, M., Kasperski, S., Wilson, R.D., Flake, A.W. and Howell, L.J.: Bipolar umbilical cord cauterization for selective termination of complicated monochorionic pregnancies. Amer. J. Obstet. Gynecol. **185**:246 (abstract 606), 2001.

Johnson, K.L., Nelson, J.L., Furst, D.E., McSweeney, P.A., Roberts, D.J., Zhen, D.K. and Bianchi, D.W.: Fetal cell microchimerism in tissue from multiple sites in women with systemic sclerosis. Arthritis Rheumatol. **44**:1848–1854, 2001.

Johnson, S., Barss, V. and Driscoll, S.: Incidence and impact of single intrauterine death in multiple gestation. Lab. Invest. **54**:29A, 1986 (abstract).

Jones, J.M., Sbarra, A.J., Dilillo, L., Cetrulo, C.L. and D'Alton, M.E.: Indomethacin in severe twin-to-twin transfusion syndrome. Amer. J. Perinatol. **10**:24–26, 1993.

Jones, K.L.: Smith's Recognizable Patterns of Human Malformation. 4th ed., pp. 600–601. Saunders, Philadelphia, 1988.

Jones, W.S.: Obstetric significance of female genital anomalies. Obstet. Gynecol. **10**:113–127, 1957.

Joseph, T.J. and Vogt, P.J.: Placental teratomas. Obstet. Gynecol. **41**:574–578, 1973.

Jou, H.-J., Ng, K.-Y., Teng, R.-J. and Hsieh, F.-J.: Doppler sonographic detection of reverse twin-twin transfusion after intrauterine death of the donor. J. Ultrasound Med. **5**:307–309, 1993.

Jovanovic, L., Landesman, R. and Saxena, B.B.: Screening for twin pregnancy. Science **198**:738, 1977.

Jung, J.H., Graham, J.M., Schultz, N. and Smith, D.W.: Congenital hydranencephaly/porencephaly due to vascular disruption in monozygotic twins. Pediatrics **73**:467–469, 1984.

Kadowaki, J.-I., Thompson, R.I., Zuelzer, W.W., Woolley, P.V., Brough, A.J. and Gruber, D.: XX/XY lymphoid chimaerism in congenital immunological deficiency syndrome with thymic alymphoplasia. Lancet **2**:1152–1156, 1965.

Kaelber, C.T. and Pugh, T.F.: Influence of intrauterine relations on the intelligence of twins. NEJM **280**:1030–1034, 1969. **281**:332, 1969.

Kalfayan, B. and Gundersen, J.H.: Ovarian twin pregnancy. Obstet. Gynecol. **55**:25S–27S, 1980.

Källén, B.: Congenital malformations in twins: a population study. Acta Genet. Med. Gemellol. **35**:167–178, 1986.

Kamin, L.J.: Transfusion syndrome and the heritability of IQ. Ann. Hum. Genet. **42**:161–171, 1978.

Kanhai, H.H.H., van Rijssel, E.J.C., Meerman, R.J. and Bennebroek Gravenhorst, J.: Selective termination in quintuplet pregnancy during first trimester. Lancet **1**:1447, 1986.

Kao, K.R., Masui, Y. and Elinson, R.P.: Lithium-induced respecification of pattern in *Xenopus laevis* embryos. Nature **322**:371–373, 1986.

Kaplan, C.G.: Color Atlas of Gross Placental Pathology. Igaku-Shoin, New York, 1994.

Kaplan, C. and Benirschke, K.: The acardiac anomaly: new case reports and current status. Acta Genet. Med. Gemellol. **28**:51–59, 1979.

Kaplan, C.G., Askin, F.B. and Benirschke, K.: Cytogenetics of extragonadal tumors. Teratology **19**:261–266, 1979.

Kaplan, C., Perlmutter, S. and Molinoff, S.: Epignathus with placental hydrops. Arch. Pathol. Lab. Med. **104**:374–375, 1980.

Kappelman, M.D.: Acardius amorphus. Amer. J. Obstet. Gynecol. **47**:412–416, 1944.

Kapur, R.P., Mahony, B.S., Nyberg, D.A., Resta, R.G. and Shephard, T.H.: Sirenomelia associated with a "vanishing twin." Teratology **43**:103–108, 1991.

Karam, J.A. and Baker, L.A.: True hermaphroditism. NEJM **350**:393, 2004.

Kaufman, M.H.: The embryology of conjoined twins. Childs Nerv. Syst. **20**:508–525, 2004.

Kaufman, M.H. and O'Shea, K.S.: Induction of monozygotic twinning in the mouse. Nature **276**:707–708, 1978.

Kawamura, A.: Siamese twins in the Sei whale *Balaenoptera borealis* Lesson. Nature **221**:490–491, 1969.

Kawamura, A. and Kashita, K.: A rare double monster of dolphin, *Stenella caeruleoalba*. Sci. Rep. Whales Res. Inst. No.**23**:139–140, 1971.

Keeler, C.E.: On the amount of external mirror imagery in double monsters and identical twins. Proc. Natl. Acad. Sci. (USA) **15**:839–842, 1929.

Keith, L.: Zygosity and Weinberg's rule. J. Reprod. Med. **13**:195–197, 1974.

Keith, L., Ellis, R., Berger, G.S., Depp, R., Filstead, W., Hatcher, R. and Keith, D.M.: The Northwestern University multihospital twin study. I. A description of 588 twin pregnancies and associated pregnancy loss, 1971 to 1975. Amer. J. Obstet. Gynecol. **138**:781–789, 1980.

Keith, L.G., Keith, D.M., Blickstein, I. and Oleszczuk, J.J., eds.: Triplet Pregnancies and their Consequences. Taylor and Francis Group, CRC Press, London, 2002.

Kempthorne, O. and Osborne, R.H.: The interpretation of twin data. Amer. J. Hum. Genet. **13**:320–339, 1961.

Kennedy, J.F. and Donahue, R.P.: Binucleate human oocytes from large follicles. Lancet **1**:754–755, 1969.

Kennedy, N.: Twin pregnancy in a double uterus. JAMA **169**:2064, 1959.

Kenney, A., Hall, C.A. and McGrath, J.: H.P.L. and twins. Lancet **1**:253–254, 1976.

Kerenyi, T.D. and Chitkara, U.: Selective birth in twin pregnancy with discordance for Down's syndrome. NEJM **304**:1525–1527, 1981.

Khudr, G. and Benirschke, K.: Discordant monozygous twins associated with amnion rupture: a case report. Obstet. Gynecol. **39**:713–716, 1972.

Khunda, S.: Locked twins. Obstet. Gynecol. **39**:453–459, 1972.

Kiely, J.L., Kleinman, J.C. and Kiely, M.: Triplets and higher-order multiple births. Time trends and infant mortality. Amer. J. Dis. Child. **146**:862–868, 1992.

Kilby, M.D., Platt, C., Whittle, M.J., Oxley, J. and Lindop, G.B.M.: Renin gene expression in fetal kidneys of pregnancies complicated by twin-twin transfusion syndrome. Pediatr. Devel. Pathol. **4**:175–179, 2001.

Kilpatrick, S.J., Jackson, R. and Croughan-Minihane, M.S.: Perinatal mortality in twins and singletons matched for gestational age at delivery at ≥30 weeks. Amer. J. Obstet. Gynecol. **174**:66–71, 1996.

Kim, C.K., Barr, R.J. and Benirschke, K.: Cytogenetic studies of conjoined twins: a case report. Obstet. Gynecol. **38**:877–881, 1971.

Kim, K.-R., Kwon, Y., Joung, J.Y, Kim, K.S., Ayala, A.G. and Ro, J.Y.: True hermaphroditism and mixed gonadal dysgenesis in young children: a clinicopathologic study of 10 cases. Modern Pathol. **15**:1013–1019, 2002.

Kindred, J.E.: Twin pregnancies with one twin blighted. Amer. J. Obstet. Gynecol. **48**:642–682, 1944.

King, A.D., Soothill, P.W., Montemagno, R., Young, M.P., Sams, V. and Rodeck, C.H.: Twin-to-twin blood transfusion in a dichorionic pregnancy without the oligohydramnios-polyhydramnios sequence. Brit. J. Obstet. Gynaecol. **102**:334–335, 1995.

Kirkland, J.A.: An acardiac, acephalic monster in a triplet pregnancy. Aust. N.Z. J. Obstet. Gynaecol. **22**:168–171, 1982.

Kirshon, B.: Fetal urine output in hydramnios. Obstet. Gynecol. **73**:240–242, 1989.

Klebe, J.G. and Ingomar, C.J.: The fetoplacental circulation during parturition illustrated by the interfetal transfusion syndrome. Pediatrics **49**:112–115, 1972.

Klingberg, W.G., Jones, B., Allen, W.M. and Dempsey, E.: Placental parabiotic circulation of single ovum human twins. Amer. J. Dis. Child. **90**:519–520, 1955.

Klinger, G., Merlob, P., Aloni, D., Maayan, A. and Sirota, L.: Normal pulmonary function in a monoamniotic twin discordant for bilateral renal agenesis: report and review. Amer. J. Med. Genet. **73**:76–79, 1997.

Kloosterman, G.J.: The "third circulation" in identical twins. Ned. Tijdschr. Verlosk. **63**:395–412, 1963.

Knox, G. and Morley, D.: Twinning in Yoruba women. J. Obstet. Gynaecol. Br. Emp. **67**:981–984, 1960.

Knudsen, L.B.: No association between griseofulvin and conjoined twinning. Lancet **2**:1097, 1987.

Kobak, A.J. and Cohen, M.R.: Velamentous insertion of cord with spontaneous rupture of vasa previa in twin pregnancy. Amer. J. Obstet. Gynecol. **38**:1063–1066, 1939.

Kohga, S., Nambu, T., Tanaka, K., Benirschke, K., Feldman, B.H. and Kishikawa, T.: Hypertrophy of the placenta and sacrococcygeal teratoma: report of two cases. Virchows Arch. [A] Histol. **386**:223–229, 1980.

Kohler, H.G.: An unusual case of sirenomelia. Teratology **6**:295–302, 1972.

Kohler, H.G. and MacDonald, H.N.: Discordant anencephaly in a set of triplets. Obstet. Gynecol. **40**:607–611, 1972.

Köhn, K.: Beobachtungen zur Ätiologie der Acardier. Zentralbl. Allg. Pathol. Pathol. Anat. **90**:209–218, 1953.

Komai, T. and Fukuoka, G.: A set of dichorionic identical triplets. J. Hered. **22**:233–243, 1931.

Koontz, W.L., Layman, L., Adams, A. and Lavery, J.P.: Antenatal sonographic diagnosis of conjoined twins in a triplet pregnancy. Amer. J. Obstet. Gynecol. **153**:230–231, 1985.

Koranyi, G. and Kovacs, J.: Über das Zwillingstransfusionssyndrom. Acta Paediatr. Acad. Sci. Hung. **16**:119–125, 1975.

Kormann, E.: Chang, and Eng Bunker. Schmidt's Jahrbücher **143**:281, 1869.

Kovacs, B., Shahbahrami, B., Platt, L.D. and Comings, D.E.: Molecular genetic prenatal determination of twin zygosity. Obstet. Gynecol. **72**:954–956, 1988.

Kovacs, B.W., Kirschbaum, T.H. and Paul, R.H.: Twin gestations. I. Antenatal care and complications. Obstet. Gynecol. **74**:313–317, 1989.

Kovacs, L., Geallen, J. and Falkay, G.: Amniotic chloride concentrations in twin-pregnancy after intra-amniotic injection of hypertonic saline. J. Obstet. Gynaecol. Br. Commonw. **79**:54–59. 1972.

Kraay, G.J., Menard, D.P. and Bedoya, M.: Monozygous cattle twins as a result of transfer of a single embryo. Can. Vet. J. **24**:281–283, 1983.

Krauer, F.: Das akute Hydramnion bei eineiigen Zwillingsschwangerschaften. Gynaecologia **158**:395–399, 1964.

Krause, H.G. and Goh, J.T.W.: Cord entanglement in monochorionic diamniotic twins. Aust. NZ J. Obstet. Gynaecol. **38**:341–342, 1998.

Kresky, B.: Transplacental transfusion syndrome. Clin. Pediatr. **3**:600–603, 1964.

Kreutner, A.K., Levine, J. and Thiede, H.: A double truncus arteriosus in thoracopagus twins. NEJM **268**:1388–1390, 1963.

Kreyberg, L.: A teratoma-like swelling in the umbilical cord possibly of acardius nature. J. Pathol. Bacteriol. **75**:109–112, 1958.

Kruyer, H., Milà, M., Glover, G., Carbonell, P., Ballesta, F. and Estivill, X.: Fragile X syndrome and the $(CGG)_n$ mutation: two families with discordant MZ twins. Amer. J. Hum. Genet. **54**:437–442, 1994.

Kurosawa, K., Kuromaru, R., Imaizumi, K., Nakamura, Y., Ishikawa, F., Ueda, K. and Kuroki, Y.: Monozygotic twins with discordant sex. Acta Genet. Med. Gemellol. **41**:301–310. 1992.

Laband, S.J., Cherny, W.B. and Finberg, H.J.: Heterotopic pregnancy: report of four cases. Amer. J. Obstet. Gynecol. **158**:437–438, 1988.

Lachapelle, M.F., Leduc, L., Côté, J.M., Grignon, A. and Fouron, J.C.: Potential value of fetal echocardiography in the differential diagnosis of twin pregnancy with presence of polyhydramnios-oligohydramnios syndrome. Amer. J. Obstet. Gynecol. **177**:388–394, 1997.

Lachman, R., McNabb, M., Furmanski, M. and Karp, L.: The acardiac monster. Eur. J. Pediatr. **134**:195–200, 1980.

Lack, E.E., Glaun, R.S., Hefter, L.G., Seneca, R.P., Steigman, C. and Athari, F.: Late occurrence of malignancy following resection of a histologically mature sacrococcygeal teratoma. Report of a case and literature review. Arch. Pathol. Lab. Med. **117**:724–728, 1993.

Lage, J.M., VanMarter, L.J. and Mikhail, E.: Vascular anastomoses in fused, dichorionic twin placentas resulting in twin transfusion syndrome. Placenta **10**:55–59, 1989.

Laird, E.G., Thomas, R.B. and Halabi, N.E.: Double pregnancy in a bicornuate uterus: a review of the literature with a case report. Delaware Med. J. **29**:78–83, 1957.

Lam, Y.H., Sin, S.Y., Lam, C., Lee, C.P., Tang, M.H.Y. and Tse, H.Y.: Prenatal sonographic diagnosis of conjoined twins in the first-trimester: two case reports. Ultrasound Obstet. Gynecol. **10**:1–3, 1997; **11**:289–291, 1998.

Lambalk, C.B. and Boomsma, D.I.: The endocrinology of dizygotic twinning. Twin Res. **1**:(#2) 96 (abstr. 061), 1998.

Lancaster, P.A.L.: Monozygotic twins and triplets after assisted conception. Twin Res. **7**:361 (abstract), 2004.

Land, R.B.: The expression of female sex-limited characters in the male. Nature **204**:208–209, 1973.

Land, R.B., Pelletier, J., Thimonier, J. and Mauleon, P.: A quantitative study of genetic differences in the incidence of oestrus, ovulation and plasma luteinizing hormone concentration in the sheep. J. Endocrinol. **58**:305–317, 1973.

Lander, M., Oosterhof, H. and Aarnoudse, J.G.: Death of one twin followed by extremely variable flow velocity waveforms in the surviving fetus. Gynecol. Obstet. Invest. **36**:127–128, 1993.

Landy, H.J., Keith, L. and Keith, D.: The vanishing twin. Acta Genet. Med. Gemellol. **31**:179–194, 1982.

Landy, H.J., Weiner, S., Corson, S.L., Batzer, F.R. and Bolognese R.J.: The "vanishing twin": ultrasonographic assessment of fetal disappearance in the first trimester. Amer. J. Obstet. Gynecol. **155**:14–19, 1986.

Landy, H.J., Larsen, J.W., Schoen, M., Larsen, M.E., Kent, S.G. and Weingold, A.B.: Acardiac fetus in a triplet pregnancy. Teratology **37**:1–6, 1988.

Lange, A.P., Hebjorn, S., Moth, I., Fuglsand, E., Hasch, E., Bruun Petersen, G. and Norgaard-Pedersen, B.: Twin fetus papyraceus and alpha-fetoprotein: a clinical dilemma. Lancet **2**:636, 1979.

Lange, I.R., Harman, C.R., Ash, K.M., Manning, F.A. and Menticoglou, S.: Twin with hydramnios: treating premature labor at source. Amer. J. Obstet. Gynecol. **160**:552–557, 1989.

Langer, J.C., Harrison, M.R., Schmidt, K.G., Silverman, N.H., Anderson, R.L., Goldberg, J.D., Filly, R.A., Crombleholme, T.M., Longaker, M.T. and Golbus, M.S.: Fetal hydrops and death from sacrococcygeal teratoma: rationale for fetal surgery. Amer. J. Obstet. Gynecol. **160**:1145–1150, 1989.

Laros, R.K. and Dattel, B.J.: Management of twin pregnancy: the vaginal route is still safe. Amer. J. Obstet. Gynecol. **158**:1330–1338, 1988.

Larroche, J.Cl., Droullé, P., Delezoide, A.L., Narcy, F. and Nessmann, C.: Brain damage in monozygous twins. Biol. Neonate **57**:261–278, 1990.

Larson, S.L., Kempers, R.D. and Titus, J.L.: Monoamniotic twins with a common umbilical cord. Amer. J. Obstet. Gynecol. **105**:635–636, 1969a.

Larson, S.L., Wilson, R.B. and Titus, J.L.: Monoamniotic hydrocephalic twins with survival: report of a case with cytogenetic study. Obstet. Gynecol. **34**:419–421, 1969b.

La Sala, G.B., Nucera, G., Gallinelli, A., Nicoli, A., Villani, M.T. and Blickstein, I.: Spontaneous embryonic loss following in vitro fertilization: incidence and effect on outcomes. Amer. J. Obstet. Gynecol. **191**:741–746, 2004.

Lassen, M.-T.: Nachgeburtsbefunde bei eineiigen Zwillingen und Ähnlichkeitsdiagnose. Arch. Gynäkol. **147**:48–64, 1931.

Lawce, H.: Case report. Prenatal chromosome findings in a case of XX/XY chimerism. Karyogram **11**:93–94, 1985.

Lawrence, J.M., Watkins, M.L., Chiu, V., Erickson, J.D. and Petitti, D.B.: Food fortification with folic acid and rate of multiple births, 1994–2000. Birth Defects Res. (Part A): Clin. Molec. Teratol. **70:**948–952, 2004.

Layton, W.M.: Random determination of a developmental process: reversal of normal visceral asymmetry in the mouse. J. Hered. **67**:336–338, 1976.

Layzer, R.B.: Selective reduction—a perinatal necessity? NEJM **318**:1062–1063, 1988.

Lazda, E.J.: Endocardial fibroelastosis in growth-discordant monozygotic twins. Pediat. Development. Pathol. **1**:522–527, 1998.

Lee, C.Y., Madrazo, B. and Roberson, J.: Management of mono-amniotic twins diagnosed by ultrasound. Personal communication, Flint, Michigan, 1988.

Lehndorff, H.: Intrauterines Bluten von einem Zwilling in den anderen. Neue Österr. Z. Kinderheilk. **6**:163–172, 1961.

Leidig, E., Dannecker, G., Pfeiffer, K.H., Salinas, R. and Pfeiffer, J.: Intrauterine development of posthaemorrhagic hydrocephalus. Eur. J. Pediatr. **147**:26–29, 1988.

Lemke, R.P., Machin, G., Muttitt, S., Bamforth, F., Rao, S. and Welch, R.: A case of aplasia cutis congenita in dizygotic twins. J. Perinatol. **13**:22–27, 1993.

Leonard, M.W.E.: Large twins: report of a case. Obstet. Gynecol. **9**:219–220, 1957.

Leppert, P.C., Wartel, L. and Lowman, R.: Fetus papyraceus causing dystocia: inability to detect blighted twin antenatally. Obstet. Gynecol. **54**:381–384, 1979.

Levi, S.: Ultrasonic assessment of the high rate of human multiple pregnancy in the first trimester. J. Clin. Ultrasound **4**:3–5, 1976.

Levinsky, H.V.: A case of conjoined twins in the Sprague-Dawley rat. Lab. Anim. Sci. **23**:903–904, 1973.

Leviton, A. and Paneth, N.: White matter damage in preterm newborns—an epidemiologic perspective. Early Human Devel. **24**:1–22, 1990.

Leviton, A., Stewart, J.E., Alfred, E.N., Dammann, O. and Kuban, K.: Neurological sequelae in in-vitro fertilization babies. Lancet **360**:718, 2002.

Lewis, S.H., Ryder, C. and Benirschke, K.: Omphalogopagus twins in *Chelonia mydas*. Herpetol. Review **23**:69–70, 1992.

Librach, S. and Terrin, A.J.: Monoamniotic twin pregnancy. Amer. J. Obstet. Gynecol. **74**:440–443, 1957.

Librach, C.L., Doran, T.A., Benzie, R.J. and Jones, J.M.: Genetic amniocentesis in seventy twin pregnancies. Amer. J. Obstet. Gynecol. **148**:585–591, 1984.

Liggins, G.C. and Ibbertson, H.K.: A successful quintuplet pregnancy following treatment with human pituitary gonadotrophin. Lancet **1**:114–117, 1966.

Lillie, F.R.: The free martin; a study of the action of sex hormones in the foetal life of cattle. J. Exp. Zool. **23**:371–452, 1917.

Linke, R.P. and Kuni, H.: Über unterschiedliche Blutfülle bei Parabiosepartnern: ein Beitrag zur Parabiosekrankheit. Z. Ges. Exp. Med. **149**:233–250, 1969.

Lipitz, S., Reichman, B., Paret, G., Modan, M., Shalev, J., Serr, D.M., Mashiach, S. and Frenkel, Y.: The improving outcome of triplet pregnancies. Amer. J. Obstet. Gynecol. **161**:1279–1284, 1989.

Lipitz, S., Reichman, B., Uval, J., Shalev, J., Achiron, R., Barkai, G., Lusky, A. and Mashiach, S.: A prospective comparison of the outcome of triplet pregnancies managed expectantly or by multifetal reduction to twins. Amer. J. Obstet. Gynecol. **170**:874–879, 1994.

Lipitz, S., Meizner, I., Yagel, S., Shapiro, I., Achiron, R. and Schiff, E.: Expectant management of twin pregnancies discordant for anencephaly. Obstet. Gynecol. **86**:969–972, 1995.

Lipitz, S., Uval, J., Achiron, R., Schiff, E., Lusky, A. and Reichman, B.: Outcome of twin pregnancies reduced from triplets compared with nonreduced twin gestations. Obstet. Gynecol. **87**:511–514, 1996.

Lipitz, S., Peltz, R., Achiron, R., Barkai, G., Mashiach, S. and Schiff, E.: Selective second-trimester termination of an abnormal fetus in twin pregnancies. J. Perinatol. **17**:301–304, 1997.

Litschgi, M. and Stucki, D.: Verlauf von Zwillingsschangerschaften nach intrauterinem Fruchttod eines Föten. Z. Geburtsh. Perinatol. **184**:227–230, 1980.

Litt, S. and Strauss, H.A.: Monoamniotic twins, one normal, the other anencephalic; multiple true knots in the cords. Amer. J. Obstet. Gynecol. **30**:728–730, 1935.

Littlewood, J.M.: Polycythaemia, and anaemia in newborn monozygotic twin girls. Br. Med. J. **1**:857–859, 1963.

Liu, S., Benirschke, K., Scioscia, A.L. and Mannino, F.L.: Intrauterine death in multiple gestation. Acta Genet. Med. Gemellol. **41**:5–26, 1992.

Livingston, J.E. and Poland, B.J.: A study of spontaneously aborted twins. Teratology **21**:139–148, 1980.

Loendersloot, E.W.: Twin pregnancy in double uterus. Amer. J. Obstet. Gynecol. **127**:682, 1977.

Loeschke, H.: Die Acardie, eine durch Anoxybiose und Nährstoffmangel verursachte Hemmungsbildung. Virchows Arch. [Pathol. Anat.] **315**:499–533, 1948.

Logroño, R., Garcia-Lithgow, C., Harris, C., Kent, M. and Meisner, L.: Heteropagus conjoined twins due to fusion of two embryos: report and review. Amer. J. Med. Genet. **73**:239–243, 1997.

Loos, R., Derom, C., Vlietinck, R. and Derom, R.: The East Flanders prospective twin survey (Belgium): a population-based register. Twin Research **1**:167–175, 1999.

Lopriore, E., Vandenbussche, F.P.H.A., Tiersma, E.S.M., de Beaufort, A.J. and de Leeuw, J.P.: Twin-to-twin transfusion syndrome: New perspectives. J. Pediat. **127**:675–680, 1995.

Lopriore, E., Nagel, H.T.C., Vandenbussche, F.P.H.A. and Walther, F.J.: Long-term neurodevelopmental outcome in twin-to-twin transfusion syndrome. Amer. J. Obstetr. Gynecol. **189**:1314–1319, 2003.

Loughead, J.R. and Halbert, D.R.: An acardiac amorphous twin presenting soft tissue dystocia. J. South. Med. Assoc. **62**:1140–1142, 1969.

Loughry, W.J., Prodöhl, P.A., McDonough, C.M. and Avise, J.C.: Polyembryony in armadillos. Amer. Scientist **86**:274–279, 1998.

Ludwig, E.: Über die Verteilung der Erbmasse unter eineiige Zwillinge. Schweiz. Med. Wochenschr. **57**:1041–1042, 1927.

Luke, B., Nugent, C., van de Ven, C., Martin, D., O'Sullivan, M.J., Eardley, S., Witter, F.R., Mauldin, J. and Newman, R.B.: The association between maternal factors and perinatal outcomes in triplet pregnancies. Amer. J. Obstet. Gynecol. **187**:752–757, 2002.

Lumme, R.H. and Saarikoski, S.V.: Monoamniotic twin pregnancy. Acta Genet. Med. Gemellol. **35**:99–105, 1986.

Lundstroem, A.: Tooth morphology as a basis for distinguishing monozygotic and dizygotic twins. Amer. J. Hum. Genet. **15**:34–43, 1963.

Lutz, H. and Lutz-Ostertag, Y.: Sur l'orientation des embryons jumeaux obtenus par fissuration parallèle à l'axe présumé du blastoderme non incubé de l'oef de Caille (Coturnix coturnix japonica). C. R. Proc. Acad. Sci. Paris **256**:3752–3754, 1963.

Lynch, L., Berkowitz, R.L., Chitkara, U. and Alvarez, M.: First-trimester transabdominal multifetal pregnancy reduction: a report of 85 cases. Obstet. Gynecol. **75**:735–738, 1990.

Lynch, L., Berkowitz, R.L., Stone, J., Alvarez, M. and Lapinski, R.: Preterm delivery after selective termination in twin pregnancies. Obstet. Gynecol. **87**:366–369, 1996.

MacGillivray, I., Nylander, P.P.S. and Corney, G.: Human Multiple Reproduction. Saunders, London, 1975.

MacGillivray, I., Campbell, D.M. and Thompson, B., eds.: Twinning and Twins. Wiley, Chichester, 1988.

Machin, G.A.: Malformations and chromosome anomalies in perinatal death. Ph.D. thesis, University of London, 1974. (quoted from Deacon et al., 1980).

Machin, G.A.: Twins and their zygosity. Lancet **343**:1577, 1994.

Machin, G.A.: Some causes of genotypic and phenotypic discordance in monozygotic twin pairs. Amer. J. Med. Genet. **61**:216–228, 1996.

Machin, G.A.: Velamentous cord insertion in monochorionic twin gestation. An added risk factor. J. Reprod. Med. **42**:785–789, 1997.

MacKenzie, A.P., Stephenson, C.D., Funai, E.F., Lee, M.-L. and Timor-Tritsch, I.: Three-dimensional ultrasound to differentiate epigastric heteropagus conjoined twins from a TRAP sequence. Amer. J. Obstet. Gynecol. **191**:1736–1739, 2004.

Mackenzie, T.C., Crombleholme, T.M., Johnson, M.P., Schnaufer, L., Flake, A.W., Hedrick, H.L., Howell, L.J. and Adzick, N.S.: The natural history of prenatally diagnosed twins. J. Pediatr. Surg. **37**:303–309, 2002.

MacLennan, A.H., Green, R.C., O'Shea, R., Brookes, C. and Morris, D.: Routine hospital admission in twin pregnancy between 26 and 30 weeks' gestation. Lancet **335**:267–269, 1990.

Macones, G.A., Schemmer, G., Pritts, E., Weiblatt, V. and Wapner, R.J.: Multifetal reduction of triplets to twins improves perinatal outcome. Amer. J. Obstet. Gynecol. **169**:982–986, 1993.

Mägiste, M., v. Schenck, H., Sjöberg, N.-O., Thorell, J.I. and Åberg, A.: Screening for detecting twin pregnancy. Amer. J. Obstet. Gynecol. **126**:697–698, 1976.

Magyar, E., Weiner, E., Shalev, E. and Ohel, G.: Pseudoamniotic twins with cord entanglement following genetic funipuncture. Obstet. Gynecol. **78**:915–918, 1991.

Maher, E.R., Brueton, L.A.S., Bowdin, S.C., Luahria, A., Cooper, W., Cole, T.R., Macdonald, F., Sampson, J.R., Barratt, C.L., Reik, W. and Hawkins, M.M.: Beckwith-Wiedemann syndrome and assisted reproductive technology (ART). J. Med. Genet. **40**:62–64, 2003.

Mahieu-Caputo, D., Dommergues, M., Dalezoide, A.-L., Lacoste, M., Cai, Y., Narcy, F., Dumez, Y. and Gubler, M.-C.: Twin-to-twin transfusion syndrome. Role of the fetal renin-angiotensin system. Amer. J. Pathol. **156**:629–636, 2000.

Mahone, P.R., Sherer, D.M., Abramowicz, J.S. and Woods, J.R.: Twin-twin transfusion syndrome: rapid development of severe hydrops of the donor following selective feticide of the hydropic recipient. Amer. J. Obstet. Gynecol. **169**:166–168, 1993.

Mahony, B.S., Filly, R.A. and Callen, P.W.: Amnionicity and chorionicity in twin pregnancies: prediction using ultrasound. Radiology **155**:205–209, 1985.

Mahony, B.S., Petty, C.N., Nyberg, D.A., Luthy, D.A., Hickok, D.E. and Hirsch, J.H.: The "stuck twin" phenomenon: ultrasonographic findings, pregnancy outcome, and management with serial amniocenteses. Amer. J. Obstet. Gynecol. **163**:1513–1522, 1990.

Maier, R.F., Bialobrzeski, B., Gross, A., Vogel, M., Dudenhausen, J.W. and Obladen, M.: Acute and chronic fetal hypoxia in monochorionic and dichorionic twins. Obstet. Gynecol. **86**:973–977, 1995.

Malinowski, W.: Very early and simple determination of chorionic and amniotic type in twin gestations by high-frequency transvaginal ultrasonography. Acta Genet. Med. Gemellol. **46**:167–173, 1997.

Malinowski, W. and Biskup, I.: The sonographic prenatal diagnosis of congenital defects of the anterior abdominal wall based on our own study of twin pregnancies—gastroschisis. Acta Genet. Med. Gemellol. **46**:101–104, 1997.

Malinowski, W. and Wierzba, W.: Twin reversed arterial perfusion syndrome. Acta Genet. Med. Gemellol. **47**:75–87, 1998.

Malinowski, W., Dec, W. and Biskup, I.: The assessment of the umbilical blood flow of the surviving twin after the intrauterine death of the other twin. Acta Genet. Med. Gemellol. **45**:383–386, 1996.

Malone, F.D., Craigo, S.D., Chelmow, D. and D'Alton, M.E.: Outcome of twin gestations complicated by a single anomalous fetus. Obstet. Gynecol. **88**:1–5, 1996.

Manivel, J.C., Dehner, L.P. and Burke, B.: Ovarian tumorlike structures, biovular follicles, and binucleated oocytes in children: their frequency and possible pathologic significance. Pediatr. Pathol. **8**:283–292, 1988.

Mannino, F.L., Jones, K.L. and Benirschke, K.: Congenital skin defects and fetus papyraceus. J. Pediatr. **91**:559–564, 1977.

March of Dimes. Updates. Multiple births and the rising rate of preterm delivery. Contemp. Ob/Gyn. July, pp. 67–77, 2003.

Marcus, N.H.: Developmental aberrations associated with twinning in laboratory-reared sea urchins. Dev. Biol. **70**:274–277, 1979.

Margono, F., Feinkind, L. and Minkoff, H.L.: Foot necrosis in a surviving fetus associated with twin-twin transfusion syndrome and monochorionic placenta. Obstet. Gynecol. **79**:867–869, 1992.

Mari, G., Uerpairojkit, B., Abuhamad, A., Martinez, E. and Copel, J.: Velamentous insertion of the cord in polyhydramnios-oligohydramnios twins. Amer. J. Obstet. Gynecol. **172**:291 (abstract 102), 1995.

Mari, G., Detti, L., Levi-D'Ancona and Kern, L.: "Pseudo" twin-to-twin transfusions syndrome and fetal outcome. J. Perinatol. **18**:399–403, 1998.

Marin-Padilla, M., Chin, A.J. and Marin-Padilla, T.M.: Cardiovascular abnormalities in thoracopagus twins. Teratology **23**:101–113, 1981.

Markavy, K.L. and Scanlon, J.W.: Hydrops fetalis in a parabiotic, acardiac twin. Amer. J. Dis. Child. **132**:638–639, 1978.

Marshall, J.R.: Ovulation induction. Obstet. Gynecol. **35**:963–970, 1970.

Martin, J.A., Hamilton, B.E., Sutton, P.D., Ventura, S.J., Menacker, F. and Munson, M.L.: Births: final data for 2002. Natl. Vital Stat. Rep. **52**:1–113, 2003.

Martin, N.G., Olsen, M.E., Theile, H., Beaini, J.L.E., Handelsman, D. and Bhatnagar, A.S.: Pituitary-ovarian function in mothers who have had two sets of dizygotic twins. Fertil. Steril. **41**:878–880, 1984a.

Martin, N.G., Beaini, J.L.E., Olsen, M.E., Bhatnagar, A.S. and Macourt, D.: Gonadotropin levels in mothers who have had two sets of DZ twins. Acta Genet. Med. Gemellol. **33**:131–139, 1984b.

Martin, N.G., Shanley S., Butt, K., Osborne, J. and O'Brien, G.: Excessive follicular recruitment and growth in mothers of spontaneous dizygotic twins. Acta Genet. Med. Gemellol. **40**:291–301, 1991.

Martinez-Poyer, J.L., Quintero, R.A., Carreño, C.A., King, M., Bottoms, S.F., Romero, R. and Evans, M.I.: Doppler assessment of the effect of umbilical-cord ligation of acardiac twins. Amer. J. Obstet. Gynecol. **176**:S152 (abstract 530), 1997.

Marx, W.: Akutes Hydramnion bei Drillingsschwangerschaft mit hochgradigem Hydrops einer Frucht. Zentralbl. Gynäkol. **78**:101–109, 1956.

Mas, C., Delatycki, M.B. and Weintraub, R.G.: Persistent truncus arteriosus in monozygotic twins: case report and literature review. Amer. J. Med. Genet. **82**:146–148, 1999.

Mashiach, S., Ben-Rafael, Z., Dor, J. and Serr, D.M.: Triplet pregnancy in uterus didelphys with delivery interval of 72 days. Obstet. Gynecol. **58**:519–520, 1981.

Massip, A., Zwalmen, P. and Mulnard, J.: Atypical hatching of a cow blastocyst leading to separation of complete twin half blastocysts. Vet. Rec. **112**:301, 1983.

Mastroiacovo, P. and Botto, L.: Structural congenital defects in multiple births. Acta Genet. Med. Gemellol. **43**:57–70, 1994.

Mastroiacovo, P., Castilla, E.E., Arpino, C., Botting, B., Cocchi, G., Goujard, J., Marinacci, C., Merlob, P., Métneki, J., Mutchinick, O., Ritvanen, A. and Rosano, A.: Congenital malformations in twins: an international study. Amer. J. Med. Genet. **83**:117–124, 1999.

Mauer, S.M., Dorrin, R.S. and Vernier, R.L.: Unilateral and bilateral renal agenesis in monoamniotic twins. Amer. J. Obstet. Gynecol. **84**:236–238, 1974.

Maxwell, C.V., Lieberman, E., Norton, M., Cohen, A., Seely, E. W. and Lee-Parritz, A.: Relationship of twin zygosity and risk of preeclampsia. Amer. J. Obstet. Gynecol. **185**:819–821, 2001.

Maymon, R., Halperin, R., Weinraub, Z., Herman, A. and Schneider, D.: Three-dimensional transvaginal sonography of conjoined twins at 10 weeks: a case report. Ultrasound Obstet. Gynecol. **11**:1–3, 1998; **11**:292–294, 1998.

McCracken, A.A., Daly, P.A., Zolnick, M.R. and Clark, A.M.: Twins and Q-banded chromosome polymorphisms. Hum. Genet. **45**:253–258, 1978.

McCrossin, D.B. and Roberton, N.R.C.: Congenital skin defects, twins and toxoplasmosis. J. R. Soc. Med. **82**:108–109, 1989.

McCurdy, C.M., Childers, J.M. and Seeds, J.W.: Ligation of the umbilical cord of an acardiac-acephalus twin with an endoscopic intrauterine technique. Obstet. Gynecol. **82**:708–711, 1993.

McFee, J.G., Lord, E.L., Jeffrey, R.L., O'Meara, O.P., Josepher, H.J., Butterfield, J. and Thompson, H.E.: Multiple gestations of high fetal number. Obstet. Gynecol. **44**:99–106, 1974.

McKeown, T. and Record, R.G.: Observations on fetal growth in multiple pregnancy in man. J. Endocrinol. **8**:386–401, 1952.

McLeod, F. and McCoy, D.R.: Monoamniotic twins with an unusual cord complication. Case report. Br. J. Obstet. Gynaecol. **88**:774–775, 1981.

McManus, C.: Right Hand Left Hand. The Origin of Asymmetry in Brains, Bodies, Atoms and Cultures. Harvard University Press, 2002.

McNamara, M.F., McCurdy, C.M., Reed, K.L., Philipps, A.F. and Seeds, J.W.: The relation between pulmonary hypoplasia and amniotic fluid volume: lessons learned from discordant urinary tract anomalies in monoamniotic twins. Obstet. Gynecol. **85**:867–869, 1995.

McNatty, K.P., Juengel, J.L., Wilson, T., Galloway, S.M. and Davis, G.H.: Genetic mutations influencing ovulation rate in sheep. Reprod. Fertil. Devel. **13**:549–555, 2001.

Meagher, S., Tippett, C., Renou, P., Baker, L. and Susil, B.: Twin-twin transfusion syndrome: Intraamniotic pressure measurement in the assessment of volume reduction at serial amniocenteses. Aust. NZ J. Obstet. Gynaecol. **35**:22–26, 1995.

Medearis, A.L., Jonas, H.S., Stockbauer, J.W. and Domke, H.R.: Perinatal deaths in twin pregnancy: a five-year analysis of statewide statistics in Missouri. Amer. J. Obstet. Gynecol. **134**:413–421, 1979.

Megory, E., Weiner, E., Shalev, E. and Ohel, G.: Pseudomonoamniotic twins with cord entanglement following genetic funipuncture. Obstet. Gynecol. **78**:915–917, 1991.

Melgar, C.A., Rosenfeld, D.L., Rawlinson, K. and Greenberg, M.: Perinatal outcome after multifetal reduction to twins compared with nonreduced multiple gestations. Obstet. Gynecol. **78**:763–767, 1991.

Melnick, M.: Brain damage in survivors after in-utero death of monozygous co-twin. Lancet **2**:1287, 1977.

Melnick, M. and Myrianthopoulos, N.C.: The effects of chorion type on normal and abnormal developmental variation in monozygous twins. Amer. J. Med. Genet. **4**:147–156, 1979.

Mercer, B.M., Crocker, L.G., Pierce, F. and Sibai, B.M.: Clinical characteristics and outcome of twin gestation complicated by preterm premature rupture of the membranes. Amer. J. Obstet. Gynecol. **168**:1467–1473, 1993.

Métneki, J. and Czeizel, A.: Twinning rates. Lancet **1**:935, 1983.

Metrakos, J.D., Metrakos, K. and Baxter, H.: Clefts of the lip and palate in twins: including a discordant pair whose monozygosity was confirmed by skin transplants. Plast. Reconstr. Surg. **22**:109–122, 1958.

Meulepas, E., Vlietinck, R. and van den Berghe, H.: The probability of dizygosity of phenotypically concordant twins. Amer. J. Human. Genet. **43**:817–826, 1988.

Meyer, W.R. and Meyer, W.W.: Report on a very young dizygotic human twin pregnancy. Arch. Gynecol. **231**:51–56, 1981.

Michaels, L.: Unilateral ischemia of fused twin placenta: a manifestation of the twin transfusion syndrome? Can. Med. Assoc. J. **96**:402–405, 1967.

Michaels, W.H., Schreiber, F.R., Padgett, R.J., Ager, J. and Pieper, D.: Ultrasound surveillance of the cervix in twin gestations: management of cervical incompetency. Obstet. Gynecol. **78**:739–744, 1991.

Michlewitz, H., Kennedy, J., Kawada, C. and Kennison, R.: Triplet pregnancies. J. Reprod. Med. **26**:243–246, 1981.

Mijsberg, W.A.: Genetic-statistical data on the presence of secondary oocytary twins among non-identical twins. Acta Genet. Statist. Med. **7**:39–42, 1957.

Milham, S.: Pituitary gonadotrophin and dizygotic twinning. Lancet **2**:566, 1964.

Milham, S.: Symmetrical conjoined twins: an analysis of the birth records of twenty-two sets. J. Pediatr. **69**:643–647, 1966.

Miller, D.L. and Dillon, J.: An unusual abdominal mass in an elderly woman. NEJM **321**:1613–1614, 1989.

Miller, V.L., Ransom, S.B., Shalhoub, A., Sokol, R.J. and Evans, M.I.: Multifetal pregnancy reduction: perinatal and fiscal outcomes. Amer. J. Obstet. Gynecol. **182**:1575–1580, 2000.

Mills, W.G.: Pathological changes in blighted twins. J. Obstet. Gynaecol. Br. Emp. **56**:619–624,1949.

Min, S.-J., Luke, B., Gillespie, B., Min, L., Newman, R.B., Mauldin, J.G., Witter, F.R., Salman, F.A. and O'Sullivan, M.J.: Birth weight references for twins. Amer. J. Obstet. Gynecol. **182**:1250–1257, 2000.

Mingeot, R.A. and Keirse, M.J.: Twin pregnancy in a pseudodidelphys. Amer. J. Obstet. Gynecol. **111**:1121–1122, 1971.

Mitrani, A.: Conjoined thoracopagus twins. Harefuah **74**:95–97, 1968.

Miyabara, S., Okamoto, N., Akimoto, N., Satow, Y. and Nakagawa, S.: A study on dicephalic monsters, especially with regard to embryopathology. Hiroshima J. Med. Sci. **22**:377–395, 1973.

Moestrup, J.K.: Monoamniotic twins: a case with vessel anomaly in one twin's umbilical cord. Acta Obstet. Gynecol. Scand. **49**:85–87, 1970.

Mohanty, C., Mishra, O.P., Singh, C.P., Das, B.K. and Singla, P.N.: Acardiac anomaly spectrum. Teratology **62**:356–359, 2000.

Moise, K.J.: Indomethacin therapy in the treatment of symptomatic polyhydramnios. Clin. Obstet. Gynecol. **34**:310–318, 1991.

Molnar-Nadasdy, G. and Altshuler, G.: Perinatal pathology case book. A case of twin transfusion syndrome with dichorionic placentas. J. Perinatol. **16**:507–509, 1996.

Monteagudo, A., Timor-Tritsch, I.E. and Sharma, S.: Early and simple determination of chorionic and amniotic type in multifetal gestations in the first fourteen weeks by high-frequency transvaginal ultrasonography. Amer. J. Obstet. Gynecol. **170**:824–829, 1994.

Monteiro, J., Derom, C., Vlietinck, R., Kohn, N., Derom, R. and Gregersen, K.: X chromosome inactivation patterns in monozygotic twin girls. Twin Res. **1**(2): 101 (abstr. 083), 1998a.

Monteiro, J., Derom, C., Vlietinck, R., Kohn, N., Lesser, M. and Gregersen, P.K.: Commitment to X inactivation precedes the twinning event in monochorionic MZ twins. Amer. J. Hum. Genet. **63**:339–346, 1998b.

Montgomery, G.W., Duffy, D.L., Hall, J., Haddon, B.R., Kudo, M., McGee, E.A., Palmer, J.S., Hsueh, A.J., Boomsma, D.I. and Martin, N.G.: Dizygotic twinning is not linked to variation at the alpha-inhibin locus on human chromosome 2. J. Clin. Endocrinol. Metab. **85**:3391–3395, 2000.

Montgomery, G.W., Duffy, D.L., Hall, J., Kudo, M., Martin, N.G. and Hsueh, A.J.: Mutations in the follicle-stimulating hormone receptor and familial dizygotic twinning. Lancet **357**:773–774, 2001.

Montgomery, G.W., Zhao, Z.Z., Morley, K.I., Marsh, A.J., Boomsma, D.I., Martin, N.G. and Duffy, D.L.: Dizygotic twinning is not associated with methylenetetrahydrofolate reductase haplotypes. Human Reprod. **18**:2460–2464, 2003.

Montgomery, G.W., Zhao, Z.Z., Marsh, A.J., Mayne, R., Treloar, S.A., James, M., Martin, N.G., Boomsma, D.I. and Duffy, D.L.: A deletion mutation in GDF9 in sisters with spontaneous DZ twins. Twin Res. **7**:548–555, 2004.

Moore, C.A., Buehler, B.A., McManus, B.M., Harmon, J.P., Mirkin, L.D. and Goldstein, D.J.: Brief clinical report. Acephalus-acardia in twins with aneuploidy. Amer. J. Med. Genet. [Suppl.] **3**:139–143, 1987.

Moore, C.M., McAdams, A.J. and Sutherland, J.: Intrauterine disseminated intravascular coagulation: a syndrome of multiple pregnancy with a dead twin fetus. J. Pediatr. **74**:523–528, 1969.

Moore, T.R., Gale, S.A. and Benirschke, K.: Perinatal outcome of forty-nine pregnancies complicated by acardiac twinning. Amer. J. Obstet. Gynecol. **163**:907–912, 1990.

Moreno, M.J. and Sanchez, O.: Mosaico cromosómico X0/XX/XY/XXY/, en un hermafrodita verdadero. Acta Cient. Venez. **22**:14–18, 1971.

Mortimer, G.: Zygosity and placental structure in monochorionic twins. Acta Genet. Med. Gemellol. **36**:417–520, 1987.

Morton, C.C., Corey, L.A., Nance, W.E. and Brown, J.A.: Quinacrine mustard and nucleolar organizer region heteromorphisms in twins. Acta Genet. Med. Gemellol. **30**:39–49, 1981.

Moshiri, M., Salari, A.A., Mansorian, H.R. and Shariat, R.: Lithopedion (stone baby). Ann. Saudi Med. **16**:69–70, 1996.

Mostoufi-Zadeh, M., Weiss, L.M. and Driscoll, S.G.: Nonimmune hydrops fetalis: a challenge in perinatal pathology. Hum. Pathol. **16**:785–789, 1985.

Motomura, K., Tateishi, H., Nishisho, I., Okazaki, M., Miki, T., Tonomura, A., Takai, S.-I., Mori, T. and Jeffreys, A.J.: The zygosity determination of Japanese twins using a minisatellite core probe. Jpn. J. Hum. Genet. **32**:9–14, 1987.

Moyaert, I. Bouters, R. and Bouquet, Y.: Birth of a monozygotic cattle twin following non surgical transfer of a single 7 day old embryo. Theriogenology **18**:127–132, 1982.

Mueller-Heubach, E. and Battelli, A.F.: Prolonged in utero retention and mummification of a *Macaca mulatta* fetus. J. Med. Primatol. **10**:265–268, 1981.

Munro, S.S.: Are monovular avian twins always female? J. Hered. **56**:285–288, 1965.

Munsinger, H.: The identical-twin transfusion syndrome: a source of error in estimating IQ resemblance and heritability. Ann. Hum. Genet. **40**:307–321, 1977.

Murray, J.C., Mansilla, M.A., Kimani, J., Mitchell, L., Christensen, K., Daack-Hirsch, S., Wyszynski, D.F. and Felix, T.: Discordant MZ twins with cleft lip and palate: a model for identifying genes in complex traits. Twin Res. **7**(4):(abstract), 2004.

Mutinelli, F., Nani, S. and Zampiron, S.: Conjoined twins (Thoracopagus) in a Wistar rat (*Rattus norvegicus*). Lab. Animal Sci. **42**:612–613, 1992.

Myrianthopoulos, N.C.: An epidemiological survey of twins in a large, prospectively studied population. Amer. J. Hum. Genet. **22**:611–629, 1970a.

Myrianthopoulos, N.C.: A survey of twins in the population of a prospective collaborative study. Acta Genet. Med. Gemellol. **19**:15–23, 1970b.

Naeye, R.: Parabiotic syndrome. NEJM **269**:1043, 1963.

Naeye, R.L.: The fetal and neonatal development of twins. Pediatrics **33**:546–553, 1964a.

Naeye, R.: Organ composition in newborn parabiotic twins with speculation regarding neonatal hypoglycemia. Pediatrics **34**:415–418, 1964b.

Naeye, R.: Organ abnormalities in a human parabiotic syndrome. Amer. J. Pathol. **46**:829–842, 1965.

Naeye, R.L. and Blanc, W.A.: Fetal renal structure and the genesis of amniotic fluid disorders. Amer. J. Pathol. **67**:95–105, 1972.

Naeye, R.L. and Letts, H.W.: Body measurements of fetal and neonatal twins. Arch. Pathol. **77**:393–396, 1964.

Naeye, R.L., Tafari, N., Judge, D. and Marboe, C.C.: Twins: causes of perinatal death in 12 United States cities and one African city. Amer. J. Obstet. Gynecol. **131**:267–272, 1978.

Nagashima, H., Kato, Y. and Ogawa, S.: Microsurgical bisection of porcine morulae and blastocysts to produce monozygotic twin pregnancy. Gamete Res. **23**:1–10, 1989.

Nageotte, M.P., Hurwitz, S.R., Kaupke, C.J., Vaziri, N.D. and Pandian, M.R.: Atriopeptin in the twin transfusion syndrome. Obstet. Gynecol. **73**:867–870, 1989.

Nakayama, A., Imai, S. and Takemura, T.: Intrauterine embolism syndrome: multiple infarction of co-twin caused by dead counterpart in utero. Teratology **34**:457, 1986 (abstract).

Nakayama, D.K., Killian, A., Hill, L.M., Miller, J.P., Hannakan, C., Lloyd, D.A. and Rowe, M.I.: The newborn with hydrops and sacrococcygeal teratoma. J. Pediatr. Surg. **26**:1435–1438, 1991.

Napolitani, F.D. and Schreiber, I.: The acardiac monster. Amer. J. Obstet. Gynecol. **80**:582–589, 1960.

Natori, M., Tanaka, M., Kohno, H., Ishimoto, H., Morisada, M., Kobayashi, T. and Nozawa, S.: A case of twin-twin transfusion syndrome treated with placental vessel occlusion using fetoscopic Nd:Yag laser System. Acta Obstet. Gynaecol. Jpn. **44**:117–120, 1992.

Neal, F.C. and Wilcox, C.J.: Double acardius amorphus case in a brown Swiss cow. J. Dairy Sci. **50**:236, 1967.

Nelson, J.L.: Microchimerism: expanding new horizon in human health or incidental remnant of pregnancy? Lancet **358**:2011–2012, 2001.

Neubecker, R.D., Blumberg, J.M. and Townsend, F.M.: A human monozygotic quintuplet placenta: report of a specimen. J. Obstet. Gynaecol. Br. Commonw. **69**:137–139, 1962.

Neuman, W.L., Ponto, K., Farber, R.A. and Shangold, G.A.: DNA analysis of unilateral twin ectopic gestation. Obstet. Gynecol. **75**:479–483, 1990.

Neurath, P.W., Lin, P.-S. and Low, D.A.: Quantitative karyotyping: a model twin study. Cytogenetics **11**:457–474, 1972.

Newman, H.H.: Palm-print patterns in twins: on the use of dermatoglyphics as an aid in the diagnosis of monozygotic and dizygotic twins. J. Hered. **22**:41–49, 1931a.

Newman, H.H.: Differences between conjoined twins: in relation to a general theory of twinning. J. Hered. **22**:201–215, 1931b.

Newman, H.H. and Patterson, J.T.: The development of the nine-banded armadillo from the primitive streak stage to birth; with especial reference to the question of specific polyembryony. J. Morphol. **21**:359–424, 1910.

Newton, R., Casabonne, D., Johnson, A. and Pharoah, P.: A case-control study of vanishing twin as a risk factor for cerebral palsy. Twin Res. **6**:83–84, 2003.

Nhân, V.Q. and Huisjes, H.J.: Double uterus with a pregnancy in each half. Obstet. Gynecol. **61**:115–117, 1983.

Nichols, J.B.: Quintuplet and sextuplet births in the United States. Obstet. Gynecol. **3**:124–125, 1954.

Nichols, R.C. and Bilbro, W.C.: The diagnosis of twin zygosity. Acta Genet. (Basel) **16**:265–275, 1966.

Nickerson, C.W.: Amniotic sac dystocia in twins. Amer. J. Obstet. Gynecol. **97**:867–868, 1967.

Nicolini, U., Pisoni, M.P., Cela, E. and Roberts, A.: Fetal blood sampling immediately before and within 24 hours of death in monochorionic twin pregnancies complicated by single intrauterine death. Amer. J. Obstet. Gynecol. **179**:800–803, 1998.

Nielsen, H.C., Harvey-Wilkes, K., MacKinnon, B. and Hung, S.: Neonatal outcome of very premature infants from multiple and singleton gestations. Amer. J. Obstet. Gynecol. **177**:653–659, 1997.

Nigro, M.: Considérations immunologiques et endocrinologiques à propos d'un cas d'acardie. J. Gynecol. Obstet. Reprod. **6**:963–970, 1977.

Nikkels, P.G.J., van Gemert, M.J.C., Sollie-Szarynska, K.M., Molendijk, H., Timmer, B. and Machin, G.A.: Rapid onset of severe twin-twin transfusion syndrome caused by placental venous thrombosis. Pediatr. Devel. Pathol. **5**:310–314, 2002.

Niku, M., Ilmonen, L., Pessa-Morikawa, T. and Iivanainen, A.: Limited contribution of circulating cells to the development and maintenance of nonhematopoietic bovine tissues. Stem Cells **22**:12–20, 2004.

Nkemayim, D.C., Hammadeh, M.E., Hippach, M., Rosenbaum, P. and Schmidt, W.: Complications of triple pregnancy following intracytoplasmic sperm injection: a case report. Twin Res. **3**:76–79, 2000.

Noonan, J.A.: Twins, conjoined twins, and cardiac defects. Amer. J. Dis. Child. **132**:17–18, 1978.

Noone, P.G., Bali, D., Carson, J.L., Sannuti, A., Gipson, C.L., Ostrowski, L.E., Bromberg, P.A., Boucher, R.C. and Knowles, M.R.: Discordant organ laterality in monozygotic twins with primary ciliary dyskinesia. Amer. J. Med. Genet. **82**:155–160, 1999.

Nores, J., Athanassiou, A., Elkadry, E., Malone, F.D., Craigo, S. D. and D'Alton, M.: Gender differences in twin-twin transfusion syndrome. Obstet. Gynecol. **90**:580–582, 1997.

Norman, M.G.: Bilateral encephaloclastic lesions in a 26 week gestation fetus: effect on neuroblast migration. J. Can. Sci. Neurol. **7**:191–194, 1980.

Norman, M.G.: Mechanism of brain damage in twins. J. Can. Sci. Neurol. **9**:339–344, 1982.

Norton, M.E., D'Alton, M.E. and Bianchi, D.W.: Molecular zygosity studies aid in the management of discordant multiple gestations. J. Perinatal. **17**:202–207, 1997.

Nunley, W.C., Jr.: The slippery slopes of advanced reproductive technologies. Presidential address. Amer. J. Obstet. Gynecol. **191**:588–592, 2004.

Nylander, P.P.S.: Placental forms and zygosity determination of twins in Ibadan, Western Nigeria: a study of 1475 twin maternities. Acta Genet. Med. Gemellol. **19**:49–54, 1970.

Nylander, P.P.S.: Ethnic differences in twinning rates in Nigeria. J. Biosoc. Sci. **3**:151–157, 1971a.

Nylander, P.P.S.: The incidence of triplets and higher multiple births in some rural and urban populations in Western Nigeria. Ann. Hum. Genet. **34**:409–415, 1971b.

Nylander, P.P.S.: Serum levels of gonadotrophins in relation to multiple pregnancy in Nigeria. J. Obstet. Gynaecol. Br. Commonw. **80**:651–653, 1973.

Nylander, P.P.S. and Corney, G.: Placentation and zygosity of twins in Ibadan, Nigeria. Ann. Hum. Genet. **33**:31–40, 1969.

Nylander, P.P.S. and Corney, G.: Placentation and zygosity of triplets and higher multiple births in Ibadan, Nigeria. Ann. Hum. Genet. **34**:417–426, 1971.

Nylander, P.P.S. and Osunkoya, B.O.: Unusual monochorionic placentation with heterosexual twins. Obstet. Gynecol. **36**:621–625, 1970.

Oberg, K.C., Pestaner, J.P., Bielamowicz, L. and Hawkins, E.P.: Renal tubular dysgenesis in twin-twin transfusion syndrome. Pediat. Developm. Pathol. **2**:25–32, 1999.

O'Brien, P.J. and Hay, D.A.: Birthweight differences, the transfusion syndrome, and the cognitive development of monozygotic twins. Acta Genet. Med. Gemellol. **36**:181–196, 1987.

Odibo, A.O. and Macones, G.A.: Management of twin-twin transfusion syndrome: Laying the foundation for future interventional studies. Twin Res. **5**:515–520, 2002.

O'Donnell, C.P.F., Pertile, M.D., Sheffield, L.J. and Sampson, A.: Monozygotic twins with discordant karyotypes: a case report. J. Pediatr. **145**:406–408, 2004.

Ohel, G., Granat, M., Zeevi, D., Golan, A., Wexler, S., David, M.P. and Schenker, J.G.: Advanced ultrasonic placental maturation in twin pregnancies. Amer. J. Obstet. Gynecol. **156**:76–78, 1987.

Okamura, K., Murotsuki, J., Tanigawara, S., Uehara, S. and Yajima, A.: Funipuncture for evaluation of hematologic and coagulation indices in the surviving twin following co-twin's death. Obstet. Gynecol. **83**:975–958, 1994.

O'Keane, J.A., Yuen, B.H., Farquharson, D.F. and Wittman, B.K.: Endocrine response to selective embryocide in a gonadotropin-induced quintuplet pregnancy. Amer. J. Obstet. Gynecol. **155**:364–367, 1988.

Olding, L.: The possibility of materno-foetal transfer of lymphocytes in man. Acta Paediatr. Scand. **61**:73–75, 1972.

Osborne, R.H.: Serology in physical anthropology. Amer. J. Phys. Anthropol. **16**:187–195, 1958.

O'Sullivan, J.V.: Multiple pregnancy. Proc. R. Soc. Med. **61**:235–236, 1968.

Ozturk, O. and Templeton, A.: In-vitro fertilisation and risk of multiple pregnancy. Lancet **359**:232, 2002.

Paepe, J.de: Mortalité périnatale dans une série de grossesses gémellaires. Bull. Soc. R. Belge Gynécol. Obstet. **29**:421–4433, 1959.

Parks, J. and Epstein, J.R.: Monoamniotic twin pregnancy with living infants. Amer. J. Obstet. Gynecol. **39**:140–142, 1940.

Patten, R.M., Mack, L.A., Harvey, D., Cyr, D.R. and Pretorius, D.H.: Disparity of amniotic fluid volume and fetal size: problem of the stuck twin—US studies. Radiology **172**:153–157, 1989a.

Patten, R.M., Mack, L.A., Nyberg, D.A. and Filly, R.A.: Twin embolization syndrome: prenatal sonographic detection and significance. Radiology **173**:685–689, 1989b.

Paulson, R.J., Lobo, R.A., Stein, A., Toker, R., Moegle, A. and Macaso, T.: Gestation of triplets after intrauterine implantation of two embryos. NEJM **318**:1339–1340, 1988.

Pavlica, F.: Über einen Fötus mit zahlreichen Entwicklungsanomalien. Pädiatrie Pädol. **3**:27–33, 1967.

Payne, S., Dudge, J. and Bradbury, W.: Ectopic pregnancy concomitant with twin intrauterine pregnancy: a case report. Obstet. Gynecol. **38**:905–906, 1971.

Pearlman, S.A. and Batton, D.G.: Effect of birth order on intraventricular hemorrhage in very low birth weight twins. Obstet. Gynecol. **71**:358–360, 1988.

Pedrosa, M.P., Salzano, F.M., Mattevi, M.S. and Viegas, J.: Quantitative analysis of C-bands in chromosomes 1, 9, 16, and Y of twins. Acta Genet. Med. Gemellol. **32**:257–260, 1983.

Pérez, M.L., Firpo, J.R. and Baldi, E.M.: Sobre las anastomosis circulatorias de las placentas dizigoticas. Obstet. Ginecol. Lat. **5**:5–21, 1947.

Pessa-Morikawa, T., Niku, M. and Iivanainen, A.: Persistent differences in the level of chimerism in B versus T cells of freemartin cattle. Dev. Comp. Immunol. **28**:77–87, 2004.

Petersen, B.L., Broholm, H., Skibsted, L. and Graem, N.: Acardiac twin with preserved brain. Fetal Diagn. Ther. **16**:231–233, 2001.

Pharoah, P.O.D. and Cooke, R.W.I.: A hypothesis for the etiology of spastic cerebral palsy—the vanishing twin. Developm. Med. Child Neurol. **39**:292–296, 1997.

Phillips, D.I.W.: Twin studies in medical research: can they tell us whether diseases are genetically determined? Lancet **341**:1008–1009, 1993.

Pickering, G.H.: Monovular twins. Br. Med. J. **2**:988, 1946.

Pickhardt, W.L. and Breen, J.L.: Monoamniotic twin pregnancy: report of a case. Obstet. Gynecol. **12**:471–472, 1958.

Pijpers, L., Jahoda, M.G.J., Vosters, R.P.L., Niermeijer, M.F. and Sachs, E.S.: Genetic amniocentesis in twin pregnancies. Br. J. Obstet. Gynaecol. **95**:323–326, 1988.

Pinette, M.G., Pan, Y.M.M., Pinette, S.G. and Stubblefield, P.G.: Treatment of twin-twin transfusion syndrome. Obstet. Gynecol. **82**:841–846, 1993.

Plath, H. and Hansmann, M.: Diagnostik und Therapie zwillingsspezifischer Anomalien. Gynäkologe **31**:229–244, 1998.

Platt, L.D., DeVore, G.R., Bieniarz, A., Benner, P. and Rao, R.: Antenatal diagnosis of acephalus acardia: a proposed management scheme. Amer. J. Obstet. Gynecol. **146**:857–859, 1983.

Platt, M.J., Marshall, A. and Pharoah, O.D.: The effects of assisted reproduction on the trends and zygosity of multiple births in England and Wales 1974–1999. Twin Res. **4**:417–421, 2001.

Poch, M., Luks, F.I., Carr, S.R. and De Paepe, M.E.: Intratwin arteriovenous fistula of the placenta in a case of twin-to-twin transfusion syndrome. Amer. J. Perinatol. **22**:3–6, 2005.

Popek, E.J., Strain, J.D., Neumann, A. and Wilson, H.: In utero development of pulmonary artery calcification in monochorionic twins: a report of three cases and discussion of the possible etiology. Pediat. Pathol. **13**:597–611, 1993.

Porreco, R.P.: Percutaneous ultrasonographically guided ablation of an acardiac twin. Amer. J. Obstet. Gynecol. **190**: 572–574, 2004.

Porreco, R.P., Burke, M.S. and Parker, D.W.: Selective embryocide in the nonsurgical management of combined intrauterine-extrauterine pregnancy. Obstet. Gynecol. **75**:498–501, 1990.

Porreco, R.P., Barton, S.M. and Haverkamp, A.D.: Occlusion of umbilical artery in acardiac, acephalic twin. Lancet **337**: 326–327, 1991.

Porter, R.P. and Gengozian, N.: Immunological tolerance and rejection of skin allografts in the marmoset. Transplantation **8**:653–665, 1969.

Potter, E.L.: Twin zygosity and placental form in relation to the outcome of pregnancy. Amer. J. Obstet. Gynecol. **87**:566–577, 1963.

Powers, W.F.: Twin pregnancy: complications and treatment. Obstet. Gynecol. **42**:795–808, 1973.

Powers, W.F. and Kiely, J.L.: The risks confronting twins: a national perspective. Amer. J. Obstet. Gynecol. **170**:456–461, 1994.

Powers, W.F. and Miller, T.C.: Bed rest in twin pregnancy: identification of a critical period and its cost implications. Amer. J. Obstet. Gynecol. **134**:23–29, 1979.

Preis, A. and Srubarova, M.: Cardiological findings in twins, with special references to their zygosity and peristasis. Acta Genet. Med. Gemellol. **15**:190–198, 1966.

Pretorius, D.H., Manchester, D., Barkin, S., Parker, S. and Nelson, T.R.: Doppler ultrasound of twin transfusion syndrome. J. Ultrasound Med. **7**:117–124, 1988a.

Pretorius, D.H., Leopold, G., Moore, T.R., Benirschke, K. and Sivo, J.J.: Acardiac twin: report of Doppler sonography. J. Ultrasound Med. **7**:413–416, 1988b.

Price, B.: Primary biases in twin studies: review of prenatal and natal differences-producing factors in monozygotic pairs. Amer. J. Hum. Genet. **2**:293–352, 1950.

Pridjian, G., Nugent, C.E. and Barr, M.: Twin gestation: influence of placentation on fetal growth. Amer. J. Obstet. Gynecol. **165**:1394–1401, 1991.

Puckett, J.D.: Fetal death of second twin in second trimester. Amer. J. Obstet. Gynecol. **159**:740–741, 1988.

Quigley, C.: Conjoined twins: An Historical, Biological and Ethical Issues Encyclopedia. McFarland & Co., Jefferson, North Carolina, 2003.

Quigley, J.K.: Mono-amniotic twin pregnancy: case record with review of literature. Amer. J. Obstet. Gynecol. **29**:354–362, 1935.

Quintero, R.A., Reich, H., Puder, K.S., Bardicef, M., Evans, M.I., Cotton, D.B. and Romero, R.: Brief report: umbilical-cord ligation of an acardiac twin by fetoscopy at 19 weeks of gestation. NEJM **330**:469–471, 1994.

Quintero, R.A., Lanouette, J., Carreño, C.A., King, M., Johnson, M.P., Sudz, C., Romero, R. and Evans, M.I.: Percutaneous ligation and transection of the umbilical cord in complicated monoamniotic twin gestations via operative fetoscopy. Amer. J. Obstet. Gynecol. **176**:S19 (abstract 43), 1997.

Quintero, R.A., Morales, W.J., Allen, M.H., Bornick, P.W., Johnson, P.K. and Kruger, M.: Staging of twin-twin transfusion syndrome. J. Perinatol. **19**:550–555, 1999.

Quintero, R.A., Dickinson, J.E., Morales, W.J., Bornick, P.W., Bermúdez, C., Cincotta, R., Chan, F.Y. and Allen, M.H.: Stage-based treatment of twin-twin transfusion syndrome. Amer. J. Obstetr. Gynecol. **188**:1333–1340, 2003a.

Quintero, R.A., Mueller, O.T., Martinez, J.M., Arroyo, J., Gilbert-Barness, E., Hilbelink, D., Papenhausen, P. and Sutcliffe, M.: Twin-twin transfusion syndrome in a dizygotic monochorionic-diamniotic twin pregnancy: J. Matern.-Fetal Neonatal. Med. **14**:279–281, 2003b.

Ramos-Arroyo, M.A., Ulbright, T.M. and Christian, J.C.: Twin study: relationship between birth weight, zygosity, placentation, and pathologic placental changes. Acta Genet. Med. Gemellol. **37**:229–238, 1988.

Raphael, S.I.: Monoamniotic twin pregnancy: a review of the literature and a report of 5 new cases. Amer. J. Obstet. Gynecol. **81**:323–330, 1961.

Rashad, M.N. and Kerr, M.G.: Observations on the so-called holoacardius amorphus. J. Anat. **100**:425–426, 1966.

Rausen, A.R., Seki, M. and Strauss, L.: Twin transfusion syndrome: a review of 19 cases studied at one institution. J. Pediatr. **66**:613–628, 1965.

Rayburn, W.F. and Barr, M.: Teratomas: concordance in mother and fetus. Amer. J. Obstet. Gynecol. **144**:110–112, 1982.

Rayburn, W.F., Lavin, J.P., Miodovnik, M. and Varner, M.W.: Multiple gestation: time interval between delivery of the first and second twins. Obstet. Gynecol. **63**:502–506, 1984.

Record, R.G., McKeown, T. and Edwards, J.H.: An investigation of the difference on measured intelligence between twins and single births. Ann. Hum. Genet. **34**:11–20, 1970.

Redline, R.W.: Nonidentical twins with a single placenta—disproving dogma in perinatal pathology. NEJM **349**:111–114, 2003.

Redline, R.W., Shah, D., Sakar, H., Schluchter, M. and Salvator, A.: Placental lesions associated with abnormal growth in twins. Pediatr. Developm. Pathol. **4**:473–481, 2001.

Reed, T., Sprague, F.R., Kang, K.W., Nance, W.E. and Christian, J.C.: Genetic analysis of dermatoglyphic patterns in twins. Hum. Hered. **25**:263–275, 1975.

Rehder, H., Geisler, M., Kleinbrecht, J. and Degenhardt, K.H.: Monozygotic twins with 47,XXY karyotype and discordant malformations. Teratology **17**:5a, 1978.

Reisner, D.P., Mahony, B.S., Petty, C.N., Nyberg, D.A., Porter, T.F., Zingheim, R.W., Williams, M.A. and Luthy, D.A.: Stuck twin syndrome: outcome in thirty-seven consecutive cases. Amer. J. Obstet. Gynecol. **169**:991–995, 1993.

Reisner, S.H., Forbes, A.E. and Cornblath, M.: The smaller of twins and hypoglycaemia. Lancet **1**:524–526, 1965.

Reitnauer, P.J., Callanan, N.P., Farber, R.A. and Aylsworth, A.S.: Prenatal exposure to disulfiram implicated in the cause of malformations in discordant monozygotic twins. Teratology **56**:358–362, 1997.

Renkonen, K.O.: Is Weinberg's differential rule defective? Ann. Hum. Genet. **30**:277–280, 1967.

Rhine, S.A. and Nance, W.E.: Familial twinning: a case for superfetation in man. Acta Genet. Med. Gemellol. **25**:66–69, 1976.

Rice-Wray, E., Cervantes, A., Gutierrez, J. and Marquez-Monter, H.: Pregnancy and progeny after hormonal contraceptives—genetic studies. J. Reprod. Med. **6**:101–104, 1971.

Richart, R. and Benirschke, K.: Holoacardius amorphus: report of a case with chromosome analysis. Amer. J. Obstet. Gynecol. **86**:329–332, 1963.

Ries, M., Beinder, E., Gruner, C. and Zenker, M.: Rapid development of hydrops fetalis in the donor twin following death of the recipient twin in twin-twin transfusion syndrome. J. Perinat. Med. **27**:68–73, 1999.

Rijnders, P.M. and Jansen, C.A.: Increased incidence of monozygotic twinning following the transfer of blastocysts in human IVF/ICSI. Fertil. Steril. **70**:S15–16 (abstract O-040), 1998a.

Rijnders, P.M. and Jansen, C.A.: The predictive value of day 3 embryo morphology regarding blastocyst formation, pregnancy and implantation rate after day 5 transfer following in-vitro fertilization or intracytoplasmic sperm injection. Human Reprod. **13**:2869–2873, 1998b.

Roberge, J.L.: Sympodia in identical twins: report of a case. JAMA **186**:728–729, 1963.

Roberts, S.J.: Veterinary Obstetrics and Genital Diseases. Edwards Broths, Ann Arbor, 1956.

Robertson, E.G. and Neer, K.J.: Placental injection studies in twin gestation. Amer. J. Obstet. Gynecol. **147**:170–175, 1983.

Robertson, J.G.: Twin pregnancy: morbidity and fetal mortality. Obstet. Gynecol. **23**:330–337, 1964a.

Robertson, J.G.: Twin pregnancy: influence of early admission on fetal survival. Obstet. Gynecol. **23**:854–860, 1964b.

Robertson, J.G.: Blood grouping in twin pregnancy. J. Obstet. Gynaecol. **76**:154–156, 1969.

Robie, G.F., Payne, G.G. and Morgan, M.A.: Selective delivery of an acardiac, acephalic twin. NEJM **320**:512–513, 1989.

Robinson, H.P. and Caines, J.S.: Sonar evidence of early pregnancy failure in patients with twin conceptions. Br. J. Obstet. Gynaecol. **84**:22–25, 1977.

Rodeck, C., Deans, A. and Jauniaux, E.: Thermocoagulation for the early treatment of pregnancy with an acardiac twin. NEJM **339**:1293–1295, 1998.

Rodis, J.F., Vintzileos, A.M., Campbell, W.A., Deaton, J.L., Fumia, F. and Nochimson, J.: Antenatal diagnosis and management of monoamniotic twins. Amer. J. Obstet. Gynecol. **157**:1255–1257, 1987.

Rodis, J.F., McIlveen, P.F., Egan, J.F.X., Borgida, A.F., Turner, G.W. and Campbell, W.A.: Monoamniotic twins: improved perinatal survival with accurate prenatal diagnosis and antenatal fetal surveillance. Amer. J. Obstet. Gynecol. **177**:1046–1049, 1997.

Rohmer, A., Ruch, J.-V., Schneegans, E. and Clavert, J.: Jumeaux dizygotes, l'un 47 XX 21+ et cliniquement mongolien, l'autre 46 XX/47 XX 21+ et cliniquement non mongolien. Pediatrie **26**:209–213, 1971.

Romero, R., Duffy, T.P., Berkowitz, R.L., Chang, E. and Hobbins, J.C.: Prolongation of a preterm pregnancy complicated by death of a single twin in utero and disseminated intravascular coagulation: effects of treatment with heparin. NEJM **310**:772–774, 1984.

Roos, F.J., Roter, A.M. and Molina, F.A.: A case of triplets including anomalous twins and a fetus compressus. Amer. J. Obstet. Gynecol. **73**:1342–1345, 1957.

Ropacka, M., Markwitz, W. and Blickstein, I.: Treatment options for the twin-twin transfusion syndrome: A review. Twin Res. **5**:507–514, 2002.

Rosa, F.W., Hernandez, C. and Carlo, W.A.: Griseofulvin teratology, including two thoracopagus conjoined twins. Lancet **1**:171, 1987.

Rosenfeld, C.R., Coln, C.D. and Duenhoelter, J.H.: Fetal teratomas as a cause of polyhydramnios. Pediatrics **64**:176–179, 1979.

Rosenquist, G.C.: Parabiotic syndrome. NEJM **269**:161–162, 1963.

Ross, J.R.W.: An acardius amorphus in a triplet pregnancy. J. Obstet. Gynaecol. Br. Emp. **58**:835–838, 1951.

Ross, R.K., Bernstein, L., Judd, H., Hanisch, R., Pike, M. and Henderson, B.: Serum testosterone levels in healthy young black and white men. J. Natl. Cancer Inst. **76**:45–48, 1986.

Rothman, K.J.: Fetal loss, twinning and birth weight after oral-contraceptive use. NEJM **297**:468–471, 1977.

Rouse, D.J., Skopec, G.S., Zlatnik, F.J.: Fundal height as a predictor of preterm twin delivery. Obstet. Gynecol. **81**:211–214, 1993.

Runner, M.N.: New evidence for monozygotic twins in the mouse: twinning initiated in the late blastocyst can account for mirror image asymmetries. Anat. Rec. **209**:399–406, 1984.

Russell, E.M.: Cerebral palsied twins. Arch. Dis. Child. **36**:328–336, 1961.

Ryan, K.J.: Paternity and pedigree, from superfecundation to "test-tube" babies. NEJM **299**:603, 1978.

Ryan, R.R. and Wislocki, G.B.: The birth of quadruplets, with an account of the placentas and fetal membranes. NEJM **250**:755–758, 1954.

Rydhstroem, H.: Twin pregnancy and the effects of prophylactic leave of absence on pregnancy duration and birth weight. Acta Obstet. Gynecol. Scand. **67**:81–84, 1988.

Rydhstroem, H.: The relationship of birth weight and birth weight discordance to cerebral palsy or mental retardation later in life for twins weighing less than 2500 grams. Am. J. Obstet. Gynecol. **173**:680–686, 1995.

Saade, G., Olson, G.L., Belfort, M. and Moise, K.: Amniotomy: a new approach to the "stuck twin" syndrome. Amer. J. Obstet. Gynecol. **172**:429 (abstract 622), 1995.

Sacks, M.O.: Occurrence of anemia and polycythemia in phenotypically dissimilar single-ovum human twins. Pediatrics **24**:604–608, 1959.

Saier, F., Burden, L. and Cavanagh, D.: Fetus papyraceus: an unusual case with congenital anomaly of the surviving fetus. Obstet. Gynecol. **45**:217–220, 1975.

Sala, M.A. and Matheus, M.: Placental characteristics in twin transfusion syndrome. Arch. Gynecol. Obstet. **246**:51–56, 1989.

Salat-Baroux, J., Alvarez, S. and Antoine, J.M.: A case of triple monoamniotic pregnancy combined with a bioamniotic twinning after in-vitro fertilization. Human Reprod. **9**:374–375, 1994.

Salihu, H.M., Aliyu, M.H., Kirby, R.S. and Alexander, G.R.: Effect of advanced maternal age on early mortality among quadruplets and quintuplets. Amer. J. Obstet. Gynecol. **190**:383–388, 2004a.

Salihu, H.M., Williams, A.T., McCainey, T.T.N., Kirby, R.S. and Alkexander, G.R.: Early mortality among triplets in the United States: black-white disparity. Amer. J. Obstet. Gynecol. **190**:477–484, 2004b.

Samon, L.M., Ash, K.M. and Murdison, K.A.: Aorto-pulmonary calcification an unusual manifestation of idiopathic calcification of infancy evident prenatally. Obstet. Gynecol. **85**:863–865, 1995.

Sander, C.H.: Fetus papyraceus. Amer. J. Obstet. Gynecol. **145**:895–896, 1983.

Sato, T., Kaneko, K., Konuma, S., Sato, I. and Tamada, T.: Acardiac anomalies: review of 88 cases in Japan. Asia Oceania J. Obstet. Gynaecol. **10**:45–52, 1984.

Saunders, M.C., Dick, J.S., McPherson, K. and Chalmers, I.: The effect of hospital admission for bed rest on the duration of twin pregnancy: a randomized trial. Lancet **2**:793–795, 1985.

Saunders, N.J., Snijders, R.J.M. and Nicolaides, K.H.: Therapeutic amniocentesis in twin-twin transfusion syndrome appearing in the second trimester of pregnancy. Amer. J. Obstet. Gynecol. **166**:820–824, 1992.

Schatz, F.: Zur Frage über die Quelle des Fruchtwassers und über Embryones papyracei. Arch. Gynäkol. **7**:336–338, 1875. **19**:329, 1882.

Schatz, F.: Die Gefässverbindungen der Placentarkreisläufe eineiiger Zwillinge, ihre Entwicklung und ihre Folgen. Arch. Gynäkol. **27**:1–72, 1886.

Schatz, F.: Die Acardii und ihre Verwandten. Hirschwald, Berlin, 1898.

Schatz, F.: Systematisches und alphabetisches Inhaltsverzeichniss von Friedrich Schatz: Placentakreisläufe eineiiger Zwillinge, ihre Entwicklung und ihre Folgen, in Band 19, 24, 27, 29, 30, 53, 55, 58, 60. Arch. Gynäkol. **60**:559–584, 1900. [Systematic index of Schatz's work on twins, with specific references to his citing various features of twin placentas, and authorities quoted.]

Scheller, J.M. and Nelson, K.B.: Twinning and neurologic morbidity. Amer. J. Dis. Child. **146**:110–1113, 1992.

Schenker, J.G., Yarkoni, S. and Granat, M.: Multiple pregnancies following induction of ovulation. Fertil. Steril. **35**:105–123, 1981.

Schieve, L.A., Meikle, S.F., Ferre, C., Peterson, H.B., Jeng, G. and Wilcox, L.S.: Low and very low birth weight in infants conceived with use of assisted reproductive technology. NEJM **346**:731–737, 2002.

Schinzel, A.A.G.L., Smith, D.W. and Miller, J.R.: Monozygotic twinning and structural defects. J. Pediatr. **95**:921–930, 1979.

Schmid, O., Trautmann, U., Ashour, H., Ulmer, R., Pfeiffer, R.A. and Beinder, E.: Prenatal diagnosis of heterokaryotypic twins discordant for fetal sex. Prenat. Diagn. **20**:999–1003, 2000.

Schmidt, W., Heberling, D. and Kubli, F.: Antepartum ultrasonographic diagnosis of conjoined twins in early pregnancy. Amer. J. Obstet. Gynecol. **139**:961–963, 1981.

Schneider, K.T.M., Vetter, K., Huch, R. and Huch, A.: Acute polyhydramnios complicating twin pregnancies. Acta Genet. Med. Gemellol. **34**:179–184, 1985.

Scholtes, G.: Zum Problem der Zwillingsschwangerschaft. Arch. Gynäkol. **210**:188–207, 1971.

Schwalbe, E.: Acardii und Verwandte. In, Die Missbildungen des Menschen und der Tiere. Vol. II. Die Doppelbildungen. Gustav Fischer, Jena, 1907.

Schwartz, J.L., Maniscalco, W.M., Lane, A.T. and Currao, W.J.: Twin transfusion syndrome causing cutaneous erythropoiesis. Pediatrics **74**:527–529, 1984.

Scipiades, E. and Burg, E.: Über die Morphologie der menschlichen Plazenta mit besonderer Berücksichtigung auf unsere eigenen Studien. Arch. Gynäkol. **141**:577–619, 1930.

Scott, F. and Evans, N.: Distal gangrene in a polycythemic recipient fetus in twin-twin transfusion. Obstet. Gynecol. **86**:677–679, 1995.

Scott, J.M. and Ferguson-Smith, M.A.: Heterokaryotypic monozygotic twins and the acardiac monster. J. Obstet. Gynaecol. **80**:52–59, 1973.

Sebire, N.J., Sepulveda, W., Hughes, K.S., Noble, P. and Nicolaides, K.H.: Management of twin pregnancies discordant for anencephaly. Brit. J. Obstet. Gynaecol. **104**:216–219, 1997a.

Sebire, N.J., Sherod, C., Abbas, A., Snijders, R.J.M. and Nicolaides, K.H.: Preterm delivery and growth restriction in mutifetal pregnancies reduced to twins. Human Reprod. **12**:173–175, 1997b.

Sebire, N.J., Snijders, R.J.M., Hughes, K., Sepulveda, W. and Nicolaides, K.H.: The hidden mortality of monochorionic twin pregnancies. Brit. J. Obstet. Gynaecol. **104**:1203–1207, 1997c.

Sekiya, S. and Hafez, E.S.E.: Physiomorphology of twin transfusion syndrome: a study of 86 twin gestations. Obstet. Gynecol. **50**:288–292, 1977.

Sekiya, S.-I., Akamatsu, H., Kaneko, K. and Takeishi, Y.: Report of a case: placental vascular communications between triplet fetuses; triplet transfusion syndrome. J. Jpn. Neonatol. Soc. (Nihon Shinseiji Gakkai Zasshi) **9**:89–96, 1973.

Selby, L.A., Khalili, A., Stewart, R.W., Edmonds, L.D. and Marienfeld, C.J.: Pathology and epidemiology of conjoined twinning in swine. Teratology **8**:1–10, 1973.

Selvin, S.: Twin zygosity diagnosis by blood group antigens. Hum. Hered. **20**:540–548, 1970.

Semchyshyn, S., Mangurten, H., Benawra, R., Trujillo, Y., Fernandez, B. and McKeown, J.C.: Fetal Tumor: antenatal diagnosis and its implications. J. Reprod. Med. **27**:231–234, 1982.

Semmens, J.P.: Monoamniotic twin pregnancy: delivery of living premature twins after uterine rupture; a case report. Obstet. Gynecol. **12**:75–77, 1958.

Senat, M.-V., Deprest, J., Boulvain, M., Paupe, A., Winer, N. and Ville, Y.: Endoscopic laser surgery versus serial amnioreduction for severe twin-to-twin transfusion syndrome. NEJM **351**:136–144, 2004.

Seo, J.W., Shin, S.S. and Chi, J.G.: Cardiovascular system in conjoined twins: an analysis of 14 Korean cases. Teratology **32**:151–161, 1985.

Seoud, M.A.-F., Toner, J.P., Kruithoff, C., Muasher, S.J.: Outcome of twin, triplet, and quadruplet in vitro fertilization pregnancies: the Norfolk experience. Fertil. Steril. **57**:825–834, 1992.

Sepulveda, W., Bower, S., Hassan, J. and Fisk, N.M.: Ablation of acardiac twin by alcohol injection into the intra-abdominal umbilical artery. Obstet. Gynecol. **86**:680–681, 1995.

Sepulveda, W., Sebire, N.J., Odibo, A., Psarra, A. and Nicolaides, K.H.: Prenatal determination of chorionicity in triplet pregnancy by ultrasonographic examination of the Ipsilon zone. Obstet. Gynecol. **88**:855–858, 1996.

Sepulveda, W., Surerus, E., Vandecruys, H. and Nicolaides, K.H.: Fetofetal transfusion syndrome in triplet pregnancies: Outcome after endoscopic laser surgery. Amer. J. Obstet. Gynecol. **192**:161–164, 2005.

Sergi, C. and Schmitt, H.P.: Central nervous system in twin reversed arterial perfusion sequence with special reference to examination of the brain in acardius anceps. Teratology **61**:284–290, 2000.

Seski, A.G. and Miller, L.A.: Plural pregnancies—the cause of plural problems. Obstet. Gynecol. **21**:227–233, 1963.

Shah, D.M. and Chaffin, D.: Perinatal outcome in very preterm births with twin-twin transfusion syndrome. Amer. J. Obstet. Gynecol. **161**:1111–1113, 1989.

Shahabi, S., Donner, C., Wallond, J., Schlikker, I., Avni, E.F. and Rodesch, F.: Monoamniotic twin cord entanglement. A case report with color flow Doppler ultrasonography for antenatal diagnosis. J. Reprod. Med. **42**:740–742, 1997.

Shapiro, L.R. and Farnsworth, P.G.: Down's syndrome in twins. Clin. Genet. **2**:364–370, 1972.

Shapiro, L.R., Zemek, L. and Shulman, M.J.: Familial monozygotic twinning: an autosomal dominant form of monozygotic twinning with variable penetrance. Pp 61–63. In: Progress in Clinical and Biological Research. Volume 24B. Twin Research. Part B. Biology and Epidemiology. W.E. Nance, ed., G. Allen and P. Parisi, Associate eds. A.R. Liss, Inc., New York.

Shapiro, L.R., Wilmot, P.L., Duncan, P.A., Davidian, M.M., Fakhry, J. and Capone, A.J.: Holoacardius acephalus: cytogenetic abnormalities as the principle pathogenetic mechanism. Proc. Greenwood Genet. Center **5**:128, 1986.

Sheffer-Mimouni, G., Littner, Y., Mimouni, F.B., Mandel, D., Deutsch, V. and Dollberg, S.: Nucleated red blood cells in concordant, appropriate-for-gestational age twins. Amer. J. Obstet. Gynecol. **191**:1291–1295, 2004.

Sherer, D.M., Armstrong, B., Shah, Y.G., Metlay, L.A. and Woods, J.R.: Prenatal sonographic diagnosis, Doppler velocimetric umbilical cord studies, and subsequent management of an acardiac twin pregnancy. Obstet. Gynecol. **74**:472–475, 1989.

Sherer, D.M., Abramowicz, J.S., Jaffe, R., Smith, S.A., Metlay, L.A. and Woods, J.R.: Twin-twin transfusion syndrome with abrupt onset of microcephaly in the surviving recipient following spontaneous death of the donor twin. Amer. J. Obstet. Gynecol. **169**:85–88, 1993.

Shevell, T., Malone, F.D., Weintraub, J., Thaker, H.M. and d'Alton, M.E.: Radiofrequency ablation in a monochorionic twin discordant for fetal anomalies. Amer. J. Obstet. Gynecol. **190**:575–576, 2004.

Shorland, J.: Management of the twin transfusion syndrome. Clin. Pediatr. **10**:160–163, 1971.

Short, R.V.: Testis size, ovulation rate and breast cancer. In: One Medicine. O.A. Ryder and M.L. Byrd, eds., pp. 32–44. Springer-Verlag, New York, 1984.

Sills, E.S., Tucker, M.J. and Palermo, G.D.: Assisted reproductive technologies and monozygous twins: implications for future study and clinical practice. Twin Res. **3**:217–223, 2000.

Sills, E.S., Sweitzer, C.L., Morton, P.C., Perloe, M., Kaplan, C.R. and Tucker, M.J.: Dizygotic twin delivery following in vitro fertilization and transfer of thawed blastocysts cryopreserved at day 6 and 7. Fertil. Steril. **79**:424–427, 2003.

Simonds, J.P. and Gowen, G.A.: Fetus amorphus. Surg. Gynecol. Obstet. **41**:171–179, 1925.

Simonsen, M.: Monoamniotic twins. Acta Obstet. Gynecol. Scand. **45**:43–52, 1966.

Simpson, C.W., Olatunbosun, O.A. and Baldwin, V.J.: Delayed interval delivery in triplet pregnancy: report of a single case and review of the literature. Obstet. Gynecol. **64**:8S–11S, 1984.

Simpson, J.L., Morillo-Cucci, G., Horwith, M., Stiefel, F.H., Feldman, F. and German, J.: Abnormalities of human sex chromosomes. VI. Monozygotic twins with the complement 48,XXXY. Humangenetik **21**:301–308, 1974.

Simpson, L.L., Elkadry, E.A., Marx, G.R. and D'Alton, M.E.: Cardiac dysfunction in twin-twin transfusion syndrome. Amer. J. Obstet. Gynecol. **176**:174 (abstract 609), 1997.

Simpson, P.C., Trudinger, B.J., Walker, A. and Baird, P.J.: The intrauterine treatment of fetal cardiac failure in a twin pregnancy with an acardiac, acephalic monster. Amer. J. Obstet. Gynecol. **147**:842–844, 1983.

Sinclair, J.G.: The Badgett quadruplets. J. Hered. **31**:163–164, 1940.

Sinykin, M.B.: Monoamniotic triplet pregnancy with triple survival. Obstet. Gynecol. **12**:78–82, 1958.

Sironi, M., Declich, P., Isimbaldi, G., Monguzzi, A. and Poggi, G.: Placental teratoma with three-germ layer differentiation. Teratology **50**:165–167, 1994.

Skelly, H., Marivate, M., Norman, R., Kenoyer, G. and Martin, R.: Consumptive coagulopathy following fetal death in a triplet pregnancy. Amer. J. Obstet. Gynecol. **142**:595–596, 1982.

Skupski, D.W., Nelson, S., Kowalik, A., Polaneczky, M., Smith-Levitin, M., Hutson, J.M. and Rosenwaks, Z.: Multiple gestations from in vitro fertilization: successful implantation alone is not associated with subsequent preeclampsia. Amer. J. Obstet. Gynecol. **175**:1029–1032, 1996.

Smith, J.F., Pesterfield, W., Day, L.D. and Jones, R.O.: Doppler evidence of improved fetoplacental hemodynamics following amnioreduction in the stuck twin. Obstet. Gynecol. **90**:681–682, 1997.

Smith-Levitin, M., Kowalik, A., Birnholz, J., Skupski, D.W., Hutson, J.M., Chervenak, F.A. and Rosenwaks, Z.: Selective reduction of multifetal pregnancies to twins improves outcome over nonreduced triplet gestations. Amer. J. Obstet. Gynecol. **175**:878–882, 1996.

Soma, H., Takayama, M., Kiyokawa, T., Akaeda, T. and Tokoro, K.: Serum gonadotropin levels in Japanese women. Obstet. Gynecol. **46**:311–312, 1975.

Soma, H., Saito, T., Kikuchi, K., Arai, K., Takayama, M., Yoshida, K. and Terada, K.: Sacrococcygeal teratoma in a fetus and its placenta. Rinsho Fujinka Sanka (Clin. Gynecol. Obstet. Jpn.) **33**:303–307, 1979.

Sorensen, S.A. and Fenger, K.: On the use of linked markers in the diagnosis of zygosity in twins. Hum. Hered. **24**:529–539, 1974.

Sotrel, G., Rao, R. and Scommegna, A.: Heterotopic pregnancy following Clomid treatment. J. Reprod. Med. **16**:78–80, 1976.

Souter, V.L., Kapur, R.P., Nyholt, D.R., Skogerboe, K., Myerson, D., Ton, C.C., Opheim, K.E., Easterling, T.R., Shields, L.E.,

Montgomery, G.W. and Glass, I.A.: A report of dizygous monochorionic twins. NEJM 349:154–158, 2003.

Sowards, D.L. and Monif, R.G.: Serum immunoglobulin M levels between weeks 22 and 37 of gestation. Amer. J. Obstet. Gynecol. 112:394–396, 1972.

Speiser, P. and Brezina, K.: Lithopedion in a 92-year-old woman. Lancet 345:737–738, 1995.

Spellacy, W.N., Kalra, P.S., Buggie, J. and Birk, S.A.: Gonadotropin responses to graded GNRF injections in women with prior twin pregnancies. J. Reprod. Med. 27:435–438, 1982.

Spellacy, W.N., Handler, A. and Ferre, C.D.: A case-control study of 1253 twin pregnancies from 1982–1987 perinatal data base. Obstet. Gynecol. 75:168–171, 1990.

Spencer, R.: Conjoined twins: Theoretical embryological basis. Teratology 45:591–602, 1992.

Spencer, R.: Rachipagus conjoined twins: They really do occur! Teratology 52:346–356, 1995.

Spencer, R.: Theoretical and analytical embryology of conjoined twins: Part I: embryogenesis. Clin. Anat. 13:36–53, 2000. (Part II: 97–120, 2000).

Spencer, R.: Parasitic conjoined twins: external, internal (fetuses in fetu and teratomas), and detached (acardiacs). Clin. Anat. 14:428–444, 2001.

Spencer, R.: Conjoined Twins: Developmental Malformations and Clinical Implications. Johns Hopkins University Press, Baltimore, 2003.

Spitzer, W.: Zur geburtshilflichen Bedeutung der kongenitalen Sakraltumoren. Zentralbl. Gynäkol. 56:1403–1409, 1932.

Spurway, J.H.: The fate and management of the second twin. Amer. J. Obstet. Gynecol. 83:1377–13388, 1962.

Srivatsa, B., Srivatsa, S., Johnson, K.L., Samura, O., Lee, S.L. and Bianchi, D.W.: Microchimerism of presumed fetal origin in thyroid specimens from women: a case-control study. Lancet 358:2034–2038, 2001.

Stagiannis, K.D., Sepulveda, W., Southwell, D., Price, D.A. and Fisk, N.M.: Ultrasonographic measurement of the dividing membrane in twin pregnancy during the second and third trimesters. A reproducibility study. Amer. J. Obstet. Gynecol. 173:1546–1550, 1995.

Starks, G.C.: Unilateral twin interstitial ectopic pregnancy: a case report. J. Reprod. Med. 25:79–82, 1980.

St. Clair, D.M., St. Clair, J.B., Swainson, C.P., Bamforth, F. and Machin, G.A.: Twin zygosity testing for medical purposes. Amer. J. Med. Genet. 77:412–414, 1998.

Steinman, G.: Spontaneous monozygotic quadruplet pregnancy: an obstetric rarity. Obstet. Gynecol. 91:866, 1998.

Steinman, G.: Mechanisms of twinning. I. Effect of environmental diversity on genetic expression in monozygotic multifetal pregnancies. J. Reprod. Med. 46:467–472, 2001a.

Steinman, G.: Mechanisms of twinning. II. Laterality and intercellular bonding in monozygotic twinning. J. Reprod. Med. 46:473–479, 2001b.

Steinman, G.: Mechanisms of twinning. IV. Sex preference and lactation. J. Reprod. Med. 46:1003–1007, 2001c.

Steinman, G.: Mechanisms of twinning. V. Conjoined twins, stem cells and the calcium model. J. Reprod. Med. 47:313–321, 2002a.

Steinman, G.: Mechanisms of twinning. VI. Genetics and the etiology of monozygotic twinning in in vitro fertilization. J. Reprod. Med. 48:583–590, 2002b.

Steinman, G.: Mechanisms of twinning. VI. Genetics and the etiology of monozygotic twinning in in vitro fertilization. J. Reprod. Med. 48:583–590, 2003.

Steinman, G. and Valderrama, E.: Mechanisms of twinning. IIII. Placentation, calcium reduction, and modified compaction. J. Reprod. Med. 46:995–1002, 2001.

Stephens, T.D., Spall, R., Urfer, A.G. and Martin, R.: Fetus amorphus or placental teratoma? Teratology 40:1–10, 1989.

Stoeckel, W.: Lehrbuch der Geburtshilfe. p. 258. Gustav Fischer, Jena 1945.

Stone, C.A., Quinn, M.W. and Saxby, P.J.: Congenital skin loss following Nd:YAG placental photocoagulation. Burns 24:275–277, 1998.

Stone, J., Eddleman, K., Lynch, L. and Berkowitz, R.L.: A single center experience with 1000 consecutive cases of multifetal pregnancy reduction. Amer. J. Obstet. Gynecol. 187:1163–1167, 2002.

Storch, M.P. and Petrie, R.H.: Unilateral tubal twin gestation. Amer. J. Obstet. Gynecol. 125:1148, 1976.

Strain, L., Dean, J.C.S., Hamilton, M.P.R. and Bonthron, D.T.: A true hermaphrodite chimera resulting from embryo amalgamation after in vitro fertilization. NEJM 338:166–195, 1998.

Stranc, M.F.: Skin homograft survival in a severely burned triplet: study of triplet zygotic type. Plast. Reconstr. Surg. 37:280–290, 1966.

Strauss, J.H., Ballard, J.O. and Chamlian, D.: Consumption coagulopathy associated with intrauterine fetal death: the role of heparin therapy. Int. J. Gynaecol. Obstet. 16:225–227, 1978.

Streit, J.A., Penick, G.D., Williamson, R.A., Weiner, C.P. and Benda, J.A.: Prolonged elevation of alphafetoprotein and detectable acetylcholinesterase after death of an anomalous twin. Prenat. Diagn. 9:1–6, 1989.

Strömberg, B., Dahlquist, G., Ericson, A., Finnstrom, O., Köster, M. and Stjernqvist, K.: Neurological sequelae in children born after in-vitro fertilization: a population-based study. Lancet 359:461–465, 2002.

Strong, S.J. and Corney, G.: The Placenta in Twin Pregnancy. Pergamon Press, Oxford, 1967.

Strong, T.H.: The umbilical pump: a contribution to the twin-twin transfusion. Obstet. Gynecol. 89:812–813, 1997.

Sulak, L.E. and Dodson, M.G.: The vanishing twin: pathologic conformation of an ultrasonographic phenomenon. Obstet. Gynecol. 68:811–815, 1986.

Sullivan, A.E., Varner, M.W., Ball, R.H., Jackson, M. and Silver, R.M.: The management of acardiac twins: a conservative approach. Amer. J. Obstet. Gynecol. 189:1310–1313, 2003.

Suslak, L., Mimms, G.M. and Desposito, F.: Monozygosity and holoprosencephaly: cleavage disorders of the "midline field." Amer. J. Med. Genet. 28:99–102, 1987.

Sutter, J., Arab, H. and Manning, F.A.: Monoamniotic twins: antenatal diagnosis and management. Amer. J. Obstet. Gynecol. 155:836–837, 1986.

Sutton, J.B.: An acardiac from a cow. Trans. Obstet. Soc. Lond. 41:97, 1899.

Swindle, M.M., Adams, R.J. and Craft, C.F.: Intrauterine mummified fetus in a rhesus monkey (Macaca mulatta). J. Med. Primatol. 10:269–273, 1981.

Szabuniewicz, M. and McCrady, J.D.: A case of "Siamese" twins in the turtle (Pseudemys scripta elegans). Texas J. Sci. 19:232–233, 1967.

Szendi, B.: Über die Bedeutung der Struktur der Eihäute und des Gefässnetzes der Placenta auf Grund von 112 Zwillingsgeburten. Arch. Gynäkol. **167**:108–129, 1938.

Szymonowicz, W., Preston, H. and Yu, Y.Y.H.: The surviving monozygotic twin. Arch. Dis. Child. **61**:454–458, 1986.

Tabsh, K.: Genetic amniocentesis in multiple gestation: a new technique to diagnose monoamniotic twins. Obstet. Gynecol. **75**:296–298, 1990a.

Tabsh, K.M.A.: Transabdominal multifetal pregnancy reduction: report of 40 cases. Obstet. Gynecol. **75**:739–741, 1990b.

Tabsh, K.M.A.: A report of 131 cases of multifetal pregnancy reduction. Obstet. Gynecol. **82**:57–60, 1993.

Tabsh, K.M.A., Crandall, B., Lebherz, T.B. and Howard, J.: Genetic amniocentesis in twin pregnancy. Obstet. Gynecol. **65**:843–845, 1985.

Tafeen, C.H., Freedman, H.L. and Kahane, A.J.: Monoamniotic twins. Amer. J. Obstet. Gynecol. **79**:1078–1081, 1960.

Talbert, D.G., Bajiora, R., Sepulveda, W., Bower, S. and Fisk, N.M.: Hydrostatic and osmotic pressure gradients produce manifestations of fetofetal transfusion syndrome in a computerized model of monochorial twin pregnancy. Amer. J. Obstet. Gynecol. **174**:598–608, 1996.

Tan, K.L., Goon, S.M., Salmon, Y. and Wee, J.H.: Conjoined twins. Acta Obstet. Gynecol. Scand. **50**:373–380, 1971a.

Tan, K.L., Tock, E.P.C., Dawood, M.Y. and Ratnam, S.S.: Conjoined twins in a triplet pregnancy. Amer. J. Dis. Child. **122**:455–458, 1971b.

Tan, T.Y. and Sepulveda, W.: Acardiac twin: a systematic review of minimally invasive treatment modalities. Ultrasound Obstetr. Gynecol. **22**:409–419, 2003.

Tan, T.Y., Denbow, M.L., Cox, P.M., Talbert, D. and Fisk, N.M.: Occlusion of arterio-arterial anastomosis manifesting as acute twin-twin transfusion syndrome. Placenta **25**:238–242, 2004.

Tan, T.Y., Taylor, M.J., Wee, L.Y., Vanderheyden, T., Wimalasundera, R. and Fisk, N.M.: Doppler for artery-artery anastomosis and stage-independent survival in twin-twin transfusion. Obstetr. Gynecol. **103**:1174–1180, 2004.

Tarkowski, A.K.: Mouse chimaeras developed from fused eggs. Nature **190**:875–860, 1961.

Taylor, M.B., Anderson, R.L. and Golbus, M.S.: One hundred twin pregnancies in a prenatal diagnosis program. Amer. J. Med. Genet. **18**:419–422, 1984.

Taylor, M.J.O., Denbow, M.L., Duncan, K.R., Overton, T.G. and Fisk, N.M.: Antenatal factors at diagnosis that predict outcome in twin-twin transfusion syndrome. Amer. J. Obstet. Gynecol. **183**:1023–1028, 2000a.

Taylor, M.J., Denbow, M.L., Tanawattanacharoen, S., Gannon, C., Cox, P.M. and Fisk, N.M.: Doppler detection of arterio-arterial anastomoses in monochorionic twins: feasibility and clinical application. Human Reprod. **15**:1632–1636, 2000b.

Taylor, M.J., Farquharson, D., Cox., P.M. and Fisk, N.M.: Identification of arterio-venous anastomoses in vivo in monochorionic twin pregnancies: preliminary report. Ultrasound Obstetr. Gynecol. **16**:218–222, 2000c.

Taylor, M.J., Shalev, E., Tanawattanacharoen, S., Jolly, M., Kumar, S., Weiner, E., Cox, P.M. and Fisk, N.M.: Ultrasound-guided umbilical cord occlusion using bipolar diathermy for stage III/IV twin-twin transfusion syndrome. Prenat. Diagn. **22**:70–76, 2002.

Taylor, M.J.O., Wee, L. and Fisk, N.M.: Placental types and twin-twin transfusion syndrome. Amer. J. Obstet. Gynecol. **188**:1119, 2003.

Taylor, M.J.O., Talbert, D. and Fisk, N.M.: Pseudo-arterio-arterial anastomoses in twin-twin transfusion syndrome. Placenta **25**:742–747, 2004.

Templeton, A.: The multiple gestation epidemic: the role of the assisted reproductive technologies. Amer. J. Obstet. Gynecol. **190**:894–898, 2004.

Terasaki, P.I., Gjertson, D., Bernoco, D., Perdue, S., Mickey, M.R. and Bond, J.: Twins with two different fathers identified by HLA. NEJM **299**:590–592, 1978.

Tessen, J.A. and Zlatnik, F.J.: Monoamniotic twins: a retrospective controlled study. Obstet. Gynecol. **77**:832–834, 1991.

Thiery, M., Dhont, M. and Vandekerckhove, D.: Serum hCG and hPL in twin pregnancies. Acta Obstet. Gynecol. Scand. **56**:495–497, 1976.

Thomas, D.B.: Intrauterine intraventricular haemorrhage and disseminated intravascular coagulation in a triplet pregnancy. Aust. Paediatr. J. **10**:25–27, 1974.

Thomas, J.: Untersuchungsergebnisse über die Aplasie einer Nabelarterie unter besonderer Berücksichtigung der Zwillingsschwangerschaft. Geburtsh. Frauenheilk. **21**:984–992, 1961.

Thomas, J.: Morphologische Untersuchungen über das "große Herz" des Feten. Geburtsh. Frauenheilk. **22**:1316–1323, 1962.

Thompson, J.P. and Johnson, C.E.: Survival and management of the second-born twin. Obstet. Gynecol. **27**:827–832, 1966.

Thomsen, R.J.: Delayed interval delivery of a twin pregnancy. Obstet. Gynecol. **52**:37s–40s, 1978.

Thornton, J.G. and Rout, D.J.: Hospital admission in twin pregnancy. Lancet **335**:978, 1990.

Thurin, A., Hausken, J., Hillensjö, T., Jablonowska, B., Pinborg, A., Strandell, A. and Bergh, C.: Elective single-embryo transfer versus double-embryo transfer in in vitro fertilization. NEJM **351**:2392–2402, 2004.

Timmons, J.D. and Alvarez, R.R. de: Monoamniotic twin pregnancy. Amer. J. Obstet. Gynecol. **86**:875–881, 1963.

Timonen, S. and Carpen, E.: Multiple pregnancies and photoperiodicity. Ann. Chir. Gynaecol. Fenn. **57**:135–139, 1968.

Tippett, P.: Human chimeras. In, Chimeras in Developmental Biology. N.L. Douarin and A. McLaren, eds., pp. 165–178. Academic Press, Orlando, 1984.

Tojo, R., Larripa, J., Iglesias, H. and Quiroga, E.: Sindrome de transfusion feto-fetal: a proposito de tres observaciones. Rev. Esp. Pediatr. **27**:101–112, 1971.

Tokunaga, S., Ikeda, T., Matsuo, T., Maeda, H., Kurosaki, N. and Shimoda, H.: A case of sacral parasite. Congen. Anom. (Jpn.) **26**:321–330, 1986.

Torgersen, J.: Genic factors in visceral asymmetry and in the development and pathologic changes of lungs, heart and abdominal organs. Arch. Pathol. **47**:566–593, 1949.

Torretta, G. and Cobellis, G.: Aspetti vascolari della placenta monocoriale su calchi al neoprene. Arch. Ostet. Ginecol. **71**:357–362, 1966.

Toubas, P.L., Silverman, N.H., Heyman, M.A. and Rudolph, A. M.: Cardiovascular effects of acute hemorrhage in fetal lambs. Amer. J. Physiol. **240**:H45–H48, 1981.

Tow, S.H.: Foetal wastage in twin pregnancy. J. Obstet. Gynaecol. Br. Emp. **66**:444–451, 1959.

Townsend, R.R., Simpson, G.F. and Filly, R.A.: Membrane thickness in ultrasound prediction of chorionicity of twin gestations. J. Ultrasound Med. **7**:327–332, 1988.

Trespidi, L., Boschetto, C., Caravelli, E., Villa, L., Kustermann, A. and Nicolini, U.: Serial amniocenteses in the management of twin-twin transfusion syndrome: When is it valuable? Fetal Diagn. Therapy **12**:15–20, 1997.

Tsao, K., Feldstein, V.A., Albanese, C.T., Sandberg, P.L., Lee, H., Harrison, M.R. and Farmer, D.L.: Selective reduction of acardiac twin by radiofrequency ablation. Amer. J. Obstet. Gynecol. **187**:635–640, 2002.

Tsunoda, Y. and McLaren, A.: Effect of various procedures on the viability of mouse embryos containing half the normal number of blastomeres. J. Reprod. Fertil. **69**:315–322, 1983.

Tsunoda, Y., Tokunaga, T., Sugie, T. and Katsumata, M.: Production of monozygotic twins following the transfer of bisected embryos in the goat. Theriogenology **24**:337–342, 1985.

Tuncer, M.: Placenta angiograms in the diagnosis of placental transfusion syndrome in twins. Hacettepe Bull. Med. Surg. **3**:182–191, 1970.

Turksoy, R.N., Toy, B.L., Rogers, J. and Papageorge, W.: Birth of septuplets following human gonadotropin administration in Chiari-Frommel syndrome. Obstet. Gynecol. **30**:692–697, 1967.

Turpin, R., Bocquet, L. and Grasset, J.: Étude d'un couple monozygote: fille normale—Monstre acardiaque féminin: considérations anatomo-pathologiques et cytogénétiques. Ann. Génét. (Paris) **10**:107–113, 1967.

Tüscher, H.: Zur Frage der Entscheidung über die Ein = oder Zweieiigkeit bei bichorischen biamniotischen Zwillingen mit Gefäßanastomosen in der Plazenta. Erbarzt **10**:148–149, 1936.

Tutschek, B., Reihs, T. and Crombach, G.: Diagnostik und Prognose in Mehrlingsgraviditäten im I. Trimenon. Gynäkologe **31**:209–217, 1998.

Tutschek, B., Hecher, K., Somville, T. and Bender, H.G.: Twin-to-twin transfusion syndrome complicated by spontaneous mid-trimester uterine rupture. J. Perinat. Med. **32**:95–97, 2004.

Uchida, I.A., Freeman, V.C.P., Gedeon, M. and Goldmaker, J.: Twinning rate in spontaneous abortions. Amer. J. Hum. Genet. **35**:987–993, 1983.

Umur, A., van Gemert, M.J.C. and Ross, M.G.: Amniotic fluid and hemodynamic model in monochorionic twin pregnancies and twin-twin transfusion syndrome. Amer. J. Physiol. Regulat. Integr. Physiol. **280**:R1499–R1509, 2001a.

Umur, A., van Gemert, M.J.C. and Ross, M.G.: Fetal urine and amniotic fluid in monochorionic twins with twin-twin transfusion syndrome: simulations of therapy. Amer. J. Obstet. Gynecol. **185**:996–1003, 2001b.

Umur, A., van Gemert, M.J.C. and Ross, M.G.: Does amniotic fluid volume affect fetofetal transfusion in monochorionic twin pregnancies? Modelling two possible mechanisms. Phys. Med. Biol. **47**:2165–2177, 2002.

Umur, A., van Gemert, M.J.C. and Nikkels, P.G.J.: Monoamniotic-versus diamniotic-monochorionic twin placentas: anastomoses and twin-twin transfusion syndrome. Amer. J. Obstetr. Gynecol. **189**:1325–1329, 2003a.

Umur, A., van Gemert, M.J.C., Nikkels, P.G.J. and Ross, M.G.: Monochorionic twins and twin-twin transfusion syndrome: the protective role of arterio-arterial anastomoses. Placenta **23**:201–209, 2003b.

Urig, M.A., Clewell, W.H. and Elliott J.P.: Twin-twin transfusion syndrome. Amer. J. Obstet. Gynecol. **163**:1522–1526, 1990.

Van Allen, M.I., Smith, D.W. and Shepard, T.H.: Twin reversed arterial perfusion (TRAP) sequence: a study of 14 twin pregnancies with acardius. Semin. Perinatol. **7**:285–293, 1983.

Van de Berghe, H. and Verresen, H.: Triploid-diploid mosaicism in the lymphocytes of a liveborn child with multiple malformations. Humangenetik **11**:18–21, 1970.

Van der Kolk, W.F.J.: De asymmetrische derde circulatie en haar gevolgen voor monozygote gemelli. Maandschr. Kindergenesk. **32**:186–194, 1964.

Van Gemert, M.J.C. and Sterenborg, H.J.C.M.: Haemodynamic model of twin-twin transfusion syndrome in monochorionic twin pregnancies. Placenta **19**:195–208, 1998.

Van Gemert, M.J.C., Scherjon, S.A., Major, A.L. and Borst, C.: Twin-twin transfusion syndrome. Three possible pathophysiologic mechanisms. J. Reprod. Med. **42**:708–714, 1997.

Van Gemert, M.J.C., Milanovic, Z., Vergroesen, I. and Steenbeck, A.: Polyhydramnios can beneficially affect twin-twin transfusion syndrome pregnancies. Twin Res. **1**(2): 89 (abstr. 036), 1998a.

Van Gemert, M.J.C., Zondervan, H.A., Scherjon, S.A. and Nikkels, P.J.G.: Is there a rationale for laser or amniocentesis in twin-twin transfusion syndrome pregnancies? Twin Res. **1**(2): 90 (abstr. 037), 1998b.

Van Gemert, M.J.C., Major, A.L. and Scherjon, S.A.: Placental anatomy, fetal demise and therapeutic intervention in monochorionic twins and the transfusion syndrome: new hypotheses. Eur. J. Obstet. Gynecol. Reprod. Biol. **78**:53–62, 1998c.

Van Gemert, M.J.C., Wijngaard, J.P.H.M.v.d., Vries, H.R. de and Nikkels, P.G.J.: Invited comments on the paper by M.J.O. Taylor, D. Talbert & N.M. Fisk. Pseudo-arterio-arterial anastomoses in twin-twin transfusion syndrome. Placenta **25**:742–747, 2004. Placenta **25**:748–751, 2004.

Van Verschuer, O.: Ein Fall von Monochorie bei zweieiigen Zwillingen. Münch. Med. Wochenschr. **72**:184, 1925.

Van Verschuer, O.: Die vererbungsbiologische Zwillingsforschung: Ihre biologischen Grundlagen: Studien an 102 eineiigen und 45 gleichgeschlechtlichen zweieiigen Zwillings- und 2 Drillingspaaren. Ergebn. Inn. Med. Kinderheilk. **31**:35–120, 1927.

Vayssière, C.F., Heim, N., Camus, E.P., Hillion, Y.E. and Nisand, I.F.: Determination of chorionicity in twin gestations by high-frequency abdominal ultrasonography: counting the layers of the dividing membrane. Amer. J. Obstet. Gynecol. **175**:1529–1533, 1996.

Verger, P., Martin, CL. and Cardinaud, M.-C.: Anémie-polygobulie des jumeaux univitellins et transfusion foeto-foetale. Pediatrie **18**:533–541, 1963.

Verma, R.S., Luke, S. and Dhawan, P.: Twins with different fathers. Lancet **339**:63–64, 1992.

Vermelin, H. and Ribon, M.: Quoted from Corner, G.W. (1955).

Vermesh, M. and Kletzky, O.A.: Follicle-stimulating hormone is the main determinant of follicular recruitment and development in ovulation induction with human menopausal gonadotropin. Amer. J. Obstet. Gynecol. **157**:1397–402, 1987.

Vestergaard, P.: Triplets pregnancy with a normal foetus and dicephalus dibrachius sirenomelus. Acta Obstet. Gynecol. Scand. **51**:93–94, 1972,

Vetter, K. and Schneider, K.T.M.: Iatrogenous remission of twin transfusion syndrome. Amer. J. Obstet. Gynecol. **158**:221, 1988.

Vidaeff, A.C., Racowsky, C. and Rayburn, W.F.: Blastocyst transfer in human in vitro fertilization. A solution to the multiple pregnancy epidemic. J. Reprod. Med. **45**:529–539, 2000. (Discussion pp. 539–540).

Viljoen, D.L., Nelson, M.M. and Beighton, P.: The epidemiology of conjoined twinning in Southern Africa. Clin. Genet. **24**:15–21, 1983.

Ville, Y., Hecher, K., Ogg, D., Warren, R. and Nicolaides, K.: Successful outcome after Nd:Yag laser separation of chorio-angiopagus-twins under sonoendoscopic control. Ultrasound Obstet. Gynecol. **2**:429–431, 1992.

Ville, Y., Hyett, J., Hecher, K. and Nicolaides, K.: Preliminary experience with endoscopic laser surgery for severe twin-twin transfusion syndrome. NEJM **332**:224–227, 1995.

Ville, Y., Hecher, K., Gagnon, A., Sebire, N., Hyett, J. and Nicolaides, K.: Endoscopic laser coagulation in the management of severe twin-to-twin transfusion syndrome. Br. J. Obstet. Gynaecol. **105**:446–453, 1998.

Vlietinck, R., Derom, C., Derom, R., van der Berghe, H. and Thiery, M.: The validity of Weinberg's rule in the East Flanders prospective twin survey (EFPTS). Acta Genet. Med. Gemellol. **37**:137–141, 1988.

Wachtel, S.S., Somkuti, S.G. and Schinfeld, J.S.: Monozygotic twins of opposite sex. Cytogenet. Cell Genet. **91**:293–295, 2000.

Walker, N.F.: Determination of the zygosity of twins. Acta Genet. (Basel) **7**:33–38, 1957.

Walters, D. and Whitehead, D.: Monoamniotic twin pregnancy. Amer. J. Obstet. Gynecol. **73**:1129–1131, 1957.

Wan, Y.-J., Wu, T.-C. and Damjanov, I.: Twinning and conjoined placentation in mice. J. Exp. Zool. **221**:81–86, 1982.

Wapner, R.J., Davis, G.H., Johnson, A., Weinblatt, V.J., Fischer, R.L., Jackson, L.G., Chervenak, F.A. and McCullough, L.B.: Selective reduction of multifetal pregnancies. Lancet **335**:90–93, 1990.

Wataganara, T., Gratacos, E., Jani, J., Becker, J., Lewi, L., Sullivan, L.M., Nianchi, D.W. and Deprest, J.A.: Persistent elevation of cell-free fetal DNA levels in maternal plasma after selective laser coagulation of chorionic plate anastomoses in severe midgestational twin-twin transfusion syndrome. Amer. J. Obstet. Gynecol. **192**:604–609, 2005.

Wax, J.R., Steinfeld, J.D. and Ingardia, C.J.: Fetal triploidy: a unique cause of the stuck twin sign. Obstet. Gynecol. **92**:714, 1998.

Wedberg, R., Kaplan, C., Leopold, G., Porreco, R., Resnik, R. and Benirschke, K.: Cephalothoracopagus (janiceps) twinning. Obstet. Gynecol. **54**:390–396, 1979.

Wee, L.Y., Taylor, M., Watkins, N., Franke, V., Parker, K. and Fisk, N.M.: Characterisation of deep arterio-venous anastomoses within monochorionic placenta by vascular casting. Placenta **26**:19–24, 2005.

Wei, P.Y. and Lin, C.C.: Incidence of twin births among the Chinese in Taiwan. Amer. J. Obstet. Gynecol. **98**:881–884, 1967.

Weinberg, W.: Beiträge zur Physiologie und Pathologie der Mehrlingsgeburten beim Menschen. Pflügers Arch. **88**:346–430, 1901.

Weinberg, W.: Die Anlage zur Mehrlingsgeburt beim Menschen und ihre Vererbung. Arch. Rass. Ges. Biol. **6**:322–339, 470–482, 609–630, 1909.

Weiner, C.P.: Diagnosis and treatment of twin to twin transfusion in the mid-trimester of pregnancy. Fetal Ther. **2**:71–74, 1987.

Weiner, C.P. and Ludomirski, A.: Diagnosis, pathophysiology, and treatment of chronic twin-to-twin transfusion syndrome. Fetal Diagn. **9**:283–290, 1994.

Weiner, J.: Selective first-trimester termination in octuplet and quadruplet pregnancies: clinical and ethical issues. Obstet. Gynecol. **72**:821, 1988.

Weir, P.E., Ratten, G.J. and Beischer, N.A.: Acute polyhydramnios—a complication of monozygous twin pregnancy. Br. J. Obstet. Gynaecol. **86**:849–853, 1979.

Weiss, D.B., Aboulafia, Y. and Isachson, M.: Gastroschisis and fetus papyraceus in double ovum twins. Harefuah **91**:392–394, 1976.

Wenner, R.: Les examens vasculaires des placentas gemellaires et le diagnostic des jumeaux homozygotes. Bull. Soc. R. Belge Gynecol. Obstet. **26**:773–783, 1956.

Wensinger, J.A. and Daly, R.F.: Monoamniotic twins. Amer. J. Obstet. Gynecol. **83**:1254–1256, 1962.

Wenstrom, K.D.: Midtrimester selective delivery of an acardiac twin. (Letter to Editor). Amer. J. Obstet. Gynecol. **168**:1647, 1993.

Wenstrom, K.D., Tessen, J.A., Zlatnik, F.J. and Sipes, S.L.: Frequency, distribution, and theoretical mechanisms of hematologic and weight discordance in monochorionic twins. Obstet. Gynecol. **80**:257–261, 1992.

Weston, P.A., Ives, E.J., Honoré, R.L.H., Lees, G.M., Sinclair, D.B. and Schiff, D.: Monochorionic diamniotic minimally conjoined twins: a case report. Amer. J. Med. Genet. **37**:558–561, 1990.

Westover, T., Guzman, E.R. and Shen-Schwarz, S.: Prenatal diagnosis of an unusual nuchal cord complication in monoamniotic twins. Obstet. Gynecol. **84**:689–691, 1994.

Wharton, B., Edwards, J.H. and Cameron, A.H.: Monoamniotic twins. J. Obstet. Gynaecol. Br. Commonw. **75**:158–163, 1968.

White, C. and Wyshak, G.: Inheritance in human dizygotic twinning. NEJM **271**:1003–1006, 1964.

Whitehouse, D.B.: Mono-amniotic twins with one blighted. J. Obstet. Gynaecol. Brit. Emp. **62**:610–611, 1955.

Whitehouse, D.B.B. and Kohler, H.G.: Vasa previa in twin pregnancy. J. Obstet. Gynaecol. Br. Emp. **67**:281–283, 1960.

Wiegenstein, L. and Iozzo, R.V.: Unusual findings in a conjoined ("Siamese") twin placenta. Amer. J. Obstet. Gynecol. **137**:744–745, 1980.

Willadsen, S.M.: A method for culture of micromanipulated sheep embryos and its use to produce monozygotic twins. Nature **277**:298–300, 1979.

Williams, J.W.: Note on placentation in quadruplet and triplet pregnancy. Bull. Johns Hopkins Hosp. **39**:271–280, 1926.

Willis, R.: The Borderland of Embryology and Pathology. Butterworth, London, 1958.

Wilson, J.K.: Mono-amniotic multiple pregnancy: a report of five new cases. J. Obstet. Gynaecol. Br. Emp. 62:605–609, 1955.

Wilson, R.S.: Twin growth: initial deficit, recovery, and trends in concordance from birth to nine years. Ann. Hum. Biol. 6:205–220, 1979.

Winn, H.N., Gabrielli, S., Reece, E.A., Roberts, J.A., Salafia, C. and Hobbins, J.C.: Ultrasonographic criteria for the prenatal diagnosis of placental chorionicity in twin gestations. Amer. J. Obstet. Gynecol. 161:1540–1542, 1989.

Winner, W.: Parabiotic syndrome. NEJM 269:1043, 1963.

Winsor, E.J.T., Brown, B.S.J., Luther, E.R., Heifetz, S. and Welch, J.P.: Deceased co-twin as a cause of false positive amniotic fluid AFP and AChE. Prenat. Diagn. 7:485–489, 1987.

Witschi, E.: Appearance of accessory "organizers" in overripe eggs of the frog. Proc. Soc. Exp. Biol. Med. 31:419–420, 1934.

Wittmann, B.K., Baldwin, V.J. and Nichol, B.: Antenatal diagnosis of twin transfusion syndrome by ultrasound. Obstet. Gynecol. 58:123–127, 1981.

Wittmann, B.K., Farquharson, D.F., Thomas, W.D.S., Baldwin, V.J. and Wadsworth, L.D.: The role of feticide in the management of severe twin transfusion syndrome. Amer. J. Obstet. Gynecol. 155:1023–1026, 1986.

Wittmann, B.K., Farquharson, D., Wong, G.P., Baldwin, V., Wadsworth, L.D. and Elit, L.: Delayed delivery of second twin: report of four cases and review of the literature. Obstet. Gynecol. 79:260–263, 1992.

Wolf, H.K., Macdonald, J. and Bradford, W.B: Acardius anceps with evidence of intrauterine vascular occlusion: report of a case and discussion of the pathogenesis. Pediatr. Pathol. 11:143–152, 1991.

Wolf, P.L., Jones, K.L., Longway, S.R., Benirschke, K. and Bloor, C.: Prenatal death from acute myocardial infarction and cardiac tamponade due to embolus from the placenta. Amer. Heart J. 109:603–605, 1985.

Wolf, W.: Zwei neue Fälle monoamniotischer Zwillinge. Inaug. Diss. Leipzig, 1920. (Quoted by v. Verschuer, O.: Die vererbungsbiologische Zwillingsforschung. Ergebn. Inn. Med. Kinderheilk. 31:35, 1927.)

Wood, S.L., Onge, R.St., Connors, G. and Elliott, P.D.: Evaluation of the twin peak or lambda sign in determining chorionicity in multiple pregnancy. Obstet. Gynecol. 88:6–9, 1996.

Wurzbach, F.A. and Bunkin, I.A.: Unilateral acute hydramnios in uniovular twin pregnancy. J. Obstet. Gynaecol. Br. Emp. 56:242–245, 1949.

Wylin, R.: Acardiac monster in a triplet pregnancy. J. Reprod. Med. 6:29–32, 1971.

Yamagishi, H., Ishii, C., Maeda, J., Kojima, Y., Matsuoka, R., Kimura, M., Takao, A., Momma, K. and Matsuo, N.: Phenotypic discordance in monozygotic twins with 22q11.2 deletion. Amer. J. Med. Genet. 78:319–321, 1998.

Yaron, Y., Bryant-Greenwood, P.K., Dave, N., Moldenhauer, J.S., Kramer, R.L., Johnson, M.P. and Evans, M.I.: Multifetal pregnancy reductions of triplets to twins: comparison with nonreduced triplets and twins. Amer. J. Obstet. Gynecol. 180:1268–1271, 1999.

Yoshida, K.: Absence of one umbilical artery in twins. Twin Res. 1(2):116 (abstr. 142), 1998.

Yoshida, K. and Soma, H.: Outcome of the surviving cotwin of a fetus papyraceus or of a dead baby. Acta Genet. Med. Gemellol. 35:91–98, 1986.

Yoshioka, H., Kadomoto, Y., Mino, M., Morikawa, Y, Kasabuchi, Y. and Kusunoki, T.: Multicystic encephalomalacia in liveborn twin with a stillborn macerated co-twin. J. Pediatr. 95:798–800, 1979.

Young, B.K., Suidan, J., Antoine, C., Silverman, F., Lustig, I. and Wasserman, J.: Differences in twins: the importance of birth order. Amer. J. Obstet. Gynecol. 151:915–921, 1985.

Young, P.E., Carson, K.F., Prichard, L.L. and Jones, O.W.: A technique for obtaining precise chromosome and bilirubin studies on amniotic fluid in twin pregnancy. J. Reprod. Med. 13:163–166, 1974.

Yu, N., Kruskall, M.S., Yunis, J.J., Knoll, J.H.M., Uhl, L., Alosco, S., Ohashi, M., Clavijo, O., Husain, Z., Yunis, E.J., Yunis, J.J. and Yunis, E.J.: Disputed maternity leading to identification of tetragametic chimerism. NEJM 346:1545–1544, 2002.

Zaw, W. and Stone, D.G.: Caudal regression syndrome in twin pregnancy with type II diabetes. J. Perinatol. 22:171–174, 2002.

Zeilmaker, G.H., Alberda, A.TH. and Gent, I.v.: Fertilization and cleavage of oocytes from binovular human ovarian follicle: a possible cause of dizygotic twinning and chimerism. Fertil. Steril. 40:841–843, 1983.

Zervoudakis, I.A., Lauersen, N.H. and Saary, Z.: Unusual twin pregnancy in a double uterus. Amer. J. Obstet. Gynecol. 124:659–661, 1976.

Ziomek, C.A. and Johnson, M.H.: The roles of phenotype and position in guiding the fate of 16—cell mouse blastomeres. Dev. Biol. 91:440–447, 1982.

Zorlu, C.G., Yalçin, Çaglar, T. and Gökmen, O.: Conservative management of twin pregnancies with one dead fetus: Is it safe? Acta Obstet. Gynecol. Scand. 76:128–130, 1997.

Zucchini, S., Borghesani, F., Soffriti, G., Chirico, C., Vultaggio, E. and Di Donato, P.: Transvaginal ultrasound diagnosis of twin reversed arterial perfusion syndrome at 9 weeks gestation. Ultrasound Obstet. Gynecol. 3:209–211, 1993.

Zuckerman, H. and Brzezinski, A.: Monoamniotic twin pregnancy: report of two cases with review of the literature. Gynaecologia 150:290–298, 1960.

Zuelzer, W.W., Beattie, K.M. and Reisman, L.E.: Generalized unbalanced mosaicism attributable to dispermy and probable fertilization of a polar body. Amer. J. Hum. Genet. 16:38–51, 1964.

26
Legal Considerations

Numerous litigations against hospitals and obstetricians take place in which the placental findings become an important participant in advising the disputing parties on perinatal circumstances. These litigations are initiated most often on behalf of children with cerebral palsy, occasionally with malformations, stillbirth, or with other less than optimal or expected outcomes (Rosenblatt & Hurst, 1989; Richards & Thomasson, 1992). Record keeping of the clinical circumstances and a professional placental study prove to be of great importance in many cases. Weinstein (1988), who wrote a concise review on the topic, asserted that such litigation is principally the result of the following:

1. Society's belief that all wrongs must have a reason and that the wrongs must be put right
2. The pervasive lottery mentality
3. The inability of many individuals to accept responsibility for themselves or their actions
4. An increasing incidence of true medical negligence

Many physicians who have become involved in this legal process in one way or another have witnessed that Weinstein's third point is now common reality. Physicians frequently take care of pregnant patients who continue the use of alcohol and tobacco during pregnancy despite many personal or public warnings against it. Other pregnant patients abuse themselves with cocaine, crack, and other agents and thus endanger their fetuses simultaneously. This aspect of modern society was discussed in an incisive paper on wrongful births by Fleischer (1987). Unfortunately, these facts are rarely taken into serious consideration when malpractice claims are litigated, or they are casually dismissed as not likely to be contributory. Other physicians argue that the fourth of the above statements is incorrect; they believe that there has been no true increase of medical malpractice—only the lawsuits that claim it to be true have increased. Sandmire (1989) provided cogent evidence for this view. No doubt, there has been an increase in the overall incidence of cerebral palsy as a result of the increasingly smaller babies for whom care is provided (Anonymous, 1989; Kuban & Leviton, 1994). Moreover, with increased usage of fertility assistance, more multiple births occur prematurely, and older woman have children, factors that are of importance in the determination of palsy. Conversely, older causes of cerebral palsy-like conditions, such as kernicterus, have all but disappeared, and fewer term babies now suffer this fate. But the oversimplified allegations of intrapartum hypoxia and its blanket alleged relationship to neonatal pH or Apgar score and the ultimate infant performance are often incorrectly assessed, and assumption of negligence or guilt on the part of a perinatologist is frequently not justified. The understanding of how cerebral palsy develops is still imperfect, but it is under intense scrutiny in important studies by Depp (1995) and Marin-Padilla (1997). Some aspects have been reviewed by Nelson and Leviton (1991), and others by Kuban and Leviton (1994), but cases such as the one described by Lopez-Zeno et al. (1990) should always be remembered before hasty conclusions on etiology are drawn. These authors observed the survival of a normal child, delivered by cesarean section 22 minutes after maternal cardiac arrest had occurred, which was 45 minutes after the fatal shooting occurred. Follow-up failed to show neurologic damage; the placenta was not described. This complete anoxia that was incurred by this fetus is much longer and certainly more severe than is the case for many alleged cerebral palsy hypoxia cases. Thus, careful evaluation is indicated. In a thoughtful review, Perkins (1987) examined this very complex field. It should be required reading before unwarranted conclusions are drawn. It is especially noteworthy that Perkins concluded that "the number of infants injured before labor is highly underestimated," whereas that "of infants injured during labor is highly overestimated." The placental record can help materially in sorting out these discrepancies.

"The examination of the placenta may be viewed as a diary of the pregnancy," as Gillan (1992) has aptly stated, and the placenta, therefore, has become an increasingly important organ in adjudicating medicolegal allegations (Benirschke, 1990, 1996; Kaplan, 1995). The recognition that placental examination can be of material help in adjudicating perinatal asphyxia litigations has even been recognized by the legal profession. Schindler (1991) concluded that defense verdicts were issued in the 12 cases in which both the placenta and the cord were available for presentation at court. A monograph by Fisher (1996) on risk management techniques in perinatal and neonatal practice asserts the same view. Regrettably, this aspect was not considered in the last review on cerebral palsy by Kuban and Leviton (1994). Even now, the principal reason for submitting a placenta to the scrutiny of the pathologist remains that it comes from a surgical intervention (Booth et al., 1997). This makes little sense in that a large number of such interventions are routine repeat cesarean section deliveries, not the potentially fetus-endangering gestations. Altshuler and Herman (1989) reviewed the specific needs to be addressed by pathologists, and they also considered some of the epidemiologic principles in an incisive review of this medicolegal topic. Of particular interest is their capsular review of relevant pathologic features of the placenta and the possible correlations of lesions with fetal hypoxic states. They were correct in reiterating that the placenta "is an objective diary, related to the outcome of pregnancy." Later, Altshuler (1993a,b, 1999) wrote three incisive reviews of the principal lesions of the placenta that may be of paramount importance in reflecting a prenatal onset of hypoxic insults. These papers suggested that the presence of nucleated red blood cells at term, chronic villitis, meconium damage, excessive fibrin deposits, chorioamnionitis, chorangiosis, and "placental dysmaturity" are the most important aspects to be considered in this context. These papers also provide a triage for placental study, and the third paper (Altshuler, 1999) is directed to nonpathologists as well. Furthermore, an important meeting of pathologists, perinatologists, and the legal profession resulted in a volume that attempts to address the complexity of the medicolegal aspects of placental pathology (Travers & Schmidt, 1991; Langston et al., 1997). More quantitative data to ensure that pathologic interpretations by different pathologists are meaningful can be found in Beebe et al. (2000).

The pathologist is often consulted to render specific advice on pathologic findings and on other perinatal aspects of pregnancies with poor outcomes. This consultation prominently includes considerations of findings made at placental examinations. All too often, however, the placental material available is insufficient for an expert opinion. Recommendations are made here about how to collect placentas for such possible need of the future. Altshuler and Herman (1989) suggested that one should briefly record findings from placental examination of all deliveries because cerebral palsy may also occur

with entirely normal deliveries. We agree with this view but found it to be an impractical task for most hospitals. To have placental material available for possible future study, the authors also suggested that formalin-fixed samples be embedded in paraffin and archived as uncut specimens. In our view, the value accruing to the child and pediatrician from an examination of the placenta at the time of delivery supersedes the storage of unexamined material.

It is particularly regrettable, as happens occasionally, that erroneous testimony is given in best faith because the consultants have not properly evaluated the entire facts of a given case. They may have reviewed only the slides without knowing the gross findings of the placenta, for instance, and may have based their opinions solely on those histologic findings that were available, whereas detailed study of perinatal circumstances might have provided a more educated judgment. Pathologists should not be put into the position of making judgments on monitor strips and the like. They must, however, have a general idea of the entirety of these complex cases before the placental examination can be meaningfully interpreted. Even more unfortunate still is testimony by "experts" who have little experience in placental pathology. Likewise, pathologists must be mindful not to render expert opinions on areas that are outside of their field of competence, for instance regarding the findings of heart rate monitoring.

Litigation has had an impact on the practice of perinatal medicine, without having much improved our knowledge of the cause(s) of cerebral palsy. But because the placental study often provides significant insight into prenatal life, it has become apparent to many health care providers that, when caring for problematic neonates or when difficulties in labor and delivery are encountered, the placenta should be examined professionally.

The notion that it is imperative to examine the placenta, if only to establish the cause of perinatal deaths, is not new. For instance, in efforts to understand the causes of fetal demise, Davies and Arroyo (1985) were able to ascertain the cause of perinatal death by autopsy alone in 47.6% of their cases. For the purpose of ascribing a cause of death, however, placental study was necessary in an additional 34% of their cases. We have reviewed our material of perinatal autopsies over 2 years and found that the true cause of perinatal death could not be established in 15.6% of the cases (Fig. 26.1). Thrombosis of vessels (Kraus, 1997), maternal floor infarct, villitis, and abruptio placentae are major reasons in singletons why the placenta must be studied. Driscoll (1965) found it also to be true for 16% of her case material; Salafia and Vintzileos (1990) were equally emphatic about the need to examine all placentas.

If the cause of perinatal mortality is strongly corroborated by placental findings, the same is likely to be true

Figure 26.1. Perinatal autopsy findings in 122 consecutive cases (University of California, San Diego, 1981 to 1982). Placental examination was necessary in 19 (16%) to provide the cause of death. In many others, especially the premature infants and anomalies, there were abnormal placental findings such as inflammation and single umbilical artery, but these were not the *cause* of death. HMS, hyaline membrane syndrome.

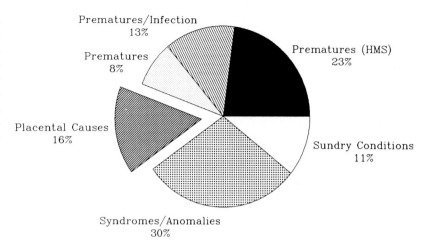

Prematures/Infection 13%

Prematures 8%

Placental Causes 16%

Prematures (HMS) 23%

Sundry Conditions 11%

Syndromes/Anomalies 30%

of possible perinatal fetal or neonatal damage, making the examination of this organ all the more mandatory. So that one may have the placentas of neonates with developing problems available for study, suggestions were made in Chapter 1 how best to store placentas. This triage for the selection and other related aspects of placental study were well detailed in tabular form by Altshuler (1993a,b). Aside from the aspect of placental storage, to facilitate examination of the placenta in cases of possible neonatal difficulties, it is our opinion that all placentas of twins, those of premature infants, and of deliveries in which meconium staining or other obvious perinatal problems are apparent should be studied by the pathologist. It is imperative that these findings then also become an entry in the patient's record. This practice is not only desirable for adjudicating many legal cases in which placental pathology can be helpful, but it may materially assist the obstetrician when counseling about future pregnancies and in the accumulation of data that may ultimately help our understanding of perinatal problems.

We have often wished in legal consults that a photograph of the placenta was available, particularly when confronted with the record of a poorly described or inadequately studied placenta. This desire has been made light of in litigations, but photography can be easily accomplished on delivery floors, where pictures of neonates are taken routinely. This has also been advocated for regions where pathologic support is inadequate (Ward, 1991). If photography is impractical, a drawing of salient findings, for example, to indicate the insertion of the umbilical cord or the presence of twin vascular anastomoses, is often more helpful than a poor description of the gross features. Ideally, all placentas would have an examination by a knowledgeable pathologist, but this is not likely to happen routinely. Those placentas that are studied, however, must be adequately sampled for histology. At least three sections of villous tissue plus at least one of cord and at least one membrane roll are optimal. When selecting the villous tissue, it is important that

more than the obviously infarcted or pathologic areas are sampled; most infarcts look alike microscopically. An estimate of the percentage of the villous tissue involved with a gross lesion or lesions is most helpful. For an appreciation of the placental status, for example, for the identification of Tenney-Parker changes in preeclampsia or chorangiosis and villitis, the more normal-appearing villous tissue is usually more informative than are sections of infarcts. In the membrane roll, the decidua capsularis must be included, as it is the best site for an analysis of maternal vessel pathology and for the appreciation of inflammatory processes. Formalin fixation of placentas before examination provides much less valuable information than the examination of a fresh organ. The sooner the placenta is studied, the better the results; however, storage in a refrigerator preserves the salient feature for many days. There is little autolysis when the placenta is refrigerated; it only loses some weight during storage by extrusion of villous water, particularly edematous organs. The pathologist must also become familiar with the artifacts produced by fixation, especially being cognizant of changes in weight after fixation (the weight increases).

As stated earlier, litigation has involved, most importantly, deliveries in which cerebral palsy became a problem in the future development of an infant. This is, in general, much more common in prematurely born infants, in multiple pregnancy, and in infants who come from prolonged pregnancies. The study of the causes of cerebral palsy is a difficult aspect of medicine, as no single etiology can possibly be assigned, despite the efforts expended in the large, prospective Collaborative Perinatal Study. Rosen and Dickinson (1992) estimated that 2.7 per 1000 children age 5 to 7 years suffered a form of this illness. Nearly 36% occurred in children with birth weights of less than 2500 g, and the authors suggested that 70% had an antenatal onset. Interestingly, Rosen and Dickinson (1993) provided evidence that electronic fetal monitoring was unable to predict the development of cerebral palsy, even though this had been the original intent for this technology. Nelson et al. (1996) also examined in a very large population whether heart rate abnormalities correlated with the development of cerebral palsy. They also found a high degree of unreliability of this procedure and indicated that, were reliance principally based on irregular heart monitor findings, an excessive and unwarranted cesarean section rate would follow. Other authors have related similar views, although employing different criteria (Yudkin et al., 1994; Depp, 1995; Goodlin, 1995; Lien et al., 1995). Because they have little relation to placental pathology, they are not discussed here, but the interested reader will want to review these contributions as well. Naeye and Peters (1987) examined the 7-year outcome of children from the aforementioned large Collaborative Perinatal Study of 56,000 pregnancies. Their overriding conclusion was that chronic, rather than acute, hypoxia has a greater influence in causing abnormal brain development (see comments by Harkavy, 1987, and those by Durant and Woodward, 1987). This study, as many others, well demonstrated how complex is the topic of the cause of cerebral palsy (see also Naeye et al., 1989; Naeye, 1992). The two reviews of Altshuler (1993a,b) cited many additional studies that should be consulted by the reader who wishes to obtain a well-rounded appreciation of this complex topic. At the same time, cerebral palsy also has great social and medical importance; the disease often represents a major tragedy to the families involved and to the child. One of the most thoughtful reviews of this complexity was provided by Perkins (1987). Additional studies from Australia were summarized in the Collaborative Perinatal Study involving 608 children reported by Aylward et al. (1989). These authors also found only weak correlations to perinatal variables. Their instructive tables showed impressively that many time-honored indicators of asphyxia have little or no bearing on cerebral outcome of the neonate. Regrettably, items such as meconium staining and many more conditions of concern were not studied. Grant et al. (1989) also concluded from their randomized study of the benefits possibly coming from intrapartum monitoring that prevention of cerebral palsy is difficult. This study and others have been succinctly annotated in editorial comments (Anonymous, 1989; Freeman, 1990).

The findings made during a competent placental examination, including histologic study frequently identify abnormal prenatal circumstances that had not been recognized clinically. Grafe (1994) made the same point after correlating placental pathology with central nervous system (CNS) necrosis, hemorrhage, and gliosis. In a large study that correlated placental features with perinatal asphyxia, Beebe et al. (1996) sought to identify specific features that were more important. Villous ischemic changes, meconium damage, and chorioamnionitis stood out as most important. Nevertheless, the authors urged that long-term follow-up is needed to ascertain precisely what the impact of certain lesions may have been. Thus, results from placental studies have often materially aided in advising the legal profession accurately. For the purpose of this chapter, we will summarize salient points that have come from our experience in this arena. More details on the conditions to be described are to be found in the relevant sections of this book. It must be reemphasized that an interpretation of the placenta alone is often insufficient to arrive at a full appreciation of the complexity of individual cases. It is frequently necessary to know many other factors than only the placental findings in order to render appropriate advice. For instance, one may need to know the identity of microorganisms in infectious cases, etc. The social history may be of considerable importance, and an accurate estimation of the length of gestation, the complications known to have occurred during pregnancy, and so on must all be weighed in the context of the placental findings. These items give valuable information with which one is in a better position to interpret subtle placental findings. Reviewed here are only some of the more common placental problems that we have encountered, and observations we have made in litigation proceedings.

Twinning Problems

Placentas from twins provide the pathologist with the unique opportunity to compare different placental features with neonatal outcome. Thus, the fetus accompanied by a velamentous insertion of the umbilical cord is usually more growth-restricted than one with a normal cord and is thus uniquely exposed also to the prenatal hazards of anomalous cord insertion. Multiple births also have not only a much higher incidence of prematurity but they also suffer a manifold increased frequency of cerebral palsy compared with singletons. Studies have suggested that some of these cerebral lesions may have a prenatal onset because cystic areas of former white matter necrosis can be evident at birth (Bejar et al., 1990). Larroche (1986) described a case that also demonstrated these prenatal lesions; she found other cases of prenatal encephalopathies with trauma and other prenatal events. Central nervous system damage of prenatal onset appears to be commoner in monozygotic, monochorionic twins than in dizygotic multiples. It is therefore imperative that the membrane relation of all twins be firmly established at the time of delivery or during placental study, if one wants to understand the origin of the lesions. This point is particularly important when one twin has died prenatally. Coagulative, destructive events in the survivor are then especially common and these are usually confined to monochorionic twins. They generally have a prenatal onset, as sonographic studies have clearly shown (Patten et al., 1989), and commence soon after the death of one fetus (Liu et al., 1992; Benirschke, 1993). A particularly illustrative case with which we have had personal connection demonstrates clearly how such problems may be inaccurately adjudicated. It was superbly summarized in a book by Werth (1998).

As stated earlier, monochorionic twins not only have a higher rate of prematurity but they suffer perinatal mortality more frequently (Baldwin, 1994). The highest mortality attends monoamnionic twins. Monoamnionic/ monochorionic (MoMo) twins entangle their cords frequently and this may cause restrictions to venous return from the placenta. This complication often kills one or both fetuses; in others one can infer venous return problems from existing thrombi. Further, vascular anastomoses between twins may allow rapid shifts of blood from one twin to the other, which may lead to acute anemia and hypotension in utero. Neonatal anemia seen in one of twins, where the other had recently died in utero has been difficult to interpret prior to detailed placental studies. It goes without saying that the umbilical cords of twins must be labeled at delivery, so that it becomes possible to assign specific placental lesions to individual infants. It is also necessary to identify and record the presence of a fetus papyraceus, as it may have great relevance in affecting the development of the surviving twin through interplacental vascular anastomoses. Perhaps the cause of the death of one twin was sublethal to the other.

Inflammatory processes also have an important impact on fetal well-being and they are frequently correlated with cerebral palsy. As was discussed in some detail in the consideration of infections (Chapter 20), in twins, chorioamnionitis much more often affects twin A, that is to say the twin closest to the cervical os. When one has knowledge of the location of twins in utero, this may lead to a better appreciation of possible aspiration pneumonia and other fetal effects.

Twins have a high frequency of velamentous and marginal insertion of their umbilical cords, and these insertional abnormalities are often correlated with single umbilical artery. The membranous vessels may have ruptured during delivery and have caused acute anemia, or they may be thrombosed, which often produces dire fetal sequelae. Cords with a single umbilical artery are more common in twins, and not only when the cords are marginally inserted. When twins are delivered by cesarean section, the twin located in the lower uterine segment may actually be delivered as the second twin. Therefore, recording the distance of membrane rupture from the edge of the placenta aids in assigning the correct position of twins in utero when labeling of cords is inadequate. This point has particular relevance with respect to inflammation and to the possible rupture of velamentous vessels.

Twins with velamentous insertion of the umbilical cord are usually smaller than those with more normal cord

position. Such discrepancy in size does not automatically affirm the diagnosis of the transfusion syndrome, as is all too readily done; that diagnosis requires the demonstration of the responsible arteriovenous (AV) shunts in the monochorionic twin placenta. The twin-to-twin transfusion syndrome (TTTS) is a most important aspect of monozygotic twinning. It is largely responsible for the frequent occurrence of hydramnios in twin pregnancy that leads to the high frequency of premature delivery of monochorionic twins. Although anemia and plethora of the neonatal twins may be obvious, this finding alone does not accurately attest to the underlying cause, the presence of an AV fistula in the placenta. Plethora can occur in one twin when for instance the first-born twin has been allowed to drain blood into the second, while this one was still in utero. This is sometimes referred to as acute rather than chronic twin-to-twin transfusion. A surviving twin also may partially and acutely exsanguinate into a stillborn twin while in utero, with resulting acute hypotension. Knowledge of the time when clamping of the cords was done may also be important when interpreting discordant hemoglobin values of twins. When one twin is small for gestational age, possibly because it had a velamentous insertion of the cord, large surface anastomoses may drain blood from the larger twin into the smaller member while still in situ, an apparent paradox to the findings of the transfusion syndrome. But this is not the equivalent of the classical transfusion syndrome. For all these reasons, it is important that the nature of interfetal placental blood vessel anastomoses be ascertained, possibly by injection of the placental vasculature. The findings are best recorded by making a drawing of these connections; they cannot otherwise be readily reconstructed.

Inflammation

As with the cause of some premature monochorionic twins, chorioamnionitis (membranitis) and funisitis are much overrepresented in children who develop cerebral palsy (Redline et al., 1998). These pathologic changes are now clearly established as being the result of ascending infection. They cannot be explained by hypoxia occurring during labor or be assigned to changes in amnionic pH, as had been previously suggested. Infections not only are much more common in premature deliveries, but also are indeed probably a main reason for most premature births before 30 weeks' gestation (see Ornoy et al., 1976, for a consideration of its importance in stillbirths). Ascending infection also correlates with prenatal cystic changes in the brain. Studies have suggested that the hypoxia may be the result of vasoconstriction, engendered by the release of prostaglandins, tumor necrosis factor, or other vasoactive agents that come either from the inflammatory exudate or from bacterial products suspended in the amnionic cavity. Indeed, the current suspicion exists that some cytokines may be the direct cause of cerebral degenerative changes (Yoon et al., 1996).

Culturing the surface of the placenta is usually not so helpful for studying the cause of chorioamnionitis as is a meticulous histologic study. The causative organisms of chorioamnionitis frequently do not grow readily in the laboratory, or they require special microbiologic attention that is not always available. Moreover, the placenta is frequently contaminated by the birth process, making most routine cultures worthless, or the patient has received antibiotics before delivery. It may be more practical to obtain material for culture from underneath the chorionic plate or to make touch preparations of the placental surface for the identification of organisms. Chorioamnionitis is also an occasional cause of thrombosis in fetal surface vessels, which can be identified macroscopically by the appearance of white-yellow streaks on the surfaces of blood vessels. Altshuler and Herman (1989) referred to the mural thrombi as "cushions," following De Sa's (1984) lead (see Chapter 12, Fig. 12.24). They must be sampled for histologic study. Their relevance to medicolegal issues has been well described by Kraus (1997).

When thrombi have developed in large fetal surface vessels, the distal fetal villous vascular bed degenerates, leading to defoliation of vascular endothelium, dispersion of blood, and disorganization of the vessels. It produces the appearance of hemorrhagic endovasculitis (HEV), which we consider to be not an inflammatory process but rather a degenerative one. It is commonly found in the main stem placental vessels of stillborn infants, but this endothelial degeneration has then usually occurred after the fetus's death. Unfortunately, much inappropriate testimony has been given in the past with this confusing entity of HEV, supposedly indicating the existence of an undiagnosed virus infection before birth. Perhaps the most informative finding for an understanding of HEV has come from finding the lesion confined to the placental portion of only the dead MZ twin of a diamnionic/monochorionic (DiMo) twin placenta. The fact that the surviving twin's placental bed did not have HEV nearly invalidates the possible inference that HEV is a specific pathologic finding of prenatal infection. In his study of placentas from stillborn fetuses, Genest (1992) depicted these changes and placed a time frame on their occurrence (see Chapter 12).

Villous tissue should be sampled for microscopy in all cases of a suspected virus infection because it must be admitted that many virus infections are difficult to identify precisely by histopathologic study alone. For instance, the immunodeficiency virus that is responsible for the acquired immunodeficiency syndrome (AIDS) leaves no characteristic alterations in the placenta. Hepatitis, Coxsackie virus infection, and other virus-caused diseases cannot be reliably diagnosed histologically from placental material alone. Therefore, these diseases cannot always be ruled out by placental study alone. Cytomegalovirus (CMV) infection is perhaps the most common prenatal virus infection of relevance to cerebral palsy-type lesions. Significant damage to fetal brain and other organs occurs frequently from CMV infection, and the placenta often shows characteristic alterations. But these changes are frequently widely scattered in the placenta, sometimes affecting only a few villi, and they may be difficult to find. It is one of the reasons why several blocks of villous tissue should be prepared for histologic study. It is probably best to obtain five blocks so as to optimally sample the suspect material. Of considerable importance is the prenatal infection with herpes virus, as it may be responsible for porencephaly and neonatal death. It is commonly assumed that the infection is only acquired during the delivery process and thus cesarean section is often practiced when genital blisters exist. Less well known is that a number of cases have been described in which the infection was acquired before birth and where neonates had blisters from herpes simplex virus (HSV) infection with positive cultures (see Chapter 20). These infants may progress to destructive encephalopathy, and when they come to autopsy, neither culture nor electron microscopy identifies the now vanished agent. For that reason, Schwartz and Caldwell (1991) proposed that in situ DNA hybridization studies be done on placental tissue for the correct diagnosis. Few absolutely specific placental changes of this virus infection exist, although Robb et al. (1986a,b) identified suggestive features.

Premature infants delivered because of chorioamnionitis are often associated with decidual hemorrhage that clinically may give the appearance of an abruptio placentae. This hemorrhage, however, is usually due to bleeding from deciduitis with thrombosis of decidual veins at the placental margins and cannot be compared with the classic abruptio placentae seen with toxemia and trauma.

Villitis of unknown etiology (VUE) is a severe alteration of villi that includes infiltration with T lymphocytes and macrophages but only rarely with plasma cells; it usually leads to destruction of villi. It may be indistinguishable from CMV-induced villitis. Considerable experience may be required to differentiate the two and it may occasionally be impossible without the use of CMV probes. Villitis of unknown etiology definitely reduces the area of placental exchange and is also often associated with fetal death and with growth restriction. The etiology of VUE is unknown at this time, but the dire significance of the entity cannot be in doubt. There are, however, also cases of VUE that have no apparent effect on fetal development. Villitis of unknown etiology has a tendency to recur in future pregnancies. Evaluation of the significance of finding VUE in the placenta of a retarded child may be difficult, and it requires much experience with placental study.

The Green Placenta

The presence of meconium at birth was a frequent reason for alleging that birth was delayed or inappropriately handled in the British examination of obstetrical malpractice claims (Capstick & Edwards, 1990). These authors doubted that preventive measures could avoid the alleged accidents and recommended that attention be paid to the immediate handling of incidents. Interestingly, meconium staining of the placental surface is not only a frequent finding in mature placentas, it is usually not associated with fetal distress or cerebral palsy. In our experience, meconium staining/discharge occurs in about 17% of all births, most often when they occur after 40 weeks' gestation. Almost all neonates are normal. One should also consider the possibility that, when a meconium-stained placenta has been standing unrefrigerated for very many hours, some of the meconium pigment may actually travel slightly into the amnion and it may perhaps even minimally discolor the chorion. Usually, however, this is then also associated with some autolysis of tissues and is thus recognizable by the pathologist as having been artifactually caused. Refrigeration minimizes this problem, an important point, as the legal profession often disputes the age of meconium presence in placental sections. Because of the nature of the hormonal control of the propulsion of intestinal content, meconium staining is more common in postmature organs and it is extremely rare in immature placentas. Some of the legal guidelines pertaining to meconium staining have been examined by Sepkowitz (1987). In his 8-year experience, 4.3% of newborns (1368) were meconium-stained. His further data suggested that, because of legal negotiations, from 1982 to 1985 there was a marked increase in the reported incidence (14.4%) of meconium staining. Therapeutic measures such as laryngoscopy and oxygen administration to the neonate were increased as a consequence of these interventions, but they did not guarantee an overall improvement of the neonatal outcome. The author concluded, "While the issuance of medical guidelines alone had little effect on the incidence and care of the meconium-stained newborn, the combination of the legal imperative with medical guidelines had a profound and corruptive effect."

Prolonged pregnancy is significantly correlated with meconium discharge, as are the complications from its aspiration and other hazards of prolonged pregnancy (Arias, 1987). The results of Arias' study suggested that "the increased incidence of complications in pregnancy prolonged beyond 40 weeks cannot be adequately predicted with antepartum electronic monitoring, and ultrasound evaluation of fetal size, placental grade, and amniotic fluid volume." It is also noteworthy that not all meconium-stained placentas are accompanied by fetal meconium aspiration (Altshuler & Herman, 1989). Sunoo and his colleagues (1989) clearly identified that meconium discharge and aspiration may occur before labor and without evidence of fetal distress. They made a detailed study of 75 cases of meconium aspiration (among 14,527 deliveries) and identified four infants in whom the aspiration occurred during early labor and in whom it was accompanied by normal fetal heart tracings. Postmaturity in itself is also often a reason for litigation when it is associated with a cerebral palsied offspring. Whether these are truly related events remains to be established. But the oligohydramnios and meconium discharge that so often occur after 40 weeks' gestation are often considered to be signs of placental insufficiency, a concept espoused by Vorherr (1975). We have not been impressed that good evidence for placental dysfunction has been identified, and Naeye (1978) agreed with this notion. Thus, a definitive deleterious influence of postmaturity on placental growth and function needs yet to be established.

When a placenta from a premature infant has a green surface, one must consider the possibility that this discoloration is not due to meconium but represents hemosiderin and related precursor pigments. Hemosiderin deposits most frequently accompany the peripheral hemorrhages of circumvallate placentas, but retromembranous hematomas, thromboses, marginal hemorrhage, and fetal hemolysis (after demise) can cause hemosiderin deposits on the placental surface because of hemolysis. An iron stain of the placenta quickly reveals the nature of the pigment when doubt exists. Other discolorations, from brown to green, may be the result of other insults, for instance the infection with fusobacteria. The nature of those pigments is not always understood. Finally, it must be cautioned that the bilirubin pigment of meconium-laden macrophages will bleach when slides lie in sunlight or fluorescent light.

Because meconium is gradually processed in macrophages, moving from the amnionic surface toward the chorion, a rough estimate of the minimum time elapsed between discharge and delivery may be available from microscopic examination of the placental surface; or when the amnion is stripped and the underlying chorion is examined and found to be green at gross examination, an approximate time frame is indicated by the depth of staining. It must be emphasized, however, that this evaluation is subject to a few errors that must be borne in mind when, as is so frequent in giving testimony, one is asked what the probability is for the meconium to have been discharged at such and such a time. And in our estimation these parameters are not really decisive in understanding cerebral palsy anyway; rather, it may be the *consequences* of meconium discharge that are relevant. Furthermore, meconium may have been discharged days before delivery, and most of it may already have been transported away from the fetal surface when the placenta becomes available for study. It is also probable that repeated meconium discharge can occur in utero, which would be most difficult to discern from placental examination alone. Thus, an estimate of time, based on the only in vitro study of meconium transport, may be misleading (Miller et al., 1985). But that is the best estimate we have at present. It is our opinion that the legal profession is overemphasizing the importance of meconium discharge, without appreciating the complexity of this process and the complex etiology of spastic quadriplegia and other features of cerebral palsy. At the same time, when a damaged infant, even a stillborn, is under consideration and its birth had not been accompanied by meconium discharge, the question why this dead baby was *not* meconium-stained is never asked. Interestingly, most stillbirths we see have no meconium staining, even though, ultimately, anoxia was the cause of their death.

Meconium may be otherwise injurious to the fetal well-being, in part because of its effect on the umbilical circulation. It also causes severe degenerative changes in the vascular walls of the placenta and cord, as it does in the amnionic epithelium. Some evidence now exists to show that vasoconstriction is a consequence of meconium exposure rather than its cause (Altshuler & Hyde, 1989). Thus, although meconium discharge has become the "red flag" in legal cases, in which it is usually suggested that the passage of meconium alone must be evidence of fetal distress, it is more likely that it is the meconium that damages the fetus by acting as a vasoconstrictive agent on the umbilical and superficial placental vessels. In so doing it perhaps reduces the venous return of oxygenated blood from the placenta; of course, there could also be constriction of arteries with reduced blood flow to the placenta (Naeye, 1995). These avenues are now being explored experimentally, but the courtroom treats the association of meconium and cerebral palsy as being causally related as given facts, unjustly in our opinion. Similar suggestions of umbilical cord vessel constriction by bacterial products in the amnionic sac infection syndrome have come from experimental studies by Hyde et al. (1989), and Mazor et al. (1995) found meconium staining and bacterial infection with poor outcomes to be linked. Finally, we speculate that the real damage of the "meconium aspiration syndrome" of neonates may be a chemical injury to the alveolar epithelium, similar to its effect on amnion and cord vessels.

Vascular Abnormalities

Abnormalities of the umbilical cord and placental surface vessels are important findings in placental examinations. It has long been obvious that it is important to record the absence of one umbilical artery, as this frequent finding correlates well with a variety of fetal congenital anomalies and with growth restriction. But it is particularly important also to look for thromboses in the fetal surface vessels of every placenta. Most surface vascular thrombi are evident macroscopically by the yellow-white streak that then accompanies a chorionic vessel, but may not be appreciated by the inexperienced observer. Thrombi are more difficult to spot in the umbilical cord unless the cord is routinely sectioned in areas of discoloration that were not caused by clamping. Thromboses have many causes. They develop usually over a long period, although we have seen fresh, occlusive thrombi in cases of recent cord entanglement with stillbirth. The thrombi definitely point to significant prenatal fetal problems. We find thrombi most frequently to be associated with excessively long and heavily spiraled umbilical cords, less often in association with maternal lupus anticoagulant, and often with chorioamnionitis. Cytomegalovirus infection also has the propensity to affect endothelium and to produce thrombi. Thrombosis of surface vessels may be a feature of diabetes complicating pregnancy and of toxoplasmosis. In banal chorioamnionitis one often finds mural thrombi and occasionally organized thrombi, the so-called cushions. We have reported that thrombi may embolize to the fetus and there they may cause infarcts. However, unless such an infant comes to autopsy, embolic sequelae are usually not evident.

Complete vascular obliteration leads to atrophy of the villous district subserved by the vessel. It is the frequent cause of avascular, apparently hyalinized villi, which may thus reduce the quantity of available "exchange membrane"; for this reason, chronic thrombosis correlates with growth restriction and hypoxia. Some fetal thrombi are found in association with lupus anticoagulant, a condition that must be actively investigated, as it may produce few maternal symptoms. There are additionally many placentas with, at times, extensive thrombosis, in which the etiology of the thrombi remains obscure. Some may well be the result of inherited coagulation disorders and then be associated with CNS damage. This was well delineated by Thorarensen et al. (1990) and speculated upon by Kraus (1997). Relevant studies are now feasible but rarely undertaken. An unknown etiology is particularly true for the arterial thrombi. For the purpose of legal adjudication, it is important to recognize this point and to acknowledge that thrombosis is a long-standing event and that it can usually not be anticipated before birth. We have seen a child with cerebral palsy in whom one umbilical artery was nearly completely occluded by an inflammatory thrombus. The pregnancy was not complicated in any way and, upon arrival at the hospital, a cesarean section was performed for fetal distress immediately. Still, the jury was led to believe that this tragedy could have been averted by better prenatal care, despite having knowledge of the placental findings. Redline (2005) has recently summarized his findings in the pathology of placental vascular lesions (thrombosis, VUE, inflammation, meconium damage) in 125 legal cases and compared these with random placentas. He found a remarkably good correlation of these lesions with neurologic impairment.

Umbilical Cord

Aside from the cord accidents that occur with monoamnionic twins, the cord displays lesions that often have a significant impact on fetal well-being. Green discoloration of the entire Wharton's jelly can be observed only macroscopically, as the relatively small number of cord macrophages in the umbilical cord does not stain prominently. The cord is also often discolored from hemolysis, especially when thrombi are present or when prenatal bleeding has occurred. At the site where the cord has been clamped, hemorrhage is frequent, but it can be distinguished from spontaneous hemorrhage by the marks of the serrated clamps that are left embedded on the cord's surface. We have seen in a child with cerebral palsy that a true cord hematoma had histologic features of an angioma, presumably secondary to its "organization." The mother had been traumatized during pregnancy. The surface of the cord may have tiny granular protuberances from candidal infection. The compression from knots or prolapsed cords may be seen macroscopically. When it is present, there may be marked distention of blood vessels on one side but not the other, betraying the prenatal compromise of the circulation. The presence of knots in the umbilical cord may be of great significance. It may be the cause of death but it also betrays the possibly long existence of an impediment to venous return. Such has at least once been clearly demonstrated in a Doppler flow study of a 23-week fetus whose cord was also wound about its neck (Gembruch & Baschat, 1996). Edematous cords occur in edematous as well as in immature infants, whereas thin cords often accompany growth-restricted infants. Angiomas are rare, but when present they are of great significance. Usually the cord is spiraled. When the twists are especially numerous, the cord is also usually excessively long. That such excessive spiraling can lead to fetal death is not in doubt. Indeed, the remarkable twisting on the fetus's abdominal surface in some abortuses testifies to this lethal effect of twists. More problematic is the chronic effect that may ensue from excessive cord twists. They are often associated with fetal surface vessel (venous) thrombi, and a reduced venous return (with oxygenated blood) from the placenta can be deduced. Future Doppler velocimetry and cordocentesis observations will have to clarify the hemodynamic aspects of cord twists. It is important, however, to be mindful of the correlation of fetal problems with excessively long umbilical cords; thus, an accurate assessment of the complete length of the cord is essential in all placental studies.

Placental Villous Color

Aside from the meconium staining of the fetal surface, the color of the villous tissue is an important notation at placental delivery, especially in problematical cases. The villous tissue is red because of its *fetal* hemoglobin content. Placentas of diabetic mothers are darker because of fetal plethora, and those of immature infants are lighter. Once a number of normal placentas have been examined with this fact in mind, the observer should be able to identify those placentas that are unusually light-colored. They may be from infants with hydrops or, more often, they are associated with infants that had a fetomaternal hemorrhage. In that case, immediate Kleihauer-Betke stains on maternal blood are mandatory. This test is important so that one may estimate the amount of fetal blood loss; it also provides information needed for the therapeutic transfusion that may have to be instituted. Although intervillous thrombi may be noted in these cases, they are not invariably present.

In hydropic infants, the cause of hydrops should be studied as best as possible. The protocol includes mandatory examination of the Rh status plus a search for nucleated red blood cells, for parvovirus inclusions in red blood cell precursors, and for the existence of other fetal infections, such as CMV. There are many other causes of fetal anemia and hydrops. For instance, cardiac arrhythmias often produce hydrops that the pathologist cannot detect at autopsy. These causes are detailed in Chapter 15. Here it is important to stress that the appreciation of an unusually light-colored placenta has relevance for legal purposes as well. Occasional hydropic infants are the result of high-output cardiac failure of the fetus that results from large placental chorioangiomas. They are readily apparent when the placenta is palpated and then sectioned. Neonatal anemia is obvious when a low hemoglobin value is found at neonatal examination. The adjustment of the fetal hematocrit may take some time after fetal blood loss but we have only the most superficial knowledge of how quickly the hematocrits adjust after fetal bleeding—information that would be useful in adjudicating the timing of fetal hemorrhage.

In patients with hepatitis and jaundice, the villous tissue may be a deep golden color, which is often difficult to visualize microscopically and is thus an important macroscopic descriptor. This discoloration also tends to bleach in the histologic slides from office lighting alone.

The maternal surface may be yellow and firmer than normal in a condition known as maternal floor infarction. This condition is strongly correlated with diffuse fibrinoid deposition throughout the placenta and with fetal growth restriction. Some observers have suggested that an increased fibrinoid deposition confirms the diagnosis of prolonged placental perfusion problems, but the maternal floor infarction syndrome has an unknown etiology, although it is a frequent cause of stillbirth. Appropriate histologic study verifies the existence of this condition. Such excessive fibrinoid deposits are frequently a repetitive event in subsequent pregnancies. It has also been associated with adverse perinatal outcome (Adams-Chapman et al., 2002). Contrary to opinions expressed in the literature, this condition is not *caused* by fetal death.

Color changes on the maternal surface and behind the membranes may disclose an unrecognized abruptio placentae. Most cases of placental separation are clinically silent and can be observed only when the maternal surface is carefully scrutinized. A fresh retroplacental hematoma with indentation of the villous tissue is obvious, however, if the hematoma is formed within an hour or so of delivery; the placenta may then appear unaffected. The clot may have dried (in contrast to the "currant jelly" clot of normal retroplacental blood), and it may be stringy and compacted. When placental separation is focal and has occurred long before delivery, the clot may have largely disappeared, or it is replaced by a brown, filmy material. Still older clots leave a greenish (hemosiderin) residue.

Infarcts at the edge of the placenta are common and, when small, are of little significance. Their age can be approximated from their initially red, then yellow, and eventually white color. Infarcts that are scattered throughout the placenta, however, signify maternal disease of some sort. This finding assumes particular importance in prematurely delivered infants in whom infarcts are generally rare. Most commonly, the cause of such infarcts is preeclampsia, but the lesions due to lupus anticoagulant have a similar appearance; and when infarcts are found in the absence of signs of pregnancy toxemia, their cause requires further study. Moreover, for the understanding of the fetal impact of infarcts, it is probably beneficial that a percentage estimate of the amount of infarcted villous tissue be recorded. Altshuler suggested that most infarcts are not associated with fetal CNS changes (Altshuler & Herman, 1989).

Chorangiosis, on the other hand, is correlated with prolonged fetal oxygen deprivation. Just how the placenta is able to adapt to changing oxygen supply was considered in detail by Kaufmann and his colleagues (1993) and in earlier chapters of this book. Vascular proliferation, mediated through a complex system, is one important feature. Chorangiosis, one such outcome, is a highly abnormal condition that must be recognized as being associated with many perinatal problems. Although minor forms of chorangiosis are reasonably common, its value for our understanding of the fetal/placental/maternal relations has so far been underestimated. Altshuler (1984, 1993a,b) found chorangiosis in about 5% of neonates admitted to

his intensive care unit—much more commonly than occurs in cases with "routine" placentas. Chorangiosis is never found in normal cases, and Altshuler made the point that chorangiosis is significantly different from congestion, and that it probably relates to chronic low-grade hypoxia. That suggestion is supported by the finding of chorangiosis in women gestating at very high altitude (Reshetnikova et al., 1996). Chorangiosis if also often seen with VUE, and we find it peripheral to atrophying villi when old vascular thrombi have occluded the fetal vascular bed. Other correlations exist to fetal death, diabetes, umbilical cord problems, etc. The recognition of chorangiosis is an important feature of placental study. Whether "grading" the degree of chorangiosis as promoted by Altshuler (1984) is truly helpful remains to be confirmed by new studies. From a legal perspective it must be emphasized that the development of chorangiosis takes time to develop. Scheffen et al. (1990) provided beautiful evidence of the capillary adaptation in the guinea pig placenta following long-standing hypoxia and indicated temporal aspects. Although this system may differ from the histology of human adaptation processes, the underlying mechanism is the same and confirms the clinical findings. Other adaptations to low oxygen saturation were discussed in the context of preeclampsia in Chapter 19. They included cytotrophoblast proliferation with syncytial excess, reduction of villous length, and the possible mediation of these processes through cytokines.

Other Types of Pathology

The fetal circulation of the placenta normally contains very few nucleated red blood cells (NRBCs). When they are found in sections of the placenta, the pathologist must seek an explanation for their presence. It may be obvious from hematologic study that there is evidence of hemolytic disease, or that transplacental bleeding or chronic infection existed, but often the cause of an excessive number of NRBCs in the fetal vessels is not immediately evident. Fox (1967) suggested that NRBCs are often found in the fetal circulation because of acute hypoxia. Presumably, the human fetus reacts to oxygen deficiency, as it does to anemia, by secreting NRBCs from the hepatic or bone marrow stores. How acutely this reaction occurs and whether it reflects a quantitative response to certain levels of oxygen deprivation is unknown. But this relationship to fetal hypoxia has now been shown to have led to elevated NRBC counts in numerous studies of which only a few recent investigations will be cited here. Thus, Baschat et al. (1999, 2003, 2004) found that elevated NRBCs at birth, and especially the persistence of these cells into neonatal life, correlate well with major neonatal complication. Phelan et al. (1995) looked upon the presence of NRBCs in term neonates as evidence of prenatal asphyxia. These investigators, as well as Minior et al. (2000a,b) also found it to accompany fetal growth restriction as the result of "placental insufficiency" (Baschat & Hecher, 2004). The finding of NRBCs in the fetal vessels merely signals to the pathologist that a careful review of the record is needed to explain this important observation that may otherwise be overlooked. As stated, how quickly such a response occurs is unknown, for which reason Shields et al. (1993) attempted to elucidate the blood replacement by experimental hemorrhage in ovine fetuses. Despite an initial increase in fetal erythropoietin (EPO) levels, a significant hemorrhage (40%) was not followed by a significant rise in the fetal reticulocyte count, nor were the former blood volume and hematocrit restored before birth. Thus, the ovine model may not be appropriate to settle this important question. Older studies have suggested that sheep fetuses marshal some response; the current understanding of all of these aspects is discussed in admirable detail in Altshuler's review (1993a). It cites the study by Ruth et al. (1988), which determined the EPO levels at birth in preeclamptic pregnancies and those of severe asphyxia. The EPO levels were elevated in most pregnancy-induced hypertension (PIH)-derived neonates, irrespective of CNS damage; the significant finding was the marked elevation of EPO levels in those infants who ultimately had CNS damage but not in others. Ferber et al. (2004) later clearly showed that the EPO levels correlate well with the neonatal NRBC counts. We can personally relate two experiences from our files that help in understanding the time course in human fetuses to some extent: One patient was at term and had a major gush of bright red blood (later identified as fetal blood from disrupted velamentous vessels) upon insertion of an intrauterine pressure catheter. She was delivered by cesarean section 48 minutes later; the infant was pale, the placenta otherwise entirely normal. The cord arterial pH was 7.05, hemoglobin 14.6 g, hematocrit 44.8%, white blood count (WBC) 28,000, and platelets 120,000 and falling to 71,000. Three transfusions of packed red blood cells were given and the hemoglobin level was then only 10.3 g, and hematocrit 29.9%. The first enumeration of NRBCs occurred 1½ hours after delivery and showed 19 NRBC/100 WBC; 6 hours later it was 32 NRBC/100 WBC. Thus, there was a continued hematologic response after the delivery of the anemic child, and some degree of an initial NRBC response was detectable within an hour. This is contrary to the rapid decline of NRBCs postnatally when the hypoxic event has been more remote; under those circumstances most NRBCs are gone on the second day. Another case that is relevant came as a consultation: the mother had a car accident with lap belt injury at 28 weeks' pregnancy. Approximately 12 hours later the fetus was born with a hematocrit of 25%. Kleihauer stains gave an estimated 40 to 50 mL fetal blood in the maternal circulation; 45

NRBCs/100 WBC were found and there was villous edema. It is entirely possible that the acute blood loss as shown in these two cases initiated a stronger response than would gradual hypoxia. This is consistent with Altshuler's (1993b) comment that "acute fetal blood loss and congenital septic hemolysis reduce the time it takes fetal hypoxia to cause fetal erythropoiesis and increased nucleated red blood cells." In another child, the 102 cm long umbilical cord had prolapsed and was hemorrhagic for half of its length. The neonate had 53 NRBCs/100 WBC, but the placenta showed chorangiosis and mural thrombi in large vessels. The latter observations indicate very long-standing fetal hypoxia, a more frequent finding in this complex situation that prevents adequate assessment of the temporal response of the fetal system. We do not know the complete answers to these questions at present, and encourage colleagues to collect case material in order to gain a better understanding of the time course of the NRBC response. It should also be cautioned that fetal growth restriction is known to be associated with an increased number of NRBCs in their circulation (Nicolini et al., 1990). These authors deduced from the blood studies by cordocentesis that the only reasonable explanation for intrauterine growth restriction with the presence of NRBCs is long-standing hypoxia. Korst et al. (1996) studied NRBCs in asphyxiated and normal neonates. They found that normal infants have 3.4 (±3.0) NRBCs/100 WBC, but that asphyxiated and neurologically damaged newborns had significantly elevated counts (30.3 ± 77.5/100 WBC). The most elevated NRBC counts were explicable only by assuming hypoxia to have occurred long before birth. More discussion of the control of NRBCs in the fetal circulation is to be found at the end of Chapter 8. It should also be related here that Korst et al. (1999) found that neonates with encephalopathy had statistically reduced platelet counts, yet another means of evaluating neonates with CNS problems.

During legal proceedings the pathologist is frequently asked to specify a time frame for the lesion under discussion (e.g., Naeye & Localio, 1995, who enumerated NRBCs and lymphocytes). He or she may be required to specify how quickly villi can become atrophic following thrombosis, or what is the exact temporal evolution of thrombi. How long has a significant phlebitis been present, and is it correlated with the length of time from rupture of membranes? These and other probing questions are often difficult to adjudicate, and the answers (with respect to best medical judgment) may present problems for a conscientious witness. It requires experience, and it may be better to state the lack of our knowledge than to express unwarranted opinions that are contradicted in the courtroom or by other experts. This uncertainty is also an indication for the pathologist to seek new information from appropriate cases in which clinical data corroborate a particular finding. It is the reason why the meticulous

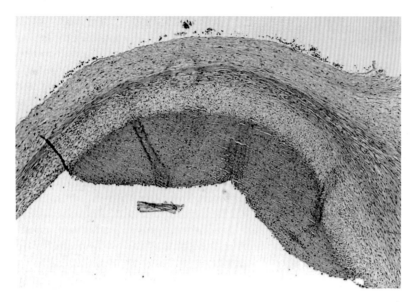

FIGURE 26.2. Mural thrombus in a placental surface vein ("cushion") of a child with unexplained cerebral palsy. Note that the vein wall is partially degenerated. The lesion was not recognized, macroscopically or microscopically, by the pathologist who signed off on the case. H&E × 160.

study of twin placentas can be so useful as it often provides a "control," a fetus who has shared the same intrauterine environment as the case under litigation but who may be normal.

Another relevant feature found in the study of abnormal infants is villous dysmaturity, the discrepancy of villous maturation with the chronologic age. This is not to say that this placenta is merely an immature one, rather that the placenta shows abnormalities, often irregularly distributed, such as an increase in fibrin, villous size, and stromal cells; decreased syncytial knots; and frequently an increased vascularity. Irregularly matured villi are frequent in the placentas of a variety of chromosomal abnormalities, for instance. Similar villous changes are found in other placental disturbances, as shown in Figure 26.2, and they may be difficult to explain. In this case, they probably resulted

from partial venous thrombosis of surface vessels (Fig. 26.3) in a child whose outcome was cerebral palsy, and which involved litigation. The ultimate cause of these lesions was not apparent, but it is clear that they were long-standing prenatal deviations from normal. Similar thromboses and degenerative changes may have taken place in the organs of the surviving fetus. We will never know. Tenney-Parker changes of villi (increased syncytial knotting) signify deficient uteroplacental blood flow of some duration, and focal villous edema may all be associated with premature delivery and neonatal hypoxia. These notations are all microscopic findings, however, that cannot be anticipated macroscopically. Their frequent presence with abnormal fetal outcomes signifies the importance of placental examination by a competent pathologist and knowledge of the spectrum of what is "normal."

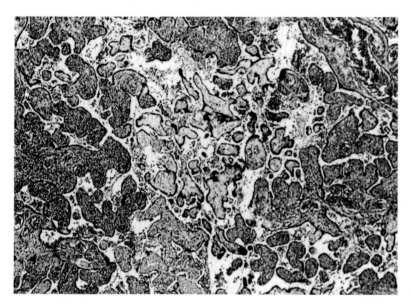

FIGURE 26.3. Irregular villous maturation and adjacent chorangiosis of the placenta in a cerebral palsy case (see Fig. 26.3). The vascularity of the central group of villi is apparent. It is presumed that this focal villous vascular loss is due to the same abnormality that was responsible for the mural thrombus. H&E × 60.

It may be pertinent to review the presence of villous edema in this context. Edema of villi has been associated with poor fetal outcome and has also played a role in the litigation process. Naeye et al. (1983) suggested that villous edema was frequent and severe in the immature placentas (more than 32 weeks) of pregnancy complications. It was believed to correlate with fetal hypoxia, and the authors postulated that the hypoxia was the result of compression of fetal villous capillaries by edema. We find villous edema exceedingly difficult to quantitate, especially when the placenta has been stored and has lost some of its fluid. Moreover, many mildly hydropic fetuses with marked villous edema have not had a hypoxic deficit from compression of villous vessels, making us uneasy to use this criterion in our evaluation of abnormal placentas. No additional studies of this topic were published until the report by Shen-Schwarz et al. (1989). These investigators found villous edema in 13% of singleton placentas during the second half of pregnancy. In 11% of term placentas, edema was associated with fetal and neonatal deaths. They also detected edema more often in prematurely delivered placentas but were unable to relate villous edema to chorioamnionitis. Altshuler (1993a,b) was also uncertain that villous edema was a *cause* of fetal hypoxia, as resulting from compressing the villous capillaries. Further studies are needed to clarify the importance of villous edema as a correlate of fetal well-being and to delineate its precise pathogenesis.

References

Adams-Chapman, I., Vaucher, Y.E., Bejar, R.F., Benirschke, K., Baergen, R.N. and Moore, T.R.: Maternal floor infarction of the placenta: Association with central nervous system injury and adverse neurodevelopmental outcome. J. Perinatol. **22**: 236–241, 2002.

Altshuler, G.: Chorangiosis: an important placental sign of neonatal morbidity and mortality. Arch. Pathol. Lab. Med. **108**:71–74, 1984.

Altshuler, G.: A conceptual approach to placental pathology and pregnancy outcome. Semin. Diagn. Pathol. **10**:204–221, 1993a.

Altshuler, G.: Some placental considerations related to neurodevelopmental and other disorders. J. Child. Neurol. **8**:78–94, 1993b.

Altshuler, G.: Placental pathology clues for interdisciplinary clarification of fetal disease—a review. Trophobl. Res. **13**:511–525, 1999.

Altshuler, G. and Herman, A.: The medicolegal imperative: placental pathology and epidemiology. In, Fetal and Neonatal Brain Injury: Mechanisms, Management and the Risk of Malpractice. D.K. Stevenson and P. Sunshine, eds., pp. 250–263. B.C. Decker, Toronto, 1989.

Altshuler, G. and Hyde, S.: Meconium induced vasoconstriction: a potential cause of cerebral and other fetal hypoperfusion and of poor pregnancy outcome. Child Neurol. **4**:137–142, 1989.

Anonymous: Cerebral palsy, intrapartum care, and a shot in the foot. Lancet **2**:1251–1252, 1989.

Arias, F.: Predictability of complications associated with prolongation of pregnancy. Obstet. Gynecol. **70**:101–106, 1987.

Aylward, G.P., Verhulst, S.J. and Bell, S.: Correlation of asphyxia and other risk factors with outcome: a contemporary view. Dev. Med. Child Neurol. **31**:329–340, 1989.

Baldwin, V.J.: Pathology of Multiple Pregnancy. Springer-Verlag, New York, 1994.

Baschat, A.A. and Hecher, K.: Fetal growth restriction due to placental disease. Semin. Perinatol. **28**:67–80, 2004.

Baschat, A.A., Gembruch, U., Reiss, I., Gortner, L., Harman, C.R. and Weiner, C.P.: Neonatal nucleated red blood cell counts in growth-restricted fetuses: relationship to arterial and venous Doppler studies. Amer. J. Obstet. Gynecol. **181**:190–195, 1999.

Baschat, A.A., Gembruch, U., Reiss, I., Gortner, L. and Harman, C.R.: Neonatal nucleated red blood count and postpartum complications in growth restricted fetuses. J. Perinatol. **31**: 323–329, 2003.

Beebe, L.A., Cowan, L.D. and Altshuler, G.: The epidemiology of placental features: association with gestational age and neonatal outcome. Obstet. Gynecol. **87**:771–778, 1996.

Beebe, L.A., Cowan, L.D., Hyde, S.R. and Altshuler, G.: Methods to improve the reliability of histopathological diagnoses in the placenta. Paediatr. Perinatl. Epidemiol. **14**:172–178, 2000.

Bejar, R., Vigliocco, G., Gramajo, H., Solana, C., Benirschke, K., Berry, C., Coen, R. and Resnik, R.: Antenatal origin of neurologic damage in newborn infants. Part II. Multiple gestations. Amer. J. Obstet. Gynecol. **162**:1230–1236, 1990.

Benirschke, K.: The placenta in the litigation process. Amer. J. Obstetr. Gynecol. **162**:1445–1450, 1990.

Benirschke, K.: Intrauterine death of a twin: Mechanisms, implications for surviving twin, and placental pathology. In, Seminars in Diagnostic Pathology, W.B. Saunders, Co. **10**: 222–231, 1993.

Benirschke, K.: The use of the placenta in the understanding of perinatal injury. In, Risk Management Techniques and Neonatal Practice. D.S.M. Fisher, ed. Futura Publishing Co., Armonk, N.Y. pp. 325–345, 1996.

Booth, V.J., Nelson, K.B., Dambrosia, J.M. and Grether, J.K.: What factors influence whether placentas are submitted for pathological examination? Amer. J. Obstet. Gynecol. **176**:567–571, 1997.

Capstick, J.B. and Edwards, P.J.: Trends in obstetric malpractice claims. Lancet **336**:931–932, 1990.

Davies, B.R. and Arroyo, P.: The importance of primary diagnosis in perinatal death. Amer. J. Obstet. Gynecol. **152**:17–23, 1985.

Depp, R.: Perinatal asphyxia: assessing its causal role and timing. Semin. Pediatr. Neurol. **2**:3–36, 1995.

De Sa, D.J.: Diseases of the umbilical cord. In, Pathology of the Placenta. E.V.D.K. Perrin, ed. Churchill Livingstone, New York, 1984.

Driscoll, S.G.: Pathology and the developing fetus. Pediatr. Clin. North Amer. **12**:493–514, 1965.

Durant, R.H. and Woodward, C.: Antenatal hypoxia and IQ values. Amer. J. Dis. Child. **141**:1150–1151, 1987.

Ferber, A., Fridel, Z., Weissmann-Brenner, A., Minior, V.K. and Divon, M.Y.: Are elevated nucleated red blood cell counts an indirect reflection of enhanced erythropoietin activity? Amer. J. Obstet. Gynecol. **190**:1473–1475, 2004.

Fisher, D.S.M. ed.: Risk Management Techniques and Neonatal Practice. Futura Publishing Co., Armonk, N.Y. 1996.

Fleischer, L.D.: Wrongful births: when is there liability for prenatal injury? Amer. J. Dis. Child. **141**:1260–1265, 1987.

Fox, H.: The incidence and significance of nucleated erythrocytes in the foetal vessels of the mature human placenta. J. Obstet. Gynaecol. Br. Commonw. **74**:40–43, 1967.

Freeman, R.: Intrapartum fetal monitoring—a disappointing story. NEJM **322**:624–626, 1990.

Gembruch, U. and Baschat, A.A.: True knot of the umbilical cord: transient constrictive effect to umbilical venous blood flow demonstrated by Doppler sonography. Ultrasound Obstet. Gynecol. **8**:53–56, 1996.

Genest, D.R.: Estimating the time of death in stillborn fetuses: II. Histologic evaluation of the placenta; a study of 71 stillborns. Obstet. Gynecol. **80**:585–592, 1992.

Gillan, J.E.: Perinatal placental pathology. Current Opinion in Obstetr. Gynecol. **4**:286–294, 1992.

Goodlin, R.C.: Do concepts of causes and prevention of cerebral palsy require revision? Amer. J. Obstet. Gynecol. **172**:1830–1836, 1995.

Grafe, M.R.: The correlation of prenatal brain damage with placental pathology. J. Neuropathol. Exp. Neurol. **53**:407–415, 1994.

Grant, A., O'Brien, N., Joy, M.-T., Hennessy, E. and MacDonald, D.: Cerebral palsy among children born during the Dublin randomized trial of intrapartum monitoring. Lancet **2**:1233–1235, 1989.

Harkavy, K.L.: Antenatal hypoxia and IQ values. Amer. J. Dis. Child. **141**:1150, 1987.

Hyde, S., Smotherman, J., Moore, J.I. and Altshuler, G.: A model of bacterially induced umbilical vein spasm, relevant to fetal hypoperfusion. Obstet. Gynecol. **73**:966–970, 1989.

Kaplan, C.G.: Forensic aspects of the placenta. In, Forensic Aspects in Pediatric Pathology, Dimmick, J.E. and Singer, D.B., eds. Perspectives of Pediatric Pathology, Vol. **19**:20–42. Karger, Basel, 1995.

Kaufmann, P., Kohnen, G. and Kosanke, G.: Wechselwirkungen zwischen Plazentamorphologie und fetaler Sauerstoffversorgung. Gynäkologe **26**:16–23, 1993.

Korst, L., Phelan, J.P., Ahn, N.O. and Martin, G.I.: Nucleated red blood cells: an update on the marker for fetal asphyxia. Amer. J. Obstet. Gynecol. **175**:843–846, 1996.

Korst, L.M., Phelan, J.P., Wang, Y.M. and Ahn, M.O.: Neonatal platelet counts in fetal brain injury. Amer. J. Perinatol. **16**:79–83, 1999.

Kraus, F.T.: Cerebral palsy and thrombi in placental vessels of the fetus: insights from litigation. Human Pathol. **28**:246–248, 1997.

Kuban, K.C.K. and Leviton, A.: Cerebral palsy. NEJM **330**:188–195, 1994.

Langston, C., Kaplan, C., Macpherson, T., Manci, E., Peevy, K., Clark, B., Murtagh, C., Cox, S. and Glenn, G.: Practice guideline for examination of the placenta. Developed by the placental pathology practice guideline development task force of the College of American Pathologists. Arch. Pathol. Lab. Med. **121**:449–476, 1997.

Larroche, J.-C.: Fetal encephalopathies of circulatory origin. Biol. Neonate. **50**:61–74, 1986.

Lien, J.M., Towers, C.V., Quilligan, E.J., Veciana, M.de, Toohey, J.S. and Morgan, M.A.: Term early-onset neonatal seizures: obstetric characteristics, etiological classifications, and perinatal care. Obstet. Gynecol. **85**:163–169, 1995.

Liu, S., Benirschke, K., Scioscia, A.L. and Mannino, F.L.: Intrauterine death in multiple gestation. Acta. Genet. Med. Gemellol. **41**:5–26, 1992.

Lopez-Zeno, J.A., Carlo, W.A., O'Grady, J.P. and Fanaroff, A.A.: Infant survival following delayed postmortem cesarean delivery. Obstet. Gynecol. **76**:991–992, 1990.

Marin-Padilla, M.: Developmental neuropathology and impact of perinatal brain damage. II: White matter lesions of the neocortex. J. Neuropathol. Exp. Neurol. **56**:219–235, 1997.

Mazor, M., Furman, B., Wiznitzer, A., Shoham-Vardi, I., Cohen, J. and Ghezzi, F.: Maternal and perinatal outcome of patients with preterm labor and meconium-stained amniotic fluid. Obstet. Gynecol. **86**:830–833, 1995.

Miller, P.W., Coen, R.W. and Benirschke, K.: Dating the time interval from meconium passage to birth. Obstet. Gynecol. **66**:459–462, 1985.

Minior, V.K., Shatzkin, E. and Divon, M.Y.: Nucleated red blood cell count in the differentiation of fetuses with pathologic growth restriction from healthy small-for-gestational-age fetuses. Amer. J. Obstet. Gynecol. **182**:1107–1109, 2000a.

Minior, V.K., Bernstein, P.S. and Divon, M.Y.: Nucleated red blood cells in growth-restricted fetuses: associations with short-term neonatal outcome. Fetal Diagn. Ther. **15**:165–169, 2000b.

Naeye, R.L.: Causes of perinatal mortality excess in prolonged gestations. Amer. J. Epidemiol. **108**:429–433, 1978.

Naeye, R.L.: Disorders of the Placenta, Fetus, and Neonate. Diagnosis and Clinical Significance. Mosby Year Book, St. Louis, 1992.

Naeye, R.L.: Can meconium in the amniotic fluid injure the fetal brain? Obstet. Gynecol. **86**:720–724, 1995.

Naeye, R.L. and Localio, A.R.: Determining the time before birth when ischemia and hypoxemia initiated cerebral palsy. Obstet. Gynecol. **86**:713–719, 1995.

Naeye, R.L. and Peters, E.C.: Antenatal hypoxia and low IQ values. Amer. J. Dis. Child. **141**:50–54, 1987.

Naeye, R., Maisels, M.J., Lorenz, R.P. and Botti, J.J.: The clinical significance of placental villous oedema. Pediatrics **71**:588–594, 1983.

Naeye, R.L., Peters, E.C., Bartholomew, M. and Landis, R.: Origins of cerebral palsy. Amer. J. Dis. Child. **143**:1154–1161, 1989.

Nelson, K.B. and Leviton, A.: How much of neonatal encephalopathy is due to birth asphyxia? Amer. J. Dis. Childr. **145**:1325–1331, 1991.

Nelson, K.B., Dambrosia, J.M., Ting, T.Y. and Grether, J.K.: Uncertain value of electronic fetal monitoring in predicting cerebral palsy. NEJM **334**:613–618, 1996.

Nicolini, U., Nicolaides, P., Fisk, N.M., Vaughan, J.I., Fusi, L., Gleeson, R. and Rodeck, C.H.: Limited role of fetal blood sampling in prediction of outcome in intrauterine growth retardation. Lancet **336**:768–772, 1990.

Ornoy, A., Crone, K. and Altshuler, G.: Pathological features of the placenta in fetal death. Arch. Pathol. Lab. Med. **100**:367–371, 1976.

Patten, R.M., Mack, L.A., Nyberg, D.A. and Filly, R.A.: Twin embolization syndrome: prenatal sonographic detection and significance. Radiology **173**:685–689, 1989.

Perkins, R.P.: Perspectives on perinatal brain damage. Obstet. Gynecol. **69**:807–819, 1987.

Phelan, J.P., Ahn, M.O., Korst, L.M. and Martin, G.I.: Nucleated red blood cells: a marker for fetal asphyxia? Amer. J. Obstet. Gynecol. **173**:1380–1384, 1995.

Redline, R.W., Wilson-Costello, D., Borawski, E., Fanaroff, A.A. and Hack, M.: Placental lesions associated with neurologic impairment and cerebral palsy in very low-birth-weight infants. Arch. Pathol. Lab. Med. **122**:1091–1098, 1998.

Redline, R.W.: Severe fetal placental vascular lesions in term infants with neurologic impairment. Amer. J. Obstet. Gynecol. **192**:452–457, 2005.

Reshetnikova, O.S., Burton, G.J., Milovanov, A.P. and Fokin, E.I.: Increased incidence of placental chorioangioma in high-altitude pregnancies: hypobaric hypoxia as a possible etiologic factor. Amer. J. Obstet. Gynecol. **174**:557–561, 1996.

Richards, B.C. and Thomasson, G.: Closed liability claims analysis and the medical record. Obstet. Gynecol. **80**:313–316, 1992.

Robb, J.A., Benirschke, K. and Barmeyer, R.: Intrauterine latent herpes simplex virus infection. I. Spontaneous abortion. Hum. Pathol. **17**:1196–1209, 1986a.

Robb, J.A., Benirschke, K., Mannino, F. and Voland, J.: Intrauterine latent herpes simplex virus infection. II. Latent neonatal infection. Hum. Pathol. **17**:1210–1217, 1986b.

Rosen, M.G. and Dickinson, J.C.: The incidence of cerebral palsy. Amer. J. Obstet. Gynecol. **167**:417–423, 1992.

Rosen, M.G. and Dickinson, J.C.: The paradox of electronic fetal monitoring: more data may not enable us to predict or prevent infant neurologic morbidity. Amer. J. Obstet. Gynecol. **168**:745–751, 1993.

Rosenblatt, R.A. and Hurst, A.: An analysis of closed obstetric malpractice claims. Obstet. Gynecol. **74**:710–714, 1989 (**75**:471–472, 1990).

Ruth, V., Autti-Rämö, I., Granström, M.-J., Korkman, M. and Raivio, K.O.: Prediction of perinatal brain damage by cord plasma vasopressin, erythropoietin, and hypoxanthine values. J. Pediatr. **113**:880–885, 1988.

Salafia, C.M. and Vintzileos, A.M.: Why all placentas should be examined by a pathologist in 1990. Amer. J. Obstet. Gynecol. **163**:1282–1293, 1990.

Sandmire, H.F.: Malpractice—the syndrome of the 80s. Obstet. Gynecol. **73**:145–146, 1989.

Scheffen, I., Kaufmann, P., Philippens, L., Leiser, R., Geisen, C. and Mottaghy, K.: Alterations of the fetal capillary bed in the guinea pig placenta following long-term hypoxia. In, Oxygen Transport to Tissue XII. J. Piiper et al., eds. Plenum Press, New York, 1990.

Schindler, N.R.: Importance of the placenta and cord in the defense of neurologically impaired infant claims. Arch. Pathol. Lab. Med. **115**:685–687, 1991.

Schwartz, D.A. and Caldwell, E.: Herpes simplex virus infection of the placenta. The role of molecular pathology in the diagnosis of viral infection of placenta-associated tissues. Arch. Pathol. Lab. Med. **115**:1141–1144, 1991.

Sepkowitz, S.: Influence of the legal imperative and medical guidelines on the incidence and management of the meconium-stained newborn. Amer. J. Dis. Child. **141**:1124–1127, 1987.

Shen-Schwarz, S., Ruchelli, E. and Brown, D.: Villous oedema of the placenta: a clinicopathological study. Placenta **10**:297–307, 1989.

Shields, L.E., Widness, J.A. and Brace, R.A.: Restoration of fetal red blood cells and plasma proteins after a moderately severe hemorrhage in the ovine fetus. Amer. J. Obstet. Gynecol. **169**:1472–1478, 1993.

Sunoo, C., Kosasa, T.S. and Hale, R.W.: Meconium aspiration syndrome without evidence of fetal distress in early labor before elective cesarean delivery. Obstet. Gynecol. **73**:707–709, 1989.

Thorarensen, O., Ryan, S., Hunter, J. and Younkin, D.P.: Factor V Leiden mutation: an unrecognized cause of hemiplegic cerebral palsy, neonatal stroke, and placental thrombosis. Ann. Neurol. **42**:372–375, 1997.

Travers, H. and Schmidt, W.A.: College of American Pathologists Conference XIX on the Examination of the Placenta. Arch. Pathol. Lab. Med. **115**:660–731, 1991. (This is a composite of many articles by numerous authors.)

Vorherr, H.: Placental insufficiency and postmaturity. Europ. J. Obstetr. Gynecol. Reprod. Biol. **5**:109–122, 1975.

Ward, C.J.: Analysis of 500 obstetric and gynecologic malpractice claims: causes and prevention. Amer. J. Obstet. Gynecol. **165**:298–306, 1991.

Weinstein, L.: Malpractice—the syndrome of the 80s. Obstet. Gynecol. **72**:130–135, 1988.

Werth, B.: Damages: One Family's Legal Struggle in the World of Medicine. Berkley Trade Publ., 1998.

Yoon, B.H., Romero, R., Yang, S.H., Jun, J.K., Kim, I.O., Choi, J.H. and Syn, H.C.: Interleukin-6 concentrations in umbilical cord plasma are elevated in neonates with white matter lesions associated with periventricular leukomalacia. Amer. J. Obstet. Gynecol. **174**:1433–1440, 1996.

Yudkin, P.L., Johnson, A., Clover, L.M. and Murphy, K.W.: Clustering of perinatal markers of birth asphyxia and outcome at age five years. Brit. J. Obstet. Gynaecol. **101**:774–781, 1994.

27
Glossary

This glossary is intended to trace the roots of the often-confusing terms used in placental pathology and perinatal development. The accents are placed for pronunciation.

Gk. = Greek; **L.** = Latin; **Fr.** = French; **OE** = Old English; **ME** = Middle English.

Abrúptio (placéntae): detachment of placenta [L. *abrumpere* = to break away]

Acárdius: malformed twin without heart, invariably one of monozygotic twins [Gk. a = without, not + *kardia* = heart]

Adventítia: outer layer of vessel wall [L. *advenire* = to add]

Allántoïs (allantóic): designation of one type of placenta, because of its roots in other mammals; thin membrane between amnion and chorion [Gk. *allantos* = sausage]

Ámnion: thin membrane surrounding the fetus; lamb's caul [Gk. *amnos* = lamb] **Note**: Because we use chorionic and not choriotic, it is here preferred to speak of amnionic, rather than amniotic. Hyrtl (1880) explored the various terminology used to describe placental structures. He concluded that amnios and amnion were both correct. It was first used by Galen, referring to skin. The reference to lamb comes from Vesalius.

Andrógenesis: development of male gender [Gk. *andros* = man + *gennan* = produce]

Anídian monster: a hideous fetus with peculiar features; a form of acardiac twin [Gk. *an* = not + *idios* = peculiar + L. *monstrum*]

Artiodáctyla: order of mammals, the even-hoofed animals, e.g., cow, deer [Gk. *artios* = even + *daktylos* = toe]

Báttledore (placenta): marginal insertion of cord [OE = flat, wooden paddle used in the game of battledore to hit the shuttlecock]

Blástocyst: early germinative vesicle [Gk. *blaste* = germ + *kystis* = vesicle]

Bosselátion: surface granulation of placenta [Fr. *bosseler* = to ornament with bosses; from *bosse* = knob]

Capillary: hair-fine blood vessel [L. *capilla* = hair]

Céllular: belonging to the cell [L. *cellula* = small cabin, cell]

   Extracellular: outside the cell

   Intercellular: between cells

   Intracellular: within cells

   Transcellular: across cells

Chiméra (Chímerism): the composite of several genotypes [Gk. *chimaira* = a monstrous beast. In Greek mythology a monster made of the head of a lion, body of a goat, and tail of a dragon.]

Chirálity: the quality of being chiral [Gk. *chiro* = the hand; a three-dimensional form, as a molecule, that cannot be superimposed on its mirror image; used in designating the twist of the umbilical cord; its first usage was discussed by McManus (2002)]

Chorioangiópagus parasíticus: a fetus, connected by blood vessels to another fetus [Gk. *chorion* = "little gut" = outer membranes around embryo + *angeios* = vessel + *pagos* = something set or fixed; *para* = next to + *sitos* = food]

Chórion: outer membrane around embryo [Gk. *chorion* = "little gut"; according to Hyrtl (1880) the term was also used by Galen as the outer shell of the membranes]

   frondósum: the placenta proper [L. *frondosus* = richly covered with leaves, as in tree]

   laéve: the membranous portion of the chorionic sac [L. *levis* = smooth, without villi]

Chorionepithelióma: malignant tumor of trophoblast = chorio-epithelioma or choriocarcinoma [Gk. *chorion* = "little gut" (outer membrane enclosing an embryo) + *epi* = on + *thele* = nipple + *oma* = tumor]

Circumvállate (placenta): an abnormal form of placenta with circumferential, old hemorrhages [L. *circum* + *vallare* = to wall around]

Cirsoid: aneurysmal dilatation of vessel [Gk. *kirsos* = enlarged vein]

Cotylédon: originally name for the single spots of placental tissue in the ruminants; lobe of the human placenta [Gk. *kotyle* = cup]

Cytotrophoblast: cellular type of the trophoblast [Gk. *kytos* = cell + *trephein* = to nourish + *blaste* = germ]

Decídua: the endometrium at end of the luteal phase [L. *decidere* = fall, die]

   basalis: basal portion of placenta [Gk. *basis* = base]

capsuláris: outer portion of membranes [L. *capsula* = little box]

parietális: endometrium of pregnancy, covering wall portion of uterus [L. *paries* = wall; parietalis = pertaining to wall]

véra: uterine decidua, contrasting it to pseudodecidua, outside of uterus, as in endometriosis [L. *verus* = true]

Désmosome: intercellular junction [Gk. *desmos* = Ligament + *soma* = body]

Dizygótic: twins of two ova, "fraternal twins" [Gk. *dis* = twice, two + *zygon* = yoke]

Eclámpsia: coma and convulsive seizure in pregnancy [Gk. *eklampsis* = shining forth; or *ek* = out + *lampein* = to shine]

Émbryoblast: embryo-forming cells of the blastocyst [Gk. *embryon* = unborn child + *blaste* = germ]

Endométrium: innermost layer of the uterus [Gk. *endon* = inside + *metra* = uterus]

Endoplásmic reticulum: a net-like, membrane-lined cell organelle [Gk. *endon* = inside + *plasma* = juice; L. *reticulum* = small net]

Endothélium: innermost layer of blood vessels [Gk. *endon* = inside + *thele* = mamilla]

Epígnathus: tumorous mass in mouth, affixed to jaw and possibly a twin [Gk. *epi* = upon, at, over + *gnathos* = jaw]

Epithelium: superficial cellular layer [Gk. *epi* = upon + *thele* = mamilla]

Fétus papyráceus: paper-like, macerated, compressed ("compressus") fetus [L. *papyrus* = plant from which paper is made]

Fíbrin: blood clot product [L. *fibra* = fiber]

Fíbrinoid: a substance similar to but not identical with fibrin [Gk: . . . *eides* = looking like]

Fíbroblast: connective tissue cell [Gk. *blaste* = germ]

Freemártin: the female of fraternal cattle twins, sterilized in utero by the male co-twin with whose placental vessels she is joined; the term presumably comes from the St. Martin's feast in England, when these animals were consumed

Funiculópagous (twins): twins joined at umbilical cord [L. *funis* = rope, cord + Gk. *pagos* = fixed]

Fúnis (funículus): umbilical cord [L. *funis* = rope, cord]

Funisítis: inflammation of umbilical cord [L. *funis* = rope]

Fúrcate (cord) ("insértio funículi furcáta"): forked insertion of the little rope [L. *furca* = fork]

Glycocálix: superficial layer of polysaccharides, covering the cell surface [Gk. *glycos* = sweet + *kalyx* = goblet]

Granulomatósis infantiséptica: neonatal disseminated listeriosis [L. *granulum* = little grain + Gk. *oma* = tumor]

Gynogénesis: female development [Gk. *gyne* = woman + *gennan* = produce]

Hemiacárdius: acardiac monster in which remnants of heart may be found [L. *hemi* = a half]

Holoacárdius: completely heartless monster (twin) [Gk. *holos* = whole]

Hydatídiform (mole): severely hydropic placenta with bulbous, villous enlargement [Gk. *hydatis* = watery vesicle + L. *forma* = shape; L. *mola* = false conception; mass]

Hydrámnios: excessive amount of amnionic fluid [Gk. *hydor* = water (*hydros* = sweat; some early authors believed that amnionic fluid was fetal sweat) + *amnion* = lamb's caul]

Implantátion: establishing of intimate fetomaternal contact in the uterus [L. *implantare* = to embed]

Intervíllous: between the placental villi, i.e., in the maternal blood space [L. *inter* = between]

Intravíllous: within a villus [L. *intra* = in]

Lacúna: [L. = hole, gap]

Lithopédion: stone-like fetus [Gk. *lithos* = stone + *paidion* = child]

Lóchia (pl.): uterine discharges after birth [Gk. *lochia*]

Mácrophage: phagocytotic and paracrine cell type [Gk. *macros* = large + *phagein* = to eat]

Mágma reticuláre: jelly-like fluid in original embryonic sac [Gk. *magma* = suspension of finely divided material in small amount of water + L. *reticulum* = little net (network)]

Mármoset: family of small South American primates that always produce fraternal twins [Old Fr. *marmouset* = grotesque figure]

Mecónium: fetal intestinal content [Gk. *mekonion* = poppy juice]

Mésenchyme: undifferentiated connective tissue [Gk. *mesos* = in the middle of + *chein* = to pour (something poured in between)]

Mésoderm: the middle germ layer [Gk. *derma* = skin]

Mésothelium: connective tissue-derived epithelial layer [Gk. *thele* = mamilla]

Microvíllus: finger-like extension of the cell surface

Mitochóndrion: rod-shaped cell organelle [Gk. *mitos* = thread + *chondros* = grain]

Mole (hydatidiform, Breus', etc.): vesicular mass of placenta [L. *mola* = false conception]

Monozygótic: single-egg-derived twins ("identical twins") [Gk. *monos* = single + *zygotos* = yoked]

Nódus spúrius vasculósus (gelatínus): false knot in umbilical cord of vascular genesis [L. *nodus* = knot + *spurius* = not genuine + *gelatina* = gelatin]

Núchal (cord): umbilical cord entwined around neck [L. *nucha* = nape of the neck]

Óctoploid: having eight sets of chromosomes [Gk. *okto* = eight + *ploos* = fold + *eidos* = form]

Oligohydrámnios: too little, or no amnionic fluid [Gk. *oligos* = little + *hydor* = water (*hydros* = Sweat) + *amnion* = lamb caul]

Ómphalo-(mesentéric): umbilicus [Gk. *omphalos* = Navel]

Páraplacénta: those parts of the chorionic sac, not belonging to the placenta, *e.g.*, membranes [Gk. *para* = beside]

Périvillous: around the placental villi [Gk. *peri* = around]

Placénta: [L. flat cake] According to Hyrtl (1880) this term, with an originally Greek root, was introduced in 1559 by Realdus Columbus; others referred to it as "secundines"

accréta: unusually adherent placenta that fails to detach [L. *accrescere* = to grow together, adhere]

incréta: placenta that has grown into the myometrium [L. *increscere* = to grow into]

membranácea: very thin placental membrane, the entire outside of which is covered with villi [L. *membrana* = from parchment, membrane]

percréta: placenta that has grown through the uterine wall [L. *percrebescere* = to crowd everywhere]

prévia: placenta that is located in the lower uterus and is in the way before the fetus can be delivered [L. *praevius* = in front of, before, leading the way]

Plasmódium: multinucleate mass of protoplasm [Gk. *plasma* = a thing formed (juice) + *eidos* = to form]

Pólyploid: having many sets of chromosomes [Gk. *polys* = much, many + *ploos* = fold + *eidos* = form]

Pólypoid: protrusion of tissue, polyp [Gk. *polys* = many + *pous* = foot + *oid* = like]

Pycnósis (pyknosis): degenerative condensation of cells or nuclei [Gk. *pyknos* = dense]

Schístocytes: broken red cells in disseminated intravascular coagulation [Gk. *schistos* = split]

Secúndines: synonymous with afterbirth [L. *secundus* = following]

Sínusoid: enlarged capillary [L. *sinus* = bight + Gk. *eides* = looking like]

Siréniform (fétus): malformed infant with fused legs [Gk. *seiren* = mermaid]

Sirenomélia: malformed infant with fused legs [Gk. *seiren* = mermaid + *melos* = limb]

Stróma: connective tissue core of an organ [L. *stroma* = cushion]

Subchórial: under the chorionic plate [L. *sub* = below + Gk. *chorion* = leather, embryonic membrane]

Succentúriate (lobe): accessory lobe of placenta [L. *succenturiare* = to substitute]

Superfecundátion: fertilization of two or more ova at different times during the same menstrual period [L. *super* = beyond, excessively + *fecundus* = fertile]

Superfetátion: pregnancy on top of already existing pregnancy [L. *superfetare* = to bring forth while already pregnant; L. *fetus* = fruit, offspring]

Sympus: fetus with fused legs [Gk. *syn* = together + *pous* = foot (same as siren)]

Syncytiotrophoblast: syncytial type of trophoblast

Syncytium: multinuclear mass, derived from cell fusion [Gk. *syn* = together + *kytos* = cell]

Synéchia (pl. synéchiae): adhesion of parts, here in the uterus [Gk. *synecheia* = continuity]

Tessellátion: irregular surface of placenta [L. *tessella* = little square stone (From Gk. *tessares* = four)]

Tétraploid: having four sets of chromosomes [Gk. *tettares* = four + *ploos* = fold]

Thalassémias: hemoglobin disorders [from Gk. *thalassa* = the sea; generally referring to the Mediterranean]

Thixotrópic (Thyxo-) gel: gel that liquefies when shaken, generally the extraembryonic fluid [Gk. *thixis* = touching + *trope* = turn]

Thoracopágus: twins, conjoined at chest [Gk. *thorax* = chest + *pagos* = fix]

Trabécula: small septum [L. small beam]

Tróphoblast: the epithelium that covers the placenta [Gk. *trophe* = nourishment + *blastos* = germ]

Trophótropism: the "wandering" of the placenta to the site of best nourishment [Gk. *trophe* = nourishment + *trope* = turn]

Urachus: connection of bladder to allantoic sac [Gk. *ourachos* ("that which has a tail") = cord that extends from bladder to navel]

Vas prévium (pl. Vása prévia): blood vessels within membranes that present before fetal parts during delivery [L. *vas* = vessel(s) that is (are) ahead ("previous") of fetal part]

Vas vasórum (Vása vasórum): blood vessels that nourish the vessels [L. *vas* = vessel]

Velaméntous (cord insertion): membranous insertion of umbilical cord [L. *velamen* = veil + *velamentum* = cover]

Vérnix caseósa: sebum, hair and other skin secretions from fetus [L. *vernix* = varnish + *caseus* = cheese]

Víllus (pl. vílli): ramifications of placenta with fetal vessels that are the "business end" of the placenta, covered with trophoblast [L. *villus* = tuft of hair]

Vitélline: belonging to the yolk sac [L. *vitellus* = yolk of an egg]

References

Hyrtl, J.: Onomatologia Anatomica. W. Braumüller, Vienna, 1880.

McManus, C.: Right Hand Left Hand. The Origins of Asymmetry in Brains, Bodies, Atoms, and Cultures. Harvard University Press, 2002.

Bibliography

Haubrich, W.S.: Medical Meanings. A Glossary of Word Origins. Harcourt, Brace, Jovanovich, San Diego, 1984.

Thomas, C.L.: Taber's Cyclopedic Medical Dictionary. 15th Ed. Davis, Philadelphia, 1985.

Webster, D.: Webster's Unabridged Dictionary. Dorset & Baber, Cleveland, 1983.

Acknowledgment. We are grateful to Professor E.N. Genovese, San Diego State University, for correcting this text.

28
Normative Values and Tables

Some quantitative structural and biochemical data concerning pregnancy, placental development, and composition of the term placenta are given in Tables 28.1 to 28.10.

When examining the tables on placental morphometry and comparing the results from different authors, it is important to note that quantitative structural data are heavily influenced by the mode of sampling and by the preparation of the material. Because of the high degree of maternal and fetal vascularization, the placenta reacts immediately to changes in intravascular pressure. Thus, the mode of birth, the time elapsing from cessation of maternal and fetal blood flows to tissue fixation (see Tables 28.6 to 28.10), and the nature of cord clamping (see Table 28.8) directly influence the volumetric relations of villi and intervillous space. In particular, parameters such as the width of fetal vessels, degree of fetal vascularization, maternal-fetal diffusion distance, and trophoblastic thickness are easily affected. Moreover, the composition of the fixative and its osmolarity (see Table 28.10), as well as the mode of fixation (immersion versus perfusion fixation) are of importance. Normally, immersion fixation of the entire placenta or of small pieces is used. The more advanced methods, such as perfusion fixation (Burton et al., 1987) or puncture biopsy of the still maternally perfused placenta during cesarean section (Schweikhart & Kaufmann, 1977; Voigt et al., 1978; Sen et al., 1979), are very time-consuming. When studying immersion fixed material, however, one should keep in mind that this material differs quantitatively and qualitatively from the in vivo conditions (see Tables 28.6 and 28.9). It is impossible to include the results of numerous other valuable contributions to placental morphometry in these tables. For further information on special issues, we refer to the following publications: placental growth development in relation to birth weight (Bouw et al., 1978; Molteni et al., 1978); relationship of placental weight to body size at 7 years of age, and to abnormalities in children (Naeye, 1987); fetal and placental weights in relation to maternal weight (Auinger & Bauer, 1974); ultrasonographic measurements of volumetric growth of the placenta (Bleker et al., 1977); weight development of placenta and membranes in early pregnancy (Abramovich, 1969); ratio of gestational sac volume to crown–rump length in early pregnancy (Goldstein et al., 1986); villous surface area and villous volume densities in various placental regions and along different levels of the chorial basal axis (Teasdale, 1978; Boyd et al., 1980; Cabezon et al., 1985; Bacon et al., 1986); local variations of villous surface, fetal vascularization, and amount of vasculosyncytial membranes in the placentone (maternal-fetal circulatory unit) (Schuhmann et al., 1986); total villous surface in relation to fetal weight, in normal and various pathologic cases (Clavero-Nunez & Botella-Llusia, 1961, 1963); morphometric data affecting placental oxygen diffusion (Mayhew et al., 1984, 1986); computer measurement of the mass of syncytiotrophoblast (Boyd et al., 1983); ultrastructural morphometric analysis of the villous syncytiotrophoblast (Sala et al., 1983); microvillous surface enlargement of the villous surface (Teasdale & Jean-Jacques, 1985); comparison of villous structure following immersion and perfusion fixation (Burton et al., 1987).

TABLE 28.1. Length and weight data for placenta and fetus; pregnancies and deliveries at sea level. (1) Data extrapolated from Boyd & Hamilton (1970) and O'Rahilly (1973); (2) data from Johannigmann et al. (1972); (3) data from Winckel (1893), Branca (1922), Naeye & Tafari (1983), and Fujinaga et al. (1990); (4) data from Weissman et al. (1994). Placental weight data published by Molteni et al. (1978) are 5% to 10% lower because fetal blood was drained from chorionic vessels before weighing. Compare with data on influence of cord clamping given in Table 28.8. Umbilical cord length as measured by ultrasound throughout the first trimester (Hill et al., 1994) amounts to only about 50% of the length measured after abortion.

Pregnancy week (postconception)	Pregnancy week (postmenstruation)	Pregnancy month (postmenstruation)	Crown–rump length (mm)[1]	Embryonic/fetal weight (g)[1]	Diameter of the chorionic sac (mm)[1]	Placental diameter (mm)[1]	Placental weight (g)[1]	Placental thickness postpartum (mm)[1]	Placental thickness including uterine wall measured by ultrasound in vivo (mm)[2]	Length of the umbilical cord (mm)[3]	Diameter of the umbilical cord measured by ultrasound (mm)[4]	Diameter of the umbilical artery measured by ultrasound (mm)[4]	Diameter of the umbilical vein measured by ultrasound (mm)[4]
	1												
	2	1											
1	3												
2	4									2			
3	5		2.5		5–11					4			
4	6	2	5		12–19					7			
5	7		9		20–25					12			
6	8		14	1.1	26–33		6			20	2.5		
7	9		20	2	34–41		8			33			
8	10	3	26	5	42–48		13			55	3.3		
9	11		33	11	49–56		19			92			
10	12		40	17	57–65		26			126	4.4		
11	13		48	23	66–73	50	32			158			
12	14	4	56	30	74–81	56	41	10		188	6.1	1.2	2.0
13	15		65	40	82–89	62	50	11		215			
14	16		75	60	90–99	69	60	12		240	7.0	1.1	2.4
15	17		88	90		75	70	12		264			
16	18	5	99	130		81	80	13		287	10.1	1.9	3.6
17	19		112	180		87	101	14		309			
18	20		125	250		94	112	15	28	330	11.1	2.0	4.1
19	21		137	320		100	126	15	29	350			
20	22	6	150	400		106	144	16	30	369	12.8	2.4	4.7
21	23		163	480		112	162	17	32	387			
22	24		176	560		119	180	18	34	404	13.9	2.6	5.4
23	25		188	650		125	198	18	35	420			
24	26	7	200	750		131	216	19	36	435	15.2	2.8	6.0
25	27		213	870		137	234	19	37	450			
26	28		226	1,000		144	252	20	38	464	15.9	3.1	6.6
27	29		236	1,130		150	270	20	39	477			
28	30	8	250	1,260		156	288	21	40	490	16.3	3.4	7.3
29	31		263	1,400		162	306	21	41	502			
30	32		276	1,550		169	324	22	42	520	17.6	3.6	7.7
31	33		289	1,700		175	342	22	42	530			
32	34	9	302	1,900		181	360	23	43	540	17.4	3.3	7.4
33	35		315	2,100		187	378	23	43	549			
34	36		328	2,300		194	396	24	44	557	17.4	3.7	7.6
35	37		341	2,500		200	414	24	44	565			
36	38	10	354	2,750		206	432	24	45	572	18.0	4.2	8.2
37	39		367	3,000		213	451	25	45	579			
38	40		380	3,400		220	470	25	45	585	17.0	3.9	7.8

TABLE 28.2. Quantitative data of various placental tissues as related to fetal weight and stage of pregnancy. (1) Data calculated from Table 28.1; (2) Data from Kloos & Vogel (1974); (3) data from Kaufmann (1981); (4) data from Knopp (1960). Fetoplacental weight ratios calculated by Molteni et al. (1978) are generally higher because these authors had drained fetal blood from chorionic vessels before weighing.

Pregnancy week (postconception)	Pregnancy week (postmenstruation)	Pregnancy month (postmenstruation)	Fetal weight (g) per 1-g of placental weight[1]	Placental weight index: placental weight (g) per 1-g of fetal weight[2]	Villous weight (g) per placenta[1] (percentage of total placental weight) placental diameter (mm)[1]	Villous surface (cm²) per placenta[1]	Fetal weight (g) per 10,000-cm² villous surface[1]	Villous surface (cm²) per 1-g of placental villi[1]	Number of villous cross sections per mm² of paraffin sections[3]	Number of villous cross sections per mm² of paraffin sections[4]	Villous diameter (mean of all peripheral villous types) (µm)[3]
	1										
	2	1									
1	3										
2	4										
3	5										
4	6	2									
5	7										
6	8		0.18	10.0–9.3	5 (83%)	830		166	15	47	204
7	9		0.25								
8	10	3	0.38								
9	11		0.58								
10	12		0.65	3.9–3.3	18 (69%)	3,020	29.8	168	20		
11	13		0.72								
12	14	4	0.73								
13	15		0.80								
14	16		1.00	2.5–1.0	28 (43%)	5,440	64.3	194	25	104	158
15	17		1.29								
16	18	5	1.63								
17	19		1.78								
18	20		2.23	0.97–0.57	63 (55%)	14,800	104.7	235	30	131	108
19	21		2.54								
20	22	6	2.78								
21	23		2.96								
22	24		3.11	0.49–0.38	102 (55%)	28,100	156.6	275	40	202	61
23	25		3.28								
24	26	7	3.47								
25	27		3.72								
26	28		3.97	0.31–0.26	135 (54%)	42,200	191.9	313	60		
27	29		4.19	0.26						205	53
28	30	8	4.38	0.242							
29	31		4.58	0.208							
30	32		4.78	0.203	191 (61%)	72,000	184.5	377	90		
32	33		4.97	0.180							
32	34	9	5.28	0.168							
33	35		5.56	0.163							
34	36		5.81	0.157	234 (60%)	101,000	198.0	432	140		
35	37		6.04	0.145						264	52
36	38	10	6.37	0.138							
37	39		6.65	0.132							
38	40		7.23	0.130	273 (58%)	125,000	230.0	458	150	321	48

TABLE 28.3. Histomorphometrical evaluation of placental villi. The data presented here are mean data for the complete villous tree including all villous types. (1) Data from Glöde (1984); (2) data from Kaufmann (1972); (3) calculated from data from Kaufmann (1981); (4) data from Kaufmann & Scheffen (1992).

Pregnancy week (postconception)	Pregnancy week (postmenstruation)	Pregnancy month (postmenstruation)	Trophoblastic volume as a percentage of the villous volume (%)[1]	Mean trophoblastic thickness (μm)[1]	Villous cytotrophoblast volume as a percentage of villous trophoblast (%)[2]	Villous stromal volume as a percentage of villous volume (%)[1]	Villous connective tissue volume as a percentage of villous volume (%)[3]	Volume of fetal vessel lumina as a percentage of villous volume (%)[3]	Percentage of the villous surface that is characterized by a double-layered trophoblast (syncytium and Langhans cells) (%)[2]	Maternofetal diffusion distance (μm)[4]
	1	1								
	2									
1	3									
2	4									
3	5									
4	6	2								
5	7		31.7	18.9		68.3	65.6	2.7		55.9
6	8				30					
7	9		33.5	19.1		66.5	63.5	3.0	85	
8	10	3								
9	11		34.5	21.6		65.8	61.8	4.0		
10	12				35				80	
11	13									
12	14	4								
13	15									
14	16				43			6.0	80	40.2
15	17									
16	18	5	24.8	11.6		75.2	68.9	6.3		
17	19									
18	20				35			6.6	60	22.4
19	21									
20	22	6								
21	23									
22	24				30				55	21.6
23	25									
24	26	7								
25	27									
26	28		30.1	9.7	25	69.9	60.8	9.1	45	
27	29									
28	30	8								
29	31									
30	32				20				35	20.6
31	33									
32	34	9								
33	35									
34	36		30.8	5.2	15	69.2	47.9	21.3	25	11.7
35	37									
36	38	10								
37	39									
38	40		32.9	4.1	14	67.1	38.7	28.4	23	4.8

TABLE 28.4. Fetal and placental weights as related to the number of pregnancies.

	Male neonates				Female neonates			
Pregnancy no.	Mat. age (years)	Neo. length (cm)	Neo. wt. (g)	Plac. wt. (g)	Mat. age (years)	Neo. length (cm)	Neo. wt. (g)	Plac. wt. (g)
First (n = 101)	22.37	51.04	3,141.3	548.7	22.42	50.96	2,974.0	560.7
Second (n = 71)	25.24	51.95	3,442.8	607.9	25.15	51.29	3,133.6	565.5
Third (n = 27)	30.21	50.29	3,495.0	603.2	26.69	50.29	3,228.1	553.9
Fourth (n = 18)	30.00	53.83	3,677.5	599.6	29.00	50.83	3,095.0	568.3

Mat. = maternal; Neo. = neonatal; Plac. = placental.
All results are given as the mean value.
From Lips (1891).

TABLE 28.5. Qualitative data for the human placenta at term. The data were taken or calculated from (1) Knopp (1960); (2) Aherne & Dunnill (1966); (3) Baur (1970); (4) Wördehoff (1971); (5) Laga et al. (1973); (6) Ehrhardt & Gerl (1970); (7) Bacon et al. (1986); (8) Mayhew et al. (1986); (9) Bouw et al. (1976); (10) Feneley & Burton (1991); (11) Voigt et al. (1978); (12) Burton & Feneley (1992).

Mean placental volume (cm³) (without cord and membranes)	448 (2)	448 (5)	540 (9)	408 (10)
Percentage of villous volume per placenta (%)	57.5 (1)	57.9 ± 5.7 (2)	45.6 (5)	62.9 ± 2.1 (7)
Mean villous volume per placenta (g)	273 (1)	214 (5)	224 (2)	239 (9)
Percentage of intervillous space per placenta (postpartum) (%)	35.8 ± 3.2 (2)	23.29 (5)	29.3 ± 2.0 (7)	37.9 (8)
Volume of intervillous space (cm³)	144 (2)	110 (5)	210 (9)	173 (8)
Percentage of intervillous fibrinoid per placenta (%)	4.3 ± 2.1 (2)	2.58 (5)		
Villous surface covered with fibrinoid (%)	0.364 (6)			
Percentage of villous tissues per placenta (chorionic plate, basal plate, septa, cell islands, infarctions) (%)	27.6 (5)			
Villous surface per placenta (m²)	13.3 ± 0.47 (4)	12.0 (3)	11.8 (6)	11.0 ± 1.3 (2)
Villous surface per 1 cm³ of villous volume (cm²)	330 (1)	248 (3)	301.2 (4)	
Inner fetal capillary surface per placenta (m²)	12.2 ± 1.5 (2)	12.0 (5)		
Total length of all villi per placenta (km)	90 (1)			
Arithmetic mean thickness of villous membrane (mean maternofetal diffusion distance) (μm)	3.5 (2)	4.5 (10)	5.0 (11)	
Harmonic mean thickness of villous membrane (μm)	10.0 (5)	4.9 (8)		

TABLE 28.6. Quantitative composition of peripheral villous types of diameter of less than 80 μm following resin embedding.

		After in situ puncture of placenta					
Parameter	All villous types after spon. del.	All villous types	SV	IIV	MIV	TV, neck	TV, no neck
Villous surface showing cytotrophoblast below the syncytium (%)	27.5	22.8	21.4	23.4	24.6	20.0	23.5
Cytotrophoblastic volume as a percentage of total villous trophoblast (%)	13.3	14.0	11.7	14.3	13.8	11.6	15.7
Percent of total villous volume {Trophoblast	41.7	37.7	30.0	33.8	38.0	46.2	29.6
Villous stroma	58.3	62.3	70.0	66.2	62.0	53.8	70.4
Fetal vessel lumens	20.0	28.4	26.0	15.7	21.0	20.2	45.2
Connective tissue including vessel walls	38.4	33.9	44.0	50.5	41.0	33.6	25.2
Mean trophoblastic thickness	4.7	4.1	4.7	5.2	4.4	4.0	3.3
Distribution of maternofetal diffusion distances in % of villous surface {-0–2 μm	10.4	21.0	9.2	10.9	13.1	21.8	37.1
2.1–5 μm	29.9	40.2	27.3	27.3	37.5	41.4	36.5
5.1–10 μm	40.3	32.4	50.5	37.7	37.8	32.6	25.1
10.1–∞ μm	19.5	6.4	13.0	24.1	11.6	4.4	1.3
Mean maternofetal diffusion distance (μm)	7.1	5.0	6.8	7.5	6.0	4.8	3.7
Macrophages (no.)/mm² of histologic section			24	730	241	83	192
Mast cells (no.)/mm² of histologic section			18	10	5	<1	<1

Spon. del. = spontaneous delivery; SV = stem villi; IIV = immature intermediate villi; MIV = mature intermediate villi; TV, neck = neck regions of terminal villi; TV, no neck = terminal villi, excluding neck regions.
The data obtained from spontaneous deliveries (fixation about 10 minutes after cord clamping, ischemic period far above 10 minutes), are compared with such obtained by puncture aspiration out of the still maternally perfused in situ placenta (ischemic period: 0 minutes) (Voigt et al., 1978). In addition, data have been separately measured and calculated for different villous types (Sen et al., 1979).

TABLE 28.7. Number of villous cross sections (%), percentages of villous surface, and percentages of villous volume in different groups of villi.

Parameter	Villous cross sections (% of total no.)	Surface of villi (% of total)	Volume of villi (% of total)	Type of villus	Mean caliber (μm)	Mean length of cross sections (μm)
Diameter of villi (μm)						
->1,500	0.003	0.1	1.2	⎫		
1,201–1,500	0.002	0.1	0.8	⎬ Trunci chorii		
901–1,200	0.007	0.1	1.4	⎭		
601–900	0.02	0.5	2.4	⎫ Rami chorii		
301–600	0.2	1.9	9.0	⎭		
226–300	0.3	1.7	6.4	⎫		
151–225	0.6	3.2	7.7	⎬ Ramuli chorii, mature and		
76–150	7.1	15.1	20.8	immature intermediate		
0–75	91.8	77.2	50.4	⎭ villi, terminal villi[a]		
Type of villus						
Ramuli	5.1	12.4	22.7		120.5	340.1
Immature intermediate	5.1	8.4	10.1		76.6	233.5
Mature intermediate	29.1	31.0	27.8		60.6	153.5
Terminal	55.1	46.3	38.7		50.8	118.4
Neck regions	5.5	2.0	0.8		34.3	46.4

[a]The villi are classified according to diameter (using data from I. Hansen & V. König, personal communication, 1978) and compared according to structure.
Modified from Sen et al. (1979).

TABLE 28.8. Influence of cord clamping on placental structure.

Parameter	Early clamped (n = 9)	Late clamped (n = 7)
Placental weight (g)	567.4 ± 114.5	407.1 ± 74.0
Birth weight (g)	3,593.5 ± 380.0	3,404.3 ± 313.5
Placental weight index	0.156 ± 0.021	0.116 ± 0.088
Villous volume (cm³)	239.1 ± 51.9	185.3 ± 39.5
Villous vessel volume (cm³)	74.9 ± 28.2	33.4 ± 18.3
Villous vessel volume (%)	30.4 ± 5.8	17.4 ± 6.9
Villous vessel surface (mm²) per mm³ of villous volume	66.9 ± 10.0	46.3 ± 10.5
Total villous surface (m²)	13.3 ± 2.6	9.3 ± 2.1
Volume of intervillous space (cm³)	210.3 ± 50.0	116.0 ± 21.7

Results are given as the mean ± SD. A group of spontaneously delivered placentas of which the cord was clamped as early as possible as compared with a group of which the cord was clamped after cessation of the arterial pulsation.
Data from Bouw et al. (1976).

TABLE 28.9. Influence of total ischemia of varying length on the structure of terminal villi.

Parameter	0 min	2 min	5 min	10 min	20 min
Fetal capillary volume (%)	45	32	19	13	17
Connective tissue volume (%)	25	42	49	54	47
Trophoblastic volume (%)	23	26	32	33	36
Mean maternofetal diffusion distance (μm)	3.2	3.7	5.2	7.1	7.4
Epithelial plates (percentage of villous surface) (%)	40.4	—	—	—	14.7
Mean mitochondrial diameter (syncytiotrophoblast) (μm)	0.30	0.34	0.51	0.63	0.61

Data from Kaufmann (1985).

TABLE 28.10. Influence of total osmolarity of the fixative (2.2% phosphate-buffered glutaraldehyde) on the volumes of syncytiotrophoblast and fetal capillary lumina in the guinea pig placenta.

Parameter	235	290	340	390	600
Trophoblastic volume (%)	39.5	39.3	33.3	32.7	24.6
Fetal capillary volume (%)	12.1	14.7	25.5	16.9	19.3
Extracellular space (%)	<1.0	<1.0	<1.0	2.3	11.7
Mean mitochondrial diameter (syncytiotrophoblast) (μm)	0.68	0.56	0.30	0.26	0.25

Data from Kaufmann (1980) can be transferred to the human.

References

Abramovich, D.R.: The weight of placenta and membranes in early pregnancy. Obstet. Gynaecol. Brit. Commonw. **76**:523–526, 1969.

Aherne, W. and Dunnill, M.S.: Morphometry of the human placenta. B. Med. Bull. **22**:5–8, 1966.

Auinger, W. and Bauer, P.: Zum Zusammenhang zwischen Kindsgewicht, Placentagewicht, Muttergewicht und Muttergröße. Arch. Gynäkol. **217**:69–83, 1974.

Bacon, B.J., Gilbert, R.D. and Longo, L.D.: Regional anatomy of the term human placenta. Placenta **7**:233–241, 1986.

Baur, R.: Über die Relation zwischen Zottenoberfläche der Geburtsplacenta und Gewicht des Neugeborenen bei verschiedenen Säugetieren. Z. Anat. Entwicklungsgesch. **131**:31–38, 1970.

Bleker, O.P., Kloosterman, G.J., Breur, W. and Mieras, D.J.: The volumetric growth of the human placenta: a longitudinal ultrasonic study. Amer. J. Obstet. Gynecol. **127**:657–661, 1977.

Bouw, G.M., Stolte, L.A.M., Baak, J.P.A. and Oort, J.: Quantitative morphology of the placenta. 1. Standardization of sampling. Eur. J. Obstet. Gynecol. Reprod. Biol. **6**:325–331, 1976.

Bouw, G.M., Stolte, L.A.M., Baak, J.P.A. and Oort, J.: Quantitative morphology of the placenta. 3. The growth of the placenta and its relationship to birth weight. Eur. J. Obstet. Gynecol. Reprod. Biol. **8**:73–76, 1978.

Boyd, J.D. and Hamilton, W.J.: The Human Placenta. Heffer & Sons, Cambridge, 1970.

Boyd, P.A., Brown, R.A. and Stewart, W.J.: Quantitative structural differences within the normal term human placenta: a pilot study. Placenta **1**:337–344, 1980.

Boyd, P.A., Brown, R.A., Coghill, G.R., Slidders, W. and Stewart, W.J.: Measurement of the mass of syncytiotrophoblast in a range of human placentae using an image analysing computer. Placenta **4**:255–262, 1983.

Branca, A.: Precis D' Embryologie. Librairie J.-B. Bailliere et Fils, Paris, 1922.

Burton, G.J. and Feneley, M.R.: Capillary volume fraction is the principal determinant of villous membrane thickness in the normal human placenta at term. J. Dev. Physiol. **17**:39–45, 1992.

Burton, G.J., Ingram, S.C. and Palmer, M.E.: The influence of mode of fixation on morphometrical data derived from terminal villi in the human placenta at term: a comparison of immersion and perfusion fixation. Placenta **8**:37–51, 1987.

Cabezon, C., De la Fuente, F., Jurado, M. and Lopez, G.: Histometry of the placental structures involved in the respiratory interchange. Acta Obstet. Gynecol. Scand. **64**:411–416, 1985.

Clavero-Nunez, J.A. and Botella-Llusia, J: Measurement of the villus surface in normal and pathologic placentas. Amer. J. Obstet. Gynecol. **86**:234–240, 1961.

Clavero-Nunez, J.A. und Botella-Llusia, J: Ergebnisse von Messungen der Gesamtoberfläche normaler und krankhafter Placenten. Arch. Gynäkol. **198**:56–60, 1963.

Ehrhardt, G. und Gerl, D.: Eine einfache Methode zur Bestimmung der Zottenoberfläche von Placenten mit Hilfe der Flächenintegration nach der "Nadelmethode." Zentralbl. Gynäkol. **92**:728–731, 1970.

Feneley, M.R. and Burton, G.J.: Villous composition and membrane thickness in the human placenta at term: a stereological study using unbiased estimators and optimal fixation techniques. Placenta **12**:131–142, 1991.

Fujinaga, M., Chinn, A. and Shepard, T.H.: Umbilical cord growth in human and rat fetuses: evidence against the "stretch hypothesis". Teratology **41**:333–339, 1990.

Glöde, B.: Morphometrische Untersuchungen zur Reifung menschlicher Placentazotten. Medical Thesis, University of Hamburg, 1984.

Goldstein, S.R., Subramanyam, B.R. and Snyder, J.R.: Ratio of gestational sac volume to crown-rump length in early pregnancy. Hum. Pathol. **31**:320–321, 1986.

Hill, L.M., DiNofrio, D.M. and Guzick, D.: Sonographic determination of first trimester umbilical cord length. J. Clin. Ultrasound **22**:435–438, 1994.

Johannigmann, J., Zahn, V. and Thieme, V.: Einführung in die Ultraschalluntersuchung mit dem Vidoson. Elektromedica **2**:1–11, 1972.

Kaufmann, P.: Untersuchungen über die Langhanszellen in der menschlichen Placenta. Z. Zellforsch. **128**:283–302, 1972.

Kaufmann, P.: Der osmotische Effekt der Fixation auf die Placentastruktur. Verh. Anat. Ges. **74**:351–352, 1980.

Kaufmann, P.: Entwicklung der Plazenta. In, Die Plazenta des Menschen. V. Becker, Th.H. Schiebler and F. Kubli, eds. Thieme Verlag, Stuttgart, 1981.

Kaufmann, P.: Influence of ischemia and artificial perfusion on placental ultrastructure and morphometry. Contrib. Gynecol. Obstet. **13**:18–26, 1985.

Kaufmann, P. and Scheffen, I.: Placental development. In, Neonatal and Fetal Medicine—Physiology and Pathophysiology. R. Polin and W. Fox, eds., pp. 47–55, Saunders, Orlando 1992.

Kloos, K. and Vogel, M.: Pathologie der Perinatalperiode. Grundlage, Methodik und erste Ergebnisse einer Kyematopathologie, 1–361. Thieme, Stuttgart, 1974.

Knopp, J.: Das Wachstum der Chorionzotten vom 2. bis 10. Monat. Z. Anat. Entwicklungsgesch. **122**:42–59, 1960.

Laga, E.M., Driscoll, S.G. and Munro, H.N.: Quantitative studies of human placenta. 1. Morphometry. Biol. Neonate **23**:231–259, 1973.

Lips, F.: Über die Gewichtsverhaeltnisse der neugeborenen Kinder zu ihren Placenten. Medical Thesis, University of Erlangen, 1891.

Mayhew, T.M., Joy, C.F. and Haas, J.D.: Structure-function correlation in the human placenta: the morphometric diffusing capacity for oxygen at full term. J. Anat. **139**:691–708, 1984.

Mayhew, T.M., Jackson, M.R. and Haas, J.D.: Microscopical morphology of the human placenta and its effects on oxygen diffusion: a morphometric model. Placenta **7**:121–131, 1986.

Molteni, R.A., Stys, S.J. and Battaglia, F.C.: Relationship of fetal and placental weight in human beings: Fetal/placental weight ratios at various gestational ages and birth weight distributions. J. Reprod. Med. **21**:327–334, 1978.

Naeye, R.L.: Do placental weights have clinical significance? Hum. Pathol. **18**:387–391, 1987.

Naeye, R.L. and Tafari N.: Noninfectious disorders of the placenta, fetal membranes and umbilical cord. In: Risk Factors in Pregnancy and Disease of the Fetus and Newborn. Williams & Wilkins, Baltimore, pp. 145–172, 1983.

O'Rahilly, R.: Developmental stages in human embryos. Part A, Publ. 631. Carnegie Institute, Washington, D.C., 1973.

Sala, M.A., Valeri, V. and Matheus, M.: Stereological analysis of syncytiotrophoblast from human mature placenta. Arch. Anat. Microsc. **72**:99–106, 1983.

Schuhmann, R., Stoz, F. and Maier, M.: Histometric studies of placentones of the human placenta. Z. Geburtsh. Perinatol. **190**:196–203, 1986.

Schweikhart, G. and Kaufmann, P.: Zur Abgrenzung normaler, artefizieller und pathologischer Strukturen in reifen menschlichen Plazentazotten. I. Ultrastruktur des Syncytiotrophoblasten. Arch. Gynäkol. **222**:213–230, 1977.

Sen, D.K., Kaufmann, P. and Schweikhart, G.: Classification of human placental villi. II. Morphometry. Cell Tissue Res. **200**:425–434, 1979.

Teasdale, F.: Functional significance of the zonal morphologic differences in the normal human placenta. Amer. J. Obstet. Gynecol. **130**:773–781, 1978.

Teasdale, F. and Jean-Jacques, G.: Morphometric evaluation of the microvillous surface enlargement factor in the human placenta from mid-gestation to term. Placenta **6**:375–381, 1985.

Voigt, S., Kaufmann, P. and Schweikhart, G.: Zur Abgrenzung normaler, artefizieller und pathologischer Strukturen in reifen menschlichen Plazentazotten. II. Morphometrische Untersuchungen zum Einfluss des Fixationsmodus. Arch. Gynäkol. **226**:347–362, 1978.

Weissman, A., Jakobi, P., Bronshtein, M. and Goldstein, I.: Sonographic measurements of the umbilical cord and vessels during normal pregnancies. J. Ultrasound Med. **13**:11–14, 1994.

Winckel, F.K.L.W.: Lehrbuch der Geburtshilfe, 2nd ed. Veit, Leipzig, 1893.

Wördehoff, B.: Zur Bestimmung der Zottenoberfläche der menschlichen Plazenta. Medical Thesis, Würzburg 1971.

Index